Andrews'
Diseases
OF
THE Skin
Clinical Dermatology

Commissioning Editor: *Russell Gabbedy*
Development Editor: *Sven Pinczewski*
Editorial Assistant: *Kirsten Lowson / Rachael Harrison*
Project Manager: *Elouise Ball*
Design: *Stewart Larking*
Illustration Manager: *Gillian Richards*
Illustrator: *Richard Tibbits, Richard Prime*
Marketing Manager: *Helena Mutak*

Andrews' Diseases OF THE Skin

Clinical Dermatology

Eleventh Edition

William D James, MD
Paul R Gross Professor of Dermatology
Department of Dermatology
University of Pennsylvania School of
Medicine
Philadelphia, Pennsylvania
USA

Dirk M Elston, MD
Director
Department of Dermatology
Geisinger Medical Center
Danville, Pennsylvania
USA

Timothy G Berger, MD
Professor of Clinical Dermatology
Executive Vice Chair and Residency
Program Director
Chair in Dermatology Medical Student
Education
University of California, San Francisco
San Francisco, California
USA

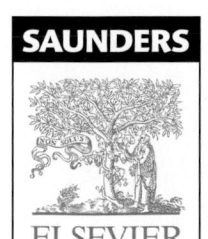

SAUNDERS

ELSEVIER

For additional online content visit
www.expertconsult.com

Expert | CONSULT

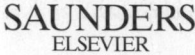

is an imprint of Elsevier Inc.

© 2011, Elsevier Inc. All rights reserved.

10th edition © 2006, Saunders Elsevier

ISBN: 978-1-4377-0314-6
International ISBN: 978-0-8089-2417-3

British Library Cataloguing in Publication Data
A catalogue record for this book is available from the British Library

Library of Congress Cataloging in Publication Data
A catalog record for this book is available from the Library of Congress

Notice
Medical knowledge is constantly changing. Standard safety precautions must be followed, but as new research and clinical experience broaden our knowledge, changes in treatment and drug therapy may become necessary or appropriate. Readers are advised to check the most current product information provided by the manufacturer of each drug to be administered to verify the recommended dose, the method and duration of administration, and contraindications. It is the responsibility of the practitioner, relying on experience and knowledge of the patient, to determine dosages and the best treatment for each individual patient. Neither the Publisher nor the author assume any liability for any injury and/or damage to persons or property arising from this publication.

The Publisher

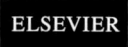
James, William D. (William Daniel), 1950–
  Andrews' Diseases of the skin : clinical dermatology. — 11th ed.
  1. Skin—Diseases. 2. Dermatology.
  I. Title   II. Diseases of the skin   III. Elston, Dirk M.   IV. Berger, Timothy G. V.
Andrews, George Clinton, 1891-1978. Diseases of the skin.
  616.5—dc22

The publisher's policy is to use **paper manufactured from sustainable forests**

Printed in China
Last digit is the print number: 9 8 7 6 5 4 3 2

CONTENTS

PREFACE AND ACKNOWLEDGEMENTS

Andrews' remains as it was from the beginning: an authored text whose one volume is filled with clinical signs, symptoms, diagnostic tests, and therapeutic pearls. The authors have remained general clinical dermatologists in an era of subspecialists in academia. They are committed to keeping *Andrews'* as an excellent tool for anyone who needs help in diagnosing a patient with a clinical conundrum or treating a patient with a therapeutically challenging disease.

Andrews' is primarily intended for the practicing dermatologist. It is meant to be used on the desktop at his or her clinic, giving consistent, concise advice on the whole gamut of clinical situations faced in the course of a busy workday. While we have been true to our commitment to a single-volume work, we provide our text in a convenient online format as well. Because of its relative brevity but complete coverage of our field, many find the text ideal for learning dermatology the first time. It has been a mainstay of the resident yearly curriculum for many programs. We are hopeful that trainees will learn clinical dermatology by studying the clinical descriptions, disease classifications, and treatment insights that define *Andrews'*. We believe that students, interns, internists or other medical specialists, family practitioners, and other health professionals who desire a comprehensive dermatology textbook will find that ours meets their needs. Long-time dermatologists will hopefully discover *Andrews'* to be the needed update that satisfies their lifelong learning desires. On our collective trips around the world, we have been gratified to see our international colleagues studying *Andrews'*. Several thousand books have been purchased by Chinese and Brazilian dermatologists alone.

Many major changes have been made to this edition. Bill James, Tim Berger and Dirk Elston, three great friends of nearly three decades, have worked closely to continue to improve the quality of our text. The surgical chapters have been updated and expanded by Isaac Neuhaus. We thank him for his efforts to enhance the procedural portion of our textbook and acknowledge the contributions of Roy Grekin in prior editions. We have tried to ensure that each entity is only discussed once, in a complete yet concise manner. In order to do this we have had to make decisions regarding the placement of disease processes in only one site. Clearly, neutrophilic eccrine hidradenitis, for example, could be presented under drug eruptions, neutrophilic reactive conditions, infection or cancer-associated disease, or with eccrine disorders. The final decisions were a team effort and made in the interest of eliminating redundancy. This allows us to present our unified philosophy in treating patients in one dense volume.

Medical science continues to progress with break-neck speed. Our understanding of the etiology of certain conditions has now led us to recategorize well-recognized disease states and dictated the addition over 70 newly described entities.

Molecular investigative techniques, technologic breakthroughs, and designer therapeutics lead the way in providing advances in our specialty. We cover the new understanding following from such innovations by discussing the mechanisms at work in genetic diseases, covering the latest in dermatopathologic staining and analysis, adding a second chapter on cosmetic surgery, and enlarging the therapeutic recommendations to include our expanded therapeutic options, such as biologic response modifiers, and biologically engineered targeted medications. We have attempted to define therapeutics in a fashion that emphasizes those interventions with the highest level of evidence, but also present less critically investigated therapeutic options. To care for our patients we need a large array of options. Not all are fully supported by formal evidence, yet are helpful to individual patients.

Extensive revisions were necessary to add this wealth of new information. We selectively discarded older concepts. By eliminating older, not currently useful information we maintain the brief but complete one-volume presentation that we and all previous authors have emphasized. Additionally, older references have been updated. The classic early works are not cited; instead we have chosen to include only new citations and let the bibliographies of the current work provide the older references as you need them. A major effort in this edition was to reillustrate the text with 567 new color images. Many have been added to the printed text; you will also find a large number only in the online version. Enjoy! We have looked to our own collections to accomplish this. These are the result of many hours of personal effort, the generosity of our patients, and a large number of residents and faculty of the programs in which we currently work or have worked in the past. Additionally, friends and colleagues from all parts of the globe have allowed us to utilize their photographs. They have given their permission for use of these wonderful educational photos to enhance your understanding of dermatology and how these diseases affect our patients. We cannot thank them enough.

All of the authors recognize the importance of our mentors, teachers, colleagues, residents, and patients in forming our collective expertise in dermatology. Dirk, Tim and Bill were all trained in military programs, and our indebtedness to this fellowship of clinicians is unbounded. The many institutions we have called home, from the East Coast of Walter Reed, to the West Coast of the University of California at San Francisco, and many in between, such as Brooke in San Antonio and the Cleveland Clinic, nurtured us and expanded our horizons. Our friendship goes well beyond the limits of our profession; it is wonderful to work with people you not only respect as colleagues, but also enjoy as closely as family. Finally we are proud to be a part of the Elsevier team and have such professionals as Claire Bonnett, Sven Pinczewski, Elouise Ball, and Russell Gabbedy supporting us every step of the way.

For my family, whose love and support sustain me and make me happy.

Bill D James

My wife Jessica and my children, Olivia and Mateo, who give me the joy and strength to undertake such a task.

Tim G Berger

To my wife and best friend, Kathy, and our wonderful children, Carly and Nate.

Dirk M Elston

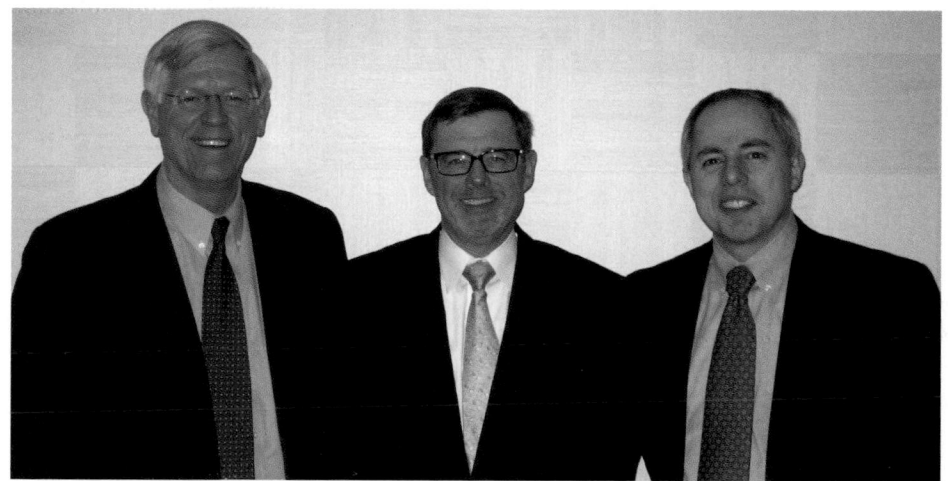

The authors: William D James, Timothy G Berger, Dirk M Elston.

Isaac M Neuhaus, MD
Assistant Professor
Dermatologic Surgery and Laser Center
University of California, San Francisco
San Francisco, California
USA

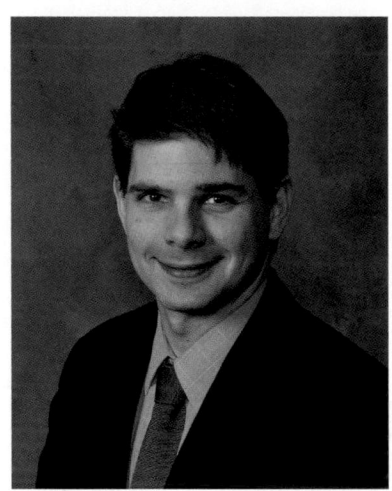

Skin: Basic Structure and Function

1

Skin is composed of three layers: the epidermis, dermis, and subcutaneous fat (panniculus) (Fig. 1-1). The outermost layer, the epidermis, is composed of viable keratinocytes covered by a layer of keratin, the stratum corneum. The principal component of the dermis is the fibrillar structural protein collagen. The dermis lies on the panniculus, which is composed of lobules of lipocytes separated by collagenous septae that contain the neurovascular bundles.

There is considerable regional variation in the relative thickness of these layers. The epidermis is thickest on the palms and soles, measuring approximately 1.5 mm. It is very thin on the eyelid, where it measures less than 0.1 mm. The dermis is thickest on the back, where it is 30–40 times as thick as the overlying epidermis. The amount of subcutaneous fat is generous on the abdomen and buttocks compared with the nose and sternum, where it is meager.

Epidermis and adnexa

During the first weeks of life, the fetus is covered by a layer of nonkeratinizing cuboidal cells called the periderm (Fig. 1-2). Later, the periderm is replaced by a multilayered epidermis. Adnexal structures, particularly follicles and eccrine sweat units, originate during the third month of fetal life as downgrowths from the developing epidermis. Later, apocrine sweat units develop from the upper portion of the follicular epithelium and sebaceous glands from the midregion of the follicle. Adnexal structures appear first in the cephalic portion of the fetus and later in the caudal portions.

The adult epidermis is composed of three basic cell types: keratinocytes, melanocytes, and Langerhans cells. An additional cell, the Merkel cell, can be found in the basal layer of the palms and soles, oral and genital mucosa, nail bed, and follicular infundibula. Merkel cells, located directly above the basement membrane zone, contain intracytoplasmic dense-core neurosecretory-like granules, and, through their association with neurites, act as slow-adapting touch receptors. They have direct connections with adjacent keratinocytes by desmosomes and contain a paranuclear whorl of intermediate keratin filaments. Both polyclonal keratin immunostains and monoclonal immunostaining for keratin 20 stain this whorl of keratin filaments in a characteristic paranuclear dot pattern. Merkel cells also label for neuroendocrine markers such as chromogranin and synaptophysin.

Keratinocytes

Keratinocytes, or squamous cells, are the principal cells of the epidermis. They are of ectodermal origin and have the specialized function of producing keratin, a complex filamentous protein that not only forms the surface coat (stratum corneum) of the epidermis but also is the structural protein of hair and nails. Multiple distinct keratin genes have been identified and

consist of two subfamilies, acidic and basic. The product of one basic and one acidic keratin gene combines to form the multiple keratins that occur in many tissues. The presence of various keratin types is used as a marker for the type and degree of differentiation of a population of keratinocytes. Keratins are critical for normal functioning of the epidermis and keratin mutations are recognized causes of skin disease. Mutations in the genes for keratins 5 and 14 are associated with epidermolysis bullosa simplex. Keratin 1 and 10 mutations are associated with epidermolytic hyperkeratosis. Mild forms of this disorder may represent localized or widespread expressions of mosaicism for these gene mutations.

The epidermis may be divided into the following zones, beginning with the innermost layer: basal layer (stratum germinativum), Malpighian or prickle layer (stratum spinosum), granular layer (stratum granulosum), and horny layer (stratum corneum). On the palms and soles a pale clear to pink layer, the stratum lucidum, is noted just above the granular layer. When the skin in other sites is scratched or rubbed, the Malpighian and granular layers thicken, a stratum lucidum forms, and the stratum corneum becomes thick and compact. Histones appear to regulate epidermal differentiation and histone deacetylation suppresses expression of profilaggrin. Slow-cycling stem cells provide a reservoir for regeneration of the epidermis. Sites rich in stem cells include the deepest portions of the rete, especially on palmoplantar skin, as well as the hair bulge. Stem cells divide infrequently in normal skin, but in cell culture they form active growing colonies. They can be identified by their high expression of β1-integrins and lack of terminal differentiation markers. Stem cells can also be identified by their low levels of desmosomal proteins, such as desmoglein 3. The basal cells divide and, as their progeny move upward, they flatten and their nucleus disappears. Abnormal keratinization can manifest as parakeratosis (retained nuclei), as corps ronds (round, clear to pink, abnormally keratinized cells), or as grains (elongated, basophilic, abnormally keratinized cells).

During keratinization, the keratinocyte first passes through a synthetic and then a degradative phase on its way to becoming a horn cell. In the synthetic phase, the keratinocyte accumulates within its cytoplasm intermediate filaments composed of a fibrous protein, keratin, arranged in an alpha-helical coiled coil pattern. These tonofilaments are fashioned into bundles, which converge on and terminate at the plasma membrane, where they end in specialized attachment plates called desmosomes. The degradative phase of keratinization is characterized by the disappearance of cell organelles and the consolidation of all contents into a mixture of filaments and amorphous cell envelopes. This programmed process of maturation resulting in death of the cell is termed terminal differentiation. Terminal differentiation is also seen in the involuting stage of keratoacanthomas, where the initial phase of proliferation gives way to terminal keratinization and involution.

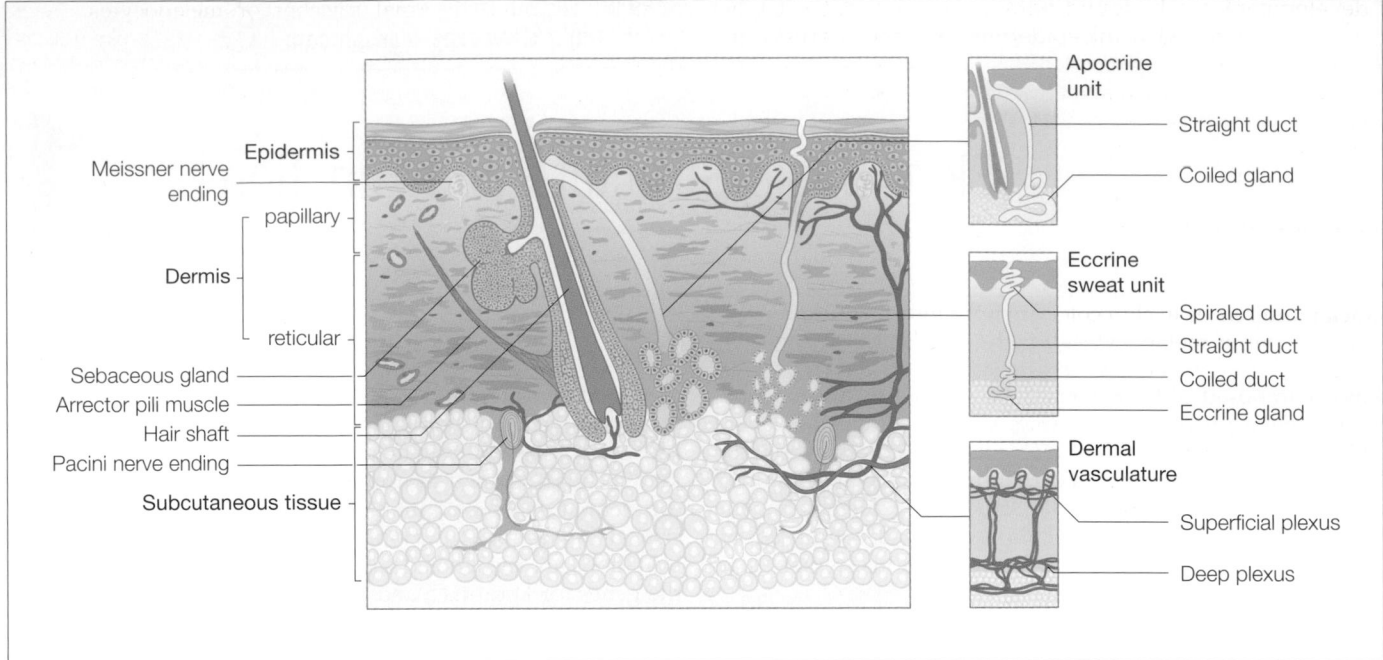

Fig. 1-1 Diagrammatic cross-section of the skin and panniculus.

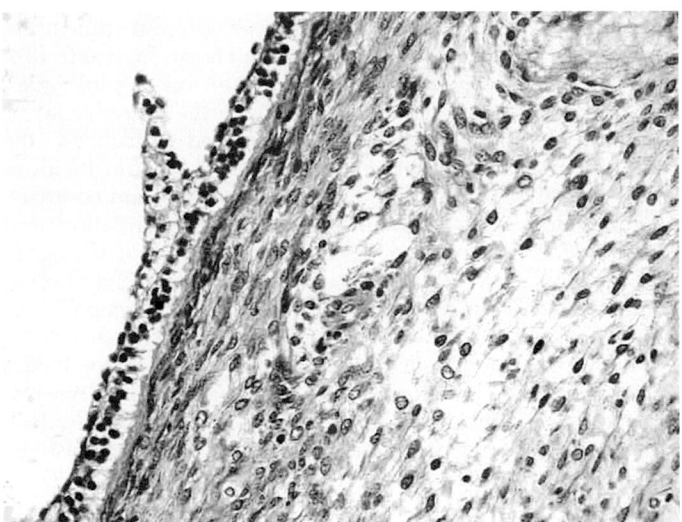

Fig. 1-2 Fetal periderm covering fetal mesenchyme.

Premature programmed cell death, or apoptosis, appears in hematoxylin and eosin (H&E)-stained sections as the presence of scattered bright red cells, some of which may contain small black pyknotic nuclei. These cells are present at various levels of the epidermis, as this form of cell death does not represent part of the normal process of maturation. Widespread apoptosis is noted in the verrucous phase of incontinentia pigmenti. It is also a prominent finding in catagen hairs, where apoptosis results in the involution of the inferior segment of the hair follicle.

In normal skin, the plasma membranes of adjacent cells are separated by an intercellular space. Electron microscopic histochemical studies have shown that this interspace contains glycoproteins and lipids. Lamellar granules (Odland bodies or membrane-coating granules) appear in this space, primarily at the interface between the granular and cornified cell layers. Lamellar granules contribute to skin cohesion and impermeability. Conditions such as lamellar ichthyosis and Flegel's hyperkeratosis demonstrate abnormal lamellar granules.

Glycolipids such as ceramides contribute a water barrier function to skin and are commonly found in topical products meant to restore the epidermal barrier. Lamellar bodies form abnormally in the absence of critical ceramides such as glucosylceramide or there is disproportion of critical lipids. Desmosomal adhesion depends upon cadherins, including the calcium-dependent desmogleins and desmocollins. Antibodies to these molecules result in immunobullous diseases.

Keratinocytes of the granular zone contain, in addition to the keratin filament system, keratohyaline granules, composed of amorphous particulate material of high sulfur–protein content. This material, called profilaggrin, is a precursor to filaggrin, so named because it is thought to be responsible for keratin filament aggregation. Conversion to filaggrin takes place in the granular layer, and this forms the electron-dense interfilamentous protein matrix of mature epidermal keratin. Keratohyaline is hygroscopic, and repeated cycles of hydration and dehydration contribute to normal desquamation of the stratum corneum. Ichthyosis vulgaris is characterized by a diminished or absent granular layer, contributing to the retention hyperkeratosis noted in this disorder. Keratohyalin results in the formation of soft, flexible keratin. Keratin that forms in the absence of keratohyaline granules is typically hard and rigid. Hair fibers and nails are composed of hard keratin.

Keratinocytes play an active role in the immune function of the skin. In conditions such as allergic contact dermatitis they participate in the induction of the immune response, rather than acting as passive victims. Keratinocytes secrete a wide array of cytokines and inflammatory mediators, including tumor necrosis factor (TNF)-α. They also can express molecules on their surface, such as intercellular adhesion molecule-1 (ICAM-1) and major histocompatibility complex (MHC) class II molecules, suggesting that keratinocytes actively respond to immune effector signals.

Melanocytes

Melanocytes are the pigment-producing cells of the epidermis. They are derived from the neural crest and by the eighth week of development can be found within the fetal epidermis. In normal, sun-protected, trunk epidermis, melanocytes reside in the basal layer at a frequency of approximately 1 in every 10 basal keratinocytes. Areas such as the face, shins, and genitalia have a greater density of melanocytes, and in heavily sun-damaged facial skin, Mart-1 immunostaining can demonstrate ratios of melanocytes to basal keratinocytes that approach 1:1. Recognition of the variation in melanocyte to keratinocyte ratio is critical in the interpretation of biopsies of suspected lentigo maligna (malignant melanoma in situ) on sun-damaged skin.

Racial differences in skin color are not caused by differences in the number of melanocytes. It is the number, size, and distribution of the melanosomes or pigment granules within keratinocytes that determine differences in skin color. Pale skin has fewer melanosomes and these are smaller and packaged within membrane-bound complexes. Dark skin has more melanosomes, and these tend to be larger and singly dispersed. Chronic sun exposure can stimulate melanocytes to produce larger melanosomes, thereby making the distribution of melanosomes within keratinocytes resemble the pattern seen in dark-skinned individuals.

In histologic sections of skin routinely stained by H&E, the melanocyte appears as a cell with ample amphophilic cytoplasm, or as a clear cell in the basal layer of the epidermis. The apparent halo is an artifact formed during fixation of the specimen. This occurs because the melanocyte, lacking tonofilaments, cannot form desmosomal attachments with keratinocytes. Keratinocytes also frequently demonstrate clear spaces, but can be differentiated from melanocytes because they demonstrate cell–cell junctions and a layer of cytoplasm peripheral to the clear space.

The melanocyte is a dendritic cell. Its dendrites extend for long distances within the epidermis and any one melanocyte is therefore in contact with a great number of keratinocytes; together they form the so-called epidermal melanin unit. Keratinocytes actively ingest the tips of the melanocytic dendrites, thus imbibing the melanosomes.

Melanosomes are synthesized in the Golgi zone of the cell and pass through a series of stages in which the enzyme tyrosinase acts on melanin precursors to produce the densely pigmented granules. Melanocytes in red-heads tend to be rounder and produce more phaeomelanin. The melanocortin 1 receptor (MC1R) is important in the regulation of melanin production. Loss-of-function mutations in the *MC1R* gene bring about a change from eumelanin to phaeomelanin production, whereas activating gene mutations can enhance eumelanin synthesis. Most red-heads are compound heterozygotes or homozygotes for a variety of loss-of-function mutations in this gene. Eumelanin production is optimal at pH 6.8 and changes in cellular pH also result in alterations of melanin production and the eumelanin to phaeomelanin ratio. Within keratinocytes, melanin typically forms a cap over the nucleus, where it presumably functions principally in a photoprotective role. Evidence of keratinocyte photodamage in the form of thymidine dimer formation can be assessed using gas chromatography–mass spectrometry or enzyme-linked immunosorbent assays. Pigment within melanocytes also serves to protect the melanocytes themselves against photodamage, such as ultraviolet (UV) A-induced membrane damage.

Areas of leukoderma or whitening of skin can be caused by very different phenomena. In vitiligo, the affected skin becomes white because of destruction of melanocytes. In albinism, the number of melanocytes is normal, but they are unable to synthesize fully pigmented melanosomes because of defects in the enzymatic formation of melanin. Local areas of increased pigmentation can result from a variety of causes. The typical freckle results from a localized increase in production of pigment by a near-normal number of melanocytes. Black "sunburn" or "ink spot" lentigines demonstrate basilar hyperpigmentation and prominent melanin within the stratum corneum. Nevi are benign proliferations of melanocytes. Melanomas are their malignant counterpart. Melanocytes and keratinocytes express neurotrophins (ectodermal nerve growth factors). Melanocytes release neurotrophin 4, but the release is downregulated by UVB irradiation, suggesting neurotrophins as possible targets for therapy of disorders of pigmentation. Melanocytes express toll-like receptors (TLRs) and stimulation by bacterial lipopolysaccharides increases pigmentation.

Langerhans cells

Langerhans cells are normally found scattered among keratinocytes of the stratum spinosum. They constitute 3–5% of the cells in this layer. Like melanocytes, they are not connected to adjacent keratinocytes by the desmosomes. The highest density of Langerhans cells in the oral mucosa occurs in the vestibular region, and the lowest density in the sublingual region, suggesting the latter is a relatively immunologically "privileged" site.

At the light microscopic level, Langerhans cells are difficult to detect in routinely stained sections; however, they appear as dendritic cells in sections impregnated with gold chloride, a stain specific for Langerhans cells. They can also be stained with CD1α or S-100 immunostains. Ultrastructurally, they are characterized by a folded nucleus and distinct intracytoplasmic organelles called Birbeck granules. In their fully developed form, the organelles are rod-shaped with a vacuole at one end and they resemble a tennis racquet. The vacuole is an artifact of processing.

Functionally, Langerhans cells are of the monocyte–macrophage lineage and originate in bone marrow. They function primarily in the afferent limb of the immune response by providing for the recognition, uptake, processing, and presentation of antigens to sensitized T lymphocytes, and are important in the induction of delayed-type sensitivity. Once an antigen is presented, Langerhans cells migrate to the lymph nodes. Hyaluronan (hyaluronic acid) plays a critical role in Langerhans cell maturation and migration. Langerhans cells express langerin, membrane ATPase (CD39), and CCR6, while CD1α[+] dermal dendritic cells express macrophage mannose receptor, CD36, factor XIIIa, and chemokine receptor 5, suggesting different functions for these two CD1α+ populations. If skin is depleted of Langerhans cells by exposure to UV radiation, it loses the ability to be sensitized until its population of Langerhans cell is replenished. Macrophages that present antigen in Langerhans cell-depleted skin can induce immune tolerance. In contrast to Langerhans cells, which make interleukin (IL)-12, the macrophages found in the epidermis 72 h after UVB irradiation produce IL-10, resulting in downregulation of the immune response. At least in mice, viral immunity appears to require priming by CD8α+ dendritic cells, rather than Langerhans cells, suggesting a complex pattern of antigen presentation in cutaneous immunity.

Ahn JH, et al: Human melanocytes express functional toll-like receptor 4. Exp Dermatol 2008 May; 17(5):412–417.

Allam JP, et al: Distribution of Langerhans cells and mast cells within the human oral mucosa: new application sites of allergens in sublingual immunotherapy? Allergy 2008 Jun; 63(6):720–727.

Baxter LL, et al: Networks and pathways in pigmentation, health, and disease. Wiley Interdiscip Rev Syst Biol Med 2009 Nov 1; 1(3):359–371.

Boulais N, et al: The epidermis: a sensory tissue. Eur J Dermatol 2008 Mar–Apr; 18(2):119–127.

Dusek RL, et al: Discriminating roles of desmosomal cadherins: beyond desmosomal adhesion. J Dermatol Sci 2007 Jan; 45(1):7–21.

Ernfors P: Cellular origin and developmental mechanisms during the formation of skin melanocytes. Exp Cell Res 2010 May 1; 316(8):1397–1407.

Imai Y, et al: Freshly isolated Langerhans cells negatively regulate naïve T cell activation in response to peptide antigen through cell-to-cell contact. J Dermatol Sci 2008 Jul; 51(1):19–29.

Jennemann R, et al: Integrity and barrier function of the epidermis critically depend on glucosylceramide synthesis. J Biol Chem 2007 Feb 2; 282(5):3083–3094.

Le Douarin NM, et al: The stem cells of the neural crest. Cell Cycle 2008 Jan; 24:7(8).

Markova NG, et al: Inhibition of histone deacetylation promotes abnormal epidermal differentiation and specifically suppresses the expression of the late differentiation marker profilaggrin. J Invest Dermatol 2007 May; 127(5):1126–1139.

Ortonne JP, et al: Latest insights into skin hyperpigmentation. J Investig Dermatol Symp Proc 2008 Apr; 13(1):10–14.

Santegoets SJ, et al: Transcriptional profiling of human skin-resident Langerhans cells and CD1α+ dermal dendritic cells: differential activation states suggest distinct functions. J Leukoc Biol 2008 Apr; 24.

Schwarz T: Regulatory T cells induced by ultraviolet radiation. Int Arch Allergy Immunol 2005; 137:187.

Dermoepidermal junction

The junction of the epidermis and dermis is formed by the basement membrane zone (BMZ). Ultrastructurally, this zone is composed of four components: the plasma membranes of the basal cells with the specialized attachment plates (hemidesmosomes); an electron-lucent zone called the lamina lucida; the lamina densa (basal lamina); and the fibrous components associated with the basal lamina, including anchoring fibrils, dermal microfibrils, and collagen fibers. At the light microscopic level, the periodic acid–Schiff (PAS)-positive basement membrane is composed of the fibrous components. The basal lamina is synthesized by the basal cells of the epidermis. Type IV collagen is the major component of the basal lamina. Type VII collagen is the major component of anchoring fibrils. The two major hemidesmosomal proteins are the BP230 (bullous pemphigoid antigen 1) and BP180 (bullous pemphigoid antigen 2, type XVII collagen).

In the upper permanent portion of the anagen follicle, plectin, BP230, BP180, α6β4-integrin, laminin 5, and type VII collagen show essentially the same expression as that found in the interfollicular epidermis. Staining in the lower, transient portion of the hair follicle, however, is different. All BMZ components diminish and may become discontinuous in the inferior segment of the follicle. Hemidesmosomes are also not apparent in the BMZ of the hair bulb. The lack of hemidesmosomes in the deep portions of the follicle may relate to the transient nature of the inferior segment, while abundant hemidesmosomes stabilize the upper portion of the follicle.

The BMZ is considered to be a porous semipermeable filter, which permits exchange of cells and fluid between the epidermis and dermis. It further serves as a structural support for the epidermis and holds the epidermis and dermis together, but also helps to regulate growth, adhesion, and movement of keratinocytes and fibroblasts, as well as apoptosis. Much of this regulation takes place through activation of integrins and syndecans. Extracellular matrix protein 1 demonstrates loss-of-function mutations in lipoid proteinosis, resulting in reduplication of the basement membrane.

Masunaga T: Epidermal basement membrane: its molecular organization and blistering disorders. Connect Tissue Res 2006; 47(2):55–66.

McMillan JR, et al: Epidermal basement membrane zone components: ultrastructural distribution and molecular interactions. J Dermatol Sci 2003; 31:169.

Schéele S, et al: Laminin isoforms in development and disease. J Mol Med 2007 Aug; 85(8):825–836.

Sercu S, et al: Interaction of extracellular matrix protein 1 with extracellular matrix components: ECM1 is a basement membrane protein of the skin. J Invest Dermatol 2008 Jun; 128(6):1397–1408.

Sugawara K, et al: Laminin-332 and 511 in skin. Exp Dermatol 2008 Jun; 17(6):473–480.

Verdolini R, et al: Autoimmune subepidermal bullous skin diseases: the impact of recent findings for the dermatopathologist. Virchows Arch 2003; 443:184.

Epidermal appendages: adnexa

Eccrine and apocrine glands, ducts, and pilosebaceous units constitute the skin adnexa. Embryologically, they originate as downgrowths from the epidermis and are therefore ectodermal in origin. Hedgehog signaling by the signal transducer known as smoothened appears critical for hair development. Abnormalities in this pathway contribute to the formation of pilar tumors and basal cell carcinoma. In the absence of hedghog signaling, embryonic hair germs may develop instead into modified sweat gland or mammary epithelium.

While the various adnexal structures serve specific functions, they all can function as reserve epidermis in that re-epithelialization after injury to the surface epidermis occurs, principally by virtue of the migration of keratinocytes from the adnexal epithelium to the skin surface. It is not surprising, therefore, that skin sites such as the face or scalp, which contain pilosebaceous units in abundance, reepithelialize more rapidly than do skin sites such as the back, where adnexae of all types are comparatively scarce. Once a wound has reepithelialized, granulation tissue is no longer produced. Deep saucerized biopsies in an area with few adnexae will slowly fill with granulation tissue until they are flush with the surrounding skin. In contrast, areas rich in adnexae will quickly be covered with epithelium. No more granulation tissue will form and the contour defect created by the saucerization will persist.

The pseudoepitheliomatous hyperplasia noted in infections and inflammatory conditions consists almost exclusively of adnexal epithelium. Areas of thin intervening epidermis are generally evident between areas of massively hypertrophic adnexal epithelium.

Eccrine sweat units

The eccrine sweat unit is composed of three sections that are modified from the basic tubular structure that formed during embryogenesis as a downgrowth of surface epidermis. The intraepidermal spiral duct, which opens directly on to the skin surface, is called the acrosyringium. It is derived from dermal duct cells through mitosis and upward migration. The acrosyringium is composed of small polygonal cells with a central round nucleus surrounded by ample pink cytoplasm. Cornification takes place within the duct and the horn cells become part of the stratum corneum of the epidermis. In the stratum corneum overlying an actinic keratosis, the lamellar spiral acrosyringeal keratin often stands out prominently against the compact red parakeratotic keratin produced by the actinic keratosis.

The straight dermal portion of the duct is composed of a double layer of cuboidal epithelial cells and is lined by an eosinophilic cuticle on its luminal side. The coiled secretory acinar portion of the eccrine sweat gland may be found within the superficial panniculus. In areas of skin, such as the back, that possess a thick dermis, the eccrine coil is found in the deep dermis, surrounded by an extension of fat from the underlying panniculus. An inner layer of epithelial cells, the secretory portion of the gland, is surrounded by a layer of flattened myoepithelial cells. The secretory cells are of two types: glycogen-rich, large pale cells; and smaller, darker-staining cells. The pale glycogen-rich cells are thought to initiate the formation of sweat. The darker cells may function in a manner similar to that of cells of the dermal duct, which actively reabsorb sodium, thereby modifying sweat from a basically isotonic solution to a hypotonic one by the time it reaches the skin surface. Sweat is similar in composition to plasma, containing the same electrolytes, though in a more dilute concentration. Physical conditioning in a hot environment results in production of larger amounts of extremely hypotonic sweat in response to a thermal stimulus. This adaptive response allows greater cooling with conservation of sodium.

In humans, eccrine sweat units are found at virtually all skin sites. Other mammals have both apocrine and eccrine glands, but the apocrine gland is the major sweat gland, and eccrine glands are generally restricted to areas such as the footpad. Ringtailed lemurs have an antebrachial organ rich in sweat glands with hybrid characteristics of eccrine and apocrine glands.

In humans, eccrine glands are abundant and serve a thermoregulatory function. They are most abundant on the palms, soles, forehead, and axillae. Some eccrine glands in the axillae, especially in patients with hyperhidrosis, may have widely dilated secretory coils that contain apocrine-appearing cells. These findings suggest the presence of hybrid glands in humans. On friction surfaces, such as the palms and soles, eccrine secretion is thought to assist tactile sensibility and improve adhesion.

Physiologic secretion of sweat occurs as a result of many factors and is mediated by cholinergic innervation. Heat is a prime stimulus to increased sweating, but other physiologic stimuli, including emotional stress, are important as well. During early development, there is a switch between adrenergic and cholinergic innervation of sweat glands. Some responsiveness to both cholinergic and adrenergic stimuli persists. Cholinergic sweating involves a biphasic response, with initial hyperpolarization and secondary depolarization mediated by the activation of calcium and chloride ion conductance. Adrenergic secretion involves monophasic depolarization and is dependent on cystic fibrosis transmembrane conductance regulator-GCl. Cells from patients with cystic fibrosis demonstrate no adrenergic secretion. Vasoactive intestinal polypeptide may also play a role in stimulating eccrine secretion.

Apocrine units

Apocrine units develop as outgrowths, not of the surface epidermis, but of the infundibular or upper portion of the hair follicle. Although immature apocrine units are found covering the entire skin surface of the human fetus, these regress and are absent by the time the fetus reaches term. The straight excretory portion of the duct, which opens into the infundibular portion of the hair follicle, is composed of a double layer of cuboidal epithelial cells.

Hidrocystomas may show focal secretory cells, but are generally composed of cuboidal cells resembling the straight portion of the apocrine duct. Various benign cutaneous tumors demonstrate differentiation resembling apocrine duct cells, including hidroacanthoma simplex, poroma, dermal duct tumor, and nodular hidradenoma. Although some of these tumors were formerly classified as "eccrine" in differentiation, each may demonstrate focal apocrine decapitation secretion, suggesting apocrine differentiation.

The coiled secretory gland is located at the junction of the dermis and subcutaneous fat. It is lined by a single layer of cells, which vary in appearance from columnar to cuboidal. This layer of cells is surrounded by a layer of myoepithelial cells. Apocrine coils appear more widely dilated than eccrine

coils, and apocrine sweat stains more deeply red in H&E sections, contrasting with the pale pink of eccrine sweat.

The apices of the columnar cells project into the lumen of the gland and in histologic cross-section appear as if they are being extruded (decapitation secretion). Controversy exists about the mode of secretion in apocrine secretory cells, whether merocrine, apocrine, holocrine, or all three. The composition of the product of secretion is only partially understood. Protein, carbohydrate, ammonia, lipid, and iron are all found in apocrine secretion. It appears milky white, although lipofuscin pigment may rarely produce dark shades of brown and gray-blue (apocrine chromhidrosis). Apocrine sweat is odorless until it reaches the skin surface, where it is altered by bacteria, which makes it odoriferous. Apocrine secretion is mediated by adrenergic innervation and by circulating catecholamines of adrenomedullary origin. Vasoactive intestinal polypeptide may also play a role in stimulating apocrine secretion. Apocrine excretion is episodic, although the actual secretion of the gland is continuous. Apocrine gland secretion in humans serves no known function. In other species it has a protective as well as a sexual function, and in some species it is important in thermoregulation as well.

Although occasionally found in an ectopic location, apocrine units of the human body are generally confined to the following sites: axillae, areolae, anogenital region, external auditory canal (ceruminous glands), and eyelids (glands of Moll). They are also generally prominent in the stroma of nevus sebaceous of Jadassohn. Apocrine glands do not begin to function until puberty.

Hair follicles

During embryogenesis, mesenchymal cells in the fetal dermis collect immediately below the basal layer of the epidermis. Epidermal buds grow down into the dermis at these sites. The developing follicle forms at an angle to the skin surface and continues its downward growth. At this base, the column of cells widens, forming the bulb, and surrounds small collections of mesenchymal cells. These papillary mesenchymal bodies contain mesenchymal stem cells with broad functionality. At least in mice, they demonstrate extramedullary hematopoietic stem cell activity, and represent a potential therapeutic source of hematopoietic stem cells and a possible source of extramedullary hematopoiesis in vivo.

Along one side of the fetal follicle, two buds are formed: an upper, which develops into the sebaceous gland, and a lower, which becomes the attachment for the arrector pili muscle. A third epithelial bud develops from the opposite side of the follicle above the level of the sebaceous gland anlage, and gives rise to the apocrine gland. The uppermost portion of the follicle, which extends from its surface opening to the entrance of the sebaceous duct, is called the infundibular segment. It resembles the surface epidermis and its keratinocytes may be of epidermal origin. The portion of the follicle between the sebaceous duct and the insertion of the arrector pili muscle is the isthmus. The inner root sheath fully keratinizes and sheds within this isthmic portion. The inferior portion includes the lowermost part of the follicle and the hair bulb. Throughout life, the inferior portion undergoes cycles of involution and regeneration.

Hair follicles develop sequentially in rows of three. Primary follicles are surrounded by the appearance of two secondary follicles; other secondary follicles subsequently develop around the principal units. The density of pilosebaceous units decreases throughout life, possibly because of dropout of the secondary follicles. In mouse models, signaling by molecules designated as ectodysplasin A and noggin is essential for the

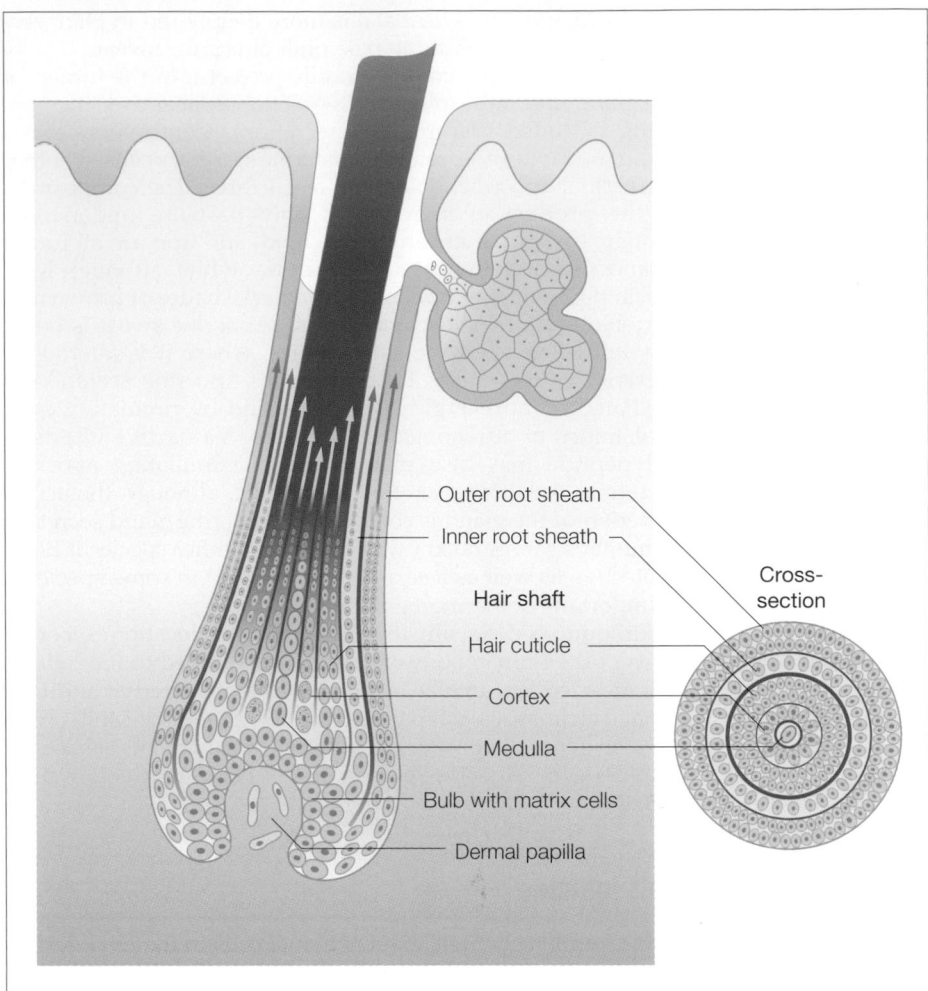

Fig. 1-3 Anatomy of the hair follicle.

Outer root sheath

Inner root sheath

Hair shaft

Hair cuticle

Cortex

Medulla

Bulb with matrix cells

Dermal papilla

Cross-section

development of primary hair follicles and induction of secondary follicles. Arrector pili muscles contained within the follicular unit interconnect at the level of the isthmus.

The actual hair shaft, as well as an inner and an outer root sheath, is produced by the matrix portion of the hair bulb (Fig. 1-3). The sheaths and contained hair form concentric cylindrical layers. The hair shaft and inner root sheath move together as the hair grows upwards until the fully keratinized inner root sheath sheds at the level of the isthmus. The epidermis of the upper part of the follicular canal is contiguous with the outer root sheath. The upper two portions of the follicle (infundibulum and isthmus) are permanent; the inferior segment is completely replaced with each new cycle of hair growth. On the scalp, anagen, the active growth phase, lasts about 3–5 years. Normally, approximately 85–90% of all scalp hairs are in the anagen phase, a figure that decreases with age and decreases faster in individuals with male-pattern baldness (as the length of anagen decreases dramatically). Scalp anagen hairs grow at a rate of about 0.37 mm/day. Catagen, or involution, lasts about 2 weeks. Telogen, the resting phase, lasts about 3–5 months. Most sites on the body have a much shorter anagen phase and much longer telogen, resulting in short hairs that stay in place for long periods of time without growing longer. Prolongation of the anagen phase results in long eyelashes in patients with acquired immunodeficiency syndrome (AIDS).

Human hair growth is cyclical, but each follicle functions as an independent unit (Fig. 1-4). Therefore, humans do not shed hair synchronously, as most animals do. Each hair follicle undergoes intermittent stages of activity and quiescence. Synchronous termination of anagen or telogen results in telogen effluvium. Most commonly, telogen effluvium is the result of early release from anagen, such as that induced by a febrile illness, surgery, or weight loss.

Various exogenous and endogenous physiologic factors can modulate the hair cycle. The hair papilla and the connective tissue sheath form a communicating network through gap junctions. This network may play a role in controlling hair cycling. Pregnancy is typically accompanied by retention of an increased number of scalp hairs in the anagen phase, as well as a prolongation of telogen. Soon after delivery, telogen loss can be detected as abnormally prolonged telogen hairs are released. At the same time, abnormally prolonged anagen hairs are converted synchronously to telogen. Between 3 and 5 months later, a more profound effluvium is noted. Patients on chemotherapy often have hair loss because the drugs interfere with the mitotic activity of the hair matrix, leading to the formation of a tapered fracture. Only anagen hairs are affected, leaving a sparse coat of telogen hairs on the scalp. As the matrix recovers, anagen hairs resume growth without having to cycle through catagen and telogen.

The growing anagen hair is characterized by a pigmented bulb (Fig. 1-5) and an inner root sheath (Fig. 1-6). Histologically, catagen hairs are best identified by the presence of many apoptotic cells in the outer root sheath (Fig. 1-7). Telogen club hairs have a nonpigmented bulb with a shaggy lower border. The presence of bright red trichilemmal keratin bordering the club hair results in a flame thrower-like appearance in vertical H&E sections (Fig. 1-8). As the new anagen hair grows, the old telogen hair is shed.

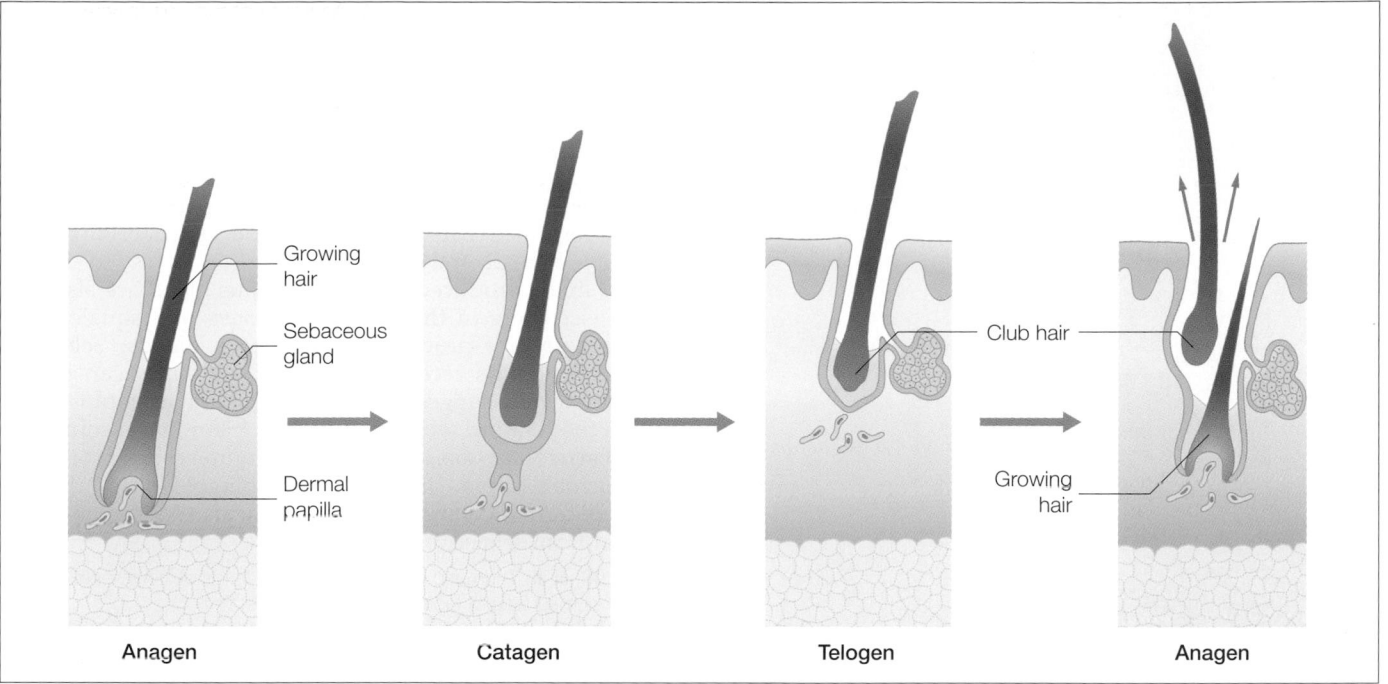

Fig. 1-4 Phases of the growth cycle of a hair.

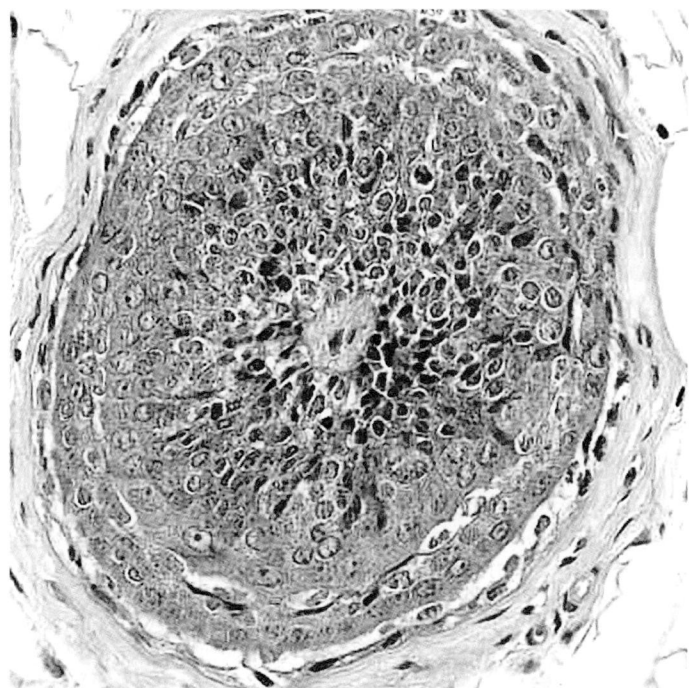

Fig. 1-5 Cross-section of anagen bulb demonstrating pigment within matrix.

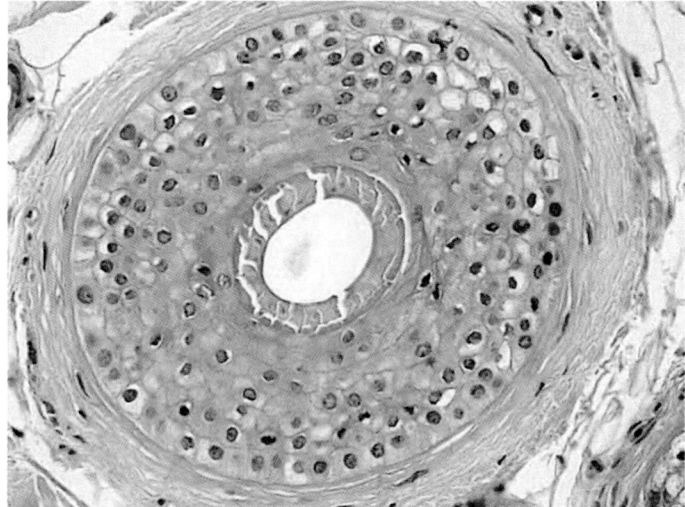

Fig. 1-6 Cross-section of isthmus of anagen follicle demonstrating glycogenated outer root sheath and keratinized inner root sheath.

The scalp hair of white people is round; pubic hair, beard hair, and eyelashes are oval. The scalp hair of black people is also oval, and it is this, plus a curvature of the follicle just above the bulb, that causes black hair to be curly. Uncombable hair is triangular with a central canal.

Hair color depends on the degree of melanization and distribution of melanosomes within the hair shaft. Melanocytes of the hair bulb synthesize melanosomes and transfer them to the keratinocytes of the bulb matrix. Larger melanosomes are found in the hair of black persons; smaller melanosomes, which are aggregated within membrane-bound complexes, are found in the hair of white persons. Red hair is character-ized by spherical melanosomes. Graying of hair is a result of a decreased number of melanocytes, which produce fewer melanosomes. Repetitive oxidative stress causes apoptosis of hair follicle melanocytes, resulting in normal hair graying. Premature graying is related to exhaustion of the melanocyte stem cell pool.

Sebaceous glands

Sebaceous glands are formed embryologically as an outgrowth from the upper portion of the hair follicle. They are composed of lobules of pale-staining cells with abundant lipid droplets in their cytoplasm. At the periphery of the lobules basaloid germinative cells are noted. These germinative cells give rise to the lipid-filled pale cells, which are continuously being extruded through the short sebaceous duct into the infundibu-lar portion of the hair follicle. The sebaceous duct is lined by a red cuticle that undulates sharply in a pattern resembling

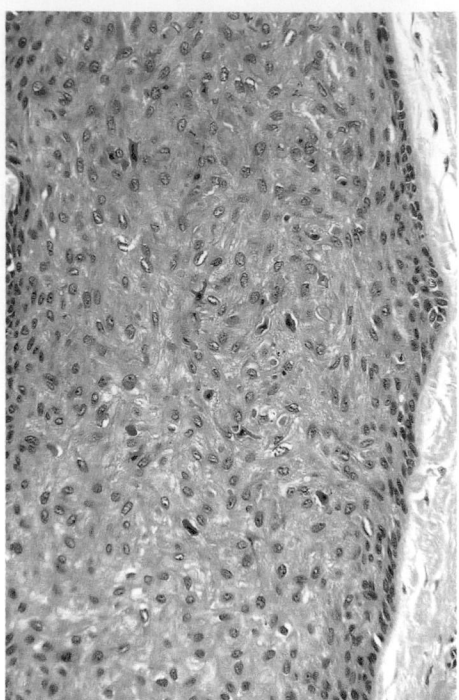

Fig. 1-7 Catagen hair with many apoptotic keratinocytes within the outer root sheath.

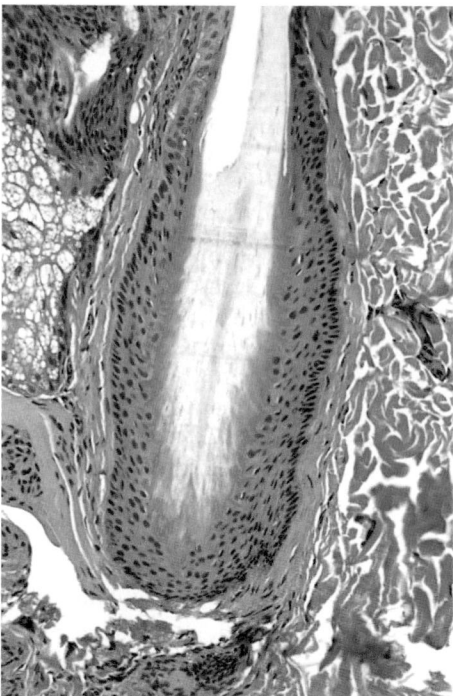

Fig. 1-8 Vertical section of telogen hair demonstrating "flame thrower" appearance of club hair.

shark's teeth. This same undulating cuticle is seen in steatocystoma and some dermoid cysts.

Sebaceous glands are found in greatest abundance on the face and scalp, though they are distributed throughout all skin sites except the palms and soles. They are always associated with hair follicles except at the following sites: tarsal plate of the eyelids (meibomian glands), buccal mucosa and vermilion border of the lip (Fordyce spots), prepuce and mucosa lateral to the penile frenulum (Tyson glands), labia minora, and female areola (Montgomery tubercles).

Although sebaceous glands are independent miniorgans in their own right, they are anatomically and functionally related to the hair follicle. Cutaneous disorders attributed to sebaceous glands, such as acne vulgaris, are really disorders of the entire pilosebaceous unit. The clinical manifestations of acne, namely the comedo, papule, pustule, and cyst, would not form, regardless of increased sebaceous gland activity, as long as the sebaceous duct and infundibular portion of the hair follicle remained patent, and lipid and cell debris (sebum) were able to reach the skin surface.

Most lipids produced by the sebaceous gland are also produced elsewhere in the body. Wax esters and squalene are unique secretory products of sebaceous glands. Sebocytes express histamine receptors and antihistamines can reduce squalene levels, suggesting that antihistamines could play a role in modulating sebum production. Skin lipids contribute to the barrier function and some have antimicrobial properties. Antimicrobial lipids include free sphingoid bases derived from epidermal ceramides and fatty acids like sapienic acid derived from sebaceous triglycerides.

Drake DR, et al: Thematic review series: skin lipids. Antimicrobial lipids at the skin surface. J Lipid Res 2008 Jan; 49(1):4–11.
Gritli-Linde A, et al: Abnormal hair development and apparent follicular transformation to mammary gland in the absence of hedgehog signaling. Dev Cell 2007 Jan; 12(1):99–112.
Kizawa K, et al: Specific citrullination causes assembly of a globular S100A3 homotetramer: a putative Ca2+ modulator matures human hair cuticle. J Biol Chem 2008 Feb 22; 283(8):5004–5013.
Novotný J, et al: Synthesis and structure-activity relationships of skin ceramides. Curr Med Chem 2010; 17(21):2301–2324.
Pelle E, et al: Identification of histamine receptors and reduction of squalene levels by an antihistamine in sebocytes. J Invest Dermatol 2008 May; 128(5):1280–1285.
Saga K: Structure and function of human sweat glands studied with histochemistry and cytochemistry. Prog Histochem Cytochem 2002; 37:323.
Smith KR, et al: Thematic review series: skin lipids. Sebaceous gland lipids: friend or foe? J Lipid Res 2008 Feb; 49(2):271–281.
Spatz KR, et al: Increased melanocyte apoptosis under stress-mediator substance P-elucidating pathways involved in stress-induced premature graying. Exp Dermatol 2008 Jul; 17(7):632.
Xu X, et al: Co-factors of LIM domains (Clims/Ldb/Nli) regulate corneal homeostasis and maintenance of hair follicle stem cells. Dev Biol 2007 Dec 15; 312(2):484–500.

Nails

Nails act to assist in grasping small objects and in protecting the fingertip from trauma. Matrix keratinization leads to the formation of the nail plate. Fingernails grow an average of 0.1 mm/day, requiring about 4–6 months to replace a complete nail plate. The growth rate is much slower for toenails, with 12–18 months required to replace the great toenail. Abnormalities of the nail may serve as important clues to cutaneous and systemic disease, and may provide the astute clinician with information about disease or toxic exposures that occurred several months in the past.

The keratin types found in the nail are a mixture of epidermal and hair types, with the hair types predominating. Nail isthmus keratinization differs from that of the nail bed in that K10 is only present in nail isthmus. Brittle nails demonstrate widening of the intercellular space between nail keratinocytes on electron microscopy.

Whereas most of the skin is characterized by rete pegs that resemble an egg crate, the nail bed has true parallel rete ridges. These ridges result in the formation of splinter hemorrhages when small quantities of extravasated red cells mark their path. The nail cuticle is formed by keratinocytes of the proximal nailfold, whereas the nail plate is formed by matrix keratinocytes. Endogenous pigments tend to follow the contour of the lunula (the distal portion of the matrix), whereas exogenous pigments tend to follow the contour of the cuticle. The dorsal nail plate is formed by the proximal matrix, and the ventral nail plate is formed by the distal matrix with some contribution from the nail bed. The location of a melanocytic lesion within the matrix can be assessed by the presence of pigment within the dorsal or ventral nail plate.

Kitamori K, et al: Weakness in intercellular association of keratinocytes in severely brittle nails. Arch Histol Cytol 2006 Dec; 69(5):323–328.

McCarthy DJ: Anatomic considerations of the human nail. Clin Podiatr Med Surg 2004; 21:477.

Perrin C: Expression of follicular sheath keratins in the normal nail with special reference to the morphological analysis of the distal nail unit. Am J Dermatopathol 2007 Dec; 29(6):543–550.

Dermis

The constituents of the dermis are mesodermal in origin except for nerves, which, like melanocytes, derive from the neural crest. Until the sixth week of fetal life, the dermis is merely a pool of acid mucopolysaccharide-containing, scattered dendritic-shaped cells, which are the precursors of fibroblasts. By the 12th week, fibroblasts are actively synthesizing reticulum fibers, elastic fibers, and collagen. A vascular network develops, and by the 24th week, fat cells have appeared beneath the dermis. During fetal development, Wnt/beta-catenin signaling is critical for differentiation of ventral versus dorsal dermis, and the dermis then serves as a scaffold for the adnexal structures identified with ventral or dorsal sites.

Infant dermis is composed of small collagen bundles that stain deeply red. Many fibroblasts are present. In adult dermis, few fibroblasts persist; collagen bundles are thick and stain pale red.

Two populations of dermal dendritic cells are noted in the adult dermis. Factor XIIIa-positive dermal dendrocytes appear to give rise to dermatofibromas, angiofibromas, acquired digital fibrokeratomas, pleomorphic fibromas, and fibrous papules. CD34+ dermal dendroctyes are accentuated around hair follicles, but exist throughout the dermis. They disappear from the dermis early in the course of morphea. Their loss can be diagnostic in subtle cases. CD34+ dermal dendrocytes reappear in the dermis when morphea responds to UVA1 light treatment.

The principal component of the dermis is collagen, a family of fibrous proteins comprising at least 15 genetically distinct types in human skin. Collagen serves as the major structural protein for the entire body; it is found in tendons, ligaments, and the lining of bones, as well as in the dermis. It represents 70% of the dry weight of skin. The fibroblast synthesizes the procollagen molecule, a helical arrangement of specific polypeptide chains that are subsequently secreted by the cell and assembled into collagen fibrils. Collagen is rich in the amino acids hydroxyproline, hydroxylysine, and glycine. The fibrillar collagens are the major group found in the skin. Type I collagen is the major component of the dermis. The structure of type I collagen is uniform in width and each fiber displays characteristic cross-striations with a periodicity of 68 nm. Collagen fibers are loosely arranged in the papillary and adventitial (periadnexal) dermis. Large collagen bundles are noted in the reticular dermis (the dermis below the level of the postcapillary venule). Collagen I mRNA and collagen III mRNA are both expressed in the reticular and papillary dermis, and are downregulated by UV light, as is the collagen regulatory proteoglycan decorin. This downregulation may play a role in photoaging.

Type IV collagen is found in the BMZ. Type VII collagen is the major structural component of anchoring fibrils and is produced predominately by keratinocytes. Abnormalities in type VII collagen are seen in dystrophic epidermolysis bullosa, and autoantibodies to this collagen type characterize acquired epidermolysis bullosa. Collagen fibers are continuously being degraded by proteolytic enzymes called spare collagenases, and replaced by newly synthesized fibers. Additional information on collagen types and diseases can be found in Chapter 25.

The fibroblast also synthesizes elastic fibers and the ground substance of the dermis, which is composed of glycosaminoglycans or acid mucopolysaccharides. Elastic fibers differ both structurally and chemically from collagen. They consist of aggregates of two components: protein filaments and elastin, an amorphous protein. The amino acids desmosine and isodesmosine are unique to elastic fibers. Elastic fibers in the papillary dermis are fine, whereas those in the reticular dermis are coarse. The extracellular matrix or ground substance of the dermis is composed of sulfated acid mucopolysaccharide, principally chondroitin sulfate and dermatan sulfate, neutral mucopolysaccharides, and electrolytes. Sulfated acid mucopolysaccharides stain with colloidal iron and with alcian blue at both pH 2.5 and 0.5. They stain metachromatically with toluidine blue at both pH 3.0 and 1.5. Hyaluronan (hyaluronic acid) is a minor component of normal dermis, but is the major mucopolysaccharide that accumulates in pathologic states. It stains with colloidal iron, and with both alcian blue and toluidine blue (metachromatically), but only at the higher pH for each stain.

Collagen is the major stress-resistant material of the skin. Elastic fibers contribute very little to resisting deformation and tearing of skin, but have a role in maintaining elasticity. Connective tissue disease is a term generally used to refer to a clinically heterogeneous group of autoimmune diseases, including lupus erythematosus, scleroderma, and dermatomyositis. Scleroderma involves the most visible collagen abnormalities, as collagen bundles become hyalinized and the space between collagen bundles diminishes. Both lupus and dermatomyositis produce increased dermal mucin, mostly hyaluronic acid. Bullous lupus has autoantibodies directed against type VII collagen.

Defects in collagen synthesis have been described in a number of inheritable diseases, including Ehlers–Danlos syndrome, X-linked cutis laxa, and osteogenesis imperfecta. Defects in elastic tissue are seen in Marfan syndrome and pseudoxanthoma elasticum.

Vasculature

The dermal vasculature consists principally of two intercommunicating plexuses. The subpapillary plexus, or upper horizontal network, contains the postcapillary venules and courses at the junction of the papillary and reticular dermis. This plexus furnishes a rich supply of capillaries, end arterioles, and venules to the dermal papillae. The deeper, lower horizontal plexus is found at the dermal–subcutaneous interface and is composed of larger blood vessels than those of the superficial plexus. Nodular lymphoid infiltrates surrounding this lower plexus are typical of early inflammatory morphea. The vasculature of the dermis is particularly well developed at sites of adnexal structures. Associated with the vascular plexus are dermal lymphatics and nerves.

Muscles

Smooth muscle occurs in the skin as arrectores pilorum (erectors of the hairs), as the tunica dartos (or dartos) of the scrotum, and in the areolas around the nipples. The arrectores pilorum are attached to the hair follicles below the sebaceous glands and, in contracting, pull the hair follicle upward, producing gooseflesh. The presence of scattered smooth muscle throughout the dermis is typical of anogenital skin.

Smooth muscle also comprises the muscularis of dermal and subcutaneous blood vessels. The muscularis of veins is composed of small bundles of smooth muscle that criss-cross at right angles. Arterial smooth muscle forms a concentric wreath-like ring. Specialized aggregates of smooth muscle cells (glomus bodies) are found between arterioles and venules, and are especially prominent on the digits and at the lateral margins of the palms and soles. Glomus bodies serve to shunt blood and regulate temperature. Most smooth muscle expresses desmin intermediate filaments, but vascular smooth muscle expresses vimentin instead. Smooth muscle actin is consistently expressed by all types of smooth muscle.

Striated (voluntary) muscle occurs in the skin of the neck as the platysma muscle and in the skin of the face as the muscles of expression. This complex network of striated muscle, fascia, and aponeuroses is known as the superficial muscular aponeurotic system (SMAS).

Nerves

In the dermis, nerve bundles are found together with arterioles and venules as part of the neurovascular bundle. In the deep dermis, nerves travel parallel to the surface, and the presence of long sausage-like granulomas following this path is an important clue to the diagnosis of Hansen's disease.

Touch and pressure are mediated by Meissner corpuscles found in the dermal papillae, particularly on the digits, palms, and soles, and by Vater–Pacini corpuscles located in the deeper portion of the dermis of weight-bearing surfaces and genitalia. Mucocutaneous end organs are found in the papillary dermis of modified hairless skin at the mucocutaneous junctions: namely, the glans, prepuce, clitoris, labia minora, perianal region, and vermilion border of the lips. Temperature, pain, and itch sensation are transmitted by unmyelinated nerve fibers which terminate in the papillary dermis and around hair follicles. Impulses pass to the central nervous system by way of the dorsal root ganglia. Histamine-evoked itch is transmitted by slow-conducting unmyelinated C-polymodal neurons. Signal transduction differs for sensations of heat and cold, and in peripheral nerve axons.

Postganglionic adrenergic fibers of the autonomic nervous system regulate vasoconstriction, apocrine gland secretions, and contraction of arrector pili muscles of hair follicles. Cholinergic fibers mediate eccrine sweat secretion.

Mast cells

Mast cells play an important role in the normal immune response, as well as immediate-type sensitivity, contact allergy, and fibrosis. Measuring 6–12 microns in diameter, with ample amphophilic cytoplasm and a small round central nucleus, normal mast cells resemble fried eggs in histologic sections. In telangiectasia macularis eruptiva perstans (TMEP mastocytosis), they are spindle-shaped and hyperchromatic, resembling large, dark fibroblasts. Mast cells are distinguished by containing up to 1000 granules, each measuring 0.6–0.7 microns in diameter. Coarse particulate granules, crystalline granules, and granules containing scrolls may be seen. On the cell's surface are 100 000–500 000 glycoprotein receptor sites for immunoglobulin E (IgE). There is heterogeneity to mast cells with type I or connective tissue mast cells found in the dermis and submucosa, and type II or mucosal mast cells found in the bowel and respiratory tract mucosa.

Mast cell granules stain metachromatically with toluidine blue and methylene blue (in the Giemsa stain) because of their high content of heparin. They also contain histamine, neutrophil chemotactic factor, eosinophil chemotactic factor of anaphylaxis, tryptase, kininogenase, and β-glucosaminidase. Slow-reacting substance of anaphylaxis (leukotrienes C4 and D4), leukotriene B4, platelet activating factor, and prostaglandin D2 are formed only after IgE-mediated release of granules. Mast cells stain reliably with the Leder ASD-chloracetase esterase stain. Because this stain does not rely on the presence of mast cell granules, it is particularly useful in situations when mast cells have degranulated. In forensic medicine, fluorescent labeling of mast cells with antibodies to the mast cell enzymes chymase and tryptase is useful in determining the timing of skin lesions in regard to death. Lesions sustained while living show an initial increase, then decline in mast cells. Lesions sustained postmortem demonstrate few mast cells.

Cutaneous mast cells respond to environmental changes. Dry environments result in an increase in mast cell number and cutaneous histamine content. In mastocytosis, mast cells accumulate in skin because of abnormal proliferation, migration, and failure of apoptosis. The terminal deoxynucleotidyl transferase-mediated deoxyuridine triphosphate-biotin nick end labeling (TUNEL) method is commonly used to assess apoptosis, and demonstrates decreased staining in mastocytomas. Proliferation is usually only moderately enhanced.

Abraham SN, et al: Mast cell-orchestrated immunity to pathogens. Nat Rev Immunol 2010 Jun; 10(6):440–452.

Charkoudian N: Skin blood flow in adult human thermoregulation: how it works, when it does not, and why. Mayo Clin Proc 2003; 78:603.

Galli SJ, et al: Mast cells: versatile regulators of inflammation, tissue remodeling, host defense and homeostasis. J Dermatol Sci 2008 Jan; 49(1):7–19.

Hendrix S, et al: Skin and hair follicle innervation in experimental models: a guide for the exact and reproducible evaluation of neuronal plasticity. Exp Dermatol 2008 Mar; 17(3):214–227.

Hoffmann T, et al: Sensory transduction in peripheral nerve axons elicits ectopic action potentials. J Neurosci 2008 Jun 11; 28(24):6281–6284.

Metz M, et al: Mast cell functions in the innate skin immune system. Immunobiology 2008; 213(3–4):251–260.

Norman MU, et al: Mast cells regulate the magnitude and the cytokine microenvironment of the contact hypersensitivity response. Am J Pathol 2008 Jun; 172(6):1638–1649.

Ohtola J, et al: β-Catenin has sequential roles in the survival and specification of ventral dermis. Development 2008 Jul; 135(13):2321–2329.

Subcutaneous tissue (fat)

Beneath the dermis lies the panniculus, lobules of fat cells or lipocytes separated by fibrous septa composed of collagen and large blood vessels. The collagen in the septa is continuous with the collagen in the dermis. Just as the epidermis and dermis vary in thickness according to skin site, so does the subcutaneous tissue. The panniculus provides buoyancy, and functions as a repository of energy and an endocrine organ. It is an important site of hormone conversions, such as that of androstenedione into estrone by aromatase. Leptin, a hormone produced in lipocytes, regulates body weight via the hypothalamus and influences how we react to flavors in food. Various substances can affect lipid accumulation within lipocytes. Obestatin is a polypeptide that reduces feed intake and weight gain in rodents. (–)-ternatin, a highly N-methylated cyclic heptapeptide that inhibits fat accumulation, produced by the mushroom *Coriolus versicolor*, has similar effects in mice. Study of these molecules provides insight into the molecular basis of weight gain and obesity. Abnormal fat distribution and insulin resistance are seen in Cushing syndrome and as a result of antiretroviral therapy. In obese children and adolescents developing diabetes, severe peripheral insulin resistance is associated with intramyocellular and intra-abdominal lipocyte lipid accumulation.

Certain inflammatory dermatoses, known as the panniculitides, principally affect this level of the skin, producing subcutaneous nodules. The pattern of the inflammation, specifically whether it primarily affects the septa or the fat lobules, serves to distinguish various conditions which may resemble one another clinically.

Nagaraj S, et al: Fragments of obestatin as modulators of feed intake, circulating lipids, and stored fat. Biochem Biophys Res Commun 2008 Feb 15; 366(3):731–737.

Shimokawa K, et al: Biological activity, structural features, and synthetic studies of (-)-ternatin, a potent fat-accumulation inhibitor of 3T3-L1 adipocytes. Chem Asian J 2008 Feb 1; 3(2):438–446.

Weiss R, et al: Prediabetes in obese youth: a syndrome of impaired glucose tolerance, severe insulin resistance, and altered myocellular and abdominal fat partitioning. Lancet 2003; 362:951.

Bonus images for this chapter can be found online at

http://www.expertconsult.com

Fig. 1-1 Electron micrograph illustrating the three basic cell types in the epidermis and their relationships.

Fig. 1-2 Ultrastructural appearance of the desmosome specialized attachment plate between adjacent keratinocytes.

Fig. 1-3 Upper portion of the epidermis.

Fig. 1-4 Portion of a melanocyte from dark skin.

Fig. 1-5 Relationship between melanocytes (M) and basal keratinocytes (K) in light skin.

Fig. 1-6 Ultrastructural appearance of the Langerhans cell.

Fig. 1-7 Ultrastructural appearance of the basement membrane zone at the junction of the epidermis and dermis.

2

Cutaneous Signs and Diagnosis

In some cases, the appearance of skin lesions may be so distinctive that the diagnosis is clear at a glance. In other cases, subjective symptoms and clinical signs in themselves are inadequate, and a complete history and laboratory examinations, including a biopsy, are essential to arrive at a diagnosis.

The same disease may show variations under different conditions and in different individuals. The appearance of the lesions may have been modified by previous treatment or obscured by extraneous influences, such as scratching or secondary infection. Subjective symptoms may be the only evidence of a disease, as in pruritus, and the skin appearance may be generally unremarkable. Although history is important, the diagnosis in dermatology is most frequently made based on the objective physical characteristics and location or distribution of one or more lesions that can be seen or felt. Therefore, careful physical examination of the skin is paramount in dermatologic diagnosis.

Cutaneous signs

Typically, most skin diseases produce or present with lesions that have more or less distinct characteristics. They may be uniform or diverse in size, shape, and color, and may be in different stages of evolution or involution. The original lesions are known as the primary lesions, and identification of such lesions is the most important aspect of the dermatologic physical examination. They may continue to full development or be modified by regression, trauma, or other extraneous factors, producing secondary lesions.

Primary lesions

Primary lesions are of the following forms: macules (or patches), papules (or plaques), nodules, tumors, wheals, vesicles, bullae, and pustules.

Macules (maculae, spots)

Macules are variously sized, circumscribed changes in skin color, without elevation or depression (nonpalpable) (Fig. 2-1). They may be circular, oval, or irregular, and may be distinct in outline or fade into the surrounding skin. Macules may constitute the whole or part of the eruption, or may be merely an early phase. If the lesions become slightly raised, they are then designated papules or, sometimes, morbilliform eruptions.

Patches

A patch is a large macule, 1 cm or greater in diameter, as may be seen in nevus flammeus or vitiligo.

Papules

Papules are circumscribed, solid elevations with no visible fluid, varying in size from a pinhead to 1 cm. They may be

acuminate, rounded, conical, flat-topped, or umbilicated, and may appear white (as in milium), red (as in eczema), yellowish (as in xanthoma), or black (as in melanoma).

Papules are generally centered in the dermis and may be concentrated at the orifices of the sweat ducts or at the hair follicles. They may be of soft or firm consistency. The surface may be smooth or rough. If capped by scales, they are known as squamous papules, and the eruption is called papulosquamous.

Some papules are discrete and irregularly distributed, as in papular urticaria, whereas others are grouped, as in lichen nitidus. Some persist as papules, whereas those of the inflammatory type may progress to vesicles and even to pustules, or may erode or ulcerate before regression takes place.

The term maculopapular should not be used. There is no such thing as a maculopapule, but there may be both macules and papules in an eruption. Most typically such eruptions are morbilliform.

Plaques

A plaque is a broad papule (or confluence of papules), 1 cm or more in diameter (Fig. 2-2). It is generally flat, but may be centrally depressed. The center of a plaque may be normal skin.

Nodules

Nodules are morphologically similar to papules, but they are larger than 1 cm in diameter. They most frequently are centered in the dermis or subcutaneous fat.

Tumors

Tumors are soft or firm and freely movable or fixed masses of various sizes and shapes (but in general greater than 2 cm in diameter). General usage dictates that the word "tumor" means a neoplasm. They may be elevated or deep-seated, and in some instances are pedunculated (fibromas). Tumors have a tendency to be rounded. Their consistency depends on the constituents of the lesion. Some tumors remain stationary indefinitely, whereas others increase in size or break down.

Wheals (hives)

Wheals are evanescent, edematous, plateau-like elevations of various sizes (Fig. 2-3). They are usually oval or of arcuate contours, pink to red, and surrounded by a "flare" of macular erythema. They may be discrete or may coalesce. These lesions often develop quickly. Because the wheal is the prototypic lesion of urticaria, diseases in which wheals are prominent are frequently described as "urticarial" (e.g. urticarial vasculitis). Dermatographism, or pressure-induced whealing, may be evident.

Vesicles (blisters)

Vesicles are circumscribed, fluid-containing, epidermal elevations, 1–10 mm in size. They may be pale or yellow from

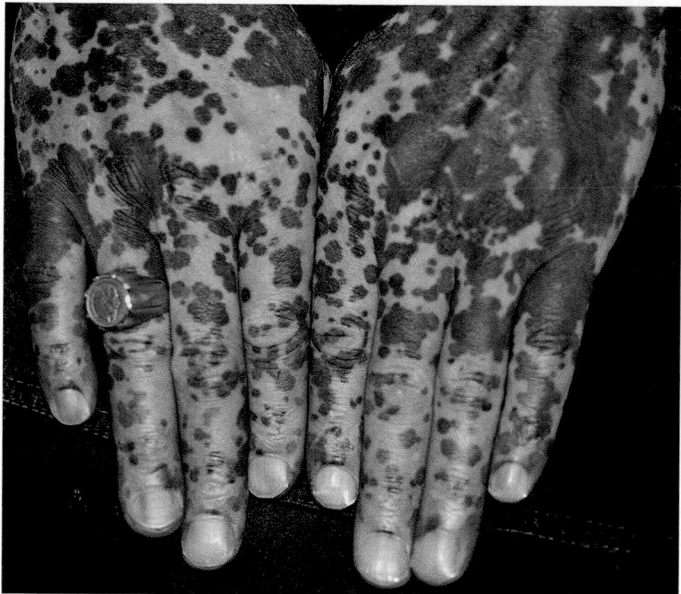

Fig. 2-1 Macular depigmentation, vitiligo.

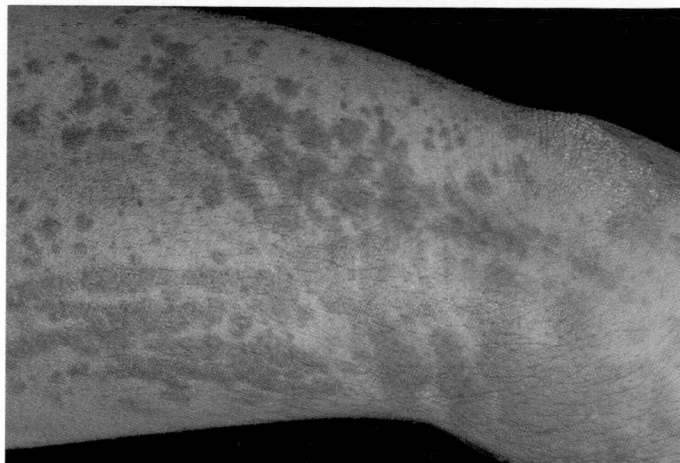

Fig. 2-3 Multiple wheals and dermatographism, urticarial vasculitis.

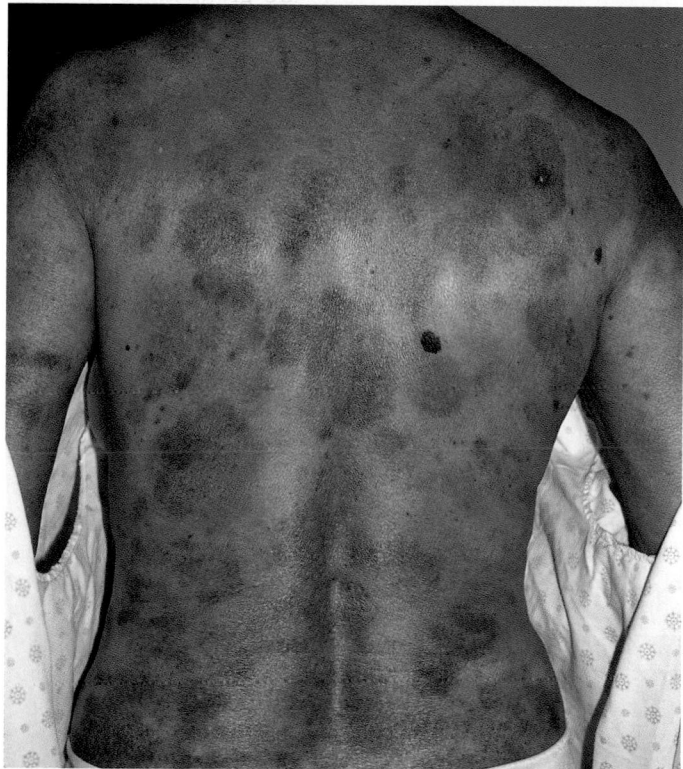

Fig. 2-2 Multiple hyperpigmented patches and plaques, cutaneous T-cell lymphoma.

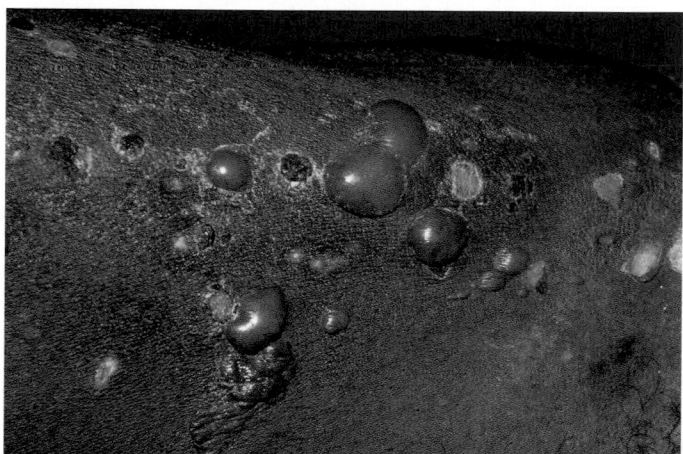

Fig. 2-4 Vesicles, bullae, and erosions, bullous pemphigoid.

Bullae

Bullae are rounded or irregularly shaped blisters containing serous or seropurulent fluid. They differ from vesicles only in size, being larger than 1 cm. They are usually unilocular but may be multilocular. Bullae may be located superficially in the epidermis, so that their walls are flaccid and thin, and subject to rupture spontaneously or from slight injury. After rupture, remnants of the thin walls may persist and, together with the exudate, may dry to form a thin crust; or the broken bleb may leave a raw and moist base, which may be covered with sero-purulent or purulent exudate. More rarely, irregular vegetations may appear on the base (as in pemphigus vegetans). When the bullae are subepidermal, they are tense, and ulceration and scarring may result.

Nikolsky's sign refers to the diagnostic maneuver of putting lateral pressure on unblistered skin in a bullous eruption and having the epithelium shear off. Asboe–Hansen's sign refers to the extension of a blister to adjacent unblistered skin when pressure is put on the top of the blister. Both of these signs demonstrate the principle that in some diseases the extent of microscopic vesiculation is more than is evident by simple inspection. These findings are useful in evaluating the severity of pemphigus vulgaris and severe bullous drug reactions. Hemorrhagic bullae are common in pemphigus, herpes zoster, severe bullous drug reactions, and lichen sclerosus. The cellular contents of bullae may be useful in cytologically confirming the diagnosis of pemphigus, herpes zoster, and herpes simplex.

serous exudate, or red from serum mixed with blood. The apex may be rounded, acuminate, or umbilicated as in eczema herpeticum. Vesicles may be discrete, irregularly scattered, grouped as in herpes zoster, or linear as in allergic contact dermatitis from urushiol (poison ivy/oak). Vesicles may arise directly or from a macule or papule, and generally lose their identity in a short time, breaking spontaneously or developing into bullae through coalescence or enlargement, or developing into pustules (Fig. 2-4). When the contents are of a seropurulent character, the lesions are known as vesicopustules. Vesicles consist of either a single cavity (unilocular) or several compartments (multilocular) containing fluid.

Pustules

Pustules are small elevations of the skin containing purulent material (usually necrotic inflammatory cells) (Fig. 2-5). They are similar to vesicles in shape and usually have an inflammatory areola. They are usually white or yellow centrally, but may be red if they also contain blood. They may originate as pustules or may develop from papules or vesicles, passing through transitory early stages, during which they are known as papulopustules or vesicopustules.

Secondary lesions

Secondary lesions are of many kinds; the most important are scales, crusts, erosions, ulcers, fissures, and scars.

Scales (exfoliation)

Scales are dry or greasy laminated masses of keratin. The body ordinarily is constantly shedding imperceptible tiny, thin fragments of stratum corneum. When the formation of epidermal cells is rapid or the process of normal keratinization is interfered with, pathologic exfoliation results, producing scales. These vary in size, some being fine, delicate, and branny, as in tinea versicolor, others being coarser, as in eczema and ichthyosis, while still others are stratified, as in psoriasis. Large sheets of desquamated epidermis are seen in toxic epidermal necrolysis, staphylococcal scalded skin syndrome, and infection-associated (toxin-mediated) desquamations, such as scarlet fever. Scales vary in color from white–gray to yellow or brown from the admixture of dirt or melanin. Occasionally, they have a silvery sheen from trapping of air between their layers; these are micaceous scales, characteristic of psoriasis. When scaling occurs, it usually implies that there is some pathologic process in the epidermis, and parakeratosis is often present histologically.

Crusts (scabs)

Crusts are dried serum, pus, or blood, usually mixed with epithelial and sometimes bacterial debris. They vary greatly in size, thickness, shape, and color, according to their origin, composition, and volume. They may be dry, golden yellow, soft, friable, and superficial, as in impetigo; yellowish, as in favus; thick, hard, and tough, as in third-degree burns; or lamellated, elevated, brown, black, or green masses, as in late syphilis. The latter have been described as oyster-shell (ostraceous) crusts and are known as rupia. When crusts become detached, the base may be dry or red and moist.

Excoriations and abrasions (scratch marks)

An excoriation is a punctate or linear abrasion produced by mechanical means, usually involving only the epidermis but not uncommonly reaching the papillary layer of the dermis. Excoriations are caused by scratching with the fingernails in an effort to relieve itching in a variety of diseases. If the skin damage is the result of mechanical trauma or constant friction, the term abrasion may be used. Frequently there is an inflammatory areola around the excoriation or a covering of yellowish dried serum or red dried blood. Excoriations may provide access for pyogenic microorganisms and the formation of crusts, pustules, or cellulitis, occasionally associated with enlargement of the neighboring lymphatic glands. In general, the longer and deeper excoriations are, the more severe was the pruritus that provoked them. Lichen planus is an exception, however, in which pruritus is severe, but excoriations are rare.

Fissures (cracks, clefts)

A fissure is a linear cleft through the epidermis or into the dermis. These lesions may be single or multiple, and vary from microscopic to several centimeters in length with sharply defined margins. They may be dry or moist, red, straight, curved, irregular, or branching. They occur most commonly when the skin is thickened and inelastic from inflammation and dryness, especially in regions subjected to frequent movement. Such areas are the tips and flexural creases of the thumbs, fingers, and palms; the edges of the heels; the clefts between the fingers and toes; at the angles of the mouth; the lips; and about the nares, auricles, and anus. When the skin is dry, exposure to cold, wind, water, and cleaning products (soap, detergents) may produce a stinging, burning sensation, indicating microscopic fissuring is present. This may be referred to as chapping, as in "chapped lips." When fissuring is present, pain is often produced by movement of the parts, which opens or deepens the fissures or forms new ones.

Erosions

Loss of all or portions of the epidermis alone, as in impetigo or herpes zoster or simplex after vesicles rupture, produces an erosion. It may or may not become crusted, but it heals without a scar.

Ulcers

Ulcers are rounded or irregularly shaped excavations that result from complete loss of the epidermis plus some portion of the dermis. They vary in diameter from a few millimeters to several centimeters (Fig. 2-6). They may be shallow, involving

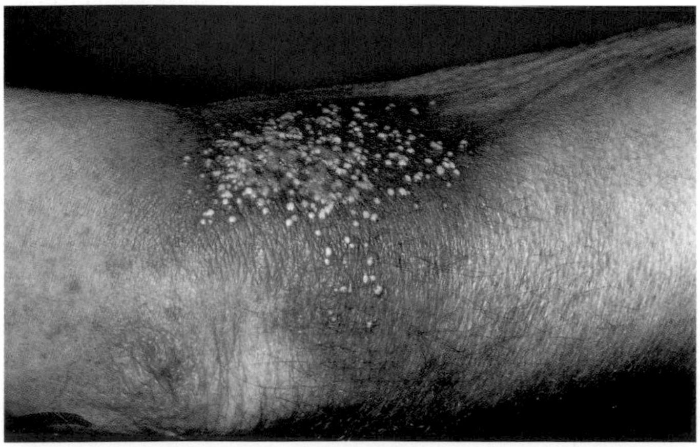

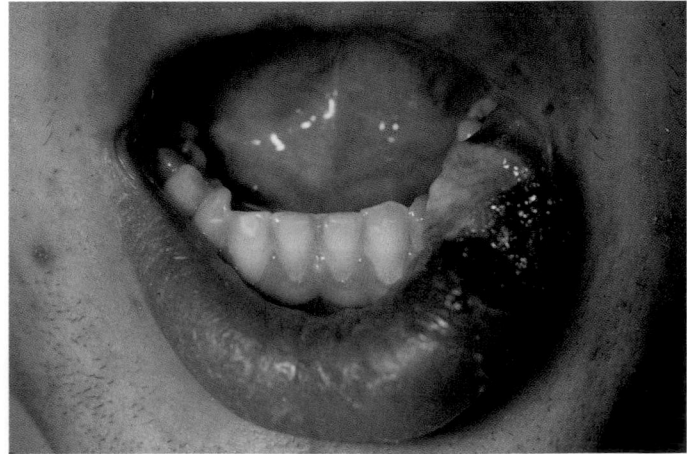

Fig. 2-5 Erythematous plaques studded with sheets of pustules, pustular psoriasis.

Fig. 2-6 Ulcer of lip, chancre of primary syphilis.

little beyond the epidermis, as in dystrophic epidermolysis bullosa, the base being formed by the papillary layer, or they may extend deep into the dermis, subcutaneous tissues, or deeper, as with leg ulcers. They heal with scarring.

Scars

Scars are composed of new connective tissue that replaced lost substance in the dermis or deeper parts as a result of injury or disease, as part of the normal reparative process. Their size and shape are determined by the form of the previous destruction. Scarring is characteristic of certain inflammatory processes and is therefore of diagnostic value. The pattern of scarring may be characteristic of a particular disease. Lichen planus and discoid lupus erythematosus, for example, have inflammation that is in relatively the same area anatomically, yet discoid lupus characteristically causes scarring as it resolves, whereas lichen planus rarely results in scarring of the skin. Both processes, however, cause scarring of the hair follicles when they occur on the scalp. Scars may be thin and atrophic, or the fibrous elements may develop into neoplastic overgrowths, as in keloids. Some individuals and some areas of the body, such as the anterior chest, are especially prone to scarring. Scars may be smooth or rough, pliable or firm, and tend at first to be pink or violaceous, later becoming white, glistening, and rarely, hyperpigmented.

Scars are persistent but tend to become less noticeable in the course of time. At times, and especially in certain anatomic locations (central chest), they grow thick, tough, and corded, forming a hypertrophic scar or keloid.

General diagnosis

Interpretation of the clinical picture may be difficult, because identical manifestations may result from widely different causes. Moreover, the same etiologic factors may give rise to a great diversity of eruptions. There is one great advantage in dermatology: namely, that of dealing with an organ that can be seen and felt. Smears and cultures may be readily made for bacteria and fungi. Biopsy and histologic examination of skin lesions are usually very minor procedures, making histopathology an important component of the evaluation in many clinical situations. Given the ease of histologic confirmation of diagnoses in skin diseases, the threshold for biopsy should be low. This is especially true of inflammatory dermatoses, potentially infectious conditions, and skin disorders in immunosuppressed and hospitalized patients where clinical morphology may be atypical. Once therapy is begun empirically, histologic features may be altered by the treatment, making pathologic diagnosis more difficult.

History

Knowledge of the patient's age, health, occupation, hobbies, and living conditions, and of the onset, duration, and course of the disease, and its response to previous treatment are important. The family history of similar disorders and other related diseases may be useful.

A complete drug history is one of the most important aspects of a thorough history. This includes prescription and over-the-counter medications, supplements, and herbal products. Drug reactions are frequently seen and may simulate many different diseases. Anti-inflammatory agents (steroidal or nonsteroidal), antibiotics, antihypertensives, antiarrhythmics, cholesterol-lowering agents, antiepileptics, and antidepressants may all produce cutaneous disorders. All may simulate entities not usually attributed to drugs. It is equally important to inquire about topical agents that have been applied to the skin and

mucous membranes for medicinal or cosmetic purposes, for these agents may cause cutaneous or systemic reactions.

Other illnesses, travel abroad, the patient's environment at home and at work, seasonal occurrences and recurrences of the disease, and the temperature, humidity, and weather exposure of the patient are all important items in a dermatologic history. Habitation in certain parts of the world predisposes to distinctive diseases for that particular geographic locale. San Joaquin Valley fever (coccidioidomycosis), Hansen's disease, leishmaniasis, and histoplasmosis are examples. Sexual orientation and practices may be relevant, as in genital ulcer diseases, human immunodeficiency virus (HIV) infection, and infestations (e.g. scabies, pubic lice).

Examination

Examination should be conducted in a well-lit room. Natural sunlight is the ideal illumination. Fluorescent bulbs that produce wavelengths of light closer to natural sunlight than standard fluorescent bulbs are commercially available. Abnormalities of melanin pigmentation, e.g. vitiligo and melasma, are more clearly visible under ultraviolet (UV) light. A Wood's light (365 nm) is most commonly used and is also valuable for the diagnosis of some types of tinea capitis, tinea versicolor, and erythrasma.

A magnifying lens is of inestimable value in examining small lesions. It may be necessary to palpate the lesion for firmness and fluctuation; rubbing will elucidate the nature of scales; scraping will reveal the nature of the lesion's base. Pigmented lesions, especially in infants, should be rubbed in an attempt to elicit Darier's sign (whealing), as seen in urticaria pigmentosa. Dermoscopy is an essential part of the examination of pigmented lesions.

The entire eruption must be seen to evaluate distribution and configuration. This is optimally done by having the patient completely undress and viewing him/her from a distance to take in the whole eruption at once. "Peek-a-boo" examination, by having the patient expose one anatomic area after another while remaining clothed, is not optimal because the examination of the skin will be incomplete and the overall distribution is hard to determine. After the patient is viewed at a distance, individual lesions are examined to identify primary lesions and to determine the evolution of the eruption and the presence of secondary lesions.

Diagnostic details of lesions

Distribution

Lesions may be few or numerous, and in arrangement they may be discrete or may coalesce to form patches of peculiar configuration. They may appear over the entire body, or follow the lines of cleavage (pityriasis rosea), dermatomes (herpes zoster), or lines of Blaschko (epidermal nevi). Lesions may form groups, rings, crescents, or unusual linear patterns. A remarkable degree of bilateral symmetry is characteristic of certain diseases such as dermatitis herpetiformis, vitiligo, and psoriasis.

Evolution

Some lesions appear fully evolved. Others develop from smaller lesions, then may remain the same during their entire existence (e.g. warts). When lesions succeed one another in a series of crops, as they do in varicella and dermatitis herpetiformis, a polymorphous eruption results with lesions in various stages of development or involution all present at the same time.

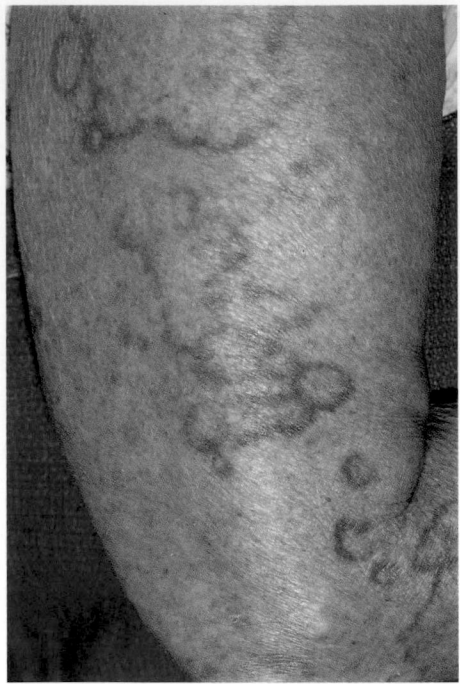

Fig. 2-7 Annular, arcuate, and polycyclic configurations on granuloma annulare.

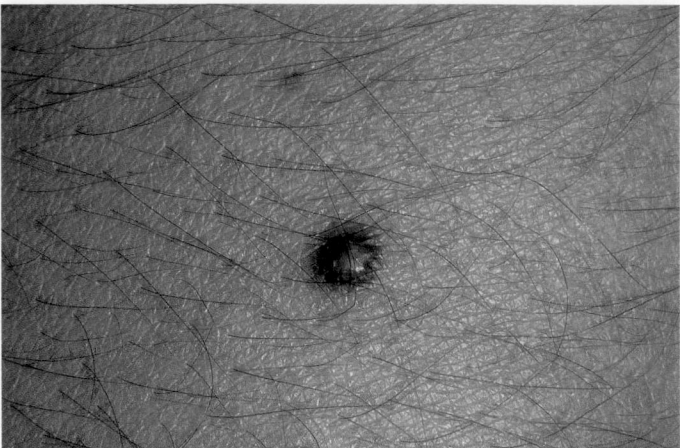

Fig. 2-8 Acral small blue papule, blue nevus.

Involution

Certain lesions disappear completely, whereas others leave characteristic residual pigmentation or scarring. Residual dyspigmentation, although a significant cosmetic issue, is not considered a scar. The pattern in which lesions involute may be useful in diagnosis, e.g. the typical keratotic papule of pityriasis lichenoides varioliformis acuta.

Grouping

Grouping is a characteristic of dermatitis herpetiformis, herpes simplex, and herpes zoster. Small lesions arranged around a large one are said to be in a corymbose arrangement. Concentric annular lesions are typical of borderline Hansen's disease and erythema multiforme. These are sometimes said to be in a cockade pattern, like the tricolor cockade hats worn by French revolutionists. Flea and other arthropod bites are usually grouped and linear (breakfast-lunch-and-dinner sign). Grouped lesions of various sizes may be termed agminated.

Configuration

Certain terms are used to describe the configuration that an eruption assumes either primarily or by enlargement or coalescence. Lesions in a line are called linear, and they may be confluent or discrete. Lesions may form a complete circle (annular) or a portion of a circle (arcuate or gyrate), or may be composed of several intersecting portions of circles (polycyclic) (Fig. 2-7). If the eruption is not straight but does not form parts of circles, it may be serpiginous . Round lesions may be small, like drops, called guttate; or larger, like a coin, called nummular. Unusual configurations that do not correspond to these patterns or to normal anatomic or embryonic patterns should raise the possibility of an exogenous dermatosis or factitia.

Color

The color of the skin is determined by melanin, oxyhemoglobin, reduced hemoglobin, and carotene. Not only do the proportions of these components affect the color, but their depth within the skin, the thickness of the epidermis, and

hydration also play a role. The Tyndall effect modifies the color of skin and of lesions by the selective scattering of light waves of different wavelengths. The blue nevus and Mongolian spots are examples of this light dispersion effect, in which brown melanin in the dermis appears blue–gray (Fig. 2-8).

The color of lesions may be very valuable as a diagnostic factor. Dermatologists should be aware that there are many shades of pink, red, and purple, each of which tends to suggest a diagnosis or disease group. Interface reactions such as lichen planus or lupus erythematosus are described as violaceous. Lipid-containing lesions are yellow, as in xanthomas or steatocystoma multiplex. The orange–red (salmon) color of pityriasis rubra pilaris is characteristic. The constitutive color of the skin determines the quality of the color one observes with a specific disorder. In dark-skinned persons, erythema is hard to perceive. Pruritic lesions in African-Americans may evolve to be small, shiny, flat-topped papules with a violaceous hue (due to the combination of erythema and pigmentary incontinence). These lichenified lesions would be suspected of being lichenoid by the untrained eye, but are in fact eczematous.

Patches lighter in color than the normal skin may be completely depigmented or have lost only part of their pigment (hypopigmented). This is an important distinction, since certain conditions are or may be hypopigmented, such as tinea versicolor, nevus anemicus, Hansen's disease, hypomelanotic macules of tuberous sclerosis, hypomelanosis of Ito, seborrheic dermatitis, and idiopathic guttate hypomelanosis. True depigmentation should be distinguished from this; it suggests vitiligo, nevus depigmentosus, halo nevus, scleroderma, morphea, or lichen sclerosus.

Hyperpigmentation may result from epidermal or dermal causes. It may be related to either increased melanin or deposition of other substances. Epidermal hyperpigmentation occurs in nevi, melanoma, café-au-lait spots, melasma, and lentigines. These lesions are accentuated when examined with a Wood's light. Dermal pigmentation occurs subsequent to many inflammatory conditions (postinflammatory hyperpigmentation) or from deposition of metals, medications, medication–melanin complexes, or degenerated dermal material (ochronosis). These conditions are not enhanced when examined by a Wood's light. The hyperpigmentation following inflammation is most commonly the result of dermal melanin deposition, but in some conditions, such as lichen aureus, is caused by iron. Dermal iron deposition appears more yellow–brown or golden than dermal melanin.

Consistency

Palpation is an essential part of the physical examination of lesions. Does the lesion blanch on pressure? If not, it may be

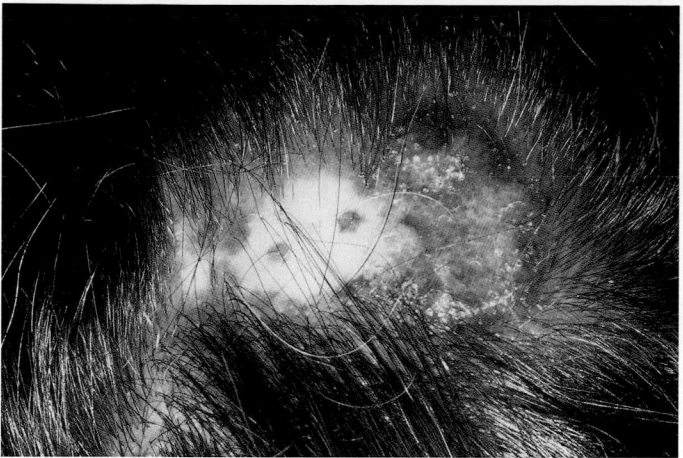

Fig. 2-9 Scalp plaque with scarring alopecia hyperpigmentation and depigmentation, discoid lupus erythematosus.

purpuric. Is it fluctuant? If so, it may have free fluid in it. Is it cold or hot? If there is a nodule or tumor, does it sink through a ring into the panniculus, like a neurofibroma? Is it hard enough for calcification to be suspected, merely very firm, like a keloid or dermatofibroma, or branny, like scleredema?

Hyperesthesia/anesthesia

Certain conditions may be associated with increased or decreased sensation. For example, the skin lesions of borderline and tuberculoid Hansen's disease typically are anesthetic in their centers. In neuropathic conditions (such as notalgia paresthetica), the patient may perceive both pruritus and hyperesthesia. Neurally mediated itch may be accompanied by other neural sensations such as heat or burning. The combination of pruritus with other neural symptoms suggests the involvement of nerves in the pathological process.

Hair, nails, and oral mucosa

Involvement of hair-bearing areas by certain skin disorders causes characteristic lesions. Discoid lupus, for example, causes scarring alopecia with characteristic dyspigmentation (Fig. 2-9). On the skin the lesions may be much less characteristic. Diffuse hair loss may be seen in certain conditions such as acrodermatitis enteropathica, and may be a clue to the diagnosis. In addition, loss of hair within a skin lesion may be suggestive of the correct diagnosis, e.g. the alopecia seen in the tumid plaques of follicular mucinosis.

Some skin disorders cause characteristic changes of the nails, even when the periungual tissue is not involved. The pitting seen in psoriasis and alopecia areata may be useful in confirming these diagnoses when other findings are not characteristic. In addition, the nails and adjacent structures may be the sole site of pathology, as in candidal paronychia.

The complete skin examination includes examination of the oral mucosa. Oral lesions are characteristically found in viral syndromes (exanthems), lichen planus, HIV-associated Kaposi sarcoma, and autoimmune bullous diseases (pemphigus vulgaris).

http://www.dermatologylexicon.org/
http://missinglink.ucsf.edu/lm/DermatologyGlossary/index.html

 Bonus images for this chapter can be found online at
http://www.expertconsult.com

Fig. 2-1 Serpiginous lesions, cutaneous larva migrans.
Fig. 2-2 Erythematous plaques studded with sheets of pustules, pustular psoriasis.
Fig. 2-3 Penile ulcer with a purulent base, chancroid.
Fig. 2-4 Erythematous papules in an annular configuration, granuloma annulare.
Fig. 2-5 Scalp plaque with scarring alopecia hyperpigmentation and depigmentation, discoid lupus erythematosus.

3

Dermatoses Resulting from Physical Factors

The body requires a certain amount of heat, but beyond definite limits, insufficient or excessive amounts are injurious. The local action of excessive heat causes burns or scalds; on the other hand, undue cold causes chilblains, frostbite, and congelation. Thresholds of tolerance exist in all body structures sensitive to electromagnetic wave radiation of varying frequencies, such as x-rays and ultraviolet (UV) rays. The skin, which is exposed to so many external physical forces, is more subject to injuries caused by them than is any other organ.

Heat injuries

Thermal burns

Injury of varying intensity may be caused by the action of excessive heat on the skin. If this heat is extreme, the skin and underlying tissue may be destroyed. The changes in the skin resulting from dry heat or scalding are classified in four degrees.

- *First-degree burns* of the skin result merely in an active congestion of the superficial blood vessels, causing erythema that may be followed by epidermal desquamation (peeling). Ordinary sunburn is the most common example of a first-degree burn. The pain and increased surface heat may be severe, and it is not rare to have some constitutional reaction if the involved area is large.

- *Second-degree burns* are subdivided into superficial and deep forms.
  - In the superficial type there is a transudation of serum from the capillaries, which causes edema of the superficial tissues. Vesicles and blebs are formed by the serum gathering beneath the outer layers of the epidermis (Fig. 3-1). Complete recovery without scarring is usual in burns of this kind.
  - The deep second-degree burn is pale and anesthetic. Injury to the reticular dermis compromises blood flow and destroys appendages, so that healing takes over 1 month to occur and results in scarring.

- *Third-degree burns* involve loss of tissue of the full thickness of the skin, and often some of the subcutaneous tissues. Since the skin appendages are destroyed, there is no epithelium available for regeneration of the skin. An ulcerating wound is produced, which in healing leaves a scar.

- *Fourth-degree burns* involve the destruction of the entire skin and subcutaneous fat with any underlying tendons.

Both third- and fourth-degree burns require grafting for closure. All third- and fourth-degree burns are followed by constitutional symptoms of varied gravity, their severity depending on the size of the involved surface, the depth of the burn, and particularly the location of the burned surface. The more vascular the involved area, the more severe the symptoms.

The prognosis is poor for any patient in whom a large area of skin surface is involved, particularly if more than two-thirds of the body surface has been burned. Women, infants, and toddlers all have an increased risk of death from burns when compared to men. Excessive scarring, with either keloid-like scars or flat scars with contractures, may produce deformities and dysfunctions of the joints, as well as chronic ulcerations due to impairment of local circulation. Delayed post-burn blistering may occur in partial-thickness wounds and skin-graft donor sites. It is most common on the lower extremities, and is self-limited. Burn scars may be the site of development of carcinoma or sarcoma. With modern reconstructive surgery these unfortunate end results can be minimized.

Treatment

Immediate first aid for minor thermal burns consists of prompt cold applications (ice water, or cold tap water if no ice is at hand), continued until pain does not return on stopping them.

The vesicles or blebs of second-degree burns should not be opened but should be protected from injury, since they form a natural barrier against contamination by microorganisms. If they become tense and unduly painful, the fluid may be evacuated under strictly aseptic conditions by puncturing the wall with a sterile needle, allowing the blister to collapse on to the underlying wound. Excision of full-thickness and deep dermal wounds that will not reepithelialize within 3 weeks reduces wound infections, shortens hospital stays, and improves survival. Additionally, contractures and functional impairment may be mitigated by such early intervention and grafting. The most superficial wounds may be dressed with greasy gauze, while silver-containing dressings are used for their antiobitic properties in intermediate wounds. Fluid resuscitation, treatment of inhalation injury and hypercatabolism, monitoring and early intervention of sepsis, and intensive care management in a burn center are all recommended in large partial-thickness wounds and full-thickness burns.

Electrical burns

Electrical burns may occur from contact or as a flash exposure.

A contact burn is small but deep, causing some necrosis of the underlying tissues. Low-voltage injuries usually occur in the home, are treated conservatively, and generally heal well. Oral commissure burns may require reconstructive procedures. High-voltage burns are often occupational; internal damage may be masked by little surface skin change, and be complicated by subtle and slowly developing sequelae. Early surgical intervention to improve circulation and repair vital tissues is helpful in limiting loss of the extremity.

Flash burns usually cover a large area and, being similar to any surface burn, are treated as such. Lightning may cause burns after a direct strike (Fig. 3-2), where an entrance and an

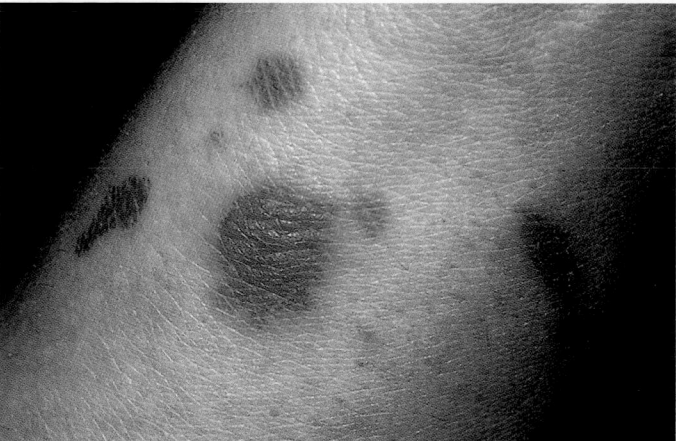

Fig. 3-1 Hot coffee burn.

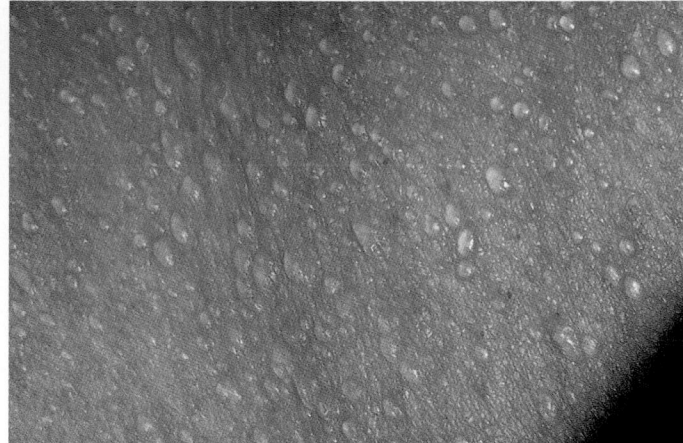

Fig. 3-3 Miliaria crystallina.

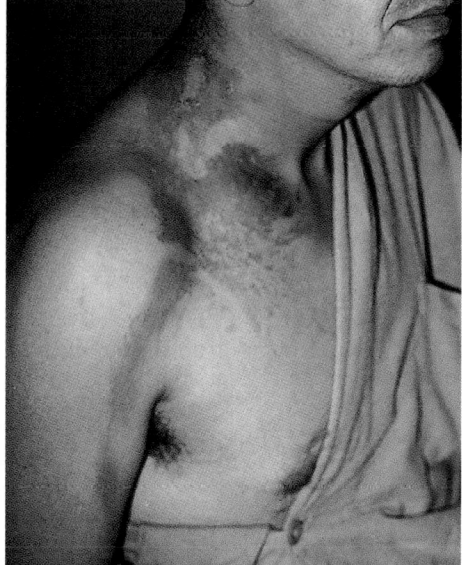

Fig. 3-2 Lightning strike.

exit wound are visible. This is the most lethal type of strike, and cardiac arrest or other internal injuries may occur. Other types of strike are indirect and result in burns that are either:

- linear in areas on which sweat was present
- in a feathery or arborescent pattern, which is believed to be pathognomonic
- punctate with multiple, deep, circular lesions
- thermal burns from ignited clothing or heated metal. These may occur if the patient was speaking on a cellphone or listening to an iPod when struck.

Hot tar burns

Polyoxyethylene sorbitan in neosporin ointment or sunflower oil is an excellent dispersing agent that facilitates the removal of hot tar from burns.

Barrow RE, et al: Mortality related to gender, age, sepsis, and ethnicity in severely burned children. Shock 2005; 23:485.

Chetty BV, et al: Blisters in patients with burns. Arch Dermatol 1992; 128:181.

Church D, et al: Burn wound infections. Clin Microbiol Rev 2006; 19:403.

Compton CC: The delayed postburn blister. Arch Dermatol 1992; 128:24.

Dega S, et al: Electrical burn injuries. Burns 2007; 33:653.

Demling R, et al: Management of hot tar burns. J Trauma 1980; 20:24.

Heffernan EJ, et al: Thunderstorms and iPods. N Engl J Med 2007; 357:198.

Kerby JD, et al: Sex differences in mortality after burn injury. Burn Care Res 2006; 27:452.

Mellemkjaer I, et al: Risks for skin and other cancers up to 25 years after burn injuries. Epidemiology 2006; 17:668.

Pham TN, Gibran NS: Thermal and electrical injuries. Surg Clin N Am 2007; 87:185.

Tennenhaus M, et al: Burn surgery. Clin Plast Surg 2007; 34:697.

Volinsky JB, et al: Picture of the month—lightning injury. Arch Pediatr Adolesc Med 1994; 148:529.

Wasaik J, et al: Minor thermal burns. Clin Evid 2005; 14:2388.

Miliaria

Miliaria, the retention of sweat as a result of occlusion of eccrine sweat ducts, produces an eruption that is common in hot, humid climates, such as in the tropics and during the hot summer months in temperate climates. *Staphylococcus epidermidis*, which produces an extracellular polysaccharide substance, induces miliaria in an experimental setting. This polysaccharide substance may obstruct the delivery of sweat to the skin surface. The occlusion prevents normal secretion from the sweat glands, and eventually pressure causes rupture of the sweat gland or duct at different levels. The escape of sweat into the adjacent tissue produces miliaria. Depending on the level of the injury to the sweat gland or duct, several different forms are recognized.

Miliaria crystallina (sudamina)

Miliaria crystallina (Fig. 3-3) is characterized by small, clear, superficial vesicles with no inflammatory reaction. It appears in bedridden patients in whom fever produces increased perspiration or in situations in which clothing prevents dissipation of heat and moisture, as in bundled children. The lesions are generally asymptomatic and their duration is short-lived because they tend to rupture at the slightest trauma. One patient with post-exercise itching was found to have miliaria crystallina; it resolved spontaneously. Drugs such as isotretinoin, bethanechol and doxorubicin may induce it. The lesions are self-limited; no treatment is required.

Miliaria rubra (prickly heat)

The lesions of miliaria rubra (Fig. 3-4) appear as discrete, extremely pruritic, erythematous papulovesicles accompanied by a sensation of prickling, burning, or tingling. They later may become confluent on a bed of erythema. The sites most

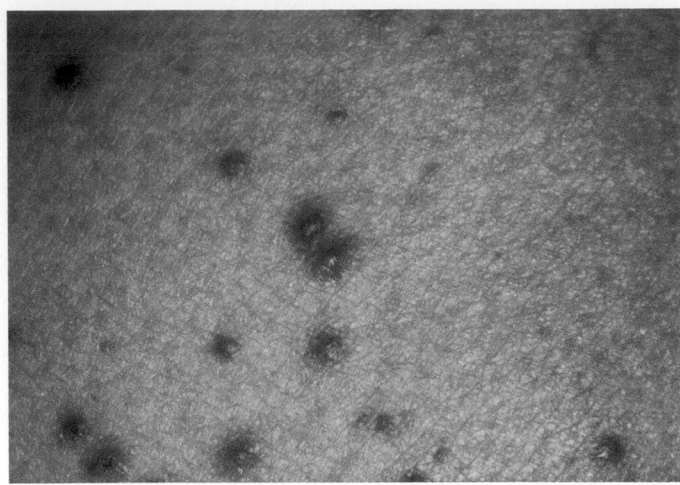

Fig. 3-4 Miliaria rubra.

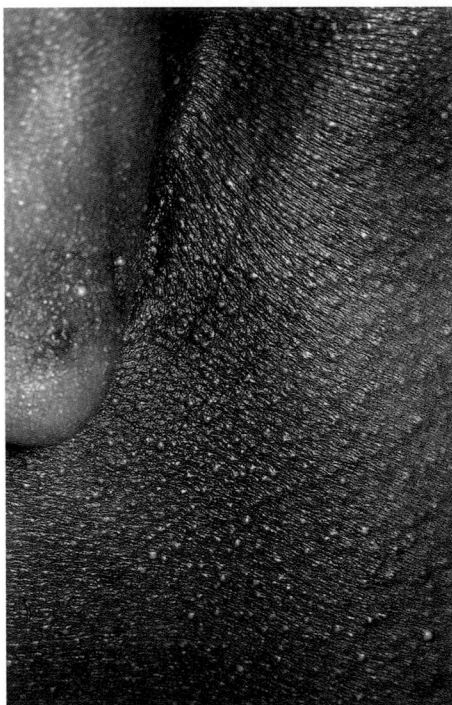

Fig. 3-5 Miliaria pustulosa. (Courtesy of Curt Samlaska, MD)

frequently affected are the antecubital and popliteal fossae, trunk, inframammary areas (especially under pendulous breasts), abdomen (especially at the waistline), and inguinal regions; these sites frequently become macerated because evaporation of moisture has been impeded. Exercise-induced itching may also be caused by miliaria rubra. The site of injury and sweat escape is in the prickle cell layer, where spongiosis is produced.

Miliaria pustulosa

Miliaria pustulosa (Fig. 3-5) is preceded by another dermatitis that has produced injury, destruction, or blocking of the sweat duct. The pustules are distinct, superficial, and independent of the hair follicle. The pruritic pustules occur most frequently on the intertriginous areas, flexure surfaces of the extremities, scrotum, and back of bedridden patients. Contact dermatitis, lichen simplex chronicus, and intertrigo are some of the associated diseases, although pustular miliaria may occur several weeks after these diseases have subsided. Recurrent episodes

may be a sign of type I pseudohypoaldosteronism, as salt-losing crises may precipitate miliaria pustulosa or rubra, with resolution after stabilization.

Miliaria profunda

Non-pruritic, flesh-colored, deep-seated, whitish papules characterize this form of miliaria. It is asymptomatic, usually lasts only 1 h after overheating has ended, and is concentrated on the trunk and extremities. Except for the face, axillae, hands, and feet, where there may be compensatory hyperhidrosis, all the sweat glands are nonfunctional. The occlusion is in the upper dermis. This form is observed only in the tropics and usually follows a severe bout of miliaria rubra.

Postmiliarial hypohidrosis

Postmiliarial hypohidrosis results from occlusion of sweat ducts and pores, and may be severe enough to impair an individual's ability to perform sustained work in a hot environment. Affected persons may show decreasing efficiency, irritability, anorexia, drowsiness, vertigo, and headache; they may wander in a daze.

It has been shown that hypohidrosis invariably follows miliaria, and that the duration and severity of the hypohidrosis are related to the severity of the miliaria. Sweating may be depressed to half the normal amount for as long as 3 weeks.

Tropical anhidrotic asthenia

This is a rare form of miliaria with long-lasting poral occlusion, which produces anhidrosis and heat retention.

Treatment

The most effective treatment for miliaria is to place the patient in a cool environment. Even a single night in an air-conditioned room helps to alleviate the discomfort. Next best is the use of circulating air fans to cool the skin. Anhydrous lanolin resolves the occlusion of pores and may help to restore normal sweat secretions. Hydrophilic ointment also helps to dissolve keratinous plugs and facilitates the normal flow of sweat. Soothing, cooling baths containing colloidal oatmeal or cornstarch are beneficial if used in moderation. Mild cases may respond to dusting powders, such as cornstarch or baby talcum powder.

Akeakus M, et al: Newborn with pseudohypaldosteronism and miliaria rubra. Int J Dermatol 2006; 45:1432.

Dimon NS, et al: Goosefleshlike lesions and hypohidrosis. Arch Dermatol 2007; 143:1323.

Godkar D, et al: Rare skin disorder complicating doxorubicin therapy: miliaria crystallina. Am J Ther 2005; 12:275.

Haas N, et al: Congenital miliaria crystallina. J Am Acad Dermatol 2002; 47:S270.

Kirk JF, et al: Miliaria profunda. J Am Acad Dermatol 1996; 35:854.

La Shell MS, et al: Pruritus, papules, and perspiration. Ann Allergy Immunol 2007; 98:299.

Mowad CM, et al: The role of extracellular polysaccharide substance produced by Staphylococcus epidermidis in miliaria. J Am Acad Dermatol 1995; 20:713.

Wenzel FG, et al: Nonneoplastic disorders of the eccrine glands. J Am Acad Dermatol 1998; 38:1.

Erythema ab igne

Erythema ab igne is a persistent erythema—or the coarsely reticulated residual pigmentation resulting from it—that is usually produced by long exposure to excessive heat without the production of a burn (Fig. 3-6). It begins as a mottling caused by local hemostasis and becomes a reticulated erythema, leaving pigmentation. Multiple colors are simultaneously present in an active patch, varying from pale pink to old rose or dark purplish-brown. After the cause is removed, the

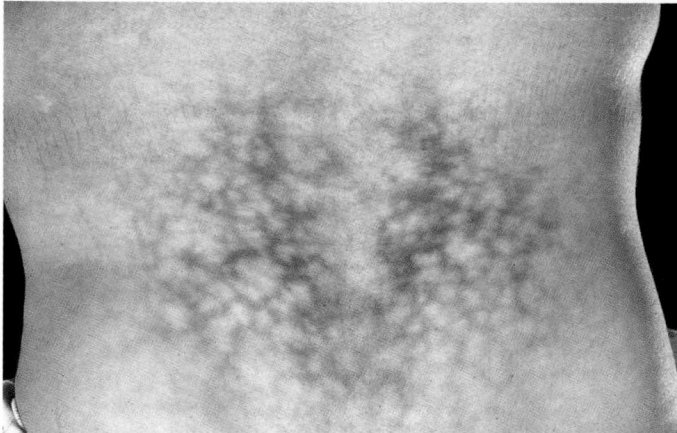

Fig. 3-6 Erythema ab igne.

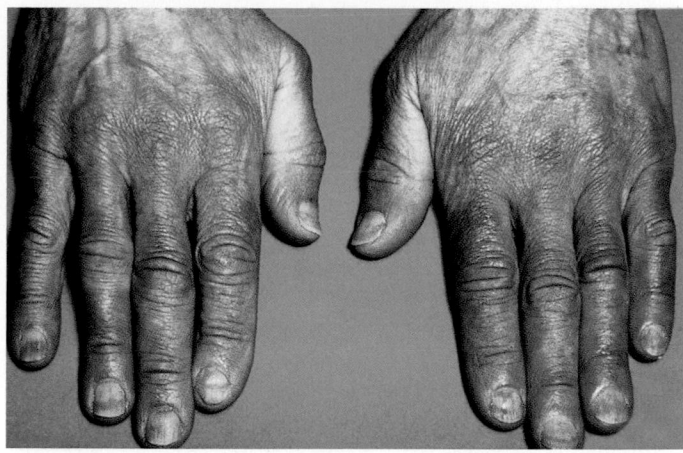

Fig. 3-7 Acrocyanosis.

affection tends to disappear gradually, but sometimes the pigmentation is permanent.

Histologically, an increased amount of elastic tissue in the dermis is noted. The changes in erythema ab igne are similar to those of actinic elastosis. Interface dermatitis and epithelial atypia may be noted.

Erythema ab igne occurs on the legs as a result of habitually warming them in front of open fireplaces, space heaters, or car heaters. Similar changes may be produced at sites of an electric heating pad application such as the low back, or the upper thighs with laptop computers. The condition occurs also in cooks, silversmiths, and others exposed over long periods to direct moderate heat.

Epithelial atypia, which may lead to Bowen's disease and squamous cell carcinoma, has rarely been reported to occur overlying erythema ab igne. Treatment with 5-fluorouracil (5-FU) or imiquimod cream may be effective in reversing this epidermal alteration.

The use of emollients containing α-hydroxy acids or a cream containing fluocinolone acetonide 0.01%, hydroquinone 4%, and tretinoin 0.05% may help reduce the unsightly pigmentation.

Chan CC, et al: Erythema ab igne. N Engl J Med 2007; 356:e8.
Chatterjee S: Erythema ab igne from prolonged use of a heating pad. Mayo Clin Proc 2005; 80:1500.
Levinbook WS, et al: Laptop computer-associated erythema ab igne. Cutis 2007; 80:319.

Cold injuries

Exposure to cold damages the skin by at least three mechanisms.

- Reduced temperature directly damages the tissue, as in frostbite and cold immersion foot.
- Vasospasm of vessels perfusing the skin prevents adequate perfusion of the tissue and causes vascular injury and consequent tissue injury (pernio, acrocyanosis, and frostbite).
- In unusual circumstances, adipose tissue is predisposed to damage by cold temperatures due to fat composition or location (cold panniculitis, see Chapter 23).

Outdoor workers and recreationalists, the armed forces, alcoholics, and the homeless are particularly likely to suffer cold injuries.

Jurkovich GJ: Environmental cold-induced injury. Surg Clin N Am 2007: 87:247.

Acrocyanosis

Acrocyanosis is a persistent blue discoloration of the entire hand or foot worsened by cold exposure. The hands and feet may be hyperhidrotic (Fig. 3-7). It occurs chiefly in young women. Cyanosis increases as the temperature decreases and changes to erythema with elevation of the dependent part. The cause is unknown. Smoking should be avoided. Acrocyanosis is distinguished from Raynaud syndrome by its persistent nature (as opposed to the episodic nature of Raynaud) and lack of tissue damage (ulceration, distal fingertip resorption).

Acrocyanosis with swelling of the nose, ears, and dorsal hands may occur after inhalation of butyl nitrite. Interferon-α 2a may induce it. Repeated injection of the dorsal hand with narcotic drugs may produce lymphedema and an appearance similar to the edematous phase of scleroderma. This so-called puffy hand syndrome may include erythema or a bluish discoloration of the digits. Patients with anorexia nervosa frequently manifest acrocyanosis as well as perniosis, livedo reticularis and acral coldness. It may improve with weight gain.

Acral vascular syndromes may also be a sign of malignancy. In 47% of the 66 reported cases the diagnosis of cancer coincided with the onset of the acral disease. These are most likely to be vasospastic or occlusive; however, acrocyanosis has also been reported.

Brown PJ, et al: The purple digit. Am J Clin Derm 2010; 11:103.
Del Giudice P, et al: Hand edema and acrocyanosis: puffy hand syndrome. Arch Dermatol 2006; 142:1084.
Nousari HC, et al: Chronic idiopathic acrocyanosis. J Am Acad Dermatol 2001; 45:S207.
Solak Y, et al: Acrocyanosis as a presenting symptom of Hodgkin lymphoma. Am J Hematol 2006; 81:149.
Strumia R: Dermatologic signs in patients with eating disorders. Am J Clin Dermatol 2005; 6:165.

Chilblains (pernio)

Chilblains constitute a localized erythema and swelling caused by exposure to cold. Blistering and ulcerations may develop in severe cases. In people predisposed by poor peripheral circulation, even moderate exposure to cold may produce chilblains. Cryoglobulins, cryofibrinogens or cold agglutinins may be present and pathogenic. Chilblain-like lesions may occur in discoid and systemic lupus erythematosus (chilblain lupus) or as a presenting sign of leukemia cutis. The chronic use of crack

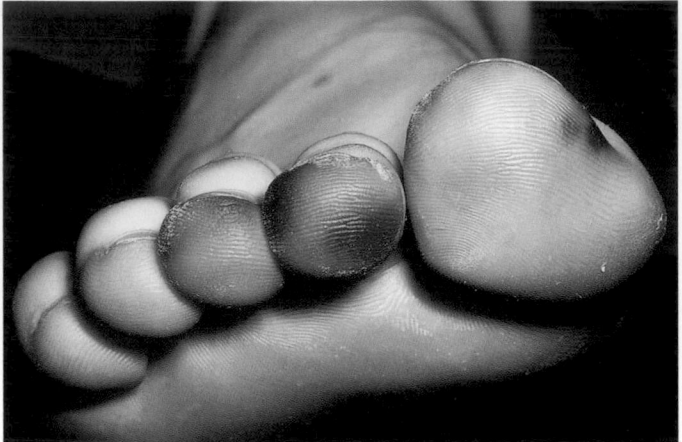

Fig. 3-8 Pernio.

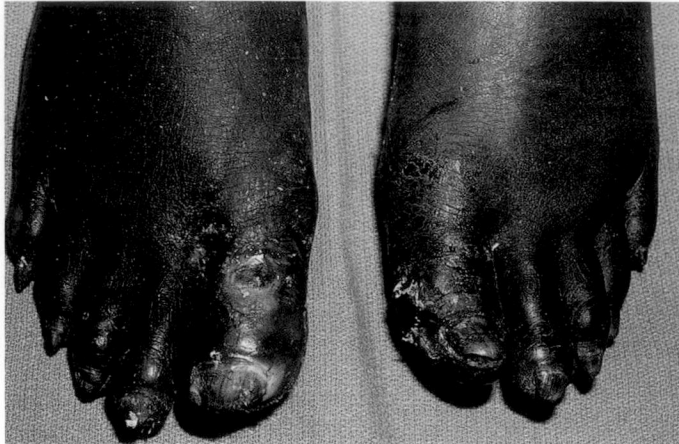

Fig. 3-9 Frostbite in a homeless person.

cocaine and its attendant peripheral vasoconstriction will lead to perniosis with cold, numb hands and atrophy of the digital fat pads, especially of the thumbs and index fingers, as well as nail curvature.

Chilblains occur chiefly on the hands, feet, ears, and face, especially in children; onset is enhanced by dampness (Fig. 3-8). A variant occurs on the lateral thighs in women equestrians who ride on cold damp days (equestrian perniosis). Tight-fitting jeans with a low waistband may produce this type of cold injury on the hips. Wading across cold streams may produce similar lesions. Erythrocyanosis crurum has been used to describe similar cases. Lesions of cold injury of the lateral thighs can be nodular.

Patients with chilblains are often unaware of the cold injury when it is occurring, but later burning, itching, and redness call it to their attention. The affected areas are bluish-red, the color partially or totally disappearing on pressure, and are decidedly cool to the touch. Sometimes the extremities are clammy because of excessive sweating. As long as the damp/cold exposure continues, new lesions will continue to appear and lesions may resolve slowly. Investigation into an underlying cause should be undertaken in cases that are recurrent, chronic, extending into warm seasons or poorly responsive to treatment.

Perniosis histologically demonstrates a lymphocytic vasculitis. There is dermal edema, and a superficial and deep perivascular, tightly cuffed, lymphocytic infiltrate. The infiltrate involves the vessel walls and is accompanied by characteristic "fluffy" edema of the vessel walls.

Treatment

The affected parts should be protected against further exposure to cold or dampness. If the feet are affected, woolen socks should be worn at all times during the cold months. Because patients are often not conscious of the cold exposure that triggers the lesions, appropriate dress must be stressed, even if patients say they do not sense being cold. Since central cooling triggers peripheral vasoconstriction, keeping the whole body (not just the affected extremity) warm is critical. Heating pads may be used judiciously to warm the parts. Smoking is strongly discouraged.

Nifedipine, 20 mg three times a day, has been effective. Vasodilators such as nicotinamide, 500 mg three times a day, or dipyridamole, 25 mg three times a day, or the phosphodiesterase inhibitor sildenafil, 50 mg twice daily, may be used to improve circulation. Pentoxifylline may be effective. Spontaneous resolution occurs without treatment in 1–3 weeks. Systemic corticoid therapy is useful in chilblain lupus erythematosus.

Affleck AG, et al: Chilblain-like leukemia cutis. Pediatr Dermatol 2007; 24:38.

Bouaziz JD, et al: Cutaneous lesions of the digits in SLE: 50 cases. Lupus 2007; 16:163.

Cribier B, et al: A histologic and immunohistochemical study of chilblains. J Am Acad Dermatol 2001; 45:924.

Long WB 3rd, et al: Cold injuries. J Long Term Eff Med Implants 2005; 15:67.

McClesky PE, et al: Tender papules on the hands. Arch Dermatol 2006; 142:1501.

Payne-James JJ, et al: Pseudosclerodermatous triad of perniosis, pulp atrophy and parrot-beaked clawing of the nails—newly recognized syndrome of chronic crack cocaine use. J Forensic Leg Med 2007; 14:65.

Price RD, Murdoch DR: Perniosis (chilblains) of the thigh: report of five cases, including four following river crossings. High Alt Med Biol 2001; 2:535.

Simon TD, et al: Pernio in pediatrics. Pediatrics 2005; 116:e472.

Viguier M, et al: Clinical and histopathologic features and immunologic variables in patients with severe chilblains. A study of the relationship to lupus erythematosus. Medicine (Baltimore) 2001; 80:180.

Weismann K, et al: Pernio of the hips in young girls wearing tight-fitting jeans with a low waistband. Acta Derm Venereol 2006; 86:558.

Yang X, et al: Adult perniosis and cryoglobulinemia. J Am Acad Dermatol 2010; 62:e21.

Frostbite

When soft tissue is frozen and locally deprived of blood supply, the damage is called frostbite. The ears, nose, cheeks, fingers, and toes are most often affected. The frozen part painlessly becomes pale and waxy. Various degrees of tissue destruction similar to those caused by burns are encountered. These are erythema and edema, vesicles and bullae, superficial gangrene, deep gangrene, and injury to muscles, tendons, periosteum, and nerves (Fig. 3-9). The degree of injury is directly related to the temperature and duration of freezing. African Americans are at increased risk of frostbite.

Treatment

Early treatment of frostbite before swelling develops should consist of covering the part with clothing or with a warm hand or other body surface to maintain a slightly warm temperature so that adequate blood circulation can be maintained. Rapid rewarming in a water bath between 37 and 43°C (100–110°F) is the treatment of choice for all forms of frostbite. Rewarming should be delayed until the patient has been removed to an area where there is no risk of refreezing. Slow thawing results in more extensive tissue damage. Analgesics, unless contraindicated, should be administered because of the considerable pain experienced with rapid thawing. When the skin flushes and is pliable, thawing is complete. The use of tissue plasminogen activator to lyse thrombi decreases the need for amputation if given within 24 h of injury. Supportive measures such as bed rest, a high-protein/high-calorie diet, wound care, and avoidance of trauma are imperative. Any rubbing of the affected part should be avoided, but gentle massage of proximal portions of the extremity that are not numb may be helpful.

After swelling and hyperemia have developed, the patient should be kept in bed with the affected limb slightly flexed, elevated, and at rest. Exposing the affected limb to air at room temperature relieves pain and helps prevent tissue damage. Protection by a heat cradle may be desirable.

The use of anticoagulants to prevent thrombosis and gangrene during the recovery period has been advocated. Pentoxifylline, ibuprofen, and aspirin may be useful adjuncts. Antibiotics should be given as a prophylactic measure against infection and tetanus immunization should be updated. Recovery may take many months. Injuries that affect the proximal phalanx or the carpal or tarsal area, especially when accompanied by a lack of radiotracer uptake on bone scan, have a high likelihood of requiring amputation. Whereas prior cold injury is a major risk factor for recurrent disease, sympathectomy may be preventative against repeated episodes. Arthritis may be a late complication.

Bruen KJ, et al: Reduction in the incidence of amputation in frostbite injury with thrombolytic therapy. Arch Surg 2007; 142:546.
Cauchy E, et al: Retrospective study of 70 cases of severe frostbite lesions. Wilderness Environ Med 2001; 12:248.
Kahn JE, et al: Frostbite arthritis. Ann Rheum Dis 2005; 64:966.

Immersion foot syndromes

Trench foot

Trench foot results from prolonged exposure to cold, wet conditions without immersion or actual freezing. The term is derived from trench warfare in World War I, when soldiers stood, sometimes for hours, in trenches with a few inches of cold water in them. Fishermen, sailors, and shipwreck survivors are sometimes seen with this condition. The lack of circulation produces edema, paresthesias, and damage to the blood vessels. Gangrene may occur in severe cases. Treatment consists of removal from the causal environment, bed rest, and restoration of the circulation. Other measures, such as those used in the treatment of frostbite, should be employed.

Warm water immersion foot

Exposure of the feet to warm, wet conditions for 48 h or more may produce a syndrome characterized by maceration, blanching, and wrinkling of the soles and sides of the feet (Fig. 3-10). Itching and burning with swelling may persist for a few days after removal of the cause, but disability is temporary. It was commonly seen in military service members in Vietnam but has also been seen in persons wearing insulated boots.

This condition should be differentiated from tropical immersion foot, seen after continuous immersion of the feet in water or mud at temperatures above 22°C (71.6°F) for 2–10 days. This was known as "paddy foot" in Vietnam. It involves erythema, edema, and pain of the dorsal feet, as well as fever and adenopathy (Fig. 3-11). Resolution occurs 3–7 days after the feet have been dried.

Warm water immersion foot can be prevented by allowing the feet to dry for a few hours in every 24 or by greasing the soles with a silicone grease once a day. Recovery is usually rapid if the feet are thoroughly dry for a few hours.

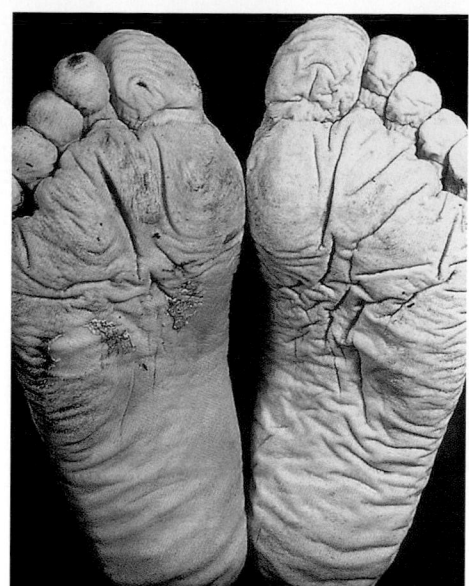

Fig. 3-10 Warm water immersion foot. (Courtesy of James WD (ed): Textbook of Military Medicine, Office of the Surgeon General, United States Army, 1994)

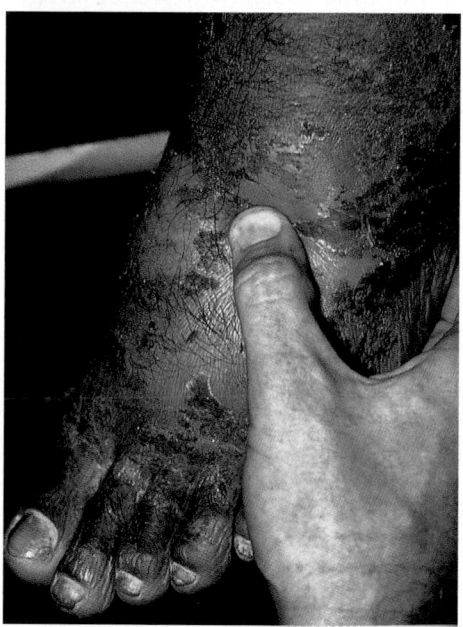

Fig. 3-11 Tropical immersion foot. (Courtesy of James WD (ed): Textbook of Military Medicine, Office of the Surgeon General, United States Army, 1994)

Adnot J, et al: Immersion foot syndromes. In: James WD (ed): Military Dermatology. Washington, DC: Office of the Surgeon General, 1994.
Wrenn K: Immersion foot. Arch Intern Med 1991; 151:785.

Actinic injury

Sunburn and solar erythema

The solar spectrum has been divided into different regions by wavelength. The parts of the solar spectrum important in photomedicine include UV radiation (below 400 nm), visible light (400–760 nm), and infrared radiation (beyond 760 nm). Visible light has limited biologic activity, except for stimulating the retina. Infrared radiation is experienced as radiant heat. Below 400 nm is the UV spectrum, divided into three

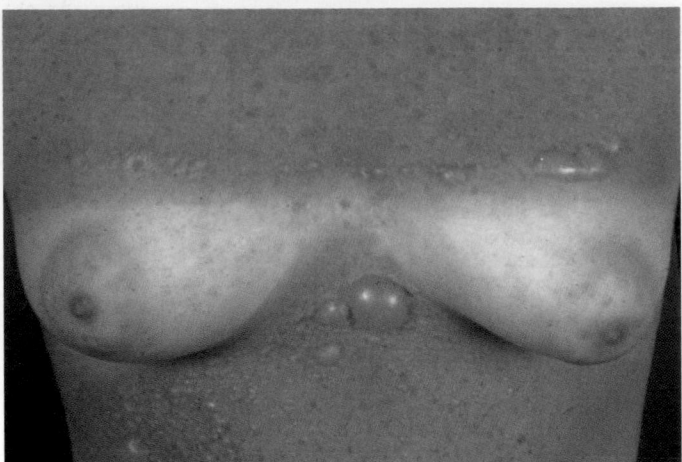

Fig. 3-12 Acute sunburn. (Courtesy of Dr L Lieblich)

Table 3-1 Skin types (phototypes)

Skin type	Baseline skin color	Sunburn and tanning history
I	White	Always burns, never tans
II	White	Always burns, tans minimally
III	White	Burns moderately, tans gradually
IV	Olive	Minimal burning, tans well
V	Brown	Rarely burns, tans darkly
VI	Dark brown	Never burns, tans darkly black

bands: UVA, 320–400 nm; UVB, 280–320 nm; and UVC, 200–280 nm. UVA is divided into two subcategories: UVA I (340–400 nm) and UVA II (320–340 nm). Virtually no UVC reaches the earth's surface because it is absorbed by the ozone layer above the earth.

The minimal amount of a particular wavelength of light capable of inducing erythema on an individual's skin is called the minimal erythema dose (MED). Although the amount of UVA radiation is 100 times greater than UVB radiation during midday hours, UVB is up to 1000 times more erythemogenic than UVA, and so essentially all solar erythema is caused by UVB. The most biologically effective wavelength of radiation from the sun for sunburn is 308 nm. UVA does not play a significant role in solar erythema and sunburn; however, in the case of drug-induced photosensitivity, UVA is of major importance.

The amount of UV exposure increases at higher altitudes, is substantially larger in temperate climates in the summer months, and is greater in tropical regions. UVA may be reflected somewhat more than UVB from sand, snow, and ice. While sand and snow reflect as much as 85% of the UVB, water allows 80% of the UV to penetrate up to 3 feet. Cloud cover, although blocking substantial amounts of visible light, is a poor UV absorber. During the middle 4–6 h of the day, the intensity of UVB is 2–4 times greater than in the early morning and late afternoon.

Clinical signs and symptoms

Sunburn is the normal cutaneous reaction to sunlight in excess of an erythema dose. UVB erythema becomes evident at around 6 h after exposure and peaks at 12–24 h, but the onset is sooner and the severity greater with increased exposure. The erythema is followed by tenderness, and in severe cases, blistering, which may become confluent (Fig. 3-12). Discomfort may be severe; edema commonly occurs in the extremities and face; chills, fever, nausea, tachycardia, and hypotension may be present. In severe cases such symptoms may last for as long as a week. Desquamation is common about a week after sunburn, even in areas that have not blistered.

After UV exposure, skin pigment undergoes two changes: immediate pigment darkening (IPD, Meirowsky phenomenon) and delayed melanogenesis. IPD is maximal within hours after sun exposure and results from metabolic changes and redistribution of the melanin already in the skin. It occurs after exposure to long-wave UVB, UVA, and visible light. With large doses of UVA, the initial darkening is prolonged and may blend into the delayed melanogenesis. IPD is not photoprotective. Delayed tanning is induced by the same wave-lengths of UVB that induce erythema, begins 2–3 days after exposure, and lasts 10–14 days. Delayed melanogenesis by UVB is mediated through the production of DNA damage and the formation of cyclobutane pyrimidine dimers (CPD). Therefore, although UVB-induced delayed tanning does provide some protection from further solar injury, it is at the expense of damage to the epidermis and dermis. Hence, tanning is not recommended for sun protection. Commercial sunbed-induced tanning, while increasing skin pigment, does not increase UVB MED, and is therefore not protective for UVB damage. An individual's inherent baseline pigmentation, ability to tan, and the ease with which he/she burns are described as his/her "skin type." Skin type (Table 3-1) is used to determine starting doses of phototherapy and sunscreen recommendations, and reflects the risk of development of skin cancer and photoaging.

Exposure to UVB and UVA causes an increase in the thickness of the epidermis, especially the stratum corneum. This increased epidermal thickness leads to increased tolerance to further solar radiation. Patients with vitiligo may increase their UV exposure without burning by this mechanism.

Treatment

Once redness and other symptoms are present, treatment of sunburn has limited efficacy. The damage is done and the inflammatory cascades are triggered. Prostaglandins, especially of the E series, are important mediators. Aspirin (ASA) and nonsteroidal anti-inflammatory drugs (NSAIDs), including indomethacin, have been studied, as well as topical and systemic steroids. Medium potency (class II) topical steroids applied 6 h after the exposure (when erythema first appears) give a small reduction in signs and symptoms. Since oral NSAIDs and systemic steroids have been tested primarily prior to or immediately after sun exposure, there is insufficient evidence to recommend their routine use, except immediately after solar over-exposure. Therefore treatment of sunburn should be supportive, with pain management (using acetaminophen, ASA, or NSAIDs), plus soothing topical emollients or corticosteroid lotions. In general, a sunburn victim experiences at least 1 or 2 days of discomfort and even pain before much relief occurs.

Prophylaxis

Sunburn is best prevented. Use of the UV index, published daily by the National Weather Service for many US cities and found in newspapers, facilitates taking adequate precautions to prevent solar injury. Numerous educational programs have been developed to make the public aware of the hazards of sun exposure. Despite this, sunburn and excessive sun exposure continue to occur in the US and Western Europe, especially in white persons under the age of 30, among whom more than 50% report at least one sunburn per year. Sun protection programs have four messages:

- Avoid midday sun.
- Seek shade.
- Wear protective clothing.
- Apply a sunscreen.

The period of highest UVB intensity, between 9 am and 3–4 pm, accounts for the vast majority of potentially hazardous UV exposure. This is the time when the angle of the sun is less than 45° or when a person's shadow is shorter than his/her height. In temperate latitudes it is almost impossible to burn if these hours of sun exposure are avoided. Trees and artificial shade provide substantial protection from UVB. Foliage in trees provides the equivalent of sun protection factor (SPF) 4–50, depending on the density of the greenery. Clothing can be rated by its ability to block UVB radiation. The scale of measure is the UV protection factor (UPF) (analogous to SPF in sunscreens). Although it is an in vitro measurement, as with SPF, it correlates well with the actual protection the product provides in vivo. In general, denser weaves, older, washed clothing, and loose-fitting clothing screen UVB more effectively. Wetting a fabric may substantially reduce its UPF. Laundering a fabric in a Tinosorb-containing material (SunGuard) will add substantially to the UPF of the fabric. Hats with at least a 4-inch brim all around are recommended.

A sunscreen's efficacy in blocking the UVB (sunburn-inducing) radiation is expressed as an SPF. This is the ratio of the number of MEDs of radiation required to induce erythema through a film of sunscreen ($2 \, mg/cm^2$), compared with unprotected skin. Most persons apply sunscreens in too thin a film, so the actual "applied SPF" is about half that on the label. Sunscreening agents include UV-absorbing chemicals (chemical sunscreens) and UV-scattering or blocking agents (physical sunscreens). Available sunscreens, especially those of high SPFs (>30), usually contain both chemical sunscreens (such as p-aminobenzoic acid [PABA], PABA esters, cinnamates, salicylates, anthranilates, benzophenones, benzylidene camphors such as ecamsule [Mexoryl], dibenzoylmethanes [Parsol 1789, in some products present as a multicompound technology Helioplex], and Tinosorb [S/M]) and physical agents (zinc oxide or titanium dioxide). They are available in numerous formulations, including sprays, gels, emollient creams, and wax sticks. Sunscreens may be water-resistant (maintaining their SPF after 40 min of water immersion) or waterproof (maintaining their SPF after 80 min of water immersion).

For skin types I–III (see Table 3-1), daily application of a sunscreen with an SPF of 30 in a facial moisturizer, foundation, or aftershave is recommended. For outdoor exposure, a sunscreen of SPF 30 or higher is recommended for regular use. In persons with severe photosensitivity and at times of high sun exposure, high-intensity sunscreens of SPF 30+ with inorganic blocking agents may be required. Application of the sunscreen at least 20 min before and 30 min after sun exposure has begun is recommended. This dual application approach will reduce the amount of skin exposure by two- to three-fold over a single application. Sunscreen should be reapplied after swimming or vigorous activity or toweling. Sunscreen failure occurs mostly in men, due to failure to apply it to all the sun-exposed skin, or failure to reapply sunscreen after swimming. Sunscreens may be applied to babies (under 6 months) on limited areas. Vitamin D supplementation may be recommended with the most stringent sun-protection practices.

Photoaging and cutaneous immunosuppression are mediated by UVA as well as UVB. For this reason, sunscreens with improved UVA coverage have been developed (Parsol 1789, Mexoryl, Tinosorb). The UVA protection does not parallel the SPF on the label. If UVA protection is sought, a combination sunscreen with inorganic agents and UVA organic sunscreens (identified by name in the list of ingredients) is recommended.

Baron ED, Stevens SR: Sunscreens and immune protection. Br J Dermatol 2002; 146:933.

Diffey BL, Diffey JL: Sun protection with trees. Br J Dermatol 2002; 147:385.

D'Souza G, et al: Mexoryl. Plast Reconstr Surg 2007; 120:1071.

Duteil L, et al: A randomized, controlled study of the safety and efficacy of topical corticosteroid treatments of sunburn in healthy volunteers. Clin Exp Dermatol 2002; 27:314.

Faurschaou A, et al: Topical corticosterids in the treatment of acute sunburn. Arch Dermatol 2008; 144:620.

Hatch KL, et al: Garments as solar ultraviolet radiation screening materials. Dermatol Clin 2006; 24:85.

Iuternschlager S, et al: Photoprotection. Lancet 2007; 370:528.

Lim HW, et al: Sunlight, tanning booths and vitamin D. J Am Acad Dermatol 2005; 52:868.

Lowe NJ: An overview of ultraviolet protection, sunscreens, and photo-induced dermatoses. Dermatol Clin 2006; 24:9.

Medeiras VL, et al: Sunscreens in the management of photodermatoses. Skin Therapy Lett 2010; 15:1.

Moehrle M, et al: UV exposure in cars. Photodermatol Photoimmunol Photomed 2003; 19:175.

Palm MD, et al: Update on photoprotection. Dermatol Ther 2007; 20:360.

Thieden E, et al: Sunburn related to UV radiation exposure, age, sex, occupation and sun bed use based on time-stamped personal dosimetry and sun behaviour diaries. Arch Dermatol 2005; 141:482.

Ephelis (freckle) and lentigo

Freckles are small (<0.5 cm) brown macules that occur in profusion on the sun-exposed skin of the face, neck, shoulders, and backs of the hands. They become prominent during the summer when exposed to sunlight and subside, sometimes completely, during the winter when there is no exposure. Blonds and red-heads with blue eyes and of Celtic origin (skin types I or II) are especially susceptible. Ephelides may be genetically determined and may recur in successive generations in similar locations and patterns. They usually appear around age 5.

Ephelis must be differentiated from lentigo simplex. The lentigo is a benign discrete hyperpigmented macule appearing at any age and on any part of the body, including the mucosa. The intensity of the color is not dependent on sun exposure. The solar lentigo appears at a later age, mostly in persons with long-term sun exposure. The backs of the hands and face (especially the forehead) are favored sites.

Histologically, the ephelis shows increased production of melanin pigment by a normal number of melanocytes. Otherwise, the epidermis is normal, whereas the lentigo has elongated rete ridges that appear to be club-shaped.

Freckles and solar lentigines are best prevented by appropriate sun protection. Cryotherapy, topical retinoids, hydroquinone, and lasers are effective in the treatment of solar lentigines.

Draelos ZD: Skin lightening preparations and the hydroquinone controversy. Dermatol Ther 2007; 20:308.

Ortonne J-P, et al: Treatment of solar lentigines. J Am Acad Dermatol 2006; 54:S262.

Photoaging (dermatoheliosis)

The characteristic changes induced by chronic sun exposure are called photoaging or dermatoheliosis. An individual's risk for developing these changes correlates with his/her skin type (see Table 3-1). Risk for melanoma and nonmelanoma skin cancer is also related to skin type. The most susceptible to the deleterious effects of sunlight are those of skin type I—blue-eyed, fair-complexioned persons who do not tan. They are frequently of Irish or other Celtic or Anglo-Saxon descent. Individuals who have developed photoaging have the genetic susceptibility and have had sufficient actinic damage to develop skin cancer, and therefore require more frequent and careful cutaneous examinations.

Chronic sun exposure and chronologic aging are additive. Cigarette smoking is also important in the development of wrinkles; hence the inability of observers to distinguish solar-induced from smoking-induced skin aging accurately. The areas primarily affected by photoaging are those regularly exposed to the sun: the V area of the neck and chest, back and sides of the neck, face, backs of the hands and extensor arms, and in women the skin between the knees and ankles. The skin becomes atrophic, scaly, wrinkled, inelastic, or leathery with a yellow hue (Milian citrine skin). In some persons of Celtic ancestry, dermatoheliosis produces profound epidermal atrophy without wrinkling, resulting in an almost translucent appearance of the skin through which hyperplastic sebaceous glands and prominent telangiectasias are seen. These persons are at high risk for nonmelanoma skin cancer. Pigmentation is uneven, with a mixture of poorly demarcated hyperpigmented and white atrophic macules observed. The photodamaged skin appears generally darker because of these irregularities of pigmentation; added to this is dermal hemosiderosis from actinic purpura. Solar lentigines occur on the face and dorsa of the hands.

Many of the textural and tinctorial changes in sun-damaged skin are caused by alterations in the upper dermal elastic tissue and collagen. This process is called solar (actinic) elastosis, which imparts a yellow color to the skin. Many clinical variants of solar elastosis have been described, and an affected individual may simultaneously have many of these changes. Small yellowish papules and plaques may develop along the sides of the neck. They have been variably named striated beaded lines (the result of sebaceous hyperplasia) or fibroelastolytic papulosis of the neck, which is caused by solar elastosis. At times, usually on the face or chest, this elastosis may form a macroscopic, translucent papule with a pearly color that may closely resemble a basal cell carcinoma (Dubreuilh elastoma, actinic elastotic plaque). Similar plaques may occur on the helix or antihelix of the ear (elastotic nodules of the ear). Poikiloderma of Civatte refers to reticulate hyperpigmentation with telangiectasia, and slight atrophy of the sides of the neck, lower anterior neck, and V of the chest. The submental area, shaded by the chin, is spared (Fig. 3-13). Poikiloderma of Civatte frequently presents in fair-skinned men and women in their mid- to late thirties or early forties. Cutis rhomboidalis nuchae (sailor's or farmer's neck) is characteristic of long-term, chronic sun exposure (Fig. 3-14). The skin on the back of the neck becomes thickened, tough, and leathery, and the normal skin markings are exaggerated. Nodular elastoidosis with cysts and comedones occurs on the inferior periorbital and malar skin (Favre–Racouchot syndrome) (Fig. 3-15) on the forearms (actinic comedonal plaque) or helix of the ear. These lesions appear as thickened yellow plaques studded with comedones and keratinous cysts.

Telangiectasias over the cheeks, ears, and sides of the neck may develop. Because of the damage to the connective tissue of the dermis, skin fragility is prominent, and patients note skin tearing from trivial injuries. Most commonly, patients complain that even minimal trauma to their extensor arms leads to an ecchymosis, a phenomenon called actinic purpura. As the ecchymoses resolve, dusky brown macules remain for

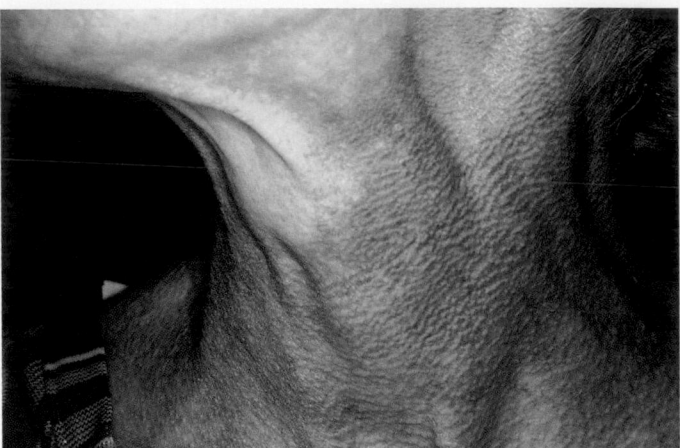

Fig. 3-13 Poikiloderma of Civatte.

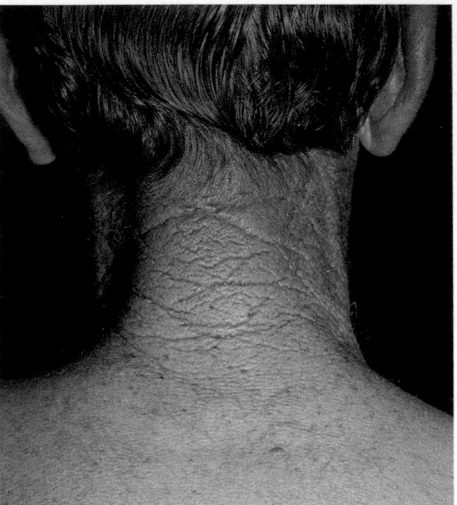

Fig. 3-14 Cutis rhomboidalis nuchae.

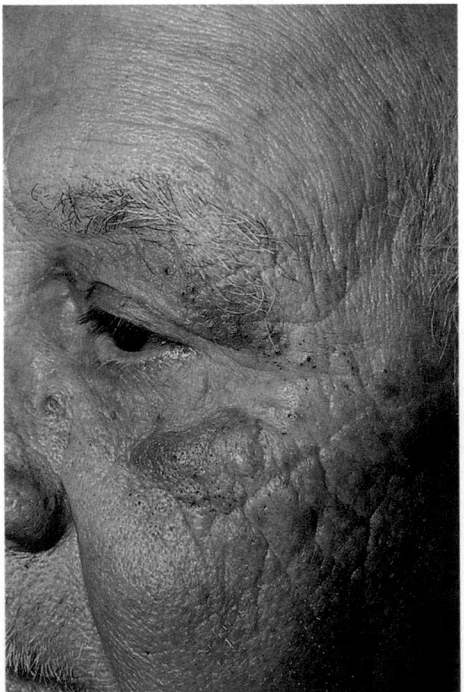

Fig. 3-15 Favre–Racouchot syndrome (nodular elastoidosis with cysts and comedones).

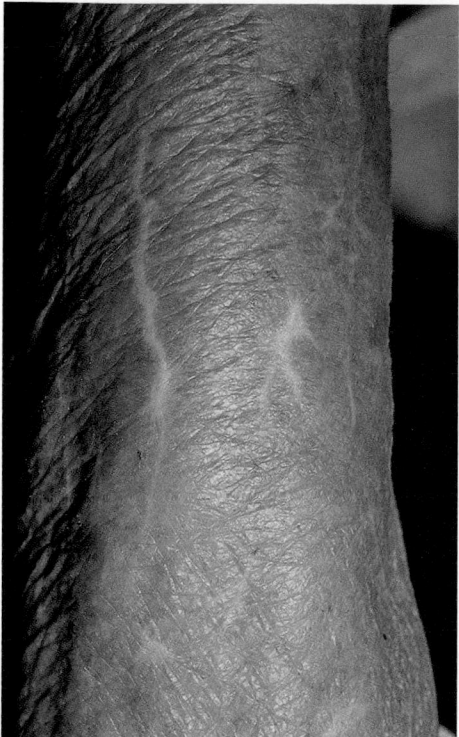

Fig. 3-16 Stellate pseudoscars.

months, increasing the mottled appearance of the skin. White stellate pseudoscars on the forearms are a frequent complication of this enhanced skin fragility (Fig. 3-16). In some patients, soft, flesh-colored to yellow papules and nodules coalesce on the forearms to form a cordlike band extending from the dorsal to the flexural surfaces (solar elastotic bands).

UVB and UVA radiation induce reactive oxygen species (ROS) and hydrogen peroxide. Acting through activator protein (AP)-1, transcription of various matrix-degrading enzymes is upregulated, specifically matrix metalloproteinase (MMP)-1 (collagenase), MMP-3 (stromelysin 1), and MMP-9 (gelatinase). MMP-1 cleaves a critical site on collagens types I and III, creating collagen fragments which are further degraded by MMP-3 and 9. Collagen fragments plus downregulation of procollagen promoters through AP-1 lead to a marked decrease in new collagen formation in UV-exposed skin. In darkly pigmented persons, UV exposure does not activate MMP-1, in part explaining the protective effect of skin pigmentation against photoaging. In chronologically aged skin, due perhaps to ROS generation, MMP-1 levels are also increased through AP-1, and collagen fragments are increased four-fold. Thus, chronologic aging and photoaging may be mediated through an identical biochemical mechanism.

Histologically, chronically sun-exposed skin demonstrates homogenization and a faint blue color of the connective tissue of the upper reticular dermis, so-called solar elastosis. This "elastotic" material is derived largely from elastic fibers, stains with histochemical stains for elastic fibers, and demonstrates marked increased deposition of fibulin-2 and its breakdown products. Types I and III collagen are decreased. Characteristically, there is a zone of normal connective tissue immediately below the epidermis and above the elastotic material.

Colloid milium

There are two forms of colloid milium: adult and juvenile. Cases of "nodular" colloid degeneration or "paracolloid" may represent severe presentations of adult colloid milium or cases of nodular amyloidosis, but these cases are few in number and reports of them occurred prior to technologies that could have better elucidated their etiology. Pigmented forms of colloid milium associated with hydroquinone use represent ochronosis-like pigmentation. In both the adult and juvenile forms of colloid milium, the primary skin lesion is a translucent, flesh-colored, or slightly yellow 1–5 mm papule. Minimal trauma may lead to purpura due to vascular fragility. Histologically, the colloid consists of intradermal, amorphous fissured eosinophilic material. In adult colloid milium lesions appear in the sun-exposed areas of the hands, face, neck, forearms, and ears in middle-aged and older adults, usually men. Lesions often coalesce into plaques, and may rarely be verrucous. Petrochemical exposures have been associated with adult colloid milium. Lesions have been induced by sunbed exposure, and can be unilateral, usually in commercial drivers. Adult colloid milium may be considered a papular variant of solar elastosis. The colloid material is derived from elastic fibers, and solar elastosis is found adjacent to the areas of colloid degeneration histologically.

Juvenile colloid milium is much rarer. It develops before puberty and there may be a family history. The lesions are similar to the adult form, but appear initially on the face, later extending to the neck and hands. Sun exposure also appears to be important in inducing lesions of juvenile colloid milium. Juvenile colloid milium, ligneous conjunctivitis, and ligneous periodontitis may appear in the same patient and are probably of similar pathogenesis. Histologically, juvenile colloid milium can be distinguished from adult colloid milium by the finding of keratinocyte apoptosis in the overlying epidermis. The colloid material in juvenile colloid milium is derived from the apoptotic keratinocytes and stains for cytokeratin. Treatment with fractional photothermolysis is effective.

Prevention and treatment

Since both UVB and UVA are capable of inducing the tissue-destructive biochemical pathways implicated in photoaging, sun protection against both portions of the UV spectrum is the primary prevention required against photoaging. Because photoaging, like other forms of radiation damage, appears to be cumulative, reducing the total lifetime UV exposure is the goal. The guidelines outlined above for sunburn prophylaxis should be followed.

The regular use of emollients or moisturizing creams on the areas of sun damage will reduce scaling and may improve fragility by making the skin more pliable. α-Hydroxy acids may improve skin texture when used in lower, nonirritating concentrations. Topical tretinoin, adapalene, and tazarotene can improve the changes of photoaging. Changes are slow and irritation may occur. Chemical peels, resurfacing techniques, laser and other light technologies for the treatment of vascular alterations, pigmented lesions, and dermal alterations, botulinum toxins and soft tissue augmentation are all used to treat the consequences of photoaging. The surgical and laser treatments of photoaging are discussed in Chapter 38.

Balus L, et al: Fibroelastolytic papulosis of the neck: a report of 20 cases. Br J Dermatol 1997; 137:461.

Calderone DC, Fenske NA: The clinical spectrum of actinic elastosis. J Am Acad Dermatol 1995; 32:1016.

Chowdhury MMU, et al: Juvenile colloid milium associated with ligneous conjunctivitis. Clin Exp Dermatol 2000; 25:138.

Desai C, et al: Colloid milium. Arch Dermatol 2006; 142:784.

Dierickx CC, et al: Visible light treatment of photoaging. Dermatol Ther 2005; 18:191.

Fisher GJ, et al: Looking older. Arch Dermatol 2008; 144:666.

Ikmeki TR, et al: Juvenile colloid milium. J Eur Acad Dermatol Venereol 2005; 19:355.

Gambichler T, et al: Cerebriform elastoma: an unusual presentation of actinic elastosis. J Amer Acad Dermatol 2005; 52:1106.

Hunzelmann N, et al: Increased deposition of fibulin-2 in solar elastosis and its colocalization with elastic fibers. Br J Dermatol 2001; 145:217.

Katoulis AC, et al: Poikiloderma of Civatte. Dermatology 2007; 214: 177.

Kwittken J: Papular elastosis. Cutis 2000; 66:81.

Lewis AT, et al: Unilateral colloid milium of the arm. J Am Acad Dermatol 2002; 46:S5.

Marra DE, et al: Fractional photothermolysis for the treatment of adult colloid milium. Arch Dermatol 2007; 143:572.

Morgan MB, et al: Multiple follicular cysts, infundibular type with vellus hairs and solar elastosis of the ears: a new dermatoheliosis? J Cutan Pathol 2003; 30:29.

Mukherjee S, et al: Retinoids in the treatment of skin aging. Clin Interv Aging 2006; 1:327.

Oskay T, et al: Juvenile colloid milium associated with conjunctival and gingival involvement. J Am Acad Dermatol 2003; 49:1185.

Pourrabbani S, et al: Colloid milium. J Drugs Dermatol 2007; 6:293.

Rabe JH, et al: Photoaging: mechanisms and repair. J Am Acad Dermatol 2006; 55:1.

Rostan EF: Laser treatment of photodamaged skin. Facial Plast Surg 2005; 21:99.

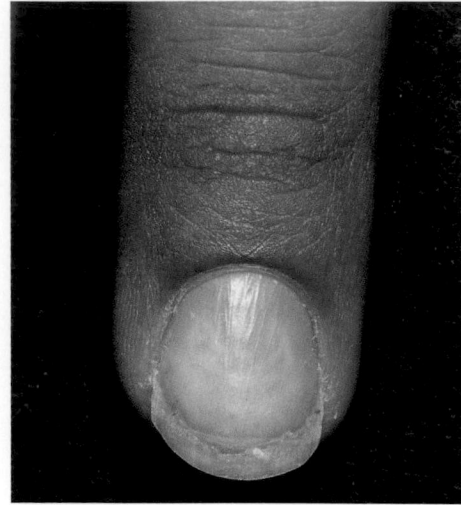

Fig. 3-17 Photo-onycholysis from minocycline.

Photosensitivity

Photosensitivity disorders include cutaneous reactions that are chemically induced (from an exogenous source), metabolic (inborn errors such as the porphyrias, resulting in the production of endogenous photosensitizers), idiopathic, and light-exacerbated (genetic and acquired). Phototoxicity and the idiopathic disorders are discussed below; the other conditions are covered elsewhere.

Chemically induced photosensitivity

A number of substances known as photosensitizers may induce an abnormal reaction in skin exposed to sunlight or its equivalent. The result may be a markedly increased sunburn response without allergic sensitization called phototoxicity. Phototoxicity may occur from both externally applied (phytophotodermatitis and berloque dermatitis) and internally administered chemicals (phototoxic drug reaction). In contrast, photoallergic reactions are true allergic sensitizations triggered by sunlight, produced either by internal administration (photoallergic drug reaction) or by external contact (photoallergic contact dermatitis). Chemicals capable of inducing phototoxic reactions may also produce photoallergic reactions.

In the case of external contactants, the distinction between phototoxicity and photoallergy is usually straightforward. The former occurs on initial exposure, has an onset of less than 48 h, occurs in the vast majority of persons exposed to the phototoxic substance and sunlight, and shows a histologic pattern similar to sunburn. By contrast, photoallergy occurs only in sensitized persons, may have a delayed onset (up to 14 days—the period of initial sensitization), and shows histologic features of allergic contact dermatitis.

Action spectrum

Chemicals known to cause photosensitivity (photosensitizers) are usually resonating compounds with a molecular weight of less than 500. Absorption of radiant energy (sunlight) by the photosensitizer produces an excited state, which in returning to a lower energy state gives off energy through fluorescence, phosphorescence, charge transfer, heat, or formation of free radicals. Each photosensitizing substance absorbs only specific wavelengths of light, called its absorption spectrum. The specific wavelengths of light that evoke a photosensitive reaction are called the action spectrum. The action spectrum is included in the absorption spectrum of the photosensitizing chemical. The action spectrum for photoallergy is mostly in the long ultraviolet (UVA) region and may extend into the visible light region (320–425 nm).

Photosensitivity reactions occur only when there is sufficient concentration of the photosensitizer in the skin, and the skin is exposed to a sufficient intensity and duration of light in the action spectrum of that photosensitizer. The intensity of the photosensitivity reaction is, in general, dose-dependent and is worse with a greater dose of photosensitizer and greater light exposure.

Phototoxic reactions

A phototoxic reaction is a nonimmunologic reaction that develops after exposure to a specific wavelength and intensity of light in the presence of a photosensitizing substance. It is a sunburn-type reaction, with erythema, tenderness, and even blistering occurring only on the sun-exposed parts. This type of reaction can be elicited in many persons who have no previous history of exposure or sensitivity to that particular substance, but individual susceptibility varies widely. In general, to elicit a phototoxic reaction, a considerably greater amount of the photosensitizing substance is necessary than that needed to induce a photoallergic reaction. The erythema begins (like any sunburn) within 2–6 h but worsens for 48–96 h before beginning to subside. Exposure of the nailbed may lead to onycholysis, called photo-onycholysis (Fig. 3-17). Phototoxic reactions, especially from topically applied photosensitizers, may cause marked hyperpigmentation, even without significant preceding erythema. The action spectrum for most phototoxic reactions is in the UVA range.

Phototoxic tar dermatitis

Coal tar, creosote, crude coal tar, or pitch, in conjunction with sunlight exposure, may induce a sunburn reaction associated with a severe burning sensation (tar "smarts" or "flashes"). Since these volatile hydrocarbons may be airborne, the patient may give no history of touching tar products. The burning and erythema may continue for 1–3 days. While up to 70% of white persons exposed to such a combination develop this reaction, persons with type V and VI skin are protected by their constitutive skin pigmentation. Following the acute reaction, hyperpigmentation occurs, which may persist for years. Coal tar or its derivatives may be found in cosmetics, drugs, dyes, insecticides, and disinfectants.

Phytophotodermatitis

Furocoumarins in many plants may cause a phototoxic reaction when they come in contact with skin that is exposed to

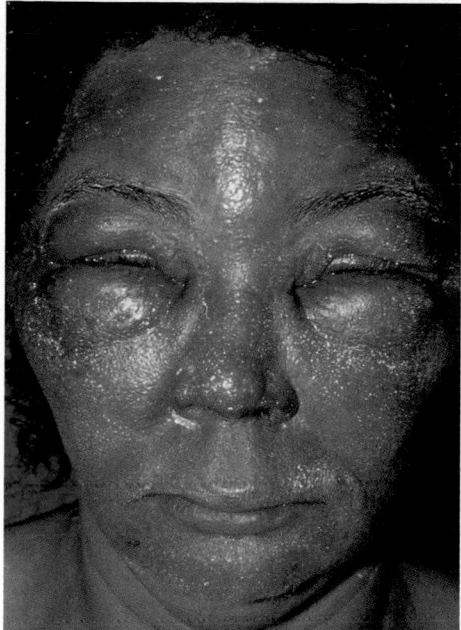

Fig. 3-18 Severe phytophototoxicity.

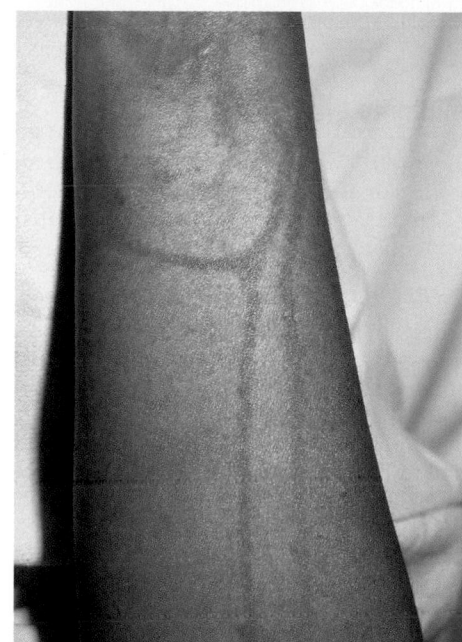

Fig. 3-19 Phytophotodermatitis; the patient had rinsed her hair with lime juice in Mexico.

UVA light. This is called phytophotodermatitis. Several hours after exposure, a burning erythema occurs, followed by edema and the development of vesicles or bullae. An intense residual hyperpigmentation results that may persist for weeks or months. The intensity of the initial phototoxic reaction may be mild and may not be recalled by the patient despite significant hyperpigmentation. Fragrance products containing bergapten, a component of oil of bergamot, will produce this reaction. If a fragrance containing this 5-methoxypsoralen or other furocoumarin is applied to the skin prior to exposure to the sun or tanning lights, berloque dermatitis may result. This hyperpigmentation, which may be preceded by redness and edema, occurs primarily on the neck and face. Artificial bergapten-free bergamot oil and laws limiting the use of furocoumarins in Europe and the US have made this a rare condition. However, "Florida Water" and "Kananga Water" colognes, formerly popular in the Hispanic, African American, and Caribbean communities, contain this potent photosensitizer and can still be ordered online, as can other aromatherapy products containing furocoumarins.

Most phototoxic plants are in the families Umbelliferae, Rutaceae (rue), Compositae, and Moraceae. Incriminated plants include agrimony, angelica, atrillal, bavachi, buttercup, common rice, cowslip, dill, fennel, fig, garden and wild carrot, garden and wild parsnip, gas plant, goose foot, zabon, lime and Persian lime, lime bergamot, masterwort, mustard, parsley, St John's wort, and yarrow. In Hawaii the anise-scented mokihana berry (*Pelea anisata*) was known to natives for its phototoxic properties (the mokihana burn). It is a member of the rue family. Home tanning solutions containing fig leaves can produce phytophotodermatitis. These may be widespread and severe enough to require burn unit management (Fig. 3-18).

Occupational disability from exposure to the pink rot fungus (*Sclerotinia sclerotiorum*), present on celery roots, occurs in celery farmers. In addition, disease-resistant celery contains furocoumarins and may produce phytophotodermatitis in grocery workers. Usually not enough sensitizing furocoumarin is absorbed from dietary exposure; however, ingested herbal remedies may cause sytemic phototoxicity.

Dermatitis bullosa striata pratensis (grass or meadow dermatitis) is a phytophotodermatitis caused by contact not with grass, but with yellow-flowered meadow parsnip or a wild, yellow-flowered herb of the rose family. The eruption consists of streaks and bizarre configurations with vesicles and bullae that heal with residual hyperpigmentation. The usual cause is sunbathing in fields containing the phototoxic plants. Similarly, tourists in the tropics will sometimes rinse their hair with lime juice outdoors and streaky hyperpigmentation of the arms and back will result where the lime juice runs down (Fig. 3-19).

Blistering phytophotodermatitis must be differentiated from rhus dermatitis. The vesicles and bullae of rhus are not necessarily limited to the sun-exposed areas, and itching is the most prominent symptom. Lesions continue to occur in rhus dermatitis for a week or more. In phytophotodermatitis the reaction is limited to sun-exposed sites, a burning pain appears within 48 h, and marked hyperpigmentation results. The asymmetry, atypical shapes, and streaking of the lesions are helpful in establishing the diagnosis. These features may, however, lead to a misdiagnosis of child abuse.

Treatment of a severe, acute reaction is similar to the management of a sunburn, with cool compresses, mild analgesics if required, and topical emollients. Use of topical steroids and strict sun avoidance immediately following the injury may protect against the hyperpigmentation. The hyperpigmentation is best managed by "tincture of time."

Carlsen K, et al: Phytophotodermatitis in 19 children admitted to hospital and their differential diagnosis. J Am Acad Dermatol 2007; 57:S88.

Derraik JG, et al: Phytophotodermatitis caused by contact with a fig tree. NZ Med J 2007; 120:U2720.

Eickhorst K, et al: Rue the herb: *Ruta graveolens*-associated phytophotodermatitis. Dermatitis 2007; 18:52.

Kaddu S, et al: Accidental bullous phototoxic reactions to bergamot aromatherapy oil. J Am Acad Dermatol 2001; 45:458.

Koh D, Ong CN: Phytophotodermatitis due to the application of *Citrus hystrix* as a folk remedy. Br J Dermatol 1999; 140:737.

Maloney FJ, et al: Iatrogenic phytophotodermatitis resulting from herbal treatment of an allergic contact dermatitis. Clin Exp Dermatol 2006; 31:39.

Pomeranz MK, et al: Phytophotodermatitis and limes. N Engl J Med 2007; 357:e1.

Wain EM, et al: Acute severe blistering in a 24-year-old man. Arch Dermatol 2006; 142:1059.

Wang L, et al: Berloque dermatitis induced by "Florida Water." Cutis 2002; 70:29.

Idiopathic photosensitivity disorders

This group includes the photosensitivity diseases for which no cause is known. They are not associated with external photosensitizers (except for some cases of chronic actinic dermatitis) or inborn errors of metabolism.

Polymorphous light eruption

Polymorphous light eruption (PLE, PMLE) is the most common form of photosensitivity. In various studies among Northern European white persons, a history of PLE can be elicited in between 5% and 20% of the adult population. It represents about one-quarter of all photosensitive patients in referral centers. All races and skin types can be affected. The onset is typically in the first four decades of life and females outnumber males by 2 or 3:1. The pathogenesis is unknown, but a family history may be elicited in between 10% and 50% of patients. It has been reported by some investigators that 10–20% of patients with PLE may have positive antinuclear antigens (ANAs) and a family history of lupus erythematosus. Photosensitive systemic lupus erythematosus (SLE) patients may give a history of PLE-like eruptions for years before the diagnosis of SLE is made. PLE patients should be followed for the development of symptoms of SLE.

Clinically, the eruption may have several different morphologies, although in the individual patient the morphology is usually constant. The papular (or erythematopapular) variant is the most common, but papulovesicular, eczematous, erythematous, and plaque-like lesions also occur (Fig. 3-20). Plaque-like lesions are more common in elderly patients and may closely simulate lupus erythematosus, with indurated, erythematous, fixed lesions. In African Americans, a pinpoint papular variant has been observed, closely simulating lichen nitidus but showing spongiotic dermatitis histologically (Fig. 3-21). Scarring and atrophy do not occur; however, in darkly pigmented races, marked postinflammatory hyper- or hypo-pigmentation may be present. In some patients, pruritus only without an eruption may be reported (PLE sine eruptione). Some of these patients will develop typical PLE later in life.

The lesions of PLE appear most typically 1–4 days after exposure to sunlight. Patients may report itching and erythema during sun exposure, and development of lesions within the first 24 h. A change in the amount of sun exposure appears to be more critical than the absolute amount of radiation. Patients living in tropical climates may be free of eruption, only to develop disease when they move to temperate zones, where there is more marked seasonal variation in UV intensity. Areas of involvement include the face, the V area of the chest, neck, and arms. In general, for each individual certain areas are predisposed. However, typically, areas protected during the winter, such as the extensor forearms, are particularly affected, whereas areas exposed all year (face and dorsa of hands) may be relatively spared. The eruption appears most commonly in the spring. Often the eruption improves with continued sun exposure (hardening) so that patients may be clear of the condition in the summer or autumn.

An unusual variant of PLE is juvenile spring eruption of the ears (Fig. 3-22). This occurs most commonly in boys aged 5–12 years, but may also be found in young adult males. It presents in the spring, often after sun exposure on cold but sunny days. Large outbreaks may occur in boys' schools. The typical lesions are grouped small papules or papulovesicles on the helices. Lesions may form visible vesicles and crusting. It is self-limited and does not scar. UVA is the inducing spectrum, and some patients also have lesions of PLE elsewhere. The histologic picture is identical to that of PLE.

Histologically, a perivascular, predominately T-cell, infiltrate is present in the upper and mid-dermis. There is often edema and endothelial swelling, with occasional neutrophils.

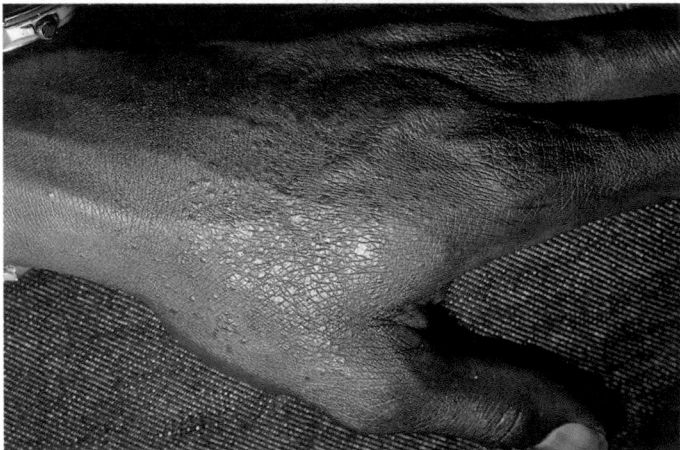

Fig. 3-21 Polymorphous light eruption, micropapular variant resembling lichen nitidus.

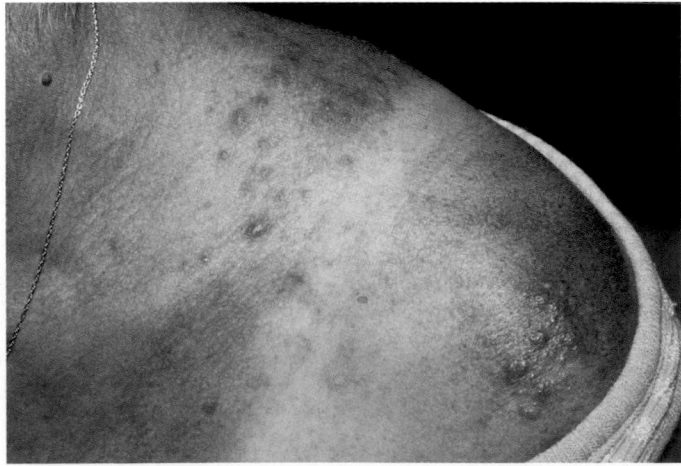

Fig. 3-20 Polymorphous light eruption, papulovesicular variant.

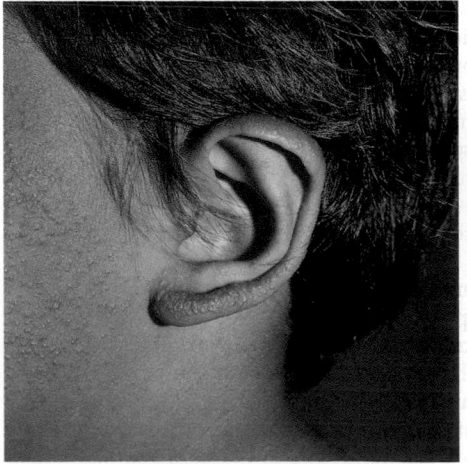

Fig. 3-22 Juvenile spring eruption of the ear.

Epidermal changes are variable, with spongiosis and exocytosis the changes most often observed. Occasionally, a virtual absence of findings microscopically may paradoxically be reported and has been referred to as pauci-inflammatory photodermatitis.

The reported action spectrum of PLE varies, possibly depending on the different ethnic backgrounds of reported populations. UVA is most often responsible; however, UVB and both wavelengths in combination are also frequently necessary. Patients often report eruptions following sun exposure through window glass. Visible light sensitivity can also occur, albeit very rarely. Women more commonly than men are sensitive to UVA only, and men are more commonly sensitive to visible light. Men, although the minority of PLE patients, tend to have more severe PLE and broader wavelengths of sensitivity. Most patients react more in affected sites, and in some, lesions can only be induced in affected areas. Phototesting produces variable results. Schornagel et al reported that one protocol, which produced positive results in 83% of tested patients, used four exposures of UVB, UVA, or a combination in previously affected sites. However, the light sources are not readily available and reported protocols vary widely. In clinical practice the diagnosis is usually made clinically.

In the differential diagnosis of PLE, the following should be considered: lupus erythematosus, photosensitive drug eruption, prurigo nodularis, and photoallergic contact dermatitis. Histopathologic examination, ANA testing, and direct immunofluorescence (DIF) are helpful in distinguishing these diseases. Serologic testing alone may not distinguish PLE from SLE, due to the possibility of positive ANA tests in PLE patients. Lupus erythematosus may present initially with photosensitivity before other features of lupus erythematosus occur.

Therapeutically, most patients with mild disease can be managed by avoiding the sun and using barrier protection and high-SPF, broad-spectrum sunscreens. It is critical that the sunblocks contain specific absorbers of long-wave UVA (Parsol 1789, Mexoryl, zinc oxide, and titanium dioxide). Sunblocks containing more than one of these agents are more effective. Since UVA is the most common triggering wavelength, good UVA coverage is critical. Most patients do not apply an adequate amount of sunscreen for it to be optimally effective. DermaGard film can be applied to windows at home and in the car to block the transmission of nearly all UBV and UVA, while allowing visible light to be transmitted. Degradation does occur so it should be replaced every 5 years. These measures of photoprotection are critical for all patients, since they are free of toxicity and reduce the amount and duration of other therapies required. Patient education is important in the management of this disease, and phototesting may be required to convince the patient that he/she is UV-sensitive. It will also determine the action spectrum.

The use of topical tacrolimus ointment at night or twice daily, combined with the above measures for sun avoidance and the use of sunscreens, controls many of these patients. At times topical steroids, frequently of super or high potency in several daily to weekly pulses, are necessary to control the pruritus and clear the eruption. Antihistamines (hydroxyzine, diphenhydramine, or doxepin) may be used for pruritus. Systemic corticosteroids in short courses may be necessary, especially in the spring. In patients whose condition is not controlled by the above measures, hardening in the spring with UVB, narrow-band UVB, or psoralen + UVA (PUVA) can dramatically decrease the sun sensitivity of patients with PLE, and up to 80% of patients can be controlled with phototherapy. In the most sensitive patients, systemic steroids may be needed at the inception of the phototherapy. Systemic hydroxychloro-quine sulfate, 200–400 mg/day, may be used. It has a delayed onset and is best instituted in the late winter to prevent spring outbreaks. Chloroquine or quinacrine may be effective if hydroxychloroquine is not, but in general antimalarials are inferior to phototherapy. In the most severe cases, management with azathioprine, cyclosporine, thalidomide, or mycophenolate mofetil may be considered. If these agents are used in a patient considered to have PLE, an evaluation for chronic actinic dermatitis should be performed, as patients with PLE rarely require these agents.

Actinic prurigo

Actinic prurigo probably represents a variant of PLE; it is most commonly seen in Native Americans of North and Central America and Colombia. The incidence in Mexico has been reported to be between 1.5% and 3.5%. It has been reported in Europe, Australia, and Japan as well. The female to male ratio is 2–6:1. Actinic prurigo in Native Americans in the US begins before age 10 in 45% of cases and before age 20 in 72%. Up to 75% of cases have a positive family history (hereditary PLE of Native Americans). In Europe, 80% of cases occur before age 10. In the Inuit Canadian population onset is later and frequently in adulthood.

In childhood, lesions begin as small papules or papulovesicles that crust and become impetiginized. They are intensely pruritic and frequently excoriated. In children, the cheeks, distal nose, ears, and lower lip are typically involved (Fig. 3-23). Cheilitis may be the initial and only feature for years. Conjunctivitis is seen in 10–20% of patients (limbal-type vernal catarrah). Lesions of the arms and legs are also common and usually exhibit a prurigo nodule-like configuration (Fig. 3-24). The eruption may extend to involve sun-protected areas, especially the buttocks, but lesions in these areas are always less severe. In adults, chronic, dry papules and plaques are most typical, and cheilitis and crusting occur less frequently. Skin lesions tend to persist throughout the year in the tropics, although they are clearly worse during periods of increased sun exposure. In temperate and high-latitude regions, lesions occur from March through the summer and substantially remit in the winter. Hardening, as seen with PLE, does not occur. In up to 60% of patients with actinic prurigo that presents before the age of 20, the condition improves or resolves within 5 years, whereas adults usually have the disease throughout life.

Initial therapy is identical to that for PLE. Thalidomide has been used effectively and safely over many years in this condition. In cases refractory to or intolerant of thalidomide, cyclosporine A can be very effective. Topical cyclosporine A

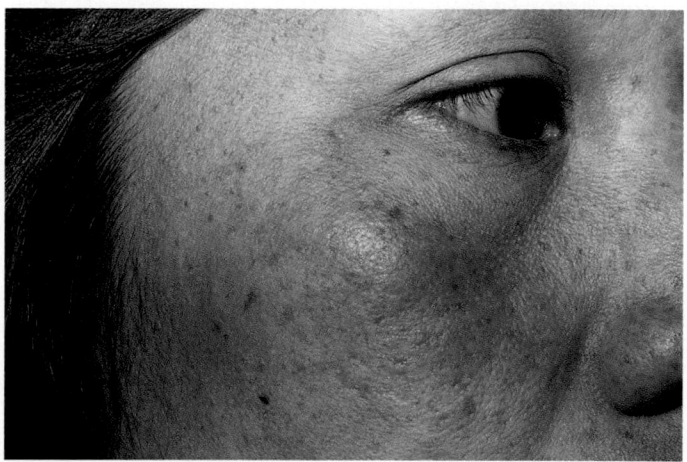

Fig. 3-23 Actinic prurigo.

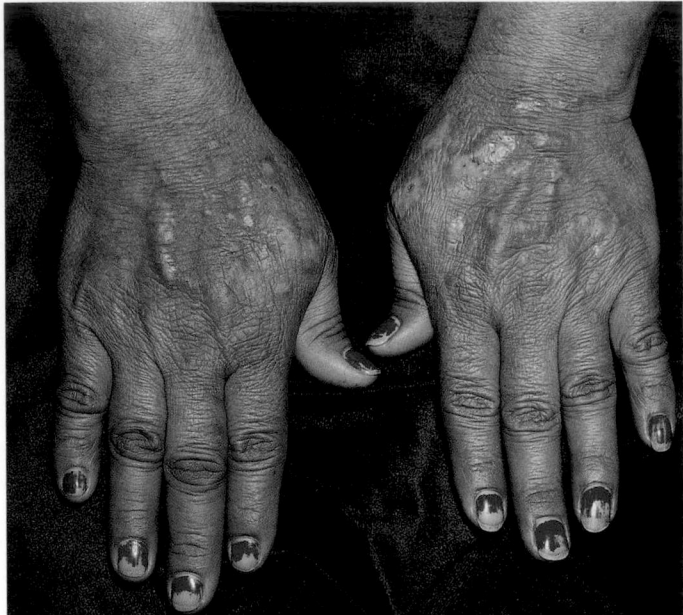

Fig. 3-24 Actinic prurigo, prurigo nodularis-like lesions.

2% was effective in controlling limbal lesions in one case of actinic prurigo-associated conjunctivitis.

Akaraphanth R, et al: Adult-onset actinic prurigo in Thailand. Photodermatol Photoimmunol Photomed 2007; 23:234.

Bansal I, et al: Pinpoint papular variant of PLE. J Eur Acad Dermatol Venereol 2006; 20:406.

Boonstra HE, et al: Polymorphous light eruption: a clinical, photo-biologic, and follow-up study of 110 patients. J Am Acad Dermatol 2000; 42:199.

Crouch RB, et al: Actinic prurigo. Australas J Dermatol 2002; 43:128.

Crouch RB, et al: Analysis of patients with suspected photosensitivity referred for investigation to an Australian photodermatology clinic. J Am Acad Dermatol 2003; 48:714.

Dummer R, et al: Clinical and therapeutic aspects of PLE. Dermatology 2003; 207:93.

Fusaro RM, Johnson JA: Hereditary polymorphic light eruption of American Indians. J Am Acad Dermatol 1996; 34:612.

Hasan T, et al: Disease associations in PMLE. Arch Dermatol 1998; 134:1081.

Hatch KL, et al: Garments as solar ultraviolet radiation screening materials. Dermatol Clin 2006; 24:85.

Kerr AC: Actinic prurigo deterioration due to degradation of DermaGard window film. Br J Dermatol 2007; 157:609.

Kerr HA, et al: Photodermatoses in African Americans. J Am Acad Dermatol 2007; 57:638.

Kontos AP, et al: PLE in African Americans: pinpoint popular variant. Photodermatol Photoimmunol Photomed 2002; 18:303.

Lehmann P: Diagnostic approach to photodermatoses. J Dtsch Dermatol Ges 2006; 4:965.

McCoombes JA, et al: Use of topical cyclosporin for conjunctival manifestations of actinic prurigo. Am J Ophthalmol 2000; 130:830.

Millard TP, et al: Familial clustering of PLE in relatives of patients with lupus erythematosus. Br J Dermatol 2001; 144:334.

Naleway AL, et al: Characteristics of diagnosed PLE. Photodermatol Photoimmunol Photomed 2006; 22:205.

Patel DC, et al: Efficacy of short-course oral prednisolone in PLE: a randomized controlled trial. Br J Dermatol 2000; 143:828.

Perrett CM, et al: Primary cutaneous B-cell lymphoma associated with actinic prurigo. Br J Dermatol 2005; 153:186.

Roelandts R: The diagnosis of photosensitivity. Arch Dermatol 2000; 136:1152.

Schornagel IJ, et al: Diagnostic phototesting in PLE. Br J Dermatol 2005; 153:1220.

Stratigos AJ, et al: Juvenile spring eruption. J Am Acad Dermatol 2004; 50:57.

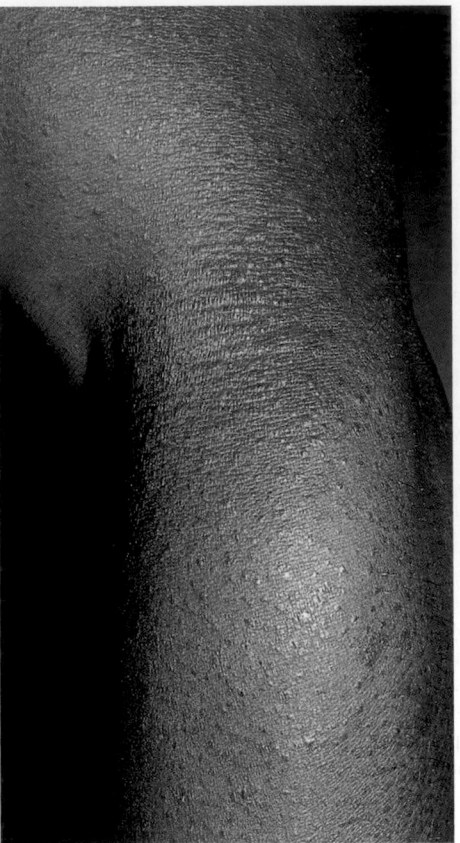

Fig. 3-25 Polymorphous light eruption, brachioradial distribution.

Su W, et al: Photodermatitis with minimal inflammatory infiltrate. Am J Dermatopathol 2006; 28:482.

Van de Pas CB, et al: An optimal method of photoprovocation of PLE. Arch Dermatol 2004; 140:286.

Wiseman MC, et al: Actinic prurigo. J Am Acad Dermatol 2001; 44:952.

Yong Gee SA, et al: Long-term thalidomide for actinic prurigo. Australas J Dermatol 2001; 42:281.

Brachioradial pruritus

PLE may present initially and only on the brachioradial area. This type of brachioradial eruption was the initial pattern of brachioradial pruritus described and was termed solar pruritus (Fig. 3-25). The majority of cases of brachioradial pruritus, and especially those characterized by severe, refractory, intractable pruritus and secondary severe lichenification, are now felt to represent a form of neuropathic pruritus, related to cervical spine disease (see Chapter 4). Sunlight may be an eliciting factor and cervical spine disease a predisposing factor in patients with brachioradial pruritus. To identify those patients in whom photosensitivity plays a prominent role, a high-SPF (UVA/UVB) sunscreen should be applied to one arm only for several weeks. In cases of PLE this usually leads to improvement of that one arm, as compared to the contralateral unprotected arm. In patients with primarily neuropathic disease, sunscreen application leads to minimal improvement.

Solar urticaria

Solar urticaria is most common in females aged 20–40 years. Within seconds to minutes after light exposure, typical urticarial lesions appear and resolve in 1–2 h, rarely lasting more than 24 h. Delayed reactions rarely occur. Chronically exposed sites may have some reduced sensitivity. In severe attacks, syncope, bronchospasm, and anaphylaxis may occur.

Patients with solar urticaria may be sensitive to wavelengths over a broad spectrum. The wavelengths of sensitivity and the minimal urticarial doses may vary with anatomic site and over time within the same patient. UVA sensitivity is the most common, but visible light sensitivity is also frequently reported. The photosensitivity can be passively transferred, and irradiation of the patient's serum with the activating wavelength followed by reinjection will create a wheal in the patient, but not in an unaffected patient. This suggests the presence of a circulating photoinducible allergen to which the individual patient with solar urticaria is sensitive. In some patients an inhibition spectrum may be identified which inhibits the binding of the endogenous photoallergen to mast cells.

Solar urticaria is virtually always idiopathic. Rarely, medications including tetracycline (but not minocycline), chlorpromazine, progestational agents, and repirinast have been reported to induce solar urticaria. Erythropoietic protoporphyria and very rarely porphyria cutanea tarda may present with lesions simulating solar urticaria. There are rare reports of solar urticaria in lupus erythematosus.

The diagnosis of solar urticaria is usually straightforward from the history. Phototesting is useful to determine the wavelengths of sensitivity, and to ascertain the minimal urticarial dose (MUD) if UVA desensitization is being considered.

Because many patients have sensitivity in the UVA or even visible range, standard sunscreens are of limited benefit but broad-spectrum sunscreens should be instituted. Antihistamines, especially the nonsedating H1 agents loratadine, cetirizine HCl, and fexofenadine, may increase the MUD 10-fold or more. Higher doses, twice or more the standard recommendation, may be required (e.g. 180 mg of fexofenadine twice a day). These, plus sun avoidance and broad-spectrum sunscreens, are the first-line therapy. PUVA or increasing UVA exposures are effective in more difficult cases, the former having greater efficacy. Rush hardening may induce UVA tolerance, allowing patients to begin PUVA therapy. PUVA is effective, even if the patient is not sensitive to UVA. Cyclosporine A (4.5 mg/kg/day) and intravenous immunoglobulin (IVIG; 0.4 g/kg/day for 5 days repeated monthly) have been anecdotally reported as effective. For the most difficult cases, plasmapheresis may be used to remove the circulating photoallergen, allowing PUVA to be given leading to remission.

Beattie PE, et al: Characteristics and prognosis of idiopathic solar urticaria: a cohort of 87 cases. Arch Dermatol 2003; 139:1149.
Beissert S, et al: UVA rush hardening for the treatment of solar urticaria. J Am Acad Dermatol 2000; 42:1030.
Fukunaga A, et al: The inhibition spectrum of solar urticaria suppresses the wheal-flare response following intradermal injection with photoactivated autologous serum but not with compound 48/80. Photodermatol Photoimmunol Photomed 2006; 22:129.
Ng JCH, et al: Changes of photosensitivity and action spectrum with time in solar urticaria. Photodermatol Photoimmunol Photomed 2002; 18:191.
Palma-Carlos AG, et al: Eur Ann Allergy Clin Immunol 2005; 37:17.
Roelandts R: Diagnosis and treatment of solar urticaria. Dermatol Ther 2003; 16:52.
Rose RF, et al: Solar angioedema. Photodermatol Photoimmunol Photomed 2005; 21:226.
Uetsu N, et al: The clinical and photobiological characteristics of solar urticaria in 40 patients. Br J Dermatol 2000; 142:32.
Wallengren J: Brachioradial pruritus is associated with a reduction in cutaneous innervation that normalizes during symptom-free periods. J Am Acad Dermatol 2005; 52:142.
Yap LM, et al: Drug-induced solar urticaria due to tetracycline. Australas J Dermatol 2000; 41:181.

Hydroa vacciniforme

Hydroa vacciniforme is a rare, chronic photodermatosis with onset in childhood. Boys and girls are equally represented, but boys present earlier and have disease on average for a longer time. There is a bimodal onset (between ages 1 and 7 and between 12 and 16). The natural history of the typical disorder is for it to remit spontaneously before age 20, but rare cases in young adults do occur. Within 6 h of exposure stinging begins. At 24 h or sooner erythema and edema appear, followed by the characteristic 2–4 mm vesicles. Over the next few days these lesions rupture, become centrally necrotic, and heal with a smallpox-like scar. Lesions tend to appear in crops with disease-free intervals. The ears, nose, cheeks, and extensor arms and hands are affected. Subungual hemorrhage or oral ulcerations may occur.

Histologically, early lesions show intraepidermal vesiculation and dermal edema that evolves into a subepidermal blister. Necrotic lesions show reticular degeneration of keratinocytes, with epidermal necrosis flanked by spongiosis with a dense perivascular infiltrate of neutrophils and lymphocytes. Dermal vessels may be thrombosed, simulating vasculitis. Lesions may be reproduced by repetitive UVA, with the action spectrum in the 330–360 nm range.

The differential diagnosis includes PLE, actinic prurigo, and erythropoietic protoporphyria. Porphyrin levels are normal in hydroa vacciniforme. In erythropoietic protoporphyria the burning typically begins within minutes of sun exposure, and over time patients develop diffuse, thickened, waxlike scarring, rather than the smallpox-like scars of hydroa vacciniforme. Histologic evaluation is useful in distinguishing these two conditions. Treatment is principally to avoid sunlight exposure and to use broad-spectrum sunscreens that block in the UVA range. Prophylactic narrow-band UVB phototherapy in the early spring may be effective.

A subset of children and, less commonly, adults with photosensitive hydroa vacciniforme-like skin lesions manifest facial swelling, indurated nodules or progressive ulcers, fever and liver damage. Hypersensitivity to mosquito bites may also be seen. These patients may develop Epstein–Barr virus (EBV)-associated NK/T-cell lymphomas and die of this or of a hemophagocytic syndrome. The hydroa vacciniforme-like skin lesions may precede the diagnosis of the lymphoma by up to a decade, and initially the patient may appear to have typical hydroa vacciniforme of the self-limited type. This, then, is a disease spectrum, with both typical and severe hydroa vacciniforme being EBV-associated. Treatment of the lymphoma may lead to clearing of these lesions.

Chen HH, et al: Hydroa vacciniforme-like primary cutaneous CD8-positive T-cell lymphoma. Br J Dermatol 2002; 147:587.
Cho KH, et al: Epstein–Barr virus-associated peripheral T-cell lymphoma in adults with hydroa vacciniforme-like lesions. Clin Exp Dermatol 2001; 26:242.
Drummond A, et al: Subungual hemorrhage in hydroa vacciniforme. Clin Exp Dermatol 2003; 28:222.
Gupta G, et al: Hydroa vacciniforme: A clinical and follow-up study of 17 cases. J Am Acad Dermatol 2000; 42:208.
Iwatsuki K, et al: Pathogenic link between hydroa vacciniforme and Epstein–Barr virus-associated hematologic disorders. Arch Dermatol 2006; 142:587.
Wierzbicka E, et al: Oral involvement in hydroa vacciniforme. Arch Dermatol 2006; 142:651.
Wong SN, et al: Late-onset hydroa vacciniforme: two case reports. Br J Dermatol 2001; 144:874.
Wu YH, et al: Hydroa-vacciniforme-like Epstein–Barr virus-associated monoclonal T-lymphoproliferative disorder in a child. Int J Dermatol 2007; 46:1081.
Yamamoto T, et al: A novel, noninvasive diagnostic probe for hydroa vacciniforme and related disorders. J Microbiol Methods 2007; 68:403.

Chronic actinic dermatitis

Chronic actinic dermatitis represents the end stage of progressive photosensitivity in some patients. It has replaced the

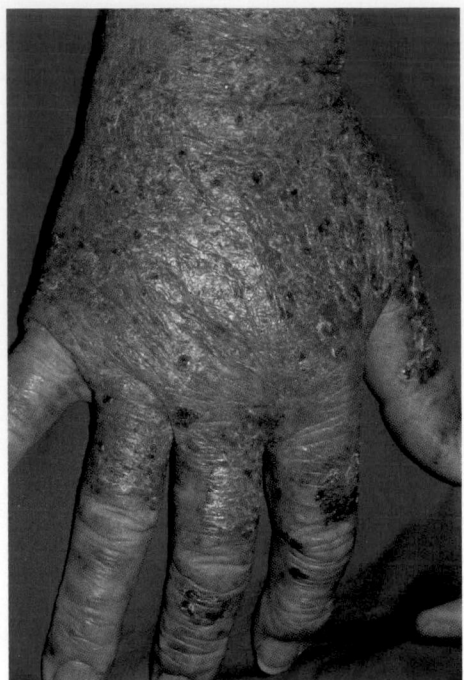

Fig. 3-26 Chronic actinic dermatitis.

terms persistent light reactivity, actinic reticuloid, photosensitive eczema, and chronic photosensitivity dermatitis. The basic components of this disease are:

- a persistent, chronic, eczematous eruption in the absence of exposure to known photosensitizers
- usually broad-spectrum photosensitivity with decreased MED to UVA and/or UVB, and at times visible light
- histology consistent with a chronic dermatitis, with or without features of lymphoma.

Clinically, the disease predominantly affects middle-aged or elderly men. In the US, patients with skin types V and VI may be disproportionately affected. Skin lesions consist of edematous, scaling, thickened patches and plaques that tend to be confluent. Lesions occur primarily or most severely on the exposed skin and may spare the upper eyelids, behind the ears, and the bottoms of wrinkles (Fig. 3-26). Involvement of unexposed sites often occurs, progressing to erythroderma in the most severe cases. Marked depigmentation resembling vitiligo may result. Patients may not realize their condition is exacerbated by exposure to light. It may persist in all seasons.

The pathogenesis of this syndrome is unknown. In some patients a preceding topical or oral photosensitizer may be implicated, but the condition fails to improve with discontinuation of the inciting agent. In about one-third of patients, photopatch testing yields a positive response to previously applied agents, especially musk ambrette, sunscreen ingredients, and hexachlorophene. Patch testing to standard agents may have a positive result in about 30% of patients, but no particular relevance is found. However, in up to 85% of European patients, sesquiterpene lactone contact sensitivity from Compositae has been identified. In addition, more than 75% of men over the age of 60 with sesquiterpene lactone sensitivity have abnormal phototesting results. CD8 (suppressor/cytotoxic) T cells are disproportionately represented in the cutaneous infiltrates in the majority of cases, and less commonly, in the peripheral blood. IgE levels may be elevated.

In this clinical setting the diagnosis of chronic actinic dermatitis is established by histologic evaluation and phototesting. Phototesting often reproduces the lesions. Around 65% of patients are sensitive to UVA, UVB, and visible light; 22% to UVA and UVB; and 5% to UVB or UVA only. The finding of photosensitivity to UVA and UVB helps to differentiate chronic actinic dermatitis from drug-induced photosensitivity, which usually exhibits only UVA photosensitivity. PLE, photoallergic contact dermatitis, airborne contact dermatitis, and mycosis fungoides or Sézary syndrome must be excluded. PLE is excluded by the broad-spectrum reduced MED in chronic actinic dermatitis, although some patients may begin with a PLE-like disease that later meets the criteria for chronic actinic dermatitis. Contact dermatitis is excluded by patch and photopatch testing. Mycosis fungoides may be difficult to differentiate from chronic actinic dermatitis in cases with atypical histology. Phototesting is critical in these cases. Mycosis fungoides will manifest a T-cell receptor rearrangement in lesional skin or peripheral blood and usually shows a CD4 (helper) T-cell predominance.

Therapy for chronic actinic dermatitis includes identifying possible topical photosensitizers by photopatch testing and scrupulously avoiding them. Maximum sun avoidance and broad-spectrum sunscreens are essential. Topical tacrolimus is useful in some patients. Topical and systemic steroids are effective in some cases, but chronic toxicity of systemic steroids limits chronic usage. Azathioprine, 50–200 mg/day, is the most reproducibly effective treatment and may be required annually during periods of increased sun intensity. Low-dose PUVA can be attempted, but is often not tolerated, even when used with topical and systemic steroids. Hydroxyurea, 500 mg twice a day, benefited one patient. Cyclosporine A, thalidomide, and mycophenolate mofetil may also be utilized. Immunosuppressive agents may allow patients to tolerate PUVA therapy. With careful management about 1 in 10 patients will lose their photosensitivity within 5 years, 1 in 5 by 10 years, and half of patients by 15 years.

Abe R, et al: Severe refractory chronic actinic dermatitis successfully treated with tacrolimus ointment. Br J Dermatol 2002; 147:1273.

Dawe RS: Chronic actinic dermatitis in the elderly. Drugs Aging 2005; 22:201.

Dawe RS, et al: The natural history of chronic actinic dermatitis. Arch Dermatol 2000; 136:1215.

Gramvussakis A, et al: Chronic actinic dermatitis (photosensitivity dermatitis/actinic reticuloid syndrome): beneficial effect from hydroxyurea. Br J Dermatol 2000; 143:1340.

Safa G, et al: Recalcitrant chronic actinic dermatitis treated with low-dose thalidomide. J Am Acad Dermatol 2005; 52:E6.

Thomson MA, et al: Chronic actinic dermatitis treated with mycophenolate mofetil. Br J Dermatol 2005; 152:784.

Photosensitivity and HIV infection

Photosensitivity resembling PLE, actinic prurigo, or chronic actinic dermatitis is seen in about 5% of human immunodeficiency virus (HIV)-infected persons. In general, photosensitivity is seen when the CD4 count is below 200 (often below 50), except in persons with a genetic predisposition (Native Americans). Photosensitivity may be the initial manifestation of HIV disease. African American patients are disproportionately represented among patients with HIV photosensitivity. Photosensitivity may be associated with ingestion of a photosensitizing medication, especially NSAIDs or trimethoprim–sulfamethoxazole, but the skin eruption often does not improve even when the medication is discontinued. Histologically, the lesions may show subacute or chronic dermatitis, often with a dense dermal infiltrate with many eosinophils. Histology identical to PLE, lichen planus or lichen nitidus may also occur. When the CD4 count is below 50, especially in black patients, chronic actinic dermatitis with features of actinic prurigo is typical. Widespread vitiliginous lesions may develop. Therapy is difficult, but thalidomide may be beneficial.

Bilu D, et al: Clinical and epidemiological characterization of photosensitivity in HIV-positive individuals. Photodermatol Photoimmunol Photomed 2004; 20:175.

Maurer TA, et al: Thalidomide treatment for prurigo nodularis in HIV-infected subjects: efficacy and risk of neuropathy. Arch Dermatol 2004; 140:845.

Vin-Christian K, et al: Photosensitivity in HIV-infected individuals. J Dermatol 2000; 27:361.

Wong SN, Khoo LSW: Chronic actinic dermatitis as the presenting feature of HIV infection in three Chinese males. Clin Exp Dermatol 2003; 28:265.

Radiodermatitis

The major target within the cell by which radiation damage occurs is the DNA. The effects of ionizing radiation on the cells depend on the amount of radiation, its intensity (exposure rate), and the characteristics of the individual cell. Rapidly dividing cells and anaplastic cells in general have increased radiosensitivity when compared with normal tissue. When radiation therapy is delivered, it is frequently fractionated—divided into small doses. This allows the normal cells to recover between doses.

When the dose is large, cell death results. In small amounts, the effect is insidious and cumulative. Mitosis is arrested temporarily, with consequent retardation of growth. The exposure rate affects the number of chromosome breaks. The more rapid the delivery of a certain amount of radiation, the greater the number of chromosome breaks. The number of breaks is also increased by the presence of oxygen.

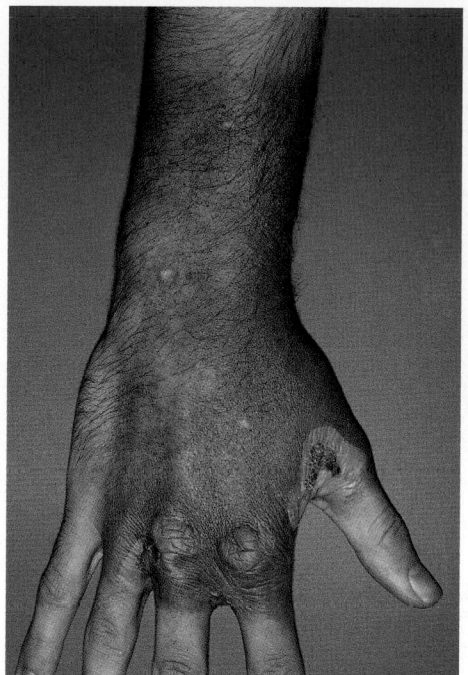

Fig. 3-27 Acute radiation burn during treatment of epithelioid sarcoma.

Acute radiodermatitis

When an "erythema dose" of ionizing radiation is given to the skin, there is a latent period of up to 24 h before visible erythema appears. This initial erythema lasts 2–3 days but may be followed by a second phase beginning up to 1 week after the exposure and lasting up to 1 month. When the skin is exposed to a large amount of ionizing radiation, an acute reaction develops, the extent of which will depend on the amount, quality, and duration of exposure. Such radiation reaction occurs in the treatment of malignancy and in accidental overexposure. The reaction is manifested by initial erythema, followed by a second phase of erythema at 3–6 days (Fig. 3-27). Vesiculation, edema, and erosion or ulceration may occur, accompanied by pain. The skin develops a dark color that may be mistaken for hyperpigmentation, but that desquamates. This type of radiation injury may subside in several weeks to several months, again depending on the amount of radiation exposure. Skin that receives a large amount of radiation will never return to normal. It will lack adnexal structures, be dry, atrophic, and smooth, and be hypopigmented or depigmented. Cutaneous necrosis may complicate yttrium-90 synovectomy, a treatment given for chronic synovitis.

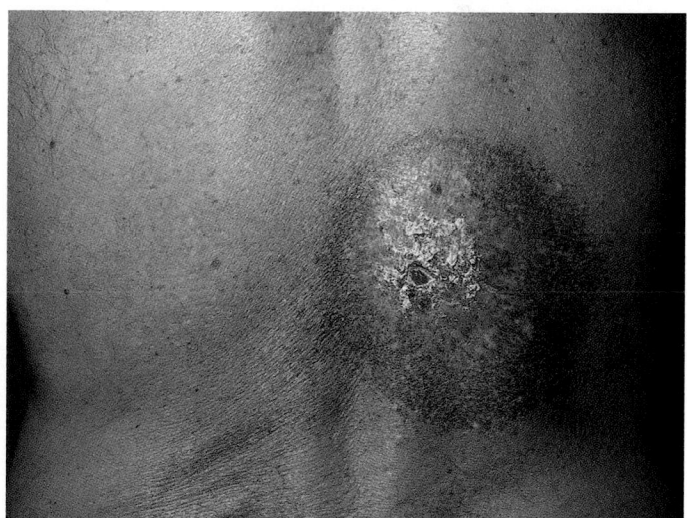

Fig. 3-28 Chronic radiodermatitis after fluoroscopy.

Eosinophilic, polymorphic, and pruritic eruption associated with radiotherapy

This polymorphic, pruritic eruption arising several days to several months after radiotherapy for cancer tends to favor the extremities. Acral excoriations, erythematous papules, vesicles, and bullae occur. It is not necessarily limited to the areas of radiation treatment. Histologically, a superficial and deep perivascular lymphohistiocytic infiltrate with eosinophils is present. Topical steroids, antihistamines, and UVB are all effective, and spontaneous resolution also occurs.

Chronic radiodermatitis

Chronic exposure to "suberythema" doses of ionizing radiation over a prolonged period will produce varying degrees of damage to the skin and its underlying parts after a variable latent period ranging from several months to several decades. It may also occur on the back or flank after fluoroscopy and roentgenography for diagnostic purposes (Fig. 3-28).

Telangiectasia, atrophy, and hypopigmentation with residual focal increased pigment (freckling) may appear (Fig. 3-29). The skin becomes dry, thin, smooth, and shiny. The nails may become striated, brittle, and fragmented. The capacity to repair injury is substantially reduced, resulting in ulceration from minor trauma. The hair becomes brittle and sparse. In more severe cases these chronic changes may be followed by radiation keratoses and carcinoma. Additionally, subcutaneous fibrosis, thickening, and binding of the surface layers to deep tissues may present as tender, erythematous plaques 6–12 months after radiation therapy (Fig. 3-30). It may resemble erysipelas or inflammatory metastases.

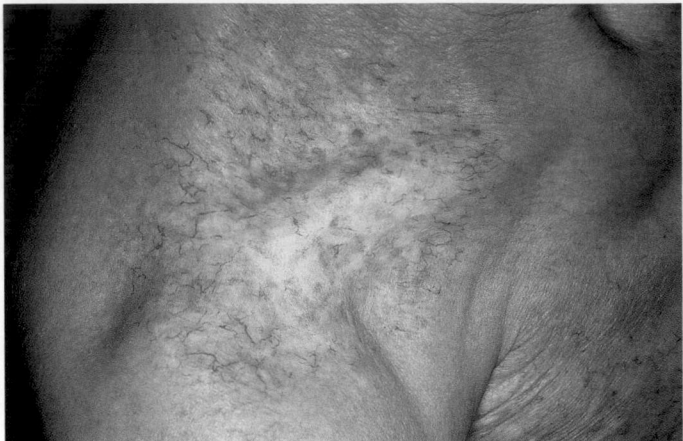

Fig. 3-29 Chronic radiodermatitis.

Radiation cancer

After a latent period averaging 20–40 years, various malignancies may develop. Most frequent are basal cell carcinoma (BCC), followed by squamous cell carcinoma (SCC). These may appear in sites of prior radiation, even if there is no evidence of chronic radiation damage. Sun damage may be additive to radiation therapy, increasing the appearance of nonmelanoma skin cancers. SCCs arising in sites of radiation therapy metastasize more frequently than purely sun-induced SCCs. In some patients, either type of tumor may predominate. Location plays some role; SCCs are more common on the arms and hands, whereas BCCs are seen on the head and neck and lumbosacral area. Other radiation-induced cancers include angiosarcoma (Fig. 3-31), malignant fibrous histiocytoma, sarcomas, and thyroid carcinoma. The incidence of malignant neoplasms increases with the passage of time.

Treatment

Acute radiodermatitis may be reduced with a topical corticosteroid ointment combined with an emollient cream applied twice a day and instituted at the onset of therapeutic radiotherapy. Chronic radiodermatitis without carcinoma requires little or no attention except protection from sunlight and the extremes of heat and cold. Careful cleansing with mild soap and water, the use of emollients, and, on occasion, hydrocortisone ointment are the only requirements for good care.

The early removal of precancerous keratoses and ulcerations is helpful in preventing the development of cancers. For radiation keratoses treatment with cryosurgery, 5-FU, imiquimod cream, or topical 5-aminolaevulinic acid–photodynamic therapy may be sufficient. If the keratosis feels infiltrated, a biopsy is indicated. Radiation ulcerations should be studied by excisional or incisional biopsy if they have been present for 3 or more months. Complete removal by excision is frequently required to obtain healing and exclude focal carcinoma in the ulceration. Radiation-induced nonmelanoma skin cancers are managed by standard methods. The higher risk of metastasis from radiation-induced SCCs mandates careful follow-up and regular regional lymph node evaluation.

Bolderston A, et al: The prevention and mangement of acute skin reactions related to radiation therapy: a systematic review and practice guideline. Support Care Cancer 2006; 14:802.

Davis MM, et al: Skin cancer in patients with chronic radiation dermatitis. J Am Acad Dermatol 1989; 20:608.

Escurdero A, et al: Chronic X-ray dermatitis treated by topical 5-aminolaevulinic acid–photodynamic therapy. Br J Dermatol 2002; 147:394.

Frazier TH, et al: Fluoroscopy-induced chronic radiation skin injury. Arch Dermatol 2007; 143:637.

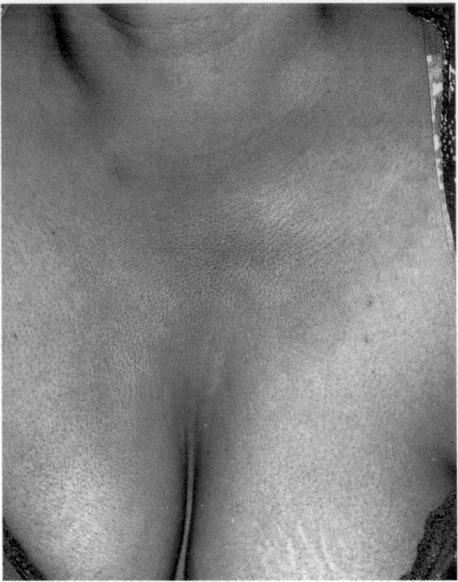

Fig. 3-30 Delayed radiation reaction 8 months after therapy.

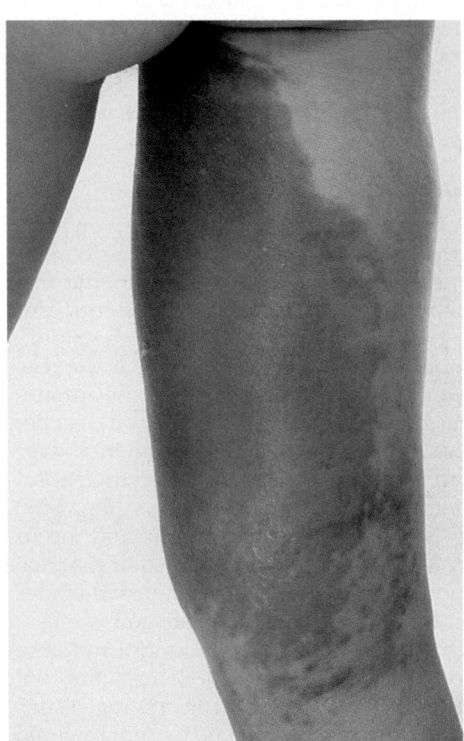

Fig. 3-31 Angiosarcoma years after radiation therapy.

James WD, et al: Late subcutaneous fibrosis following megavoltage radiotherapy. J Am Acad Dermatol 1980; 3:616.

Kiyohara T, et al: Spindle cell angiosarcoma following irradiation therapy for cervical carcinoma. J Cutan Pathol 2002; 29:96.

Lee JE, et al: Eosinophilic, polymorphic and pruritic eruption associated with radiotherpy in a patient with breast cancer. J Am Acad Dermatol 2007; 56:S60.

Sojan S, et al: Cutaneous radiation necrosis as a complication of yttrium-90 synovectomy. Hell J Nucl Med 2005; 8:58.

Mechanical injuries

Mechanical factors may induce distinctive skin changes. Pressure, friction, and the introduction of foreign substances (such as by injection) are some of the means by which skin injuries may occur.

Callus

Callus is a nonpenetrating, circumscribed hyperkeratosis produced by pressure. It occurs on parts of the body subject to intermittent pressure, particularly the palms and soles, and especially the bony prominences of the joints. Those engaged in various sports, certain occupations, or other repetitive activity develop callosities of distinctive size and location as stigmata. Examples of these are surfer's nodules, boxer's knuckle pads, jogger's toe, rower's rump, tennis toe (Fig. 3-32), jogger's nipple, prayer callus, neck callosities of violinists, bowler's hand, and Russell's sign. The latter are calluses, small lacerations or abrasions on the dorsum of the hand overlying the metacarpophalangeal and interphalangeal joints, and are seen as a clue to the diagnosis of bulimia nervosa.

The callus (Fig. 3-33) differs from the clavus in that it has no penetrating central core and it is a more diffuse thickening. It tends to disappear spontaneously when the pressure is removed. Most problems are encountered with calluses on the soles. Ill-fitting shoes, orthopedic problems of the foot caused by aging or a deformity of the foot exerting abnormal pressure, and high activity level are some of the etiologic factors to be considered in painful callosities of the feet.

Padding to relieve the pressure, paring of the thickened callus, and the use of keratolytics, such as 40% salicylic acid plasters, are some of the effective means of relieving painful callosities. Twelve percent ammonium lactate lotion or a urea-containing cream is often helpful.

Clavus (corns)

Corns are circumscribed, horny, conical thickenings with the base on the surface and the apex pointing inward and pressing on subjacent structures. There are two varieties: the hard corns, which occur on the dorsa of the toes or on the soles, and the soft corns, which occur between the toes and are softened by the macerating action of sweat. In a hard corn, the surface is shiny and polished and, when the upper layers are shaved off, a core is noted in the densest part of the lesion. It is this core that causes a dull/boring or sharp/lancinating pain by pressing on the underlying sensory nerves. Corns arise at sites of friction or pressure, and when these causative factors are removed, they spontaneously disappear. Frequently, a bony spur or exostosis is present beneath both hard and soft corns of long duration, and unless this exostosis is removed cure is unlikely. The soft interdigital corn usually occurs in the fourth interdigital space of the foot. Frequently, there is an exostosis at the metatarsal–phalangeal joint that causes pressure on the adjacent toe. These are soft, soggy, and macerated so that they appear white. Treatment by simple excision may be effective.

Plantar corns must be differentiated from plantar warts, and in most cases this can be done with confidence only by paring off the surface keratin until either the pathognomonic elongated dermal papillae of the wart with its blood vessels, or the clear horny core of the corn can be clearly seen. Porokeratosis plantaris discreta is a sharply marginated, cone-shaped, rubbery lesion that commonly occurs beneath the metatarsal heads. Multiple lesions may occur. It has a 3:1 female predominance, is painful, and is frequently confused with a plantar wart or corn. Keratosis punctata of the creases may be seen in the creases of the digits of the feet, where it may be mistaken for a corn.

The relief of pressure or friction by corrective footwear or the application of a ring of soft felt wadding around the region of the corn will often bring a good result. Soaking the feet in hot water and paring the surface by means of a scalpel blade or pumice stone leads to symptomatic improvement. Salicylic acid is successful when carefully and diligently used. After careful paring of the corn with emphasis on removing the center core, 40% salicylic acid plaster is applied. Soaking the foot for half an hour before reapplying the medication enhances

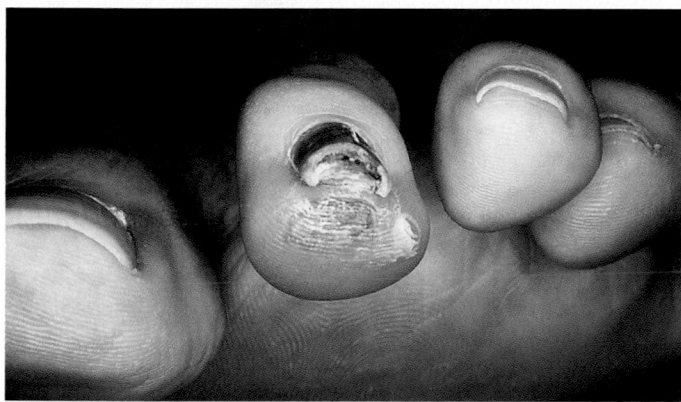

Fig. 3-32 Tennis toe.

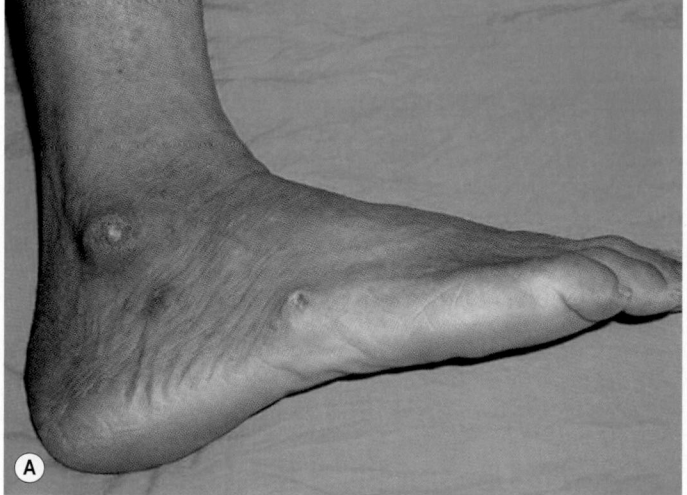

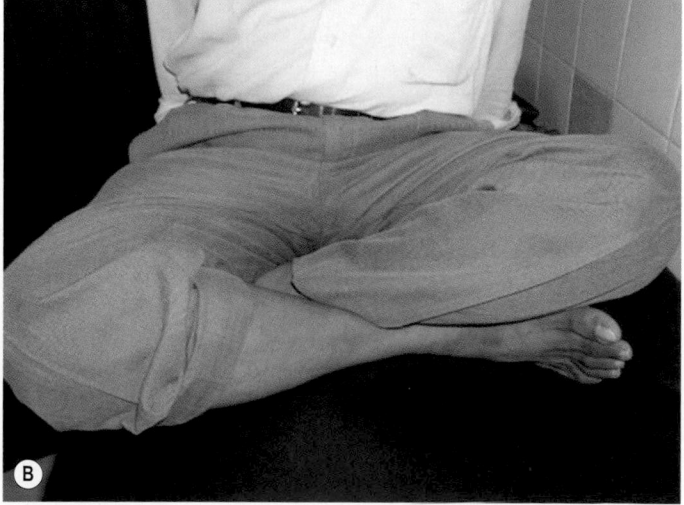

Fig. 3-33 A and B, Calluses from sitting in yoga position. (Courtesy of Dr Shyam Verma)

the effect. After 48 h the plaster is removed, the white macerated skin is rubbed off, and a new plaster is reapplied. This is continued until the corn is gone. It should be stressed that removal of any underlying bony abnormality, if present, is often necessary to effect a cure.

Pseudoverrucous papules and nodules

These striking 2–8 mm, shiny, smooth, red, moist, flat-topped, round lesions in the perianal area of children are considered to be a result of encopresis or urinary incontinence. There is a similarity to lesions affecting urostomy patients. Protection of the skin will help eliminate them. Similar lesions have been described in women who repeatedly apply Vagisil to the groin area.

Coral cuts

A severe type of skin injury may occur from the cuts of coral skeletons (Fig. 3-34). The abrasions and cuts are painful, and local therapy may sometimes provide little or no relief. Healing may take months. As a rule, if secondary infection is guarded against, such cuts heal as well as any others. The possibility of *Mycobacterium marinum* infection must be considered in persistent lesions.

Pressure ulcers (decubitus)

The bedsore, or decubitus, is a pressure ulcer produced anywhere on the body by prolonged pressure. The pressure sore is caused by ischemia of the underlying structures of the skin, fat, and muscles as a result of sustained and constant pressure. Usually, it occurs in chronically debilitated persons who are unable to change position in bed. The bony prominences of the body are the most frequently affected sites. Around 95% of all pressure ulcers develop on the lower body, with 65% in the pelvic area and 30% on the legs. The ulcer usually begins with erythema at the pressure point; in a short time a "punched-

out" ulcer develops. Necrosis with a grayish pseudomembrane is seen, especially in the untreated ulcer. Potential complications of pressure ulcers include sepsis, local infection, osteomyelitis, fistulas, and SCC.

Over 100 risk factors have been identified, with diabetes mellitus, peripheral vascular disease, cerebrovascular disease, sepsis, and hypotension being prominent. Pressure ulcers are graded according to a four-stage system, with the earliest being recognized by changes in one or more of the following: skin temperature, tissue consistency, and/or sensation. The lesion first appears as an area of persistent redness. Stage II is a superficial ulcer involving the epidermis and/or dermis, with the deeper stage III ulcers damaging the subcutaneous fat, and in stage IV, the muscle, bone, tendon, or joint capsule.

Prevention relies on redistributing pressure at a minimum interval of 2 h. Treatment consists of relief of the pressure on the affected parts by frequent change of position, meticulous nursing care, and the use of air-filled products, liquid-filled flotation devices, or foam products. Other measures include ulcer care, management of bacterial colonization and infection, operative repair if necessary, continual education, the ensuring of adequate nutrition, management of pain, and provision of psychosocial support.

Ulcer care is critical. Debridement may be accomplished by sharp, mechanical, enzymatic, and/or autolytic measures. In some cases operative care will be required. Stable heel ulcers are an exception; they do not need debridement if only a dry eschar is present. Wounds should be cleaned initially and each dressing changed by a nontraumatic technique. Normal saline rather than peroxide or povidone–iodine is best. Selection of a dressing should ensure that the ulcer tissue remains moist and the surrounding skin dry.

Occlusive dressings include over 300 marketed products. They are generally classified as film, alginates, foams, hydrogels, hydrofibers, and hydrocolloid dressings. Transparent films are only used for stage II ulcers, as they only provide light drainage, while hydrofibers are utilized only for full-thickness stage III and IV ulcers. Surgical debridement with reconstructive procedures may be necessary. Adjuvant therapies such as ultrasound, laser, UV, hyperbaric oxygen, electrical stimulation, radiant heat, the application of growth factors, cultured keratinocyte grafts, skin substitutes, and miscellaneous topical and oral agents are being investigated to determine their place in the treatment of these ulcers.

At times anaerobic organisms colonize these ulcers and cause a putrid odor. The topical application of metronidazole eliminates this odor within 36 h.

Friction blisters

The formation of vesicles or bullae may occur at sites of combined pressure and friction, and may be enhanced by heat and moisture. The feet of military recruits in training, the palms of oarsmen who have not yet developed protective calluses, and the fingers of drummers ("drummer's digits") are examples of those at risk. The size of the bulla depends on the site of the trauma. If the skin is tense and uncomfortable, the blister should be drained, but the roof should not be completely removed as it may act as its own dressing.

In studies focusing on the prevention of friction blister of the feet in long-distance runners and soldiers, acrylic fiber socks with drying action have been found to be effective. Additionally, pretreatment with a 20% solution of aluminum chloride hexahydrate for at least 3 days has been shown to reduce foot blisters significantly after prolonged hiking, but at the expense of skin irritation. Emollients decrease the irritation, but reduce the overall effectiveness of the treatment.

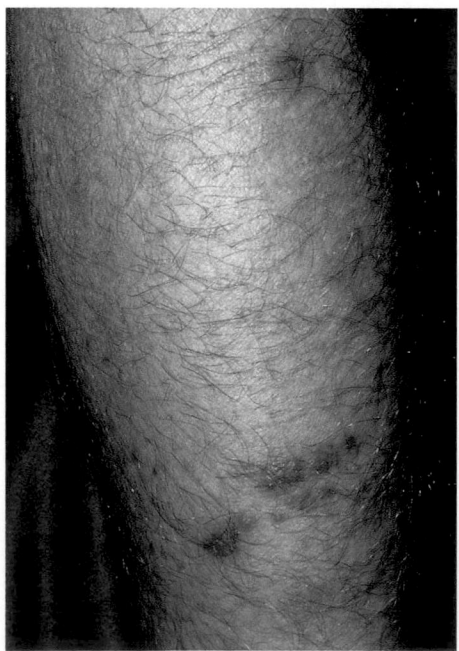

Fig. 3-34 Fire coral stings.

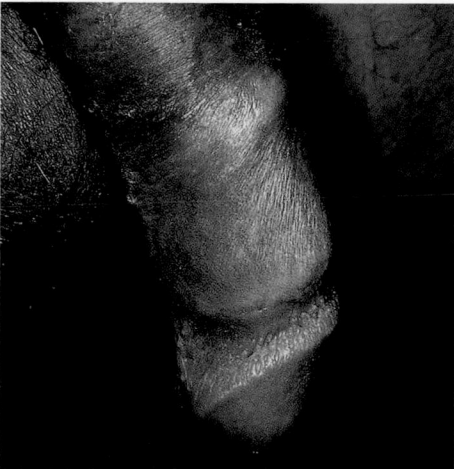

Fig. 3-35 Sclerosing lymphangiitis of the penis.

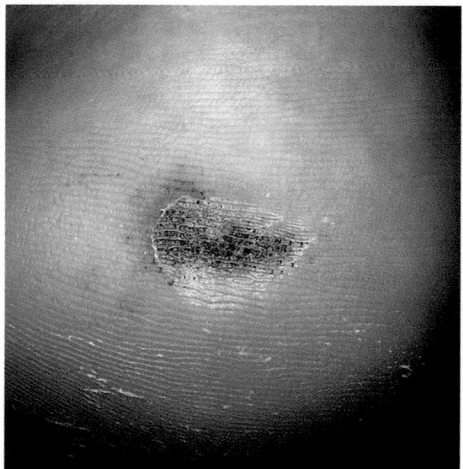

Fig. 3-36 Black heel.

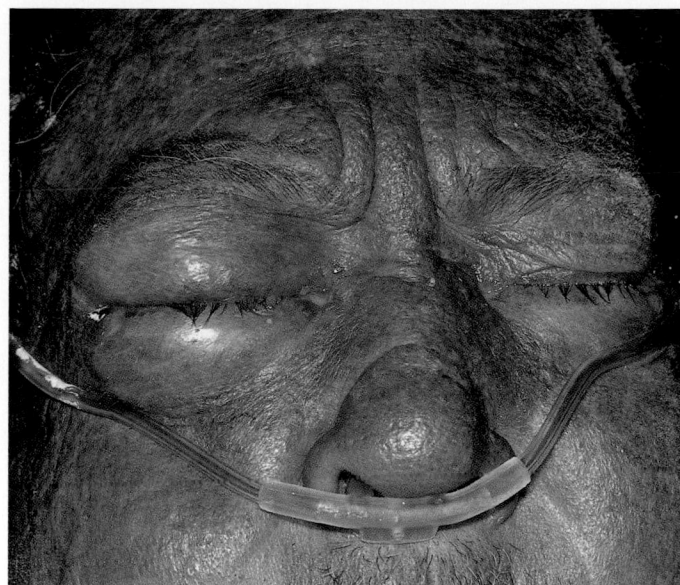

Fig. 3-37 Subcutaneous emphysema. (Courtesy of C Samlaska, MD)

Fracture blisters

These blisters overlie sites of closed fractures, especially the ankle and lower leg. They appear a few days to 3 weeks after the injury, and are felt to be caused by vascular compromise. They may create complications such as infection and scarring, especially if blood-filled or when present in diabetics. They generally heal spontaneously in 5–14 days but may cause delay of surgical reduction of the fracture.

Sclerosing lymphangiitis

This lesion is a cordlike structure encircling the coronal sulcus of the penis, or running the length of the shaft, that has been attributed to trauma during vigorous sexual play (Fig. 3-35). It results from a superficial thrombophlebitis and thus has been renamed Mondor's disease of the penis. Treatment is not necessary; it follows a benign, self-limiting course.

Black heel

Synonyms for black heel include talon noir and calcaneal petechiae. A sudden shower of minute, black, punctate macules occurs most often on the posterior edge of the plantar surface of one or both heels (Fig. 3-36), but sometimes distally on one or more toes. Black heel is often seen in basketball, volleyball, tennis, or lacrosse players. Seeming confluence may lead to

mimicry of melanoma. The bleeding is caused by shearing stress of sports activities. Paring with a No 15 blade and performing a guaiac test will confirm the diagnosis. Treatment is unnecessary.

Subcutaneous emphysema

Free air occurring in the subcutaneous tissues is detected by the presence of cutaneous crepitations. Gas-producing organisms, especially *Clostridia*, and leakage of free air from the lungs or gastrointestinal tract are the most common causes (Fig. 3-37). Samlaska et al reviewed the wide variety of causes of subcutaneous emphysema, including penetrating and non-penetrating injuries, iatrogenic causes occurring during various procedures in hospitalized patients, spontaneous pneumomediastinum such as may occur with a violent cough, childbirth, asthma, Boerhaave syndrome (esophageal rupture after vomiting), or the Heimlich maneuver, intra-abdominal causes, such as inflammatory bowel disease, cancer, perirectal abscess, pancreatitis, or cystitis, dental procedures when using air pressure instruments and high-speed drills, and factitial disease.

Traumatic asphyxia

Cervicofacial cyanosis and edema, multiple petechiae of the face, neck, and upper chest, and bilateral subconjunctival hemorrhage may occur after prolonged crushing injuries of the thorax or upper abdomen. Such trauma reverses blood flow in the superior vena cava or its tributaries.

Painful fat herniation

Also called painful piezogenic pedal papules, this rare cause of painful feet represents fat herniations through thin fascial layers of the weight-bearing parts of the heel (Fig. 3-38). These dermatoceles become apparent when weight is placed on the heel and disappear as soon as the pressure is removed. These fat herniations are present in many people but the majority experience no symptoms. However, extrusion of the fat tissue together with its blood vessels and nerves may initiate pain on prolonged standing. Avoidance of prolonged standing will

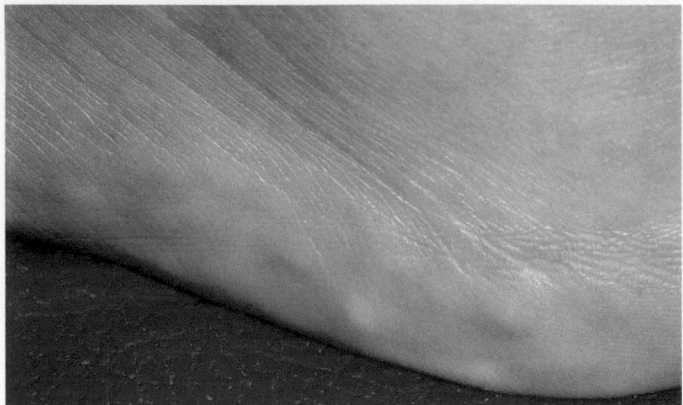

Fig. 3-38 Piezogenic papules.

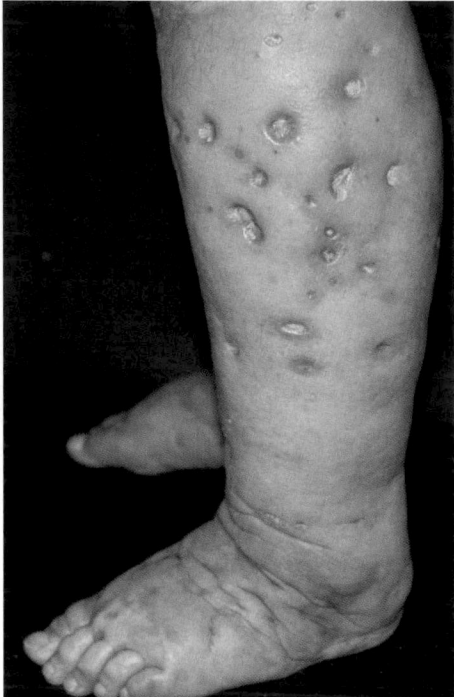

Fig. 3-39 Scars caused by "skin popping."

with it. These lesions may ulcerate. Chronic persistent, firm nodules, a combination of scar and foreign body reaction, may result. If cocaine is being injected, it may cause ulcers because of its direct vasospastic effect. Addicts will continue to inject heroin and cocaine into the chronic ulcer bed.

The cutaneous manifestations of injection of heroin and other drugs also include camptodactylia, edema of the eyelids, persistent nonpitting edema of the hands, urticaria, abscesses, atrophic scars, and hyperpigmentation. Pentazocine abuse leads to a typical clinical picture of tense, woody fibrosis, irregular punched-out ulcerations, and a rim of hyperpigmentation at the sites of injections. Extensive calcification may occur within the thickened sites.

Bauer J, et al: MOC-PSSM CME article: Pressure sores. Plast Reconstr Surg 2008; 121:1.
Booth J, et al: The aetiology and management of plantar callus formation. J Wound Care 1997; 6:427.
Borglund E, et al: Classification of peristomal skin changes in patients with urostomy. J Am Acad Dermatol 1988; 19:623.
Del Giudice P: Cutaneous complications of intravenous drug abuse. Br J Dermatol 2004; 150:1.
Goldberg NS, et al: Perianal pseudoverrucous papules and nodules on children. Arch Dermatol 1992; 128:240.
Herring KM, et al: Friction blisters and sock fiber composition. J Am Podiatr Med Assoc 1990; 80:63.
Knapik JJ, et al: Influence of an antiperspirant on foot blister incidence during cross-country hiking. J Am Acad Dermatol 1998; 39:202.
Kumar B, et al: Mondor's disease of penis. Sex Transm Infect 2005; 81:480.
Laing VB, et al: Piezogenic wrist papules. J Am Acad Dermatol 1991; 24:415.
Leventhal LC, et al: An asymptomatic penile lesion (circular indurated lymphangitis). Arch Dermatol 1993; 129:365.
Levi B, et al: Diagnosis and management of pressure ulcers. Clin Plast Surg 2007; 34:735.
Lowe L, et al: Traumatic asphyxia. J Am Acad Dermatol 1990; 23:972.
Lyder CH: Pressure ulcer prevention and management. JAMA 2003; 289:223.
Magee KL, et al: Extensive calcinosis as a late complication of pentazocine injections. Arch Dermatol 1991; 127:1591.
Mailler-Savage EA, et al: Skin manifestations of running. J Am Acad Dermatol 2006; 55:290.
Patel N, et al: Cervicofacial subcutaneous emphysema. J Oral Maxillofac Surg 2010; 68:1976.
Rimmer S, et al: Dermatologic problems of musicians. J Am Acad Dermatol 1990; 22:657.
Samlaska CP, et al: Subcutaneous emphysema. Adv Dermatol 1996; 11:117.
Strauss EJ, et al: Blisters associated with lower-extremity fracture. J Orthop Surg 2006; 20:618.
Strumia R: Dermatologic signs in patients with eating disorders. Am J Clin Dermatol 2005; 6:165.

obviously relieve this pain. Other options include taping of the foot, use of compression stockings, or use of plastic heel cups or padded orthotics to restrict the herniations. Laing et al found 76% of 29 subjects had pedal papules, and interestingly, by placing pressure on the wrists, found 86% to have piezogenic wrist papules.

Narcotic dermopathy

Heroin (diacetylmorphine) is a narcotic prepared for injection by dissolving the heroin powder in boiling water and then injecting it. The favored route of administration is intravenous. This results in thrombosed, cordlike, thickened veins at the sites of injection. Subcutaneous injection ("skin popping") can result in multiple, scattered ulcerations, which heal with discrete atrophic scars (Fig. 3-39). In addition, amphetamines, cocaine, and other drugs may be injected. Subcutaneous injection may result in infections, complications of bacterial abscess and cellulites, or sterile nodules, apparently acute foreign body reactions to the injected drug, or the adulterants mixed

Foreign body reactions

Tattoo

Tattoos result from the introduction of insoluble pigments into the skin. They may be traumatic, cosmetic, or medicinal in nature, and be applied by a professional or an amateur. Pigment is applied to the skin and then needles pierce the skin to force the material into the dermis. Pigments utilized may be carmine, indigo, vermilion, India ink, chrome green, magnesium (lilac color), Venetian red, aluminum, titanium (white color) or zinc oxide, lead carbonate, copper, iron, logwood, cobalt blue, cinnabar (mercuric sulfide), and cadmium sulfide. Cadmium, cobalt, mercury, and lead are not often used; however, occasional photosensitive reactions to cadmium, which was used for yellow color or to brighten the cinnabar red, are still seen.

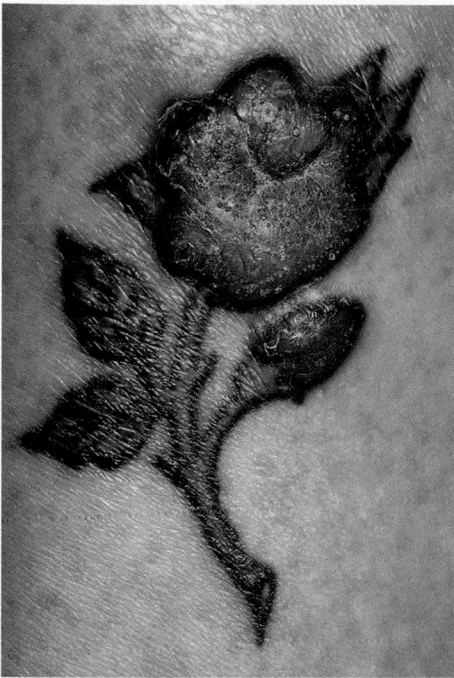

Fig. 3-40 Red tattoo reaction. (Courtesy of Curt Samlaska, MD)

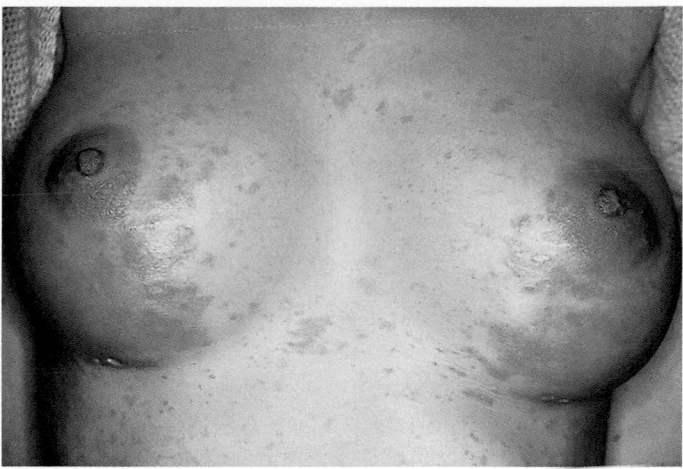

Fig. 3-41 Silicone reaction.

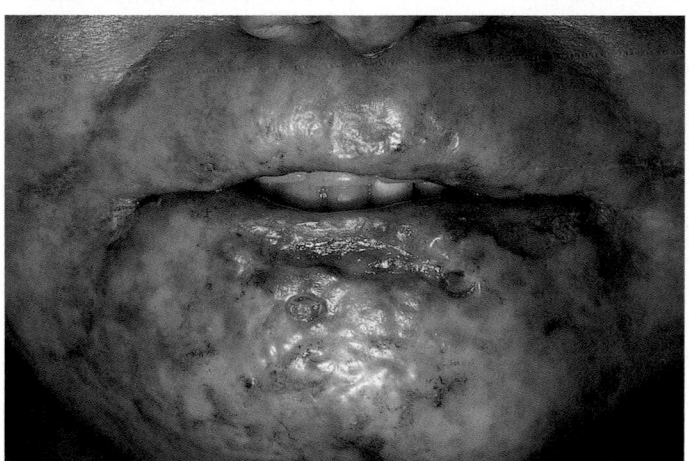

Fig. 3-42 Silicone granuloma.

Tattoo-associated dermopathies may be reactive (allergic, lichenoid, granulomatous, or photosensitive) (Fig. 3-40) or infective (inoculation of syphilis, infectious hepatitis, tuberculosis, HIV, warts, molluscum and Hansen's disease), or may induce a Koebner response in patients with active lichen planus or psoriasis. Discoid lupus erythematosus has been reported to occur in the red-pigmented portion of tattoos. Occasionally, the tattoo marks may become keloidal. Severe allergic reactions to "temporary tattoos" (painting of pigments such as henna on the surface of the skin) occur when the allergen p-phenylenediamine is added to make the color more dramatic.

Red tattoos are the most common cause of delayed reactions, with the histologic findings typically showing a lichenoid process. Occasionally, a pseudolymphomatous reaction may occur in red tattoos. Dermatitis in areas of red (mercury), green (chromium), or blue (cobalt) have been described in patients who are patch test-positive to these metals. Sarcoidal, foreign body, and allergic granulomatous reactions may also occur within tattoos. Aluminum may induce such reactions.

Treatment of such reactions is with topical or intralesional steroids. Excision is also satisfactory when the lesions are small enough and situated so that ellipsoid excisions are feasible. They may also be successfully treated with the Q-switched 532 nm neodymium:YAG laser, although generalized allergic reactions occasionally occur with this modality; prevention by treatment with oral steroids and antihistamines has been suggested. Tattoo darkening and nonresponse to laser treatment are not uncommon. Caution must be used when treating flesh-colored and pink–red tattoos, as they may darken after treatment. This is likely due to the reduction of ferric oxide to ferrous oxide. White ink, composed mostly of titanium dioxide, is commonly used to brighten green, blue, yellow, and purple tattoos. Laser irradiation reduces titanium to a blue-colored pigment. Test areas are recommended when treating light-colored facial tattoos. CO_2 resurfacing lasers used conservatively are an alternative to the Q-switched lasers in such patients. A full discussion of laser treatment of tattoos appears in Chapter 38.

Paraffinoma (sclerosing lipogranuloma)

At one time the injection of oils into the skin for cosmetic purposes, such as the smoothing of wrinkles and the augmentation of breasts, was popular. Paraffin, camphorated oil, cottonseed or sesame oil, mineral oil, and beeswax may produce plaquelike indurations with ulcerations after a time lapse of months up to as many as 40 years. Several reports document penile paraffinomas caused by self-injection. When vaseline gauze or a topical ointment is used to dress unsutured wounds, lipogranulomas or inflammatory mild erysipelas-like lesions with marked tenderness may occur. Present treatment methods for sclerosing lipogranuloma are unsatisfactory. Surgical removal must be wide and complete.

Granulomas

Silicone granuloma

Liquid silicones, composed of long chains of dimethyl siloxy groups, are biologically inert. They have been used for the correction of wrinkles, for the reduction of scars, and for the building up of atrophic depressed areas of the skin. Many case reports detail granulomatous reactions to silicone, some with migration and reactive nodules at points distant from the injection site (Figs 3-41 and 3-42). As acupuncture needles are coated with silicone, granulomas may occur at the entry points of the needle. The incidence of the nodular swellings, which may be quite destructive and treatment-resistant, remains

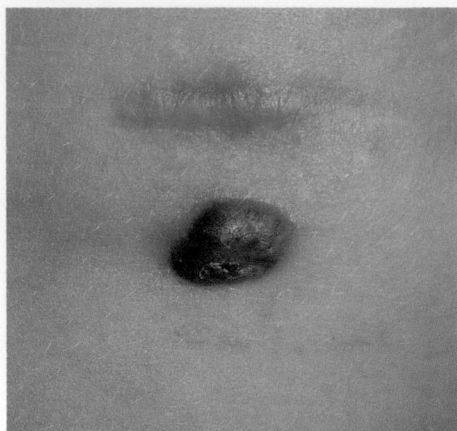

Fig. 3-43 Mercury granuloma.

unknown. It is clear that, if used, medical-grade silicone injected in small volumes should be the rule and that it should not be injected into the penis or the glandular tissue of the breast.

For breast augmentation, silicone may be used as silastic implants. If trauma causes rupture of the bag, subcutaneous fibrotic nodules often develop. Human adjuvant disease and sclerodermatous reactions after such events have been reported; however, large reviews have failed to establish an etiologic link to silicone and connective tissue disease.

Treatment of silicone granulomas is often not successful. Surgical removal may lead to fistulas, abscesses, and marked deformity. Both minocycline, 100 mg twice a day for several months, and imiquimod cream have been anecdotally useful.

Bioplastique consists of polymerized silicone particles dispersed in a gel carrier. When used for lip augmentation, nodules may develop. Histologically, these are foreign body granulomas.

Mercury granuloma

Mercury may cause foreign body giant cell or sarcoidal-type granulomas (Fig. 3-43), pseudolymphoma, or membranous fat necrosis. It is usually identifiable as egg-shaped, extracellular, dark grey to black irregular globules. The gold lysis test is positive in tissues. Energy-dispersive radiographic spectroscopy may be done and will identify mercury by the characteristic emission spike. Such testing may be helpful in identifying any foreign substance suspected to have been implanted accidentally or intentionally by the patient. Systemic toxicity or embolus may develop from mercury and may result in death. Therefore excision is necessary and can be accomplished under x-ray guidance.

Beryllium granuloma

This is seen as a chronic, persistent, granulomatous inflammation of the skin with ulceration that may follow accidental laceration, usually in an occupational setting.

Zirconium granuloma

A papular eruption involving the axillae is sometimes seen as an allergic reaction in those shaving their armpits and using a deodorant containing zirconium (Fig. 3-44). Although zirconium was eliminated from aerosol-type deodorants in 1978, aluminum–zirconium complex is present in some antiperspirants. Additionally, various poison ivy lotions contain zirconium compounds. The lesions are brownish-red, dome-shaped, shiny papules. This is an acquired, delayed-type, allergic reaction resulting in a granuloma of the sarcoidal type. After many months the lesions involute spontaneously.

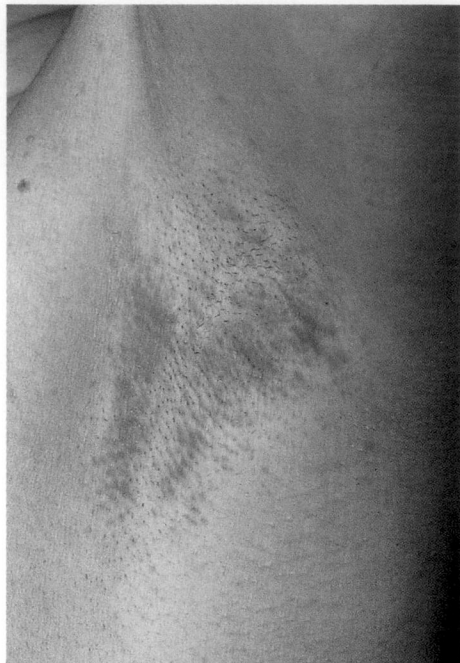

Fig. 3-44 Aluminum–zirconium granuloma secondary to antiperspirant use.

Silica granuloma

Automobile and other types of accidents may produce tattooing of dirt (silicon dioxide) into the skin, which induces silica granulomas (Fig. 3-45). These present commonly as black or blue papules or macules arranged in a linear fashion. At times the granulomatous reaction to silica may be delayed for many years, with the ensuing reaction being both chronic and disfiguring. They may be caused by amorphous or crystalline silicon dioxide (quartz), magnesium silicate (talcum), or complex polysilicates (asbestos). Talc granulomas of the skin and peritoneum may develop after surgical operations from the talcum powder used on surgical gloves. Silica granulomas have a statistical association with systemic sarcoidosis, and silica may act as a stimulus for granuloma formation in patients with latent sarcoidosis.

Removal of these granulomas is fraught with difficulties. The best method of care is immediate and complete removal to prevent these reactions. Excision and systemic steroids have been used but recurrences are common. Some reactions may subside spontaneously after 1–12 months. Dermabrasion is a satisfactory method for the removal of dirt accidentally embedded into the skin of the face or scalp.

Carbon stain

Discoloration of the skin from embedded carbon usually occurs in children from the careless use of firearms or firecrackers, or from a puncture wound by a pencil, which may leave a permanent black mark of embedded graphite, easily mistaken for a metastatic melanoma (Figs 3-46 and 3-47). Narcotic addicts who attempt to clean needles by flaming them with a lighted match may tattoo the carbon formed on the needle as it is inserted into the skin. The carbon is deposited at various depths, which produces a connective tissue reaction and even keloids.

Carbon particles may be removed immediately after their deposition using a toothbrush and forceps. This expeditious and meticulous early care results in the best possible cosmetic result. If the particles are left in place long enough, they are

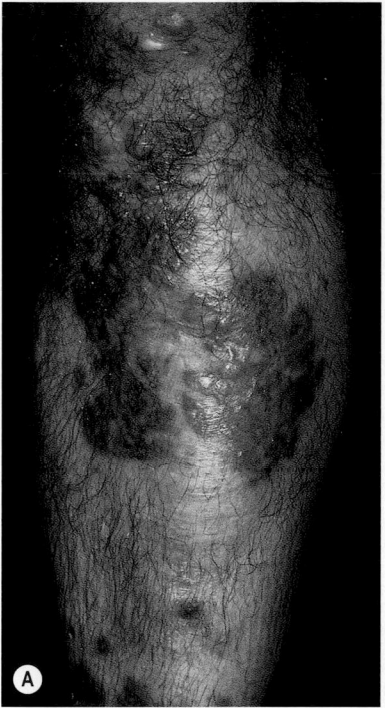

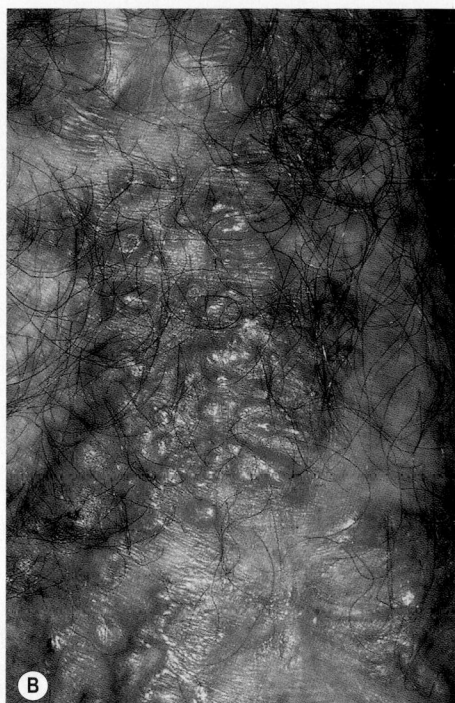

Fig. 3-45 A and B, Silica granuloma years after a motorcycle accident.

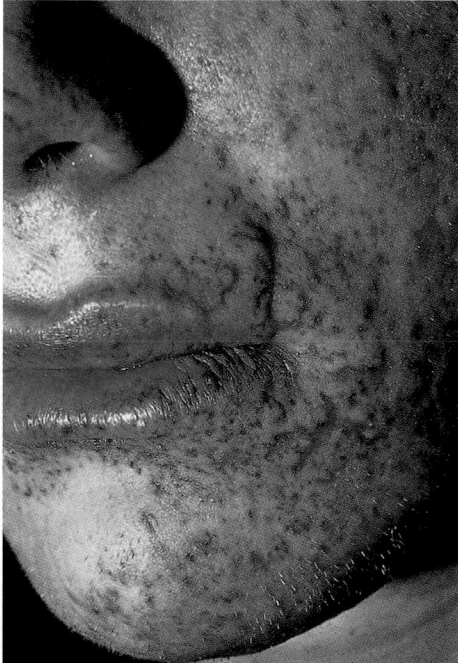

Fig. 3-46 Gunshot tattoo.

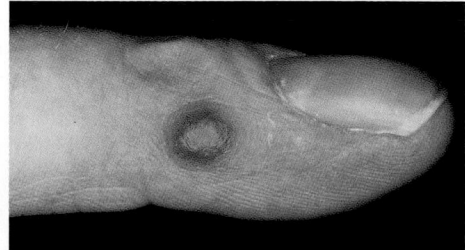

Fig. 3-47 Graphite granuloma.

best removed using the Q-switched neodymium:YAG laser at 1064 nm. Suzuki reported success in 50 of 51 treated tattoos with an average of 1.7 treatments. However, microexplosions producing poxlike scars have occurred with each laser pulse. Alternatively, dermabrasion may be used.

Injected filler substances

Injected or implanted filler substances utilized for facial rejuvenation may produce foreign body or sarcoidal granulomas. Palpable thickening and nodules, which may occasionally be painful, have been reported to collagen, hyaluronic acid and acrylic hydrogels, polylactic acid, polyalkylimide and polymethylmethacrylate microspheres. The reaction may be delayed for years; at times patients are reluctant to admit to these prior cosmetic interventions and frequently cannot name the filler used. Topical, intralesional, or systemic steroids, at times augmented by tacrolimus, or minocycline or doxycycline have been reported to be helpful medical interventions.

Akkus E, et al: Paraffinoma and ulcer of the external genitalia after self-injection of vaseline. J Sex Med 2006; 3:170.

Alani RM, et al: Acupuncture granulomas. J Am Acad Dermatol 2001; 45:S225.

Alijotas-Reig J, et al: Delayed immune-mediated adverse effects of polyalkylimide dermal fillers. Arch Dermatol 2008; 144:637.

Angus JE, et al: Two cases of delayed granulomatous reactions to the cosmetic filler Dermalive. Br J Dermatol 2006; 154:1074.

Antonovitch DD, et al: Development of sarcoidosis in cosmetic tattoos. Arch Dermatol 2005; 141:869.

Baumann LS, et al: Lip silicone granulomatous foreign body reaction treated with aldara. Dermatol Surg 2003; 29:429.

Bigata X, et al: Adverse granulomatous reaction after cosmetic dermal silicone injection. Dermatol Surg 2001; 27:198.

Boyd AS, et al: Mercury exposure and cutaneous disease. J Am Acad Dermatol 2000; 43:81.

Boztepe G, et al: Cutaneous silica granuloma. Eur J Dermatol 2005; 15:194.

Chung W-H, et al: Clinicopathologic features of skin reactions to temporary tattoos and analysis of possible causes. Arch Dermatol 2002; 138:88.

England RW, et al: Immediate cutaneous hypersensitivity after treatment of tattoo with Nd:Yag laser. Ann Allergy Asthma Immunol 2002; 89:215.

Fusade T, et al: Treatment of gunpowder traumatic tattoo by Q-switched Nd:YAG laser. Dermatol Surg 2000; 26:1057.

Gormley RH, et al: Role for trauma in introducing pencil "lead" granuloma in the skin. J Am Acad Dermatol 2010; 62:1074.

Hamzavi I, et al: Removing skin-colored cosmetic tattoos with carbon dioxide resurfacing lasers. J Am Acad Dermatol 2002; 46:764.

Ho WS, et al: Management of paraffinoma of the breast. Br J Plast Surg 2001; 54:232.

Kazandjieva J, et al: Tattoos: dermatological complications. Clin Dermatol 2007; 25:375.

Kenmochi A, et al: Silica granuloma induced by indwelling catheter. J Am Acad Dermatol 2007; 57:S54.

Klontz KL, et al: Adverse effects of cosmetic tattooing. Arch Dermatol 2005; 141:918.

Lazaro C, et al: Foreign body post-varicella granulomas due to talc. J Eur Acad Dermatol Venereol 2006; 20:75.

Lloret P, et al: Successful treatment of granulomatous reactions secondary to injection of esthetic implants. Dermatol Surg 2005; 31:486.

Lombardi T, et al: Orofacial granulomas after injection of cosmetic fillers. J Oral Pathol Med 2004; 33:115.

Lowe NJ, et al: Adverse reactions to dermal fillers. Dermatol Surg 2005; 31:1616.

Mafong EA, et al: Removal of cosmetic tattooing with the pulsed carbon dioxide laser. J Am Acad Dermatol 2003; 48:271.

Matulich J, et al: A temporary henna tattoo causing hair dye and clothing dye dermatitis 2005; 53:33.

Moody BR, et al: Topical tacrolimus in the treatment of bovine collagen hypersensitivity. Dermatol Surg 2001; 27:789.

Montemarano AD, et al: Cutaneous granulomas caused by an aluminum–zirconium complex. J Am Acad Dermatol 1997; 37:496.

Mortimer NJ, et al: Red tattoo reactions. Clin Exp Dermatol 2003; 28:508.

Mouzopoulos G, et al: Cutanous mercury deposits after henna dye application in the arm. Br J Dermatol 2007; 175:394.

Ramdial PK, et al: Membraneous fat necrosis due to subcutaneous elemental mercury injections. Am J Forensic Med Pathol 1999; 20:369.

Rosenberg E, et al: Three cases of penile paraffinoma. Urology 2007; 70:372.

Ross EV, et al: Tattoo darkening and nonresponse after laser treatment. Arch Dermatol 2001; 137:33.

Rossman MD: Chronic beryllium disease. Appl Occup Environ Hyg 2001; 16:615.

Sclafarni AP, et al: Treatment of injectable soft tissue filler complications. Dermatol Surg 2009; 35 Suppl 2:1672.

Senet P, et al: Minocycline for the treatment of cutaneous silicone granulomas. Br J Dermatol 1999; 140:963.

Timko AL, et al: In vitro quantitative chemical analysis of tattoo pigments. Arch Dermatol 2001; 137:143.

Uchida Y, et al: Facial paraffinoma after cosmetic paraffin injection. J Dermatol 2007; 34:798.

Vagefi MR, et al: Adverse reactions to eyeliner tattoo. Ophthal Plast Reconstr Surg 2006; 22:48.

Vargas-Machuca I, et al: Facial granulomas secondary to Dermalive microimplants. Am J Dermatopathol 2006; 28:173.

Wolfram D, et al: Surgery for foreign body reactions to injectable fillers. Dermatology 2006; 213:300.

Zimmermann US, et al: The histopathological aspects of filler complications. Semin Cutan Med Surg 2004; 23:24.

Zwad J, et al: Treatment modalities for allergic reactions in pigmented tattoos. J Dtsch Dermatol Ges 2007; 5:8.

Bonus images for this chapter can be found online at
http://www.expertconsult.com

Pruritus and Neurocutaneous Dermatoses

4

Pruritus

Pruritus, commonly known as itching, is a sensation exclusive to the skin. It may be defined as the sensation that produces the desire to scratch. Pruritogenic stimuli are first responded to by keratinocytes, which release a variety of mediators, and fine intraepidermal C-neuron filaments. Approximately 5% of the afferent unmyelinated C neurons respond to pruritogenic stimuli. Itch sensations in these nerve fiber endings in the subepidermal area are transmitted via the lateral spinothalamic tract to the brain. Here a variety of foci generate both stimulatory and inhibitory responses. The sum of this complicated set of interactions appears to determine the quality and intensity of itch.

Itching may be elicited by many normally occurring stimuli, such as light touch, temperature change, and emotional stress. Chemical, mechanical, and electrical stimuli may also elicit itching. The brain may reinterpret such sensations as being painful or causative of burning or stinging sensations. A large group of neuromediators have been identified. Some of the most important mediators are histamine, serotonin, tryptate, opioid peptides, substance P, prostaglandins such as PGE2, acetylcholine, cytokines such as interleukin (IL)-2, and a variety of neuropeptides and vasoactive peptides. Investigation is ongoing to discover the relative importance of each of these and to determine under which clinical circumstances therapeutic targeting of these molecules will lead to relief of symptoms.

Itch has been classified into four primary categories: pruritoceptive, or that initiated by skin disorders, itch caused by systemic disorders, neuropathic itch due to disorders of the central or peripheral nervous systems, and psychogenic itch (the type observed in parasitophobia). An overlap or mixture of these may be causative in any individual patient.

Patterns of itching

There are wide variations from person to person, and in the same person there may be a variation in reactions to the same stimulus. Heat will usually aggravate preexisting pruritus. Stress, absence of distractions, anxiety, and fear may all enhance itching. It is apt to be most severe at the time of undressing for bed.

Severe pruritus, with or without prior skin lesions, may be paroxysmal in character with a sudden onset, often severe enough to awaken the patient. It may stop instantly and completely as soon as pain is induced by scratching. However, the pleasure of scratching is so intense that the patient—despite the realization that he/she is damaging the skin—is often unable to stop short of inflicting such damage (Fig. 4-1). Itching of this distinctive type is characteristic of a select group of dermatoses: lichen simplex chronicus, atopic dermatitis, nummular eczema, dermatitis herpetiformis, neurotic excoriations, eosinophilic folliculitis, uremic pruritus, subacute prurigo,

paraneoplastic itch (usually secondary to lymphoma), and prurigo nodularis. In general, only these disorders produce such intense pruritus and scratching as to induce bleeding. In individual cases, other diseases may manifest such severe symptoms.

Treatment

General guidelines for therapy of the itchy patient include keeping cool, and avoidance of hot baths or showers and of wool clothing. The latter is a nonspecific irritant, as is xerosis. Many patients note itching increases after showers, when they wash with soap and then dry roughly. Using soap only in the axilla and inguinal area, patting dry, and applying a moisturizer will often help avoid such exacerbations. Patients often use an ice bag or hot water to calm pruritus; however, hot water can irritate the skin, is effective only for short periods, and over time exacerbates the condition.

Relief of pruritus with topical remedies may be achieved with topical anesthetic preparations. Many contain benzocaine, which may produce contact sensitization. Pramoxine in a variety of vehicles, lidocaine 5% ointment, EMLA ointment (a eutectic mixture of lidocaine and prilocaine) and lidocaine gel are preferred anesthetics that may be quite useful in localized conditions. EMLA and lidocaine may be toxic if applied to large areas. Topical antihistamines are generally not recommended, although doxepin cream may be effective for mild pruritus when used alone. Doxepin cream may cause contact allergy or a burning sensation, and somnolence may occur when doxepin is used over large areas. Topical lotions that contain menthol or camphor feel cool and improve pruritus. Others with specific ceramide content designed to mimic that of the normal epidermal barrier are useful. Capsaicin, by depleting substance P, can be effective, but the burning sensation present during initial use frequently causes patients to discontinue its use. Topical steroids and calcineurin inhibitors effect a decrease in itching via their anti-inflammatory action, and therefore are of limited efficacy in neurogenic, psychogenic and systemic disease-related pruritus.

Phototherapy with ultraviolet (UV) B, UVA, and PUVA may be useful in a variety of dermatoses and pruritic disorders. Many oral agents are available to treat pruritus. The most frequently utilized by nondermatologists are the antihistamines. First-generation H_1 antihistamines, such as hydroxyzine and diphenhydramine, may be helpful in nocturnal itching, but their efficacy as antipruritics in many disorders, with the exception of urticaria and mastocytosis, is disappointing. Doxepin is an exception in that it has the ability to reduce anxiety and depression, and has utility in several pruritic disorders. Sedating antihistamines should be prescribed cautiously because of their impairment of cognitive ability. The nonsedating antihistamines and H_2 blockers are only effective in urticaria and mast cell disease. Opioids are involved in

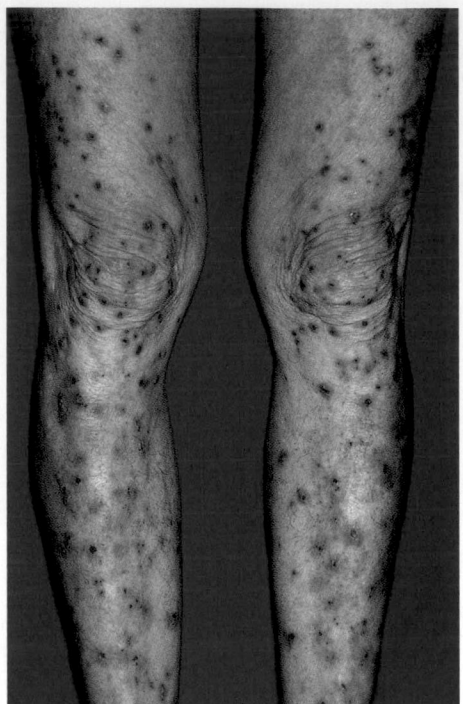

Fig. 4-1 Severe pruritus with excoriations.

itch induction. In general, activation of μ-opioid receptors stimulates itch, while κ-opioid receptor stimulation inhibits itch perception; however, the interaction is complex. Additionally, opioid-altering agents such as naltrexone, naloxone, nalfurafine, and butorphanol have significant side effects and varying modes of delivery (intravenous, intranasal, and oral). Initial reports of utility in one condition are often followed by conflicting reports on further study. Specific recommendations in selected pruritic conditions are detailed in those sections. They appear most useful for cholestatic pruritus. Central reduction of itch perception may be effected by anticonvulsants and antidepressants. Gabapentin and pregabalin are examples of the former, while mirtazapine, paroxetine, sertraline, and fluoxetine are examples of the latter. Ondansetron, a serotonin receptor antagonist, had initial reports of efficacy in some pruritic disorders; however, more detailed investigation has revealed its utility to be minimal. Finally thalidomide, through a variety of direct neural effects, immunomodulatory actions and hypnosedative effects, is also useful in selected patients.

Bernard JD: Itch and pruritus. Dermatol Ther 2005; 18:288.
Greaves MW: Recent advances in pathophysiology and current management of itch. Ann Acad Med Singapore 2007; 36:788.
Hundley JL, et al: Mirtazapine for reducing nocturnal itch in patients with chronic pruritus: a pilot study. J Am Acad Dermatol 2004; 50:889.
Ikoma A, et al: The neurobiology of itch. Nat Rev Neurosci 2006; 7:535.
Lynde CB, et al: Novel agents for intractable itch. Skin Therapy Lett 2008; 13:6.
Patel T, et al: Therapy of pruritus. Expert Open Pharmacother 2010; 11:1673.
Rivard J, et al: Ultraviolet phototherapy for pruritus. Dermatol Ther 2005; 18:344.
Schmelz M, et al: Opioids and the skin. J Invest Dermatol 2007; 127:1287.
Shaw RJ, et al: Psychiatric medications for the treatment of pruritus. Psychosom Med 2007; 69:970.
Steinhoff M, et al: Neurophysiological, neuroimmunological and neuroendocrine basis of pruritus. J Invest Dermatol 2006; 126:1705.
Summey BT Jr, et al: Pharmacologic advances in the systemic treatment of itch. Dermatol Ther 2005; 18:328.
Yosipovitch G, et al: Chronic itch and chronic pain. Pain 2007; 131:4.

Internal causes of pruritus

Itching may be present as a symptom in a number of internal disorders. The intensity and duration of itching vary from one disease to another. Among the most important internal causes of itching are liver disease, especially obstructive and hepatitis C (with or without evidence of jaundice or liver failure), renal failure, hypo- and hyperthyroidism, hematopoietic diseases such as iron deficiency anemia, polycythemia vera, neoplastic diseases such as lymphoma (especially Hodgkin disease), leukemia, and myeloma, internal solid tissue malignancies, intestinal parasites, carcinoid, multiple sclerosis, acquired immunodeficiency syndrome (AIDS), and neuropsychiatric diseases, with anorexia nervosa prominent among the latter. Diabetes mellitus is frequently listed as an internal cause of pruritus but most individuals with diabetes do not itch. If a diabetic patient has pruritus with no primary skin lesions, other causes of pruritus should be investigated.

The pruritus of Hodgkin disease is usually continuous and at times is accompanied by severe burning. The incidence of pruritus is between 10% and 30% and is the first symptom of this disease in 7% of patients. Its cause is unknown. The pruritus of leukemia, except for chronic lymphocytic leukemia, has a tendency to be less severe than in Hodgkin disease.

Internal organ cancer may be found in patients with generalized pruritus that is unexplained by skin lesions. However, no significant overall increase of malignant neoplasms can be found in patients with idiopathic pruritus. A suggested work-up for chronic, generalized pruritus includes taking a complete history, performing a thorough physical examination and carrying out the following laboratory tests: a complete blood count (CBC) and differential, thyroid, liver, and renal panels, hepatitis C serology, an human immunodeficiency virus (HIV) antibody (if risk factors are present), urinalysis, stool for occult blood, serum protein electrophoresis, and chest x-ray evaluation. Presence of eosinophilia on the CBC is a good screen for parasitic diseases, but if the patient has been on systemic corticosteroids, blood eosinophilia may not be a reliable screen for parasitic diseases and stool samples for ova and parasites should be submitted. Additional radiologic studies or specialized testing, as indicated for the patient's age and as dictated by the history and physical findings, should be performed. A biopsy for direct immunofluorescence can occasionally be helpful to detect dermatitis herpetiformis or pemphigoid.

Etter L, et al: Pruritus in systemic disease. Dermatol Clin 2002; 20:459.
Fisher DA, et al: Pruritus as a symptom of hepatitis C. J Am Acad Dermatol 1995; 32:629.
Greaves MW: Itch in systemic disease. Dermatol Ther 2005; 18:323.
Lidsone V, et al: Pruritus in cancer patients. Cancer Treat Rev 2001; 27:305.

Chronic kidney disease

Chronic kidney disease (CKD) is the most common systemic cause of pruritus; 20–80% of patients with chronic renal failure itch. The pruritus is often generalized, intractable, and severe; however, dialysis-associated pruritus may be episodic, mild, or localized to the dialysis catheter site, face, or legs.

The mechanism of pruritus associated with CKD is multifactorial. Xerosis, secondary hyperparathyroidism, increased serum histamine levels, hypervitaminosis A, iron deficiency anemia, and neuropathy have been implicated. Complications such as Kyrle disease, acquired perforating disease, lichen simplex chronicus, and prurigo nodularis may develop and contribute to the degree and severity of pruritus (Fig. 4-2).

CKD-associated pruritus responds well to narrow-band UVB phototherapy but often recurs after discontinuation. Many patients have concomitant xerosis, and aggressive use

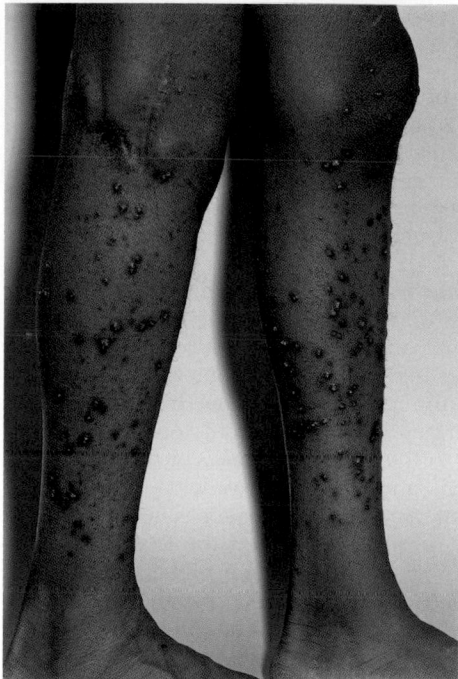

Fig. 4-2 Acquired perforating dermatosis of uremia.

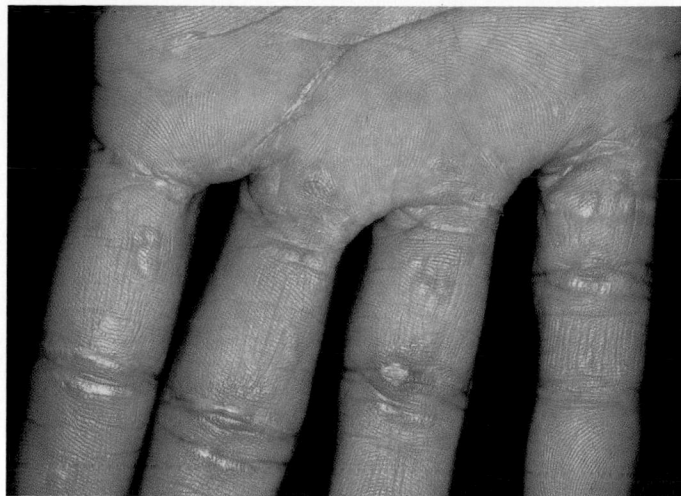

Fig. 4-3 Primary biliary cirrhosis with plane xanthomas.

of emollients, including soaking and smearing, may help them. Gabapentin given three times weekly at the end of hemodialysis sessions can be effective, but its renal excretion is decreased in CKD so a low initial dose of 100 mg after each session with slow upward titration is recommended. In recalcitrant disease, the options include colestyramine, 5 g twice a day, or activated charcoal, 6 g/day. Naltrexone, topical tacrolimus and ondansetron were reported to be useful in initial trials, but subsequent studies indicate they are ineffective. Thalidomide, topical capsaicin, intranasal butorphanol, and intravenous lidocaine are less practical options. Renal transplantation will eliminate pruritus.

Ada S, et al: Treatment of uremic pruritus with narrow band UVB. J Am Acad Dermatol 2005; 53:149.

Gutman A, et al: Soak and smear. Arch Dermatol 2005; 141:1556.

Lugon JR: Uremic pruritus. Hemodial Int 2005; 9:180.

Murtagh FE, et al: Symptoms in advanced renal disease. J Palliat Med 2007; 10:1266.

Patel TS, et al: An update on pruritus associated with CKD. Am J Kid Dis 2007; 50:11.

Robinson-Bostom L, et al: Cutaneous manifestations of end-stage renal disease. J Am Acad Dermatol 2002; 43:975.

Biliary pruritus

Chronic liver disease with obstructive jaundice may cause severe generalized pruritus, and 20–50% of patients with jaundice have pruritus. This itching is probably caused by central mechanisms, as suggested by elevated central nervous system (CNS) opioid peptide levels, downregulation of opioid peptide CNS receptors, and the reported therapeutic effectiveness of naloxone, butorphanol, naltrexone, or nalmefene. Opioid withdrawal-type reactions may occur. The serum-conjugated bile acid levels do not correlate with the severity of pruritus.

Primary biliary cirrhosis

Primary biliary cirrhosis occurs almost exclusively in women older than 30 years of age. Itching may begin insidiously and be the presenting symptom in a quarter to one-half of patients. With time, extreme pruritus develops in nearly 80% of patients. This almost intolerable itching is accompanied by jaundice and a striking melanotic hyperpigmentation of the entire skin; the

patient may turn almost black, except for a hypopigmented "butterfly" area in the upper back. Eruptive xanthomas, plane xanthomas of the palms (Fig. 4-3), xanthelasma, and tuberous xanthomas over the joints may be seen.

Dark urine, steatorrhea, and osteoporosis occur frequently. Serum bilirubin, alkaline phosphatase, serum ceruloplasmin, serum hyaluronate, and cholesterol values are increased. The antimitochondrial antibody test is positive. The disease is usually relentlessly progressive with the development of hepatic failure. Several cases have been accompanied by scleroderma.

To treat the pruritus, opioid antagonists, such as naltrexone, 50 mg/day, have proven efficacy but significant side effects. Additionally, colestyramine, 4 g 1–3 times a day, UVB twice weekly, and rifampin, 300–450 mg/day, have been reported to be effective. The latter should be used with caution as it may cause hepatitis. Ondansetron was not effective in a controlled trial. Liver transplantation is the definitive treatment for end-stage disease and provides dramatic relief from the severe pruritus.

Bergasa NV: Medical palliation of the jaundiced patient with pruritus. Gastroenterol Clin N Am 2006; 35:113.

Cies JJ, et al: Treatment of cholestatic pruritus in children. Am J Health Syst Pharm 2007; 64:1157.

Gong Y, et al: Colchicine for primary biliary cirrhosis. Am J Gastroenterol 2005; 100:1876.

Gong Y, et al: Methotrexate for primary biliary cirrhosis. Cochrane Database Syst Rev 2005; 20:CD4385.

Gong Y, et al: Ursodeoxycholic acid for patients with primary biliary cirrhosis. Am J Gastroenterol 2007; 103:1799.

Kaplan MM, et al: Primary biliary cirrhosis. N Engl J Med 2005; 353:1261.

Lindor K: Ursodeoxycholic acid for the treatment of primary biliary cirrhosis. N Engl J Med 2007; 375:1524.

Tandon P, et al: The efficacy and safety of bile acid binding agents, opioid antagonists or rifampin in the treatment of cholestasis-associated pruritus. Am J Gastroenterol 2007; 102:1528.

Polycythemia vera

More than one-third of patients with polycythemia vera report pruritus; it is usually induced by temperature changes or several minutes after bathing. The cause is unknown.

Aspirin has been shown to provide immediate relief from itching; however, there is a risk of hemorrhagic complications, and low doses are recommended. PUVA and narrow-band UVB are also effective. A marked improvement is noted after an average of six treatments, while a complete remission occurs within 2–10 weeks in 8 of 10 treated patients. Paroxetine,

20 mg/day, produced clearing or near-complete clearing in a series of nine patients. Interferon (IFN)-α2 has been shown to be effective for treating the underlying disease and associated pruritus. Myelosuppressive therapy is useful for long-term control of symptoms.

Baldo A, et al: Narrowband (TL-01) ultraviolet B phototherapy for pruritus in polycythaemia vera. Br J Dermatol 2002; 147:979.

Hernandez-Nunez A, et al: Water-induced pruritus in haematologically controlled polycythaemia vera. J Dermatol Treat 2001; 12:107.

Muller EW, et al: Long-term treatment with interferon-alpha 2b for severe pruritus in patients with polycythaemia vera. Br J Haematol 1995; 89:313.

Rivard J, et al: Ultraviolet therapy for pruritus. Derm Ther 2005; 18:344.

Tefferi A, et al: Selective serotonin reuptake inhibitors are effective in the treatment of polycythemia vera-associated pruritus. Blood 2002; 99:2627.

Pruritic dermatoses

Winter itch

Asteatotic eczema, eczema craquelé, and xerotic eczema are other names given to this pruritic condition. It is characterized by pruritus that usually first manifests and is most severe on the legs and arms. Extension to the body is common; however, the face, scalp, groin, axilla, palms and soles are spared. The skin is dry with fine flakes (Fig. 4-4). The pretibial regions are particularly susceptible and may develop eczema craquelé, exhibiting fine cracks in the eczematous area that resemble the cracks in old porcelain dishes.

Frequent and lengthy bathing with plenty of soap during the winter is the most frequent cause. This is especially prevalent in elderly persons, whose skin has a decreased rate of repair of the epidermal water barrier and whose sebaceous glands are less productive. Low humidity in overheated rooms during cold weather contributes to this condition. In a study of 584 elderly individuals, the prevalence of asteatosis (28.9%) was second only to seborrheic dermatitis as the most common finding.

Treatment consists of educating the patient regarding using soap only in the axilla and inguinal area, and lubrication of the skin with emollients immediately after showering. Lactic acid- or urea-containing preparations are helpful after-bath applications for some patients; however, they may cause irritation and worsening of itching in patients with erythema and eczema.

For those with more severe symptoms, long-standing disease, or a significant inflammatory component, a regimen referred to as "soaking and smearing" is dramatically effective. The patient soaks in a tub of plain water at a comfortable temperature for 20 min prior to bedtime. Immediately on exiting the tub, without drying, triamcinolone, 0.025–0.1% ointment, is applied to the wet skin. This will trap the moisture, lubricate the skin, and allow for excellent penetration of the steroid component. An old pair of pajamas is then donned and the patient will note relief even on the first night. The night-time soaks are repeated for several nights, after which the ointment alone suffices, with the maintenance therapy of limiting soap use to the axilla and groin, and moisturization after showering. Plain petrolatum may be used as the lubricant after the soaking if simple dryness without inflammation is present.

Gutman A, et al: Soak and smear therapy. Arch Dermatol 2005; 141:1556.

Pruritus ani

Pruritus is often centered on the anal or genital area (less commonly in both), with little or no pruritus elsewhere. Anal neurodermatitis is characterized by paroxysms of violent itching, at which time the patient may tear at the affected area until bleeding is induced. Manifestations are identical to those of lichen simplex chronicus elsewhere on the body. There should always be a thorough search for specific etiologic factors.

Allergic contact dermatitis occurs from various medicaments, fragrance in toilet tissue, or preservatives in moist toilet tissue, with one study reporting 18 of 40 consecutive patients being patch test-positive. Also, irritant contact dermatitis from gastrointestinal contents, such as hot spices or cathartics, or failure to cleanse the area adequately after bowel movements may be causes. Anatomic factors may lead to leakage of rectal mucus on to perianal skin and thus promote irritation. Physical changes such as hemorrhoids, anal tags, fissures, and fistulas may aggravate or produce pruritus. Anal warts and condyloma latum (syphilis) may be causative agents, although these rarely itch. Anal gonorrhea, especially in men, is frequently overlooked when pruritus is the only symptom.

Mycotic pruritus ani is characterized by fissures and a white, sodden epidermis. Scrapings from the anal area are examined directly with potassium hydroxide mounts for fungi. Cultures for fungi are also taken. *Candida albicans*, *Epidermophyton floccosum*, and *Trichophyton rubrum* are frequent causative fungi in this area. Other sites of fungal infection, such as the groin, toes, and nails, should also be investigated. Erythrasma in the groin and perianal regions may also occasionally produce pruritus. The diagnosis is established by coral red fluorescence under the Wood's light. Beta-hemolytic streptococcal infections have also been implicated. The use of tetracyclines may cause pruritus ani, most often in women, by inducing candidiasis. Diabetic patients are susceptible to perianal candidiasis.

Pinworm infestations may cause pruritus ani, especially in children and sometimes in their parents. Nocturnal pruritus is

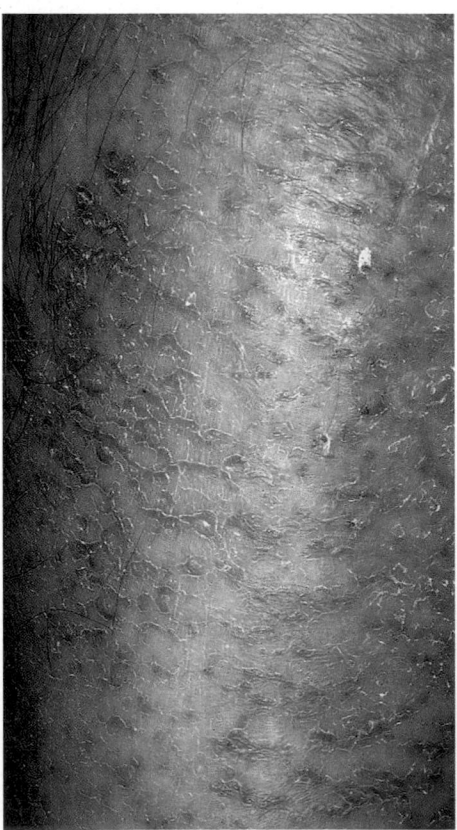

Fig. 4-4 Eczema craquelé.

most prevalent. Other intestinal parasites such as *Taenia solium*, *T. saginata*, amebiasis, and *Strongyloides stercoralis* may produce pruritus. Pediculosis pubis may cause anal itching; however, attention is focused by the patient on the pubic area, where itching is most severe. Scabies may be causative, but will usually also involve the finger webs, wrists, axillae, areolae, and genitals.

Seborrheic dermatitis of the anal area may cause pruritus ani. It usually also involves other areas, such as the inguinal regions, scalp, chest, and face. Similarly, lichen planus may involve the perianal region. Anal psoriasis may cause itching. The perianal lesions are usually sharply marginated, and psoriatic lesions may be present on other parts of the body. Other frequent sites for psoriasis should be examined, such as the fingernails.

A thorough examination for malignancies should be carried out; extramammary Paget's disease is easily overlooked. Lumbosacral radiculopathy may be present, as assessed by radiographs and nerve conduction studies; paravertebral blockade may help these patients.

Treatment

Meticulous toilet care should be followed, no matter what the cause of the itching. After defecation, the anal area should be cleansed with soft cellulose tissue paper and, whenever possible, washed with mild soap and water. Cleansing with wet toilet tissue is advisable in all cases. Medicated cleansing pads, such as Tucks, should be used regularly. A variety of moist toilet tissue products are now available. Contact allergy to preservatives in these products is occasionally a problem. An emollient lotion, Balneol, is helpful for cleansing without producing irritation.

Except in psychogenic pruritus ani, once the etiologic agent has been identified, a rational and effective treatment regimen may be started. Topical corticosteroids are effective for most noninfectious types of pruritus ani; however, use of topical tacrolimus ointment will frequently suffice and is safer. Pramoxine hydrochloride, a nonsteroidal topical anesthetic, is also often effective, especially in a lotion form combined with hydrocortisone. In pruritus ani, as well as in pruritus scroti and vulvae, it is sometimes best to discontinue all topical medications and treat with plain water sitz baths at night, followed immediately by plain petrolatum applied over wet skin. This soothes the area, provides a barrier, and eliminates contact with potential allergens and irritants.

Al-Ghnaniem R, et al: 1% hydrocortisone ointment is an effective treatment of pruritus ani. Int J Colorectal Dis 2007; 22:1463.

Dasan S, et al: Treatment of persistent pruritus ani in a combined colorectal and dermatological clinic. Br J Surg 1999; 86:1337.

Farage MA, et al: Incontinence in the aged. Contact Dermatitis 2007; 57:211.

Markell KW, et al: Pruritus ani: etiology and management. Surg Clin North Am 2010; 90:125.

Redondo P, et al: Pruritus ani in an elderly man. Extramammary Paget's disease. Arch Dermatol 1995; 131:952.

Zuccati G, et al: Pruritus ani. Dermatol Ther 2005; 18:355.

Pruritus scroti

The scrotum of an adult is relatively immune to dermatophyte infection, but it is a favorite site for circumscribed neurodermatitis (lichen simplex chronicus) (Fig. 4-5). Psychogenic pruritus is probably the most frequent type of itching seen. Why it preferentially affects this area, or in women the vulva, is unclear. Lichenification may result, be extreme, and persist for many years despite intensive therapy.

Infectious conditions may complicate or cause pruritus on the scrotum but are less common than idiopathic scrotal pru-

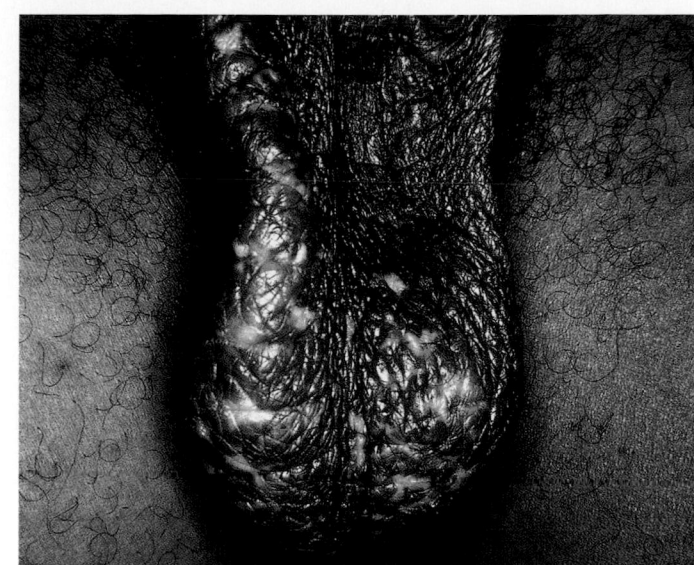

Fig. 4-5 Pruritus scroti.

ritus. Fungal infections, except candidiasis, usually spare the scrotum. When candidal infection affects the scrotum, burning rather than pruritus is frequently the primary symptom. The scrotum is eroded, weepy, or crusted. The scrotum may be affected to a lesser degree in cases of pruritus ani, but this pruritus usually affects the midline, extending from the anus along the midline to the base of the scrotum, rather than the dependent surfaces of the scrotum, where pruritus scroti usually occurs. Scrotal pruritus may be associated with allergic contact dermatitis from topical medications, including topical steroidal agents.

Topical corticosteroids are the mainstay of treatment, but caution should be exercised. The "addicted scrotum syndrome" may be caused by the use of high-potency topical steroidal agents. Although this is usually seen after chronic use, even short-term high-potency steroid medications may produce it. The scrotum is frequently in contact with inner thigh skin, producing areas of occlusion, which increases the penetration of topical steroidal agents. If topical steroids are utilized in this area, those of low potency are favored. As with facial skin, high-potency steroids used on the scrotum can result in addictive skin; every time the patient attempts to taper off the steroid, severe burning and redness occur. Topical tacrolimus ointment is useful in overcoming the effects of overuse of potent topical steroids. Another alternative is gradual tapering to less and less potent corticosteroids. Other useful nonsteroidal alternatives include topical pramoxine, doxepin, or simple petrolatum, the latter applied after a sitz bath as described for pruritus ani.

Cohen AD, et al: Neuropathic scrotal pruritus. J Am Acad Dermatol 2005; 52:61.

Pruritus vulvae

The vulva is a common site for pruritus of different causes. Pruritus vulvae is the counterpart of pruritus scroti. In a prospective series of 141 women with chronic vulvar symptoms, the most common causes were unspecified dermatitis (54%), lichen sclerosus (13%), chronic vulvovaginal candidiasis (10%), dysesthetic vulvodynia (9%), and psoriasis (5%). In prepubertal children such itching is most frequently irritant in nature and they generally benefit from education about improved hygienic measures.

Vaginal candidiasis is a frequent cause of pruritus vulvae. This is true especially during pregnancy and when oral

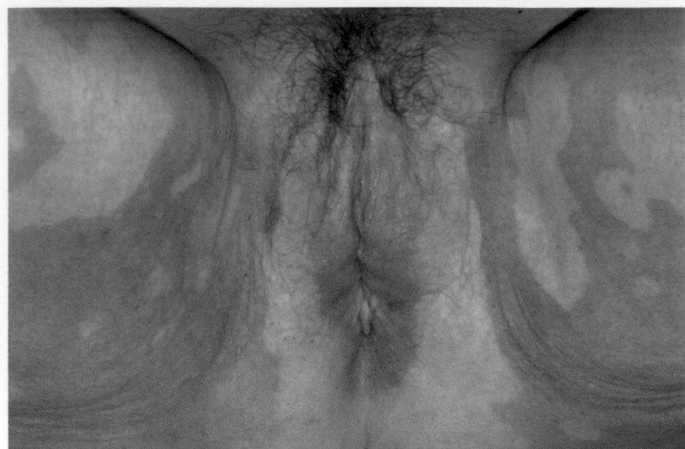

Fig. 4-6 Lichen sclerosus in a woman with vitiligo.

antibiotics are taken. The inguinal, perineal, and perianal areas may be affected. Microscopic examination for *Candida albicans* and cultures for fungus should be performed. *Trichomonas vaginitis* may cause vulvar pruritus. For the detection of *T. vaginalis*, examination of vaginal secretions is often diagnostic. The organism is recognized by its motility, size (somewhat larger than a leukocyte), and piriform shape.

Contact dermatitis from sanitary pads, contraceptives, douche solutions, fragrance, colophony, corticosteroids, and a partner's condoms may account for vulvar pruritus. Urinary incontinence should also be considered. Lichen sclerosus is another frequent cause of pruritus in the genital area in middle-aged and elderly women (Fig. 4-6). Lichen planus may involve the vulva, resulting in pruritus and mucosal changes, including resorption of the labia minora and atrophy.

When burning rather than itching predominates, the patient should be evaluated for signs of sensory neuropathy.

Treatment

Candidiasis is treated with topical anticandidal agents. A single 150 mg dose of fluconazole is effective for acute candidiasis, but chronic disease with pruritus may require 150 mg/day for 5 days, followed by 150 mg/week for several months. *Trichomonas* infection is best treated with oral metronidazole or by vaginal gel or inserts. Lichen sclerosus responds best to pulsed dosing of high-potency topical steroids or to topical tacrolimus or pimecrolimus. Topical steroidal agents and topical tacrolimus may be used to treat psychogenic pruritus or irritant or allergic reactions. High-potency topical steroids are effective in treating lichen planus, but other options are also available (see Chapter 12). Topical lidocaine, topical pramoxine, or an oral tricyclic antidepressant may be helpful in select cases. Any chronic skin disease that does not appear to be responding to therapy should prompt a biopsy. Referral to a physician specializing in vulvar diseases should be considered for patients whose condition is unresponsive to therapy. In chronic idiopathic forms hypnosis therapy may be useful.

Bohl TG, et al: Overview of vulvar pruritus through the life cycle. Clin Obstet Gynecol 2005; 48:786.

Foster DC: Vulvar disease. Obstet Gynecol 2002; 100:145.

Lewis FM, et al: Contact sensitivity in pruritus vulvae: a common and manageable problem. Contact Dermat (Denmark) 1994; 31:264.

Paek SC, et al: Pruritus vulvae in prepubertal children. J Am Acad Dermatol 2001; 44:795.

Sarifakioglu E, et al: Efficacy of topical pimecrolimus in the treatment of chronic vulvar pruritus. J Dermatolog Treat 2006; 17:276.

Weichert GF: An approach to the treatment of anogenital itch. Dermatol Ther 2004; 17:129.

Puncta pruritica (itchy points)

"Itchy points" consists of one or two intensely itchy spots in clinically normal skin, sometimes followed by the appearance of seborrheic keratoses at exactly the same site. Others believe puncta pruritica is a variant of notalgia paresthetica. Curettage, cryosurgery, or punch biopsy of the itchy points may cure the condition.

Boyd AS, et al: Puncta pruritica. Int J Dermatol 1992; 31:370.

Crissey JT: Puncta pruritica. Int J Dermatol 1992; 31:166.

Aquagenic pruritus and aquadynia

Aquagenic pruritus is itching evoked by contact with water of any temperature. Degranulation of mast cells and increased concentration of histamine and acetylcholine in the skin after contact with water are found. In most cases there is severe, prickling discomfort within minutes of exposure to water or on cessation of exposure to water, and there is often a family history of similar symptoms.

Aquagenic pruritus must be distinguished from xerosis or asteatosis and an initial trial of "soaking and smearing," as described for winter itch above, is recommended. The condition may be associated with polycythemia vera, hypereosinophilic syndrome, juvenile xanthogranuloma, and myelodysplastic syndrome. Treatment options include the use of antihistamines, systemic steroids, sodium bicarbonate dissolved in bath water, propranolol, naltrexone, and UVB or psoralen + UVA (PUVA) phototherapy. One patient found tight-fitting clothing settled the symptoms after only 5 minutes.

Shelley et al reported two patients with widespread burning pain that lasted 15–45 min after water exposure. They called this reaction aquadynia and consider the disorder a variant of aquagenic pruritus. Clonidine and propranolol seemed to provide some relief.

Goodkin R, et al: Repeated PUVA treatment of aquagenic pruritus. Clin Exp Dermatol 2002; 27:164.

Ingber S, et al: Successful treatment of refractory aquagenic pruritus with naltrexone. J Cutan Med Surg 2005; 9:215.

Shelley WB, et al: Aquadynia. J Am Acad Dermatol 1998; 38:357.

Xifra A, et al: Narrow-band UVB in aquagenic pruritus. Br J Dermatol 2005; 153:1220.

Scalp pruritus

Pruritus of the scalp, especially in elderly persons, is rather common. Lack of excoriations, scaling, or erythema excludes inflammatory causes of scalp pruritus such as seborrheic dermatitis, psoriasis, dermatomyositis or lichen simplex chronicus. Most such cases remain idiopathic, but some represent chronic folliculitis. Treatment is challenging. Topical tar shampoos, salicylic acid shampoos, corticosteroid topical gels, mousse, shampoos, and liquids, and in severe cases with localized itch, an intralesional injection of corticosteroid suspension can sometimes provide relief. Minocycline or oral antihistamines may be helpful. In other patients, low doses of antidepressants, such as doxepin, are useful.

Elewski BE: Clinical diagnosis of common scalp disorders. J Investig Dermatol Symp Proc 2005; 10:190.

Hoss D, et al: Scalp dysesthesia. Arch Dermatol 1998; 134:327.

Drug-induced pruritus

Medications should be considered a possible cause of protracted pruritus with or without a skin eruption. For instance, pruritus is frequently present after opioid use. Also chloroquine and amodiaquine produce pruritus in many patients treated for malaria.

Hydroxyethyl starch (HES) is used as a volume expander, a substitute for human plasma. One-third of all patients treated will develop severe pruritus with long latency of onset (3–15 weeks) and persistence. Up to 30% of patients have localized symptoms. Antihistamines are ineffective. HES deposits are found in the skin of all patients tested, distributed in dermal macrophages, endothelial cells of blood and lymph vessels, perineural cells, endoneural macrophages of larger nerve fascicles, keratinocytes, and Langerhans cells. Substance P release from macrophages is not increased, and basophil degranulation test results are negative, suggesting that the actions of HES-induced pruritus result from the direct stimulation of cutaneous nerves.

Gall H, et al: Clinical and pathophysiological aspects of hydroxyethyl starch-induced pruritus: evaluation of 96 cases. Dermatology (Switz) 1996; 192:222.

Ganesh A, et al: Pathophysiology and management of opioid-induced pruritus. Drugs 2007; 67:2323.

Osifo NG: Chloroquine-induced pruritus among patients with malaria. Arch Dermatol 1984; 120:80.

Chronic pruritic dermatoses of unknown cause

Prurigo simplex is the preferred term for the chronic itchy idiopathic dermatosis described below. Papular dermatitis, subacute prurigo, "itchy red bump" disease, and Rosen papular eruption in black men most likely represent variations of prurigo simplex. The term prurigo continues to lack nosologic precision.

Prurigo is characterized by the lesion known as the prurigo papule, which is dome-shaped and topped with a small vesicle. The vesicle is usually present only transiently because of its immediate removal by scratching, so that a crusted papule is more frequently seen. Prurigo papules are present in various stages of development and are seen mostly in middle-aged or elderly persons of both sexes. The trunk and extensor surfaces of the extremities are favorite sites, symmetrically distributed. Other areas include the face, neck, lower trunk, and buttocks. The lesions usually appear in crops, so that papulovesicles and the late stages of scarring may be seen at the same time.

The histopathology of prurigo simplex is nonspecific, but often suggests an arthropod reaction. Spongiosis accompanied by a perivascular mononuclear infiltrate with some eosinophils is often found.

Many conditions may cause pruritic erythematous papules. Scabies, atopic dermatitis, insect bite reactions, papular urticaria, dermatitis herpetiformis, contact dermatitis, pityriasis lichenoides et varioliformis acuta (PLEVA), transient acantholytic dermatosis (TAD), papuloerythroderma of Ofuji, dermatographism, and physical urticarias should be considered. Biopsy may be helpful in differentiating dermatitis herpetiformis, PLEVA, TAD, and, on occasion, unsuspected scabies.

Treatment

The medications for initial treatment of prurigo simplex and its variants should be topical corticosteroids and oral antihistamines. Early in the disease process, moderate-strength steroids should be used; if the condition is found to be unresponsive, a change to high-potency forms is indicated. Rebound may occur. Intralesional injection of triamcinolone will eradicate individual lesions. For more recalcitrant disease, UVB or PUVA therapy may be beneficial.

Clark AR, et al: Papular dermatitis (subacute prurigo, "itchy red bump" disease). J Am Acad Dermatol 1998; 38:929.

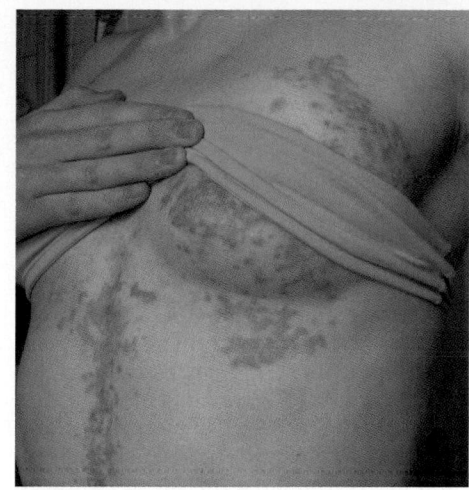

Fig. 4-7 Prurigo pigmentosa.

Streit V, et al: Foil bath PUVA in the treatment of prurigo simplex subacuta. Acta Dermatol Venereol (Norway) 1996; 76:319.

Prurigo pigmentosa

Prurigo pigmentosa is a rare dermatosis of unknown cause characterized by the sudden onset of erythematous papules or vesicles that leave reticulated hyperpigmentation when they heal (Fig. 4-7). The condition mainly affects Japanese. Only a few cases have been reported in white persons. Men outnumber women 2:1. The mean age of onset is 25. It is associated with weight loss, dieting, anorexia, diabetes, and ketonuria. It is exacerbated by heat, sweating, and friction, and thus occurs most commonly in the winter and spring. The areas most frequently involved are the upper back, nape, clavicular region, and chest. Mucous membranes are spared. Histology of early lesions shows neutrophils in the dermal papillae and epidermis. Following this, a lichenoid dermatitis with variable psoriasiform hyperplasia occurs. Direct immunofluorescence yields negative findings. The cause is unknown. Minocycline, 100–200 mg/day, is the treatment of choice. Dapsone and alteration of the diet are also effective but topical steroids are not. Recurrence and exacerbations are common.

Boer A, et al: Prurigo pigmentosa. Am J Dermatopathol 2003; 25:117.

DeGrancesco V, et al: Bullous prurigo pigmentosa. Eur J Dermatol 2006; 16:184.

Roehr P, et al: A pruritic eruption with reticular pigmentation. Arch Dermatol 1993; 129:370.

Yanguas I, et al: Prurigo pigmentosa in a white woman. J Am Acad Dermatol 1996; 35:473.

Papuloerythroderma of Ofuji

A rare disorder most commonly found in Japan, papuloerythroderma of Ofuji is characterized by pruritic papules that spare the skinfolds, producing bands of uninvolved cutis, the so-called deck-chair sign. Frequently there is associated blood eosinophilia. This condition is considered by some to be a form of erythroderma in the elderly and by others to be a paraneoplastic syndrome. Skin biopsies reveal a dense lymphohistiocytic infiltrate, eosinophils in the papillary dermis, and increased Langerhans cells. Reported malignancies include T-cell lymphomas, B-cell lymphomas, Sézary syndrome, and visceral carcinomas. Not enough cases have been reported to determine a true association with cancer. Other associations are hepatitis C infection and medication reactions to aspirin, ranitidine, and furosemide.

The differential diagnosis is the same as for prurigo simplex. Systemic steroids are the treatment of choice, and may result in long-term remissions. Topical steroids, tar derivatives, emollients, systemic retinoids, cyclosporine, and PUVA may also be therapeutic.

DeVries JH, et al: Ofuji papuloerythroderma associated with Hodgkin's lymphoma. Br J Dermatol 2002; 147:186.

Nomura T, et al: Papuloerythroderma of Ofuji associated with early gastric cancer. Int J Dermatol 2008; 47:590.

Sugita K, et al: Papuloerythroderma caused by aspirin. Arch Dermatol 2006; 142:792.

Sugita K, et al: Papuloerythroderma of Ofuji induced by furosemide. J Am Acad Dermatol 2008; 58:S554.

Lichen simplex chronicus

This is also known as circumscribed neurodermatitis. As a result of long-continued rubbing and scratching, more vigorously than a normal pain threshold would permit, the skin becomes thickened and leathery (Fig. 4-8). The normal markings of the skin become exaggerated, so that the striae form a criss-cross pattern, and between them a mosaic is produced composed of flat-topped, shiny, smooth, quadrilateral facets. This change, known as lichenification, may originate on seemingly normal skin or may develop on skin that is the site of another disease, such as atopic or allergic contact dermatitis or ringworm. Such underlying etiologies should be sought and, if found, treated specifically. Paroxysmal pruritus is the main symptom.

Circumscribed, lichenified, pruritic patches may develop on any part of the body; however, the disease has a predilection for the back and sides of the neck, and the extremities, especially the wrists and ankles. At times, the eruption is decidedly papular, resembling lichen planus; in other instances, the patches are excoriated, slightly scaly or moist, and, rarely, nodular.

Several distinctive types are recognized. Lichen simplex nuchae often occurs on the back of the neck. It is not unusual to find this area excoriated and bleeding. Nodular neurodermatitis of the scalp consists of multiple pruritic and excoriated papules and may be called prurigo of the scalp. The nodules or papules may ooze and form crusts and scales. The vulva, scrotum, and anal area can be sites of severe neurodermatitis. Genital and anal areas, however, are seldom involved at the same time. An upper eyelid, the orifice of one or both ears, or a palm or sole may also be involved; the ankle flexure is also a favorite site. Persistent rubbing of the shins or upper back may result in dermal deposits of amyloid and the subsequent development of lichen and macular amyloidosis, respectively.

To what extent mechanical trauma plays a role in producing the original irritation is not known. The onset of this dermatosis is usually gradual and insidious. Chronic scratching of a localized area is a response to unknown factors; however, stress and anxiety have long been thought important.

Treatment

Essentially, cessation of pruritus is the goal. It is important to stress the need for the patient to avoid scratching the areas involved if the sensation of itch is ameliorated. Recurrences are frequent, even after the most thorough treatment, and there are instances in which the clearance of one lesion will see the onset of another elsewhere.

High-potency agents, such as clobetasol propionate, diflorasone diacetate, or betamethasone dipropionate cream or ointment, should be used initially but not indefinitely because of the potential for steroid-induced atrophy. Occlusion of medium-potency steroids may be beneficial. Use of a steroid-containing tape to provide both occlusion and anti-inflammatory effects may have benefit. Treatment can be shifted to the use of medium- to lower-strength topical steroid creams as the lesions resolve. Topical doxepin, capsaicin, or pimecrolimus cream or tacrolimus ointment provides significant antipruritic effects and is a good adjunctive therapy. Botulinum toxin type A injection was curative in three patients within 2–4 weeks.

Intralesional injections of triamcinolone suspension, using a concentration of 5 or (with caution) 10 mg/mL, may be required. Too superficial injection invites the twin risks of epidermal and dermal atrophy and depigmentation, which may last for many months. The suspension should not be injected into infected lesions for fear of causing abscesses. In the most severe cases, complete occlusion with an Unna boot may break the cycle.

Aschoff R, et al: Topical tacrolimus for the treatment of lichen simplex chronicus. J Dermatolog Treat 2007; 18:15.

Goldstein AT, et al: Pimecrolimus cream 1% for treatment of vulvar lichen simplex chronicus. Gynecol Obstet Invest 2007: 64:180.

Heckmann M, et al: Botulinum toxin type A injection in the treatment of lichen simplex. J Am Acad Dermatol 2002; 46:617.

Lotti T, et al: Prurigo nodularis and lichen simplex chronicus. Dermatol Ther 2008; 21:42.

Prurigo nodularis

Prurigo nodularis is a disease with multiple itching nodules situated chiefly on the extremities (Fig. 4-9), especially on the anterior surfaces of the thighs and legs. A linear arrangement is common. The individual lesions are pea-sized or larger, firm, and erythematous or brownish. When fully developed, they become verrucous or fissured. The course of the disease is chronic and the lesions evolve slowly. Itching is severe but usually confined to the lesions themselves. Bouts of extreme pruritus often occur when these patients are under stress. Prurigo nodularis is one of the disorders in which the pruritus is characteristically paroxysmal: intermittent, unbearably severe, and relieved only by scratching to the point of damaging the skin, usually inducing bleeding and often scarring.

The cause of prurigo nodularis is unknown; multiple factors may contribute, including atopic dermatitis, anemia, hepatic diseases (including hepatitis C), HIV disease, pregnancy, renal failure, lymphoproliferative disease, photodermatitis, gluten enteropathy, stress, and insect bites. Pemphigoid nodularis may be confused with prurigo nodularis clinically.

The histologic findings are those of compact hyperkeratosis, irregular acanthosis, and a perivascular mononuclear cell infiltrate in the dermis. Dermal collagen may be increased, especially in the dermal papillae, and subepidermal fibrin may be seen, both evidence of excoriation. In cases associated with renal failure, transepidermal elimination of degenerated collagen may be found.

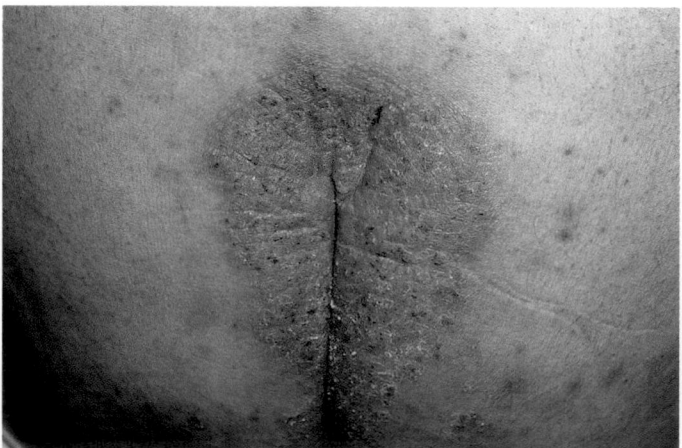

Fig. 4-8 Lichen simplex chronicus.

Treatment

Treatment is challenging. Local measures include antipruritic lotions and emollients. Administration of antihistamines, antidepressants or anxiolytics is of moderate benefit in allaying symptoms. The initial treatment of choice is intralesional or topical administration of steroids. Usually, superpotent topical products are required, but at times lower-strength preparations used with occlusion may be beneficial. The use of steroids in tape (Cordran) and prolonged occlusion with semipermeable dressings, such as are used for treating non-healing wounds, can be useful in limited areas. Intralesional steroids will usually eradicate individual lesions, but unfortunately many patients have too extensive disease for these local measures. PUVA has also been shown to be effective in some cases. Vitamin D_3 ointment, calcipotriene ointment, or tacrolimus ointment applied topically twice a day may be therapeutic and steroid-sparing. Isotretinoin, 1 mg/kg/day for 2–5 months, may benefit some patients.

Good results have been obtained with thalidomide and cyclosporine. With thalidomide the onset may be rapid or slow and sedation may occur. The initial dose is 100 mg/day, titered to the lowest dose required. Patients treated with thalidomide are at risk of developing a dose-dependent neuropathy at cumulative doses of 40–50 g. Combination therapy with sequential UVB and thalidomide may be better than either alone. Cyclosporine at doses of 3–4.5 mg/kg/day has also been shown to be effective in treating recalcitrant disease. Cryotherapy has been used adjunctively.

Alfadley A, et al: Treatment of prurigo nodularis with thalidomide. Int J Dermatol 2003; 42:372.

Berth-Jones J, et al: Nodular prurigo responds to cyclosporin. Br J Dermatol 1995; 132:795.

Lee MR, et al: Prurigo nodularis. Austral J Dermatol 2005; 46:211.

Lotti T, et al: Prurigo nodularis and lichen simplex chronicus. Dermatol Ther 2008; 21:42.

Matthews SN, et al: Prurigo nodularis in HIV-infected individuals. Int J Dermatol 1998; 37:401.

Neri S, et al: Hyde's prurigo nodularis and chronic HCV hepatitis. J Hepatol 1998; 28:161.

Setoyama M, et al: Prurigo as a clinical prodrome to adult T-cell leukaemia/lymphoma. Br J Dermatol 1998; 138:137.

Wong S-S, et al: Double-blind, right/left comparison of calcipotriol ointment and betamethasone ointment in the treatment of prurigo nodularis. Arch Dermatol 2000; 36:807.

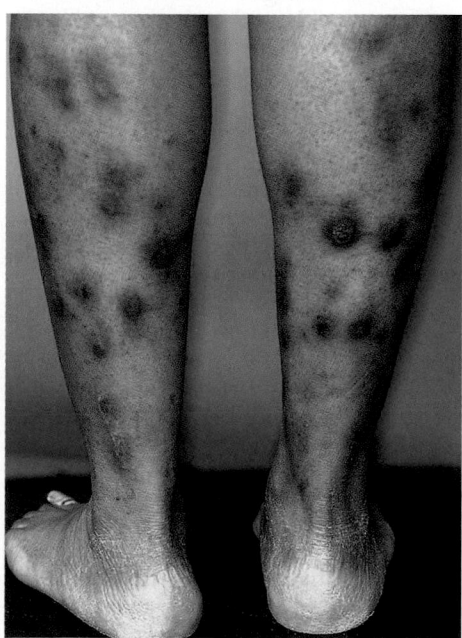

Fig. 4-9 Prurigo nodularis. (Courtesy of Lawrence Lieblich, MD)

Psychodermatology

There are purely cutaneous disorders that are psychiatric in nature, their cause being directly related to psychopathologic causes in the absence of primary dermatologic or other organic causes. Delusions of parasitosis, neurotic excoriations, factitial dermatitis, and trichotillomania compose the major categories of psychodermatology. The differential diagnosis for these four disorders is two-fold, requiring the exclusion of organic causes and the definition of a potential underlying psychologic disorder. Other delusional disorders include bromidrosiphobia and body dysmorphic disorder.

Psychosis is characterized by the presence of delusional ideation, which is defined as a fixed misbelief that is not shared by the patient's subculture. Monosymptomatic hypochondriacal disorder is a form of psychosis characterized by delusions regarding a particular hypochondriacal concern. In contrast to schizophrenia, there are no other mental deficits, such as auditory hallucination, loss of interpersonal skills, or presence of other inappropriate actions. Patients with monosymptomatic hypochondriacal psychosis often function appropriately in social settings, except for a single fixated belief that there is a serious problem with their skin or other parts of their body.

Buljan D, et al: Psychodermatology. Psychiatr Danub 2005; 17:76.

Elmer KB, et al: Therapeutic update: use of risperidone for the treatment of monosymptomatic hypochondriacal psychosis. J Am Acad Dermatol 2000; 43:683.

Fried RG: Nonpharmacologic treatments in psychodermatology. Dermatol Clin 2002; 20:177.

Koblenzer CS: Psychotropic drugs in dermatology. Adv Dermatol 2000; 15:183.

Lorenzo R, et al: Pimozide in dermatologic practice. Am J Clin Dermatol 2004; 5:339.

Poot F, et al: Basic knowledge in psychodermatology. J Eur Acad Dermatol Venereol 2007; 21:227.

Tennyson H, et al: Neurotropic and psychotropic drugs in dermatology. Dermatol Clin 2001; 19:179.

Walling HW, et al: Psychocutaneous syndromes. Clin Exper Dermatol 2007; 32:317.

Skin signs of psychiatric illness

The skin is a frequent target for the release of emotional tension. Self-injury by prolonged, compulsive repetitious acts may produce various mutilations, depending on the act and site of injury.

Self-biting may be manifested by biting the nails (onychophagia) (Fig. 4-10), skin (most frequently the forearms, hands, and fingers) and lip. Dermatophagia is a habit or

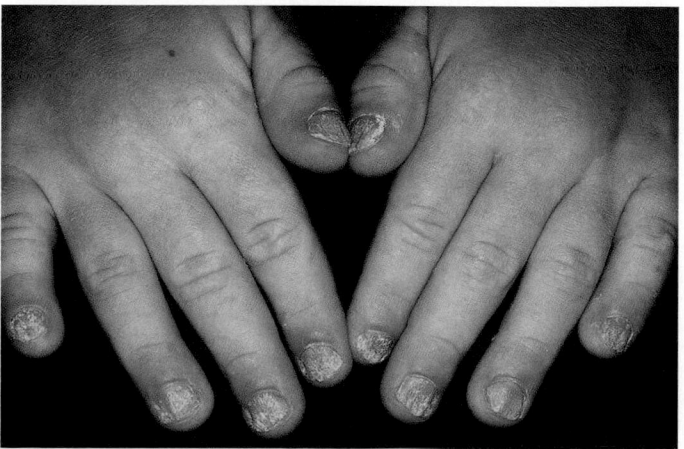

Fig. 4-10 Onychophagia. (Courtesy of Curt Samlaska, MD)

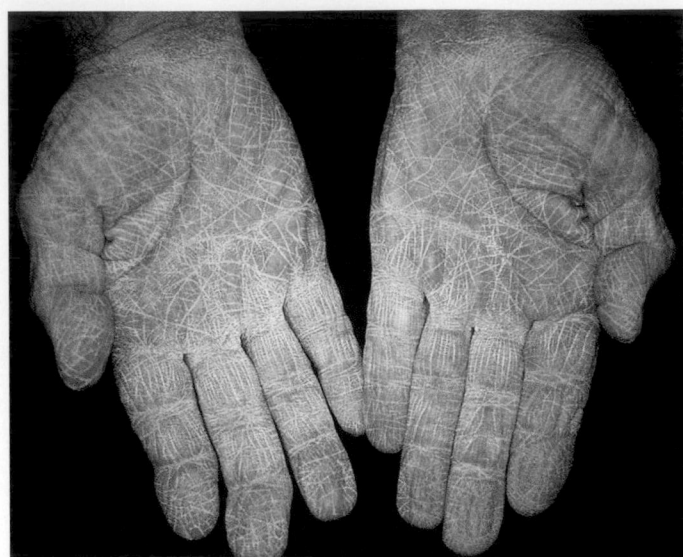

Fig. 4-11 Irritant dermatitis from chronic handwashing.

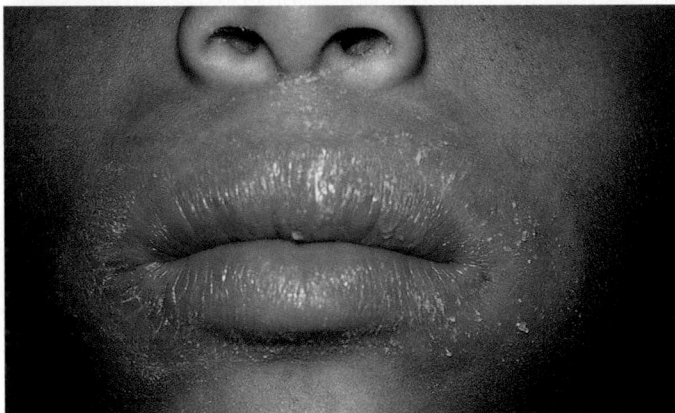

Fig. 4-12 Dermatitis caused by lip-licking.

compulsion, which may be conscious or subconscious. Bumping of the head produces lacerations and contusions, which may be so severe as to produce cranial defects and life-threatening complications. Compulsive repetitive handwashing may produce an irritant dermatitis of the hands (Fig. 4-11).

Bulimia, with its self-induced vomiting, results in Russell's sign—crusted papules on the dorsum of the dominant hand from cuts by the teeth. Clenching of the hand produces swelling and ecchymosis of the fingertips and subungual hemorrhage. Self-inflicted lacerations may be of suicidal intent. Lip-licking produces increased salivation and thickening of the lips. Eventually the perioral area becomes red and produces a distinctive picture resembling the exaggerated mouth make-up of a clown (Fig. 4-12). Pressure produced by binding the waistline tightly with a cord will eventually lead to atrophy of the subcutaneous tissue.

Psychopharmacologic agents, especially the newer atypical antipsychotic agents, and behavioral therapy alone or in combination with these agents are the treatments of choice.

Strumia R: Dermatologic signs in patients with eating disorders. Am J Clin Dermatol 2005; 6:165.

Delusions of parasitosis

Delusions of parasitosis (delusional parasitosis, Ekbom syndrome, acarophobia, dermatophobia, parasitophobia, entomo-

phobia, or pseudoparasitic dysesthesia) are firm fixations in a person's mind that he or she suffers from a parasitic infestation of the skin. At times close contacts may share the delusion. The belief is so fixed that the patient may pick small pieces of epithelial debris from the skin and bring them to be examined, always insisting that the offending parasite is contained in such material. Samples of alleged parasites enclosed in assorted containers, paper tissue, or sandwiched between adhesive tape are so characteristic that it is referred to as the "matchbox sign." Usually, the only symptom is pruritus or a stinging, biting, or crawling sensation. Intranasal formication, or a crawling sensation of the nasal mucosa, is common in this condition. Cutaneous findings may range from none to excoriations, prurigo nodularis, and frank ulcerations.

Frequently, these patients have paranoid tendencies. Women are affected 2:1 over men, often during middle or old age. The condition has been reported to be associated with schizophrenia, bipolar disorders, depression, anxiety disorders, and obsessional states, but is usually a monosymptomatic hypochondriacal disorder. A variety of organic causes have been suggested, including cocaine and amphetamine abuse, dementia, malignancies, cerebrovascular disease, multiple sclerosis, and vitamin B_{12} deficiency. Some of these may produce cutaneous symptoms, particularly pruritus, which may contribute to the delusion.

The differential diagnosis is influenced by the cutaneous findings and history. Initial steps should be directed at excluding a true infestation, such as scabies, or an organic cause. A thorough history, particularly in reference to therapeutic and recreational drug use (amphetamines and cocaine), review of systems, and physical examination should be performed. Morgellons disease is considered by many simply to be another name for delusions of parasitosis. Patients complain of crawling, biting, burning or other sensations which cause them to be intensely anxious. Often granules or fibers are provided by the patient for analysis. Many patients have associated psychiatric conditions.

A skin biopsy is frequently performed, more to reassure the patient than to uncover occult skin disease. Screening laboratory tests to exclude systemic disorders should be obtained: a CBC, urinalysis (UA), liver function tests (LFTs), thyroid function tests (TFTs), iron studies, and serum B_{12}, folate, and electrolyte levels. Multiple sclerosis may present with dysesthesia, which may at times be mistaken for infestation. Once organic causes have been eliminated, the patient should be evaluated to determine the cause of the delusions. Schizophrenia, monosymptomatic hypochondriacal psychosis, psychotic depression, dementia, and depression with somatization are considerations in the differential diagnosis.

Management of this difficult problem varies. While referral to a psychiatrist may be considered best for the patient, most frequently the patient will reject suggestions to seek psychiatric help. The dermatologist is cautioned against confronting the patient with the psychogenic nature of the disease. It is preferable to develop trust, which will usually require several visits. If pharmacologic treatment is undertaken, the patient may accept it if the medication is presented as one which will alter the perception of this bothersome sensation. Pimozide was the long-standing treatment of choice, but is associated with a variety of side effects, including stiffness, restlessness, prolongation of the Q–T interval, and extrapyramidal signs. Patients often respond to relatively low dosages, in the 1–4 mg range, which limits these problems. Pimozide is an antipsychotic medication approved for the treatment of Tourette syndrome and patients should understand the labeling prior to obtaining the drug. Newer atypical antipsychotic agents, such as risperidone, and olanzapine, have fewer side effects and are now considered the appropriate first-line agents for the treatment of delusions of parasitosis. With appropriate pharmacologic intervention it is likely that 25–50% of patients will remit.

Accordino RE, et al: Morgellons disease? Dermatol Ther 2008; 21:8.

Aw DC, et al: Delusional parasitosis. Ann Acad Med Singapore 2004; 13:89.

Friedman AC, et al: Delusional parasitosis presenting as folie à trois. Br J Dermatol 2006; 155:841.

Koblenzer CS: The challenge of Morgellons disease. J Am Acad Dermatol 2006; 55:920.

Koo J, et al: Delusions of parasitosis. Am J Clin Dermatol 2001; 2:285

Lepping P, et al: Antipsychotic treatment of primary delusional parasitosis: systematic review. Br J Psychiatry 2007; 191:198.

Meehan WJ, et al: Successful treatment of delusions of parasitosis with olanzapine. Arch Dermatol 2006; 142:352.

Nicolato R, et al: Delusional parasitosis or Ekbom syndrome. Gen Hospital Psychiatr 2006; 28:78.

Walling HW, et al: Intranasal formication correlates with diagnosis of delusions of parasitosis. J Am Acad Dermatol 2008; 58:S35.

Neurotic excoriations

Many persons have unconscious compulsive habits of picking at themselves, and at times the tendency is so persistent and pronounced that excoriations of the skin are produced. The lesions are caused by picking, digging, or scraping, and they usually occur on parts readily accessible to the hands. These patients admit their actions induce the lesions, but cannot control their behavior.

The excavations may be superficial or deep and are often linear. The bases of the ulcers are clean or covered with a scab. Right-handed persons tend to produce lesions on their left side and left-handed persons on their right side. There is evidence of past healed lesions, usually with linear scars, or rounded hyper- or hypopigmented lesions, in the area of the active excoriations. The face, upper arms, and upper back (Fig. 4-13) are favorite sites for these excoriations. Sometimes the focus is on acne lesions, producing acne excoriée.

Most of these patients are otherwise healthy adults. They usually lead normal lives. The organic differential diagnosis is vast and includes any condition that may manifest with excoriations. The most common psychopathologies associated with neurotic excoriations are depression, obsessive–compulsive disorder, and anxiety.

The treatment of choice is doxepin because of its antidepressant and antipruritic effects; doses are slowly increased to 100 mg or higher, if tolerated. Many alternatives to doxepin may be indicated, especially in those affected by an obsessive–compulsive component. These include clomipramine, paroxetine, fluoxetine, and sertraline. Other drugs with utility include

desipramine, buspirone, and quick-acting benzodiazepines. Treatment is difficult, often requiring a combined psychiatric and pharmacologic intervention. It is important to establish a constructive patient–therapist alliance. Training in diversion strategies during "scratching episodes" may be helpful. An attempt should be made to identify specific conflicts or stressors preceding onset. The therapist should concentrate on systematic training directed at the behavioral reaction pattern. There should be support and advice given with regard to the patient's social situation and interpersonal relations.

Arnold LM, et al: Psychogenic excoriation. CNS Drugs 2001; 15:351.

Mustasim DF, et al: The psychiatric profile of patients with psychogenic excoriation. J Am Acad Dermatol 2009; 61:611.

Factitious dermatitis (dermatitis artefacta)

Factitious dermatitis is the term applied to self-inflicted skin lesions made consciously and often with the intent to elicit sympathy, escape responsibilities, or collect disability insurance (Fig. 4-14). Most patients are adults in midlife, with women more often affected than men by a 3:1 ratio. The vast majority have multiple lesions and are unemployed or on sick leave. These skin lesions are provoked by mechanical means or by the application or injection of chemical irritants and caustics. The lesions may simulate other dermatoses but usually have a distinctive, geometric, bizarre appearance (Fig. 4-15), whose shape and arrangement frequently are not encountered in any other affection. The lesions are generally distributed on parts easily reached by the hands and have a

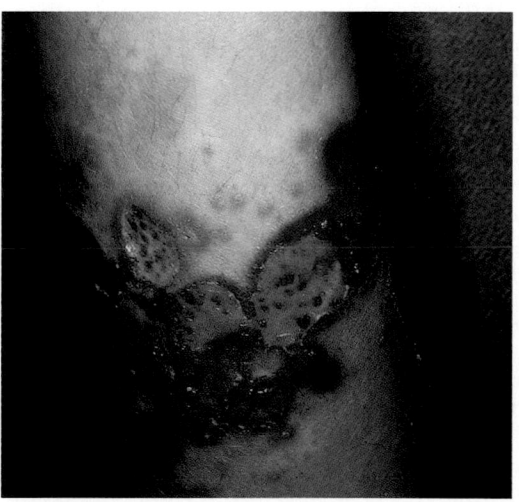

Fig. 4-14 Cigarette burns.

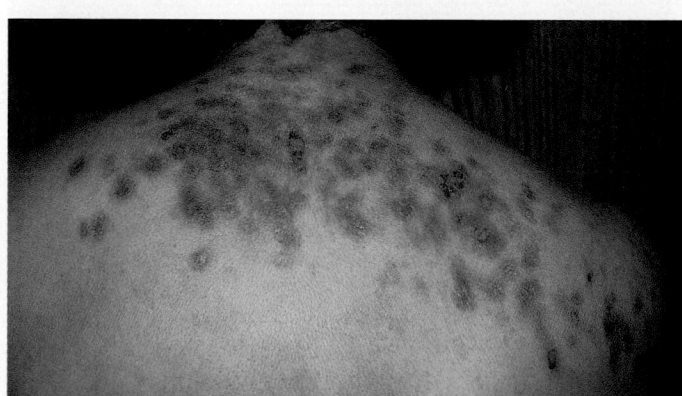

Fig. 4-13 Neurotic excoriations. (Courtesy of Lawrence Lieblich, MD)

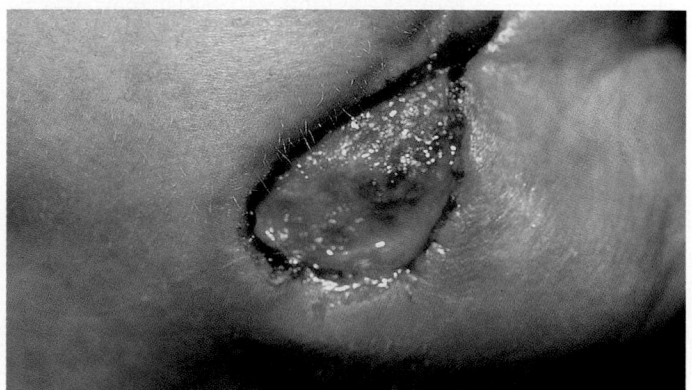

Fig. 4-15 Factitial ulcers.

tendency to be linear and arranged regularly and symmetrically. They are rarely seen on the right hand, right wrist or right arm unless the patient is left-handed.

When chemicals are used, red streaks or guttate marks are often seen beneath the principal patch, where drops of the chemical have accidentally run or fallen on the skin. According to the manner of production, the lesions may be erythematous, vesicular, bullous, ulcerative, or gangrenous. The more common agents of destruction used are the fingernails, pointed instruments, hot metal; chemicals such as carbolic, nitric, or acetic acid; caustic potash or soda, turpentine, table salt, urine, and feces. The lesions are likely to appear in crops. At times the only sign may be the indefinitely delayed healing of an operative wound, which is purposely kept open by the patient. Tight cords or clothing tied around an arm or leg may produce factitious lymphedema, which may be mistaken for postphlebitic syndrome or nerve injury, as well as other forms of chronic lymphedema.

Subcutaneous emphysema, manifesting as cutaneous crepitations, may be factitial in origin. Recurrent migratory subcutaneous emphysema involving the extremities, neck, chest, or face can be induced through injections of air into tissue with a needle and syringe. Circular pockets and bilateral involvement without physical findings that suggest a contiguous spread from a single source suggest a factitial origin. Puncturing the buccal mucosa through to facial skin with a needle and puffing out the cheeks can produce alarming results. Neck and shoulder crepitation is also a complication in manic patients that results from hyperventilation and breath-holding.

The organic differential diagnosis depends on the cutaneous signs manifested (e.g. gas gangrene for patients with factitious subcutaneous emphysema, and the various forms of lymphedema for factitious lymphedema). Considerations for psychopathology include malingering, borderline personality disorders, and psychosis.

Proof of diagnosis is sometimes difficult. Occlusive dressings may be necessary to protect the lesions from ready access by the patient. It is usually best not to reveal any suspicion of the cause to the patient and to establish the diagnosis definitely without the patient's knowledge. If the patient is hospitalized, a resourceful, cooperative nurse may be useful in helping to establish the diagnosis. When injection of foreign material is suspected, examination of biopsy material by spectroscopy may reveal talc or other foreign material.

Treatment should ideally involve psychotherapy, but most frequently the patient promptly rejects the suggestion and goes to another physician to seek a new round of treatment. It is best for the dermatologist to maintain a close relationship with the patient and provide symptomatic therapy and nonjudgmental support. Pimozide or atypical antipsychotic agents in low dose have been used with some success. High doses of selective serotonin reuptake inhibitors (SSRIs) may also be beneficial. Consultation with an experienced psychiatrist is prudent.

Angus J, et al: Dermatitis artefacta in a 12-year-old girl mimicking CTCL. Pediatr Dermatol 2007; 24:327.

Finore ED, et al: Dermatitis artefacta in a child. Pediatr Dermatol 2007; 24:E51.

Heydendael VMR, et al: Acute blue patch on the forearm. Arch Dermatol 2007; 143:937.

Nielsen K, et al: Self-inflicted skin diseases. Acta Derm Venereol 2005; 85:512.

Koblenzer CS: Dermatitis artefacta. Am J Clin Dermatol 2000; 1:47.

Koo J, et al: Delusions of parasitosis. Am J Clin Dermatol 2001; 2:285.

Shah KN, et al: Facticial dermatoses in children. Curr Opin Pediatr 2006; 18:403.

Ugurlu S, et al: Factitious disease of periocular and facial skin. Am J Ophthalmol 1999; 127:196.

Trichotillomania

Trichotillomania (trichotillosis or neuromechanical alopecia) is a neurosis characterized by an abnormal urge to pull out the hair. The sites involved are generally the frontal region of the scalp, eyebrows, eyelashes, and the beard. There are irregular areas of hair loss, which may be linear or bizarrely shaped. Uncommonly, adults may pull out pubic hair. The classic presentation is the "Friar Tuck" form of vertex and crown alopecia. Hairs are broken and show differences in length (Fig. 4-16). The pulled hair may be ingested and occasionally the trichobezoar will cause obstruction. When the tail extends from the main mass in the stomach to the small or large intestine, Rapunzel syndrome is the diagnosis. The nails may show evidence of onychophagy (nail biting), but no pits are present. The disease is seven times more common in children than in adults, and girls are affected 2.5 times more often than boys.

This disease often develops in the setting of psychosocial stress in the family, which may revolve around school problems, sibling rivalry, moving to a new house, hospitalization of a parent, or a disturbed parent–child relationship.

Differentiation from alopecia areata is possible because of the varying lengths of broken hairs present, the absence of nail pitting, and the microscopic appearance of the twisted or broken hairs as opposed to the tapered fractures of alopecia areata. Other organic disorders to consider are androgenic alopecia, tinea capitis, monilethrix, pili torti, pseudopelade of Brocq, traction alopecia, syphilis, nutritional deficiencies, and systemic disorders such as lupus and lymphoma. If necessary, a biopsy can be performed and is usually quite helpful. It reveals traumatized hair follicles with perifollicular hemorrhage, fragmented hair in the dermis, empty follicles, and deformed hair shafts (trichomalacia). Multiple catagen hairs are typically seen. An alternative technique to biopsy, particularly for children, is to shave a part of the involved area and observe for regrowth of normal hairs. The differential diagnosis for underlying psychopathology is obsessive–compulsive disorder (most common), depression, and anxiety.

In children the diagnosis should be addressed openly, and referral to a child psychiatrist for behavioral therapy should be encouraged. In adults with the problem, psychiatric impairment may be severe. Pharmacotherapy with clomipramine was found most effective of the studied medications, but

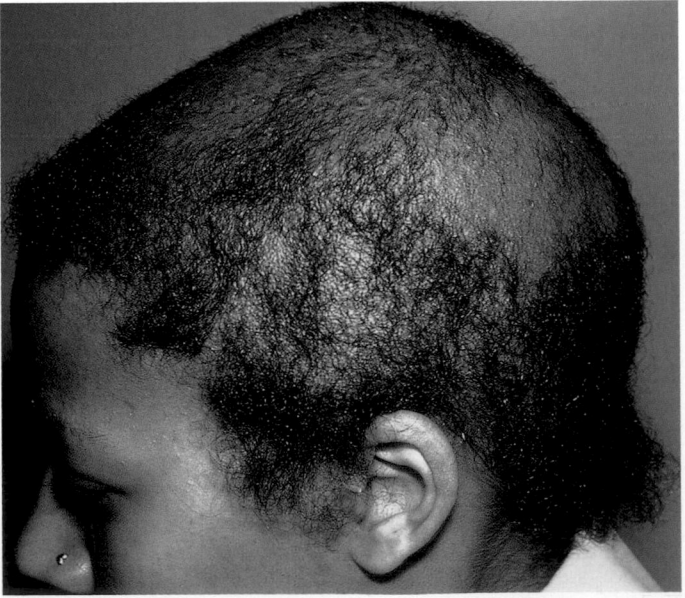

Fig. 4-16 Trichotillomania.

fluoxetine, venlafaxine, and olanzapine have proven effective in some patients. Trichobezoars require surgical removal.

Bergeld W, et al: The combined utilization of clinical and histological findings in the diagnosis of trichotillomania. J Cutan Pathol 2002; 29:207.

Bloch MH, et al: Systematic review: pharmacological and behavioral treatment for trichotillomania. Biol Psychiatry 2007; 62:839.

Hautmann G, et al: Trichotillomania. J Am Acad Dermatol 2002; 46:807.

Keuthen NJ, et al: Retrospective review of treatment outcome for 63 patients with trichotillomania. Am J Psychiatry 1998; 155:560.

Shegal VN, et al: Trichotillomania ± trichobezoar. J Eur Acad Dermatol Venereol 2006: 20:911.

Tay YK, et al: Trichotillomania in childhood. Pediatrics 2004; 113:e494.

Walsh KH, et al: Trichotillomania. Am J Clin Dermatol 2001; 2:327.

Dermatothlasia

Dermatothlasia is a cutaneous neurosis characterized by a patient's uncontrollable desire to rub or pinch themselves to form bruised areas on the skin, sometimes as a defense against pain elsewhere.

Bromidrosiphobia

Bromidrosiphobia (delusions of bromhidrosis) is a monosymptomatic delusional state in which a person is convinced that his or her sweat has a repugnant odor that keeps other people away. The patient is unable to accept any evidence to the contrary. Three-quarters of patients with bromidrosiphobia are male, with an average age of 25. Atypical antipsychotic agents or pimozide may be beneficial. It may be an early symptom of schizophrenia.

Body dysmorphic disorder (dysmorphic syndrome, dysmorphophobia)

Body dysmorphic disorder is the delusion of having an ugly body part. It is most common in young adults of either sex. The concern is frequently centered about the nose, mouth, genitalia, breasts, or hair. Objective evaluation will reveal a normal appearance or slight defect. Patients may manifest obsessional features, spending large amounts of time inspecting the area. Depression may present a risk of suicide. Therapy with SSRIs may help those who manifest this obsessive-compulsive disease. Those more severely affected have delusions that may lead to requests for repeated surgeries of the site, and require antipsychotic medications.

Albertini RS, et al: Thirty-three cases of body dysmorphic disorder in children and adolescents. J Am Acad Child Adolesc Psychiatry 1999; 38:453.

Cotterill JA: Body dysmorphic disorder. Dermatol Clin 1996; 14:457.

Mackley CL: Body dysmorphic disorder. Dermatol Surg 2005; 31:S53.

Phillips KA, et al: Body dysmorphic disorder. A guide for dermatologists and cosmetic surgeons. Am J Clin Dermatol 2000; 1:235.

Neurocutaneous dermatoses

Scalp dysesthesia

Cutaneous dysesthesia syndromes are characterized by pain and burning sensations without objective findings. Many patients report coexisting pruritus or transient pruritus associated with the dysesthesia. Scalp dysesthesia occurs primarily in middle-aged to elderly women. A psychiatric cause or overlay is frequently associated and treatment with low-dose antidepressants is often helpful.

Hoss D, et al: Scalp dysesthesia. Arch Dermatol 1998; 134:327.

Burning mouth syndrome (glossodynia, burning tongue)

Burning mouth syndrome (BMS) is divided into two forms: a primary type characterized by a burning sensation of the oral mucosa without a dental or medical cause, and secondary BMS. A number of conditions, such as lichen planus, candidiasis, vitamin or nutritional deficiencies such as low B_{12}, iron or folate, hypoestrogenism, parafunctional habits, diabetes, dry mouth, contact allergies, cranial nerve injuries, and medication side effects, may cause secondary BMS. Identification of such underlying conditions and treatment directed at them will result in relief of secondary BMS.

Primary BMS occurs most commonly in postmenopausal women. They are particularly prone to a feeling of burning of the tongue, mouth, and lips, with no objective findings. Symptoms vary in severity but are more or less constant. Patients with burning mouth syndrome often complain that multiple oral sites are involved. Management with topical applications of clonazepam, capsaicin, doxepin, or lidocaine can help. Oral administration of α-lipoic acid, SSRIs or tricyclic antidepressants, amisulpride, anticonvulsants, or benzodiazepines has been reported to be effective. The most commonly used, best studied, and most often successful therapy is provided by the antidepressant medications, and many patients have other symptoms of depression as well.

Burning lips syndrome may be a separate entity; it appears to affect both men and women equally and occurs in individuals between the ages of 50 and 70 years. The labial mucosa may be smooth and pale, and the minor salivary glands of the lips are frequently dysfunctional. Treatment with α-lipoic acid showed improvement in 2 months in a double-blind controlled study.

Drage LA, et al: Burning mouth syndrome. Dermatol Clin 2003; 21:135.

Minguez Serra MO, et al: Pharmacological treatment of burning mouth syndrome. Med Oral Patol Oral Cir Buchal 2007; 12:E299.

Patton LL, et al: Management of burning mouth syndrome. Oral Surg Oral Med Oral Pathol Oral Radio Endod 2007; 103:S39.e1

Sardella A: An up-to-date view on burning mouth syndrome. Minerva Stomatol 2007; 56:327.

Zakrzewska JM, et al: Interventions for the treatment of burning mouth syndrome. Cochrane Database Syst Rev 2005; 25:CD002779.

Vulvodynia

Vulvodynia is defined as vulvar discomfort, usually described as burning pain, occurring without medical findings. It is chronic, defined as lasting 3 months or longer. Two subtypes are seen, the localized and generalized subsets. Both may occur only when provoked by physical contact, as a spontaneous pain, or mixed in type. Vulvar pain secondary to many underlying disorders may occur, but when candidal infections, endometriosis, neoplastic conditions, referred pain from myalgic muscles, contact dermatitis, hypoestrogenism, neurologic etiologies, or prior radiotherapy are the cause, these are treated appropriately and the patient's condition is not categorized as vulvodynia.

The typical patient is a nulligravid married woman in her late thirties. Up to 15% of women seen in some gynecologic practices may be affected. Dyspareunia may completely prevent sexual intercourse. This problem and the chronic pain may lead to compromise of interpersonal relations. They may be exacerbated by stress, depression, or anxiety, or may lead to such conditions over time. A male counterpart may be seen and has been called the burning genital skin syndrome or dysesthetic peno-/scrotodynia.

Treatment should always include patient education and psychological support. Topical anesthetics and lubricants, such as petrolatum, applied before intercourse may be tried initially. Elimination of irritants, treatment of atopy with topical tacrolimus (allowing for the discontinuance of topical steroids which have usually been tried without success), and the use of antihistamines for dermatographism may be helpful. Vulvodynia is considered among the chronic pain syndromes that can have a psychological impact. Treatment then centers on the use of tricyclic and SSRI antidepressants, and neuroleptics, chiefly gabapentin or pregabalin. Other interventions such as botulinum toxin A, montelukast, and surgery may be considered in individual cases, but the evidence for any of the above therapies is limited.

Bachmann GA, et al: Vulvodynia. J Reprod Med 2006; 51:447.

Gunter J: Vulvodynia. Obstet Gynecol Surv 2007; 62:812.

Harris G, et al: Evaluation of gabapentin in the treatment of generalized vulvodynia, unprovoked. J Reprod Med 2007; 52:103.

Hoffstetter S, et al. Vulvodynia. Mo Med 2007; 104:522.

Jerome L: Pregabalin-induced remission in a 62-year-old woman with a 20-year history of vulvodynia. Pain Res Manag 2007; 12:212.

Kamdar N, et al: Improvement in vulvar vestibulitis with montelukast. J Reprod Med 2007, 52:912.

Markos AR: The male genital skin burning syndrome. Int J STD AIDS 2002; 13:271.

Reed BD, et al: Treatment of vulvodynia with tricyclic antidepressants. J Low Genit Tract Dis 2006; 10:245.

Sadownick LA: Clinical profile of vulvodynia patients. J Reprod Med 2000; 45:679.

Trebo MJ, et al: Clinical characteristics and psychopathological profile of patients with vulvodynia. Dermatology 2008; 216:24.

Yoon H, et al: Botulinum toxin A for the management of vulvodynia. Int J Impot Res 2007; 19:84.

Notalgia paresthetica

Notalgia paresthetica is a unilateral sensory neuropathy characterized by infrascapular pruritus, burning pain, hyperalgesia, and tenderness, often in the distribution of the second to sixth thoracic spinal nerves. A pigmented patch localized to the area of pruritus is often found. This is due to postinflammatory change. Macular amyloidosis may be produced by chronic scratching. In the majority of cases, degenerative changes in the corresponding vertebrae leading to spinal nerve impingement are seen.

Topical capsaicin has been shown to be effective; however, relapse occurs in most patients within 4 weeks of discontinuing its use. The area of involvement may be injected intradermally with 4 U of botulinum toxin type A spaced 2 cm apart. Excellent long-term results may occur and injections may be repeated as necessary. The topical lidocaine patch may provide relief. Paravertebral blocks, oxycarbazepine, ultrasound, and physiotherapy are useful interventions when a structural change in the vertebrae is found to be the cause.

Goulden V, et al: Successful treatment of notalgia paresthetica with a paravertebral local anesthetic block. J Am Acad Dermatol 1998; 38:114.

Savk E, et al: Investigation of spinal pathology in notalgia paresthetica. J Am Acad Dermatol 2005; 52:1085.

Wallengren J: Successful treatment of notalgia paresthetica with topical capsaicin: vehicle-blind, crossover study. J Am Acad Dermatol 1995; 32:287.

Weinfeld PK, et al: Successful treatment of notalgia paresthetica with botulinum toxin type A. Arch Dermatol 2007; 143:980.

Wisenberg E, et al: Notalgia paresthetica associated with nerve root impingement. J Am Acad Dermatol 1997; 37:998.

Brachioradial pruritus

This condition is characterized by itching localized to the brachioradial area of the arm. To relieve the burning, stinging, or even painful quality of the itch, patients will frequently use ice packs. Cervical spine pathology is frequently found on radiographic evaluation. Searching for causes of the abnormality should include discussion of spinal injury, such as trauma, arthritis, or chronic repetitive microtrauma, whiplash injury, or assessment for a tumor in the cervical spinal column. Patients often present in the spring and report that UV light precipitates the pruritus. Cervical spine disease may then be a predisposing factor, with sunlight the eliciting factor.

Interventions of value include gabapentin, carbamazepine, topical capsaicin, cervical spine manipulation, neck traction, anti-inflammatory medications, physical therapy, or surgical resection of a cervical rib.

Bernhard JD, et al: The ice-pack sign in brachioradial pruritus. J Am Acad Dermatol 2005; 52:1073.

Cohen AD, et al: Brachioradial pruritus. J Am Acad Dermatol 2003; 48:825.

Kanitakis JK: Brachioradial pruritus. Eur J Dermatol 2006; 16:311.

Wallengren J, et al: Brachioradial pruritus is associated with a reduction in cutaneous innervation that normalizes during the symptom-free remissions. J Am Acad Dermatol 2005; 52:142.

Meralgia paresthetica (Roth–Bernhardt disease)

This affection is a variety of paresthesia, with persistent numbness and periodic transient episodes of burning or lancinating pain on the anterolateral surface of the thigh. The lateral femoral cutaneous nerve innervates this area and is subject to entrapment and compression along its course. Sensory mononeuropathies besides notalgia and meralgia paresthetica include mental and intercostal neuropathy and cheiralgia, gonyalgia, and digitalgia paresthetica.

Meralgia paresthetica occurs most frequently in middle-aged, obese men. Alopecia localized to the area innervated by the lateral femoral nerve may be a skin sign of this disease. External compression may occur from tight-fitting clothing, cell phones or other heavy objects in the pockets or worn on belts, or seat-belt injuries from automobile accidents. Internal compression from arthritis of the lumbar vertebrae, a herniated disk, pregnancy, intra-abdominal disease that increases intrapelvic pressure, iliac crest bone graft harvesting, diabetes, neuroma, and rarely, a lumbar spine or pelvic tumor have been reported causes in individual cases.

The diagnostic test of choice is somatosensory evoked potentials of the lateral femoral cutaneous nerve. Local anesthetics, such as use of a lidocaine patch, nonsteroidal anti-inflammatories, rest, and avoidance of aggravating factors may lead to improvement. Gabapentin is useful in various neuropathic pain disorders. If such interventions fail and a nerve block rapidly relieves symptoms, then local infiltration with corticosteroids is indicated. Surgical decompression of the lateral femoral cutaneous nerve can produce good to excellent outcomes, but should be reserved for patients with intractable symptoms who responded to nerve blocks but not corticosteroids. If the nerve block does not result in symptom relief, CT scans of the lumbar spine and pelvic and lower abdominal ultrasound examinations to assess for tumors are indicated.

Devers A, et al: Topical lidocaine patch relieves a variety of neuropathic pain conditions. Clin J Pain 2000; 16:205.

Haim A, et al: Meralgia paresthetica. Acta Orthop 2006; 77:482.

Harney D, et al: Meralgia paresthetica. Pain Med 2007; 8:669.

Complex regional pain syndrome

Encompassing the descriptors reflex sympathetic dystrophy, causalgia, neuropathic pain, and Sudek syndrome, complex regional pain syndrome (CRPS) is characterized by burning pain, hyperesthesia, and trophic disturbances resulting from injury to a peripheral nerve. It most commonly occurs in one of the upper extremities, although leg involvement is frequent. The most common symptom is burning pain aggravated by movement or friction. The skin of the involved extremity becomes shiny, cold, and atrophic, and may profusely perspire. Additional cutaneous manifestations include bullae, erosions, edema, telangiectases, hyperpigmentation, ulcerations, and brownish-red patches with linear fissures (Fig. 4-17).

The intensity of the pain varies from trivial burning to a state of torture accompanied by extreme hyperesthesia and, frequently, hyperhidrosis. The part not only is subject to an intense burning sensation, but also a touch or a tap of the finger causes exquisite pain. Exposure to the air is avoided with a care that seems absurd, and the patient walks carefully, carrying the limb tenderly with the sound hand. Patients are tremulous and apprehensive, and keep the hand constantly wet, finding relief in the moisture rather than in the temperature of the application. A condition resembling permanent chilblains or even trophic ulcers may be present.

CRPS usually begins with severe, localized, burning pain, focal edema, muscle spasm, stiffness or restricted mobility, and vasospasm affecting skin color and temperature. This may be followed by a diffusion of the pain and edema, diminished hair growth, brittle nails, joint thickening, and onset of muscle atrophy. Finally, irreversible trophic changes, intractable pain involving the entire limb, flexor contractures, marked atrophy of the muscles, severe limitation in joint and limb mobility, and severe osteoporosis result.

There may be a precipitating event, such as a crush injury, laceration, fracture, sprain, burn, or surgery that produces some degree of soft-tissue or nerve complex injury. Causes include fractures, peripheral revascularization of the extremities, hypothermic insult, myocardial infarction, peripheral nerve injury, and multiple sclerosis. Associations with Munchausen syndrome and factitial ulcerations have also been reported.

Not all patients will have all of the features of CRPS, and an early diagnosis improves the chance of cure. The five major components are pain, edema, dysregulation of autonomic function, alterations in motor function, and dystrophic changes. A three-phase technetium bone scan is helpful in confirming the diagnosis of CRPS in patients who fail to meet all five of these criteria.

Consultation with a neurologist or an anesthesiologist specializing in pain is advisable. Osteoporosis is a frequent complication, and studies using pamidronate, a powerful inhibitor of bone absorption, have been shown to improve symptoms of pain, tenderness, and swelling significantly. Tricyclic antidepressants and antipsychotic agents are often helpful. Transcutaneous electrical nerve stimulation and deep brain stimulation may also be useful. Paravertebral block or sympathectomy is most effective, but not without potential complications.

Birklein F: Complex regional pain syndrome. J Neurol 2005; 252:131.
Koblenzer CS, et al: Chronic cutaneous dysesthesia syndrome: a psychotic phenomenon or a depressive symptom? J Am Acad Dermatol 1994; 30:370.
Kubalek I, et al: Treatment of reflex sympathetic dystrophy with pamidronate. Rheumatology 2001; 40:1394.
Littlejohn G: Regional pain syndrome. Nat Clin Pract Rheumatol 2007; 3:504.
Lipp KE, et al: Reflex sympathetic dystrophy with mutilating ulcerations suspicious of a factitial origin. J Am Acad Dermatol 1996; 35:843.
Nelson DV, et al: Interventional therapies in the management of complex regional pain syndrome. Clin J Pain 2006; 22:438.
Schurmann M, et al: Early diagnosis in post-traumatic complex regional pain syndrome. Orthopedics 2007; 30:450.
Sharma A, et al: Advances in treatment of complex regional pain syndrome. Curr Opin Anesthesiol 2006; 19:566.
Sundaram S, et al: Vascular diseases are the most common cutaneous manifestations of reflex sympathetic dystrophy. J Am Acad Dermatol 2001; 44:1050.

Trigeminal trophic lesions

Interruption of the peripheral or central sensory pathways of the trigeminal nerve may result in a slowly enlarging, unilateral, uninflamed ulcer on ala nasi or adjacent cheek skin (Fig. 4-18). The nasal tip is spared. It may infrequently occur elsewhere on the face. Onset of ulceration varies from weeks to several years after trigeminal nerve injury. Biopsy to exclude tumor or a variety of granulomatous or infective etiologies is usually indicated. Self-inflicted trauma to the

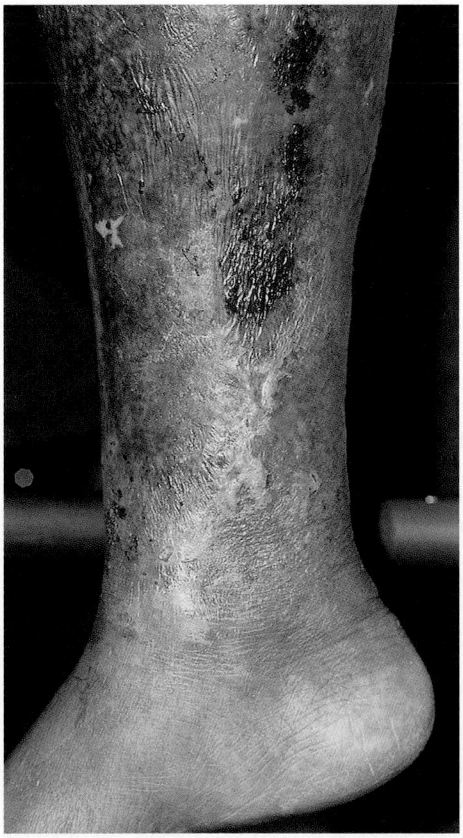

Fig. 4-17 Complex regional pain syndrome.

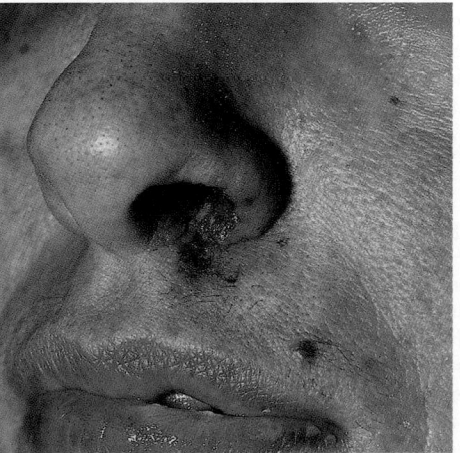

Fig. 4-18 Trigeminal trophic syndrome.

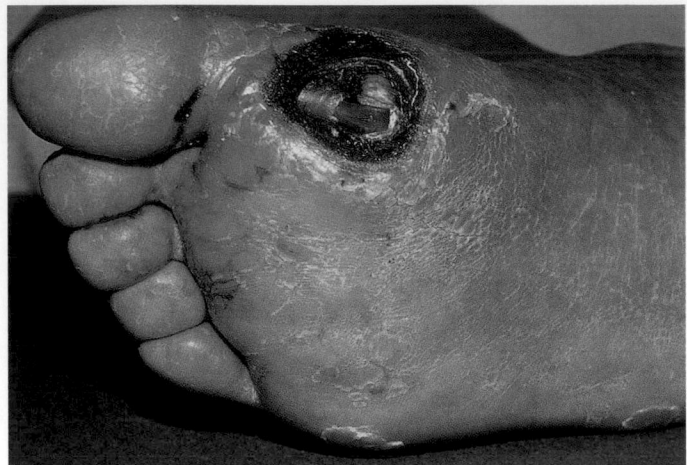

Fig. 4-19 Diabetic foot ulcer.

anesthetic skin is believed to be the cause, and the appropriate treatment is to prevent this by occlusion or with the initiation of psychotropic medicine. It is usually successful, but scarring may be severe.

Luksic I, et al: Trigeminal trophic syndrome of all three nerve branches. J Neurosurg 2008; 108:170.

Setyadi HG, et al: Trigeminal trophic syndrome. S Med J 2007; 100:43.

Shea CR, et al: Herpetic trigeminal trophic syndrome. Arch Dermatol 1996; 132:613.

Mal perforans pedis

Also known as neuropathic ulceration or perforating ulcer of the foot, mal perforans is a chronic ulcerative disease seen on the sole in conditions that result in loss of pain sensation at a site of constant trauma (Fig. 4-19). The primary cause lies in either the posterolateral tracts of the cord (in arteriosclerosis and tabes dorsalis), lateral tracts (in syringomyelia), or peripheral nerves (in diabetes or Hansen's disease).

In most cases, mal perforans begins as a circumscribed hyperkeratosis, usually on the ball of the foot. This lesion becomes soft, moist, and malodorous, and later exudes a thin, purulent discharge. A slough slowly develops and an indolent, necrotic ulcer is left that lasts indefinitely. Whereas the neuropathy renders the ulceration painless and walking continues, plantar ulcers in this situation have a surrounding thick callus. Deeper perforation and secondary infection often lead to osteomyelitis of the metatarsal or tarsal bones.

Treatment should consist of relief of pressure on the ulcer through use of a total-contact cast and debridement of the surrounding callosity. Removable cast walkers and half-shoes were significantly less effective means of off-loading in a randomized clinical trial. Administration of local and systemic antibiotics is sometimes helpful.

Armstrong DG, et al: Off-loading the diabetic foot wound. Diabetes Care 2001; 24:1019.

Sciatic nerve injury

Serious sciatic nerve injury can result from improperly performed injections into the buttocks. Older patients are more susceptible to injection-induced sciatic nerve injury because of their decreased muscle mass and/or debilitating diseases. The most common scenario for nerve damage is improper needle placement. Other common causes of sciatic neuropathy are hip surgery complications, hip fracture and dislocation, and compression by benign and malignant tumors. A paralytic foot drop is the most common finding. There is sensory loss and absence of sweating over the distribution of the sciatic nerve branches. The skin of the affected extremity becomes thin, shiny, and often edematous.

Surgical exploration, guided by nerve action potentials, with repair of the sciatic nerve is worthwhile in selected cases.

Ramtahal J, et al: Sciatic nerve injury following intramuscular injection. J Neurosci Nurs 2006; 38:238.

Syringomyelia

Also known as Morvan's disease, syringomyelia results from cystic cavities inside the cervical spinal cord, due to alterations of cerebrospinal fluid flow. Compression of the lateral spinal tracts produces sensory and trophic changes on the upper extremities, particularly in the fingers. The disease begins insidiously and gradually causes muscular weakness, hyperhidrosis, and sensory disturbances, especially in the thumb and index and middle fingers. The skin changes are characterized by dissociated anesthesia with loss of pain and temperature sense but with retention of tactile sense. Burns are the most frequent lesions noted. Bullae, warts, and trophic ulcerations occur on the fingers and hands, and ultimately there are contractures and gangrene. Other unusual features may be hypertrophy of the limbs, hands, or feet, and asymmetric scalp hair growth with a sharp midline demarcation. The disease must be differentiated chiefly from Hansen's disease. Unlike Hansen's disease, syringomyelia does not interfere with sweating or block the flare around a histamine wheal. Early surgical treatment allows for improvement of symptoms and prevents progression of neurologic deficits.

DiLorenzo N, et al: Adult syringomyelia. J Neurosurg Sci 2005; 49:65.

Hereditary sensory and autonomic neuropathies (HSAN)

A number of inherited conditions are characterized by sensory dysfunctions and varying degrees of autonomic alterations. From a dermatologic standpoint, altered pain and temperature sensation, self-mutilating behavior, and sweating abnormalities may be present. Two of them are discussed below.

Familial dysautonomia (Riley–Day syndrome)

Familial dysautonomia (HSAN III) is characterized by defective lacrimation, decreased pain sensation, impaired temperature and blood pressure regulation, and absent tendon reflexes. Skin and oral manifestations include hyperhidrosis, a transient erythema, predominantly on the trunk, acrocyanosis of the hands, absence of fungiform and circumvallate papillae of the tongue, and measurable deficiencies in taste from water and sweet, bitter, and salty stimuli. Dental features may be prominent and include hypersalivation and orodental trauma progressing to self-mutilation.

This neurodegenerative disease is inherited as an autosomal-recessive trait, most often in Jewish families. The Schirmer test for lacrimal dysfunction is positive. The intradermal histamine test shows a diminished flare, and immersion of the hands in water at 40°C (104°F) causes erythematous mottling of the skin. The mutation in Riley–Day syndrome is in the Iκ-B (IKBKAP) associated protein, a subunit of *Elongator*. This leads to a tissue-specific abnormality in splicing of pre-mRNA. Splicing defects are estimated to be responsible for up to 15% of human diseases. Treatment is supportive; however, there is hope that kinetin, a cytokinin, will prove to be a helpful treatment, as in vitro studies have shown it can rescue the mRNA splicing defect of Riley–Day syndrome.

Congenital insensitivity to pain with anhidrosis

HSAN type IV is an autosomal-recessive disorder characterized by anhidrosis, recurrent hyperpyrexia, absence of the pain sensation, self-mutilating behavior, and mental retardation. Repeated injuries produce ulcers, most commonly of the acral and oral tissues. Secondary infection of the digits with osteomyelitis is not an infrequent complication.

The disease has been found to be caused by mutations and polymorphisms in the *TRKA* (*NTRK1*) gene, which is present on chromosome 1 and encodes for the receptor tyrosine kinase for nerve growth factor. Treatment of this disorder is supportive. Care should be taken to avoid burning, scratching, and the various other traumatic events that can happen in ordinary living.

Amano A, et al: Oral manifestations of hereditary sensory and autonomic neuropathy type IV. Oral Surg Oral Med Oral Pathol Oral Radiol Endod 1998; 86:425.

Axelrod FB, et al: Pediatric autonomic disorders. Pediatrics 2006; 118:309.

Hims MM, et al: Therapeutic potential and mechanism of kinetin as a treatment for the human splicing disease familial dysautonomia. J Mol Med 2007; 85:149.

Luft FC: Better days are coming for Riley–Day patients. J Mol Med 2007; 85:99.

Bonus images for this chapter can be found online at

http://www.expertconsult.com

Fig. 4-1 Dry skin of the leg.
Fig. 4-2 Factitial ulcers.
Fig. 4-3 Mal perforans ulcer.

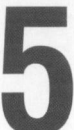
5 | Atopic Dermatitis, Eczema, and Noninfectious Immunodeficiency Disorders

Atopic dermatitis

Atopic dermatitis (AD) is a chronic, inflammatory skin disease that is characterized by pruritus and a chronic course of exacerbations and remissions. It is associated with other allergic conditions, including asthma and allergic rhinoconjunctivitis. Recent studies have cast doubt on the importance of AD in the subsequent development of asthma, refuting the concept of the "atopic march." However, a common genetic defect predisposes patients to the development of AD, asthma, and allergic rhinoconjunctivitis—the "atopic" disorders.

Epidemiology

The prevalence of AD, asthma, and allergic rhinoconjunctivitis increased dramatically in the last half of the twentieth century, becoming a major health problem in many countries. The increase began first in the most developed nations, and as nations' standards of living have increased worldwide, so has the prevalence of AD. Rates of AD are around 30% in the most developed nations and exceed 10% in many countries, resulting in a worldwide cumulative prevalence of 15–20%. In the most developed nations, the rates of AD plateaued in the 1990s, whereas developing nations have rates that continue to increase. Other factors associated with high rates of AD are high latitude (perhaps associated with low levels of annual sun exposure) and lower mean annual temperature. A role for exposure to allergens thought to "trigger" AD is not supported by epidemiological studies. Iceland has a very high rate of AD (27%) yet has no dust mites, few trees, and low pet ownership. Children in Iceland, none the less, often have positive skin prick tests to environmental allergens (24%). This brings into question the value of such tests in predicting causal environmental allergens in AD. In some studies maternal smoking and the fact that two or more members of the household smoke are associated with higher rates of AD. Girls are slightly more likely to develop AD. In the US, an increased risk of AD during the first 6 months of life is noted in infants with African and Asian race/ethnicity, male gender, greater gestational age at birth, and a family history of atopy, particularly a maternal history of eczema.

About 50% of cases of AD appear in the first year of life, the vast majority within the first 5 years of life, and the remaining cases of "adult" AD usually before age 30. Atopy is now so common in the population that most individuals have a family history of atopy. Elevated IgE levels are not diagnostic of atopic disease in the adult. Therefore, elevated IgE and a family history of "atopy" in an adult with new-onset dermatitis should not be used to confirm the diagnosis of "adult" AD. Rather, a dermatologist should uncommonly make the diagnosis of adult "atopic dermatitis" for a dermatitis appearing for the first time after age 30. Adult AD should only be considered when the dermatitis has a characteristic distribution and other significant diagnoses, such as allergic contact dermatitis, photodermatitis, and cutaneous T-cell lymphoma, have been excluded.

Genetic basis of atopic dermatitis

Eighty percent of identical twins show concordance for AD. A child is at increased risk of developing AD if either parent is affected. More than one-quarter of offspring of atopic mothers develop AD in the first 3 months of life. If one parent is atopic, more than half his/her children will develop allergic symptoms by age 2. This rate rises to 79% if both parents are atopic. All these findings strongly suggested a genetic cause for AD. Filaggrin is a protein encoded by the gene *FLG*, which resides in the "epidermal differentiation complex" on chromosome 1q21. Ichthyosis vulgaris is caused by mutations in the *FLG* gene, and is frequently associated with AD. Large population-based studies have identified more than 35 mutations in *FLG* that are associated with AD. Inheriting one null *FLG* mutation slightly increases one's risk of developing AD, and inheriting two mutations (either as a homozygote or a compound heterozygote) dramatically increases one's risk. Between 42% and 79% of persons with one or more *FLG* null mutations will develop AD. *FLG* mutations account for between 11% and 15% of AD cases in Europe. However, 40% of carriers with *FLG* null mutations never have AD. *FLG* mutations are associated with AD that presents early in life, tends to persist into childhood and adulthood, and is associated with wheezing in infancy, and asthma. *FLG* mutations are also associated with allergic rhinitis and keratosis pilaris, independent of AD. Hyperlinear palms are strongly associated with *FLG* mutations, with a 71% positive predictive value for marked palmar hyperlinearity.

Not all cases of AD are associated with *FLG* mutations, and AD patients often demonstrate clinical findings consistent with a T-helper 2 (Th2) phenotype. Polymorphisms/mutations in genes expressed by Th2 cells, especially the interleukin (IL)-4 gene promoter region, have been identified in patients with AD. Other immunomodulatory genes in which mutations have been observed in AD patients include *RANTES* and eotaxin, IL-13, and the β-subunit of high-affinity Fc IgE receptor on mast cells. These mutations, in and of themselves, could potentially be causal in AD. In addition, however, over-expression of Th2 cytokines downregulates filaggrin protein expression in patients with AD. This could lead to an "acquired" filaggrin deficiency, resulting in or exacerbating AD.

Prevention of atopic dermatitis

Extensive studies have been undertaken to determine whether it is possible to prevent the development of AD in children at high risk—those with parents or siblings with atopy. Maternal antigen avoidance during pregnancy does not reduce the incidence of AD. Some studies have suggested that hydrolyzed protein formula milks (and even better, extensively hydrolyzed formulas) may delay the onset of AD, but a Cochrane review found no clear evidence of protective effect for AD. Soy formulas do not appear to reduce the risk of developing AD. Early introduction of solids does, in a dose-dependent fashion, increase the risk of AD. Prolonged breast feeding (>4–6 months) appears to reduce the risk of AD. In two independent cohorts, cat ownership at birth substantially increases the risk of developing AD within the first year of life in children with *FLG* loss-of-function mutations, but not in those without. Dog and dust mite exposure was NOT associated with the development of AD. Filaggrin-deficient individuals should avoid cat exposure early in life.

Food allergy and AD

The role of food allergy in AD is complicated, and the purported role of foods in AD has changed in recent years. Parents may use older Internet resources and be misinformed about food allergy. Approximately 35% of children with moderate to severe AD have food allergy. Food allergy in adults is rare. However, 85% of children with AD will have elevated IgE to food or inhalant allergens, making a diagnosis of food allergy with serum or prick tests alone inadvisable. Before food allergy testing is embarked upon, the treatment of the AD should be optimized. Parents are often seeking a "cause" for the child's AD, when in fact it could be controlled with appropriate topical measures. Since food restriction diets can be difficult and could potentially put the child at risk for malnourishment, food allergy should only be pursued in younger children or infants with more severe AD when standard treatments have failed. Prick tests have a high negative predictive value (>95%) but a positive predictive value of only 30–65%. For example, more than 8% of the US population has a positive prick test to peanut, but only 0.4% are actually clinically allergic. Possible food allergy detected by testing should be confirmed by clinical history. For instance, a positive radioallergosorbent test (RAST) or skin prick test for a food that the child rarely or never ingests is probably not causally relevant to their AD. Higher serum IgE levels and larger wheal sizes (>8–10 mm) are associated with greater likelihood of reacting to these foods when challenged. Around 90% of food allergy is due to a limited number of foods:

- infants: cow's milk, egg, soybean, wheat
- children (2–10 years): cow's milk, egg, peanut, tree nuts, fish, crustacean shellfish, sesame, and kiwi fruit
- older children: peanut, tree nuts, fish, shellfish, sesame, pollen-associated foods.

Breast-feeding mothers must avoid the incriminated foods if their infant has been diagnosed with a food allergy.

Clinical manifestations

AD can be divided into three stages: infantile AD, occurring from 2 months to 2 years of age; childhood AD, from 2 to 10 years; and adolescent/adult AD. In all stages, pruritus is the hallmark. Itching often precedes the appearance of lesions; hence the concept that AD is "the itch that rashes." Useful diagnostic criteria include those of Hannifin and Rajka, the UK Working Party, and the American Academy of Dermatology's Consensus Conference on Pediatric Atopic Dermatitis (Boxes 5-1 and 5-2). These criteria have specificity at or above 90%, but have much lower sensitivities (40–100%). Therefore, they are useful for enrolling patients in studies and insuring that they have AD, but are not so useful in diagnosing a specific patient with AD.

Infantile atopic dermatitis

Fifty percent or more of cases of AD present in the first year of life, but usually not until after 2 months of age. Eczema in

Box 5-1 Criteria for atopic dermatitis

Major criteria

Must have three of the following:
1. Pruritus
2. Typical morphology and distribution
   - Flexural lichenification in adults
   - Facial and extensor involvement in infancy
3. Chronic or chronically relapsing dermatitis
4. Personal or family history of atopic disease (asthma, allergic rhinitis, atopic dermatitis)

Minor criteria

Must also have three of the following:
1. Xerosis
2. Ichthyosis/hyperlinear palms/keratosis pilaris
3. IgE reactivity (immediate skin test reactivity, RAST test positive)
4. Elevated serum IgE
5. Early age of onset
6. Tendency for cutaneous infections (especially *Staphylococcus aureus* and herpes simplex virus)
7. Tendency to nonspecific hand/foot dermatitis
8. Nipple eczema
9. Cheilitis
10. Recurrent conjunctivitis
11. Dennie–Morgan infraorbital fold
12. Keratoconus
13. Anterior subcapsular cataracts
14. Orbital darkening
15. Facial pallor/facial erythema
16. Pityriasis alba
17. Itch when sweating
18. Intolerance to wool and lipid solvents
19. Perifollicular accentuation
20. Food hypersensitivity
21. Course influenced by environmental and/or emotional factors
22. White dermatographism or delayed blanch to cholinergic agents

Box 5-2 Modified criteria for children with atopic dermatitis

Essential features
1. Pruritus
2. Eczema
   - Typical morphology and age-specific pattern
   - Chronic or relapsing history

Important features
1. Early age at onset
2. Atopy
3. Personal and/or family history
4. IgE reactivity
5. Xerosis

Associated features
1. Atypical vascular responses (e.g. facial pallor, white dermatographism)
2. Keratosis pilaris/ichthyosis/hyperlinear palms
3. Orbital/periorbital changes
4. Other regional findings (e.g. perioral changes/periauricular lesions)
5. Perifollicular accentuation/lichenification/prurigo lesions

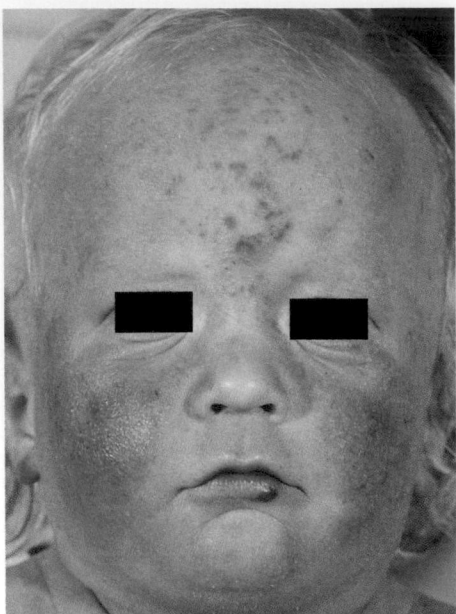

Fig. 5-1 Involvement of the cheeks in infantile atopic dermatitis.

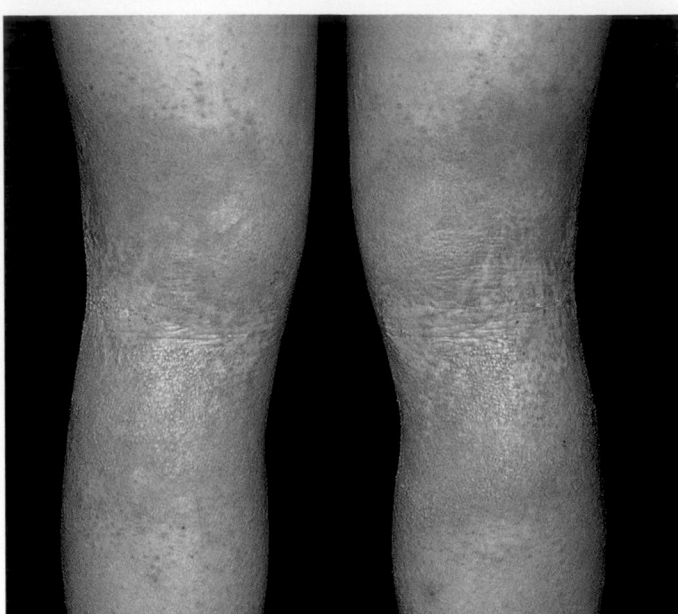

Fig. 5-2 Flexural involvement in childhood atopic dermatitis.

infancy usually begins as erythema and scaling of the cheeks (Fig. 5-1). The eruption may extend to the scalp, neck, forehead, wrists, and extensor extremities. The areas involved correlate with the capacity of the child to scratch or rub the site, and the activities of the infant, such as crawling. There may be a significant amount of exudate, and there are many secondary effects from scratching, rubbing, and infection: crusts, infiltration, and pustules, respectively. The infiltrated plaques eventually take on a characteristic lichenified appearance. The infantile pattern of AD usually disappears by the end of the second year of life.

Worsening of AD is often observed in infants after immunizations and viral infections. Partial remission may occur during the summer, with relapse in winter. This may relate to the therapeutic effects of ultraviolet (UV) B and humidity in many atopic patients, and the aggravation by wool and dry air in the winter.

Childhood atopic dermatitis

During childhood, lesions are apt to be less exudative. The classic locations are the antecubital and popliteal fossae (Fig. 5-2), flexor wrists, eyelids, face, and around the neck. Lesions are often lichenified, indurated plaques, and in African-American patients may have a lichenoid appearance and favor the extensor surfaces. These are intermingled with isolated, excoriated 2–4 mm papules that are scattered more widely over the uncovered parts.

Pruritus is a constant feature and most of the cutaneous changes are secondary to it. Itching is paroxysmal. Scratching induces lichenification and may lead to secondary infection. A vicious cycle may be established (the itch–scratch cycle), as pruritus leads to scratching, and scratching causes secondary changes that in themselves cause itching. Instead of scratching causing pain, in the atopic patient the "pain" induced by scratching is perceived as itch and induces more scratching. The scratching impulse is beyond the control of the patient. Severe bouts of scratching occur during sleep, leading to poor rest and chronic tiredness in atopic children. This can affect their school performance.

Severe AD involving a large percentage of the body surface area can be associated with growth retardation. Restriction diets and steroid usage may exacerbate growth retardation. Aggressive management of such children with phototherapy or systemic immunosuppressives may allow for rebound growth. Children with severe AD may also have substantial psychological disturbances. Parents should be questioned with regard to school performance and socialization.

Atopic dermatitis in adolescents and adults

Most adolescents and adults with AD will give a history of childhood disease. In only 6–14% of patients diagnosed with AD will it begin after age 18. One exception is the patient who moves from a humid, tropical region to a more temperate one of higher latitude. This climatic change is often associated with the appearance of AD. In older patients, AD may occur as localized erythematous, scaly, papular, exudative, or lichenified (Fig. 5-3) plaques. In adolescents, the eruption often involves the classic antecubital and popliteal fossae, front and sides of the neck, forehead, and area around the eyes. In older adults the distribution is generally less characteristic, and localized dermatitis may be the predominant feature, especially hand, nipple, or eyelid eczema). At times the eruption may generalize, with accentuation in the flexures. The skin, in general, is dry and somewhat erythematous. Lichenification and prurigo-like papules are common (Fig. 5-4). Papular lesions tend to be dry, slightly elevated, and flat-topped. They are nearly always excoriated and often coalesce to form plaques. Staphylococcal colonization is nearly universal. In darker-skinned patients, the lesions are often dramatically hyperpigmented, frequently with focal hypopigmented areas related to healed excoriations.

Itching usually occurs in crises or paroxysms, often during the evening when the patient is trying to relax, or during the night. Adults frequently complain that flares of AD are triggered by acute emotional upsets. Stress, anxiety, and depression reduce the threshold at which itch is perceived and result in damage to the epidermal permeability barrier, further exacerbating AD. Atopic persons may sweat poorly, and may complain of severe pruritus related to heat or exercise. Physical conditioning and liberal use of emollients improve this component, and atopic patients can participate in competitive sports.

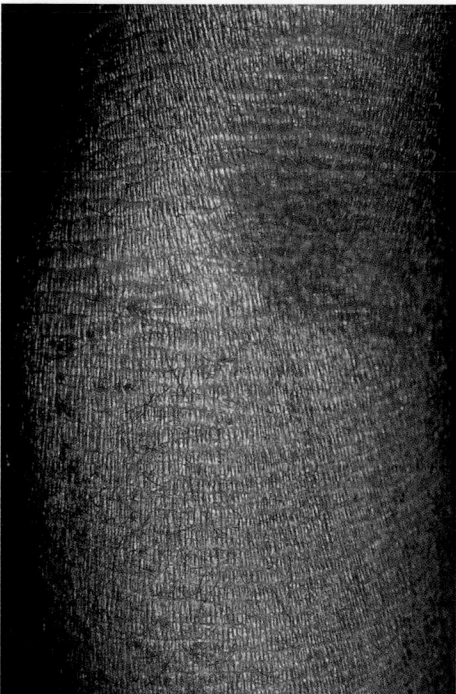

Fig. 5-3 Flexural lichenification in adult atopic dermatitis.

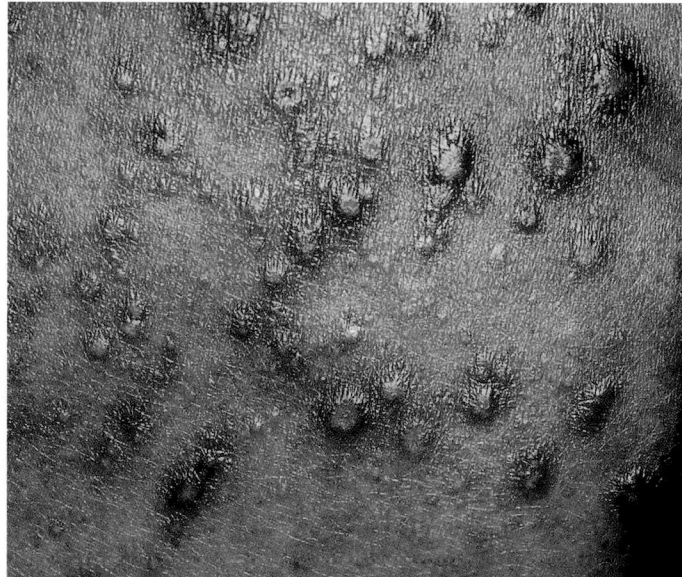

Fig. 5-4 Prurigo-like papules in adult atopic dermatitis.

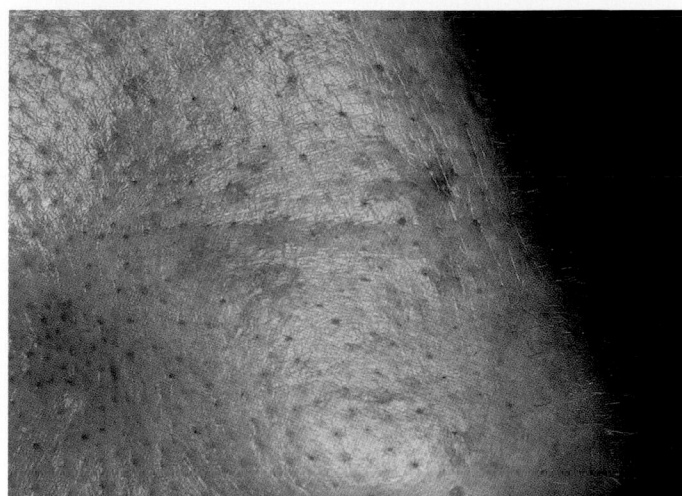

Fig. 5-5 Nasal crease.

Even in patients with AD in adolescence or early adulthood, improvement usually occurs over time, and dermatitis is uncommon after middle life. In general, these patients retain mild stigmata of the disease, such as dry skin, easy skin irritation, and itching in response to heat and perspiration. They remain susceptible to a flare of their disease when exposed to the specific allergen or environmental situation. Some will flare in response to aeroallergens, and a few patients will develop flexural dermatitis in response to niacin-induced flushing. Photosensitivity develops in approximately 3% of AD patients, and may manifest as either a polymorphous light eruption-type reaction or simply exacerbation of the AD by UV exposure. Most patients (65%) are sensitive to UVA and UVB, but about 17% are sensitive to only UVA or UVB. The average age for photosensitive AD is the mid- to late thirties. Human immunodeficiency virus (HIV) infection can also serve

as a trigger, and new-onset AD in an at-risk adult should lead to counseling and testing for HIV if warranted.

The hands, including the wrists, are frequently involved in adults, and hand dermatitis is a common problem for adults with a history of AD. It is extremely common for atopic hand dermatitis to appear in young women after the birth of a child, when increased exposure to soaps and water triggers their disease. Wet work is a major factor in hand eczema in general, including those patients with AD. Atopic hand dermatitis can affect both the dorsal and palmar surfaces. Keratosis punctata of the creases, a disorder seen almost exclusively in black persons, is also more common in atopics. Patients with AD have frequent exposure to preservatives and other potential allergens in the creams and lotions that are continually applied to their skin. Contact allergy may manifest as chronic hand eczema. Patch testing with clinical correlation is the only certain way to exclude contact allergy in an atopic patient with chronic hand dermatitis.

Eyelids are commonly involved. In general, the involvement is bilateral and the condition flares with cold weather. As in hand dermatitis, irritants and allergic contact allergens must be excluded by a careful history and patch testing.

Associated features and complications

Cutaneous stigmata

A linear transverse fold just below the edge of the lower eyelids, known as the Dennie–Morgan fold, is widely believed to be indicative of the atopic diathesis, but may be seen with any chronic dermatitis of the lower lids. In atopic patients with eyelid dermatitis, increased folds and darkening under the eyes is common. When taken together with other clinical findings, they remain helpful clinical signs. A prominent nasal crease may also be noted (Fig. 5-5).

The less involved skin of atopic patients is frequently dry and slightly erythematous, and may be scaly. Histologically, the apparently normal skin of atopics is frequently inflamed subclinically. The dry, scaling skin of AD may represent low-grade dermatitis. Filaggrin is processed by caspase 14 during terminal keratinocyte differentiation into highly hydroscopic pyrrolidone carboxylic acid and urocanic acid, collectively known as the "natural moisturizing factor" or NMF. Null mutations in *FLG* lead to reduction in NMF, which probably contributes to the xerosis that is almost universal in AD. Transepidermal water loss (TEWL) is increased. This may be due to subclinical dermatitis, but is also caused by abnormal

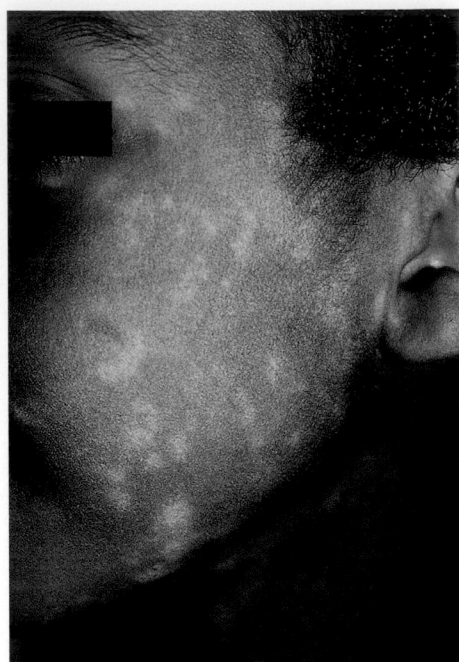

Fig. 5-6 Pityriasis alba.

delivery of lamellar body epidermal lipids (especially ceramide) to the interstices between the terminally differentiated keratinocytes. The defective lipid bilayers that result retain water poorly, leading to increased TEWL and clinical xerosis. Pityriasis alba is a form of subclinical dermatitis, frequently atopic in origin. It presents as poorly marginated, hypopigmented, slightly scaly patches on the cheeks (Fig. 5-6), upper arms, and trunk, typically in children and young adults. It usually responds to emollients and mild topical steroids, preferably in an ointment base.

Keratosis pilaris (KP), horny follicular lesions of the outer aspects of the upper arms, legs, cheeks, and buttocks, is commonly associated with AD. The keratotic papules on the face may be on a red background, a variant of KP called keratosis pilaris rubra facei. KP is often refractory to treatment. Moisturizers alone are only partially beneficial. Some patients will respond to topical lactic acid, urea, or retinoids. Retinoids can easily irritate the skin of atopics, and treatment should begin with applications only once or twice a week. KP must be distinguished from follicular eczema, as AD and other eczemas are commonly folliculocentric, especially in black patients.

Thinning of the lateral eyebrows, Hertoghe's sign, is sometimes present. This apparently occurs from chronic rubbing due to pruritus and subclinical dermatitis. Hyperkeratosis and hyperpigmentation, which produce a "dirty neck" appearance, are also frequent in AD.

Vascular stigmata

Atopic individuals often exhibit perioral, perinasal, and periorbital pallor ("headlight sign"). White dermatographism is blanching of the skin at the site of stroking with a blunt instrument. This reaction differs from the triple response of Lewis, in that it typically lacks a wheal, and the third response (flaring) is replaced by blanching to produce a white line. When 0.1 mL of a 1:100 000 solution of histamine is injected intradermally, the flare phase of the triple response is absent or diminished.

Atopics are at increased risk of developing various forms of urticaria, including contact urticaria. Episodes of contact urticaria may be followed by typical eczematous lesions at the affected site.

Ophthalmologic abnormalities

Up to 10% of patients with AD develop cataracts, either anterior or posterior subcapsular ones. Posterior subcapsular cataracts in atopic individuals are indistinguishable from corticosteroid-induced cataracts. Development of cataracts is more common in patients with severe dermatitis. Keratoconus is an uncommon finding, occurring in approximately 1% of atopic patients. Contact lenses, keratoplasty, and intraocular lenses may be required to treat this condition.

Susceptibility to infection

More than 90% of chronic eczematous lesions contain *S. aureus*, often in large numbers. In addition, the apparently normal nonlesional skin of atopic patients is also commonly colonized by *S. aureus*. The finding of increasing numbers of pathogenic staphylococci on the skin of a patient with AD is frequently associated with weeping and crusting of skin lesions, retro- and infra-auricular and perinasal fissures, folliculitis, and adenopathy. In any flaring atopic the possibility of secondary infection must be considered. IgE antibodies directed against *Staphylococcus* and its toxins have been documented in some atopic individuals. Staphylococcal production of superantigens is another possible mechanism for staphylococcal flares of disease. Treatment of lesions of AD with topical steroids is associated with reduced numbers of pathogenic bacteria on the surface, even if antibiotics are not used. Despite the frequent observation that the presence of staphylococcal infection of lesions of AD is associated with worsening of disease, it has been impossible to prove that oral antibiotic therapy makes a long-term difference in the course of the AD. None the less, treatment of the "infected" AD patient with oral antibiotics is a community standard of dermatologists worldwide. With the widespread presence of antibiotic-resistant *S. aureus*, dermatologists have shifted from the chronic use of oral antibiotics in managing patients with frequent flares of AD associated with staphylococcal infection. Rather, bleach baths and reduction of nasal carriage have become the basis for controlling infection-triggered AD. In an occasional patient with AD and frequent infections, chronic suppressive oral antibiotic therapy may stabilize the disease. Options include cephalosporins, trimethoprim–sulfamethoxazole, clindamycin, and (in older patients) doxycycline. Identifying and treating *S. aureus* carriers in the family may also be of benefit. An unusual complication of *S. aureus* infection in patients with AD is subungual infection, with osteomyelitis of the distal phalanx. In atopic patients with fever who appear very toxic, the possibility of streptococcal infection must be considered. These children may require hospital admission and intravenous antibiotics.

AD patients have increased susceptibility to generalized herpes simplex infection (eczema herpeticum), as well as widespread vaccinia infection (eczema vaccinatum) and complicated varicella. Eczema herpeticum is seen most frequently in young children and is usually associated with herpes simplex virus (HSV)-1 transmitted from a parent or sibling. Once infected, the atopic may have recurrences of HSV and repeated episodes of eczema herpeticum. Eczema herpeticum presents as the sudden appearance of vesicular, pustular, crusted, or eroded lesions concentrated in the areas of dermatitis. The lesions may continue to spread and most of the skin surface may become involved. Secondary staphylococcal infection is frequent, and local edema and regional adenopathy commonly occur. If lesions of eczema herpeticum occur on or around the eyelids, ophthalmologic evaluation is recommended. The severity of eczema herpeticum is quite variable, but most cases requires systemic antiviral therapy and an antistaphylococcal antibiotic.

Vaccination against smallpox is contraindicated in persons with AD, even when the dermatitis is in remission. Widespread and even fatal vaccinia can occur in patients with an atopic diathesis.

Atopic individuals may also develop extensive flat warts or molluscum contagiosum. Because the skin is very easily irritated, chemical treatments such as salicylic acid and cantharidin are poorly tolerated. Destruction with curettage (for molluscum), cryosurgery, or electrosurgery may be required to clear the lesions.

Pathogenesis

Immunologic events noted early in the development of atopic lesions include activation of the Th2 immune response, with synthesis of cytokines IL-4, IL-5, IL-10, and IL-13. These immunological propensities are already evident in newborns. Neonatal cord blood mononuclear cells stimulated with phytohemagglutinin show significantly higher IL-13 levels in children who subsequently develop AD. IL-4 and IL-5 produce elevated IgE levels and eosinophilia in tissue and peripheral blood. IL-10 inhibits delayed-type hypersensitivity. IL-4 downregulates interferon (IFN)-γ production. Early lesions of AD are often urticarial in character, a manifestation of Th2 hyperreactivity. These immunologic alterations result in the reduced production of antimicrobial peptides (AMP), specifically LL-37 (cathelicidin) and β-defensins 2 and 3. This loss of AMP production may predispose atopics to widespread skin infections due to viruses (herpes, molluscum, and vaccinia) and bacteria, especially *Staphylococcus*. AD patients who develop eczema herpeticum are more likely to be Th2-polarized, supporting the causal relationship between reduced AMP production and cutaneous viral infection. Epicutaneous exposure to staphylococcal superantigens, to which AD patients develop IgE antibodies, further skews the immune response toward Th2 cytokine production, explaining the association of staphylococcal infection with exacerbations of AD. Staphylococcal superantigens, such as SEB, SEE, and TSST-1, cause profound reduction in steroid responsiveness of T cells. This is another possible mechanism for flares of AD associated with staphylococcal skin infection or colonization. While AD begins as a Th2-mediated disorder, in its chronic phase, cutaneous inflammation is characterized by Th1 cytokines. This explains why chronic AD histologically resembles other chronic dermatoses.

Monocytes in the peripheral blood of patients with AD produce elevated levels of prostaglandin E2 (PGE2). PGE2 reduces IFN-γ production but not IL-4 from helper T cells, enhancing the Th2 dominance. PGE2 also directly enhances IgE production from B cells.

Abnormalities of cutaneous nerves and the products they secrete (neuropeptides) have been identified in atopic patients. These may explain the abnormal vascular responses, reduced itch threshold, and perhaps some of the immunologic imbalances seen in atopic skin. Decreased activation of peripheral pruriceptors has been demonstrated in patients with atopy, suggesting that itch in lesional skin might have a central component (central sensitization) based on altered spinal impulses rather than in primary afferent neurons. The acetylcholine content of atopic skin is markedly elevated, and acetylcholine may play a role in atopic signs and symptoms. In subjects with AD, acetylcholine injected intradermally will produce marked pruritus, while it produces pain in control patients. Epidermal nerve fibers are "stretched" in the acanthotic, lichenified lesions of AD, reducing their threshold for stimulation. Fissures in the skin in AD expose these epidermal nerve fibers, perhaps triggering pruritus, and explaining the rapid reduction of pruritus by simple emollients in some lesions. In addition, in chronic AD, mu opiate receptors are absent from the surface of keratinocytes. This may allow endogenous opiates in the epidermis to bind directly to epidermal nerves, triggering itch. In fact, topical opiate antagonists can reduce itch in AD.

In atopic patients, the epidermal barrier is abnormal, even in apparently normal skin. An increase in TEWL correlates with the severity of the disease. AD usually worsens in the winter due to decreased ambient humidity. Stress also results in poor formation of epidermal lipid bilayers, worsening TEWL. This is mediated by endogenous corticoid production, and systemic corticosteroid therapy of AD results in similar abnormalities in epidermal lipid bilayer synthesis. This could explain the flares of AD seen with stress and following systemic steroid therapy. Correction of barrier dysfunction is critical to improving AD; hence the value of skin hydration, ointments, and occlusion. Optimizing this component of AD treatment appears to have the greatest benefit in reducing the severity of AD.

Differential diagnosis

Typical AD in infancy and childhood is not difficult to diagnose because of its characteristic morphology, predilection for symmetric involvement of the face, neck, and antecubital and popliteal fossae, and association with food allergy, asthma, and allergic rhinoconjunctivitis. Dermatoses that may resemble AD include seborrheic dermatitis (especially in infants), irritant or allergic contact dermatitis, nummular dermatitis, photodermatitis, scabies, and cases of psoriasis with an eczematous morphology. Certain immunodeficiency syndromes (see below) may exhibit a dermatitis remarkably similar or identical to AD.

Histopathology

The histology of AD varies with the stage of the lesion, with many of the changes induced by scratching. Hyperkeratosis, acanthosis, and excoriation are common. Staphylococcal colonization may be noted histologically. Although eosinophils may not be seen in the dermal infiltrate, staining for eosinophil major basic protein (MBP) reveals deposition in many cases. Heavy MBP deposition is often seen in specimens from patients with AD and a personal or family history of respiratory atopy.

General management

Education and support

Parental and patient education is of critical importance in the management of AD. In the busy clinic setting dermatologists frequently have insufficient time to educate patients adequately regarding the multiple factors that are important in managing AD. Educational formats that have proved effective have been immediate nursing education on the correct use of medications, weekly evening educational sessions, and multidisciplinary day treatment venues. In all cases, "written action plans" outlining a "stepwise approach" have been important for parent/patient education. In addition, patients with chronic disease often become disenchanted with medical therapies or simply "burn out" from having to spend significant amounts of time managing their skin disease. The psychological support that can be piggy-backed into educational sessions can help motivate parents/patients and keep them engaged in the treatment plan. Having a child with AD is extremely stressful and generates significant stress within the family. Sleep is lost by both the patient and the parents. Supportive educational techniques can help the family cope with this burden. Finally, the dermatologist must consider the complexity and time commitment of any prescribed regimen and make sure the parents/patient both understand and are committed to undertaking the treatments proposed.

Barrier repair

In virtually all cases of AD, there is xerosis and an impaired epidermal barrier. The cornerstone of treatment and prevention of AD lies in addressing this problem. Patients should moisturize daily, especially after bathing. This may be with petrolatum or a petrolatum-based product, an oil-based product, vegetable shortening, or a "barrier repair" moisturizer that contains the essential lipids of the epidermal barrier. These special barrier repair moisturizers have similar benefits in AD to low-potency topical steroids. They are easier to apply and, if they are available to the patient, may enhance compliance. Petrolatum and petrolatum-based moisturizers are most commonly recommended and are the cheapest and most effective for most patients. However, men with significant body hair, AD patients triggered by heat, and the rare patient with true allergic contact dermatitis to petrolatum may not be able to tolerate petrolatum-based agents. Patients should be instructed on the barrier-damaging properties of soaps, hot water, and scrubbing. Synthetic detergents that have a more acidic pH are preferred to harsh soaps. Detergent use should be restricted to the axilla, groin, face, soles, and scalp. Oil-based cleansers can be used to "wash" the skin without water. For flares of AD, the soak and smear technique (soak in a tub then seal in the water with a heavy moisturizer or medicated ointments) or wet dressings (wet wraps) with topical steroids can be very effective. In dry climates, AD patients may note some benefit with humidifiers. Alpha-hydroxy acid-containing products (lactic acid, glycolic acid) can be irritating and can exacerbate inflamed AD. These products should only be used for the xerosis of AD when there is absolutely no inflammation or pruritus.

Antimicrobial therapy

When there is evidence of infection, treatment with topical or systemic antibiotics may be appropriate. Rather than treating once an infection occurs, it appears that the key in AD is to reduce nasal staphylococcal carriage pre-emptively and to keep the skin decolonized from *Staphylococcus*. Bleach bathes have rapidly become a mainstay in AD patients. Twice-weekly bathing in a tepid bath with ½ cup of standard household bleach (6%) diluted into 40 gallons of water dramatically improves AD on the trunk and extremities, but less so on the face. This treatment combines decolonization of the skin with hydration, addressing two of the major factors in worsening of AD. Adequate moisturization following bathing is critical. Intranasal application of mupirocin is beneficial in reducing nasal carriage and improving the AD. In 80% of families, at least one parent is carrying the same staphylococcal strain as a colonized AD child. If recurrent infections afflict a patient with AD, look for other carriers in the family and treat them aggressively. Recurrent infections, especially furunculosis, are a cardinal feature of children and adults with AD who have systemic immunological abnormalities, especially hyper-IgE syndrome.

Environmental factors

Stress, heat, sweating, and external irritants may precipitate an attack of itching and flare AD. Wool garments should be avoided. Addressing these triggers may improve the AD. Exercise may need to be limited in patients with significant flares to swimming or walking during cool times of the day to avoid triggering sweating. Itch nerves are more active at higher temperatures, so overheating should be avoided. Irritants and allergens in the numerous products that AD patients may use can lead to flares of AD. Patients should avoid products that contain common allergens, and should be evaluated for allergic contact dermatitis if a topical agent is associated with worsening of their AD.

Antipruritics

Sedating antihistamines are optimally used nightly (not as needed) for their antipruritic and sedative effects. Diphenhydramine, hydroxyzine, and Sinequan can all be efficacious. Cetirizine and fexofenadine have both demonstrated efficacy in managing the pruritus of AD in children and adults, respectively. These can be added without significant sedation if standard first-generation antihistamines are not adequate in controlling pruritus. Applying ice during intense bouts of itch may help to "break" an itch paroxysm. Moisturizing lotions containing menthol, phenol, or pramocaine can be used between steroid applications to moisturize and reduce local areas of severe itch. More widespread use of topical Sinequan is limited by systemic absorption and sedation.

Specific treatment modalities

Topical corticosteroid therapy

Topical corticosteroids are the most commonly used class of medications, along with moisturizers, for the treatment of AD. They are effective and economical. In infants, low-potency steroid ointments, such as hydrocortisone 1% or 2.5%, are preferred. Emphasis must be placed on regular application of emollients. Once corticosteroid receptors are saturated, additional applications of a steroid preparation contribute nothing more than an emollient effect. In most body sites, once-a-day application of a corticosteroid is almost as effective as more frequent applications, at lower cost and with less systemic absorption. In some areas, twice-a-day applications may be beneficial, but more frequent applications are almost never of benefit. Steroid phobia is common in parents and patients with AD. Less frequent applications of lower-concentration agents, with emphasis on moisturizing, address these concerns. Application of topical corticosteroids under wet wraps or vinyl suit occlusion (soak and smear) can increase efficiency. For refractory areas, a stronger corticosteroid, such as desonide, aclomethasone, or triamcinolone, may be used. A more potent molecule is more appropriate than escalating concentrations of a weaker molecule because the effect of the latter plateaus rapidly as receptors become saturated. Do not undertreat! This leads to loss of faith on the part of the patient/parents and prolongs the suffering of the patient. For severe disease, use more potent topical steroids in short bursts of a few days to a week to gain control of the disease. In refractory and relapsing AD, twice-weekly steroid application may reduce flares.

In older children and adults, medium-potency steroids such as triamcinolone are commonly used, except on the face, where milder steroids or calcineurin inhibitors are preferred. For thick plaques and lichen simplex chronicus-like lesions, very potent steroids may be necessary. These are generally applied on weekends, with a milder steroid used during the week. Ointments are more effective, due to their moisturizing properties, and require no preservatives, reducing the likelihood of allergic contact dermatitis. If an atopic patient worsens or fails to improve after the use of topical steroids and moisturizers, the possibility of allergic contact dermatitis to a preservative or the corticosteroids must be considered. Contact allergy to the corticosteroid itself is not uncommon.

Corticosteroid allergy seldom manifests as acute worsening of the eczema. Instead, it manifests as a flare of eczema whenever the corticosteroid is discontinued, even for a day. This may be difficult to differentiate from stubborn AD.

Although the potential for local and even systemic toxicity from corticosteroids is real, the steroid must be strong enough to control the pruritus and remove the inflammation. Even in small children, strong topical steroids may be necessary in weekly pulses to control severe flares. Weekend pulses are always preferable to daily application of a potent steroid. Monitoring of growth parameters should be carried out in infants and young children.

Topical calcineurin inhibitors (TCIs)

Topical calcineurin inhibitors, such as tacrolimus or pimecrolimus, offer an alternative to topical steroids. Systemic absorption is generally not significant with either of these agents. Although a 0.03% tacrolimus ointment is marketed for use in children, it is unclear whether it really offers any safety advantage over the 0.1% formulation. Tolerability is improved if the ointment is applied to bone-dry skin. Patients experience less burning if eczematous patches are treated initially with a corticosteroid, with transition to a calcineurin inhibitor after partial clearing. Improvement tends to be steady, with progressively smaller areas requiring treatment. These agents are particularly useful on the eyelids and face, in areas prone to steroid atrophy, when steroid allergy is a consideration, or when systemic steroid absorption is a concern. Tacrolimus is more effective than pimecrolimus, with tacrolimus 0.1% ointment equivalent to triamcinolone acetonide 0.1%, and pimecrolimus equivalent to a class V or VI topical corticosteroid.

Tar

Crude coal tar 1–5% in white petrolatum or hydrophilic ointment USP, or liquor carbonis detergens (LCD) 5–20% in hydrophilic ointment USP, is sometimes helpful for an area of refractory AD. Tar preparations are especially beneficial when used for intensive treatment for adults in an inpatient or daycare setting, especially in combination with UV phototherapy.

Phototherapy

If topical modalities fail to control AD, phototherapy is the next option on the therapeutic ladder. Narrow-band UVB (NB-UVB) is highly effective and has replaced broadband UV for treating AD. When acutely inflamed, AD patients may tolerate UV poorly. Initial treatment with a systemic immunosuppressive can cool off the skin enough to institute UV treatments. Patients with significant erythema must be introduced to UV at very low doses to avoid nonspecific irritancy and flaring of the AD. Often the initial dose is much lower and the dose escalation much slower than in patients with psoriasis. In acute flares of AD, UVA-1 can be used. In patients in whom NB-UVB fails, photochemotherapy (PUVA) can be effective. It requires less frequent treatments, and can be given either topically (soak/bath PUVA) or systemically (oral PUVA). Goeckerman therapy with tar and UVB in a day treatment setting will lead to improvement in more than 90% of patients with refractory AD, and a prolonged remission can be induced.

Systemic therapy

Systemic corticosteroids

In general, systemic steroids should be used only to control acute exacerbations. In patients requiring systemic steroid therapy, short courses (3 weeks or less) are preferred. If repeated or prolonged courses of systemic corticosteroids are required to control the AD, phototherapy or a steroid-sparing agent should be considered. Chronic corticosteroid therapy for AD frequently results in significant corticosteroid-induced side effects. Osteoporosis in women requires special consideration and should be addressed with a bisphosphonate early in the course of therapy when bone loss is greatest. Preventive strategies, such as calcium supplements, vitamin D supplementation, bisphosphonates, regular exercise, and stopping smoking, should be strongly encouraged. Dual energy x-ray absorptiometry (DEXA) scans are recommended.

Cyclosporine

Cyclosporine is highly effective in the treatment of severe AD, but the response is rarely sustained after the drug is discontinued. It is very useful to gain rapid control of severe AD. It has been shown to be safe and effective in both children and adults, although probably tolerated better in children. Potential long-term side effects, especially renal disease, require careful monitoring, with attempts to transition the patient to a potentially less toxic agent if possible. The dose range is 3–5 mg/kg, with a better and more rapid response at the higher end of the dose range.

Other immunosuppressive agents

Several immunosuppressive agents have demonstrated efficacy in patients with AD. There are no comparative trials, so the relative efficacy of these agents is unknown. They do not appear to be as effective or quick to work as cyclosporine. However, over the long term, they may have a better safety profile, so patients requiring long-term immunosuppression may benefit from one of these agents. They include azathioprine (Immuran), mycophenolate mofetil (Cellcept), and methotrexate (Rheumatrex). The dosing of azathioprine is guided by the serum thiopurine methyltransferase level. Mycophenolate mofetil is generally well tolerated and, like azathioprine, takes about 6 weeks to begin to reduce the AD. Low-dose weekly methotrexate is very well tolerated in the elderly and may have special benefit in that population. Intravenous immunoglobulin (IVIG) has had some limited success in managing AD, but its high cost precludes it use, except when other reasonable therapeutic options have been exhausted. IFN-γ given by daily injection has demonstrated efficacy in both children and adults with severe AD. The onset of response can be delayed. It is well tolerated but can cause flu-like symptoms. Omalizumab can be considered in refractory cases, but only 20% of patients achieve a 50% or greater reduction of their AD. Infliximab has not been beneficial in AD.

Traditional Chinese herb mixtures have shown efficacy in children and in animal models for AD. The active herbs appear to be ophiopogon tuber and schisandra fruit. Chinese herbs are usually delivered as a brewed tea to be drunk daily. Their bitter taste makes them unpalatable to most Western patients. However, this option should be considered in patients who might accept this treatment approach.

Management of an acute flare

Initially, the precipitating cause of the flare should be sought. Recent stressful events may be associated with flares. Secondary infection with *S. aureus* should be assumed in most cases. Less commonly, herpes simplex or coxsackie virus may be involved. Pityriasis rosea may also cause AD to flare. The development of contact sensitivity to an applied medication or photosensitivity must be considered.

In the setting of an acute flare, treating triggers (see above) may lead to improvement. A short course of systemic steroids may be of benefit, but patients should be counseled that prolonged systemic corticosteroid therapy must be avoided. "Home hospitalization" may be useful. The patient goes home to bed, isolated from work and other stressors; large doses of an antihistamine are given at bedtime; the patient soaks in the tub twice daily, then applies a topical steroid ointment under wet pajamas and a sauna suit (soak and smear). Often, 3–4 days of such intensive home therapy will break a severe flare.

Akhavan A, et al: Atopic dermatitis: systemic immunosuppressive therapy. Semin Cutan Med Surg 2008; 27:151.

Allen HB, et al: Lichenoid and other clinical presentations of atopic dermatitis in an inner city practice. J Am Acad Dermatol 2008; 58:503.

Annesi-Maesano I, et al: Time trends in prevalence and severity of childhood asthma and allergies from 1995 to 2002 in France. Allergy 2009; 64:798.

Ashcroft DM, et al: Efficacy and tolerability of topical pimecrolimus and tacrolimus in the treatment of atopic dermatitis: meta-analysis of randomised controlled trials. BMJ 2005; 330:516.

Barker JN, et al: Null mutations in the filaggrin gene (FLG) determine major susceptibility to early-onset atopic dermatitis that persists into adulthood. J Invest Dermatol 2007; 127:564.

Beck LA, et al: Phenotype of atopic dermatitis subjects with a history of eczema herpeticum. J Allergy Clin Immunol 2009; 124:260.

Bigliardi PL, et al: Treatment of pruritus with topically applied opiate receptor antagonist. J Am Acad Dermatol 2007; 56:979.

Bisgaard H, et al: Gene-environment interaction in the onset of eczema in infancy: filaggrin loss-of-function mutations enhanced by neonatal cat exposure. PLoS Med 2008; 5:e131.

Boguniewicz M, et al: A multidisciplinary approach to evaluation and treatment of atopic dermatitis. Semin Cutan Med Surg 2008; 27:115.

Bonness S, et al: Pulsed-field gel electrophoresis of *Staphylococcus aureus* isolates from atopic patients revealing presence of similar strains in isolates from children and their parents. J Clin Microbiol 2008; 46:456.

Bremmer MS, et al: Are biologics safe in the treatment of atopic dermatitis? A review with a focus on immediate hypersensitivity reactions. J Am Acad Dermatol 2009.

Brenninkmeijer EE, et al: Diagnostic criteria for atopic dermatitis: a systematic review. Br J Dermatol 2008; 158:754.

Brown SJ, et al: Atopic eczema and the filaggrin story. Semin Cutan Med Surg 2008; 27:128.

Chisolm SS, et al: Written action plans: potential for improving outcomes in children with atopic dermatitis. J Am Acad Dermatol 2008; 59:677.

Clausen M, et al: High prevalence of allergic diseases and sensitization in a low allergen country. Acta Paediatr 2008; 97:1216.

Clayton TH, et al: The treatment of severe atopic dermatitis in childhood with narrowband ultraviolet B phototherapy. Clin Exp Dermatol 2007; 32:28.

Diepgen TL: Long-term treatment with cetirizine of infants with atopic dermatitis: a multi-country, double-blind, randomized, placebo-controlled trial (the ETAC trial) over 18 months. Pediatr Allergy Immunol 2002; 13:278.

Eichenfield LF, et al: Consensus conference on pediatric atopic dermatitis. J Am Acad Dermatol 2003; 49:1088.

Hata TR, et al: Antimicrobial peptides, skin infections, and atopic dermatitis. Semin Cutan Med Surg 2008; 27:144.

Howell MD, et al: Cytokine modulation of atopic dermatitis filaggrin skin expression. J Allergy Clin Immunol 2007; 120:150.

Huang JT, et al: Treatment of *Staphylococcus aureus* colonization in atopic dermatitis decreases disease severity. Pediatrics 2009; 123:e808.

Jolles S, et al: Use of IGIV in the treatment of atopic dermatitis, urticaria, scleromyxedema, pyoderma gangrenosum, psoriasis, and pretibial myxedema. Int Immunopharmacol 2006; 6:579.

Kawashima M, et al: Addition of fexofenadine to a topical corticosteroid reduces the pruritus associated with atopic dermatitis in a 1-week randomized, multicentre, double-blind, placebo-controlled, parallel-group study. Br J Dermatol 2003; 148:1212.

Leung D: Superantigens, steroid insensitivity and innate immunity in atopic eczema. Acta Derm Venereol Suppl (Stockh) 2005:11.

Makino T, et al: Effect of bakumijiogan, an herbal formula in traditional Chinese medicine, on atopic dermatitis-like skin lesions induced by mite antigen in NC/Jic mice. Biol Pharm Bull 2008; 31:2108.

Meduri NB, et al: Phototherapy in the management of atopic dermatitis: a systematic review. Photodermatol Photoimmunol Photomed 2007; 23:106.

Moore E, et al: Nurse-led clinics reduce severity of childhood atopic eczema: a review of the literature. Br J Dermatol 2006; 155:1242.

Morales Suarez-Varela M, et al: Parents' smoking habit and prevalence of atopic eczema in 6–7 and 13–14 year-old schoolchildren in Spain. ISAAC phase III. Allergol Immunopathol (Madr) 2008; 36:336.

Morar N, et al: Filaggrin mutations in children with severe atopic dermatitis. J Invest Dermatol 2007; 127:1667.

Murray ML, et al: Mycophenolate mofetil therapy for moderate to severe atopic dermatitis. Clin Exp Dermatol 2007; 32:23.

Naldi L, et al: Prevalence of atopic dermatitis in Italian schoolchildren: factors affecting its variation. Acta Derm Venereol 2009; 89:122.

O'Regan GM, et al: Filaggrin in atopic dermatitis. J Allergy Clin Immunol 2008; 122:689.

Ozkaya E: Adult-onset atopic dermatitis. J Am Acad Dermatol 2005; 52:579.

Paller AS, et al: Tacrolimus ointment is more effective than pimecrolimus cream with a similar safety profile in the treatment of atopic dermatitis: results from 3 randomized, comparative studies. J Am Acad Dermatol 2005; 52:810.

Rance F, et al: New visions for atopic eczema: an iPAC summary and future trends. Pediatr Allergy Immunol 2008; 19(Suppl 19):17.

Ricci G, et al: Three years of Italian experience of an educational program for parents of young children affected by atopic dermatitis: improving knowledge produces lower anxiety levels in parents of children with atopic dermatitis. Pediatr Dermatol 2009; 26:1.

Schmitt J, et al: Cyclosporin in the treatment of patients with atopic eczema—a systematic review and meta-analysis. J Eur Acad Dermatol Venereol 2007; 21:606.

Selnes A, et al: Diverging prevalence trends of atopic disorders in Norwegian children. Results from three cross-sectional studies. Allergy 2005; 60:894.

Sugarman JL: The epidermal barrier in atopic dermatitis. Semin Cutan Med Surg 2008; 27:108.

ten Berge O, et al: Throwing a light on photosensitivity in atopic dermatitis: a retrospective study. Am J Clin Dermatol 2009; 10:119.

van Os-Medendorp H, et al: Costs and cost-effectiveness of the nursing program 'Coping with itch' for patients with chronic pruritic skin disease. Br J Dermatol 2008; 158:1013.

Verhoeven EW, et al: Biopsychosocial mechanisms of chronic itch in patients with skin diseases: a review. Acta Derm Venereol 2008; 88:211.

Weiland SK, et al: Climate and the prevalence of symptoms of asthma, allergic rhinitis, and atopic eczema in children. Occup Environ Med 2004; 61:609.

Williams HC: Clinical practice. Atopic dermatitis. N Engl J Med 2005; 352:231.

Zoller L, et al: Low dose methotrexate therapy is effective in late-onset atopic dermatitis and idiopathic eczema. Isr Med Assoc J 2008; 10:413.

Eczema

The word eczema seems to have originated in AD 543 and is derived from the Greek work *ekzein*, meaning to "to boil forth" or "to effervesce." In its modern use, the term refers to a broad range of conditions that begin as spongiotic dermatitis and may progress to a lichenified stage. The term encompasses such disorders as dyshidrotic eczema and nummular eczema. The acute stage generally presents as a red edematous plaque that may have grossly visible, small, grouped vesicles. Subacute lesions present as erythematous plaques with scale or crusting. Later, lesions may be covered by a dryer scale or become lichenified. In most eczematous reactions, severe pruritus is a prominent symptom. The degree of irritation at which itching begins (the itch threshold) is lowered by stress. Itching is often prominent at bedtime and commonly results in insomnia. Heat and sweating may also provoke episodes of itching.

Histologically, the hallmark of all eczematous eruptions is a serous exudate between cells of the epidermis (spongiosis), with an underlying dermal perivascular lymphoid infiltrate and exocytosis (lymphocytes noted within spongiotic foci in the dermis). Spongiosis is generally out of proportion to the lymphoid cells in the epidermis. This is in contrast to mycosis fungoides, which demonstrates minimal spongiosis confined to the area immediately surrounding the lymphocytes.

In most eczematous processes, spongiosis is very prominent in the acute stage, where it is accompanied by little acanthosis or hyperkeratosis. Subacute spongiotic dermatitis demonstrates epidermal spongiosis with acanthosis and hyperkeratosis. Chronic lesions may have little accompanying spongiosis, but it is not uncommon for acute and chronic stages to overlap, as episodes of eczematous dermatitis follow one another. Scale corresponds to foci of parakeratosis produced by the inflamed epidermis. A crust is composed of serous exudate, acute inflammatory cells, and keratin. Eczema, regardless of cause, will manifest similar histologic changes if allowed to persist chronically. These features are related to chronic rubbing or scratching, and correspond clinically to lichen simplex chronicus or prurigo nodularis. Histologic features at this stage include compact hyperkeratosis, irregular acanthosis, and thickening of the collagen bundles in the papillary portion of the dermis. The dermal infiltrate at all stages is predominantly lymphoid, but an admixture of eosinophils may be noted. Neutrophils generally appear in secondarily infected lesions. Spongiosis with many intraepidermal eosinophils may be seen in the early spongiotic phase of pemphigoid, pemphigus, and incontinentia pigmenti, as well as some cases of allergic contact dermatitis.

Regional eczemas

Ear eczema

Eczema of the ears or otitis externa may involve the helix, postauricular fold, and external auditory canal. By far the most frequently affected site is the external canal, where it is often a manifestation of seborrheic dermatitis or allergic contact dermatitis (Fig. 5-7). Secretions of the ear canal derive from the

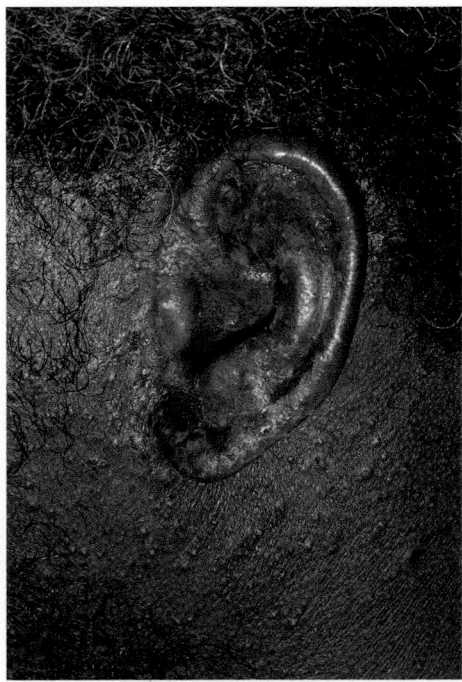

Fig. 5-7 Ear eczema secondary to allergic contact dermatitis.

specialized apocrine and sebaceous glands, which form cerumen. Rubbing, wiping, scratching, and picking exacerbate the condition. Secondary bacterial colonization or infection is common. Infection is usually caused by staphylococci, streptococci, or *Pseudomonas*. Contact dermatitis from neomycin, benzocaine, and preservatives may be caused by topical remedies. *Pseudomonas aeruginosa* can result in malignant external otitis with ulceration and sepsis. Earlobe dermatitis is virtually pathognomonic of metal contact dermatitis (especially nickel) and occurs most frequently in women who have pierced ears.

Treatment should be directed at removal of causative agents, such as topically applied allergens. Scales and cerumen should be removed by gentle lavage with an ear syringe. Antibiotic–corticoid preparations, such as Cortisporin otic suspension, have frequently been prescribed, and ingredients such as neomycin are therefore frequently found as relevant contact allergens. A combination of ciprofloxacin plus a topical steroid (Ciprodex) is preferred to neomycin-containing products. Corticosteroids alone can be effective for noninfected dermatitis. For very weepy lesions, Domeboro optic solution may be drying and beneficial.

Eyelid dermatitis

Eyelid dermatitis is most commonly related to atopic dermatitis or allergic contact dermatitis, or both (see Chapter 6). Allergic conjunctivitis in an atopic patient may lead to rubbing and scratching of the eyelid and result in secondary eyelid dermatitis. Seborrheic dermatitis, psoriasis, and airborne dermatitis are other possible causes. Ninety percent of patients with eyelid dermatitis are female. When an ocular medication contains an allergen, the allergen passes through the nasolacrimal duct, and dermatitis may also be noted below the nares in addition to the eyelids. Some cases of eyelid contact dermatitis are caused by substances transferred by the hands to the eyelids. If eyelid dermatitis occurs without associated atopic dermatitis, an allergen is detected in more than 50% of cases. More than 25% of patients with atopic dermatitis and eyelid dermatitis will also have allergic contact dermatitis contributing to the condition. Fragrances and balsam of Peru, metals (nickel and gold), paraphenylenediamine, thiomersal, quaternium 15, oleamidopropyl dimethlyamine, thiuram (in rubber pads used to apply eyelid cosmetics), and tosylamide formaldehyde (in nail polish) are common environmental allergens causing eyelid dermatitis. In medications, preservatives such as cocamidopropyl betaine and active agents such as phenylephrine hydrochloride, sodium cromoglycate, papaine, and idoxuridine have all been implicated.

Eyelid dermatitis requires careful management, often in collaboration with an ophthalmologist. The most important aspect is to identify and eliminate any possible triggering allergens as noted above. Patch testing for standard allergens, as well as the patient's ocular medications, is required. Preservative-free eye medications should be used. The ophthalmologist should monitor the patient for conjunctival complications, measure the intraocular pressure, and monitor for the development of cataracts, especially in patients with atopic dermatitis who have an increased risk for cataracts. Initially, topical corticosteroids and petrolatum-based emollients are recommended. If the dermatitis is persistent, the patient may be transitioned to TCIs to reduce the long-term risk of ocular steroid complications. The TCIs are often not initially tolerated on inflamed eyelids due to the burning. If there is an associated allergic conjunctivitis, or in patients who fail treatment with topical medications applied to the eyelid, ocular instillation of cyclosporine ophthalmic emulsion (Restasis) can be beneficial. Cromolyn sodium ophthalmic drops may be used to stabilize mast cells in the eyelid and reduce pruritus. In balsam of Peru-allergic patients, a balsam of Peru elimination diet may benefit.

Breast eczema (nipple eczema)

Eczema of the breasts usually affects the areolae, and may extend on to the surrounding skin (Fig. 5-8). The area around the base of the nipple is usually spared, and the nipple itself is less frequently affected. The condition is rarely seen in men. Usually, eczema of the nipples is of the moist type with oozing and crusting. Painful fissuring is frequently seen, especially in nursing mothers. Atopic dermatitis is a frequent cause, and nipple eczema may be the sole manifestation of atopic dermatitis in adult women. It frequently presents during breastfeeding. The role of secondary infection with bacteria and *Candida* should be considered in breastfeeding women. Other causes of nipple eczema are allergic contact dermatitis and irritant dermatitis. Irritant dermatitis occurs from friction (jogger's nipples), or from ill-fitting brassieres with seams in women with asymmetrical and large breasts. In patients in whom eczema of the nipple or areola has persisted for more than 3 months, especially if it is unilateral, a biopsy is mandatory to rule out the possibility of Paget's disease of the breast. Topical corticosteroids or TCIs are often effective in the treatment of non-Paget eczema of the breast. Nevoid hyperkeratosis of the nipples is a chronic condition that may mimic nipple eczema, but is not steroid-responsive.

Nipple eczema in the breastfeeding woman is a therapeutic challenge. The dermatitis may appear in an atopic woman when her child begins to ingest solid foods. This may signal contact dermatitis to a food. Allergic contact dermatitis may develop to topically applied protective creams (containing vitamin A and E, aloe, chamomile, or preservatives). Staphylococcal superinfection may develop, and can be identified by culture. Oral antibiotics are the preferred treatment for bacterial secondary infection. Candidal infection of the areola may present as normal skin, erythema, or an acute or chronic eczema. The area of the areola immediately adjacent to the nipple tends to be involved, sometimes with fine hairline cracks. Patients frequently complain of severe pain, especially with nursing. Analgesia may be required, and breastfeeding

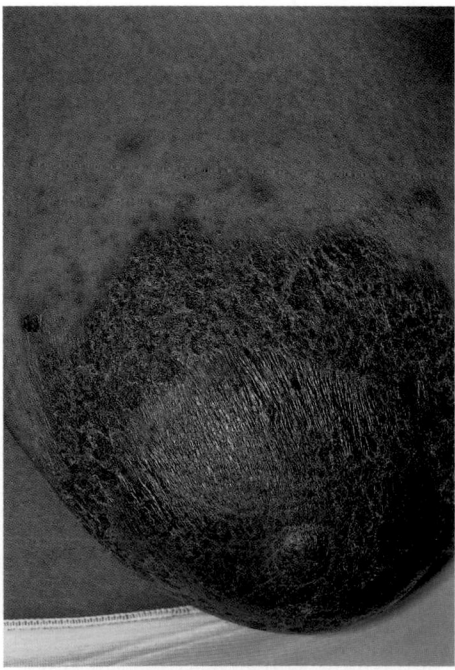

Fig. 5-8 Nummular eczema of the breast.

may need to be suspended for a period. Pumping and the use of a silicone nipple shield may be helpful. Associated conditions include oral thrush in the infant, antibiotic use, and a personal history of vaginal candidiasis. Cultures may or may not be positive from the affected areola/nipple. The child's mouth should also be cultured, even if the examination is completely normal, as candidal colonization of the breastfeeding infant's mouth may be asymptomatic with no findings on clinical examination. A positive culture from the infant in the setting of nipple eczema in the mother would warrant therapy of the mother and infant. Therapy with topical or systemic antifungal agents may be required to determine whether *Candida* is pathogenic. Oral fluconazole can be dramatically effective in these patients. Topical gentian violet 0.5%, applied once daily to the nipple, or all-purpose nipple ointment [(mupirocin 2% (10 g), nystatin 100 000 units/mL ointment (10 g), clotrimazole 10% (vaginal cream) (10 g), and betamethasone 0.1% ointment (10 g)] is an effective topical agent. The child's thrush should also be treated. A lactation consultant or nurse may be helpful in managing these patients, since poor positioning during breastfeeding is a common cofactor in the development of nipple eczema.

Hand eczema

Hand eczema is a common and important skin condition. Every year, about 10% of the population has at least one episode of hand dermatitis, and at any time about 5% of the population is affected. The genetic risk factors for the development of hand dermatitis are unknown. Even among patients with atopic dermatitis, it is unclear whether patients with null mutations for *FLG* are at increased risk. Hand eczema is the most common occupational skin condition, accounting for more than 80% of all occupational dermatitis. Tobacco smoking and alcohol consumption do not appear to be risk factors for the development of hand eczema. Women are at increased risk for the development of hand eczema. Most of this increased risk is accounted for by a "spike" in the rate of hand eczema in the 20–29-year age group, when increased environmental exposures increase women's risk (childcare, housecleaning, etc). Chronic hand eczema, especially if severe, significantly reduces the patient's quality of life and is associated with symptoms of depression. A significant portion of patients with hand eczema will still be affected 15 years later. The risk for persistence of the hand eczema is doubled if there is associated eczema at other sites at presentation, if there is a childhood history of atopic dermatitis, and if the onset of the hand eczema was before age 20. Preventive interventions have been successful on two fronts:

1. Persons at high risk for hand eczema can be identified and counseled to avoid high-risk occupations.
2. Once occupational hand eczema develops, there are some occupation-specific strategies that can lead to improvement and prevent recurrence.

The evaluation and management of hand eczema have been hampered by the lack of a uniform classification system and a dearth of controlled therapeutic trials. The diagnostic dilemma in hand dermatitis is in part related to two factors. The clinical appearance of the skin eruption on the palms and soles may be very similar, independent of the etiology. In addition, virtually all chronic hand dermatitis demonstrates a chronic dermatitis histologically, again independent of pathogenic cause. Psoriasis, specifically, on the palms and soles, may show spongiosis and closely resemble a dermatitis (Fig. 5-9). As a consequence, the proposed classification schemes rely on a combination of morphological features, history of coexistent illnesses, occupational exposure, and results of patch testing. The different types of hand eczema are:

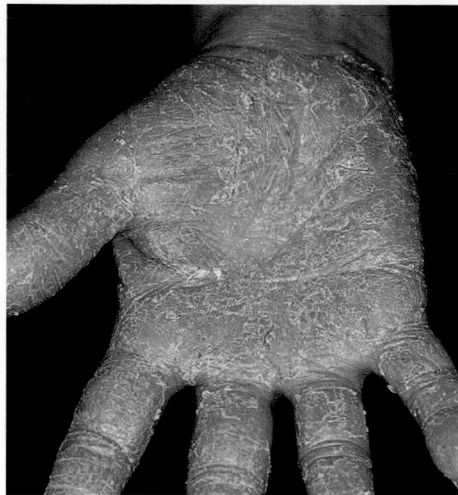

Fig. 5-9 Hand eczema.

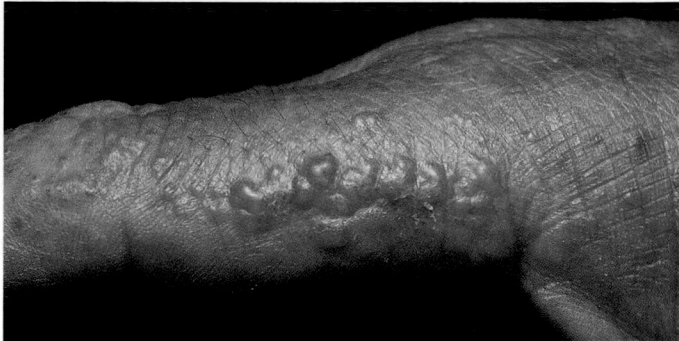

Fig. 5-10 Acute vesiculobullous hand eczema.

1. allergic contact dermatitis (with or without an additional irritant component)
2. irritant hand dermatitis
3. atopic hand eczema (with or without an additional irritant component)
4. vesicular (or vesiculobullous) endogenous hand eczema
5. hyperkeratotic endogenous hand eczema.

A complete history, careful examination of the rest of the body surface, and, at times, patch testing are essential in establishing a diagnosis. The importance of patch testing cannot be overemphasized. Allergens in the environment (especially shower gels and shampoos), in the workplace, and in topical medications may be important in any given patient. Patch testing must include broad screens of common allergens or cases of allergic contact dermatitis will be missed.

The role of ingested nickel in the development of hand eczema in nickel-allergic patients is controversial. Some practitioners treat such patients with low-nickel diets and even disulfiram chelation with reported benefit. However, the risk of development of hand eczema in adulthood is independent of nickel allergy. Similarly, the role of low-balsam diets in the management of balsam of Peru-allergic patients with hand eczema is unclear.

Wet work (skin in liquids or gloves for more than 2 hours per day, or handwashing more than 20 times per day) is a strong risk factor for hand eczema. High-risk occupations include those that entail wet work, and those with exposure to potential allergens. These nine "high-risk" occupations include bakers, hairdressers, dental surgery assistants, kitchen workers/cooks, butchers, healthcare workers, cleaners, doctors/dentists/veterinarians, and laboratory technicians. In about 5% of patients with hand eczema, especially if this is severe, it is associated with prolonged missed work, job change, and job loss. In healthcare workers, the impaired barrier poses a risk for infection by blood-borne pathogens.

Almost one-third of baker's apprentices develop hand dermatitis within 12 months of entering the profession. Among hairdressers, the incidence approaches 50% after several years. Both irritant dermatitis and allergic contact dermatitis are important factors, with glyceryl monothioglycolate and ammonium persulfate being the most common allergens among hairdressers. Among those with preservative allergy, the hands are preferentially involved in patients allergic to isothiazolinones and formaldehyde, while the hands and face are equally involved with paraben allergy. Cement workers have a high rate of hand dermatitis related to contact allergy, alkalinity, and hygroscopic effects of cement. Dorsal hand dermatitis in a cement worker suggests contact allergy to chromate or cobalt. The addition of ferrous sulfate to cement has no effect on irritant dermatitis, but reduces the incidence of allergic chromate dermatitis by two-thirds.

Among patients with occupational hand dermatitis, atopic patients are disproportionately represented. Hand dermatitis is frequently the initial or only adult manifestation of an atopic diathesis. The likelihood of developing hand eczema is greatest in patients with atopic dermatitis, more common if the atopic dermatitis was severe, but still increased in incidence in patients with only respiratory atopy. Atopic patients should receive career counseling in adolescence to avoid occupations that are likely to induce hand dermatitis.

Contact urticaria syndrome may present as immediate burning, itching, or swelling of the hands, but a chronic eczematous phase may also occur. Latex is an important cause of the syndrome, but raw meat, lettuce, garlic, onion, carrot, tomato, spinach, grapefruit, orange, radish, fig, parsnip, cheese, or any number of other foods may be implicated.

Vesiculobullous hand eczema (pompholyx, dyshidrosis)

Idiopathic acute vesicular hand dermatitis is not related to blockage of sweat ducts, although palmoplantar hyperhidrosis is common in these patients and control of hyperhidrosis improves the eczema. Acute pompholyx, also known as cheiropompholyx if it affects the hands, presents with severe, sudden outbreaks of intensely pruritic vesicles. Primary lesions are macroscopic, deep-seated multilocular vesicles resembling tapioca on the sides of the fingers (Fig. 5-10), palms, and soles. The eruption is symmetrical and pruritic, with pruritus often preceding the eruption. Coalescence of smaller lesions may lead to bulla formation severe enough to prevent ambulation. Individual outbreaks resolve spontaneously over several weeks. Bullous tinea or an id reaction from a dermatophyte should be excluded, and patch testing should be considered to rule out allergic contact dermatitis.

Chronic vesiculobullous hand eczema

In chronic cases the lesions may be hyperkeratotic, scaling, and fissured, and the "dyshidrosiform" pattern may be recognized only during exacerbations. There is a tendency for the pruritic 1–2 mm vesicles to be most pronounced at the sides of the fingers. In long-standing cases the nails may become dystrophic. The distribution of the lesions is, as a rule, bilateral and roughly symmetrical.

Hyperkeratotic hand dermatitis

Males outnumber females by 2:1, and the patients are usually older adults. The eruption presents as hyperkeratotic, fissure-prone, erythematous areas of the middle or proximal palm. The volar surfaces of the fingers may also be involved (Fig. 5-11). Plantar lesions occur in about 10% of patients.

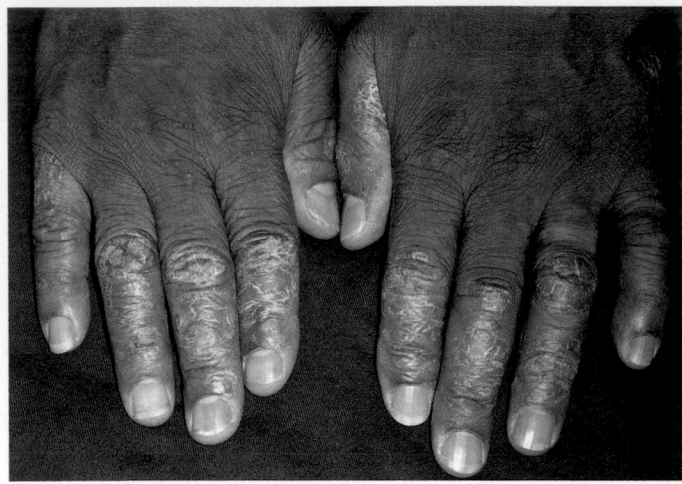

Fig. 5-11 Hyperkeratotic hand dermatitis.

Histologically, the lesions show chronic spongiotic dermatitis. The most important differential diagnosis is psoriasis, and some of the patients with chronic hyperkeratotic hand dermatitis will ultimately prove to be psoriatic. The presence of sharply demarcated plaques, nail pitting, or occasional crops of pustules is an important clue to psoriatic hand involvement.

Treatment

The hands are essential for work both in and out of the home. Treatment regimens must be practical and allow patients to function as normally as possible. There are few controlled treatment trials for hand dermatitis, and only recently has the type of hand eczema been identified in the trial. As one might suspect, the efficacy of some of the treatments depends on the morphology of the eruption and the diagnostic classification (see above).

Protection Vinyl gloves may be worn during wet work, especially when detergents are used. Although vinyl gloves protect against chemicals, they do not prevent exposure to heat through the glove or the macerating effect of sweat, which accumulates under the gloves. They are also far less durable than rubber gloves. Rubber gloves may be used at home if patients do not exhibit allergy to rubber chemicals or latex. Wearing white cotton gloves under the vinyl gloves is beneficial. For rough work, such as gardening, wearing protective cloth or leather gloves is essential. Cotton can adsorb allergens in the environment, and cotton gloves worn throughout the day offer little protection from many allergens.

Barrier repair Moisturizing is a critical component of the management of hand dermatitis. Application of a protective moisturizing cream or ointment after each handwashing or water exposure is recommended. Creams require a preservative and have a higher risk of contact sensitivity. Ointments tend to have few ingredients and do not generally require a preservative. At night, even during periods of remission, a heavy moisturizing ointment should be applied to the hands after soaking in water. If palmar dryness is present, occlusion of the moisturizer with a plastic bag or vinyl gloves is recommended. White petrolatum is cheap and nonsensitizing, and remains a valuable agent in the treatment of hand dermatitis.

Topical agents Superpotent and potent topical steroid agents are first-line pharmacologic therapy. Their efficacy is enhanced by presoaking and occlusion (soak and smear technique or wet dressings). A single application with occlusion at night is often more effective than multiple daytime applications. As in the treatment of atopic dermatitis, once steroid receptors are saturated, additional applications of a corticos-

teroid contribute only an emollient effect. Triamcinolone 0.1% ointment is available in a nonsensitizing white petrolatum base. It is fairly potent and inexpensive, does not irritate, and has a low incidence of sensitization. In refractory cases, superpotent steroids may be used for a period of 2–3 weeks, then on weekends, with a milder corticosteroid applied during the week. The addition of 2.5% zinc sulfate to clobetasol seemed to enhance efficacy of the topical steroid. Chronic use of potent fluorinated corticosteroids may be associated with skin atrophy.

TCIs may be of benefit in some mildly affected patients. Soaks with a tar bath oil or applications of 20% liquor carbonis detergens or 2% crude coal tar in an ointment base may be of benefit, especially in those patients with the hyperkeratotic type of hand eczema. Bexarotene gel can be beneficial in up to 50% of patients with refractory hand eczema.

Phototherapy Phototherapy in the form of high-dose UVA-1, soak or cream PUVA, and oral PUVA can be effective. Given the thickness of the palms, UVA irradiation should be delivered 30 min after soaking, as opposed to bath PUVA, which can be done immediately after bathing. Relatively few phototoxic reactions are seen with regimens that use a 15–20 min soak in a 3 mg/L solution of 8-methoxypsoralen, starting with 0.25–0.5 J/cm^2 and increasing by 0.25–0.5 J/cm^2 three times a week.

Superficial Grenz ray radiotherapy remains a viable modality, but well-maintained machines are few in number. The depth of penetration is limited, so it is best used after acute crusting and vesiculation have been cleared with other treatment. Doses of 200 cG are delivered at weekly intervals for a total of 800–1000 cG. Therapy may be repeated after 6 months. The total lifetime dose should not exceed 5000 cG.

Botulinum toxin In patients with palmoplantar hyperhidrosis and associated hand eczema, treatment of the hyperhidrosis with intradermal injections of botulinum toxin leads to both dramatic resolution of the sweating and clearing of the hand eczema. The hand eczema returns when the sweating returns. Iontophoresis, which also reduces sweating, can similarly improve hand dermatitis. This illustrates the importance of wetness in the exacerbation of hand eczema.

Systemic agents The systemic agents used to treat severe chronic hand dermatitis are identical to those used for atopic dermatitis. The use of systemic corticosteroids usually results in dramatic improvement. Unfortunately, relapse frequently occurs almost as rapidly, so systemic steroids are recommended only to control acute exacerbations. For instance, patients with infrequent, but severe, outbreaks of pompholyx may benefit from a few weeks of systemic steroids, starting at about 1 mg/kg/day. Patients with persistent severe hand dermatitis should be considered for alternative, steroid-sparing therapy.

Methotrexate, in psoriatic doses, azathioprine, and mycophenolate mofetil (in doses of 1–1.5 g twice a day for an adult) can all be considered. Cyclosporine can be effective, but given the chronicity of hand eczema, its use is best reserved for severe outbreaks. Oral retinoids may have a place in the management of hand dermatitis. Alitretinoin, at a dose of 30 mg per day, will lead to complete or near-complete clearance of chronic refractory hand eczema in about 50% of cases. The onset of response is delayed, with some patients achieving optimal benefit only after more than 6 months of treatment.

Workplace modifications The incidence of hand dermatitis in the workplace can be reduced by identifying major irritants and allergens, preventing exposure through engineering controls, substituting less irritating chemicals when possible, enforcing personal protection and glove use, and instituting organized worker education. Hand eczema classes have been documented to reduce the burden of occupational dermatitis. It is important to note that prevention of exposure to a weak but frequent irritant can have more profound effects than removal of a strong but infrequently contacted irritant. Proper gloves are essential in industrial settings. Nitrile gloves are generally less permeable than latex gloves. Gloves of ethylene vinyl alcohol copolymer sandwiched with polyethylene are effective against epoxy resin, methyl methacrylate, and many other organic compounds. Latex and vinyl gloves offer little protection against acrylates. The 4H (4 h) glove and nitrile are best in this setting. As hospitals transition to nonlatex gloves, it is important to note that even low-protein, powder-free latex gloves reduce self-reported skin problems among health workers.

Barrier products can improve hand dermatitis if used in the appropriate setting. Foams containing dimethicone and glycerin can reduce hand dermatitis related to wet work.

Diaper (napkin) dermatitis

Diaper dermatitis has dramatically decreased due to highly absorbable disposable diapers. None the less, dermatitis of the diaper area in infants remains a common cutaneous disorder. The highest prevalence occurs between 6 and 12 months of age. Diaper dermatitis is also seen in adults with urinary or fecal incontinence who wear diapers.

Irritant diaper dermatitis is an erythematous dermatitis limited to exposed surfaces. The folds remain unaffected, in contrast to intertrigo, inverse psoriasis, and candidiasis, where the folds are frequently involved. In severe cases of irritant dermatitis there may be superficial erosion or even ulceration. The tip of the penis may become irritated and crusted, with the result that the baby urinates frequently and spots of blood appear on the diaper.

Complications of diaper dermatitis include punched-out ulcers or erosions with elevated borders (Jacquet erosive diaper dermatitis); pseudoverrucous papules and nodules; and violaceous plaques and nodules (granuloma gluteale infantum).

The importance of ammonia in common diaper dermatitis has been overstated, but constant maceration of the skin is critical. The absence of diaper dermatitis in societies in which children do not wear diapers clearly implicates the diaper environment as the cause of the eruption. Moist skin is more easily abraded by friction of the diaper as the child moves. Wet skin is more permeable to irritants. Skin wetness also allows the growth of bacteria and yeast. Bacteria raise the local pH, increasing the activity of fecal lipases and proteases. *Candida albicans* is frequently a secondary invader and, when present, produces typical satellite erythematous lesions or pustules at the periphery as the dermatitis spreads.

Napkin psoriasis (Fig. 5-12), seborrheic dermatitis, atopic dermatitis, Langerhans cell histiocytosis, tinea cruris, allergic contact dermatitis, acrodermatitis enteropathica, aminoacidurias, biotin deficiency, and congenital syphilis should be included in the differential diagnosis. Given the skill of most pediatricians in the management of diaper dermatitis, dermatologists should think about these conditions in infants who have failed the standard interventions used by pediatricians. Refractory diaper dermatitis may require a biopsy to exclude some of the above conditions.

Prevention is the best treatment. Diapers that contain superabsorbent gel have been proved effective in preventing diaper dermatitis in both neonates and infants. They work by absorbing the wetness away from the skin and by buffering the pH. Cloth diapers and regular disposable diapers are equal to each other in their propensity to cause diaper dermatitis and are inferior to the superabsorbent gel diapers. The frequent changing of diapers is also critical.

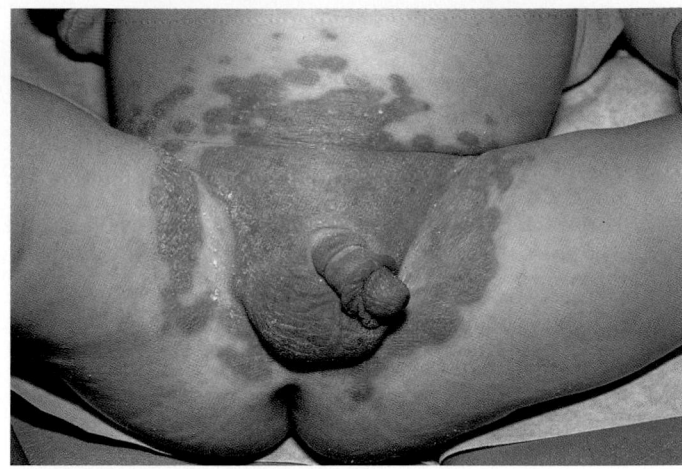

Fig. 5-12 Napkin psoriasis.

Protecting the skin of the diaper area is of great benefit in all forms of diaper dermatitis. Zinc oxide paste is excellent. Zinc oxide paste with 0.25% miconazole may be considered if *Candida* may be present. If simple improved hygiene and barrier therapy are not effective, the application of a mixture of equal parts nystatin ointment and 1% hydrocortisone ointment at each diaper change offers both anticandidal activity and an occlusive protective barrier from urine and stool, and can be very effective.

Circumostomy eczema

Eczematization of the surrounding skin frequently occurs after an ileostomy or colostomy. It is estimated that some 75% of ileostomy patients have some postoperative sensitivity as a result of the leakage of intestinal fluid on to unprotected skin. As the consistency of the intestinal secretion becomes viscous, the sensitization subsides. Proprietary medications containing karaya powder have been found to be helpful. Twenty percent cholestyramine (an ion-exchange resin) in Aquaphor, and topical sucralfate as a powder or emollient at 4 g% concentration, are both effective treatments. Psoriasis may also appear at ostomy sites. Topical treatment may be difficult, as the appliance adheres poorly after the topical agents are applied. A topical steroid spray may be used, and will not interfere with appliance adherence. Contact dermatitis to the ostomy bag adhesive can be problematic, as even supposed hypoallergenic ostomy bags may still trigger dermatitis in these patients.

Autosensitization and conditioned irritability

The presence of a localized, chronic, and usually severe focus of dermatitis may affect distant skin in two ways. Patients with a chronic localized dermatitis may develop dermatitis at distant sites from scratching or irritating the skin. This is called "conditioned irritability." The most common scenario is distant dermatitis in a patient with a chronic eczematous leg ulcer. Autoeczematization refers to the spontaneous development of widespread dermatitis or dermatitis distant from a local inflammatory focus. The agent causing the local inflammatory focus is not the direct cause of the dermatitis at the distant sites. Autoeczematization most commonly presents as a generalized acute vesicular eruption with a prominent dyshidrosiform component on the hands. The most common associated condition is a chronic eczema of the legs, with or without ulceration. The "angry back" or "excited skin" syndrome observed with strongly positive patch tests, and the local dermatitis seen around infectious foci (infectious eczematoid dermatitis), may represent a limited form of this reaction.

Id reactions

Patients with a variety of infectious disorders may present with eczematous dermatitis. The classic example is the vesicular id reactions of the hands in response to an inflammatory tinea of the feet. Similarly, inflammatory tinea capitis is often associated with a focal or diffuse dermatitis, primarily of the upper half of the body. Nummular eczematous lesions or pityriasis rosea-like lesions may occur in patients with head or pubic louse infestation. Id reactions clear when the focus of infection or infestation is treated.

Juvenile plantar dermatosis

Juvenile plantar dermatosis is an eczematous disorder of children, first described by Enta and Moller in 1972, and named by Mackie in 1976. It is probably the same disease as symmetrical lividity of the soles described by Pernet in 1925. It usually begins as a patchy, symmetrical, smooth, red, glazed macule on the base or medial surface of the great toes, sometimes with fissuring and desquamation, in children aged 3 to puberty. Lesions evolve into red scaling patches involving the weight-bearing and frictional areas of the feet, usually symmetrically (Fig. 5-13). The forefoot is usually much more involved than the heel. Toe webs and arches are spared. The eruption is disproportionately more common in atopic children. In some patients, a similar eruption occurs on the fingers.

The disease is caused by the repeated maceration of the feet by occlusive shoes, especially athletic shoes, or by the abrasive effects of pool surfaces or diving boards. The affected soles remain wet in the rubber bottoms of the shoes or are macerated by pool water. Thin, nonabsorbent, synthetic socks contribute to the problem.

Histologically, there is psoriasiform acanthosis and a sparse, largely lymphocytic infiltrate in the upper dermis, most dense around sweat ducts at their point of entry into the epidermis. Spongiosis is commonly present and the stratum corneum is thin but compact.

The diagnosis is apparent on inspection, especially if there is a family or personal history of atopy and the toe webs are spared. Allergic contact dermatitis to shoes and dermatophytosis should be considered in the differential diagnosis.

Allergic shoe dermatitis usually involves the dorsal foot, but some patients with rubber allergy have predominant involvement of the soles. Treatment involves avoidance of maceration. Foot powders, thick absorbent socks, absorbent insoles, and having alternate pairs of shoes to wear to allow the shoes to dry out are all beneficial. Topical steroid medications are of limited value and often are no more effective than occlusive barrier protection. Petrolatum or urea preparations can sometimes be of benefit. Most cases clear within 4 years of diagnosis.

Xerotic eczema

Xerotic eczema is also known as winter itch, eczema craquelé, and asteatotic eczema. These vividly descriptive terms are all applied to dehydrated skin showing redness, dry scaling, and fine crackling that may resemble crackled porcelain or the fissures in the bed of a dried lake or pond. The primary lesion is an erythematous patch covered with an adherent scale. As the lesion enlarges, fine cracks in the epidermis occur (Fig. 5-14). Nummular lesions may occur. Xerotic "nummular" eczema is less weepy than classic nummular dermatitis. Favored sites are the anterior shins, extensor arms, and flank. Elderly persons are particularly predisposed, and xerosis appears to be the most common cause of pruritus in older individuals. Xerotic eczema is seen most frequently during the winter, when there is low relative humidity. Bathing with hot water and harsh soaps contributes. The epidermal water barrier is impaired and TEWL is increased. Epidermal barrier repair begins to decrease after age 55. It is correlated with an increase in epidermal pH. This is why older patients complain that they have not changed their bathing routine or soaps, yet have developed xerotic dermatitis. The loss of barrier repair ability is improved by acidifying the epidermis; hence the benefit of mild acids in treating xerosis.

Short tepid baths, limitation of the use of soap to soiled and apocrine-bearing areas, avoiding harsh soaps and using acid pH synthetic detergents, and prompt application of an emollient after bathing are usually effective. White petrolatum and emollients containing 10% urea or 5% lactic acid are effective.

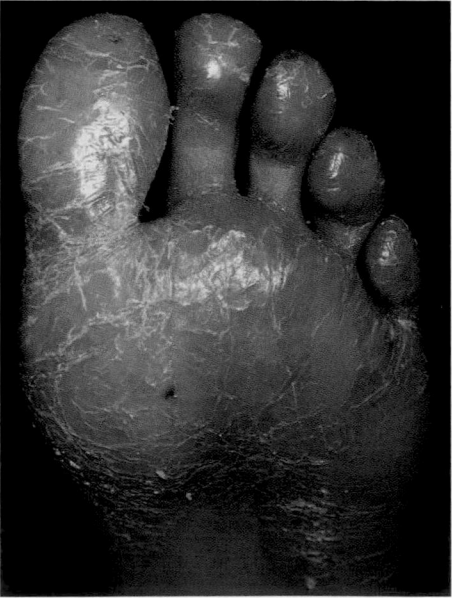

Fig. 5-13 Glazed appearance of the weight-bearing surfaces in juvenile plantar dermatosis.

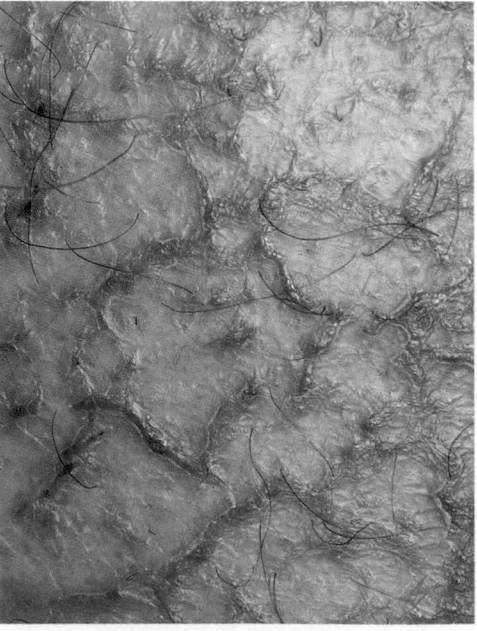

Fig. 5-14 Fine network of epidermal fissures in eczema craquelé.

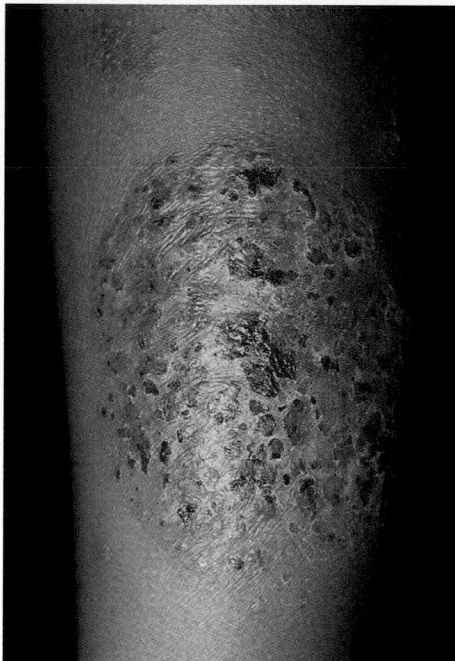

Fig. 5-15 Nummular eczema.

Topical steroids in ointment vehicles are useful for inflamed areas.

Nummular eczema (discoid eczema)

Nummular eczema usually begins on the lower legs, dorsa of the hands, or extensor surfaces of the arms. A single lesion often precedes the eruption and may be present for some time before other lesions appear. The primary lesions are discrete, coin-shaped, erythematous, edematous, vesicular, and crusted patches (Fig. 5-15). Most lesions are 2–40 cm in diameter. Lesions may form after trauma (conditioned hyperirritability). As new lesions appear, the old lesions expand as tiny papulovesicular satellite lesions appear at the periphery and fuse with the main plaque. In severe cases the condition may spread into palm-sized or larger patches. Pruritus is usually severe and of the same paroxysmal, compulsive quality and nocturnal timing seen in atopic dermatitis and prurigo nodularis.

Atopic dermatitis frequently has nummular morphology in adolescents, but in atopy the lesions tend to be more chronic and lichenified. Histologically, nummular eczema is characterized by acute or subacute spongiotic dermatitis.

Initial treatment consists of simple soaking and greasing with an occlusive ointment, and once or twice a day application of a potent or superpotent topical steroid cream or ointment. Ointments are more effective and occlusion may be necessary. If secondary staphylococcal infection is present, an antibiotic with appropriate coverage is recommended. Sedating antihistamines at bedtime are useful to help with sleep and reduce night-time scratching. In some cases refractory to topical agents, intralesional or systemic corticosteroid therapy may be required. In cases failing topical steroids, phototherapy with NB-UVB, or soak or oral PUVA can be effective. For refractory plaques, the addition of topical tar as 2% crude coal tar or 20% LCD may be beneficial.

Pruritic dermatitis in the elderly

Pruritic skin conditions are common in elderly patients. They begin to appear around age 60 and increase in severity with age. Males are more commonly affected. The dermatoses seen in this age group are typically either eczematous or papular. The eczematous plaques may resemble nummular dermatitis, a feature recognized by Marion Sulzberger when he coined the phrase "exudative discoid and lichenoid chronic dermatitis" or "oid-oid disease." The pathogenic basis of this component of dermatitis in the elderly may be related to barrier failure due to loss of acidification of the epidermis. In addition, patients often have urticarial papules on the trunk and proximal extremities that resemble insect bites. These lesions are termed "subacute prurigo." Histologically, they demonstrate features of an arthropod assault, with superficial and deep perivascular lymphohistiocytic infiltrates, dermal edema, and at times interstitial eosinophils. Lesions may also show features of transient acantholytic dermatitis or eosinophilic folliculitis. This component of the eruption may be related to the tendency of the elderly to have immune systems that skew toward Th2, due to loss of Th1 function. At times patients will have both types of eruption, either simultaneously or sequentially. The combination of barrier failure and an immune system skewed toward Th2 is parallel to what occurs in the setting of atopic dermatitis. For this reason, some practitioners consider this "adult atopic dermatitis." However, it is unknown whether these conditions have a genetic basis, or more likely, given the time of onset, are due to acquired barrier and immune system abnormalities. In these patients, allergic contact dermatitis and photodermatitis may be present or develop. Patch testing may identify important allergens, avoidance of which leads to improvement. Calcium channel blockers may be associated with this condition, but stopping them will clear only about one-quarter of patients on that class of medication. Treatment for these patients is similar to treatment of atopic dermatitis, with antihistamines, emollients, and topical steroids (soak and smear) as the first line. In refractory cases, phototherapy (UVB or PUVA), Goeckerman therapy (UVB plus crude coal tar) in a day-treatment setting, and immunosuppressive agents can be effective. Inadvertent use of phototherapy in the patient with coexistent photosensitivity will lead to an exacerbation of the disorder.

Hormone-induced dermatoses

Autoimmune progesterone dermatitis may appear as urticarial papules, deep gyrate lesions, papulovesicular lesions, an eczematous eruption, or targetoid lesions. Urticarial and erythema multiforme-like lesions are most characteristic. Lesions typically appear 5–7 days before menses, and improve or resolve a few days following menses. Biopsies show dense superficial and deep dermal lymphocytic infiltration, with involvement of the follicles, and an admixture of eosinophils. There may be an accompanying mild interface component, as seen in drug eruptions. Pruritus is common. Onset is typically in the third and fourth decades. Familial cases have been reported. When urticaria is the predominant skin lesion, there is a generalized distribution, and it may be accompanied by laryngospasm. Anaphylactoid reactions may occur. Oral erosions may be present. The eruption typically appears during the luteal phase of the menstrual period, and spontaneously clears following menstruation, only to return in the next menstrual period. Many of the reported patients had received artificial progestational agents before the onset of the eruption. In some it appeared during a normal pregnancy. The eruption may worsen or clear during pregnancy. Rarely, it can occur in males and adolescent females. Progesterone luteal phase support during in vitro fertilization has exacerbated the disease.

In most cases, diagnosis has been confirmed by intradermal testing with 0.01 mL of aqueous progesterone suspension (50 mg/mL). A positive test may be immediate (30 min) or delayed (24–96 h). Flares may be induced by intramuscular or oral progesterone. The most commonly used treatment is an oral contraceptive to suppress ovulation, thereby reducing progesterone levels. Topical steroids, antihistamines (cetirizine plus hydroxyzine), conjugated estrogen, leuprolide acetate, danazol, and tamoxifen may be effective in some cases.

Autoimmune estrogen dermatitis also presents as a cyclic skin disorder that may appear eczematous, papular, bullous, or urticarial. Pruritus is typically present. Skin eruptions may be chronic but are exacerbated premenstrually or occur only immediately before the menses. Characteristically, the dermatosis clears during pregnancy and at menopause. Intracutaneous skin testing with estrone produces a papule lasting longer than 24 h or an immediate urticarial wheal (in cases with urticaria). Injections of progesterone yield negative results, ruling out autoimmune progesterone dermatitis. Tamoxifen is effective in some cases.

Agner T, et al: Hand eczema severity and quality of life: a cross-sectional, multicentre study of hand eczema patients. Contact Dermatitis 2008; 59:43.

Amato L, et al: Atopic dermatitis exclusively localized on nipples and areolas. Pediatr Dermatol 2005; 22:64.

Amin KA, et al: The aetiology of eyelid dermatitis: a 10-year retrospective analysis. Contact Dermatitis 2006; 55:280.

Aydin O, et al: Non-pustular palmoplantar psoriasis: is histologic differentiation from eczematous dermatitis possible? J Cutan Pathol 2008; 35:169.

Barankin B, et al: Nipple and areolar eczema in the breastfeeding woman. J Cutan Med Surg 2004; 8:126.

Behrens S, et al: PUVA-bath photochemotherapy (PUVA-soak therapy) of recalcitrant dermatoses of the palms and soles. Photodermatol Photoimmunol Photomed 1999; 15:47.

Chawla SV, et al: Autoimmune progesterone dermatitis. Arch Dermatol 2009; 145:341.

Cvetkovski RS, et al: Prognosis of occupational hand eczema: a follow-up study. Arch Dermatol 2006; 142:305.

Diepgen TL, et al: Hand eczema classification: a cross-sectional, multicentre study of the aetiology and morphology of hand eczema. Br J Dermatol 2009; 160:353.

Elston DM, et al: Hand dermatitis. J Am Acad Dermatol 2002; 47:291.

Faghihi G, et al: The efficacy of '0.05% clobetasol + 2.5% zinc sulphate' cream vs. '0.05% clobetasol alone' cream in the treatment of the chronic hand eczema: a double-blind study. J Eur Acad Dermatol Venereol 2008; 22:531.

Feser A, et al: Periorbital dermatitis—a recalcitrant disease: causes and differential diagnoses. Br J Dermatol 2008; 159:858.

Guillet MH, et al: A 3-year causative study of pompholyx in 120 patients. Arch Dermatol 2007; 143:1504.

Halevy S, et al: Autoimmune progesterone dermatitis manifested as erythema annulare centrifugum: confirmation of progesterone sensitivity by in vitro interferon-gamma release. J Am Acad Dermatol 2002; 47:311.

Hanifin JM, et al: Novel treatment of chronic severe hand dermatitis with bexarotene gel. Br J Dermatol 2004; 150:545.

Jacob SE: Ciclosporin ophthalmic emulsion—a novel therapy for benzyl alcohol-associated eyelid dermatitis. Contact Dermatitis 2008; 58:169.

Jarvikallio A, et al: Mast cells, nerves and neuropeptides in atopic dermatitis and nummular eczema. Arch Dermatol Res 2003; 295:2.

Jenkins J, et al: Autoimmune progesterone dermatitis associated with infertility treatment. J Am Acad Dermatol 2008; 58:353.

Kontochristopoulos G, et al: Letter: regression of relapsing dyshidrotic eczema after treatment of concomitant hyperhidrosis with botulinum toxin-A. Dermatol Surg 2007; 33:1289.

Kucharekova M, et al: A randomized comparison of an emollient containing skin-related lipids with a petrolatum-based emollient as adjunct in the treatment of chronic hand dermatitis. Contact Dermatitis 2003; 48:293.

Lerbaek A, et al: Incidence of hand eczema in a population-based twin cohort: genetic and environmental risk factors. Br J Dermatol 2007; 157:552.

Meding B, et al: Fifteen-year follow-up of hand eczema: persistence and consequences. Br J Dermatol 2005; 152:975.

Meding B, et al: Fifteen-year follow-up of hand eczema: predictive factors. J Invest Dermatol 2005; 124:893.

Modak S, et al: A topical cream containing a zinc gel (allergy guard) as a prophylactic against latex glove-related contact dermatitis. Dermatitis 2005; 16:22.

Mutasim DF, et al: Bullous autoimmune estrogen dermatitis. J Am Acad Dermatol 2003; 49:130.

Nivenius E, et al: Tacrolimus ointment vs steroid ointment for eyelid dermatitis in patients with atopic keratoconjunctivitis. Eye 2007; 21:968.

Oskay T, et al: Autoimmune progesterone dermatitis. Eur J Dermatol 2002; 12:589.

Petering H, et al: Comparison of localized high-dose UVA1 irradiation versus topical cream psoralen-UVA for treatment of chronic vesicular dyshidrotic eczema. J Am Acad Dermatol 2004; 50:68.

Pozo-Roman T, et al: Psoralen cream plus ultraviolet A photochemotherapy (PUVA cream): our experience. J Eur Acad Dermatol Venereol 2006; 20:136.

Rasi A, et al: Autoimmune progesterone dermatitis. Int J Dermatol 2004; 43:588.

Robertson L: New and existing therapeutic options for hand eczema. Skin Therapy Lettercom, 2009.

Ruzicka T, et al: Efficacy and safety of oral alitretinoin (9-cis retinoic acid) in patients with severe chronic hand eczema refractory to topical corticosteroids: results of a randomized, double-blind, placebo-controlled, multicentre trial. Br J Dermatol 2008; 158:808.

Salam TN, et al: Balsam-related systemic contact dermatitis. J Am Acad Dermatol 2001; 45:377.

Shackelford KE, et al: The etiology of allergic-appearing foot dermatitis: a 5-year retrospective study. J Am Acad Dermatol 2002; 47:715.

Snyder JL, et al: Autoimmune progesterone dermatitis and its manifestation as anaphylaxis: a case report and literature review. Ann Allergy Asthma Immunol 2003; 90:469.

Swartling C, et al: Treatment of dyshidrotic hand dermatitis with intradermal botulinum toxin. J Am Acad Dermatol 2002; 47:667.

Temesvari E, et al: Periocular dermatitis: a report of 401 patients. J Eur Acad Dermatol Venereol 2009; 23:124.

Veien NK, et al: Hand eczema: causes, course, and prognosis I. Contact Dermatitis 2008; 58:330.

Veien NK, et al: Hand eczema: causes, course, and prognosis II. Contact Dermatitis 2008; 58:335.

Walling HW, et al: Autoimmune progesterone dermatitis. Case report with histologic overlap of erythema multiforme and urticaria. Int J Dermatol 2008; 47:380.

Immunodeficiency syndromes

Primary immunodeficiency diseases (PIDs), although rare, are important to the dermatologist. They may present with skin manifestations, and the dermatologist may be instrumental in referring appropriate patients for immunodeficiency evaluations. These conditions have also given us tremendous insight into the genetic makeup and functioning of the immune system. The PIDs are still classified as those with predominantly antibody deficiency, impaired cell-mediated immunity (cellular immunodeficiencies, T cells, natural killer (NK) cells), combined B- and T-cell deficiencies, defects of phagocytic function, complement deficiencies, and well-characterized syndromes with immunodeficiency. More than 120 PIDs were identified, as of the 2005 classification. While many PIDs will present within the first year of life, adult presentations can occur.

The dermatologist should suspect a PID in certain situations. Skin infections, especially chronic and recurrent bacterial skin infections, are often the initial manifestation of a PID. Fungal (especially *Candida*) and viral infections (warts, molluscum) less commonly are the dermatological presentation of a PID.

Eczematous dermatitis and erythroderma, at times closely resembling severe atopic dermatitis or seborrheic dermatitis, may affect the skin of PID patients. They may be refractory to standard therapies. Granuloma formation, autoimmune disorders, and vasculitis are other cutaneous manifestations seen in some forms of primary immunodeficiency. The PIDs in which a specific infection or finding is the more common presentation are discussed in other chapters (for example, chronic mucocutaneous candidiasis in Chapter 15; Hermansky–Pudlak, Chédiak–Higashi, and Griscelli syndromes with pigmentary anomalies (Chapter 36), and cartilage–hair hypoplasia syndrome with disorders of hair (Chapter 33). The conditions described below are the most important PID conditions with which dermatologists should be familiar.

Abrams M, et al: Genetic immunodeficiency diseases. Adv Dermatol 2007; 23:197.
Notarangelo L, et al: Primary immunodeficiency diseases: an update from the International Union of Immunological Societies Primary Immunodeficiency Diseases Classification Committee Meeting in Budapest, 2005. J Allergy Clin Immunol 2006; 117:883.
Ozcan E, et al: Primary immune deficiencies with aberrant IgE production. J Allergy Clin Immunol 2008; 122:1054.
Sillevis Smitt JH, et al: The skin in primary immunodeficiency disorders. Eur J Dermatol 2005; 15:425.

Disorders of antibody deficiency

X-linked agammaglobulinemia (XLA)

Also known as Bruton syndrome, this rare hereditary immunologic disorder usually only becomes apparent between 4 and 12 months of life, since the neonate obtains adequate immunoglobulin from the mother to protect it from infection in young infancy. The affected boys present with infections of the upper and lower respiratory tracts, gastrointestinal tract, skin, joints, and central nervous system (CNS). The infections are usually due to *Streptococcus pneumoniae*, *Staphylococcus aureus*, *Haemophilus influenzae*, and *Pseudomonas*. Recurrent skin staphylococcal infection may be a prominent component of this condition. Atopic-like dermatitis and pyoderma gangrenosum have been described. Hepatitis B, enterovirus, and rotavirus infections are common in XLA patients and one-third develop a rheumatoid-like arthritis. Enterovirus infection may result in a dermatomyositis–meningoencephalitis syndrome. An absence of palpable lymph nodes is characteristic.

IgA, IgM, IgD, and IgE are virtually absent from the serum, although IgG may be present in small amounts. The spleen and lymph nodes lack germinal centers, and plasma cells are absent from the lymph nodes, spleen, bone marrow, and connective tissues. In XLA B cells usually only make up 0.1% of circulating peripheral blood lymphocytes (normal 5–20%). More than 500 different mutations have been identified in the *Btk* gene in XLA patients. Some of these mutations only partially compromise the gene, so some patients may have milder phenotype and up to 7% circulating B cells, making differentiation from common variable immunodeficiency difficult. The Bruton tyrosine kinase (Btk) is essential for the development of B lymphocytes.

Treatment with relatively high-dose gamma globulin has enabled many patients to live into adulthood. Chronic sinusitis and pulmonary infection remain problematic due to the lack of IgA. Chronic pulmonary disease affects 76% of XLA patients over the age of 20 years.

Hunter HL, et al: Eczema and X-linked agammaglobulinaemia. Clin Exp Dermatol 2008; 33:148.
Lin MT, et al: De novo mutation in the BTK gene of atypical X-linked agammaglobulinemia in a patient with recurrent pyoderma. Ann Allergy Asthma Immunol 2006; 96:744.

Isolated IgA deficiency

An absence or marked reduction of serum IgA occurs in approximately 1 in 600, making it the most common immunodeficiency state. Autosomal-dominant, autosomal-recessive, and sporadic cases have been reported. Certain medications appear to induce selective IgA deficiency, including phenytoin, sulfasalazine, cyclosporine, nonsteroidal anti-inflammatory drugs (NSAIDs), and hydroxychloroquine. The genetic cause in most cases is unknown, but a few cases have a mutation in the tumor necrosis factor (TNF) receptor family member TACI. Common variable immunodeficiency (CVID) may develop in patients with IgA deficiency, or other members of IgA-deficient patients' families may have CVID.

Ten to fifteen percent of all symptomatic immunodeficiency patients have IgA deficiency. Most IgA-deficient patients are entirely well, however. Of those with symptoms, half have repeated infections of the gastrointestinal and respiratory tracts, and one-quarter have autoimmune disease. Allergies such as anaphylactic reactions to transfusion or IVIG, asthma, and atopic dermatitis are common in the symptomatic group. There is an increased association of celiac disease, dermatitis herpetiformis, and inflammatory bowel disease. Vitiligo, alopecia areata, and other autoimmune diseases such as systemic lupus erythematosus, dermatomyositis, scleroderma, thyroiditis, rheumatoid arthritis, polyarteritis-like vasculitis and Sjögren syndrome have all been reported to occur in these patients. Malignancy is increased in adults with IgA deficiency.

Mellemkjaer L, et al: Cancer risk among patients with IgA deficiency or common variable immunodeficiency and their relatives: a combined Danish and Swedish study. Clin Exp Immunol 2002; 130:495.
Paradela S, et al: Necrotizing vasculitis with a polyarteritis nodosa-like pattern and selective immunoglobulin A deficiency: case report and review of the literature. J Cutan Pathol 2008; 35:871.
Samolitis NJ, et al: Dermatitis herpetiformis and partial IgA deficiency. J Am Acad Dermatol 2006; 54:S206.
Uram R, et al: Isolated IgA deficiency after chemotherapy for acute myelogenous leukemia in an infant. Pediatr Hematol Oncol 2003; 20:487.

Common variable immunodeficiency

Common variable immunodeficiency (CVID), also known as acquired hypogammaglobulinemia, is a heterogeneous disorder and is the most common immunodeficiency syndrome after IgA deficiency. Patients have low levels of IgG and IgA, and 50% also have low levels of IgM. The genetic defect is unknown. These patients do not form antibodies to bacterial antigens, and have recurrent sinopulmonary infections. They have a predisposition to autoimmune disorders, such as vitiligo and alopecia areata, gastrointestinal abnormalities, lymphoreticular malignancy, and gastric carcinoma. Cutaneous, as well as visceral, granulomas have been reported in as many as 22% of patients. These can involve both the skin and the viscera, creating a sarcoidosis-like clinical syndrome. Replacement of the reduced immunoglobulins with IVIG may help reduce infections. Topical, systemic, and intralesional corticosteroids may be used for the granulomas, depending on their extent. Infliximab and etanercept have been effective in steroid-refractory cases.

Artac H, et al: Sarcoid-like granulomas in common variable immunodeficiency. Rheumatol Int 2009 (Epub ahead of print).
Fernandez-Ruiz M, et al: Fever of unknown origin in a patient with common variable immunodeficiency associated with multisystemic granulomatous disease. Intern Med 2007; 46:1197.
Lin JH, et al: Etanercept treatment of cutaneous granulomas in common variable immunodeficiency. J Allergy Clin Immunol 2006; 117:878.

5

Lun KR, et al: Granulomas in common variable immunodeficiency: a diagnostic dilemma. Australas J Dermatol 2004; 45:51.

Mazzatenta C, et al: Granulomatous dermatitis in common variable immunodeficiency with functional T-cell defect. Arch Dermatol 2006; 142:783.

Mitra A, et al: Cutaneous granulomas associated with primary immunodeficiency disorders. Br J Dermatol 2005; 153:194.

Class-switch recombination defects (formerly immunodeficiency with hyper-IgM)

This group of diseases includes disorders which are combined T- and B-cell abnormalities, such as CD40 deficiency and CD40 ligand deficiency, and disorders of primary B cells, such as cytidine deaminase and uracil-DNA glycosylase deficiencies. They are rare, and the different genetic diseases included in this group appear to have different clinical manifestations. These patients experience recurrent sinopulmonary infections, diarrhea, and oral ulcers. Neutropenia may be associated with the ulcers. Recalcitrant human papillomavirus infections may occur.

Chang MW, et al: Mucocutaneous manifestations of the hyper-IgM immunodeficiency syndrome. J Am Acad Dermatol 1998; 38:191.

Gilmour KC, et al: Immunological and genetic analysis of 65 patients with a clinical suspicion of X-linked hyper-IgM. Mol Pathol 2003; 56:256.

Kasahara Y, et al: Hyper-IgM syndrome with putative dominant negative mutation in activation-induced cytidine deaminase. J Allergy Clin Immunol 2003; 112:755.

Kutukculer N, et al: Disseminated *Cryptosporidium* infection in an infant with hyper-IgM syndrome caused by CD40 deficiency. J Pediatr 2003; 142:194.

Thymoma with immunodeficiency

Thymoma with immunodeficiency, also known as Good syndrome, occurs in adults in whom profound hypogammaglobulinemia and benign thymoma appear almost simultaneously. It is now classified predominantly as an antibody deficiency disorder. There is a striking deficiency of B and pre-B cells. One patient developed vulvovaginal gingival lichen planus. Myelodysplasia and pure red cell aplasia may occur. Patients are at risk for fatal opportunistic pulmonary infections with fungi and *Pneumocystis*. Thymectomy does not prevent the development of the infectious or lymphoreticular complications. Supportive therapy with IVIG, GM-CSF, and transfusions may be required.

Di Renzo M, et al: Myelodysplasia and Good syndrome. A case report. Clin Exp Med 2008; 8:171.

Jian L, et al: Fatal *Pneumocystis* pneumonia with Good syndrome and pure red cell aplasia. Clin Infect Dis 2004; 39:1740.

Moutasim KA, et al: A case of vulvovaginal gingival lichen planus in association with Good's syndrome. Oral Surg Oral Med Oral Pathol Oral Radiol Endod 2008; 105:e57.

Ohuchi M, et al: Good syndrome coexisting with leukopenia. Ann Thorac Surg 2007; 84:2095.

Disorders with T-cell deficiency

T-cell deficiency states can occur due to lack of thymic tissue, enzyme defects toxic to T lymphocytes (purine nucleoside phosphorylase deficiency), failure to express surface molecules required for immune interactions (CD3, major histocompatibility complex (MHC) class I and II), or defects in signaling molecules (ZAP-70).

DiGeorge syndrome

DiGeorge syndrome is also called congenital thymic hypoplasia, the velocardiofacial syndrome, and III and IV pharyngeal pouch syndrome. It is an autosomal-dominant disorder, which, in 50% of cases, is due to hemizygous deletion of 22q11-pter and rarely due to deletions in 10p. Many cases are sporadic. Most DiGeorge syndrome patients have the congenital anomalies and only minor thymic anomalies. They present with hypocalcemia or congenital heart disease. The syndrome includes congenital absence of the parathyroids and an abnormal aorta. Aortic and cardiac defects are the most common cause of death. DiGeorge syndrome is characterized by a distinctive facies: notched, low-set ears, micrognathia, shortened philtrum, and hypertelorism. Patients with these DiGeorge congenital malformations and complete lack of thymus are deemed to have "complete DiGeorge syndrome." Cell-mediated immunity is absent or depressed, and few T cells with the phenotype of recent thymus emigrants are found in the peripheral blood or tissues. Opportunistic infections commonly occur despite normal immunoglobulin levels. Maternally derived graft-versus-host disease (GVHD) may occur in these patients. A small subset of patients with complete DiGeorge syndrome develop an eczematous dermatitis, lymphadenopathy, and an oligoclonal T-cell proliferation. The condition may present as an atopic-like dermatitis, severe and extensive seborrheic dermatitis, or an erythroderma. This is called "atypical complete DiGeorge syndrome." Biopsies show features of a spongiotic dermatitis with eosinophils, necrotic keratinocytes with satellite necrosis, and characteristically peri- and intraeccrine inflammation. This resembles the histology of grade 1–2 GVHD, lichen striatus, and some cases of mycosis fungoides. One African American patient with DiGeorge syndrome developed a granulomatous dermatitis. The treatment for complete DiGeorge syndrome is thymic transplantation.

Jyonouchi H, et al: SAPHO osteomyelitis and sarcoid dermatitis in a patient with DiGeorge syndrome. Eur J Pediatr 2006; 165:370.

Patel JY, et al: Thymus transplantation advances in DiGeorge syndrome. Curr Allergy Asthma Rep 2005; 5:348.

Selim MA, et al: The cutaneous manifestations of atypical complete DiGeorge syndrome: a histopathologic and immunohistochemical study. J Cutan Pathol 2008; 35:380.

Purine nucleoside phosphorylase deficiency

This very rare autosomal-recessive enzyme defect leads to greatly reduced T-cell counts and depressed cell-mediated immunity. B-cell numbers are normal, but immunoglobulins may be normal or decreased. Mutation in the gene for the enzyme located on chromosome 14q13 is responsible. Accumulation of purines in cells of the lymphoid system and CNS leads to the clinical findings of T-cell deficiency and neurological impairment. Patients usually present at between 3 and 18 months of age with recurrent infections involving the upper and lower respiratory tracts, spasticity, ataxia, developmental delay, and autoimmune hemolytic anemia. They usually die from overwhelming viral infections. Bone marrow transplant may be life-saving.

Aytekin C, et al: An unconditioned bone marrow transplantation in a child with purine nucleoside phosphorylase deficiency and its unique complication. Pediatr Transplant 2008; 12:479.

Delicou S, et al: Successful HLA-identical hematopoietic stem cell transplantation in a patient with purine nucleoside phosphorylase deficiency. Pediatr Transplant 2007; 11:799.

Gregoriou S, et al: Cutaneous granulomas with predominantly CD8(+) lymphocytic infiltrate in a child with severe combined immunodeficiency. J Cutan Med Surg 2008; 12:246.

Liao P, et al: Lentivirus gene therapy for purine nucleoside phosphorylase deficiency. J Gene Med 2008; 10:1282.

Ozkinay F, et al: Purine nucleoside phosphorylase deficiency in a patient with spastic paraplegia and recurrent infections. J Child Neurol 2007; 22:741.

Miscellaneous T-cell deficiencies

TAP 1 and *TAP 2* gene deficiencies are very, very rare autosomal-recessive disorders that result in severe reduction of MHC class I expression on the surface of cells. CD8 cells are decreased but CD4 cells are normal, as are B-cell numbers and serum immunoglobulins. Three forms of disease occur. One phenotype develops severe bacterial, fungal, and parasitic infection, and dies by age 3. The second phenotype is completely asymptomatic. The third group is the most common. Group 3 patients present in childhood with recurrent and chronic bacterial respiratory infections. These lead to bronchiectasis and eventually fatal respiratory failure in adulthood. The skin abnormalities appear in late childhood or more commonly in young adulthood (after age 15). Necrotizing granulomatous lesions appear as plaques or ulcerations on the lower legs and on the midface around the nose. The perinasal lesions are quite destructive and resemble "lethal midline granuloma" or Wegener's granulomatosis. Nasal polyps with necrotizing granulomatous histology also occur. One patient also developed leukocytoclastic vasculitis.

MHC class II deficiency is due to mutations in transcription factors for MHC class II proteins (*C2TA, RFX5, RFXAP, RFSANK* genes). It is inherited in an autosomal-recessive manner and results in decreased CD4 cells.

ZAP-70 deficiency is an autosomal-recessive disorder of considerable heterogeneity. This enzyme is required for T-cell receptor intracellular signaling. Patients present before age 2 with recurrent bacterial, viral, and opportunistic infections, diarrhea, and failure to thrive. They have a lymphocytosis with normal CD4 cells and decreased CD8 cells. Some patients develop an exfoliative erythroderma, eosinophilia, and elevated IgE levels.

Omenn syndrome is a rare autosomal-recessive disorder that presents at birth or in the neonatal period. Clinical features are exfoliative erythroderma, eosinophilia, diarrhea, hepatosplenomegaly, lymphadenopathy, hypogammaglobulinemia with elevated IgE, recurrent infections, and early death (usually by 6 months of age). Both antibody production and cell-mediated immune function are impaired. T-cell receptor rearrangements are severely restricted in patients with Omenn syndrome. Mutations in *RAG1, RAG2, Artemis,* and *IL-7Ralpha* genes may result in Omenn syndrome.

Anhidrotic ectodermal dysplasia with immunodeficiency is an X-linked recessive disorder with lymphocytosis and elevated CD3 and CD4 cells, and low levels of NK cells. It is due to a mutation in the gene that codes for nuclear factor κ B essential modulator (NEMO). The mother may have mild stigmata of incontinentia pigmentii. The mutations are hypomorphic (some NEMO function is preserved). These male infants present within the first few months of life with hypohidrosis, delayed tooth eruption, and immunodeficiency. Hair may be absent. Frequent infections of the skin and respiratory tract are common. The eruption has been characterized as an "atopic dermatitis-like eruption," although some cases may have prominent intertriginous lesions resembling seborrheic dermatitis. Treatment is bone marrow transplantation. A similar autosomal-dominant syndrome is caused by a mutation in the gene IKBA (inhibitory κ B kinase γ).

IPEX syndrome (immune dysregulation, polyendocrinopathy, enteropathy, X-linked syndrome) is a rare disorder with neonatal autoimmune enteropathy, diabetes, thyroiditis, food allergies, and skin eruptions. IPEX is caused by mutations in *FOXP3*, the master control gene for regulatory T-cell (Treg) development. Patients present with diffuse and severe erythematous exudative plaques resembling atopic dermatitis. The skin eruption may be follicularly based or lead to prurigo nodularis. The scalp develops hyperkeratotic psoriasiform plaques. Cheilitis and onychodystrophy can occur. Staphylococcal sepsis may develop.

Severe combined immunodeficiency disease

This heterogeneous group of genetic disorders is characterized by severely impaired humoral and cellular immunity. Moniliasis of the oropharynx and skin, intractable diarrhea, and pneumonia are the triad of findings that commonly lead to the diagnosis of severe combined immunodeficiency disease (SCID). In addition, severe recurrent infections may occur, caused by *Pseudomonas, Staphylococcus,* Enterobacteriaceae, or *Candida.* Overwhelming viral infections are the usual cause of death. Engraftment of maternally transmitted or transfusion-derived lymphocytes can lead to GVHD. The initial seborrheic dermatitis-like eruption may represent maternal engraftment GVHD. This cutaneous eruption may be asymptomatic but tends to generalize. More severe eczematous dermatitis and erythroderma may develop with alopecia. Cutaneous granulomas have been reported in a *Jak-3*-deficient SCID patient.

SCID is characterized by deficiency or total absence of circulating T lymphocytes. Immunoglobulin levels are consistently very low, but B-cell numbers may be reduced, normal, or increased. The thymus is very small; its malformed architecture at autopsy is pathognomonic.

The inheritance may be autosomal-recessive or X-linked; the most common type of SCID is X-linked. A deficiency of a common γ-chain that is an essential component of the IL-2 receptor is responsible for the profound lymphoid dysfunction in X-linked SCID. This abnormality also causes defects in IL-4, 7, 9, 15, and 21. The mutation has been mapped to Xq13.1. About half the autosomal-recessive cases have a deficiency of adenosine deaminase, the gene for which is located on chromosome 20q13. Mutations in *Jak-3, IL-7Ralpha, CD45, CD3delta/CD3epsilon, RAG1* or *RAG2,* and *Artemis* (*DCLREC1C*) can all also cause the SCID phenotype. Reticular dysgenesis causes SCID, granulocytopenia, and thrombocytopenia.

Prenatal diagnosis and carrier detection are possible for many forms of SCID. The definitive treatment is hematopoietic stem cell transplantation (HSCT, bone marrow transplantation). This should ideally be carried out before 3 months of age for optimal outcome. The success rate is less than 90%. In utero hematopoietic stem cell transplantation has been successful in X-linked SCID. SCID patients rarely live longer than 2 years without transplantation. On average, 8 years after successful HSCT, SCID patients may develop severe human papillomavirus (HPV) infection with common warts, flat warts, or even epidermodysplasia verruciformis. The development of HPV infections in SCID patients following HSCT is only seen in patients with either *JAK-3* or γ-chain (gamma c) deficiency, but in those patients more than 50% may develop this complication.

Gadola SD, et al: TAP deficiency syndrome. Clin Exp Immunol 2000; 121:173.

Gaspar HB, et al: Severe cutaneous papillomavirus disease after haematopoietic stem-cell transplantation in patients with severe combined immunodeficiency. Br J Haematol 2004; 127:232.

Halabi-Tawil M, et al: Cutaneous manifestations of immune dysregulation, polyendocrinopathy, enteropathy, X-linked (IPEX) syndrome. Br J Dermatol 2009; 160:645.

Katugampola RP, et al: Omenn's syndrome: lessons from a red baby. Clin Exp Dermatol 2008; 33:425.

Laffort C, et al: Severe cutaneous papillomavirus disease after haemopoietic stem-cell transplantation in patients with severe combined immune deficiency caused by common gamma c cytokine receptor subunit or JAK-3 deficiency. Lancet 2004; 363:2051.

Mancini AJ, et al: X-linked ectodermal dysplasia with immunodeficiency caused by NEMO mutation: early recognition and diagnosis. Arch Dermatol 2008; 144:342.

Moins-Teisserenc HT, et al: Association of a syndrome resembling Wegener's granulomatosis with low surface expression of HLA class-I molecules. Lancet 1999; 354:1598.

O'Shea JJ, et al: Jak3 and the pathogenesis of severe combined immunodeficiency. Mol Immunol 2004; 41:727.

Plebani A, et al: Defective expression of HLA class I and CD1a molecules in boy with Marfan-like phenotype and deep skin ulcers. J Am Acad Dermatol 1996; 35:814.

Turul T, et al: Clinical heterogeneity can hamper the diagnosis of patients with ZAP70 deficiency. Eur J Pediatr 2009; 168:87.

Zimmer J, et al: Clinical and immunological aspects of HLA class I deficiency. QJM 2005; 98:719.

WHIM syndrome

WHIM (warts, hypogammaglobulinemia, infections, myelokathexis) syndrome is an autosomal-dominant syndrome with hypogammaglobulinemia, reduced B cell numbers, and neutropenia. The most common genetic cause is a truncation mutation of *CXCR4*, which leads to gain of function in that gene. Additional mutations that are not in the *CXCR4* gene can also cause WHIM, but all of them lead to functional hyperactivity of *CXCR4*. *CXCR4* causes retention of neutrophils in the bone marrow and is the basis of the neutropenia and myelokathexis (increased apoptotic neutrophils in the bone marrow). There is profound loss of circulating CD27+ memory B cells, resulting in hypogammaglobulinemia, and the observation that WHIM patients have normal antibody response to certain antigens, but fail to maintain this antibody production. However, normal immunoglobulin levels do not exclude the diagnosis of WHIM. Almost 80% of WHIM patients have warts at the time of their diagnosis. These include common and genital wart types. A significant number of female WHIM patients have cervical and vulval dysplasia, which can progress to carcinoma. WHIM patients have disproportionately more HPV infections than SCID patients, yet WHIM patients have little problem resolving other viral infections. They may develop Epstein–Barr virus (EBV)-induced lymphomas, however. The vast majority of patients in early childhood suffer recurrent sinopulmonary infections, skin infections, osteomyelitis, and urinary tract infections. Recurrent pneumonias lead to bronchiectasis. Treatment is G-CSF, IVIG, prophylactic antibiotics, and aggressive treatment of infections. The HPV infections can progress to fatal carcinomas and therefore male patients must be regularly examined by dermatologists and female ones by gynecologists; a low threshold for biopsy of genital lesions is required.

Hagan JB, et al: WHIM syndrome. Mayo Clin Proc 2007; 82:1031.

Kawai T, et al: WHIM syndrome: congenital immune deficiency disease. Curr Opin Hematol 2009; 16:20.

Wiskott–Aldrich syndrome

Wiskott–Aldrich syndrome, an X-linked recessive syndrome, consists of a triad of chronic eczematous dermatitis resembling atopic dermatitis (Fig. 5-16); increased susceptibility to bacterial infections, such as pyoderma or otitis media; and thrombocytopenic purpura with small platelets. There are normal levels of IgM and IgG, but elevated levels of IgA and IgE. T cells progressively decline in number and activity. Untreated survival is about 15 years, with death from infection, bleeding, or lymphoma.

The genetic cause of Wiskott–Aldrich syndrome is a mutation in the *WASP* gene. This gene codes for a protein called WASP, which is universally expressed in hematopoietic cells and is critical in the reorganization of the actin cytoskeleton in

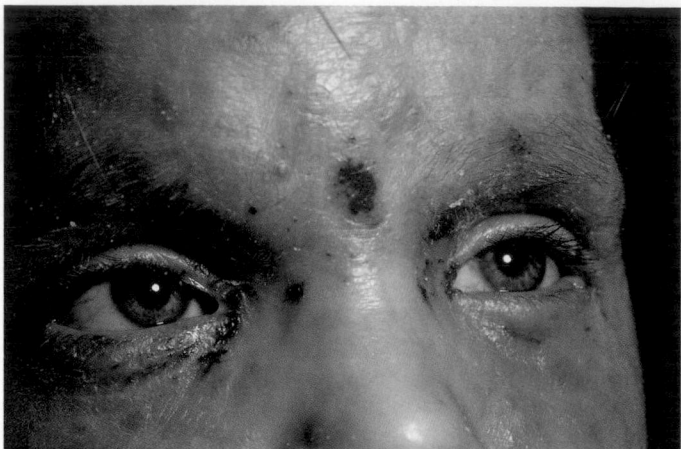

Fig. 5-16 Eczematous eruption with purpura in Wiskott–Aldrich syndrome.

hematopoietic cells in response to external stimuli. The hematopoietic cells of affected patients cannot polarize or migrate in response to physiologic stimuli, accounting for the protean clinical features of the syndrome. Wiskott–Aldrich syndrome occurs when mutations in *WASP* lead to absence or truncation of the WASP protein (WASP– mutations). Mutations that result in normal length but some loss of function in the WASP protein (WASP+ mutations) result in three different syndromes: X-linked thrombocytopenia (XLT), intermittent X-linked thrombocytopenia, and X-linked neutropenia. Patients with XLT may also have an atopic-like dermatitis, but this is usually milder than the severe and difficult to control eczema affecting patients with the full Wiskott–Aldrich syndrome. WASP/XLT patients may also develop autoimmune disease, especially autoimmune hemolytic anemia, vasculitis, Henoch–Schönlein-like purpura, and inflammatory bowel disease. High IgM is associated with the development of autoimmune disease.

Treatment is with platelet transfusions, antibiotics, and IVIG, if required. Often splenectomy is performed to help control bleeding, but this leads to increased risk of sepsis and is not routinely recommended. Immunosuppressive therapy or rituximab may be used to control autoimmune complications. Bone marrow transplantation from a human leukocyte antigen (HLA)-identical sibling as early as possible in the disease course provides complete reversal of the platelet and immune dysfunction, as well as improvement or clearing of the eczematous dermatitis. Survival at 7 years with a matched sibling donor transplant approaches 90%.

Ochs HD, et al: Wiskott–Aldrich syndrome: diagnosis, clinical and laboratory manifestations, and treatment. Biol Blood Marrow Transplant 2008; 15:84.

Ataxia telangiectasia

Ataxia telangiectasia is an autosomal-recessive condition that is due to mutations in a single gene on chromosome 11 (*ATM*), which encodes a protein called ATM. This protein is critical in cell cycle control. When ATM is absent, the cell cycle does not stop to repair DNA breaks or for B(D)J recombination of immunoglobulin and T-cell receptor genes. This results in immunodeficiency and an increased risk for malignancy. The clinical features of the patients are progressive ocular and cutaneous telangiectasias, premature aging, and progressive neurodegeneration. Skin changes that are characteristic are cutaneous non-infectious granulomas (which can be ulcerative and painful), loss of subcutaneous fat, premature gray hair, large irregular café-au-lait spots, vitiligo, seborrheic dermatitis, atopic dermatitis, recurrent impetigo, and acanthosis nigricans. Late tightening of the skin can occur and resembles acral sclerosis. Sinopulmonary infections are common, especially otitis media, sinusitis, bronchitis, and pneumonia. Varicella, at times severe, herpes simplex, molluscum contagiosum, and herpes zoster can occur. Refractory warts occur in more than 5% of patients. Aside from candidal esophagitis, unusual opportunistic infections are rare. Childhood immunizations, including liver viral vaccines, are well tolerated. Lymphopenia is common, with reduction of both B and T cells occurring in the majority of patients. Helper T-cell counts can be below 200. IgA, IgG4, IgG2, and IgE deficiencies can all be present. Paradoxically, IgM, IgA, and IgG can be elevated in some patients, including the presence of monoclonal gammopathy in more than 10% of cases. The immunological abnormalities are not progressive. Lymphoma risk is increased more than 200-fold (especially B-cell lymphoma), and leukemia (especially T-cell chronic lymphocytic leukemia) is increased 70-fold. Treatment includes high vigilance for infection and malignancy. In patients with low CD4 counts, prophylaxis to prevent *Pneumocystis* pneumonia can be considered. When IgG deficiency is present and infections are frequent, IVIG may be beneficial. IVIG and intralesional corticosteroids may be used for the cutaneous granulomas. Carriers of ataxia telangiectasia have an increased risk for hematologic and breast malignancies. Due to the accumulation of chromosomal breaks following radiation exposure, both the ataxia telangiectasia patients and the carriers should minimize radiation exposure.

Nowak-Wegrzyn A, et al: Immunodeficiency and infections in ataxia-telangiectasia. J Pediatr 2004; 144:505.

Defects of phagocyte number, function, or both

Chronic granulomatous disease

Chronic granulomatous disease (CGD) is a rare disorder caused by mutations in one of the genes that encode the subunits of the superoxide-generating phagocyte NADPH oxidase system responsible for the respiratory burst involved in organism killing. CGD is characterized by repeated and recurrent bacterial and fungal infections of the lungs, skin, lymph nodes, and bones. Gingivostomatitis (aphthous-like ulcerations) and a seborrheic dermatitis of the periauricular, perinasal, and perianal area are characteristic. The dermatitis is frequently infected with *S. aureus*, and regional adenopathy and abscesses may complicate the infections. The term "suppurative dermatitis" is used in the immunology literature to describe this seborrheic-like dermatitis with secondary infection (very analogous to the "infective dermatitis" seen in human T-cell lymphotropic virus (HTLV)-1 infection). In addition to *S. aureus*, *Serratia* species are commonly isolated from skin abscesses, liver abscesses, and osteomyelitis. *Aspergillus* is the most common agent causing pneumonia in CGD patients. In tuberculosis-endemic areas, CGD patients frequently develop active tuberculosis or prolonged scarring, abscesses, or disseminated infection following BCG immunization.

There are four types of CGD, one X-linked and three autosomal-recessive. The X-linked form is the most common (65–75% of CGD patients) and is due to a mutation in the *CYBB* gene, which leads to absence of the high molecular weight subunit of cytochrome b 558 (gp 91-phox) and a total absence of NADPH oxidase activity. In autosomal-recessive forms, mutations in the genes encoding for the remaining three oxidase components have been described: p22-phox (*CYBA*), p47-phox (*NCF-1*), and p67-phox (*NCF-2*). The X-linked variant has the most severe phenotype. Compared to the autosomal-recessive CGD patients, the X-linked patients present at an

earlier age (14 months vs 30 months), and are diagnosed at an earlier age (3 years vs 6 years). The lack of superoxide generation apparently causes disease, not because the bacteria are not being killed by the superoxide, but because the superoxide is required to activate proteases in phagocytic vacuoles that are needed to kill infectious organisms.

Granuloma formation is characteristic of CGD and can occur in the skin, gastrointestinal tract, liver, bladder, bone, and lymph node. Up to 40% of biopsies from these organs will demonstrate granulomas, at times with identifiable fungal or mycobacterial organisms. Since these patients are often on prophylactic antibiotics, organisms are frequently not found, however. Subcorneal pustular eruptions can also be seen in CGD patients. In the intestinal tract an inflammatory bowel disease-like process occurs, with granulomas in the colon. This can cause significant gastrointestinal symptoms.

The diagnosis of CGD is made by demonstrating low reduction of yellow nitro-blue tetrazolium (NBT) to blue formazan in the "NBT test." Dihydrorhodamine 123 flow cytometry, chemiluminescence production, and the ferricytochrome C reduction assay are also confirmatory and may be more accurate.

Female carriers of the X-linked form of CGD have a mixed population of normal and abnormal phagocytes, and therefore show intermediate NBT reduction. The majority of carriers have skin complaints. Raynaud phenomenon can occur. More than half will report a photosensitive dermatitis, 40% have oral ulcerations, and a third have joint complaints. Skin lesions in carriers have been described as DLE-like (Discoid lupus erythematosus), but histologically there is often an absence of the interface component and they resemble tumid lupus. DIF examination is usually negative, as is common in tumid lupus erythematosus (LE). Less commonly, CGD patients themselves have been described as having similar LE-like lesions, or "arcuate dermal erythema." Despite these findings, the vast majority of patients with LE-like skin lesions, both carriers and CGD patients, are antinuclear antibody (ANA)-negative.

Treatment of infections should be early and aggressive. There should be a low threshold to biopsy skin lesions, as they may reveal important and potentially life-threatening infections. Patients usually receive chronic trimethoprim–sulfamethoxazole prophylaxis, chronic oral itraconazole or another anti-*Aspergillus* agent, and IFN-γ injections. Bone marrow or stem cell transplantation has been successful in restoring enzyme function, reducing infections, and improving the associated bowel disease. However, survival is NOT increased with bone marrow transplantation, so it is not routinely undertaken.

Cale CM, et al: Cutaneous and other lupus-like symptoms in carriers of X-linked chronic granulomatous disease: incidence and autoimmune serology. Clin Exp Immunol 2007; 148:79.

Gallin JI, et al: Itraconazole to prevent fungal infections in chronic granulomatous disease. N Engl J Med 2003; 348:2416.

Holland SM: Chronic granulomatous disease. Clin Rev Allergy Immunol 2010; 38:3.

Lee PP, et al: Susceptibility to mycobacterial infections in children with X-linked chronic granulomatous disease: a review of 17 patients living in a region endemic for tuberculosis. Pediatr Infect Dis J 2008; 27:224.

Levine S, et al: Histopathological features of chronic granulomatous disease (CGD) in childhood. Histopathology 2005; 47:508.

Luis-Montoya P, et al: Chronic granulomatous disease: two members of a single family with different dermatologic manifestations. Skinmed 2005; 4:320.

Martire B, et al: Clinical features, long-term follow-up and outcome of a large cohort of patients with chronic granulomatous disease: an Italian multicenter study. Clin Immunol 2008; 126:155.

Vieira AP, et al: Lymphadenopathy after BCG vaccination in a child with chronic granulomatous disease. Pediatr Dermatol 2004; 21:646.

Leukocyte adhesion molecule deficiency

This rare autosomal-recessive disorder has three types. Leukocyte adhesion molecule deficiency (LAD) type I is due to a mutation in the common chain (CD18) of the β2 integrin family. It is characterized by recurrent bacterial infections of the skin and mucosal surfaces, especially gingivitis and periodontitis. Skin ulcerations from infection may continue to expand. Cellulitis and necrotic abscesses, especially in the perirectal area, can occur. Minor injuries may lead to pyoderma gangrenosum-like ulcerations that heal slowly. Infections begin at birth, and omphalitis with delayed separation of the cord is characteristic. Neutrophilia is marked, usually 5–20 times normal, and the count may reach up to 100 000 during infections. Despite this, there is an absence of neutrophils at the sites of infection, demonstrating the defective migration of neutrophils in these patients. LAD type I patients are either severely (<1% normal CD18 expression) or moderately affected (2.5–10% of normal expression.) Patients with moderate disease have less severe infections and survive into adulthood, whereas patients with severe disease often die in infancy.

LAD type II is due to a mutation in *FUCT1*, which results in a general defect in fucose metabolism and causes the absence of SLeX and other ligands for the selectins. Severe mental retardation, short stature, a distinctive facies, and the rare hh blood phenotype are the features. Initially, these patients have recurrent cellulitis with marked neutrophilia, but the infections are not life-threatening. After age 3 years, infections become less of a problem and patients suffer from chronic periodontitis.

LAD type III is due to mutation in the gene *KINDLIN3* (*FERMT3*) and is characterized by severe recurrent infections, bleeding tendency (due to impaired platelet function), and marked neutrophilia.

Bone marrow transplantation is required for patients with severe LAD type I and LAD type III.

Dababneh R, et al: Periodontal manifestation of leukocyte adhesion deficiency type I. J Periodontol 2008; 79:764.
Etzioni A: Leukocyte adhesion deficiencies: molecular basis, clinical findings, and therapeutic options. Adv Exp Med Biol 2007; 601:51.
Qasim W, et al: Allogeneic hematopoietic stem-cell transplantation for leukocyte adhesion deficiency. Pediatrics 2009; 123:836.
Svensson L, et al: Leukocyte adhesion deficiency-III is caused by mutations in *KINDLIN3* affecting integrin activation. Nat Med 2009; 15:306.

Hyperimmunoglobulinemia E syndrome

There are at least two types of hyperimmunoglobulin E syndrome (HIES): an autosomal-dominant form caused by mutations in *STAT3*, and an autosomal-recessive form, for which the genetic cause is still unknown. The two forms of HIES are clinically somewhat different and will be described separately.

Autosomal-dominant HIES was first called Job's syndrome. The classic triad is eczema, recurrent skin and lung infections, and high serum IgE. The skin disease is the first manifestation of STAT3 deficiency and begins at birth in 19% of cases, within the first week of life in more than 50%, and in the first month in 80%. The initial eruption is noted first on the face or scalp, but quickly generalizes to affect the face, scalp, and body. Dermatitis of the body only is distinctly uncommon. The body rash favors the shoulder, arms, chest, and buttocks. The newborn rash begins as pink papules that may initially be diagnosed as "neonatal acne." The papules develop quickly into pustules, then coalesce into crusted plaques. Histologically, these papules are intraepidermal eosinophilic pustules. The dermatitis evolves to bear a close resemblance to atopic dermatitis, often very severe. Staphylococcal infec-

tion of the dermatitis is frequent, and treatment of the staphylococcal infection with antibiotics and bleach baths leads to improvement. Since only about 8% of children with IgE levels below 2000 actually have HIES, other features must be used to confirm the diagnosis. Abscesses, sometimes cold, are characteristic. Recurrent pyogenic pneumonia is the rule, starting in childhood. Due to the lack of neutrophilic inflammation in the pneumonia, symptoms may be lacking and lead to a delay in diagnosis. Although antibiotic treatment clears the pneumonia, healing is abnormal, with the formation of bronchiectasis and pneumatoceles, a characteristic feature of HIES. Mucocutaneous candidiasis is common, typically thrush, vaginal candidiasis, and candida onychomycosis. Musculoskeletal abnormalities are common, including scoliosis, osteopenia, minimal trauma fractures, and hyperextensibility, leading to premature degenerative joint disease. Retention of some or all of the primary teeth is a characteristic feature. Other oral manifestations include median rhomboid glossitis, high-arch palate, and abnormally prominent wrinkles on the oral mucosa. Arterial aneurysms are common, including berry and coronary aneurysms. The coronary aneurysms can cause myocardial infarction. Autosomal-dominant HIES patients have a characteristic facies, developing during childhood and adolescence. Features include facial asymmetry, broad nose, deep-set eyes, and a prominent forehead. The facial skin is rough, with large pores. There is an increased risk of malignancy, predominantly B-cell non-Hodgkin lymphoma. Laboratory abnormalities are limited to eosinophilia and an elevated IgE. In adults, the IgE levels may become normal. Th17 cells are lacking from the peripheral blood of *STAT3* mutation patients. A scoring system developed at the National Institutes of Health (NIH) can accurately identify patients with HIES, selecting those in whom genetic testing could be considered.

Autosomal-recessive HIES is much less common. These patients also suffer from severe eczema and recurrent skin and lung infections. The lung infections resolve without pneumatoceles, however. Autosomal-recessive HIES patients are predisposed to cutaneous viral infections, especially molluscum contagiosum, herpes simplex, and varicella zoster. They also contract mucocutaneous candidiasis. Neurological disease is much more common in autosomal-recessive HIES, ranging from facial paralysis to hemiplegia. Autosomal-recessive HIES has normal facies, no fractures, and normal shedding of primary dentition.

Treatment for HIES is currently traditional. Infections are suppressed with bleach baths and chronic antibiotic prophylaxis (usually with trimethoprim/sulfamethoxazole); antifungal agents may be used for candidal infections of the skin and nails. Topical anti-inflammatories are used to manage the eczema, and in severe cases cyclosporine can be considered. Bisphosphonates are used for osteopenia. The role of IVIG, antihistamines, omalizumab (antibody against IgE) and bone marrow transplantation in HIES is unknown.

Eberting CL, et al: Dermatitis and the newborn rash of hyper-IgE syndrome. Arch Dermatol 2004; 140:1119.
Freeman AF, et al: The hyper-IgE syndromes. Immunol Allergy Clin North Am 2008; 28:277.
Freeman AF, et al: Hyper IgE (Job's) syndrome: a primary immune deficiency with oral manifestations. Oral Dis 2009; 15:2.
Grimbacher B, et al: Genetic linkage of hyper-IgE syndrome to chromosome 4. Am J Hum Genet 1999; 65:735.
Holland SM, et al: *STAT3* mutations in the hyper-IgE syndrome. N Engl J Med 2007; 357:1608.
Joshi AY, et al: Elevated serum immunoglobulin E (IgE): when to suspect hyper-IgE syndrome—a 10-year pediatric tertiary care center experience. Allergy Asthma Proc 2009; 30:23.
Lei XB, et al: Unusual coexistence of molluscum contagiosum and verruca plana in a hyper-IgE syndrome. Int J Dermatol 2006; 45:1199.

Ling JC, et al: Coronary artery aneurysms in patients with hyper IgE recurrent infection syndrome. Clin Immunol 2007; 122:255.

Ohameje NU, et al: Atopic dermatitis or hyper-IgE syndrome? Allergy Asthma Proc 2006; 27:289.

Renner ED, et al: Novel signal transducer and activator of transcription 3 (*STAT3*) mutations, reduced T(H)17 cell numbers, and variably defective STAT3 phosphorylation in hyper-IgE syndrome. J Allergy Clin Immunol 2008; 122:181.

Complement deficiency

The complement system is an effector pathway of proteins that results in membrane damage and chemotactic activity. Four major functions result from complement activation: cell lysis, opsonization/phagocytosis, inflammation, and immune complex removal. In the "classic" complement pathway, complement is activated by an antigen–antibody reaction involving IgG or IgM. Some complement components are directly activated by binding to the surface of infectious organisms; this is called the "alternate" pathway. The central component common to both pathways is C3. In the classic pathway, antigen–antibody complexes sequentially bind and activate three complement proteins, C1, C4, and C2, leading to the formation of C3 convertase, an activator of C3. The alternate pathway starts with direct activation of C3. From activated C3, C5–C9 are sequentially activated. Cytolysis is induced mainly via the "membrane attack complex," which is made up of the terminal components of complement. Opsonization is mainly mediated by a subunit of C3b, and inflammation by subunits of C3, C4, and C5.

Inherited deficiencies of complement are usually autosomal-recessive traits. Deficiencies of all 11 components of the classic pathway, as well as inhibitors of this pathway, have been described. Genetic deficiency of the C1 inhibitor is the only autosomal-dominant form of complement deficiency and results in hereditary angioedema (see Chapter 7). In general, deficiencies of the early components of the classic pathway result in connective tissue disease states, while deficiencies of the late components of complement lead to recurrent neisserial sepsis or meningitis. Overlap exists, and patients with late-component deficiencies may exhibit connective tissue disease, while patients with deficiencies of early components, such as C1q, may manifest infections. Deficiency of C3 results in recurrent infections with encapsulated bacteria such as *Pneumococcus*, *H. influenzae*, and *Streptococcus pyogenes*. C3 inactivator deficiency, like C3 deficiency, results in recurrent pyogenic infections. Properdin (a component of the alternate pathway) dysfunction is inherited as an X-linked trait and predisposes to fulminant meningococcemia. Deficiency of C9 is the most common complement deficiency in Japan but is uncommon in other countries. Most patients appear healthy. MASP2 deficiency, resulting in absent hemolytic activity by the lectin pathway, is considered a complement deficiency and results in a syndrome resembling systemic lupus erythematosus (SLE) and increased pyogenic infection. Factor I deficiency results in recurrent infections, including *Neisseria meningitides*. Partially deficient family members may also have increased infections.

C2 deficiency is the most common complement deficiency in the US and Europe. Most patients are healthy, but SLE-like syndromes, disseminated cutaneous lupus erythematosus, frequent infections, anaphylactoid purpura, dermatomyositis, vasculitis, and cold urticaria may be seen. C1q-, C4-, and C2-deficient patients have SLE at rates of 90%, 75%, and 15% respectively. Complement deficiency-associated SLE typically has early onset, photosensitivity, less renal disease, and Ro/La autoantibodies in two-thirds. C2- and C4-deficient patients with LE commonly have subacute annular morphology,

Sjögren syndrome, arthralgias, and oral ulcerations. Renal disease, anti-dsDNA antibodies, and anticardiolipin antibodies are uncommon. Patients with C4 deficiency may have lupus and involvement of the palms and soles.

Many of the complement component deficiencies can be acquired as an autoimmune phenomenon or a paraneoplastic finding. Examples include acquired angioedema, as when C1 inhibitor is the target, or lipodystrophy and nephritis, when C3 convertase is the target.

When complement deficiency is suspected, a useful screening test is a CH50 (total hemolytic complement) determination, because deficiency of any of the complement components will usually result in CH50 levels that are dramatically reduced or zero.

Grumach AS, et al: Recurrent infections in partial complement factor I deficiency: evaluation of three generations of a Brazilian family. Clin Exp Immunol 2006; 143:297.

Jamal S, et al: The role of complement testing in dermatology. Clin Exp Dermatol 2005; 30:321.

Graft-versus-host disease

Graft-versus-host disease (GVHD) occurs most frequently in the setting of hematopoietic stem cell transplantation (HSCT), but may also occur following organ transplantation or in the rare situation of transfusion of active lymphoid cells into an immunodeficient child postpartum or even in utero. Blood transfusions with active lymphocytes (non-radiated whole blood) from family members or in populations with minimal genetic variability, given to an immunodeficient patient, can result in GVHD. HSCT from a monozygotic twin (syngeneic) or even from the patient's own stem cells (autologous) can induce a mild form of GVHD.

GVHD requires three elements. First, the transplanted cells must be immunologically competent. Second, the recipient must express tissue antigens that are not present in the donor and therefore are recognized as foreign. Third, the recipient must be unable to reject the transplanted cells. Immunological competence of the transplanted cells is important, since ablating them too much may lead to failure of engraftment, or more commonly incomplete eradication of the recipient's malignancy (graft vs tumor effect). Therefore, some degree of immunological competence of the transplanted cells is desired. For this reason, the prevalence of GVHD still remains about 50% following HSCT. Another important factor in determining the development and severity of the GVHD is the preconditioning regimen. Chemotherapy and radiation cause activation of dendritic cells (antigen-presenting cells, APCs) in tissues with high cell turnover—the skin, gut, and liver. These APCs increase their expression of HLA and other minor cell surface antigens, priming them to interact with transplanted lymphoid cells. Host APCs are important in presenting these antigens to the active lymphoid donor cells. Cytokines, especially IL-2, TNF-α, and IFN-γ, are important in enhancing this host–donor immunological interaction. Reducing this early inflammatory component in GVHD can delay the onset of the GVHD, but may not reduce the prevalence. The indications for HSCT, the age limits, and the degree of HLA incompatibility allowed have all increased over the last decade, increasing the number of persons at risk for GVHD.

While initially only reactions that occurred within the first 100 days after transplantation were considered acute GVHD, it is now recognized that classical acute GVHD can occur up to a year or more following HSCT. Acute GVHD is based on the clinical presentation, NOT the duration following transplantation. In acute GVHD the cutaneous eruption (Fig. 5-17) typically begins between the 14th and 42nd days after transplantation, with a peak at day 30. Acute GVHD is

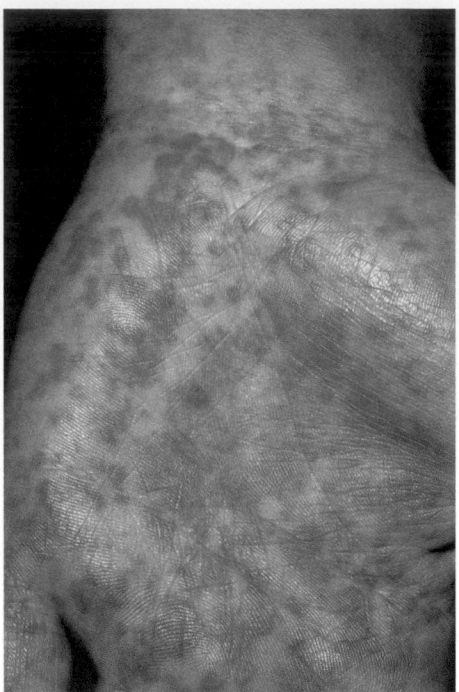

Fig. 5-17 Acute graft-versus-host disease.

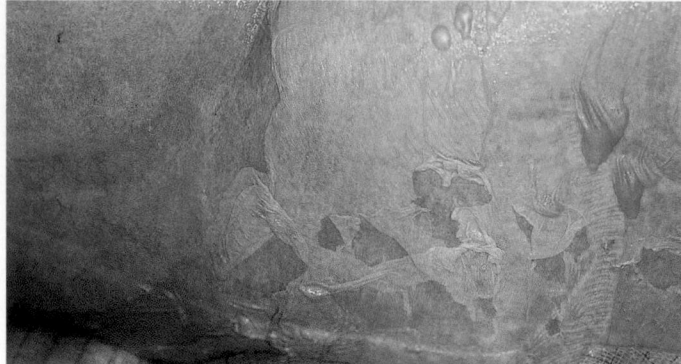

Fig. 5-18 Grade IV graft-versus-host disease with full-thickness slough of skin resembling toxic epidermal necrolysis.

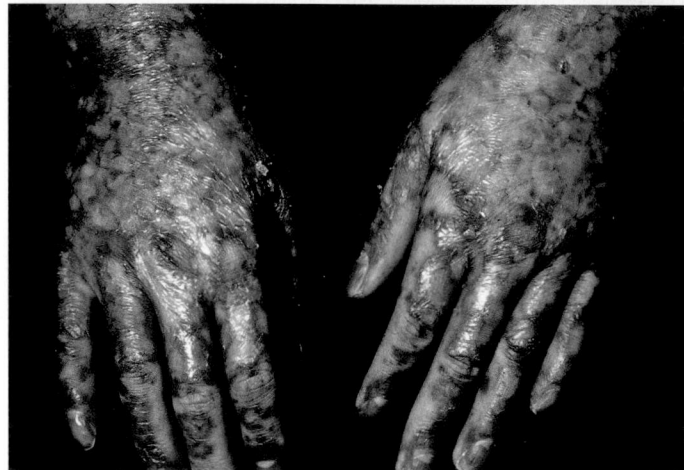

Fig. 5-19 Chronic graft-versus-host disease.

characterized by an erythematous morbilliform eruption of the face and trunk, which may become confluent and result in exfoliative erythroderma. It often begins with punctate lesions corresponding to hair follicles and eccrine ducts. Even when morbilliform, darker punctate areas are a helpful clinical sign. In children, the diaper area is often involved. The eruption may appear papular and eczematous, involving web spaces, periumbilical skin, and ears. The appearance bears some resemblance to scabies. The differential diagnosis for the eruption of acute GVHD includes the eruption of lymphocyte recovery, engraftment syndrome (see below), a viral exanthema, and a drug eruption. The cutaneous histology in the early phases of acute GVHD may not be able to distinguish these entities. Grade IV GVHD is characterized by full-thickness slough and may resemble toxic epidermal necrolysis (Fig. 5-18). The mucous membranes and the conjunctivae can be involved as well, which can be difficult to distinguish from chemotherapy-induced and infectious mucositis. Often around the same time, the patient develops the other characteristic features of acute GVHD, a cholestatic hepatitis with elevated bilirubin and a high-volume diarrhea. Syngeneic/autologous GVHD usually involves only the skin and is self-limited. The preconditioning regimens are felt to result in loss of "self-tolerance."

Engraftment syndrome is a combination of symptoms that occur around the time of engraftment and neutrophil recovery. Patients develop fever (without an infectious source), diarrhea, pulmonary infiltrates with hypoxia, and capillary leak syndrome with edema and weight gain. It occurs as soon as 7 days after autologous HSCT, and between 11 and 16 days after allogeneic transplants. The associated skin eruption is clinically and histologically identical to acute.GVHD, but at the time of presentation is usually diagnosed as a "drug eruption" and antibiotic therapy is frequently changed. Ocular involvement with keratitis can occur. This syndrome occurs in 7–59% of patients following HSCT, and is a significant cause of morbidity and mortality in the setting of autologous peripheral blood progenitor cell transplants. In one series it accounted for 45% of all transplant-related mortality. It is mediated by cytokine production and neutrophil infiltration of the organs

damaged by the conditioning chemotherapy, especially the lungs. Administration of G-CSF and autologous transplantation are risk factors for the development of engraftment syndrome. The relationship of engraftment syndrome to eruption of lymphocyte recovery is unclear. The treatment of engraftment syndrome is high-dose systemic steroids.

With improved support for patients following HSCT, more people are surviving and developing chronic GVHD. It is the second most common cause of death in HSCT patients. It is unclear whether chronic GVHD is mediated by the same pathological mechanisms as acute GVHD. Chronic GVHD has features more typical of an "autoimmune" disease. Diagnostic criteria have been adopted. There are "diagnostic" and "distinctive" cutaneous manifestations. The most common diagnostic feature, which occurs in 80% of patients who develop chronic GVHD, is a lichen planus-like eruption. It typically occurs 3–5 months after grafting, usually beginning on the hands and feet, but becoming generalized. It may present with a malar rash resembling LE. The chronic interface dermatitis can leave the skin with a poikilodermatous appearance. Similar lichen planus-like lesions may occur on the oral mucosa and can result in pain and poor nutrition. Sclerosis is the other "diagnostic" family of skin lesions. This can include lesions resembling superficial morphea/lichen sclerosus. The morphea-like lesions demonstrate an isomorphic response, favoring areas of pressure, especially the waist-band and brassiere-band areas. Sclerosis can occur on the genital mucosa, and complete fusion of the labia minora may occur, requiring surgical correction. Deeper sclerotic lesions resembling eosinophilic fasciitis (resulting in joint contractures, Fig. 5-19) and restriction of the oral commissure due to sclerosis can occur. These sclerotic plaques may ulcerate, especially during therapy with PUVA. The extent of involvement of the deep tissues, such as muscle and fascia, cannot be easily defined by clinical examination, and may be aided by magnetic resonance imaging (MRI). Rarely, the myositis of chronic GVHD may be accompanied by a skin eruption very similar to dermatomyositis. The "distinctive" features include depigmentation resembling vitiligo; scarring or non-scarring alopecia; nail dystrophy (longitudinal ridging, brittle thin nails, pterygium, and nail loss); and xerostomia and other Sjögren-like mucosal symptoms.

Histologically, acute GVHD demonstrates vacuolar interface dermatitis. Individual keratinocyte necrosis with adjacent lymphocytes (satellite necrosis) is typically present, suggesting cell-mediated cytotoxicity. The extent of necrosis, bulla formation, and slough is used in grading schemes. In early acute GVHD, the findings may be focal and restricted to hair follicles and sweat ducts. The histologic findings in very early disease may be nonspecific, and many treatment protocols do not depend on histologic features to initiate therapy. A background of epidermal disorder and atypia resembling bowenoid actinic keratosis is almost universally present in later lesions of acute GVHD, and is a helpful diagnostic feature. Similar epidermal changes may be seen with cancer chemotherapy, especially in acral erythema or after busulfan. Chronic GVHD demonstrates lichenoid dermatitis or dermal sclerosis with hyalinization of collagen bundles and narrowing of the space between the collagen bundles.

Prevention of post-transfusion GVHD is most safely achieved by irradiating the blood before transfusion in high-risk individuals. Acute GVHD is managed on the skin with topical steroids, TCIs, and UV phototherapy. When systemic symptoms appear, a glucocorticoid, cyclosporine, or tacrolimus is instituted. Blocking the cytokine storm with monoclonal antibodies such as etanercept, infliximab, and others can be beneficial in some patients. Extracorporeal photopheresis can be considered in acute and chronic GVHD that fails to respond to these first-line therapies. Bath PUVA, with or without isotretinoin, can improve sclerodermatous chronic GVHD. Imatinib can be beneficial in refractory sclerodermatous chronic GVHD.

GVHD in solid organ transplantation

Transplantation of a solid organ into a partially immunosuppressed host may result in GVHD, since the organ may contain immune cells. The prevalence of GVHD following transplantation is related to the type of organ transplanted and is dependent upon the amount of lymphoid tissue that the organ contains. The risk profile is small intestine > liver > kidney > heart. In liver and small intestine transplants the risk is 1–2%, but when it occurs the mortality is 85%. Close matching increases the risk of GVHD in organ transplantation, since the immunocompetent recipient cells are less likely to recognize the donor lymphocytes as "non-self" and destroy them. The onset is usually 1–8 weeks following transplantation, but can be delayed for years. Fever, rash, and pancytopenia are the cardinal features. The skin is the first site of involvement and only cutaneous disease occurs in 15% of cases. Both acute and chronic GVHD skin findings can occur. Skin biopsies tend to show more inflammation than in HSCT-associated GVHD. In GVHD accompanying liver transplantation, the liver is unaffected, since it is syngeneic with the donor lymphocytes. In these patients pancytopenia can occur and is a frequent cause of mortality. The diagnosis of GVHD in the setting of organ transplantation can be aided by documenting macrochimerism in the peripheral blood and skin after the first month of transplantation.

Alkhatib AA, et al: Colitis secondary to engraftment syndrome in a patient with autologous peripheral blood stem cell transplant. Dig Dis Sci 2009.

Calzavara Pinton P, et al: Prospects for ultraviolet A1 phototherapy as a treatment for chronic cutaneous graft-versus-host disease. Haematologica 2003; 88:1169.

Carcagni MR, et al: Extracorporeal photopheresis in graft-versus-host disease. J Dtsch Dermatol Ges 2008; 6:451.

Carpenter PA: Late effects of chronic graft-versus-host disease. Best Pract Res Clin Haematol 2008; 21:309.

Dai E, et al: Bilateral marginal keratitis associated with engraftment syndrome after hematopoietic stem cell transplantation. Cornea 2007; 26:756.

Ferrara JL: Novel strategies for the treatment and diagnosis of graft-versus-host disease. Best Pract Res Clin Haematol 2007; 20:91.

Ferrara JL, et al: Graft-versus-host disease. Lancet 2009; 373:1550.

Flowers ME, et al: A multicenter prospective phase 2 randomized study of extracorporeal photopheresis for treatment of chronic graft-versus-host disease. Blood 2008; 112:2667.

Foncillas MA, et al: Engraftment syndrome emerges as the main cause of transplant-related mortality in pediatric patients receiving autologous peripheral blood progenitor cell transplantation. J Pediatr Hematol Oncol 2004; 26:492.

Ghoreschi K, et al: PUVA-bath photochemotherapy and isotretinoin in sclerodermatous graft-versus-host disease. Eur J Dermatol 2008; 18:667.

Goiriz R, et al: Cutaneous lichenoid graft-versus-host disease mimicking lupus erythematosus. Lupus 2008; 17:591.

Gorak E, et al: Engraftment syndrome after nonmyeloablative allogeneic hematopoietic stem cell transplantation: incidence and effects on survival. Biol Blood Marrow Transplant 2005; 11:542.

Hausermann P, et al: Cutaneous graft-versus-host disease: a guide for the dermatologist. Dermatology 2008; 216:287.

Horger M, et al: Musculocutaneous chronic graft-versus-host disease: MRI follow-up of patients undergoing immunosuppressive therapy. AJR Am J Roentgenol 2009; 192:1401.

Katzel JA, et al: Engraftment syndrome after hematopoietic stem cell transplantation in multiple myeloma. Clin Lymphoma Myeloma 2006; 7:151.

Kuykendall TD, et al: Lack of specificity in skin biopsy specimens to assess for acute graft-versus-host disease in initial 3 weeks after bone-marrow transplantation. J Am Acad Dermatol 2003; 49:1081.

Magro L, et al: Efficacy of imatinib mesylate in the treatment of refractory sclerodermatous chronic GVHD. Bone Marrow Transplant 2008; 42:757.

Miano M, et al: Early complications following haematopoietic SCT in children. Bone Marrow Transplant 2008; 41(Suppl 2):S39.

Moreno-Romero JA, et al: Imatinib as a potential treatment for sclerodermatous chronic graft-vs-host disease. Arch Dermatol 2008; 144:1106.

Nellen RG, et al: Eruption of lymphocyte recovery or autologous graft-versus-host disease? Int J Dermatol 2008; 47(Suppl 1):32.

Norian JM, et al: Labial fusion: a rare complication of chronic graft-versus-host disease. Obstet Gynecol 2008; 112:437.

Patel AR, et al: Rippled skin, fasciitis, and joint contractures. J Am Acad Dermatol 2008; 59:1070.

Perfetti P, et al: Extracorporeal photopheresis for the treatment of steroid refractory acute GVHD. Bone Marrow Transplant 2008; 42:609.

Rapoport AP, et al: Rapid immune recovery and graft-versus-host disease-like engraftment syndrome following adoptive transfer of costimulated autologous T cells. Clin Cancer Res 2009; 15:4499.

Scarisbrick JJ, et al: U.K. consensus statement on the use of extracorporeal photopheresis for treatment of cutaneous T-cell lymphoma and chronic graft-versus-host disease. Br J Dermatol 2008; 158:659.

Schaffer JV: The changing face of graft-versus-host disease. Semin Cutan Med Surg 2006; 25:190.

Bonus images for this chapter can be found online at
http://www.expertconsult.com

Fig. 5-1 Dennie–Morgan folds.
Fig. 5-2 Perioral pallor.
Fig. 5-3 Napkin psoriasis.
Fig. 5-4 Eczematous eruption with purpura in Wiskott–Aldrich syndrome.
Fig. 5-5 Early punctate eruption of graft-versus-host disease.
Fig. 5-6 Involvement of the diaper area in graft-versus-host disease.

6

Contact Dermatitis and Drug Eruptions

Contact dermatitis

There are two types of dermatitis caused by substances coming in contact with the skin: irritant dermatitis and allergic contact dermatitis. Irritant dermatitis is an inflammatory reaction in the skin resulting from exposure to a substance that causes an eruption in most people who come in contact with it. Allergic contact dermatitis is an acquired sensitivity to various substances that produce inflammatory reactions in those, and only those, who have been previously sensitized to the allergen.

Irritant contact dermatitis

Many substances act as irritants that produce a nonspecific inflammatory reaction of the skin. This type of dermatitis may be induced in any person if a sufficiently high concentration is used. No previous exposure is necessary and the effect is evident within minutes, or a few hours at most. The concentration and type of the toxic agent, the duration of exposure, and the condition of the skin at the time of exposure produces the variation in the severity of the dermatitis from person to person, or from time to time in the same person. The skin may be more vulnerable by reason of maceration from excessive humidity, or exposure to water, heat, cold, pressure, or friction. Dry skin is less likely to react to contactants. Thick skin is less reactive than thin. Repeated exposure to some of the milder irritants may, in time, produce a hardening effect. This process makes the skin more resistant to the irritant effects of a given substance. Symptomatically, pain and burning are more common in irritant dermatitis, contrasting with the usual itch of allergic reactions.

Alkalis

Irritant dermatitis is often produced by alkalis such as soaps, detergents, bleaches, ammonia preparations, lye, drain pipe cleaners, and toilet bowl and oven cleansers. Alkalis penetrate and destroy deeply because they dissolve keratin. Strong solutions are corrosive and immediate application of a weak acid such as vinegar, lemon juice, or 0.5% hydrochloric acid solution will lessen their effects.

The principal compounds are sodium, potassium, ammonium, and calcium hydroxides. Occupational exposure is frequent among workers in soap manufacturing. Alkalis in the form of soaps, bleaching agents, detergents, and most household cleansing agents figure prominently in the causes of hand eczema. Sodium silicate (water glass) is a caustic used in soap manufacture and paper sizing, and for the preservation of eggs. Alkaline sulfides are used as depilatories (Fig. 6-1). Calcium oxide (quicklime) forms slaked lime when water is added. Severe burns may be caused in plasterers.

Acids (Fig. 6-2)

The powerful acids are corrosive, whereas the weaker ones are astringent. Hydrochloric acid produces burns that are less deep and more liable to form blisters than injuries from sulfuric and nitric acids. Hydrochloric acid burns are encountered in those who handle or transport the product, and in plumbers and those who work in galvanizing or tin-plate factories. Sulfuric acid produces a brownish charring of the skin, beneath which is an ulceration that heals slowly. Sulfuric acid is used more widely than any other acid in industry; it is handled principally by brass and iron workers and by those who work with copper or bronze. Nitric acid is a powerful oxidizing substance that causes deep burns; the tissue is stained yellow. Such injuries are observed in those who manufacture or handle the acid or use it in the making of explosives in laboratories.

Hydrofluoric acid is used widely in rust remover, in the semiconductor industry, and in germicides, dyes, plastics, and glass etching. It may act insidiously at first, starting with erythema and ending with vesiculation, ulceration, and, finally, necrosis of the tissue. It is one of the strongest inorganic acids, capable of dissolving glass. Oxalic acid may produce paresthesia of the fingertips, with cyanosis and gangrene. The nails become discolored yellow. Oxalic acid is best neutralized with limewater or milk of magnesia to produce precipitation.

Phenol (carbolic acid) is a protoplasmic poison that produces a white eschar on the surface of the skin. It can penetrate deep into the tissue. If a large surface of the skin is treated with phenol for cosmetic peeling effects, the absorbed phenol may produce glomerulonephritis and arrhythmias. Locally, temporary anesthesia may also occur. Phenol is readily neutralized with 65% ethyl or isopropyl alcohol. Titanium hydrochloride is used in the manufacture of pigments. Application of water to the exposed part will produce severe burns. Therefore, treatment consists only of wiping away the noxious substance.

Other strong acids that are irritants include acetic, trichloracetic, arsenious, chlorosulfonic, chromic, fluoroboric, hydriodic, hydrobromic, iodic, perchloric, phosphoric, salicylic, silicofluoric, sulfonic, sulfurous, tannic, and tungstic acids.

Treatment of acid burns consists of immediate rinsing with copious amounts of water and alkalization with sodium bicarbonate, calcium hydroxide (limewater), or soap solutions. Some chemicals require unusual treatment measures. Fluorine is best neutralized with magnesium oxide. Periungual burns should be treated intralesionally with 10% calcium gluconate solution, which deactivates the fluoride ion and averts more tissue damage. Hypocalcemia, hypomagnesemia, hyperkalemia, and cardiac dysrhythmias may complicate hydrofluoric acid burns. Phosphorus burns should be rinsed off with water followed by application of copper sulfate to produce a precipitate.

Airbag dermatitis

Airbags are deployed as a safety feature on cars when rapid deceleration occurs. Activation of a sodium azide and cupric oxide propellant cartridge releases nitrogen gas, which expands the bag at speeds exceeding 160 km/h. Talcum

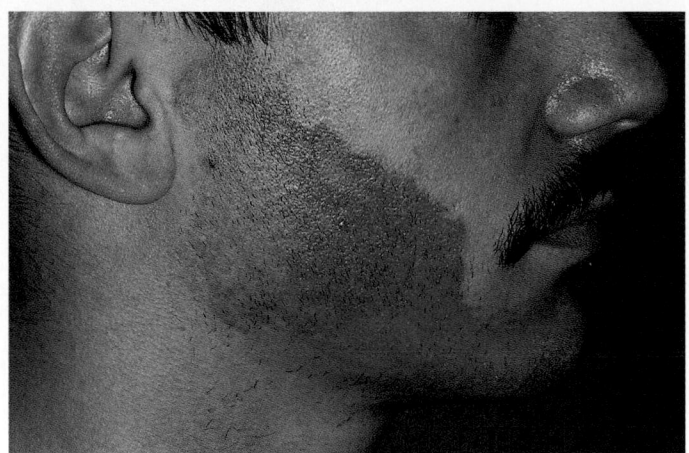

Fig. 6-1 Alkali burn from depilatory.

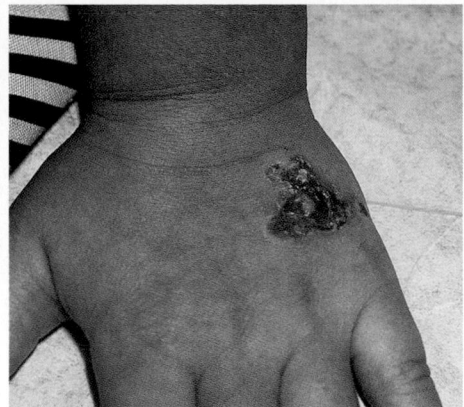

Fig. 6-2 Acid burn.

powder, sodium hydroxide, and sodium carbonate are released into the bag. Abrasions, thermal, friction, and chemical burns, and an irritant contact dermatitis may result. Superficial erythema may respond well to topical steroids, but full-thickness burns may occur and require debridement and grafting.

Other irritants

Some metal salts that act as irritants are the cyanides of calcium, copper, mercury, nickel, silver, and zinc, and the chlorides of calcium and zinc. Bromine, chlorine, fluorine, and iodine are also irritants. Occupational exposure to methyl bromide may produce erythema and vesicles in the axillary and inguinal areas. Insecticides, including 2,2-dichlorovinyl dimethyl phosphate used in roach powder and fly repellents and killers, can act as irritants.

Fiberglass dermatitis

Fiberglass dermatitis is seen after occupational or inadvertent exposure. The small spicules of glass penetrate the skin and cause severe irritation with tiny erythematous papules, scratch marks, and intense pruritus. Usually, there is no delayed hypersensitivity reaction. Wearing clothes that have been washed together with fiberglass curtains, handling air conditioner filters, or working in the manufacture of fiberglass material may produce severe folliculitis, pruritus, and eruptions that may simulate scabies or insect or mite bites. Fiberglass is also used in thermal and acoustic installations, padding, vibration isolation, curtains, draperies, insulation for automobile bodies, furniture, gasoline tanks, and spacecraft. Talcum powder dusted on the flexure surfaces of the arms prior to exposure makes the fibers slide off the skin. A thorough washing of the skin after handling fiberglass is helpful. Patch testing to epoxy resins should be done when evaluating workers in fiberglass/reinforced plastics operations, as an allergic contact dermatitis may be difficult to discern from fiberglass dermatitis.

Dusts

Some dusts and gases may irritate the skin in the presence of heat and moisture, such as perspiration. The dusts of lime, zinc, and arsenic may produce folliculitis. Dusts from various woods, such as teak, may incite itching and dermatitis. Dusts from cinchona bark, quinine, and pyrethrum produce widespread dermatitis. Tobacco dust in cigar factories, powdered orris root, lycopodium, and dusts of various nutshells may cause swelling of the eyelids and dermatitis of the face, neck, and upper extremities, the distribution of an airborne contact dermatitis. Dusts formed during the manufacture of high explosives may cause erythematous, vesicular, and eczema-

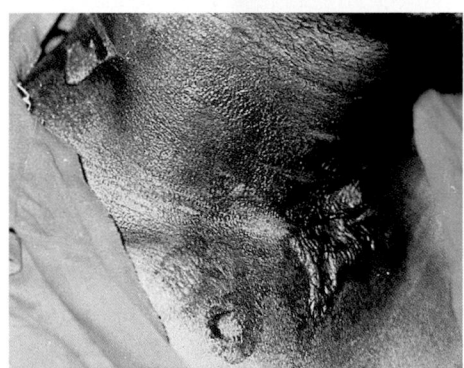

Fig. 6-3 Mustard gas burn. (Courtesy of James WD [ed]: Textbook of Military Medicine. Office of the Surgeon General, United States Army, 1994.)

tous dermatitis that may lead to generalized exfoliative dermatitis.

Capsaicin

Hand irritation produced by capsaicin in hot peppers used in Korean and North Chinese cuisine (Hunan hand) may be severe and prolonged. Pepper spray, used by police in high concentrations, and by civilians in less concentrated formulas, contains capsaicin and may produce severe burns. Cold water is not much help; capsaicin is insoluble in water. Acetic acid 5% (white vinegar) or antacids (Maalox) may completely relieve the burning even if applied an hour or more after the contact. Application should be continued until the area can be dried without return of the discomfort.

Tear gas dermatitis

Lacrimators such as chloroacetophenone in concentrated form may cause dermatitis, with a delayed appearance some 24–72 h after exposure. Irritation or sensitization, with erythema and severe vesiculation, may result. Treatment consists of lavage of the affected skin with sodium bicarbonate solution and instillation of boric acid solution into the eyes. Contaminated clothing should be removed.

Sulfur mustard gas, also known as yperite, has been used in chemical warfare such as in the Iraq–Iran war. Erythema, vesicles, and bullae, followed by healing with hyperpigmentation over a 1-week period, result from mild to moderate exposure (Fig. 6-3). Toxic epidermal necrolysis (TEN)-like appearance may follow more concentrated contact. The earliest and most frequently affected sites are areas covered by clothing and humidified by sweat, such as the groin, axilla, and genitalia.

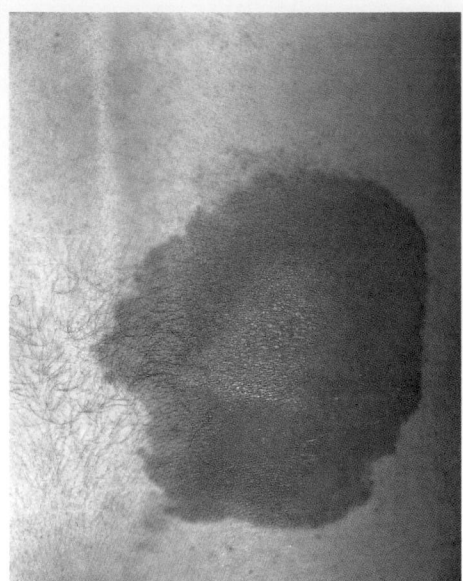

Fig. 6-4 Mace reaction.

Mace is a mixture of tear gas (chloroacetophenone) in trichloroethane and various hydrocarbons resembling kerosene. It is available in a variety of self-defense sprays. It is a potent irritant (Fig. 6-4) and may cause allergic sensitization. Treatment consists of changing clothes, then washing with oil or milk, followed by washing with copious amounts of water.

Chloracne

Workers in the manufacture of chlorinated compounds may develop chloracne, with small straw-colored follicular plugs and papules, chiefly on the malar crescent, retroauricular areas, earlobes, neck, shoulders, and scrotum. The synthetic waxes chloronaphthalene and chlorodiphenyl, used in the manufacture of electric insulators and in paints, varnishes, and lacquers, similarly predispose workers engaged in the manufacture of these synthetic waxes to chloracne. Exposure to 2,6-dichlorobenzonitrile during the manufacture of a herbicide, and to 3,4,3',4'-tetrachloroazooxybenzene, which is an unwanted intermediate byproduct in the manufacture of a pesticide, may also produce chloracne.

A contaminant in the synthesis of herbicides and hexachlorophene, 2,3,7,8-tetracholorodibenzo-p-dioxin, produces a chemical burn in the acute stage, but chloracne, hyperpigmentation, hirsutism, and skin fragility (with or without criteria for porphyria cutanea tarda) are manifestations of chronic toxicity. Gastrointestinal tract cancer and malignancies of the lymphatic and hematopoietic systems are suspected to result but the studies are still inconclusive. While contact is the usual method of exposure, inhalation, ingestion, or contact with contaminated clothing may also result in chloracne. Chloracne may persist for long periods because dioxin is stored in the liver and released slowly into the circulation. Treatment is with medications used in acne vulgaris, including isotretinoin.

Hydrocarbons

Many hydrocarbons produce skin eruptions. Crude petroleum causes generalized itching, folliculitis, or acneiform eruptions. The irritant properties of petroleum derivatives are directly proportional to their fat-solvent properties and inversely proportional to their viscosity. Oils of the naphthalene series are more irritating than those of the paraffin series. Refined fractions from petroleum are less irritating than the unrefined products, although benzene, naphtha, and carbon disulfide may cause a mild dermatitis.

Lubricating and cutting oils are causes of similar cutaneous lesions. They represent a frequent cause of occupational dermatoses in machine tool operators, machinists, layout men, instrument makers, and set-up men. Insoluble (neat) cutting oils are responsible for a follicular acneiform eruption on the dorsa of the hands, the forearms, face, thighs, and back of the neck. Hyperpigmentation, keratoses, and scrotal cancer have been found in those exposed to insoluble cutting oils. Soluble oils and synthetic fluids used in metalworking do not result in acne, but rather an eczematous dermatitis, usually of the dorsal forearms and hands. Approximately 50% of the time it is irritant and in the remainder it is allergic. Allergic contact dermatitis arises from various additives, such as biocides, coloring agents, and deodorizers.

Coal briquette makers develop dermatitis as a result of a tarry residue from petroleum used in their trade. Paraffin exposure leads to pustules, keratoses, and ulcerations. Shale oil workers develop an erythematous, follicular eruption that eventually leads to keratoses, which may become the sites of carcinoma. It is estimated that 50% of shale oil workers have skin problems.

Impure and low-grade paraffins and mineral oils cause similar skin eruptions. Initially, the skin changes are similar to those in chloracne. In due time, a diffuse erythema with dappled pigmentation develops. Gradually, keratoses appear, and after many years some of these are the sites of carcinoma. Melanoderma may occur from exposure to mineral oils and lower-grade petroleum, from creosote, asphalt, and other tar products. Photosensitization may play a role. Creosote is a contact irritant, sensitizer, and photosensitizer. Allergy is demonstrated by patch testing with 10% creosote in oil.

Petrolatum dermatitis may appear as a verrucous thickening of the skin caused by prolonged contact with impure petroleum jelly or, occasionally, lubricating oil. A follicular centered process may occur in which erythematous horny nodules are present, usually on the anterior and inner aspects of the thighs. There are no comedones and the lesions are separated by apparently normal skin.

Acne corne consists of follicular keratosis and pigmentation resulting from crude petroleum, tar oils, and paraffin. The dorsal aspects of the fingers and hands, the arms, legs, face, and thorax are the areas usually involved. The lesions are follicular, horny papules, often black, and are associated at first with a follicular erythema and later with a dirty brownish or purplish spotty pigmentation, which in severe cases becomes widespread and is especially marked around the genitals. This syndrome may simulate pityriasis rubra pilaris or lichen spinulosus.

Coal tar and pitch and many of their derivatives produce photosensitization and an acneiform folliculitis of the forearms, legs, face, and scrotum. Follicular keratoses (pitch warts) may develop and later turn into carcinoma. Soot, lamp black, and the ash from peat fires produce dermatitis of a dry, scaly character, which in the course of time forms warty outgrowths and cancer. Chimney sweep's cancer occurs under a soot wart and is usually located on the scrotum, where soot, sebum, and dirt collect in the folds of the skin. This form of cancer has virtually disappeared.

Acquired perforating disease may occur in oil field workers who use drilling fluid containing calcium chloride. Patients develop tender, umbilicated papules of the forearms that microscopically show transepidermal elimination of calcium.

Solvents

These cause approximately 10% of occupational dermatitis. When they are applied to the hands to cleanse them, the surface oil is dissolved and a chronic fissured dermatitis results. Additionally, peripheral neuropathy and chemical lymphangitis may occur after the solvents are absorbed through the fissured skin. Solvent sniffers may develop an eczematous eruption about the mouth and nose. There is erythema and edema. It is a direct irritant dermatitis caused by the inhalation of the solvent placed on a handkerchief.

Trichloroethylene is a chlorinated hydrocarbon solvent and degreasing agent, and is also used in the dry-cleaning and refrigerant industry. Inhalation may produce exfoliative erythroderma, mucous membrane erosions, eosinophilia, and hepatitis.

Allergic contact dermatitis caused by alcohol is rarely encountered with lower aliphatic alcohols. A severe case of bullous and hemorrhagic dermatitis on the fingertips and deltoid region was caused by isopropyl alcohol. Though rare, ethyl alcohol dermatitis may also be encountered. Cetyl and stearyl alcohols may provoke contact urticaria.

Amshel CE, et al: Anhydrous ammonia burns. Burns 2000; 26:493.

Bordel-Gomez MT, et al: Fiberglass dermatitis. Contact Dermatitis 2008; 59:120.

Bourke J, et al: Guidelines for the management of contact dermatitis. Br J Dermatol 2009; 160:946.

Bullman T, et al: A 50 year mortality follow-up study of veterans exposed to low level chemical warfare agent, mustard gas. Ann Epidemiol 2000; 10:333.

Edlich RF, et al: Modern concepts of treatment and prevention of chemical injuries. J Long Term Eff Med Implants 2005; 15:303.

Finkelstein E, et al: Oil acne. J Am Acad Dermatol 1994; 30:491.

Flammiger A, et al: Sulfuric acid burns. Cutan Ocul Toxicol 2006: 25:55.

Fyhrquist-Vanni N, et al: Contact dermatitis. Dermatol Clin 2007; 25:615.

Goon AT, et al: A case of trichloroethylene hypersensitivity syndrome. Arch Dermatol 2001; 137:274.

Herzemans-Boer M, et al: Skin lesions due to methyl bromide. Arch Dermatol 1988; 124:917.

Jia X, et al: Adverse effects of gasoline on the skin of gasoline workers. Contact Dermatitis 2002; 46:44.

Minamoto K, et al: Occupational dermatoses among fibreglass-reinforced plastics factory workers. Contact Dermatitis 2002; 46:339.

Momeni AZ, et al: Skin manifestations of mustard gas. Arch Dermatol 1992; 128:775.

Panteleyev AA, et al: Dioxin-induced chloracne. Exp Dermatol 2006: 15:705.

Salzman M, et al: Updates on the evaluation and management of caustic exposures. Emerg Med Clin N Am 2007; 25:459.

Sanz-Gallen P, et al: Hypocalcaemia and hypomagnesaemia due to hydrofluoric acid. Occup Med 2001; 51:294.

Stuke LE, et al: Hydrofluoric acid burns. J Burn Care Res 2008; 29:893.

Suchard JR: Treatment of capsaicin dermatitis. Am J Emerg Med 1999; 17:210.

Treudler R, et al: Occupational contact dermatitis due to 2-chloracetophenone tear gas. Br J Dermatol 1999; 140:531.

Ueno S, et al: Metalworking fluid hand dermatitis. Ind Health 2002; 40:291.

Varma S, et al: Severe cutaneous reaction to CS gas. Clin Exp Dermatol 2001; 26:248.

Williams SR, et al: Contact dermatitis associated with capsaicin: Hunan hand syndrome. Ann Emerg Med 1995; 25:713.

Wu JJ, et al: A case of air bag dermatitis. Arch Dermatol 2002; 138:1383.

Allergic contact dermatitis

Allergic contact dermatitis results when an allergen comes into contact with previously sensitized skin. It is due to a specific acquired hypersensitivity of the delayed type, also known as cell-mediated hypersensitivity or immunity. Occasionally, dermatitis may be induced when the allergen is taken internally by a patient first sensitized by topical application; this occurs, for example, with substances such as cinnamon oil or various medications. The anamnestic response is termed systemic contact dermatitis. It may appear first at the site of the prior sensitization or past positive patch test, but may spread to a generalized morbilliform or eczematous eruption.

Additional morphologic patterns include vesicular hand eczema, urticaria, erythema multiforme, vasculitis, or the baboon syndrome. The latter is a deep red–violet eruption on the buttocks, genital area, inner thighs, and sometimes axilla.

The most common causes of contact dermatitis in the US are: toxicodendrons (poison ivy, oak, or sumac), nickel, balsam of Peru (*Myroxylon pereirae*), neomycin, fragrance, thimerosal, gold, formaldehyde and the formaldehyde-releasing preservatives, bacitracin, and rubber compounds. Frequent positive reactions to thimerosal do not often correlate with clinical exposure histories. These reactions are probably related to its use as a preservative in commonly administered vaccines and skin-testing material. It also serves as a marker for piroxicam photosensitivity. These sensitizers do not cause demonstrable skin changes on initial contact. Persons may be exposed to allergens for years before finally developing hypersensitivity. Once sensitized, however, subsequent outbreaks may result from extremely slight exposure.

When allergens are applied to the skin, Langerhans cells in the epidermis process them and display them in a complex with human leukocyte antigen (HLA)-DR on their surface. This is presented to a CD4+ T cell, interaction with the T-cell receptor–CD3 complex occurs, and the allergen is recognized. This leads to proliferation and recruitment of lymphocytes with release of vasoactive substances and direct inflammatory mediators. Genetic variability in these processes and other factors, such as concentration of the allergen applied, its vehicle, timing and site of the exposure, presence of occlusion, age, sex, and race of the patient, and presence of other skin or systemic disorders, likely determine whether any given exposure will result in sensitization.

Eczematous delayed-type hypersensitivity reaction, as exemplified by allergic contact dermatitis and the patch test, must be distinguished from immediate-type hypersensitivity reactions. The latter presents within minutes of exposure with urticaria and is proven with a scratch test. It should be kept in mind, however, that persons who develop contact urticaria to a substance may concomitantly have a type IV delayed-type sensitization and eczema from the same allergen.

In some instances, impetigo, pustular folliculitis, and irritations or allergic reactions from applied medications are superimposed on the original dermatitis. A particularly vexing situation is when allergy to topical steroids complicates an eczema, in which case the preexisting dermatitis usually does not flare, but simply does not heal as expected. The cutaneous reaction may also provoke a hypersusceptibility to various other previously innocuous substances, which continues the eczematous inflammatory response indefinitely.

These eruptions resolve when the cause is identified and avoided. For acute generalized allergic contact dermatitis treatment with systemic steroidal agents is effective, beginning with 40–60 mg/day prednisone in a single oral dose, and tapering slowly to topical steroids. When the eruption is limited in extent and severity, local application of topical corticosteroid creams, lotions, or aerosol sprays is preferred.

Testing for sensitivity

Patch test

The patch test is used to detect hypersensitivity to a substance that is in contact with the skin so that the allergen may be determined and corrective measures taken. So many allergens can cause allergic contact dermatitis that it is impossible to test a person for all of them. In addition, a good history and observation of the pattern of the dermatitis, its localization on the body, and its state of activity are all helpful in determining the cause. The patch test is confirmatory and diagnostic, but only within the framework of the history and physical findings; it is rarely helpful if it must stand alone. Interpretation of the relevance of positive tests and the subsequent education of patients are challenging in some cases. The Contact Allergen Avoidance Database (CARD) provides names of alternative products that may be used by patients when an allergen is identified. This is available through the American Contact Dermatitis Society.

The patch test consists of application of substances suspected to be the cause of the dermatitis to intact uninflamed skin. Patch testing may be administered by the thin-layer rapid-use epicutaneous (TRUE) test or by individually prepared aluminum (Finn) chambers mounted on Scanpor tape. The TRUE test has resulted in more screening for allergic contact dermatitis than in the past; however, if this test does not reveal the allergen for a highly suspect dermatitis, testing with an expanded series by the Finn chamber technique may yield relevant allergens in more than half of these patients.

Test substances are applied usually to the upper back, although if only one or two are applied, the upper outer arm may be used. Each patch should be numbered to avoid confusion. The patches are removed after 48 h (or sooner if severe itching or burning occurs at the site) and read. The patch sites need to be evaluated again at day 4 or 5 because positive reactions may not appear earlier. Some allergens may take up to day 7 to show a reaction and the patient should be advised to return if such a delayed reaction occurs. Erythematous papules and vesicles with edema are indicative of allergy (Fig. 6-5). Occasionally, patch tests for potassium iodide, nickel, or mercury will produce pustules at the site of the test application. Usually no erythema is produced; therefore, the reaction has no clinical significance.

Strong patch-test reactions may induce a state of hyperirritability ("excited skin syndrome") in which negative tests appear as weakly positive. Weakly positive tests in the presence of strong ones do not prove sensitivity. There is wide variation in the ability of the skin and mucous membranes to react to antigens. The oral mucosa is more resistant to primary irritants and is less liable to be involved in allergic reactions. This may be because the keratin layer of the skin more readily combines with haptens to form allergens. Also, the oral mucosa

is bathed in saliva, which cleanses and buffers the area and dilutes irritants. However, patch testing for various types of oral signs and symptoms, such as swelling, tingling and burning, perioral dermatitis, and the appearance of oral lichen planus, is useful in determining a cause in many cases.

The ability of the skin to react to allergens also depends on the presence of functional antigen-presenting cells, the Langerhans cells. Potent topical steroids, ultraviolet (UV) light, various immunosuppressants such as oral prednisone and the acquired immunodeficiency syndrome (AIDS) have been reported to interfere with the number and function of these key cells. False-negative reactions may result; the value of testing in such circumstances is that if a positive reaction occurs, a diagnosis may be made. Vitiliginous skin is less reactive than normally pigmented adjacent skin.

Provocative use test

The provocative use test will confirm a positive closed patch-test reaction to ingredients of a substance, such as a cosmetic; it is used to test products that are made to stay on the skin once applied. The material is rubbed on to normal skin of the inner aspect of the forearm several times a day for 5 days.

Photopatch test

The photopatch test is used to evaluate for contact photo-allergy to such substances as sulfonamides, phenothiazines, p-aminobenzoic acid, oxybenzone, 6-methyl coumarin, musk ambrette, or tetrachlorsalicylanilide. A standard patch test is applied for 48 h; this is then exposed to 5–15 J/m^2 of UVA and read after another 48 h. To test for 6-methyl coumarin sensitivity, the patch is applied in the same manner but for only 30 min before light exposure, rather than for 48 h. A duplicate set of nonirradiated patches is used in testing for the presence of routine delayed hypersensitivity reactions. Also, a site of normal skin is given an identical dose of UVA to test for increased sensitivity to light without prior exposure to chemicals. There is a steady increase in incidence of photoallergy to sunscreening agents and a falling incidence of such reactions to fragrance.

Regional predilection

Familiarity with certain contactants and the typical dermatitis they elicit on specific parts of the body will assist in diagnosis of the etiologic agent.

Head and neck

The scalp is relatively resistant to the development of contact allergies; however, involvement may be caused by hair dye, hair spray, shampoo, or permanent wave solutions. The surrounding glabrous skin, including the ear rims and backs of the ears, may be much more inflamed and suggestive of the cause. Persistent otitis of the ear canal may be caused by sensitivity to the neomycin that is an ingredient of most aural medications. The eyelids are the most frequent site for nail polish dermatitis. Volatile gases, false-eyelash adhesive, fragrances, preservatives, mascara, rubber in sponges used to apply cosmetics, and eyeshadow are also frequently implicated (Fig. 6-6). Perioral dermatitis and cheilitis may be caused by flavoring agents in dentifrices and gum, as well as fragrances, shellac, medicaments, and sunscreens in lipstick and lip balms. Perfume dermatitis may cause redness just under the ears or on the neck. Earlobe dermatitis is indicative of nickel sensitivity. Photocontact dermatitis may involve the entire face and may be sharply cut off at the collar line or extend down on to the sternum in a V shape. There is a typical clear area under the chin where there is little or no exposure to sunlight. In men, in whom shaving lotion fragrances may

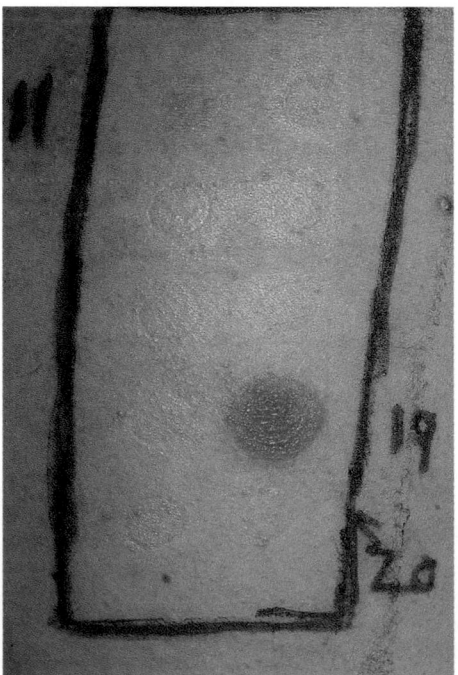

Fig. 6-5 Positive patch-test reaction.

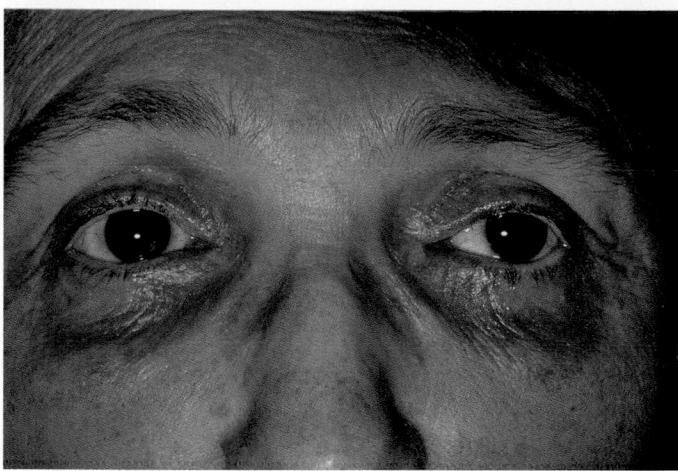

Fig. 6-6 Eyelid dermatitis.

be responsible, the left cheek and left side of the neck (from sun exposure while driving) may be the first areas involved.

Trunk

The trunk is an infrequent site; however, the dye or finish of clothing may cause dermatitis. The axilla may be the site of deodorant and clothing-dye dermatitis. Involvement of the axillary vault suggests the former; of the axillary folds, the latter. In women, brassieres cause dermatitis from either the material itself, the elastic, or the metal snaps or underwires.

Arms

The wrists may be involved because of jewelry or the backs of watches and clasps, all of which may contain nickel. Wristbands made of leather are a source of chrome dermatitis.

Hands

Innumerable substances may cause allergic contact dermatitis of the hands, which typically occurs on the backs of the hands and spares the palms. Florists will often develop fingertip or palmar lesions. A hand dermatitis that changes from web spaces to fingertips or from palms to dorsal hands should trigger patch testing. Poison ivy and other plant dermatitides frequently occur on the hands and arms. Rubber glove sensitivity must be kept constantly in mind. Usually irritancy is superimposed on allergic contact dermatitis of the hands, altering both the morphologic and histologic clues to the diagnosis.

Abdomen

The abdomen, especially the waistline, may be the site of rubber dermatitis from the elastic in pants and undergarments. The metallic rivets in blue jeans may lead to periumbilical dermatitis in nickel-sensitive patients, as may piercings of the umbilicus.

Groin

The groin is usually spared, but the buttocks and upper thighs may be sites of dermatitis caused by dyes. The penis is frequently involved in poison ivy dermatitis. Condom dermatitis may also occur. The perianal region may be involved from the "caine" medications in suppositories, as well as preservatives and fragrances in cleansing materials. Nearly half of women with pruritus vulvae have one or more relevant allergens; often these are medicaments, fragrances, or preservatives.

Lower extremities

The shins may be the site of rubber dermatitis from elastic stockings. Feet are sites for shoe dermatitis, most often attrib-

utable to rubber sensitivity, chrome-tanned leather, dyes, or adhesives. Application of topical antibiotics to stasis ulcers commonly leads to sensitivity and allergic contact dermatitis.

Bryden AM, et al: Photopatch testing of 1155 patients. Br J Dermatol 2006; 155:737.

Diepgen TL, et al: Management of chronic hand eczema. Contact Dermatitis 2007; 57:203.

Duarte I, et al: Excited skin syndrome: study of 39 patients. Am J Contact Dermat 2002; 13:59.

Feser A, et al: Periorbital dermatitis. Br J Dermatol 2008; 159:858.

Guin JD: Eyelid dermatitis. J Am Acad Dermatol 2002; 47:755.

Kockentiet B, et al: Contact dermatitis in athletes. J Am Acad Dermatol 2007; 56:1048.

Lazzarini R, et al: Contact dermatitis of the feet. Dermatitis 2004; 15:125.

Marks JG Jr, et al: Contact and Occupational Dermatology, 3rd edn. St Louis: Mosby, 2002.

Mowad CM: Patch testing. Curr Opin Allergy Clin Immunol 2006; 6:340.

Nardelli A, et al: Contact allergic reactions of the vulva. Dermatitis 2004; 15:131.

Prakash AV, et al: Contact dermatitis in older adults. Am J Clin Dermatol 2010; epub.

Rietschel RL, Fowler JF Jr: Fisher's Contact Dermatitis, 6th edn. Hamilton, BC: Decker, 2008.

Saary J, et al: A systematic review of contact dermatitis treatment and prevention. J Am Acad Dermatol 2005; 53:845.

Schena D, et al: Contact allergy in chronic eczematous lip dermatitis. Eur J Dermatol 2008: 18:688.

Sheman A, et al: Contact allergy alternatives. Dis Mon 2008: 54:7.

Thyssen JP, et al: The epidemiology of contact allergy in the general population. Contact Dermatitis 2007; 57:287.

Torgerson RR, et al: Contact allergy in oral disease. J Am Acad Dermatol 2007; 57:315.

Uter W, et al: Patch test results with patients' own perfumes, deodorants and shaving lotions. J Eur Acad Dermatol Venereol 2007; 21:374.

Warshaw EM, et al: Shoe allergens. Dermatitis 2007: 18:191.

Zug KA, et al: Contact allergy in children referred for patch testing. Arch Dermatol 2008; 144:1329.

Zug KA, et al: Patch-test results of the North American Contact Dermatitis Group 2005–2006. Dermatitis 2009; 20:149.

Dermatitis resulting from plants

A large number of plants, including trees, grasses, flowers, vegetables, fruits, and weeds, are potential causes of dermatitis. Eruptions from them vary considerably in appearance but are usually vesicular and accompanied by marked edema. After previous exposure and sensitization to the active substance in the plant, the typical dermatitis results from re-exposure. The onset is usually a few hours or days after contact. The characteristic linearly grouped lesions are probably produced by brushing the skin with a leaf edge or a broken twig, or by carriage of the allergen under the nails. Contrary to general belief, the contents of vesicles are not capable of producing new lesions.

Toxicodendron (poison ivy)

Toxicodendron dermatitis includes dermatitis from members of the Anacardiaceae family of plants: poison ivy (Fig. 6-7), poison oak, poison sumac, Japanese lacquer tree, cashew nut tree (the allergen is in the nutshell), mango (the allergen is in the rind, leaves, or sap), Rengas tree, and Indian marking nut tree. The ginkgo (the allergen is in the fruit pulp), spider flower or silver oak, *Gluta* species of trees and shrubs in Southeast Asia, Brazilian pepper tree, also known as Florida holly, and poisonwood tree contain nearly identical antigens.

Toxicodendron dermatitis appears within 48 h of exposure of a person previously sensitized to the plant. It usually begins on the backs of the fingers, interdigital spaces, wrists, and eyelids, although it may begin on the ankles or other parts that have been exposed. Marked pruritus is the first symptom; then

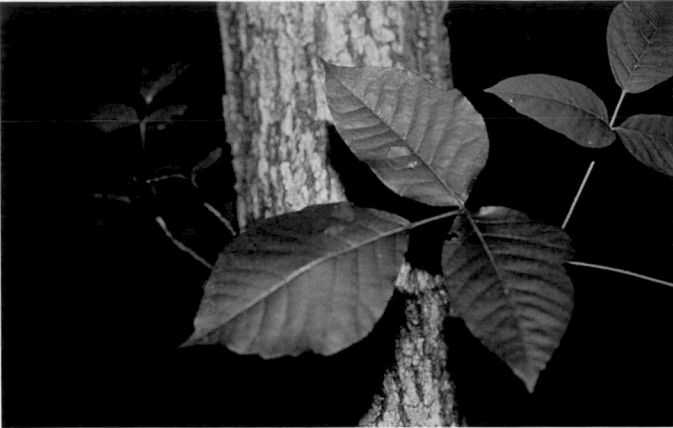

Fig. 6-7 *Toxicodendron radicans* subsp *radicans*. Poison ivy species found commonly in the eastern US. (Courtesy of James WD [ed]: Textbook of Military Medicine. Office of the Surgeon General, United States Army, 1994)

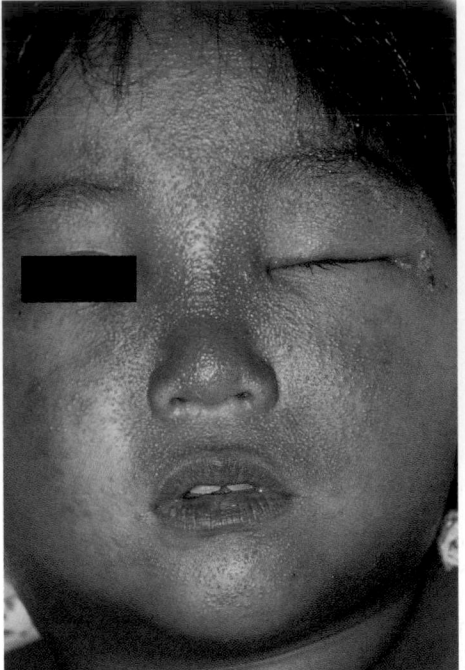

Fig. 6-9 Acute poison ivy reaction.

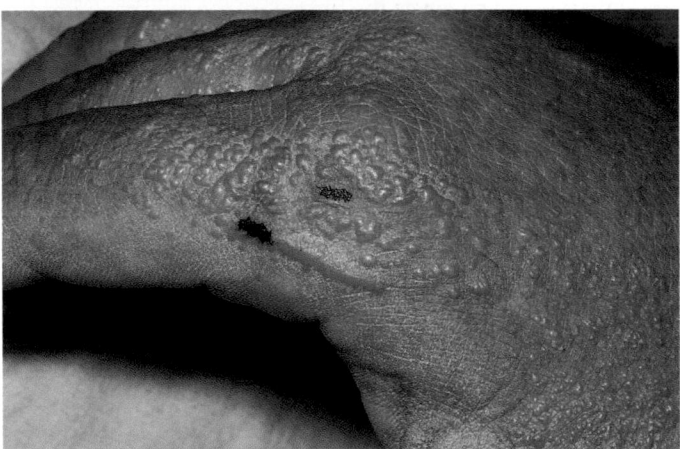

Fig. 6-10 Black dot sign in poison ivy reaction.

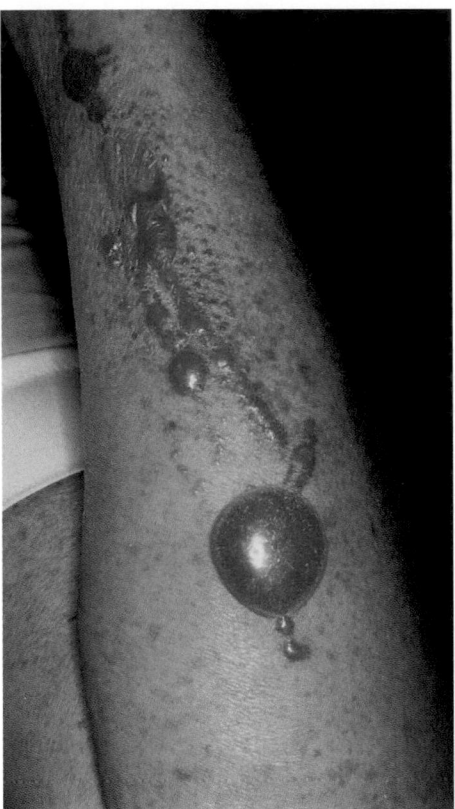

Fig. 6-8 Acute poison ivy reaction.

inflammation, vesicles, and bullae may appear. The vesicles are usually grouped and often linear (Fig. 6-8). Large bullae may be present, especially on the forearms and hands. The eyelids are puffy; they will be worst in the morning and improve as the day progresses (Fig. 6-9). Pruritus ani and involvement of the genital areas occur frequently. A black lacquer deposit may occur in which the sap of the plant has been oxidized after being bound to the stratum corneum (Fig. 6-10). Untreated toxicodendron dermatitis usually lasts 2–3 weeks.

The fingers transfer the allergen to other parts, especially the forearms and the male prepuce, which become greatly swollen. However, once the causative oil has been washed off, there is no spreading of the allergen and no further spread of the dermatitis. Some persons are so susceptible that direct contact is

not necessary, the allergen apparently being carried by the fur of their pets or by the wind. It can also be acquired from golf clubs or fishing rods, or even from furniture that a dog or cat might have occupied after exposure to the catechol. Occasionally, eating the allergen, as occurred in a patient who ingested raw cashew nuts in an imported pesto sauce, may result in the baboon syndrome (a deep red–violet eruption on the buttocks, genital area, inner thighs, and sometimes axilla), or a systematized allergic contact dermatitis with the morphology of a generalized erythematous papular eruption.

The cause is an oleoresin known as urushiol, of which the active agent is a mixture of catechols. This and related resorcinol allergens are present in many plants and also in philodendron species, wood from *Persoonia elliptica*, wheat bran, and marine brown algae.

The most striking diagnostic feature is the linearity of the lesions. It is rare to see vesicles arranged in a linear fashion except in plant-induced dermatitis. A history of exposure in the country or park to plants that have shiny leaves in groups of three, followed by the appearance of vesicular lesions within 2 days, usually establishes the diagnosis. Persons with known susceptibility not only should avoid touching plants having the grouped "leaves-of-three," but should also exercise care in handling articles of clothing, tools, toys, and pets that have come in contact with such plants.

Eradication of these plants growing in frequented places is one easy preventive measure, as is recognition of the plants to avoid. An excellent resource is a pamphlet available from the American Academy of Dermatology. If the individual is exposed, washing with soap and water within 5 min may prevent an eruption. Protective barrier creams are available that are somewhat beneficial. Quaternium-18 bentonite has been shown to prevent or diminish experimentally produced poison ivy dermatitis.

Innumerable attempts have been made to immunize against poison ivy dermatitis by oral administration of the allergen, or subcutaneous injections of oily extracts. To date, no accepted method of immunization is available. Repeated attacks do not confer immunity, although a single severe attack may achieve this by what has been called massive-dose desensitization.

When the diagnosis is clear and the eruption severe or extensive, systemic steroidal agents are effective, beginning with 40–60 mg of prednisone in a single oral dose daily, tapered off over a 3-week period. When the eruption is limited in extent and severity, local application of topical corticosteroid creams, lotions, or aerosol sprays is preferred. Time-honored calamine lotion without phenol is helpful and does no harm. Antihistaminic ointments should be avoided because of their sensitization potential. This also applies to the local application of the "caine" topical anesthetics.

Other toxicodendron-related dermatitis

Lacquer dermatitis is caused by a furniture lacquer made from the Japanese lacquer tree, used on furniture, jewelry, or bric-a-brac. Antique lacquer is harmless, but lacquer less than 1 or 2 years old is highly antigenic. Cashew nutshell oil is extracted from the nutshells of the cashew tree (*Anacardium occidentale*). This vesicant oil contains cardol, a phenol similar to urushiol in poison ivy. The liquid has many commercial applications, such as the manufacture of brake linings, varnish, synthetic glue, paint, and sealer for concrete.

Mango dermatitis is uncommon in natives of mango-growing countries (the Philippines, Guam, Hawaii, Cuba) who have never been exposed to contact with toxicodendron species. Many persons who have been so exposed, however, whether they had dermatitis from it or not, are sensitized by one or a few episodes of contact with the peel of the mango fruit. The palms carry the allergen, so the eyelids and the male prepuce are often early sites of involvement. Sponging all contaminated or itchy areas meticulously and systematically with equal parts of ether and acetone at the outset will often remove the oleoresin and ameliorate any worsening of the dermatitis, which can be treated with topical or oral steroids as needed.

Ginkgo tree dermatitis simulates toxicodendron dermatitis with its severe vesiculation, erythematous papules, and edema. The causative substances are ginkgolic acids from the fruit pulp of the ginkgo tree. Ingestion of the ginkgo fruit may result in perianal dermatitis. Ginkgo biloba given orally for cerebral disturbances is made from a leaf extract so it does not elicit a systemic contact allergy when ingested.

Flowers and houseplants

Among the more common houseplants, the velvety-leafed philodendron, *Philodendron crystallinum* (and its several variants), known in India as the money plant, is a frequent cause of contact dermatitis. The eruption is often seen on the face, especially the eyelids, carried there by hands that have watered or cared for the plant. English ivy follows philodendron in frequency of cases of occult contact dermatitis. Primrose derma-

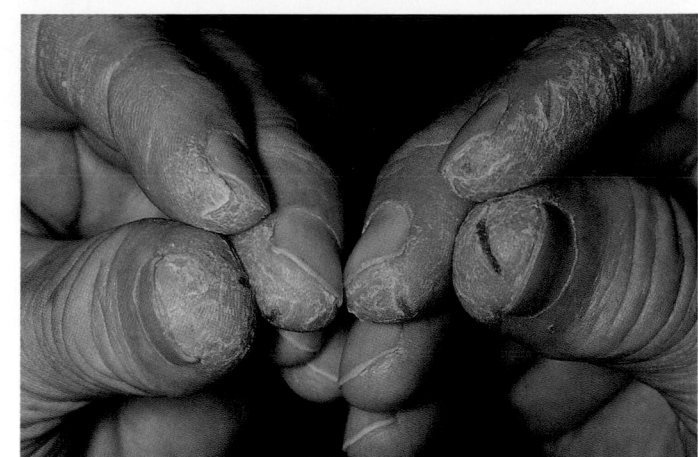

Fig. 6-11 Chronic fissured fingertip dermatitis in a florist.

titis affects the fingers, eyelids, and neck with a punctate or diffuse erythema and edema. It was formerly most frequently encountered in Europe; however, the primrose is now a common houseplant in the US. Primin, a quinone, is the causative oleoresin abounding in the glandular hairs of the plant *Primula obconica*.

The popular cut flower, the Peruvian lily, is the most common cause of allergic contact dermatitis in florists. When handling flowers of the genus *Alstroemeria* the florist utilizes the thumb, and second and third digits of the dominant hand. Since it is chronic, fissured hyperkeratotic dermatitis results and is identical to the so-called tulip fingers seen among sensitized tulip workers (Fig. 6-11). Testing is done with the allergen tuliposide A. It does not penetrate nitrile gloves.

Chrysanthemums frequently cause dermatitis, with the hands and eyelids of florists most commonly affected. The α-methylene portion of the sesquiterpene lactone molecule is the antigenic site, as it is in the other genera of the Compositae family.

A severe inflammatory reaction with bulla formation may be caused by the prairie crocus (*Anemone patens L*), the floral emblem of the province of Manitoba. Several species of ornamental "bottle brush" from Queensland, *Grevillea banksii*, *G. Robyn Gordon*, and *G. robusta*, may cause allergic contact dermatitis. It is exported to the US and other Western countries. The allergen is a long-chain alkyl resorcinol. A cross-sensitivity to toxicodendron has been demonstrated.

Contact dermatitis may be caused by handling many other flowers, such as the geranium, scorpion flower (*Phacelia crenulata* or *campanularia*), hydrangea, creosote bush (*Larvia tridentata*), *Heracula*, daffodil, foxglove, lilac, lady slipper, magnolia, and tulip and narcissus bulbs. The poinsettia and oleander almost never cause dermatitis, despite their reputation for it, although they are toxic if ingested. Treatment of all these plant dermatitides is the same as that recommended for toxicodendron dermatitis.

Parthenium hysterophorus, a photosensitizing weed, was accidentally introduced into India in 1956 and has spread over most of the country; it is also spreading in Australia, China, and Argentina. The well-deserved reputation for harmfulness of dieffenbachia, a common, glossy-leafed house plant, rests on the high content of calcium oxalate crystals in its sap, which burn the mouth and throat severely if any part of the plant is chewed or swallowed. Severe edema of the oral tissues may result in complete loss of voice; hence its common nickname, "dumb cane." It does not appear to sensitize. The castor bean, the seed of *Ricinus communis*, contains ricin, a poisonous substance (phytotoxin). Its sap contains an antigen that may cause anaphylactic hypersensitivity and also dermatitis.

Fruit and vegetables

Many vegetables may cause contact dermatitis, including asparagus, carrot, celery, cow-parsnip, cucumber, garlic, Indian bean, mushroom, onion, parsley, tomato, and turnip. Onion and celery, among other vegetables, have been incriminated in the production of contact urticaria and even anaphylaxis. Several plants, including celery, fig, lime, and parsley, can cause a phototoxic dermatitis because of the presence of psoralens.

Trees

Trees whose timber and sawdust may produce contact dermatitis include ash, birch, cedar, cocobolo, elm, Kentucky coffee tree, koa, mahogany, mango, maple, mesquite, milo, myrtle, pine, and teak. The latex of fig and rubber trees may also cause dermatitis, usually of the phototoxic type. Melaleuca oil (tea tree oil), which may be applied to the skin to treat a variety of maladies, can cause allergic contact dermatitis, primarily through the allergen D-limonene. The exotic woods, especially cocobolo and rosewood, and tea tree oil are prominent among allergens that may produce erythema multiforme after cutaneous exposure. Toxicodendron, various medicaments, and a variety of other allergens may induce this reaction.

Tree-associated plants

Foresters and lumber workers can be exposed to allergenic plants other than trees. Lichens are a group of plants composed of symbiotic algae and fungi. Foresters and wood choppers exposed to these lichens growing on trees may develop severe allergic contact dermatitis. Exposure to the lichens may also occur from firewood, funeral wreaths, and also fragrances added to aftershave lotions (oak moss and tree moss). Sensitization is produced by D-usnic acid and other lichen acids contained in lichens. The leafy liverwort (*Frullania nisquallansis*), a forest epiphyte growing on tree trunks, has produced allergic dermatitis in forest workers. The eruption is commonly called cedar poisoning. It resembles toxicodendron dermatitis; its attacks are more severe during wet weather. The allergen is sesquiterpene lactone.

Pollens and seeds

The pollens in ragweed are composed of two antigens. The protein fraction causes the respiratory symptoms of asthma and hay fever, and the oil-soluble portion causes contact dermatitis. Ragweed oil dermatitis is a seasonal disturbance seen mainly during the ragweed growing season from spring to fall. Contact with the plant or with wind-blown fragments of the dried plant produces the typical dermatitis. The oil causes swelling and redness of the lids and entire face, and a red blotchy eruption on the forearms that, after several attacks, may become generalized, with lichenification. It closely resembles chronic atopic dermatitis, with lichenification of the face, neck, and major flexures, and severe pruritus. The distribution also mimics that of photodermatitis, the differentiating point being that in ragweed dermatitis there is involvement of the upper eyelids and the retroauricular and submental areas. Chronic cases may continue into the winter; however, signs and symptoms are most severe at the height of the season. Sesquiterpene lactones are the cause. Coexistent sensitization to pyrethrum may account for prolongation of ragweed dermatitis. Men outnumber women in hypersensitivity reactions; farmers outnumber patients of all other occupations.

Marine plants

Numerous aquatic plants are toxic or produce contact dermatitis. Algae are the worse offenders. Freshwater plants are rarely of concern. Seaweed dermatitis is a type of swimmer's eruption produced by contact with a marine blue–green alga, which has been identified as *Lyngbya majuscula Gomont*. The onset is within a few minutes of leaving the ocean, with severe itching and burning, followed by dermatitis, blisters, and deep and painful desquamation that affects the areas covered by the bathing suit (in men, especially the scrotum, perineum, and perianal areas; occasionally, in women, the breasts). Patch tests with the alga are neither necessary nor helpful, since it is a potent irritant. Bathing in fresh water within 10 or 15 min of leaving the ocean may prevent the dermatitis. The Bermuda fire sponge may produce contact erythema multiforme. Trawler fishermen in the Dogger Bank area of the North Sea develop allergic dermatitis after contact with *Alcyonidium hirsutum*. This is a seaweed-like animal colony that becomes caught in the fishermen's net and produces erythema, edema, and lichenification on the hands and wrists.

Plant-associated dermatitis

Phototoxic contact dermatitis from plants is discussed in Chapter 3 (Fig. 6-12).

The residua of various insecticides on plants may also produce dermatitis. This is especially true of arsenic- and malathion-containing sprays. Randox (2-chloro-N, N-diallyl-acetamide) has been reported as the cause of hemorrhagic bullae on the feet of farmers. Lawn-care companies spray herbicides and fungicides throughout the spring, summer, and fall. Dryene, thiuram, carbamates, and chlorothalonil are potential sensitizers in these workers, whose clothing frequently becomes wetted while spraying.

Barbs, bristles, spines, thorns, spicules, and cactus needles are some of the mechanical accessories of plants that may produce dermatitis. Sabra dermatitis is an occupational dermatitis resembling scabies. It is seen among pickers of the prickly pear cactus plant. It also occurs in persons handling Indian figs in Israel, where the condition is seen from July to November. The penetration of minute, invisible thorns into the skin is the cause. *Agave americana* is a low-growing plant grown for ornamental purposes in many Southwestern communities. Trimming during landscaping can induce an irritant dermatitis caused by calcium oxalate crystals. The stinging

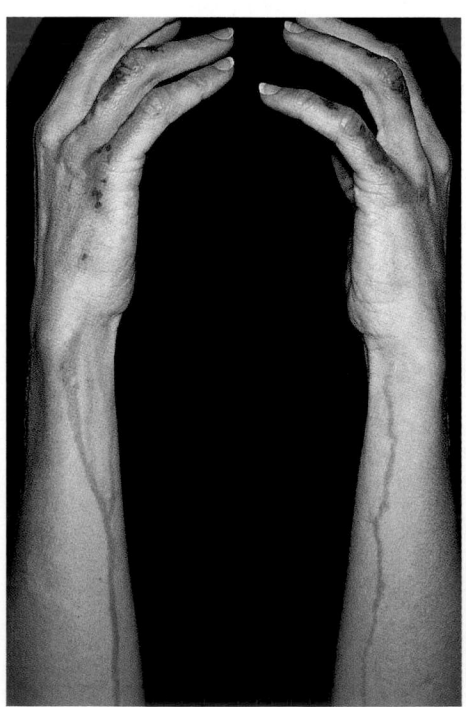

Fig. 6-12 Photosensitivity caused by dripping fruit juice.

nettle is a common weed that bears tiny spines with biologically active substances such as histamine that produce itching and urticaria within minutes of contact.

Plant derivatives

Sensitizing substances derived from plants are found in the oleoresin fractions that contain camphors, essential oils, phenols, resins, and terpenes. The chief sensitizers are the essential oils. They may be localized in certain parts of the plant, such as in the peel of citrus fruits, leaves of the eucalyptus tree, and bark of the cinnamon tree. Aromatherapy, an increasingly popular treatment for relief of stress, involves either inhaling or massaging with essential oils; this may cause allergic contact dermatitis in therapists or clients. Exposure to botanical extracts through many cosmetics and homeopathic remedies has resulted in an increasing number of reports of allergic contact sensitivity to individual ingredients, especially tea tree oil.

Cinnamon oil (cassia oil) is a common flavoring agent, especially in pastries. Hand dermatitis in pastry bakers is often caused by cinnamon. It is also used as a flavor for lipstick, bitters, alcoholic and nonalcoholic beverages, toothpaste, and chewing gum. Perioral dermatitis may be caused by cinnamon in chewing gum. A 5% cinnamon solution in olive oil is used for patch testing. Eugenol, clove oil, and eucalyptus oil are used by dentists, who may acquire contact dermatitis from them. Anise, peppermint, and spearmint oils may cause sensitization.

Nutmeg, paprika, and cloves are causes of spice allergy. Fragrance-mix is a useful indicator allergen. Lemon oil from lemon peel or lemon wood may cause sensitization in the various handlers of these substances. Citric acid may cause dermatitis in bakers. Lime oil in lime-scented shaving cream or lotion may cause photoallergy. *Myroxylon pereirae* contains numerous substances, among which are essential oils similar to the oil of lemon peel. It is known to cross-react with vanilla and cinnamon, among many others. Vanillin is derived from the vanilla plant and frequently produces contact dermatitis, vanillism, in those connected with its production and use.

Turpentine frequently acts as an irritant and as an allergic sensitizer (carene). It is contained in paints, paint thinners, varnishes, and waxes.

Testing for plant allergens

The method of testing for plant hypersensitivity is the application of the crushed plant leaf, stem, and petal, and then covering with micropore tape. The plant should be washed thoroughly as infection with fungi from the soil may complicate testing. A test should also be performed on several controls to make sure that the leaf is not an irritant. It must be remembered that some of the plants are photosensitizers. Test sites for these must be done in duplicate, with one set kept covered and the other exposed to artificial light or sunlight for the detection of photosensitivity.

Anderson BE, et al: Stinging nettle dermatitis. Am J Contact Dermat 2003; 14:44.

Arberer W: Contact allergy and medicinal plants. J Dtsch Dermatol Ges 2008; 6:15.

Bedi MK, et al: Herbal therapy in dermatology. Arch Dermatol 2002; 138:232.

Crawford GH, et al: Tea tree oil. Am J Contact Dermat 2004; 15:59.

Crawford GH, et al: Use of aromatherapy products and increased risk of hand dermatitis in massage therapists. Arch Dermatol 2004; 140:991.

Gladman AC: Toxicodendron dermatitis. Wilderness Environ Med 2006; 17:120.

Gordon LA: Compositae dermatitis. Australas J Dermatol 1999; 40:123.

Guanche AD, et al: Generalized eczematous contact dermatitis from cocobolo wood. Am J Contact Dermat 2003; 14:90.

Gutman AB, et al: Liverworts—*Frullania* species. Cutis 2005; 75:262.

Hamilton TK, et al: Systemic contact dermatitis to raw cashew nuts in a pesto sauce. Am J Contact Dermat 1998; 9:51.

Hershko K, et al: Exploring the mango–poison ivy connection. Contact Dermatitis 2005; 52:3.

High WA: Agave contact dermatitis. Am J Contact Dermat 2003; 14:213.

Kurlan JG, et al: Black spot poison ivy. J Am Acad Dermatol 2001; 45:246.

LeSuer BW, et al: Necrotizing cellulites caused by *Apophysomyces elegans* at a patch test site. Am J Contact Dermat 2002; 13:140.

Marks JG Jr, et al: Prevention of poison ivy and poison ash allergic contact dermatitis by quaternium-18 bentonite. J Am Acad Dermatol 1995; 33:212.

McGovern TW, et al: Is it, or isn't it? Poison ivy look-a-likes. Am J Contact Dermat 2000; 11:104.

Paulsen E: Contact sensitisation from Compositae-containing herbal remedies and cosmetics. Contact Dermatitis 2002; 47:189.

Rutherford T, et al: Allergy to tea tree oil. Australas J Dermatol 2007; 48:83.

Sharma VK, et al: Parthenium dermatitis. Dermatitis 2007; 18:183.

Simpson EL, et al: Prevalence of botanical extract allergy in patients with contact dermatitis. Am J Contact Dermat 2004; 15:67.

Dermatitis from clothing

A predisposition to contact dermatitis from clothing occurs in persons who perspire freely or who are obese and wear clothing that tends to be tight. Depending on the offending substance, various regions of the body will be affected. Regional location is helpful in identifying the sensitizing substance. The axillary folds are commonly involved; the vaults of the axillae are usually spared. Sites of increased perspiration and sites where evaporation is impeded, such as the intertriginous areas, will tend to leach dyes from fabrics to produce dermatitis. Areas where the material is tight against the skin, such as the waistband or neck, are frequently involved (Fig. 6-13). The thighs are commonly affected when pants contain the offending allergen. Sparing of the hands, face, and undergarment sites is usual, but otherwise these reactions may be scattered and generalized. Secondary changes of lichenification and infection occur frequently because of the chronicity of exposure.

Cotton, wool, linen, and silk fabrics were used exclusively before the advent of synthetic fabrics. Most materials are now blended in definite proportions with synthetics to produce superior lasting and esthetic properties. Dermatitis from cotton is virtually nonexistent. In most instances there is no true sensitization to wool. Wool acts as an irritant because of the barbs on its fibers. These barbs may produce severe

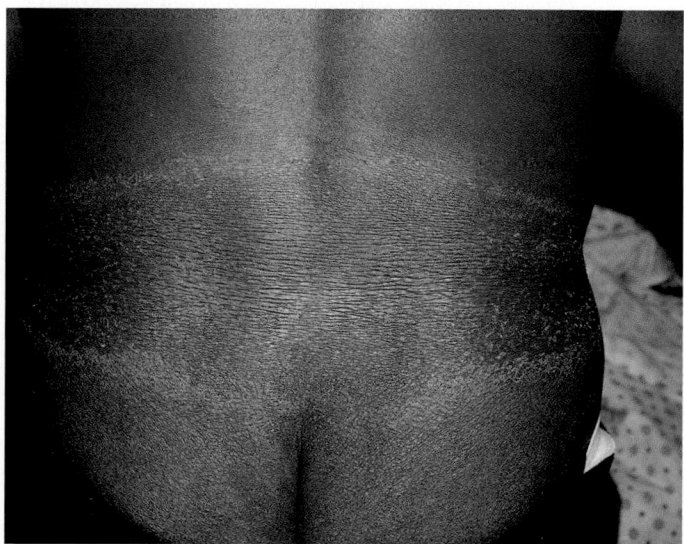

Fig. 6-13 Waistband clothing dermatitis.

pruritus at points of contact with the skin, especially in the intertriginous areas. In sensitive-skinned persons, such as those with atopic dermatitis, the wearing of wool is not advisable because of its mechanical irritative properties. Silk is a sensitizer, but rarely; the nature of the allergen is not known. Many patients believe their detergent is the source of a dermatitis, but this is rarely the case.

Numerous synthetic fibers are available for clothing and accessory manufacture, all of which again are remarkably free of sensitizing properties. Polyvinyl resins are the plastics used in such apparel as raincoats, rainhoods, wristbands, suspenders, plastic mittens, and gloves. These again are only infrequently found to be causes of contact dermatitis.

The most common causes of clothing dermatitis are the fabric finishers, dyes, and rubber additives. Fabric finishers are used to improve the durability, appearance, and feel of a material. Antiwrinkling and crease-holding chemicals are mostly resins, which are incorporated into the fibers as they are being manufactured or applied to the completed (finished) fabric. Fabrics are treated to make them less vulnerable to the effects of perspiration and ironing. Clothing may be treated with these substances to make it dry rapidly after washing. They are used to make clothing fabrics shrink-resistant, and water- and stain-repellent. When all these uses are taken into consideration, the low incidence of dermatitis from these formaldehyde resin materials is remarkable.

Ethylene urea melamine formaldehyde resin and dimethylol dihydroxyethylene urea formaldehyde resin are the best screening agents. Many also react to formaldehyde and the formaldehyde-releasing preservatives such as quaternium-15. Avoidance of exposure of the skin to formaldehyde resin is most difficult. New clothes should be thoroughly washed twice before wearing the first time. Even with this precaution, however, allergens may still be present in sufficient quantities to continue the dermatitis. Jeans, Spandex, silk, 100% linen, 100% nylon, and 100% cotton that is not wrinkle-resistant or colorfast are best tolerated. T-shirts, sweat shirts, sweat pants, white underclothes suitable for bleaching, and any type of mixed synthetic fibers with cotton fibers that are added to make them drip-dry are most likely to cause problems in these patients.

An increasing number of patients allergic to clothing dye are being reported. Synthetic fabrics such as polyester and acetate liners in women's clothing are prime causes, and affected patients are more commonly women than men. Even infants may be affected, however, with dyes in diapers accounting for five cases reported by Alberta et al. In many cases patients do not react to paraphenylene diamine, but only to the disperse dye allergens. The best screening agents are disperse blue 106 and 124. Suspected fabrics may be soaked in water for 15 min and applied under a patch for 72–96 h.

Spandex is a nonrubber (but elastic) polyurethane fiber. It is widely used for garments such as girdles, brassieres, and socks, but is generally safe in the US, as it is free of rubber additives.

Alberta L, et al: Diaper dye dermatitis. Pediatrics 2005; 116:e450.
Carlson RM, et al: Diagnosis and treatment of dermatitis due to formaldehyde resin in clothing. Dermatitis 2004; 15:169.
Cohen D, et al: Clothes make the woman: diagnosis and management of clothing dermatitis. Am J Contact Dermat 2001; 12:229.
Donovan J, et al: Allergic contact dermatitis from formaldehyde textile resins in surgical uniforms and nonwoven textile masks. Dermatitis 2007; 18:40.
Hatch K, et al: Textile dye dermatitis. J Am Acad Dermatol 1995; 32:631.
Hatch KL, et al: Disperse dyes in fabrics of patients patch-test-positive to disperse dyes. Am J Contact Dermat 2003; 14:205.
Nedorost S, et al: Allergens retained in clothing. Dermatitis 2007; 18:212.

Reich HC, et al: Allergic contact dermatitis from formaldehyde textile resins. Dermatitis 2010; 21:65.
Ryberg K, et al: Contact allergy to textile dyes in southern Sweden. Contact Dermatitis 2006; 54:313.
Zug KA, et al: The value of patch testing patients with a scattered generalized distribution of dermatitis. J Am Acad Dermatol 2008; 59:426.

Shoe dermatitis

Footwear dermatitis may begin on the dorsal surfaces of the toes and may remain localized to that area indefinitely (Fig. 6-14). There is erythema, lichenification, and, in severe cases, weeping and crusting. Secondary infection is frequent. In severe cases an id reaction may be produced on the hands similar to the reaction from fungus infection of the feet. A diagnostic point is the normal appearance of the skin between the toes, which has no contact with the offending substance. In fungus infections the toe webs are usually involved. Another pattern seen is involvement of the sole with sparing of the instep and flexural creases of the toes. Also purpuric reactions to components of black rubber mix may occur. Hyperhidrosis and atopy predispose to the development of shoe allergy.

Shoe dermatitis is most frequently caused by the rubber accelerators mercaptobenzothiazole, carbamates, and tetramethylthiuram disulfide. Potassium dichromate in leather and the adhesives used in synthetic materials (especially p-tert-butylphenol formaldehyde resin) are also common shoe allergens. Diisocyanates are used in making foam rubber padding for athletic shoes and may cause allergy. Other causative agents are felt, cork liners, formaldehyde, dyes, asphalt, dimethyl fumarate and tar. Patch testing with pieces of various shoe parts may be done by soaking them for 15 min in water and applying them to the back for 72–96 h. Once the allergen has been identified, selection of shoes without the offending substance will lead to resolution. This is, unfortunately, a difficult process, as most shoes are made in areas without mandatory labeling requirements, and plastic, wooden, or fabric shoes which contain fewer allergens are often impractical.

Castando-Tardan MP, et al: Allergic contact dermatitis to Crocs. Contact Dermatitis 2008; 58:248.
Chowdhuri S, et al: Epidemio-allergological study in 155 cases of footwear dermatitis. Indian J Dermatol Venereol Leprol 2007; 73:319.
Fraga A, et al: Allergic contact dermatitis to dimethyl fumarate in footwear. Contact Dermatitis 2010; 62:121.
Oztas P, et al: Shoe dermatitis from para-tertiary butylphenol formaldehyde. Contact Dermatitis 2007; 56:294.
Van Coevorden AM, et al: Contact allergens in shoe leather among patients with foot eczema. Contact Dermatitis 2002; 46:145.
Washaw EM, et al: Shoe allergens. Dermatitis 2007; 18:191.

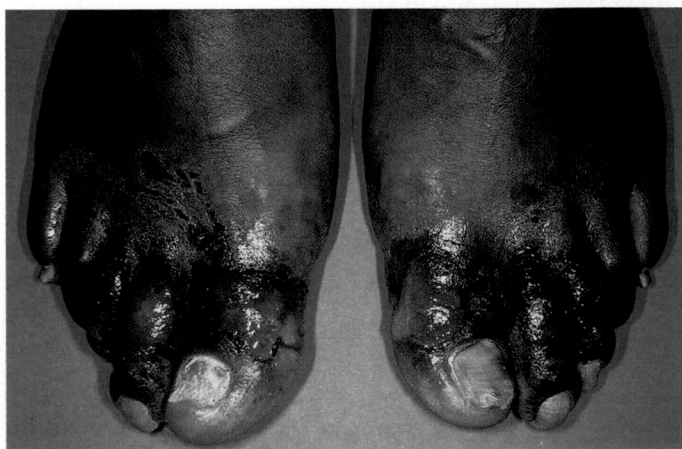

Fig. 6-14 Shoe dermatitis.

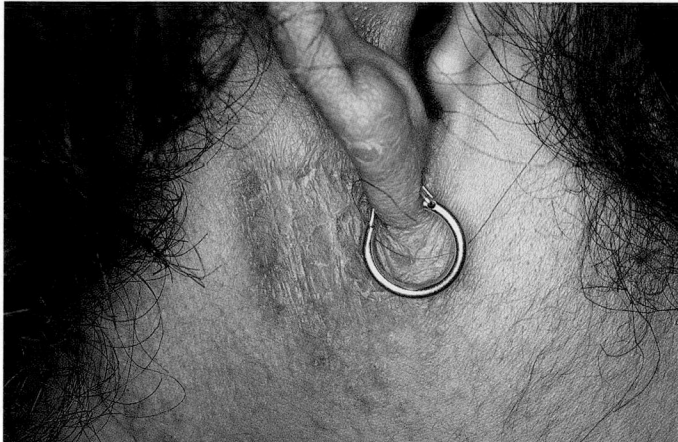

Fig. 6-15 Nickel dermatitis from earring.

Dermatitis from metals and metal salts

Metal dermatitis is most frequently caused by nickel and chromates. Usually, with the exception of nickel, the pure metals generally do not cause hypersensitivity; it is only when they are incorporated into salts that they cause reactions. Most objects containing metal or metal salts are combinations of several metals, some of which may have been used to plate the surface, thereby enhancing its attractiveness, durability, or tensile strength. For this reason suspicion of a metal-caused dermatitis should be investigated by doing patch tests to several of the metal salts.

Patients have been reported who developed a variety of dermatoses, most often eczematous in type, after placement of an orthopedic implant or an endovascular device. Reed et al and Honari et al have published recent reviews of these two situations. In general, patch testing prior to placement may help guide the specific type of device to be utilized. However, patch testing after placement to evaluate a new eruption is rarely useful. A positive diagnosis of allergy requires at a minimum the appearance of a chronic dermatitis after placement, no other cause, a positive patch test for the suspected metal (or in the case of drug-eluting stents, the drug), and healing after removal. This scenario is exceedingly uncommon; removal of a foreign material rarely results in cure.

Black dermatographism

Black or greenish staining under rings, metal wristbands, bracelets, and clasps is caused by the abrasive effect of cosmetics or other powders containing zinc or titanium oxide on gold jewelry. This skin discoloration is black because of the deposit of metal particles on skin that has been powdered and that has metal, such as gold, silver, or platinum, rubbing on it. Abrasion of the metal results from the fact that some powders are hard (zinc oxide) and are capable of abrading the metal.

Nickel

Because we are all constantly exposed to nickel, nickel dermatitis is a frequent occurrence. While still most frequent among women, sensitization is increasing among men. A direct relationship between prevalence of nickel allergy and number of pierced sites has been documented. Nickel produces more cases of allergic contact dermatitis than all other metals combined. Erythematous and eczematous eruptions, sometimes with lichenification, appear beneath earrings (Fig. 6-15), bracelets, rings, wrist watches, clasps, and blue-jeans buttons (Figs 6-16 and 6-17). The snaps on clothing have been implicated in producing allergy in children; nickel is the most common cause of allergic contact dermatitis in children as well as

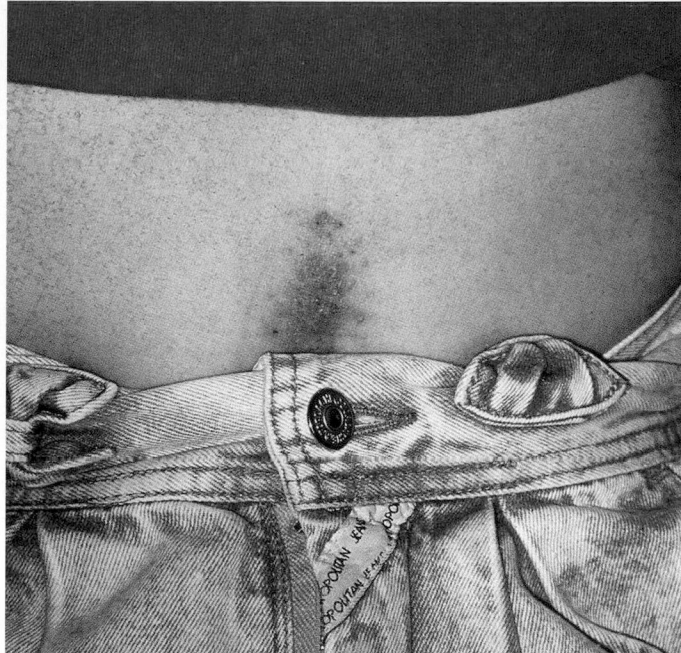

Fig. 6-16 Jeans button nickel dermatitis.

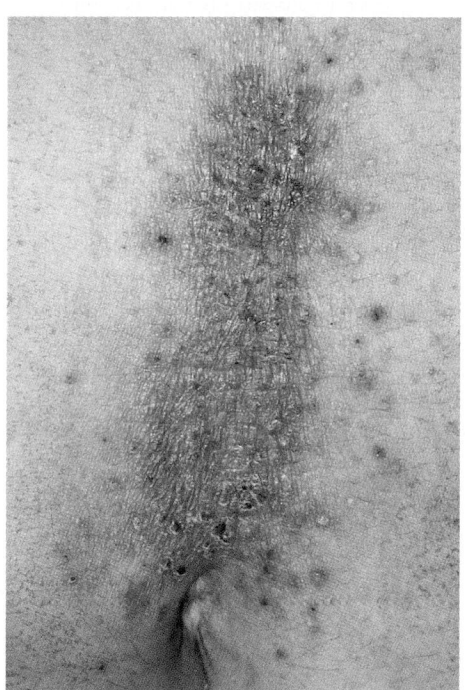

Fig. 6-17 Close-up of Fig. 6-16.

adults. Several patients with dermatitis on one ear or the preauricular area have been reported to be allergic to their cell phone. The metal portion is often nickel-containing, with this being the implicated allergen. Euro coins have enough nickel in them to elicit allergic responses in nickel-sensitive individuals; however, coins are rarely a cause of hand dermatitis. Nickel ranks highly on lists of occupationally induced allergic contact dermatitis.

Nickel dermatitis is seen most frequently on the earlobes. Piercing the earlobes with nickel-plated instruments or wearing nickel-plated jewelry readily induces nickel sensitivity. Earlobes should be pierced only with stainless steel instruments, and only stainless steel earrings should be worn until the ears have healed. Exposure to the metal may not be readily apparent most of the time. Even in gold jewelry the clasps and solder may contain nickel. Nickel objects may be plated with chrome and yet cause nickel dermatitis through the leaching of some of the nickel through the small pores of the chromium plating.

Nickel oxides in green paints may produce nickel dermatitis. Homeopathic and complementary medicaments may also contain enough nickel to produce a contact allergy. Sweat containing sodium chloride may combine with nickel to form nickel chloride. This affects the degree of nickel dermatitis, it being more severe in persons who perspire profusely.

The diagnosis is established by a positive patch-test reaction to nickel sulfate. Nickel may be detected by applying a freshly prepared 1% alcohol solution of dimethylglyoxime and a 10% aqueous solution of ammonia separately in equal amounts to the test object. In the presence of nickel, the cotton swab used to apply the solution will turn orange–pink. A positive test always means that nickel is present, but a negative test does not rule out its presence. Sweat, blood, or saline may leach nickel from stainless steel.

Prophylactic measures should include the reduction of perspiration in those sensitive to nickel. Topical corticosteroids applied before exposure to nickel, such as before putting on a wrist band, may be successful. Clasps and other objects are available in plastic material so that some of the exposure to nickel may be decreased. Polyurethane varathane 91 (Flecto) applied in three coats will give protection for several months. Treatment of nickel dermatitis consists of the application of topical corticosteroids. In Europe laws regulating the maximum content of nickel in jewelry are in force; this has led to a marked decrease in sensitization. Efforts to enact a similar standard in the US are under way.

Hand eczema and pompholyx in nickel- or cobalt-sensitive patients has rarely been aggravated by orally ingested metals in the diet. In severe, treatment-resistant dermatitis a specific diet low in nickel and cobalt may be tried.

Chromium

The chromates are strongly corrosive and irritating to the skin; they may act as primary irritants or as sensitizers to produce allergic contact dermatitis. Aside from occurrence among employees in chromate works, chrome dermatitis is encountered among tanners, painters, dyers, photographers, polishers, welders, aircraft workers, diesel engine workers, and those involved with the bleaching of crude oils, tallows, and fats. Traces of dichromates in shoe leather and gloves may cause eczema of the feet and hands. Many zippers are chromium-plated, and the nickel underneath the plate may be the causative agent. Chromium metal and stainless steel do not produce contact dermatitis.

Zinc chromate paint is a source of dermatitis. Matches, hide glues, chrome alloys, cigarette lighters, and leather hatbands, sandals, or camera cases may cause chrome dermatitis. Anticorrosion solutions used for refrigeration and other recirculation systems often contain chromates that produce dermatitis. Most individuals in the cement industry suffering from cement eczema show positive patch tests to dichromates. Cement eczema is often a primary irritant dermatitis complicated by allergic contact dermatitis to the hexavalent chromates. The incidence of cement dermatitis has decreased significantly over the years, which is believed to be because of the addition of ferrous sulfate, delivery of premixed cement to the job site, and improved education.

The skin changes are multiform, ranging from a mild follicular dermatitis to widespread nodular and crusted eruptions, all being worse on exposed parts. Often they are slow to clear up, lasting from a few weeks to 6 months after contact has ceased. Heavy exposure of industrial workers to chromates may produce chrome ulcers on the backs of the hands and forearms, usually beginning around a hair follicle, or in the creases of the knuckles or finger webs. The hole begins as a small abrasion that deepens and widens as its edges grow thick, eventually forming a conical indolent ulceration. Chrome ulcers may also arise on—and perforate—the nasal septum. Arsenic exposure may result in similar ulcers.

Diagnosis of chrome sensitivity is made by a positive patch test to potassium dichromate in petrolatum. The hexavalent chrome compounds are the most frequent cause of chrome dermatitis since they penetrate the skin more easily than the trivalent form. Both forms are sensitizers. Even with avoidance of chromate-containing materials, chromate-induced dermatitis is often persistent.

Mercury

The mercurials may act not only as irritants but also as sensitizers. Thimerosal is a mercuric-containing preservative; it is an allergen that is rarely relevant. Allergy to this compound is likely to have been caused by exposure during childhood vaccinations and to tincture of merthiolate antiseptic. In general, these patients tolerate repeated vaccinations well. Most individuals are sensitized to the ethyl mercuric component of thimerosal; however, those who react to the thiosalicylic acid portion develop photodermatitis to piroxicam. Mercury in amalgam dental fillings has been shown in multiple large studies to cause oral lichoid eruptions. The relationship is especially strong when the oral lesion, often with a painful erosion present, is apposed to a gold or amalgam filling. In many cases where sensitivity is proven by patch testing and fillings are replaced, involution of the oral findings occurs.

Cobalt

Cobalt is frequently combined with nickel as a contaminant and patients allergic to cobalt are commonly also allergic to nickel. The metals have similar properties but do not produce cross-reactions. Cobalt dermatitis may occur in those involved in the manufacture of polyester resins and paints, in the manufacture of hard metal used for cutting and drilling tools, and in the manufacture and use of cement. Cobalt dermatitis may also occur in producers of pottery, ceramics, metal alloys, glass, carbides, and pigments. Individuals may be exposed to cobalt in hair dye, flypaper, and vitamin B_{12}. Blue tattoo pigment contains cobalt oxide. Rarely, cobalt chloride may cause nonimmunologic local release of vasoreactive materials, with a local urticarial response.

Gold

Gold dermatitis may rarely occur from the wearing of gold jewelry. A predisposing factor in such patients is the presence of dental gold. Oral lichoid eruptions have also been reported with gold, similar to the situation with mercury-containing amalgams. It is not uncommon to see positive reactions to gold when patch-testing patients with facial, eyelid, or widespread dermatitis of unknown cause. Although it is difficult to make a direct clinical correlation with any one piece of jewelry, occasional patients will clear if they stop wearing all gold jewelry. However, in most patients there is a lack of relevance.

A number of cases of dermatitis resulting from gold jewelry, especially gold rings, contaminated with radon and its decay products have been reported. This may eventuate in radiation dermatitis and squamous cell carcinoma of the finger. Evidently, the source of contaminated gold for the rings had been reclaimed decayed radon gold seeds.

Other metals

Most other commonly used metals are not important in causing contact dermatitis. Platinum dermatitis may occur from exposure to platinum salts and sprays in industry. Platinum rings, earrings, white gold spectacles, clasps, and other jewelry cause eruptions resembling those caused by nickel. Zinc, aluminum, copper sulfate, titanium, and antimony dermatitis rarely occur; these metals may, however, act as irritants.

Belsito DV: Thimerosal: contact (non)allergen of the year. Am J Contact Dermat 2002; 13:1.

De Medeiros LM, et al: Complementary and alternative remedies: an additional source of potential systemic nickel exposure. Contact Dermatitis 2008; 58:97.

Filan FL, et al: Sensitization to palladium chloride. Am J Contact Dermat 2003; 14:78.

Fowler J Jr, et al: Gold. Am J Contact Dermat 2001; 12:1.

Fowler J Jr, et al: Gold allergy in North America. Am J Contact Dermat 2001; 12:3.

Freiman A, et al: Patch testing with thimerosal in a Canadian center. Am J Contact Dermat 2003; 14:138.

Heim KE, et al: Children's clothing fasteners as a potential source of exposure to releasable nickel ions. Contact Dermatitis 2009; 60:100.

Honari G, et al: Hypersensitivity reactions associated with endovascular devices. Contact Dermatitis 2008; 59:7.

Kornick R, et al: Nickel. Dermatitis 2008; 19:3.

Reed KB, et al: Retrospective evaluation of patch testing before or after metal device implantation. Arch Dermatol 2008; 144:999.

Seishma M, et al: Cellular phone dermatitis with chromate allergy. Dermatology 2003; 207:48.

Shah M, et al: Nickel as an occupational allergen. Arch Dermatol 1998; 134:1231.

Stuckert J, et al: Low cobalt diet for dyshidrotic eczema. Contact Dermatitis 2008; 59:361.

Suneja T, et al: Blue-jean button nickel. Dermatitis 2007; 18:208.

Thyssen JP, et al: Patch test reactivity to metal allergens following regulatory intervention. Contact Dermatitis 2010; 63:102.

Thyssen JP, et al: The outcome of dimethylglyoxime testing in a sample of cell phones in Denmark. Contact Dermatitis 2008; 59:38.

Torgerson RR, et al: Contact allergy in oral disease. J Am Acad Dermatol 2007; 57:315.

Wong L, et al: Oral lichenoid lesions and mercury in amalgam fillings. Contact Dermatitis 2003; 48:74.

Contact stomatitis

The role of contact allergy in oral symptomatology is significant. Approximately 30% of patients with oral symptoms will have relevant allergens; these are most commonly metals used in dental fillings, food additives (flavorings and antioxidants), and dental products such as acrylic monomers, epoxy resins, and hardeners used in prosthedontics and dental impression materials. Chewing gums and dentifrices may also produce contact stomatitis. Ingredients responsible for this are hexylresorcinol, thymol, dichlorophen, oil of cinnamon, and mint.

Clinical signs may be bright erythema of the tongue and buccal mucosa with scattered erosions. Angular cheilitis may also develop. Oral lichenoid lesions may be caused by sensitization to metals in dental fillings or gold caps or crowns.

Ditrichova D, et al: Oral lichenoid lesions and allergy to dental materials. Biomed Pap Med Fac Univ Palacky Olomouc Czech Repub 2007; 151:333.

Kanerva L, et al: A multicenter study of patch test reactions with dental screening series. Am J Contact Dermat 2001; 12:83.

Torgerson RR, et al: Contact allergy in oral disease. J Am Acad Dermatol 2007; 57:315.

Zug KA, et al: Patch-testing North American lip dermatitis patients. Dermatitis 2008; 19:202.

Rubber dermatitis

Rubber dermatitis generally occurs on the hands from wearing rubber gloves (surgeons, nurses, homemakers). The eruption is usually sharply limited to the gloved area but may spread up the forearms. Rubber dermatitis also develops from exposure to condoms, diaphragms, swim goggles, caps and scuba masks, wet suits, bandages for chronic leg ulcers, respirators, gas masks, rubber sheets, and cosmetic sponges. Shoe dermatitis may be caused by rubber allergy to insoles or sneakers (see above).

Natural and synthetic rubbers are used separately or in combination to make the final rubber product. It is the chemicals added in the rubber manufacturing process, most importantly the accelerators and antioxidants, which are the common causes of allergic contact dermatitis. A similar list of additives is present in neoprene, a synthetic rubber. One particular class of additive in neoprene is causing an increasing number of reactions: the dialkyl thioureas. These are not in the standard patch trays and thus may escape detection unless they are applied as a supplemental allergen. Elastic in underwear is chemically transformed by laundry bleach, such as Clorox, into a potent sensitizing substance. The allergen is permanent and cannot be removed by washing. The offending garments must be thrown out and the use of bleaches interdicted.

Accelerators

During the manufacturing process, chemicals are used to hasten the vulcanization of rubber. Among the numerous chemicals available, tetramethylthiuram disulfide, mercaptobenzothiazole, and diphenylguanidine are frequently used. Tetramethylthiuram disulfide and its analogs, known as disulfiram and thiuram, may produce contact dermatitis when moist skin is exposed to the finished rubber product. In one 10-year study of 636 cases of allergy to rubber additives, thiuram mix was by far the most common sensitizer. Mercaptobenzothiazole is most often the cause in shoe allergy and thiuram in glove allergy.

Antioxidants

Antioxidants are used to preserve rubber. Among antioxidants the amine type, such as phenyl-α-naphthylamine, is most effective. Hydroquinone antioxidants may cause depigmentation of the skin, as well as allergic contact dermatitis. A frequent antioxidant sensitizer, propyl p-phenylenediamine, is used in tires, heavy-duty rubber goods, boots, and elastic underwear.

Adams AK, et al: Allergic contact dermatitis from mercapto compounds. Dermatitis 2006; 17:56.

Cravo M, et al: Allergic contact dermatitis to rubber-containing bandages in patients with leg ulcers. Contact Dermatitis 2008; 58:371.

Gibbon KL, et al: Changing frequency of thiuram allergy in healthcare workers with hand dermatitis. Br J Dermatol 2001; 144:347.

Militello G, et al: Dialkyl thioureas. Dermatitis 2008; 19:E42.

Warshaw EM, et al: Positive patch-test reactions to mixed dialkyl thioureas. Dermatitis 2008; 19:190.

Woo DK, et al: Neoprene. Dermatitis 2004; 15:206.

Adhesive dermatitis

Cements, glues, and gums may cause adhesive dermatitis. Formaldehyde resin adhesives contain free formaldehyde, naphtha, glue, and disinfectants. Synthetic resin adhesives contain plasticizers; hide glues may contain chromates from the tanned leather while other glues incorporate preservatives such as formaldehyde. Dental bonding adhesives may contain acrylic monomers and epoxy resins and hardeners. Pressure-sensitive adhesives contain rubber and acrylates, and anaerobic adhesives primarily acrylates.

Vegetable gums, such as gum tragacanth, gum arabic, and karaya, may be used in denture adhesives, hair wave lotions, topical medications, toothpastes, and depilatories, and many cause contact dermatitis. Resins are used in adhesive tapes and in various adhesives such as tincture of benzoin. Turpentine is frequently found in rosin; abietic acid in the rosin is the causative sensitizer.

Adhesive tape reactions are frequently irritant in nature. Allergic reactions to adhesive tape itself are caused by the rubber components, accelerators, antioxidants, and various resins or turpentine. Some adhesive tapes contain acrylate polymers rather than rubber adhesives. These acrylates may cause allergic contact dermatitis. Pressure-sensitive adhesives are in widespread use in the tape and label industries. Allergens present in these adhesives include rosin, rubber accelerators, antioxidants, acrylates, hydroquinones, lanolin, thiourea compounds, and N-dodecylmaleamic compounds.

Howard BK, et al: Contact dermatitis from Dermabond. Contact Dermatitis 2010; 62:314.

Kanerva L, et al: Patch-test reactions to plastic and glue allergens. Acta Dermatol Venereol 1999; 79:296.

Sharma PR: Allergic contact stomatitis from colophony. Dent Update 2006; 33:440.

Volz A, et al: Mastix, a known herbal allergen, as a causative agent in occupation-related dermatitis. Contact Dermatitis 2006; 54:346.

Widman TJ, et al: Allergic contact dermatitis from medical adhesive bandages in patients who report having a reaction to medical bandages. Dermatitis 2008; 19:32.

Synthetic resin dermatitis

The many varieties of synthetic resins preclude adequate discussion of each. The reactions incurred during the manufacture of these substances are more frequent than those encountered in their finished state.

Epoxy resins

The epoxy resins in their liquid (noncured, monomer) form may produce severe dermatitis, especially during the manufacturing process. The fully polymerized or cured product is nonsensitizing. Nonindustrial exposure is usually to epoxy resin glues, nail lacquers, and artificial nails. Epoxy resins are used in the home as glues and paints (bathtub and refrigerator). Artists and sculptors frequently use epoxy resins.

Epoxy resins consist of two or more components, the resin and the curing agent. Approximately 90% of allergic reactions are to the resin and 10% to the hardener. There are numerous curing agents such as the amines, phenolic compounds, peroxides, and polyamides. These may be irritants and/or allergens. The resin, based on an acetone and phenol compound known as bisphenol A, in its raw state may cause allergic contact dermatitis. BIS-GMA, a combination of bisphenol A and glycidyl methacrylate, is the main allergen in dental bonding agents. Epoxy resins are used also as stabilizers and plasticizers. Their use in the manufacture of polyvinyl chloride (plastic) film has caused dermatitis from plastic handbags, beads, gloves, and panties.

Polyester resins

Ordinarily, completely cured or polymerized resins are not sensitizers. The unsaturated polyester resins are dissolved and later copolymerized with vinyl monomers. Such polyester resins are used for polyester plasticizers, polyester fibers (Dacron), and polyester film (Mylar). The unsaturated polyester resins, on the other hand, will produce primary irritation in their fabrication or among sculptors. The dermatitis occurs typically as an eczematous eruption on the back of the hands, wrists, and forearms. Polyester resins are commonly incorporated into other plastic material as laminates to give them strength; applications include boat hulls, automobile body putty, safety helmets, fuel tanks, lampshades, and skylights.

Acrylic monomers

Cyanoacrylates are used widely as adhesives in a variety of home and commercial products. They are generally a rare cause of contact dermatitis. With the advent of skin bonding agents, reports of allergy may increase. Multifunctional acrylic monomers may produce allergic or irritant contact dermatitis. Pentaerythritol triacrylate, trimethylolpropane triacrylate, and hexanediol diacrylate are widely used acrylic monomers. Printers handling multifunctional acrylic monomers in printing inks and acrylic printing plates may present with an erythematous, pruritic eruption, mainly of the hands and arms, swelling of the face, and involvement of the eyelids.

Orthopedic surgeons experience contact dermatitis from the use of acrylic bone cement (methyl methacrylate monomer) used in mending hip joints. Dentists and dental technicians are exposed when applying this to teeth. The sensitizer passes through rubber and polyvinyl gloves and may additionally cause paresthesias. In patients who are allergic to their acrylate dental prosthesis, coating this with UV light-cured acrylate lacquer may allow it to be worn without adverse effects.

Benzoyl peroxide is a popular acne remedy. It is also used for bleaching flour and edible oils, and for curing plastics, such as acrylic dentures. Infrequently, an allergic contact dermatitis may be caused.

Aalto-Korte K, et al: Methacrylate and acrylate allergy in dental personnel. Contact Dermatitis 2007; 57:324.

Hivnor CM, et al: Allergic contact dermatitis after postsurgical repair with 2-octylcyanoacrylate. Arch Dermatol 2008; 144:814.

Lazarov A: Sensitization to acrylates is a common adverse reaction to artificial fingernails. J Eur Acad Dermatol Venereol 2007; 21:169.

Militello G, et al: Allergic contact dermatitis from isocyanates among sculptors. Dermatitis 2004; 15:150.

Cosmetic dermatitis

Cutaneous reactions to cosmetics may be divided into irritant, allergic hypersensitivity, and photosensitivity reactions. More than half of the reactions occur on the face and are due primarily to skin-care products, nail cosmetics, shaving preparations, and deodorants. The leading cause of allergic contact dermatitis associated with cosmetics is from fragrance. A close second is preservatives, such as Bronopol (2-bromo-2-nitropropane-1-3-diol), Kathon CG, quarternium-15, Euxyl K 400, and imidazolidinyl urea. Third is *p*-phenylenediamine in hair dye. It is recommended that patch testing with the patient's own product, as long as it is applied to the skin as a leave-on product, be part of the evaluation.

Fragrances

Almost all cosmetic preparations, skin-care products, and many medications contain fragrance; even those labeled non-scented often contain a "masking" fragrance that may be a sensitizer. Even "fragrance-free" products have been documented to contain the raw fragrance ingredients, e.g. rose oil in "all-natural" products. Fragrances are the most common cosmetic ingredient causing allergic contact dermatitis. Photodermatitis, irritation, contact urticaria, and dyspigmentation are other types of reactions they may produce.

The most common individual allergens identified are cinnamic alcohol, oak moss, cinnamic aldehyde, hydroxy citronellal, musk ambrette, isoeugenol, geraniol, coumarin, lyral, and eugenol. Frequently, unspecified allergens are the cause, as they are not listed on labels and fragrances are combinations of many different ingredients. *Myroxylon pereirae* (balsam of Peru) will identify approximately half of those often unsuspected cases of allergic dermatitis, and additional testing with the fragrance mixes will identify over 90%. Additionally, a natural fragrance mixture of jasmine absolute, ylang-ylang oil, narcissus absolute, spearmint oil, and sandalwood oil is recommended. New products should be tested for tolerance in those with a history of fragrance sensitivity.

Around 1% of the population has fragrance sensitivity. Women still outnumber men, but as the frequency of fragrance contact reactions has increased over the years, men have shown a steeper increase in sensitivity. Ingestion of balsam-related foods, such as tomatoes, citrus fruits, and spices, may cause a flare in some sensitive patients. In particularly difficult-to-treat patients, balsam-restricted diets may be beneficial but are not easy to follow.

Hair dyes

Permanent hair dyes incorporate *p*-phenylenediamine (PPDA), a popular but potent sensitizer that may cross-react with many chemicals. In rinses and tints the azo dyes, acid violet 6B, water-soluble nigrosine, and ammonium carbonate may sensitize and cross-react with PPDA. Those engaged in the manufacture of PPDA, furriers, hairdressers, and those in the photographic and rubber vulcanization industries develop eruptions at first on the backs of the hands, wrists, forearms, eyelids, and nose, consisting of an eczematous, erythematous, oozing dermatitis. Lichenification and scaling are seen in the chronic type. In those whose hair has been dyed, sensitivity is manifested by itching, redness, and puffiness of the upper eyelids, tops of the ears, temples, and back of the neck. Beard dermatitis may be due to coloring of the facial hair and eyelid dermatitis from dying eyelashes. PPDA added to temporary henna tattoos to make them darker has resulted in a large number of acute vesicular allergic reactions, some with scarring and hyperpigmentation. Kumkum is a commonly used cosmetic in India, primarily smeared on the forehead of women to denote their marital status; one of many reported allergens in the product is PPDA.

For those sensitive to this type of hair dye, use of semipermanent or temporary dyes might be the solution. In the case of sensitivity to the latter, vegetable dyes such as henna may be tried. Metallic dyes are usually not favored by women but are frequently used by men as "hair color restorers." The metallic hair dyes may contain nickel, cobalt, chromium, or lead. Hair dyes containing FD&C and D&C dyes often do not cross-react with PPDA.

Other hair products

Hair bleach products incorporate peroxides, persulfates, and ammonia, which may act as primary irritants. Hair bleaches that contain ammonium persulfate, a primary irritant, may produce a local urticarial and a generalized histamine reaction.

Several types of permanent wave preparations exist. The alkaline permanent wave preparations, which use ammonium thioglycolate, are rarely, if ever, sensitizers, and usually cause only hair breakage and irritant reactions. The hot type, or acid perm, is a common sensitizer, the allergen being glyceryl monothioglycolate. Cosmetologists are at risk for development of hand dermatitis. The glyceryl monothioglycolate persists in the hair for at least 3 months after application and may cause a long-lasting dermatitis. It readily penetrates rubber and vinyl gloves. A more neutral pH permanent wave solution is less allergenic than the acid perms; however, allergy to cysteamine hydrochloride found in neutral permanent wave products may occur. This allergen does not penetrate household-weight latex gloves and hair waved with it does not produce allergic reactions in sensitized individuals. Also, it is an amine salt and not a thioglycolate, so cross-reactivity is unlikely.

Hair straighteners using greases and gums are not sensitizers; however, the perfume incorporated in these preparations

can be. Thioglycolates are also used, and hair breakage may occur with these products.

Hair sprays may contain shellac, gum arabic, sunscreens, and synthetic resins as sensitizers, and allergic reactions occur infrequently. Lanolin is frequently incorporated into aerosol sprays.

Chemical depilatories containing calcium thioglycolate and the sulfides and sulfhydrates may cause primary irritant dermatitis. Mechanical hair removers are the mercaptans, waxes, and resins. The latter may produce allergic dermatitis.

Hair tonics and lotions with tincture of cinchona produce allergic sensitization; tincture of cantharidin and salicylic acid, primary irritation. Resorcin, quinine sulfate, and perfumes such as bay rum are also sensitizers.

Nail products

Nail lacquers may contain tosylamide/formaldehyde resin and are a frequent cause of eyelid and neck dermatitis. Polishes free of this resin are available. Nail polish removers are solvents such as acetone, which can cause nail brittleness. The acrylic monomers in artificial nails, as well as the ethyl cyanoacrylate glue required to attach the prosthetic nail, may produce allergic sensitivity. Photoinitiating agents, such as benzophenone, used in photobonded acrylic sculptured nails are other potential allergens.

Lipsticks

Various R and C dyes, sunscreens, shellac, flavoring agents, preservative, and lipstick perfumes may cause sensitization reactions. Lipsticks are tested as is. Lip plumpers may cause contact urticaria in those being kissed. Propolis is found in many so-called natural products, including lip balms, toothpastes, lotions, shampoos, and other cosmetics. Its main allergens are two types of caffeates.

Eye make-up

In mascara, eye shadow, and eyeliners, the preservative, shellac, metals, base wax, and perfumes are the components that may produce sensitization, but this occurs rarely. False-positive reactions to some mascaras occur when a closed patch test is used. This is caused by the irritative qualities of the solvents. An open or nonocclusive patch test is recommended. A provocative use test in the antecubital fossae may ultimately be necessary. The rubber sponges used to apply eye make-up also cause eyelid dermatitis.

Sunscreens

p-Aminobenzoic acid (PABA) and its derivatives, such as padimate O, padimate A, and glycerol PABA, and dibenzoylmethanes, salicylates, cinnamates, and benzophenones are photosensitizers as well as sensitizers. If allergy to PABA exists, its derivatives should be avoided and there should be an awareness that thiazides, sulfonylurea antidiabetic medication, azo dyes, *p*-aminosalicylic acid, benzocaine, and *p*-phenylenediamine all may cause dermatitis from cross-reactions. Oxybenzone is the most common sunscreen allergen.

Bleaching creams

Hydroquinones are occasional sensitizers. Ammoniated mercury is a sensitizing agent formerly used in bleaching creams.

Lanolin

The fatty alcohol lanolin is rarely a sensitizer on normal skin and most cosmetic and skin-care products do not cause dermatitis. It provokes allergic reactions more frequently in therapeutic agents used by atopic patients and in emollient products which may be used postsurgically.

Dentifrices and mouthwashes

Dentifrices and mouthwashes contain sensitizers, such as the essential oils used as flavoring agents, preservatives, formalin, antibiotics, and antiseptics. Beacham et al reported 20 women who developed circumoral dermatitis and cheilitis from tartar-control types of dentifrice.

Axillary antiperspirants

Aluminum salts, such as aluminum chloride and chlorhydroxide, and zinc salts, such as zinc chloride, act as primary irritants, and may rarely produce a folliculitis. Aluminum chlorhydrate is considered to be the least irritating antiperspirant. Zirconium salt preparations, now removed from all antiperspirants, produced a granulomatous reaction. Zirconium–aluminum complexes, however, are commonly used as the active ingredient in topical antiperspirants and may produce granulomas. Quaternary ammonium compounds in some roll-on deodorants may produce allergic contact dermatitis.

Axillary deodorants and feminine hygiene sprays

Fragrances, bacteriostats, and propellants cause the majority of the reactions seen with these products. Deodorants that contain cinnamic aldehyde can induce irritation on axillary skin even when tolerated on healthy skin in other sites.

Cosmetic intolerance syndrome

Occasionally, a patient will complain of intense burning or stinging after applying any cosmetic. Usually there are only subjective symptoms, but objective inflammation may also be present. The underlying cause may be difficult to document, even though thorough patch testing, photopatch testing, and contact urticaria testing are completed. Endogenous disease, such as seborrheic dermatitis, rosacea, or atopic dermatitis, may complicate the assessment. Avoidance of all cosmetics, with only glycerin being allowed, for 6–12 months is often necessary to calm the reactive state. Adding back cosmetics one at a time, no more frequently than one a week, may then be tolerated.

Baran R: Nail cosmetics: allergies and irritations. Am J Clin Dermatol 2002; 3:547.

Beacham BE, et al: Circumoral dermatitis and cheilitis caused by tartar control dentifrices. J Am Acad Dermatol 1990; 22:1029.

Biebl KA, et al: Allergic contact dermatitis to cosmetics. Dermatol Clin 2006; 24:215.

Bruze M, et al: Deodorants. J Am Acad Dermatol 2003; 48:194.

Castanedo-Tardan MP, et al: Patterns of contact allergy. Dermatol Clin 2009; 27:265.

Diepgen TL, et al: Contact dermatitis: epidemiology and frequent sensitizers to cosmetics. J Eur Acad Dermatol Venereol 2007; 21(Suppl 2):9.

Firoz EF, et al: Lip plumper contact urticaria. J Am Acad Dermatol 2009; 60:861.

Francalanci S, et al: Multicentre study of allergic contact cheilitis from toothpastes. Contact Dermatitis 2000; 43:216.

Hartford O, et al: Tea tree oil. Cutis 2005; 76:178.

Jacob SE, et al: Benzyl alcohol: a covert fragrance. Dermatitis 2007; 18:232.

Jacob SE, et al: Sensitivity to para-phenylenediamine and intolerance to hydrochlorothiazide. Dermatitis 2008; 19:E44.

Jovanovic DL, et al: Allergic contact dermatitis from temporary henna tattoo. J Dermatol 2009; 36:63.

Khumalo NP, et al: Prevalence of cutaneous adverse effects of hairdressing. Arch Dermatol 2006; 142:377.

Landers MC, et al: Permanent wave dermatitis. Am J Contact Dermat 2003; 14:157.

LeCoz CJ, et al: Allergic contact dermatitis to shellac in mascara. Contact Dermatitis 2002; 46:149.

Lee B, et al: Lanolin allergy. Dermatitis 2008; 19:63.

Militello G: Contact and primary irritant dermatitis of the nail unit. Dermatol Ther 2007; 20:47.

Militello G, et al: Lyral: a fragrance allergen. Dermatitis 2005; 16:41.

Nath AK, et al: Kumkum-induced dermatitis. Clin Expert Dermatol 2007; 32:385.

Nguyen JC, et al: Allergic contact dermatitis caused by lanolin (wool) alcohol contained in an emollient in three post surgical patients. J Am Acad Dermatol 2010; 62:1064.

Salam TN, et al: Balsam-related systemic contact dermatitis. J Am Acad Dermatol 2002; 45:377.

Scheuer E, et al: Sunscreen allergy. Dermatitis 2006; 17:3.

Thyssen JP, et al: Epidemiological data on consumer allergy to p-phenylenediamine. Contact Dermatitis 2008; 59:327.

Turchin I, et al: Cross-reactions among parabens, para-phenyldiamine, and benzocaine. Dermatitis 2006; 17:192.

Uter W, et al: Contact allergy to fragrances. Contact Dermatitis 2010; epub.

Valks R, et al: Contact dermatitis in hairdressers, ten years later. Dermatitis 2005; 16:28.

Walgrave SE, et al: Allergic contact dermatitis from propolis. Dermatitis 2005; 16:209.

Warshaw EM, et al: Positive patch test reactions to lanolin. Dermatitis 2009; 20:79.

Waters AJ, et al: Photocontact allergy to PABA in sunscreens: the need for continued vigilance. Contact Dermatitis 2009; 60:172.

Preservatives

Preservatives are added to any preparation that contains water to kill microorganisms and prevent spoilage. Such products include moist materials such as baby wipes, which when used in either infants or adults can produce reactions caused by preservatives. The most important class is formaldehyde and the formaldehyde-releasing compounds, including quaternium-15 (the leading preservative sensitizer in the US), imidazolidinyl urea, diazolidinyl urea, DMDM hydantoin, and 2-bromo-2 nitropropane-1,3-diol.

Kathon CG or methylchloroisothiazolinone/methyl isothiazolinone (MCI/MI) and Euxyl K 400 (methyldibromoglutaronitrile and phenoxyethanol in a 1:4 ratio) are other important preservative allergens. In the latter it is the methyldibromoglutaronitrile component that produces the allergic response. This preservative may produce false-negatives on testing, so repeat open testing is indicated if a specific leave-on product is suspected of causing allergy. Methyldibromoglutaronitrile has been the subject of a European regulation limiting exposure to it. As with similar laws regulating nickel in Europe, allergy to this preservative is also lowering in incidence over time.

Tea tree oil is an additive to some natural products that may serve as an antimicrobial. Developing data show it to be a sensitizer as well. Sorbic acid is a rare sensitizer among the preservatives; however, it is a cause of facial flushing and stinging through its action as an inducer of nonimmunologic contact urticaria. Benzalkonium chloride is widely used but a rare sensitizer. Finally, triclosan and benzyl alcohol are weak sensitizers. Thimerosal is discussed above.

Formaldehyde and formaldehyde-releasing agents

Formaldehyde is used rarely, primarily in shampoos. Because it is quickly diluted and washed away, sensitization through this exposure is rare. Formaldehyde releasers are polymers of formaldehyde that may release small amounts of formaldehyde under certain conditions. Allergy may be to the formaldehyde-releasing preservatives (which act as antibacterial and antifungal agents in their own right) and/or to the released formaldehyde. Cross-reactivity among them is common, so when allergy is proven to one compound and avoidance does not clear the eruption, screening for clinically relevant reactions to the others is indicated. This may be done by repetitive open application testing to the leave-on product, or by extended patch testing.

Parabens

Allergic contact dermatitis may develop from parabens, which are used in cosmetics, foods, drugs, dentifrices, and suppositories. The paraben esters (methyl, ethyl, propyl, and butyl p-hydroxybenzoates) are used in low concentrations in cosmetics and rarely cause dermatitis. They are found in higher concentration in topical medicaments and may be the cause of allergic reactions. Perpetuation of a dermatitis, despite effective topical medication, suggests the possibility of paraben or corticosteroid sensitivity, or that another sensitizer may be present. Parabens, which are frequently used as bacteriostatic agents, are capable of producing immunologically mediated immediate systemic hypersensitivity reactions. Cross-reactivity to para-phenylenediamine and benzocaine occurs in some individuals.

p-Chloro-meta-xylenol (PCMX)

This chlorinated phenol antiseptic is used in many over-the-counter products with the disinfectant properties of p-chloro-metacresol. Sensitization occurs primarily through exposure to betamethasone-containing cream. There is cross-reactivity to p-chloro-metacresol.

Askari SK, et al: Parabens. Dermatitis 2006; 17:215.
Berthelot C, et al: Allergic contact dermatitis to choroxylenol. Dermatitis 2006; 17:156.
Campbell L, et al: Triclosan. Dermatitis 2006; 17:204.
Cashman AL, et al: Parabens. Dermatitis 2005; 16:57.
Curry EJ, et al: Benzyl alcohol allergy. Dermatitis 2005; 16:203.
Fields KS, et al: Contact dermatitis caused by baby wipes. J Am Acad Dermatol 2006; 54(Suppl):S230.
Isaksson M, et al: Repeated open application tests with methyldibromoglutaronitrile in dermatitis patients with and without hypersensitivity to methyldibromoglutaronitrile. Dermatitis 2007; 18:203.
Johansen JD, et al: Decreasing trends in methyldibromoglutaronitrile contact allergy following regulatory intervention. Contact Dermatitis 2008; 59:48.
Jong CT, et al: Contact sensitivity to preservatives in the UK 2004–2005. Contact Dermatitis 2007; 57:165.
Marcano ME, et al: Occupational allergic contact dermatitis to methyldibromoglutaronitrile in hand degreasing toilet paper. Contact Dermatitis 2007; 57:126.
Sanchez-Perez J, et al: Allergic and systemic contact dermatitis to methylparaben. Contact Dermatitis 2006; 54:117.
Williams JD, et al: Dermatologically tested baby toilet tissues: a cause of allergic contact dermatitis in adults. Contact Dermatitis 2007; 57:97.
Wilson M, et al: Chloroxylenol. Dermatitis 2007; 18:120.
Zug KA, et al: Patch test results of the North American Contact Dermatitis Group 2005–2006. Dermatitis 2009; 20:149.

Vehicles

Formulation of topically applied products is complex and additives are blended to make a pleasing base for carriage of the active ingredient to the skin. Various emulsifiers, humectants, stabilizers, surfactants, and surface active agents are used to make esthetically pleasing preparations. These may cause irritation, erythema, and allergy. The surfactant cocamidopropyl betaine produces dermatitis of the head and neck in consumers and the hands in hairdressers, often due to its presence in shampoos. Propolis and lanolin are discussed within the cosmetic portion above.

Propylene glycol

Propylene glycol is widely used as a vehicle for topical medications, cosmetics (especially antiperspirants), and various emollient lotions. It is used in the manufacture of automobile brake fluid and alkyd resins, as a lubricant for food machinery, and as an additive for food colors and flavoring agents. Propylene glycol must be considered as a sensitizer able to produce contact dermatitis, and it can cause a flare of the contact dermatitis when ingested. It is tested as a 4% aqueous solution, but irritant reactions or false-negatives are common. A use test of the implicated propylene glycol-containing products may be required.

Ethylenediamine

Ethylenediamine is used as a stabilizer in medicated creams. It may cause contact dermatitis and cross-react with internally taken aminophylline, which consists of theophylline and ethylenediamine. Hydroxyzine is a piperazine derivative that is structurally based on a dimer of ethylenediamine, to which patients sensitive to the stabilizer may develop a generalized itchy, red eruption that recurs each time hydroxyzine is taken orally.

Ash S, et al: Systemic contact dermatitis to hydroxyzine. Am J Contact Dermat 1997; 8:2.
Jacob SE, et al: Cocamidopropyl betaine. Dermatitis 2008; 19:157.
Lessman H, et al: Skin-sensitizing and irritant properties of propylene glycol. Contact Dermatitis 2005; 53:247.
Lowther A, et al: Systemic contact dermatitis from propylene glycol. Dermatitis 2008; 19:105.
Pereira F, et al: Contact dermatitis due to emulsifiers. Contact Dermatitis 1997; 36:114.

Topical drug contact dermatitis

Drugs, in addition to their pharmacologic and possible toxic action, also possess sensitizing properties. Sensitization may occur not only from topical application but also from ingestion, injection or inhalation. Some, such as the antihistamines, including topical doxepin, sensitize much more frequently when applied topically than when taken orally. With the advent of transdermal patches for delivery of medications such as nitroglycerin, hormones, nicotine, clonidine, fentanyl, lidocaine, and scopolamine, reports of sensitization are increasing. Clonidine induces the highest rate of allergic reactions. At times erythema multiforme-like reactions may occur with transdermally applied drugs.

Some drugs may produce sensitization of the skin when applied topically; if the medication is taken later internally, an acute flare at the site of the contact dermatitis may result. This so-called anamnestic (recalled) eruption or systemic contact dermatitis can occur with antihistamines, sulfonamides, and penicillin. The same is true of the local anesthetic ointments containing "caine" medications. Usually, if sensitization occurs when using transdermal patches, the drugs do not cause systemic contact dermatitis when taken orally.

Although it is impossible to mention all topical medications that cause irritation or allergic contact dermatitis, some are important enough to be dealt with individually.

Local anesthetics

Physicians and dentists may develop allergic contact dermatitis from local anesthetics. In addition, the continued use of these local anesthetics as antipruritic ointments and lotions causes sensitization of the skin. Benzocaine is a frequently used topical antipruritic and is the most common topical sensitizer of this group. Itchy dermatitis of the anogenital area may be due to a topically applied anesthetic.

Local anesthetics may be divided into two groups. The first includes the p-aminobenzoic acid esters, such as benzocaine, butethamine, chloroprocaine, procaine (Novacaine), and tetracaine (Pantocaine). The second, which sensitizes much less frequently, includes the amides, such as dibucaine (Nupercainal), lidocaine (Lido-Mantle, EMLA, Lidoderm patch, LMX, Xylocaine), mepivacaine (Carbocaine), and prilocaine (Citanest). In addition, the preservative methylparaben, frequently found in these prepared solutions, may cause hypersensitivity reactions that can easily be misattributed to the local anesthetics. It should be kept in mind that numerous cross-reactions are seen in benzocaine-sensitive individuals. These are discussed in the section on sunscreens and preservatives. Lidocaine can induce contact urticaria as well.

Antimicrobials

Physicians, dentists, nurses, and other medical personnel, as well as patients, especially those suffering from chronic leg ulcers, may develop contact dermatitis from various antibiotics. Neomycin and bacitracin are only behind nickel, fragrances (and the related *Myroxylon pereirae*), and quaternium-15 as the most frequent sensitizers in the US. As a topical antibiotic, neomycin sulfate has been incorporated into innumerable ointments, creams, and lotions. It is present in such preparations as underarm deodorants, otic and ophthalmologic preparations, and antibiotic creams and ointments available without prescription. The signs of neomycin sensitivity may be those of a typical contact dermatitis but are often those of a recalcitrant skin eruption that has become lichenified and even hyperkeratotic. This may be because many topical agents contain several types of antibiotic but also often have corticosteroids present. This picture may be seen in persistent external otitis, lichen simplex chronicus of the nuchal area, or dermatophytosis between the toes. A late-appearing reaction on patch testing is not uncommon, so an assessment at day 7 is recommended.

There has been a dramatic rise in allergy to bacitracin. Its use after minor surgical procedures may account for this. After clean surgical procedures white petrolatum is as effective in aiding wound healing as antibiotic ointment, allows no more infection, and of course does not carry the allergenic potential. Petrolatum should be used after clean cutaneous surgery; antibiotic ointments are not necessary and contribute to the overall increasing problem of allergy to these medications. There is a high rate of coreaction (not cross-reaction) with neomycin because of simultaneous exposures. Contact urticaria and anaphylaxis are reported more often with bacitracin than with other antibiotics.

Mafenide acetate, the topical antimicrobial found in Sulfamylon, a burn remedy, may cause allergic contact dermatitis, as can metronidazole.

Antifungal agents

Allergic contact dermatitis to imidazole and other antifungal agents may occur. There is a high cross-reactivity rate between miconazole, isoconazole, clotrimazole, and oxiconazole because of their common chemical structure.

Phenothiazine drugs

Handling injectable solutions and tablets may produce dermatitis in those sensitized to chlorpromazine and other phenothiazine derivatives. The reactions may be photoallergic or nonphotoallergic.

Corticosteroids

Numerous reports of large series of patients who have developed allergy to these commonly used preparations emphasize the need for a high index of suspicion when treating patients with chronic dermatitis who fail to improve, or who worsen, when topical steroidal agents are used. Once sensitized to one type of corticosteroid, cross-sensitization may occur. The corticosteroids have been separated into four structural classes:

- Class A is the hydrocortisone, tixocortol pivalate group.
- Class B is the triamcinolone acetonide, budesonide group.
- Class C is the betamethasone group.
- Class D is the hydrocortisone-17-butyrate group.

There are frequent cross-reactions between classes B and D. Tixocortol pivalate and budesonide have been found to be the best screening agents, finding 93% of steroid allergies. In the absence of having these materials, patch testing to the implicated product may be useful. An empiric trial of desoximetasone (Topicort) or mometasone (Elocon) in the absence of patch testing will give the best chance of selecting a topical steroid with an extremely low risk of sensitization.

Cronin H, et al: Anaphylactic reaction to bacitracin ointment. Cutis 2009; 83:127.

Chaudari PR, et al: Allergic contact dermatitis from ophthalmics. Contact Dermatitis 2007; 57:11.

Firoz EF: Allergic contact dermatitis to mafenide acetate. J Drug Dermatol 2007; 6:825.

Foti C, et al: Allergic contact dermatitis from ciclopirox olamine. Australas J Dermatol 2001; 42:145.

Foti C, et al: Contact allergy to topical corticosteroids. Recent Pat Inflamm Allergy Drug Discov 2009; 3:33.

Gehrig KA, et al: Allergic contact dermatitis to topical antibiotics. J Am Acad Dermatol 2008; 58:1.

Green CM, et al: Contact allergy to topical medicaments becomes more common with advancing age. Contact Dermatitis 2007; 56:229.

Isaksson M: Systemic contact allergy to corticosteroids revisited. Contact Dermatitis 2007; 57:368.

Javanovic M, et al: Contact urticaria and allergic contact dermatitis to lidocaine in a patient sensitive to benzocaine and propolis. Contact Dermatitis 2006; 54:124.

Mackley CL, et al: Delayed type hypersensitivity to lidocaine. Arch Dermatol 2003; 139:343.

Madsen JT, et al: Allergic contact dermatitis to topical metronidazole. Contact Dermatitis 2007; 56:364.

Musel AL, et al: Cutaneous reactions to transdermal therapeutic systems. Dermatitis 2006; 17:109.

Sidhu SK, et al: A 10-year retrospective study on benzocaine allergy in the UK. Am J Contact Dermat 1999; 10:57.

Smack DP, et al: Infection and allergy incidence in ambulatory surgery patients using white petrolatum vs. bacitracin ointment. JAMA 1996; 276:972.

Sood A, et al: Bacitracin: allergen of the year. Am J Contact Dermat 2003; 14:3.

Warshaw EM, et al: Patch-test reactions to topical anesthetics. Dermatitis 2008; 19:81.

Occupational contact dermatitis

Workers in various occupations are prone to contact dermatitis from primary irritants and allergic contactants. In certain occupations it is a common occurrence. Irritant contact dermatitis is more frequent in the workplace, but it tends to be less severe and less chronic than allergic contact dermatitis. Occupational skin disease has declined over the past 30 years but still constitutes approximately 10% of all occupational disease cases. Agriculture, forestry, and fishing have the highest incidence of occupational skin disease, with the manufacturing and healthcare sectors contributing many cases as well.

Irritant contact dermatitis is commonly present in wet-work jobs, and allergy occurs in hairdressers, machinists, and many others with unique exposures to multiple sensitizing chemicals. The hands are the parts most affected, being involved in 60% of allergic reactions and 80% of irritant dermatitis. Epoxy resin is an allergen overrepresented when evaluating occupational patients. The allergens most frequently encountered in occupational cases are carba mix, thiuram mix, epoxy resin, formaldehyde, and nickel.

Management

Occupational contact dermatitis is managed by eliminating contact of the skin with irritating and sensitizing substances.

The work environment should be carefully controlled, with use of all available protective devices to prevent accidental and even planned exposures. Personal protective measures, such as frequent clothing changes, cleansing showers, protective clothing, and protective barrier creams should be used as appropriate. Hand-cleansing procedures should be thoroughly surveyed, with particular attention paid to the soaps available and also what solvents may be used.

Treatment of the dermatitis follows closely that recommended for toxicodendron dermatitis. Topical corticosteroid preparations are especially helpful in the acute phase. For dry, fissured hands, soaking them in water for 20 min at night followed immediately upon removing (without drying them) with triamcinolone 0.1% ointment will help hydrate and heal them. Topical tacrolimus ointment and pimecrolimus cream may assist in maintenance therapy. When rubber and polyvinyl gloves cannot be used against irritant and allergenic substances, skin protective creams may offer a solution, although they are often impractical. A wide variety is available, but two main types are used. One is for "wet work"—to protect against acids, alkalis, water-base paints, coolants, and cutting oils with water; and the other type is for "dry work"—to protect against oils, greases, cutting oils, adhesive, resins, glues, and wood preservatives.

Unfortunately, despite the best efforts at treatment and prevention, the prognosis for occupational skin disease is guarded. One-third to one-quarter heal, and another one-third to one-half improve, with the remainder the same or worse. A change or discontinuance of the job does not guarantee relief, as many individuals continue to have persistent postoccupational dermatitis. The importance of thorough patient education cannot be overemphasized. Atopics, males with chromate allergy, females with nickel allergy, those with a delay in diagnosis before institution of treatment, and construction industry workers fare the worst, while irritation from metalworking fluids, reactions to urushiols in foresters, and allergic contact dermatitis to acrylic monomers or amine-curing agents is usually short-lived.

Adisesh A, et al: Prognosis and work absence due to occupational contact dermatitis. Contact Dermatitis 2002; 46:273.

Bauer A, et al: Intervention for preventing occupational irritant hand dermatitis. Cochrane Database Syst Rev 2010; 6:CD004414.

Belsito DV: Occupational contact dermatitis. J Am Acad Dermatol 2005; 53:303.

Bourrain JL: Occupational contact urticaria. Clin Rev Allergy Immunol 2006; 30:39.

Diepgen TL, et al: Management of chronic hand eczema. Contact Dermatitis 2007; 57:203.

Elsner P: Skin protection in the prevention of skin diseases. Curr Probl Dermatol 2007; 34:1.

Emmitt EA: Occupational contact dermatitis. Am J Contact Dermat 2003; 14:21.

Mai Konen T, et al: Long-term follow-up study of occupational hand eczema. Br J Dermatol 2010; epub.

Marks JG Jr, et al: Contact and Occupational Dermatology, 3rd edn. St Louis: Mosby, 2002.

Meding B: Differences between the sexes with regard to work-related skin disease. Contact Dermatitis 2000; 42:65.

Nettis E, et al: Occupational irritant and allergic contact dermatitis among healthcare workers. Contact Dermatitis 2002; 46:101.

Rietschel RL, et al: Relationship of occupation to contact dermatitis. Am J Contact Dermat 2002; 13:170.

Rietschel RL, Fowler JF Jr: Fisher's Contact Dermatitis, 6th edn. Hamilton: Lippincott, BC Decker, 2008.

Saary J, et al: A systematic review of contact dermatitis treatment and prevention. J Am Acad Dermatol 2005; 53:845.

Shalock PC, et al: Protection from occupational allergens. Curr Probl Dermatol 2007; 34:58.

Slodownik D, et al: Occupational factors in skin diseases. Curr Prob Dermatol 2007; 35:173.

Sohrabian S, et al: Contact dermatitis in agriculture. J Agromedicine 2007; 12:3.

Suneja T, et al: Occupational dermatoses in health care workers evaluated for suspected allergic contact dermatitis. Contact Dermatitis 2008; 58:285.

Uter W, et al: Contact allergy to hairdressing allergens in female hairdressers and clients. J Dtsch Dermatol Ges 2007; 5:993.

Zhai H, et al: Protection from irritants. Curr Prob Dermatol 2007; 34:47.

Contact urticaria

Contact urticaria may be defined as a wheal and flare reaction occurring when a substance is applied to the intact skin. Urticaria is only one of a broad spectrum of immediate reactions, including pruritus, dermatitis, local or general urticaria, bronchial asthma, orolaryngeal edema, rhinoconjunctivitis, gastrointestinal distress, headache, or an anaphylactic reaction. Any combination of these is subsumed under the expression "syndrome of immediate reactions."

It may be nonimmunologic (no prior sensitization), immunologic, or of unknown mechanism. The nonimmunologic type is the most common, and may be caused by direct release of vasoactive substances from mast cells. The allergic type tends to be the most severe, as anaphylaxis is possible. The third type has features of both.

Nonimmunologic mechanism

This type of reaction occurs most frequently and may produce contact urticaria in almost all exposed individuals. Examples of this type of reaction are seen with nettle rash (plants), dimethyl sulfoxide (DMSO), sorbic acid, benzoic acid, cinnamic aldehyde, cobalt chloride, and Trafuril.

Immunologic mechanism

This reaction is of the immediate (IgE-mediated) hypersensitivity type. Latex, potatoes, phenylmercuric propionate, and many other allergens have been reported to cause this.

Uncertain mechanism

This type of reaction occurs with those agents that produce contact urticaria and a generalized histamine type of reaction but lack a direct or immunologic basis for the reaction.

Substances causing contact urticaria

Many different substances can elicit such a reaction. It is seen in homemakers and food handlers who handle raw vegetables, raw meats and fish, shellfish, and other foods. Raw potatoes have been shown to cause not only contact urticaria but also asthma at the same time. It has been seen in hairdressers who handle bleaches and hair dyes containing ammonium persulfate, in whom the contact urticaria is accompanied by swelling and erythema of the face, followed by unconsciousness. Caterpillars, moths, and hedgehogs may cause contact urticaria just by touching the skin.

Additional substances inducing this reaction are oatmeal, flour, meat, turkey skin, calf liver, banana, lemon, monoamylamine, benzophenone, nail polish, tetanus antitoxin, streptomycin, cetyl alcohol, stearyl alcohol, estrogenic cream, cinnamic aldehyde, sorbic acid, benzoic acid, castor bean, lindane, carrots, spices, wool, silk, dog and cat saliva, dog hairs, horse serum, ammonia, sulfur dioxide, formaldehyde, acrylic monomers, exotic woods, wheat, cod liver oil, and aspirin.

Bacitracin ointment may cause anaphylactic reactions when applied topically, especially to chronic leg ulcers; however, it may rarely occur after application to acute wounds.

Universal precautions not only led to a marked increase in delayed-type hypersensitivity reaction to rubber additives, but also to a large number of reports of contact urticaria and anaphylaxis to latex. Most of these reactions occur in health professionals. Reactions are characterized by itching and swelling of the hands within a few minutes of donning the gloves, and will usually resolve within an hour after removing them. In patients with continued exposures the eruption may eventually appear as chronic eczema. Glove powder may aerosolize the allergen and produce more generalized reactions. While these reactions may occur on the job, many cases present as death or near-death events when sensitized individuals undergo operations or other procedures, especially when there is mucosal exposure (dental care, rectal examination, childbirth).

In addition to healthcare workers, who have a reported incidence of between 3% and 10%, atopics and spina bifida patients are other risk groups for the development of type I allergy to latex protein. The sensitized individual should also be aware that up to 50% of them will have a concomitant fruit allergy to foods such as banana, avocado, kiwi, chestnut, and passion fruit.

Testing

The usual closed patch tests do not show sensitivity reactions. Instead, open patch tests are performed for eliciting immediate-type hypersensitivity. The substance is applied to a 1 cm^2 area on the forearm and observed for 20–30 min for erythema that evolves into a wheal and flare response. When foods are tested, a small piece of the actual food is placed on the skin. Rubber glove testing can be done by applying one finger of a latex glove to a moistened hand for 15 min. If no reaction is observed, the entire glove is worn for another 15–20 min. Radioallergosorbent testing (RAST) detects 75% of latex-allergic individuals. There is no standard allergen available for prick testing. Prick, scratch, or intradermal testing is resorted to only when there are problems of interpretation of the open patch tests. These tests have produced anaphylactic reactions and should only be attempted when support for this complication is available.

Management

Avoidance of the offending substance is best, but if this is not possible, antihistamines are of benefit. If generalized urticaria or asthmatic reactions occur, then systemic glucocorticoids are best. For anaphylaxis, epinephrine and supportive measures are needed.

Adachi A, et al: Anaphylaxis to polyvinylpyrrolidone after vaginal application of povidone-iodine. Contact Dermatitis 2003; 48:133.
Bourrain JL: Occupational contact urticaria. Clin Rev Allergy Immunol 2006; 30:39.
Bourrain JL, et al: Contact urticaria photoinduced by benzophenones. Contact Dermatitis 2003; 48:45.
Bousquet J, et al: Natural rubber latex allergy among health care workers. J Allergy Clin Immunol 2006; 118:447.
Cronin H, et al: Anaphylactic reaction to bacitracin ointment. Cutis 2009; 83:127.
Doutre MS: Occupational contact urticaria and protein contact dermatitis. Eur J Dermatol 2005; 15:419.
Fairley JA, et al: Hedgehog hives. Arch Dermatol 1999; 135:561.
Firoz EF, et al: Lip plumper contact urticaria. J Am Acad Dermatol 2009; 60:861.
Kim KT, et al: Prevalence of food allergy in 137 latex-allergic patients. Allergy Asthma Proc 1999; 20:95.
Konstantinou GN, et al: Food contact hypersensitivity syndrome. Clin Exp Dermatol 2008; 33:383.
Stutz N, et al: Anaphylaxis caused by contact urticaria because of epoxy resins. Contact Dermatitis 2008; 58:307.
Tan BM, et al: Severe food allergies by skin contact. Ann Allergy Asthma Immunol 2001; 86:583.
Williams JD, et al: Occupational contact urticaria. Br J Dermatol 2008; 159:125.

Drug reactions

Epidemiology

Adverse drug reactions (ADRs) are a common cause of dermatologic consultation. In a large French study, about 1 in 200 inpatients on medical services developed a drug eruption, as compared to 1 in 10 000 on surgical services. In the US, similar studies have shown a reaction rate of 2–3 in 100 for medical inpatients. In only about 55% of patients who were carefully evaluated was it possible to attribute a specific medication definitely as the cause of the eruption. Simple exanthems (75–95%) and urticaria (5–6%) account for the vast majority of drug eruptions. The risk for development of a drug eruption is related to the following factors: age, gender, dose, and the nature of the medication itself. Females are 1.3–1.5 times more likely to develop drug eruptions, except in children under the age of 3 where boys are more likely to be affected. Not all drugs cause reactions at the same rate. Aminopenicillins cause drug eruptions in between 1.2% and 8% of exposures, and the combination of trimethoprim–sulfamethoxazole at a rate of 2.8–3.7%. About 20% of emergency room (ER) visits for adverse events due to medications were caused by antibiotics, largely penicillins and cephalosporins. This is estimated to have accounted for more than 28 000 visits annually in the US. Up to 20 ER visits occurred per 10 000 prescriptions written for certain antibiotics. Nonsteroidal anti-inflammatory drugs (NSAIDs) have a reaction rate of about 1 in 200. In contrast, reaction rates for digoxin, lidocaine, prednisone, codeine, and acetaminophen are less than 1 in 1000.

In addition, the immune status and genetic make-up of the patient strongly determine the risk of developing certain drug eruptions. For example, patients with human immunodeficiency virus (HIV) infection and Epstein–Barr virus (EBV) infection have dramatically increased rates of exanthematous reactions to certain antibiotics. Hypersensitivity syndromes from multiple drug classes have been associated with reactivation of latent viral infections, primarily human herpes virus (HHV)-6 and 7, but also EBV and cytomegalovirus. In addition, the status of the immune system, as measured by helper T-cell count in the case of HIV, defines a window of immune dysfunction in which this enhanced risk for ADRs occurs. Certain hypersensitivity syndromes are closely associated with genetic differences in the ability of the patient to metabolize a specific medication or a toxic metabolite of the medication. In addition, HLA type, in a race-specific manner, may increase risk for drug reactions for specific medications. Therefore, drug eruptions are not simply drug "allergy," but result from variations in drug metabolism, immune status, coexistent viral disease, the patient's racial background, the patient's HLA status, and the inherent chemical structure (allergenicity) and dosage of the medication itself (see below).

Evaluation

Four basic rules should always be applied in evaluating the patient with a suspected drug reaction.

- First, the patient is probably on unnecessary medications, and all of these should be stopped. Pare down the medication list to the bare essentials.
- Second, the patient must be asked about non-prescription medications and pharmaceuticals delivered by other means (eye drops, suppositories, implants, injections, patches, and recreational drugs).
- Third, no matter how atypical the patient's cutaneous reaction, always consider medication as a possible cause. In patients with unusual reactions, searching the medical

literature and calling the manufacturer for prior reports may be very useful.

- Fourth, the timing of drug administration must correlate with the appearance of the eruption. A drug chart lists all the drugs given to the patient in the left column, with the dates along the lower axis, and the course of the drug eruption at the top. Lines extend from left to right for the dates of administration of each medication. These are directly below the course of the eruption. This graphic representation of the timing of medication administration and eruption is a very handy tool in assigning plausibility to a certain medication causing an eruption. The nurses' notes and patient history are most useful in determining exactly when the eruption first appeared.

An important step in evaluating a patient with a potential drug reaction is to diagnose the cutaneous eruption by clinical pattern (e.g. urticaria, exanthem, vasculitis, hypersensitivity syndrome, etc.). In determining whether the patient's current eruption could be related to a specific medication, two basic questions should be asked. Which of this patient's medications cause this pattern of reaction? How commonly does this medication cause this reaction pattern? Bigby reviewed how to use this information to make clinical decisions about stopping possible reaction-inducing medications. A regularly updated manual (such as Litt) or similar databases on the web are strongly recommended as ready reference sources for this information. An algorithm by which the likelihood can be evaluated of a certain medication causing a particular reaction has been developed. This algorithm, summarized below, can be used as a framework for the evaluation of a given patient:

1. Previous general experience with the drug: Has the suspected medication been reported to cause the reaction the patient is experiencing? If so, how commonly? Also ask the patient if he/she has had a previous reaction to any medications, as the current eruption may represent a cross-reaction from a prior exposure.
2. Alternative etiologic candidates: What are other possible causes of the patient's eruption? An exanthem, for instance, could be related to an associated viral illness, not the medication.
3. Timing of events: When did the eruption appear relative to the administration of the suspected medication? A detailed history from the patient and a careful review of the patient record, including the nursing notes, are useful to establish the chronologic sequence of all drug therapy. A drug chart as described above is very useful
4. Drug levels and evidence of overdose: Certain reactions are known to be related to rate of administration (vancomycin red man syndrome) or cumulative dose (lichenoid reactions to gold).
5. Response to discontinuation (dechallenge): Does the eruption clear when the suspected medication is stopped? Because certain eruptions may clear in the face of continuation, this is a useful, but not irrefutable criterion to ascribe a specific reaction to a medication.
6. Rechallenge: If the offending medication reproduces the reaction on readministration, this is strong evidence that the medication did indeed cause the reaction. Reactions associated with an increase in dosage may also be considered in this category. In certain reaction patterns (e.g. exanthems), even a fraction of the original dose may reproduce the reaction. It may be impossible to rechallenge if the reaction was severe.

In addition to the clinical evaluations noted above, complete evaluation may include special testing for confirmation. Skin testing is most useful in evaluating type I (immediate) hypersensitivity. It is most frequently used in evaluating adverse reactions to penicillin, local anesthetics, insulin, and vaccines. RAST has a 20% false-negative rate in penicillin type I allergy, so it must be followed by skin testing. In their current form, RAST tests cannot replace skin testing. Intradermal, prick skin, and patch testing are also reported to be beneficial in some cases of morbilliform reactions or fixed drug reaction. The patient's metabolism of certain drugs in lymphocytotoxicity assays may be associated with an adverse reaction. Such testing is commercially available, but is expensive and time-consuming, and its value is limited to certain situations such as anticonvulsant or sulfonamide hypersensitivity reactions.

The patient should be given concrete advice about his/her reaction. What was the probability that the patient's reaction was caused by the medication? Can the patient take the medication again, and if so, what may occur? What cross-reactions are known? What other medications must the patient avoid? Unusual reactions should be reported to regulatory agencies and the manufacturer.

Pathogenesis

T cells, specifically Th1 cells, are felt to be important inducers of ADRs. These T cells act in two ways to induce reactions. They can directly secrete biologically active molecules, resulting in direct tissue effects (epidermal necrosis, for example), or they can act by secreting chemokines that recruit the effector cells (eosinophils or neutrophils, for example). In biopsies from ADRs, the cytokines produced by helper T cells in the skin parallel the reaction pattern observed. For example, T cells in the dermis in acute generalized exanthematous pustulosis (AGEP) secrete interleukin (IL)-8, a neutrophil-attracting chemokine. In drug rash with eosinophils and systemic symptoms (DRESS), they secrete IL-5 and eotaxin, recruiting eosinophils. As a consequence of helper T-cell activation, memory T cells are produced, resulting in recurrence of the eruption upon rechallenge. Since Th1 cells are mediators of these eruptions, interferon (IFN)-γ release assays using peripheral blood lymphocytes are being evaluated for confirming the inciting medication in ADRs. The sensitivity appears to be drug class-dependent, and specifically of low sensitivity for ADRs induced by anticonvulsants, antibiotics, and cardiovascular medications.

The medications that induce ADRs can create immune-mediated reactions by several mechanisms. Large molecules, such as rat- or mouse-derived antibodies, can be immunogenic. Most medications, however, are too small to be recognized as antigens by immunologically active cells. They must bind to a larger molecule, usually a protein, to form an immunogenic product. The medication is the hapten, and the immunologically active molecule is a medication–protein complex, or hapten–carrier complex. Some medications, such as penicillin, are active enough to bind directly to proteins. Most, however, need to be metabolized to more active or more immunogenic forms in order to bind to proteins and cause an immunologic reaction. The drug metabolites can also be toxic to cells, causing direct cell damage. This metabolism occurs in the cytochrome P450 system in the liver, and perhaps in lower amounts in other organs. These active immunogenic molecules are inactivated through metabolism. This model of immune-mediated ADR explains why the drug itself, the metabolism and breakdown of the medication by the patient, and the patient's immune status all determine the likelihood of developing an ADR.

There has also been a proposed model for ADRs in which the drug or a metabolite binds directly to T cells or Langerhans cells in close opposition to sentinel T cells in the skin. This direct binding could activate the T cell–Langerhans cell interactive unit, resulting in the production of biologically active molecules. This would explain how some drug eruptions occur soon after exposure or with the first exposure to a medication. It could also explain a dose-dependent effect in drug eruptions. Also, a systemic viral infection would have already activated the immune cells in the skin, reducing their threshold for activation by drug binding. This could also explain why many drug eruptions occur only on the skin, apparently sparing other organs. The skin may uniquely have T cells that are sensitive to activation corresponding to a "sentinel" activity appropriate for cells residing on a surface that interacts with the environment. Since the avidity with which drugs directly bind to T cells would vary considerably, this could account for the wide variation in the rate of exanthems from different medications (from 30% for gemifloxacin to <1% for acetaminophen).

Once the T cell is activated, it chooses among one of four programs (or some combination) to create the specific reaction pattern the dermatologist observes. Since it might be possible for several different programs to be chosen, there could be a significant pleomorphism in the clinical and histological pattern observed with any ADR. The four options are as follows:

1. T cells stimulate IFN-γ production and a Th1 response, simulating contact dermatitis. This type of reaction could be "bullous" but without extensive epidermal necrosis.
2. T cells could be activated to function in a Th2 manner and stimulate eosinophil ingress through Th2 cytokines (morbilliform and urticarial drug eruptions).
3. T cells could activate cytotoxic (CD8+) T cells which would secrete perforin/granzyme B and Fas ligand, resulting in keratinocyte apoptosis. This could explain bullous reaction, the observation that occasional necrotic keratinocytes are seen in patients with exanthems, and the rare eruption that begins as an exanthem then progresses to a bullous eruption. Drug eruptions containing activated CD8+ T cells are more dangerous, since CD8+ cells attack all major histocompatibility complex (MHC) class I-expressing cells (including keratinocytes), resulting in more severe reactions.
4. T cells, via granulocyte–macrophage colony-stimulating factor (GM-CSF) and IL-8 local production, call in neutrophils, resulting in pustular exanthems and AGEP.

Dermal CD4+CD25+Foxp3 regulatory T cells (T-regs) are reduced in severe bullous drug eruptions (TEN). Circulating T-regs expressing skin-homing molecules are increased in early drug-induced hypersensitivity syndromes. They are immunologically active early on in the course of the eruption, enter the skin, and can effectively suppress the immune response. However, they become functionally deficient later, perhaps explaining the occasional development of autoimmune phenomena months following drug-induced hypersensitivity syndromes (DIHS), and the tendency of DIHS reactions to relapse, recur, or fail to resolve. In addition, peripheral blood mononuclear cells are stimulated by the incriminated drug (in a lymphocyte transformation test [LTT]) for only the first week in TEN and exanthems. However, in DIHS, the LTT test is negative until 5–6 weeks following the eruption and remains positive for 1 year or more. This supports the observation that DIHS reactions are long-lived. In addition, the LTT is essentially only useful in diagnosing DIHS, since it is rarely performed during the first week of an ADR.

Clinical morphology

Cutaneous drug reactions will initially be discussed by their morphologic pattern. In addition to the cutaneous eruption, some reactions may be associated with other systemic symptoms or findings. The modifier "simple" is used to describe reactions without systemic symptoms or internal organ involvement. "Complex" reactions are those with systemic findings. Complex reactions are also called DIHS, since the ancillary features of complex reactions are often a characteristic syndrome of findings (e.g. an infectious mononucleosis-like picture with anticonvulsant hypersensitivity reactions). DIHS or complex reaction is synonymous with DRESS.

Drug reactions may cause cutaneous lesions and findings identical to a known disease or disorder. These may be of similar or disparate pathogenesis. For example, true serum sickness caused by the injection of foreign proteins, such as antithymocyte globulin, is associated with circulating immune complexes. Medications, notably cefaclor, induce a serum sickness-like illness, clinically extremely similar to, but not associated with, circulating immune complexes. The suffix "-like" is used to describe these syndromes with different or unknown pathogenesis but similar clinical features.

Exanthems (morbilliform or maculopapular reactions)

Exanthems are the most common form of adverse cutaneous drug eruption. They are characterized by erythema, often with small papules throughout. They tend to occur within the first 2 weeks of treatment but may appear later, or even up to 10 days after the medication has been stopped. Lesions tend to appear first proximally, especially in the groin and axilla, generalizing within 1 or 2 days. The face may be spared. Pruritus is usually prominent, helping to distinguish a drug eruption from a viral exanthem. Antibiotics, especially semisynthetic penicillins and trimethoprim–sulfamethoxazole, are the most common causes of this reaction pattern (Fig. 6-18). Ampicillin–amoxicillin given during EBV causes an exanthem in 29–69% of adults and 100% of children. Trimethoprim–sulfamethoxazole given to AIDS patients causes exanthems in a large proportion of patients (about 40%). Certain quinolones (gemfloxacin) cause exanthems at a high rate (4% overall and 30% in young women).

Morbilliform eruptions may rarely be restricted to a previously sunburned site, the so-called "UV recall-like" phenomenon. It occurs during antibiotic therapy from various antibiotics. The sunburn may have occurred 1–7 months before the drug eruption. This pattern of eruption must be distinguished from a true UV recall caused by antimetabolites and

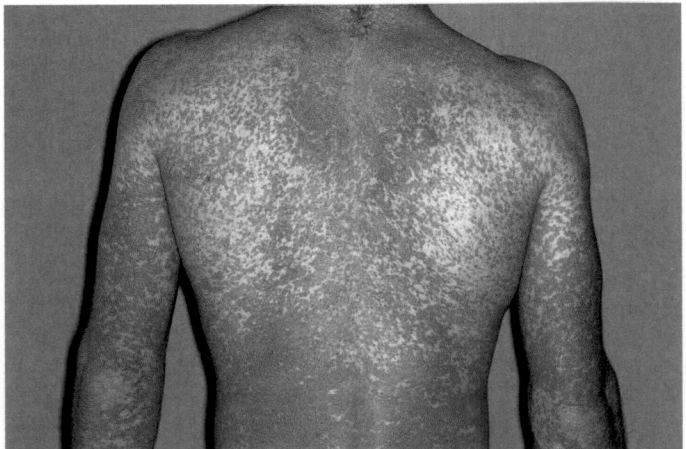

Fig. 6-18 Morbilliform (exanthematous) drug eruption due to an antibiotic.

true radiation recall (see adverse reactions to chemotherapy below).

In the case of simple exanthems, treatment is supportive. The eruption will clear within 2 weeks of stopping the offending medication, and may clear even if it is continued. Topical steroids and antihistamines may benefit and allow the course of therapy to be completed. Rechallenge usually results in the reappearance of the eruption, except in the setting of HIV. In many HIV-infected patients with simple reactions to trimethoprim–sulfamethoxazole, re-exposure by slow introduction or full-dose re-exposure may be tolerated. Uncommonly in HIV infection, however, and rarely in persons with normal immune function, rechallenge may result in a more severe blistering reaction. The use of patch and intradermal testing for the confirmation of the incriminated drug in morbilliform exanthems is not standardized. Only between 2% and 10% of patients who experience the eruption on rechallenge will have a positive patch or intradermal test, making such testing not very useful clinically.

Cutaneous findings identical to simple exanthems may occur as part of DIHS or DRESS. As opposed to simple exanthems, in complex exanthems the inciting agent must be stopped immediately and rechallenge should rarely be undertaken.

Aihara Y, et al: Carbamazepine-induced hypersensitivity syndrome associated with transient hypogammaglobulinaemia and reactivation of human herpesvirus 6 infection demonstrated by real-time quantitative polymerase chain reaction. Br J Dermatol 2003; 149:165.

Azukizawa H, et al: Prevention of toxic epidermal necrolysis by regulatory T cells. Eur J Immunol 2005; 35:1722.

Bigby M: Rates of cutaneous reactions to drugs. Arch Dermatol 2001; 137:765.

Cotliar, J: Approach to the patient with a suspected drug eruption. Semin Cutan Med Surg 2007; 26:147.

Descamps V, et al: Drug-induced hypersensitivity syndrome associated with Epstein–Barr virus infection. Br J Dermatol 2003; 148:1032.

Fiszenson-Albala F, et al: A 6-month prospective survey of cutaneous drug reactions in a hospital setting. Br J Dermatol 2003; 149:1018.

Gueant JL, et al: Pharmacogenetic determinants of immediate and delayed reactions of drug hypersensitivity. Current Pharmaceu Design 2008; 14:2770.

Halevy S, et al: Clinical implications of in vitro drug-induced interferon gamma release from peripheral blood lymphocytes in cutaneous adverse drug reactions. J Am Acad Dermatol 2005; 52:254.

Kano Y, et al: HLA-N allele associations with certain drugs are not confirmed in Japanese patients with severe cutaneous drug reactions. Acta Derm Venereol 2008; 88:616.

Keno Y, et al: Utility of the lymphocyte transformation test in the diagnosis of drug sensitivity: dependence on its timing and the type of drug eruption. Allergy 2007; 62:1439.

Lerch M, Pichler WJ: The immunological and clinical spectrum of delayed drug-induced exanthems. Curr Opin Allergy Clin Immunol 2004; 4:411.

Renn CN, et al: Amoxicillin-induced exanthema in young adults with infectious mononucleosis: demonstration of drug-specific lymphocyte reactivity. Br J Dermatol 2002; 147:1166.

Shehab N, et al: Emergency department visits for antibiotic-associated adverse events. Clin Infec Dis 2008; 47:735.

Sullivan JR, Shear NH: What are some of the lessons learnt from in vitro studies of severe unpredictable drug reactions? Br J Dermatol 2000; 142:206.

Svensson CK, et al: Cutaneous drug reactions. Pharmacol Rev 2000; 53:357.

Takahashi R, et al: Defective regulatory T cells in patients with severe drug eruptions: timing of the dysfunction associated with the pathological phenotype and outcome. J Immunol 2009; 188071.

Torres MJ, et al: Nonimmediate allergic reactions induced by drugs: pathogenesis and diagnostic tests. J Investig Allergol Clin Immunol 2009; 19:80.

Yagami A, et al: Drug-induced hypersensitivity syndrome due to mexiletine hydrochloride associated with reactivation of human herpesvirus 7. Dermatol 2006; 213:341.

Drug-induced hypersensitivity syndrome (DIHS or DHS) or drug reaction with eosinophilia and systemic symptoms (DRESS)

Hypersensitivity syndromes are discussed by the class of medication that causes them. Each class of medication appears to cause a constellation of features characteristic of that medication class, although all cases of DIHS or DRESS share the characteristic features of fever, rash, and internal organ involvement. The characteristic (and according to some authors) diagnostic features of DRESS include:

1. Rash developing late (more than 3 weeks) after the inciting medication is started. It often occurs with the first exposure to the medication.
2. Long-lasting symptoms (>2 weeks) after the discontinuation of the causative drug.
3. Fever (over 38°C).
4. Multiorgan involvement.
5. Eosinophilia (>1500 absolute eosinophilia).
6. Lymphocyte activation (lymphocytosis, atypical lymphocytosis, lymphadenopathy).
7. Frequent reactivation of herpesviruses HHV-6, HHV-7, EBV, and cytomegalovirus.

The vast majority of DRESS cases are caused by a limited number of medications, although more than 200 medications have been incriminated. Only 7 medications/classes of medication are implicated:

1. anticonvulsants (phenobarbital, lamotrigine, and phenytoin)
2. long-acting sulfonamides (sulfamethoxazole, sulfadiazine, and sulfasalazine but NOT related medications—sulfonylureas, thiazine diuretics, furosemide, and acetazolamide)
3. allopurinol
4. nevirapine
5. abacavir
6. dapsone
7. minocycline.

Vancomycin has also recently been recognized as a cause.

The skin eruption accompanying DRESS (DIHS) is typically morbilliform and can vary from faint and mild to severe with exfoliative erythroderma. Facial edema often accompanies the skin eruption, and the eruption may evolve to demonstrate superficial pustules (especially on the face). Some patients with Stevens–Johnson syndrome (SJS)/TEN may have some of the features of DRESS, specifically fever, eosinophilia, and internal organ involvement. How to classify these cases is controversial, but from a pragmatic point of view, the management is that of SJS/TEN and they are best given that diagnosis. The relative frequency of internal organ involvement and other features of DRESS differs depending on the medication which causes the reaction. The variants of DRESS/DIHS are outlined below.

The internal organ involvement described in DRESS can be divided into two types: organ dysfunction occurring during or immediately associated with the acute episode; and late sequelae, possibly with an autoimmune basis. The first category includes colitis/intestinal bleeding, encephalitis/aseptic meningitis, hepatitis, interstitial nephritis, interstitial pneumonitis/respiratory distress syndrome, sialadenitis, and myocarditis. Late sequelae include syndrome of inappropriate secretion of antidiuretic hormone (ADH), thyroiditis/Graves' disease, and diabetes mellitus. Systemic lupus erythematosus (SLE) can rarely occur. In one series, 5% of patients with DRESS died, usually due to complications of liver or renal involvement.

The pathogenesis of DRESS has been studied extensively. Three factors appear to play a role, to various degrees depending on the medication class inducing the DRESS. These are:

1. Certain HLA types put individuals from specific genetic backgrounds at risk of developing DRESS from specific medications.

2. Genetic or acquired inadequate metabolism of toxic or immunogenic breakdown products of certain classes of medication increases the risk for DRESS.

3. Reactivation of herpes viruses (especially HHV-6, but also cytomegalovirus, EBV, and HHV-7) is associated with the development of DRESS. HHV-6 may reactivate during the transient hypogammaglobulinemia that often accompanies DRESS. The mononucleosis-like syndrome accompanying DRESS could be analogous to the mononucleosis-like syndrome accompanying primary HHV-6 infection. In severe DRESS cases, HHV-6 can also be found in the liver and cerebrospinal fluid associated with hepatitis and encephalitis. Certain drugs known to induce DRESS, e.g. sodium valproate, directly induce HHV-6 replication. In one series all fatal cases of DRESS were associated with HHV-6 reactivation. During the acute phase of DRESS, regulatory T cells (T-regs) are expanded and functionally more robust. T-regs become functionally deficient as DRESS resolves, perhaps allowing for the development of autoimmune disease.

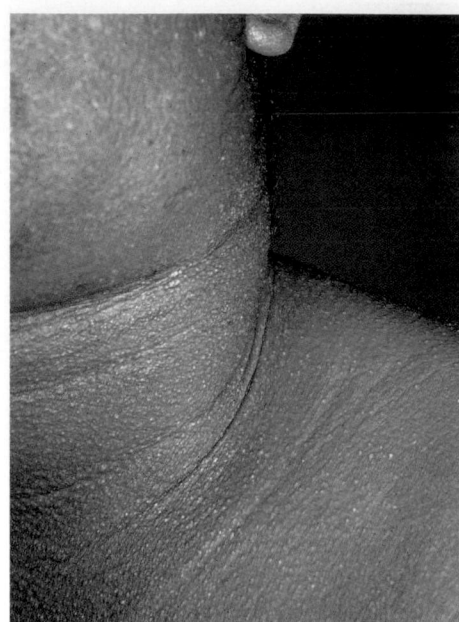

Fig. 6-19 Erythroderma with papulopustules and lymphadenopathy, dilantin-induced hypersensitivity syndrome. (Courtesy of Dr L Lieblich)

Anticonvulsant hypersensitivity syndrome

Anticonvulsant hypersensitivity syndrome can be seen with phenytoin, phenobarbital, carbamazepine, lamotrigine, zonisamide, and other anticonvulsants, so the general term "anticonvulsant hypersensitivity syndrome" is preferred to the original descriptive term "dilantin hypersensitivity syndrome." The incidence of this condition has been estimated at between 1 in 1000 and 1 in 10 000 patients treated with these medications, but is ten times that rate for lamotrigine. Carbamazepine is currently the most common anticonvulsant causing DRESS, because it is also used to treat neuropathic pain, bipolar disorder, and schizophrenia. Medication dosage does not determine risk for this syndrome. HHV-6 and 7 reactivation are observed in about 30% of anticonvulsant hypersensitivity syndrome patients, much more commonly in carbamazepine-induced cases.

The DRESS begins on average 30–40 days after starting the anticonvulsant. Low-grade fever and pharyngitis may precede the eruption by a few days. The skin eruption is typically morbilliform initially, and associated with marked facial and neck edema (Fig. 6-19). The eruption begins on the trunk and face, spreading centrifugally. As the eruption becomes more severe, it may evolve to confluent plaques with purpura. The intense dermal edema accompanying the eruption may lead to bulla formation. Commonly associated findings include fever (in more than 50%), adenopathy (in about 20% of cases), and elevated liver function tests (in between two-thirds and three-quarters of cases). Atypical lymphocytosis can occur, completing a mononucleosis-like picture. Lung and renal involvement is uncommon. Lamotrigine DRESS is somewhat different than that induced by the other anticonvulsants. It has eosinophilia in only 19% of cases, lymphadenopathy in only 12%, and multiorgan involvement in only 45%—lower rates than seen with the other anticonvulsants. Lamotrigine DRESS occurs within 4 weeks in most patients, but may not occur for up to 6 months in 10% of cases. Coadministration of valproate increases the risk of lamotrigine DRESS. Slow introduction reduces the risk for lamotrigine DRESS.

In anticonvulsant hypersensitivity syndrome, as the eruption evolves, it is typical for widespread pinpoint pustules to appear on the face, trunk, and extremities, especially in dark-skinned patients. The syndrome may continue to progress, even after the inciting medication has been stopped. The associated hepatitis can be life-threatening.

Because many of the anticonvulsants are metabolized through the same pathway, cross-reactions are frequent, making selection of an alternative agent quite difficult. The rate of cross-reactivity between phenytoin, phenobarbital, and carbamazepine is 70%. In vitro tests are commercially available and may aid in selecting an agent to which the patient will not cross-react. Valproate is a safe alternative.

The management of anticonvulsant hypersensitivity syndrome begins with considering it in the appropriate setting and ruling out other possible explanations for the patient's findings. The offending medication must be immediately discontinued. Because cross-reactivity among these drugs is high, the therapeutic benefit of a medication from this class must be carefully reconsidered. If the treatment is for depression, prophylaxis after closed head injury, or atypical pain syndromes, medication from another class can often be substituted. Treatment is initially supportive until the extent and severity of the syndrome are assessed. Some patients clear if the medication is simply discontinued. If there is liver or renal involvement, or if the patient appears ill or requires hospitalization, and there is no contraindication, systemic steroids are given. The usually starting dose is between 1 and 1.5 mg/kg/day. N-acetylcysteine may be added if hepatitis is present. Steroid therapy is continued at doses required for control then gradually tapered. It may require months to wean the patient off steroids successfully. If steroids are tapered too rapidly, the syndrome may recur. Intravenous immunoglobulin (IVIG) and other immunosuppressives, such as azathioprine or cyclosporine, have been successfully used in steroid-refractory cases.

Allopurinol hypersensitivity syndrome

Allopurinol hypersensitivity syndrome typically occurs in persons with preexisting renal failure. Often, affected patients are treated unnecessarily for asymptomatic hyperuricemia, with clear indications for therapy present in only about one-third of patients suffering this syndrome. They are often given

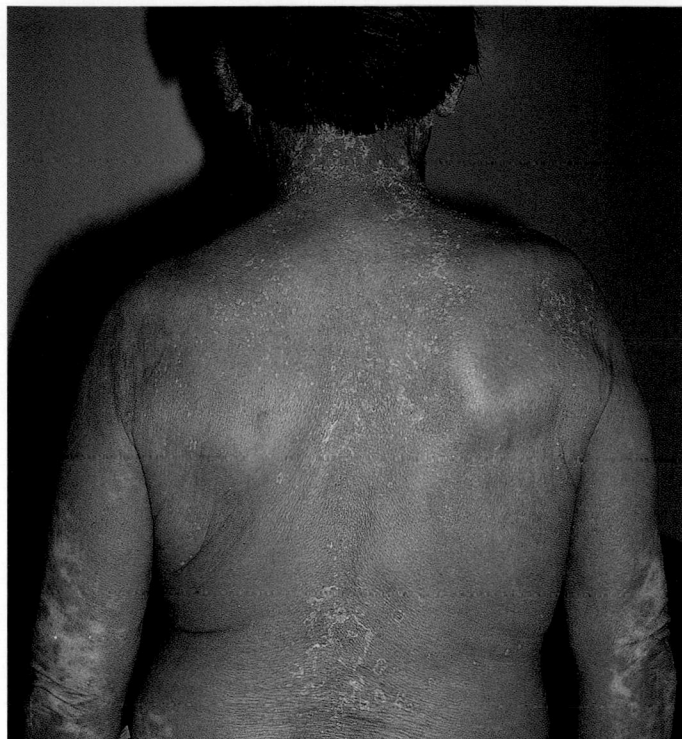

Fig. 6-20 Allopurinol hypersensitivity syndrome.

a dose not adjusted for their coexisting renal disease. They are frequently on a thiazide diuretic. Weeks to many months (average 7 weeks) after the allopurinol is begun, the patient develops a morbilliform eruption (50% of cases) that often evolves to an exfoliative erythroderma (20%) (Fig. 6-20). Bullae as a consequence of severe dermal edema may occur, especially on the palms and soles. Occasional oral ulcers may occur. Associated with the dermatitis are fever, eosinophilia, sometimes hepatitis (70% of cases), and typically worsening of renal function (40–80% of cases, the higher percentage in those with pre-existing renal disease). Lung involvement and adenopathy are uncommon. About 25% of patients die as a consequence of this syndrome, often from cardiovascular complications of the syndrome. Pancreatitis and subsequent insulin-dependent diabetes may occur as a complication. Dialysis does not appear to accelerate the resolution of the eruption, suggesting that if a drug metabolite is responsible, it is not dialyzable. It has been suggested that adjusting the allopurinol dose to compensate for the patient's impaired renal function might reduce the risk of developing this reaction. There is a strong association between HLA-B-5801 and the development of allopurinol hypersensitivity syndrome in the Han Chinese, but not in other races. HHV-6 reactivation may be associated. This syndrome may be steroid-responsive, but is extremely slow to resolve, frequently lasting for months after allopurinol has been stopped. Very gradual tapering of systemic steroids with monitoring of eosinophil count and renal function is essential. Too rapid tapering may lead to relapse of the syndrome.

Sulfonamide hypersensitivity syndrome

Fewer than 0.1% of treatment courses with sulfonamides are complicated by a hypersensitivity syndrome. Sulfonamide hypersensitivity syndrome is similar to that seen with the anticonvulsants, including the characteristic facial and periorbital edema. It typically begins 3 weeks after starting the medication, but may occur as soon as 1 week after. The skin eruption is usually morbilliform or an erythroderma. Patients with this

syndrome are often slow acetylators unable to detoxify the toxic and immunogenic metabolites generated during the metabolism of the sulfonamides. Patients with sulfonamide hypersensitivity syndrome may develop antibodies that recognize microsomal proteins to which the reactive metabolite of the sulfonamides binds. Hepatitis, nephropathy, pneumonitis, pericarditis, myocarditis, pancreatitis, and pleural effusion can all occur as a part of the syndrome. The hepatitis can be life-threatening. Sulfonamide hypersensitivity syndrome is treated with topical treatments appropriate for the skin eruption, and systemic steroids for systemic complications. Zonisamide, a sulfonamide anticonvulsant, cross-reacts with sulfonamides but not other anticonvulsants.

Minocycline hypersensitivity syndrome

Minocycline hypersensitivity syndrome occurs in young adults, usually in the context of acne therapy. Females are favored, as are those of Afro-Caribbean ancestry. Deficiency of glutathione S-transferases is common in affected individuals, and is more common in persons of Afro-Caribbean descent. In patients with minocycline hypersensitivity syndrome, minocycline may be detected in the blood up to 17 months after discontinuation of the medication, suggesting that slow metabolism and persistent levels of medication may play a role. The syndrome begins usually 2–4 weeks after starting the minocycline. Fever, a skin eruption, and adenopathy occur in more than 80% of cases. Headache and cough are common complaints. The eruption can be morbilliform, erythrodermic, or pustular. Facial edema is common. Liver involvement occurs in 75% of cases, and renal disease in 17%. Minocycline hypersensitivity is particularly associated with interstitial pneumonia with eosinophilia. This may progress to respiratory distress syndrome. It can be life-threatening, but most patients survive. Myocarditis has also been reported. Treatment is systemic steroids.

Dapsone hypersensitivity syndrome

Dapsone hypersensitivity syndrome occurs in <1% of patients given this medication. It usually begins 4 weeks or more after starting the drug. Hemolytic anemia and methemoglobinemia may be present. A morbilliform eruption that heals with desquamation is most characteristic. Icterus and lymphadenopathy occur in 80% of patients. Eosinophilia is typically NOT present. Liver involvement is a mixture of hepatocellular and cholestatic. The bilirubin is elevated in 85%, partly attributable to the hemolysis. Liver involvement may be fatal. Hypoalbuminemia is characteristic.

Abecassis S, et al: Severe sialadenitis: a new complication of drug reaction with eosinophilia and systematic symptoms. J Am Acad Dermatol 2004; 51:827.

Aota A, et al: Systematic lupus erythematosus presenting with Likuchi-Fujimoto's disease as a long-term sequela of drug-induced hypersensitivity syndrome. Dermatol 2009; 218:275.

Augusto JF, et al: A case of sulphasalazine-induced DRESS syndrome with delayed acute interstitial nephritis. Nephrol Dial Transplant 2009; 24:2940.

Balci DD, et al: Sulfasalazine-induced hypersensitivity syndrome in a 15-year-old boy associated with human herpesvirus-6 reactivation. Cutan Ocular Toxicol 2009; 18:45.

Ben m'rad M, et al: Drug-induced hypersensitivity syndrome. Clinical and biologic disease patterns in 24 patients. Med 2009; 88:131.

Boccara O, et al: Association of hypogammaglobulinemia with DRESS (drug rash with eosinophilia and systemic symptoms). Eur J Dermatol 2006; 16:666.

Brown RJ, et al: Minocycline-induced drug hypersensitivity syndrome followed by multiple autoimmune sequelae. Arch Dermatol 2009; 145:63.

Chan YC, et al: Allopurinol hypersensitivity syndrome and acute myocardial infarction—two case reports. Ann Acad Med Singapore 2002; 31:231.

Chen YC, et al: Drug reaction with eosinophilia and systemic symptoms. Arch Dermatol 2010; 198.

Eshki M, et al: Twelve-year analysis of severe cases of drug reaction with eosinophilia and systemic symptoms. Arch Dermatol 2009; 145:67.

Hung SL, et al: Genetic susceptibility to carbamazepine-induced cutaneous adverse drug reactions. Pharmacogenetics Genomics 2006; 16:297.

Kano Y, Shiohara T: The variable clinical picture of drug-induced hypersensitivity syndrome/drug rash with eosinophilia and systematic symptoms in relations to the eliciting drug. Immunol Allergy Clin N Am 2009; 29:481.

Komatsuda A, et al: Sulfasalazine-induced hypersensitivity syndrome and hemophagocytic syndrome associated with reactivation of Epstein–Barr virus. Clin Rheumatol 2008; 27:395.

Lee HY, et al: Allopurinol hypersensitivity syndrome: a preventable severe cutaneous adverse reaction. Singapore Med J 2008; 49:384.

Maubec E, et al: Minocycline-induced DRESS: evidence for accumulation of the culprit drug. Dermatol 2008; 216:200.

Neuman MG, et al: Predicting possible zonisamide hypersensitivity syndrome. Experimental Dermatol 2008; 17:1045.

Ohtani T, et al: Slow acetylator genotypes as a possible risk factor for infectious mononucleosis-like syndrome induced by salazosulfapyridine. Br J Dermatol 2003; 148:1035.

Oskay T, et al: Association of anticonvulsant hypersensitivity syndrome with herpesvirus 6, 7. Epilepsy Res 2006; 70:27.

Peyriere H, et al: Variability in the clinical pattern of cutaneous side-effects of drugs with systemic symptoms: does a DRESS syndrome really exist? Br J Dermatol 2006; 155:422.

Ragucci MV, et al: Gabapentin-induced hypersensitivity syndrome. Clin Neuropharmacol 2001; 24:103.

Robles DT, et al: Severe drug-hypersensitivity reaction in a young woman treated with doxycycline. Dermatol 2008; 217:23.

Scheuerman O, et al: Successful treatment of antiepileptic drug hypersensitivity syndrome with intravenous immune globulin. Pediatrics 2001; 107:E14.

Sommers LM, et al: Allopurinol hypersensitivity syndrome associated with pancreatic exocrine abnormalities and new-onset diabetes mellitus. Arch Dermatol 2002; 162:1190.

Tohyama M, et al: Association of human herpesvirus 6 reactivation with the flaring and severity of drug-induced hypersensitivity syndrome. Br J Dermatol 2007; 157:934.

Vauthey L, et al: Vancomycin-induced DRESS syndrome in a female patient. Dermatol 2008; 82:138.

Watanabe T, et al: Detection of human herpesvirus-6 transcripts in carbamazepine-induced hypersensitivity syndrome by in situ hybridization. J Dermatol Science 2009; 54:134.

Bullous drug reactions (Stevens–Johnson syndrome [SJS] and toxic epidermal necrolysis [TEN])

Skin blistering may complicate drug reactions in many ways. Medications may induce known autoimmune bullous diseases such as pemphigus (penicillamine) or linear IgA disease (vancomycin). Acute generalized exanthematous pustulosis may be so extensive as to cause a positive Nikolsky sign, and have a background of purpura and targetoid lesions, simulating SJS/TEN. Pseudoporphyria and other photodermatoses from drugs may form bullae. Cytokines may produce widespread bullous eruptions, perhaps through physiologic mechanisms. The term bullous drug reaction, however, most commonly refers to a drug reaction in the erythema multiforme group (Fig. 6-21). (For a complete discussion of other forms of erythema multiforme see Chapter 7.)

These are fortunately uncommon reactions to medications, with an incidence of 0.4–1.2 per million person-years for TEN and 1.2–6.0 per million person-years for SJS. These drug-induced forms of erythema multiforme are usually more extensive than herpes-associated erythema multiforme or mycoplasma-associated SJS, but at times the distinction may be difficult. The more severe the reaction, the more likely it is to be drug-induced (50% of cases of SJS and 80% of cases of TEN). The exact definitions of SJS and TEN remain arbitrary

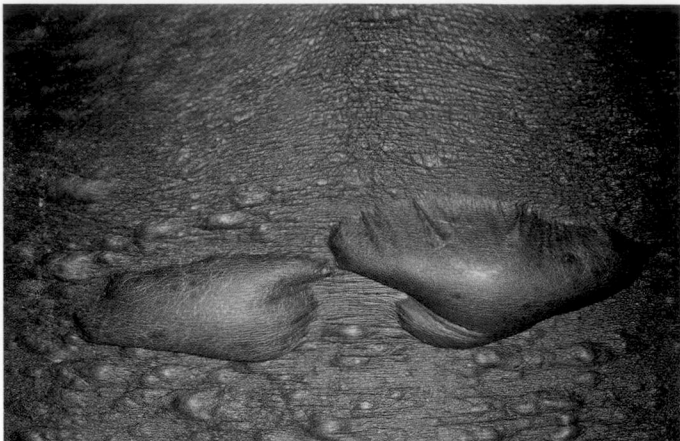

Fig. 6-21 Bullous drug reaction.

as a result of overlap in some cases. The following definitions are useful to classify cases: SJS has less than 10% body surface area (BSA) involved, cases with 10–30% are SJS–TEN overlap cases, and more than 30% BSA erosion is called TEN. SJS and TEN are considered by some as parts of a disease spectrum based on the following:

- They are most commonly induced by the same medications.
- Patients initially presenting with SJS may progress to extensive skin loss resembling TEN.
- The histologic findings are indistinguishable.
- Both are increased by the same magnitude in HIV infection.

However, recently, genetic evaluations of Caucasians with SJS and TEN showed distinct genetic predispositions for these conditions, allowing for consideration of them as distinct disorders.

The cause of SJS/TEN is not established. In Taiwan carbamazepine causes up to one-third of cases, but only 5% of cases in Europe. In Han Chinese the HLA haplotype HLA-B*1502 is present in the vast majority of cases of carbamazepine-induced SJS/TEN patients and is present in about 10% of the Han Chinese population in general. This HLA association is NOT found, however, in patients with carbamazepine-induced SJS/TEN of other ethnicities, suggesting that this marker for risk is specific for Asians. HLA typing should be performed in all Asians before starting carbamazepine, since the prevalence of HLA-B*1502 is 5–10% in Asians in the USA and Asia. HHV-6 reactivation may also be seen in SJS/TEN patients.

More than 100 medications have been reported to cause SJS and TEN. In adults, common inciting medications are trimethoprim–sulfamethoxazole (1–3 in 100 000), Fansidar-R, sulfadoxine plus pyrimethamine (10 in 100 000), nevirapine, lamotrigine (1 in 1000 adults and 3 in 1000 children), and carbamazepine (14 in 100 000). Antibiotics (especially long-acting sulfa drugs and penicillins), other anticonvulsants, anti-inflammatories (NSAIDs), and allopurinol are also frequent causes. Currently, in Europe, allopurinol is the most common cause of SJS and TEN. In children SJS/TEN is most commonly caused by sulfonamides and other antibiotics, antiepileptics, and acetaminophen. SJS/TEN from trimethoprim–sulfamethoxazole is significantly more common in the spring. If the inciting drug has a short half-life, and the drug is promptly stopped, the mortality is reduced from 26% to 5%. This suggests that the use of agents with short half-lives and the prompt discontinuation of the medication when the first signs of an adverse reaction appear may be very important ways to reduce the mortality from TEN.

Fever and influenza-like symptoms often precede the eruption by a few days. Skin lesions appear on the face and trunk and rapidly spread (usually within 4 days) to their maximum extent. Initial lesions are macular and may remain so, followed by desquamation, or may form atypical targets with purpuric centers that coalesce, form bullae, then slough. Patients with purpuric atypical targets may evolve more slowly, and usually the skin lesions are clinically inflammatory. In SJS, virtually always, two or more mucosal surfaces are also eroded, the oral mucosa and conjunctiva being most frequently affected. There may be photophobia, difficulty with swallowing, rectal erosions, painful urination, and cough, indicative of ocular, alimentary, urinary, and respiratory tract involvement, respectively. Over time more than 10% of the skin surface may be sloughed, leading to SJS/TEN overlap; if more than 30% of the skin is lost, a case is classified as TEN. In other patients, macular erythema is present in a local or widespread distribution over the trunk. Mucosal involvement may not be found. The epidermis in the areas of macular erythema rapidly becomes detached from the dermis, leading to extensive skin loss, often much more rapidly than occurs in the patients with atypical targets and extensive mucosal involvement. "Pure TEN" is a conceptual way of thinking of such patients. Rarely, SJS/TEN patients may present with lesions predominantly in sun-exposed areas, with a clear history of a recent significant sun exposure. This suggests that, in rare cases, SJS/TEN may be photo-induced or photo-exacerbated. Patients with SJS/TEN may have internal involvement very similar to patients with DRESS/DIHS induced by the same medication (see above). These most commonly include eosinophilia, hepatitis, and worsening renal function.

A skin biopsy is usually performed. Frozen-section analysis may lead to a rapid diagnosis. This is to exclude other diseases (such as staphylococcal scalded skin syndrome, pemphigus, graft versus host disease (GVHD), etc.) and to confirm the diagnosis. Independent of the extent of the slough, the clinical morphology (atypical targets as opposed to simple erythema), or the clinical diagnosis (SJS or TEN), the histology is similar. There is a lymphocytic infiltrate at the dermoepidermal junction with necrosis of keratinocytes that at times may be full-thickness. The infiltrate may be marked or very scant. Paraneoplastic pemphigus also shows changes of erythema multiforme and may be excluded with direct immunofluorescence. Patients with GVHD may also demonstrate a TEN-like picture with identical histology.

Management of these patients is similar to those with an extensive burn. They suffer fluid and electrolyte imbalances, bacteremia from loss of the protective skin barrier, hypercatabolism, and sometimes acute respiratory distress syndrome. Their metabolic and fluid requirements are less than in burn victims, however. Survival is improved if patients are cared for in a specialized "burn unit," or on a special dermatology unit with skill in managing these patients. Hospital dermatologists have greatly improved the care of such patients. Nutritional support is critical. Patients who are very ill or with more than 30–50% loss of epidermis should be transferred for such care. In addition to extent of skin loss, age, known malignancy, tachycardia, renal failure, hyperglycemia, and low bicarbonate are all risk factors for having a higher mortality with SJS/TEN. The SCORTEN gives one point for each of these findings. The SCORTEN total predicts mortality, with a 3.2% mortality for 0–1 points, and a 90% mortality for 5 or more points. However, respiratory tract involvement, not included in the SCORTEN, is also a bad prognostic sign. About one-quarter of TEN patients have bronchial involvement. In TEN, epithelial detachment of the respiratory mucosae and associated acute respiratory distress syndrome are associated with a mortality of 70%. Pre-existing diabetes mellitus and concurrent tuberculosis may also increase mortality.

The use of systemic agents to treat SJS/TEN is very controversial due to the rarity of these cases and the lack of controlled interventional trials. One important point appears to be that, whatever therapy is considered, it should be given early and in adequate doses. Low doses are associated with either lack of efficacy or medication complications without benefit. IVIG is now frequently used to manage the more severe adult and pediatric patients with bullous drug eruptions (TEN). A dose of 1 g/kg/day for the first 4 days following admission is effective. It is best used when detachment has not become extensive, as total BSA of skin loss is an important predictor of mortality.

Keratinocyte death in SJS and TEN is proposed to occur via two potential mechanisms, and the relative importance of each of these mechanisms in SJS and TEN is not known. Activated cytotoxic T cells and natural killer (NK) cells produce granulysin, perforin, and granzyme B, all of which can induce keratinocyte necrosis. In addition, keratinocyte necrosis can be induced by the binding of soluble Fas ligand (sFasL) to Fas (also known as the death receptor or CD95). Soluble Fas ligand is elevated in the blood of patients with TEN, and its level correlates with BSA involvement. In addition, the peripheral blood mononuclear cells of patients with TEN secrete Fas ligand upon exposure to the incriminated drug. The sera of patients with TEN induce necrosis of cultured keratinocytes, and a monoclonal antibody to Fas ligand in a dose-dependent fashion inhibits keratinocyte necrosis exposed to TEN patient sera. This strongly supports Fas expression by keratinocytes, and Fas ligand production by immune cells, as the mechanisms by which TEN is mediated. The proposed mechanism of action of IVIG in TEN is by IVIG blocking the binding of sFasL to Fas, stopping keratinocyte apoptosis.

The presence of cytotoxic T lymphocytes and NK cells within the dermis subjacent to the necrotic epidermis suggests that immunosuppressive agents that block immune function could also be effective in SJS or TEN. The role of immunosuppressive therapy, however, is very controversial. The benefit of immunosuppressives would be to stop the process very quickly and thereby reduce the ultimate amount of skin lost. Once most of the skin loss has occurred, immunosuppressives only add to the morbidity and perhaps mortality of the disorder. In children with SJS, this adverse effect has been documented, probably since their mortality is low and immunosuppressives only add risk for infection. Because SJS and TEN evolve rapidly (average 4 days to maximum extent), very early treatment would be required to observe benefit. Patients have developed TEN while undergoing systemic corticosteroid therapy in moderate to high doses (40–60 mg of prednisone equivalent daily), suggesting that this level of immunosuppression is insufficient to alter the evolution of SJS or TEN. If immunosuppressive treatment is considered, it should be used as soon as possible, given as a short trial to see if the process may be arrested, and then tapered rapidly to avoid the risk of immunosuppression in a patient with substantial loss of skin. High-dose corticosteroids given intravenously with reported success have included 100 mg of dexamethasone per day for 3 or 4 days and methylprednisolone, 30 mg/kg/day for 3 days. Cyclosporine in doses of 3–5 mg/kg/day for 8–24 days, with or without an initial burst of systemic steroids, has also been reported to stop SJS and TEN abruptly. Anecdotally, both etanercept, 25 mg twice, and infliximab, 5 mg/kg intravenously once, have led to rapid termination of skin sloughing. Systemic and topical steroid therapy for ocular involvement also appears to improve outcomes. In patients with SJS/TEN who also have systemic involvement as seen in DIHS (considered by some as SJS/TEN representing the cutaneous eruption of DIHS), systemic steroids should be considered.

For patients who survive, the average time for epidermal regrowth is 3 weeks. The most common sequelae are ocular scarring and vision loss. The only predictor of eventual visual complications is the severity of ocular involvement during the acute phase. A sicca-like syndrome with dry eyes may also result, even in patients who never had clinical ocular involvement during the acute episode. Other complications include cutaneous scarring, eruptive melanocytic lesions, and nail abnormalities. Transient, widespread verrucous hyperplasia resembling confluent seborrheic keratoses has also been reported.

Abe R: Toxic epidermal necrolysis and Stevens–Johnson syndrome: soluble Fas ligand involvement in the pathomechanisms of these diseases. J Dermatol Science 2008; 52:151.

Aihara Y, et al: Toxic epidermal necrolysis in a child successfully treated with cyclosporine A and methylprednisolone. Ped Int 2007; 49:659.

Araki Y, et al: Successful treatment of Stevens–Johnson syndrome with steroid pulse therapy at disease onset. Am J Ophthalmol 2009; 147:1004.

Assler H, et al: EM with mucous membrane involvement and SJS are clinically different disorders with distinct causes. Arch Dermatol 1995; 131:539.

Blitz JB, et al: Possible environment effects of sunscreen run-off. J Am Acad Dermatol 2008; 59:898.

Callaly EL, et al: Hydroxychloroquine-associated, photo-induced toxic epidermal necrolysis. Clin Exp Dermatol 2008; 33:572.

Chung WH, et al: Human leukocyte antigens and drug hypersensitivity. Current Opinion Allergy Clin Immunol 2007; 7:317.

Chung WH, et al: Granulysin is a key mediator for disseminated keratinocyte death in Stevens–Johnson syndrome and toxic epidermal necrolysis. Nature Med 2008; 14:1343.

Ferrell PB, et al: Carbamazepine, HLA-B*1502 and risk of Stevens–Johnson syndrome and toxic epidermal necrolysis: US FDA recommendations. Pharmacogenomics 2008; 9:1543.

Garcia-Doval I, et al: Toxic epidermal necrolysis and Stevens–Johnson syndrome: does early withdrawal of causative drugs decrease the risk of death? Arch Dermatol 2000; 136:323.

Garcia-Doval I, et al: Transient verrucous hyperplasia after toxic epidermal necrolysis. Br J Dermatol 2003; 149:1082.

Giuseppe F, et al: Etanercept for toxic epidermal necrolysis. Annals Pharmacother 2007; 41:1083.

Gueudry J, et al: Risk factors for the development of ocular complications of Stevens–Johnson syndrome and toxic epidermal necrolysis. Arch Dermatol 2009; 145:157.

Hague JS, et al: Respiratory involvement in toxic epidermal necrolysis portends a poor prognosis that may not be reflected in Scorten. Br J Dermatol 2007; 157:1294.

Hallgren J, et al: Stevens–Johnson syndrome associated with ciprofloxacin: a review of adverse cutaneous events reported in Sweden as associated with this drug. J Am Acad Dermatol 2003; 49:S267.

Hung SL, et al: Genetic susceptibility to carbamazepine-induced cutaneous adverse drug reactions. Pharmacogenetics Genom 2006; 16:297.

Hynes AY, et al: Controversy in the use of high-dose systematic steroids in the acute care of patients with Stevens–Johnson syndrome. Int Ophthalmol Clin 2005; 45:25.

Kardaun SH, et al: Dexamethasone pulse therapy for Stevens–Johnson syndrome/toxic epidermal necrolysis. Acta Derm Venereol 2007; 87:144.

Laffitte E, et al: Severe Stevens–Johnson syndrome induced by contrast medium iopentol (Imagopaque). Br J Dermatol 2004; 150:367.

Levi N, et al: Medications as risk factors of Stevens–Johnson syndrome and toxic epidermal necrolysis in children: a pooled analysis. Ped 2009; 123:e297.

Lonjou C, et al: A marker for Stevens–Johnson syndrome ethnicity matters. Pharmagenomics J 2006; 6:265.

Mayes T, et al: Energy requirements of pediatric patients with Stevens–Johnson syndrome and toxic epidermal necrolysis. Nutri Clin Prac 2008; 23:547.

Murata J, Abe R: Soluble Fas ligand: is it a critical mediator of toxic epidermal necrolysis and Stevens–Johnson syndrome? J Invest Dermatol 2007; 127:744.

Murata J, et al: Increased soluble Fas ligand levels in patients with Stevens–Johnson syndrome and toxic epidermal necrolysis preceding skin detachment. J Allergy Clin Immunol 2008; 122:992.

Petkov T, et al: Toxic epidermal necrolysis as a dermatological manifestation of drug hypersensitivity syndrome. Eur J Dermatol 2007; 17:422.

Pirmohamed M, et al: Investigation into the multidimensional genetic basis of drug-induced Stevens–Johnson syndrome and toxic epidermal necrolysis. Pharmacogenomics 2007; 12:1661.

Sevketoglu E, et al: Toxic epidermal necrolysis in a child after carbamazepine dosage increment. Pediatr Emer Care 2009; 25:93.

Sotozono C, et al: Diagnosis and treatment of Stevens–Johnson syndrome and toxic epidermal necrolysis with ocular complications. Am Acad Ophthal 2009; 116:685.

Srinivas RR: Suprapharmacologic doses of intravenous dexamethasone followed by cyclosporine in the treatment of toxic epidermal necrolysis. Indian J Dermatol Venereol Leprol 2008; 74:263.

Tay TL, et al: Stevens–Johnson syndrome and toxic epidermal necrolysis: efficacy of intravenous immunoglobulin and a review of treatment options. Singapore Med J 2009; 50:29.

Teraki Y, et al: Toxic epidermal necrolysis due to zonisamide associated with reactivation of human herpesvirus 6. Arch Dermatol 2008; 144:232.

Vaishampayan CSS, et al: Scorten: does it need modification? Indian J Dermatol Venereol Leprol 2008; 74:35.

Wanat KA, et al: Seasonal variation of Stevens–Johnson syndrome and toxic epidermal necrolysis associated with trimethoprim–sulfamethoxazole. J Am Acad Dermatol 2009; 60:589.

Wojtkiewics A, et al: Beneficial and rapid effect of infliximab on the course of toxic epidermal necrolysis. Acta Dermatol Venereol 2008; 88:420.

Yeung CK, et al: The timing of intravenous immunoglobulin therapy in Stevens–Johnson syndrome and toxic epidermal necrolysis. Clin Exp Dermatol 2005; 30:578.

Radiation-induced erythema multiforme

If phenytoin is given prophylactically in neurosurgical patients who are receiving whole-brain radiation therapy and systemic steroids, an unusual reaction occurs. As the dose of steroids is being reduced, erythema and edema initially appear on the head in the radiation ports. This evolves over 1 or 2 days to lesions with the clinical appearance and histology of SJS or even TEN. The eruption spreads caudad and mucosal involvement may occur (Fig. 6-22). A similar syndrome has been reported with the use of amifostine during radiation for head and neck cancers. This syndrome can rarely be seen with radiation therapy alone. If amifostine is used to reduce head and neck radiation-associated acute and chronic xerostomia, there is a significant risk of SJS/TEN.

Allanore LV, et al: Stevens–Johnson syndrome and toxic epidermal necrolysis induced by amifostine during head and neck radiotherapy. Radiotherapy Oncol 2008; 87:300.

Barbosa LA, Teixeira CB: Erythema multiforme associated with prophylactic use of phenytoin during cranial radiation therapy. Am J Health-Syst Pharm 2008; 65:1048.

Duncan KO, et al: SJS limited to multiple sites of radiation therapy in a patient receiving phenobarbital. J Am Acad Dermatol 1999; 40:493.

Metro G, et al: Brain radiotherapy during treatment with anticonvulsant therapy as a trigger for toxic epidermal necrolysis. Anticancer Res 2007; 27:1167.

HIV disease and drug reactions

HIV-infected patients, especially those with helper T-cell counts between 25 and 200, are at increased risk for the development of adverse reactions to medications. Morbilliform reactions to trimethoprim–sulfamethoxazole occur in 45% or

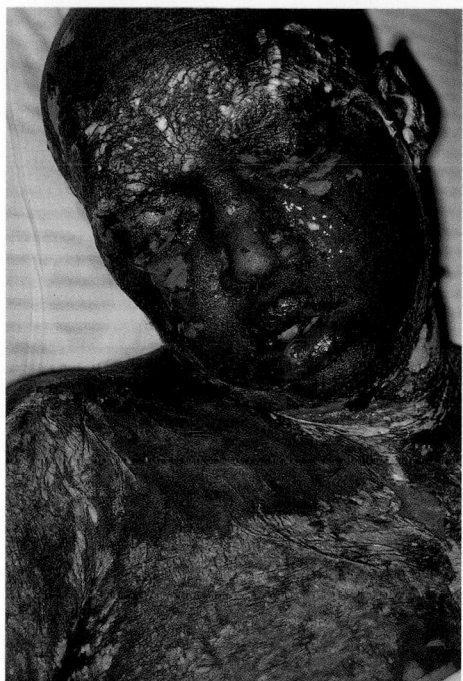

Fig. 6-22 Radiation-induced reaction.

more of AIDS patients being treated for *Pneumocystis jirovecii* (formerly *carinii*) pneumonia. In two-thirds of patients without life-threatening reactions, trimethoprim–sulfamethoxazole treatment can be continued with simple conservative support, and the eruption may resolve. Associated hepatitis or neutropenia may require discontinuation of the drug. A similar increased rate of reaction to amoxicillin–clavulanate in HIV is also seen. If the dermatitis is treatment-limiting but the eruption is not life-threatening, low-dose rechallenge/desensitization may be attempted. It is successful in 65–85% of patients in the short term, and in more than 50% in the long term. In fact, initial introduction of trimethoprim-sulfamethoxazole for prophylaxis by dose escalation reduces the rate of adverse reactions as well. However, rechallenge at full dose may have the same rate of recurrent eruptions as does introduction by dose escalation. Although low-dose rechallenge is usually safe, severe, acute reactions including marked hypotension may occur. Although most adverse reactions occur in the first few days of rechallenge, adverse reactions may appear months after restarting trimethoprim-sulfamethoxazole, and may be atypical in appearance. The mechanism of this increased adverse reaction to trimethoprim-sulfamethoxazole is unknown.

Severe bullous reactions, SJS, and TEN are between 100 and 1000 times more common per drug exposure in patients with AIDS. These reactions are usually caused by sulfa drugs, especially long-acting ones, but may be caused by many agents. Nevirapine, a non-nucleoside reverse transcriptase inhibitor, has been associated with a high rate of severe drug eruptions including SJS/TEN. Most of these adverse reactions are cutaneous and occur in the first 6 weeks of treatment. This high rate of reaction can be reduced by starting with a lower lead-in dose, and by concomitant treatment with prednisone during the induction period. Nevirapine hypersensitivity syndrome presents with fever, hepatitis, or rash. Over 1% of patients will develop SJS/TEN. HLA-DRB1*0101 patients are at increased risk for cutaneous reactions to nevirapine if not associated with hepatotoxicity. Hepatitis, but not cutaneous reactions, is seen more commonly in patients with CD4 counts above 200–250. Fixed drug eruptions are also frequently seen in patients with HIV infection. Abacavir is associated with a potentially life-threatening adverse reaction in 8% of patients. The syndrome includes fever, rash, gastrointestinal, or respiratory symptoms. It usually occurs in the first 6 weeks of treatment, but can happen within hours of the first dose. Rechallenge in these patients may lead to life-threatening hypotension and death. Abacavir hypersensitivity is increased in patients who are HLA-B*5701 positive, and screening of patients for this HLA type and not exposing patients with this HLA type to abacavir have decreased the number of cases of abacavir hypersensitivity syndrome. Adverse drug reactions to abacavir can also occur in HLA-B*5701-negative patients.

Aciclovir, nucleoside and non-nucleoside reverse transcriptase inhibitors (except nevirapine), and protease inhibitors are uncommon causes of ADRs. Many reactions attributed to these agents may actually be coexistent HIV-associated pruritic disorders, especially folliculitis, which are very common in patients with AIDS.

Borras-Blasco J, et al: Adverse cutaneous reactions associated with the newest antiretroviral drugs in patients with human immunodeficiency virus infection. J Antimicrob Chemot 2008; 62:879.

Capparelli EV, Syed SS: Nitazoxanide treatment of *Cryptosporidium parvum* in human immunodeficiency virus-infected children. Pediatr Infec Dis 2008; 27:1041.

Dolev J, et al: Treatment of recurring cutaneous drug reactions in patients with human immunodeficiency virus 1 infection. Arch Dermatol 2004; 140:1051.

Eliaszewicz M, et al: Prospective evaluation of risk factors of cutaneous drug reactions to sulfonamides in patients with AIDS. J Am Acad Dermatol 2002; 47:40.

Fox J, et al: An unusual abacavir reaction. J Acquir Immune Defic Syndr 2008; 22:1520.

Leng K, et al: Fatal outcome of nevirapine-associated toxic epidermal necrolysis. Int J STD and AIDS 2008; 19:642.

Metry DW, et al: Stevens–Johnson syndrome caused by the antiretroviral drug nevirapine. J Am Acad Dermatol 2001; 44:354.

Phanuphak N, et al: Nevirapine-associated toxicity in HIV-infected Thai men and women, including pregnant women. HIV Med 2007; 8:357.

Tebruegge M, et al: Human immunodeficiency virus-infected boy with Stevens–Johnson syndrome caused by nevirapine. Ped Infec Dis J 2008; 27:1041.

Vitezica ZG, et al: HLA-DRB1*01 associated with cutaneous hypersensitivity induced by nevirapine and efavirenz. J Acquir Immune Defic Syndr 2008; 22:540.

Fixed drug reactions

Fixed drug reactions (FDE) are common. Fixed drug eruptions are so named because they recur at the same site with each exposure to the medication. The time from ingestion of the offending agent to the appearance of symptoms is between 30 minutes and 8 hours, averaging 2 hours. In most patients, six or fewer lesions occur, and frequently only one. Uncommonly, fixed eruptions may be multifocal with numerous lesions (Fig. 6-23). They may present anywhere on the body, but half occur on the oral and genital mucosa. Fixed eruptions represent 2% of all genital ulcers evaluated at clinics for sexually transmitted diseases, and are not infrequent in young boys. In males lesions are usually unifocal and can affect the glans or shaft of the penis. FDE of the vulva is often symmetrical, presenting as an erosive vulvitis, with lesions on the labia minora and majora and extending on to the perineum. Other unusual variants of FDE include eczematous, urticarial, papular, purpuric, linear, giant, and psoriasiform. At times, some lesions of FDE will not reactivate with exposure due to a presumed "refractory period" which may last from weeks to months.

Clinically, an FDE begins as a red patch that soon evolves to an iris or target lesion similar to erythema multiforme, and may eventually blister and erode. Lesions of the genital and oral mucosa usually present as erosions. Most lesions are 1 to several cm in diameter, but larger plaques may occur,

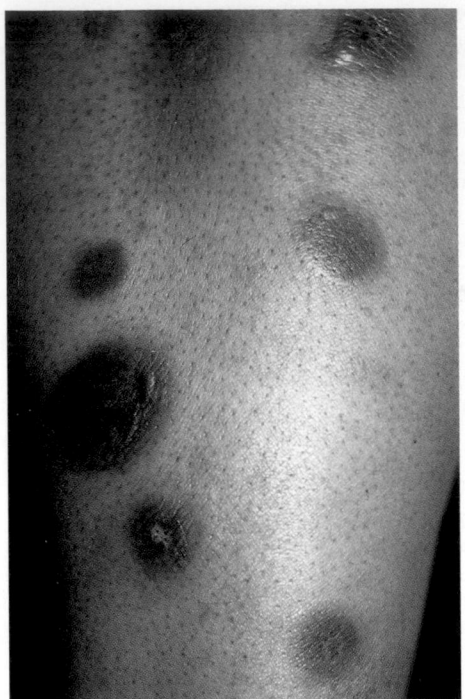

Fig. 6-23 Fixed drug reactions. (Courtesy of Dr L Lieblich)

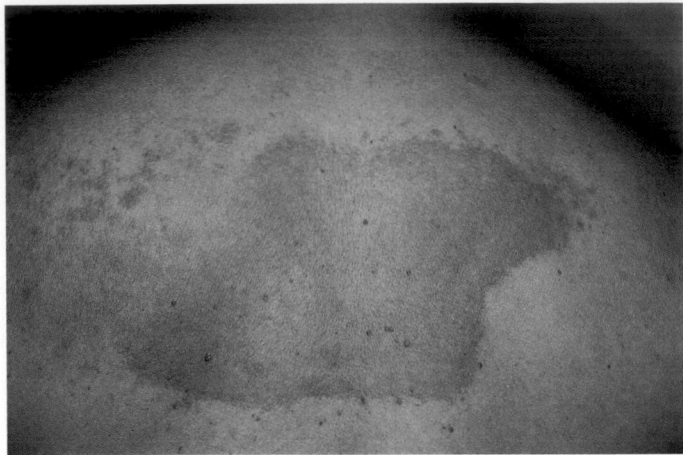

Fig. 6-24 Fixed drug eruption, nonpigmenting variant due to pseudoephedrine.

resembling cellulitis. Characteristically, prolonged or permanent postinflammatory hyperpigmentation results, although a nonpigmenting variant of an FDE is recognized. With repeated or continued ingestion of the offending medication, new lesions may be added, sometimes eventuating in a clinical picture similar to SJS. Histologically, an interface dermatitis occurs with subepidermal vesicle formation, necrosis of keratinocytes, and a mixed superficial and deep infiltrate of neutrophils, eosinophils, and mononuclear cells. Pigment incontinence is usually marked, correlating with the pigmentation resulting from FDEs. As biopsies are generally performed during the acute stage of a recurrence, the stratum corneum is normal. Papillary dermal fibrosis and deep perivascular pigment incontinence are commonly present from prior episodes. This contrast between a normal stratum corneum (suggesting an acute process) and chronic dermal changes is virtually pathognomonic of FDE.

Medications inducing FDEs are usually those taken intermittently. Many of the NSAIDs, especially pyrazolone derivatives, paracetamol, naproxen, oxicams, and mefenamic acid, cause FDE, with a special predilection for the lips. Sulfonamides, trimethoprim, or the combination are now responsible for the majority of genital FDEs. Barbiturates, tetracyclines, phenolphthalein (in laxatives), acetaminophen, cetirizine, celecoxib, dextromethorphan, hydroxyzine, quinine, lamotrigine, phenylpropanolamine, erythromycin, and Chinese and Japanese herbs are other possible causes. The risk of developing an FDE has been linked to HLA-B22. Patch tests with various concentrations of the offending medication can reproduce the lesion on affected but not unaffected skin. Tape-stripping the skin before applying the suspected medication in various vehicles may increase the likelihood of a positive patch test. This technique appears to be most useful in pyrazolone derivative-related reactions that are reproduced in 85% or more of cases.

Occasionally, FDEs do not result in long-lasting hyperpigmentation. The so-called nonpigmenting FDE is distinctive, and has two variants. One is the pseudo-cellulitis or scarlatiniform type which is characterized by large, tender, erythematous plaques that resolve completely within weeks, only to recur on reingestion of the offending drug (Fig. 6-24).

Pseudoephedrine hydrochloride is by far the most common culprit. The second variant is the baboon syndrome, also called symmetrical drug-related intertriginous and flexural exanthema (SDRIFE). SDRIFE preferentially affects the buttocks, groin, and axilla with erythematous, fixed plaques. Histologically, a giant cell lichenoid dermatitis can be seen in this setting.

The diagnosis of FDE is often straightforward and is elucidated by the history. However, confirmation with provocation tests can be performed. Due to the "refractory period," provocation tests need to be delayed at least 2 weeks from the last eruption. If an oral provocation test is considered, the initial challenge should be 10% of the standard dose, and patients with widespread lesions (SJS/TEN-like) should not be challenged. Patch testing using a drug concentration of 10–20% in petrolatum or water applied to a previously reacted site is the recommended approach. In most patients the treatment is simply to stop the medication. Desensitization can be successful.

Lesions of an FDE contain intraepidermal CD8+ T cells with the phenotypic markers of effector memory T cells. These epidermal-resident T cells produce IFN-γ. Such cells are found in resolved lesions of HSV, suggesting they are a defense mechanism preventing viral reactivation in the epidermis. Once the medication is stopped, the abundant CD4+ Fox P3+ T cells (T-regs) in lesions of FDE are felt to downregulate the eruption. In SJS/TEN patients, such T-regs are found in much fewer numbers than in FDE, explaining the progression of SJS/TEN despite stopping of the medication. Resident mast cells in lesions of FDE may be the cells initially activated with drug exposure, explaining the rapid onset of the lesion.

Abad RL, et al: Fixed drug eruption induced by phenylephrine: a case of polysensitivity. J Investig Allergol Clin Immunol 2009; 19:321.

Bandyopadhyay D: Celecoxib-induced fixed drug eruption. Clin Exp Dermatol 2003; 28:447.

Choonhakarn C: Non-pigmenting fixed drug eruption: a new case due to eperisone hydrochloride. Br J Dermatol 2001; 144:1288.

Drummond C, Fischer G: Vulval fixed drug eruption due to paracetamol. Aus J Dermatol 2009; 50:118.

Escobosa MC, et al: Exanthema and fixed drug eruption caused by trimethoprim. J Investig Allergol Clin Immunol 2009; 19:237.

Fujimoto N, Tajima S: Extensive fixed drug eruption due to the Japanese herbal drug "kakkon-to." Br J Dermatol 2003; 149:1292.

Gazquez V, et al: A case of fixed drug eruption due to quinine. Clin Exp Dermatol 2009; 34:95.

Handisurya A, et al: SDRIFE (baboon syndrome induced by penicillin). Clin Exp Dermatol 2008; 34:355.

Hayashi H, et al: Multiple fixed drug eruption caused by acetaminophen. Clin Exp Dermatol 2003; 28:447.

Heikkila H, et al: Fixed drug eruption due to phenylpropanolamine hydrochloride. Br J Dermatol 2000; 142:845.

Helmbold P, et al: Symmetric psychotropic and nonpigmenting fixed drug eruption due to cimetidine (so-called baboon syndrome). Dermatology 1998; 197:402.

Hsiao CJ, et al: Extensive fixed drug eruption due to lamotrigine. Br J Dermatol 2001; 144:1262.

Inamadar AC, et al: Multiple fixed drug eruptions due to cetirizine. Br J Dermatol 2002; 147:1020.

Katoulis AC, et al: Psoriasiform fixed drug eruption cause by nimesulide. Clin Exp Dermatol 2009; 34:e360.

Kawakami A, et al: Dextromethorphan induces multifocal fixed drug eruption. Int J Dermatol 2003; 42:501.

Khelifa-Hamdani E, et al: Giant cell lichenoid dermatitis in a patient with baboon syndrome. J Cutan Pathol 2008; 35:17.

Konotey-Ahulu FID, et al: Fixed drug eruptions. Br Med J 2009; 339:b2924.

Matsumoto K, et al: Nonpigmenting solitary fixed drug eruption caused by a Chinese traditional herbal medicine, ma huang (*Ephedra hebra*), mainly containing pseudoephedrine and ephedrine. J Am Acad Dermatol 2003; 48:629.

Min JA, et al: Fixed drug eruption caused by pamabrom. Clin Exp Dermatol 2009; 34:e455.

Mizukawa Y, et al: In vivo dynamics of intraepidermal CD8+ T cells and CD4+ T cells during the evolution of fixed drug eruption. Br J Dermatol 2008; 158:1230.

Nussinovitch M, et al: Fixed drug eruption in the genital area in 15 boys. Pediatr Dermatol 2002; 19:216.

Oyama N, Kanero F: Solitary fixed drug eruption caused by finasteride. J Am Acad Dermatol 2009; 60:168.

Ozkaya-Bayazit E: Specific site involvement in fixed drug eruption. J Am Acad Dermatol 2003; 49:1003.

Patriarca G, et al: Desensitization to co-trimoxazole in a patient with fixed drug eruption. J Investig Allergol Clin Immunol 2008; 18:309.

Rodriguez-Jimenez B, et al: Dimenhydrinate-induced fixed drug eruption in a patient who tolerated other antihistamines. J Investig Allergol Clin Immunol 2009; 19:321.

Ruiz-Genao DP, et al: Fixed drug eruption due to loratadine. Br J Dermatol 2002; 146:524.

Savin JA: Current causes of fixed drug eruption in the U.K. Br J Dermatol 2001; 145:667.

Sentruk N, et al: Topotecan-induced cellulitis-like fixed drug eruption. J Eur Acad Dermatol Venereol 2002; 16:411.

Shiohara T: Fixed drug: pathogenesis and diagnostic tests. Curr Opin Allergy Clin Immunol 2009; 9:316.

Short KA, et al: Fixed drug eruption following metronidazole therapy and the use of topical provocation testing in diagnosis. Clin Exp Dermatol 2002; 27:464.

Zedlitz S, et al: Reproducible identification of the causative drug of a fixed drug eruption by oral provocation and lesional patch testing. Contact Dermatitis 2002; 46:352.

Acute generalized exanthematous pustulosis

Acute generalized exanthematous pustulosis (AGEP), also known as toxic pustuloderma and pustular drug eruption, is an uncommon reaction with an incidence of 1–5 cases per million per year. The average age in Europe is in the fifties, and about one decade younger in Israel and Taiwan. Children can be affected. Women have been slightly more commonly affected until recently, when a strong female predominance has been identified. Drugs are the most common cause of this reaction pattern, but it has also been reported following mercury exposure. AGEP following viral and bacterial infections has been reported, but a causal association has not been validated. Similarly, *Loxoceles* bites have been followed by AGEP, but these patients in some cases have also received antibiotics. Recent reports of "acute localized exanthematous pustulosis" (ALEP) appear to be acneiform eruptions which occur acutely following antibiotic exposure. Their relationship to AGEP is unclear.

The eruption is of sudden onset, within 1 day in many cases associated with antibiotics, and averaging 11 days in other

Fig. 6-25 Acute generalized exanthematous pustulosis.

cases. The rash is accompanied by fever in most cases. Facial edema may be present. Initially, there is a scarlatiniform erythema. The eruption evolves and disseminates rapidly, consisting usually of more than 100 nonfollicular pustules less than 5 mm in diameter (Fig. 6-25). The Nikolsky sign may be positive. Mucous membrane involvement is common, but usually only affects one surface and is non-erosive. Laboratory abnormalities typically include a leukocytosis with neutrophilia (90%), and at times an eosinophilia (30%). Typically, the entire self-limited episode lasts up to 15 days. Characteristically, widespread superficial desquamation occurs as the eruption clears. The reported mortality is 5%. AGEP can recur with a second exposure to the medication.

In over 90% of cases, drugs are the cause of AGEP. Commonly implicated medications include ampicillin/amoxicillin, pristinamycin, quinolones, hydroxychloroquine, sulfonamide antibiotics, terbinafine, imatinib, and diltiazem. Corticosteroids, macrolides, oxicam, NSAIDs, pseudoephedrine, terazosin, omeprazole, sennoside, and antiepileptics have also caused AGEP. In some cases contact sensitivity has been implicated as a cause, with corticosteroids, mercury, bufexamac, and lacquer chicken the triggering agents. Recently radiocontrast material has been shown to cause AGEP. In 5% of cases, no trigger can be identified.

In the classic case, the diagnosis is straightforward, with the characteristic sudden and rapid onset, widespread pustulation, and self-limited course. The facial edema and pustulation can simulate DRESS/DIHS from anticonvulsants. In anticonvulsant hypersensitivity syndrome, eosinophilia, lymphadenopathy, atypical lymphocytosis, and liver dysfunction are often found. Recently, cases of AGEP have been reported with a prolonged course, widespread erosive mucosal lesions, and systemic involvement identical to DRESS/DIHS, suggesting that AGEP can be the eruption seen in anticonvulsant hypersensitivity syndrome. In about 1% or less of AGEP cases, skin lesions similar to SJS/TEN are seen. These include purpuric atypical targets and widespread skin loss. Biopsies may show AGEP with or without additional features of SJS/TEN. These cases are termed AGEP/TEN overlap. Pustular psoriasis, especially pustular psoriasis of pregnancy, can be difficult to differentiate from AGEP. If there are no characteristic lesions of psoriasis elsewhere, and no prior personal or family history of psoriasis, distinguishing these two entities may be impossible, and the patient may need to be followed for a final diagnosis to be made. Amicrobial pustulosis in the setting of a connective tissue disease can also resemble AGEP, but lesions are usually localized to the flexors and the course is more chronic.

Histologically, early lesions show marked papillary edema, neutrophil clusters in the dermal papillae, and perivascular eosinophils. There may be an associated leukocytoclastic vasculitis. Well-developed lesions show intraepidermal or subcorneal spongiform pustules. If there is a background of erythema multiforme clinically, the histologic features of erythema multiforme may be superimposed. The presence of eosinophils and the marked papillary edema help to distinguish this eruption from pustular psoriasis. However, pustular psoriasis of pregnancy is often associated with tissue eosinophilia.

Patch testing with the suspected agent may reproduce a pustular eruption on an erythematous base at 48 h in about 50% of cases. Patch testing rarely will result in a recrudescence of AGEP. AGEP is mediated by T cells, which produce high levels of IL-8, IFN-γ, IL-4 and 5, and GM-CSF. IL-8 is also produced by keratinocytes in lesions of AGEP.

Most patients with AGEP can be managed with topical steroids and antihistamines. In many cases, systemic steroids are also given. In severe cases infliximab and etanercept have rapidly stopped the pustulation and appeared to have hastened the resolution of the eruption. This approach has also been used in AGEP/TEN cases with success. Cyclosporine, as used for pustular psoriasis, has been used effectively in an AGEP case that relapsed as systemic steroids were tapered.

Attili SK, Ferguson J: Varenicline-induced acute generalized exanthematous pustulosis. Clin Exp Dermatol 2009; 34:e362.

Betto P, et al: Acute localized exanthematous pustulosis caused by amoxicillin-clavulanic acid. Int J Dermatol 2008; 47:295.

Cannistraci C, et al: Acute generalized exanthematous pustulosis in cystic echinococcosis: immunological characterization. Br J Dermatol 2003; 148:1245.

Gencoglan G, et al: The molecular mechanism of etanercept, an anti-tumor necrosis factor-α receptor-fusion protein, in the treatment of acute generalized exanthematous pustulosis. J Dermatol Treatment 2009; 20:241.

Gibbon KL, et al: Mesalazine-induced pustular drug eruption. J Am Acad Dermatol 2001; 45:S220.

Goh TK, et al: Acute generalized exanthematous pustulosis and toxic epidermal necrolysis induced by carbamazepine. Singapore Med J 2008; 49:507.

Golberg M, et al: Pustular psoriasis of pregnancy in a patient whose dermatosis showed features of acute generalized exanthematous pustulosis. Int J Dermatol 2009; 48:299.

Guevara-Gutierrez E, et al: Acute generalized exanthematous pustulosis: report of 12 cases and literature review. Int J Dermatol 2009; 48:253.

Halevy S: Acute generalized exanthematous pustulosis. Curr Opin Allergy Clin Immunol 2009; 9:322.

Hammerbeck AA, et al: Ioversol-induced acute generalized exanthematous pustulosis. Arch Dermatol 2009; 145:683.

Lateo S, et al: Localized toxic pustuloderma associated with nimesulide therapy confirmed by patch testing. Br J Dermatol 2002; 147:624.

Leclair MA, et al: Acute generalized exanthematous pustulosis with severe organ dysfunction. Canadian Med Assoc J 2009; 181:393.

Lernia VD, et al: Rapid clearing of acute generalized exanthematous pustulosis after administration of ciclosporin. Clin Exp Dermatol 2009; Jul 29 (Epub ahead of print).

Lim CSH, Lim SL: Acute generalized exanthematous pustulosis associated with asymptomatic *Mycoplasma pneumoniae* infection. Arch Dermatol 2009; 145:848.

Makris M, et al: Acute generalized exanthematous pustulosis triggered by a spider bite. Allergol Int 2009; 58:301.

Mashiah J, et al: A systemic reaction to patch testing for the evaluation of acute generalized exanthematous pustulosis. Arch Dermatol 2003; 139:1181.

Meiss F, et al: Overlap of acute generalized exanthematous pustulosis and toxic epidermal necrolysis: response to antitumour necrosis factor-α antibody infliximab: report of three cases. J Eur Acad Dermatol Venereol 2007; 21:717.

Oskay T, et al: Acute generalized exanthematous pustulosis induced by simvastatin. Clin Exp Dermatol 2003; 28:554.

Padial MA, et al: Acute generalized exanthematous pustulosis associated with pseudoephedrine. Br J Dermatol 2004; 150:139.

Pippirs U, et al: Acute generalized exanthematous pustulosis following a *Loxosceles* bite in Great Britain. Br J Dermatol 2009; 161:208.

Sadighha A: Etanercept in the treatment of a patient with acute generalized exanthematous pustulosis/toxic epidermal necrolysis: definition of a new model based on translational research. Int J Dermatol 2009; 48:908.

Sidoroff A, et al: Risk factors for acute generalized exanthematous pustulosis (AGEP)—results of a multinational case-control study (EuroScar). Br J Dermatol 2007; 157:989.

Son CH, et al: Acute generalized exanthematous pustulosis as a manifestation of carbamazepine hypersensitivity syndrome. J Investig Allergol Clin Immunol 2008; 18:461.

Treudler R, et al: Prolonged course of acute generalized exanthematous pustulosis with liver involvement due to sensitization to amoxicillin and paracetamol. Acta Derm Venereol 2009; 89:314.

Drug-induced pseudolymphoma

At times, exposure to medication may result in cutaneous inflammatory patterns that resemble lymphoma. These pseudolymphomatous drug eruptions may resemble either T-cell or B-cell lymphomas. The most common drug-induced pseudolymphoma is one resembling cutaneous T-cell lymphoma (CTCL) clinically and histologically. The most frequent setting in which they occur is that of a drug-induced hypersensitivity syndrome (DRESS/DIHS) as described above, in which, uncommonly, the histology may resemble cutaneous T-cell lymphoma. More rarely, medications may induce plaques or nodules, usually in elderly white men after many months of treatment. Lymphadenopathy and circulating Sézary cells may also be present. CD30-positive cells may be present in the infiltrate. Usually, other features such as keratinocyte necrosis and dermal edema help to distinguish these reactions from true lymphoma. Importantly, T-cell receptor gene rearrangements in the skin and blood may be positive (or show pseudoclones) in these drug-induced cases, representing a potential pitfall for the unwary physician. Pseudolymphoma resolves with discontinuation of the medication. The medication groups primarily responsible are anticonvulsants, sulfa drugs (including thiazide diuretics), dapsone, and antidepressants. Vaccinations and herbal supplements can also induce pseudolymphoma.

Boer A, et al: Pseudoclonality in cutaneous pseudolymphomas: a pitfall in interpretation of rearrangement studies. Br J Dermatol 2008; 159:394.

Choi TS, et al: Clinicopathological and genotypic aspects of anticonvulsant-induced pseudolymphoma syndrome. Br J Dermatol 2003; 148:730.

Cogrel O, et al: Sodium valproate-induced cutaneous pseudolymphoma followed by recurrence with carbamazepine. Br J Dermatol 2001; 144:1235.

Fine A, et al: Drug-associated lymphoma and pseudolymphoma: recognition and management. Dermatol Clin 2007; 2:233.

Gatti FR, et al: Pseudolymphoma as an adverse reaction to tamoxifen. J Eur Acad Dermatol Venereol 2008; 22:1004.

Maubec E, et al: Vaccination-induced cutaneous pseudolymphoma. J Amer Acad Dermatol 2005; 52:623.

Meyer S, et al: Cutaneous pseudolymphoma induced by *Cimicifuga racemosa*. Dermatol 2007; 214:94.

Stavrianeas NG, et al: Cutaneous pseudolymphoma following administration of lornoxicam. Acta Dermatol Venereol 2007; 87:453.

Welsh JP, et al: Lymphomatoid drug reaction secondary to methyl phenidate hydrochloride. Cutis 2008; 81:61.

Werner B, et al: Large CD30-positive cells in benign atypical lymphoid infiltrates of the skin. J Cutan Pathol 2008; 83:1100.

Urticaria/angioedema

Medications may induce urticaria by immunologic and non-immunologic mechanisms. In either case, clinically the lesions

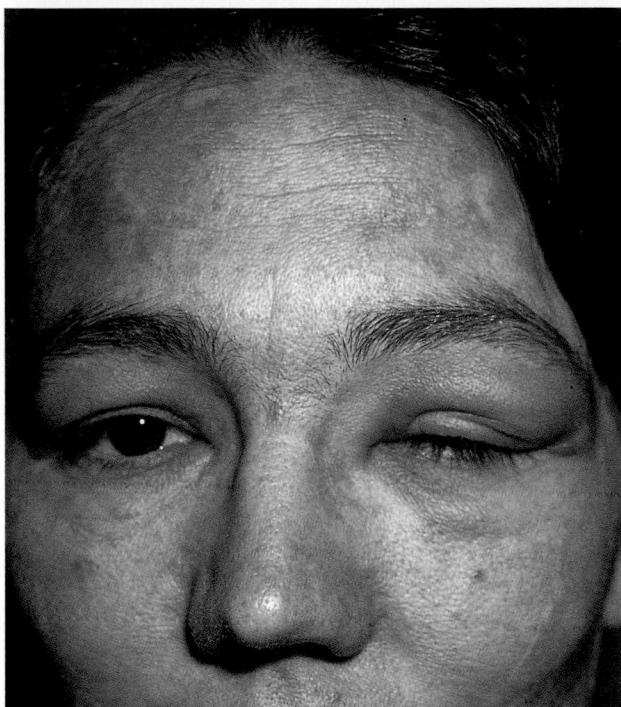

Fig. 6-26 Angioedema and urticaria.

are pruritic wheals or angioedema (Fig. 6-26). Urticaria may be part of a more severe anaphylactic reaction with broncho-spasm, laryngospasm, or hypotension. Immediate hypersensi-tivity skin testing and sometimes RAST is useful in evaluating risk for these patterns of reaction.

Aspirin and the NSAIDs are the most common causes of nonimmunologic urticarial reactions. They alter prostaglandin metabolism, enhancing degranulation of mast cells. They may therefore also exacerbate chronic urticaria of other causes. The nonacetylated salicylates (trilisate and salsalate) do not cross-react with aspirin in patients experiencing bronchospasm and may be safe alternatives. Some patients have urticaria to only one medication in this family, without cross-reaction with other NSAIDs, suggesting that specific IgE-mediated mecha-nisms may also be possible in NSAID-induced urticaria. Other agents causing nonimmunologic urticaria include radiocon-trast material, opiates, tubocurarine, and polymyxin B. Pretesting does not exclude the possibility of anaphylactoid reaction to radiocontrast material. The use of low-osmolarity radiocontrast material and pretreatment with antihistamines, systemic steroids, and in those with a history of asthma, theo-phylline, may reduce the likelihood of reaction to radiocon-trast material.

Immunologic urticaria is most commonly associated with penicillin and related β-lactam antibiotics. It is associated with IgE antibodies to penicillin or its metabolites. Skin testing with penicillin and its major and minor determinants is useful in evaluating patients with a history of urticaria associated with penicillin exposure. If the patient is skin test-positive, an alternative antibiotic must be considered, or the patient should be given penicillin in a desensitization protocol. Most patients with a history of penicillin "allergy" are skin test-negative. These patients can be treated with penicillin with a low likeli-hood of a severe adverse event. If a semisynthetic penicillin is associated with the initial reaction, the patient may be skin test-negative to the standard penicillin-derived reagents and still suffer anaphylaxis. This may be caused by IgE antibodies directed against the acyl side chain, in the case of amoxicillin. Patients with penicillin allergy have an increased rate of reac-

tion to cephalosporins. In the case of cefaclor, half of anaphy-lactic reactions occur in patients with a history of penicillin allergy. Third-generation cephalosporins are much less likely to induce a reaction in a penicillin-allergic patient than are first- or second-generation ones.

Bupropion is commonly used for depression and smoking cessation. It can induce urticaria, which may be associated with hepatitis and a serum sickness-like syndrome. Two anti-histamines, cetirizine and hydroxyzine, may induce urticaria, an apparent paradox which may lead to confusion in the clini-cal setting.

Angioedema is a known complication of the use of angiotensin-converting enzyme (ACE) inhibitors and angio-tensin II antagonists. Black persons are at nearly five times greater risk than white persons. Lisinopril and enalapril produce angioedema more commonly than captopril. Angioedema typically occurs within a week of starting therapy, but may begin after months of treatment. The episodes may be severe, requiring hospitalization in up to 45% of patients, intensive care in up to 27%, and intubation in up to 18%. One-quarter of patients affected give a history of previous angioedema. Captopril enhances the flare reaction around wheals. The angioedema appears to be dose-dependent, as it may resolve with decreased dose. All these factors suggest that the angioedema may represent a consequence of a normal pharmacologic effect of the ACE inhibitors. The blocking of kininase II by ACE inhibitors may increase tissue kinin levels, enhancing urticarial reactions and angioedema. Although this is dose-dependent, ACE inhibitor users with one episode of angioedema have a ten-fold risk of a second episode, and the recurrent episodes may be more severe. The treatment of urti-caria is discussed in Chapter 7.

Red man syndrome

The intravenous infusion of vancomycin is frequently compli-cated, especially if the infusion is rapid, by a characteristic reaction called "red man syndrome." At any time during the infusion, a macular eruption appears initially on the back of the neck, sometimes spreading to the upper trunk, face, and arms. Angioedema has been described. There is associated pruritus and "heat," as well as hypotension. The hypotension may be severe enough to cause cardiac arrest. Oral vanco-mycin has caused a similar reaction in a child. Children with systemic juvenile idiopathic arthritis (JIA) may suffer poten-tially fatal macrophage activation syndrome (MAS) during or after a red man reaction from vancomycin. The red man reac-tion is caused by elevated blood histamine. Red man syn-drome can be prevented in most patients by reducing the rate of infusion of the antibiotic, or by pretreatment with H_1 and H_2 antihistamines. While typically reported with vancomycin, similar "anaphylactoid" reactions have been seen with ciprofloxacin, amphotericin B, rifampin, infliximab, and teicoplanin.

Brown NJ, et al: Recurrent angiotensin-converting enzyme inhibitor-associated angioedema. JAMA 1997; 278:232.

Calista D, et al: Urticaria induced by cetirizine. Br J Dermatol 2001; 144:196.

Fays S, et al: Bupropion and generalized acute urticaria: eight cases. Br J Dermatol 2003; 148:177.

Lobel EZ, et al: Red man syndrome and infliximab. J Clin Gastroenterol 2003; 36:186.

Loo WJ, et al: Bupropion and generalized acute urticaria: a further case. Br J Dermatol 2003; 149:660.

Olgar S, et al: Does red-man reaction stimulate macrophage activation syndrome in children with systemic juvenile idiopathic arthritis? J Rheumatol 2007; 34:2491.

Renz CL, et al: Antihistamine prophylaxis permits rapid vancomycin infusion. Crit Care Med 1999; 27:9.

Sivagnanam S, et al: Red man syndrome. Crit Care 2003; 7:119.
Warner K, et al: Angiotensin II receptor blockers in patients with ACE inhibitor-induced angioedema. Ann Pharmacother 2000; 34:526.

Photosensitivity reactions (photosensitive drug reactions)

Medications may cause phototoxic, photoallergic, and lichenoid reactions, and photodistributed telangiectasias, as well as pseudoporphyria. The mechanisms of photosensitivity are discussed in Chapter 3. In many cases the mechanism for drug-induced photosensitivity is unknown. Most medication-related photosensitivity is triggered by radiation in the UVA range, partly for two reasons. First, most photosensitizing drugs have absorption spectra in the UVA and short-visible range (315–430 nm), and second, UVA penetrates into the dermis where the photosensitizing drug is present. The most common causes of photosensitivity are NSAIDs, trimethoprim–sulfamethoxazole, thiazide diuretics and related sulfonyl-ureas, quinine and quinidine, phenothiazines, and certain tetracyclines; numerous other medications in many classes induce photosensitivity less commonly.

Phototoxic reactions are related to the dose of both the medication and the UV irradiation. They potentially could occur in anyone if sufficient thresholds are reached, and do not require prior exposure or participation by the immune system. Persons of higher skin types are at lower risk of developing phototoxic eruptions in some studies. There is individual variation in the amount of photosensitivity created by a standard dose of medication, independent of serum concentration. This remains unexplained, but reflects the clinical setting, where interindividual variability in development of phototoxic eruptions is seen. Reactions can appear from hours to days after exposure. Tetracyclines (especially demeclocycline), amiodarone, and the NSAIDs are common culprits. The reaction may present as immediate burning with sun exposure (amiodarone, chlorpromazine) or exaggerated sunburn (fluoroquinolone antibiotics, chlorpromazine, amiodarone, thiazide diuretics, quinine, tetracyclines). Hyperpigmentation may complicate phototoxic reactions and may last for many months. Treatment may include dose reduction and photoprotection, with a sunblock with strong coverage through the whole UVA spectrum.

Photoallergic reactions are typically eczematous and pruritic, and may first appear weeks to months after drug exposure. They involve the immune system. Unfortunately, in the case of photoallergy to systemic medications, photopatch testing is infrequently positive and is of limited clinical value. In general, photoallergic reactions are not as drug dose-dependent as phototoxic reactions. Photosensitivity of both the phototoxic and photoallergic types may persist for months to years after the medication has been stopped. Photosensitivity reactions to various drugs are discussed individually below, emphasizing the characteristic patterns seen with each medication group.

Amiodarone photosensitivity develops in up to 75% of treated patients, and occurs after a cumulative dose of 40 g. A reduced minimal erythema dose (MED) to UVA, but not UVB, occurs, and gradually returns to normal between 12 and 24 months after stopping the medication. Stinging and burning may occur as soon as 30 min after sun exposure. Less commonly, a dusky, blue–red erythema of the face and dorsa of the hands occurs (Fig. 6-27). At times papular reactions are also seen. Desquamation, as seen following sunburn, is not observed following amiodarone photosensitivity reactions. This reaction may be dose-dependent and acute burning may be relieved by dose reduction. Narrow-band UVB may desensitize patients with persistent phototoxicity after stopping amiodarone.

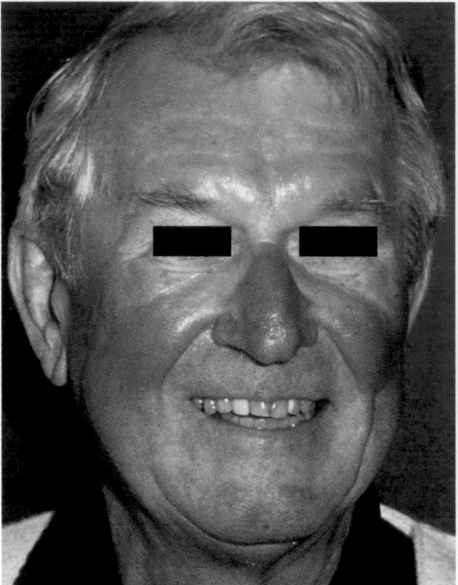

Fig. 6-27 Amiodarone pigmentation.

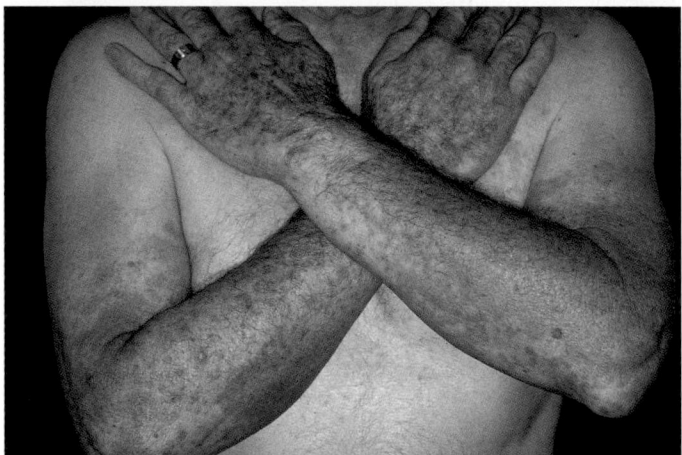

Fig. 6-28 Piroxicam photosensitivity.

NSAIDs, especially piroxicam, are frequently associated with photosensitivity (Fig. 6-28). The characteristic reaction is a vesicular eruption of the dorsa of the hands, sometimes associated with a dyshidrosiform pattern on the lateral aspects of the hands and fingers. In severe cases even the palms may be involved. Histologically, this reaction pattern shows intraepidermal spongiosis, exocytosis, and perivascular inflammatory cells—a pattern typical of photoallergy. However, this reaction may occur on the initial exposure to the medication, but phototoxicity tests in animals and humans have been negative. Patients with photosensitivity to piroxicam may also react to thiosalicylic acid, a common sensitizer in thimerosal. Half of patients having a positive patch test to thimerosal with no prior exposure to piroxicam are photopatch test-positive to piroxicam. This suggests that piroxicam reactions seen on initial exposure to the medication may be related to sensitization during prior thimerosal exposure. Topical exposure to ketoprofen (Orudis gel) can lead to a photoallergic contact dermatitis, and contamination of personal objects may lead to persistence despite stopping the use of the product.

Sulfonamide antibiotics, related hypoglycemic agents, and the sulfonylurea diuretics may all be associated with photosensitivity reactions. In addition, patients may tolerate one of the medications from this group, but when additional members of the group are added, clinical photosensitivity occurs. The typical pattern is erythema, scale, and in chronic cases, lichenification and hyperpigmentation.

Fluoroquinolone antibiotics are frequently associated with photosensitivity reactions. Sparfloxacin is highly photosensitizing; enoxacin, ciprofloxacin, and sitafloxacin are mildly photosensitizing; and levofloxacin rarely, if ever, causes photosensitivity.

Photodistributed lichenoid reactions have been reported most commonly from thiazide diuretics, quinidine, and NSAIDs, but also occur from diltiazem and clopidogrel bisulfate. They present as erythematous patches and plaques. Sometimes, typical Wickham's striae are observed in the lesions. Histologically, photodistributed lichenoid reactions are often indistinguishable from idiopathic lichen planus. Marked hyperpigmentation may occur, especially in persons of higher skin types (IV–VI), and especially in diltiazem-induced cases. The lichenoid nature of the eruption may not be clinically obvious, and histology is required to confirm the diagnosis. This hyperpigmentation may persist for months.

Voriconazole, a second-generation triazole, has been associated with an unusual combination of photosensitive phenomena. Photosensitivity occurs in 1–2% or more of patients taking voriconazole for more than 12 weeks. It appears to be UVA-induced, and is not dose-dependent. Usually, the photosensitivity is mild and with the use of sun protection and topical treatment the voriconazole can be continued. Cheilitis and facial erythema are typical initial manifestations. In a few patients, however, significant complications occur. Pseudoporphyria (with foot erosions as well), eruptive lentigines and atypical nevi, premature aging, and even the development of highly aggressive and potentially fatal squamous cell carcinomas in sun-exposed sites have been reported. Affected patients can closely resemble patients with xeroderma pigmentosa. Photodistributed granuloma annulare has also been seen by one of the authors (TB). This severe form of photosensitivity rapidly resolves with stopping of the voriconazole. Posaconazole can be an effective alternative.

Photodistributed telangiectasias are a rare complication of calcium channel blockers (nifedipine, felodipine, and amlodipine). UVA appears to be the action spectrum. Cefotaxime has also been reported to produce this reaction. Corticosteroids, oral contraceptives, isotretinoin, interferons (IFNs), lithium, thiothixene, lithium, methotrexate, and other medications may induce telangiectasias, but not via photosensitivity.

Pseudoporphyria is a photodistributed bullous reaction clinically and histologically resembling porphyria cutanea tarda (Fig. 6-29). Patients present with blistering on sun-exposed skin of the face and hands, and skin fragility. Varioliform scarring occurs in 70% of patients. Facial scarring is especially common in children with pseudoporphyria. Hypertrichosis is very rarely found; dyspigmentation and sclerodermoid changes are not reported. Porphyrin studies are normal. The blistering usually resolves gradually once the offending medication is stopped. However, skin fragility may persist for years. Naproxen is the most commonly reported cause. Up to 12% of children with JIA treated with NSAIDs may develop pseudoporphyria. Pseudoporphyria has also been reported to other NSAIDs (oxaprozin, nabumetone, ketoprofen, mefenamic acid [but not piroxicam]), tetracycline, furosemide, nalidixic acid, isotretinoin, acitretin, 5-fluorouracil, bumetanide, dapsone, oral contraceptives, rofecoxib, celecoxib, cyclosporine, voriconazole, and pyridoxine. Sunbed exposure and even excessive sun exposure can produce pseudoporphyria. Cases in women outnumber men by 24:1. Some women with sunbed-induced pseudoporphyria are on oral contraceptives. Patients on dialysis may develop pseudoporphyria, and N-acetylcysteine in doses up to 600 mg twice a day may lead to improvement in these cases. Histologically, a pauci-inflammatory subepidermal vesicle is seen. Direct immunofluorescence may show immunoglobulin and complement deposition at the dermoepidermal junction and perivascularly, as seen in porphyria cutanea tarda.

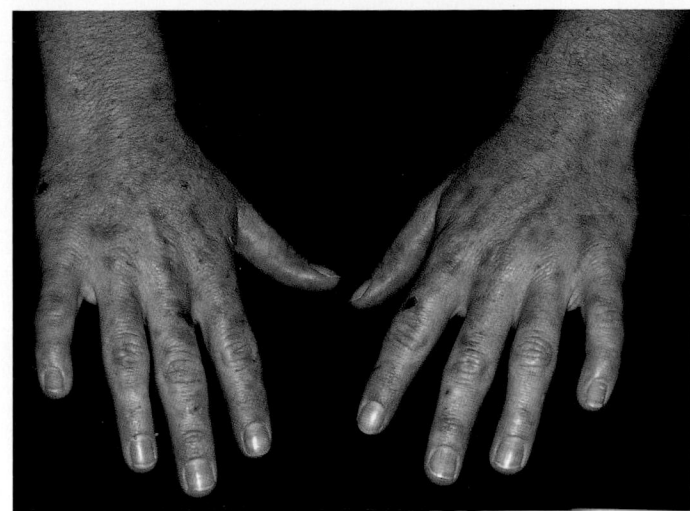

Fig. 6-29 Sixteen-year-old with scarring from pseudo-porphyria cutanea tarda reaction to tetracycline.

Borgia F, et al: Photodistributed telangiectasia following use of cefotaxime. Br J Dermatol 2000; 143:674.

Bryant P, Lachman P: Pseudoporphyria secondary to non-steroidal anti-inflammatory drugs. Arch Dis Child 2003; 88:961.

Conilleau V, et al: Photoscratch testing in systemic drug-induced photosensitivity. Photodermatol Photoimmunol Photomed 2000; 16:62.

Cummins R, et al: Pseudoporphyria induced by celecoxib in a patient with juvenile rheumatoid arthritis. J Rheumatol 2000; 27:2938.

Dawe RS, et al: A randomized controlled trial (volunteer study) of sitafloxacin, enoxacin, levofloxacin and sparfloxacin phototoxicity. Br J Dermatol 2003; 149:1232.

De Silva B, et al: Pseudoporphyria and nonsteroidal anti-inflammatory agents in children with juvenile idiopathic arthritis. Pediatr Dermatol 2000; 17:480.

Dogra S, Kanwar AJ: Clopidogrel bisulphate-induced photosensitive lichenoid eruption: first report. Br J Dermatol 2003; 148:593.

Dolan CK, et al: Pseudoporphyria as a result of voriconazole use: a case report. Int J Dermatol 2004; 43:768.

Ferguson J: Photosensitivity due to drugs. Photodermatol Photoimmunol Photomed 2002; 18:262.

Grabczynska SA, Cowley N: Amlodipine-induced photosensitivity presenting as telangiectasia. Br J Dermatol 2000; 142:1255.

Green JJ, Manders SM: Pseudoporphyria. J Am Acad Dermatol 2001; 44:100.

Hindsen M, et al: Photoallergic contact dermatitis from ketoprofen induced by drug-contaminated personal objects. J Am Acad Dermatol 2004; 50:215.

Hivnor C, et al: Cyclosporine-induced pseudoporphyria. Arch Dermatol 2003; 139:1373.

Janssen A, et al: Ann Dermatol Venereol 2006; 133:330.

Johnston GA, Coulson GA: Thiazide-induced lichenoid photosensitivity. Clin Exp Dermatol 2002; 27:670.

LaDuca JR, et al: Nonsteroidal anti-inflammatory drug-induced pseudoporphyria: a case series. J Cutan Med Surg 2002; 6:320.

Lim DS, Murphy GM: High-level ultraviolet A photoprotection is needed to prevent doxycycline phototoxicity: lessons learned in East Timor. Br J Dermatol 2003; 149:193.

Malani AN, et al: Voriconazole-induced photosensitivity. Clin Med Res 2008; 6:83.

McCarthy K, et al: Severe photosensitivity causing multifocal squamous cell carcinomas secondary to prolonged voriconazole therapy. Clin Infect Dis 2007; 44:e55.

Racette AJ, et al: Photoaging and phototoxicity from long-term voriconazole treatment in a 15-year-old girl. J Am Acad Dermatol 2005; 52:S81.

Schanbacher CF, et al: Pseudoporphyria: a clinical and biochemical study of 20 patients. Mayo Clin Proc 2001; 76:488.

Scherschun L, et al: Diltiazem-associated photodistributed hyperpigmentation: a review of 4 cases. Arch Dermatol 2001; 137:179.

Sharp MT, et al: Pseudoporphyria induced by voriconazole. J Am Acad Dermatol 2005; 53:341.

Silver EA, et al: Pseudoporphyria induced by oral contraceptive pills. Arch Dermatol 2003; 139:227.

Tolland JP, et al: Voriconazole-induced pseudoporphyria. Photodermatol Photoimmunol Photomed 2007; 23:29.

Tremblay JF, Veilleux B: Pseudoporphyria associated with hemodialysis treated with N-acetylcysteine. J Am Acad Dermatol 2003; 49:1189.

Anticoagulant-induced skin necrosis

Both warfarin and heparin induce lesions of cutaneous necrosis, albeit by different mechanisms. Obese, postmenopausal women are predisposed, and lesions tend to occur in areas with abundant subcutaneous fat such as the breast, abdomen, thigh, or buttocks

Warfarin-induced skin necrosis (WISN) usually occurs 3–5 days after therapy is begun, and a high initial dose increases the risk. Cases with a much more delayed onset (up to 15 years) are ascribed to noncompliance, drug–drug interactions, and liver dysfunction. WISN occurs in 1 in 1000 to 1 in 10 000 persons treated with warfarin. Lesions begin as red, painful plaques that develop petechiae, then form a large bulla. Necrosis follows (Fig. 6-30). Priapism can complicate warfarin necrosis. A less common variant seen in patients with a deep venous thrombosis (DVT) of an extremity is necrosis of a distal extremity, usually the one in which the patient has the DVT. Hereditary or acquired deficiency of protein C, and less commonly protein S, antithrombin III, or factor V Leiden and lupus anticoagulant syndrome are associated. Early in warfarin treatment the serum levels of the vitamin K-dependent antithrombotic protein C fall. Since the half-life of antithrombotic protein C is shorter than those of the vitamin K-dependent prothrombotic factors II, X, and IX, an acquired state of reduced protein C level occurs before the clotting factors are reduced. This creates a temporary prothrombotic state. This is more likely to occur if the levels of protein C are already low, if other antithrombotic proteins are deficient, or if the patient has an associated hypercoagulable state. This explains why the syndrome does not always recur with gradual reinstitution of warfarin, and has been reported to resolve with continued warfarin treatment. Histologically, noninflammatory thrombosis with fibrin in the subcutaneous and dermal vessels is seen. Treatment is to stop the warfarin, administer vitamin K to reverse the warfarin, and begin heparin or low molecular weight heparin. Administration of purified protein C can rapidly reverse the syndrome, as well as associated priapism. Untreated, the reaction can be fatal.

Heparin induces necrosis both at the sites of local injections and in a widespread pattern when infused intravenously or given by local injection. Local reactions are the most common. Heparin can also induce local allergic reactions at injection sites, which are distinct from the necrosis syndrome. Independent of its method of delivery, heparin-induced skin necrosis lesions present as tender red plaques that undergo necrosis, usually 6–12 days after the heparin treatments are started. Unfractionated heparin is more likely to cause this complication than fractionated low molecular weight heparin, and postoperative surgical patients are at greater risk than medical patients. Even the heparin used for dialysis may be associated with cutaneous necrosis, simulating calciphylaxis. Some necrotic reactions to local injections, and most disseminated reactions occurring with intravenous heparin, are associated with heparin-induced thrombocytopenia (HIT). Patients with underlying prothrombotic conditions, such as factor V Leiden and prothrombin mutations or elevated levels of factor VIII, may develop severe skin lesions if they develop HIT and heparin necrosis. A heparin-dependent antiplatelet antibody is the pathogenic basis of HIT and apparently of heparin-induced skin necrosis. This antibody causes both the thrombocytopenia and the aggregation of platelets in vessels, leading to thrombosis (white clot syndrome). The antibody may appear up to 3 weeks after the heparin has been discontinued, so the onset of the syndrome may be delayed. Histologically, fibrin thrombi are less reproducibly found in affected tissues, since the vascular thrombosis is the result of platelet aggregation, not protein deposition. The process may not only produce infarcts in the skin, but also may cause arterial thrombosis of the limbs, heart, lung, and brain, resulting in significant morbidity or mortality. Bilateral adrenal necrosis due to hemorrhagic infarction can occur and, if not detected early, may lead to death due to acute Addisonian crisis. The syndrome must be recognized immediately in anyone receiving heparin with late-developing thrombocytopenia. The treatment is to stop the heparin and give a direct thrombin inhibitor and vitamin K. After the platelet count has returned to normal, warfarin therapy is commonly given for 3–6 months. Patients with HIT cannot be treated with warfarin immediately, as the warfarin would be ineffective in stopping the thrombosis (it is NOT antithrombotic) and may worsen the thrombosis by enhancing coagulation. The diagnosis of HIT can be delayed because the antiplatelet antibody may not be present while the platelet count is falling. Adding warfarin at this time can lead to disastrous widespread acral thrombosis resembling disseminated intravascular coagulopathy (DIC).

Patients with cancer, an acquired prothrombotic state, are at increased risk for DVT. If they are treated with heparin and develop heparin-induced thrombocytopenia, they are at extreme risk for the development of a prothrombotic state if treated with warfarin. In this setting, digital and limb gangrene has occurred in the face of normal peripheral pulses and super-therapeutic anticoagulation by standard measures (INR). The consumptive coagulopathy induced by the cancer is the underlying trigger.

Abdel-Wahab O, et al: Warfarin-induced skin necrosis in a patient with heparin-induced thrombocytopenia: two diseases or one? Acta Haematol 2008; 120:117.

Barginear MF, et al: Heparin-induced thrombocytopenia complicating hemodialysis. Clin Applied Thrombosis/Hemostasis 2008; 14:105.

Nadir Y, et al: A fatal case of enoxaparin-induced skin necrosis and thrombophilia. Eur J Haematol 2006; 77:166.

Nazarian R, et al: Warfarin-induced skin necrosis. J Am Acad Dermatol 2009; 61:325.

Ng T, et al: Warfarin-induced skin necrosis associated with factor V Leiden and protein S deficiency. Clin Lab Haem 2001; 23:261.

Parsi K, et al: Warfarin-induced skin necrosis associated with acquired protein C deficiency. Australas J Dermatol 2003; 44:57.

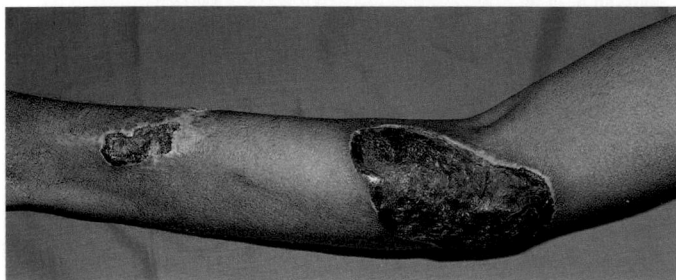

Fig. 6-30 Warfarin necrosis

Rafiei N, et al: Warfarin-induced skin necrosis of the eyelids. Arch Ophthalmol 2007; 125:421.

Simbelman J, et al: Unusual complications of warfarin therapy: skin necrosis and priapism. J Pediatr 2000; 137:266.

Takwale A, et al: British Society for Paediatric Dermatology 17th Annual Symposium, Bristol, 8–9 November 2002. Summaries of papers: heparin skin necrosis in a child. Br J Dermatol 2003; 148:1292.

Ward CT, et al: A typical warfarin-induced skin necrosis. Pharmacotherapy 2006; 26:1175.

Warkentin TE: Venous limb gangrene during warfarin treatment of cancer-associated deep venous thrombosis. Ann Intern Med 2001; 135:589.

Warkentin TE: Think of HIT. Hematol Am Soc Hematol Edu Program 2006; 408.

Warkentin TE, et al: Warfarin-associated multiple digital necrosis complicating heparin-induced thrombocytopenia and Raynaud's phenomenon after aortic valve replacement for adenocarcinoma-associated thrombotic endocarditis. Am J Hematol 2001; 75:56.

Warkentin TE, et al: Delayed-onset heparin-induced thrombocytopenia and cerebral thrombosis after a single administration of unfractionated heparin. N Engl J Med 2003; 348:1067.

Vitamin K reactions

Several days to 2 weeks after injection of vitamin K, an allergic reaction at the site of injection may occur (Fig. 6-31). Most affected persons have liver disease and are being treated for elevated prothrombin times. The lesions are pruritic red patches or plaques that can be deep-seated, involving the dermis and subcutaneous tissue. There may be superficial vesiculation. Lesions occur most commonly on the posterior arm and over the hip or buttocks. Plaques on the hip tend to progress around the waist and down the thigh, forming a "cowboy gunbelt and holster" pattern. Generalized eczematous small papules may occur on other skin sites in severe reactions. These reactions usually persist for 1–3 weeks, but may persist much longer, or resolve only to recur spontaneously. On testing, patients with this pattern of reaction are positive on intradermal testing to the pure vitamin K_1.

In Europe, a second pattern of vitamin K reaction has been reported. Subcutaneous sclerosis with or without fasciitis appears at the site of injections many months after vitamin K treatment. There may have been a preceding acute reaction as described above. Peripheral eosinophilia may be found. These pseudosclerodermatous reactions have been termed Texier's disease, and last several years.

The addition of vitamin K_1 to cosmetics has led to allergic contact dermatitis due to the vitamin K, confirmed by patch testing.

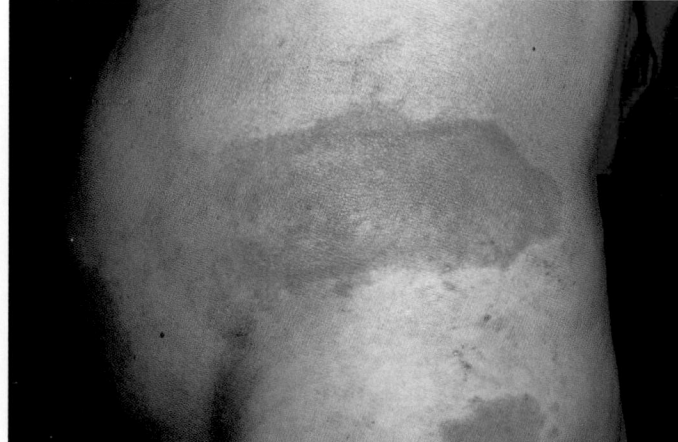

Fig. 6-31 Vitamin K allergy.

Injection site reactions

In addition to allergic reactions, as described with vitamin K, cutaneous necrosis may occur at sites of medication injections. These are of two typical forms: those associated with intravenous infusions and those related to intramuscular injections. Pharmacologic agents that extravasate into tissue during intravenous infusion may cause local tissue necrosis resulting from inherent tissue-toxic properties. These include chemotherapeutic agents, calcium salts, radiocontrast material, and nafcillin.

Intramuscular injections may produce a syndrome called embolia cutis medicamentosa, livedoid dermatitis, or Nicolau syndrome. Immediately after injection there is local intense pain and the overlying skin blanches (ischemic pallor). Within minutes to hours the site develops an erythematous macule that evolves into a livedoid violaceous patch with dendrites. This becomes hemorrhagic, then ulcerates, often forming a deep ulcer of many centimeters in diameter. Eventually (over weeks to months) the ulcer heals with an atrophic scar. Muscle and liver enzymes may be elevated, and neurologic symptoms and sequelae occur in a third of patients. The circulation of the limb may be affected, rarely leading to amputation. This syndrome has been seen with injection of many unrelated agents, including NSAIDs, local anesthetics, corticosteroids, antibiotics, IFN-α, sedatives, vaccines, and Depo-Provera. It appears to be caused by periarterial injection leading to arterial thrombosis. IFN-β injections into subcutaneous tissue of the abdomen, buttocks, or thighs of patients with multiple sclerosis has resulted in similar lesions. Patient education and auto-injectors can prevent this complication. Biopsy of the interferon injection site reactions resembles lupus panniculitis. Treatment of Nicolau syndrome is conservative: dressing changes, debridement, bed rest, and pain control. Surgical intervention is rarely required.

Arrue I, et al: Lupus-like reaction to interferon at the injection site: report of five cases. J Cutan Pathol 2007; 34:18.

Clark SM, et al: Acute necrotic skin reaction to intramuscular Depo-Provera. Br J Dermatol 2000; 143:1356.

Conroy M, et al: Interferon-beta injection site reaction: review of the histology and report of a lupus-like pattern. J Am Acad Dermatol 2008; 59:S48.

Corrazza M, et al: Five cases of livedo-like dermatitis (Nicolau's syndrome) due to bismuth salts and various other non-steroidal anti-inflammatory drugs. J Eur Acad Dermatol Venereol 2001; 15:585.

De Sousa R, et al: Nicolau syndrome following intramuscular benzathine penicillin. J Postgrad Med 2008; 54:332.

Ezzedine K, et al: Nicolau syndrome following diclofenac administration. Br J Dermatol 2004; 150:367.

Gettler SL, et al: Off-center fold: indurated plaques on the arms of a 52-year-old man. Diagnosis: cutaneous reaction to phytonadione injection. Arch Dermatol 2001; 137:957.

Gimenez-Arnau AM, et al: Immediate cutaneous hypersensitivity response to phytomenadione induced by vitamin K, in procedure. Contact Dermatitis 2005; 52:284.

Gono T, et al: Lupus erythematosus profundus (lupus panniculitis) induced by interferon-β in a multiple sclerosis patient. J Clin Neurosci 2007; 14:997.

Guarneri C, et al: Embolia cutis medicamentosa following thiocolchicoside injection. J Eur Acad Dermatol Venereol 2008; 22:1005.

Hamilton B, et al: Nicolau syndrome in an athlete following intramuscular diclofenac injection. Acta Orthop Belg 2008; 74:860.

Kienast AK, et al: Nicolau's syndrome induced by intramuscular vaccinations in children: report of seven patients and review of the literature. Clin Exp Dermatol 2008; 33:555.

Koontz D, Alshekhlee A: Embolia cutis medicamentosa following interferon beta injection. Multiple Sclerosis 2007; 13:1203.

Luton K, et al: Nicolau syndrome: three cases and review. Int J Dermatol 2006; 45:1326.

Ruiz-Hornillos FJ, et al: Allergic contact dermatitis due to vitamin K, contained in a cosmetic cream. Contact Dermatitis 2006; 55:246.

Drug-induced pigmentation

Pigmentation of the skin may occur as a consequence of drug administration. The mechanism may be postinflammatory hyperpigmentation in some cases but frequently is related to actual deposition of the offending drug in the skin.

Minocycline induces many types of hyperpigmentation, which may occur in various combinations in the affected patient. Classically, three types of pigmentation are described. Type I is a blue–black discoloration appearing in areas of prior inflammation, often acne or surgical scars (Fig. 6-32). This may be the most common type seen by dermatologists. It does not appear to be related to the total or daily dose of exposure. In all other types of pigmentation resulting from minocycline, the incidence increases with total dose, with up to 40% of treated patients experiencing hyperpigmentation with more than 1 year of therapy. The second type (type II) is the appearance of a similar-colored pigmentation on the normal skin of the anterior shins, analogous to that seen in antimalarial-induced hyperpigmentation. It is initially mistaken for ecchymoses, but does not fade quickly. In most cases, types I and II minocycline pigmentation occur after 3 months to several years of treatment. Generalized black hyperpigmentation has occurred after several days or a few weeks of treatment in Japanese patients. In type I and II minocycline hyperpigmentation, histologic evaluation reveals pigment granules within macrophages in the dermis (and at times in the fat), very similar to a tattoo. These granules usually stain positively for both iron and melanin, the usual method for confirming the diagnosis. At times the macrophages containing minocycline are found only in the subcutaneous fat. Stains for iron may be negative in some cases. Calcium stains may also be positive, as minocycline binds calcium. In unusual cases electron microscopy or sophisticated chemical analysis can confirm the presence of minocycline in the granules. The least common type (type III) is generalized, muddy brown hyperpigmentation, accentuated in sun-exposed areas. Tigecycline may produce similar hyperpigmentation. Histologic examination reveals only increased epidermal and dermal melanin. This may represent the consequence of a low-grade photosensitivity reaction.

In addition to the skin, minocycline type I and II pigmentation may also involve the sclera, conjunctiva, bone, thyroid, ear cartilage (simulating alkaptonuria), nailbed, oral mucosa, and permanent teeth. Tetracycline staining of the teeth is usually related to childhood or fetal exposure, is brown, and is accentuated on the gingival third of the teeth. Dental hyperpigmentation due to minocycline in contrast occurs in adults, is gray or gray–green, and is most marked in the midportion of the tooth. Some patients with affected teeth do not have hyperpigmentation elsewhere. Cutaneous hyperpigmentation from minocycline fades slowly and the teeth may remain pigmented for years. The blue–gray pigmentation of the skin may be improved with the Q-switched ruby laser or fractional photothermolysis.

Chloroquine, hydroxychloroquine, and quinacrine all may cause a blue–black pigmentation of the face, extremities, ear cartilage, oral mucosa, and nails. Pretibial hyperpigmentation is the most common pattern and is very similar to that induced by minocycline. The gingiva or hard palate may also be discolored. Quinidine may also rarely cause such a pattern of hyperpigmentation. Quinacrine is yellow and is concentrated in the epidermis. Generalized yellow discoloration of the skin and sclera (mimicking jaundice) occurs reproducibly in patients but fades within 4 months of stopping the drug. In dark-skinned patients this color is masked and not so significant cosmetically. Histologically, in both forms of pigmentation, pigment granules are present within macrophages in the dermis.

Amiodarone after 3–6 months causes photosensitivity in 30–57% of treated patients. In 1–10% of patients, a slate-gray hyperpigmentation develops in the areas of photosensitivity. The pigmentation gradually fades after the medication is discontinued. Histologically, periodic acid–Schiff-positive, yellow–brown granules are seen within the cytoplasm of macrophages in the dermis. Electron microscopy reveals membrane-bound structures resembling lipid-containing lysosomes. It responds to treatment with the Q-switched ruby laser.

Clofazimine treatment is reproducibly complicated by the appearance of a pink discoloration that gradually becomes reddish-blue or brown and is concentrated in the lesions of patients with Hansen's disease. This pigmentation may be very disfiguring and is a major cause of noncompliance with this drug in the treatment of Hansen's disease. Histologically, a periodic acid–Schiff-positive, brown, granular pigment is variably seen within foamy macrophages in the dermis. This has been called "drug-induced lipofuscinosis."

Zidovudine causes a blue or brown hyperpigmentation that is most frequently observed in the nails. The lunula may be blue or the whole nail plate may become dark brown. Diffuse hyperpigmentation of the skin, pigmentation of the lateral tongue, and increased tanning are less common. It occurs in darkly pigmented persons, is dose-dependent, and clears after the medication is discontinued. Hydroxyurea causes a very similar pattern of hyperpigmentation.

Chlorpromazine, thioridazine, imipramine, and clomipramine may cause a slate-gray hyperpigmentation in sun-exposed areas after long periods of ingestion. Frequently, corneal and lens opacities are also present, so all patients with hyperpigmentation from these medications should have an ophthalmologic evaluation. The pigmentation from the phenothiazines fades gradually over years, even if the patient is treated with another phenothiazine. The corneal, but not the lenticular, changes also resolve. Imipramine hyperpigmentation has been reported to disappear within a year. Histologically, in sun-exposed but not sun-protected skin, numerous refractile golden-brown granules are present within macrophages in the dermis, along with increased dermal melanin. The slate-gray color comes from a mixture of the golden-brown pigment of the drug and the black color of the melanin viewed in the dermis.

The heavy metals gold, silver, and bismuth produce blue to slate-gray hyperpigmentation. Pigmentation occurs after years of exposure, predominantly in sun-exposed areas, and is permanent. Silver is by far the commonest form of heavy metal-induced pigmentation seen by dermatologists. It occurs in two forms, local or systemic. Local argyria most commonly follows

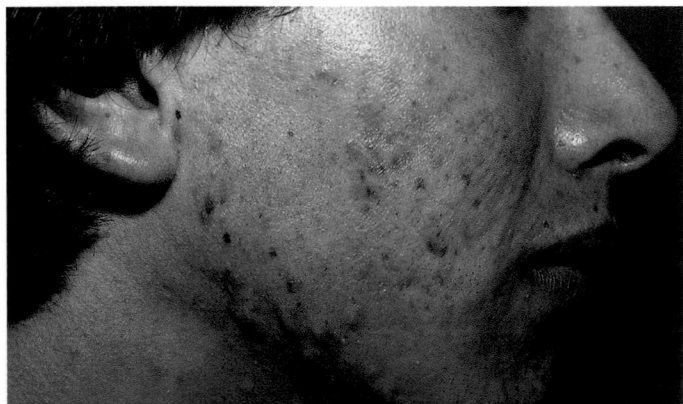

Fig. 6-32 Minocycline hyperpigmentation.

the topical use of silver sulfadiazine or silver-containing dressings (Acticoat). Blue–gray pigmentation occurs at the site of application. Implantation into the skin by needles or pierced jewelry may lead to focal areas of argyria. Systemic argyria can also arise from topical application to the skin (in burn and epidermolysis bullosa patients), by inhalation, by mucosal application (nose drops or eye drops), or by ingestion. Patients may purchase or build devices which allow them to make colloidal silver solutions which they then ingest for arthritis, infections, or general health. After several months of such exposures the skin becomes slate-gray or blue–gray, primarily in areas of sun exposure. Histologically, granules of silver are found in basement membranes at the dermoepidermal junction and around adnexal (especially eccrine) and vascular structures. Sun exposure leads to the silver binding to either sulfur or selenium in the skin, increasing deposition. The deposited silver activates tyrosinase, increasing pigmentation. Most patients with argyria have no systemic symptoms or consequences of the increased silver in their body. In one patient, the use of a Q-switched 1064 Nd:YAG laser improved the condition. Gold deposition was more common when gold was used as a treatment for rheumatoid arthritis. Cutaneous chrysiasis also presents as blue–gray pigmentation, usually after a cumulative dose of 8 g. Chrysiasis is also more prominent in sun-exposed sites. Dermatologists should remain aware of this condition, since patients treated with gold, even decades before, may develop disfiguring hyperpigmentation following Q-switched laser therapy for hair removal or lentigines lightening. Chrysiasis has been treated effectively in one patient using repeated 595 nm pulsed dye laser therapy. Bismuth also pigments the gingival margin. Histologically, granules of the metals are seen in the dermis and around blood vessels. Arsenical melanosis is characterized by black, generalized pigmentation or by a pronounced truncal hyperpigmentation that spares the face, with depigmented scattered macules that resemble raindrops.

Diltiazem can cause a severe photodistributed hyperpigmentation. This is most common in African American or Hispanic women, and occurs about 1 year after starting therapy. The lesions are slate-gray or gray–blue macules and patches on the face, neck, and forearms. Perifollicular accentuation is noted. Histology shows a sparse lichenoid dermatitis with prominent dermal melanophages. The action spectrum of the drug appears to be in the UVB range, but hyperpigmentation is induced by UVA irradiation. The mechanism appears to be post-inflammatory hyperpigmentation from a photosensitive lichenoid eruption rather than drug or drug metabolite deposition. Treatment is broad-spectrum sunscreens, stopping the diltiazem, and bleaching creams if needed. Other calcium channel blockers can be substituted without the reappearance of the hyperpigmentation.

Periocular hyperpigmentation occurs in patients treated with prostaglandin analogs for glaucoma. These agents also cause pigmentation of the iris. Eyelash length increases. The periocular hyperpigmentation may gradually resolve when the medications are discontinued.

Pigmentary changes induced by chemotherapeutic agents are discussed later in this chapter.

Alm A, et al: Side effects associated with prostaglandin analog therapy. Surv Ophthalmol 2008; 53:S93.

Almoallim H, et al: Laser-induced chrysiasis: disfiguring hyperpigmentation following Q-switched laser therapy in a woman previously treated with gold. J Rheumatol 2006; 33:620.

Anderson EL, et al: Argyria as a result of somatic delusions. Am J Psychiatry 2008; 165:649.

Aste N, et al: Nail pigmentation caused by hydroxyurea: report of 9 cases. J Am Acad Dermatol 2002; 47:146.

Bianchi L, et al: Familial generalized argyria. Arch Dermatol 2006; 143:79

Bowen AR, et al: The histopathology of subcutaneous minocycline pigmentation. J Am Acad Dermatol 2007; 57:836.

Brandt D, et al: Argyria secondary to ingestion of homemade silver solution. J Am Acad Dermatol 2005; 53:S105.

Chang AL, et al: A case of argyria after colloidal silver ingestion. J Cutan Pathol 2006; 33:809.

Chatterjee S: Hyperpigmentation associated with minocycline therapy. Can Med Assoc J 2007; 176:322.

Cho EA, et al: Occupational generalized argyria after exposure to aerosolized silver. J Dermatol 2008; 35:759.

D'Agostino ML, et al: Imipramine-induced hyperpigmentation: a case report and review of the literature. J Cutan Pathol 2009; 36:799.

eSilva LP, et al: Facial hyperpigmentation. Amiodarone-induced hyperpigmentation. Am Fam Physician 2008; 78:1297.

Fay B, et al: Minocycline-induced hyperpigmentation in rheumatoid arthritis. J Clin Rheumatol 2008; 14:17.

Flohr C, et al: Topical silver sulfadiazine-induced systemic argyria in a patient with severe generalized dystrophic epidermolysis bullosa. Br J Dermatol 2008; 159:740.

Gangnon A, et al: A study of histopathological features of latanoprost-treated irides with or without darkening compared with non-latanoprost irides. Arch Ophthalmol 2008; 126:1403.

Geist DE, Phillips TJ: Development of chrysiasis after Q-switched ruby laser treatment of solar lentigines. J Am Acad Dermatol 2006; 55:S59.

Greenberg JE, et al: Mucocutaneous pigmented macule as a result of zinc deposition. J Cutan Pathol 2002; 29:613.

Griffiths MR, et al: Penile argyria. Br J Dermatol 2006; 155:1074.

Huq F, Durso SC: Spurious bruising in a patient taking warfarin: minocycline-induced skin hyperpigmentation. J Am Geriatr Soc 2008; 56:1156.

Izikson L, Anderson RR: Resolution of blue minocycline pigmentation of the face after fractional photothermolysis. Lasers in Surg Med 2008; 40:399.

Jeevankumar B, et al: Blue lunula due to hydroxyurea. J Dermatol 2003; 30:628.

Kim Y, et al: A case of generalized argyria after ingestion of colloidal silver solution. Am J Ind Med 2009; 52:246.

Knueppel RC, Rahimian J: Diffuse cutaneous hyperpigmentation due to tigecycline or polymyxin B. Clin Infect Dis 2007; 45:136.

Madan V, Lear JT: Minocycline-induced pigmentation of pre-existing capillaritis. Br J Dermatol 2007; 156:575.

Mouton RW, et al: A new type of minocycline-induced cutaneous hyperpigmentation. Clin Exp Dermatol 2004; 29:8.

Nakamura S, et al: Acute pigmentation due to minocycline therapy in atopic dermatitis. Br J Dermatol 2003; 148:1058.

Oh ST, et al: Hydroxyurea-induced melanonychia concomitant with a dermatomyositis-like eruption. J Am Acad Dermatol 2003; 49:339.

Rahman Z, et al: Minocycline hyperpigmentation isolated to the subcutaneous fat. J Cutan Pathol 2005; 32:516.

Rhee DY, et al: Treatment of argyria after colloidal silver ingestion using Q-switched 1,064-nm Nd:YAG laser. Dermatol Surg 2008; 34:1427.

Roberts G, Capell HA: The frequency and distribution of minocycline-induced hyperpigmentation in a rheumatoid arthritis population. J Rheumatol 2006; 33:1254.

Sakai N, et al: A case of generalized argyria caused by the use of silver protein as a disinfection medicine. Acta Dermatol Venereol 2007; 87:186.

Saladi RN, et al: Diltiazem induces severe photodistributed hyperpigmentation. Arch Dermatol 2006; 142:206.

Suwannarat P, et al: Minocycline-induced hyperpigmentation masquerading as alkaptonuria in individuals with joint pain. Arthritis Rheuma 2004; 50:3698.

Trop M, et al: Silver-coated dressing acticoat caused raised liver enzymes and argyria symptoms in burn patient. J Trauma 2006; 60:648.

Utikal J, et al: Local cutaneous argyria mimicking melanoma metastases in a patient with disseminated melanoma. J Am Acad Dermatol 2006; 55:S92.

Wadhera A, Fung M: Systematic argyria associated with ingestion of colloidal silver. Dermatol Online J 2005; 11:12.

Wang XQ, et al: A silver deposit in cutaneous burn scar tissue is a common phenomenon following application of a silver dressing. J Cutan Pathol 2009; 36:788.

Wu JJ, et al: Generalized chrysiasis improved with pulsed dye laser. Dermatol Surg 2009; 35:538.

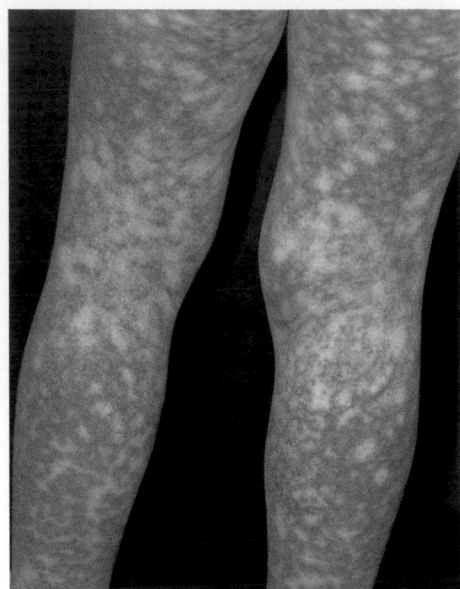

Fig. 6-33 Cefaclor reaction.

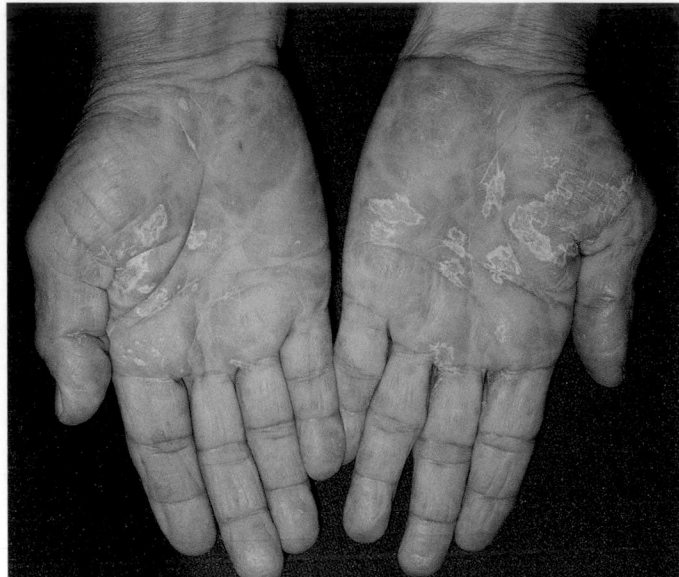

Fig. 6-34 Lichenoid drug eruption due to gold.

Vasculitis and serum sickness-like reactions

True leukocytoclastic vasculitis can be induced by many medications, but these events are rare, except in the case of propylthiouracil. True serum sickness is caused by foreign proteins such as antithymocyte globulin. They are produced by circulating immune complexes. In the case of true serum sickness there is a tendency for purpuric lesions to be accentuated along the junction between palmoplantar and glabrous skin (Wallace line).

Serum sickness-like reactions refer to adverse reactions that have similar symptoms to serum sickness, but in which immune complexes are not found. This reaction was particularly common with cefaclor. Patients present with fever, an urticarial rash and arthralgias 1–3 weeks after starting the medication (Fig. 6-33). Minocycline, bupropion and rituximab have been reported to cause serum sickness-like reactions.

King BA, et al: Adverse skin and joint reactions associated with oral antibiotics in children: the role of cefaclor in serum sickness-like reactions. J Paediatr Child Health 2003; 39:677.

Knowles SR, Shear NH: Recognition and management of severe cutaneous drug reactions. Dermatol Clin 2007; 25:245

Lichenoid reactions

Lichenoid reactions can be seen with many medications, including gold (Fig. 6-34), hydrochlorothiazide, furosemide, NSAIDs, aspirin, antihypertensives (ACE inhibitors, β-blockers, and calcium channel blockers), terazosin, quinidine, proton pump inhibitors, pravastatin, phenothiazines, anticonvulsants, anti-tuberculous drugs, ketoconazole, sildenafil, imatinib, and the antimalarials. Hepatitis B immunization may trigger a lichenoid eruption. Reactions may be photodistributed (lichenoid photoeruption) or generalized, and those drugs causing lichenoid photoeruptions may also induce more generalized ones. In either case, the lesions may be plaques (very occasionally with Wickham striae), small papules, or exfoliative erythema. Photolichenoid reactions favor the extensor extremities, including the dorsa of the hands. Oral involvement is less common in lichenoid drug reactions than in idiopathic lichen planus but can occur (and with imatinib may be quite severe). It appears as either plaques or erosions. The lower lip is frequently involved in photolichenoid reactions. The nails may also be affected, and can be the only site of involvement. Lichenoid drug eruptions can occur within months to years of starting the offending medication, and may take months to years to resolve once the medication has been stopped. Histologically, there is inflammation along the dermoepidermal junction, with necrosis of keratinocytes and a dermal infiltrate composed primarily of lymphocytes. Eosinophils are useful, if present, but are not common in photolichenoid reactions. The histology is often very similar to idiopathic lichen planus, and a clinical correlation is required to determine if the lichenoid eruption is drug-induced.

Lichenoid reactions may be restricted to the oral mucosa, especially if induced by dental amalgam. In these cases the lesions are topographically related to the dental fillings or to metal prostheses. Patients may be patch test-positive to mercury, or less commonly gold, cobalt, or nickel, in up to two-thirds of cases. Amalgam replacement will result in resolution of the oral lesions in these cases. Patients with cutaneous lesions of lichen planus and oral lesions do not improve with amalgam removal. An unusual form of eruption is the "drug-induced ulceration of the lower lip." Patients present with a persistent erosion of the lower lip that is tender but not indurated. It is induced by diuretics and resolves slowly once they are discontinued.

Al-Hashimi I, et al: Oral lichen planus and oral lichenoid lesions: diagnostics and therapeutic considerations. Oral Surg Oral Med Oral Pathol Oral Radiol Endod 2007; 103:S25.e1.

Antiga E, et al: A case of lichenoid drug eruption associated with sildenafil citratus. J Dermatol 2005; 32:972.

Armour K, Lowe P: Complicated lichenoid drug eruption. Aus J Dermatol 2005; 46:21.

Bong JL, et al: Lichenoid drug eruption with proton pump inhibitors. BMJ 2000; 320:283.

Ko MJA, et al: Lichenoid drug eruption to terazosin. Br J Dermatol 2008; 158:405.

Majmudar V, et al: Lichenoid drug eruption secondary to treatment with nicorandil. Clin Exp Dermatol 2007; 33:193.

Perez-Perez L, et al: Photosensitive lichenoid eruption and inhaled tiotropium bromide. Dermatol 2007; 214:97.

Pua VSC, et al: Pravastatin-induced lichenoid drug eruption. Aus J Dermatol 2006; 47:57.

Saito M, et al: Lichenoid drug eruption of nails induced by propylthiouracil. J Dermatol 2007; 34:696.

Shalders K, Gach JE: Photodistributed lichenoid drug eruption secondary to solifenacin. Clin Exp Dermatol 2007; 33:340.

Swale VJ, McGregor JM: Amlodipine-associated lichen planus. Br J Dermatol 2001; 144:901.

Usman A, et al: Lichenoid eruption following hepatitis B vaccination: first North American case report. Pediatr Dermatol 2001; 18:123.

Villaverde RR, et al: Generalized lichen planus-like eruption due to acetylsalicylic acid. J Eur Acad Dermatol Venereol 2003; 17:469.

Wahidussaman M, et al: Oral and cutaneous lichenoid reaction with nail changes secondary to imatinib: report of a case and literature review. Dermatol Online J 2008; 14:14.

Adverse reactions to chemotherapeutic agents

Chemotherapeutic agents can cause adverse reactions by multiple potential mechanisms. Adverse reactions may be related to toxicity either directly to the mucocutaneous surfaces (stomatitis, alopecia), or to some other organ system, and reflected in the skin, such as purpura resulting from thrombocytopenia. Being organic molecules or monoclonal antibodies, they can act as antigens inducing classic immunologic reactions. In addition, since they are inherently immunosuppressive, they can cause skin reactions associated with alterations of immune function. Some of these patterns may be overlapping and clinically difficult to distinguish. For example, oral erosions may occur as a toxic effect of chemotherapy and also by immunosuppression-associated activation of herpes simplex virus.

Dermatologists are rarely confronted with the relatively common acute hypersensitivity reactions seen during infusion of chemotherapeutic agents. These reactions resemble type I allergic reactions, with urticaria and hypotension. Although the type I reactions are IgE-mediated in only some cases, they can be prevented with premedication with systemic steroids and antihistamines in most cases.

Numerous macular and papular eruptions have been described with chemotherapeutic agents as well. Many of these occur at the time of the earliest recovery of the bone marrow, as lymphocytes return to the peripheral circulation. They are associated with fever. Horn et al have termed this phenomenon cutaneous eruptions of lymphocyte recovery. Histologically, these reactions demonstrate a nonspecific superficial perivascular mononuclear cell infiltrate, composed primarily of T lymphocytes. Treatment is not required and the eruption spontaneously resolves.

Radiation enhancement and recall reactions

Radiation dermatitis, in the form of intense erythema and vesiculation of the skin, may be observed in radiation ports. Administration of many chemotherapeutic agents, during or in close proximity to the time of radiation therapy, may induce an enhanced radiation reaction. However, in some cases, months to years following radiation treatment the administration of a chemotherapeutic agent may induce a reaction within the prior radiation port with features of radiation dermatitis. This phenomenon has been termed "radiation recall." It has been reported with numerous chemotherapeutic agents, high-dose IFN-α, and simvastatin. Not only the skin, but also internal structures such as the gut may be affected. A similar reaction of reactivation of a sunburn after methotrexate therapy also occurs. Exanthems restricted to prior areas of sunburn are not true radiation recall.

Chemotherapy-induced acral erythema (palmoplantar erythrodysesthesia syndrome, hand-foot syndrome)

This is a relatively common syndrome induced most frequently by 5-fluorouracil (5-FU), doxorubicin, and cytosine arabinoside, but also seen with docetaxel, capecitabine, and high-dose liposomal doxorubicin and daunorubicin. A localized plaque of fixed erythrodysesthesia has been described proximal to the infusion site of docetaxel. The reaction may occur in as many as 40% or more of treated patients. The reaction is dose-dependent, and may appear with bolus short-term infusions or low-dose, long-term infusions. It may present days to months after the treatments are started. It is probably a direct toxic effect of the chemotherapeutic agents on the skin. The large number of sweat glands on the palms and soles that may concentrate the chemotherapeutic agents may explain the localization of the toxicity. In the case of pegylated liposomal doxorubicin localization of the chemotherapeutic agent to the sweat glands has been demonstrated, and the sweat glands appear to be the organ by which the chemotherapy is delivered on to the surface of normal skin. A flexural eruption in the groin and axilla may accompany acral erythema, again from sweat gland accumulation of the drug in these regions. Cases of neutrophilic eccrine hidradenitis and syringometaplasia all induced by the same agents suggest that the eccrine glands are unique targets for adverse reactions to antineoplastic agents.

The initial manifestation is often dysesthesia or tingling of the palms and soles. This is followed in a few days by painful, symmetric erythema and edema most pronounced over the distal pads of the digits. The reaction may spread to the dorsal hands and feet, and can be accompanied by a morbilliform eruption of the trunk, neck, scalp, and extremities. Over the next several days the erythema becomes dusky, develops areas of pallor, blisters, desquamates, then re-epithelializes. The desquamation is often the most prominent part of the syndrome. Blisters developing over pressure areas of the hands, elbows, and feet are a variant of this syndrome. The patient usually recovers without complication, although rarely full-thickness ischemic necrosis occurs in the areas of blistering.

The histopathology is nonspecific, with necrotic keratinocytes and vacuolar changes along the basal cell layer. Acute GVHD is in the differential diagnosis. Histologic evaluation may not be useful in the acute setting to distinguish these syndromes. Most helpful are gastrointestinal or liver findings of GVHD.

Most cases require only local supportive care. Cold compresses and elevation are helpful, and cooling the hands during treatment may reduce the severity of the reaction. Modification of the dose schedule can be beneficial. Pyridoxine, 100–150 mg daily, decreases the pain of 5-FU-induced acral erythema. IVIG has been reported to be beneficial in a methotrexate-induced case of acral erythema.

Sorafenib and sunitinib are multikinase-inhibiting small molecules with blocking activity for numerous tyrosine kinases, including vascular endothelial growth factor (VEGF), platelet-derived growth factor (PDGFRβ), and c-KIT. They both induce a condition very similar to acral erythema, called "hand-foot skin reaction" (HFSR). Patients also present with acral pain and dysesthesia, but usually less severe and with less edema than with classic chemotherapeutic agents. As opposed to classic acral erythema, multikinase inhibitor-induced HFSR causes patchy marked hyperkeratotic plaques over areas of friction. The HFSR is dose-dependent, high-grade in 9% of cases (with blisters, ulceration, and function loss), and results in the sorafenib being stopped in about 1% of patients. The addition of another VEGF inhibitor, bevacizumab, leads to worse HFSR. Painful distal subungual splinter hemorrhages can also occur 2–4 weeks after the onset of treatment. It has been suggested that the blocking of VEGF may be pathogenically important in causing HFSR splinter hemorrhages. Histologically, there are horizontal layers of necrotic keratinocytes within the epidermis (if the biopsy is taken in the first 30 days) or in the stratum corneum (later biopsies). Topical tazarotene, 40% urea, and fluorouracil cream have been used to treat HFSR from multikinase inhibitors.

Neutrophilic eccrine hidradenitis is discussed in Chapter 33.

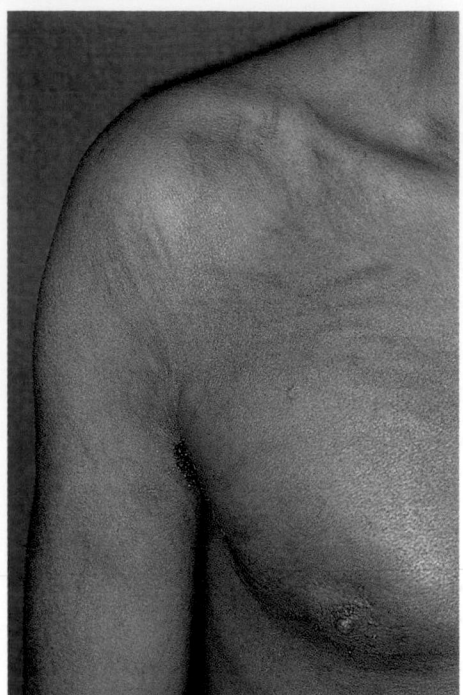

Fig. 6-35 Flagellate hyperpigmentation, bleomycin.

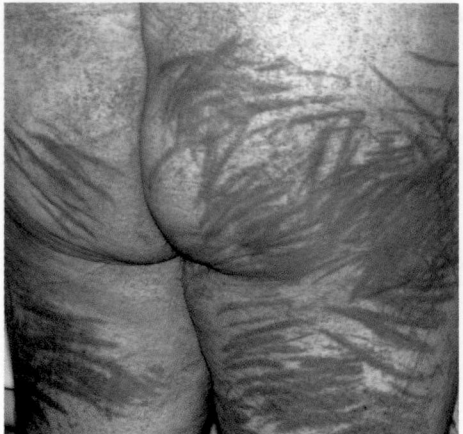

Fig. 6-36 Shiitake mushroom dermatitis. (Courtesy of Don Adler, DO)

Chemotherapy-induced dyspigmentation

Many chemotherapeutic agents (especially the antibiotics bleomycin, doxorubicin, and daunorubicin) and the alkylating agents (cyclophosphamide and busulfan) cause various patterns of cutaneous hyperpigmentation. Adriamycin (doxorubicin) causes marked hyperpigmentation of the nails, skin, and tongue. This is most common in black patients and appears in locations where constitutional hyperpigmentation is sometimes seen. Hydroxyurea can also cause this pattern of hyperpigmentation. It is very similar to zidovudine-associated pigmentation seen in pigmented persons. Cyclophosphamide causes transverse banding of the nails or diffuse nail hyperpigmentation beginning proximally. Bleomycin and 5-FU cause similar transverse bands. Busulfan and 5-FU induce diffuse hyperpigmentation that may be photoaccentuated. Paradoxical hyperpigmentation of the skin, nails, and hair has been reported due to imatinib. Eruptive melanocytic nevi and lentigines with an acral predisposition have been seen with sorafenib therapy.

Bleomycin induces characteristic flagellate erythematous urticarial wheals associated with pruritus within hours or days of infusion (Fig. 6-35). Lesions continue to appear for days to weeks. While investigators have not always been able to induce lesions, the pattern strongly suggests scratching is the cause of the erythematous lesions. A similar characteristic pattern of flagellate hyperpigmentation occurs following bleomycin treatment. It may have been preceded by the erythematous reaction or simply pruritus. Bleomycin hyperpigmentation may be accentuated at areas of pressure, strongly supporting trauma as the cause of the peculiar pattern.

Patients may present with linear erythematous wheals (Fig. 6-36) 1–2 days after eating raw or cooked shiitake mushrooms. This so-called toxicodermia, or shiitake flagellate dermatitis, is thought to be caused by a toxic reaction to lentinan, a polysaccharide component of the mushrooms. It is self-limited and resolves within days to weeks of its appearance, but can be treated with topical steroids to relieve the associated pruritus some patients experience. Other associations with flagellate eruptions include adult-onset Still's disease, dermatomyositis, and docetaxel therapy.

5-FU, and less commonly other chemotherapeutic agents, may produce a serpentine hyperpigmentation overlying the veins proximal to an infusion site. This represents postinflammatory hyperpigmentation from a direct cytotoxic effect of the chemotherapeutic agent.

Imatinib in doses of 400–600 mg daily leads to generalized or localized depigmentation in 40% or more of pigmented persons. It starts an average of 4 weeks after treatment and progresses over time if treatment with imatinib is continued. Patients also complain of an inability to tan and "photosensitivity". One patient with vitiligo had significant progression with imatinib therapy. The proposed mechanism is inhibition of c-KIT and its ligand "stem cell factor," which are implicated in melanogenesis. By a similar mechanism, sunitinib leads to depigmentation of the hair after 5–6 weeks of treatment. Sunitinib may lead to yellow pigmentation of the skin due to drug or its metabolites being deposited.

Exudative hyponychial dermatitis

Nail toxicity is common (26–40%) during chemotherapy for breast cancer, especially if docetaxel is in the chemotherapeutic regimen. Subungual hemorrhage, subungual abscesses, paronychia, subungual hyperkeratosis, and onychomadesis all occur. In its most severe form, severe exudation and onycholysis may result. All these reactions probably represent various degrees of toxicity to the nailbed. Capecitabine has caused a similar reaction.

Palifermin-associated papular eruption

Palifermin is a recombinant human keratinocyte growth factor that is used to reduce the severity and duration of mucositis in patients undergoing preparative regimens for hematopoietic stem cell transplantation. An intertriginous erythema accompanied by oral confluent white plaques and small lichenoid papules developed in one patient while on palifermin therapy. The papules resembled flat warts clinically and histologically, but were human papillomavirus (HPV)-negative by in situ hybridization studies. A direct hyperproliferative effect of the keratinocyte growth factor is the proposed mechanism.

Scleroderma-like reactions to taxanes

Patients treated with docetaxel or paclitaxel may develop an acute, diffuse, infiltrated edema of the extremities and head. This occurs after one to several courses of the taxane. The affected areas, specifically the lower extremities, evolve over months to become sclerotic and at times painful. Flexion contractures of the palm, digits, and large joints may occur.

Biopsies of the initial lesion show lymphangiectasia and a diffuse infiltration with mononuclear cells in the superficial dermis. Late fibrotic lesions demonstrate marked dermal fibrosis. Discontinuation of the taxane therapy leads to resolution in most cases.

Adverse reactions to immunosuppressants used in dermatology

Azathioprine is commonly used as a steroid-sparing agent for dermatological conditions. It can cause a hypersensitivity syndrome. In addition, neutrophilic dermatoses resembling Sweet syndrome appear with azathioprine therapy and resolve with its discontinuation. Patients with inflammatory bowel disease appear to be at particular risk. Photosensitivity can also occur with azathioprine, despite its frequent use in severe photodermatoses. Methotrexate can cause erosive skin lesions in two patterns. Rarely, patients with psoriasis will develop ulceration or erosion of their plaques. This can be associated with methotrexate marrow toxicity or can be an apparently idiosyncratic but reproducible phenomenon in rare patients. If coexistent renal failure is present or occurs during low-dose methotrexate therapy, a severe bullous eruption resembling TEN can occur. This apparently represents severe cutaneous toxicity from the prolonged blood and skin levels of methotrexate that result from reduced excretion due to coexistent renal disease and drug–drug interactions. If this scenario is recognized, leucovorin rescue should be given immediately.

Agarwal KK, et al: Methotrexate toxicity presenting as ulceration of psoriatic plaques: a report of two cases. Indian J Dermatol Venereol Leprol 2008;74:481.

Camidge DR: Methotrexate-induced radiation recall. Am J Clin Oncol 2001; 24:211.

Camidge DR, Kunkler IH: Docetaxel-induced radiation recall dermatitis and successful rechallenge without recurrence. Clin Oncol 2000; 12:272.

Camidge R, Price A: Characterizing the phenomenon of radiation recall dermatitis. Radiother Oncol 2001; 59:237.

Chen GY, et al: Onychomadesis and onycholysis associated with capecitabine. Br J Dermatol 2001; 145:521.

Chen GY, et al: Exudative hyponychial dermatitis associated with capecitabine and docetaxel combination chemotherapy for metastatic breast carcinoma: report of three cases. Br J Dermatol 2003; 148:1071.

Chu CY, et al: Docetaxel-induced recall dermatitis on previous laser treatment sites. Br J Dermatol 2005; 153:441.

Dabaja MAK, et al: Radiation recall dermatitis induced by methotrexate in a patient with Hodgkin's disease. Am J Clin Oncol 2000; 23:531.

El-Azhary RA, et al: Sweet syndrome as a manifestation of azathioprine hypersensitivity. Mayo Clin Proc 2008; 83:1026.

Gaigal Z, et al: Methotrexate-induced toxic epidermal necrolysis-like skin toxicity. Eur J Dermatol 2007; 17:169.

Heidary N, et al: Chemotherapeutic agents and the skin: an update. J Am Acad Dermatol 2008; 58:545.

Hornreich G, et al: Doxil-induced radiation recall: a cause for false-positive PET scan findings. Gynecol Oncol 2001; 80:422.

Hui YF, et al: Chemotherapy-induced palmar-plantar erythrodysesthesia syndrome: recall following different chemotherapy agents. Invest New Drugs 2002; 20:49.

Kaya AO: Acute erythema and edematous skin reaction and ectropion following docetaxel in a patient with non-small cell lung cancer. Cutan Ocular Toxicol 2008; 27:327.

Krishnan RS, et al: Ultraviolet recall-like phenomenon occurring after piperacillin, tobramycin and ciprofloxacin therapy. J Am Acad Dermatol 2001; 44:1045.

Kroumpouzos G, et al: Generalized hyperpigmentation with daunorubicin chemotherapy. J Am Acad Dermatol 2002; 46:S1.

Kupfer I, et al: Scleroderma-like cutaneous lesions induced by paclitaxel: a case study. J Am Acad Dermatol 2003; 48:279.

Lauchli S, et al: Scleroderma-like drug reaction to paclitaxel (Taxol). Br J Dermatol 2002; 147:604.

Mangana J, et al: Skin problems associated with pegylated liposomal doxorubicin—more than palmoplantar erythrodysesthesia syndrome. Eur J Dermatol 2008; 18:566.

Marcoux D, et al: Persistent serpentine supravenous hyperpigmented eruption as an adverse reaction to chemotherapy combining actinomycin and vincristine. J Am Acad Dermatol 2000; 43:540.

O'Branski EE, et al: Skin and nail changes in children with sickle cell anemia receiving hydroxyurea therapy. J Am Acad Dermatol 2001; 44:859.

Tezer H, et al: Intravenous immunoglobulin in the treatment of severe methotrexate-induced acral erythema. J Pediatr Hematol Oncol 2008; 30:391.

von Hilsheimer GE, Norton SA: Delayed bleomycin-induced hyperpigmentation and pressure on the skin. J Am Acad Dermatol 2002; 46:642.

von Moos R, et al: Pegylated liposomal doxorubicin-associated hand-foot syndrome: recommendation of an international panel of experts. Eur J Cancer 2008; 44:781.

Yiasemides E, Thom G: Azathioprine hypersensitivity presenting as a neutrophilic dermatosis in a man with ulcerative colitis. Aus J Dermatol 2009; 50:48.

Cutaneous side effects of epidermal growth factor receptor (EGFR) inhibitors

EGFR is expressed by basal keratinocytes, sebocytes, and the outer root sheath, explaining why up to 90% of patients treated with these agents may develop cutaneous side effects. Xerosis is often seen. Painful periungual or finger pulp fissures and paronychia (with or without periungual pyogenic granulomas) may develop. The most common and characteristic adverse skin reaction is a papulopustular eruption that is dose-dependent. The eruption begins 7–10 days after therapy is begun and the maximum severity is reached in the second week. The seborrheic areas of the scalp, central face, upper back, and retroauricular regions are primarily affected. The primary lesion is a follicular papule or pustule with few or no comedones. Hemorrhagic crusting and confluence can occur, resembling rosacea fulminans (pyoderma faciale) in the most severely affected patients. Telangiectasia may be prominent. The eruption may itch. The presence and severity of this skin eruption are correlated with survival, so some oncologists will increase the dose to induce the eruption. Radiation therapy during EGFR inhibitor therapy will enhance the EGFR skin toxicity, but previously radiated skin is often spared from EGFR inhibitor toxicity. Effective topical therapies have included metronidazole, clindamycin, hydrocortisone, pimecrolimus, and tretinoin. Oral tetracyclines can treat or prevent the eruption. In the most severe cases isotretinoin or acitretin can be used. Tumor necrosis factor (TNF)-α and IL-1 are involved in the pathogenesis of EGFR inhibitor toxicity. Etanercept and kineret can, therefore, also be therapeutically useful. Long eyelashes and curlier scalp hair may also occur.

Cutaneous side effects of multikinase inhibitors

In addition to the reactions listed above, multikinase inhibitors may cause other skin reactions. Psoriasis exacerbation, acral psoriasiform hyperkeratosis, and pityriasis rosea-like eruptions have been described with imatinib. Both imatinib and sunitinib cause facial edema, with a periocular predilection. Increased vascular permeability due to PDGFR inhibition has been the proposed mechanism. Dasatinib has caused a lobular panniculitis. Bevacizumab, a VEGF inhibitor, causes bleeding and wound healing complications. Extensive cutaneous surgery should probably be delayed for 60 days after bevacizumab therapy, and 28 days should pass from the time of surgery until bevacizumab therapy is initiated. Sorafenib has been associated with the rapid development of multiple squamoproliferative lesions called keratoacanthomas or squamous cell carcinomas. Bexarotene was therapeutic in one case.

Multiple, monomorphous, follicular, keratotic, skin-colored papules resembling keratosis pilaris can develop during sorafenib treatment. Histologically, these papules show hyperplasia of the follicular isthmus or follicular hyperkeratosis with plugging. Facial and scalp erythema and dysesthesia occur in about 60% of sorafenib-treated patients.

Adverse reactions to cytokines

Cytokines, which are normal mediators of inflammation or cell growth, are increasingly used in the management of malignancies and to ameliorate the hematologic complications of disease or its treatment. Skin toxicity is a common complication of the use of these agents. Many of them cause local inflammation and/or ulceration at the injection sites in a large number of the patients treated. More widespread papular eruptions are also frequently reported, but these have been poorly studied in most cases and are of unclear pathogenesis.

Granulocyte colony-stimulating factor (G-CSF) has been associated with the induction of several neutrophil-mediated disorders, most commonly Sweet syndrome or bullous pyoderma gangrenosum. These occur about a week after cytokine therapy is initiated and are present despite persistent neutropenia in peripheral blood. A rare complication of G-CSF is a thrombotic and necrotizing panniculitis. Both G-CSF and granulocyte–macrophage (GM)-CSF may exacerbate leukocytoclastic vasculitis. IFN-α, IFN-γ, and G-CSF have been associated with the exacerbation of psoriasis. G-CSF can also cause cutaneous eruptions containing histiocytes. Anakinra and rarely erythropoietin can cause similar granulomatous skin reactions.

IL-2 commonly causes diffuse erythema followed by desquamation, pruritus, mucositis (resembling aphthosis), glossitis, and flushing. While the majority of erythema reactions with IL-2 treatment are mild to moderate, some may be quite severe. Erythroderma with blistering or TEN-like reactions can occur, and be dose-limiting. Administration of iodinated contrast material within 2 weeks of IL-2 therapy will be associated with a hypersensitivity reaction in 30% of cases. Fever, chills, angioedema, urticaria, and hypotension may occur. Subcutaneous injections of IL-2 can lead to injection site nodules or necrosis. Histologically, a diffuse panniculitis with noninflammatory necrosis of the involved tissue is present. Rarely, linear IgA disease can be induced by IFN-α.

Adverse reactions to biologic agents

TNF inhibitors

Injection site reactions (ISRs) are common with etanercept therapy for rheumatologic disease, with 20–40% of patients developing ISR. ISRs present as erythematous, mildly swollen plaques, appearing 1–2 days after the injection. Pruritus occurs in 20% of cases. ISR is most common early in the treatment course (median number of injections was four), and stops appearing with continued treatment. Individual lesions resolve over 2–3 days. Recall ISR (reappearance of the eruption at a site of a previous ISR) occurs in 40% of patients. This adverse reaction appears to be mediated by CD8+ T cells. Cytokine therapy with TNF and IFN-α, β, and γ also causes ISRs.

The paradoxical appearance of psoriasis or a psoriasiform dermatitis is now a well-recognized complication of TNF inhibitor therapy. It occurs with all three of the commonly used TNF inhibitors: infliximab, etanercept, and adalimumab. The risk may be slightly higher for adalimumab. The psoriasis can appear from days to years following anti-TNF therapy. There is no age or gender predisposition. Several clinical patterns have been described. Palmoplantar pustulosis represents

about 40% of cases. Generalized pustular disease may accompany the palmoplantar lesions. Plaque-type psoriasis occurs in about one-third of TNF inhibitor-induced psoriasis. New-onset guttate psoriasis occurs in 10% of cases. Stopping the TNF inhibitor led to improvement or resolution in the vast majority of patients. In some cases therapy was continued and the eruption resolved. There is controversy among experts as to whether switching to a different anti-TNF agent may be tolerated in these patients. Many patients have been rechallenged with other TNF inhibitors. In severe cases this is probably not prudent, but in milder or localized cases this could be considered. The psoriasis caused by anti-TNF agents can be treated with topical steroids, UV phototherapy, topical vitamin D analogs, methotrexate, acitretin, or cyclosporine. The proposed mechanism for the appearance with psoriasis with anti-TNF therapy is either overactivity of Th1 cells or increased IFN-α production by skin-resident plasmacytoid dendritic cells. Systemic IFN-α and topical imiquimod (an interferon inducer) have been reported to exacerbate psoriasis, supporting this hypothesis. Sarcoidosis induced by anti-TNF agents could also be related to increased Th1 function.

Around 11% of patients treated for rheumatoid arthritis with etanercept develop new antinuclear antibodies (ANAs) and 15% anti-double-stranded DNA (dsDNA) antibodies. Anti-Sm antibodies can also occur. Similarly, patients treated with infliximab may develop new ANAs, anti-dsDNA (14%), and anticardiolipin antibodies. All of the three commonly used TNF inhibitors have caused drug-induced lupus (DIL) with features of SLE. It begins on average after 41 weeks of treatment. As compared to DIL from other medications, the TNF inhibitors cause more skin disease with malar rash, discoid lesions, and photosensitivity. Many of the patients will fulfill the American Rheumatology Association (ARA) criteria for SLE, and significant internal organ involvement can occur, including renal and CNS involvement. Etanercept, specifically, seems to cause skin lesions more commonly. Etanercept patients also developed vasculitis more frequently. The vast majority of patients improve about 10 months after therapy has been discontinued. Switching from one TNF inhibitor to another has been reported to be successful. Dermatomyositis has also been caused by TNF inhibitor treatment.

Vasculitis is also a well-recognized complication of treatment with TNF inhibitors. Etanercept is the most common agent to induce vasculitis. The lesions of vasculitis may begin around the injection sites in some etanercept-induced vasculitis cases. More than 85% of patients present with skin lesions, usually a leukocytoclastic vasculitis. Ulcerations, nodules, digital lesions, chilblains, livedo, and other morphologies have also been described. Visceral vasculitis occurs in about one-quarter of the patients. They may be ANA- or antineutrophil cytoplasmic antibody (ANCA)-positive (usually p-ANCA), or have cryoglobulins. Drug-induced antiphospholipid syndrome with TNF inhibitors can be associated with DIL or vasculitis, and presents with thrombosis as well as cutaneous lesions. Some patients with TNF inhibitor-induced vasculitis have died. Stopping the TNF inhibitor leads to resolution of the vasculitis in more than 90% of cases. Rechallenge leads to new vasculitic lesions in three-quarters of cases.

Lichenoid drug eruptions have been reported from all three commonly used anti-TNF agents. They are typically pruritic and affect areas commonly involved by lichen planus: the flexor wrists. However, gluteal cleft lesions are also common. In some cases, the lichenoid eruption superimposes itself on psoriatic lesions presenting as an exacerbation of the "psoriasis." Biopsies show features of both lichen planus and psoriasis, and stopping the anti-TNF therapy leads to improvement of the "psoriasis." Despite these agents' immunosuppressive properties, patients can still develop allergic contact dermatitis while taking them, and patch testing while on anti-TNF treatment may identify relevant allergens. It appears that patients on anti-TNF agents are at slightly increased risk for the development of non-melanoma skin cancers, especially if they also have used methotrexate.

Agero AL, et al: Dermatologic side effects associated with the epidermal growth factor receptor inhibitors. J Am Acad Dermatol 2006; 55:657.

Alexandrescu DT, et al: Persistent cutaneous hyperpigmentation after tyrosine kinase inhibition with imatinib for GIST. Dermatol Online J 2008; 14:7.

Alexandrescu DT, et al: Persistent hair growth during treatment with the EGFR inhibitor erlotinib. Dermatol Online J 2009; 15:4.

Asarch A, et al: Lichen planus-like eruptions: an emerging side effect of tumor necrosis factor and antagonists. J Am Acad Dermatol 2009; 61:104.

Beldner M, et al: Localized palmar-plantar epidermal hyperplasia: a previously undefined dermatologic toxicity to sorafenib. Oncol 2007; 12:1178.

Boone SL, et al: Blackberry-induced hand-foot skin reaction to sunitinib. Invest New Drugs 2009; 24:389.

Boone SL, et al: Impact and management of skin toxicity associated with anti-epidermal growth factor receptor therapy: survey results. Oncol 2007; 72:152.

Bovenschen HJ, et al: Etanercept-induced lichenoid reaction pattern in psoriasis. J Dermatolog Treatment 2006; 17:381.

Brazzelli V, et al: Pityriasis rosea-like eruption during treatment with imatinib mesylate: description of 3 cases. J Am Acad Dermatol 2005; 53:S240.

Brazzelli V, et al: Vitiligo-like lesions and diffuse lightening of the skin in a pediatric patient treated with imatinib mesylate: a noninvasive colorimetric assessment. Ped Dermatol 2006; 23:175.

Brazzelli V, et al: A long-term time course of colorimetric assessment of the effects of imatinib mesylate on skin pigmentation: a study of five patients. Eur Acad Dermatol Venereol 2007; 21:384.

Cario-Andre M, et al: Imatinib mesylate inhibits melanogenesis in vitro. Br J Dermatol 2006; 155:477.

Chakravarty EF, et al: Skin cancer, rheumatoid arthritis, and tumor necrosis factor inhibitors. J Rheumatol 2005; 32:2130.

Collamer AN, et al: Psoriatic skin lesions induced by tumor necrosis factor antagonist therapy: a literature review and potential mechanism of action. Arthritis Rheumatism 2008; 59:996.

De Gannes G, et al: Psoriasis and pustular dermatitis trigged by TNF and inhibitors in patients with rheumatologic conditions. Arch Dermatol 2007; 143:223.

Dereure O, et al: Thrombotic and necrotizing panniculitis associated with recombinant human granulocyte colony-stimulating factor treatment. Br J Dermatol 2000; 142:834.

D'Souza AD, et al: Granulocyte colony-stimulating factor administration adverse events. Transfusion Med Reviews 2008; 22:280.

Eliling E, et al: Pimecrolimus: a novel treatment for cetuximab-induced papulopustular eruption. Arch Dermatol 2008; 144:1236.

Ena P, et al: Oral lichenoid eruption secondary to imatinib (Glivec). J Dermatolog Treatment 2004; 15:253.

Feyerabend S, et al: Toxic dermatolysis, tissue necrosis and impaired wound healing due to sunitinib treatment leading to forefoot amputation. Urol Int 2009; 82:246.

Florentino DF: The yin and yang of TNF and inhibition. Arch Dermatol 2007; 143:233.

Galaria NA, et al: Leukocytoclastic vasculitis due to etanercept. J Rheumatol 2000; 27:2041.

Gressett S, Shah SR: Intricacies of bevacizumab-induced toxicities and their management. Annals Pharmacoth 2009; 43:490.

Hague JS, Ilchyshyn A: Lichenoid photosensitive eruption due to capecitabine chemotherapy for metastatic breast cancer. Clin Exp Dermatol 2006; 32:102.

Harrison MJ, et al: Rates of new-onset psoriasis in patients with rheumatoid arthritis receiving anti-tumor necrosis factor and therapy: results from the British Society for Rheumatology biologics register. Ann Rheum Dis 2009; 68:209.

Heidary N, et al: Chemotherapeutic agents and the skin: an update. J Am Acad Dermatol 2008; 58:545.

Hong DS, et al: Multiple squamous cell carcinomas of the skin after therapy with tipifarnib. Arch Dermatol 2008; 144:779.

Hu JC, et al: Cutaneous side effects of epidermal growth factor receptor inhibitors: clinical presentation, pathogenesis and management. J Am Acad Dermatol 2007; 56:317.

King B, et al: Palifermin-associated papular eruption. Arch Dermatol 2009; 145:179.

Ko JM, et al: Induction and exacerbation of psoriasis with TNF-blockade therapy: a review and analysis of 127 cases. J Dermatolog Treat 2009; 20:100.

Kocharla L, et al: Is the development of drug-related lupus a contraindication for switching from one TNF alpha inhibitor to another? Lupus 2009; 18:169.

Kocyigit P, et al: Linear Iga bullous dermatosis induced by interferon-α 2a. Clin Exp Dermatol 2009; 34:e123.

Kong HH, et al: Sorafenib-induced eruptive melanocytic lesions. Arch Dermatol 2008; 144:820.

Kong HH, et al: Array of cutaneous adverse effects associated with sorafenib. J Am Acad Dermatol 2008; 61:360.

Jarrett SJ, et al: Anti-tumor necrosis factor-alpha therapy-induced vasculitis: case series. J Rheumatol 2003; 30:2287.

Lacouture ME, et al: Hand foot skin reaction in cancer patients treated with the multikinase inhibitors sorafenib and sunitinib. Annal Oncol 2008; 19:1955.

Lepore L, et al: Drug-induced systemic lupus erythematosus associated with etanercept therapy in a child with juvenile idiopathic arthritis. Clin Exp Rheumatol 2003; 21:276.

Li T, Perez-Soler R: Skin toxicities associated with epidermal growth factor receptor inhibitors. Targ Oncol 2009; 4:107.

Lopez V, et al: Follicular hyperplasia on the face subsequent to therapy with sorafenib: a new skin side effect. J Eur Acad Dermatol Venereol 2009; 23:959.

Lunne J, et al: Generalized xerotic dermatitis with neutrophilic spongiosis induced by erlotinib (Tarceva). Dermatol 2008; 216:247.

Marques CB, et al: Multiple keratoacanthomas arising in the setting of sorafenib therapy: novel chemoprophylaxis with bexarotene. J Moffit Cancer Center 2009; 16:66.

Melosky B, et al: Management of skin rash during EGFR-targeted monoclonal antibody treatment for gastrointestinal malignancies: Canadian recommendations. Current Oncol 2009; 16:16.

Michael TE, et al: Severe acneiform skin reaction during therapy with erlotinib (Tarceva), an epidermal growth factor receptor (EGFR) inhibitor. EJD 2007; 17:552.

Pomerantz RG, et al: Acitretin for treatment of EGFR inhibitor induced cutaneous toxic effects. Arch Dermatol 2008; 144:949.

Ramos-Casals M, et al: Autoimmune diseases induced by TNF-targeted therapies. Best Practice Res Clin Rheumatol 2008; 22:847.

Regula CG, et al: Interstitial granulomatous drug reaction to anakinra. J Am Acad Dermatol 2008; 59:S25.

Richetta AG, et al: A case of infliximab-induced psoriasis. Dermatol Online J 2008; 14:9.

Robert C, et al: Dermatologic symptoms associated with the multikinase inhibitor sorafenib. J Am Acad Dermatol 2009; 60:299.

Rodeck U, et al: Skin toxicity caused by EGFR antagonists: an autoinflammatory condition trigged by deregulated IL-1 signaling. J Cell Physiol 2009; 218:32.

Rosmarin D, et al: Patch testing a patient with allergic contact hand dermatitis who is taking infliximab. J Am Acad Dermatol 2008; 59:145.

Shakoor N, et al: Drug-induced systemic lupus erythematosus associated with etanercept therapy. Lancet 2002; 359:579.

Stanley CY, et al: Development of new-onset psoriasis in a patient receiving infliximab for treatment of rheumatoid arthritis. Dermatol Online J 2008; 14:9.

Surguladze D, et al: Tumor necrosis factor and interleukin-1 antagonists alleviate inflammatory skin changes associated with epidermal growth factor receptor antibody therapy in mice. Cancer Res 2009; 69:5643.

Swale VJ, et al: Etanercept-induced systemic lupus erythematosus. Clin Exp Dermatol 2003; 28:604.

Talwar V, et al: Imatinib mesylate induced skin hypopigmentation. J Assoc Physician India 2007; 55:527.

Thomas R, Stea B: Radiation recalls dermatitis from high-dose interferon alfa-2b. J Clin Oncol 2002; 20:355.

Tsimboukis S, et al: Erlotinib-induced skin rash in patients with non-small cell lung cancer: pathogenesis, clinical significance, and management. Clin Lung Cancer 2009; 10:106.

Van De Voorde K, et al: Imatinib-induced eccrine squamous syringometaplasia. J Am Acad Dermatol 2006; 55:s58.

Verscheuren K, et al: Development of sarcoidosis in etanercept-treated rheumatoid arthritis patients. Clin Rheumatol 2007; 26:1969.

Werth VP, Levinson AI: Etanercept-induced injection site reactions. Arch Dermatol 2001; 137:953.

Wolf IH, et al: Erythroderma with lichenoid granulomatous features induced by erythropoietin. J Cutan Pathol 2005; 32:371.

Woo SM, et al: Exacerbation of psoriasis in a chronic myelogenous leukemia patient treated with imatinib. J Dermatol 2007; 34:724.

Zeltser R, et al: Clinical, histological and immunophenotypic characteristics of injection site reactions associated with etanercept: a recombinant tumor necrosis factor-α receptor:Fc fusion protein. Arch Dermatol 2001; 137:893.

Mercury

Mercury may induce multiple cutaneous syndromes. The classic syndrome is acrodynia, also known as calomel disease, pink disease, and erythrodermic polyneuropathy. Acrodynia is caused by mercury poisoning, usually in infancy. The skin changes are characteristic and almost pathognomonic. They consist of painful swelling of the hands and feet, sometimes associated with considerable itching of these parts. The hands and feet are also cold, clammy, and pink or dusky red. The erythema is usually blotchy but may be diffuse. Hemorrhagic puncta are frequently evident. Over the trunk a blotchy macular or papular erythema is usually present. Stomatitis and loss of teeth may occur. Constitutional symptoms consist of moderate fever, irritability, marked photophobia, increased perspiration, and a tendency to cry most of the time. There is always moderate upper respiratory inflammation with soreness of the throat. There may be hypertension, hypotonia, muscle weakness, anorexia, and insomnia. Albuminuria and hematuria are usually present. The diagnosis is made by finding mercury in the urine.

An exanthem may occur from inhalation of mercury vapors or absorption by direct contact. A diffuse, symmetrical erythematous morbilliform eruption in the flexors and proximal extremities begins within a few days of exposure. Accentuation in the groin and medial thighs produces a "baboon syndrome" appearance. The eruption burns or itches, and small follicular pustules appear. Extensive desquamation occurs with resolution. Old broken thermometers or the application of mercury-containing creams and herbal medications are potential sources. In Haiti elemental mercury is applied to surfaces for religious purposes and may result in contamination of those coming in contact.

Mercury is also a possible cause of foreign body granulomas and hyperpigmentation at the sites of application. An eruption of 1–2 mm, minimally pruritic papules and papulovesicles on the palms (all patients) and soles, arms, and trunk has also been ascribed to levels of mercury in the blood at near the upper limits considered to be safe. Treatment with a seafood-free diet and chelation with succimer led to resolution of the eruption in some patients. Nummular dermatitis improved in two mercury patch test-positive patients when their dental amalgam was removed.

Bromoderma

Bromides produce distinctive follicular eruptions, acneiform, papular, or pustular. Vegetative, exudative plaques studded with pustules may develop, resembling Sweet syndrome, pyoderma gangrenosum, or an orthopox virus infection. Characteristically, there are coalescent pustules on a raised border at the periphery of the lesion—the diagnostic clue. Histologically, the lesions show epidermal hyperplasia with intraepidermal and dermal neutrophilic abscesses. There is rapid involution of the lesions on cessation of bromide inges-

tion. Excessive cola or soft-drink ingestion, or the ingestion of bromine-containing medications (ipratropium bromide, dextromethorphan hydrobromide, potassium bromide, pipobroman, Medecitral) may be the cause of a bromoderma. Serum bromide is elevated and confirms the diagnosis.

Iododerma

Iodides may cause a wide variety of skin eruptions. The most common sources of exposure are oral and intravenous contrast materials, and when iodides are used to treat thyroid disease. Application of povidone-iodine to the skin, or as a soak in the tub has produced iododerma. The most common type is the acneiform eruption with numerous acutely inflamed follicular pustules (Fig. 6-37), each surrounded by a ring of hyperemia. Dermal bullous lesions are also common and may become ulcerated and crusted, resembling pyoderma gangrenosum or Sweet syndrome. The eruption may involve the face, upper extremities, trunk, and even the buccal mucosa. Acne vulgaris and rosacea are unfavorably affected by iodides. Acute iododerma may follow intravenous radiocontrast studies in patients with renal failure. The lesions may be associated with severe leukocytoclastic vasculitis, intraepidermal spongiform pustules, and suppurative folliculitis. Iodine is removed quickly by hemodialysis. Forced diuresis with sodium chloride and furosemide can be used to "wash out" the iodide. The lesions respond to prednisone.

Adachi A, et al: Mercury-induced nummular dermatitis. J Am Acad Dermatol 2000; 43:383.

Anzai S, et al: Bromoderma. Int J Dermatol 2003; 42:370.

Audicana M, et al: An unusual case of baboon syndrome due to mercury present in a homeopathic medicine. Contact Dermatitis 2001; 45:185.

Aydingoz IE, et al: Iododerma following sitz bath with povidone-iodine. Aus J Dermatol 2007; 48:102.

Bel S, et al: Vegetant bromoderma in an infant. Pediatr Dermatol 2001; 18:336.

Boyd AS, et al: Mercury exposure and cutaneous disease. J Am Acad Dermatol 2000; 43:81.

Dantzig PI: A new cutaneous sign of mercury poisoning? J Am Acad Dermatol 2003; 49:1109.

Garcia-Menaya JM, et al: Baboon syndrome: 2 simultaneous cases in the same family. Contact Dermatitis 2008: 58:108.

Hafiji J, et al: A case of bromoderma and bromism. Br J Dermatol 2008; 158:405.

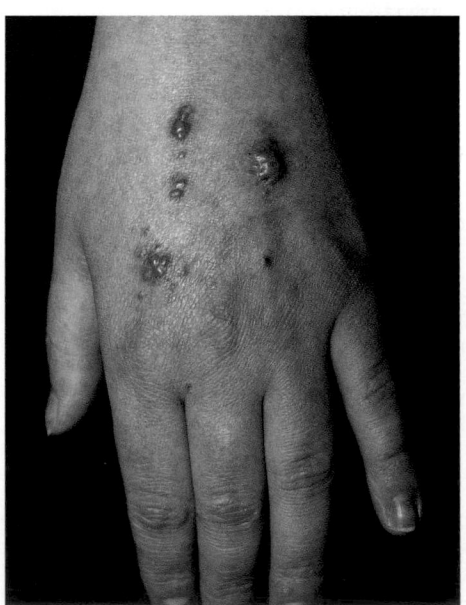

Fig. 6-37 Iododerma.

Jih DM, et al: Bromoderma after excessive ingestion of Ruby Red Squirt. N Engl J Med 2003; 348:1932.

Maffeis L, et al: Single-plaque vegetating bromoderma. J Am Acad Dermatol 2008; 58:682.

Masse M, et al: Use of topical povidone-iodine resulting in an iododerma-like eruption. J Dermatol 2008; 35:744.

Ozkaya E, et al: Mercury-induced systemic allergic dermatitis caused by "white precipitate" in a skin lightening cream. Contact Dermatitis 2009: 60:61.

van der Linde AAA, et al: A previously healthy 11-year-old girl with behavioural disturbances, desquamation of the skin and loss of teeth. Eur J Pediatr 2009; 168:509.

Drug-induced autoimmune diseases

Lupus erythematosus

Drug-induced SLE is rarely associated with skin lesions. It occurs in older patients and affects men as commonly as women. The symptoms are generally mild and include fever, myalgias/arthralgias, and serositis. This form of DIL is associated with a positive ANA, homogenous pattern, and antihistone antibodies, but a negative anti-dsDNA antibody and normal complement levels. Procainamide, hydralazine, quinidine, captopril, isoniazid, minocycline, carbamazepine, propylthiouracil, sulfasalazine, and the statins are among the reported agents triggering this form of DIL. The TNF inhibitors, especially etanercept, may also cause an SLE-like syndrome but with prominent skin lesions. Women are favored, and nephropathy and CNS involvement can occur. Again, the affected patients are ANA-positive, but also anti-dsDNA antibody-positive, and more than half are hypocomplementemic.

Numerous medications have been reported to produce cutaneous lesions characteristic of subacute cutaneous lupus erythematosus (SCLE). The eruption begins days to years after starting the medications. Hydrochlorthiazide, diltiazem (and other calcium channel blockers), and terbinafine are the most common causative agents, but ACE inhibitors, proton pump inhibitors, statins, NSAIDS, and even agents used to treat lupus, such as hydroxychloroquine and leflunomide, can induce SCLE. These patients may also be ANA-positive and have antihistone antibodies, but in addition have positive anti-SSA antibodies. Cutaneous lesions are photosensitive, but not photodistributed, annular or papulosquamous plaques. Chilblain-like lesions are rarely seen. Treatment is as for SCLE, with sun avoidance, and topical and systemic steroids as required. Drug withdrawal results in resolution over weeks to months. The positive serologies may decrease as the eruption improves. The pathogenesis of drug-induced SCLE is unknown, but most agents that cause it are also agents that cause both photosensitive and lichenoid drug eruptions. Etanercept can produce both classic drug-induced SLE and drug-induced SCLE (see above).

Hydroxyurea dermopathy

Chronic use of hydroxyurea for chronic myelogenous leukemia, thrombocythemia, or psoriasis may be associated with the development of cutaneous lesions characteristic of dermatomyositis. Scaly, linear erythema of the dorsal hands, accentuated over the knuckles, is noted. There may be marked acral atrophy and telangiectasia. Elbow and eyelid involvement characteristic of dermatomyositis may also be seen. Biopsy shows vacuolar degeneration of the basal cells and an interface lymphocytic infiltrate. The skin lesions tend to improve over months, although the atrophy may not improve.

Linear IgA bullous dermatosis

Linear IgA disease is frequently associated with medication exposure, especially vancomycin. Men and women are equally affected, and the eruption usually begins within 2 weeks of vancomycin therapy. Clinical morphology is variable and can include flaccid or tense bullae, vesicles, erythematous papules or plaques, exanthematous morbilliform eruptions typical of a drug exanthem, and targetoid papules. TEN or severe SJS may be simulated, but mucosal involvement is not universal (30–45%) and conjunctival involvement is uncommon (10%). Histology will show subepidermal blistering with neutrophils and eosinophils in biopsies taken from bullous lesions. In nonbullous and TEN/SJS-like lesions, there is a vacuolar/lichenoid dermatitis with eosinophils. Unless a direct immunofluorescence (DIF) test is performed, this would be interpreted as erythema multiforme or a drug eruption, and the diagnosis of linear IgA disease would be missed. Treatment is to stop the offending drug and to give dapsone at 100–200 mg daily, as needed.

Leukotriene receptor antagonist-associated Churg–Strauss syndrome

Asthma patients being treated with leukotriene receptor antagonists may develop a syndrome resembling Churg–Strauss vasculitis. It occurs 2 days to 10 months after the leukotriene receptor antagonist has been started. Inhaled fluticasone has also been reported to produce this syndrome. Involvement may be limited to the skin. Features of the syndrome include peripheral eosinophilia, pulmonary infiltrates, and less commonly neuropathy, sinusitis, pericardial effusion, and cardiomyopathy. Skin lesions occur in about half the patients and are usually purpuric and favor the lower legs. Histologically, the skin lesions show leukocytoclastic vasculitis with significant tissue eosinophilia. In one case cutaneous perivascular granulomas with eosinophils were found in the skin with surrounding necrobiotic collagen. Antibodies to neutrophilic cytoplasmic antigens (p-ANCA) may be positive. Withdrawal of the leukotriene receptor antagonist therapy may lead to improvement, but systemic therapy with prednisone and cyclophosphamide may be required. The neuropathy may be permanent. The pathogenesis of this drug-induced syndrome is unknown. Some cases occur as steroids are tapered, but others have occurred in steroid-naïve asthmatics. Unopposed leukotriene B4 activity, a potent chemoattractant for eosinophils and neutrophils, may explain the clinical findings.

Arm JP, Mark EJ: Case 30-2000: a 25-year-old man with asthma, cardiac failure, diarrhea, and weakness of the right hand. N Engl J Med 2000; 343:953.

Billet SE, et al: A morbilliform variant of vancomycin-induced linear IgA bullous dermatosis. Arch Dermatol 2008; 144:774.

Black JG, et al: Montelukast-associated Churg–Strauss vasculitis: another associated report. Ann Allergy Asthma Immunol 2009; 102:351.

Bonsmann G, et al: Terbinafine-induced subacute cutaneous lupus erythematosus. J Am Acad Dermatol 2001; 44:925.

Ching JC, et al: Childhood linear IgA bullous disease triggered by amoxicillin-clavulanic acid. Pediatr Dermatol 2007; 24:E40.

Currie GP, et al: Histological appearances of putative montelukast-related Churg–Strauss syndrome. Thorax 2008; 63:1120.

Dacey MJ, Callen JP: Hydroxyurea-induced dermatomyositis-like eruption. J Am Acad Dermatol 2003; 48:439.

Dam C, Bygum A: Subacute cutaneous lupus erythematosus induced or exacerbated by proton pump inhibitors. Acta Dermatol Venereol 2008; 88:87.

Dellavalle RP, et al: Vancomycin-associated linear IgA bullous dermatosis mimicking toxic epidermal necrolysis. J Am Acad Dermatol 2003; 48:S56.

Eming SA, et al: Lichenoid chronic graft-versus-host disease-like acrodermatitis induced by hydroxyurea. J Am Acad Dermatol 2001; 45:321.

Gal AA, et al: Cutaneous lesions of Churg–Strauss syndrome associated with montelukast therapy. Br J Dermatol 2002; 147:604.

Hauser T, et al: The leucotriene receptor antagonist montelukast and the risk of Churg–Strauss syndrome: a case crossover study. Thorax 2008; 63:677.

Keogh KA, Specks U: Churg–Strauss syndrome: clinical presentation, antineutrophil cytoplasmic antibodies, and leukotriene receptor antagonists. Am J Med 2003; 115:284.

Konig C, et al: Linear IgA bullous dermatosis induced by atorvastatin. J Am Acad Dermatol 2001; 44:689.

Marzano AV, et al: Leflunomide-induced subacute cutaneous lupus erythematosus with erythema multiforme-like lesions. Lupus 2008; 17:329.

Oh ST, et al: Hydroxyurea-induced melanonychia concomitant with a dermatomyositis-like eruption. J Am Acad Dermatol 2003; 49:339.

Oskay T, et al: Dermatomyositis-like eruption after long-term hydroxyurea therapy for polycythemia vera. Eur J Dermatol 2002; 12:586.

Palmer RA: Vancomycin-induced linear IgA disease with autoantibodies to BP180 and LAD285. Br J Dermatol 2001; 145:816.

Plunkett RW, et al: Linear IgA bullous dermatosis in one of two piroxicam-induced eruptions: a distinct direct immunofluorescence trend revealed by the literature. J Am Acad Dermatol 2001; 45:691.

Ruiz-Genao DP, et al: Dermatomyositis-like reaction induced by chemotherapeutical agents. Int J Dermatol 2002; 41:885.

Shapiro LE, et al: Minocycline, perinuclear antineutrophilic cytoplasmic antibody, and pigment: the biochemical basis. J Am Acad Dermatol 2001; 45:787.

Sontheimer RD, et al: Drug-induced subacute cutaneous lupus erythematosus: a paradigm for bedside-to-bench patient-oriented translational clinical investigation. Arch Dermatol Res 2009; 301:65.

Tang MBY, Yosipovitch G: Acute Churg–Strauss syndrome in an asthmatic patient receiving montelukast therapy. Arch Dermatol 2003; 139:715.

Vedove CD, et al: Drug-induced lupus erythematosus. Arch Dermatol Res 2009; 301:99.

Adverse reactions to corticosteroids

Cutaneous reactions may result from topical, intralesional, subcutaneous, or systemic delivery of corticosteroids.

Topical application

The prolonged topical use of corticosteroid preparations may produce distinctive changes in the skin. The appearance of these side effects is dependent on four factors: the strength of the steroid, the area to which it is applied, the amount of coexistent sun damage at the site of application, and the individual's predisposition to certain side effects. Atrophy, striae, telangiectasia, skin fragility, and purpura are the most frequent changes seen (Fig. 6-38). The most striking changes of telangiectasia are seen in fair-skinned individuals who use fluorinated corticosteroids on the face. The changes in the skin are enhanced by occlusion. When these side effects occur, the strength of the steroid should be reduced or substituted with pimecrolimus or tacrolimus. Weekly pulse dosing of a potent topical steroid can also reduce the incidence of side effects. Adjunctive measures to reduce steroid requirement could include addition of topical doxepin, pramoxine, or menthol and camphor to the regimen. Usually, the telangiectases disappear a few months after corticosteroid applications are stopped.

When corticosteroid preparations are applied to the face over a period of weeks or months, persistent erythema with telangiectases, and often small pustules, may occur. Perioral dermatitis and rosacea are in some cases caused by the use of topical corticosteroids. Steroid rosacea has been reported from long-term use of 1% hydrocortisone cream. For this reason, the authors do not recommend chronic topical steroid preparations of any strength in the adjunctive treatment of rosacea. A

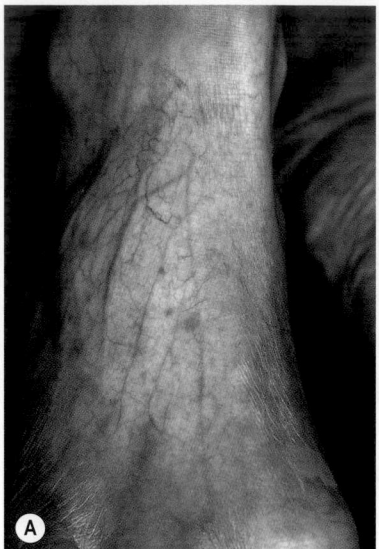

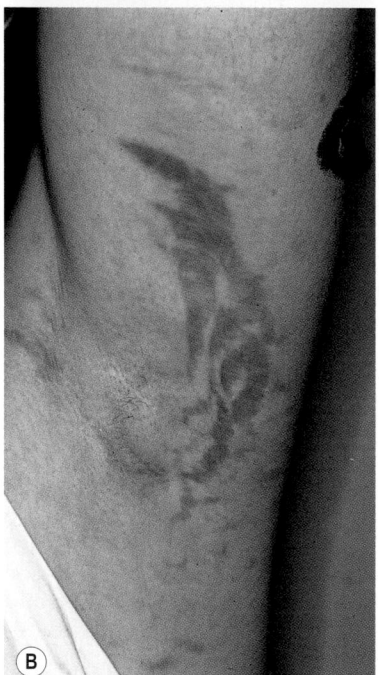

Fig. 6-38 A, Steroid atrophy. B, Steroid-induced striae.

topical calcineurin inhibitor may be used instead as an anti-inflammatory, although it can also induce a rosacea-like eruption. When a rosacea-like eruption appears in the setting of a topical anti-inflammatory, a pustule should be opened and the contents examined for overgrowth of *Demodex* mites.

Repeated application of corticosteroids to the face, scrotum, or vulva may lead to marked atrophy of these tissues. The tissues become "addicted" to the topical steroid, so that withdrawing the topical steroid treatment results in severe itching or burning and intense erythema. Topical application of corticosteroids can produce epidermal atrophy with hypopigmentation. If used over large areas, sufficient topical steroids may be absorbed to suppress the hypothalamic–pituitary axis. This may affect the growth of children with atopic dermatitis and has led to Addisonian steroid dependency and also Cushing syndrome. Atopic children with more than 50% body surface area involvement have short stature. This may be related to their increased use of potent topical steroids. In addition, bone mineral density is reduced in adults with chronic atopic dermatitis severe enough to require corticosteroid preparations stronger than hydrocortisone.

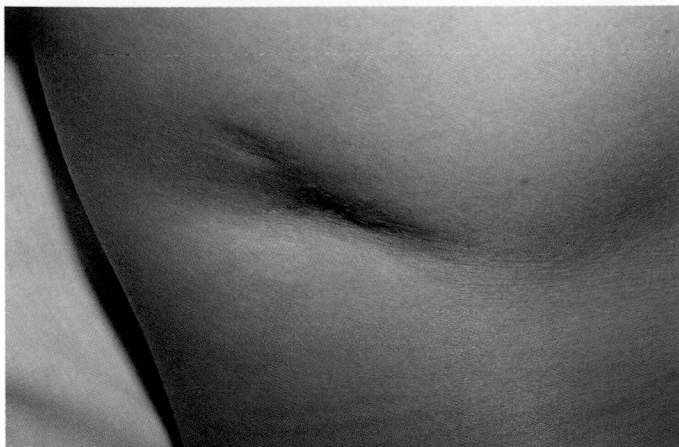

Fig. 6-39 Fat atrophy due to superficial corticosteroid injection.

Injected corticosteroids

Intralesional injection of corticosteroids is valuable in the management of many dermatoses. The injection of corticosteroids may produce subcutaneous atrophy at the site of injection (Fig. 6-39). The injected corticosteroid may also migrate along lymphatics, causing not only local side effects but also linear atrophic hypopigmented hairless streaks. These may take years to resolve. These complications are best avoided by injecting directly into the lesion, not into the fat, and using only the minimal concentration and volume required. Triamcinolone acetonide, not hexacetonide, should be used for injecting cutaneous lesions.

Intramuscular steroid injections should always be given into the buttocks with a long needle (at least 1½ inches in adults). Injection of corticosteroids into the deltoid muscle sometimes causes subcutaneous atrophy. The patient becomes aware of the reaction by noticing depression and depigmentation at the site of injection. There is no pain, but it is bothersome cosmetically. The patient may be assured that this will fill in but it may take several years to do so.

Systemic corticosteroids

Prolonged use of corticosteroids may produce numerous changes of the skin. In addition, they have a profound effect on the metabolism of many tissues, leading to predictable, and sometimes preventable, complications. Intramuscular injections are not a safer delivery method than oral administration.

Purpura and ecchymosis

The skin may become thin and fragile. Spontaneous tearing may occur from trivial trauma. Purpura and ecchymoses are especially seen over the dorsal forearms in many patients over the age of 50. It is aggravation of actinic purpura.

Cushingoid changes

The most common change is probably the alteration in fat distribution. Buffalo hump, facial and neck fullness, increased supraclavicular and suprasternal fat, gynecomastia, protuberant or pendulous abdomen, and flattening of the buttocks may occur. Aggressive dietary management with reduction in carbohydrate and caloric intake may ameliorate these changes.

Steroid acne

Small, firm follicular papules on the forehead, cheeks, and chest may occur. Even inhaled corticosteroids for pulmonary disease can cause acne. Steroid acne can persist as long as the corticosteroids are continued. The management is similar to acne vulgaris with topical preparations and oral antibiotics. Acne from androgen use closely resembles steroid acne.

Striae

These may be widely distributed, especially over the abdomen, buttocks, and thighs.

Other skin changes

There may be generalized skin dryness (xerosis); the skin may become thin and fragile; keratosis pilaris may develop; persistent erythema of the skin in sun-exposed areas may occur, and erythromelanosis may rarely occur.

Hair changes

Hair loss occurs in about half of patients on long-term corticosteroids in large doses. There may be thinning and brittle fracturing along the hair shaft. There may be increased hair growth on the bearded area and on the arms and back with fine vellus hairs.

Systemic complications

Hypertension, cataracts, aseptic necrosis of the hip, and osteoporosis are potential consequences of therapy with systemic steroids. Bone loss can occur early in the course of corticosteroid therapy, so it should be managed preemptively. Effective management can reduce steroid-induced osteoporosis. All patients with anticipated treatment courses longer than 1 month should be supplemented with calcium and vitamin D (1.0–1.5 g calcium and 400–800 U cholecalciferol a day) and a bisphosphonate, such as alendronate or risedronate. Smoking should be stopped and alcohol consumption minimized. Bone mineral density can be accurately measured at baseline via dual energy x-ray absorptiometry (DEXA) scan, and followed during corticosteroid therapy. Hypogonadism, which contributes to osteoporosis, can be treated in men and women with testosterone or estrogen, respectively. Implementation of bone loss prevention strategies by dermatologists is unacceptably low.

Aalto-Korte K, et al: Bone mineral density in patients with atopic dermatitis. Br J Dermatol 1997; 136:172.

Coureau B, et al: Cushing's syndrome induced by misuse of moderate-to-high-potency topical corticosteroids. Ann Pharmacother 2008; 42:1903.

Gul U, et al: A case of granulomatous rosacea successfully treated with pimecrolimus cream. J Dermatol Treat 2008; 19:313.

Massarano AA, et al: Growth in atopic eczema. Arch Dis Child 1993; 68:677.

Monk B, et al: Acne induced by inhaled corticosteroids. Clin Exp Dermatol 1993; 18:48.

Papadopoulos PJ, et al: The clinical picture: soft tissue atrophy after corticosteroid injection. Cleveland Clin J Med 2009; 76:373.

Rapaport MJ, Lebwohl M: Corticosteroid addiction and withdrawal in the atopic: the red burning skin syndrome. Clin Dermatol 2003; 21:201.

Summey BT, et al: Glucocorticoid-induced bone loss in dermatologic patients: an update. Arch Dermatol 2006; 142:300.

Bonus images for this chapter can be found online at

http://www.expertconsult.com

Fig. 6-1 Argyria.

7

Erythema and Urticaria

Flushing

Flushing presents with transient erythema, usually localized to the face, neck, and upper trunk. Menopausal flushing may be associated with perspiration, as is that induced by high ambient temperature, fever, or consumption of hot or spicy food and beverages. Flushing associated with medications, histamine, or serotonin is generally dry.

Menopausal flushing may be age-related, may be induced by oophorectomy or medication (tamoxifen, leuprolide acetate), and may begin long before menses cease. Men may also experience climacteric flushing following surgery or antiandrogen therapy (flutamide).

Blushing, or emotional flushing, may be either emotionally or physiologically induced. Simple facial redness may occur in individuals with translucent skin and is called anatomically predisposed blushing. Intense flushing may be associated with rosacea. In patients with rosacea, spicy foods, alcohol, and hot beverages are frequent triggers for flushing. Drugs associated with flushing include niacin, calcium channel blockers, cyclosporine, chemotherapeutic agents, vancomycin, bromocriptine, intravenous contrast material, sildenafil and related drugs for erectile dysfunction, and high-dose methylprednisolone. Severe serotonin toxicity with flushing can be precipitated by the combination of a monoamine oxidase inhibitor and a serotonin reuptake inhibitor. Reduced to absent methylnicotinate-induced flushing has been noted in patients with schizophrenia. This lack of flushing in response to methylnicotinate has been used for diagnostic psychiatric testing. Flushing after induction of general anesthesia with agents such as thiopental and muscle relaxants is more common in patients prone to blushing. It appears to be neuronally mediated, rather than related to histamine release. Endogenous vasoactive substances are associated with flushing in carcinoid syndrome, mastocytosis, medullary thyroid carcinoma, and pheochromocytoma.

Food-associated flushing may be caused by capsaicin (red pepper), sodium nitrate, or alcohol. Alcohol may produce flushing in patients using topical calcineurin inhibitors. Sulfites are found in wine, dried fruit, prepared foods, and fresh grapes and potatoes. Ciguatera or scombroid fish poisoning is a form of histamine-related food poisoning, caused by histamine within the flesh of the fish. Dietary histamine is normally detoxified by amine oxidases, and those with low amine oxidase activity are at greater risk for histamine toxicity. Individuals who flush without an identifiable cause should be investigated for dietary triggers and subtle manifestations of rosacea. Urine catecholamines, and serotonin and histamine metabolites should be measured if an endogenous cause is suspected. Many cases of flushing remain idiopathic. These patients may be managed with avoidance of dietary triggers and by sipping iced water to break the flush. Menopausal flushing responds to low-dose estrogen given orally or transdermally. The Women's Health Initiative studies concerning hormone replacement therapy (HRT) suggested that breast cancer risk is increased by combinations of estrogen and progestogen taken for longer than 5 years. Unopposed estrogen can increase the risk of endometrial carcinoma in premenopausal women. HRT does not appear to lower the risk of cardiac events, and the risks of long-term therapy often outweigh the benefits. Short-term HRT may still be very helpful in the management of perimenopausal flushing, although alternatives, including serotonin reuptake inhibitors, adrenergic agents, gabapentin, and phytoestrogens, have generally been disappointing. Flushing can be reduced by avoidance of alcohol, caffeine, and spicy foods. Niacin-induced flushing is mediated by prostaglandin D2. It shows some response to aspirin, as well as the prostaglandin D(2) receptor 1 antagonist, laropiprant. Topical oxymetazoline, an α-adrenergic receptor agonist, shows some promise for the treatment of flushing associated with rosacea.

Isbister GK, et al: Serotonin toxicity: a practical approach to diagnosis and treatment. Med J Aust 2007 Sep 17; 187(6):361–365.

Kademian M, et al: Case reports: new onset flushing due to unauthorized substitution of niacin for nicotinamide. J Drugs Dermatol 2007 Dec; 6(12):1220–1221.

Lubbe J, et al: Tacrolimus ointment, alcohol, and facial flushing. N Engl J Med 2004; 351:2740.

Maintz L, et al: Histamine and histamine intolerance. Am J Clin Nutr 2007 May; 85(5):1185–1196.

Mattsson LA, et al: Efficacy and tolerability of continuous combined hormone replacement therapy in early postmenopausal women. Menopause Int 2007 Sep; 13(3):124–131.

Ogunleye T, et al: Ethanol-induced flushing with topical pimecrolimus use. Dermatitis 2008 Mar–Apr; 19(2):E1–E2.

Paolini JF, et al: Effects of laropiprant on nicotinic acid-induced flushing in patients with dyslipidemia. Am J Cardiol 2008 Mar 1; 101(5):625–630.

Sassarini J, et al: Hot flushes: are there effective alternatives to estrogen? Menopause Int 2010 Jun; 16(2):81–88.

Shanler SD, et al: Successful treatment of the erythema and flushing of rosacea using a topically applied selective alpha1-adrenergic receptor agonist, oxymetazoline. Arch Dermatol 2007 Nov; 143(11):1369–1371.

Erythemas

The term erythema means blanchable redness (hyperemia) of the skin. A number of reactive skin conditions are referred to as erythemas. These include toxic erythemas related to viral and bacterial infections, erythema multiforme (EM), erythema nodosum, and the gyrate (figurate) erythemas.

Erythema palmare

Erythema palmare, persistent palmar erythema, is usually most marked on the hypothenar areas, and is associated with an elevated level of circulating estrogen. Cirrhosis, hepatic metastases, and pregnancy are common causes.

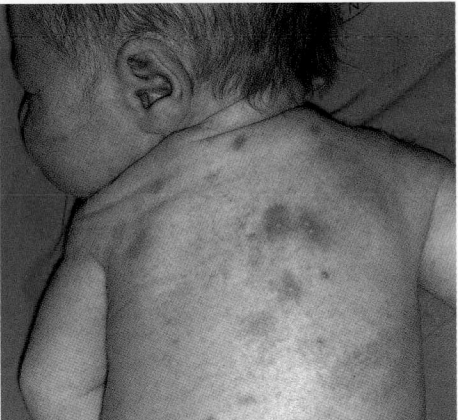

Fig. 7-1 Erythema toxicum neonatorum.

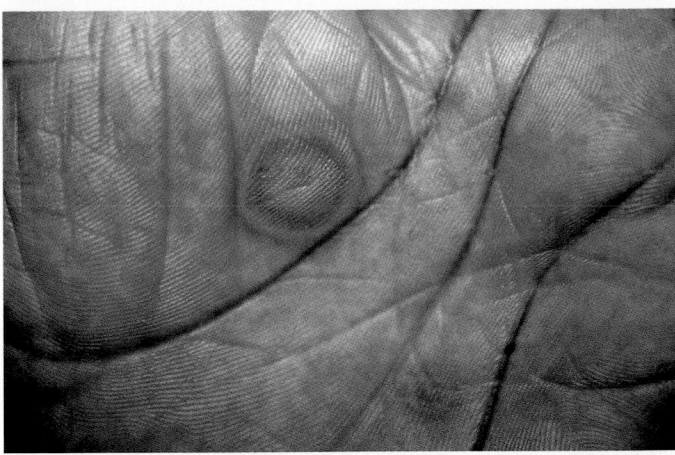

Fig. 7-2 Erythema multiforme, target lesions.

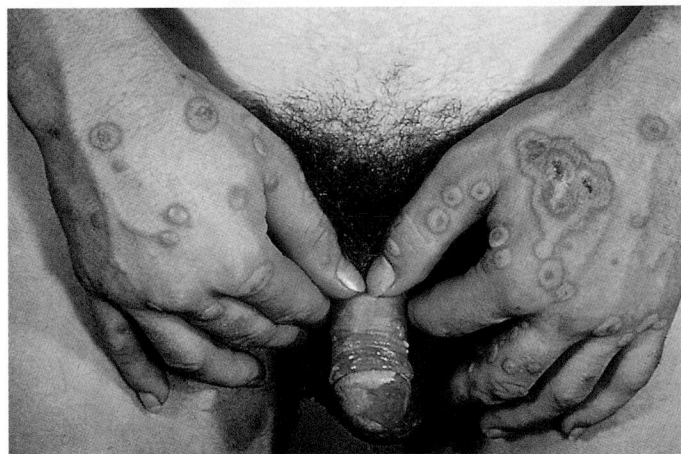

Fig. 7-3 Erythema multiforme involving the dorsal hands and penis.

Generalized erythema

Generalized erythema may be caused by medications, bacterial toxins, or viral infection. It is often uneven in distribution, being most noticeable on the chest, proximal extremities, and face. In general, these reactions are self-limited and resolve when the offending medication is stopped or the associated infection is treated or resolves. Specific exanthems associated with bacterial or viral infections are discussed in Chapters 14 and 19.

Erythema toxicum neonatorum

Erythema toxicum neonatorum (Fig. 7-1) occurs in just under half of healthy full-term newborns, usually on the second or third day. Because it is so common, dermatologists are usually consulted only for the most florid or atypical cases. Characteristically, the broad erythematous flare is much more prominent than the small follicular papule or pustule it surrounds. Lesions involve the face, trunk, and proximal extremities, and appear only rarely on the soles or palms. There may be confluent erythema on the face. Fever is absent and the eruption generally disappears by the 10th day. It must be distinguished from miliaria, bacterial folliculitis, neonatal herpes, and scabies. When the rash is atypical, smears of the pustules demonstrating eosinophils are adequate to confirm the diagnosis. Rarely, a biopsy will be required. Biopsy demonstrates a folliculitis containing eosinophils and neutrophils. Tryptase-expressing mast cells are also noted in lesional skin. Macrophages may play a pathogenic role through secretion of high-mobility group box chromosomal protein 1, a pro-inflammatory cytokine.

Erythema multiforme

In 1860, von Hebra first described erythema exudativum multiforme. The original disease described by von Hebra is now called erythema multiforme minor or herpes simplex-associated erythema multiforme (HAEM). It is strongly associated with a preceding herpetic infection. In contrast, Stevens–Johnson syndrome (SJS) and toxic epidermal necrolysis (TEN) usually represent adverse reactions to medications (see Chapter 6). There is, however, overlap in this spectrum of diseases, with herpes being causative in 6–10% of cases of SJS, and in some series *Mycoplasma* causing up to 25%. As treatment and prognosis are related in part to the inciting agent, it is useful to classify EM as follows:

- herpes simplex-associated EM (HAEM)
- chronic oral EM
- mycoplasma-induced EM/SJS (see Chapter 6)
- contact dermatitis-induced EM (see Chapter 6)
- drug-induced EM (see Chapter 6)
- radiation-induced EM (see Chapter 6)
- idiopathic.

Clinical features

EM minor is a self-limited, recurrent disease, usually of young adults, occurring seasonally in the spring and fall, with each episode lasting 1–4 weeks. The individual clinical lesions begin as sharply marginated, erythematous macules, which become raised, edematous papules over 24–48 h. The lesions may reach several centimeters in diameter. Typically, a ring of erythema forms around the periphery, and centrally the lesions become flatter, more purpuric, and dusky. This lesion is the classic "target" or "iris" lesion with three zones—central dusky purpura; an elevated, edematous, pale ring; and surrounding macular erythema (Figs 7-2 to 7-4). The central area may be bullous. Typical targets are best observed on the palms and soles. Lesions generally appear symmetrically and acrally, with initial involvement most frequently on the dorsal hands. The dorsal feet, extensor limbs, elbows, knees, palms and soles typically become involved. In about 10% of cases, more widespread lesions occur on the trunk. The Koebner phenomenon or photoaccentuation may be observed. Mucosal involvement occurs 25% of the time and is usually limited to the oral mucosa. Oral lesions may appear as indurated plaques, target lesions, or erosions (Fig. 7-5). An atypical variant of HAEM has been described in women. It consists of outbreaks of

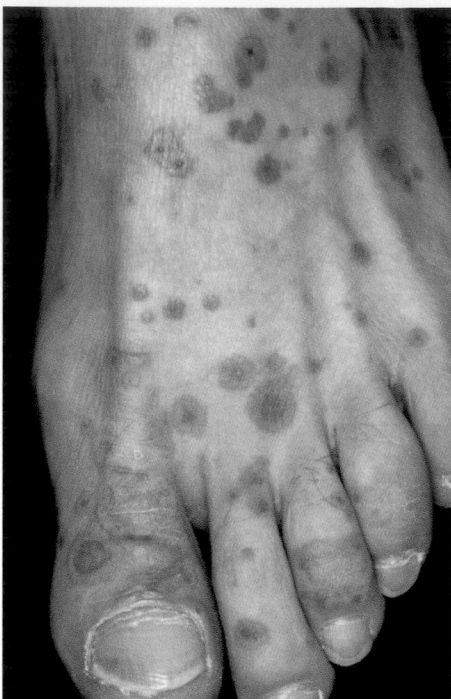

Fig. 7-4 Erythema multiforme, target lesions.

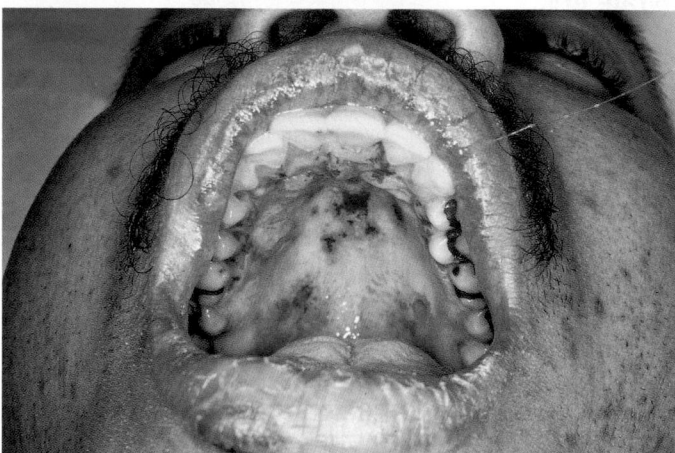

Fig. 7-5 Mucosal lesions of erythema multiforme.

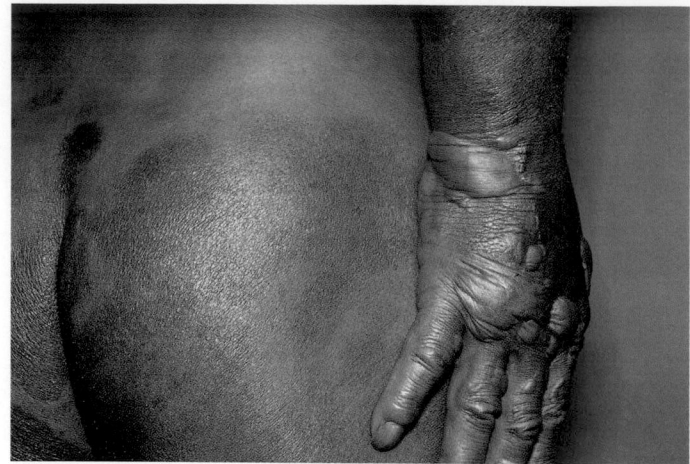

Fig. 7-6 Atypical target lesion in Stevens–Johnson syndrome.

Etiologic factors

Typical EM minor is usually associated with a preceding oro-labial HSV infection. HAEM lesions appear 1–3 weeks (average 10 days) after the herpes outbreak. Episodes of EM minor may not follow every episode of herpes, and some EM outbreaks will not be preceded by a clinically recognizable herpetic lesion. Using PCR and in situ hybridization techniques, HSV DNA and antigens have been found in the lesions of EM minor. The majority of "idiopathic" cases of EM minor are associated with recurrent HSV, and may be successfully treated with suppressive antiviral regimens. SJS is associated with medications and *Mycoplasma* infections. The most common implicated drugs are sulfonamides and other antibiotics, nonsteroidal anti-inflammatory drugs (NSAIDs), allopurinol, and anticonvulsants (see Chapter 6).

Histopathology

The histologic features are similar in all entities within the spectrum, from EM minor to TEN, and are not predictive of etiology. The extent of epidermal involvement depends on the duration of the lesion and where in the lesion the biopsy is taken. All lesions are characterized by cellular necrosis, and the concept of dermal EM is no longer accepted. Biopsies of EM demonstrate a normal basket-weave stratum corneum, suggesting an acute process that has not had time to produce abnormal keratin. Vacuolar interface dermatitis is present, with vacuoles and foci of individual cell necrosis out of proportion to the number of lymphocytes. With time, the necrosis becomes confluent. The dermal infiltrate is largely mononuclear and tends to be primarily around the upper dermal vessels and along the dermoepidermal junction. Activated T lymphocytes are present in lesions of EM, with cytotoxic or suppressor cells more prominent in the epidermis and helper T cells in the dermis. Leukocytoclastic vasculitis is not observed. Eosinophils may sometimes be present, but are rarely prominent. The presence of eosinophils is not predictive of the etiology. Histologically, EM must be distinguished from fixed drug eruption (which often has a deeper infiltrate, eosinophils and neutrophils, papillary dermal fibrosis, and melanophages around postcapillary venules), graft versus host disease (which typically has a more compact stratum corneum and epithelial disorder resembling Bowen's disease), pityriasis lichenoides (which characteristically has a lymphocyte in every vacuole, erythrocyte extravasation, and neutrophil margination within dermal vessels), and lupus erythematosus (which has compact hyperkeratosis, a deeper periadnexal infiltrate, dermal mucin, and basement membrane zone thickening).

unilateral or segmental papules and plaques that may be few in number or solitary. Lesions may be up to 20 cm in diameter. The plaques are erythematous and evolve to have a dusky center, which desquamates. Subcutaneous nodules resembling erythema nodosum may be simultaneously present. Histologic examination shows features of EM, and herpes simplex virus (HSV) DNA is identified in the lesions by polymerase chain reaction (PCR). Acyclovir suppression prevents the lesions, and prednisone therapy seems to increase the frequency of attacks.

Mycoplasma-induced SJS is frequently accompanied by a febrile prodrome. The eruption occurs at all ages; it begins diffusely or on the trunk and mucous membranes. The individual lesions are flat, erythematous, or purpuric macules that form incomplete "atypical targets." Lesions tend to become confluent (Fig. 7-6). Mucous membrane disease is prominent and multiple mucous membranes are generally involved.

In children, polycyclic urticarial lesions often become dusky centrally and are frequently misdiagnosed as EM. This presentation of urticaria has been dubbed "urticaria multiforme." It represents urticaria, and histologic changes of EM are never present.

Differential diagnosis

When characteristic target lesions are present, the diagnosis is established clinically. When bullae are prominent, EM must be distinguished from bullous arthropod reactions and auto-immune bullous diseases (pemphigus if mucous membrane involvement is prominent, and bullous pemphigoid if lesions are small and erythema is prominent at the periphery of the bulla). Paraneoplastic pemphigus may produce atypical target lesions, mucosal involvement, and a vacuolar interface derma-titis, and appear very similar to EM major. Use of direct immunofluorescence may be necessary to exclude this possibility.

Treatment

Treatment of EM is determined by its cause and extent. EM minor is generally related to HSV, and prevention of herpetic outbreaks is central to control of the subsequent episodes of EM. A sunscreen lotion and sunscreen-containing lip balm should be used daily on the face and lips to prevent ultraviolet (UV) B-induced outbreaks of HSV. If this does not prevent recurrences or if genital HSV is the cause, chronic suppressive doses of an oral antiviral drug (acyclovir, valacyclovir, or fam-ciclovir) may be used. This will prevent recurrences in up to 90% of HSV-related cases. Intermittent treatment with sys-temic antivirals or the use of topical antivirals is of little benefit in preventing HSV-associated EM. In patients whose condition fails to respond adequately to antiviral suppression, dapsone, cyclosporine, or thalidomide may occasionally be helpful. It should be noted that most cases of EM minor (HAEM) are self-limited and symptomatic treatment may be all that is required. Symptoms related to oral lesions often respond to topical "swish and spit" mixtures containing lidocaine, bena-dryl, and kaolin. In extensive cases of EM minor, systemic steroids have been used, but because they theoretically may reactivate HSV, they are best given concurrently with an anti-viral drug. The response to systemic corticosteroids is often disappointing. For patients with widespread EM unrespon-sive to the above therapies, management is as for severe drug-induced EM (see Chapter 6).

Abe R, et al: Toxic epidermal necrolysis and Stevens–Johnson syndrome are induced by soluble Fas ligand. Am J Pathol 2003; 162:1515.

Bakis S, et al: Intermittent oral cyclosporin for recurrent herpes simplex-associated erythema multiforme. Australas J Dermatol 2005; 14:18.

Chen CW, et al: Persistent erythema multiforme treated with thalidomide. Am J Clin Dermatol 2008; 9(2):123–127.

Mahendran R, et al: Dapsone-responsive persistent erythema multiforme. Dermatology 2000; 200:281.

Majorana A, et al: Oral mucosal lesions in children from 0 to 12 years old: ten years' experience. Oral Surg Oral Med Oral Pathol Oral Radiol Endod 2010 Jul; 110(1):e13–e18.

Marzano AV, et al: Immunohistochemical expression of apoptotic markers in drug-induced erythema multiforme, Stevens–Johnson syndrome and toxic epidermal necrolysis. Int J Immunopathol Pharmacol 2007 Jul–Sep; 20(3):557–566.

Nelson A, et al: Urticaria neonatorum: accumulation of tryptase-expressing mast cells in the skin lesions of newborns with erythema toxicum. Pediatr Allergy Immunol 2007 Dec; 18(8):652–658.

Quaglino P, et al: Serum levels of the Th1 promoter IL-12 and the Th2 chemokine TARC are elevated in erythema multiforme and Stevens–Johnson syndrome/toxic epidermal necrolysis and correlate with soluble Fas ligand expression. An immunoenzymatic study from the Italian Group of Immunopathology. Dermatology 2007; 214(4):296–304.

Shah KN, et al: "Urticaria multiforme": a case series and review of acute annular urticarial hypersensitivity syndromes in children. Pediatrics 2007 May; 119(5):e1177–1183.

Sun Y, et al: Detection and genotyping of human herpes simplex viruses in cutaneous lesions of erythema multiforme by nested PCR. J Med Virol 2003; 71:423.

Weston WL: Herpes-associated erythema multiforme. J Invest Dermatol 2005; 124:15.

Wetler DA, et al: Recurrent erythema multiforme. J Am Acad Dermatol 2010; 62:45.

Oral erythema multiforme

A unique subset of EM is limited to or most prominent in the oral cavity. Clinically, patients are otherwise well; 60% are female, with a mean age of 43 years. The minority (about one-quarter) have recurrent, self-limited, cyclical disease. The oral cavity is the only site of involvement in 45%, in 30% there is oral and lip involvement, and in 25% the skin is also involved. All portions of the oral cavity may be involved, but the tongue, gingiva, and buccal mucosa are usually most severely affected. Lesions are almost universally eroded, with or without a pseudomembrane. There are no well-designed trials of treat-ment for this subgroup, but the treatments listed above for EM minor are commonly used. "Swish and spit" mixtures contain-ing lidocaine, benadryl, and kaolin are helpful for sympto-matic relief. Patients should be warned to chew carefully, as the anesthetic effect may dampen their gag reflex.

Al-Johani KA, et al: Erythema multiforme and related disorders. Oral Surg Oral Med Oral Pathol Oral Radiol Endod 2007 May; 103(5):642–654.

Scully C, Bagan J: Oral mucosal diseases: erythema multiforme. Br J Oral Maxillofac Surg 2008 Mar; 46(2):90–95.

Gyrate erythemas (figurate erythemas)

The gyrate erythemas are characterized by clinical lesions that are round (circinate), ring-like (annular), polycyclic (figurate), or arcuate. The primary lesions are erythematous and slightly elevated. There may be a trailing scale, as in erythema annu-lare centrifugum. In some of these diseases the lesions are transient and migratory, and in some they are fixed. Gyrate erythemas often represent the cutaneous manifestations of an infection, malignancy, or drug reaction. Certain diseases in this group have specific causes and are discussed in the rele-vant chapters (erythema marginatum of rheumatic fever; the carrier state of chronic granulomatous disease; and erythema migrans of Lyme borreliosis).

Erythema annulare centrifugum

Erythema annulare centrifugum (EAC) is the most common gyrate erythema. It is characterized by annular or polycyclic lesions that grow slowly (2–3 mm/day), rarely reaching more than 10 cm in diameter. Characteristically, there is a trailing scale at the inner border of the annular erythema (Fig. 7-7). The surface is typically devoid of crusts or vesicles, although

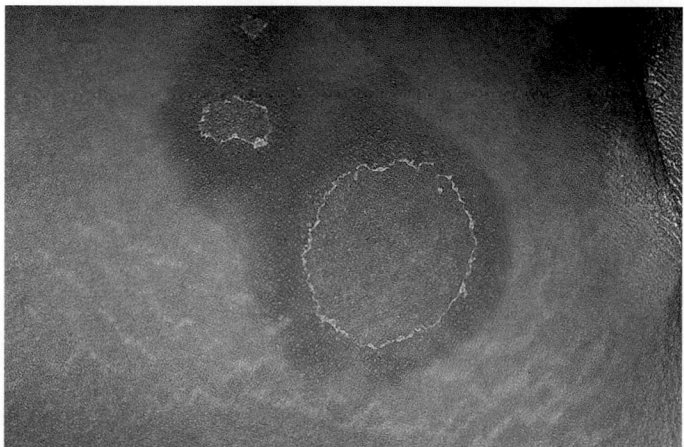

Fig. 7-7 Erythema annulare centrifugum.

atypical cases with telangiectasia and purpura have been described. Lesions commonly occur on the trunk and proximal extremities. Mucosal lesions are absent.

Histologically, the epidermis will show mild focal spongiosis and parakeratosis. Within the superficial dermis and at times the deep dermis, lymphocytes are organized tightly around the blood vessels in a pattern described as a "coat sleeve" arrangement. Histologically, the gyrate erythemas are divided into the superficial and deep types, but these histologic types do not correlate with etiology.

EAC tends to be recurrent over months to years, waxing and waning in severity. Most cases eventually subside spontaneously. While active, the eruption is sometimes responsive to topical steroids. Topical macrolide therapy and topical calcipotriol have also been reported to be successful.

The majority of cases are idiopathic. Some cases are clearly associated with dermatophytosis or the ingestion of molds, such as those in blue cheese. Other foods, such as tomatoes, are sometimes implicated, and a dietary journal may be helpful. Medications are implicated in some cases, and internal cancer has been found. Laboratory tests should be dictated by the physical examination and associated signs and symptoms. In one study of 66 patients, 48% were found to have an associated cutaneous fungal infection such as tinea pedis, and 13% to have internal malignancies.

The differential diagnosis includes those conditions that can have annular configuration, including granuloma annulare, secondary syphilis, tinea, subacute cutaneous lupus erythematosus sarcoidosis, Hansen's disease, erythema marginatum, erythema migrans, annular urticaria, and mycosis fungoides. Histologic examination, clinical features, and basic laboratory examinations will usually allow these diseases to be excluded.

Erythema gyratum repens

Erythema gyratum repens (EGR) is a rare disease that is striking and unique in appearance. Lesions consist of undulating wavy bands of slightly elevated erythema with trailing scale over the entire body. Lesions migrate rapidly (up to 1 cm/day) and are characteristically concentric, giving the skin a "wood grain" appearance (Fig. 7-8).

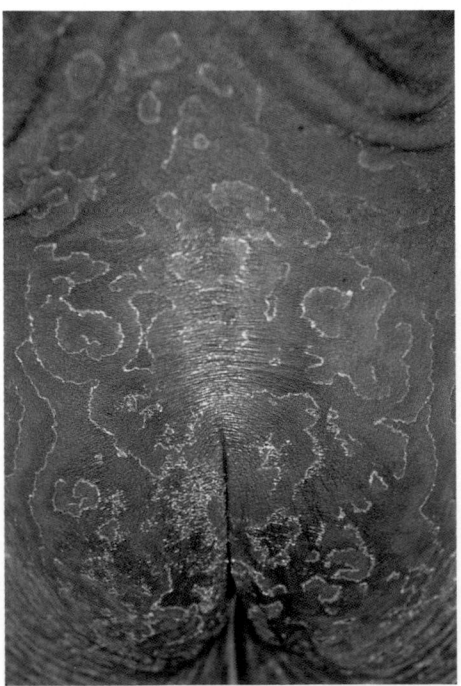

Fig. 7-8 Erythematous gyratum repens.

Pruritus may be severe and blood eosinophilia is often found. In more than 80% of cases, an underlying malignancy is found. Lung cancer is the most common associated malignancy, although a wide range of neoplasms has been described. The skin eruption precedes the detection of the malignancy by an average of 9 months. Given the high frequency of malignant disease, patients with EGR should have extensive evaluations to exclude internal malignancy. If the carcinoma is removed, the lesions clear. Otherwise, the eruption is generally resistant to treatment, although a tumor-associated case responsive to cetirizine has been reported. Rarely, EGR may be associated with pulmonary tuberculosis, a pre-existing papulosquamous disorder, or drug therapy. These cases respond to treatment of the underlying condition or discontinuation of the implicated medication.

Annular erythema of infancy

Peterson and Jarratt reported a case in a 6-month-old boy; lesions were transient (36–48 h), and the eruption stopped without treatment at age 11 months. They called it annular erythema of infancy. A similar case, with more persistent lesions, was reported in a 6-month-old girl; it lasted 11 months without treatment.

Neutrophilic figurate erythema of infancy is a variant of annular erythema of infancy, with a dermal neutrophilic infiltrate and karyorrhexis on biopsy.

Al Hammadi A, et al: Erythema annulare centrifugum secondary to treatment with finasteride. J Drugs Dermatol 2007 Apr; 6(4):460–463.
De Aloe G, et al: Erythema annulare centrifugum successfully treated with metronidazole. Clin Exp Dermatol 2005; 30:583.
Eubanks LE, et al: Erythema gyratum repens. Am J Med Sci 2001; 321:302.
Gniadecki R: Calcipotriol for erythema annulare centrifugum. Br J Dermatol 2002; 146:317.
Kim KJ, et al: Clinicopathologic analysis of 66 cases of erythema annulare centrifugum. J Dermatol 2002; 29:61.
Kreft B, et al: Lupus erythematosus gyratus repens. Eur J Dermatol 2007 Jan–Feb; 17(1):79–82.
Minni J, et al: A novel therapeutic approach to erythema annulare centrifugum. J Am Acad Dermatol 2006 Mar; 54(3 Suppl 2):S134–135.
Miyagawa F, et al: Erythema gyratum repens responding to cetirizine hydrochloride. J Dermatol 2002; 29:731.
Rao NG, et al: Annular erythema responding to tacrolimus ointment. J Drugs Dermatol 2003; 2:421.
Senel E, et al: Erythema annulare centrifugum in pregnancy. Indian J Dermatol 2010; 55(1):120–121.

Eosinophilic cellulitis (Wells syndrome)

In 1971, Wells described four patients with acute onset of plaques resembling cellulitis that persisted for many weeks. Wells syndrome occurs at all ages and pruritus is common. The condition is typically recurrent, and individual episodes may be prolonged. Degranulation of dermal eosinophils produces the flame figures seen in histologic sections. These consist of dermal collagen with adherent eosinophil granules. Eosinophilic panniculitis may also be present.

It is unclear whether Wells syndrome is a distinct disorder sui generis, or a reaction pattern to many possible allergic stimuli. Many (perhaps most) cases represent arthropod reactions. It has also been associated with onchocerciasis, intestinal parasites, varicella, mumps, immunization, drug reactions, myeloproliferative diseases, angioimmunoblastic lymphadenopathy, atopic diathesis, inflammatory bowel disease, hypereosinophilic syndrome, the Churg–Strauss syndrome, anti-tumor necrosis factor (TNF)-α biologic agents, and fungal infection. Expression of the α chain of the interleukin (IL)-2 receptor (CD25) on eosinophils appears to be important in determining the extent of eosinophil degranulation and the degree of tissue damage in eosinophil-mediated disorders, including Wells syndrome. Treatment includes topical and intralesional corticosteroids, oral antihistamines, minocycline, UVB, PUVA, dapsone, and low-dose prednisone. Any triggering factor, such as arthropod bites, should be eliminated.

Boura P, et al: Eosinophilic cellulitis (Wells' syndrome) as a cutaneous reaction to the administration of adalimumab. Ann Rheum Dis 2006 Jun; 65(6):839–840.

Davis RF, et al: Eosinophilic cellulitis as a presenting feature of chronic eosinophilic leukaemia, secondary to a deletion on chromosome 4q12 creating the FIP1L1-PDGFRA fusion gene. Br J Dermatol 2006 Nov; 155(5):1087–1089.

Hirsch K, et al: Eosinophilic cellulitis (Wells' syndrome) associated with colon carcinoma. J Dtsch Dermatol Ges 2005; 3:530.

Karabudak O, et al: Eosinophilic cellulitis presented with semicircular pattern. J Dermatol 2006 Nov; 33(11):798–801.

Renner R, et al: Eosinophilic cellulitis (Wells' syndrome) in association with angioimmunoblastic lymphadenopathy. Acta Derm Venereol 2007; 87(6):525–528.

Sakaria SS, et al: Wells' syndrome associated with ulcerative colitis: a case report and literature review. J Gastroenterol 2007 Mar; 42(3):250–252.

Winfield H, et al: Eosinophilic cellulitislike reaction to subcutaneous etanercept injection. Arch Dermatol 2006 Feb; 142(2):218–220.

Reactive neutrophilic dermatoses

Like the gyrate erythemas, the reactive neutrophilic dermatoses tend to follow certain stimuli, such as acute upper respiratory infections, or are associated with underlying diseases, such as inflammatory bowel disease and hematologic malignancy. Some of the neutrophilic dermatoses share common triggers, and clinical features may overlap. Patients may exhibit the simultaneous or sequential appearance of two or more of the conditions. In some cases, it may be difficult to establish the diagnosis firmly as one or the other of these disorders. For these reasons, it is clinically useful to think of these diseases as forming a spectrum of conditions expressed in certain individuals by a group of stimuli with various overlapping morphologies.

Erythema nodosum

Erythema nodosum (EN) is the most commonly diagnosed form of inflammatory panniculitis, with most cases occurring in young adult women. The eruption consists of bilateral, symmetrical, deep, tender, bruise-like nodules, 1–10 cm in diameter, located pretibially (Fig. 7-9). Initially, the skin over the nodules is red, smooth, slightly elevated, and shiny. The onset is generally acute, and frequently associated with malaise, leg edema, and arthritis or arthralgias. Over a few days, the lesions flatten, leaving a purple or blue–green color resembling a resolving bruise. The natural history is for the nodules to last a few days or weeks, appearing in crops, and then to involute slowly.

EN is a reactive process. Specific causes, histopathology, and other features of EN are discussed in Chapter 23. The disorder is grouped with the other neutrophilic dermatoses because it shares common triggers, and the acute phase of the disorder is characterized by neutrophils within subcutaneous septae.

Sweet syndrome (acute febrile neutrophilic dermatosis)

Since its first description in 1964 by Dr Robert Sweet, as a recurrent febrile dermatosis in women, the spectrum of this syndrome has expanded. Sweet syndrome primarily affects adults, and females outnumber males by about 3:1. In younger

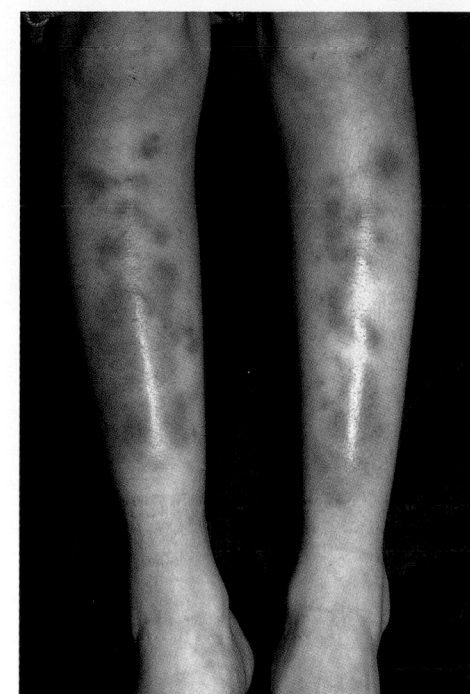

Fig. 7-9 Erythema nodosum.

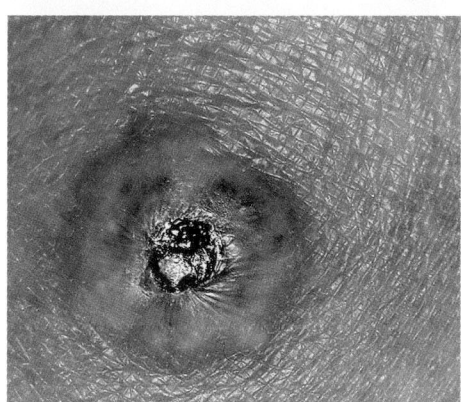

Fig. 7-10 Sweet syndrome, intensely edematous lesion.

adults, female predominance is marked, but in persons older than 50 years of age, the sex ratio is more equal, as cases associated with malignancy have a sex ratio of 1:1. In children, males and females are equally affected. In Europe, cases are more common in the spring and fall. Four subtypes of Sweet syndrome have been described, based on their pathogenesis: the classic type (71%); cases associated with neoplasia (11%); cases associated with inflammatory disease (16%); and cases associated with pregnancy (2%).

The clinical features of all four subtypes are similar, although dusky bullous and necrotic lesions that overlap with pyoderma gangrenosum are more common in patients with associated leukemia. The primary skin lesion is a sharply marginated, rapidly extending, tender, erythematous or violaceous, painful, elevated plaque, 2–10 cm in diameter. Lesions may appear intensely edematous (Fig. 7-10) or merely indurated (Fig. 7-11). They typically involve the face, neck, upper trunk, and extremities. They may burn, but do not itch. The surface of the plaques may develop vesiculation or pustulation as a result of an intense dermal inflammatory infiltrate and accompanying dermal edema. Localized Sweet syndrome has been used to describe cases in which lesions are present only on the face, usually the cheeks. Pathergy and koebnerization after trauma or UVB uncommonly occur.

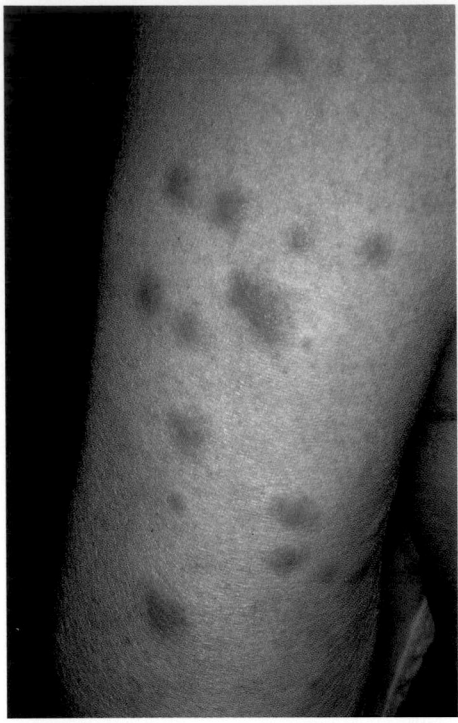

Fig. 7-11 Sweet syndrome, erythematous lesions.

More than three-quarters of patients have systemic findings. The most common is fever, occurring in 50–80% of patients. Arthritis, arthralgias, or myalgias occur in one-third to two-thirds of cases. Conjunctivitis or episcleritis occurs in about 30% of cases. Other ocular manifestations include periorbital inflammation, dacryoadenitis, limbal nodules, peripheral ulcerative keratitis, glaucoma, iritis, and choroiditis. Oral lesions resembling aphthae occur in 2% or 3% of classic cases, but in 10% or more of those associated with hematologic malignancy. Cough, dyspnea, and pleuritis may represent pulmonary involvement. Pulmonary infiltrates and effusions are often seen on chest x-rays of such patients. Rarely, there may be cardiac, renal, hepatic, intestinal, and neurologic involvement. Multifocal sterile osteomyelitis may occur.

Laboratory findings include an elevated sedimentation rate (90%), neutrophilia (70%), leukocytosis (60%), and a left shift (increased bands; 50%). Antineutrophilic cytoplasmic antibodies have been reported. In most cases, an attack lasts 3–6 weeks and then resolves. Recurrences may be seen with the same precipitating cause, such as upper respiratory infection. Persistent cases, with new lesions erupting before the old lesions resolve, may continue for many years.

The hallmark of Sweet syndrome is a nodular and diffuse dermal infiltrate of neutrophils with karyorrhexis and massive papillary dermal edema. Leukocytoclastic vasculitis may be present focally, and this does not exclude a diagnosis of Sweet syndrome. Upper dermal edema may be so intense as to form subepidermal bullae. A mononuclear variant has been described. Leukemic cells may be present in the infiltrate, and it should be noted that clonal restriction of neutrophils has even been seen in Sweet syndrome not associated with malignancy.

The majority of cases of Sweet syndrome follow an upper respiratory tract infection and are therefore acute and self-limited. Other associated conditions include infections with *Yersinia*, toxoplasmosis, histoplasmosis, salmonellosis, tuberculosis, tonsillitis, or vulvovaginal infections. Sweet syndrome has been reported in association with inflammatory bowel disease, and overlaps with the bowel bypass or "blind loop"

syndrome. Cases have also been associated with peripheral ulcerative keratitis and Behçet syndrome.

Hematologic malignancies or solid tumors are present in about 10% of reported cases. Sweet syndrome often presents early in the course of the cancer, when therapy is more efficacious. Associated malignancies are usually hemoproliferative and include leukemias (usually acute myelogenous), lymphomas, anemias, or polycythemias. Solid tumors are of any type but are most commonly genitourinary, breast (in women), or gastrointestinal (in men). Anemia is found in 93% of men and 71% of women with malignancy-associated Sweet syndrome. Thrombocytopenia is seen in half. Solitary or ulcerative lesions are more frequently associated with malignancy.

Pregnancy-associated Sweet syndrome typically presents in the first or second trimester with lesions on the head, neck, trunk, and less commonly on the upper extremities. Lower-extremity lesions resembling EN may occur. The condition may resolve spontaneously or clear with topical or systemic steroids. It may recur with subsequent pregnancies but there does not seem to be any risk to the fetus.

Many medications have been associated with Sweet-like reactions in the skin, although the strongest association exists for granulocyte colony-stimulating factor and all-trans-retinoic acid. Oral contraceptives, vaccines, trimethoprim–sulfamethoxazole, and minocycline have also been implicated, but the evidence is not as compelling. All-trans-retinoic acid causes terminal differentiation of some leukemic clones, and is used to treat promyelocytic leukemia. After about 2 weeks of treatment, Sweet-like syndrome lesions may appear. Initially, these skin lesions may contain immature blasts, making it difficult to distinguish them from leukemia cutis. Later, the lesions contain more mature neutrophils. Induction of the skin lesions appears to be related to the desired pharmacologic effect of the medication.

The two major criteria for the diagnosis of Sweet syndrome are the presence of red edematous plaques and a biopsy demonstrating neutrophils, karyorrhexis, and marked papillary dermal edema. Minor criteria include associated symptoms or conditions, laboratory findings, and response to therapy. Patients should have both of the major and two of the minor criteria for diagnosis (Box 7-1). EM can be distinguished by its typical morphology and histologic features. Clinically, both diseases can have red plaques, and central vesiculation can occur. True target lesions are not seen in Sweet syndrome.

Box 7-1 Revised diagnostic criteria for the diagnosis of Sweet syndrome*

Major criteria

1. Abrupt onset of erythematous plaques or nodules, occasionally with vesicles, pustules, or bullae
2. Nodular and diffuse neutrophilic infiltration in the dermis with karyorrhexis and massive papillary dermal edema

Minor criteria

1. Preceded by a respiratory infection, gastrointestinal tract infection or vaccination, or associated with:
   - Inflammatory disease or infection
   - Myeloproliferative disorders or other malignancy
   - Pregnancy
2. Malaise and fever (>38°C)
3. Erythrocyte sedimentation rate >20 mm; C-reactive protein positive; peripheral leukocytosis, and left shift
4. Excellent response to treatment with systemic corticosteroids

*Both major and two minor criteria are needed for diagnosis.

Bowel bypass syndrome has skin lesions that, on histologic examination, are identical to those of Sweet syndrome; fever and arthritis also accompany this condition. Although it is easy to distinguish classic EN from Sweet syndrome, these two conditions share many features. They occur most often in young adult women and frequently follow upper respiratory infections. They may be associated with pregnancy, underlying malignancy, and inflammatory bowel disease. In both, fever and arthritis may occur, along with leukocytosis with neutrophilia. There are many reports of simultaneous or sequential EN and Sweet syndrome in the same patient. Leukemia-associated Sweet syndrome may overlap with pyoderma gangrenosum. A search for an underlying cause should be undertaken, especially in persons over the age of 50 and those with anemia, thrombocytopenia, or lesions that are bullous or necrotic. The standard treatment is systemic corticosteroids (approximately 1 mg/kg/day oral prednisone). This will result in resolution of fever and skin lesions within days. Potassium iodide has been reported to be effective. Colchicine, dapsone, doxycycline, clofazimine, cyclosporine, and NSAIDs may be helpful in chronic or refractory disease. Medication should be continued for several weeks to prevent relapse.

Neutrophilic dermatosis of the dorsal hands

Lesions of neutrophilic dermatosis of the dorsal hands present as edematous, pustular, or ulcerative nodules or plaques localized to the dorsal hands (Fig. 7-12). Histologically, papillary dermal edema and a nodular and diffuse neutrophilic infiltrate with karyorrhexis are noted. As in Sweet syndrome, leukocytoclastic vasculitis may be present focally. Individual flares respond to prednisone and dapsone, but recurrences are common. As the clinical appearance, tendency to relapse, response to treatment, and histologic features overlap with those of Sweet syndrome and pyoderma gangrenosum, this condition illustrates the close relationship of the various neutrophilic dermatoses. It is best considered a localized variant of Sweet syndrome.

Neutrophilic eccrine hidradenitis

Neutrophilic eccrine hidradenitis is discussed in Chapter 33.

Marshall syndrome

This rare syndrome is characterized by skin lesions resembling Sweet syndrome, which are followed by acquired cutis laxa. Cases occur primarily in children. Small red papules expand

to urticarial, targetoid plaques with hypopigmented centers. Histologic evaluation of the skin lesions usually shows a neutrophilic dermatosis virtually identical to Sweet syndrome. Occasionally, an eosinophilic infiltrate will be found. The lesions resolve with destruction of the elastic tissue at the site, producing soft, wrinkled, skin-colored, protuberant plaques that can be pushed into the dermis. Elastic tissue in other organs may also be affected, especially the heart and lungs. Some cases may be associated with α1-antitrypsin deficiency.

Cohen PR: Sweet's syndrome—a comprehensive review of an acute febrile neutrophilic dermatosis. Orphanet J Rare Dis 2007 Jul 26; 2:34.
Cook-Norris RH, et al: Neutrophilic dermatosis of the hands: an under-recognized hematological condition that may result in unnecessary surgery. Am J Hematol 2009; 84(1):60.
Del Pozo J, et al: Neutrophilic dermatosis of the hands: presentation of eight cases and review of the literature. J Dermatol 2007 Apr; 34(4):243–247.
Glendenning J, et al: Sweet's syndrome in prostate cancer. Prostate Cancer Prostatic Dis 2008 Jan 29 (Epub).
Gottlieb CC, et al: Ocular involvement in acute febrile neutrophilic dermatosis (Sweet syndrome): new cases and review of the literature. Surv Ophthalmol 2008 May–June; 53(3):219–226.
Kaune KM, et al: Bullous sweet syndrome in a patient with t(9; 22)(q34; q11)-positive chronic myeloid leukemia treated with the tyrosine kinase inhibitor nilotinib: interphase cytogenetic detection of BCR-ABL-positive lesional cells. Arch Dermatol 2008 Mar; 144(3):361–364.
Magro CM, et al: Clonality in the setting of Sweet's syndrome and pyoderma gangrenosum is not limited to underlying myeloproliferative disease. J Cutan Pathol 2007 Jul; 34(7):526–534.
Malone JC, et al: Sweet's syndrome: a disease in histologic evolution? Arch Dermatol 2005; 141:893.
Neoh CY, et al: Sweet's syndrome: a spectrum of unusual clinical presentations and associations. Br J Dermatol 2007 Mar; 156(3):480–485.
Ratzinger G, et al: Acute febrile neutrophilic dermatosis: a histopathologic study of 31 cases with review of literature. Am J Dermatopathol 2007 Apr; 29(2):125–133.
Requena L, et al: Histiocytoid Sweet syndrome: a dermal infiltration of immature neutrophilic granulocytes. Arch Dermatol 2005; 141:837.
Tabanlioğlu D, et al: Sweet's syndrome and erythema nodosum: a companionship or a spectrum?—a case report with review of the literature. Int J Dermatol 2010 Jan; 49(1):62–66.
Thompson DF, et al: Drug-induced Sweet's syndrome. Ann Pharmacother 2007 May; 41(5):802–811.
Wallach D, et al: From acute febrile neutrophilic dermatosis to neutrophilic disease: forty years of clinical research. J Am Acad Dermatol 2006 Dec; 55(6):1066–1071.

Pyoderma gangrenosum

Brunsting is credited with the initial clinical description of pyoderma gangrenosum (PG) in 1930. Classic PG begins as an inflammatory pustule with a surrounding halo that enlarges and begins to ulcerate. A primary lesion may not always be seen, and a substantial proportion of lesions appear at sites of trauma (pathergy). Satellite violaceous papules may appear just peripheral to the border of the ulcer and break down to fuse with the central ulcer. Fully developed lesions are painful ulcers with sharply marginated, undermined, blue to purple borders (Fig. 7-13). PG most commonly occurs in adults aged 40–60 years, and typically presents on the lower extremities and trunk. Lesions heal with characteristic thin, atrophic scars. "Malignant pyoderma" is no longer used as a diagnosis, according to the investigators at the Mayo Clinic who originally described it. Although ulcerative PG may occur on the head and neck, most cases described originally as malignant pyoderma are c-ANCA (antibodies to neutrophilic cytoplasmic antigens)-positive, and represent cutaneous presentations of Wegener's granulomatosis. Pustular PG consists of pustular lesions that generally do not progress to ulcerative lesions.

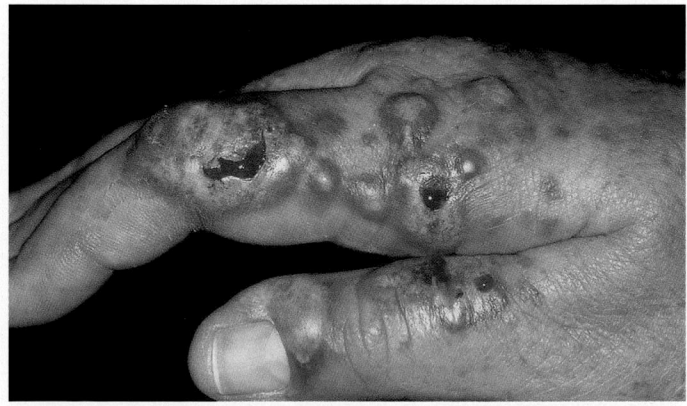

Fig. 7-12 Neutrophilic dermatosis of the dorsal hands.

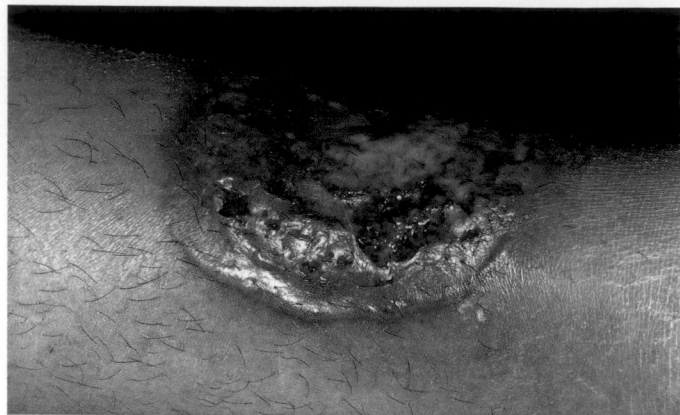

Fig. 7-13 Enlarging ulcer of pyoderma gangrenosum.

This forme fruste of PG is often seen in patients with inflammatory bowel disease. Pyostomatitis vegetans and subcorneal pustular dermatosis are two other pustular neutrophilic diseases reported in association with PG, sometimes in patients with IgA gammopathy.

"Bullous" PG is more superficial and less destructive than the ulcerative type. These lesions have considerable overlap with what has been called bullous Sweet syndrome, and are usually seen in patients with leukemia or polycythemia vera. These red plaques become dusky and develop superficial erosions. They are not deep, usually are not undermined, and are less painful than ulcerative PG.

"Vegetative" PG is the least aggressive form of PG. It is synonymous with "superficial granulomatous pyoderma." Lesions present as cribriform chronic superficial ulcerations usually of the trunk. They enlarge slowly and have elevated borders and clean bases. They are rarely painful, generally respond to relatively conservative treatments, and are usually not associated with underlying systemic disease. PG is rare in children. More than 40% of these patients have underlying inflammatory bowel disease, and another 18% have leukemia. An association of childhood acquired immunodeficiency syndrome (AIDS) and PG has been documented. About one-quarter of children with PG have no underlying disease. Genital and head and neck lesions are not uncommon in children.

Overall, approximately 50% of patients with PG have an associated disease. The most common is inflammatory bowel disease, both Crohn's and ulcerative colitis. Between 1.5% and 5% of patients with inflammatory bowel disease develop PG. The two diseases may flare together or run an independent course. Surgical removal of the diseased intestine may lead to complete remission of PG, or lesions may persist or first appear after removal of the affected bowel. Most patients with PG and inflammatory bowel disease have involvement of the colon. The ulcerative and pustular types of PG are most commonly seen in patients with associated inflammatory bowel disease.

Many other associated conditions have been reported. Leukemia (chiefly acute or chronic myelogenous leukemia), myeloma, monoclonal gammopathy (chiefly IgA), polycythemia vera, myeloid metaplasia, chronic active hepatitis, hepatitis C, human immunodeficiency virus (HIV) infection, systemic lupus erythematosus, pregnancy, PAPA syndrome, and Takayasu arteritis are among the many diseases seen in conjunction with PG. PAPA syndrome is discussed with the other autoinflammatory disorders (see below). More than one-third of PG patients have arthritis, most commonly an asymmetrical, seronegative, monoarticular arthritis of the large joints. Monoclonal gammopathy, usually IgA, is found in 10% of PG patients. Children with congenital deficiency of leukocyte-adherence glycoproteins (LAD) develop PG-like lesions.

Early biopsies of PG show a suppurative folliculitis. The affected follicle is often ruptured. As the lesions evolve, they demonstrate suppurative inflammation in the dermis and subcutaneous fat. Massive dermal edema and epidermal neutrophilic abscesses are present at the violaceous undermined border. These features are not diagnostic and infectious causes must still be excluded.

The clinical picture of PG, in the classic ulcerative form, is very characteristic. Because there are no diagnostic serologic or histologic features, however, PG remains a diagnosis of exclusion. Multiple infections, including mycobacteria, deep fungi, gummatous syphilis, synergistic gangrene, and amebiasis, must be excluded with cultures and special studies. Other disorders frequently misdiagnosed as PG include vascular occlusive or chronic venous disease, vasculitis, cancer, and exogenous tissue injury including factitial disease.

PG may be misdiagnosed as a spider bite if there is only a solitary lesion on an extremity. Spider bites tend to evolve more rapidly and may be associated with other systemic symptoms or findings, such as disseminated intravascular coagulation. Various forms of cutaneous large-vessel vasculitis may produce similar clinical lesions; they are excluded by histologic evaluation and ancillary studies, such as ANCA and antiphospholipid antibody tests.

The most difficult diagnosis to exclude is factitial disease. The clinical lesions may be strikingly similar, evolving from small papulopustules to form ulcerations that do not heal. Histologic evaluation will often simply show suppurative dermatitis, since the injected or applied caustic substance may not be identifiable (urine, disinfectants, drain cleaner). Even the most experienced clinician may misdiagnose factitial disease as PG.

Management of PG is challenging. The initial step is to classify the lesion by type. Underlying conditions should be sought, even if no symptoms are found. Treatment of underlying inflammatory bowel disease may lead to improvement. In general, the vegetative type will respond to topical or local measures. The treatment is determined by the severity of the disease and by its rate of progression. In rapidly progressive cases, aggressive early management may reduce morbidity.

Local treatment includes compresses or whirlpool baths, followed by the use of ointment or hydrophilic occlusive dressings. In mild cases, application of potent topical steroidal medications, intralesional steroid injections, or topical 4% cromolyn or tacrolimus may be beneficial, although pathergy may sometimes be seen at sites of injection. Hyperbaric oxygen therapy has been successful in some patients. Systemic steroids can be very effective. Initial doses are in the range of 1 mg/kg or higher. If control is achieved, the dose may be rapidly tapered. If steroid reduction is not possible, a steroid-sparing agent may be added. In cases that are unresponsive to oral corticosteroids, the use of pulse methylprednisolone may be beneficial.

In general, when the disease is aggressive and use of steroidal medications does not lead to rapid resolution, an immunosuppressive agent is added. Azathioprine, cyclophosphamide, and chlorambucil have been used effectively; however, cyclosporine and infliximab result in faster healing and are the immunosuppressives of choice for PG. The lesions often respond dramatically to these agents, including many that have not responded adequately to corticosteroid therapy. Initial doses of cyclosporine of approximately 5 mg/kg/day are effective in most cases. In failures, the dose can be raised to 10 mg/kg/day. The response is independent of any underlying cause. Infliximab is given as intravenous infusions in doses of about 5 mg/kg every few weeks. In very aggressive, rapidly progressive cases, consideration should be given to starting cyclosporine or infliximab treatment early to gain control of the disease. Etanercept, adalimumab, and alefacept have also been used.

Tacrolimus and mycophenolate mofetil are also effective in some cases, but experience with these agents is much more limited. Sulfapyridine, sulfasalazine, salicylazosulfapyridine, and dapsone may be helpful, either as single agents or in combination with corticosteroids. Clofazimine, in doses of 200–400 mg/day, has been useful in some patients. Minocycline and rarely other antibiotics have anecdotally been successful. Epidermal allografts or autografts may be applied soon after the disease is controlled. Pathergy is rarely noted at the donor site when patients are on adequate immunosuppressive therapy.

Adişen E, et al: Treatment of idiopathic pyoderma gangrenosum with infliximab: induction dosing regimen or on-demand therapy? Dermatology 2008; 216(2):163–165.

Callen JP, et al: Pyoderma gangrenosum: an update. Rheum Dis Clin North Am 2007 Nov; 33(4):787–802.

Hubbard VG, et al: Systemic pyoderma gangrenosum responding to infliximab and adalimumab. Br J Dermatol 2005; 152:1059.

Kikuchi N, et al: Pyoderma gangrenosum following surgical procedures. Int J Dermatol 2010 Mar; 49(3):346–348.

Miller J, et al: Pyoderma gangrenosum: a review and update on new therapies. J Am Acad Dermatol 2010 Apr; 62(4):646–654.

Reichrath J, et al: Treatment recommendations for pyoderma gangrenosum: an evidence-based review of the literature based on more than 350 patients. J Am Acad Dermatol 2005; 53:273.

Rogge FJ, et al: Treatment of pyoderma gangrenosum with the anti-TNFalpha drug—etanercept. J Plast Reconstr Aesthet Surg 2008; 61(4):431–433.

Turner RB, et al: Rapid resolution of pyoderma gangrenosum after treatment with intravenous cyclosporine. J Am Acad Dermatol 2010 Sep; 63(3):e72–e74.

Zaccagna A, et al: Anti-tumor necrosis factor alpha monoclonal antibody (infliximab) for the treatment of pyoderma gangrenosum associated with Crohn's disease. Eur J Dermatol 2003; 13:258.

Autoinflammatory syndromes

The autoinflammatory syndromes are a group of inherited disorders characterized by bouts of inflammation and periodic fevers. Inflammatory skin lesions are often prominent manifestations, especially acne, PG, and erysipelas- and urticaria-like lesions.

Familial Mediterranean fever (FMF) is an autosomal-recessive syndrome characterized by recurrent attacks of fever, peritonitis, pleuritis, arthritis, and erysipelas-like erythema. It is caused by mutation in the *MEFV* gene, which produces pyrin, but a significant number of patients with a similar phenotype lack a detectable gene defect. Incomplete penetrance is common and many patients with paired mutations lack symptoms or have attenuated symptoms. Colchicine is the mainstay of treatment for these patients and it can reduce the risk of associated amyloidosis. Thalidomide was reported as successful in a colchicine-resistant patient. An herbal remedy (a combination of *Andrographis paniculata* Nees with *Eleutherococcus senticosus* Maxim, *Schizandra chinensis* Bail, and *Glycyrrhiza glabra* L extracts) was shown to be effective in a small double-blind, randomized, placebo-controlled study.

The PAPA syndrome is an autosomal-dominant syndrome characterized by pyogenic arthritis, PG, and acne, and is caused by proline serine threonine phosphatase-interacting protein 1 (PSTPIP1) or CD2-binding protein 1 (CD2BP1) mutations. PSTPIP1/CD2BP1, a tyrosine-phosphorylated protein involved in cytoskeletal organization, interacts with pyrin, the gene product important in the pathogenesis of FMF.

The TNF receptor-associated periodic syndrome (TRAPS) is similar to FMF, but shows autosomal-dominant inheritance,

longer attacks, and a lack of response to colchicine. TRAPS is associated with mutations in the *TNFRSF1A* gene, resulting in decreased serum-soluble TNF receptor. The hyper-IgD syndrome (HIDS), associated with mutations in the mevalonate kinase (*MVK*) gene, leading to MVK deficiency, also presents with hereditary periodic fever.

Cryopyrin, the product of the *CAIS1* locus, is associated with familial cold urticaria (familial cold autoinflammatory syndrome), an autosomal-dominant syndrome characterized by fever, rash, conjunctivitis, and arthralgia elicited by generalized exposure to cold. The defect has been mapped to a 10-cM region on chromosome 1q44. The same gene and product are associated with the Muckle–Wells syndrome and chronic infantile neurologic and articular syndrome/neonatal-onset multisystem inflammatory disease (CINCA/NOMID). The Muckle–Wells syndrome is an autosomal-dominant syndrome associated with acute febrile inflammatory episodes comprising abdominal pain, arthritis, urticaria, and multiorgan amyloidosis. The cryopyrin-related diseases often respond to anakinra, a recombinant human IL-1 receptor antagonist that appears promising for other autoinflammatory diseases. Patients with the CINCA syndrome have fever, chronic meningitis, uveitis, sensorineural hearing loss, urticarial rash, and a deforming arthritis. They may also have dysmorphic facial appearance, clubbing of the fingers, mild mental retardation, and papilledema. The Blau syndrome, an autosomal-dominant syndrome with arthritis, uveitis, granulomatous inflammation, and camptodactyly, is associated with mutations in the *NOD2/CARD15* gene, which also predisposes to Crohn's disease. Schnitzler syndrome (urticaria, periodic fever, bone pain, and monoclonal gammopathy) may respond to anakinra and is classified by some as an autoinflammatory syndrome.

Farasat S, et al: Autoinflammatory diseases: clinical and genetic advances. Arch Dermatol 2008 Mar; 144(3):392–402.

Jéru I, et al: Mutations in *NALP12* cause hereditary periodic fever syndromes. Proc Natl Acad Sci U S A 2008 Feb 5; 105(5):1614–1619.

Jesus AA, et al: Phenotype-genotype analysis of cryopyrin-associated periodic syndromes (CAPS): description of a rare non-exon 3 and a novel *CIAS1* missense mutation. J Clin Immunol 2008 Mar; 28(2):134–138.

Kanazawa N, et al: Autoinflammatory syndromes with a dermatological perspective. J Dermatol 2007 Sep; 34(9):601–618.

Maksimovic L, et al: New *CIAS1* mutation and anakinra efficacy in overlapping of Muckle–Wells and familial cold autoinflammatory syndromes. Rheumatology (Oxford) 2008 Mar; 47(3):309–310.

Ross JB, et al: Use of anakinra (Kineret) in the treatment of familial cold autoinflammatory syndrome with a 16-month follow-up. J Cutan Med Surg 2008 Jan–Feb; 12(1):8–16.

Shinkai K, et al: Cryopyrin-associated periodic syndromes and autoinflammation. Clin Exp Dermatol 2008 Jan; 33(1):1–9.

Stankovic K, et al: Autoinflammatory syndromes: diagnosis and treatment. Joint Bone Spine 2007 Dec; 74(6):544–550.

Yamazaki T, et al: Anakinra improves sensory deafness in a Japanese patient with Muckle–Wells syndrome, possibly by inhibiting the cryopyrin inflammasome. Arthritis Rheum 2008 Mar; 58(3):864–868.

Urticaria (hives)

Urticaria is a vascular reaction of the skin characterized by the appearance of wheals (Fig. 7-14), generally surrounded by a red halo or flare and associated with severe itching, stinging, or pricking sensations. These wheals are caused by localized edema. Clearing of the central region may occur and lesions may coalesce, producing an annular or polycyclic pattern. Subcutaneous swellings (angioedema) may accompany the wheals. Angioedema may target the gastrointestinal and respiratory tracts, resulting in abdominal pain, coryza, asthma, and respiratory problems. Respiratory tract involvement can

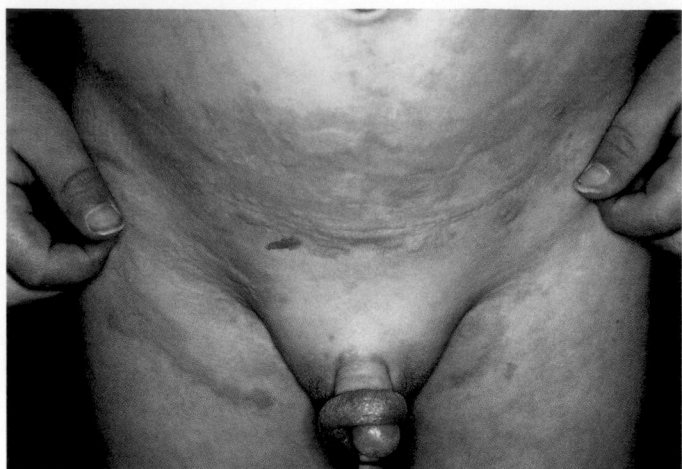

Fig. 7-14 Annular and polycyclic urticaria.

produce airway obstruction. Anaphylaxis and hypotension may also occur.

Classification

Acute urticaria evolves over days to weeks, producing evanescent wheals that individually rarely last more than 12 h, with complete resolution of the urticaria within 6 weeks of onset. Daily episodes of urticaria and/or angioedema lasting more than 6 weeks are designated chronic urticaria. Chronic urticaria predominantly affects adults and is twice as common in women as in men.

Nonimmunologic mechanisms can produce mast cell degranulation. Common triggers include opiates, polymyxin B, tubocurarine, radiocontrast dye, aspirin, other NSAIDs, tartrazine, and benzoate. More than 50% of chronic urticaria is idiopathic. Physical stimuli may produce urticarial reactions and represent 7–17% of cases of chronic urticaria. The physical urticarias include dermatographic, cold, heat, cholinergic, aquagenic, solar, vibratory, and exercise-induced cases. Physical urticaria commonly occurs in patients with chronic urticaria.

Etiologic factors

Drugs

Drugs are probably the most frequent cause of acute urticaria. Penicillin and related antibiotics are the most frequent offenders (see Chapter 6). A frequently overlooked factor is that penicillin sensitivity may become so exquisite that reactions can occur from penicillin in dairy products. The incidence of aspirin-induced urticaria has fallen, most likely related to the availability of alternative anti-inflammatory agents. Aspirin-sensitive persons tend to have cross-sensitivity with tartrazine, the yellow azo-benzone dye, and other azo dyes, natural salicylates, and benzoic acid and its derivatives. These are common food additives and preservatives. Aspirin exacerbates chronic urticaria in at least 30% of patients. Patients may have allergic rhinitis or asthma, nasal polyps, and food-induced anaphylaxis. Mite-contaminated wheat flour has been implicated as an allergen. The nature of the association between aspirin intolerance and mite-induced respiratory allergies is unknown.

Food

Foods are a frequent cause of acute urticaria, whereas in chronic urticaria food is a less frequent factor. The most aller-

genic foods are chocolate, shellfish, nuts, peanuts, tomatoes, strawberries, melons, pork, cheese, garlic, onions, eggs, milk, and spices. Food allergens that may cross-react with latex include chestnuts, bananas, passion fruit, avocado, and kiwi. Exposure to safely cooked fish and shellfish parasitized by *Anisakis simplex* can result in angioedema and urticaria, suggesting that some seafood allergies may be related to exposure to parasite antigens.

If the urticaria is acute and recurrent, food allergy may be suggested by a food diary. Serum radioallergosorbent tests (RASTs) can be used to detect specific IgE, and elimination diets can be of benefit in some patients. One such diet permits inclusion of the following: lamb, beef, rice, potatoes, carrots, string beans, peas, squash, apple sauce, tapioca, preserved pears, peaches, or cherries, Ry-Krisp crackers, butter, sugar, tea without milk or lemon, and coffee without cream. This diet is followed for 3 weeks. If urticaria does not occur, then suspected foods are added one by one and reactions observed. It should be noted that potatoes often contain sulfites, and that some patients may be allergic to the foods contained in the above diet. It is best tried only after a careful history.

The use of food challenges and of scratch and intradermal tests can be misleading. False-positive food challenges are common and an offending food may give a negative prick or intradermal test. Moreover, food additives and preservatives may be responsible.

Food additives

Fewer than 10% of cases of chronic urticaria are caused by food additives. Natural food additives that may be implicated in urticaria include yeasts, salicylates, citric acid, egg, and fish albumin. Synthetic additives include azo dyes, benzoic acid derivatives, sulfite, and penicillin. Yeast is widely used in foods. When it is suspected of being the causative agent, bread and breadstuffs, sausages, wine, beer, grapes, cheese, vinegar, pickled foods, catsup, and yeast tablets should be avoided. Foods containing azo dyes and benzoic acid include candy, soft drinks, jelly, marmalade, custards, puddings, various cake and pancake mixes, mayonnaise, ready-made salad dressings and sauces, packaged soups, anchovies, and colored toothpastes. With the exception of sulfite and penicillin, most food additives can be avoided by eating only meat, produce, and dairy products (the outer aisles of the grocery store). Packaged foods found in the interior aisles are largely off limits.

Infections

Acute urticaria may be associated with upper respiratory infections, especially streptococcal infections. The incidence of streptococcal infection in pediatric cases of acute urticaria varies greatly in reported series. The possibility of localized infection in the tonsils, a tooth, the sinuses, gallbladder, prostate, bladder, or kidney should be considered as a possible cause in cases of acute or chronic urticaria. In some patients, treatment with antibiotics for *Helicobacter pylori* has led to resolution of the urticaria.

Chronic viral infections, such as hepatitis B (Fig. 7-15) and C, may cause urticaria. Acute infectious mononucleosis and psittacosis may also be triggering conditions. Helminths may cause urticaria. Among these are *Ascaris*, *Ankylostoma*, *Strongyloides*, *Filaria*, *Echinococcus*, *Schistosoma*, *Trichinella*, *Toxocara*, and liver fluke.

Emotional stress

Persons under severe emotional stress may have more marked urticaria, no matter what the primary cause is. In cholinergic urticaria emotional stress is a particularly well-documented inciting stimulus.

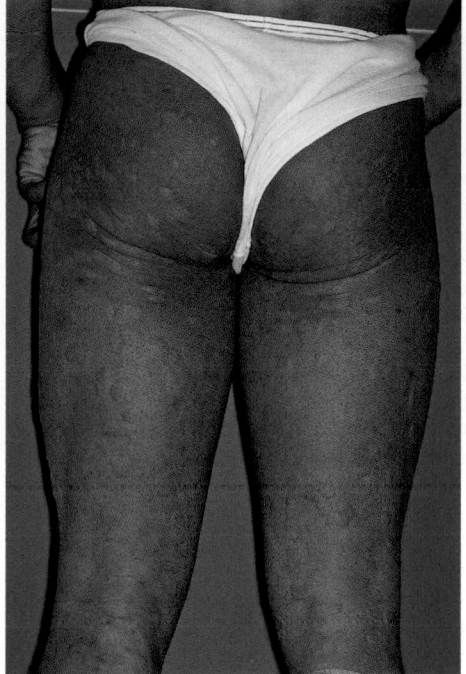

Fig. 7-15 Urticaria secondary to hepatitis B.

Menthol

Rarely, menthol may cause urticaria. It is found in mentholated cigarettes, candy and mints, cough drops, aerosol sprays, and topical medications.

Neoplasms

Urticaria has been associated with carcinomas and Hodgkin disease. Cold urticaria with cryoglobulinemia has been reported as being associated with chronic lymphocytic leukemia.

Inhalants

Grass pollens, house dust mites, feathers, formaldehyde, acrolein (produced when frying with lard or by smoking cigarettes containing glycerin), castor bean or soybean dust, cooked lentils, cottonseed, animal dander, cosmetics, aerosols, pyrethrum, and molds have been known to cause urticaria.

Alcohol

Urticaria may be induced by the ingestion of alcohol. The mechanism of alcohol-induced indirect mast cell stimulation is unknown. Wines generally contain sulfites, which may produce flushing or urticaria.

Hormonal imbalance

Chronic urticaria is approximately twice as common among women than men and low levels of dehydroepiandrosterone (DHEA)-S have been noted, suggesting a possible role for hormone imbalance.

Genetics

Polymorphisms in the β2 adrenergic receptor (*ADRB2*) gene have been identified in aspirin-intolerant acute urticaria.

Pathogenesis/histopathology

Capillary permeability results from the increased release of histamine from the mast cells situated around the capillaries. The mast cell is the primary effector cell in urticarial reactions. Other substances besides histamine may cause vasodilation and capillary permeability, and thereby may possibly become mediators of urticaria and angioedema. These include serotonin, leukotrienes, prostaglandins, proteases, and kinins. The major basic protein of eosinophil granules is abnormally high in the blood of more than 40% of patients with chronic urticaria, even when peripheral blood eosinophil counts are normal, and there are extracellular deposits of it in the skin in about the same proportion of patients.

About one-third of patients with chronic idiopathic urticaria have circulating functional histamine-releasing IgG autoantibodies that bind to the high-affinity IgE receptor. Some patients have IgG that does not bind the IgE receptor, but causes mast-cell degranulation. Thyroid autoantibodies are often present in women with chronic idiopathic urticaria, but clinically relevant thyroid disease is seldom present. Even in those with thyroid disease, treatment of the thyroid disorder generally does not affect the course of the urticaria.

The histopathologic changes in acute urticaria include mild dermal edema and margination of neutrophils within postcapillary venules. Later, neutrophils migrate through the vessel wall into the interstitium, and eosinophils and lymphocytes are also noted in the infiltrate. Karyorrhexis and fibrin deposition within vessel walls are absent, helping to differentiate urticaria from vasculitis.

A subset of patients has long-lasting, refractory lesions and this has been dubbed "neutrophilic urticaria." Lesions in these patients often persist for longer than 24 h, and biopsies demonstrate a neutrophil-rich perivascular infiltrate that lacks karyorrhexis or fibrin deposition within vessels walls. Eosinophils and mononuclear cells are noted in varying proportions. Patients with neutrophilic urticaria may present with acute urticaria, chronic urticaria, or physical urticaria. Lesional skin demonstrates increased expression of TNF-α and IL-3, whereas IL-8 expression is only minor. As neutrophils are commonly present in urticaria in general, it is likely that cases of neutrophilic urticaria simply represent urticaria with upregulation of some mast cell-derived cytokines.

Diagnosis

Diagnosis of urticaria and angioedema is usually made on clinical grounds. Lesions in a fixed location for more than 24 h suggest the possibility of urticarial vasculitis, the urticarial phase of an immunobullous eruption, EM, granuloma annulare, sarcoidosis, or cutaneous T-cell lymphoma. If individual wheals last for longer than 24 h, a skin biopsy should be performed.

Clinical evaluation

Laboratory evaluation should be driven by associated signs and symptoms. Random tests in the absence of a suggestive history or physical findings are rarely cost-effective. A practical evaluation is limited to a detailed history (foods, drugs, including aspirin, physical causes) and physical examination. Angioedema in the absence of urticaria may be related to hereditary angioedema or an angiotensin-converting enzyme (ACE) inhibitor. C1 esterase deficiency does not cause hives, only angioedema. If there is a history of sinus difficulties, particularly if there is palpable tenderness over the maxillary or ethmoid sinuses, radiologic sinus evaluation is recommended. In areas where parasitic disease is common, a blood count to detect eosinophilia is an inexpensive screening test with a fair yield. The blood count may be unreliable if the patient has been on a systemic corticosteroid.

In patients with chronic urticaria, a review of medications, including over-the-counter products, supplements, aspirin, and other NSAIDs, should be obtained. If the history suggests a physical urticaria, then the appropriate challenge test should be used to confirm the diagnosis. Lesions that burn rather than itch, resolve with purpura, or last longer than 24 h should prompt a biopsy to exclude urticarial vasculitis.

A directed history and physical examination should elicit signs or symptoms of thyroid disease, connective tissue disease, changes in bowel or bladder habits, vaginal or urethral discharge, other localized infection, jaundice, or risk factors for hepatitis or Lyme disease. Positive findings should prompt appropriate screening tests. Although sinus x-ray films, a Panorex dental film, a streptococcal throat culture, abdominal ultrasonography, and urinalysis with urine culture (in men, with prostatic massage) may reveal the most common occult infections triggering urticaria, positive cases are almost always associated with some signs or symptoms suggestive of the diagnosis. In patients with chronic angioedema, without classic wheals or symptoms of pruritus, a careful drug history and evaluation of C4 level should be ordered. If C4 is low, an evaluation of C1 esterase inhibitor is appropriate.

Anaphylaxis

Anaphylaxis is an acute and often life-threatening immunologic reaction, frequently heralded by scalp pruritus, diffuse erythema, urticaria, or angioedema. Bronchospasm, laryngeal edema, hyperperistalsis, hypotension, and cardiac arrhythmia may occur. Antibiotics, especially penicillins, other drugs, and radiographic contrast agents are the most common causes of serious anaphylactic reactions. Hymenoptera stings are the next most frequent cause, followed by ingestion of crustaceans and other food allergens. Atopic dermatitis is commonly associated with anaphylaxis regardless of origin. Causative agents can be identified in up to two-thirds of cases and recurrent attacks are the rule. Exercise-induced anaphylaxis is often dependent on priming by prior ingestion of a specific food, or food in general, and aspirin may be an additional exacerbating factor.

Treatment

Acute urticaria

The mainstay of treatment of acute urticaria is administration of antihistamines. In adults, nonsedating antihistamines pose a lower risk of psychomotor impairment. If the cause of the acute episode can be identified, avoiding that trigger should be stressed. In patients with acute urticaria that does not respond to antihistamines, systemic corticosteroids are generally effective. Less rebound is seen with a 3-week tapered course of systemic corticosteroid therapy as compared with shorter courses.

For severe reactions, including anaphylaxis, respiratory and cardiovascular support is essential. A 0.3 mL dose of a 1:1000 dilution of epinephrine is administered every 10–20 min as needed. In young children, a half-strength dilution is used. In rapidly progressive cases, intubation or tracheotomy may be required. Adjunctive therapy includes intramuscular antihistamines (25–50 mg hydroxyzine or diphenhydramine every 6 h as needed) and systemic corticosteroids (250 mg hydrocortisone or 50 mg methylprednisolone intravenously every 6 h for 2–4 doses).

Chronic urticaria

The mainstay of treatment for chronic urticaria is, again, administration of antihistamines. These should be taken on a daily basis; they should not be prescribed to be taken only as needed. The patient should be warned about driving an automobile when first-generation antihistamines are used.

Second-generation H_1 antihistamines (cetirizine, levocetirizine, famotidine, loratadine, acrivastine, and azelastine) are large, lipophilic molecules with charged side chains that bind extensively to proteins, preventing the drugs from crossing the blood–brain barrier; thus they produce less sedation in most patients. Long-acting forms are available, and the long half-life of these antihistamines and reduced sedation result in improved compliance and efficacy. Cetirizine (Zyrtec) and some of the other second-generation antihistamines can cause drowsiness in some individuals, particularly in higher doses or when combined with other antihistamines. Doxepin, a tricyclic antidepressant with potent H_1 antihistaminic activity, may be useful and can be added to the existing antihistamine. Doxepin is frequently dosed at bedtime, so much of the drowsiness and dry mouth are gone by morning. In stubborn cases, dosages of antihistamines that exceed drug labeling are sometimes required. Even second-generation antihistamines may become sedating at higher doses. Fexofenadine is generally well tolerated, even at doses that exceed product labeling. The authors have found escalating doses of antihistamines to be helpful in management, but in one published study of 22 adult patients with refractory urticaria, tripling the dose of cetirizine resulted in adequate control in only one patient. The others required alternate systemic agents such as cyclosporine. The combination of H_1 and H_2 antihistamines, such as hydroxyzine and cimetidine or ranitidine, may be effective in some cases. Cimetidine or ranitidine should not be used alone for treatment of urticaria, as they may interfere with feedback inhibition of histamine release. Other second-line treatments include phototherapy, calcium channel antagonists (nifedipine), antimalarial medications, leukotriene and 5-lipoxygenase inhibitors, gold, azathioprine, low-dose cyclosporine, terbutaline, omalizumab, and methotrexate. Dapsone and colchicines may be helpful in neutrophil-rich urticaria. Unfortunately, although systemic corticosteroids are effective in suppressing most cases of chronic urticaria, their long-term side effects make their extended use impractical. As soon as the corticosteroid is stopped, hives recurs. In addition, if an infection is the trigger, this could be exacerbated by long-term steroid therapy. Topical corticosteroids, topical antihistamines, and topical anesthetics have no role in the management of chronic urticaria. For local treatment, tepid or cold tub baths or showers may be freely advocated. Topical camphor and menthol can provide symptomatic relief. Sarna lotion contains menthol, phenol, and camphor.

In about one-third of cases of chronic idiopathic urticaria, patients have autoantibodies that bind to high-affinity IgE receptors. Such patients may require more aggressive management to include chronic immunosuppressive therapy, plasmapheresis, or intravenous immunoglobulin (IVIG).

Other urticarial variants

Angioedema

Angioedema is an acute, evanescent, circumscribed edema that usually affects the most distensible tissues, such as the eyelids, lips (Fig. 7-16), lobes of the ears, and external genitalia, or the mucous membranes of the mouth, tongue, or larynx. The swelling occurs in the deeper parts of the skin or in the subcutaneous tissues and as a rule is only slightly tender, with the overlying skin unaltered, edematous, or, rarely, ecchymotic. There may be a diffuse swelling on the hands, forearms, feet, and ankles. Frequently, the condition begins during the night and is found on awakening.

There are two distinct subsets of angioedema. The first is considered a deep form of urticaria and may be observed as solitary or multiple sites of angioedema alone or in

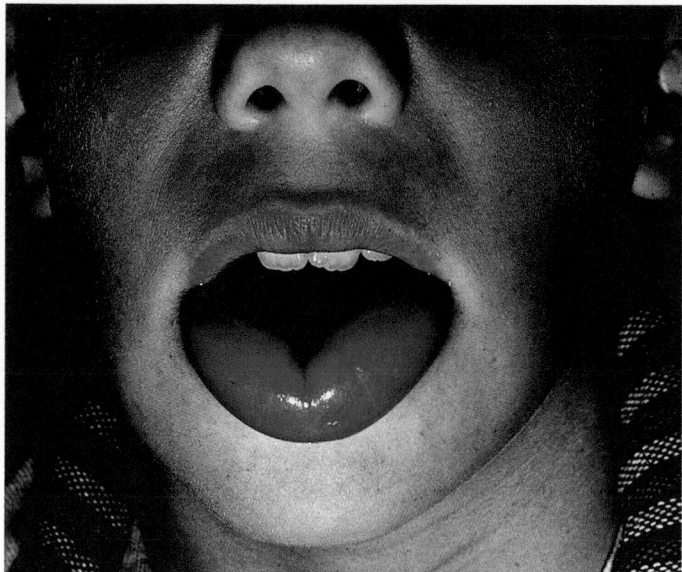

Fig. 7-16 Angioedema of the lips.

combination with urticaria. The action of histamine or similar substances creates vasomotor lability, and pruritus may be a significant feature. The second, angioedema associated with C1 esterase inhibitor deficiency, is not associated with hives and there is no pruritus. Symptoms of pain predominate.

Angioedema may be related to ACE inhibitors.

Hereditary angioedema

Also known as Quincke edema, hereditary angioedema (HAE) was originally described and named by Osler in 1888. HAE characteristically appears in the second to fourth decade. Sudden attacks of angioedema occur as frequently as every 2 weeks throughout the patient's life, lasting for 2–5 days. Swelling is typically asymmetrical, and urticaria or itching does not occur. The presentation may overlap with that of the autoinflammatory syndromes.

Patients may experience local swelling in subcutaneous tissues (face, hands, arms, legs, genitals, and buttocks); abdominal organs (stomach, intestines, bladder), mimicking surgical emergencies; and the upper airway (larynx), which can be life-threatening. There is little response to antihistamines, epinephrine, or steroids. The mortality rate is high, with death often caused by laryngeal edema. Gastrointestinal edema is manifested by nausea, vomiting, and severe colic, and it may simulate appendicitis so closely that appendectomy is mistakenly performed. The factors that trigger attacks are minor trauma, surgery, sudden changes of temperature, or sudden emotional stress.

Inherited in an autosomal-dominant fashion, HAE is estimated to occur in 1 in 50 000–150 000 persons. There are three phenotypic forms of the disease. Type I is characterized by low antigenic and functional plasma levels of a normal C1 esterase inhibitor protein (C1-EI). Type II is characterized by the presence of normal or elevated antigenic levels of a dysfunctional protein. Type III demonstrates normal C1-EI function and normal complement. It has been described only in female members of affected families. Criteria for type III include a long history of recurrent attacks of skin swelling, abdominal pain, or upper airway obstruction; absence of urticaria; familial occurrence; normal C1-EI and C4 concentrations; and failure of treatment with antihistamines, corticosteroids, and C1-EI concentrate.

The screening test of choice for types I and II is a C4 level. C4 will be low (<40% of normal) as a result of continuous activation and consumption. In addition to depressed C4 levels, patients with types I and II also have low C1, C1q, and C2 levels. If the clinical picture and screening tests are positive, a titer of C1-EI should be ordered. C1-EI is a labile protein and sample decay is common. A low C1-EI in the presence of normal C4 levels should raise the suspicion of sample decay, rather than true HAE.

The treatment of choice for acute HAE types I and II is replacement therapy with concentrates or fresh frozen plasma. Short-term prophylaxis (e.g. for patients undergoing dental care, endoscopy, or intubation for surgery) can be obtained from stanozolol, an attenuated androgen. Estrogens in oral contraceptives, in contrast, may precipitate attacks. Antifibrinolytic tranexamic acid, a drug related to e-aminocaproic acid, has been used to treat acute and chronic disease. Type III does not respond to C1-EI replacement, but may respond to danazol.

Acquired C1 esterase inhibitor deficiency

Some patients present with symptoms indistinguishable from HAE, but with onset after the fourth decade of life and lacking a family history. As in HAE, there is no associated pruritus or urticaria. This condition is subdivided into acquired angioedema-I and II, and an idiopathic form. Acquired angioedema-I is a rare disorder associated with lymphoproliferative diseases. These associations include lymphomas (usually B-cell), chronic lymphocytic leukemia, monoclonal gammopathy, myeloma, myelofibrosis, Waldenström macroglobulinemia, and breast carcinoma. Some patients have detectable autoantibodies to C1-EI. Worsening of stable hereditary angioedema has been the presenting sign of lymphoma.

Acquired angioedema-II is an extremely rare disease defined by the presence of autoantibodies to C1-EI. It is important to realize that autoantibodies directed against C1-EI may also be found in acquired angioedema-I, particularly in patients with B-cell lymphomas, so the diagnosis of acquired angioedema-II is made only when no such underlying condition exists.

The pathophysiology of acquired angioedema-I is unknown but may be related to increased catabolism of C1-EI, since many patients with the disorder have been shown to produce normal amounts of C1-EI. In acquired angioedema-II, hepatocytes and monocytes are able to synthesize normal C1-EI; however, a subpopulation of B cells secretes autoantibodies to the functional region of the C1-EI molecule.

Management of acute attacks in acquired angioedema-I is directed toward replacement of C1-EI with fresh frozen plasma, plasma-derived C1 inhibitor, or recombinant human C1 inhibitor. Some patients develop progressive resistance to the infusions. Antifibrinolytic agents, such as aminocaproic acid or tranexamic acid, may be beneficial, and are more effective than antiandrogen therapy. Synthetic androgens, such as danazol, may be helpful in angioedema-I; however, androgens are ineffective in treating patients with acquired angioedema-II, stressing the importance of identifying these patients. Immunosuppressive therapy has been shown to be effective in the treatment of acquired angioedema-II by decreasing autoantibody production. Systemic corticosteroids may be temporarily effective. Plasmapheresis, the B2 bradykinin receptor antagonist HOE-140, and the kallikrein inhibitor DX-88 are promising therapies for patients refractory to other treatments.

Episodic angioedema with eosinophilia

Episodic angioedema or isolated facial edema may occur with fever, weight gain, eosinophilia, and elevated eosinophil major basic protein. The disorder is not uncommon, and there is no underlying disease. Increased levels of IL-5 have been documented during periods of attack. Treatment options include administration of systemic steroidal medications, antihistamines, and IVIG.

Schnitzler syndrome

The rare disorder, Schnitzler syndrome, is a combination of chronic, non-pruritic urticaria, fever of unknown origin, disabling bone pain, hyperostosis, increased erythrocyte sedimentation rate, and monoclonal IgM gammopathy. Pruritus is not generally a feature. The age of onset ranges from 29 to 77 years, without gender predilection. In some cases the IgM gammopathy progresses to neoplasia, especially Waldenström macroglobulinemia. Effective therapy has not been determined, although the bone pain and urticarial lesions respond to systemic corticosteroids in some patients. Others have responded to anakinra.

Physical urticarias

Specific physical stimuli are the cause of approximately 20% of all urticarias. They occur most frequently in persons between the ages of 17 and 40. The most common form is dermatographism followed by cholinergic and cold urticaria. Several forms of physical urticaria may occur in the same patient. Physical urticarias, particularly dermatographism, delayed pressure, cholinergic, and cold urticaria, are frequently found in patients with chronic idiopathic urticaria.

Dermatographism

Dermatographism is a sharply localized edema or wheal with a surrounding erythematous flare occurring within seconds to minutes after the skin has been stroked (Fig. 7-17). It affects 2–5% of the population. Dermatographism may arise spontaneously after drug-induced urticaria and persist for months. It has also been reported to be associated with the use of the H$_2$ blocker, famotidine. It may occur in hypothyroidism and hyperthyroidism, infectious diseases, diabetes mellitus, and during onset of menopause. It may be a cause of localized or generalized pruritus. Antihistamines suppress this reaction. The addition of an H$_2$ antihistamine may be of benefit.

Cholinergic urticaria

Cholinergic urticaria, produced by the action of acetylcholine on the mast cell, is characterized by minute, highly pruritic, punctate wheals or papules 1–3 mm in diameter and surrounded by a distinct erythematous flare (Fig. 7-18). These lesions occur primarily on the trunk and face. The condition spares the palms and soles. Lesions persist for 30–90 min and are followed by a refractory period of up to 24 h. Bronchospasm may occur. Familial cases have been reported.

The lesions may be induced in the susceptible patient by exercise, emotional stress, increased environmental temperature, or intradermal injection of nicotine picrate or methacholine. Sometimes an attack may be aborted by rapid cooling of the body, as by taking a cold shower. A refractory period with no lesions occurs for approximately 24 h after an attack. Cholinergic dermatographism is noted in some patients.

Treatment with antihistamines is often effective if dosage is adequate. Antihistamines have been combined with other agents, such as montelukast and propranolol. Attenuated androgens, such as danazol, may be of benefit in refractory cases. Provocative tests include exercise, a warm bath to raise core temperature by 0.7–1.0°C (1.2–1.8°F), or a methacholine skin test.

Adrenergic urticaria

Adrenergic urticaria may occur by itself or coexist with cholinergic urticaria. Bouts of urticaria are mediated by norepinephrine. The eruption consists of small (1–5 mm) red macules and papules with a pale halo, appearing within 10–15 min of emotional upset, coffee, or chocolate. Serum catecholamines, norepinephrine, dopamine, and epinephrine may rise markedly during attacks, whereas histamine and serotonin levels remain normal. Propranolol, in a dosage of 10 mg four times a day, is effective; atenolol has been ineffective. A provocative test consists of intradermal administration of 3–10 ng of norepinephrine.

Cold urticaria

Exposure to cold may result in edema and whealing on the exposed areas, usually the face and hands. The urticaria does not develop during chilling, but on rewarming. This heterogenous group of disorders is classified into primary (essential), secondary, and familial cold urticaria.

Primary (essential) cold urticaria is not associated with underlying systemic diseases or cold reactive proteins. Symptoms are usually localized to the areas of cold exposure, although respiratory and cardiovascular compromise may develop. Fatal shock may occur when these persons go swimming in cold water or take cold showers. This type of cold urticaria usually begins in adulthood. It is usually ice cube test-positive.

The treatment of primary cold urticaria is with doxepin, in doses from 25 mg at bedtime to 50 mg twice a day, or cyproheptadine, 4 mg three times a day. Good therapeutic responses to the second-generation antihistamines acrivastine and cetirizine have been reported, and these agents are less likely to result in sedation. Cetirizine and zafirlukast in combination

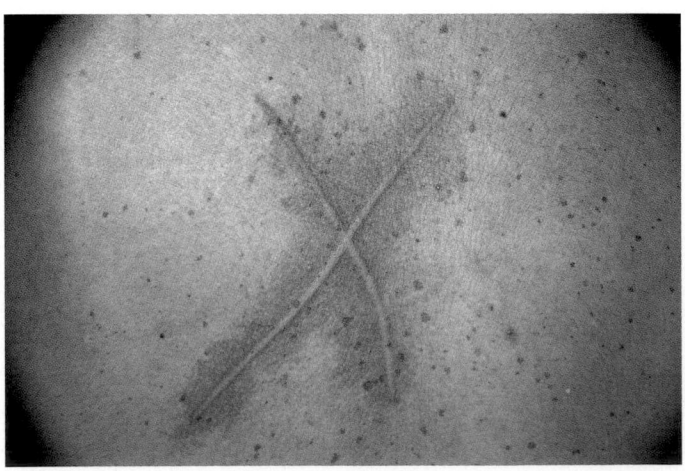

Fig. 7-17 Dermatographism.

Fig. 7-18 Cholinergic urticaria, small papules with surrounding large erythematous flare.

are more effective than either drug given alone. Ketotifen may also be effective, but is not marketed in the US. Corticosteroid medications are ineffective.

Desensitization by repeated, increased exposures to cold has been effective in some cases. In one report, successful desensitization was induced in an 18-year-old patient with severe cold urticaria. Tolerance in a small area of the skin was achieved by repeated applications of an ice cube at 30-min intervals for 7 h, followed by forearm immersion in cold water hourly for 4 h. The other limbs were then treated one at a time, and finally the trunk. After a week, the patient was able to tolerate whole-body immersion in cold water for 5 min without urticaria. He maintained this "desensitization" with a 5-min cold shower every 12 h. He was free from urticaria for 6 months, continuing his daily cold showers. This sort of regimen is only suitable in rare cases. In many patients cold urticaria will resolve after months, although about 50% of patients have symptomatic disease for years.

As a provocative test, a plastic-wrapped ice cube is applied to the skin for 5–20 min. If no wheal develops, the area should be fanned for an additional 10 min. The use of a combination of cold and moving air is, in some cases, more effective in reproducing lesions than cold alone. The provocative test is not performed if secondary cold urticaria is being considered.

Secondary cold urticaria is associated with an underlying systemic disease, such as cryoglobulinemia. Other associations include cryofibrinogenemia, multiple myeloma, secondary syphilis, hepatitis, and infectious mononucleosis. Patients may have headache, hypotension, laryngeal edema, and syncope. An ice cube test is not recommended, since it can precipitate vascular occlusion and tissue ischemia.

Familial cold urticaria is grouped with the other autoinflammatory syndromes. The lesions produce a burning sensation rather than itching. They may have cyanotic centers and surrounding white halos, and last for 24–48 h. They may be accompanied by fever, chills, headache, arthralgia, myalgia, and abdominal pain. A prominent feature is leukocytosis, which is the first observable response to cold. Familial cold urticaria will yield a negative result to an ice cube test. Stanozolol therapy has been shown to be effective in treating 3 of 8 patients.

Heat urticaria

Within 5 min of the skin being exposed to heat above 43°C (109.4°F), the exposed area begins to burn and sting, and becomes red, swollen, and indurated. This rare type of urticaria may also be generalized and is accompanied by cramps, weakness, flushing, salivation, and collapse. Heat desensitization may be effective. As a provocative test, apply a heated cylinder, 50–55°C (122–131°F), to a small area of skin on the upper body for 30 min.

Solar urticaria

Solar urticaria appears soon after unshielded skin is exposed to sunlight. It is classified by the wavelengths of light that precipitate the reaction. Visible light can trigger solar urticaria, and sunscreens may not prevent it. Angioedema may occasionally occur. Solar urticaria may be a manifestation of porphyria, leukocytoclastic vasculitis, and the Churg–Strauss syndrome. Treatment is sun avoidance, sunscreens, antihistamines, repetitive phototherapy, and PUVA. (Solar urticaria is reviewed more extensively in Chapter 3.)

Pressure urticaria (delayed pressure urticaria)

Pressure urticaria is characterized by the development of swelling with pain that occurs 3–12 h after local pressure has been applied. It occurs most frequently on the feet after walking and on the buttocks after sitting. It is unique in that

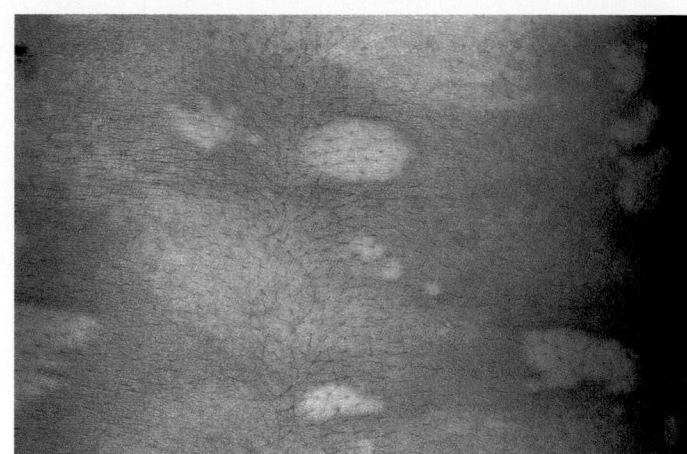

Fig. 7-19 Exercise-induced urticaria.

there may be a latent period of as much as 24 h before lesions develop. Arthralgias, fever, chills, and leukocytosis can occur. The pain and swelling last for 8–24 h. Pressure urticaria may be seen in combination with other physical urticarias. As a provocative test, a 15 lb weight is applied to the skin for 20 min and the area inspected after 4–8 h. The combination of montelukast and an antihistamine has been used effectively. Systemic corticosteroids are often therapeutic, but are generally unsuitable for long-term use. Tranexamic acid, high-dose IVIG, or an anti-TNF biologic may be effective in cases refractory to other treatment, and the disease has remitted after eradication of *Blastocystis hominis*.

Exercise-induced urticaria

Although both cholinergic urticaria and exercise urticaria are precipitated by exercise, they are distinct entities. Raising the body temperature passively will not induce exercise urticaria, and the lesions of exercise urticaria are larger (Fig. 7-19) than the tiny wheals of cholinergic urticaria. Urticarial lesions appear 5–30 min after the start of exercise. Anaphylaxis may be associated. Atopy is common in these patients and some have documented food allergy. Avoiding these allergens may improve symptoms.

Therapy with H_1 and H_2 antihistamines may be partially effective. Self-injectable epinephrine kits are recommended for those rare patients with episodes of anaphylaxis manifesting with respiratory symptoms. Exercise is a provocative test, but may require priming with the identified food allergens.

Vibratory angioedema

Vibratory angioedema, a form of physical urticaria, may be an inherited autosomal-dominant trait, or may be acquired after prolonged occupational vibration exposure. Dermatographism, pressure urticaria, and cholinergic urticaria may occur in affected patients. Plasma histamine levels are elevated during attacks. The appearance of the angioedema is usually not delayed. The treatment is antihistamines. As a provocative test, laboratory vortex vibration is applied to the forearm for 5 min.

Aquagenic urticaria

This rare condition is elicited by water or seawater at any temperature. Pruritic wheals develop immediately or within minutes at the sites of contact of the skin with water, irrespective of temperature or source, and clear within 30–60 min. Sweat, saliva, and even tears can precipitate a reaction. Aquagenic urticaria may be familial in some cases, or associated with atopy or cholinergic urticaria. Systemic symptoms have been reported to include wheezing, dysphagia, and respiratory distress. The pathogenesis is unknown but may be associated with water-soluble antigens that diffuse into the dermis and cause histamine release from sensitized mast cells.

Whealing may be prevented by pretreatment of the skin with petrolatum. Many antihistamines have been effective. PUVA appears to prevent skin lesions but may not prevent the symptoms of pruritus. The provocative test is to apply water compresses (35°C [95°F]) to the skin of the upper body for 30 min.

Galvanic urticaria

Galvanic urticaria has been described after exposure to a galvanic device used to treat hyperhidrosis. The relationship of this condition to other forms of physical urticaria remains to be established.

Asero R: Chronic unremitting urticaria: is the use of antihistamines above the licensed dose effective? A preliminary study of cetirizine at licensed and above-licensed doses. Clin Exp Dermatol 2007 Jan; 32(1):34–38.

Aversano M, et al: Improvement of chronic idiopathic urticaria with L-thyroxine: a new TSH role in immune response? Allergy 2005; 60:489.

Belsito DV: Second-generation antihistamines for the treatment of chronic idiopathic urticaria. J Drugs Dermatol 2010 May; 9(5):503–512.

Bernstein IL: Hereditary angioedema: a current state-of-the-art review, II: historical perspective of non-histamine-induced angioedema. Ann Allergy Asthma Immunol 2008 Jan; 100(1 Suppl 2):S2–S6.

Brodell LA, et al: Pathophysiology of chronic urticaria. Ann Allergy Asthma Immunol 2008 Apr; 100(4):291–297.

Cascavilla N, et al: Successful treatment of Schnitzler's syndrome with anakinra after failure of rituximab trial. Int J Immunopathol Pharmacol 2010 Apr–Jun; 23(2):633–636.

Craig TJ: Appraisal of danazol prophylaxis for hereditary angioedema. Allergy Asthma Proc 2008 May–Jun; 29(3):225–231.

Criado RF, et al: Urticaria unresponsive to antihistaminic treatment: an open study of therapeutic options based on histopathologic features. J Dermatolog Treat 2008; 19(2):92–96.

Davis AE 3rd: New treatments addressing the pathophysiology of hereditary angioedema. Clin Mol Allergy 2008 Apr 14; 6:2.

Dubuske LM: Levocetirizine: the latest treatment option for allergic rhinitis and chronic idiopathic urticaria. Allergy Asthma Proc 2007 Nov–Dec; 28(6):724–734.

Engin B, et al: Treatment of chronic urticaria with narrowband ultraviolet B phototherapy: a randomized controlled trial. Acta Derm Venereol 2008; 88(3):247–251.

Feinberg JH, et al: Successful treatment of disabling cholinergic urticaria. Mil Med 2008 Feb; 173(2):217–220.

Fromer L: Treatment options for the relief of chronic idiopathic urticaria symptoms. South Med J 2008 Feb; 101(2):186–192.

Gorman PJ: Hereditary angioedema and pregnancy: a successful outcome using C1 esterase inhibitor concentrate. Can Fam Physician 2008 Mar; 54(3):365–366.

Guilarte M, et al: Acquired angioedema associated with hereditary angioedema due to C1 inhibitor deficiency. J Investig Allergol Clin Immunol 2008; 18(2):126–130.

Irinyi B, et al: Clinical and laboratory examinations in the subgroups of chronic urticaria. Int Arch Allergy Immunol 2007; 144(3):217–225.

Jáuregui I, et al: Antihistamines in the treatment of chronic urticaria. J Investig Allergol Clin Immunol 2007; 17(Suppl 2):41–52.

Khakoo G, et al: Clinical features and natural history of physical urticaria in children. Pediatr Allergy Immunol 2008 Jun; 19(4):363–366.

Khalaf AT: Current advances in the management of urticaria. Arch Immunol Ther Exp 2008 Mar–Apr; 56(2):103–114.

Kim HA, et al: Association of beta 2-adrenergic receptor polymorphism with the phenotype of aspirin-intolerant acute urticaria. Yonsei Med J 2007 Dec 31; 48(6):1079–1081.

Klote MM: Autoimmune urticaria response to high-dose intravenous immunoglobulin. Ann Allergy Asthma Immunol 2005; 94:307.

Kobza-Black A: Delayed pressure urticaria. J Investig Dermatol Symp Proc 2001; 6:148.

Komarow HD, et al: Office-based management of urticaria. Am J Med 2008 May; 121(5):379–384.

Kröpfl L, et al: Treatment strategies in urticaria. Expert Opin Pharmacother 2010 Jun; 11(9):1445–1450.

La Shell MS, et al: Severe refractory cholinergic urticaria treated with danazol. J Drugs Dermatol 2006 Jul–Aug; 5(7):664–667.

Magerl M, et al: Successful treatment of delayed pressure urticaria with anti-TNF-alpha. J Allergy Clin Immunol 2007 Mar; 119(3):752–754.

Mihara S, et al: Adrenergic urticaria in a patient with cholinergic urticaria. Br J Dermatol 2008 Mar; 158(3):629–631.

Morita E, et al: Food-dependent exercise-induced anaphylaxis. J Dermatol Sci 2007 Aug; 47(2):109–117.

Ohtsuka T: Response to oral cyclosporine therapy and high sensitivity-CRP level in chronic idiopathic urticaria. Int J Dermatol 2010 May; 49(5):579–584.

Pereira C, et al: Low-dose intravenous gammaglobulin in the treatment of severe autoimmune urticaria. Eur Ann Allergy Clin Immunol 2007 Sep; 39(7):237–242.

Serhat Inaloz H, et al: Low-dose and short-term cyclosporine treatment in patients with chronic idiopathic urticaria: a clinical and immunological evaluation. J Dermatol 2008 May; 35(5):276–282.

Shedden C, et al: Delayed pressure urticaria controlled by tranexamic acid. Clin Exp Dermatol 2006 Mar; 31(2):295–296.

Shimauchi T, et al: Solar urticaria as a manifestation of Churg–Strauss syndrome. Clin Exp Dermatol 2007 Mar; 32(2):209–210.

Sloane DE, et al: Hereditary angioedema: safety of long-term stanozolol therapy. J Allergy Clin Immunol 2007 Sep; 120(3):654–658.

Soubrier M: Schnitzler syndrome. Joint Bone Spine 2008 May; 75(3):263–266.

Temiño VM, et al: The spectrum and treatment of angioedema. Am J Med 2008 Apr; 121(4):282–286.

Torchia D, et al: Multiple physical urticarias. Postgrad Med J 2008 Jan; 84(987):e1–e2.

Varadarajulu S: Urticaria and angioedema. Controlling acute episodes, coping with chronic cases. Postgrad Med 2005; 117:225.

Verneuil L, et al: Association between chronic urticaria and thyroid autoimmunity: a prospective study involving 99 patients. Dermatology 2004; 208:98.

Weinstein ME, et al: Efficacy and tolerability of second- and third-generation antihistamines in the treatment of acquired cold urticaria: a meta-analysis. Ann Allergy Asthma Immunol 2010 Jun; 104(6):518–522.

Zuraw BL, et al: New promise and hope for treating hereditary angioedema. Expert Opin Investig Drugs 2008 May; 17(5):697–706.

Bonus images for this chapter can be found online at http://www.expertconsult.com

Fig. 7-1 Erythema multiforme involving the lips.

Fig. 7-2 Cold urticaria after an ice cube had been applied to the site for 3 min.

Fig. 7-3 Erythema multiforme, target lesions.

Fig. 7-4 Erythema multiforme, target lesions.

Fig. 7-5 Mucosal lesions of erythema multiforme.

Fig. 7-6 Atypical target lesion in Stevens–Johnson syndrome.

Fig. 7-7 Erythema nodosum.

Fig. 7-8 Sweet syndrome, erythema lesions.

Fig. 7-9 Enlarging ulcer of pyoderma gangrenosum.

Fig. 7-10 Annular and polycyclic urticaria.

Fig. 7-11 Dermatographism.

Fig. 7-12 Cholinergic urticaria, small papules with surrounding large erythematous flare.

Fig. 7-13 Cold urticaria after an ice cube had been applied to the site for 3 min.

Connective Tissue Diseases

8

Lupus erythematosus (LE), dermatomyositis, scleroderma, rheumatoid arthritis, Sjögren syndrome, eosinophilic fasciitis, mixed connective tissue disease, and relapsing polychondritis are classified as connective tissue diseases. Basic to them all is a complex array of autoimmune responses that target or affect collagen or ground substance.

Lupus erythematosus

LE may manifest as a systemic disease or in purely cutaneous forms. Significant overlap occurs and chronic skin lesions do not equate with purely cutaneous disease. Chronic discoid lesions may be seen in patients with severe systemic lupus erythematosus (SLE). A number of patients with verrucous LE or lupus panniculitis have systemic disease, and most patients with subacute cutaneous LE have at least some systemic symptoms, although most do not meet the current American College of Rheumatology (ACR) criteria for SLE. Cutaneous manifestations of LE are classified as in Box 8-1.

Chronic cutaneous lupus erythematosus

Discoid lupus erythematosus

Discoid lupus erythematosus (DLE) generally occurs in young adults, with women outnumbering men 2:1. Lesions begin as dull red macules or indurated plaques that develop an adherent scale, and evolve with atrophy, scarring, and pigment changes (Fig. 8-1). In darker-skinned individuals, lesions typically demonstrate areas of both hyperpigmentation and depigmentation. In lighter-skinned patients, the plaques may appear gray or have little pigment alteration. The hyperkeratosis characteristically extends into patulous follicles, producing carpet tack-like spines on the undersurface of the scale. These spines have been called carpet tacks or langue du chat (cat's tongue).

Very small lesions of DLE may be mistaken for actinic keratoses. Some early discoid lesions are very superficial, resembling mild seborrheic dermatitis. Others may be brightly erythematous or even urticarial. Sometimes erythema is minimal, especially in scalp lesions. This may produce the clinical appearance of a noninflammatory alopecia, although a biopsy demonstrates deep nodular and perifollicular lymphoid infiltrates.

Localized discoid lupus erythematosus

Discoid lesions are usually localized above the neck. Favored sites are the scalp, bridge of the nose, malar areas, lower lip, and ears (Fig. 8-2). The concha of the ear and external canal are frequently involved. Some patients present with periorbital edema and erythema. On the scalp most lesions begin as erythematous patches or plaques that evolve into white, often depressed, hairless patches. Perifollicular erythema and the presence of easily extractable anagen hairs are signs of active disease and are helpful in monitoring the response to therapy. Scarred areas may appear completely smooth, or may demonstrate dilated follicular openings in the few remaining follicles. Itching and tenderness are common and may rarely be severe. On the lips lesions may be gray or red and hyperkeratotic. They may be eroded and are usually surrounded by a narrow, red inflammatory zone (Fig. 8-3). In one study, 24% of DLE patients had mucosal involvement of the mouth, nose, eye, or vulva. Rarely, aggressive squamous cell carcinoma arises in long-standing lesions of DLE.

Generalized discoid lupus erythematosus

Generalized DLE is less common than localized DLE. All degrees of severity are encountered. Most often the thorax and upper extremities are affected in addition to the head and neck (Fig. 8-4). The scalp may become quite bald with striking patterns of hyperpigmentation and depigmentation. Diffuse scarring may involve the face and upper extremities. Laboratory abnormalities, such as an elevated erythrocyte sedimentation rate (ESR), elevated antinuclear antibodies (ANAs), single-stranded (ss)DNA antibodies, or leukopenia, are more common with this form of LE than with localized DLE.

The course of DLE is variable, but 95% of cases confined to the skin at the outset will remain so. Progression from purely cutaneous DLE to SLE is uncommon. However, patients with SLE frequently have discoid lesions. These patients generally have systemic involvement early in the course of their disease, rather than evolving from chronic cutaneous LE to SLE. Fever and arthralgia are common in patients with SLE and discoid lesions. In patients with systemic symptoms, abnormal laboratory tests, such as elevation of ANAs, antibodies to double-stranded (ds)DNA and C1q, leukopenia, hematuria, and proteinuria, help to identify patients with SLE and give an indication of prognosis.

Childhood discoid lupus erythematosus

Among children with DLE, a low frequency of photosensitivity and a higher rate of association with SLE have been noted. In most other respects, the clinical presentation and course are similar to those in adults.

Histology

The epidermis is usually thin with effacement of the rete ridge pattern. Compact hyperkeratosis without parakeratosis is characteristic, and follicular plugging is typically prominent. Hydropic degeneration of the basal layer of the epidermis and follicular epithelium results in pigmentary incontinence. A patchy perivascular and periadnexal lymphoid inflammatory infiltrate occurs in the superficial and deep dermis. The infiltrate characteristically surrounds vessels, follicles, and the eccrine coil. Increased mucin is often present, and may be visible as deposition of a blue to amphophilic substance between collagen bundles, or merely as a widening of the

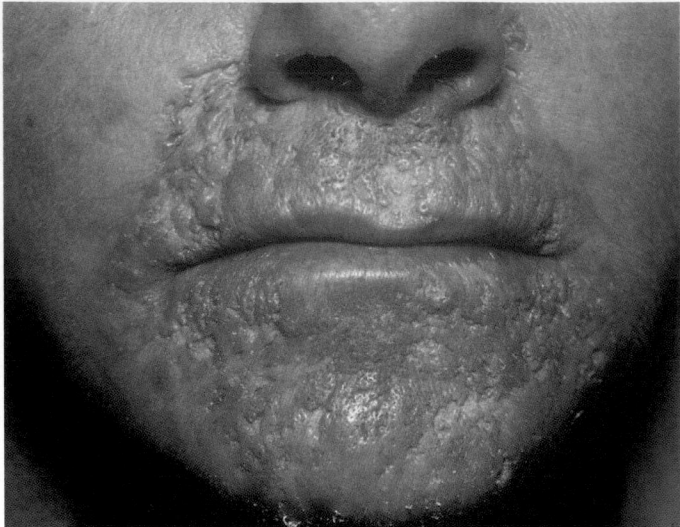

Fig. 8-1 Discoid lupus erythematosus.

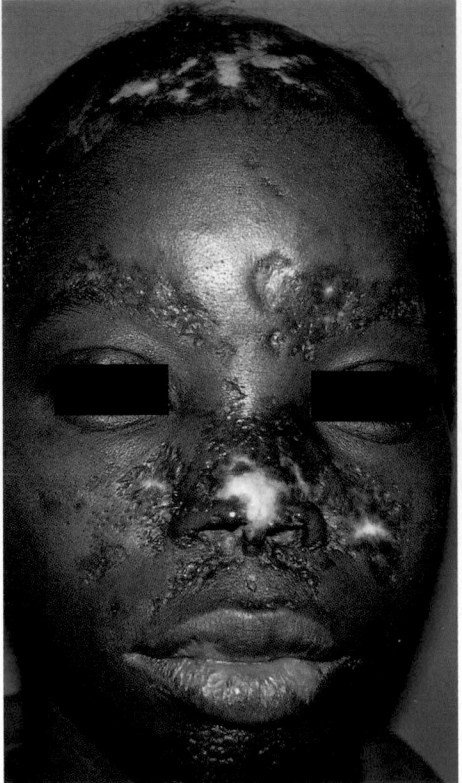

Fig. 8-2 Extensive scarring from discoid lupus erythematosus.

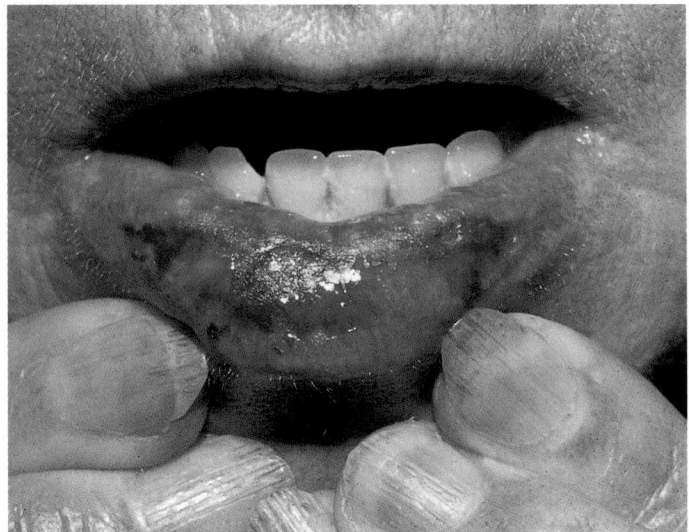

Fig. 8-3 Lupus of the lip.

Box 8-1 Classification of cutaneous manifestations of lupus erythematosus

I. Chronic cutaneous LE
  A. Discoid LE
    1. Localized
    2. Disseminated
  B. Verrucous (hypertrophic) LE (Behçet): usually acral and often lichenoid
  C. Lupus erythematosus–lichen planus overlap
  D. Chilblain LE
  E. Tumid lupus
  F. Lupus panniculitis (LE profundus)
    1. With no other involvement
    2. With overlying discoid LE
    3. With systemic LE

II. Subacute cutaneous LE
  A. Papulosquamous
  B. Annular
  C. Syndromes commonly exhibiting similar morphology
    1. Neonatal LE
    2. Complement deficiency syndromes
    3. Drug-induced

III. Acute cutaneous LE: localized or generalized erythema or bullae, generally associated with SLE

---

space between the bundles. Thickening of the basement membrane zone may be prominent.

The histology varies with the stage of the lesion. Acute lesions show only patchy lymphoid inflammation and vacuolar interface dermatitis. Lesions established for several months begin to show hyperkeratosis, basement membrane thickening, and dermal mucin. Chronic, inactive lesions show atrophy, with postinflammatory pigmentation and scarring throughout the dermis. At this stage, the inflammatory infiltrate is sparse to absent. Pilosebaceous units, except for "orphaned" arrector muscles, are destroyed. At this stage, the dermis appears fibrotic, but an elastic tissue stain can still distinguish the diffuse dermal scar of lupus from the focal wedge-shaped superficial scars of lichen planopilaris or folliculitis decalvans. Direct immunofluorescence (DIF) testing of lesional skin is positive in more than 75% of cases, providing that the lesions have been active for at least several months. Transporting specimens in normal saline may result in a

higher yield than freezing or Michel's transport medium, if the specimen can reach the laboratory within 24 h. Early lesions usually have negative or nonspecific immunofluorescent findings, whereas established lesions usually demonstrate strong continuous granular deposition of immunoglobulin and complement located at the dermoepidermal junction. Uninvolved skin is negative, and the biopsy should always be from lesional skin of a well-established inflammatory lesion.

Differential diagnosis

DLE must often be differentiated from seborrheic dermatitis, rosacea, lupus vulgaris, sarcoidosis, drug eruptions, actinic keratosis, Bowen's disease, lichen planus, tertiary syphilis, polymorphous light eruption (PMLE), and lymphocytic infiltration (Jessner). Immunoglobulin deposits distinguish DLE

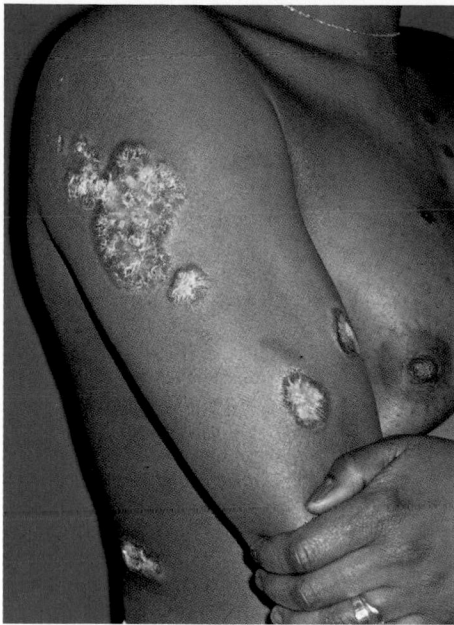

Fig. 8-4 Generalized discoid lupus erythematosus.

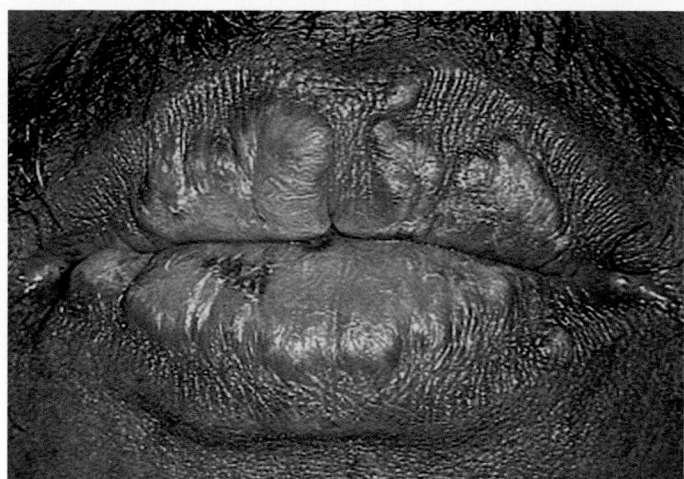

Fig. 8-5 Lip involvement in hypertrophic lupus erythematosus.

from the latter conditions. LE also demonstrates predominantly CD4+ lymphocytes, whereas Jessner's infiltrate may be composed largely of CD8+ lymphocytes. Seborrheic dermatitis does not show atrophy, alopecia, or dilated follicles, and has greasy, yellowish scale without follicular plugs. Acral, lip, and scalp lesions of chronic cutaneous LE may demonstrate lichenoid dermatitis histologically. In these cases, the presence of continuous granular immunoglobulin in addition to cytoid bodies is a helpful distinguishing feature.

In rosacea, atrophy does not occur and pustules are nearly always found. Apple-jelly nodules (granulomas) are seen with diascopy in lupus vulgaris. Sunlight-sensitizing agents, such as sulfonamides, may produce lesions similar to LE, as phototoxic reactions demonstrate vacuolar interface dermatitis. It may be necessary to differentiate syphilis and sarcoid by biopsy and serologic testing. PMLE is distinguished by the absence of scarring and the presence of intensely edematous plaques and papules. DIF is generally negative or nonspecific in PMLE.

Hypertrophic lupus erythematosus

Non-pruritic papulonodular lesions may occur on the arms and hands, resembling keratoacanthoma or hypertrophic lichen planus (LP). Some of these patients have SLE, while some have only cutaneous involvement. The lips (Fig. 8-5) and scalp may also demonstrate lesions that resemble LP or lichen planopilaris (LPP). Histologic sections of these lesions typically demonstrate a lichenoid dermatitis, and a careful examination for other characteristic skin lesions of LE or LP, as well as DIF testing, may be critical in establishing a diagnosis. Basement membrane zone thickening, dermal mucin, eccrine coil involvement, and subcutaneous nodular lymphoid infiltrates are features of LE that are not found in LP. DIF may demonstrate continuous granular immunoglobulin deposition in cases of lichenoid LE. In cases where only cytoid bodies are present, they tend to be restricted to the dermoepidermal junction rather than extending deep into the follicle or fibrous tract remnants. Shaggy fibrin may be seen in both LPP and LE, but tends to extend deep into the follicle in cases of LPP.

Lupus erythematosus–lichen planus overlap syndrome

In addition to the cases of hypertrophic LE with lichenoid histology discussed above, there are patients with a true overlap syndrome with features of both LE and LP. The lesions are usually large, atrophic, hypopigmented, red or pink patches and plaques. Pigment abnormalities become prominent over time, and fine telangiectasia and scaling are usually present. The extensor aspects of the extremities and midline back are typically affected. Prominent palmoplantar involvement is characteristic and tends to be the most troublesome feature for these patients. Nail dystrophy and anonychia may occur. Scarring alopecia and oral involvement have been noted in some patients. The histology of individual lesions has features of LP and/or LE. DIF usually suggests the former, but immunofluorescence may demonstrate a continuous granular deposition of immunoglobulin. Response to treatment is poor, though potent topical corticosteroids, dapsone, thalidomide, or isotretinoin may be effective. Some patients require immunosuppressive therapy with agents such as mycophenolate mofetil or azathioprine. It should also be noted that antimalarials can occasionally produce a lichenoid drug eruption in patients with LE.

Chilblain lupus erythematosus

Chilblain LE (Hutchinson) is a chronic, unremitting form of LE with the fingertips, rims of ears, calves, and heels affected, especially in women. It is usually preceded by DLE on the face. Systemic involvement is sometimes seen. Mimicry of sarcoidosis may be striking. Cryoglobulins and antiphospholipid antibody should also be sought.

Tumid lupus erythematosus

Tumid LE is a rare but distinctive entity. Patients present with edematous erythematous plaques, usually on the trunk (Fig. 8-6). Histologically, the lesions demonstrate a patchy superficial and deep perivascular and periadnexal lymphoid infiltrate that frequently affects the eccrine coil. Dermal mucin deposition is typical and may be striking. The lesions generally respond readily to antimalarials. Tumid LE shares may features with reticular erythematous mucinosis, and some authorities consider them to be closely related entities.

Lupus erythematosus panniculitis (lupus erythematosus profundus)

Patients with this type of LE develop subcutaneous nodules that are commonly firm, sharply defined, and nontender. The proximal extremities are usually involved. Usually the overlying skin is normal, but overlying discoid or tumid lesions may occur (Fig. 8-7). Some cases are discovered incidentally when an unrelated lesion is biopsied. The lesions may heal with deep

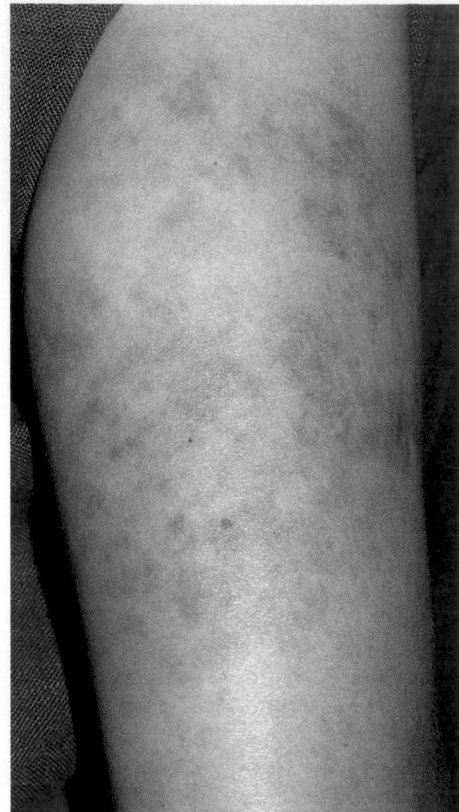

Fig. 8-6 Tumid lupus.

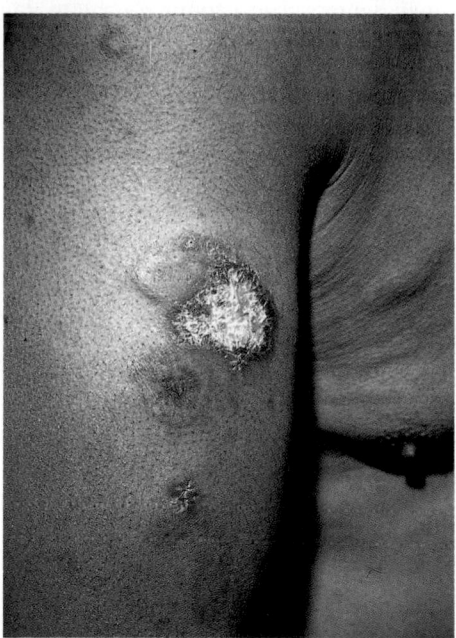

Fig. 8-7 Lupus panniculitis with overlying discoid lupus erythematosus.

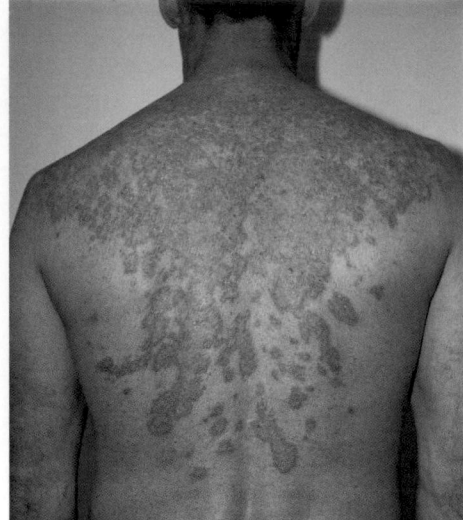

Fig. 8-8 Subacute cutaneous lupus erythematosus involving the "V" portion of the back.

depressions from loss of the panniculus. LE panniculitis is characteristically chronic and occurs most often in women between the ages of 20 and 45. Many patients have DLE at other sites, or less typically in the overlying skin.

Histologic sections demonstrate lymphoid nodules in the subcutaneous septae, necrosis of the fat lobule, and fibrinoid or hyaline degeneration of the remaining lipocytes. Lipomembranous change, resembling frost on a window pane, is more typical of stasis panniculitis (lipodermatosclerosis), but may be noted focally in LE panniculitis. The overlying

epidermis may show basal liquefaction and follicular plugging, or may be normal. It is not uncommon to see dermal lymphoid nodules or vertical columns of lymphoid cells in fibrous tract remnants. Dermal mucin may be prominent and dermal collagen hyalinization (resembling that seen in morphea) may be present. Continuous granular deposition of immunoglobulin and C3 may be seen at the dermoepidermal junction. In active cases, abundant fibrin is usually noted in the panniculus.

The most important entity to consider in the differential diagnosis is subcutaneous panniculitis-like lymphoma. Important clues include the presence of lipocytes rimmed by atypical lymphocytes, and the presence of constitutional symptoms. Erythrophagocytosis may be present focally, and T-cell clonality can usually be demonstrated. The infiltrate may be CD8-dominant, or may label strongly for CD56 (as in natural killer cell lymphoma) or CD30 (as in anaplastic lymphoma). CD5 and CD7 expression may be reduced (aberrant loss of pan-T-markers). Unfortunately, T-cell clonality, erythrophagocytosis, CD8 predominance, and loss of CD5 or CD7 may also be seen in cases of LE panniculitis that respond to antimalarials or corticosteroids and do not progress to clinical lymphoma. Taken together, these data suggest that some cases of lymphoma may be virtually indistinguishable from LE panniculitis or that some cases of LE panniculitis represent an abortive lymphoid dyscrasia.

Subacute cutaneous lupus erythematosus

Sontheimer, Thomas, and Gilliam in 1979 described a clinically distinct subset of cases of LE to which they gave the name subacute cutaneous lupus erythematosus (SCLE). Patients are most often white women aged 15–40. SCLE patients make up approximately 10–15% of the LE population. Lesions are scaly and evolve as polycyclic annular lesions) or psoriasiform plaques. The lesions vary from red to pink with faint violet tones. The scale is thin and easily detached, and telangiectasia or dyspigmentation may be present. Follicles are not involved, the lesions tend to be transient or migratory, and there is no scarring. Lesions tend to occur on sun-exposed surfaces of the face and neck, the V portion of the chest and back (Fig. 8-8), and the sun-exposed areas of the arms. Photosensitivity is prominent in about half of patients. Concomitant DLE is present in 20% of cases.

Roughly three-quarters of patients have arthralgia or arthritis, 20% have leukopenia, and 80% have a positive ANA test (usually in a particulate pattern). Roughly one-third of patients meet the ARA criteria for a diagnosis of SLE. The majority of cases have antibodies to Ro/SSA antigen, and most are positive for human leukocyte antigen (HLA)-DR3. La/SSB may also be present and many patients have overlap features with Sjögren syndrome. The disease generally runs a mild course, and renal, central nervous system (CNS), or vascular complications are unusual. An association with autoimmune thyroid disease has been noted. Most cases respond to sun protection and antimalarial agents. Drug-induced SCLE is most commonly related to hydrochlorothiazide, but may also be seen with angiotensin-converting enzyme (ACE) inhibitors, calcium channel-blockers, interferons (IFNs), anticonvulsants, griseofulvin, glyburide, piroxicam, penicillamine, spironolactone, terbinafine and statins.

Histopathology

Vacuolar interface dermatitis is a universal finding in active lesions. Mild hyperkeratosis and parakeratosis may be present. Chronic changes of DLE, such as follicular plugging, basement membrane zone thickening, and heavy lymphoid aggregates, are usually lacking. Dermal mucin is variable. DIF is positive in lesions in only about one-third of cases. A dustlike particulate deposition of IgG in epidermal nuclei of Ro-positive patients may be present and is a helpful diagnostic finding.

Neonatal lupus erythematosus

Most infants with neonatal lupus are girls, born to mothers who carry the Ro/SSA antibody. These infants have no skin lesions at birth, but develop them during the first few weeks of life. Annular erythematous macules, and plaques may appear on the head and extremities. Periocular involvement (raccoon eyes) may be prominent. With time, the lesions fade and become atrophic. Telangiectasia or dermal mucinosis in an acral papular pattern may be the predominant findings in some cases. Telangiectatic macules or angiomatous papules may be found in sun-protected sites such as the diaper area, may occur independently of active lupus skin lesions, and may be persistent (Fig. 8-9). The skin lesions usually resolve spontaneously by 6 months of age, and usually heal without significant scar-

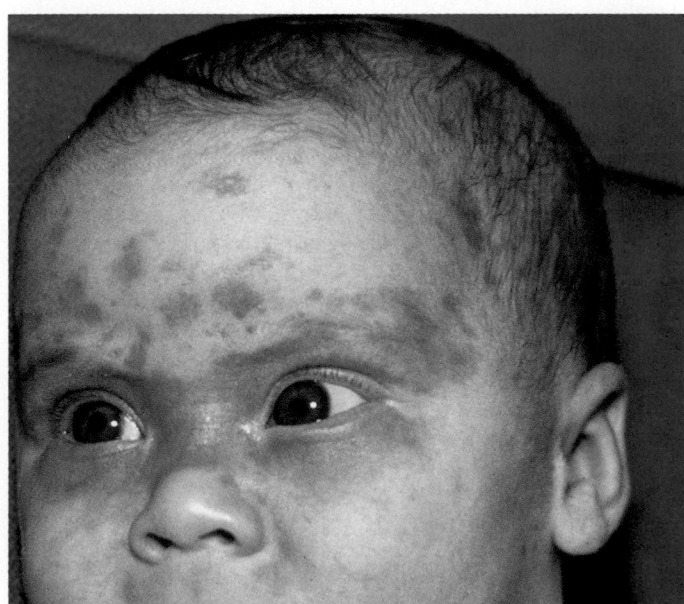

Fig. 8-9 Periocular neonatal lupus erythematosus.

ring, although atrophy may be present. Dyspigmentation and persistent telangiectasias may remain for months to years. Half of the mothers are asymptomatic at the time of delivery, although many will subsequently develop arthralgia, Sjögren syndrome, or other mild systemic findings.

Although the skin lesions are transient, half the patients have an associated isolated congenital heart block, usually third-degree, which is permanent. Some infants have only this manifestation of LE, and for cardiac lesions alone there is no female predominance. In children with cutaneous involvement, thrombocytopenia and hepatic disease may occur as frequently as cardiac disease.

There is a strong association with Ro/SSA autoantibody. Nearly all mothers, and hence nearly all infants, are positive for this antibody, although some mothers are also positive for La/SSB and some with only U1RNP antibodies have been described. Infants with only U1RNP antibodies have not developed heart block. There is linkage to HLA-DR3 in the mother. The risk that a second child will have neonatal LE is approximately 25%. Japanese infants apparently differ in that they may express anti-dsDNA antibodies and 8% progress to SLE. In unselected women with anti-Ro antibodies, only 1–2% will have an infant with neonatal LE.

Complement deficiency syndromes

Although deficiency of many complement components may be associated with LE-like conditions, deficiencies of the early components, especially C2 and C4, are most characteristic. Many such cases are found to have photosensitive annular SCLE lesions and Ro/SSA antibody formation. Patients with C4 deficiency often have hyperkeratosis of the palms and soles. Heterozygous deficiency of either complement component C4A or C4B has a frequency of approximately 20% in white populations. Homozygous deficiency of both is rare, and affected patients may present with SLE with mesangial glomerulonephritis, membranous nephropathy, and severe skin lesions. Although frequently asymptomatic, homozygous C2 deficiency can cause severe infections, SLE, and atherosclerosis.

Systemic lupus erythematosus

Young to middle-aged women are predominantly affected by SLE, manifesting a wide range of symptoms and signs. Skin involvement occurs in 80% of cases and is often helpful in arriving at a diagnosis. Its importance is suggested by the fact that four of the ACR's 11 criteria for the diagnosis of SLE are mucocutaneous findings. The diagnostic criteria are as follows:

- malar rash
- discoid rash
- photosensitivity
- oral ulcers (21%)
- arthritis
- proteinuria >0.5 g/day or casts
- neurologic disorders (seizures or psychosis in the absence of other known causes)
- pleuritis/pericarditis
- blood abnormalities (including hemolytic anemia, leukopenia, thrombocytopenia)
- immunologic disorders such as anti-dsDNA antibody, anti-Sm, antiphospholipid antibodies (based on IgG or IgM anticardiolipin antibodies, lupus anticoagulant or a false-positive serologic test for syphilis known for at least 6 months)
- positive ANA blood test.

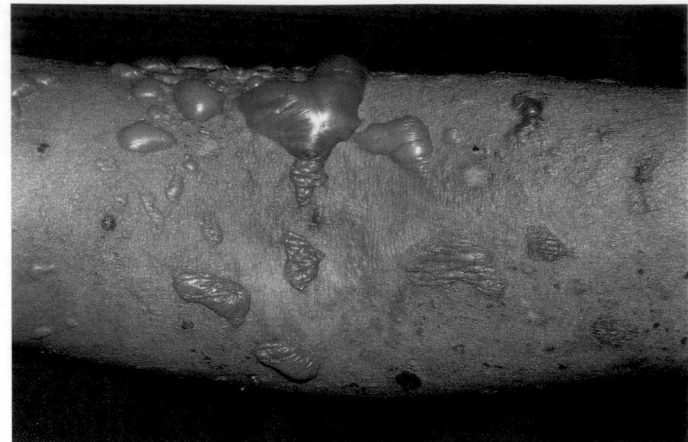

Fig. 8-10 Bullous lupus erythematosus.

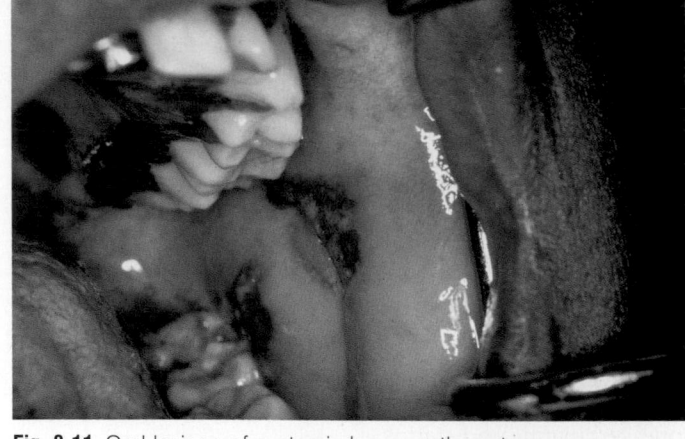

Fig. 8-11 Oral lesions of systemic lupus erythematosus.

For identification of patients in clinical studies, a patient may be said to have SLE if four or more of the above criteria are satisfied, serially or simultaneously. It is important to note that many patients present with autoantibodies, arthralgia, and constitutional signs, but do not meet ACR criteria for SLE. With time, patients may evolve to meet all criteria.

Cutaneous manifestations

The characteristic butterfly facial erythema seen in patients with SLE is a common manifestation of acute cutaneous LE. The eruption usually begins on the malar area and the bridge of the nose. There may be associated edema. The ears and chest may also be the sites of early lesions. Biopsies at all sites show interface dermatitis and a scant perivascular lymphoid infiltrate. The eruption may last from a day to several weeks, and resolves without scarring. There may be more widespread erythema in some cases.

Bullous lesions of LE (BLE) (Fig. 8-10) occur as single or grouped vesicles or bullae, often widespread, with a predilection for sun-exposed areas. Rarely, they may itch. Most sets of published criteria require that patients with BLE meet ACR criteria for SLE, but patients exist who have identical bullous lesions and fewer than four ACR criteria. ACR criteria are critical to ensure that patients with similar severity are enrolled in clinical trials, but they sometimes fall short in the evaluation of a given patient. Histologically, neutrophils accumulate at the dermoepidermal junction and within dermal papillae. In bullous lesions, there is a subepidermal bulla containing neutrophils. Fluorescence with IgG, IgM, IgA, or C3 is commonly present in a continuous granular pattern at the basement membrane zone on DIF testing. They are found in or below the lamina densa on immunoelectron microscopy. Most of these patients are HLA-DR2-positive. The recognition of this subset as a distinct one is made clear by its often dramatic therapeutic response to dapsone. Epidermolysis bullosa acquisita is histopathologically and immunopathologically identical since both diseases are mediated by circulating antibodies against type VII collagen. Dapsone is usually ineffective in epidermolysis bullosa acquisita. Bullous lesions may also occasionally arise as a result of liquefactive degeneration of the basal cell layer or full-thickness epidermal necrosis resembling toxic epidermal necrolysis.

A variety of vascular lesions occur in 50% of cases of SLE. Often the fingertips or toes show edema, erythema, or telangiectasia. Nailfold capillary loops in LE are more likely to show wandering glomeruloid loops, whereas dermatomyositis and scleroderma capillary loops demonstrate symmetrical dilatation and dropout of vessels. Capillary loops in the Osler–

Weber–Rendu syndrome demonstrate ectasia of half of the capillary loop. Erythema multiforme-like lesions may predominate; this has been termed Rowell syndrome. Rarely, toxic epidermal necrolysis may be associated with lupus.

In addition to periungual telangiectasia, red or spotted lunulae may be present in patients with SLE. The palms, soles, elbows, knees, or buttocks may become persistently erythematous or purplish, sometimes with overlying scale. Diffuse, nonscarring hair loss is common. Short hairs in the frontal region are referred to as lupus hairs. These hairs result from a combination of chronic telogen effluvium and increased hair fragility.

Mucous membrane lesions are seen in 20–30% of SLE patients, and chronic cutaneous lupus may be localized to the eyelid or oral mucosa. Conjunctivitis, episcleritis, and nasal and vaginal ulcerations may occur. Oral mucosal hemorrhages, erosions, shallow angular ulcerations (Fig. 8-11) with surrounding erythema, and gingivitis occur commonly. Erythema, petechiae, and ulcerations may occur on the hard palate.

Multiple eruptive dermatofibromas have been described in SLE. Leg ulcers, typically deeply punched out and with very little inflammation, may be seen on the pretibial or malleolar areas. Many of these patients present with a livedoid pattern and many have an antiphospholipid antibody. Sneddon syndrome is composed of livedo reticularis and strokes related to a hyalinizing vasculopathy. Both erythema multiforme-like and toxic epidermal necrolysis-like presentations have been described.

Calcinosis cutis is uncommon but may be dramatic. Also seen infrequently are plaque-like or papulonodular depositions of mucin. These reddish-purple to skin-colored lesions are often present on the trunk and arms or head and neck (Fig. 8-12). Finally, a symmetrical papular eruption of the extremities may occur (Fig. 8-13). These skin-colored to erythematous lesions with a smooth, ulcerated, or umbilicated surface may show vasculitis or, in older lesions, a palisaded granulomatous inflammation. These occur in patients with SLE, rheumatoid arthritis, or other immune complex-mediated disease. This eruption has been referred to as palisaded neutrophilic and granulomatous dermatitis of immune complex disease.

Systemic manifestations

Most organs can be involved; the symptoms and findings are often due to immune complex disease, especially vasculitis. The earliest changes noted may be transitory or migratory arthralgia, often with periarticular inflammation. Fever, weight loss, pleuritis, adenopathy, or acute abdominal pain

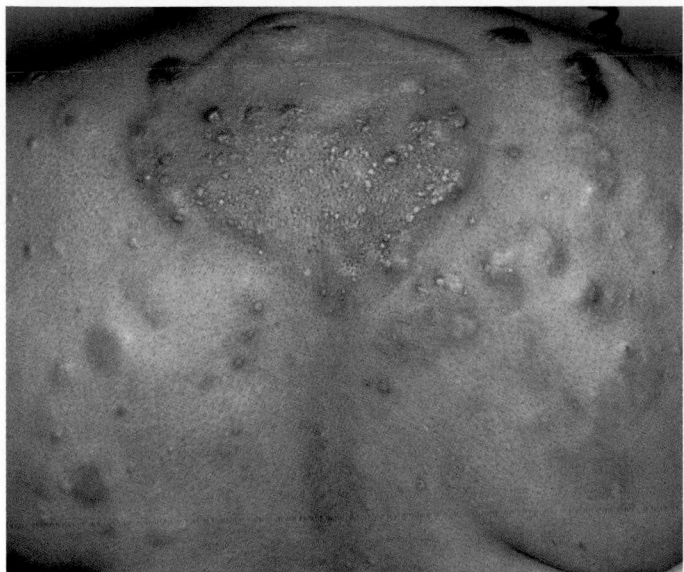

Fig. 8-12 Papulonodular mucinosis.

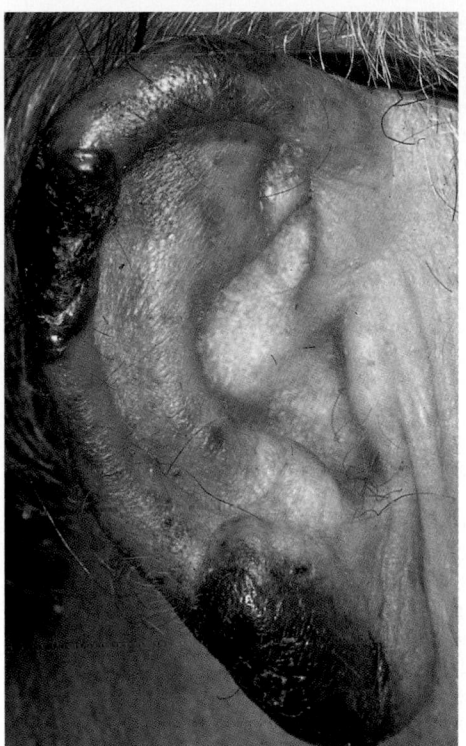

Fig. 8-14 Cutaneous thrombosis in antiphospholipid antibody syndrome.

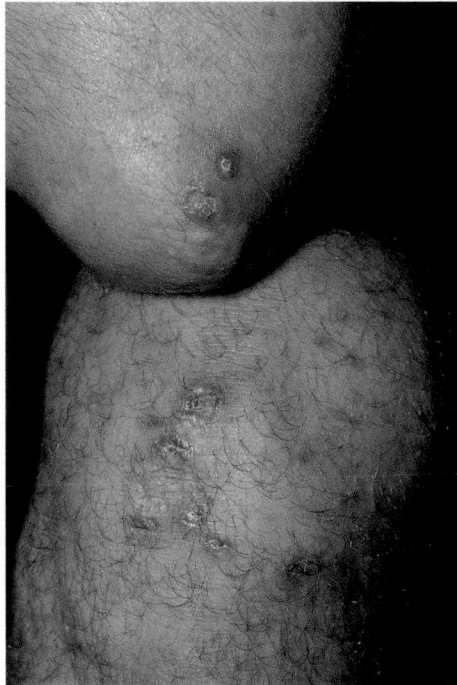

Fig. 8-13 Palisaded neutrophilic granulomatous dermatitis.

may occur. Arthralgia is often the earliest abnormality and may remain the sole symptom for some time. Around 95% of SLE patients will manifest this symptom. Arthralgia, deforming arthropathy, and acute migratory polyarthritis resembling rheumatoid arthritis may all occur as manifestations of SLE. Avascular necrosis of the femoral head has been observed. Although this is a known complication of systemic corticosteroid therapy, it has also occurred in patients with SLE who have never had corticosteroids.

Thrombosis in vessels of various sizes and thromboembolism may be a recurring event (Fig. 8-14). It may be attributed to a plasma constituent paradoxically called lupus anticoagulant (LA) because it causes prolonged coagulation studies in vitro, but thrombosis in vivo. The finding of a lupus anticoagulant is usually associated with antiphospholipid antibodies. These may be anticardiolipin antibodies, but other types of antiphospholipid antibody (antiphosphatidylserine, antiphosphatidylinositol, and antiphosphatidylethanolamine) may occur. Antiphospholipid antibodies and elevated homocysteine may each increase the risk of thrombosis. Antiphospholipid antibodies are associated with early-onset organ damage. Many, but not all, patients have a false-positive blood test for syphilis. In one study, inflammatory lesions of SLE and infections were the most common causes of death during the initial 5 years of disease, while thromboses were the most common cause of death after the first 5 years.

Renal involvement may be of either nephritic or nephrotic type, leading in either case to chronic renal insufficiency with proteinuria and azotemia. Active nephritis is unlikely in the absence of anti-dsDNA. Both anti-dsDNA antibody and anti-C1q antibody are of relatively high specificity for active nephritis. Hypercholesterolemia and hypoalbuminemia may occur. Immunoglobulin and complement components have been found localized to the basement membrane of glomeruli, where vasculitis produces the characteristic "wire-loop" lesion.

Myocarditis is indicated by cardiomegaly and gallop rhythm, but the electrocardiographic changes are usually not specific. Pericarditis (the most frequent cardiac manifestation) and endocarditis also occur. Raynaud phenomenon occurs in about 15% of patients; these individuals have less renal disease and consequently lower mortality.

The CNS may be involved with vasculitis, manifested by hemiparesis, convulsions, epilepsy, diplopia, retinitis, choroiditis, psychosis, and other personality disorders. Livedo reticularis is a marker for patients at risk for CNS lesions (Sneddon syndrome, see above).

Idiopathic thrombocytopenic purpura is occasionally the forerunner of SLE. Coombs-positive hemolytic anemia, neutropenia, and lymphopenia are other hematologic findings. Gastrointestinal involvement may produce symptoms of nausea, vomiting, and diarrhea. Frequently, the intestinal wall and the mesenteric vessels show vasculitis. Pulmonary involvement with pleural effusions, interstitial lung disease, and acute lupus pneumonitis may be present. Sjögren syndrome (keratoconjunctivitis sicca) and Hashimoto thyroiditis are associated with SLE. Overlap with any of the connective tissue diseases may be seen, and occurs in approximately 25% of patients. Muscular atrophy may accompany extreme weakness so that dermatomyositis may be suspected. Myopathy of the vacuolar type may produce muscular weakness, myocardial disease, dysphagia, and achalasia of the esophagus. Steroid myopathy may also occur. The serum aldolase level may be elevated with a normal creatine phosphokinase. Type B insulin resistance syndrome with insulin receptor antibodies accompanied by pancytopenia has been reported in the setting of chronic discoid LE evolving to SLE.

A history of exposure to excessive sunlight before the onset of the disease or before an exacerbation is sometimes obtained. Some patients may suffer only mild constitutional symptoms for weeks or months, but immediately after exposure to strong sunlight they may develop the facial eruption and severe disease complications.

Hydralazine, procainamide, sulfonamides, penicillin, anticonvulsants, minocycline, and isoniazid have been implicated as causes of drug-induced LE. Most drug-induced lupus is associated with a positive ANA test, antihistone antibodies, and sometimes serositis. Penicillamine induces (or unmasks) true SLE, and etanercept has produced a range of findings, including SLE. Anti-tumor necrosis factor (TNF) agents have produced a shift to a lupus profile of autoantibodies in patients with rheumatoid arthritis.

Childhood systemic lupus erythematosus

The onset of childhood SLE occurs between the ages of 3 and 15, with girls outnumbering boys 4:1. The skin manifestations may be the typical butterfly eruption on the face and photosensitivity. In addition, there may be morbilliform, bullous, purpuric, ulcerating, or nodose lesions. The oral mucosa is frequently involved.

Skin eruptions may be associated with joint, renal, neurologic, and gastrointestinal disease. Weight loss, fatigue, hepatosplenomegaly, lymphadenopathy, and fever are other manifestations. Pediatric patients with SLE and antiphospholipid antibodies, specifically lupus anticoagulants, are at high risk of developing thromboembolic events.

Pregnancy

Women with LE may have successful pregnancies, although there might be difficulty in conceiving, and miscarriages occur with greater frequency, especially among those with antiphospholipid antibodies. The course of pregnancy may be entirely normal, with remission of the LE, or the symptoms of LE may become worse. Risk of fetal death is increased in women with a previous history of fetal loss and anticardiolipin or anti-Ro antibodies. Low-dose aspirin is often used in the former instance. For the patient with these antibodies but without a history of previous fetal loss, the risk of fetal loss or neonatal lupus is low. In most cases, the pregnancy itself is well tolerated, although a flare of SLE may occur during the postpartum period. Several studies have failed to demonstrate a clinically significant association between oral contraceptive use and flares of SLE. There is a high incidence of thromboses in women with antiphospholipid antibodies, and oral contraceptives containing second- or third-generation progestogens may induce a higher risk.

Etiology

A family history of connective tissue disease is a strong risk factor for all forms of LE. HLA and gene linkage studies suggest a strongly heritable component, and some skin lesions

of LE follow lines of Blaschko, suggesting postzygotic mutation or loss of heterozygosity for a genetic locus. The C-reactive protein (CRP) response is defective in patients with flares of SLE, and the gene locus for CRP maps to 1q23.2 within an interval linked with SLE. Gene polymorphisms in APRIL, a member of the TNF family, have also been linked with SLE. Increased expression of TNF-α and IFN-inducible protein myxovirus protein A is noted in cutaneous LE. Polymorphisms of the *C1qA* gene are associated with both systemic and cutaneous LE. Strong linkage has been found with SLE at 5p15.3, 1q23, 1q31, 11q14, 12q24, and 16q12, as well as other candidate sites. Linkage varies in different ethnic groups and different clinical subsets of lupus. Taken together, these data suggest polygenetic susceptibility to LE.

Both ultraviolet (UV) B and UVA can upregulate antigen expression and cytokines, and cause release of sequestered antigens and free radical damage. All of these mechanisms may contribute to photosensitivity and UV-induced flares of systemic disease.

Several aspects of the altered immune response are worth particular attention. T-suppressor cell function is reduced in patients with LE. Overproduction of γ-globulins by B cells and reduced clearance of immune complexes by the reticuloendothelial system may contribute to complement-mediated damage. Externalization of cellular antigens, such as Ro/SSA in response to sunlight, may lead to cell injury by way of antibody-dependent cellular cytotoxicity. Abnormal apoptosis or reduced clearance of apoptotic cells may lead to increased exposure of nucleosome antigens and antinucleosome antibodies. HLA-DR4 individuals, who are slow acetylators, are predisposed to develop hydralazine-induced LE. Antibody to the histone complex H2A–H2B is closely associated with disease. In most drug-induced LE, antibodies are directed against histones. Exceptions include penicillamine and etanercept, which may induce or unmask native disease with anti-dsDNA antibodies. Pegylated IFN-α and ribavirin have also produced systemic LE during treatment for chronic hepatitis C. Drugs implicated in SCLE are listed earlier in this chapter. L-Canavanine, an amino acid found in alfalfa sprouts and tablets, can also induce or worsen SLE. There is little credible data regarding other possible aggravating dietary factors, but some reports have implicated excess calories, excess protein, high fat (especially saturated and ω-6 polyunsaturated fatty acids), excess zinc, and excess iron. Well-designed studies are needed. Cigarette smoking is associated with increased disease activity in SLE, and can interfere with the effects of antimalarial drugs.

Laboratory findings

There may be hemolytic anemia, thrombocytopenia, lymphopenia, or leukopenia; the ESR is usually markedly elevated during active disease, Coombs test may be positive, there is a biologic false-positive test for syphilis, and a rheumatoid factor may be present. Levels of IgG may be high, the albumin to globulin ratio is reversed, and the serum globulin is increased, especially the γ-globulin or α2 fraction. Albumin, red blood cells, and casts are the most frequent findings in the urine.

Immunologic findings

1. *ANA test.* This is positive in 95% of cases of SLE. Human substrates, such as Hep-2 or KB tumor cell lines, are far more sensitive than mouse substrates. ANA pattern has some correlation with clinical subsets, such as a shrunken peripheral pattern in SLE with renal disease, a fine particulate pattern in subacute cutaneous LE, and a homogeneous pattern with antihistone antibodies.

2. *Lupus erythematosus cell test.* This is specific but not very sensitive and has been deleted from the ACR criteria.

3. *Double-stranded DNA. Anti-dsDNA, anti-native DNA.* This is specific, but not very sensitive. It indicates a high risk of renal disease, and correlates with a shrunken peripheral ANA pattern and positive DIF in sun-protected skin.

4. *Anti-Sm antibody.* Sensitivity is less than 10% but there is very high specificity.

5. *Antinuclear ribonucleic acid protein (anti-nRNP).* Very high titers are present in mixed connective tissue disease. Lower titers may be seen in SLE.

6. *Anti-La antibodies.* These are common in SCLE and Sjögren syndrome, and occasionally found in SLE.

7. *Anti-Ro antibodies.* These are found in about 25% of SLE and 40% of Sjögren cases. They are more common in patients with SCLE (70%), neonatal LE (95%), C2- and C4-deficient LE (50–75%), late-onset LE (75%), and Asian patients with LE (50–60%). Photosensitivity may be striking, and externalization of the antigen is seen after UV exposure.

8. *Serum complement.* Low levels indicate active disease, often with renal involvement.

9. *Lupus band test. Direct cutaneous immunofluorescence.* Continuous granular deposits of immunoglobulins and complement along the dermoepidermal junction occur in more than 75% of well-established lesions of DLE. In SLE, it is commonly positive in sun-exposed skin. A positive test in normal protected skin correlates with the presence of anti-dsDNA antibodies and renal disease. The test is seldom performed, as the same population of patients can be detected with anti-dsDNA antibodies.

10. *Anti-ssDNA antibody.* This test is sensitive but not specific. Many are photosensitive. An IgM isotype seen in DLE may identify a subset of patients at risk for developing systemic symptoms.

11. *Antiphospholipid antibodies.* Both the anticardiolipin antibody and the lupus anticoagulant are subtypes of these. They are associated with a syndrome that includes venous thrombosis, arterial thrombosis, spontaneous abortions, and thrombocytopenia. Livedo reticularis is a frequent skin finding and nonfading acral microlivedo, small cyanotic pink lesions on the hands and feet, is a subtle clue to the presence of these antibodies. Antiphospholipid antibodies may occur in association with lupus and other connective tissue disease, or as a solitary event. In the latter case it is referred to as the primary antiphospholipid syndrome.

Differential diagnosis

SLE must be differentiated from dermatomyositis, erythema multiforme, polyarteritis nodosa, acute rheumatic fever, rheumatoid arthritis, pellagra, pemphigus erythematosus (Senear–Usher syndrome), drug eruptions, hyperglobulinemic purpura, Sjögren syndrome, necrotizing angiitis, and myasthenia gravis. In SLE there may be fever, arthralgia, weakness, lassitude, diagnostic skin lesions, an increased ESR, cytopenias, proteinuria, immunoglobulin deposition at the dermoepidermal junction, and a positive ANA test. Biopsies of skin lesions and involved kidney may also be diagnostic.

Treatment

Some general measures are important for all patients with LE. Exposure to sunlight must be avoided, and a high sun-protection factor (SPF) sunscreen should be used daily. Photosensitivity is frequently present even if the patient denies it, and all patients must be educated about sun avoidance and sunscreen use. The patient should also avoid exposure to excessive cold, to heat, and to localized trauma. Biopsies and scar revision will often provoke a flare of the disease. Women with SLE have an increased risk of osteoporosis, independent of the use of corticosteroids. Bone density should be monitored, and calcium and vitamin D supplementation should be considered. Some women will benefit from bisphosphonate therapy, especially if corticosteroids are used. The most rapid bone loss with corticosteroid therapy occurs at the onset of treatment, so bisphosphonate therapy should not be delayed. Patients who will be treated with immunosuppressive agents should receive a tuberculin skin test as well as a thorough physical examination. Aggressive treatment is often necessary for discoid lesions and scarring alopecia. The slowly progressive nature of these lesions, and the lack of systemic involvement, may lead to inappropriate therapeutic complacency. The result is slow, progressive disfigurement.

Local treatment

The application of potent or superpotent topical corticosteroids is beneficial. Occlusion may be necessary and may be enhanced by customized vinyl appliances (especially for oral lesions) or surgical dressings. Tape containing corticosteroid (Cordran) is sometimes helpful. The single most effective local treatment is the injection of corticosteroids into the lesions. Triamcinolone acetonide, 2.5–10 mg/mL, is infiltrated into the lesion through a 30-gauge needle at intervals of 4–6 weeks. No more than 40 mg of triamcinolone should be used at one time. Steroid atrophy is a valid concern, but so are the atrophy and scar produced by the disease. The minimal intralesional dose needed to control the disease should be used; when the response is poor, however, it is generally better to err on the slightly more aggressive side of treatment than to undertreat. Topical calcineurin inhibitors (topical macrolactams) may also be useful as second-line topical therapy. Photodynamic therapy has been reported as effective.

Systemic treatment

The safest class of systemic agent for LE is the antimalarials. Retinoids are second-line agents and are particularly helpful in treating hypertrophic LE. Systemic immunosuppressive agents are often required to manage the systemic manifestations of LE, and are third-line systemic agents for cutaneous LE. Thalidomide can be effective but its use is limited by the risk of teratogenicity and neuropathy. Dapsone is the drug of choice for bullous systemic LE, and may be effective in some cases of SCLE and DLE. Oral prednisone is generally reserved for acute flares of disease.

Antimalarials Hydroxychloroquine (Plaquenil), at a dose equal to or less than 6.5 mg/kg/day, has an excellent safety profile and is generally used as first-line systemic therapy in most forms of cutaneous LE. If no response occurs after 3 months, another agent should be considered. Chloroquine (Aralen) is effective in a dose of 250 mg/day for an average adult, but is difficult to procure. Quinacrine (Atabrine), 100 mg/day, may be added to hydroxychloroquine, since this adds no increased risk of retinal toxicity. Quinacrine is also difficult to procure and carries a higher risk of disfiguring pigmentation than the other antimalarials. Systemic treatment can sometimes be reduced or stopped during the winter months. A Cochrane group review of randomized controlled trials concluded that hydroxychloroquine and acitretin appear to be of similar efficacy, although adverse effects are more severe and occur more commonly with acitretin.

Ocular toxicity is rare with doses of hydroxychloroquine equal to or less than 6.5 mg/kg/day. Ophthalmologic consultation should be obtained before, and at 4- to 6-month intervals during, treatment. Constriction of visual fields to a red object and paracentral scotomas are rare at the recommended dose, but even a small risk of loss of vision must be taken seriously. The finding of any visual field defect or pigmentary abnormality is an indication to stop antimalarial therapy.

Other reported side effects with antimalarials include erythroderma, erythema multiforme, purpura, urticaria, nervousness, tinnitus, abducens nerve paralysis, toxic psychoses, leukopenia, and thrombocytopenia. Antimalarials, except in very small doses, will exacerbate skin disease or cause hepatic necrosis in patients with porphyria cutanea tarda. They may also worsen or induce psoriasis. Quinacrine produces a yellow discoloration of the skin and conjunctivae. Quinacrine has also been known to produce blue–black pigmentation of the hard palate, nailbeds, cartilage of the ears, alae nasi, and sclerae. Other antimalarials may also rarely produce a blue–black pigmentation of skin. Bullous erythema multiforme, lichenoid drug eruption, nausea, vomiting, anorexia, and diarrhea may develop. Aplastic anemia has rarely been noted in long-term therapy. A patient's brown or red hair may turn light blond.

Corticosteroids Systemic corticosteroids are highly effective for widespread or disfiguring lesions, but disease activity often rebounds quickly when the drug is discontinued. Because of long-term side effects, corticosteroid treatment should be limited to short (generally 3 weeks or less) courses to treat flares of disease or to obtain initial control while antimalarial therapy is being initiated. In cases with renal or neurologic involvement, corticosteroids should be administered in doses adequate to control the disease, while treatment with a steroid-sparing regimen is initiated. Treatment with 1000 mg/day intravenous methylprednisolone for 3 days, followed by oral prednisone, 0.5–1 mg/kg/day, is effective in quickly reversing most clinical and serologic signs of activity of lupus nephritis. In general, the corticosteroid dose should be optimized to the lowest possible that controls symptoms and laboratory abnormalities.

Immunosuppressive therapy Aggressive treatment protocols with agents such as pulse cyclophosphamide (with hydration and MESNA to prevent bladder toxicity) have greatly improved the outcome of renal LE. Other immunosuppressive agents, including azathioprine, methotrexate, and mycophenolate mofetil, are often employed as steroid-sparing agents for refractory cutaneous disease. Some authorities have suggested that azathioprine is inferior to mycophenolate mofetil in the treatment of cutaneous lesions. IL-6 receptor inhibition with tocilizumab appears promising but may cause neutropenia.

Other therapy

Isotretinoin therapy, in doses of 1 mg/kg/day may be effective, especially in hypertrophic or lichenoid lesions of LE. Rapid relapse may be noted when the drug is discontinued. Dapsone, clofazimine, acitretin, IFN-α 2a, auranofin (oral gold), high-dose intravenous γ-globulin, efalizumab, and thalidomide have all been reported as effective in anecdotal use or limited trials. Pulsed dye laser has been shown to be effective for some erythematous lesions of cutaneous LE, but should be used cautiously, as it may also cause flares of disease. Flares of disease are also common with surgical modalities used to improve scarring or alopecia. Anti-CD20 monoclonal antibody (rituximab) has been used successfully to treat life-threatening refractory SLE with renal and CNS involvement, as well as for hypocomplementemic urticarial vasculitis and refractory cutaneous lesions. Although lupus is a photosensitive disorder, UVA-1 therapy appears to be a useful adjuvant treatment modality in some patients, and photodynamic therapy has been effective in some patients.

Albrecht J, et al: Dermatology position paper on the revision of the 1982 ACR criteria for systemic lupus erythematosus. Lupus 2004; 13:839.

Bonilla-Martinez ZL, et al: The cutaneous lupus erythematosus disease area and severity index: a responsive instrument to measure activity and damage in patients with cutaneous lupus erythematosus. Arch Dermatol 2008 Feb; 144(2):173–180.

Cavazzana I, et al: Treatment of lupus skin involvement with quinacrine and hydroxychloroquine. Lupus 2009 Jul; 18(8):735–739.

Cervera R, et al: Morbidity and mortality in systemic lupus erythematosus during a 10-year period: a comparison of early and late manifestations in a cohort of 1,000 patients. Medicine (Baltimore) 2003; 82:299.

Costa MF, et al: Drug-induced lupus due to anti-tumor necrosis factor alpha agents. Semin Arthritis Rheum 2008 Jun; 37(6):381–387.

Fusconi M, et al: Etanercept and infliximab induce the same serological autoimmune modifications in patients with rheumatoid arthritis. Rheumatol Int 2007 Nov; 28(1):47–49.

Garcia-Carrasco M, et al: Anti-CD20 therapy in patients with refractory systemic lupus erythematosus: a longitudinal analysis of 52 Hispanic patients. Lupus 2010 Feb; 19(2):213–219.

Hamprecht A, et al: Successful treatment of recalcitrant malar rash in a patient with cutaneous lupus erythematosus with efalizumab. Clin Exp Dermatol 2008 May; 33(3):347–348.

Hivnor CM, et al: Terbinafine-induced subacute cutaneous lupus erythematosus. Cutis 2008 Feb; 81(2):156–157.

Ho V, et al: Severe systemic lupus erythematosus induced by antiviral treatment for hepatitis C. J Clin Rheumatol 2008 Jun; 14(3):166–168.

Illei GG, et al: Tocilizumab in systemic lupus erythematosus: data on safety, preliminary efficacy, and impact on circulating plasma cells from an open-label phase I dosage-escalation study. Arthritis Rheum 2010 Jan 28; 62(2):542–552.

Jessop S, et al: Drugs for discoid lupus erythematosus. Cochrane Database Syst Rev 2009 Oct 7; (4):CD002954.

Kalia S, et al: New concepts in antimalarial use and mode of action in dermatology. Dermatol Ther 2007 Jul–Aug; 20(4):160–174.

Kallel-Sellami M, et al: Pediatric systemic lupus erythematosus with C1q deficiency. Ann N Y Acad Sci 2007 Jun; 1108:193–196.

Kuhn A, et al: Cutaneous lupus erythematosus: molecular and cellular basis of clinical findings. Curr Dir Autoimmun 2008; 10:119–140.

Kuhn A, et al: Pathogenesis of cutaneous lupus erythematosus. Lupus 2008; 17(5):389–393.

Kuhn A, et al: Photosensitivity, phototesting, and photoprotection in cutaneous lupus erythematosus. Lupus 2010 Aug; 19(9):1036–1046.

Kuhn A, et al: Treatment of cutaneous lupus erythematosus. Lupus 2010 Aug; 19(9):1125–1136.

Lin JH, et al: Pathophysiology of cutaneous lupus erythematosus. Clin Rev Allergy Immunol 2007 Oct; 33(1–2):85–106.

Lourenço SV, et al: Lupus erythematosus: clinical and histopathological study of oral manifestations and immunohistochemical profile of the inflammatory infiltrate. J Cutan Pathol 2007 Jul; 34(7):558–564.

Marzano AV, et al: Drug-induced lupus: an update on its dermatologic aspects. Lupus 2009 Oct; 18(11):935–940.

Mok CC: Mycophenolate mofetil for non-renal manifestations of systemic lupus erythematosus: a systematic review. Scand J Rheumatol 2007 Sep–Oct; 36(5):329–337.

Muller S, et al: Pathogenic anti-nucleosome antibodies. Lupus 2008; 17(5):431–436.

Obermoser G, et al: Overview of common, rare and atypical manifestations of cutaneous lupus erythematosus and histopathological correlates. Lupus 2010 Aug; 19(9):1050–1070.

Paradela S, et al: Toxic epidermal necrolysis-like acute cutaneous lupus erythematosus. Lupus 2007; 16(9):741–745.

Park HS, et al: Lupus erythematosus panniculitis: clinicopathological, immunophenotypic, and molecular studies. Am J Dermatopathol 2010; 32(1):24–30.

Petri M, et al: Classification criteria for systemic lupus erythematosus: a review. Lupus 2004; 13:829.

Saarialho-Kere U: Clinical and laboratory characteristics of Finnish lupus erythematosus patients with cutaneous manifestations. Lupus 2008;17(4): 337–347.

Saito K, et al: Successful treatment with anti-CD20 monoclonal antibody (rituximab) of life-threatening refractory systemic lupus erythematosus with renal and central nervous system involvement. Lupus 2003; 12:798.

Sampaio MC, et al: Discoid lupus erythematosus in children—a retrospective study of 34 patients. Pediatr Dermatol 2008 Mar–Apr; 25(2):163–167.

Sato N, et al: Type B insulin resistance syndrome with systemic lupus erythematosus. Clin Nephrol 2010; 73(2):157–162.

Sfikakis PP, et al: Rituximab anti-B-cell therapy in systemic lupus erythematosus: pointing to the future. Curr Opin Rheumatol 2005; 17:550.

Shadid NH, et al: Lupus erythematosus associated with erythema multiforme: Rowell's syndrome. Int J Dermatol 2007 Nov; 46(Suppl 3):30–32.

Sticherling M, et al: Diagnostic approach and treatment of cutaneous lupus erythematosus. J Dtsch Dermatol Ges 2008 Jan; 6(1):48–59.

Uthman I, et al: Successful treatment of refractory skin manifestations of systemic lupus erythematosus with rituximab: report of a case. Dermatology 2008; 216(3):257–259.

Walling HW, et al: Cutaneous lupus erythematosus: issues in diagnosis and treatment. Am J Clin Dermatol 2009; 10(6):365–381.

Weide R, et al: Successful long-term treatment of systemic lupus erythematosus with rituximab maintenance therapy. Lupus 2003; 12:779.

Wenzel J, et al: Efficacy and safety of methotrexate in recalcitrant cutaneous lupus erythematosus: results of a retrospective study in 43 patients. Br J Dermatol 2005; 153:157.

Wenzel J, et al: Pathogenesis of cutaneous lupus erythematosus: common and different features in distinct subsets. Lupus 2010 Aug; 19(9):1020–1028.

Werth VP: Cutaneous lupus: insights into pathogenesis and disease classification. Bull NYU Hosp Jt Dis 2007; 65(3):200–204.

Wollina U, et al: The use of topical calcineurin inhibitors in lupus erythematosus: an overview. J Eur Acad Dermatol Venereol 2008 Jan; 22(1):1–6.

Wozniacka A, et al: Optimal use of antimalarials in treating cutaneous lupus erythematosus. Am J Clin Dermatol 2005; 6:11.

Wozniacka A, et al: Chloroquine treatment reduces the number of cutaneous HLA-DR+ and CD1a+ cells in patients with systemic lupus erythematosus. Lupus 2007; 16(2):89–94.

Yang Y, et al: Complete complement components C4A and C4B deficiencies in human kidney diseases and systemic lupus erythematosus. J Immunol 2004; 173:2803.

Zuppa AA, et al: Infants born to mothers with anti-SSA/Ro autoantibodies: neonatal outcome and follow-up. Clin Pediatr (Phila) 2008 Apr; 47(3):231–236.

Dermatomyositis

Dermatomyositis (DM) is typically characterized by inflammatory myositis and skin disease, although amyopathic DM (DM with subclinical or absent myopathy) also occurs. Muscle involvement without skin changes is called polymyositis (PM). With or without skin lesions, weakness of proximal muscle groups is characteristic.

Skin findings

Usually the disease begins with erythema and edema of the face and eyelids. Eyelid involvement (Fig. 8-15) may be charac-terized by pruritic and scaly pink patches, edema, and pinkish-violet (heliotrope) discoloration or bullae. Pruritic scaly pink patches are often seen in amyopathic DM. Edema and pinkish-violet discoloration are often signs of inflammation in the underlying striated orbicularis oculi muscle, rather than the skin itself. In such cases, the eyelids may be tender to the touch. Bullous DM may portend a poor prognosis, and patients often have severe inflammatory myopathy or lung disease.

Other skin changes include erythema, scaling, and swelling of the upper face, often with involvement of the hairline and eyebrows. Extensor surfaces of the extremities are often pink, red or violaceous with an atrophic appearance or overlying scale. The similarity to psoriasis can be striking, and patients may suffer severe flares of DM if they are inappropriately treated with phototherapy for presumed psoriasis. Photosensitivity to natural sunlight is common as well. Firm, slightly pitting edema may be seen over the shoulder girdle, arms, and neck. Associated erythema and scale (with or without poikiloderma) over the shoulder regions is known as the shawl sign. Pruritus may be severe in some cases, and is much more common in DM than in psoriasis or LE.

Over time, more widespread skin changes are typically seen. Skin lesions become more prominent on the neck, thorax, shoulders, and arms. Characteristic areas include nape of the neck, upper chest (V) pattern, and upper back, neck, and shoulder (shawl) pattern (Fig. 8-16). Occasionally, a flagellate pattern mimicking bleomycin-induced linear edematous streaks or erythroderma may be seen.

On the hands, telangiectatic vessels often become prominent in the proximal nailfolds. Enlarged capillaries of the nailfold appear as dilated, sausage-shaped loops with adjacent avascular regions (Fig. 8-17), similar to those changes observed in scleroderma. There may be cuticular overgrowth with an irregular frayed appearance. A pink to reddish-purple atrophic (Fig. 8-18) or scaling eruption often occurs over the knuckles, knees, and elbows (Gottron's sign). Flat-topped, polygonal, violaceous papules over the knuckles (Gottron's papules) are less common, but are highly characteristic of DM. Hyperkeratosis, scaling, fissuring, and hyperpigmentation over the fingertips, sides of the thumb, and fingers with occasional involvement of the palms is referred to as mechanic's hands (Fig. 8-19) and has been reported in 70% of patients with antisynthetase antibodies. Intermittent fever, malaise, anorexia, arthralgia, and marked weight loss are commonly present at this stage.

Telangiectasia and erythema may become more pronounced with time. Mottled hyperpigmentation and hypopigmentation, atrophy, and telangiectasia (poikiloderma) eventually develop in many patients. In some patients with disease remission, the residual hyperpigmentation simulates the bronze

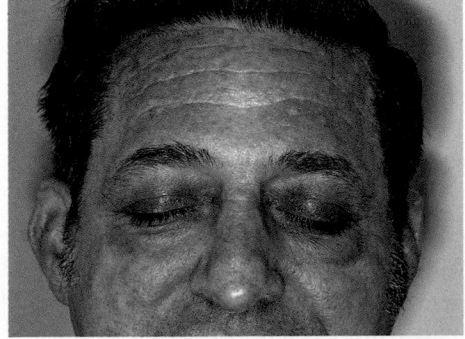

Fig. 8-15 Heliotrope rash in a patient with dermatomyositis.

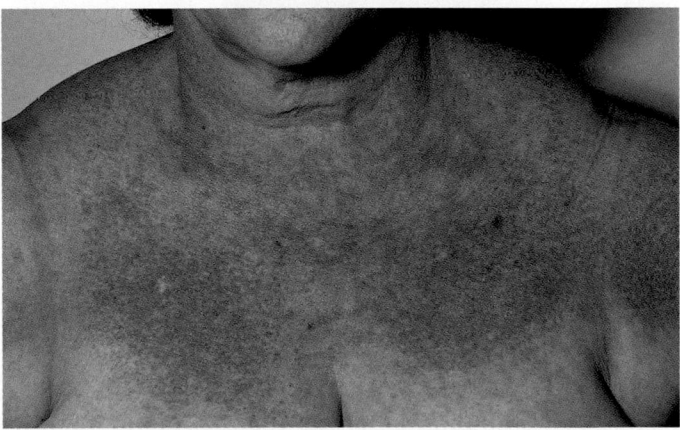

Fig. 8-16 "V" of neck with poikiloderma in dermatomyositis.

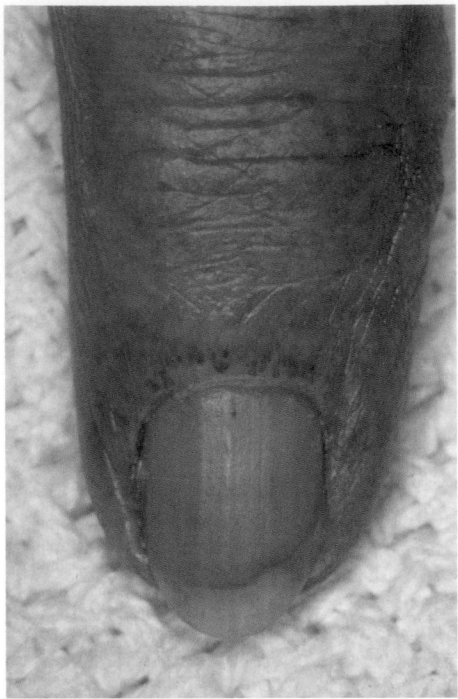

Fig. 8-17 Dilated vessels and avascular regions of the proximal nailfold.

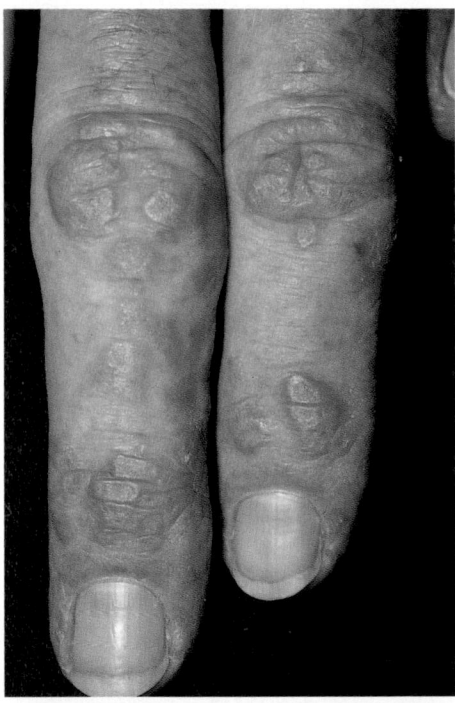

Fig. 8-18 Gottron's papules of dermatomyositis involving the knuckles.

discoloration of Addison's disease. Rarely, large, persistent ulcerations in flexural areas or over pressure points may develop. Ulceration in the early stages of disease has been reported to be associated with a higher incidence of cancer and a poor prognosis, but the authors have seen many patients with ulcerative DM without associated cancer. In later stages, ulceration may merely be a manifestation of pressure or trauma to atrophic areas. Rarely, DM may be associated with clinical findings of pityriasis rubra pilaris (Wong variant of DM) or generalized subcutaneous edema.

Calcium deposits in the skin and muscles occur in more than half of children with DM; they are found rather infrequently in adults. Calcification is related to duration of disease activity

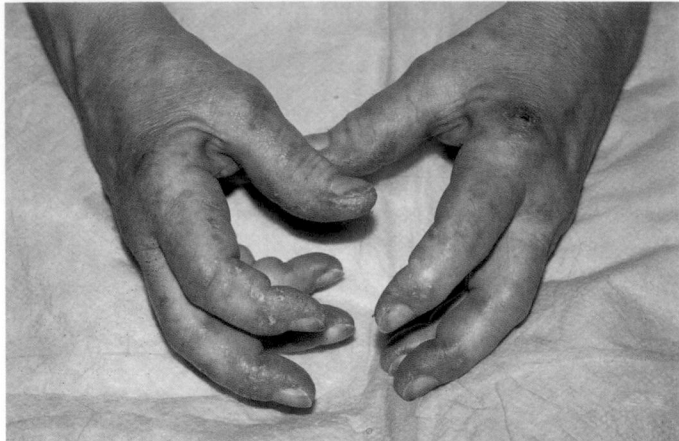

Fig. 8-19 Mechanic's hands.

and its severity. Calcinosis of the dermis, subcutaneous tissue, and muscle occurs mostly on the upper half of the body around the shoulder girdle, elbows, and hands. Ulcerations and cellulitis are frequently associated with this debilitating and disabling complication of DM.

Muscle changes

In severe cases, early and extensive muscular weakness occurs, with acute swelling and pain. The muscle weakness is seen symmetrically, most frequently involving the shoulder girdle and sometimes the pelvic region, as well as the hands. The patients may notice difficulty in lifting even the lightest objects. They may be unable to raise their arms to comb their hair, and rising from a chair may be impossible without "pushing off" with the arms. Patients often complain of pain in the legs when standing barefoot or of being unable to climb stairs. Difficulty in swallowing, talking, and breathing, caused by weakness of the involved muscles, may be noted early in the disease. Some patients with severe diaphragmatic disease require mechanical ventilation. Cardiac failure may be present in the terminal phase of the disease.

Skin involvement commonly precedes muscle involvement, but some patients have typical skin findings of DM but never develop clinically apparent muscle involvement. These cases have been termed amyopathic DM or DM sine myositis. It is common, however, for muscle inflammation to be present but not symptomatic. Muscle enzymes (to include both creatine kinase and aldolase), electromyogram (EMG), and magnetic resonance imaging (MRI) may be required to detect subtle involvement.

Diagnostic criteria

The following criteria are commonly used to define DM/PM:
- skin lesions
- heliotrope rash (red–purple edematous erythema on the upper palpebra)
- Gottron's papules or sign (red–purple flat-topped papules, atrophy, or erythema on the extensor surfaces and finger joints)
- proximal muscle weakness (upper or lower extremity and trunk)
- elevated serum creatine kinase or aldolase level
- muscle pain on grasping or spontaneous pain
- myogenic changes on EMG (short-duration, polyphasic motor unit potentials with spontaneous fibrillation potentials)

- positive anti-Jo-1 (histadyl tRNA synthetase) antibody
- nondestructive arthritis or arthralgias
- systemic inflammatory signs (fever >37°C at axilla, elevated serum CRP level or accelerated ESR of >20 mm/h by the Westergren method)
- pathologic findings compatible with inflammatory myositis.

Patients with the first criterion and four of the remaining criteria have DM. Patients lacking the first criterion but with at least four of the remaining criteria have PM. Some patients with DM have little evidence of myopathy, and drug eruptions may mimic the characteristic rash. In particular, hydroxyurea has been associated with a DM-like eruption.

Associated diseases

DM may overlap with other connective tissue diseases. Sclerodermatous changes are the most frequently observed. This is called sclerodermatomyositis. Antibodies such as anti-Ku and anti-PM/scl may be present in this subgroup. Mixed connective tissue disease (associated with high anti-ribonucleoprotein [RNP]), rheumatoid arthritis, LE, and Sjögren syndrome may occur concomitantly. DM may be associated with interstitial lung disease, which is frequently the cause of death. The presence of anti-Jo-1 antibody, as well as other antisynthetase antibodies, such as anti-PL-7, anti-PL-12, anti-DJ, and anti-EJ, correlates well with the development of pulmonary disease. Even those patients without anti-Jo-1 should routinely be screened for interstitial lung disease, as up to 69% of patients with interstitial lung disease are seronegative for the anti-Jo-1 antibody in published reports.

Neoplasia with dermatomyositis

In adults, malignancy is frequently associated with DM. The malignancy is discovered before, simultaneously, or after the DM in almost equal proportions. The highest probability of finding an associated tumor occurs within 2 years of the diagnosis. Factors associated with malignancy include age, constitutional symptoms, rapid onset of DM, the lack of Raynaud phenomenon, and a grossly elevated ESR or creatine kinase level. Malignancy is most frequently seen in patients in the fifth and sixth decades of life. Routine "age-appropriate screening" may be inadequate to uncover a significant number of malignancies. In addition to history and physical examination, a stool hemoccult test, mammography, pelvic examination, chest x-ray, and computed tomographic (CT) scans of the abdominal, pelvic, and thoracic areas may be indicated. Periodic rescreening may be of value, but the appropriate interval for screening has not been established. The presence of leukocytoclastic vasculitis might indicate a higher potential for malignancy.

Childhood dermatomyositis

Several features of childhood dermatomyositis differ from the adult form. Two childhood variants exist. The more common Brunsting type has a slow course, progressive weakness, calcinosis, and steroid responsiveness (Fig. 8-20). Calcinosis may involve intermuscular fascial planes or be subcutaneous. The second type, the Banker type, is characterized by a vasculitis of the muscles and gastrointestinal tract, rapid onset of severe weakness, steroid unresponsiveness, and a high death rate. Internal malignancy is seldom seen in children with either type, but insulin resistance may be present. Calcinosis cutis is more common in children with severe disease.

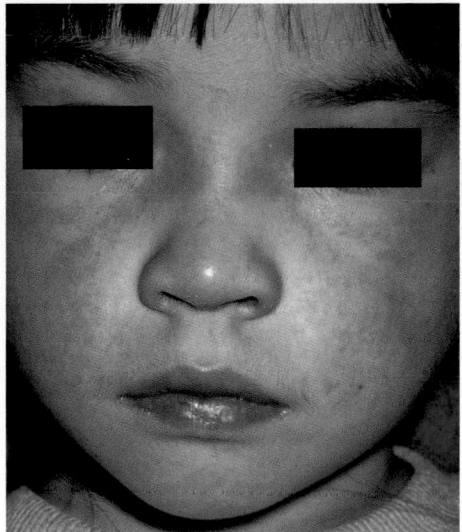

Fig. 8-20 Childhood DM.

Etiology

There is mounting evidence that muscle findings in DM are related to humoral immunity, a vasculopathy mediated by complement deposition, lysis of endomysial capillaries, and resulting muscle ischemia. In contrast, PM and inclusion-body myositis are related to clonally expanded CD8+ cytotoxic T cells invading muscle fibers and causing necrosis via the perforin pathway. The initial immune response in DM is an IFN-α/β-induced cascade with secondary stimulation of IFN-γ. Many autoantibodies may be present in DM, some of which are disease-specific and can identify specific subgroups. In addition to the antisynthetase antibodies previously discussed, the anti-Mi-2 antibody is present in some patients with acute onset of classic DM and a good prognosis. An association with bovine collagen dermal implants has been reported but may reflect a referral bias, rather than a true statistical association.

Both healthy individuals and children with juvenile DM may demonstrate persistence of maternal microchimerism, but the incidence is higher in children with juvenile DM. This has also been demonstrated in patients with other connective tissue diseases such as scleroderma. The finding may be an epiphenomenon, or may be part of a pathogenic alloimmune response. An inherited predisposition has been demonstrated, and studies of juvenile DM gene expression have shown DQA1*0501 in 85% of patients.

Viral or bacterial infections may produce an abnormal immune response. Fulminant disease may be related to an endotheliotropic viral infection. Epitopes of group A β-hemolytic streptococcal M protein have sequence homology with myosin, and can elicit both cell-mediated cytotoxicity and TNF-α production when incubated with mononuclear cells from children with active juvenile DM. The TNF-α-308A allele is associated with increased TNF-α synthesis in juvenile DM patients, and with increased thrombospondin-1 (an antiangiogenic agent) and small vessel occlusion. In adults with PM and DM, endothelial damage occurs early. Pathogenic factors in adults include IL-1α, transforming growth factor (TGF)-β, and myoblast production of IL-15. Cases associated with terbinafine may be related to apoptosis induced by the drug.

Incidence

DM is relatively rare. It is twice as prevalent in women as in men and four times as common in black as in white patients.

There is a bimodal peak, the smaller one seen in children and the larger peak in adults between the ages of 40 and 65.

Histopathology

The histologic changes in DM are similar to those of LE. The two may be indistinguishable, although lesions of DM have more of a tendency to become atrophic. Lesions typically demonstrate thinning of the epidermis, hydropic degeneration of the basal layer, basement membrane thickening, papillary dermal edema, and a perivascular and periadnexal lymphocytic infiltrate in the superficial and deep dermis with increased dermal mucin. Scattered melanophages are present in the superficial dermis. As compared with LE, DM shows less eccrine coil involvement and fewer vertical columns of lymphocytes in fibrous tract remnants. Subcutaneous lymphoid nodules and panniculitis are rarely seen in DM. Characteristic changes are found in the muscles. The deltoid, trapezius, and quadriceps muscles seem to be almost always involved, and are good biopsy sites. Muscle bundles demonstrate lymphoid inflammation and atrophy, which preferentially affects the periphery of the muscle bundle. Muscle biopsy is directed to those areas found to be most tender or in which EMG demonstrates myopathy. MRI is a useful aid in identifying active sites for muscle biopsy, and may obviate the need for biopsy in some cases. The MRI short transition interval recovery (STIR) images are best. They can be used to localize disease and longitudinally assess results of treatment.

Laboratory findings

The serum levels of creatine kinase are elevated in most patients. Aldolase, lactic dehydrogenase, and transaminases are other indicators of active muscle disease. There may be leukocytosis, anemia with low serum iron, and an increased ESR. Positive ANA tests are seen in 60–80% of patients if a human diploid substrate is used; 35–40% have myositis-specific antibodies.

Cutaneous DIF is positive in at least one-third of cases, with a higher yield in well-established (at least 3–6 months old) lesions. Cytoid bodies are commonly seen, although continuous granular staining with IgG, IgM, and IgA may be seen.

X-ray studies with barium swallow may show weak pharyngeal muscles and a collection of barium in the pyriform sinuses and valleculae. MRI of the muscles is an excellent way to assess activity of disease noninvasively.

EMG studies for diagnosis show spontaneous fibrillation, polyphasic potential with voluntary contraction, short duration potential with decreased amplitude, and salvos of muscle stimulation.

Differential diagnosis

DM must be differentiated from erysipelas, SLE, angioedema, drug eruptions, trichinosis, and erythema multiforme. Aldosteronism, with adenoma of adrenal glands and hypokalemia, may also cause puffy heliotrope eyelids and face. Hydroxyurea may produce an eruption resembling DM.

Treatment

Prednisone is the mainstay of acute treatment, at doses beginning with 1 mg/kg/day until the severity decreases and muscle enzymes are almost normal. The dosage is reduced with clinical response. The aspartate aminotransferase (AST)/serum glutamic-oxaloacetic transaminase (SGOT) and creatine phosphokinase return to normal levels as remission occurs. Methotrexate and mycophenolate mofetil are commonly used as steroid-sparing agents, and should be started early in the course of treatment to reduce steroid side effects. Some data favor methotrexate as a steroid-sparing agent, but because of the increased risk of interstitial lung disease with methotrexate, some authors avoid this agent in patients with pulmonary disease or anti-Jo-1 antibodies. Azathioprine is less expensive than mycophenolate mofetil, but skin disease may not respond as well. If patients do not respond adequately to the combination of prednisone and methotrexate, mycophenolate mofetil, or azathioprine, a trial of intravenous immunoglobulin (IVIG) (1 g/kg/day for 2 days each month), cyclosporine, or tacrolimus may be beneficial. IVIG has been associated with thromboembolic events, including deep venous thrombosis, pulmonary embolism, myocardial infarction, and stroke, and this risk must be weighed against the benefits of the drug. Anti-TNF-α treatment with infliximab has proved a rapidly effective therapy for some patients with myositis. Etanercept and infliximab have also been used, but some studies have found little improvement or flares of muscle disease. Because anti-TNF therapy has resulted in a shift to a lupus antibody profile in some patients, patients should be monitored carefully. Cyclophosphamide is generally reserved for refractory cases. Leflunomide, an immunomodulatory drug used to treat rheumatoid arthritis, has been effective as adjuvant therapy.

In severe juvenile DM, pulse intravenous methylprednisone (30 mg/kg/day) or high-dose prednisone has been reported as highly effective. Patients who fail to respond within 6 weeks should be started on an alternative agent such as methotrexate. IVIG has been reported as effective, but products with a high level of immunoglobulin A are less well tolerated. A retrospective study of 38 patients treated at a tertiary care children's hospital suggested that corticosteroids may not be necessary in many children treated with IVIG or methotrexate. Rituximab appears promising in the treatment of refractory disease. Onset of calcinosis is associated with delays in diagnosis and treatment, as well as longer disease duration. Calcinosis related to DM has been treated with aluminum hydroxide, diphosphonates, diltiazem, probenecid, colchicine, low doses of warfarin, and surgery with variable, but usually poor, results. Autologous stem cell transplantation has been reported as successful.

The skin lesions may respond to systemic therapy; however, response is unpredictable and skin disease may persist despite involution of the myositis. Because DM is photosensitive, sunscreens with high SPF (>30) should be used daily, and patients should be counseled about sun avoidance. Topical steroids may be helpful in some patients. Antimalarials, such as hydroxychloroquine given in doses of 200–400 mg/day (2–5 mg/kg/day in children), have been shown to be useful in abating the eruption of DM; however, adverse cutaneous reactions are common. Non-life-threatening cutaneous reactions occur in approximately one-third of patients, and up to one-half of those who react to hydroxychloroquine will also react to chloroquine.

Prognosis

Major causes of death are cancer, ischemic heart disease, and lung disease. Independent risk factors include failure to induce clinical remission, white blood cell count above 10 000/mm^3, temperature greater than 38°C at diagnosis, older age, shorter disease history, and dysphagia. Early aggressive therapy in juvenile cases is associated with a lower incidence of disabling calcinosis cutis.

András C, et al: Dermatomyositis and polymyositis associated with malignancy: a 21-year retrospective study. J Rheumatol 2008 Mar; 35(3):438–444.

Boswell JS, et al: Leflunomide as adjuvant treatment of dermatomyositis. J Am Acad Dermatol 2008 Mar; 58(3):403–406.

Callen JP: Cutaneous manifestations of dermatomyositis and their management. Curr Rheumatol Rep 2010 Jun; 12(3):192–197.

Choy E, et al: Immunosuppressant and immunomodulatory treatment for dermatomyositis and polymyositis. Cochrane Database Syst Rev 2005; 3:CD003643.

Chung L, et al: A pilot trial of rituximab in the treatment of patients with dermatomyositis. Arch Dermatol 2007 Jun; 143(6):763–767.

Cooper MA, et al: Rituximab for the treatment of juvenile dermatomyositis: a report of four pediatric patients. Arthritis Rheum 2007 Sep; 56(9):3107–3111.

Dastmalchi M, et al: A high incidence of disease flares in an open pilot study of infliximab in patients with refractory inflammatory myopathies. Ann Rheum Dis 2008 Feb 13 (Epub ahead of print).

Fisler RE, et al: Aggressive management of juvenile dermatomyositis results in improved outcome and decreased incidence of calcinosis. J Am Acad Dermatol 2002; 47:505.

Franks AG Jr: Skin manifestations of internal disease. Med Clin North Am 2009 Nov; 93(6):1265–1282.

Hengstman GJ, et al: Open-label trial of anti-TNF-alpha in dermato- and polymyositis treated concomitantly with methotrexate. Eur Neurol 2008; 59(3–4):159–163.

Holzer U, et al: Successful autologous stem cell transplantation in two patients with juvenile dermatomyositis. Scand J Rheumatol 2010; 39(1):88–92.

Krathen MS, et al: Dermatomyositis. Curr Dir Autoimmun 2008; 10:313–332.

Lee KH, et al: Acute dermatomyositis associated with generalized subcutaneous edema. Rheumatol Int 2008 Jun; 28(8):797–800.

Levy DM, et al: Favorable outcome of juvenile dermatomyositis treated without systemic corticosteroids. J Pediatr 2010 Feb; 156(2):302–307.

Lobo IM, et al: Calcinosis cutis: a rare feature of adult dermatomyositis. Dermatol Online J 2008 Jan 15; 14(1):10.

Lyons R, et al: Effective use of autoantibody tests in the diagnosis of systemic autoimmune disease. Ann NY Acad Sci 2005; 1050:217.

Magro CM, et al: Terbinafine-induced dermatomyositis: a case report and literature review of drug-induced dermatomyositis. J Cutan Pathol 2008 Jan; 35(1):74–81.

Magro CM, et al: Fulminant and accelerated presentation of dermatomyositis in two previously healthy young adult males: a potential role for endotheliotropic viral infection. J Cutan Pathol 2009; 36:853–858.

Manlhiot C, et al: Safety of intravenous immunoglobulin in the treatment of juvenile dermatomyositis: adverse reactions are associated with immunoglobulin A content. Pediatrics 2008 Mar; 121(3):e626–630.

Mendese G, et al: Histopathology of Gottron's papules: utility in diagnosing dermatomyositis. J Cutan Pathol 2007 Oct; 34(10):793–796.

Pelle MT, et al: Adverse cutaneous reactions to hydroxychloroquine are more common in patients with dermatomyositis than in patients with cutaneous lupus erythematosus. Arch Dermatol 2002; 138:1231.

Polat M, et al: Dermatomyositis with a pityriasis rubra pilaris-like eruption: an uncommon cutaneous manifestation in dermatomyositis. Pediatr Dermatol 2007 Mar–Apr; 24(2):151–154.

Reed AM: Microchimerism in children with rheumatic disorders: what does it mean? Curr Rheumatol Rep 2003; 5:458.

Riley P, et al: Effectiveness of infliximab in the treatment of refractory juvenile dermatomyositis with calcinosis. Rheumatology (Oxford) 2008 Jun; 47(6):877–880.

Rouster-Stevens KA, et al: Pharmacokinetic study of oral prednisolone compared with intravenous methylprednisolone in patients with juvenile dermatomyositis. Arthritis Rheum 2008 Feb 15; 59(2):222–226.

Saito E, et al: Efficacy of high-dose intravenous immunoglobulin therapy in Japanese patients with steroid-resistant polymyositis and dermatomyositis. Mod Rheumatol 2008; 18(1):34–44.

Schmidt E, et al: Rituximab in treatment-resistant autoimmune blistering skin disorders. Clin Rev Allergy Immunol 2008 Feb; 34(1):56–64.

Sparsa A, et al: Routine vs extensive malignancy search for adult dermatomyositis and polymyositis: a study of 40 patients. Arch Dermatol 2002; 138:885.

Wedderburn LR, et al: Juvenile dermatomyositis: new developments in pathogenesis, assessment and treatment. Best Pract Res Clin Rheumatol 2009 Oct; 23(5):665–678.

Scleroderma

Scleroderma is characterized by the appearance of circumscribed or diffuse, hard, smooth, ivory-colored areas that are immobile and give the appearance of hidebound skin. It occurs in both localized and systemic forms. Cutaneous types may be categorized as morphea (localized, generalized, profunda, atrophic, and pansclerotic types) or linear scleroderma (with or without melorheostosis or hemiatrophy). Progressive systemic sclerosis and the Thibierge–Weissenbach syndrome (commonly referred to as the CREST syndrome) are the two types of systemic scleroderma.

Cutaneous types

Localized morphea

This form of scleroderma is twice as common in women as in men and occurs in childhood as well as in adult life. It presents most often as macules or plaques a few centimeters in diameter, but also may occur as bands or in guttate lesions or nodules. Rose or violaceous macules may appear first, followed by smooth, hard, somewhat depressed, yellowish-white or ivory lesions. They are most common on the trunk but also occur on the extremities.

The margins of the areas are generally surrounded by a light violaceous zone or by telangiectases. Within the patch skin elasticity is lost, and when it is picked up between the thumb and index finger it feels rigid. The follicular orifices may be unusually prominent, leading to a condition that resembles pigskin. In guttate morphea multiple small, chalk-white, flat or slightly depressed macules occur over the chest, neck, shoulders, or upper back. The lesions are not very firm and may be difficult to separate clinically from guttate lichen sclerosus et atrophicus.

Morphea–lichen sclerosus et atrophicus overlap

There are patients who present with lesions of both morphea and lichen sclerosus et atrophicus (LSA). They are commonly women with widespread morphea who have typical LSA lesions either separated from morphea or overlying morphea. When the changes are seen above dermal changes of morphea, the characteristic inflammatory lymphoid band of LSA is lacking, suggesting that the superficial homogenization is really a manifestation of morphea rather than representing a separate disease process.

Generalized morphea

Widespread involvement by indurated plaques with pigmentary change characterizes this variety. Muscle atrophy may be present, but there is no visceral involvement (Fig. 8-21). Patients may lose their wrinkles as a result of the firmness and contraction of skin. Spontaneous involution is less common with generalized morphea than with localized lesions.

Atrophoderma of Pasini and Pierini

In 1923, Pasini described a peculiar form of atrophoderma now thought to be in the spectrum of morphea. The disease consists of brownish-gray, oval, round or irregular, smooth atrophic lesions depressed below the level of the skin with a well-demarcated, sharply sloping border. Some of the appearance of depression is an optical illusion related to the color change. Atrophoderma occurs mainly on the trunk of young individuals, predominately females (Fig. 8-22). The lesions are usually

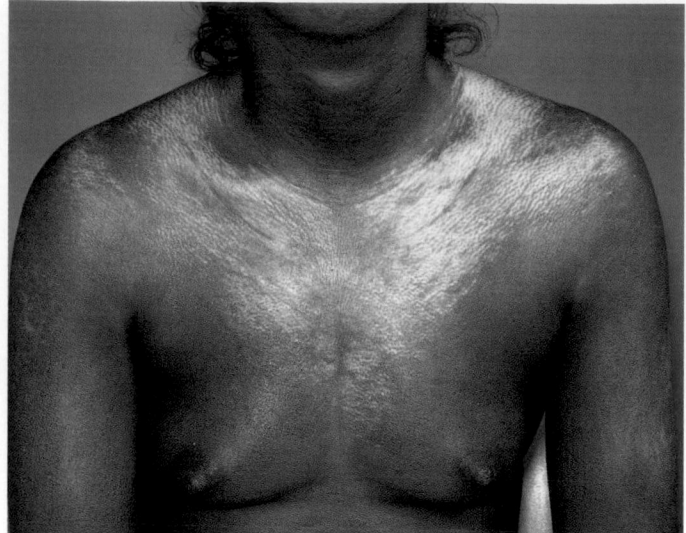

Fig. 8-21 Generalized morphea.

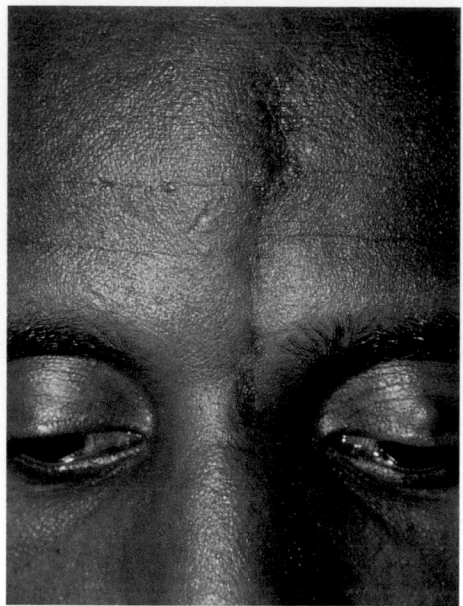

Fig. 8-23 En coup de sabre.

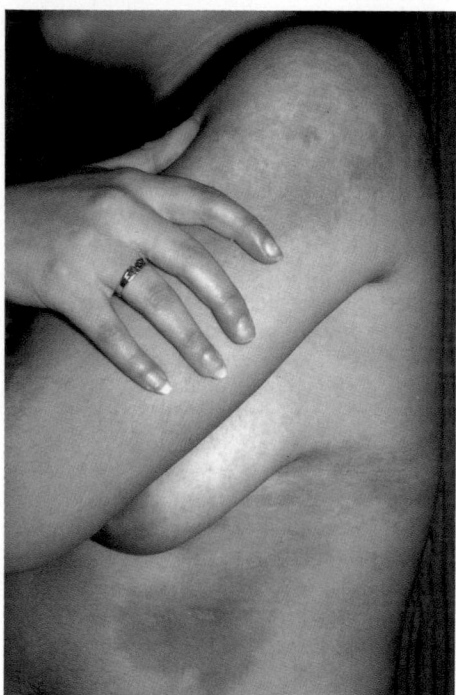

Fig. 8-22 Atrophoderma of Pasini and Pierini.

asymptomatic, and may measure 20 cm or more in diameter. Linear atrophoderma of Moulin is a related condition that follows lines of Blaschko.

Biopsies of atrophoderma demonstrate a reduction in the thickness of the dermal connective tissue. Some widening and hyalinization of collagen bundles may be noted. Because the changes may be subtle, a biopsy should include normal-appearing skin so that a comparison may be made.

Pansclerotic morphea

This variant is manifested by sclerosis of the dermis, panniculus, fascia, muscle, and at times, bone. There is disabling limitation of motion of joints.

Morphea profunda

Morphea profunda involves deep subcutaneous tissue, including fascia. There is clinical overlap with eosinophilic fasciitis,

eosinophilia myalgia syndrome, and the Spanish toxic oil syndrome. The latter two conditions were related to contaminants found in batches of tryptophan or cooking oil. Unlike eosinophilic fasciitis, morphea profunda shows little response to corticosteroids and tends to run a more chronic debilitating course.

Linear scleroderma

These linear lesions may extend the length of the arm or leg, and may follow lines of Blaschko. The condition often begins during the first decade of life. Lesions may also occur parasagittally on the frontal scalp and extend part way down the forehead (en coup de sabre) (Fig. 8-23). The Parry–Romberg syndrome, which manifests as progressive hemifacial atrophy, epilepsy, exophthalmos, and alopecia, may be a form of linear scleroderma. When the lower extremity is involved, there may be associated spina bifida, faulty limb development, hemiatrophy, or flexion contractures. Melorheostosis, seen in roentgenograms as a dense linear cortical hyperostosis, may occur. At times linear lesions of the trunk merge into more generalized involvement. Generally, the only type that shows spontaneous improvement is the childhood type involving the extremities. Physical therapy of the involved limb is of paramount importance to prevent contractures and frozen joints.

Systemic types

CREST syndrome

This variant of systemic scleroderma has the most favorable prognosis, owing to the usually limited systemic involvement. Patients with the syndrome develop calcinosis cutis (Fig. 8-24), Raynaud phenomenon, esophageal dysmotility, sclerodactyly, and telangiectasia. Patients may present with sclerodactyly, severe heartburn, or telangiectatic mats. The mats tend to have a smooth outline, in contrast to the mats of the Osler–Weber–Rendu syndrome, which tend to exhibit an irregular outline with more radiating vessels. This form of scleroderma generally lacks serious renal or pulmonary involvement. Anticentromere antibodies are highly specific for the CREST syndrome, being positive in 50–90% of cases and only 2–10% of patients with progressive sclerosis.

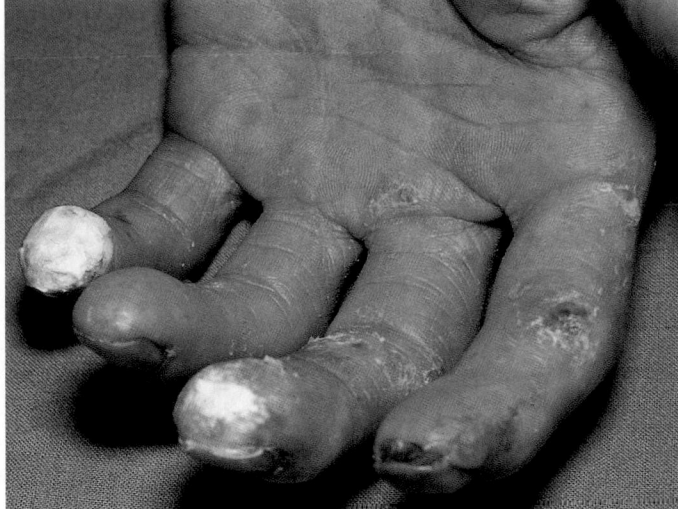

Fig. 8-24 Calcinosis in CREST syndrome.

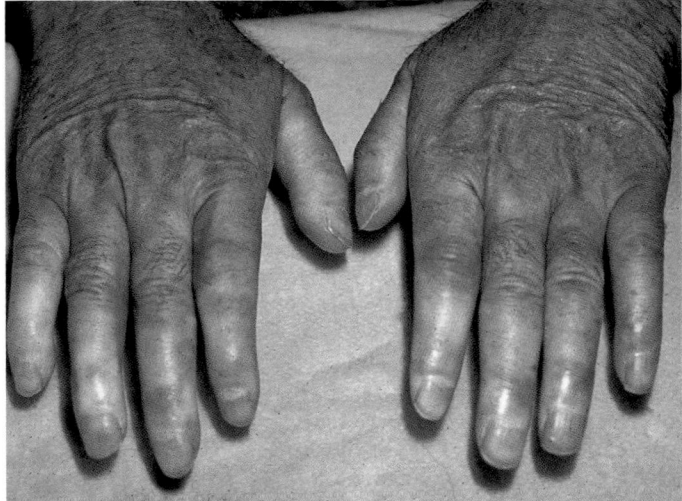

Fig. 8-25 Sclerodactyly.

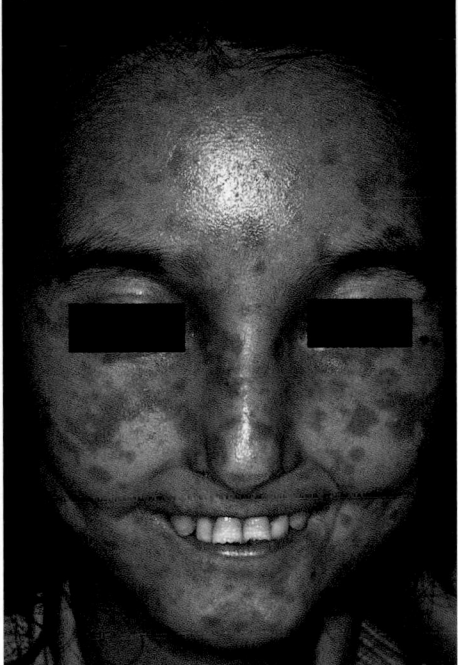

Fig. 8-26 Facial involvement in scleroderma.

Progressive systemic sclerosis

Progressive systemic sclerosis (PSS) is a generalized disorder of connective tissue in which there is thickening of dermal collagen bundles, and fibrosis and vascular abnormalities in internal organs. Raynaud phenomenon is the first manifestation of PSS in more than half the cases. Other patients present with "woody edema" of the hands. The heart, lungs, gastrointestinal tract, kidney, and other organs are frequently involved. Women are affected three times more commonly than men, with the peak age of onset being between the third and fifth decades.

Classic criteria include either proximal sclerosis or two or all of the following:

1. sclerodactyly (Fig. 8-25)
2. digital pitting scars of the fingertips or loss of substance of the distal finger pad
3. bilateral basilar pulmonary fibrosis.

Localized forms of scleroderma must be excluded. These criteria have been shown to be 97% sensitive and 98% specific for the diagnosis. The ACR has proposed an expanded list of criteria, including:

1. *Skin changes*: tightness, thickening, and nonpitting induration, sclerodactyly, proximal scleroderma; changes proximal to the metacarpophalangeal or metatarsophalangeal joints, and affecting other parts of the extremities, face, neck, or trunk (thorax or abdomen), digital pitting, loss of substance from the finger pad, bilateral firm but pitting finger or hand edema, abnormal skin pigmentation (often "pepper and salt"). The changes are usually bilateral and symmetrical, and almost always include sclerodactyly.
2. *Raynaud phenomenon*: at least two-phase color change in fingers and often toes consisting of pallor, cyanosis, and reactive hyperemia.
3. *Visceral manifestations*: bibasilar pulmonary fibrosis not attributable to primary lung disease, lower (distal) esophageal dysphagia, lower (distal) esophageal dysmotility, colonic sacculations.

Skin findings

In the earlier phases of scleroderma the affected areas are erythematous and swollen. Patients are frequently misdiagnosed as having carpal tunnel syndrome and may even have positive EMGs. Raynaud phenomenon is often present, and suggests the correct diagnosis. Over time, sclerosis supervenes. The skin becomes smooth, yellowish, and firm, and shrinks so that the underlying structures are bound down. The earliest changes often occur insidiously on the face and hands, and in more advanced stages these parts become hidebound, so that the face is expressionless, the mouth is constricted (Fig. 8-26), and the hands are clawlike. The skin of the face appears drawn, stretched, and taut, with loss of lines of expression. The lips are thin, contracted, and radially furrowed, the nose appears sharp and pinched, and the chin may be puckered. Barnett described the "neck sign" as a ridging and tightening of the neck on extension, which occurs in 90% of patients with scleroderma.

The disease may remain localized to the hands and feet for long periods (acrosclerosis). The fingers become semiflexed, immobile, and useless, the skin over them being hard, inelastic, incompressible, and pallid. The terminal phalanges are boardlike and indurated. Mizutani described the "round finger-pad sign." The fingers lose the normal peaked contour, but rather appear as a rounded hemisphere when viewed from the side. This process may lead to loss of pulp on the distal digit. Trophic ulcerations and gangrene may occur on the tips of the fingers and knuckles, which may be painful or insensitive. Pterygium inversum unguis, in which the distal part of the nailbed remains adherent to the ventral surface of the nail plate, may be seen in scleroderma and LE, or may be idiopathic. Dilated nailfold capillary loops are present in 75% of systemic scleroderma patients. Symmetrically dilated capillaries are seen adjacent to avascular areas. This differs from the nailfold capillaries of the Osler–Weber–Rendu syndrome, which typically have dilatation of only one-half of the loop and no avascular areas. Nailfold capillary hemorrhage in two or more fingers is highly specific for scleroderma and correlates with the anticentromere antibody.

Keloid-like nodules may develop on the extremities or the chest, and there may be a widespread diffuse calcification of the skin, as shown by radiographs. A diffuse involvement of the chest may lead to a cuirasse-like restraint of respiration. Late in the course of the disorder, hyperpigmented or depigmented spots or a diffuse bronzing may be present. The most characteristic pigmentary change is a loss of pigment in a large patch with perifollicular pigment retention within it. Perifollicular pigmentation may appear in response to UV light exposure. Pigment may also be retained over superficial blood vessels. The affected areas become hairless, and atrophy is often associated with telangiectasia. Bullae and ulcerations may develop, especially on the distal parts of the extremities.

Internal involvement

PSS may involve most of the internal organs. Esophageal involvement is seen in more than 90% of patients. The distal two-thirds are affected, leading to dysphagia and reflux esophagitis. Small intestinal atonia may lead to constipation, malabsorption, or diarrhea. Pulmonary fibrosis with arterial hypoxia, dyspnea, and productive cough may be present. Progressive nonspecific interstitial fibrosis, with bronchiectasis and cyst formation, is the most frequent pathologic change. Pulmonary hypertension and right-sided heart failure are ominous signs, occurring in 5–10% of patients. The cardiac involvement produces dyspnea and other symptoms of congestive heart failure. Sclerosis of the myocardium also produces conduction changes and may result in arrhythmia. Pericarditis, hypertension, and retinopathy may be present.

The skeletal manifestations include articular pain, swelling, and inflammation. Polyarthritis may be the first symptom in systemic sclerosis. There is limitation of motion, as a result of skin tautness, followed by ankylosis and severe contractual deformities. The hand joints are involved most frequently. There may be resorption and shortening of the phalanges, and narrowing of the joint spaces. Osteoporosis and sclerosis of the bones of the hands and feet may occur, as well as decalcification of the vault of the skull.

Childhood PSS has identical cutaneous manifestations. Raynaud phenomenon is less frequent, while cardiac wall involvement is more common and is responsible for half the deaths. Renal disease is unusual. Familial scleroderma rarely occurs.

Prognosis

The course of PSS is variable. Renal disease accounts for some early mortality, but pulmonary disease remains the major cause of death. The patient's age at disease onset is a significant risk factor for pulmonary arterial hypertension. Cardiac disease also correlates with a poor prognosis, while gastrointestinal involvement contributes mainly to morbidity. ANA patterns predict different subsets of disease with varying prognosis. Anticentromere antibodies correlate with CREST syndrome and a good prognosis, while Scl-70 and ANA correlate with a poorer prognosis. Malignancy may be associated with systemic sclerosis in up to 10% of patients, with lung and breast cancer as the most frequent associated malignancies. The presence of many telangiectases is strongly associated with the presence of pulmonary vascular disease.

Laboratory findings

ANA testing is positive in more than 90% of patients with systemic scleroderma. As noted above, several of these antibodies identify specific clinical subsets of patients. The antinucleolar pattern is considered most specific for scleroderma, and when present as the only pattern, it is highly specific for scleroderma. When antibodies to such nucleolar antigens as RNA polymerase t and fibrillarin are present, diffuse sclerosis, generalized telangiectasia, and internal organ involvement are often seen. The homogeneous ANA pattern is seen in those patients with PM–Scl antibodies, the marker for PM-scleroderma overlap. The true speckled or anticentromere pattern is sensitive and specific for the CREST variant. Patients with antibodies to Scl-70 tend to have diffuse truncal involvement, pulmonary fibrosis, and digital pitted scars, but a lower incidence of renal disease. Antibodies to nuclear RNP are found in patients with Raynaud phenomenon, polyarthralgia, arthritis, and swollen hands. Very high RNP titers define mixed connective tissue disease. These patients are fairly homogeneous and the term is not synonymous with connective tissue overlap. Anti-ssDNA antibodies are common in linear scleroderma.

Radiographic findings

The gastrointestinal tract is commonly involved. The esophagus may have decreased peristalsis and dilation. Esophagograms and esophageal manometry may be helpful. In early esophageal involvement, a barium swallow in the usual upright position may be reported as normal. If the patient is supine, however, barium will often be seen to pool in the flaccid esophagus. The stomach may be dilated and atonic, resulting in delayed emptying time. Involvement of the small intestine may cause extreme dilation of the duodenum and jejunum, producing a characteristic roentgenographic picture of persistently dilated intestinal loops long after the barium has passed through. Colonic or small intestinal sacculations may be present.

Histology

Systemic and localized forms of scleroderma show similar histologic changes, although lymphoid infiltrates tend to be heavier in the acute phase of morphea. In the acute phase there is a perivascular lymphocytic infiltrate with plasma cells that is heaviest at the junction of the dermis and subcutaneous fat. Collagen bundles become hyalinized and the space between adjacent bundles is lost. Loss of CD34+ dermal dendritic cells is an early finding.

Dermal sclerosis typically results in a rectangular punch biopsy specimen. As the dermis replaces the subcutaneous tissue, eccrine glands appear to be in the midportion of the thickened dermis. The subcutaneous fat is quantitatively reduced and adventitial fat (the fat that normally surrounds the adnexal structures on the trunk) is lost. Collagen abuts directly on the adnexal structures. Elastic fibers in the reticular dermis may be prominent and stain bright red, and the papillary dermis may appear pale and edematous. In advanced lesions, the inflammatory infiltrate may be minimal. Pilosebaceous units are absent, and eccrine glands and ducts are compressed by surrounding collagen.

On DIF testing of skin the nucleolus may be stained in the keratinocytes if antinucleolar circulating antibodies are present, and a "pepper-dot" epidermal nuclear reaction pattern may be seen in CREST patients who have anticentromere antibodies in their serum.

Differential diagnosis

Myxedema is softer and associated with other signs of hypothyroidism. Diabetic scleredema tends to be erythematous and affects the central back in a pebbly pattern. Scleromyxedema begins with discrete papules, but may assume an appearance very similar to systemic sclerosis. A paraprotein is typically present. Sclerodactyly may be confused with digital changes of Hansen's disease and syringomyelia. Eosinophilic fasciitis is more steroid-responsive. The skin is thickened, edematous, and erythematous, and has a coarse peau d'orange appearance, as opposed to its sclerotic, taut appearance in scleroderma. The hands and face are usually spared in eosinophilic fasciitis, and when the arms are involved, the blood vessels draw inward when the arms are raised, producing a "dry riverbed appearance."

In vitiligo the depigmentation is the sole change in the skin, and sclerosis is absent. Scleroderma in the atrophic stage may closely resemble acrodermatitis chronica atrophicans (ACA), but ACA shows more attenuation of collagen fibers and a diffuse lymphohistiocytic infiltrate. Lyme titers may be positive.

Dermal fibrosis is a major feature of chronic sclerodermoid graft versus host disease, porphyria cutanea tarda, phenylketonuria, carcinoid syndrome, juvenile-onset diabetes, progeria, and the Werner, Huriez, and Crow–Fukase (POEMS) syndromes. Occupational exposure to silica, epoxy resins, polyvinyl chloride, and vibratory stimuli (jackhammer or chain saw) may produce sclerodermoid conditions. Chemicals such as polyvinyl chloride, bleomycin, isoniazid, pentazocine, valproate sodium, epoxy resin vapor, vitamin K (after injection), contaminated Spanish rapeseed oil (toxic oil syndrome), contaminated tryptophan (eosinophilia–myalgia syndrome), nitrofurantoin, and hydantoin may also induce various patterns of fibrosis. The "stiff skin syndrome," also known as congenital fascial dystrophy, is characterized by stony-hard induration of the skin and deeper tissues of the buttocks, thighs, and legs, with joint limitation and limb contractures. The disease begins in infancy. Scleroderma-like symptoms may be the presenting features of multiple myeloma and amyloidosis.

Pathogenesis

The pathogenesis of scleroderma and morphea involves vascular damage, autoimmune mechanisms, and possibly microchimerism resulting in alloimmune graft versus host reactions. Both anticardiolipin and anti-β(2) glycoprotein I antibodies appear to play roles in pathogenesis. The plasma D-dimer concentration correlates with macrovascular complications. *Borrelia afzelii* and *Borrelia garinii* are related to the development of morphea-like lesions in some cases. Other environmental agents may be involved. Epidemiologic studies support the role of organic solvents and certain chemicals. In women, there is an association with teaching and working in the textile industry.

The immune mechanisms involved are complex. Upregulated proteins and mRNAs include monocyte chemoattractant protein-1, pulmonary and activation-regulated chemokine, macrophage inflammatory protein-1, IL-8, platelet-derived growth factor receptor β-subunit (PDGFR-β), and TGF-β (although the latter has not correlated well in some studies).

These factors may stimulate extracellular matrix production, TGF-β production and activation, and chemoattraction of T cells. Various target antigens have been proposed, including a protein termed "protein highly expressed in testis" (PHET), which is ectopically overexpressed in scleroderma dermal fibroblasts. Serum antibodies to a recombinant PHET fragment have been detected in 9 (8.4%) of 107 scleroderma patients, but in none of 50 SLE patients or 77 healthy controls. The presence of anti-PHET antibodies was associated with diffuse cutaneous scleroderma and lung involvement.

Expression of CD40 is increased on fibroblasts in lesional skin, and ligation of CD40 by recombinant human CD154 results in increased production of IL-6, IL-8, and monocyte chemoattractant protein-1 in a dose-dependent manner. These phenomena are not shown in normal fibroblasts with the addition of CD154. Lesion skin of early-stage scleroderma contains T cells preferentially producing high levels of IL-4. CD4+ Th2-like cells can inhibit collagen production by normal fibroblasts and the inhibition is mediated by TNF-α. The inhibition is dominant over the enhancement induced by IL-4 and TGF-β. To be inhibitory, Th2 cells require activation by CD3 ligation. Th2 cells are less potent than T-helper 1 (Th1) cells in inhibiting collagen production by normal fibroblasts, and fibroblasts from involved skin are resistant to inhibition. Etanercept has been shown to decrease serum TGF-β1, tissue hydroxyproline, dermal fibrosis, and the number of α-SMA-positive cells. However, because Th2 cells reduce type I collagen synthesis through the effect of TNF-α, TNF-α blockade by new biologics should be approached with caution. Drug-induced morphea has been related to the cathepsin K inhibitor balicatib used for osteoporosis. Capecitabine, an oral prodrug of 5-fluorouracil used in the treatment of metastatic colon and breast carcinoma, has been associated with a hand-foot syndrome with sclerodactyly. Onset of systemic sclerosis with digital ulcers has been reported during IFN-β therapy for multiple sclerosis.

Treatment

Although effective treatment is available for many of the visceral complications of scleroderma, treatment for the skin disease remains unsatisfactory. Spontaneous improvement may be seen in some children and in some cases of localized scleroderma. Physical therapy emphasizing range of motion for all joints as well as the mouth is important. Exposure to cold is to be avoided, and smoking is forbidden. Among patients with scleroderma, smokers are 3–4 times more likely than never-smokers to incur digital vascular complications.

Vasodilating drugs (calcium-channel blockers, angiotensin II receptor antagonists, topical nitrates, and prostanoids) remain the mainstay of medical therapy for Raynaud phenomenon. Antioxidants, such as vitamin C, have been used, but the data are mixed. Both sildenafil (Viagra) and intravenous or inhaled iloprost are useful in the treatment of both pulmonary hypertension and Raynaud phenomenon. Ginkgo biloba has been shown to have some efficacy in a double-blinded trial. Oral L-arginine has reversed digital necrosis in some patients with Raynaud phenomenon and improved symptoms in others. Calcium-channel blockers, such as nifedipine (Procardia XL), 30–60 mg/day, are commonly used as first-line therapy. Some patients who experience worsening of esophageal reflux with nifedipine do better with diltiazem (Cardizem CD), 120–180 mg/day. Botulinum toxin, topical nitroglycerin, and simple hand warming on a regular basis may also be effective.

Cyclophosphamide has shown some promising results in the treatment of cutaneous disease, improving skin scores, maximal oral opening, flexion index, forced vital capacity (FVC) and carbon monoxide diffusing capacity (DLCO). Results with cyclophosphamide have been superior to those obtained with D-penicillamine. Oral methotrexate or cyclophosphamide has been used with prednisolone in some trials. Oral cyclophosphamide must be given in the morning with vigorous hydration. Many rheumatologists prefer intravenous pulse cyclophosphamide with MESNA and hydration to reduce bladder toxicity. Cyclophosphamide has been used together with antithymocyte globulin and hematopoietic stem cell infusion. Other evolving therapies include agents that target TGF-β1 signaling, tyrosine kinase inhibitors including imatinib, and inhibitors of histone deacetylase.

Phototherapy and photochemotherapy, especially with UVA1, have also shown some efficacy. Methotrexate may have some efficacy for the skin thickening of diffuse scleroderma, although better trials are needed. Widespread morphea has been treated with oral calcitriol, and calcipotriene may have some efficacy as a topical agent. Halofuginone, an inhibitor of collagen type I synthesis, can decrease collagen synthesis in the tight skin mouse and murine graft versus host disease. Application of halofuginone caused a reduction in skin scores in a pilot study with scleroderma patients. CO_2 laser vaporization has produced remission of symptoms in cutaneous calcinosis of CREST syndrome. Some data suggest that minocycline may be effective in the control of calcinosis in systemic sclerosis. Oral type I collagen has been disappointing overall, but may be of some limited benefit for skin findings in late-phase disease.

Although there is strong evidence that the ACE inhibitors are disease-modifying for scleroderma renal crisis, better randomized controlled trials are still needed. Epoprostenol is used to treat pulmonary hypertension in scleroderma, based largely on evidence that it can be life-saving in the treatment of primary pulmonary hypertension. Other promising drugs for visceral involvement include bosentan (for pulmonary hypertension and ischemic ulcers), cyclophosphamide (for alveolitis), IFN-γ (for interstitial pulmonary fibrosis), intravenous prostaglandins (for vascular disease), and sildenafil (for pulmonary hypertension and Raynaud phenomenon).

The future lies with early aggressive intervention before the development of fibrosis and organ damage. Bone marrow and nonmyeloablative allogeneic hematopoietic stem cell transplantation has shown dramatic and sustained benefits in some patients. It should be noted that increased renal and pulmonary toxicity, as well as parenchymal fibrosis, has been reported in some patients with scleroderma, and this treatment should still be considered experimental. Objective measures of improvement of skin sclerosis can be obtained by means of durometer measurements and high-resolution ultrasound. The course of microangiopathic changes can be evaluated with serial nailfold videocapillaroscopy.

Arkachaisri T, et al: Development and initial validation of the localized scleroderma skin damage index and physician global assessment of disease damage: a proof-of-concept study. Rheumatology (Oxford) 2010; 49(2):373–381.

Boin F, et al: Scleroderma-like fibrosing disorders. Rheum Dis Clin North Am 2008 Feb; 34(1):199–220.

Brenner M, et al: Phototherapy and photochemotherapy of sclerosing skin diseases. Photodermatol Photoimmunol Photomed 2005; 21:157.

Diab M, et al: Treatment of recalcitrant generalized morphea with infliximab. Arch Dermatol 2010 Jun; 146(6):601–604.

Distler J, et al: Novel treatment approaches to fibrosis in scleroderma. Rheum Dis Clin North Am 2008 Feb; 34(1):145–159; vii.

García de la Peña-Lefebvre P, et al: Long-term experience of bosentan for treating ulcers and healed ulcers in systemic sclerosis patients. Rheumatology (Oxford) 2008 Apr; 47(4):464–466.

Gilliam AC: Scleroderma. Curr Dir Autoimmun 2008; 10:258–279.

Hachulla E, et al: Natural history of ischemic digital ulcers in systemic sclerosis: single-center retrospective longitudinal study. J Rheumatol 2007 Dec; 34(12):2423–2430.

Hasegawa M, et al: The roles of chemokines in leukocyte recruitment and fibrosis in systemic sclerosis. Front Biosci 2008 May 1; 13:3637–3647.

Henness S, et al: Current drug therapy for scleroderma and secondary Raynaud's phenomenon: evidence-based review. Curr Opin Rheumatol 2007 Nov; 19(6):611–618.

Hesselstrand R, et al: High-frequency ultrasound of skin involvement in systemic sclerosis reflects oedema, extension and severity in early disease. Rheumatology (Oxford) 2008 Jan; 47(1):84–87.

Hudson M, et al: Improving the sensitivity of the American College of Rheumatology classification criteria for systemic sclerosis. Clin Exp Rheumatol 2007 Sep–Oct; 25(5):754–757.

Koca SS, et al: Effectiveness of etanercept in bleomycin-induced experimental scleroderma. Rheumatology (Oxford) 2008 Feb; 47(2):172–175.

Kreuter A, et al: Pulsed high-dose corticosteroids combined with low-dose methotrexate in severe localized scleroderma. Arch Dermatol 2005; 141:847.

Marie I, et al: Anticardiolipin and anti-beta2 glycoprotein I antibodies and lupus-like anticoagulant: prevalence and significance in systemic sclerosis. Br J Dermatol 2008 Jan; 158(1):141–144.

Marie I, et al: Plasma D-dimer concentration in patients with systemic sclerosis. Br J Dermatol 2008 Feb; 158(2):392–395. (Epub 2007 Nov 19)

Moore SC, et al: Treatment of complications associated with systemic sclerosis. Am J Health Syst Pharm 2008 Feb 15; 65(4):315–321.

Neumeister MW, et al: Botox therapy for ischemic digits. Plast Reconstr Surg 2009; 124:191.

Nihtyanova SI, et al: Autoantibodies as predictive tools in systemic sclerosis. Nat Rev Rheumatol 2010 Feb; 6(2):112–116.

Pendergrass SA, et al: Understanding systemic sclerosis through gene expression profiling. Curr Opin Rheumatol 2007 Nov; 19(6):561–567.

Peroni A, et al: Drug-induced morphea: report of a case induced by balicatib and review of the literature. J Am Acad Dermatol 2008 Apr 12 (Epub ahead of print).

Pines M, et al: Halofuginone to treat fibrosis in chronic graft-versus-host disease and scleroderma. Biol Blood Marrow Transplant 2003; 9:417.

Poole JL: Musculoskeletal rehabilitation in the person with scleroderma. Curr Opin Rheumatol 2010 Mar; 22(2):205–212.

Postlethwaite AE, et al: A multicenter, randomized, double-blind, placebo-controlled trial of oral type I collagen treatment in patients with diffuse cutaneous systemic sclerosis: I. Oral type I collagen does not improve skin in all patients, but may improve skin in late-phase disease. Arthritis Rheum 2008 May 31; 58(6):1810–1822.

Rembold CM, et al: Oral L-arginine can reverse digital necrosis in Raynaud's phenomenon. Mol Cell Biochem 2003; 244:139.

Reyes CM, et al: Scleroderma-like illness as a presenting feature of multiple myeloma and amyloidosis. J Clin Rheumatol 2008 Jun; 14(3):161–165.

Rombold S, et al: Efficacy of UVA1 phototherapy in 230 patients with various skin diseases. Photodermatol Photoimmunol Photomed 2008 Feb; 24(1):19–23.

Rosenkranz S, et al: Sildenafil improved pulmonary hypertension and peripheral blood flow in a patient with scleroderma-associated lung fibrosis and the Raynaud phenomenon. Ann Intern Med 2003; 139:871.

Shah AA, et al: Telangiectases in scleroderma: a potential clinical marker of pulmonary arterial hypertension. J Rheumatol 2010; 37(1):98–104.

Shiratsuchi M, et al: Long-term follow-up after nonmyeloablative allogeneic hematopoietic stem cell transplantation for systemic sclerosis. Clin Rheumatol 2008 May 16 (Epub ahead of print).

Soria A, et al: The effect of imatinib (Glivec) on scleroderma and normal dermal fibroblasts: a preclinical study. Dermatology 2008; 216(2):109–117.

Steen VD: Autoantibodies in systemic sclerosis. Semin Arthritis Rheum 2005; 35:35.

Steen VD: The many faces of scleroderma. Rheum Dis Clin North Am 2008 Feb; 34(1):1–15.

Sulli A, et al: Scoring the nailfold microvascular changes during the capillaroscopic analysis in systemic sclerosis patients. Ann Rheum Dis 2008 Jun; 67(6):885–887.

Tehlirian CV, et al: High-dose cyclophosphamide without stem cell rescue in scleroderma. Ann Rheum Dis 2008 Jun; 67(6):775–781.

Trindade F, et al: Hand-foot syndrome with sclerodactyly-like changes in a patient treated with capecitabine. Am J Dermatopathol 2008 Apr; 30(2):172–173.

Valentini G, et al: Disease-specific quality indicators, guidelines and outcome measures in scleroderma. Clin Exp Rheumatol 2007 Nov–Dec; 25(6 Suppl 47):159–162.

Varga JA, et al: Fibrosis in systemic sclerosis. Rheum Dis Clin North Am 2008 Feb; 34(1):115–143.

Villela R, et al: Assessment of unmet needs and the lack of generalizability in the design of randomized controlled trials for scleroderma treatment. Arthritis Rheum 2008 May 15; 59(5):706–713.

Walker JG, et al: Update on autoantibodies in systemic sclerosis. Curr Opin Rheumatol 2007 Nov; 19(6):580–591.

Wooten M: Systemic sclerosis and malignancy: a review of the literature. South Med J 2008 Jan; 101(1):59–62. Review.

Zulian F: Systemic sclerosis and localized scleroderma in childhood. Rheum Dis Clin North Am 2008 Feb; 34(1):239–255; ix.

Eosinophilic fasciitis

In 1974, Lawrence Shulman described a disorder that he called diffuse eosinophilic fasciitis. Classically, patients had engaged in strenuous muscular activity for a few days or weeks before the acute onset of weakness, fatigability, and pain and swelling of the extremities. The prodrome was followed by severe induration of the skin and subcutaneous tissues of the forearms and legs. A favorable response to corticosteroids was noted. Since the initial description, environmental exposures have been reported as possible triggers for the syndrome, including L-tryptophan contaminated with 1,1′-ethylidenebis, *Borrelia*, and exposure to trichloroethylene. Alterations in L-tryptophan metabolism have been described with elevated levels of L-kynurenine and quinolinic acid. Some consider this disease to be a variant of scleroderma. Polycythemia vera, metastatic colorectal carcinoma, and multiple myeloma have been associated in a limited number of patients, suggesting that some cases may represent a paraneoplastic phenomenon.

The skin is commonly edematous and erythematous, with a coarse peau d'orange appearance, most noticeable inside the upper arms, thighs, or flanks. The hands and face are usually spared. When the patient holds the arms laterally or vertically, linear depressions occur within the thickened skin. This "groove sign" or "dry riverbed sign" (Fig. 8-27) follows the course of underlying vessels. This contrasts with scleroderma, in which the skin remains smooth and taut. Limitation of flexion and extension of the limbs and contracture may develop, and patients are often unable to stand fully erect. In contrast to scleroderma, Raynaud phenomenon is usually absent. Associated systemic abnormalities have included carpal tunnel syndrome, peripheral neuropathy, seizures, posterior ischemic optic neuropathy, pleuropericardial effusion, pancytopenia, anemia, antibody-mediated hemolytic anemia, thrombocytopenia, Sjögren syndrome, lymphadenopathy, pernicious anemia, and IgA nephropathy. Detected cytokine abnormalities are similar to those in atopic patients, but with a striking elevation of TGF-β1. Considerable evidence supports a Th17-mediated pathway. The ESR is generally increased and hypergammaglobulinemia is common. Increased production of IL-5 and clonal populations of circulating T cells have been reported.

Biopsy shows a patchy lymphohistiocytic and plasma cell infiltrate in the fascia and subfascial muscle with massive thickening of the fascia and deep subcutaneous septae. Peripheral blood eosinophilia of 10–40% is the rule, but eosinophils may or may not be present in the affected fascia. The inflammatory infiltrate is mainly composed of macrophages

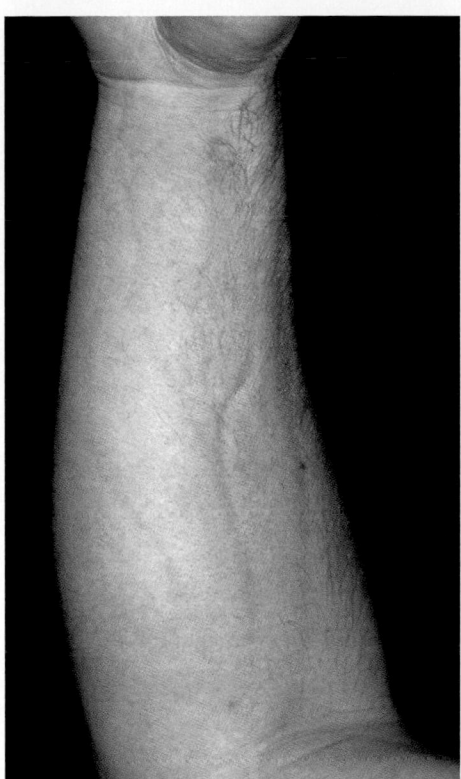

Fig. 8-27 Dry riverbed sign in eosinophilic fasciitis.

and lymphocytes, often with a CD8+ T lymphocyte predominance. Few eosinophils are typically present in tissue, although they may be numerous in some cases. Cytotoxic CD8+ T lymphocytes may be demonstrated by granzyme B staining. Major histocompatibility complex (MHC) class I antigens are upregulated in muscle fibers, but MHC class II antigens are not usually expressed by muscle fibers. C5b9 membrane attack complex (MAC) deposits are generally not detected. CT and MRI have both been used to demonstrate fascial thickening, and may obviate the need for biopsy in some cases.

The response to systemic corticosteroids is generally excellent. In responders, complete recovery is usual within 1–3 years. Some patients have also demonstrated a response to histamine blockers, including hydroxyzine and cimetidine. Patients with a prolonged course unresponsive to systemic steroids are being recognized with increasing frequency. Many of these poorly responsive cases overlap with morphea profunda. In refractory cases, plaquenil, cyclosporine, methotrexate, azathioprine, psoralen + UVA (PUVA), bath PUVA, extracorporeal photochemotherapy, IVIG, rituximab, and other immunosuppressive regimens have been used with variable success. The increased synthesis of IL-5 may be blocked by IFN-α, suggesting a possible role for IFN in the treatment of this disorder. Both infliximab and intravenous cyclophosphamide used with moderate- to high-dose prednisolone have been reported as effective in refractory cases.

Al Hammadi A, et al: Groove sign and eosinophilic fasciitis. J Cutan Med Surg 2008 Jan–Feb; 12(1):49.

Bischoff L, et al: Eosinophilic fasciitis: demographics, disease pattern and response to treatment: report of 12 cases and review of the literature. Int J Dermatol 2008 Jan; 47(1):29–35.

Kato T, et al: Therapeutic efficacy of intravenous cyclophosphamide concomitant with moderate- to high-dose prednisolone in two patients with fasciitis panniculitis syndrome. Mod Rheumatol 2008 Apr; 18(2):193–199.

Khanna D, et al: Infliximab may be effective in the treatment of steroid-resistant eosinophilic fasciitis: report of three cases. Rheumatology (Oxford) 2010 Jun; 49(6):1184–1188.

Philpott H, et al: Eosinophilic fasciitis as a paraneoplastic phenomenon associated with metastatic colorectal carcinoma. Australas J Dermatol 2008 Feb; 49(1):27–29.

Pimenta S, et al: Intravenous immune globulins to treat eosinophilic fasciitis: a case report. Joint Bone Spine 2009 Oct; 76(5):572–574.

Ronneberger M, et al: Can MRI substitute for biopsy in eosinophilic fasciitis? Ann Rheum Dis 2009 Oct; 68(10):1651-1652.

Silny W, et al: Eosinophilic fasciitis: a report of two cases treated with ultraviolet A1 phototherapy. Photodermatol Photoimmunol Photomed 2009 Dec; 25(6):325–327.

Tahara K, et al: Long-term remission by cyclosporine in a patient with eosinophilic fasciitis associated with primary biliary cirrhosis. Clin Rheumatol 2008 Sep; 27(9):1199–1201.

Tzaribachev N, et al: Infliximab effective in steroid-dependent juvenile eosinophilic fasciitis. Rheumatology (Oxford) 2008 Jun; 47(6):930–932.

Distler JH, et al: Tyrosine kinase inhibitors for the treatment of fibrotic diseases such as systemic sclerosis: towards molecular targeted therapies. Ann Rheum Dis 2010 Jan; 69(Suppl 1):i48–51.

Greidinger EL, et al: CD4+ T cells target epitopes residing within the RNA-binding domain of the U1-70-kDa small nuclear ribonucleoprotein autoantigen and have restricted TCR diversity in an HLA-DR4-transgenic murine model of mixed connective tissue disease. J Immunol 2008 Jun 15; 180(12):8444–8454.

Kim P, et al: Treatment of mixed connective tissue disease. Rheum Dis Clin N Am 2005; 31:549.

Lage LV, et al: Proposed disease activity criteria for mixed connective tissue disease. Lupus 2010 Feb; 19(2):223–224.

Lundberg IE: The prognosis of mixed connective tissue disease. Rheum Dis Clin N Am 2005; 31:535.

Perkins K, et al: A Rasch analysis for classification of systemic lupus erythematosus and mixed connective tissue disease. J Appl Meas 2008; 9(2):136–150.

Mixed connective tissue disease

Mixed connective tissue disease (MCTD) has overlapping features of scleroderma, SLE, and DM, and high U1RNP antibodies in the absence of anti-Sm antibodies. Patients often have severe arthralgia, swelling of the hands, tapered fingers, Raynaud phenomenon, abnormal esophageal motility, pulmonary fibrosis, and muscle pain, weakness, and tenderness. Occasionally, mucosal lesions occur, Pulmonary arterial hypertension is the major life-threatening complication. Hyperglobulinemia and lymphadenopathy are present in some cases. MCTD is a distinct disorder with a characteristic serologic marker. The term is not synonymous with "overlap syndrome," a combination of diseases where each disease complies with the diagnostic criteria for that disorder. MCTD is also not synonymous with undifferentiated connective tissue disease (UCTD) — patients with connective tissue disease who have not yet developed a defined disease. Only about 4% of patients with UCTD go on to develop MCTD.

The ANA test typically demonstrates a particulate pattern in MCTD, reflecting the high titers of nuclear RNP antibodies (anti-RNP antibodies). This ANA pattern generally persists through periods of remission and is a valuable diagnostic test. In addition, particulate epidermal nuclear IgG deposition on DIF study of skin is a distinctive finding in MCTD. Anti-TS1-RNA antibodies appear to define a subpopulation with predominance of lupus-like clinical features. Lung disease may be a cause of death in patients with MCTD. The pulmonary disease has many similarities to that seen in DM or scleroderma, but differences in pathogenesis may exist. Pulmonary lavage usually demonstrates a significantly higher CD4:CD8 ratio, with more CD4+ lymphocytes in MCTD patients than in PM–DM patients. MCTD patients have a significantly lower percentage of CD71+ alveolar macrophages as compared with scleroderma patients.

For acute treatment, corticosteroids (like prednisone at a daily dose of 1 mg/kg) are effective for inflammatory features such as arthritis and myositis. Like LE, MCTD may be associated with an independent risk of osteoporosis, and the long-term morbidity associated with corticosteroid treatment can be significant. Bisphosphonate therapy and therapy with a steroid-sparing agent should be considered early. In general, the LE features of MCTD are the most likely to improve with therapy, while the scleroderma features are the least likely to improve. Generally, the prognosis is better than that of scleroderma, largely related to the lower incidence of renal disease. Small-molecule tyrosine kinase inhibitors such as imatinib, dasatinib, and nilotinib target TGF-β and PDGF signaling and are being investigated as therapeutic options.

Aringer M, et al: Mixed connective tissue disease: what is behind the curtain? Best Pract Res Clin Rheumatol 2007 Dec; 21(6):1037–1049.

Nephrogenic systemic fibrosis

Nephrogenic systemic fibrosis (NSF) is a recently recognized fibrosing skin condition that resembles scleromyxedema histologically. It usually develops in patients with renal insufficiency on hemodialysis, although it has been noted in patients with acute renal failure who had never undergone dialysis. Epidemiologic and x-ray emission spectroscopic studies have implicated gadolinium-containing MRI contrast agents and the incidence of disease has decreased since their use has been limited in patients with renal failure. Concurrent infection, increased serum phosphate and calcium concentrations, and acidosis may play important roles in pathogenesis of the disease. Clinical findings include thickened sclerotic or edematous papules and plaques involving the extremities (Fig. 8-28) and trunk. Yellow scleral plaques and scleral telangiectasia resembling conjunctivitis have been described. Soft tissue calcification is rare, but may be extensive when it occurs. Clinically, the condition differs from scleromyxedema by the lack of involvement of the face, absence of plasma cells, and lack of paraproteinemia. Systemic involvement is generally absent, but may occur with fibrosis and calcification of the diaphragm, psoas muscle, renal tubules, and rete testes.

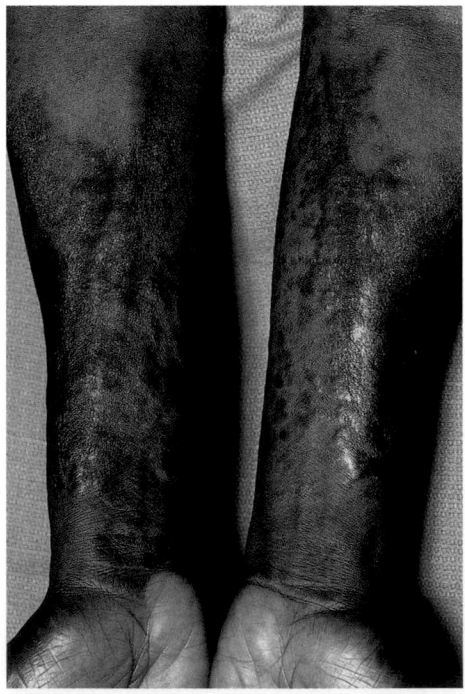

Fig. 8-28 Hyperpigmented sclerotic plaques of nephrogenic fibrosing dermopathy.

Circulating antiphospholipid antibodies have been noted in some patients. Histologic sections demonstrate plump bipolar CD34+ spindle cells with dendrites extending along both sides of elastic fibers (tram track sign), many new collagen bundles, and increased mucin. With time, thickened collagen bundles become prominent in the reticular dermis. Myofibroblasts have been noted in lesional skin. Immunohistochemical staining for CD34 and procollagen I in the spindle cells of NFD suggests that many of the dermal cells of NFD may represent circulating fibrocytes recruited to the dermis. The CD34 positivity in NFD contrasts with the loss of CD34+ cells in morphea.

Effective therapy remains elusive. Topical retinoids, steroids, and vitamin D analogs are not effective. Immunosuppressive therapy appears to be of little benefit. In three cases that have evolved after liver transplantation, treatment with basiliximab, mycophenolate mofetil, calcineurin inhibitor, and prednisone did not stop the development of "woody" skin induration of the distal extremities, erythematous papules, and contractures. The most effective treatment strategy appears to be optimization of renal function through medical therapy or transplantation. Some data support a beneficial effect from phototherapy, extracorporeal photopheresis, or intravenous sodium thiosulfate tyrosine kinase inhibitors, and rapamycin. The proliferating fibrocytes of NSF express phospho-70-S6 kinase, a protein downstream from the mammalian target of rapamycin. All patients should be referred for physical therapy.

Abraham JL, et al: Tissue distribution and kinetics of gadolinium and nephrogenic systemic fibrosis. Eur J Radiol 2008 May; 66(2):200–207.

Chen AY, et al: Nephrogenic systemic fibrosis: a review. J Drugs Dermatol 2010 Jul; 9(7):829–834.

Cowper SE: Nephrogenic systemic fibrosis: an overview. J Am Coll Radiol 2008 Jan; 5(1):23–28.

Golding LP, et al: Nephrogenic systemic fibrosis: possible association with a predisposing infection. AJR Am J Roentgenol 2008 Apr; 190(4):1069–1075.

Kallen AJ, et al: Gadolinium-containing magnetic resonance imaging contrast and nephrogenic systemic fibrosis: a case-control study. Am J Kidney Dis 2008 Jun; 51(6):966–975.

Knopp EA, et al: Nephrogenic systemic fibrosis: early recognition and treatment. Semin Dial 2008 Mar–Apr; 21(2):123–128.

Kucher C, et al: Histopathologic comparison of nephrogenic fibrosing dermopathy and scleromyxedema. J Cutan Pathol 2005; 32:484.

High WA, et al: Gadolinium is quantifiable within the tissue of patients with nephrogenic systemic fibrosis. J Am Acad Dermatol 2007 Apr; 56(4):710–712.

Idée JM, et al: Possible involvement of gadolinium chelates in the pathophysiology of nephrogenic systemic fibrosis: a critical review. Toxicology 2008 Jun 27; 248(2–3):77–88.

Linfert DR, et al: Treatment of nephrogenic systemic fibrosis: limited options but hope for the future. Semin Dial 2008 Mar–Apr; 21(2):155–159.

Marckmann P: Nephrogenic systemic fibrosis: epidemiology update. Curr Opin Nephrol Hypertens 2008 May; 17(3):315–319.

Martin DR, et al: Decreased incidence of NSF in patients on dialysis after changing gadolinium contrast-enhanced MRI protocols. J Magn Reson Imaging 2010 Feb; 31(2):440–446.

Shabana WM, et al: Nephrogenic systemic fibrosis: a report of 29 cases. AJR Am J Roentgenol 2008 Mar; 190(3):736–741.

Swaminathan S, et al: Rapid improvement of nephrogenic systemic fibrosis with rapamycin therapy: possible role of phospho-70-ribosomal-S6 kinase. J Am Acad Dermatol 2010; 62(2):343–345.

Sjögren syndrome (sicca syndrome)

Keratoconjunctivitis sicca and xerostomia (mouth dryness) are commonly associated with rheumatoid arthritis and other connective tissue diseases. Dry eyes and mouth may occur as primary Sjögren syndrome. Most patients are aged 50 or older and more than 90% are women. Sjögren syndrome is a chronic autoimmune disorder characterized by lymphocytic infiltration of the exocrine glands, particularly the salivary and lacrimal glands. One-third of patients present with extraglandular manifestations, such as vasculitis.

Xerostomia may produce difficulty in speech and eating, increased tooth decay, thrush, and decreased taste (hypogeusia). Patients frequently suck on sour candies to stimulate what little salivary secretions remain, and those unfamiliar with the condition may blame the habit of sucking lemon drops for the ensuing tooth decay. Sjögren syndrome alters the composition of saliva, producing a decrease in salivary amylase and carbonic anhydrase, along with an increase in lactoferrin, $\beta(2)$-microglobulin, cystatin C, sodium, and lysozyme C.

Rhinitis sicca (dryness of the nasal mucous membranes) may induce nasal crusting and decreased olfactory acuity (hyposmia). Vaginal dryness and dyspareunia may develop. Dry eyes are painful, feel gritty or scratchy, and produce discharge and blurry vision. Fatigue is a prominent symptom. In addition, there may be laryngitis, gastric achlorhydria, thyroid enlargement resembling Hashimoto thyroiditis, malignant lymphoma, thrombotic thrombocytopenic purpura, painful distal sensory axonal neuropathy, and splenomegaly.

Skin manifestations of Sjögren syndrome include vasculitis, xerosis, pruritus, and annular erythema. Decreased sweating occurs. Asian patients have been described who develop erythematous, indurated, annular dermal plaques primarily on the face. This is different from the annular lesions of SCLE, which show epidermal change and histologic changes of lupus. Patients may also present with an overlap of Sjögren syndrome and LE. A common finding in these patients is Ro/SSA antibody positivity. SCLE patients with Sjögren syndrome have a worse prognosis than patients with SCLE unassociated with Sjögren syndrome.

Patients with Sjögren syndrome and cutaneous vasculitis also have a significant incidence of peripheral, renal, or CNS vasculitis. Cutaneous vasculitis may present as purpura of the legs, which may be palpable or nonpalpable. Sjögren vasculitis accounts for most patients with Waldenström benign hypergammaglobulinemic purpura. Approximately 30% of benign hypergammaglobulinemic purpura patients will have or will develop Sjögren syndrome, and a high percentage have SSA and SSB antibodies. Other cutaneous vascular manifestations are urticarial vasculitis, digital ulcers, and petechiae. Histologically, a leukocytoclastic vasculitis is found at the level of the postcapillary venule with expansion of the vascular wall, fibrin deposition, and karyorrhexis, but no necrosis of the endothelium.

Labial salivary gland biopsy from inside the lower lip is regarded by many as the most definitive test for Sjögren syndrome. Typically, there is a dense lymphocytic infiltrate with many plasma cells and fewer histiocytes in aggregates within minor salivary glands. More than one focus of 50 or more lymphocytes is typically present per 4 mm^2 of the tissue biopsy. Lymphoepithelial islands predominate early, while glandular atrophy predominates in the late stages. At this stage, few lymphoid aggregates are present. Xerostomia is diagnosed by the Schirmer test and reflects diminished glandular secretion from the lacrimal glands. Imaging studies are also helpful.

Classically, the diagnosis is made when there is objective evidence for two of the following three major criteria:

1. xerophthalmia
2. xerostomia
3. an associated autoimmune, rheumatic, or lymphoproliferative disorder.

These criteria may be too restrictive, as patients are increasingly being identified with predominantly extraglandular disease. The lack of sicca symptoms or anti-SSA or SSB antibodies does not exclude Sjögren syndrome. Numerous serologic abnormalities are associated with Sjögren syndrome or its associated conditions. Antibodies to fodrin, a major component of the membrane cytoskeleton of most eukaryotic cells, are present in some populations with primary and secondary Sjögren syndrome. IgA and IgG antibodies against α-fodrin are detected in 88% and 64% respectively in some studies. In other populations, fodrin antibodies are less helpful. Around 80% of patients have anti-Ro/SSA antibodies; half as many have anti-La/SSB antibodies. The rheumatoid factor is commonly positive, and an elevated ESR, serum globulin, and CRP, and high titers of IgG, IgA, and IgM are common. Cryoglobulins may be demonstrated. Dendritic cells are increased in tissue during the early phases of the disease.

The aquaporin family of water channels (proteins freely permeated by water but not protons) appears to be an important target in the pathogenesis of Sjögren syndrome. Both duct and secretory cells are targets for the activation of CD4+ T cells. IL-12 and IFN-γ are upregulated. It appears that Th1 cytokines mediate the functional interactions between antigen-presenting cells and CD4+ T cells in early lesions.

Patients with Sjögren syndrome are predisposed to the development of lymphoreticular malignancies, especially non-Hodgkin B-cell lymphoma. Both malignant and nonmalignant extraglandular lymphoproliferative processes occur. Cases of pseudolymphoma have the potential for regression, or for progression to overt B-cell lymphoma. Patients with palpable purpura, low C4, and mixed monoclonal cryoglobulinemia are at higher risk for lymphoma.

The differential diagnosis of Sjögren syndrome includes sarcoidosis, lymphoma, amyloidosis, and human immunodeficiency virus (HIV) disease. The latter produces diffuse infiltrative lymphocytosis syndrome (DILS), which is characterized by massive parotid enlargement; prominent renal, lung, and gastrointestinal manifestations; and a low frequency of autoantibodies.

Treatment for Sjögren syndrome has largely been symptomatic, but disease-modifying therapy is also becoming a reality. Artificial lubricants are helpful for eye symptoms, as well as oral, nasal, and vaginal dryness. Topical lubricants are useful for xerosis. In hot climates, patients with impaired sweating must be counseled to avoid heat stroke. Pharmacologic agents, such as pilocarpine and cevimeline, are helpful to stimulate salivation. These agents may also have a role in the treatment of dry eyes. Topical cyclosporine A looks promising for local treatment of Sjögren syndrome, as does topical human IFN therapy for oral lesions. In all trials, the mechanical stimulation by the lozenge may play a significant role in the improvement of symptoms. This is reflected in a high placebo response. Acid maltose lozenges are cheaper and remain useful for symptomatic relief. For patients with systemic disease, biologic TNF inhibitors such as infliximab show some promise. Pilocarpine, in doses of 10 mg/day, has been shown to have a beneficial effect on subjective eye symptoms, as well as improvement of rose bengal staining. An increase in tear production, as measured by the Schirmer-I test, was not substantiated. Gene therapy also looks promising, at least in animal models. IL-10 genes can be transferred via adenovirus vectors, and can have disease-modifying effects in the salivary glands of a mouse model. Severe systemic vasculitis causing renal disease has responded to corticosteroids with or without cyclophosphamide. Mycophenolate sodium and rituximab have both been used to treat severe manifestations associated with Sjögren syndrome. Rituximab has proved effective in double-blind, placebo-controlled, randomized studies, and rituximab plus cyclophosphamide, vincristine, and prednisone

have been used to treat Sjögren syndrome-associated B-cell non-Hodgkin lymphoma.

Atkinson JC, et al: Salivary hypofunction and xerostomia: diagnosis and review. Dent Clin North Am 2005; 49:309.

Carbone J, et al: Combined therapy with rituximab plus cyclophosphamide/vincristine/prednisone for Sjögren's syndrome-associated B-cell non-Hodgkin's lymphoma. Clin Rev Allergy Immunol 2008 Feb; 34(1):80–84.

Dass S, et al: Reduction of fatigue in Sjögren's syndrome with rituximab: results of a randomised, double-blind, placebo controlled pilot study. Ann Rheum Dis 2008 Feb 14 (Epub ahead of print).

Fox RI: Sjögren's syndrome. Lancet 2005; 366:321.

Hansen A, et al: Immunopathogenesis of primary Sjögren's syndrome: implications for disease management and therapy. Curr Opin Rheumatol 2005; 17:558.

Jain AK, et al: Effect of topical cyclosporine on tear functions in tear-deficient dry eyes. Ann Ophthalmol 2007 Spring; 39(1):19–25.

Kagami H, et al: Restoring the function of salivary glands. Oral Dis 2008 Jan; 14(1):15–24.

Mavragani CP, et al: Conventional therapy of Sjögren's syndrome. Clin Rev Allergy Immunol 2007 Jun; 32(3):284–291.

Meijer JM, et al: The future of biologic agents in the treatment of Sjögren's syndrome. Clin Rev Allergy Immunol 2007 Jun; 32(3):292–297.

Ng KP, et al: Sjögren's syndrome: diagnosis and therapeutic challenges in the elderly. Drugs Aging 2008; 25(1):19–33.

Ozaki Y, et al: Decrease of blood dendritic cells and increase of tissue-infiltrating dendritic cells are involved in the induction of Sjögren's syndrome but not in the maintenance. Clin Exp Immunol 2010; 159(3):315–326.

Pers JO, et al: B-cell depletion and repopulation in autoimmune diseases. Clin Rev Allergy Immunol 2008 Feb; 34(1):50–55.

Voulgarelis M, et al: Clinical, immunologic, and molecular factors predicting lymphoma development in Sjögren's syndrome patients. Clin Rev Allergy Immunol 2007 Jun; 32(3):265–274.

Willeke P, et al: Mycophenolate sodium treatment in patients with primary Sjögren syndrome: a pilot trial. Arthritis Res Ther 2007; 9(6):R115.

Yilmaz I, et al: Parotid magnetic resonance imaging, sialography, and parotid biopsy for diagnosis of Sjögren's syndrome in a patient with negative serology. J Otolaryngol 2005; 37:199.

Rheumatoid arthritis

The majority of skin manifestations of rheumatoid arthritis (RA) are consequences of neutrophil-mediated injury. There may be annular erythemas, purpura, bullae, shallow ulcers, and gangrene of the extremities. Many diseases have been reported to occur in association with RA, such as erythema elevatum diutinum, pyoderma gangrenosum, Felty syndrome, IgA vasculitis, linear IgA disease, Sjögren syndrome, bullous pemphigoid, and yellow nail syndrome. Treatment of RA with disease-modifying drugs has reduced the burden of destructive disease for patients with this disorder. Biologic agents are being used with increasing frequency, although older drugs like methotrexate still have a role. Methotrexate-treated patients with RA have an increased incidence of melanoma, as well as non-Hodgkin lymphoma, and lung cancer. They should be followed for the development of cutaneous lesions. Of interest to dermatologists, extracts from the *Rhus* family of plants have been shown to have some benefit in limited studies. Ofatumumab, a new anti-CD20 human monoclonal antibody, shows promise in early clinical trials.

Rheumatoid nodules

Subcutaneous nodules (Fig. 8-29) are seen in 20–30% of patients. They may arise anywhere on the body but most frequently are found over the bony prominences, especially on the extensor surface of the forearm just below the elbow and

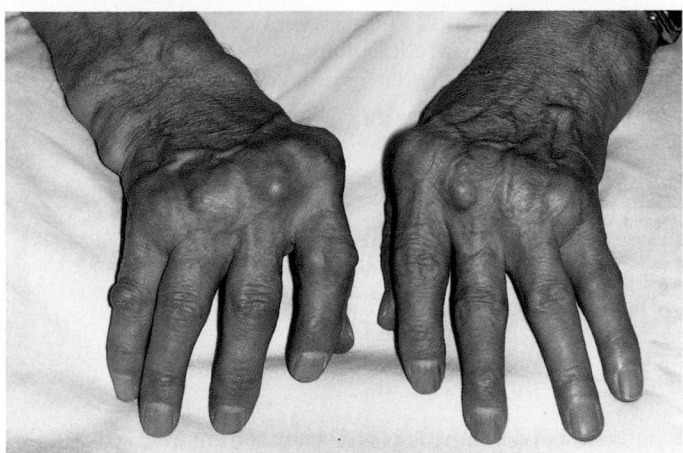

Fig. 8-29 Rheumatoid nodules.

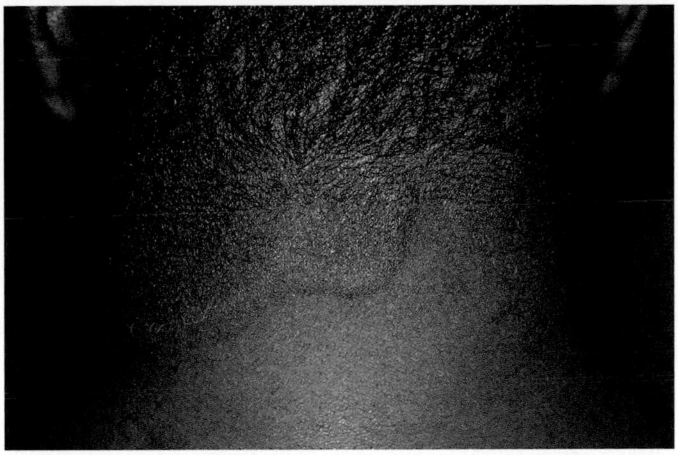

Fig. 8-30 Rheumatoid neutrophilic dermatosis presents with urticarial plaques.

the dorsal hands. The lesions are nontender, firm, skin-colored, round nodules, which may or may not be attached to the underlying tissue. Frequently, they are attached to the fibrous portions of the periarticular capsule, or they may be free in the subcutaneous tissue. Rheumatoid nodules can easily be mistaken for xanthomas because of a yellow color (pseudoxanthomatous variant). They also occur in 5–7% of patients with SLE, especially around small joints of the hands. Rheumatoid factor may or may not be present. Histologic examination of the rheumatoid nodule shows intensely staining foci of fibrin surrounded by histiocytes in palisade arrangement. Neutrophils and neutrophilic debris may be noted in association with the fibrin, and with time, the surrounding histiocytes are replaced by fibrosis.

Rheumatoid nodules are differentiated from Heberden nodes, which are tender, hard, bony exostoses on the dorsolateral aspects of the distal interphalangeal joints of patients with degenerative joint disease. Nodules or tophi of gout are characterized by masses of feathery urate crystals surrounded by a chronic inflammatory infiltrate often containing foreign body giant cells.

Rare patients present with multiple ulcerated nodules and high rheumatoid factors, but no active joint disease. This variant of rheumatoid disease without destructive joint disease is designated rheumatoid nodulosis.

Rheumatoid vasculitis

Peripheral vascular lesions appear as typical features of RA. These are localized purpura, cutaneous ulceration, and gangrene of the distal parts of the extremities. Additionally, papular lesions located primarily on the hands have been described as rheumatoid papules. These show a combination of vasculitis and palisading granuloma formation. A rheumatoid factor is typically present. Peripheral neuropathy is frequently associated with the vasculitis. The presence of rheumatoid nodules may help to distinguish these lesions of vasculitis from SLE, polyarteritis nodosa, Buerger's disease, and the dysproteinemias. Prednisone and cytotoxic agents are commonly used as in other forms of vasculitis. Rituximab has also been used successfully.

Rheumatoid neutrophilic dermatosis

Chronic urticaria-like plaques (Fig. 8-30) characterized histologically by a dense neutrophilic infiltrate have been described in patients with debilitating RA. The differential diagnosis includes erythema elevatum diutinum and Sweet syndrome.

Related palisading granulomas

Interstitial granulomatous dermatitis with arthritis is a condition that most commonly presents with symmetrical round-to-oval erythematous or violaceous plaques on the flanks, axillae, inner thighs, and lower abdomen. Linear, slightly red or skin-colored cords extending from the upper back to the axilla may occur. The presence of these linear bands has been called the rope sign. When the lesions resolve they may leave behind hyperpigmentation and a slightly wrinkled appearance. Arthritis may occur before, concurrently, or after the eruption, and tends to affect multiple joints of the upper extremities. While serologic findings of connective tissue disease are common, most patients do not have a well-defined associated condition. A moderate to dense inflammatory infiltrate is seen through the reticular dermis, composed mostly of histiocytes distributed interstitially around discrete bundles of sclerotic collagen. Variable numbers of neutrophils and/or eosinophils are seen. Mucin, necrobiosis, vasculitis, and vacuolar change are usually absent or mild. The eruption is usually asymptomatic and may spontaneously involute after many months or years. If therapy is required, methotrexate, etanercept, cyclosporine, or a steroid is needed.

Palisaded neutrophilic and granulomatous dermatitis is usually associated with a well-defined connective tissue disease (LE or RA, most commonly). It often presents with eroded or ulcerated symmetrically distributed umbilicated papules or nodules on the elbows, knuckles, and knees. The biopsy may reveal leukocytoclastic vasculitis and collagen degeneration in early lesions, or palisaded granulomatous infiltrates with dermatofibrosis and scant neutrophilic debris in older lesions. Interstitial granulomatous dermatitis has been reported in RA during treatment with etanercept but has also been reported to respond to etanercept.

Methotrexate-induced papular eruption appears in patients with rheumatic diseases during treatment with this medication. They present with erythematous indurated papules, usually located on the proximal extremities. Histopathologic examination reveals an inflammatory infiltrate composed of histiocytes interstitially arranged between collagen bundles of the dermis, intermingled with few neutrophils. At times, small rosettes composed of clusters of histiocytes surrounding a thick central collagen bundle are present in the deep reticular dermis.

Buchbinder R, et al: Incidence of melanoma and other malignancies among rheumatoid arthritis patients treated with methotrexate. Arthritis Rheum 2008 May 30; 59(6):794–799.

Hellmann M, et al: Successful treatment of rheumatoid vasculitis-associated cutaneous ulcers using rituximab in two patients with rheumatoid arthritis. Rheumatology (Oxford) 2008 Jun; 47(6):929–930.

Hu S, et al: Interstitial granulomatous dermatitis in a patient with rheumatoid arthritis on etanercept. Cutis 2008 Apr; 81(4):336–338.

Navarro-Sarabia F, et al: Adalimumab for treating rheumatoid arthritis. Cochrane Database Syst Rev 2005; 3:CD005113.

Robak T: Ofatumumab, a human monoclonal antibody for lymphoid malignancies and autoimmune disorders. Curr Opin Mol Ther 2008 Jun; 10(3):294–309.

Sacre SM, et al: Molecular therapeutic targets in rheumatoid arthritis. Expert Rev Mol Med 2005; 7:1.

Sanchez E, et al: Polymorphisms of toll-like receptor 2 and 4 genes in rheumatoid arthritis and systemic lupus erythematosus. Tissue Antigens 2004; 63:54.

Zoli A, et al: Interstitial granulomatous dermatitis in rheumatoid arthritis responsive to etanercept. Clin Rheumatol 2010 Jan; 29(1):99–101.

Juvenile rheumatoid arthritis (juvenile idiopathic arthritis)

Juvenile RA is not a single disease but a group of disorders characterized by arthritis and young age of onset. The subset called Still's disease accounts for only 20% of the patients. It shows skin manifestations in some 40% of young patients ranging in age from 7 to 25 years. An eruption consisting of evanescent, non-pruritic, salmon-pink, macular, or papular lesions on the trunk and extremities (Fig. 8-31) may precede the onset of joint manifestations by many months. Neutrophilic panniculitis has been described. The systemic symptoms of fever and serositis usually recur over weeks each afternoon. Most remit permanently by adulthood. IL-1β, IL-6, and IL-18 are implicated in the pathogenesis of the disease, as are phagocyte-specific S100-proteins, such as S100A8, S100A9, and S100A12. Steroid-sparing agents are useful to decrease steroid-associated toxicity. The dose–response curve for methotrexate plateaus with parenteral administration of 15 mg/m^2/week. The full therapeutic effect may not be evident for 12 months. Refractory disease has been treated with pulse methylprednisolone and cyclophosphamide. Anakinra has shown modest efficacy.

Adams A, et al: Update on the pathogenesis and treatment of systemic onset juvenile rheumatoid arthritis. Curr Opin Rheumatol 2005; 17:612.

Dyer JA, et al: Neutrophilic panniculitis in infancy: a cutaneous manifestation of juvenile rheumatoid arthritis. J Am Acad Dermatol 2007 Nov; 57(5 Suppl):S65–68.

Lequerré T, et al: Interleukin-1 receptor antagonist (anakinra) treatment in patients with systemic-onset juvenile idiopathic arthritis or adult onset Still disease: preliminary experience in France. Ann Rheum Dis 2008 Mar; 67(3):302–308.

Relapsing polychondritis

Relapsing polychondritis is characterized by intermittent episodes of inflammation of the articular and nonarticular cartilage eventuating in chondrolysis and collapse of the involved cartilage. The course of the disease is chronic and variable, with episodic flares. Both sexes are equally affected, with the usual age at onset being in the fourth to fifth decade. Dissolution of the cartilage involves the ears, nose, and respiratory tract. During bouts of inflammation, the bright red involvement of the ears is confined to the cartilaginous portion while the ear lobes remain conspicuously normal (Fig. 8-32). The affected areas are swollen and tender. There may be conductive deafness as a result of the obstruction produced by the swollen cartilage. The nasal septal cartilage is similarly involved to produce rhinitis, with crusting and bleeding, and, eventually, a saddle-nose deformity. Involvement of the bronchi, larynx, and epiglottis produces hoarseness, coughing, and dyspnea. Migratory arthralgia and atypical chest pain are often present. Patients evaluated for chest pain are often released without treatment and with a diagnosis of costochondritis. Ocular disease most often presents as conjunctivitis, scleritis, or iritis. Perforation of the globe may occur. Complete heart block has been reported as a presenting sign. The MAGIC syndrome is a combination of Behçet's disease and relapsing polychondritis (mouth and genital ulcers with inflamed cartilage).

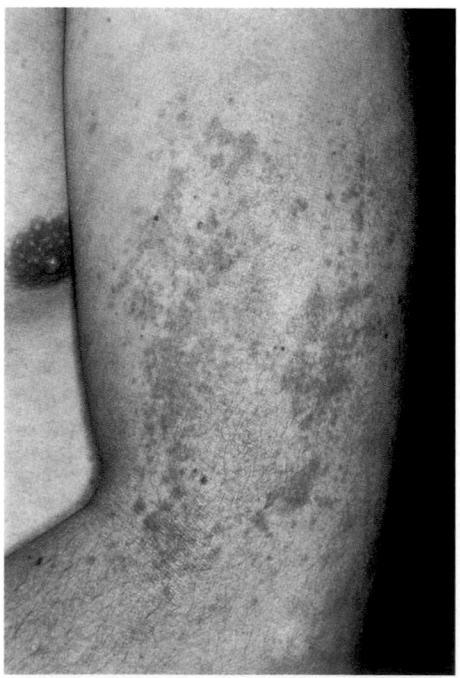

Fig. 8-31 Evanescent eruption of Still's disease.

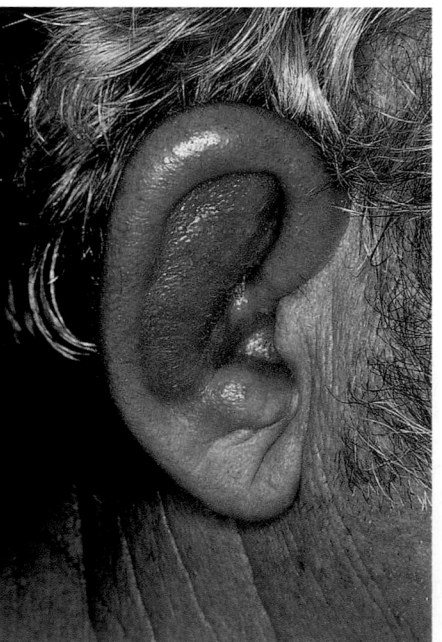

Fig. 8-32 Relapsing polychondritis characteristically involves cartilaginous portions of the ear but spares the lobe.

Autoimmune mechanisms appear to be responsible for this disease. Cell-mediated immunity to cartilage has been demonstrated in vitro, with a degree of response correlated with disease activity. IgG anti-type II collagen antibodies have been documented, again in titers corresponding with disease activity. Elevations in ESR, CRP levels, and urinary type II collagen neoepitope levels correlate with disease activity. A second connective tissue disease or other autoimmune disease is present in about one-third of patients, and some cases appear to be paraneoplastic, occurring in association with hematopoietic malignancies. Limited data suggest that serum levels of Th1 cytokines (IFN-γ, IL-12, and IL-2) may correlate better with disease activity than those of Th2 cytokines (IL-4, IL-5, IL-6, and IL-10).

Histologically, a predominantly neutrophilic infiltrate is noted in the perichondrium. Varying degrees of chondrolysis may be present. DIF often demonstrates a lupus-like continuous granular band of immunoglobulin and complement in the perichondrium.

Dapsone, 100 mg once or twice a day for an adult, reduces the frequency of flares, but is usually inadequate to control the disease. Colchicine, leflunomide, or hydroxychloroquine may also be helpful. Systemic corticosteroids should be used to treat acute flares, but most patients require a steroid-sparing immunosuppressive drug. Azathioprine, methotrexate, mycophenolate mofetil, cyclophosphamide, IVIG, anakinra, and TNF-α inhibitors have been used. Sustained response to etanercept has been reported, even after failure to respond to infliximab. Endobronchial ultrasonography has been used to facilitate the diagnosis and estimate the size of the involved airway for placement of stents.

Carter JD: Treatment of relapsing polychondritis with a TNF antagonist. J Rheumatol 2005; 32:1413.

Gergely P Jr, et al: Relapsing polychondritis. Best Pract Res Clin Rheumatol 2004; 18:723.

Goldenberg G, et al: Successful treatment of relapsing polychondritis with mycophenolate mofetil. J Dermatolog Treat 2006; 17(3):158–159.

Hojaili B, et al: Relapsing polychondritis presenting with complete heart block. J Clin Rheumatol 2008 Feb; 14(1):24–26.

Marie I, et al: Sustained response to infliximab in a patient with relapsing polychondritis with aortic involvement. Rheumatology (Oxford) 2009 Oct; 48(10):1328–1329.

Mark KA, et al: Colchicine and indomethacin for the treatment of relapsing polychondritis. J Am Acad Dermatol 2002; 46(2 Suppl Case Reports):S22.

McCarthy EM, et al: Treatment of relapsing polychondritis in the era of biological agents. Rheumatol Int 2010 Apr; 30(6):827–828.

Subrahmanyam P, et al: Sustained response to etanercept after failing infliximab, in a patient with relapsing polychondritis with tracheomalacia. Scand J Rheumatol 2008 May–Jun; 37(3):239–240.

Terrier B, et al: Complete remission in refractory relapsing polychondritis with intravenous immunoglobulins. Clin Exp Rheumatol 2008 Jan–Feb; 26(1):136–138.

Vounotrypidis P, et al: Refractory relapsing polychondritis: rapid and sustained response in the treatment with an IL-1 receptor antagonist (anakinra). Rheumatology (Oxford) 2006 Apr; 45(4):491–492.

Yanagi T, et al: Relapsing polychondritis and malignant lymphoma: is polychondritis paraneoplastic? Arch Dermatol 2007 Jan; 143(1):89–90.

Bonus images for this chapter can be found online at http://www.expertconsult.com

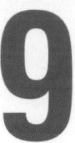
9 | Mucinoses

Within the dermis is a fibrillar matrix, termed ground substance, which is composed of proteoglycans and glycosaminoglycans. These acid mucopolysaccharides, produced by fibroblasts, are highly hygroscopic, binding about 1000 times their own volume in water. They are critical in holding water in the dermis and are responsible for dermal volume and texture. Normally, the sulfated acid mucopolysaccharide chondroitin sulfate and heparin are the primary dermal mucins. In certain diseases, fibroblasts produce abnormally large amounts of acid mucopolysaccharides, usually hyaluronic acid. These acid mucopolysaccharides (mucin) accumulate in large amounts in the dermis, and may be visible as pale blue granular or amorphous material between collagen bundles. They are often not visualized with hematoxylin eosin stains, since the water they bind is removed in processing, so the presence of increased mucin is suspected by the presence of large empty spaces between the collagen bundles. They can be detected by special stains, such as colloidal iron, alcian blue, and toluidine blue. Incubation of the tissue with hyaluronidase eliminates the staining, confirming the presence of hyaluronic acid.

Increased dermal mucin may result from many diseases and is a normal component of wound healing. The mucinoses are those diseases in which the production of increased amounts of mucin is the primary process. Mucin may also accumulate in the skin as a secondary phenomenon, such as when it is present in lupus erythematosus, dermatomyositis, Degos' disease, granuloma annulare, and cutaneous tumors, or after therapies such as psoralen and ultraviolet A (PUVA) or retinoids. The genetic diseases in which mucin accumulates as a result of inherited metabolic abnormalities are termed the mucopolysaccharidoses (see Chapter 26). Myxedema and pretibial myxedema are reviewed in Chapter 24.

Jackson EM, et al: Diffuse cutaneous mucinosis. Dermatol Clin 2002; 20:493.

Rongioletti F, et al: The new cutaneous mucinoses. J Am Acad Dermatol 1991; 24:265.

Rongioletti F, et al: Cutaneous mucinoses: microscopic criteria for diagnosis. Am J Dermatopathol 2001; 23:257.

Lichen myxedematosus

The terminology used to describe disorders in this disease group has varied widely over the years. We will use the 1991 classification of Rongioletti and Rebora. A generalized form, scleromyxedema, is accompanied by a monoclonal gammopathy and may have systemic organ involvement. Five localized forms are recognized, these being characterized by a lack of a monoclonal antibody and systemic disease. Finally, patients may have disease that does not fit into these subsets, and their condition is termed atypical or intermediate in type. Thyroid disease should not account for the findings in any category.

Generalized lichen myxedematosus

Scleromyxedema affects adults of both sexes and appears from ages 30 to 80. It is chronic and progressive. The primary lesions are multiple waxy, 2–4 mm, dome-shaped or flat-topped papules (Fig. 9-1). They may coalesce into plaques (Fig. 9-2) or be arranged in linear array. Less commonly, urticarial, nodular, or even annular lesions are seen. The dorsal hands, face, elbows, and extensor extremities are most frequently affected (Fig. 9-3). Mucosal lesions are absent.

A diffuse infiltration develops, leading to woody sclerosis of the skin. A reduced range of motion of the mouth, hands, and extremities may follow. On the glabella and forehead, coalescence of lesions leads to the prominent furrowing of a "leonine facies". At the proximal interphalangeal joint, induration surrounding a centrally depressed area has been termed the doughnut sign. Pruritus may occur.

Scleromyxedema is often associated with visceral disease. Gastrointestinal findings are most frequent. Dysphagia resulting from involvement of the esophagus is most common, but the stomach or intestine may also be affected. Pulmonary complications with dyspnea caused by restrictive or obstructive disease are the second most common visceral problem. Proximal muscle weakness with an inflammatory myopathy or a nonspecific vacuolar change may occur. Carpal tunnel syndrome occurs in 10% of patients. Arthralgia or inflammatory arthritis is not uncommon. Peripheral neuropathies and central nervous system (CNS) disturbances, including confusion, dizziness, dysarthria, ascending paralysis, seizures, syncope, and coma, can occur. The latter has been termed the dermatoneuro syndrome. Visceral disease can be fatal.

Criteria for inclusion in this disease category include mucin deposition, fibroblast proliferation and fibrosis, normal thyroid function tests, and the presence of a monoclonal gammopathy. Approximately 10% of patients do not have this latter finding on initial evaluation. The gammopathy is usually an IgG-λ type, suggesting an underlying plasma cell dyscrasia. Bone marrow examination may be normal or reveal increased numbers of plasma cells or frank myeloma.

Clinical and histologic features are usually diagnostic. Skin biopsies of early papular lesions demonstrate a proliferation of fibroblasts with mucin and many small collagen fibers. The papules generally appear more fibrotic than mucinous. Over time, fibroblast nuclei become less numerous and collagen fibers become thickened.

Many of the clinical findings seen in scleromyxedema are also found in systemic scleroderma, including cutaneous sclerosis, Raynaud phenomenon, dysphagia, and carpal tunnel syndrome. This distinction in some cases may be difficult without a biopsy. Other infiltrative disorders, such as amyloidosis, must be excluded. Association with hepatitis C has been reported frequently. Nephrogenic systemic fibrosis

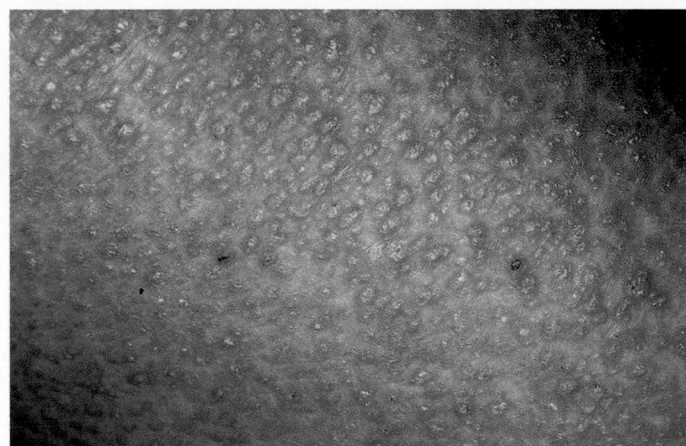

Fig. 9-1 Shiny papules of early scleromyxedema.

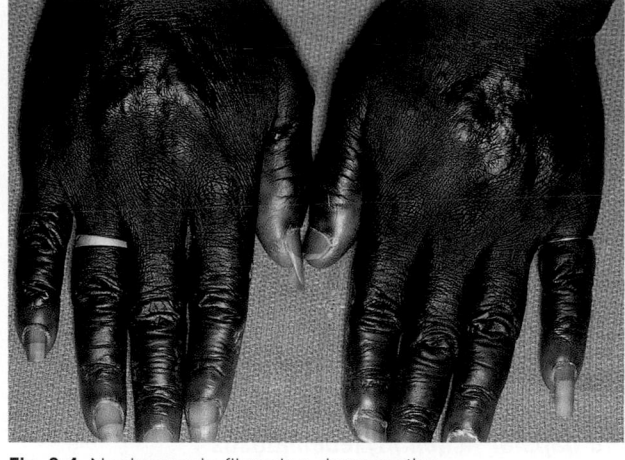

Fig. 9-4 Nephrogenic fibrosing dermopathy.

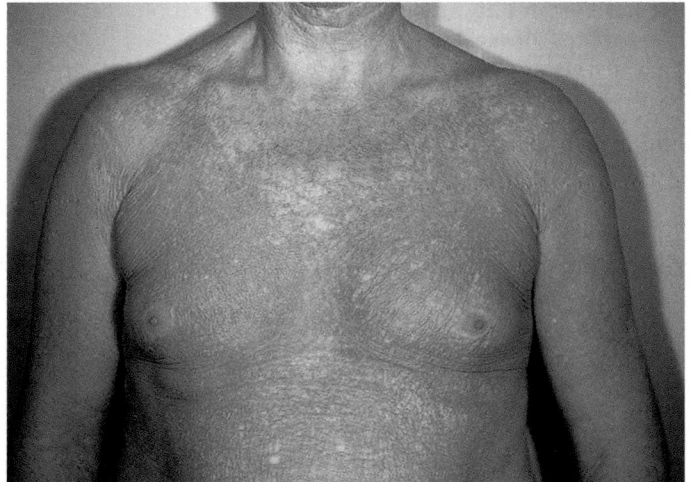

Fig. 9-2 Scleromyxedema.

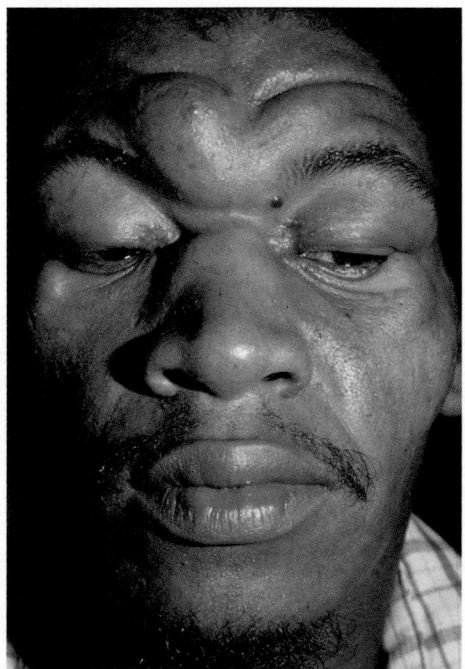

Fig. 9-3 Scleromyxedema. (Courtesy of Marshall Guill, MD)

presents with skin thickening in the setting of renal failure (Fig. 9-4). In its earliest form, it includes mucin along with collagen deposition with a proliferation of CD34+ cells in the dermis. The histologic findings are identical to those of scleromyxedema, and the first report by Cowper et al was termed a scleromyxedema-like illness associated with renal failure. The clinical findings are dominated by fibrosis, so this entity is fully discussed in Chapter 8.

Treatment of scleromyxedema is difficult and usually undertaken in concert with an oncologist. Many patients are treated with immunosuppressive agents, especially melphalan or cyclophosphamide with or without plasma exchange and prednisone. Temporary remission of progressive visceral disease may occur. These short-term benefits must be weighed against the increase in malignancies and sepsis complicating such therapy. Chances of remission are enhanced by the use of autologous stem cell transplantation with high-dose melphalan.

Skin-directed therapy may also be utilized. Physical therapy is indicated. Moderate doses of systemic steroids are not usually helpful, but high doses alone may temporarily arrest progressive cutaneous and visceral disease. Retinoids, plasmapheresis, extracorporeal photochemotherapy, intravenous immunoglobulins, Grenz ray and electron beam therapy, PUVA, thalidomide, interferon (IFN)-α, cyclosporine, topical dimethyl sulfoxide, and topical and intralesional hyaluronidase and corticosteroids have all produced improvement in the skin of selected patients. Many others, however, have not benefited and visceral disease is usually not affected. UVB and IFN-α have exacerbated scleromyxedema.

Occasional patients are reported who spontaneously remit even after many years of disease; however, scleromyxedema remains a therapeutic challenge, and the overall prognosis is poor.

Localized lichen myxedematosus

The localized variants of lichen myxedematosus lack visceral involvement or an associated gammopathy. As a group, they are benign, but often persistent. No therapy is reliably effective in any of the localized forms of lichen myxedematosus. Since there is no gammopathy, visceral involvement, or associated thyroid disease in any of the variants, often no treatment is needed. Shave excision or CO_2 ablation is an option for individual lesions, and spontaneous resolution may occur in all varieties.

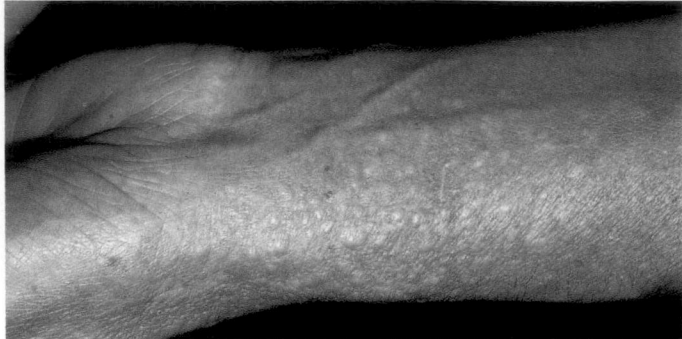

Fig. 9-5 Acral persistent papular mucinosis.

Discrete papular lichen myxedematosus

Discrete papular lichen myxedematosus is characterized by the occurrence of waxy, 2–5 mm, firm, flesh-colored papules, usually confined to the limbs or trunk. The papules may have an erythematous or yellowish hue, may coalesce into nodules or plaques, and may number into the hundreds. Nodules may occasionally be the predominant lesion present, with few or absent papules. The underlying skin is not indurated and there is no associated gammopathy or internal involvement. Biopsy reveals the presence of mucin in the upper and mid-dermis. Fibroblast proliferation is variable, but collagen deposition is minimal. The slow accumulation of papules is the usual course, without the development of a gammopathy or internal manifestations. Occasional cases may spontaneously involute.

Many patients with acquired immunodeficiency syndrome (AIDS) have been reported to develop mucinous papules, usually widespread, unassociated with a paraprotein. It is virtually always seen in advanced human immunodeficiency virus (HIV) disease, in patients with multiple infectious complications. These lesions may occur in association with an eczematous dermatitis or on normal skin. If associated with an eczematous dermatitis, the lesions often clear if the eczema is controlled. Those cases occurring on normal skin may respond to systemic retinoid therapy. At times spontaneous remission occurs. The authors have also seen one case of a patient with AIDS and true scleromyxedema with visceral involvement, and two patients have been reported with acral persistent papular mucinosis.

Acral persistent papular mucinosis

Patients with acral persistent papular mucinosis have a few to over 100 bilaterally symmetrical, 2–5 mm, flesh-colored papules localized to the hands and wrists (Fig. 9-5). The knees, calves, or elbows may also be involved in a minority of patients. The face and trunk are spared. Women outnumber men by 5:1. The course is one of persistence and slow progression. Two involved sisters have been reported. Histologically, there is a collection of upper dermal mucin with minimal or no increase in fibroblasts.

Self-healing papular mucinosis

Self-healing papular mucinosis occurs in a juvenile and an adult form. The juvenile variant, also called self-healing juvenile cutaneous mucinosis, is a rare, but distinct disorder, characterized by the sudden onset of skin lesions and polyarthritis. Children, most commonly between the ages of 5 and 15, are affected. Familial cases are reported. Skin lesions are ivory-white papules of the head, neck, trunk, and typically the periarticular regions; deep nodules on the face and periarticular sites; and hard edema of the periorbital area and face. An acute arthritis affects the knees, elbows, and hand joints. In the adult form, papular lesions occur, usually without the associated

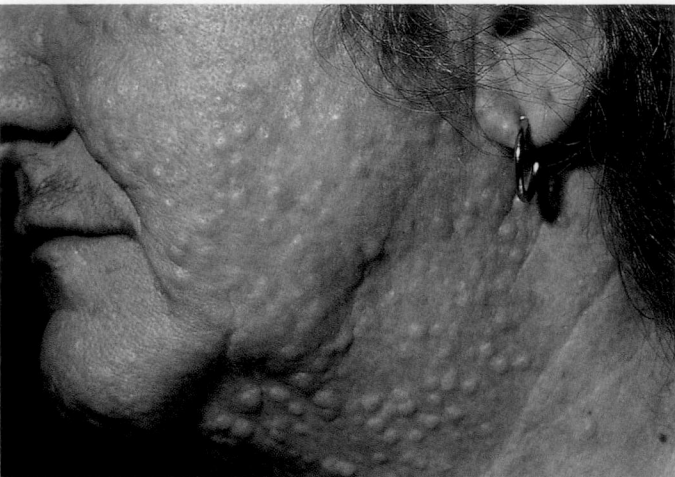

Fig. 9-6 Self-healing papular mucinosis.

joint symptoms (Fig. 9-6). Histology of the skin lesions reveals dermal mucin with little fibroblastic proliferation or collagen deposition. Although the initial presentation is worrisome, the prognosis is excellent. Spontaneous resolution without sequelae occurs over several months.

Papular mucinosis of infancy

This is also referred to as cutaneous mucinosis of infancy and is a rare syndrome that occurs at birth or within the first few months of life. Skin-colored or translucent, grouped or discrete, 2–8 mm papules develop on the trunk or upper extremities, especially the back of the hands. Biopsies show very superficial upper dermal mucin without proliferation of fibroblasts. Existing lesions remain static; new lesions continue to accumulate gradually. Similar lesions may sometimes be noted in association with neonatal lupus erythematosus.

Atypical or intermediate lichen myxedematosus

The cutaneous mucinoses are all relatively uncommon. In a literature dominated by case reports, individual patients have been found who do not fit well into the above scheme, e.g. patients exist with acral persistent papular mucinosis who have had a paraprotein, and others with apparently classic scleromyxedema with visceral lesions may not have a detectable circulating paraprotein.

Berger JR, et al: The neurologic complications of scleromyxedema. Medicine 2001; 80:313.

Blum M, et al: Scleromyxedema: a case series highlighting long-term outcomes of treatment with IVIG. Medicine (Baltimore) 2008; 87:10.

Carder KR, et al: Self-healing juvenile cutaneous mucinosis. Pediatr Dermatol 2003; 20:35.

Cheng T, et al: Complete and durable remission in a patient with life-threatening scleromyxedema treated with high-dose melphalan and BU with auto-SCT. Bone Marrow Transplant 2008 (Epub).

Cokonis Georgakis CD, et al: Scleromyxedema. Clin Dermatol 2006; 24:493.

Cowen EW, et al: Self-healing juvenile cutaneous mucinosis. J Am Acad Dermatol 2004; 50:S97.

Cowper SE, et al: Scleromyxedema-like cutaneous diseases associated with renal failure. Lancet 2000; 356:1000.

Donato ML, et al: Scleromyxedema: role of high-dose melphalan with autologous stem cell transplantation. Blood 2006; 107:463.

Efthimiou P, et al: IVIG and thalidomide may be an effective therapeutic combination in refractory scleromyxedema. Semin Arthritis Rheum 2008 (Epub).

Giron J, et al: Resolution of papular mucinosis in a person with HIV Infection. AIDS Read 2007; 17:418.

Gonzalez J, et al: Scleromyxedema with dermato-neuro syndrome. J Am Acad Dermatol 2000; 42:927.

Harris JE, et al: Acral persistent papular mucinosis. J Am Acad Dermatol 2004; 51:982.

Horn KB, et al: A complete and durable clinical response to high-dose dexamethasone in a patient with scleromyxedema. J Am Acad Dermatol 2004; 51:S120.

Illa I, et al: Steady remission of scleromyxedema 3 years after autologous stem cell transplantation. Blood 2006; 15:773.

Nagaraj LV, et al: Self-healing juvenile cutaneous mucinosis. J Am Acad Dermatol 2006; 55:1036.

Posswig A, et al: Discrete papular mucinosis—a rare subtype of lichen myxoedematosus. Clin Exp Dermatol 2000; 25:289.

Rampino M, et al: Scleromyxedema: treatment of widespread cutaneous involvement by total skin electron beam therapy. Int J Dermatol 2007; 46:864.

Rongioletti F, et al: Treatment of localized lichen myxedematosus of discrete type with tacrolimus ointment. J Am Acad Dermatol 2008; 58:530.

Sansbury JG, et al: Treatment of recalcitrant scleromyxedema with thalidomide in three patients. J Am Acad Dermatol 2004; 51:126.

Sperber BR, et al: Self-healing papular mucinosis in an adult. J Am Acad Dermatol 2004, 50.121.

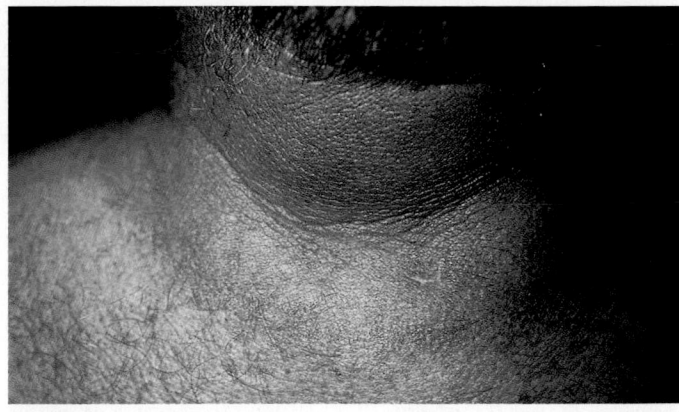

Fig. 9-7 Scleredema.

Scleredema

Scleredema is a skin disease characterized by a stiffening and hardening of the subcutaneous tissues, as if they were infiltrated with paraffin. It occurs in two forms—with and without diabetes mellitus. In the more generalized, non-diabetic condition, a sudden onset following an infection, typically streptococcal in nature, may occur. This reactive variant may also present as a drug eruption. In others the onset is insidious and chronic in nature, and has no preceding infection. In the more common diabetes-associated disease, a long-lasting induration of the upper back is characteristic.

In cases not associated with diabetes, females outnumber males by 2:1. The age at onset is from childhood through adulthood. Skin tightness and induration begins on the neck and/or face, spreading symmetrically to involve the arms, shoulders, back, and chest. The distal extremities are spared. There may be difficulty opening the mouth or eyes, and a masklike expression as a result of the infiltration. The involved skin, which is waxy and of woodlike consistency, gradually transitions into normal skin with no clear demarcation. Associated findings occur in variable numbers of patients and can include dysphagia caused by tongue and upper esophageal involvement, cardiac arrhythmias, and an associated paraprotein, usually an IgG type. Myeloma may be present. There may be pleural, pericardial, or peritoneal effusion.

In about half the patients in whom the condition follows an infection, spontaneous resolution will occur in months to a few years. In one patient whose disease had a sudden onset after beginning infliximab treatment for rheumatoid arthritis, the condition resolved quickly after discontinuation of the medicine and did not recur after etanercept was initiated. The remaining patients with nondiabetic scleredema have a prolonged course. Therapy is generally of no benefit, but patients may live with the disease for many years. Cyclosporine, UVA1, pulsed dexamethasone, and extracorporeal photopheresis have been reported to be beneficial in individual patients.

In the second group, which in most dermatologists' experience is the more common, there is an association with late-onset, insulin-dependent diabetes. Men outnumber women by 10:1. Affected men tend to be obese. The lesions are of insidious onset and long duration, presenting as woody induration and thickening of the skin of the mid-upper back, neck, and shoulders (Fig. 9-7). There is a sharp step-off from the involved to the normal skin. Persistent erythema and folliculitis may involve the affected areas. The associated diabetes is of long duration and is difficult to control. Further, patients have frequently suffered complications of their diabetes, such as nephropathy, atherosclerotic disease, retinopathy, and neuropathy. Control of the diabetes does not affect the course of the scleredema. No paraprotein is detected, and visceral involvement is not seen. Lesions are persistent and usually unresponsive to treatment. Intravenous penicillin, electron beam alone or in combination with photon irradiation, narrow-band UVB, and both bath and systemic PUVA have each been effective in individual patients. While low-dose methotrexate was successful in one patient, it was ineffective in a case series of seven patients.

The histology of both forms is identical. The skin is dramatically thickened, with the dermis often expanded two- to three-fold. There is no hyalinization such as that seen in scleroderma, but rather the thick dermal collagen bundles are separated by clear spaces that may contain visible mucin (hyaluronic acid). The amount of mucin is variable and usually only prominent in early lesions. In late lesions, slightly widened spaces between thick collagen bundles are the sole finding, as the amount of mucin is scant.

Beers WH, et al: Scleredema adultorum of Buschke: a case report and review of the literature. Semin Arthritis Rheum 2006; 35:355.

Bowen AF, et al: Scleredema adultorum of Buschke treated with radiation. Arch Dermatol 2003; 139:780.

Dogra S, et al: Dexamethasone pulse therapy for scleredema. Pediatr Dermatol 2004; 21:280.

Ioannidou DI, et al: Scleredema adultorum of Buschke presenting as periorbital edema. J Am Acad Dermatol 2005; 52:41.

Malhotra AK, et al: Scleredema following scabies infestation. Pediatr Dermatol 2008; 25:136.

Nakajima K, et al: Two cases of diabetic scleredema that responded to PUVA therapy. J Dermatol 2006; 33:820.

Ranganathan P: Infliximab-induced scleredema in a patient with rheumatoid arthritis. J Clin Rheumatol 2005; 11:319.

Stables GI, et al: Scleredema associated with paraproteinaemia treated by extracorporeal photopheresis. Br J Dermatol 2000; 142:781.

Tamburin LM, et al: Scleredema of Buschke successfully treated with electron beam therapy. Arch Dermatol 1998; 134:419.

Xiao T, et al: Scleredema adultorum treated with narrow band ultraviolet B phototherapy. J Dermatol 2007; 34:270.

Reticular erythematous mucinosis (REM syndrome, plaque-like cutaneous mucinosis)

Reticular erythematous mucinosis (REM) favors women in the third and fourth decades of life. The eruption frequently appears after intense sun exposure. Clinical lesions are erythematous plaques or reticulated patches that are several centimeters in diameter, and are most common in the midline of the chest and back (Fig. 9-8). Evolution is gradual, photosensitivity is common, and lesions may be induced with UVB. Onset or exacerbation with oral contraceptives, menses, and

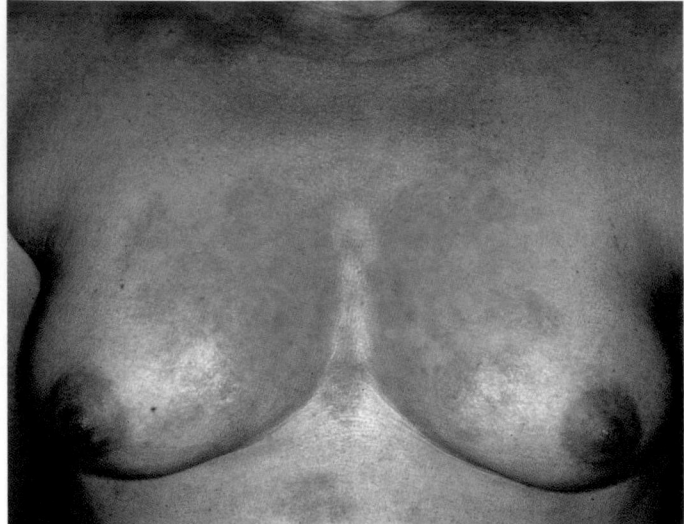

Fig. 9-8 Reticulated erythematous mucinosis.

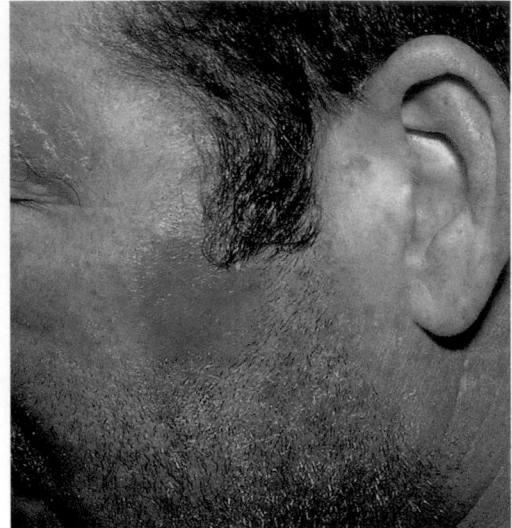

Fig. 9-9 Alopecia mucinosa.

pregnancy is another feature. Serologic tests for lupus erythematosus are negative.

Histologically, there are varying degrees of lymphocytic infiltration around dermal vessels, and deposits of mucin in the dermis. Direct immunofluorescence is negative, but focal vacuolar interface dermatitis is sometimes seen, suggesting a relationship to lupus erythematosus. Treatment with antimalarials is successful in most cases. The pulsed dye laser has led to resolution in two patients.

Lesions of REM have also been reported to occur on the face, arms, abdomen, and groin. When evaluating patients with mucinous smooth-surfaced erythematous lesions it is important to consider the possibility of connective tissue disease. Plaque-like or papulonodular lesions in sites away from the central chest and back may infrequently herald the development of systemic lupus erythematosus, discoid lupus erythematosus, dermatomyositis or scleroderma.

Tumid lupus erythematosus is a subset of chronic cutaneous lupus that is characterized by erythematous papules, nodules, and plaques that most often involve the face, extensor aspects of the arms, shoulders, V of the neck, and upper back. Histology is identical to REM. It is photoinducible and responsive to antimalarials. While serologic abnormalities occur in a small percentage of patients, this is usually a skin-limited condition. Thus, there is considerable overlap with REM and some authors consider the two to be closely related or identical.

Alexiades-Armenakas MR, et al: Tumid lupus erythematosus. Arthritis Rheum 2003; 49:494.

Caputo R, et al: Reticular erythematous mucinosis occurring in a brother and sister. Dermatology 2006; 28:482.

Greve B, et al: Treating REM syndrome with the pulsed dye laser. Lasers Surg Med 2001; 29:248.

Kaufmann R, et al: Dermatomyositis presenting as plaque-like mucinosis. Br J Dermatol 1998; 138:889.

Kuhn A, et al: Lupus erythematosus tumidus. Arch Dermatol 2000; 136:1033.

Van Zander J, et al: Papular and nodular mucinosis as a presenting sign of progressive systemic sclerosis. J Am Acad Dermatol 2002; 46:304.

Follicular mucinosis (alopecia mucinosa)

In 1957, Pinkus applied the name alopecia mucinosa to a series of patients with inflammatory plaques with alopecia characterized histologically by mucinous deposits in the outer root sheaths of the hair follicles. The plaques may be simply hypopigmented or erythematous and scaly, eczematous, or composed of flesh-colored, follicular papules (Fig. 9-9). There may be only one lesion, especially on the head and neck, or multiple sites may be present. The plaques are firm and coarsely rough to the palpating finger. They are distributed mostly on the face, neck, and scalp but may appear on any parts of the body. Itching may or may not be present. Alopecia occurs regularly in lesions on the scalp and frequently in lesions located elsewhere. Some papules show a comedo-like black central dot that corresponds to a broken hair or the mucin itself. These may cause the surface of a patch to look like keratosis pilaris. Sensory dissociation, with hot–cold perception alterations or anesthesia to light touch, has been reported in some lesions, with a resultant misdiagnosis of Hansen's disease.

The term alopecia mucinosa may be used to describe the disease process, and follicular mucinosis to describe the histologic features. The disease may be skin-limited and benign (primary follicular mucinosis) or may be associated with follicular mycosis fungoides. When lesions are solitary or few in number and cluster on the head and neck of individuals younger than 40 years of age, the condition usually follows a benign, chronic course, even in cases where the infiltrate is found to be clonal in nature. Widespread lesions in an older patient, however, will usually be found to be cutaneous T-cell lymphoma (CTCL) at initial presentation or will progress to lymphoma within 5 years. These two subsets are not exclusive, however, and no clinical or histologic criteria absolutely distinguish them in the absence of diagnostic findings of CTCL.

Histologically, follicular mucinosis demonstrates large collections of mucin within the sebaceous gland and outer root sheath. The mucin typically stains as hyaluronic acid. A mixed dermal infiltrate is present. When the condition occurs in association with CTLC, the perifollicular infiltrate is atypical but not generally epidermotropic, and a considerable admixture of eosinophils and plasma cells is present. The additional finding of the presence of syringolymphoid hyperplasia should raise concern that lymphoma is or will become evident. T-cell receptor gene rearrangement studies that indicate clonity are also supportive but do not alone predict an aggressive course.

Spontaneous involution of primary follicular mucinosis may occur, especially in young children. Topical corticosteroids produce improvement. Hydroxychlorquine cured six patients. Dapsone, PUVA, radiation therapy, IFN-α 2b, minocycline, isotretinoin, photodynamic therapy, and indomethacin have been effective in individual cases. Follicular mycosis fungoides, with or without associated mucin, is more refractory to treatment and has a worse prognosis than classic CTCL.

Brown HA, et al: Primary follicular mucinosis. J Am Acad Dermatol 2002; 47:856.

Ceroni L, et al: Follicular mucinosis. Arch Dermatol 2002; 138:182.

Dalle S, et al: Neonatal follicular mucinosis. Br J Dermatol 2007; 157:609.

Fernandez-Guarino M, et al: Primary follicular mucinosis. J Eur Acad Dermatol Venereol 2008; 22:393.

Gerami P, et al: The spectrum of histopathologic and immunohistochemical findings in folliculotropic mycosis fungoides. Am J Surg Pathol 2007; 31:1430.

Gibson LE, et al: Follicular mucinosis. Arch Dermatol 2002; 138:1615.

Lehman JS, et al: Folliculotropic mycosis fungoides. Arch dermatol 2010; 146:662.

Schneider SW, et al: Treatment of so-called idiopathic follicular mucinosis with hydroxychloroquine. Br J Dermatol 2010; 163:420.

Van Doorn R, et al: Follicular mycosis fungoides, a distinct disease entity with or without associated follicular mucinosis. Arch Dermatol 2002; 138:191.

Cutaneous focal mucinosis

Focal mucinosis is characterized by a solitary nodule or papule. Lesions are asymptomatic and usually occur on the face, neck, trunk, or extremities. They appear in adulthood. Histologically, the lesion is characterized by a loose dermal stroma containing large quantities of mucin together with numerous dendritic-shaped fibroblasts. The clinical appearance is not distinctive and may at times be suggestive of a cyst, a basal cell carcinoma, or a neurofibroma. The treatment is surgical excision.

Chen HH, et al: A solitary soft fibroma-like polypoid mucinosis. Dermatol Surg 2004; 30:400.

Takemura N, et al: Cutaneous focal mucinosis. J Dermatol 2005; 32:1051.

Myxoid cysts

These lesions occur most commonly on the dorsal or lateral terminal digits of the hands but may also occur on the toes. They present as solitary, 5–7 mm, opalescent or skin-colored cysts. They may occur as asymptomatic swellings of the proximal nailfold, as subungual growths, or over the distal interphalangeal joint. Women are more frequently affected, and osteoarthritis is frequently present in the adjacent distal interphalangeal joint. Myxoid cysts that can be reduced with pressure communicate directly with the joint space.

Multiple myxoid cysts are associated with connective tissue disease. Young children, even infants, may present with multiple myxoid cysts as the initial manifestation of juvenile rheumatoid arthritis. An adult with systemic sclerosis has also been reported. Two patients whose jobs entailed placing repeated pressure on the fingertips developed multiple myxoid cysts.

When a myxoid cyst is present beneath the proximal nailfold, a characteristic groove may be formed in the nail plate by pressure of the lesion on the nail matrix (Fig. 9-10). Those located beneath the nail cause a transverse nail curvature, a red or blue discoloration of the lunula is common, and nail integrity is typically compromised, leading to distal or longi-

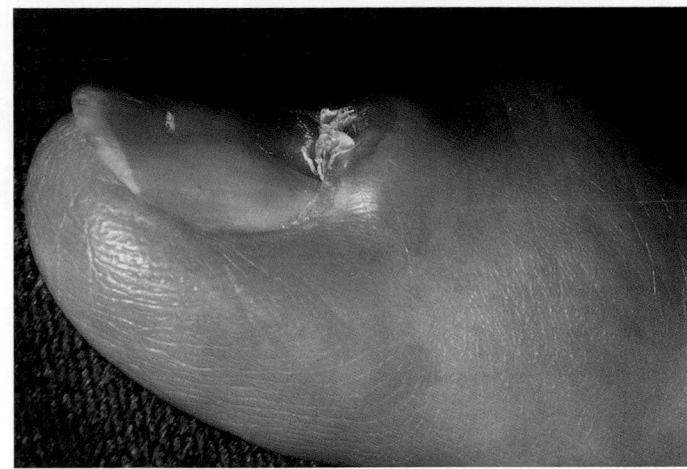

Fig. 9-10 Distortion of nail distal to a synovial cyst.

tudinal splitting or onycholysis. The diagnosis can be confirmed by magnetic resonance imaging (MRI) or surgical exploration. They contain a clear, viscous, sticky fluid that may spontaneously drain. These cysts do not have an epithelial lining but a compacted fibrous wall.

Treatment depends on the site of the cyst. The repeated puncture technique for the two accessible types may achieve a cure rate of up to 70%, but multiple punctures (>40) may be required. This technique may be complicated by local tissue or joint infection. Steroids may be injected into the tissue after draining the cyst. Destruction by cryotherapy, CO_2 laser ablation, curettage, and fulguration are alternatives with similar cure rates, but these result in scarring.

Surgical approaches that reflect the skin overlying the cyst and either excise or tie off the communication to the joint, which may be visualized by injecting the cyst with methylene blue, have a cure rate of over 90%.

Connolly M, et al: Multiple myxoid cysts secondary to occupation. Clin Exp Dermatol 2006; 31:404.

de Berker DAR, et al: Treatment of myxoid cysts. Dermatol Surg 2001; 27:296.

de Berker DAR, et al: Ganglion of the distal interphalangeal joint (myxoid cyst). Arch Dermatol 2001; 137:607.

de Berker DAR, et al: Subungual myxoid cysts. J Am Acad Dermatol 2002; 46:394.

Epstein E: A simple technique for managing digital mucous cysts. Arch Dermatol 1979; 115:1315.

 Bonus images for this chapter can be found online at

http://www.expertconsult.com

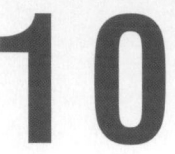

10

Seborrheic Dermatitis, Psoriasis, Recalcitrant Palmoplantar Eruptions, Pustular Dermatitis, and Erythroderma

Seborrheic dermatitis

Clinical features

Seborrheic dermatitis is common, occurring in 2–5% of the population. It is a chronic, superficial, inflammatory disease with a predilection for the scalp, eyebrows, eyelids, nasolabial creases, lips, ears (Fig. 10-1), sternal area, axillae, submammary folds, umbilicus, groins, and gluteal crease. The disease is characterized by scaling on an erythematous base. The scale often has a yellow, greasy appearance. Itching may be severe. Dandruff (pityriasis sicca) represents a mild form of seborrheic dermatitis. An oily type, pityriasis steatoides, is accompanied by erythema and an accumulation of thick crusts.

Other types of seborrheic dermatitis on the scalp include arcuate, polycyclic, or petaloid patches, and psoriasiform, exudative, or crusted plaques. The disease frequently spreads beyond the hairy scalp to the forehead, ears, postauricular regions, and neck. On these areas the patches have convex borders and are reddish-yellow or yellowish. In dark-skinned individuals, arcuate and petaloid lesions commonly involve the hairline. In extreme cases the entire scalp is covered by a greasy, dirty crust with an offensive odor. In infants, yellow or brown scaling lesions on the scalp, with accumulated adherent epithelial debris, are called cradle cap.

Erythema and scaling are often seen in the eyebrows. The lids may show yellowish-white, fine scales and faint erythema. The edges of the lids may be erythematous and granular (marginal blepharitis), and the conjunctivae may be injected. If the glabella is involved, fissures in the wrinkles at the inner end of the eyebrow may accompany the fine scaling. In the nasolabial creases and on the alae nasi, there may be yellowish or reddish-yellow scaling macules, sometimes with fissures. In men, folliculitis of the beard area is common.

In the ears, seborrheic dermatitis may be mistaken for an infectious otitis externa. There is scaling in the aural canals, around the auditory meatus, usually with marked pruritus. The postauricular region and skin under the lobe may be involved. In these areas the skin often becomes red, fissured, and swollen. In the axillae the eruption begins in the apices, bilaterally, and later progresses to neighboring skin. This pattern resembles that of allergic contact dermatitis to deodorant, but differs from that of clothing dermatitis (which involves the periphery of the axillae but spares the vault). The involvement may vary from simple erythema and scaling to more pronounced petaloid patches with fissures. The inframammary folds and the umbilicus may be involved. The presternal area is a favored site on the trunk.

Seborrheic dermatitis is common in the groin and gluteal crease, where its appearance may closely simulate tinea cruris or candidiasis. In these areas, the appearance often overlaps with that of inverse psoriasis. In fact, many of these patients have an overlap of the two conditions (sebopsoriasis or seborrhiasis) in the groin, as well as the scalp. The lesions may also become generalized and progress to a generalized exfoliative erythroderma (erythroderma desquamativum), especially in infants. A minority of these infants will have evidence of immunosuppression. In adults, generalized eruptions may be accompanied by adenopathy and may simulate mycosis fungoides or psoriatic erythroderma.

Seborrheic dermatitis may be associated with several internal diseases. Parkinson's disease is often accompanied by severe refractory seborrheic dermatitis involving the scalp and face, with waxy, profuse scaling. A unilateral injury to the innervation of the face, or a stroke, may lead to unilateral localized seborrheic dermatitis. Patients with acquired immunodeficiency syndrome (AIDS) have an increased incidence of seborrheic dermatitis. An increased incidence has also been noted in patients who are seropositive for human immunodeficiency virus (HIV), but have not developed other signs of clinical disease. Diabetes mellitus, especially in obese persons; sprue; malabsorption disorders; epilepsy; neuroleptic drugs, such as haloperidol; and reactions to arsenic and gold have all produced seborrheic dermatitis-like eruptions.

Etiology and pathogenesis

The etiology of this common disorder is complex, but may be related to the presence of the lipophilic yeast *Pityrosporum ovale*, which produces bioactive indoles. The density of yeast has been correlated with the severity of the disease, and reduction of the yeast occurs with response to therapy. *P. ovale* may also be abundant on the scalps of patients who have no clinical signs of the disease, and the yeast may only be pathogenic in predisposed individuals.

Patients with seborrheic dermatitis may show upregulation of interferon (IFN)-gamma, expressed interleukin (IL)-6, expressed IL-1β, and IL-4. Expression of cytotoxicity-activating ligands and recruitment of natural killer (NK) cells have also been noted.

Histology

The epidermis demonstrates regular acanthosis with some thinning of the suprapapillary plates. Varying degrees of spongiosis and lymphocyte exocytosis are noted. A characteristic finding is the presence of a focal scale crust adjacent to the follicular ostia.

Differential diagnosis

Some cases of seborrheic dermatitis bear a close clinical resemblance to psoriasis, and the two conditions may overlap. Psoriasis tends to have more pronounced erythema and heavier silvery scales that peel in layers. Removal of scales in psoriasis may disclose bleeding points (Auspitz sign). This sign is

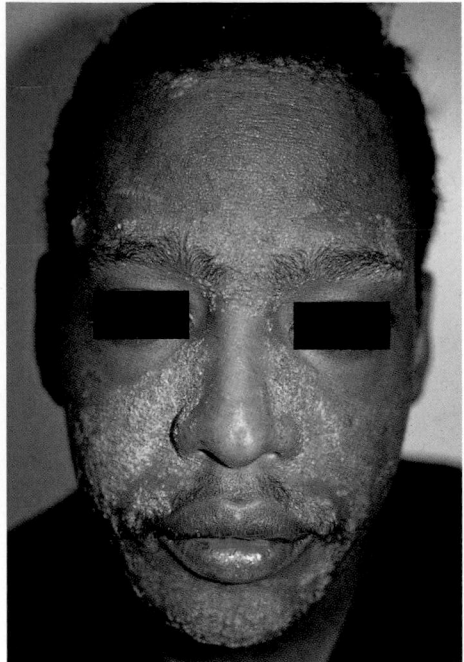

Fig. 10-1 Seborrheic dermatitis.

common but lacks great specificity. Severe itching favors seborrheic dermatitis. Characteristic psoriasis elsewhere (nail pitting, balanitis) may resolve the question. Impetigo of the scalp, especially when associated with pediculosis, may cause difficulty in differentiation. Scalp impetigo can be an indolent crusted dermatosis associated with failure to thrive. Langerhans cell histiocytosis may also resemble seborrheic dermatitis, but typically demonstrates yellow–brown perifollicular papules and groin fissuring. Crusted scabies of the scalp can also be confused with seborrheic dermatitis, and *Trichophyton tonsurans* often produces a subtle seborrheic scale. In subtle cases of tinea, a moist gauze pad rubbed vigorously on the scalp will typically dislodge short, broken KOH-positive hairs. This can be the fastest way to make the diagnosis.

Treatment

Agents suitable for use on glabrous skin include corticosteroid creams, gels, sprays and foam. Corticosteroids tend to produce a rapid effect, but on the face even mid-potency corticosteroids can produce steroid rosacea. For this reason, antifungal agents and topical calcineurin inhibitors are often preferred. Ketoconazole, ciclopirox, tacrolimus, zinc pyrithione, and pimecrolimus preparations are all effective alone and in combination. The antifungals are now available in a wide range of vehicles to include foams, gels, and liquids. Bifonazole shampoo has been shown to be effective in treating infants and small children. Topical calcineurin inhibitors may be associated with a burning sensation, especially on moist skin, and may produce flushing if patients consume alcohol. Patients generally tolerate these agents better after initial treatment with a corticosteroid. An open, randomized, prospective, comparative study of topical pimecrolimus 1% cream vs topical ketoconazole 2% cream found the two to be equally effective, but side effects were somewhat more common with pimecrolimus. Preliminary studies suggest oral itraconazole and oral terbinafine may show some efficacy. Oral fluconazole showed marginal benefit. Study results with topical metronidazole have been mixed.

When secondary bacterial infection is present, a topical or oral antibiotic may be required. In patients infected with HIV,

lithium succinate ointment (Efalith) has been used for facial disease. Lithium gluconate 8% ointment has also been shown to compare favorably with ketoconazole 2% emulsion in healthy adults and was more effective in terms of control of scaling and symptoms. Sodium sulfacetamide products, with or without sulfur, are effective in some refractory patients.

For scalp disease, selenium sulfide, ketoconazole, tar, zinc pyrithione, fluocinolone, and resorcin shampoos are effective. In many patients, these agents may be used 2–3 times a week, with a regular shampoo used in between as required. Antifungal foams and gels, as well as corticosteroid solutions, foams, gels, and sprays, are often preferred by Caucasian patients, while ointment or oil preparations are preferred by some black patients.

Itching of the external ear canal usually responds to a topical corticosteroid, calcineurin inhibitors, or antifungals such as ketoconazole or ciclopirox. Some patients require the use of a class 1 corticosteroid on weekends to control refractory pruritus. Cortisporin otic suspension can bring about prompt clearing, but contact dermatitis to neomycin may complicate the use of some Cortisporin products. Desonide otic lotion (0.05% desonide and 2% acetic acid) is also effective and may be better tolerated than Domeboro otic solution.

Sodium sulfacetamide drops or ointment may be effective for seborrheic blepharitis. Oral tetracyclines can also be effective, and have been shown to decrease the density of microorganisms in the affected follicles. Steroid preparations are suitable for short-term use, but may induce glaucoma and cataracts. Daily gentle cleansing with a cotton-tipped applicator and baby shampoo in water can reduce symptoms. In severe cases, oral antibiotics or oral antifungals may be combined with topical agents.

Berk T, et al: Seborrheic dermatitis. P.T. 2010 Jun; 35(6):348–352.
Cömert A, et al: Efficacy of oral fluconazole in the treatment of seborrheic dermatitis: a placebo-controlled study. Am J Clin Dermatol 2007; 8(4):235–238.
Dawson TL Jr: *Malassezia globosa* and *restricta*: breakthrough understanding of the etiology and treatment of dandruff and seborrheic dermatitis through whole-genome analysis. J Investig Dermatol Symp Proc 2007; 12(2):15–19.
Elewski B, et al: Efficacy and safety of a new once-daily topical ketoconazole 2% gel in the treatment of seborrheic dermatitis: a phase III trial. J Drugs Dermatol 2006; 5(7):646–650.
Firooz A, et al: Pimecrolimus cream, 1%, vs hydrocortisone acetate cream, 1%, in the treatment of facial seborrheic dermatitis: a randomized, investigator-blind, clinical trial. Arch Dermatol 2006; 142(8):1066–1067.
Food and Drug Administration, HHS: Dandruff, seborrheic dermatitis, and psoriasis drug products containing coal tar and menthol for over-the-counter human use; amendment to the monograph. Final rule. Fed Regist 2007; 72(43):9849–9852.
Gaitanis G, et al: AhR ligands, malassezin, and indolo[3,2-b]carbazole are selectively produced by *Malassezia furfur* strains isolated from seborrheic dermatitis. J Invest Dermatol 2008; 128(7):1620–1625.
Gee BC: Seborrhoeic dermatitis. Clin Evid 2004; 12:2344.
High WA, et al: Pilot trial of 1% pimecrolimus cream in the treatment of seborrheic dermatitis in African American adults with associated hypopigmentation. J Am Acad Dermatol 2006; 54(6):1083–1088.
Jackson WB: Blepharitis: current strategies for diagnosis and management. Can J Ophthalmol 2008; 43(2):170–179.
Kircik L: The evolving role of therapeutic shampoos for targeting symptoms of inflammatory scalp disorders. J Drugs Dermatol 2010; 9(1):41–48.
Koc E, et al: An open, randomized, prospective, comparative study of topical pimecrolimus 1% cream and topical ketoconazole 2% cream in the treatment of seborrheic dermatitis. J Dermatolog Treat 2008; 1:1–5.
Ozcan H, et al: Is metronidazole 0.75% gel effective in the treatment of seborrhoeic dermatitis? A double-blind, placebo controlled study. Eur J Dermatol 2007; 17(4):313–316.
Seckin D, et al: Metronidazole 0.75% gel vs. ketoconazole 2% cream in the treatment of facial seborrheic dermatitis: a randomized, double-blind study. J Eur Acad Dermatol Venereol 2007; 21(3):345–350.

Shemer A, et al: Treatment of moderate to severe facial seborrheic dermatitis with itraconazole: an open non-comparative study. Isr Med Assoc J 2008; 10(6):417–418.

Siadat AH, et al: The efficacy of 1% metronidazole gel in facial seborrheic dermatitis: a double blind study. Indian J Dermatol Venereol Leprol 2006; 72(4):266–269.

Tajima M, et al: Molecular analysis of *Malassezia* microflora in seborrheic dermatitis patients: comparison with other diseases and healthy subjects. J Invest Dermatol 2008; 128(2):345–351.

Vena GA, et al: Oral terbinafine in the treatment of multi-site seborrheic dermatitis: a multicenter, double-blind placebo-controlled study. Int J Immunopathol Pharmacol 2005; 18(4):745–753.

Waldroup W, et al: Medicated shampoos for the treatment of seborrheic dermatitis. J Drugs Dermatol 2008; 7(7):699–703.

Warshaw EM, et al: Results of a randomized, double-blind, vehicle-controlled efficacy trial of pimecrolimus cream 1% for the treatment of moderate to severe facial seborrheic dermatitis. J Am Acad Dermatol 2007; 57(2):257–264.

Psoriasis

Clinical features

Psoriasis is a common, chronic, and recurrent inflammatory disease of the skin characterized by circumscribed, erythematous, dry, scaling plaques of various sizes. The lesions are usually covered by silvery white lamellar scales. The lesions have a predilection for the scalp, nails, extensor surfaces of the limbs, umbilical region, and sacrum. The eruption is usually symmetrical. It usually develops slowly but may be exanthematous, with the sudden onset of numerous guttate (droplike) lesions (Fig. 10-2). Subjective symptoms, such as itching or burning, may be present and may cause extreme discomfort.

The early lesions are small erythematous macules, which from the beginning are covered with dry, silvery scales. The lesions increase in size by peripheral extension and coalescence. The scales are micaceous, meaning that they peel in layers. They are looser toward the periphery and adherent centrally. When removed, bleeding points appear (Auspitz sign). Although plaques typically predominate, lesions may be annular or polycyclic. Old patches may be thick and covered with tough lamellar scales like the outside of an oyster shell (psoriasis ostracea). Various other descriptive terms have in the past been applied to the diverse appearances of the lesions: psoriasis guttata, in which the lesions are the size of water drops; psoriasis follicularis, in which tiny, scaly lesions are located at the orifices of hair follicles; psoriasis figurata, psoriasis annulata, and psoriasis gyrata, in which curved linear patterns are produced by central involution; psoriasis discoi-

dea, in which central involution does not occur and solid patches persist; and psoriasis rupioides, in which crusted lesions occur, resembling syphilitic rupia. The term chronic plaque psoriasis is often applied to stable lesions of the trunk and extremities. Inverse psoriasis predominates in intertriginous areas. Pustular variants of psoriasis may be chronic on the palms and soles (Fig. 10-3), or may be eruptive and accompanied by severe toxicity and hypocalcemia.

Involved nails (Fig. 10-4) can demonstrate distal onycholysis, random pitting (the result of parakeratosis from the proximal matrix), oil spots (yellow areas of subungual parakeratosis from the distal matrix), or salmon patches (nailbed psoriasis). Thick subungual hyperkeratosis may resemble onychomycosis.

Types

Seborrheic-like psoriasis

Some cases of psoriasis overlap with seborrheic dermatitis. Seborrheic lesions may predominate on the face, under the

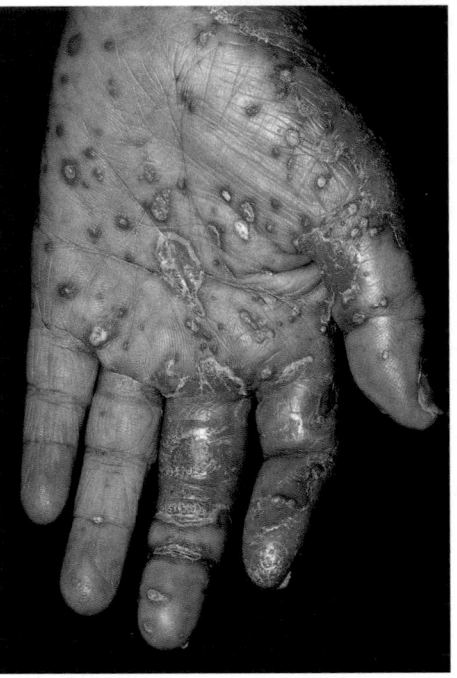

Fig. 10-3 Pustular psoriasis of the hand.

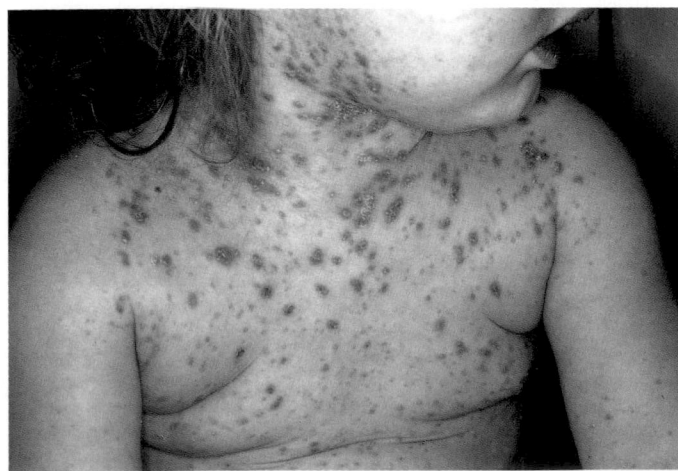

Fig. 10-2 Psoriasis.

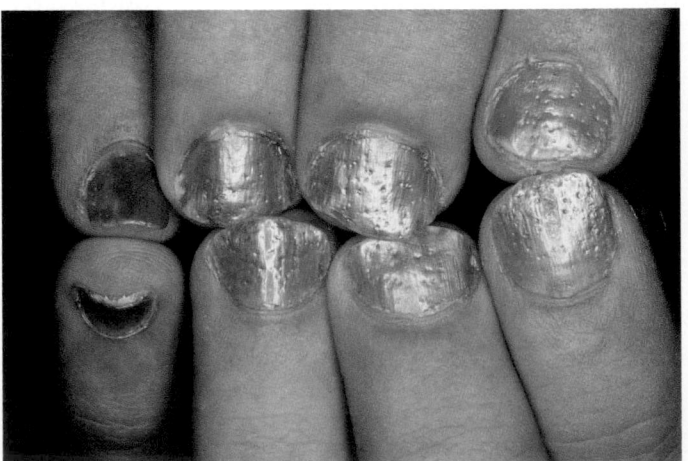

Fig. 10-4 Nail pitting and distal onycholysis in psoriasis.

breasts, and in the scalp, flexures, and axillae. Lesions in these areas are moist and erythematous, with yellow, greasy, soft scales, rather than dry and micaceous scales. Terms such as sebopsoriasis and seborrhiasis may be used to describe the condition of such patients.

Inverse psoriasis

This form selectively and often exclusively involves folds, recesses, and flexor surfaces such as the ears, axillae, groins, inframammary folds, navel, intergluteal crease, penis (Fig. 10-5), lips, and web spaces. Other areas, such as the scalp and nails, may be involved.

"Napkin" psoriasis

Napkin psoriasis, or psoriasis in the diaper area, is characteristically seen in infants between 2 and 8 months of age. Lesions appear as brightly erythematous, sharply demarcated patches of skin involving much of the diaper area. The lesions typically clear with topical therapy, but psoriasis may reappear in adulthood.

Psoriatic arthritis

Five clinical patterns of arthritis occur:

1. asymmetrical distal interphalangeal joint involvement with nail damage (16%)
2. arthritis mutilans with osteolysis of phalanges and metacarpals (5%) (Fig. 10-6)
3. symmetrical polyarthritis-like rheumatoid arthritis, with claw hands (15%)

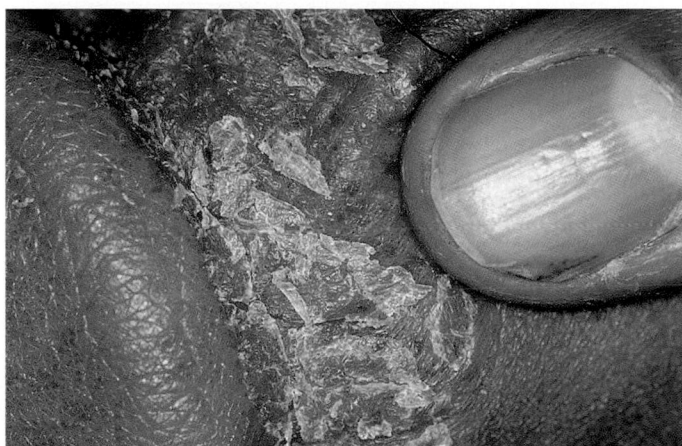

Fig. 10-5 Penile psoriasis with erythema and silver scale.

4. oligoarthritis with swelling and tenosynovitis of one or a few hand joints (70%)
5. ankylosing spondylitis alone or with peripheral arthritis (5%).

Most radiographic findings resemble those in rheumatoid arthritis, but certain findings are highly suggestive of psoriasis. These include erosion of terminal phalangeal tufts (acrosteolysis), tapering or "whittling" of phalanges or metacarpals with "cupping" of proximal ends of phalanges (pencil in a cup deformity), bony ankylosis, osteolysis of metatarsals, predilection for distal interphalangeal and proximal interphalangeal joints, relative sparing of metacarpal phalangeal and metatarsal phalangeal joints, paravertebral ossification, asymmetrical sacroiliitis, and rarity of "bamboo spine" when the spine is involved. Nearly half the patients with psoriatic arthritis have type human leukocyte antigen (HLA)-B27.

Rest, splinting, passive motion, and nonsteroidal anti-inflammatory drugs (NSAIDs) may provide symptomatic relief but do not prevent deformity. Methotrexate, cyclosporine, tacrolimus, and biologic agents are disease-modifying drugs that prevent deformity.

Guttate psoriasis

In this distinctive form of psoriasis typical lesions are the size of water drops, 2–5 mm in diameter. Lesions typically occur as an abrupt eruption following some acute infection, such as a streptococcal pharyngitis. Guttate psoriasis occurs mostly in patients under age 30. This type of psoriasis usually responds rapidly to broad-band ultraviolet (UV) B at erythemogenic doses. Suberythemogenic doses often have little impact on the lesions. This is one of the few forms of psoriasis where broad-band UVB may have an advantage over narrow-band UVB. Minimal erythemogenic dose (MED) testing is recommended to allow for appropriately aggressive treatment. Recurrent episodes may be related to pharyngeal carriage of the responsible streptococcus by the patient or a close contact. A course of a semisynthetic penicillin (such as dicloxacillin, 250 mg four times a day for 10 days) with rifampin (600 mg/day for an adult) may be required to clear chronic streptococcal carriage.

Generalized pustular psoriasis (von Zumbusch)

Typical patients have had plaque psoriasis and often psoriatic arthritis. The onset is sudden, with formation of lakes of pus periungually, on the palms, and at the edge of psoriatic plaques. Erythema occurs in the flexures before the generalized eruption appears. This is followed by a generalized erythema and more pustules (Fig. 10-7). Pruritus and intense

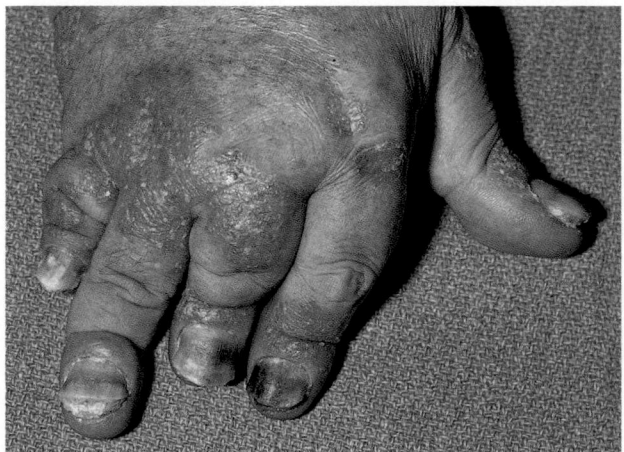

Fig. 10-6 Psoriatic arthritis.

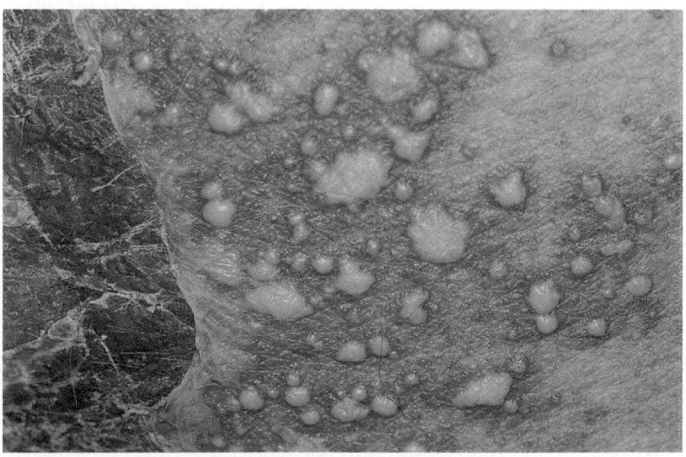

Fig. 10-7 Pustular psoriasis.

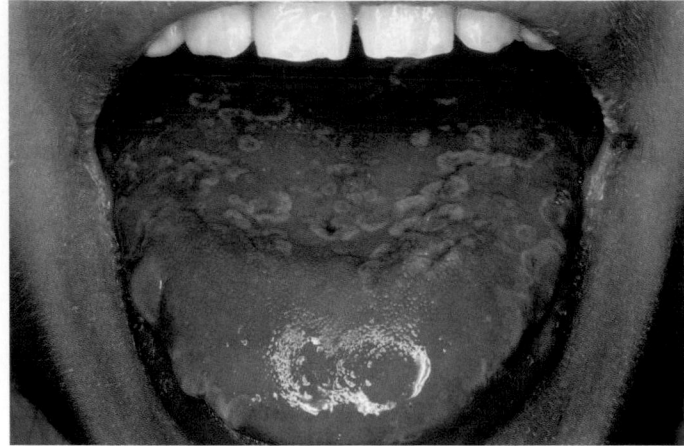

Fig. 10-8 Geographic tongue in pustular psoriasis.

burning are often present. Mucous membrane lesions are common. The lips may be red and scaly, and superficial ulcerations of the tongue and mouth occur. Geographic or fissured tongue frequently occurs (Fig. 10-8).

The patient is frequently ill with fever, erythroderma, hypocalcemia, and cachexia. A number of cases of acute respiratory distress syndrome associated with pustular and erythrodermic psoriasis have been reported. Other systemic complications include pneumonia, congestive heart failure, and hepatitis.

Episodes are often provoked by withdrawal of systemic corticosteroids. The authors have also observed generalized pustular psoriasis as the presenting sign of Cushing's disease. Other implicated drugs include iodides, coal tar, terbinafine, minocycline, hydroxychloroquine, acetazolamide, and salicylates. There is usually a strong familial history of psoriasis. Generalized pustular psoriasis may occur in infants and children with no implicated drug. It may also occur as an episodic event punctuating the course of localized acral pustular psoriasis.

Acitretin is the drug of choice in this severe disease. The response is generally rapid. Isotretinoin is also effective. Cyclosporine, methotrexate, and biologicals are alternatives. Sometimes dapsone is effective in doses of 50–100 mg/day.

Acrodermatitis continua of Hallopeau

Typical patients develop acral erythematous plaques studded with pustules. The nailbeds are heavily involved, and the fingernails float away on lakes of pus, resulting in anonychia. Hyperkeratosis often ensues, and the fingertips become increasingly painful, tapering to long keratotic points. Occasionally, patients may develop generalized pustular flares (Fig. 10-9). Acrodermatitis continua is discussed in more detail below.

Impetigo herpetiformis

This term has been applied to generalized pustular psoriasis of pregnancy. Flexural erythema, studded with pustules, often occurs initially, followed by a generalized pustular flare and increasing toxicity. As the patients are pregnant, systemic retinoids are not appropriate. Many patients only respond to delivery, and early delivery should be strongly considered as soon as it is safe for the infant. Alternatively, patients may respond to prednisone at a dose of 1 mg/kg/day. The corticosteroid can also contribute to neonatal lung maturity.

Keratoderma blennorrhagicum (Reiter syndrome)

Keratoderma blennorrhagicum resembles psoriasis both histologically and clinically, except for its tendency for thicker kera-

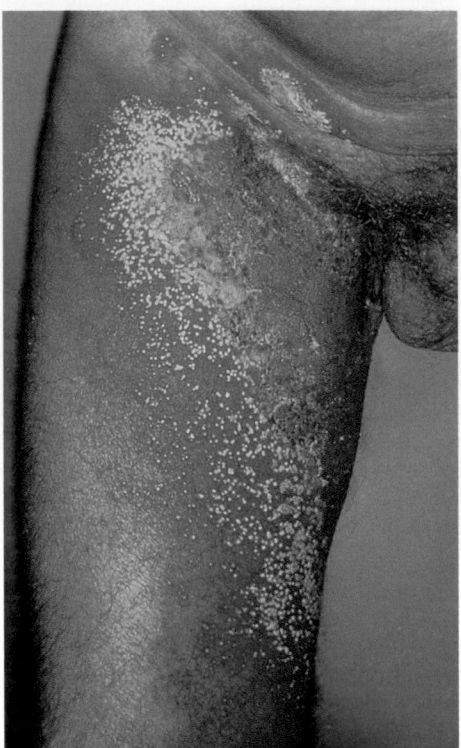

Fig. 10-9 Generalized pustular flare in a patient with acrodermatitis continua.

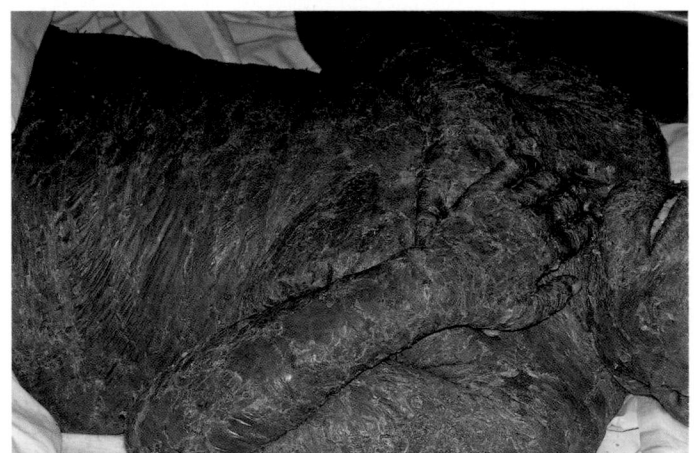

Fig. 10-10 Erythrodermic psoriasis.

totic lesions. Patients are often positive for HLA-B27 and develop reactive arthritis and skin disease after a bout of urethritis or enteritis.

Erythrodermic psoriasis

Patients with psoriasis may develop a generalized erythroderma (Fig. 10-10). Erythrodermic psoriasis is covered in greater detail under exfoliative dermatitis.

Course

The course of psoriasis is unpredictable. It usually begins on the scalp or elbows, and may remain localized in the original region for years. Chronic disease may also be almost entirely limited to the fingernails. Involvement over the sacrum may easily be confused with candidiasis or tinea. Onset may also be sudden and widespread.

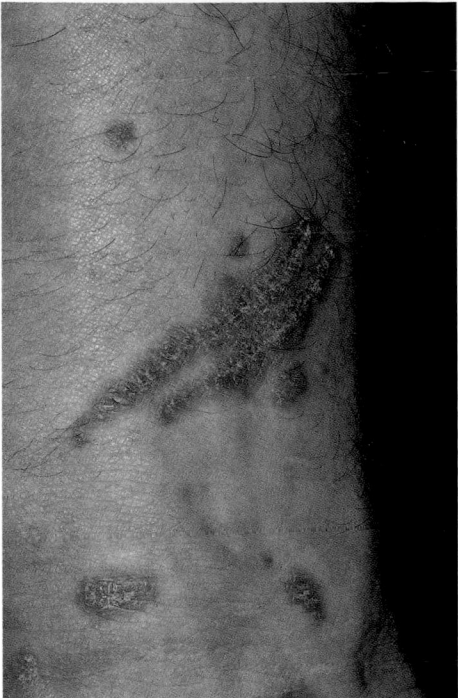

Fig. 10-11 Koebner phenomenon in psoriasis.

Two of the chief features of psoriasis are its tendency to recur and its persistence. The isomorphic response (Koebner phenomenon) is the appearance of typical lesions of psoriasis at sites of even trivial injury (Fig. 10-11). Lesions may occur at sites of scratches, incisions, and burns. Lesions may first appear after a viral exanthema or following pityriasis rosea. The isomorphic response may occur if psoriatic lesions are severely burned during phototherapy. With a reduction in light dosage, the erythema and burning resolve, and the plaques begin to clear. Woronoff's ring is concentric blanching of the erythematous skin at or near the periphery of a healing psoriatic plaque. It is often the first sign that the patient's psoriasis is responding to phototherapy.

The palms and soles are sometimes exclusively affected, showing discrete erythematous dry scaling patches, circumscribed verrucous thickenings, or pustules on an erythematous base. The patches usually begin in the mid-portions of the palms or on the soles, and gradually expand. Psoriasis of the palms and soles is typically chronic and extremely resistant to treatment.

Many studies report an association between hepatitis C and psoriasis, and hepatitis C has also been implicated in psoriatic arthritis. If treatment of psoriasis is to include a potentially hepatotoxic drug, such as methotrexate, a hepatitis C serology should be obtained. It should also be noted that interferon treatment of the hepatitis can further exacerbate or induce psoriasis. Anti-tumor necrosis factor (TNF)-α therapy shows promise in the treatment of psoriasis, even in the setting of chronic hepatitis C infection.

Inheritance

In a large study of psoriasis in monozygotic twins, heritability was high and environmental influence low. Patients with psoriasis often have relatives with the disease, and the incidence typically increases in successive generations. Multifactorial inheritance is likely. Analysis of population-specific HLA haplotypes has provided evidence that susceptibility to psoriasis is linked to the class I and II major histocompatibility complex (MHC) on human chromosome 6. A number of genetic loci are linked to psoriasis, including *PSORS1* on chromosome 6 and within the MHC, and *PSORS2* on chromosome 17q. It has also been shown that there are two subsets that differ in age of onset and in the frequency of HLA associations. Early onset is type I psoriasis and is associated mostly with Cw6, B57, and DR7. Late onset is type II and this predominantly features Cw2. *PSORS9* has also been confirmed as a susceptibility locus for psoriasis.

A variety of other HLA associations have been reported. It is believed that any individual who has B13 or B17 carries a five-fold risk of developing psoriasis. In pustular psoriasis HLA-B27 may be seen, whereas B13 and B17 are increased in guttate and erythrodermic psoriasis. In palmoplantar pustulosis, there is an association with HLA-B8, Bw35, Cw7, and DR3. HLA typing is a research tool for population-based studies, but is of limited value in assessing an individual patient.

Epidemiology

Psoriasis occurs with equal frequency in both sexes. Between 1 and 2% of the US population has psoriasis. It occurs less frequently in the tropics. It is less common in North American and West African black persons. Native Americans and native Fijians rarely have psoriasis. The onset of psoriasis is at a mean age of 27 years, but the range is wide, from the neonatal period to the seventies. Severe emotional stress tends to aggravate psoriasis in almost half of those studied.

In pregnancy there is a distinct tendency for improvement or even temporary disappearance of lesions in the majority of women studied. After childbirth there is a tendency for exacerbation of lesions. Paradoxically, pregnancy is also the milieu for impetigo herpetiformis, and psoriasis may behave differently from one pregnancy to another in the same patient.

A high prevalence of celiac disease has been noted in patients with psoriasis. Lymphoma also has an increased incidence in these patients, and psoriasis has been linked to the metabolic syndrome and a higher risk of cardiovascular disease.

Pathogenesis

Psoriasis is a hyperproliferative disorder, but the proliferation is driven by a complex cascade of inflammatory mediators. Psoriasis appears to represent a mixed T-helper (Th)1 and Th17 inflammatory disease. Th17 cells appear to be more proximal in the inflammatory cascade. T cells and cytokines play pivotal roles in the pathophysiology of psoriasis. Overexpression of type 1 cytokines, such as IL-2, IL-6, IL-8, IL-12, IFN-γ and TNF-α, has been demonstrated, and overexpression of IL-8 leads to the accumulation of neutrophils. The main signal for Th1 development is IL-12, which promotes intracellular IFN-γ production. In animal models, shifting from Th1 to Th2 responses improves psoriasis. IL-4 is capable of inducing Th2 responses and improving psoriasis. Reduced expression of the anti-inflammatory cytokines IL-1RA and IL-10 has been found, and polymorphisms for IL-10 genes correlate with psoriasis. IL-10 is a type 2 cytokine with major influences on immunoregulation, inhibiting type 1 proinflammatory cytokine production. Patients on established traditional therapies show rising levels of IL-10 mRNA expression, suggesting that IL-10 may have antipsoriatic capacity.

The response to biologic agents has demonstrated that CD2+ lymphocytes, CD-11a and TNF-α are important in the pathogenesis of psoriasis. IL-15 triggers inflammatory cell recruitment, angiogenesis, and production of inflammatory cytokines, including IFN-γ, TNF-α, and IL-17, all of which are upregulated in psoriatic lesions. The interplay is complex, but IL-17 appears to be proinflammatory, while IL-22 may serve to retard keratinocyte differentiation. IL-23 stimulates survival, as well as proliferation of Th17 cells. Circulating NK cells are reduced in psoriasis.

Specific targets for therapy include TNF-α, leukocyte function-associated antigen-1 (LFA-1)/intercellular adhesion molecule-1 (ICAM-1) binding, and LFA-3/CD2 binding. An IL-15 monoclonal antibody has been shown to be effective in a mouse model of psoriasis.

Streptococci

Streptococci play a role in some patients. Patients with psoriasis report sore throat more often than controls. Beta-hemolytic streptococci of Lancefield groups A, C, and G can cause exacerbation of chronic plaque psoriasis. Th1 cells recognize cell-wall extract isolated from group A streptococci. HLA variation has a significant effect on the immune response to group A streptococci.

Stress

Various studies have shown a positive correlation between stress and severity of disease. In almost half of patients studied, stress appears to play a significant role.

Drug-induced psoriasis

Psoriasis may be induced by β-blockers, lithium, antimalarials, terbinafine, calcium channel blockers, captopril, glyburide, granulocyte colony-stimulating factor, interleukins, interferons, and lipid-lowering drugs. Systemic steroids may cause rebound or pustular flares. Antimalarials are associated with erythrodermic flares, but patients traveling to malaria-endemic regions should take appropriate prophylaxis. Often, drugs such as doxycycline or mefloquine are appropriate for the geographic area, but when a quinine derivative offers the best protection, it is generally better to take the prophylactic doses of a quinine derivative than to risk disease and full-dose treatment.

Pathology

Histologically, all psoriasis is pustular. The microscopic pustules include spongiform intraepidermal pustules, and Munro microabscesses within the stratum corneum. In early guttate lesions, focal parakeratosis is noted within the stratum corneum. The parakeratotic focus typically has an outline resembling a child's rendition of a seagull. Neutrophils are generally noted immediately above the focus of parakeratosis, but in some sections, the neutrophils will not be visible as a result of sampling error. In plaque psoriasis, neutrophilic foci are so numerous that they are rarely missed. Neutrophilic microabscesses are generally present at multiple levels in the stratum corneum, usually on top of small foci of parakeratosis. These foci generally alternate with areas of orthokeratotic stratum corneum, suggesting that the underlying spongiform pustules arise in a rhythmic fashion. The granular layer is absent focally, corresponding to areas producing foci of parakeratosis. In well-developed plaques, there is regular epidermal acanthosis with long, bulbous rete ridges, thinning over the dermal papillae, and dilated capillaries within the dermal papillae. The last two findings correlate with the Auspitz sign. The stratum corneum may be entirely parakeratotic but still shows multiple small neutrophilic microabscesses at varying levels. Spongiosis is typically scant, except in the area immediately surrounding collections of neutrophils.

In pustular psoriasis, geographic tongue, and Reiter syndrome, intraepidermal spongiform pustules tend to be much larger. Grossly pustular lesions often have little associated acanthosis. In Reiter syndrome, the stratum corneum is often massively thickened, with prominent foci of neutrophils above parakeratosis, alternating with orthokeratosis.

Acral lesions often demonstrate nondiagnostic features histologically. Spongiosis is typically prominent in these lesions and often leads to a differential diagnosis of psoriasis or chronic psoriasiform spongiotic dermatitis. Foci of neutrophils often contain serum and may be interpreted as impetiginized crusting.

On direct immunofluorescence testing, the stratum corneum demonstrates intense fluorescence with all antibodies, complement, and fibrin. This fluorescence may be partially independent of the fluorescent label, as it has been noted in hematoxylin and eosin (H&E)-stained sections and frozen unstained sections. The same phenomenon of stratum corneum autofluorescence has been noted in some cases of candidiasis that demonstrate a psoriasiform histology.

Psoriasis can generally be distinguished from dermatitis by the paucity of edema, the relative absence of spongiosis, the tortuosity of the capillary loops, and the presence of neutrophils above foci of parakeratosis. Neutrophils in the stratum corneum are commonly seen in tinea, impetigo, candidiasis, and syphilis, but rarely are found atop parakeratosis alternating with orthokeratosis in a rhythmic fashion. In psoriasiform syphilis the rete are typically long and slender, a vacuolar interface dermatitis is commonly present, dermal blood vessels appear to have no lumen because of endothelial swelling, and plasma cells are present in the dermal infiltrate. About one-third of biopsies of syphilis lack plasma cells, but the remaining characteristics still suggest the correct diagnosis. Psoriasiform lesions of mycosis fungoides exhibit epidermotropism of large lymphocytes with little spongiosis. The lymphocytes are typically larger, darker, and more angulated than the lymphocytes in the dermis. There is associated papillary dermal fibrosis, and the superficial perivascular infiltrate is asymmetrically distributed around the postcapillary venules, favoring the epidermal side (bare underbelly sign).

Clinical differential diagnosis

Psoriasis must be differentiated from dermatomyositis, lupus erythematosus, seborrheic dermatitis, pityriasis rosea, lichen planus, eczema, and psoriasiform syphilid. The distribution in psoriasis is on the extensor surfaces, especially of the elbows and knees, and on the scalp; dermatomyositis shares this distribution, whereas lupus erythematosus generally lacks involvement of the extensor surfaces. Patients with dermatomyositis may exhibit a heliotrope sign, atrophy, poikiloderma, and nailfold changes. Advanced lesions of discoid lupus erythematosus often demonstrate follicular hyperkeratosis (carpet tack sign). Seborrheic dermatitis has a predilection for the eyebrows, nasolabial angle, ears, sternal region, and flexures. The scales in psoriasis are dry, white, and shiny, whereas those in seborrheic dermatitis are greasy and yellowish. On removal of the scales in psoriasis there is an oozing of blood from the capillaries (Auspitz sign), whereas this does not occur in seborrheic dermatitis.

In pityriasis rosea the eruption is located on the upper arms, trunk, and thighs, and the duration is a matter of weeks. Lesions are typically oval and follow skin tension lines. Individual lesions show a crinkling of the epidermis and collarette scaling. A herald patch is frequently noted. Lichen planus chiefly affects the flexor surfaces of the wrists and ankles. Often the violaceous color is pronounced. In darker-skinned individuals, the lesions have a tendency to pronounced hyperpigmentation. The nails are not pitted as in psoriasis, but longitudinally ridged, rough, and thickened. Pterygium formation is characteristic of lichen planus.

Hand eczema may resemble psoriasis. In general, psoriatic lesions tend to be more sharply marginated, but at times the lesions are indistinguishable. Psoriasiform syphilid has infiltrated copper-colored papules, often arranged in a figurate pattern. Serologic tests for syphilis are generally positive, but prozone reactions may occur, and the serum may have to be diluted in order to obtain a positive test. Generalized lymphadenopathy and mucous patches may be present.

Treatment

Topical therapy is generally suitable for limited plaques. Localized treatments, such as the excimer laser or other forms of intense pulsed light, may be suitable for limited plaques. Phototherapy remains highly cost-effective for widespread psoriasis. Cyclosporine has a rapid onset of action, but is generally not suitable for sustained therapy. Methotrexate remains the systemic agent against which others are compared. Biologic agents can produce dramatic responses at dramatic expense. Rotating therapeutic agents that have varying toxicities have conceptual appeal, and combination therapy may reduce toxicity and reduce the incidence of neutralizing antibodies to agents such as infliximab. Attention should be paid to comorbidities including metabolic syndrome, cardiac risk, and joint manifestations.

Topical treatment

Corticosteroids

Topical application of corticosteroids in creams, ointments, lotions, foams, and sprays is the most frequently prescribed therapy for psoriasis. Class I steroids are suitable for 2-week courses of therapy on most body areas. Therapy can be continued with pulse applications on weekends to reduce the incidence of local adverse effects. On the scalp, corticosteroids in propylene glycol, gel, foam, and spray bases are preferred by most white patients. Black patients may find them drying, and may prefer oil and ointment preparations. Low to mid-strength creams are preferred in the intertriginous areas and on the face. To augment effectiveness of topical corticosteroids in areas with thick keratotic scale, the area should be hydrated prior to application, and covered with an occlusive dressing of a polyethylene film (Saran wrap) or a sauna suit. Unfortunately, there is typically a rapid recurrence of disease when topical corticosteroid therapy is discontinued. Side effects include epidermal atrophy, steroid acne, miliaria, and pyoderma.

Intralesional injections of triamcinolone are helpful for refractory plaques. Triamcinolone acetonide (Kenalog) suspension, 10 mg/mL, may be diluted with sterile saline to make a concentration of 2.5–5 mg/mL. Good results are also obtained in the treatment of psoriatic nails by injecting triamcinolone into the region of the matrix and the lateral nailfold. A digital block can be performed prior to injection to provide anesthesia. Injections are given once a month until the desired effect is achieved.

Tars

Crude coal tar, and tar extracts such as liquor carbonis detergens, can be compounded into agents for topical use. Tar bath oils and shampoos are readily available. Oil of cade (pine tar) or birch tar in concentrations of 5–10% may also be incorporated into ointments. The odor of all tars may be offensive.

Anthralin

Anthralin is effective, but is irritating and stains skin, clothing, and bedding. To avoid these drawbacks, short-contact anthralin treatment (SCAT) can be helpful, with anthralin washed off after 15–30 min. In warmer climates, SCAT is often done outdoors to keep the mess out of the house. Anthralin exerts a direct effect on keratinocytes and leukocytes by suppressing neutrophil superoxide generation and inhibiting monocyte-derived IL-6, IL-8, and TNF-α.

Tazarotene

Tazarotene is a nonisomerizable retinoic acid receptor-specific retinoid. It appears to treat psoriasis by modulating keratinocyte differentiation and hyperproliferation, as well as by suppressing inflammation. Combining its use with a topical corticosteroid and weekend pulse therapy can decrease irritation.

Calcipotriene

Vitamin D_3 affects keratinocyte differentiation partly through its regulation of epidermal responsiveness to calcium. Treatment with the vitamin D analog calcipotriene (Dovonex) in ointment, cream, or solution form has been shown to be very effective in the treatment of plaque-type and scalp psoriasis. Combination therapy with calcipotriene and high-potency steroids may provide greater response rates, fewer side effects, and steroid-sparing. Calcipotriene is unstable in the presence of many other topical agents and degrades in the presence of UV light. Monitoring of serum calcium levels in adults is not required. Calcipotriene plus betamethasone dipropionate (Taclonex) is more effective than either agent alone.

Macrolactams (calcineurin inhibitors)

Topical macrolactams such as tacrolimus and pimecrolimus are especially helpful for thin lesions in areas prone to atrophy or steroid acne. The burning commonly associated with these agents can be problematic, but may be avoided by prior treatment with a corticosteroid, and by application to dry skin, rather than after bathing.

Salicylic acid

Salicylic acid is used as a keratolytic agent in shampoos, creams, and gels. It can promote the absorption of other topical agents. Widespread application may lead to salicylate toxicity manifesting with tinnitus, acute confusion, and refractory hypoglycemia, especially in patients with diabetes and those with compromised renal function.

Ultraviolet light

Phototherapy is a cost-effective and underutilized modality for psoriasis. In most instances sunlight improves psoriasis. However, severe burning of the skin may cause the Koebner phenomenon and an exacerbation. Artificial UVB light is produced by fluorescent bulbs in broad-band or narrow-band spectrums. Maximal effect is usually achieved at MEDs. Although suberythemogenic doses can be effective, the response is slower than with erythemogenic regimens. With treatment, a tanning response occurs, and the dose must be increased to maintain efficacy. Maintenance UVB phototherapy after clearing contributes to the duration of remission and is justified for many patients.

Using a monochromator, it has been shown that wavelengths of 254, 280, and 290 nm are ineffective; at 296, 300, 304, and 313 nm there is clearing. Narrow-band UVB (peak emission around 311 nm) has been shown to be more effective in treating psoriasis than broad-band UVB. Erythemogenic doses are not required in order to achieve a response. The response rates are better than 70% and close to those achievable with PUVA therapy.

Goeckerman technique

The Goeckerman technique remains an effective and cost-effective method of treatment. In its modern form, a 2–5% tar preparation is applied to the skin, and a tar bath is taken at least once a day. The excess tar is removed with mineral or vegetable oil, and UV light is given. In psoriasis daycare centers, patients clear in an average of 18 days, and 75% remain free of disease for extended periods. The addition of a topical corticosteroid to the Goeckerman regimen shortens the time required for remission. Phototoxic reactions (tar smarts) may occur as a result of UVA generated by the predominantly UVB bulbs.

Ingram technique

The Ingram technique consists of a daily coal tar bath in a solution such as 120 mL liquor carbonis detergens to 80 L of warm water. This is followed by daily exposure to UV light for increasing periods. An anthralin paste is then applied to each psoriatic plaque. Talcum powder is sprinkled over the lesions and stockinette dressings are applied. Modern versions of the technique employ SCAT.

PUVA therapy

High-intensity longwave UV radiation (UVA) given 2 h after ingestion of 8-methoxypsoralen (Oxsoralen-Ultra), twice a week, is highly effective, even in severe psoriasis. Most patients clear in 20–25 treatments, but maintenance treatment is needed.

Although PUVA therapy is highly effective, in patients with less than 50% of the skin surface affected, UVB may be as good. Polyethylene sheet bath PUVA is another therapeutic alternative to oral psoralen-UVA. The patient is immersed in a psoralen solution contained in plastic sheeting that conforms to the patient's body.

Oral psoralen can produce cataracts, and protective eyewear must be used. PUVA therapy is a risk factor for skin cancer, including squamous cell carcinoma and melanoma. Arsenic exposure is a more significant cofactor than prior exposure to methotrexate, UVB, or concomitant use of topical tar. Men treated without genital protection are at an increased risk of developing squamous cell carcinomas of the penis and scrotum. Although the risk of cancer is dose-related, there is no definitive threshold dose of cumulative PUVA exposure above which carcinogenicity can be predicted.

Surgical treatment

In patients with pharyngeal colonization by streptococci, an excellent response has been reported after tonsillectomy. More effective antibiotic regimens, such as a 10-day course of dicloxacillin combined with rifampin (600 mg/day for an adult), have largely replaced tonsillectomy.

Hyperthermia

Local hyperthermia can clear psoriatic plaques, but relapse is usually rapid. Microwave hyperthermia may produce significant complications, such as pain over bony prominences and tissue destruction.

Occlusive treatment

Occlusion with surgical tape or dressings can be effective as monotherapy or when combined with topical drugs.

Systemic treatment

Corticosteroids

The hazards of the injudicious use of systemic corticosteroids must be emphasized. There is great risk of "rebound" or induction of pustular psoriasis when therapy is stopped. Corticosteroid use is generally restricted to unique circumstances, such as impetigo herpetiformis when expeditious delivery is not possible.

Methotrexate

This folic acid antagonist remains the standard against which other systemic treatments are measured. Methotrexate has a greater affinity for dihydrofolic acid reductase than has folic acid. The indications for the use of methotrexate include psoriatic erythroderma, psoriatic arthritis, acute pustular psoriasis (von Zumbusch type), or widespread body surface involvement. Localized pustular psoriasis or palmoplantar psoriasis that impairs normal function and employment may also require systemic treatment.

It is important to make sure that the patient has no history of liver or kidney disease. Methotrexate can be toxic to the liver and decreased renal clearance can enhance toxicity. Other important factors to consider are alcohol abuse, cryptogenic cirrhosis, severe illness, debility, pregnancy, leukopenia, thrombocytopenia, active infectious disease, immunodeficiency, anemia, colitis, and ability to comply with directions. Hepatic enzymes, bilirubin, serum albumin, creatinine, alkaline phosphatase, complete blood count (CBC), platelet count, hepatitis serology (B and C), HIV antibody, and urinalysis should all be evaluated before starting treatment. Patients with hypoalbuminemia have a higher risk of developing pulmonary complications.

The need for liver biopsy remains controversial. Biopsy is not without risks and is not commonly performed in the setting of methotrexate therapy for rheumatic disease. However, patients with psoriasis have a greater risk of liver disease than other patient populations. In most patients with no risk factors for liver disease, the first liver biopsy is commonly obtained at approximately 1.0–1.5 g of cumulative methotrexate and repeated every subsequent 1.5–2.0 g until a total of 4.0 g is reached. The frequency then changes to every 1.0–1.5 g cumulative intervals. These recommendations are likely to change as more data are evaluated. Weekly blood counts and monthly liver enzyme assessment are recommended at the onset of therapy or when the dosage is changed. Monitoring of aminoterminal procollagen III peptide and metabolic panels that predict the risk of fibrosis (NASH Fibrosure) may reduce the need for liver biopsy.

Numerous treatment schedules have evolved. The authors recommend either three divided oral doses (12 h apart) weekly, weekly single doses orally, or single weekly subcutaneous injections. The weekly dose varies from 5 mg to more than 50 mg, with most patients requiring 15–30 mg a week. Once a single dose exceeds 25 mg, oral absorption is unpredictable and subcutaneous injections are recommended. Mid-week doses can result in severe toxicity and must be avoided. Oral or cutaneous ulceration may be a sign that the patient has taken a mid-week dose. Oral folic acid has been reported to decrease side effects, especially nausea, and doses of 1–4 mg/day are used. Oral folic acid is not adequate for the treatment of overdosage and leukovorin must be used in such cases.

Cyclosporine

The therapeutic benefit of cyclosporine in psoriatic disease may be related to downmodulation of proinflammatory epidermal cytokines. The microemulsion formulation Neoral has greater bioavailability and is now standard. Doses of 2–5 mg/kg/day generally produce rapid clearing of psoriasis. Unfortunately, the lesions recur rapidly as well, and transition to another form of therapy is required. Treatment durations of up to 6 months are associated with a low incidence of renal complications, but blood pressure and serum creatinine must be monitored and doses adjusted accordingly. Usually, the dose is reduced if the baseline creatinine increases by one-third.

Diet

The anti-inflammatory effects of fish oils rich in n-3 polyunsaturated fatty acids have been demonstrated in rheumatoid arthritis, inflammatory bowel disease, psoriasis, and asthma. n-3 and n-6 polyunsaturated fatty acids affect a variety of cytokines, including IL-1, IL-6, and TNF. Herbal remedies have also been used with variable effects. Many of these products are unpalatable, and their efficacy does not compare favorably to pharmacologic agents.

Oral antimicrobial therapy

The association of streptococcal pharyngitis with guttate psoriasis is well established. *Staphylococcus aureus* and streptococci secrete exotoxins that act as superantigens, producing massive T-cell activation. Oral antibiotic therapy for patients with psoriasis infected with these organisms is imperative. The efficacy of antimicrobial agents in other subsets of psoriasis is unclear. Oral bile acid supplementation has been shown to improve psoriasis, presumably by affecting the microflora and endotoxins in the gut. Oral ketoconazole, itraconazole, and other antibiotics have shown efficacy in a limited number of patients with psoriasis.

Retinoids

Oral treatment with the aromatic retinoid ethylester, etretinate, was effective in many patients with psoriasis, especially in pustular disease. Because of its long half-life, the drug has been replaced by acitretin. Alcohol ingestion can convert acitretin to etretinate and is strongly discouraged. 13-*Cis*-retinoic acid can also produce good results in some patients with pustular psoriasis. All of these drugs are potent teratogens and elevations in triglycerides may complicate therapy. Combinations of retinoic acids with photochemotherapy can be effective in chronic plaque psoriasis, resulting in lowered cumulative doses of light.

Dapsone

Dapsone use is limited largely to palmoplantar pustulosis or other variants of pustular psoriasis. Even in this setting, it is a second- or third-line agent with limited efficacy.

Biologic agents

A number of biologic agents are available that can produce dramatic responses in some patients with psoriasis; all are expensive. Three agents block TNF-α. Infliximab is a chimeric monoclonal antibody to TNF-α and requires intravenous infusion; etanercept is a fusion protein of human TNF type II receptor and the Fc region of IgG1; and adalimumab is a recombinant, fully human IgG1 monoclonal antibody to TNF-α. Alefacept is a fusion protein of the external domain of LFA-3 and the Fc region of IgG1; it blocks T-cell activation and triggers apoptosis of pathogenic T cells. Efalizumab, a humanized monoclonal antibody to the CD11a portion of LFA-1, has been withdrawn from the market. Ustekinumab, a human monoclonal antibody against IL-12 and 23, is the first of a new class of agents that appear highly effective. They block the inflammatory pathway at a more proximal point than TNF agents. Neutralizing antibodies may decrease the effectiveness of many of the biologic agents.

Percentage of patients clearing with each drug

Published data allow for various comparisons between biologic agents, but as trials are designed by the manufacturer to demonstrate the efficacy of the agent, the endpoints of some trials differ. In controlled trials of infliximab, the percentage of patients reaching at least 75% improvement from baseline in the psoriasis area and severity index (PASI 75) at week 10 is about 70% with infliximab 3 mg/kg and 90% with 5 mg/kg, as compared to 6% with placebo. About 35% of patients receiving etanercept, 25 mg subcutaneously twice a week, achieve PASI 75 at 12 weeks and 45% at 24 weeks. With the 50 mg induction dose administered twice a week, about 46% of patients achieve PASI 75 at 12 weeks and 50% at 24 weeks. About 14% of patients receiving 12 weekly intramuscular or intravenous injections of alefacept will achieve PASI 75, and about 38% PASI 50. After two 12-injection courses, about 26% of patients reach PASI 75 and 55% PASI 50. The onset of action is somewhat slower than with other agents, but ultimate clearing can be excellent. The data available suggest that about 53% of patients taking 40 mg of adalimumab every other week achieve PASI 75 by week 12, and about 80% of those taking 40 mg a week achieve PASI 75. An analysis of 24 randomized controlled trials including 9384 patients suggested that infliximab was superior to the other agents studied, and that adalimumab was superior to etanercept, 50 mg twice weekly, and cyclosporine. Ustekinumab was included in the study.

A phase III, parallel, double-blind, placebo-controlled study of ustekinumab for moderate to severe psoriasis (45 mg or 90 mg at weeks 0 and 4, and then every 12 weeks) showed that 67.1% of those who received 45 mg and 66.4% receiving 90 mg achieved PASI 75 at week 12. In a second multicenter, phase III, double-blind, placebo-controlled trial of ustekinumab in patients with moderate to severe psoriasis, 66.7% of patients receiving 45 mg and 75.7% receiving 90 mg achieved PASI 75.

Rapidity of clearing and relapse

The effects of infliximab are rapid and similar to those achieved with cyclosporine. In contrast to cyclosporine, clinical improvement after three intravenous infusions of infliximab is maintained for as long as 6 months in approximately half the patients. Adalimumab is also rapid in onset, with many patients demonstrating a response within the first week of treatment. About 15% of patients treated with alefacept will maintain benefits for more than 6 months.

Risks

TNF agents may induce flares of psoriasis through upregulation of plasmacytoid dendritic cells. This may be a class effect. The biologic agents all suppress the normal immune response. Infliximab has been associated with reactivation of tuberculosis, demyelinating disease, and serious systemic opportunistic infection. It may also lose its effect because of neutralizing antibodies. Methotrexate or azathioprine may be needed as concomitant therapy to reduce the incidence of neutralizing antibodies and infusion reactions. Even though adalimumab is a fully human antibody, it may also induce an antibody response. Serious infections have been reported in patients with rheumatoid arthritis treated with this agent. Etanercept has been associated with infection, onset, or exacerbation of multiple sclerosis, vasculitis, and lupus erythematosus-like manifestations. All these manifestations are rare, and may not be statistically increased from the general population. A single 12-week course of alefacept does not appear to impair primary or secondary antibody responses to a neoantigen or memory responses to a recall antigen, but roughly 10% of patients have to interrupt therapy because CD4 counts fall below 250/mm^3, and CD4 counts must be monitored with this agent. Many of the reported complications, such as lymphoma, demyelinating disease, and infection, are not unique to any one biologic agent.

The National Psoriasis Foundation has endorsed a recommendation that all patients be screened for latent tuberculosis infection prior to any immunologic therapy. They recommend delaying immunologic therapy until prophylaxis for latent tuberculosis infection is completed, although they note that patients with severe disease may be treated after 1–2 months of prophylaxis. IFN-γ assays have greater specificity than tuberculin skin tests and are being used along with imaging studies to confirm tuberculosis in patients with positive skin tests.

Combination therapy

In more severe forms of psoriasis a combination of treatment modalities may be employed. In treating patients with methotrexate, for example, concomitant topical agents may be used to minimize the dose. Methotrexate has been combined with infliximab to reduce the incidence of neutralizing antibodies, and has been used with acitretin in managing patients with severe, generalized pustular psoriasis. The use of PUVA and retinoids is called Re-PUVA and has been studied extensively. Acitretin has been combined with biologic agents to treat refractory psoriasis. Combination systemic therapy has the potential to reduce overall toxicity if the toxicities of each agent are different. However, new regimens should be used with caution because the potential for cumulative toxicity or drug interaction exists.

Alternative therapies

Alternative therapies for psoriasis include mycophenolate mofetil, sulfasalazine, paclitaxel, azathioprine, fumaric acid esters, climatotherapy, and Grenz ray therapy. Nail disease can respond to systemic agents, topical retinoids, local triamcinolone injections, and topical 5-fluorouracil. The latter agent can cause onycholysis if applied to the free edge of the nail.

Akaraphanth R, et al: Efficacy of a far erythemogenic dose of narrowband ultraviolet B phototherapy in chronic plaque-type psoriasis. J Dermatol 2010; 37(2):140–145.

Asarch A, et al: Th17 cells: a new paradigm for cutaneous inflammation. J Dermatolog Treat 2008; 19(5):259–266.

Bartlett BL, et al: Ustekinumab for chronic plaque psoriasis. Lancet 2008; 371(9625):1639–1640.

Benoit S, et al: Childhood psoriasis. Clin Dermatol 2007; 25(6):555–562.

Berends MA, et al: Reliability of the Roenigk classification of liver damage after methotrexate treatment for psoriasis: a clinicopathologic study of 160 liver biopsy specimens. Arch Dermatol 2007; 143(12):1515–1519.

Berneburg M, et al: Phototherapy with narrowband vs. broadband UVB. Acta Derm Venereol 2005; 85:98.

Beyer V, et al: Recent trends in systemic psoriasis treatment costs. Arch Dermatol 2010; 146(1):46–54.

Blauvelt A: T-helper 17 cells in psoriatic plaques and additional genetic links between IL-23 and psoriasis. J Invest Dermatol 2008; 128(5):1064–1067.

Boehncke WH, et al: Managing comorbid disease in patients with psoriasis. BMJ 2010 Jan 15; 340:b5666.

Bos JD, et al: Topical treatments in psoriasis: today and tomorrow. Clin Dermatol 2008; 26(5):432–437.

Brimhall AK, et al: Safety and efficacy of alefacept, efalizumab, etanercept and infliximab in treating moderate to severe plaque psoriasis: a meta-analysis of randomized controlled trials. Br J Dermatol 2008; 159(2):274–285.

Cather JC, et al: Combining traditional agents and biologics for the treatment of psoriasis. Semin Cutan Med Surg 2005; 24:37.

Conaghan PG, et al: Improving recognition of psoriatic arthritis. Practitioner 2009; 253(1724):15–18, 2–3.

Davis MD, et al: Goeckerman treatment: neglected in the consensus approach for critically challenging case scenarios in moderate to severe psoriasis. J Am Acad Dermatol 2010; 62(3):508.

Doherty SD, et al: National Psoriasis Foundation consensus statement on screening for latent tuberculosis infection in patients with psoriasis

treated with systemic and biologic agents. J Am Acad Dermatol 2008; 59(2):209–217.

Duffin KC, et al: Genetics of psoriasis and psoriatic arthritis: update and future direction. J Rheumatol 2008; 35(7):1449–1453.

Evers AW, et al: Treatment nonadherence and long-term effects of narrowband UV-B therapy in patients with psoriasis. Arch Dermatol 2010; 146(2):198–199.

Feuchtenberger M, et al: Psoriatic arthritis: therapeutic principles. Clin Dermatol 2008; 26(5):460–463.

Fluhr JW, et al: Emollients, moisturizers, and keratolytic agents in psoriasis. Clin Dermatol 2008; 26(4):380–386.

Gori A, et al: Unusual presentation of tuberculosis in an infliximab-treated patient—which is the correct TB screening before starting a biologic? Dermatol Ther 2010 Jan–Feb; 23(Suppl 1):S1–3.

Gottlieb A, et al: Guidelines of care for the management of psoriasis and psoriatic arthritis: section 2. Psoriatic arthritis: overview and guidelines of care for treatment with an emphasis on the biologics. J Am Acad Dermatol 2008; 58(5):851–864.

Gottlieb AB, et al: Psoriasis and the metabolic syndrome. J Drugs Dermatol 2008; 7(6):563–572.

Halverstam CP, et al: Nonstandard and off-label therapies for psoriasis. Clin Dermatol 2008; 26(5):546–553.

Hernandez C, et al: Tuberculosis in the age of biologic therapy. J Am Acad Dermatol 2008; 59(3):363–380.

Heydendael VM, et al: Methotrexate versus cyclosporine in moderate-to-severe chronic plaque psoriasis. N Engl J Med 2003; 349:658.

Homey B, et al: Chemokines and other mediators as therapeutic targets in psoriasis vulgaris. Clin Dermatol 2008; 26(5):539–545.

Huang W, et al: To test or not to test? An evidence-based assessment of the value of screening and monitoring tests when using systemic biologic agents to treat psoriasis. J Am Acad Dermatol 2008; 58(6):970–977.

Lebwohl M, et al: The evolving role of topical treatments in adjunctive therapy for moderate to severe plaque psoriasis. Cutis 2007; 80(5 Suppl):29–40.

Lebwohl M, et al: From the Medical Board of the National Psoriasis Foundation: monitoring and vaccinations in patients treated with biologics for psoriasis. J Am Acad Dermatol 2008; 58(1):94–105.

Lecluse LL, et al: Extent and clinical consequences of antibody formation against adalimumab in patients with plaque psoriasis. Arch Dermatol 2010; 146(2):127–132.

Leonardi CL, et al: Efficacy and safety of ustekinumab, a human interleukin-12/23 monoclonal antibody, in patients with psoriasis: 76-week results from a randomised, double-blind, placebo-controlled trial (PHOENIX 1). Lancet 2008; 371(9625):1665–1674.

Li YY, et al: Targeting leukocyte recruitment in the treatment of psoriasis. Clin Dermatol 2008; 26(5):527–538.

MacDonald A, et al: Psoriasis: advances in pathophysiology and management. Postgrad Med J 2007; 83(985):690–697. Review.

Maurice PD, et al: Monitoring patients on methotrexate: hepatic fibrosis not seen in patients with normal serum assays of aminoterminal peptide of type III procollagen. Br J Dermatol 2005; 152:451.

Menter A, et al: Guidelines of care for the management of psoriasis and psoriatic arthritis: section 1. Overview of psoriasis and guidelines of care for the treatment of psoriasis with biologics. J Am Acad Dermatol 2008; 58(5):826–850.

Mössner R, et al: Tumor necrosis factor antagonists in the therapy of psoriasis. Clin Dermatol 2008; 26(5):486–502.

Neyns B, et al: Cetuximab treatment in a patient with metastatic colorectal cancer and psoriasis. Curr Oncol 2008; 15(4):196–197.

Nolan BV, et al: A review of home phototherapy for psoriasis. Dermatol Online J 2010; 16(2):1.

Papp KA: Monitoring biologics for the treatment of psoriasis. Clin Dermatol 2008; 26(5):515–521.

Papp KA, et al: Efficacy and safety of ustekinumab, a human interleukin-12/23 monoclonal antibody, in patients with psoriasis: 52-week results from a randomised, double-blind, placebo-controlled trial (PHOENIX 2). Lancet 2008; 371(9625):1675–1684.

Qureshi AA, et al: Psoriatic arthritis screening tools. J Rheumatol 2008; 35(7):1423–1425.

Ritchlin CT: From skin to bone: translational perspectives on psoriatic disease. J Rheumatol 2008; 35(7):1434–1437.

Schneider LA, et al: Phototherapy and photochemotherapy. Clin Dermatol 2008; 26(5):464–476.

Schön MP: Treatment of psoriasis: a journey from empiricism to evidence. Clin Dermatol 2008; 26(5):417–418.

Singh SK, et al: Th17 cells in the pathogenesis of psoriasis. Curr Allergy Asthma Rep 2008; 8(5):382–385.

Taylor WJ, et al: Drug use and toxicity in psoriatic disease: focus on methotrexate. J Rheumatol 2008; 35(7):1454–1457.

Tesmer LA, et al: Th17 cells in human disease. Immunol Rev 2008; 223:87–113.

Thaçi D: Long-term data in the treatment of psoriasis. Br J Dermatol 2008; 159(Suppl 2):18–24.

Warren RB, et al: Systemic therapies for psoriasis: methotrexate, retinoids, and cyclosporine. Clin Dermatol 2008; 26(5):438–447.

Weiss SC, et al: An assessment of the cost-utility of therapy for psoriasis. Ther Clin Risk Manag 2006; 2(3):325–328.

Wozel G: Psoriasis treatment in difficult locations: scalp, nails, and intertriginous areas. Clin Dermatol 2008; 26(5):448–459.

Zell D, et al: Genetic alterations in psoriasis. J Invest Dermatol 2008; 128(7):1614.

Reactive arthritis with conjunctivitis/urethritis/diarrhea (Reiter syndrome)

Reiter syndrome is a characteristic clinical triad of urethritis, conjunctivitis, and arthritis. The disease occurs chiefly in young men of HLA-B27 genotype, generally following a bout of urethritis or diarrheal illness. Systemic involvement can include the gastrointestinal tract, kidneys, central nervous system, and cardiovascular system. As few patients present with the classic triad, the American College of Rheumatology recognizes criteria for limited manifestations of the syndrome, including peripheral arthritis of more than 1 month's duration in association with urethritis, cervicitis, or bilateral conjunctivitis.

Hans Reiter was a Nazi war criminal, involved with or having knowledge of involuntary sterilization, as well as a study of an experimental typhus vaccine that resulted in hundreds of deaths of concentration camp internees. Several authors have suggested that he no longer be afforded the recognition of using his name to designate the syndrome.

Clinical features

Any part of the triad may occur first, often accompanied by fever, weakness, and weight loss. Although the inciting urethritis may be bacterial, later manifestations include a nonbacterial urethritis with painful urination and pyuria. Cystitis, prostatitis, and seminal vesiculitis may be accompaniments. Vulvar ulceration has been reported. About one-third of patients develop conjunctivitis, which may be bulbar, tarsal, or angular. Keratitis is usually superficial and extremely painful. Iritis is common, especially in recurrent cases. Infrequently, optic neuritis may occur. An asymmetric arthritis affects peripheral joints, especially those that are weight-bearing. Its onset is usually sudden. Pain in one or both heels is a frequent symptom. Sacroiliitis may develop in up to two-thirds of patients, most of whom are of HLA-B27 type.

The skin involvement commonly begins with small, guttate, hyperkeratotic, crusted or pustular lesions of the genitals (Fig. 10-12), palms, or soles. Involvement of the glans penis (balanitis circinata) occurs in 25% of patients. Lesions on the soles and trunk often become thickly crusted or hyperkeratotic. The eruption on the soles is known as keratoderma blennorrhagicum (Fig. 10-13), and occurs in 10% of patients. The buccal, palatal, and lingual mucosa may show painless, shallow, red erosions. The nails become thick and brittle, with heavy subungual keratosis. Children are much more likely to have the post-dysenteric form, often with conjunctivitis and arthritis as the most prominent complaints.

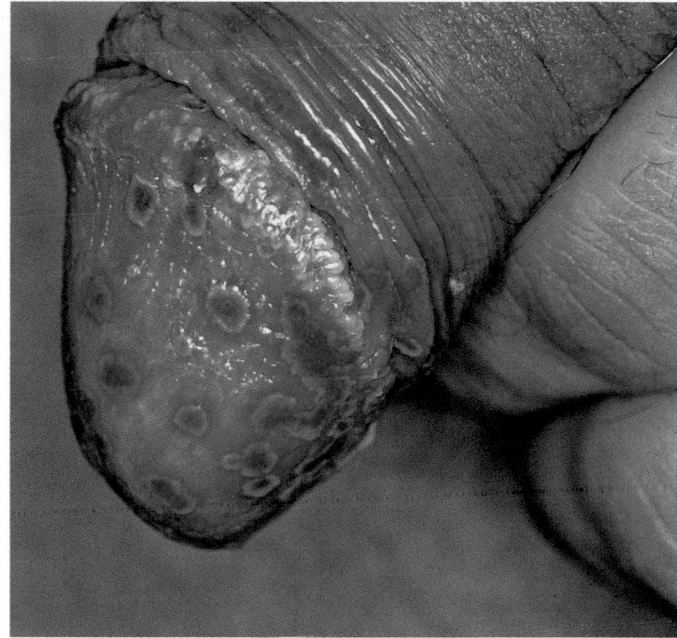

Fig. 10-12 Genital involvement in reactive arthritis.

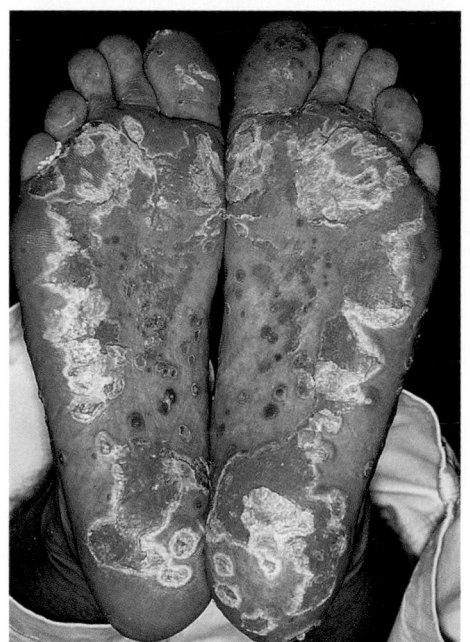

Fig. 10-13 Keratoderma blennorrhagicum.

The syndrome generally follows an infectious urethritis or diarrheal illness. Implicated organisms include *Chlamydia, Shigella, Salmonella, Yersinia, Campylobacter, Ureaplasma, Borrelia, Cryptosporidium*, gonococci, and bacillus Calmette–Guérin (BCG). *Chlamydia trachomatis* and *Ureaplasma urealyticum* have been isolated from the synovial fluid of affected joints, and some patients respond to antibiotic therapy. Reiter syndrome has also been observed in HIV disease, but may not be directly related to the virus, as it frequently occurs under treatment as the immune response improves. The disease has also been triggered by adalimumab and leflunomide in the setting of ankylosing spondyloarthropathy and Crohn disease.

The syndrome involves both infection and the resulting immunologically mediated tissue injury in a genetically predisposed patient. HLA-B27 is present in about 80% of cases. A positive family history is often noted.

Peripheral leukocytosis of 10 000–20 000/mm³ and elevated sedimentation rate are the most consistent findings. There is no specific test for Reiter syndrome.

The differential diagnosis includes rheumatoid arthritis, ankylosing spondylitis, gout, psoriatic arthritis, gonococcal arthritis, acute rheumatic fever, chronic mucocutaneous candidiasis, and serum sickness. The presence of associated mucocutaneous lesions establishes the diagnosis. Some cases of Lyme disease overlap with the syndrome. Individual skin lesions may be indistinguishable from those in psoriasis. Hyperkeratotic lesions generally have a thicker scale crust than most psoriatic plaques, but are otherwise identical.

Mucocutaneous lesions are generally self-limited and clear with topical steroids. Joint disease is managed with rest and NSAIDs. Antibiotics, such as doxycycline, have been effective in some cases. Immunosuppressive agents, such as methotrexate, are commonly employed for refractory joint disease. Infliximab has been successful in treating severe disease. Refractory skin lesions are treated like refractory psoriasis, and severely affected patients have responded to acitretin or cyclosporine.

Panush RS, et al: Retraction of the suggestion to use the term "Reiter's syndrome" sixty-five years later: the legacy of Reiter, a war criminal, should not be eponymic honor but rather condemnation. Arthritis Rheum 2007; 56(2):693–694.

Sampaio-Barros PD, et al: Frequency of HLA-B27 and its alleles in patients with Reiter syndrome: comparison with the frequency in other spondyloarthropathies and a healthy control population. Rheumatol Int 2008; 28(5):483–486.

Thielen AM, et al: Reiter syndrome triggered by adalimumab (Humira) and leflunomide (Arava) in a patient with ankylosing spondylarthropathy and Crohn disease. Br J Dermatol 2007; 156(1):188–189.

Townes JM: Reactive arthritis after enteric infections in the United States: the problem of definition. Clin Infect Dis 2010; 50(2):247–242.

Wallace DJ, et al: The physician Hans Reiter as prisoner of war in Nuremberg: a contextual review of his interrogations (1945–1947). Semin Arthritis Rheum 2003; 32:208.

Yu D, et al: Role of bacteria and HLA-B27 in the pathogenesis of reactive arthritis. Rheum Dis Clin North Am 2003; 29:21.

Subcorneal pustular dermatosis (Sneddon–Wilkinson disease)

In 1956, Sneddon and Wilkinson described a chronic pustular disease, which occurred chiefly in middle-aged women. The pustules are superficial and arranged in annular and serpiginous patterns, especially on the abdomen, axillae, and groins. Cultures from the pustules are sterile. Oral lesions are rare. Some cases are associated with a monoclonal gammopathy (usually IgA). The condition is chronic, with remissions of variable duration.

Histologically, the pustules form below the stratum corneum, as in impetigo. Acantholysis is absent, but spongiform pustules may be noted in the upper epidermis. The histologic differential diagnosis includes pustular psoriasis, and superficial fungal and bacterial infections. Some cases will show upper epidermal intercellular IgA staining.

IgA pemphigus shows significant overlap with subcorneal pustular dermatosis. Presentations of IgA pemphigus include subcorneal pustular dermatosis and intraepidermal neutrophilic IgA dermatosis types. Using immunoblotting techniques, Hashimoto et al have shown that human desmocollin 1 is an autoantigen for the subcorneal pustular dermatosis type of IgA pemphigus.

Localized cases may respond well to topical corticosteroids. Dapsone, 50–200 mg/day (for an adult), is effective for most of the remaining cases. Some patients have responded better to sulfapyridine therapy. Acitretin, narrow-band UVB phototherapy, colchicine, azithromycin, biologicals, and tetracycline with niacinamide may also be effective.

Bedi MKL: Successful treatment of long-standing, recalcitrant subcorneal pustular dermatosis with etanercept. Skinmed 2007 Sep–Oct; 6(5):245–247.

Bliziotis I, et al: Regression of subcorneal pustular dermatosis type of IgA pemphigus lesions with azithromycin. J Infect 2005; 51:E31.

Cheng S, et al: Subcorneal pustular dermatosis: 50 years on. Clin Exp Dermatol 2008; 33(3):229–233.

Howell SM, et al: Rapid response of IgA pemphigus of the subcorneal pustular dermatosis subtype to treatment with adalimumab and mycophenolate mofetil. J Am Acad Dermatol 2005; 53:541.

Eosinophilic pustular folliculitis

Eosinophilic pustular folliculitis (EPF) was first described in 1970 by Ofuji but is also referred to as sterile eosinophilic pustulosis. It occurs more commonly in males, and is mostly reported in Asia. The mean age of onset is 35. It is characterized by pruritic, follicular papulopustules that measure 1–2 mm. The lesions tend to be grouped and plaques commonly form. New lesions may form at the edges of the plaques, leading to peripheral extension, while central clearing takes place. The most frequent site is the face, particularly over the cheeks. The trunk and upper extremities are commonly affected, and 20% have palmoplantar pustules. The distribution is commonly asymmetrical, and the typical course is one of spontaneous remissions and exacerbations lasting several years. The condition must be distinguished from HIV-associated eosinophilic folliculitis, which is discussed in Chapter 19. A similar condition has occurred in association with hepatitis C virus infection, with allopurinol, and during pregnancy.

Histologically, there is spongiosis and vesiculation of the follicular infundibulum and heavy infiltration with eosinophils. Follicular mucinosis may be present. There is a peripheral eosinophilia in half the cases, and pulmonary eosinophilia has been described. The cause is unknown; but numerous studies have implicated chemotactic substances, ICAM-1, and cyclooxygenase-generated metabolites. Tryptase-positive and chymase-negative mast cells have also been implicated.

Indomethacin is effective in the vast majority of patients. Topical and intralesional corticosteroids, clofazimine, minocycline, isotretinoin, UVB therapy, dapsone, colchicine, cyclosporine, and cetirizine have also been reported as effective.

Childhood cases have been described. This subset differs from the typical cases in Asian males. Pediatric patients develop sterile pustules and papules preferentially over the scalp, although scattered clusters of pustules may occur over the trunk and extremities. Leukocytosis and eosinophilia are often present. Recurrent exacerbations and remissions usually occur, with eventual spontaneous resolution. High-potency topical steroids are the treatment of choice in pediatric patients.

Gul U, et al: Eosinophilic pustular folliculitis: the first case associated with hepatitis C virus. J Dermatol 2007; 34(6):397–399.

Kus S, et al: Eosinophilic pustular folliculitis (Ofuji's disease) exacerbated with pregnancies. J Eur Acad Dermatol Venereol 2006; 20(10):1347–1348.

Sufyan W, et al: Eosinophilic pustular folliculitis. Arch Pathol Lab Med 2007; 131(10):1598–1601.

Yoneda K, et al: Eosinophilic pustular folliculitis associated with pulmonary eosinophilia. J Eur Acad Dermatol Venereol 2007 Sep; 21(8):1122–1124.

Dermatitis repens

Dermatitis repens, also known as acrodermatitis continua and acrodermatitis perstans, is a chronic inflammatory disease of the hands and feet. It usually remains stable on the extremities, but in rare cases generalized pustular flares may occur. The disease usually begins distally on a digit, either as a pustule in the nailbed or as a paronychia. Extension takes place by eruption of fresh pustules with subsequent hyperkeratosis and crusting. The disease is usually unilateral in its beginning and asymmetrical throughout its entire course. As the disease progresses, one or more of the nails may become dystrophic or float away on lakes of pus. Anonychia is common in chronic cases. Some have used the term dermatitis repens to refer to more indolent involvement of the distal fingers.

Involvement of the mucous membranes may occur, even when the eruption of the skin is localized. Painful, circular, white plaques surrounded by inflammatory areolae are found on the tongue and may form a fibrinous membrane. Fissured or geographic tongue may occur.

Histologically, intraepithelial spongiform pustules identical to those of psoriasis are seen in the acute stage. Later stages show hyperkeratosis with parakeratosis or atrophy.

Numerous treatment options have been used, including topical corticosteroids, calipotriene, dapsone, sulfapyridine, methotrexate, PUVA, acitretin, cyclosporine, and topical mechlorethamine. The decision regarding which agent to use should take into consideration the severity of disease, and the patient's age and functional impairment.

Palmoplantar pustulosis (pustular psoriasis of the extremities)

Chronic palmoplantar pustulosis is essentially a bilateral and symmetrical dermatosis (Fig. 10-14). The favorite locations are the thenar or hypothenar eminences or the central portion of the palms and soles. The patches begin as erythematous areas in which minute intraepidermal pustules form. At the beginning these are pinhead-sized; then they may enlarge and coalesce to form small lakes of pus. As the lesions resolve, denuded areas, crusts, or hyperkeratosis may persist. Palmoplantar pustulosis is strongly associated with thyroid disorders and cigarette smoking. Medications such as lithium, which aggravate psoriasis, have also been reported to induce palmoplantar pustular psoriasis.

In 1968, Kato described the first case of bilateral clavicular osteomyelitis with palmar and plantar pustulosis. In 1974, Sonozaki described persistent palmoplantar pustulosis and sternoclavicular hyperostosis. These conditions belong to the spectrum of skin and joint involvement designated by Kahn as the SAPHO syndrome (synovitis, acne, pustulosis, hyperostosis, and osteitis). Common features include palmoplantar pustulosis, acneiform eruption, and pain and swelling of a sternoclavicular joint, or sternomanubrial or costochondral junctions. There is shoulder, neck, and back pain, and limitation of motion of the shoulders and neck is common. Brachial plexus neuropathy and subclavian vein occlusion may occur. The lumbar spine and sacroiliac joints are usually spared. Chronic multifocal osteomyelitis in children may be a pediatric variant. Others have described an association between palmoplantar pustulosis and arthritis or osteitis. SAPHO syndrome may coexist with features of Behçet's disease. The knees, spine, and ankles may be involved. Ivory vertebrae have been described.

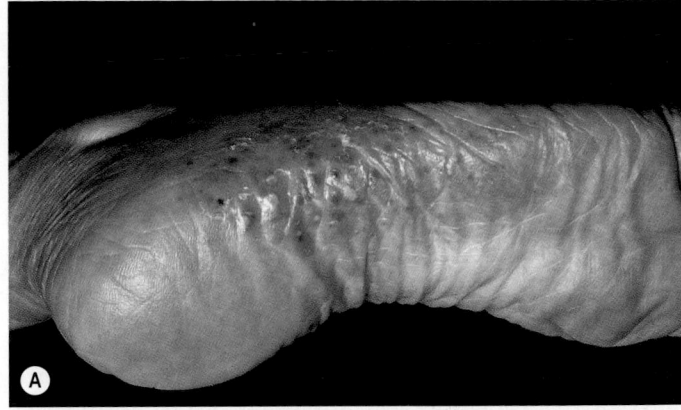

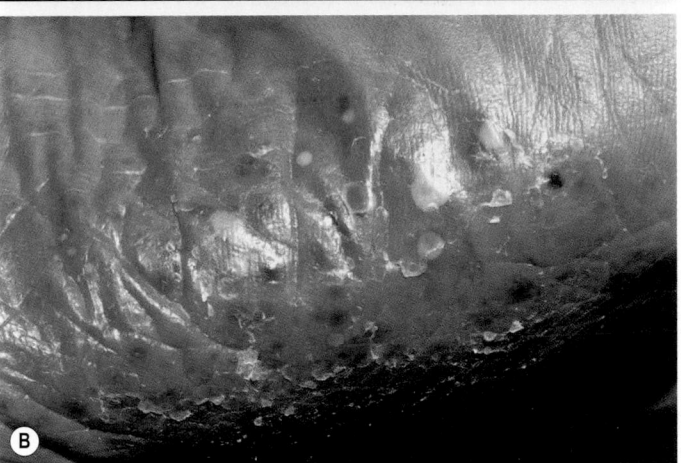

Fig. 10-14 A. Plantas pustulosis; B. Pustules and hyperkeratosis are typical.

The disease is commonly resistant to treatment. Topical steroids, retinoids, calcipotriene, or macrolactams are of some benefit. Acitretin is generally extremely effective at a dose of 1 mg/kg/day, although rebound occurs more quickly than with etretinate. Low-dose cyclosporine, in doses ranging from 1.25 to 5 mg/kg/day, has also been very effective, but it is not suitable for long-term treatment. Dapsone, colchicine, leflunomide, and mycophenolate mofetil may be effective. Oral 8-methoxypsoralen and high-intensity UVA irradiation or soak PUVA can both be helpful, and Grenz ray therapy can induce prolonged remissions in some patients. Chronic osteomyelitis in SAPHO syndrome has been reported to respond to bisphosphonates.

Blanco JF, et al: Ivory vertebra and palmoplantar pustulosis. J Rheumatol 2007 Apr; 34(4):896–899.

Hurtado-Nedelec M, et al: Characterization of the immune response in the synovitis, acne, pustulosis, hyperostosis, osteitis (SAPHO) syndrome. Rheumatology (Oxford) 2008; 47(8):1160–1167.

Nikkels AF, et al: Breaking the relentless course of Hallopeau's acrodermatitis by dapsone. Eur J Dermatol 1999; 9:126.

Piquero-Casals J, et al: Using oral tetracycline and topical betamethasone valerate to treat acrodermatitis continua of Hallopeau. Cutis 2002; 70:106.

Proença NG: Acropustulosis repens. Int J Dermatol 2006; 45(4):389–393.

Skov L, et al: IL-8 as antibody therapeutic target in inflammatory diseases: reduction of clinical activity in palmoplantar pustulosis. J Immunol 2008; 181(1):669–679.

Yabe H, et al: Two cases of SAPHO syndrome accompanied by classic features of Behçet's disease and review of the literature. Clin Rheumatol 2008; 27(1):133–135.

Pustular bacterid

Pustular bacterid was first described by George Andrews. It is characterized by a symmetric, grouped, vesicular, or pustular eruption on the palms and soles, marked by exacerbations and remissions over long periods. Andrews regarded the discovery of a remote focus of infection, and cure on its elimination, as crucial to the diagnosis.

The primary lesions are pustules. Tiny hemorrhagic puncta intermingled with the pustules are frequently seen. When lesions are so numerous as to coalesce, they form a honeycomb-like structure in the epidermis. The disease usually begins on the mid-portions of the palms or soles, from which it spreads outwardly until it may eventually cover the entire flexor aspects of the hands and feet. There is no involvement of the webs of the fingers or toes, as in tinea pedis.

When the eruption is fully developed, both palms and soles are completely covered, and the symmetry is pronounced. During fresh outbreaks, the white blood count may show a leukocytosis that ranges from 12 000 to 19 000/mm^3 with 65–80% neutrophils. As a rule, scaling is present in fully evolved lesions, and the scales are adherent, tough, and dry. During exacerbations, crops of pustules or vesicles make their appearance, and there is often severe itching of the areas. Tenderness may be present. Many regard this condition as a variant of psoriasis, triggered by infection.

Bacharach-Buhles M, et al: The pustular bacterid (Andrews): are there clinical criteria for differentiating from psoriasis pustulosa palmaris et plantaris? Hautarzt (Germany) 1993; 44:221.
Worret WI: Pustular bacterid of Andrews. Am J Dermatopathol 1985; 7:200.

Infantile acropustulosis

Infantile acropustulosis is an intensely itchy vesicopustular eruption of the hands and feet (Fig. 10-15). Most cases begin by 10 months of age. Lesions often predominate at the edges of the palms and soles. Individual crops of lesions clear in a few weeks, but recurrences may continue for months or years. Scabies, tinea, and herpetic infection can produce similar lesions, and must be excluded.

Histologically, a subcorneal pustule with neutrophils is noted. Eosinophils may be numerous. As the lesions are easily punctured to produce smears of the inflammatory cells, biopsies are seldom employed.

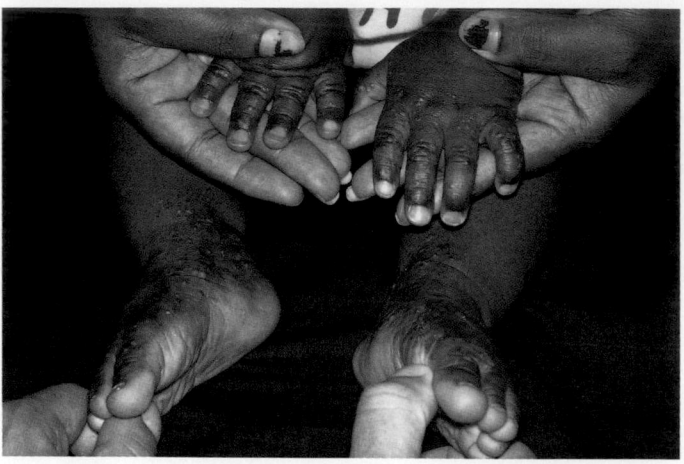

Fig. 10-15 Acropustulosis of infancy. (Courtesy of Curt Samlaska, MD)

Lesions often respond to topical corticosteroids. Refractory lesions may respond to dapsone at doses of 1–2 mg/kg/day.

Vicente J, et al: Are eosinophilic pustular folliculitis of infancy and infantile acropustulosis the same entity? Br J Dermatol 1996; 135:807.
Wagner A: Distinguishing vesicular and pustular disorders in the neonate. Curr Opin Pediatr 1997; 9:396.

 Bonus images for this chapter can be found online at

http://www.expertconsult.com

Fig. 10-1 Seborrheic dermatitis.
Fig. 10-2 Seborrheic dermatitis involving the chest and axillae.
Fig. 10-3 Psoriasis.
Fig. 10-4 Psoriasis plaque, red plaque with silver scale on the knee.
Fig. 10-5 Inverse psoriasis.
Fig. 10-6 Nail pitting and distal onycholysis in psoriasis.
Fig. 10-7 Fissured and geographic tongue in a patient with generalized pustular psoriasis.
Fig. 10-8 Nailbed involvement in acrodermatitis continua.
Fig. 10-9 Anonychia in acrodermatitis continua.
Fig. 10-10 Erythrodermic psoriasis.
Fig. 10-11 Hyperkeratotic lesions of the reactive arthritis syndrome.
Fig. 10-12 Plantar pustulosis.
Fig. 10-13 Psoriasis.

Pityriasis Rosea, Pityriasis Rubra Pilaris, and Other Papulosquamous and Hyperkeratotic Diseases

11

Small plaque parapsoriasis

Small plaque parapsoriasis (SPP) is characterized by hyperpigmented or yellowish-red scaling patches, round to oval in configuration, with sharply defined, regular borders. Most lesions occur on the trunk, and all are between 1 and 5 cm in diameter. In the digitate variant, yellowish-tan, elongated, fingerprint-like lesions are oriented along the cleavage lines, predominately on the flank (Fig. 11-1). These lesions may at times be longer than 5 cm. There is an absence of the induration, erythematous to purplish-red, large lesions, and poikiloderma that characterize small patches of cutaneous T-cell lymphoma in its early stages. The eruption may be mildly itchy or asymptomatic, and has a definite male preponderance. Typical SPP rarely progresses to mycosis fungoides (MF), although the histologic changes can overlap and clonality may be demonstrated. Debate continues on this issue. SPP has been reported in the setting of liposarcoma, with resolution of the eruption after resection of the tumor.

The histologic findings of SPP are characterized by an infiltrate in the superficial dermis composed predominantly of lymphocytes. The overlying epidermis demonstrates mild acanthosis, spongiosis, and focal overlying parakeratosis. SPP is considered to be a type of chronic spongiotic dermatitis. Lesional skin also demonstrates an increase in CD1a(+), Langerhans cells, CD1a-positive dermal dendritic cells, and CD68(+) macrophages.

SPP may be refractory to topical steroids alone, but usually responds to phototherapy. Treatment with ultraviolet (UV) B, narrow-band UVB, or natural sunlight, alone or in combination with a low-strength topical steroid or simple lubricant, will usually clear SPP. Without treatment, the patches of SPP may persist for years to decades and rarely, if ever, progress to lymphoma.

Aydogan K: Narrowband UVB phototherapy for small plaque parapsoriasis. J Eur Acad Dermatol Venereol 2006 May; 20(5):573–577.

Belousova IE, et al: A patient with clinicopathologic features of small plaque parapsoriasis presenting later with plaque-stage mycosis fungoides: report of a case and comparative retrospective study of 27 cases of "nonprogressive" small plaque parapsoriasis. J Am Acad Dermatol 2008 Sep; 59(3):474–482.

Tartaglia F, et al: Retroperitoneal liposarcoma associated with small plaque parapsoriasis. World J Surg Oncol 2007 Jul 9; 5:76.

Zeybek ND, et al: Immunohistochemical analysis of small plaque parapsoriasis: involvement of dendritic cells. Acta Histochem 2008; 110(5):380–387.

Confluent and reticulated papillomatosis (Gougerot and Carteaud)

This eruption typically begins on the intermammary and upper lateral trunk as slightly scaly macules that slowly spread to involve the remainder of the trunk (Fig. 11-2). In white

patients, the lesions vary from skin-colored or faintly erythematous to hyperpigmented; in pigmented persons, lesions usually show hyperpigmentation, although a non-pigmenting form with fine white scale has been described. There may be severe itching or the lesions may be entirely asymptomatic. Familial cases have been reported. An actinomycete, dubbed *Dietzia papillomatosis*, has been isolated from lesional skin.

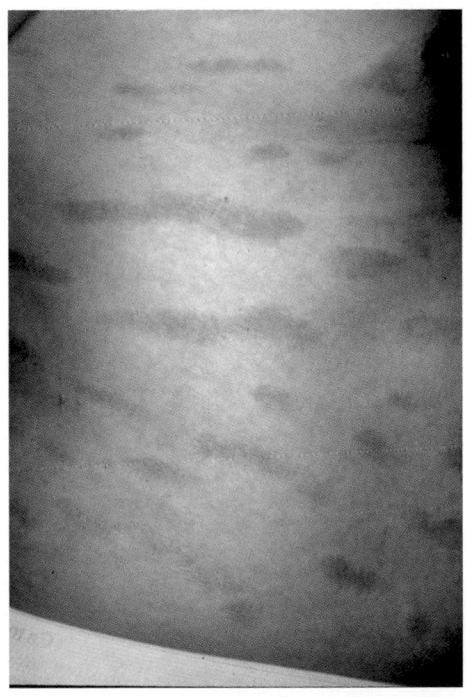
Fig. 11-1 Digitate parapsoriasis. (Courtesy of Thomas Nicotori, MD)

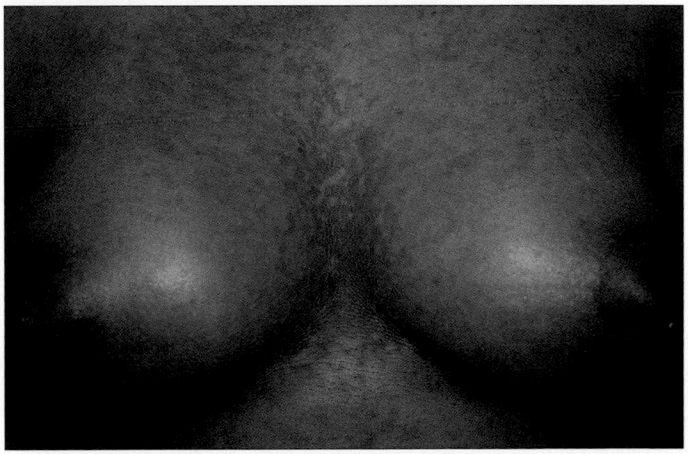
Fig. 11-2 Confluent and reticulated papillomatosis.

Histologically, hyperkeratosis, acanthosis, and papillomatosis are generally seen. The histologic changes resemble those seen in acanthosis nigricans, and the two conditions may occur together.

A variety of antibiotics have been successful in treating the disorder. Minocycline, 100 mg twice a day for 6 weeks, is used most commonly. Successful treatment has also been reported with oral fusidic acid, clarithromycin, amoxicillin, erythromycin, azithromycin, and topical mupirocin. Topical and oral retinoids have also been used successfully, either alone or in combination with topical lactic acid or urea. Confluent and reticulated papillomatosis associated with polycystic ovarian syndrome has responded to contraceptive therapy. Low-dose isotretinoin has also been used.

Pseudo-atrophoderma colli may be a related condition that occurs on the neck. It manifests as papillomatous, pigmented, and atrophic glossy lesions with delicate wrinkling. They tend to have a vertical orientation and may respond to minocycline.

Cannavò SP: Confluent and reticulated papillomatosis and acanthosis nigricans in an obese girl: two distinct pathologies with a common pathogenetic pathway or a unique entity dependent on insulin resistance? J Eur Acad Dermatol Venereol 2006 Apr; 20(4):478–480.

Davis MD, et al: Confluent and reticulate papillomatosis (Gougerot–Carteaud syndrome): a minocycline-responsive dermatosis without evidence for yeast in pathogenesis. A study of 39 patients and a proposal of diagnostic criteria. Br J Dermatol 2006 Feb; 154(2):287–293.

Davis RF, et al: Confluent and reticulated papillomatosis successfully treated with amoxicillin. Br J Dermatol 2007 Mar; 156(3):583–584.

Erkek E, et al: Confluent and reticulated papillomatosis: favourable response to low-dose isotretinoin. J Eur Acad Dermatol Venereol 2009; 23(11):1342–1343.

Jones AL, et al: *Dietzia papillomatosis* sp. nov., a novel actinomycete isolated from the skin of an immunocompetent patient with confluent and reticulated papillomatosis. Int J Syst Evol Microbiol 2008 Jan; 58(Pt 1):68–72.

Treat JR, et al: Nonpigmenting confluent and reticulated papillomatosis. Pediatr Dermatol 2006 Sep–Oct; 23(5):497–499.

Pityriasis rosea

Clinical features

Pityriasis rosea is a mild inflammatory exanthem characterized by salmon-colored papular and macular lesions that are at first discrete but may become confluent (Fig. 11-3). The individual patches are oval or circinate, and are covered with finely crinkled, dry epidermis, which often desquamates, leaving a collarette of scaling. When stretched across the long axis, the scales tend to fold across the lines of stretch, the so-called "hanging curtain" sign. The disease most frequently begins with a single herald or mother patch (Fig. 11-4), usually larger than succeeding lesions, which may persist a week or longer before others appear. By the time involution of the herald patch has begun, the efflorescence of new lesions spreads rapidly (Fig. 11-5), and after 3–8 weeks they usually disappear spontaneously. Relapses and recurrences are observed infrequently. The incidence is highest between the ages of 15 and 40, and the disease is most prevalent in the spring and autumn. Women are more frequently affected than men.

The fully developed eruption has a striking appearance because of the distribution and definite characteristics of the individual lesions. These are arranged so that the long axis of the macules runs parallel to the lines of cleavage. The eruption is usually generalized, affecting chiefly the trunk and sparing sun-exposed surfaces. At times it is localized to a certain area, such as the neck, thighs, groins, or axillae. In these regions confluent circinate patches with gyrate borders may be formed; these may strongly resemble tinea corporis. Rarely, the eyelids, palms and soles, scalp, or penis may be involved. Oral lesions are relatively uncommon. They are asymptomatic,

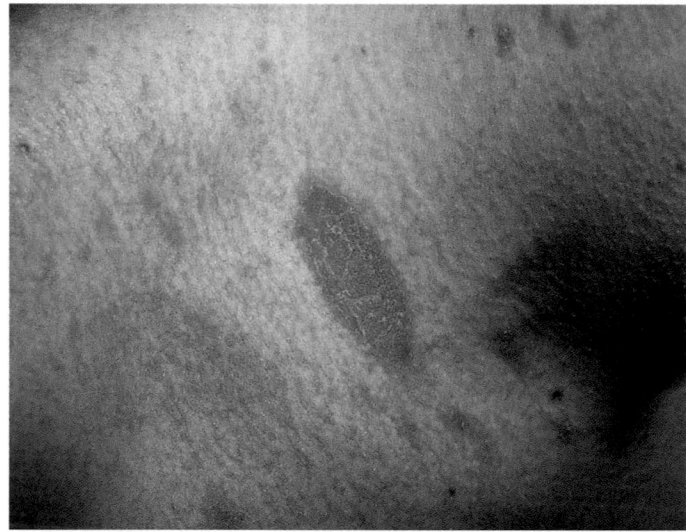

Fig. 11-4 Herald patch of pityriasis rosea.

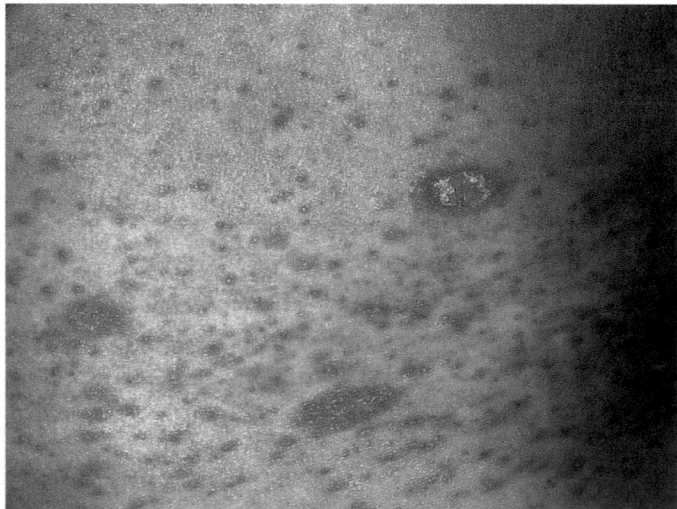

Fig. 11-3 Pityriasis rosea.

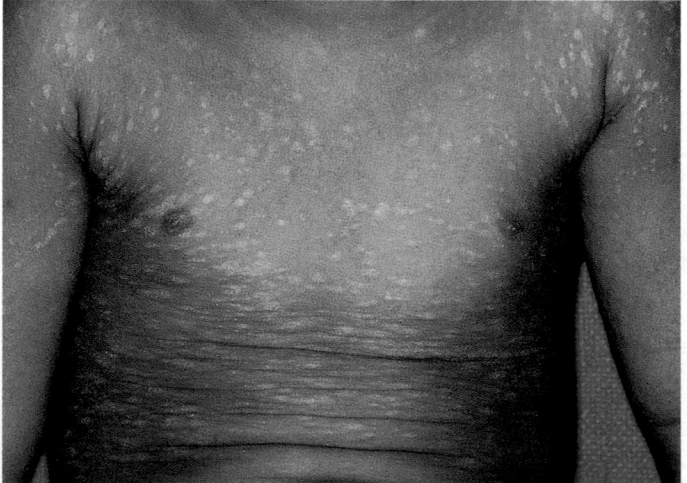

Fig. 11-5 Pityriasis rosea.

erythematous macules with raised borders and clearing centers or aphthous ulcer-like lesions. They involve simultaneously with the skin lesions. Moderate pruritus may be present, particularly during the outbreak, and there may be mild constitutional symptoms before the onset.

Variations in the mode of onset, course, and clinical manifestations are extremely common. An unusual form, common in children under age 5, is papular pityriasis rosea, occurring in the typical sites and running a course similar to that of the common form of pityriasis rosea. Black children are particularly predisposed to this papular variant, and are also more prone to facial and scalp involvement. The lesions often heal, leaving hypopigmented macules. An inverse distribution, sparing covered areas, is not rare and is common in papular cases. A vesicular variant has also been described. Purpuric pityriasis rosea may manifest with petechiae and ecchymoses along Langer lines of the neck, trunk, and proximal extremities, and may occasionally be a sign of an underlying acute myeloid leukaemia. Pityriasis rosea occurring during pregnancy may be associated with premature delivery, neonatal hypotonia, and fetal loss, especially if the eruption occurs within the first 15 weeks of gestation.

Etiology

Watanabe et al have provided evidence for the long-held belief that pityriasis rosea is a viral exanthem. They demonstrated active replication of human herpesvirus (HHV)-6 and 7 in mononuclear cells of lesional skin, as well as identifying the viruses in serum samples of patients. Although these viruses are nearly universally acquired in early childhood and remain in a latent phase as mononuclear cells, the eruption is likely secondary to reactivation leading to viremia.

A pityriasis rosea-like eruption may occur as a reaction to captopril, imatinib mesylate, interferon, ketotifen, arsenicals, gold, bismuth, clonidine, methoxypromazine, tripelennamine hydrochloride, ergotamine, lisinopril, acyclovir, lithium, adalimumab, or barbiturates.

Histology

The histologic features of pityriasis rosea include mild acanthosis, focal parakeratosis, and extravasation of erythrocytes into the epidermis. Spongiosis may be present in acute cases. A mild perivascular infiltrate of lymphocytes is found in the dermis. Histologic evaluation is especially helpful in excluding the conditions with which pityriasis rosea may be confused.

Differential diagnosis

Pityriasis rosea may closely mimic seborrheic dermatitis, tinea corporis, macular syphilid, drug eruption, other viral exanthema, and psoriasis. In seborrheic dermatitis, the scalp and eyebrows are usually scaly; there is a predilection for the sternal and interscapular regions, and the flexor surfaces of the articulations, where the patches are covered with greasy scales. Tinea corporis is rarely so widespread. Tinea versicolor may also closely simulate pityriasis rosea. A positive KOH examination serves well to differentiate these last two. In macular syphilid, the lesions are of a uniform size and assume a brownish tint. Scaling and itching are absent or slight, and there are generalized adenopathy, mucous membrane lesions, palmoplantar lesions, positive nontreponemal and treponemal tests, and often the remains of a chancre. Scabies and lichen planus may be confused with the papular type.

Treatment

Most patients require no therapy, as they are asymptomatic; however, the duration of the eruption may be notably reduced by several interventions. A Cochrane database review cited inadequate evidence for efficacy for most published treatments, but it should be noted that lack of evidence does not equate to lack of efficacy. They cited some evidence that oral erythromycin may be effective for both the rash and the itch, although this is based on only one small randomized controlled trial (see below).

UVB in erythema exposures may be used to expedite the involution of the lesions after the acute inflammatory stage has passed. The erythema produced by UV treatment is succeeded by superficial exfoliation. In a comparison study by Leenutaphong et al, using a "placebo" of 1 J UVA on the untreated side compared with the UVB-treated side, there was significant improvement in the severity of the disease on the treated side. However, there was no difference in itchiness or the course of the disease. Corticosteroid lotions or creams provide some relief from itching. One study found erythromycin, 250 mg four times a day for adults and 25–40 mg/kg in four divided doses a day for children, over a 2-week period resulted in complete clearance of all lesions. This response in 33 of 45 patients contrasted with the fact that none of the 45 placebo patients had the same response. Other studies have challenged the effectiveness of erythromycin, and more research is needed. For dryness and irritation, simple emollients are advised.

Balci DD, et al: Vesicular pityriasis rosea: an atypical presentation. Dermatol Online J 2008 Mar 15; 14(3):6.

Broccolo F, et al: Additional evidence that pityriasis rosea is associated with reactivation of human herpes 6 and 7. J Invest Dermatol 2005; 127:1234.

Chuh AA, et al: Interventions for pityriasis rosea. Cochrane Database Syst Rev 2007 Apr 18; (2):CD005068.

Drago F, et al: Pregnancy outcome in patients with pityriasis rosea. J Am Acad Dermatol 2008 May; 58(5 Suppl 1):S78–83.

Drago F, et al: Pityriasis rosea: an update with a critical appraisal of its possible herpesviral etiology. J Am Acad Dermatol 2009; 61(2):303–318.

Gündüz O, et al: Childhood pityriasis rosea. Pediatr Dermatol 2009; 26(6):750–751.

Rajpara SN, et al: Adalimumab-induced pityriasis rosea. J Eur Acad Dermatol Venereol 2007 Oct; 21(9):1294–1296.

Rasi A, et al: Oral erythromycin is ineffective in the treatment of pityriasis rosea. J Drugs Dermatol 2008 Jan; 7(1):35–38.

Singal A, et al: Purpuric pityriasis rosea-like eruption: a cutaneous marker of acute myeloid leukaemia. J Eur Acad Dermatol Venereol 2007 Jul; 21(6):822–823.

Pityriasis rubra pilaris

Clinical features

Pityriasis rubra pilaris (PRP) is a chronic skin disease characterized by small follicular papules, disseminated yellowish-pink scaling patches, and, often, solid confluent palmoplantar hyperkeratosis. The papules are the most important diagnostic feature, being more or less acuminate, reddish-brown, about pinhead-sized, and topped by a central horny plug (Fig. 11-6). A hair, or part of one, is usually embedded in the horny center. The highest incidence of onset is during the first 5 years of life or between the ages of 51 and 55. The classic disease generally manifests first by scaliness and erythema of the scalp. The eruption is limited in the beginning, having a predilection for the sides of the neck and trunk, and the extensor surfaces of the extremities, especially the backs of the first and second phalanges. Then, as new lesions occur, extensive areas are

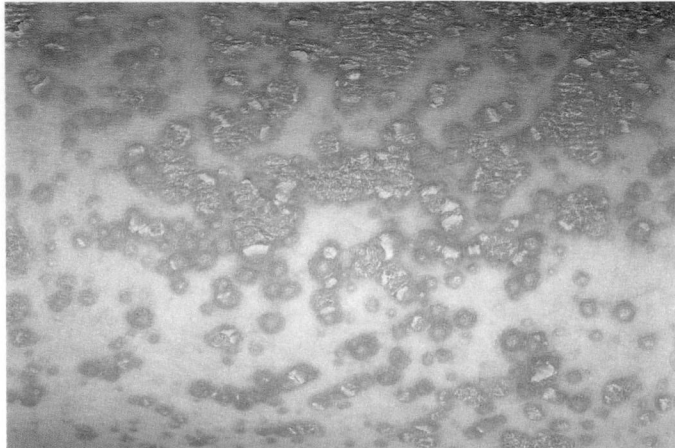

Fig. 11-6 Pityriasis rubra pilaris.

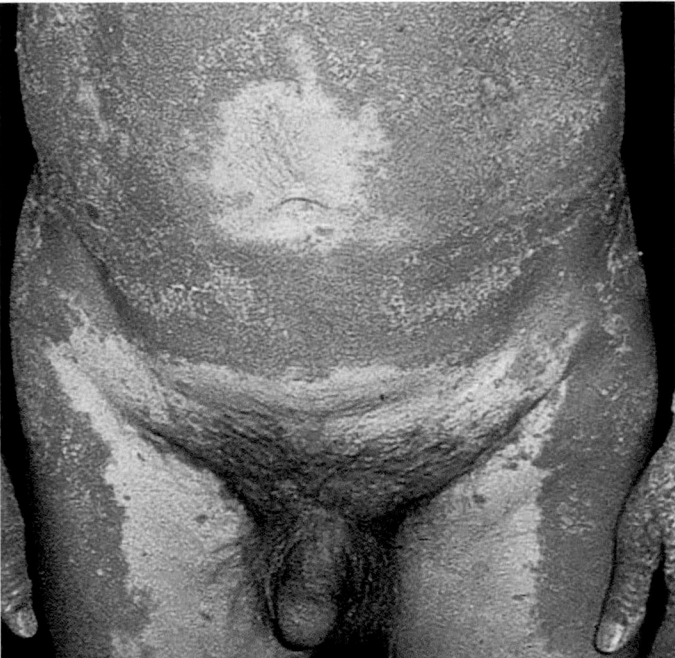

Fig. 11-7 Islands of sparing in pityriasis rubra pilaris.

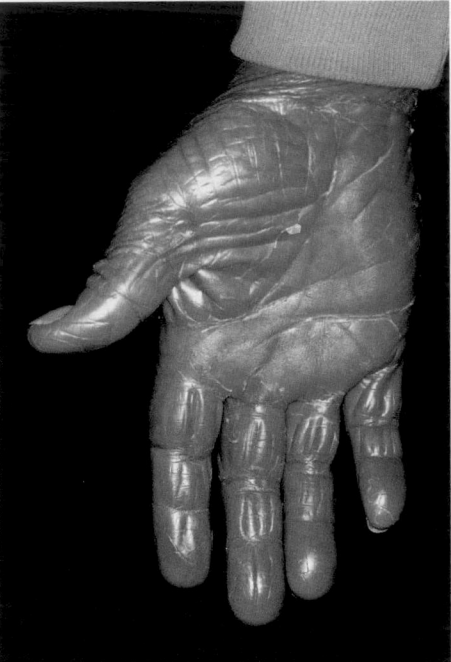

Fig. 11-8 Palmar hyperkeratosis in pityriasis rubra pilaris.

findings. Protein-losing enteropathy may occur. Both hypothyroidism and hypoparathyroidism have been reported, as has the combination of sacroiliitis and autoimmune thyroiditis.

PRP may be classified with respect to familial or acquired types, and to the onset of the disease in childhood or in adulthood. Griffith's classification is useful in this regard. Type I, the classic adult type, is seen most commonly and carries a good prognosis, with 80% involuting over a 3-year period. Likewise, most patients with the classic juvenile type (type III) have clearing of the disease in 1 year, although it may recur, even into adulthood. The atypical adult and juvenile variants and the circumscribed juvenile-onset form account for up to 35% of cases and carry a poorer prognosis for spontaneous recovery. Human immunodeficiency virus (HIV) patients may develop PRP and have associated acne conglobata, hidradenitis suppurativa, or lichen spinulosus.

Etiology

The etiology is unknown. Familial cases are uncommon. Either sex may be affected, with equal frequency. Both clinically and histologically, the disease has many features that suggest it is a vitamin deficiency disorder, particularly of vitamin A. Some reports of patients with low serum levels of retinol-binding protein have appeared, but this is not a reproducible finding.

Histology

There is hyperkeratosis, follicular plugging, and focal parakeratosis at the follicular orifice. Parakeratosis may alternate both vertically and horizontally, producing a checkerboard pattern. Acantholysis is an uncommon finding but may be present. The inflammatory infiltrate in the dermis is composed of mononuclear cells and is generally mild. Specimens should be obtained from skin sites where hair follicles are numerous. Although there may be difficulty in making an unequivocal histologic diagnosis of PRP, the findings of psoriasis, which is the most common clinical entity in the differential diagnosis, are not present.

converted into sharply marginated patches of various sizes, which look like exaggerated goose-flesh and feel like a nutmeg grater. Any part or the entire skin surface may be affected.

The involvement is generally symmetrical and diffuse, with characteristic small islands of normal skin within the affected areas (Fig. 11-7). There is a hyperkeratosis of the palms (Fig. 11-8) and soles, with a tendency to fissures. On the soles especially, the hyperkeratosis typically extends up the sides, the so-called "sandal." The nails may be dull, rough, thickened, brittle, and striated, and are apt to crack and break. They are rarely, if ever, pitted. The exfoliation may become generalized and the follicular lesions less noticeable, finally disappearing and leaving a widespread dry, scaly erythroderma. The skin becomes dull red, glazed, atrophic, sensitive to slight changes in temperature, and, over the bony prominences, subject to ulcerations.

There are no subjective symptoms except itching in some cases. The Koebner phenomenon may be present. The general health of most patients is not affected, although occasionally arthritis may accompany the eruption. A number of cases of associated malignancy have recently been reported. It remains to be established whether these are true associations or chance

Diagnosis

The diagnosis of fully developed PRP is rarely difficult because of its distinctive features, such as the peculiar orange or salmon–yellow color of the follicular papules, containing a horny center, on the backs of the fingers, sides of the neck, and extensor surfaces of the limbs; the thickened, rough, and slightly or moderately scaly, harsh skin; the sandal-like palmoplantar hyperkeratosis; and the islands of normal skin in the midst of the eruption. It is distinguished from psoriasis by the scales, which in the latter are silvery and light, and overlap like shingles, and by the papules, which extend peripherally to form patches. Phrynoderma caused by vitamin A deficiency gives a somewhat similar appearance to the skin, as may eczematous eruptions caused by vitamin B deficiency. Rheumatologic disorders, such as subacute cutaneous lupus erythematosus and dermatomyositis, may present with similar cutaneous findings.

Treatment

The management of PRP is generally with systemic retinoids, although topical tazarotene has also been reported to be of benefit. Isotretinoin, in doses of 0.5–1 mg/kg/day, may induce prolonged remissions or cures. It may take 6–9 months for full involution to occur, and tapering of the drug may prevent recurrence. Acitretin, in doses of 10–75 mg, is also effective over a course of several months. Methotrexate has been used with good results in doses of 2.5–30 mg, either alone or in combination with oral retinoids. UV light may flare some patients, but in others PUVA, UVA1, or narrow-band UVB, alone or in combination with retinoids, may be effective. Phototesting prior to instituting light treatment is recommended. Extracorporeal photochemotherapy, cyclosporine, anti-tumor necrosis factor (TNF) agents, and azathioprine have been reported to be effective in resistant and severe cases. Both improvement and flare have been reported with efalizumab.

Topical applications of calcineurin inhibitors, lactic acid, or urea-containing preparations may be helpful. Responses to topical corticosteroids are not very effective as a rule. Systemic steroids are beneficial only for acute short-term management, but are not recommended for chronic use. In HIV-related disease, multiagent antiviral therapy may be useful alone or in combination with retinoids.

Barth D, et al: Successful treatment of pityriasis rubra pilaris (type 1) under combination of infliximab and methotrexate. J Dtsch Dermatol Ges 2009; 7(12):1071–1073.

Davis KF, et al: Clinical improvement of pityriasis rubra pilaris with combination etanercept and acitretin therapy. Arch Dermatol 2007 Dec; 143(12):1597–1599.

Greene R: PRP support group. Dermatol Nurs 2006 Feb; 18(1):28.

Gül U, et al: A case of pityriasis rubra pilaris associated with sacroileitis and autoimmune thyroiditis. J Eur Acad Dermatol Venereol 2008 Jul; 22(7):889–890.

Hong JB, et al: Recurrence of classical juvenile pityriasis rubra pilaris in adulthood: report of a case. Br J Dermatol 2007 Oct; 157(4):842–844.

Karimian-Teherani D, et al: Response of juvenile circumscribed pityriasis rubra pilaris to topical tazarotene treatment. Pediatr Dermatol 2008 Jan–Feb; 25(1):125–126.

Klein A, et al: Exacerbation of pityriasis rubra pilaris under efalizumab therapy. Dermatology 2007; 215(1):72–75.

Müller H, et al: Infliximab monotherapy as first-line treatment for adult-onset pityriasis rubra pilaris: case report and review of the literature on biologic therapy. J Am Acad Dermatol 2008; 59(Suppl):S65–70.

Ruiz-Genao DP, et al: Pityriasis rubra pilaris successfully treated with infliximab. Acta Derm Venereol 2007; 87(6):552–553.

Ruzzetti M, et al: Type III juvenile pityriasis rubra pilaris: a successful treatment with infliximab. J Eur Acad Dermatol Venereol 2008 Jan; 22(1):117–118.

Sato T, et al: Protein-losing gastroenteropathy in a patient with pityriasis rubra pilaris. Digestion 2007; 75(2–3):98.

Seckin D, et al: Successful use of etanercept in type I pityriasis rubra pilaris. Br J Dermatol 2008 Mar; 158(3):642–644.

Walling HW, et al: Pityriasis rubra pilaris responding rapidly to adalimumab. Arch Dermatol 2009; 145(1):99–101.

Palmoplantar keratoderma

The term keratoderma is frequently used synonymously with keratosis palmaris et plantaris (KPP) and tylosis. This group of conditions is characterized by excessive formation of keratin on the palms and soles. Some varieties exist as part of a syndrome. Acquired types include keratoderma climactericum, arsenical keratoses, corns, calluses, porokeratosis plantaris discreta, porokeratotic eccrine ostial and dermal duct nevus, glucan-induced keratoderma in acquired immunodeficiency syndrome (AIDS), keratosis punctata of the palmar creases, and many skin disorders that are associated with palmoplantar keratoderma, such as psoriasis, paraneoplastic syndromes, PRP, lichen planus, and syphilis. A high incidence of melanoma has been noted in Japanese patients with palmoplantar keratoderma. Palmoplantar keratoderma has been described with sorafenib, an oral multikinase inhibitor used in the treatment of renal cell carcinoma. Arsenical keratoses can occur from tainted water supplies, intentional poisoning, and medications containing arsenic. Arsenical keratoses have been treated with a combination of keratolytics and low-dose acitretin.

The hereditary types include hereditary palmoplantar keratoderma (Unna–Thost), punctate palmoplantar keratosis, Papillon–Lefèvre syndrome, mal de Meleda, familial keratoderma with carcinoma of the esophagus (Howell–Evans), autosomal-dominant hereditary punctate keratoderma associated with malignancy (Buschke–Fisher–Brauer), KPP of Sybert (palmoplantar hyperkeratosis with transgrediens, autosomal-dominant inheritance, and a lack of associated systemic features), acrokeratoelastoidosis, focal acral hyperkeratosis, and several inherited disorders that have palmoplantar keratoderma as an associated finding, such as pachyonychia congenita, tyrosinemia II (Richner–Hanhart), Darier's disease, Naxos syndrome (keratoderma, wooly hair, and cardiomyopathy), and dyskeratosis congenita. Many disorders that have palmoplantar keratoderma as a feature will be discussed in other chapters.

A number of mutations in keratin genes have been found. American patients with nonepidermolytic palmoplantar keratoderma associated with malignancy are linked to abnormalities of 17q24 distal to the keratin cluster. Pachyonychia congenita is associated with mutations in the helical initiation peptide of K6a, K16, or K17. Epidermolytic palmoplantar keratoderma (EPPK) is an autosomal-dominant disease caused by mutations of the *keratin 9* gene. The mutations localize to sequences encoding the highly conserved 1 A rod domain. Acantholysis of epidermal keratinocytes suggests the presence of *desmoglein 1* mutations.

Keratolysis exfoliativa (lamellar dyshidrosis, recurrent palmar peeling)

Keratolysis exfoliativa is a superficial exfoliative dermatosis of the palms and sometimes soles. Clinically, there is little to no inflammation, but white spots appear and gradually extend peripherally. The lesions rupture to produce an annular adherent collarette (Fig. 11-9), but remain largely asymptomatic. The

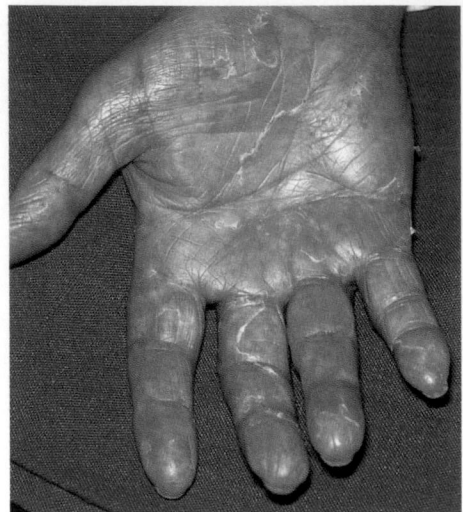

Fig. 11-9 Keratolysis exfoliativa.

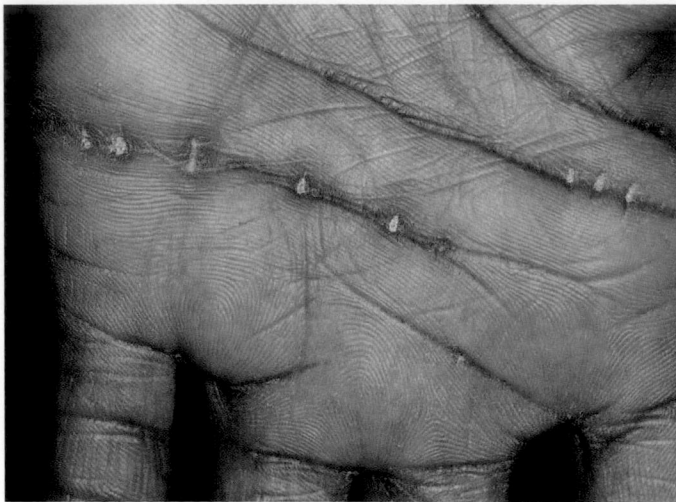

Fig. 11-10 Keratosis punctata of the palmar creases.

eruption is often exacerbated by environmental factors. Many patients have an atopic background and some have lesions of dyshidrotic eczema. Although some authors have suggested it is a disorder of cohesion of the stratum corneum, it is more likely that the condition represents subclinical eczema. The condition must be differentiated from dermatophytosis, and a KOH examination is recommended.

Because the condition is generally asymptomatic, no treatment may be necessary. In some patients, spontaneous involution occurs in a few weeks. For patients who require treatment, emollients, corticosteroid preparations, tar, urea and lactic acid or ammonium lactate may be effective.

Keratosis punctata of the palmar creases

Keratosis punctata of the palmar creases has also been referred to as keratotic pits of the palmar creases, punctate keratosis of the palmar creases, keratosis punctata, keratodermia punctata, hyperkeratosis penetrans, lenticular atrophia of the palmar creases, and hyperkeratosis punctata of the palmar creases. This common disorder occurs most often in black patients. The primary lesion is a 1–5 mm depression filled with a comedo-like keratinous plug. The lesions localize to the creases of the palms or fingers (Fig. 11-10). The soles may be involved. An autosomal-dominant inheritance pattern has been suggested, but onset is often delayed until adulthood.

Keratosis punctata of the palmar creases has been reported to be associated with atopic dermatitis, Dupuytren contractures, pterygium inversum unguis, dermatitis herpetiformis, knuckle pads, striate keratoderma, and psoriasis. Keratolytic agents and topical retinoids have provided temporary relief. Very painful lesions respond to punch excision.

Punctate keratoses of the palms and soles

Punctate keratoses of the palms and soles has also been referred to as punctate keratoderma, keratodermia punctata, keratosis punctata palmaris et plantaris, keratoma hereditarium dissipatum palmare et plantare, keratoderma disseminatum palmaris et plantaris, palmar keratoses, and palmar and plantar seed dermatoses. Spiny keratoderma of the palms and soles, known as "music box spines," is a distinct variant (Fig. 11-11).

There may be from 1 to over 40 papules, with an average in one series of 8.3. The main symptom is pruritus. The onset is between ages 15 and 68. Black individuals predominate, and it most frequently afflicts men. There have been reports of

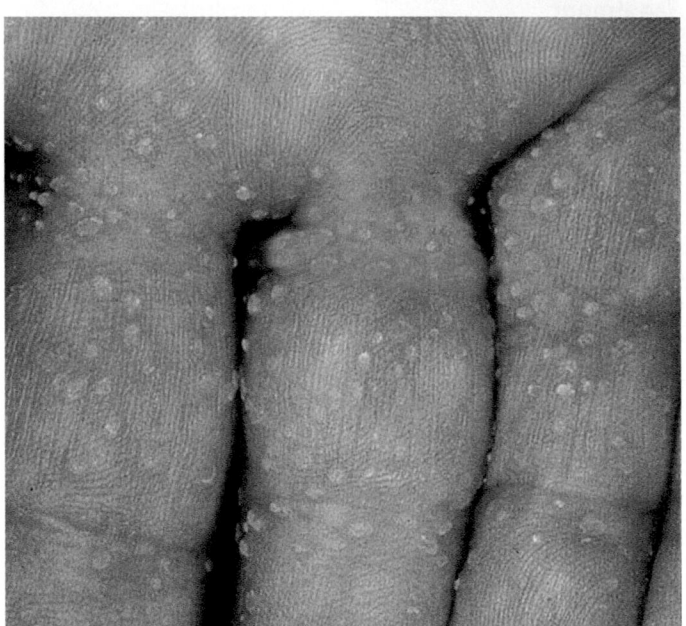

Fig. 11-11 "Music box" spine keratoderma.

autosomal-dominant inheritance. The histology demonstrates hyperkeratosis and parakeratosis, pyknotic, vacuolated epithelium, basal layer spongiosis, and dilated, occluded sweat ducts, blood vessels, and lymph vessels. Only mechanical debridement and excision have achieved any permanent results.

Porokeratosis plantaris discreta

Porokeratosis plantaris discreta occurs in adults, with a 4:1 female preponderance. It is characterized by a sharply marginated, rubbery, wide-based papule that on blunt dissection reveals an opaque plug without bleeding on removal. Lesions are multiple, painful, and usually 7–10 mm in diameter. They are usually confined to the weight-bearing area of the sole, beneath the metatarsal heads. Treatment may begin with fitted foot pads to redistribute the weight. Surgical excision, blunt dissection, and cryotherapy have been successful.

Keratoderma climactericum

Keratoderma climactericum is characterized by hyperkeratosis of the palms and soles (especially the heels) beginning at

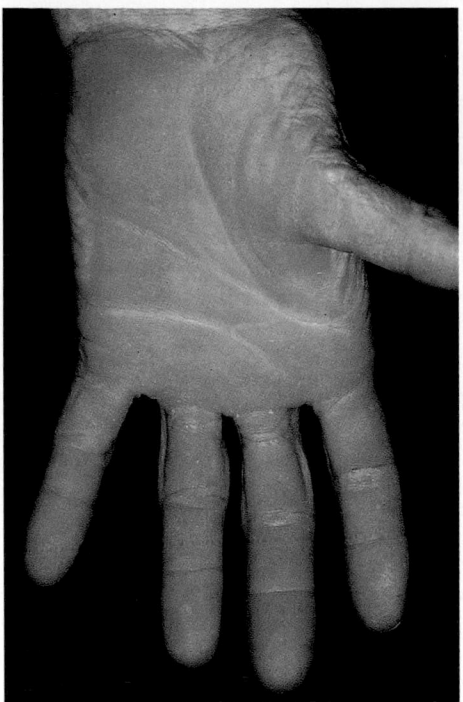

Fig. 11-12 Unna–Thost keratoderma.

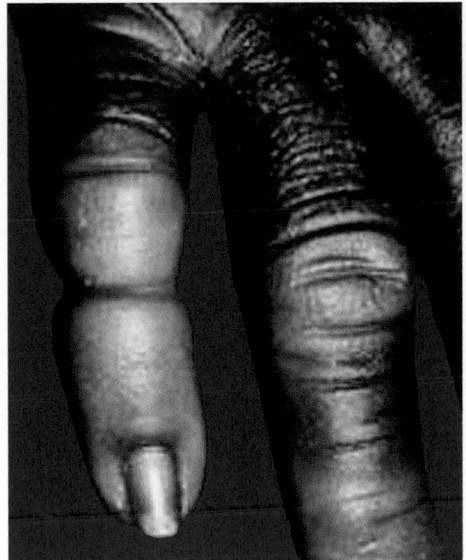

Fig. 11-13 Vohwinkel keratoderma.

about the time of the menopause. The discrete, thickened, hyperkeratotic patches are most pronounced at sites of pressure such as around the rim of the sole. Fissuring of the thickened patches may be present. There is a striking resemblance to plantar psoriasis, and indeed, keratoderma climactericum may represent a form of psoriasis. Therapy consists of keratolytics such as 10% salicylic acid ointment, lactic acid creams, or 20–30% urea mixtures. The response to topical corticosteroids is often disappointing. Acitretin is more effective than isotretinoin.

Hereditary palmoplantar keratoderma

Hereditary palmoplantar keratoderma (Unna–Thost) is characterized by a dominantly inherited, marked congenital thickening of the epidermal horny layer of the palms and soles, usually symmetrically and affecting all parts equally (Fig. 11-12). At times the thickening extends to the lateral or dorsal surfaces, especially over the knuckles. The arches of the feet are generally spared. The epidermis is thick, yellowish, and horny. The uniform thickening forms a rigid plate, which ends with characteristic abruptness at the periphery of the palm. Hyperhidrosis may cause a sodden appearance.

The condition is poorly responsive to therapy. Five percent salicylic acid, 12% ammonium lactate, and 40% urea have been used. Systemic retinoid therapy is impractical because of bone toxicity, and topical retinoids are generally not effective.

Palmoplantar keratodermas and malignancy

Howell–Evans reported a diffuse, waxy keratoderma of the palms and soles occurring as an autosomal-dominant trait associated with esophageal carcinoma. Other related features are oral leukoplakia, esophageal strictures, squamous cell carcinoma of tylotic skin, and carcinoma of the larynx and stomach. The tylosis esophageal cancer gene has been localized to chromosome 17q25. Acquired forms of palmoplantar keratodermas have also been associated with cancers of the esophagus, lung, breast, urinary bladder, and stomach.

Mutilating keratoderma of Vohwinkel

Vohwinkel described honeycomb palmoplantar hyperkeratosis, associated with starfish-like keratoses on the backs of the hands and feet, linear keratoses of the elbows and knees, and annular constriction (pseudo-ainhum) of the digits (Fig. 11-13), which may progress to autoamputation. Inheritance is mostly autosomal-dominant, although a recessive type exists. The disease is more frequent in women and in whites, with onset in infancy or early childhood. Reported associations include deafness, deaf–mutism, high-tone acoustic impairment, congenital alopecia universalis, pseudopelade-type alopecia, acanthosis nigricans, ichthyosiform dermatoses, spastic paraplegia, myopathy, nail changes, mental retardation, and bullous lesions on the soles. Vohwinkel keratoderma maps to chromosome 1q21 and represents a mutation of loricrin. There have been some reports of a response to acitretin (or etretinate) therapy. Mutations in *connexin 26* produce a similar phenotype.

Other forms of mutilating keratoderma also occur. They lack the constricting bands, honeycomb palmoplantar hyperkeratosis, and starfish-like keratoses of Vohwinkel syndrome. The affected digits are often shortened, narrow, rigid, and tapered (Fig. 11-14).

Olmsted syndrome

Olmsted syndrome is characterized by mutilating palmoplantar keratoderma and periorificial keratotic plaques. The distinctive features of this syndrome include a congenital, sharply marginated palmoplantar keratoderma; constriction of the digits; linear keratotic streaks on the flexural aspects of the wrists; onychodystrophy; and periorificial keratoses. Constriction of digits may result in spontaneous amputations. Extensive grafting has sometimes been necessary. Most cases of Olmsted syndrome are sporadic. Associated abnormalities have included hyperhidrosis of the palms and soles and congenital deafness. Histologically, there is acanthosis, papillomatosis, and orthokeratotic hyperkeratosis. The finding of Ki-67 staining of suprabasal keratinocytes suggests that Olmsted syndrome is a hyperproliferative disorder of the epidermis.

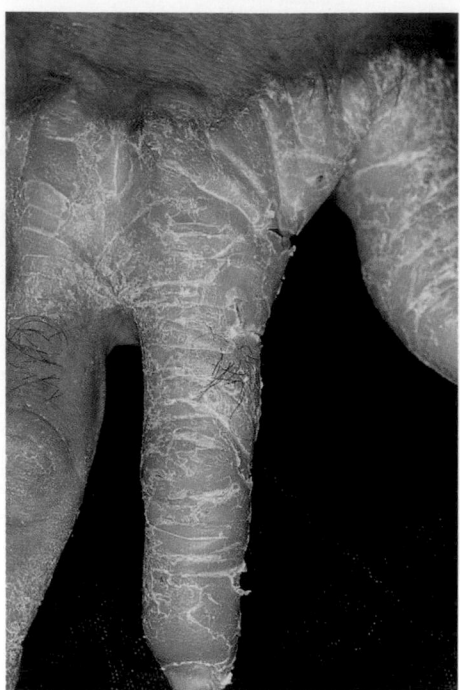

Fig. 11-14 Mutilating keratoderma.

Acrokeratoelastoidosis of Costa

This autosomal-dominantly inherited condition is more common in women. Small, round, firm papules occur over the dorsal hands, knuckles, and lateral margins of the palms and soles. The lesions appear in early childhood and progress slowly. They are most often asymptomatic. The characteristic histologic feature is dermal elastorrhexis.

Mal de Meleda

Mal de Meleda is a rare, autosomal-recessive form of palmoplantar keratoderma seen in individuals from the island of Meleda. The hyperkeratosis does not remain confined to the palms, and the extensor surfaces of the arms are frequently affected. The disease has been mapped to chromosome 8q, and mutations in the *ARS* (component B) gene have been identified in families with this disorder. Mutations in the gene encoding secreted lymphocyte antigen-6/urokinase-type plasminogen activator receptor-related protein-1 (*SLURP-1*) have been found.

"Nagashima-type" keratosis is a nonprogressive, autosomal-recessive palmoplantar keratoderma that resembles a mild form of mal de Meleda.

Papillon–Lefèvre syndrome

The Papillon–Lefèvre syndrome is inherited in an autosomal-recessive fashion and presents with palmoplantar keratoderma and destructive periodontitis usually beginning in young childhood. Well-demarcated, erythematous, hyperkeratotic lesions on the palms and soles may extend to the dorsal hands and feet. Hyperkeratosis may also be present on the elbows, knees, and Achilles tendon areas. Transverse grooves of the fingernails may occur. Severe gingival inflammation with loss of alveolar bone is typical. Histology reveals a psoriasiform pattern. Mutations in the *cathepsin C* gene have been detected. The condition usually has an early age of onset, but a late-onset variant has been reported. Some patients with late-onset disease have not shown mutations in the *cathepsin C* gene.

The early onset of periodontal disease has been attributed to alterations in polymorphonuclear leukocyte function caused by *Actinomyces actinomycetemcomitans*, although a variety of other bacteria have also been implicated. Acro-osteolysis and pyogenic liver abscesses may occur. There are asymptomatic ectopic calcifications in the choroid plexus and tentorium. Some patients have responded to acitretin, etretinate, or isotretinoin.

The stocking–glove distribution of the hyperkeratosis is similar to that seen in mal de Meleda. Haim–Munk syndrome is autosomal-recessive with periodontal disease, keratoderma, and onychogryphosis, linked to *cathepsin C* mutations.

Striate keratodermas

The striate keratodermas are a group of autosomal-dominant palmoplantar keratodermas with streaking hyperkeratosis involving the fingers and extending on to the palm of the hand. In some patients, a heterozygous C to A transversion involving the *desmoglein 1* gene has been found. Mutations in the *desmoplakin* gene have also been described. Brunauer–Fohs–Siemens syndrome is one form with diminished desmosomes, clumping of keratin filaments, and enlarged keratohyalin granules. Mutations in *desmoglein 1*, *desmoplakin*, and *keratin 1* have been described in these patients. In other patients, desmosome numbers are normal, but their inner plaques are attenuated. Striate keratoderma has also been reported in association with Rubinstein–Taybi syndrome.

Richner–Hanhart syndrome

Richner–Hanhart syndrome (tyrosinemia type 2) is characterized by corneal opacities and keratosis palmoplantaris. The skin manifestations usually develop after the first year of life, and relate to defects in tyrosine aminotransferase. Newborn screening can allow early intervention with dietary restriction.

Aquagenic wrinkling of the palms (acquired aquagenic syringeal acrokeratoderma)

Patients with this disorder, also called papulotranslucent acrokeratoderma, develop white papules on the palms after water exposure. The lesions are sharply demarcated from the surrounding skin and appear white. There may be a central prominent pore within each white lesion (Fig. 11-15). The lesions appear 3–5 min after exposure to water and resolve within a short time of drying. Sometimes the white skin can be peeled off. It may be a marker for cystic fibrosis and has also been reported in patients taking aspirin or rofecoxib. Autosomal-dominant inheritance has been suggested in some cases, and abnormal aquaporin 5 has been described in sweat glands.

Bédard MS, et al: Palmoplantar keratoderma and skin grafting: postsurgical long-term follow-up of two cases with Olmsted syndrome. Pediatr Dermatol 2008 Mar–Apr; 25(2):223–229.

Bergman R, et al: Disadhesion of epidermal keratinocytes: a histologic clue to palmoplantar keratodermas caused by *DSG1* mutations. J Am Acad Dermatol 2010; 62(1):107–113.

Bowden PE: Mutations in a keratin 6 isomer (K6c) cause a type of focal palmoplantar keratoderma. J Invest Dermatol 2010; 130(2):336–338.

Kabashima K, et al: "Nagashima-type" keratosis as a novel entity in the palmoplantar keratoderma category. Arch Dermatol 2008 Mar; 144(3):375–379.

Kabashima K, et al: Aberrant aquaporin 5 expression in the sweat gland in aquagenic wrinkling of the palms. J Am Acad Dermatol 2008 Aug; 59(2 Suppl 1):S28–S32.

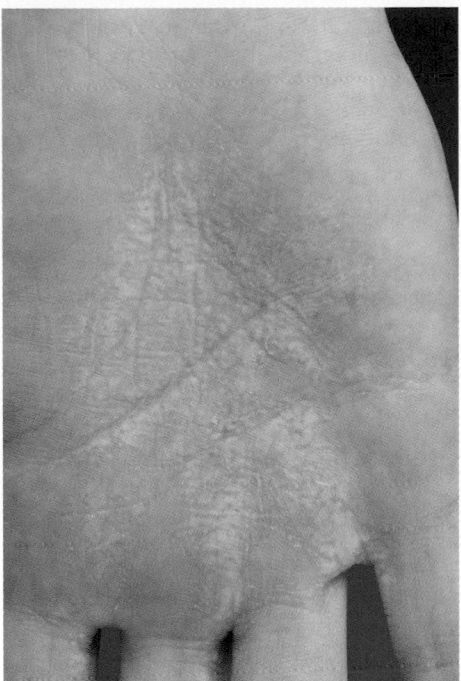

Fig. 11-15 Acquired aquagenic syringeal acrokeratoderma.

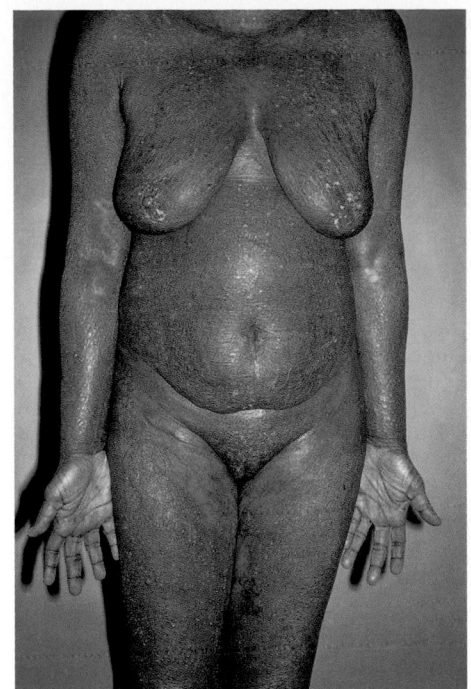

Fig. 11-16 Erythroderma.

Katz KA, et al: Aquagenic wrinkling of the palms in patients with cystic fibrosis homozygous for the delta F508 *CFTR* mutation. Arch Dermatol 2005 May; 141(5):621–624.

Khandpur S, et al: Chronic arsenic toxicity from Ayurvedic medicines. Int J Dermatol 2008 Jun; 47(6):618–621.

Lountzis NI, et al: Sorafenib-induced palmoplantar hyperkeratosis. J Drugs Dermatol 2008 Jun; 7(6):588–589.

Meissner T, et al: Richner–Hanhart syndrome detected by expanded newborn screening. Pediatr Dermatol 2008 May–Jun; 25(3):378–380.

Nakajima K, et al: Papillon–Lefèvre syndrome and malignant melanoma. A high incidence of melanoma development in Japanese palmoplantar keratoderma patients. Dermatology 2008; 217(1):58–62.

Exfoliative dermatitis (erythroderma)

Exfoliative dermatitis is also known as dermatitis exfoliativa, pityriasis rubra (Hebra), and erythroderma (Wilson–Brocq). Patients present with extensive erythema and scaling (Fig. 11-16). Ultimately, the entire body surface is dull scarlet and covered by small, laminated scales that exfoliate profusely. Vesiculation and pustulation are usually absent. An extensive telogen effluvium is often noted. In both PRP and mycosis fungoides, distinctly spared islands of skin are frequently noted. Patients with PRP also commonly have thickened, orange palms and "nutmeg grater" follicular papules on the dorsa of the fingers (see above).

Itching of the erythrodermic skin may be severe and the onset is often accompanied by symptoms of general toxicity, including fever and chills. Secondary infections by pyogenic organisms often complicate the course of the disease in the absence of treatment. Severe complications include sepsis, high-output cardiac failure, acute respiratory distress syndrome, and capillary leak syndrome. The mortality rate attributable to the erythroderma approaches 7% in some series.

Etiology

Erythroderma is frequently the result of generalization of a pre-existing chronic dermatosis such as psoriasis or atopic dermatitis. Many other cases are related to a medication, and some occur as a manifestation of an internal malignancy, erythrodermic mycosis fungoides, or the Sézary syndrome. In children, immune defects must be considered. Internal malignancies, pemphigus foliaceus, generalized dermatophytosis, and even Norwegian scabies may show the picture of generalized exfoliative dermatitis. There have been reports of inadequate intake of branched-chain amino acids in infants with maple syrup urine disease producing exfoliative erythroderma. However, in a significant number of patients the cause remains idiopathic, even after extensive evaluation.

In several reported series the largest group of patients had pre-existing dermatoses, including atopic dermatitis, chronic actinic dermatitis, psoriasis, seborrheic dermatitis, PRP, and allergic contact dermatitis. Drug eruptions are generally the next most common group, followed by idiopathic cases, cutaneous T-cell lymphoma, paraneoplastic erythroderma, and leukemia cutis. Common implicated drugs include allopurinol, sulfa drugs, gold, phenytoin, phenobarbital, isoniazid, carbamazepine, cisplatin, dapsone, mefloquine, tobramycin, minocycline, nifedipine, and iodine.

In a study of erythrodermic patients managed in the community, exacerbation of pre-existing dermatoses accounted for 61% as compared to 51% of those evaluated at a university medical; idiopathic cases for 14% and 31%, respectively; and cutaneous T-cell lymphoma for 1% and 6%, respectively. In a study of 51 children with erythroderma, immunodeficiency was diagnosed in 30%, ichthyosis in 24%, Netherton syndrome in 18%, and eczematous or papulosquamous dermatitis in 20%. Five of the 51 patients remained idiopathic. A biopsy established the diagnosis in only 19 (45%) of 42 cases. The mortality rate was 16%, usually related to an immunodeficiency disorder.

In a comparison of patients with and without HIV infection, erythroderma in the HIV-positive group was most commonly related to drug reactions (40.6%), with ethambutol accounting for 30.8%. In the non-HIV group, drug reactions accounted for only 22.5%. HIV-positive patients did not have an overall increase in the number of episodes of erythroderma.

Mycosis fungoides can be erythrodermic without meeting the criteria for the Sézary syndrome. Sézary syndrome consists of generalized exfoliative dermatitis with intense pruritus, leonine facies, alopecia, palmoplantar hyperkeratosis, and onychodystrophy. The criteria for a diagnosis of Sézary syndrome include an absolute Sézary cell count of at least 1000 cells/mm^3; a CD4/CD8 ratio of 10 or higher by flow cytometry, caused by an increase in circulating T cells or loss of expression of pan-T-cell markers; increased lymphocyte counts with evidence of a T-cell clone by Southern blot or polymerase chain reaction; or a chromosomally abnormal T-cell clone. Prognosis is poor and similar to that of patients with nodal involvement.

Hodgkin disease may show generalized exfoliative dermatitis. Fever, lymphadenopathy, splenomegaly, and hepatomegaly are frequently present. The erythrocyte sedimentation rate is elevated in most of these patients.

Histopathology

Exfoliative dermatitis may retain the histologic features of the original disease process. This is particularly true in psoriasis and mycosis fungoides. Often, however, the histology is nonspecific, with hyperkeratosis, mild acanthosis, and focal parakeratosis.

Treatment

In drug-induced erythroderma, the offending drug must be stopped. Application of a mid-strength corticosteroid after soaking, and occlusion under a sauna suit are often helpful, regardless of the cause of the erythroderma. Wet pajamas can be added under the sauna suit. Acitretin, cyclosporine, and methotrexate are useful in psoriatic erythroderma. Isotretinoin, acetretin, and methotrexate are useful in erythroderma caused by PRP. Immunosuppressive agents, such as azathioprine and methotrexate, may occasionally be necessary in idiopathic erythroderma not responding to therapy.

Kotrulja L, et al: Differential diagnosis of neonatal and infantile erythroderma. Acta Dermatovenerol Croat 2007; 15(3):178–190.

Milavec-Pureti V, et al: Exfoliative erythroderma. Acta Dermatovenerol Croat 2007; 15(2):103–107.

Okoduwa C, et al: Erythroderma: review of a potentially life-threatening dermatosis. Indian J Dermatol 2009; 54(1):1–6.

Sehgal VN, et al: Erythroderma/exfoliative dermatitis: a synopsis. Int J Dermatol 2004 Jan; 43(1):39–47.

Sehgal VN, et al: Erythroderma/generalized exfoliative dermatitis in pediatric practice: an overview. Int J Dermatol 2006 Jul; 45(7): 831–839.

Bonus images for this chapter can be found online at

http://www.expertconsult.com

Lichen Planus and Related Conditions

12

Lichen planus

Lichen planus (LP) is a pruritic, inflammatory disease of the skin, mucous membranes, and hair follicles. It occurs throughout the world, in all races. It is a common disorder, comprising more than 0.5% of all dermatological visits. It may be familial in 1–2% of cases. The pattern of LP detected and the age distribution vary among various genetic and geographic groups. In persons of European descent, it appears largely after the age of 20, and peaks between 40 and 70 years. Very few cases appear after age 80. Childhood LP typically accounts for 5% or less of cases. However, in some regions, childhood cases are responsible for more than 10% of all LP cases. These areas include the Indian subcontinent, Arab countries, and Mexico. Race appears to be the critical factor, since in the UK 80% of childhood LP is seen in Indians.

The primary lesions of LP are characteristic, almost pathognomonic, small, violaceous, flat-topped, polygonal papules (Fig. 12-1). The color of the lesions initially is erythematous. Well-developed lesions are violaceous, and resolving lesions are often hyperpigmented, especially in persons of color. The surface is glistening and dry, with scant, adherent scales. On the surface, gray or white puncta or streaks (Wickham striae) cross the lesions. Dermoscopy may enhance the visualization of this critical diagnostic element. Lesions begin as pinpoint papules and expand to 0.5–1.5 cm plaques. Infrequently, larger lesions are seen. There is a predilection for the flexor wrists, trunk, medial thighs, shins, dorsal hands, and glans penis (Fig. 12-2). The face is only rarely involved, and when it is, lesions are usually confined to the eyelids and/or lips. The palms and soles may be affected with small papules or hyperkeratotic plaques (Fig. 12-3). Certain morphologic patterns favour certain locations, e.g. annular lesions favoring the penis (Fig. 12-4), and keratotic lesions favoring the anterior shins. The Koebner phenomenon occurs in LP.

Pruritus is often prominent in LP. The pruritus may precede the appearance of the skin lesions, and, as with scabies, the intensity of the itch may seem out of proportion to the amount of skin disease. It may be almost intolerable in acute cases. Most patients react to the itching of LP by rubbing rather than scratching, and consequently scratch marks are usually not present.

The natural history of LP is highly variable and dependent on the site of involvement and the clinical pattern. Two-thirds of patients with skin lesions will have LP for less than 1 year and many patients spontaneously clear in the second year. Mucous membrane disease is much more chronic. Recurrences are common.

Nail changes are present in approximately 5–10% of patients. Involvement of the nail can occur as an initial manifestation, especially in children. Longitudinal ridging and splitting are most common. Onycholysis may be present and the lunula may be red. Involvement of the entire matrix may lead to obliteration of the whole nail plate (idiopathic atrophy of the

nail). Yellow nail syndrome may be simulated by LP of the nails. Pterygium formation is very characteristic of LP of the nails (Fig. 12-5). The nail matrix is destroyed by the inflammation and replaced by fibrosis. The proximal nailfold fuses with the proximal portion of the nailbed. LP may be a cause of some cases of twenty-nail dystrophy of childhood. Twenty-nail dystrophy in the absence of periungual lesions or pterygium

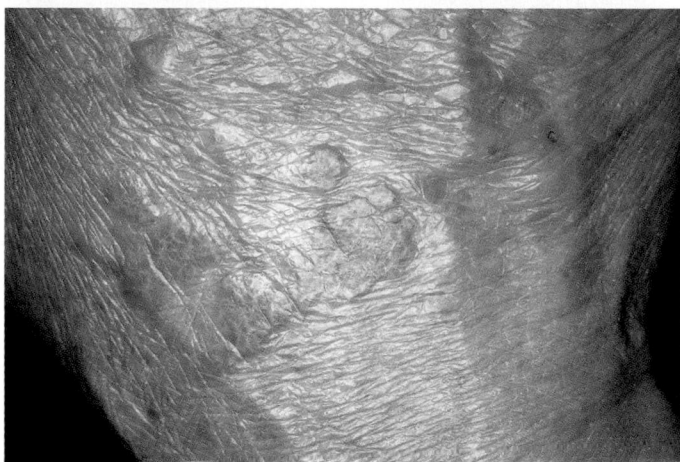

Fig. 12-1 Lichen planus, violaceous, flat-topped papules with minimal scale.

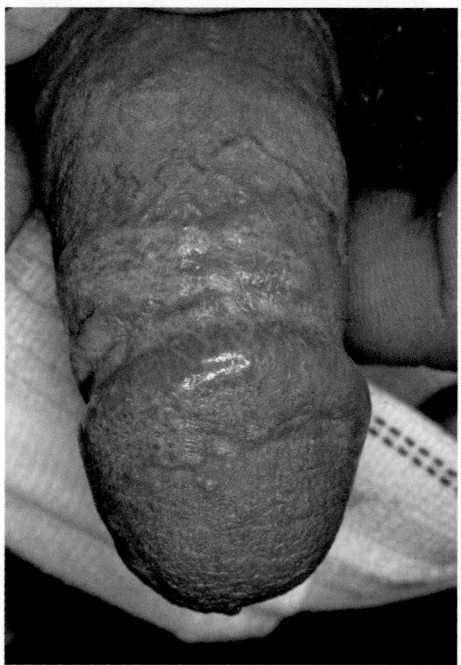

Fig. 12-2 Lichen planus of the penis.

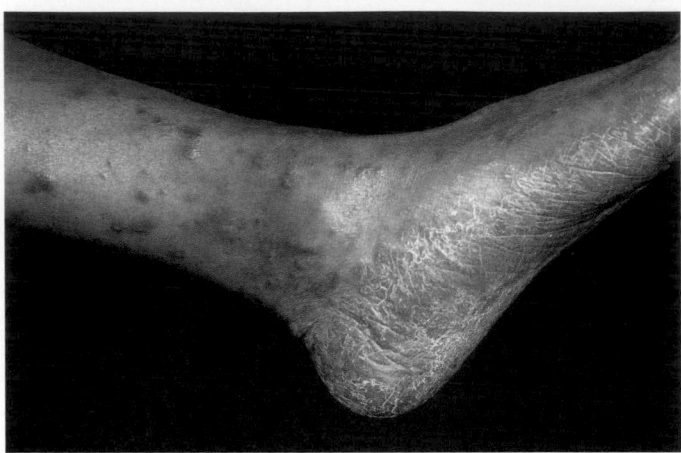

Fig. 12-3 Lichen planus of the soles.

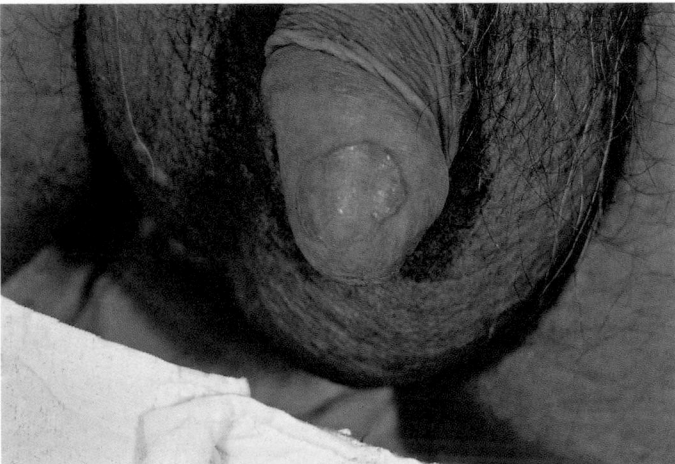

Fig. 12-4 Annular lichen planus of the penis.

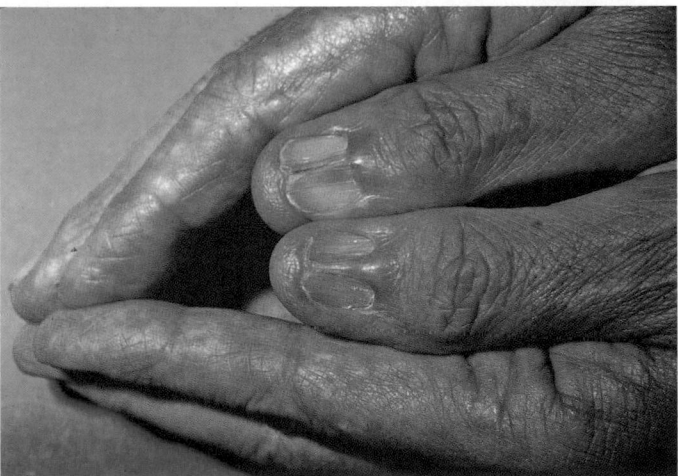

Fig. 12-5 Lichen planus, nail involvement with pterygium. (Courtesy of Lawrence Lieblich, MD)

formation usually resolves spontaneously, and frequently in these cases, no other stigmata of cutaneous or mucosal LP are found. Rarely, nailbed LP can result in onychopapilloma, a localized distal subungual hyperkeratosis.

Involvement of the genitalia, with or without lesions at other sites, is common. On the glans or shaft of the penis the lesions may consist of flat, polygonal papules, or these may be annular. Erosive LP can occur on the glans. Simultaneous involvement of the gingival and penile mucosa may occur. On the labia and anus similar lesions are observed; they are generally whitish, owing to maceration. In the vulvovaginal areas, erosive or ulcerative disease is common and may coexist with typical reticulate lesions. Vulval splitting may be caused by LP.

Conjunctival involvement is a very rare complication of LP. It occurs in patients with oral and gingival involvement. Cicatrization and subepithelial scarring can occur, as well as keratitis. It may closely simulate mucous membrane pemphigoid. Routine histology and direct immunofluorescence (DIF) may be required to confirm the diagnosis.

LP of the esophagus is increasingly being recognized, but still occurs in only 1% of cases of LP. The diagnosis is frequently delayed. Dysphagia, odynophagia, and weight loss are typical manifestations. The mid-esophagus is primarily affected. Virtually all the patients have coexistent oral disease. Esophageal involvement is much more common in women with vulvovaginal and oral disease, in whom 15% develop esophageal lesions. Stricture formation occurs in 80% of esophageal LP and may require frequent dilatations. Esophageal squamous cell carcinoma may complicate esophageal LP, suggesting that, once this diagnosis is made, routine gastrointestinal evaluation is required.

There are many clinical variants of LP. Whether these represent separate diseases or part of the LP spectrum is unknown. They all demonstrate typical LP histologically. They are described separately, since their clinical features are distinct from classic LP. Some patients with these clinical variants may have typical skin lesions of classic LP as well. The more common or better-known variants are described below.

Linear lichen planus

Small linear lesions caused by the Koebner phenomenon often occur in classic LP. Limitation of LP to one band or streak has also been described in less than 1% of patients, except in Japan, where up to 10% of reported cases are linear. Although originally described as following dermatomes (zosteriform), the lesions actually follow lines of Blaschko. It is more common in children, but also occurs in adults. Papules with varying degrees of overlying hyperkeratosis, or simple hyperpigmentation may be the presenting manifestations. There are often skip areas of normal skin between the individual lesions.

Annular/annular atrophic lichen planus

Men represent 90% of patients with annular LP. Lesions with this configuration favour the axilla, penis/scrotum, and groin. LP lesions of the mucosae, scalp, and nails are rare in patients with annular LP. Patients usually have fewer than 10 lesions. Most patients with annular LP are asymptomatic. The ringed lesions are composed of small papules and measure about 1 cm in diameter. Central hyperpigmentation may be the dominant feature. They may coalesce to form polycyclic figures. Annular lesions may also result from central involution of flat papules or plaques, forming lesions with violaceous, elevated borders and central hyperpigmented macules.

Hypertrophic lichen planus (lichen planus verrucosus)

Hypertrophic LP occurs most commonly on the shins, although it may be situated anywhere. The typical lesions are verrucous plaques with variable amounts of scale. At the edges of the plaques, small, flat-topped, polygonal papules may at times be discovered. Superficial inspection of the lesion often suggests psoriasis or a keratinocytic neoplasm rather than LP, but the typical appearance resembling rapidly cooled igneous rock (igneous rock sign) may be useful in suspecting LP over keratinocytic neoplasms. The lesions are of variable size, but are frequently several centimeters in diameter and larger than the lesions of classic LP. The anterior lower leg below the knee is the sole area of involvement in the majority of patients. Clinical diagnosis may be difficult and biopsy is often required. Histologically, the pseudoepitheliomatous keratinocyte hyperplasia may be marked, leading to the erroneous diagnosis of squamous cell carcinoma. True squamous cell carcinoma may also evolve from longstanding hypertrophic LP, and over 50% of cutaneous squamous cell carcinoma arising in LP occurs below the knee in lesions of hypertrophic LP. In addition, keratoacanthoma-like proliferations may occur in lesions of hypertrophic LP. This has also been called "hypertrophic lichen planus-like reactions combined with infundibulocystic hyperplasia." Hypertrophic LP is chronic and often refractory to topical therapy. Hypertrophic lupus erythematosus resembles hypertrophic LP both clinically and histologically. Hypertrophic lupus tends to affect the distal extremities, face, and scalp. The finding of continuous granular immunoglobulin on DIF strongly suggests a diagnosis of hypertrophic lupus erythematosus rather than LP.

Ulcerative/mucosal lichen planus

Ulcerative LP is rare on the skin but common on the mucous membranes. Typical skin lesions of LP rarely ulcerate. A rare ulcerative variant of cutaneous LP, or lupus erythematosus/LP overlap syndrome, affects the feet and toes, causing bullae, ulcerations, and permanent loss of the toenails. These chronic ulcerations on the feet are painful and disabling. Cicatricial alopecia may be present on the scalp and the buccal mucosa may also be affected. Skin grafting of the soles has produced successful results.

Oral mucosal LP is the most common form of mucosal LP, and it is usually chronic. Between 10 and 15% of patients with oral LP will also have skin lesions. Women represent 75% of patients with oral LP. Oral LP in women begins 10 years later than in men (57 years vs 47 years). Oral lesions may be reticulate (reticular) (Fig. 12-6), erythematous (atrophic), or ulcerative (erosive). The most common pattern in oral LP is the ulcerative form (40% of patients). Usually, reticulate and erythematous lesions are found adjacent to the ulcerative areas. The erythematous pattern is the predominant pattern in 37% of patients, but almost always reticulate lesions are also seen

in these patients. In oral LP the "classic" reticulate lesions are most prominent in 23% of patients. Symptoms are least common in patients with reticulate lesions; 23% are symptomatic and then only when the tongue is involved. All patients with erosive lesions are symptomatic, usually with burning or pain. Patients may simultaneously have several patterns, so patients are characterized by the primary form they exhibit. Lesions appear on any portion of the mouth, and multisite involvement is common. The buccal mucosa is involved in 90%, the gingiva in more than half, and the tongue in about 40%. On the gingiva, LP may produce desquamative gingivitis (Fig. 12-7). Oral LP may involve any portion of the mouth. The buccal mucosa is involved in 90% of cases, and the gingiva in more than 50%. Gingival involvement is particularly hard to diagnose, and often requires biopsy for both histology and DIF to confirm the diagnosis and exclude autoimmune causes of desquamative gingivitis. Gingival involvement is associated with accelerated gingival recession and aggressive management of oral hygiene, and control of candidal overgrowth is critical in the management of oral LP patients. Mechanical injury from dental procedures and poor-fitting appliances, as well as increased plaque from an inability to clean teeth due to pain, may trigger or exacerbate gingival LP. On the tongue and palate, lesions are often mistaken for leukoplakia (Fig. 12-8). The lower lip is involved in 15% of oral LP patients, but

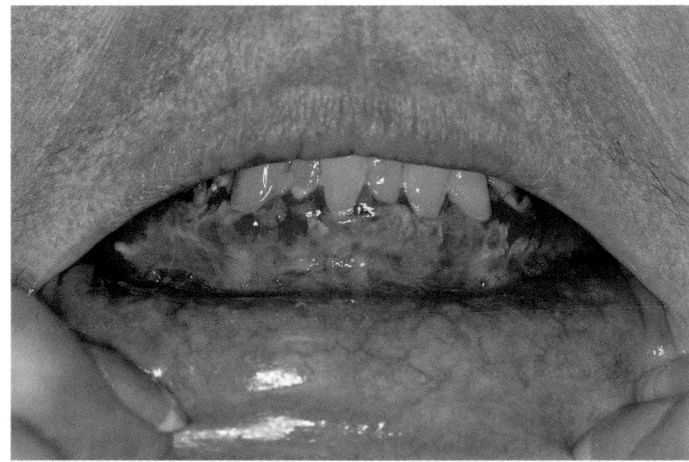

Fig. 12-7 Desquamative gingivitis secondary to lichen planus.

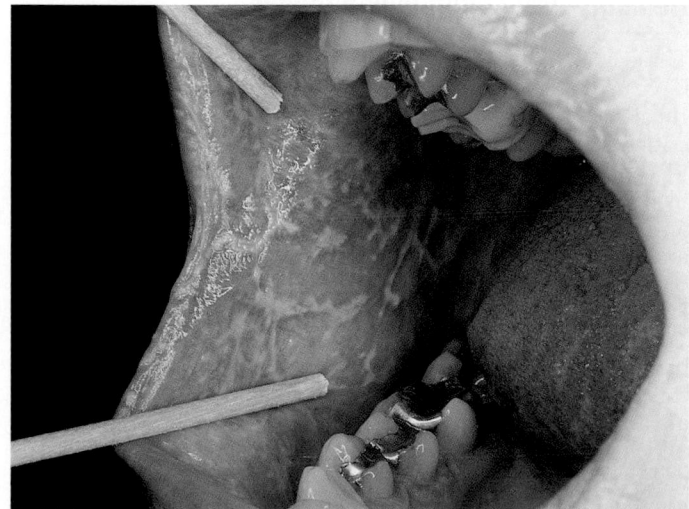

Fig. 12-6 Lichen planus, reticulate white lesions of the buccal mucosa.

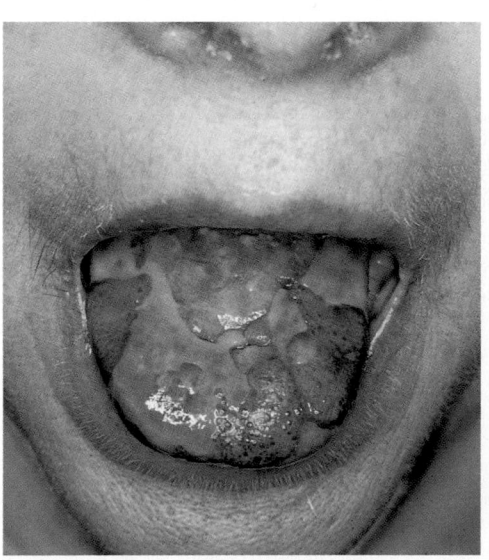

Fig. 12-8 Lichen planus of the tongue.

the upper lip in only 2%. Oral LP is stable but chronic, with less than 3% of patients having a spontaneous remission in an average 5-year follow-up. Aggressive oral hygiene plays an important role in the management of gingival LP.

Mercury, gold, cobalt, indium, manganese, chromate, nickel, or palladium sensitivity may be found by patch testing in up to 60–75% of patients with oral LP or oral lichenoid reactions. In patients with positive patch tests to metals, these tests appear relevant in at least 44% of patients, and removal of the offending amalgam leads to improvement of the oral lichenoid process in 60–100% of patch test-positive patients (more than 60% of patients who did not remove their amalgam also improved). Patch testing, however, may not identify all patients whose oral lichenoid lesions improve with removal of the oral metal. Neither can histopathological evaluation identify the metal-induced patients. This has made the role of metals in the induction of oral lichenoid lesions and oral LP very controversial. Rarely, patients with metal sensitivity will also have skin and nail lesions that improve with removal of the oral metal. Metal sensitivity as a cause of an oral lichenoid reaction should be considered, especially in those patients whose oral involvement is directly adjacent to amalgam fillings. If patch testing is positive for amalgam or metals, removal of the amalgam should be considered. Oral lichenoid reactions to cinnamates and spearmint have also been reported.

Involvement of the vulva and vagina with LP, along with the gingiva, has been called the vulvovaginal–gingival (VVG) syndrome. Although all three of these mucous membranes may be involved, only one or two sites may be involved at any one time. The prevalence of erosive vulvar LP has been underappreciated until recently, simply because many women with LP will not volunteer their vulvovaginal complaints unless specifically asked. Women affected with vulvar LP have vulvar pain or burning. Vulvar LP produces lesions very similar to oral lichen planus, with erythema, leukokeratosis, and erosion. Surrounding the red or eroded lesions is a narrow rim of white reticulation. This rim is the most fruitful area to biopsy in order to confirm the diagnosis. Scarring (Fig. 12-9) of the vagina and vulva with adhesions, vestibular bands, and atrophy of the labia minora or prepuce occurs, making the morphology similar to vulvar lichen sclerosus. In one-third, typical reticulate buccal LP is seen, and in up to 80% the oral mucosa is also involved. Cutaneous lesions occur in between 20% and 40% of VVG patients. The course of the vulvovaginal syndrome is protracted and patients frequently have sequelae, including chronic pain, dyspareunia, and even scarring of the conjunctiva, urethra, and oral, laryngeal, pharyngeal, and esophageal mucosae. Nails are involved in about 15% of patients with VVG (as compared to only 2% of patients with oral LP). The VVG syndrome is now considered to be a separate subgroup of mucosal LP that is particularly disabling, scarring, and refractory to therapy.

While the pathogenesis of LP is unknown, there is evidence that erosive LP of the vulva (and lichen sclerosus) may have an autoimmune basis. A personal and family history of autoimmune disorders (usually thyroid disease) is present in up to 30% of patients with vulvar LP, and up to 40% have circulating autoantibodies. The prevalence of autoimmune phenomena is NOT increased in patients with classic cutaneous LP. The autoantibodies do not appear to be pathogenic, as the disease seems to be caused by cytotoxic T cells. Erosive LP has significant impact on quality of life, and patients with erosive LP have high levels of depression, anxiety, and stress.

Cancer risk and lichen planus

Rare cases of squamous cell carcinoma of the skin occurring on the lower leg in lesions of hypertrophic LP have been reported. There is no statistical increase in cutaneous or visceral carcinoma in patients with cutaneous LP, and cutaneous LP alone is not considered to be a condition with increased cancer risk. Oral and vulvovaginal LP does appear, however, to increase the risk of developing squamous cell carcinoma. Between 0.4% and 5% (on average about 1–2%) of patients with oral LP will develop oral squamous cell carcinoma. Squamous cell carcinoma only occurs in patients with erythematous or ulcerative LP, not in patients with only the reticulate pattern. Of the oral LP patients who develop oral squamous cell carcinomas, about 45% have only one cancer. The majority develop multiple cancers, and close vigilance is recommended in these patients. LP patients with erosive penile and vaginal disease also have developed squamous cell carcinoma. The number of penile cases is too low to determine the frequency of this consequence, but in the case of vulvar LP, the frequency of development of SCC may be as high as 3%. Clinicians should have a low threshold to biopsy fixed erosive or leukokeratotic lesions in patients with mucosal LP. The use of oral and topical calcineurin inhibitors for LP has been associated with the appearance of squamous cell carcinoma on the genitalia. There is no evidence that the medications caused the neoplasia, but if these agents are used, regular follow-up and careful examination are required.

Hepatitis-associated lichen planus

Three liver conditions have been associated with LP: hepatitis C virus (HCV), HBV immunization, and primary biliary cirrhosis. HCV infection was found in proportionately more patients with LP than in controls in 20 of 25 studies. The prevalence of HCV infection in patients with LP varies from 1.6% to 20%. There is an association with the human leukocyte antigen (HLA)-DR6 allele. The association of HCV infection and LP has been questioned. In a large series of patients with oral LP from the US, none of the 195 patients was infected with HCV, while 29% of patients with oral LP from Italy had HCV. Twenty percent of patients infected with HCV in Scotland had oral LP, as compared to 1% of seronegative patients. Although the data are conflicting, screening for HCV appears appropriate in persons from a geographic region or population in which HCV infection is commonly associated with LP. The clinical features of LP in patients with hepatitis C infection are identical to classic LP, but LP patients with HCV infection are reported as being more likely to have erosive mucous membrane disease. The existence of underlying hepatitis cannot be

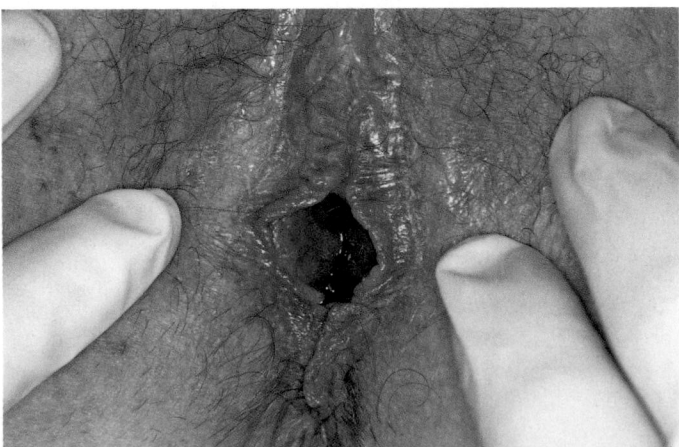

Fig. 12-9 Scarring and erosions in the vulvovaginal–gingival syndrome.

predicted by clinical pattern or the results of liver function tests. Treatment of hepatitis C with interferon-α may be associated with the initial appearance of LP or exacerbation of pre-existing LP. LP may occur at the sites of interferon injections, and skin testing may reproduce LP-like lesions. LP may improve or not change with interferon and ribavirin treatment for hepatitis C. Improvement is usually seen towards the end of the treatment course. Most patients do not completely clear their LP. The HCV genome is not found in lesions of LP associated with HCV infection.

HBV immunization may be associated with the appearance of LP in both children and adults. More than 30 cases have been reported. Lesions are typical of LP and the oral mucosa may be affected. Most typically, the first lesions of LP appear about 1 month after the second dose of vaccine. Lesions typically resolve after some time.

Primary biliary cirrhosis and LP may coexist. Patients with this liver abnormality, in addition, have a marked propensity to develop a lichenoid eruption while on d-penicillamine therapy. Xanthomas in patients with primary biliary cirrhosis may appear initially in lesions of LP, and the infiltrate, while lichenoid, may contain xanthomatous cells. Primary sclerosing cholangitis has been associated with oral LP in at least five patients.

Bullous lichen planus

Two forms of LP may be accompanied by bullae. In classic LP, usually on the lower extremities, individual lesions will vesiculate centrally (Fig. 12.10). This represents macroscopic exaggeration of the subepidermal space formed by the lichenoid interface reaction destroying the basal keratinocytes. These lesions often spontaneously resolve.

Lichen planus pemphigoides describes a rare subset of patients who usually have typical LP, then develop blistering on their LP lesions and on normal skin. Less commonly, the blistering antedates the LP. Clinically, they appear to be a combination of LP and bullous pemphigoid. Oral disease may occur and resemble either LP or mucous membrane pemphigoid. Lichen planus pemphigoides has been triggered by

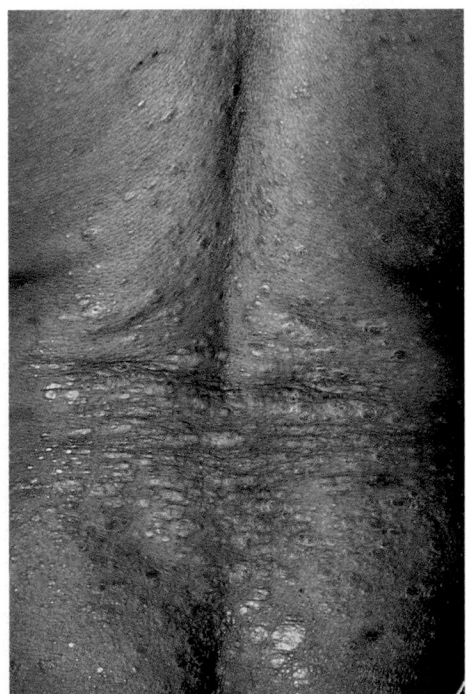

Fig. 12-10 Generalized lichen planus.

medications and PUVA. Pruritus may be severe and lesions may evolve to resemble pemphigoid nodularis. Bullous pemphigoid affects an older age group than lichen planus pemphigoides (typical onset for lichen planus pemphigoides is between age 30 and 50). Histologically, the LP lesions show LP and the bullous lesions show the features of bullous pemphigoid. DIF is positive in a linear pattern, with IgG and C3 along the basement membrane zone, at the roof of saline split skin. The antigen targeted by the autoantibody in lichen planus pemphigoides is located in the same region as the bullous pemphigoid antigen (at the basal hemidesmosome). Antibodies from patients with lichen planus pemphigoides typically bind the 180 kD bullous pemphigoid antigen, but in a different region from bullous pemphigoid sera. Lichen planus pemphigoides tends to follow a benign and chronic course, even when compared to bullous pemphigoid. Treatment is similar to bullous pemphigoid, with potent topical steroids, systemic steroids, tetracycline, nicotinamide, intravenous immunoglobulin, and immunosuppressives all being variably effective.

Pathogenesis and histology

LP is characterized by an immunologic reaction mediated by T cells. These cells induce keratinocytes to undergo apoptosis by an unknown mechanism. Recently, there have been reports of insulin resistance and frank type 2 diabetes mellitus being increased in patients with LP compared to controls.

Lichen planus pemphigoides is hypothesized to result from exposure to the immune system of epitopes in the BP180 antigen as keratinocytes are destroyed by the lichenoid inflammation. Epitope spreading can occur, and lichen planus pemphigoides patients may also have autoantibodies to the same epitopes as bullous pemphigoid patients.

The histologic features of LP are distinctive and vary with the stage of the lesion. In early lesions there is an interface dermatitis along the dermoepidermal junction. As the lesion evolves, the epidermis takes on a characteristic appearance. There is destruction of the basal layer with a "saw-tooth" pattern of epidermal hyperplasia, orthokeratosis, and beaded hypergranulosis. The basal cells are lost, so the basal layer is described as "squamatized." In the superficial dermis there is a dense, bandlike infiltrate composed of lymphocytes and melanophages. "Civatte bodies" (cytoid bodies, colloid bodies) represent necrotic keratinocytes in the superficial dermis. Hypertrophic LP shows marked epidermal hyperplasia (pseudoepitheliomatous hyperplasia). Old lesions of LP show effacement of the rete ridge pattern, melanophages in the upper dermis, and occasional Civatte bodies. LP rarely demonstrates parakeratosis or eosinophils. The presence of either of these suggests a different cause of lichenoid tissue reaction, such as lichenoid drug eruption.

Lichen planopilaris, frontal fibrosing alopecia, and Graham–Little–Piccardi–Lassueur syndrome show the findings of LP, centered on the superficial follicular epithelium. On DIF, clumps of IgM, and less frequently IgA, IgG, and C3, are commonly present subepidermally, corresponding to the colloid bodies. Dense shaggy staining for fibrinogen along the basement membrane zone is characteristic of LP. A lichenoid drug eruption may be difficult to differentiate from LP. The presence of eosinophils or parakeratosis supports the diagnosis of lichenoid drug eruption. Although LP virtually never has eosinophils or parakeratosis, they are not universally present in other lichenoid eruptions such as lichenoid drug eruption. Graft versus host disease tends to have a sparser infiltrate. Hypertrophic lupus may be histologically identical to LP, and the diagnosis is best made by clinical correlation and DIF. In most other forms of lupus erythematosus, there is a greater tendency for epidermal atrophy with parakeratosis, dermal mucin is found, and follicular plugging is more prominent. The infiltrate in lupus tends to surround and involve deep portions of the appendageal structures, such as the follicular isthmus and eccrine coil. Deep nodular perivascular lymphoplasmacytic infiltrates and necrosis of the fat lobule with fibrin or hyalin rings are also findings characteristic of lupus erythematosus.

Differential diagnosis

Classic LP displays lesions that are so characteristic that clinical examination is often adequate to lead to suspicion of the diagnosis. Lichenoid drug eruptions may be difficult to distinguish. A lichenoid drug reaction should be suspected if the eruption is photodistributed, scaly but not hypertrophic, and confluent or widespread—clinical features that are unusual for idiopathic LP. The presence of oral mucosa involvement may prompt suspicion of LP, but oral lesions may occasionally occur in lichenoid drug eruptions as well. Pityriasis rosea, guttate psoriasis, the small papular or lichenoid syphilid, and pityriasis lichenoides et varioliformis acuta are dermatoses that may resemble generalized LP. Mucous membrane lesions may be confused with leukoplakia, lupus erythematosus, mucous patches of syphilis, candidiasis, cancer, and the oral lesions of autoimmune bullous diseases, such as pemphigus or cicatricial pemphigoid. On the scalp the atrophic lesions may be mistaken for other cicatricial alopecias, such as lupus erythematosus, folliculitis decalvans, and pseudopelade of Brocq. Hypertrophic LP type may simulate psoriasis and squamous cell carcinoma in situ. Isolated patches of LP may resemble lichen simplex chronicus or, if heavily pigmented, may suggest a fixed drug eruption.

Treatment

Limited lesions may be treated with superpotent topical steroids or intralesional steroid injections. In patients with widespread disease, these treatments are usually unsatisfactory. Widespread lesions respond well to systemic corticosteroids but tend to relapse as the dose is reduced. Monthly pulse dosing has been championed by dermatologists in India. Phototherapy may be effective for cutaneous LP, including narrow-band ultraviolet (UV) B, UVA1, and PUVA. Topical cream PUVA has been used effectively in genital LP. Isotretinoin and acitretin, in doses similar to or slightly lower than those used for psoriasis, may also be useful and avoid the long-term complications of systemic steroids. They are especially helpful in cases of hypertrophic LP. Retinoid therapy may be combined with phototherapy in refractory cases. Photodynamic therapy with topical 5-aminolevulinic acid can be effective in penile LP. Low molecular weight heparin (enoxaparin), 3 mg injected subcutaneously once a week, led to remission of cutaneous and reticulate oral LP in 61% of patients and improvement in 11%. Erosive oral LP responded variably and lichen planopilaris not at all. For erosive skin lesions topical tacrolimus or pimecrolimus can be effective. Oral immunosuppressive agents may be effective for cutaneous LP, but their potential toxicity limits use to the most severe cases. Cyclosporine in typical psoriasis doses is very beneficial. Similarly, mycophenolate mofetil can induce remission in severe cases of cutaneous and oral LP.

For oral lesions, superpotent steroids in Orabase or gel form are useful. Vinyl dental trays may be used to apply steroid ointments to the gingiva. Begin with 30 min applications three times a day and reduce to maintenance of 20 min every evening. Addition of nystatin to clobetasol in Orabase may be especially effective. Overall, more than 70% of patients with vulvar LP have their symptoms relieved with topical clobetasol. Intralesional injections may be used for focal unresponsive lesions. Topical tacrolimus 0.1% ointment has become standard treatment in erosive LP of the oral and genital mucosa. While burning may occur initially, this can be reduced by concomitant use of topical steroids or initial use of a lower strength. Higher concentrations, up to 0.3%, may be used. Most patients have a partial but significant response, with increased ability to eat with much less pain. Blood levels can be detected, independent of area of involvement, but tend to decrease over time as the oral erosions heal. Pimecrolimus can be used successfully in patients intolerant of topical tacrolimus. Sustained remissions are rare, and chronic use is usually required to maintain remission. Topical cyclosporine is ineffective. Topical isotretinoin, in concentrations up to 0.18%, can be effective. PUVA, photodynamic therapy, and 308 nm excimer laser have been effective in oral LP. Hydroxychloroquine, 200–400 mg/day for 6 months, was reported to produce an excellent response in 9 of 10 patients with oral LP. Thalidomide has also proven effective in doses of 50–150 mg/day. The systemic agents recommended above to treat cutaneous LP may also improve oral disease. For VVG syndrome, corticosteroids topically and systemically are beneficial. Topical therapy with corticosteroids may be enhanced by mixing the steroid in vaginal bioadhesive moisturizer (Replens). Iontophoresis may improve delivery. Methotrexate, mycophenolate mofetil, and cyclosporine are usually effective in the most refractory cases. Extracorporeal photochemotherapy (photopheresis) has proven effective in refractory oral LP.

Aghahosseini F, et al: Methylene blue mediated photodynamic therapy: a possible alternative treatment for oral lichen planus. Lasers Surg Med 2006; 38:33.

Al-Khenaizan S: Lichen planus occurring after hepatitis B vaccination: a new case. J Am Acad Dermatol 2001; 45:614.

Al-Khenaizan S, et al: Ulcerative lichen planus of the sole: excellent response to topical tacrolimus. Int J Dermatol 2008; 47:626.

Ang P, et al: Pruritic linear eruption on a child. Arch Dermatol 2001; 137:85.

Balasubramaniam P, et al: Lichen planus in children: review of 26 cases. Clin Exp Dermatol 2008; 33:457.

Bansal R: Segmental lichen planus. Intl J Dermatol 2004; 43:985.

Baran R: Lichen planus of the nails mimicking the yellow nail syndrome. Br J Dermatol 2000; 143:1117.

Belfiore P, et al: Prevalence of vulval lichen planus in a cohort of women with oral lichen planus: an interdisciplinary study. Br J Dermatol 2006; 155:994.

Berk D, et al: Dermatologic disorders associated with chronic hepatitis C: effect of interferon therapy. Clin Gastro and Hepato 2007; 5:142.

Bermejo-Fenoll A, et al: Familiar oral lichen planus: presentation of six families. Oral Surg Oral Med Oral Pathol Oral Radiol Endod 2006; 102:e12.

Bezanis G, et al: Verrucous plaques on the leg. Arch Dermatol 2003; 139:933.

Camisa C, Popovsky JL: Effective treatment of oral erosive lichen planus with thalidomide. Arch Dermatol 2000; 136:1442.

Carbone M, et al: Systemic and topical corticosteroid treatment of oral lichen planus: a comparative study with long-term follow-up. J Oral Pathol Med 2003; 32:323.

Chandan V, et al: Esophageal lichen planus. Arch Pathol Lab Med 2008; 132:1026.

Chave TA, Graham-Brown RAC: Keratoacanthoma developing in hypertrophic lichen planus. Br J Dermatol 2003; 148:592.

Chryssostalis A, et al: Esophageal lichen planus: a series of eight cases including a patient with esophageal verrucous carcinoma. A case series. Endo 2008; 40:764.

Chu CY, et al: Lichen planus with xanthomatous change in a patient with primary biliary cirrhosis. Br J Dermatol 2000; 142:377.

Cooper S, et al: The association of lichen sclerosus and erosive lichen planus of the vulva with autoimmune disease. Arch Dermatol 2008; 144:1432.

Copper S, Wojnarowska F: Influence of treatment of erosive lichen planus of the vulva on its prognosis. Arch Dermatol 2006; 142:289.

Cunha K, et al: Prevalence of oral lichen planus in Brazilian patients with HCV infection. Oral Surg Oral Med Oral Pathol Oral Radio Endod 2005; 100:330.

Di Fede O, et al: Unexpectedly high frequency of genital involvement in women with clinical and histological features of oral lichen planus. Acta Derm Venereol 2006; 86:433.

Ditrichova D, et al: Oral lichenoid lesions and allergy to dental materials. Biomed Pap Med Fac Univ Palacky Olomuc Czech Repub 2007; 151:333.

Durrani O, et al: Bicanalicular obstruction in lichen planus. A characteristic pattern of disease. Ophthal 2008; 115:386.

Eisen D: The clinical features, malignant potential, and systemic associations of oral lichen planus: a study of 723 patients. J Am Acad Dermatol 2002; 46:207.

Fiveson D, et al: Treatment of generalized lichen planus with alefacept. Arch Dermatol 2006; 142:151.

Frieling U, et al: Treatment of severe lichen planus with mycophenolate mofetil. J Am Acad Dermatol 2003; 49:1063.

Gonzalez-Moles MA, et al: Treatment of severe erosive gingival lesions by topical application of clobetasol propionate in custom trays. Oral Surg Oral Med Oral Pathol Oral Radiol Endod 2003; 95:688.

Guiglia R, et al: A combined treatment regimen for desquamative gingivitis in patients with oral lichen planus. J Oral Patholo Med 2007; 36:110.

Guyot AD, et al: Treatment of refractory erosive oral lichen planus with extracorporeal photochemotheraphy: 12 cases. Br J Dermatol 2007; 156:553.

Hamada T, et al: Lichen planus pemphigoides and multiple keratoacanthomas associated with colon adenocarcinoma. Br J Dermatol 2004; 151:232.

Harden D, et al: Lichen planus associated with hepatitis C virus: no viral transcripts are found in the lichen planus, and effective therapy for hepatitis C virus does not clear lichen planus. J Am Acad Dermatol 2003; 49:847.

Harting M, Hsu S, et al: Lichen planus pemphigoides: a case report and review of the literature. Dermatol Online J 2006; 12:10.

Hopsu E, Pitkaranta A: Idiopathic, inflammatory, medial meatal, fibrotising otitis presenting with lichen planus. J Laryn Oto 2007; 121:796.

Hoskyn J, Guin J: Contact allergy to cinnamil in a patient with oral lichen planus. Contact Dermatitis 2005; 52:161.

Hoshi A, et al: Penile carcinoma originating from lichen planus on glans penis. J Urology 2008; 71:816.

Issa Y, et al: Oral lichenoid lesions related to dental restorative materials. Br Dent J 2005; 198:361.

Kaliakatsou F, et al: Management of recalcitrant ulcerative oral lichen planus with topical tacrolimus. J Am Acad Dermatol 2002; 46:35.

Kato Y, et al: A case of lichen planus caused by mercury allergy. Br J Dermatol 2003; 148:1268.

Kirby B, et al: Treatment of lichen planus of the penis with photodynamic therapy. Br J Dermatol 1999; 141:765.

Kirtschig G, et al: Successful treatment of erosive vulvovaginal lichen planus with topical tacrolimus. Br J Dermatol 2002; 147:625.

Kollner K, et al: Treatment of oral lichen planus with the 308-nm UVB excimer laser—early preliminary results in eight patients. Lasers Surg Med 2003; 33:158.

Kortekangas-Savolainen O, Kiilholma P: Treatment of vulvovaginal erosive and stenosing lichen planus by surgical dilatation and methotrexate. Acta Obstetricia et Gynecol Scandinavica 2007; 86:339.

Kossard S, et al: Hypertrophic lichen planus-like reactions combined with infundibulocystic hyperplasia. Arch Dermatol 2004; 140:1262.

Krasowska D, et al: Development of squamous cell carcinoma with lesions of cutaneous lichen planus. Eur J Dermatol 2007; 17:447.

Kuramoto N, et al: PUVA-induced lichen planus pemphigoides. Br J Dermatol 2000; 142:509.

Kyriakis KP, et al: Sex and age distribution of patients with lichen planus. Eur Acad Dermatol Venereol 2006; 18:625.

Laeijendecker R, et al: Oral lichen planus and allergy to dental amalgam restorations. Arch Dermatol 2004; 140:1434.

Laeijendecker R, et al: Oral lichen planus and hepatitis C virus infection. Arch Dermatol 2005; 141:906.

Lener EV, et al: Successful treatment of erosive lichen planus with topical tacrolimus. Arch Dermatol 2001; 137:419.

Level NJ: No evidence for therapeutic effect of topical ciclosporin in oral lichen planus. Br J Dermatol 2006; 155:477.

Limas C, Limas CJ: Lichen planus in children: a possible complication of hepatitis B vaccines. Pediatr Dermatol 2002; 19:204.

Lodi G, et al: Lichen planus and hepatitis C virus: a multicentre study of patients with oral lesions and a systematic review. Br Assoc Dermatol 2004; 151:1172.

Lodi G, et al: Current controversies in oral lichen planus: report of an international consensus meeting. Part 1. Infections and etiopathogenesis. Oral Surg Oral Med Oral Pathol Oral Endod 2005; 100:40.

Lonsdale-Eccles AA, Velangi S: Topical pimecrolimus in the treatment of genital lichen planus: a prospective case series. Br J Dermatol 2005; 153:390.

Lozada-Nur F, Sroussi H: Tacrolimus powder in Orabase 0.1% for the treatment of oral lichen planus and oral lichenoid lesions: an open clinical trial. Oral Surg Oral Med Oral Pathol Oral Endod 2006; 102:744.

Luis-Montaya P, et al: Lichen planus in 24 children with review of the literature. Ped Dermatol 2005; 22:295.

Lundqvist EN, et al: Psychological health in patients with genital and oral erosive lichen planus. Eur Acad Dermatol Venereol 2006; 20:661.

Maender J, et al: Complete resolution of generalized lichen planus after treatment with thalidomide. J Drugs Dermatol 2005; 4:86.

Malhotra A, et al: Betamethasone oral mini-pulse therapy compared with topical triamcinolone acetonide (0.1%) paste in oral lichen planus: a randomized comparative study. J Am Acad Dermatol 2008; 58:596.

Maluf R, et al: Bilateral lower eyelid margin erosion associated with lichen planus. Ophth Plastic Recon Surg 2006; 22:310.

Mansura A, et al: Ultraviolet A-1 as a treatment for ulcerative lichen planus of the feet. Photodermatol Photoimmunol Photomed 2006; 22:164.

Maticic M, et al: Lichen planus and other cutaneous manifestations in chronic hepatitis C: pre- and post-interferon-based treatment prevalence vary in a cohort of patients from low hepatitis C virus endemic area. Eur Acad Dermatol Venereol 2008; 22:779.

Mignogna M, et al: Dysplasia/neoplasia surveillance in oral lichen planus patients: a description of clinical criteria adopted at a single centre and their impact on prognosis. Oral Oncol 2006; 42:819.

Mohrenschlager M, et al: Primary manifestation of a zosteriform lichen planus: isotopic response following herpes zoster sine herpete. Br J Dermatol 2008; 158:1145.

Morales-Callaghan A Jr, et al: Annular atrophic lichen planus. J Am Acad Dermatol 2005; 52:906.

Nagao Y, et al: Exacerbation of oral erosive lichen planus by combination of interferon and ribavirin therapy for chronic hepatitis C. Int J Molecul Med 2005; 15:237.

Nagao Y, et al: Insulin resistance and lichen planus in patients with HCV-infectious liver diseases. J Gastroenterol Hepatol 2008; 23:580.

Nakova I, et al: Psychological profile in oral lichen planus. J Clin Periodontol 2005; 32:1034.

Neville JA, et al: Treatment of severe cutaneous ulcerative lichen planus with low molecular weight heparin in a patient with hepatitis C. Cutis 2007; 79:37.

Nousari HC, et al: Successful treatment of resistant hypertrophic and bullous lichen planus with mycophenolate mofetil. Arch Dermatol 1999; 135:1420.

Okiyama N, et al: Squamous cell carcinoma arising from lichen planus of nail matrix and nail bed. J Am Acad Dermatol 2005; 53:908.

Ortiz-Ruiz A, et al: Oral lichen planus and sensitization to manganese in a dental prosthesis. Contact Dermatitis 2006; 54:214.

Pakravan M, et al: Isolated lichen planus of the conjunctiva. Br J Ophthalmol 2006; 90:1325.

Parodi A, et al: Prevalence of stratified epithelium-specific antinuclear antibodies in 138 patients with lichen planus. J Am Acad Dermatol 2007; 56:974.

Passeron T, et al: Treatment of erosive oral lichen planus by the 308 nm excimer laser. Lasers Surg Med 2004; 34:205.

Passeron T, et al: Treatment of oral erosive lichen planus with 1% pimecrolimus cream. Arch Dermatol 2007; 143:472.

Perez A, et al: Occupational contact dermatitis from 2,4-dinitrofluorobenzene. Contact Dermatitis 2004; 51:314.

Petropoulou H, et al: Effective treatment of erosive lichen planus with thalidomide and topical tacrolimus. Intl J Dermatol 2006; 45:1244.

Pigatto P, et al: Oral lichen planus: mercury and its kin. Arch Dermatol 2005; 141:1472.

Pinto JM, et al: Lichen planus and leukocytoclastic vasculitis induced by interferon alpha-2b in a subject with HCV-related chronic active hepatitis. J Eur Acad Dermatol Venereol 2003; 17:193.

Polderman MC, et al: Ultraviolet A1 in the treatment of generalized lichen planus: a report of 4 cases. J Am Acad Dermatol 2004; 50:646.

Quispel R, et al: High prevalence of esophageal involvement in lichen planus: a study using magnification chromoendoscopy. Endo 2009; 41:187.

Radfar L, et al: A comparative treatment study of topical tacrolimus and clobetasol in oral lichen planus. Oral Surg Oral Med Oral Pathol Oral Radiol Endod 2008; 105:187.

Rahman SB, et al: Unilateral blaschkoid lichen planus involving the entire half of the body, a unique presentation. Dermatol Online J 2007; 13:36.

Rahnama Z, et al: The relationship between lichen planus and hepatitis C in dermatology outpatients in Kerman, Iran. Int J Dermatol 2005; 44:746.

Reich HL, et al: Annular lichen planus: a case series of 20 patients. J Am Acad Dermatol 2004; 50:595.

Reichrath J, et al: Treatment of genito-anal lesions in inflammatory skin diseases with PUVA cream photochemotherapy: an open pilot study in 12 patients.

Richert B, et al: Nail bed lichen planus associated with onychopapilloma. Br J Dermatol 2007; 156:1071.

Rogers RS, Bruce AJ: Lichenoid contact stomatitis. Arch Dermatol 2004; 140:1524.

Sakuma-Oyama Y, et al: Lichen planus pemphigoides evolving into pemphigoid nodularis. Clin Exp Dermatol 2003; 28:613.

Salem CB, et al: Captopril-induced lichen planus pemphigoides. Pharmacoepidemiol Drug Safety 2008; 17:722.

Sanchez-Perez J, et al: Lichen planus with lesions on the palms and/or soles: prevalence and clinicopathological study of 36 patients. Br J Dermatol 2000; 142:310.

Saricaoglu H, et al: Narrowband UVB therapy in the treatment of lichen planus. Photodermatol Photoimmunol Photomed 2003; 19:265.

Scalf LA, et al: Dental metal allergy in patients with oral cutaneous, and genital lichenoid reactions. Am J Contact Dermatitis 2001; 12:146.

Scardina GA, et al: A randomized trial assessing the effectiveness of different concentrations of isotretinoin in the management of lichen planus. Int J Oral Maxillofac Surg 2006; 35:67.

Schwartz M, et al: Two siblings with lichen planus and squamous cell carcinoma of the oesophagus. Eur J Gastroenterol Hepatol 2006; 10:1111.

Setterfield JF, et al: The vulvovaginal gingival syndrome: a severe subgroup of lichen planus with characteristic clinical features and a novel association with the class II HLA DQb1* 0201 allele. J Am Acad Dermatol 2006; 55:98.

Seyhan M, et al: High prevalence of glucose metabolism disturbance in patients with lichen planus. Diabetes Research Clin Practice 2007; 77:198.

Shichinohe R, et al: Successful treatment of severe recalcitrant erosive oral lichen planus with topical tacrolimus. Eur Acad Dermatol Venereol 2006; 20:66.

Sing SK, et al: Squamous cell carcinoma arising from hypertrophic lichen planus. Eur Acad Dermatol Venereol 2006; 20:745.

Singal A: Familial mucosal lichen planus in three successive generations. Int J Dermatol 2005; 44:81.

Swift J, et al: The effectiveness of 1% pimecrolimus cream in the treatment of oral erosive lichen planus. J Periodontol 2005; 76:627.

Thongprasom K, et al: Clinical evaluation in treatment of oral lichen planus with topical fluocinolone acetonide: a 2-year follow-up. J Oral Pathol Med 2003; 32:315.

Thorne JE, et al: Lichen planus and cicatrizing conjunctivitis: characterization of five cases. Am J Ophthalmol 2003; 136:239.

Thornhill M, et al: The role of histopathological characteristic in distinguishing amalgam-associated oral lichenoid reactions and oral lichen planus. J Oral Pathol Med 2006; 35:233.

Tilly J, et al: Lichenoid eruptions in children. J Am Acad Dermatol 2004; 51:606.

Tong DC, Ferguson MM: Concurrent oral lichen planus and primary sclerosing cholangitis. Br J Dermatol 2002; 147:356.

Torti D, et al: Oral lichen planus. Arch Dermatol 2007; 143:511.

Tosti A, et al: Nail changes in lichen planus may resemble those of yellow nail syndrome. Br J Dermatol 2000; 142:848.

Tosti A, et al: Nail lichen planus in children: clinical features, response to treatment, and long-term follow-up. Arch Dermatol 2001; 137:1027.

Vazques-Lopez F, et al: Dermoscopy of active lichen planus. Arch Dermatol 2007; 143:1092.

Verma S: Lichen planus affecting eyelid alone: a rare entity. Indian J Dermatol Venereol Leprol 2006; 72:398.

Walsh DS, et al: A vaginal prosthetic device as an aid in treating ulcerative lichen planus of the mucous membrane. Arch Dermatol 1995; 131:265.

Welsh JP, et al: A novel visual clue for the diagnosis of hypertrophic lichen planus. Arch Dermatol 2006; 142:954

Westbrook R, Stuart R: Esophageal lichen planus: case report and literature review. Dysphagia 2008; 23:331.

Wong CS, et al: Isolated vulval splitting—is this normal or pathological? J Obstet Gynaecol 2004; 24:899.

Xia J, et al: Short-term clinical evaluation of intralesional triamcinolone acetonide injection for ulcerative oral lichen planus. J Oral Pathol Med 2006; 35:327.

Yashar S, et al: Lichen sclerosus–lichen planus overlap in a patient with hepatitis C virus infection. Br J Dermatol 2004; 150:168.

Yokozeki H, et al: Twenty-nail dystrophy (trachyonychia) caused by lichen planus in a patient with gold allergy. Br J Dermatol 2005; 152:1089.

Zakrzewska JM, et al: A systematic review of placebo-controlled randomized clinical trials of treatments used in oral lichen planus. Br J Dermatol 2005; 153:336.

Zillikens D, et al: Autoantibodies in lichen planus pemphigoides react with a novel epitope within the C-terminal NC16A domain of BP180. J Invest Dermatol 1999; 113:117.

Follicular lichen planus (lichen planopilaris)

Lichen planopilaris is lichen planus involving the follicular apparatus (Fig. 12-11). Most cases involve the scalp and it is an important cause of cicatricial alopecia (see Chapter 33). Seventy to 80% of affected patients are women, usually around the age of 50. The oral mucosa is involved, with reticulate lichen planus in 7–27% of patients, and between 20% and 40% of patients have cutaneous involvement. Graham–Little–Piccardi–Lassueur syndrome describes patients with lichen planopilaris of the scalp with coexistent keratosis pilaris-like lichen planopilaris lesions and nonscarring alopecia of the eyebrows, axillae, and pubic area. Thalidomide and cyclosporine have been reported to be effective.

Cooper S, et al: The association of lichen sclerosus and erosive lichen planus of the vulva with autoimmune disease. Arch Dermatol 2008; 144:1432.

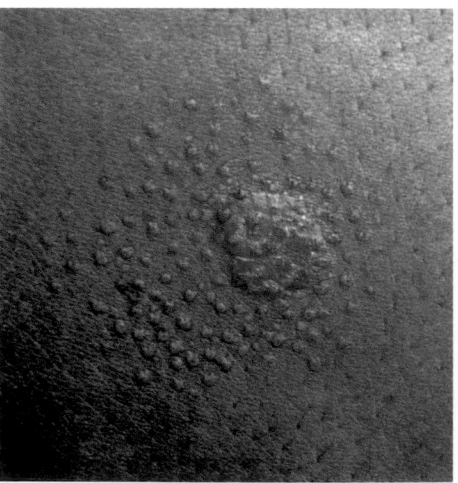

Fig. 12-11 Follicular lichen planus surrounding a classic lichen planus papule.

Lichen planus pigmentosus/actinicus

Lichen planus pigmentosus is seen primarily in Central America, the Indian subcontinent, the Middle East, and Japan. It appears to be a form of LP restricted to certain racial groups. The persons from these genetic groups can develop the condition when they move to North America and Europe, but Caucasians from Europe and North America do not develop lichen planus pigmentosus when they move to tropical areas where the disease is common. Lichen planus pigmentosus patients are young (between 20 and 45 in most cases), and men and women are equally represented. Men present a decade earlier (mean age 26 vs 34). The face and neck are primarily involved, but the axilla, inframammary region, and groin may also be affected. Lesions may be unilateral. The condition is usually mild (<10% body surface area), and while patients may have associated pruritus, it is usually much milder than in patients with classic LP. Sometimes classic LP papules occur at other sites or at the periphery of the lesions. In the US, persons of color may demonstrate this pattern of LP. Individual lesions are typically several millimeters to several centimeters in size, are oval in shape, and may follow lines of Blaschko. Some patients with lichen planus pigmentosus may have lesions predominantly in sun-exposed areas, and the diagnosis of lichen planus actinicus can be used in these cases. Lichen planus actinicus is reported most frequently in Africa, the Middle East, and the Indian subcontinent, and represents a substantial proportion of LP diagnosed in these geographic areas (36% of all LP patients in a recent Egyptian series). Most cases reported as lichen planus actinicus occur in childhood through young adulthood, 20–30 years being the primary decade of presentation. The disease presents in the spring or summer, and is frequently quiescent during the winter. Lesions favor the sun-exposed parts of the body, especially the face, which is almost always the most severely affected site. Most lesions occur on the forehead, cheeks, eyelids, and lips. Outside the face, the V area of the chest, the neck, the backs of the hands, and the lower extensor forearms are involved. Associated pruritus, the hallmark of LP, is usually described as mild or absent. Lesions are usually annular but may be reticulate or diffuse. Individual lesions are often macular but may be plaques with peripheral violaceous papules. Characteristically, lesions are hyperpigmented, sometimes with the blue–gray tinge of dermal melanin. They may resemble melasma. Since overlap cases between lichen planus pigmentosus and lichen planus actinicus do occur, it is best to think of these conditions as a single disorder that may or may not be photoexacerbated. It is important to recognize the lichen planus actinicus variant of lichen planus pigmentosus, as these patients do respond to sun protection, with gradual fading of their hyperpigmentation. Mucous membrane disease is significantly less common in patients with lichen planus pigmentosus/actinicus. Histologically, any papular element will usually show features of LP. Even macular areas may show subtle evidence of an interface dermatitis, with prominent dermal melanophages.

Erythema dyschromicum perstans

Erythema dyschromicum perstans is also known as ashy dermatosis or dermatosis cinicienta. The age of onset is virtually always before 40, but since it is a chronic disease, patients of all ages have been described. Prepubertal children have been reported. Lesions are typically several centimeters in size and affect primarily the trunk. A characteristic very fine (several millimeters), erythematous, palpable, nonscaling border is seen at the periphery of the lesions. This is described as feeling like a small cord. Unfortunately, this leading edge (and diag-

nostic feature) of the disorder is only present early in the disease course (a few months). Pruritus is not reported, and typical lichenoid papules are said not to occur. Nail and mucosal involvement is not found. An association with HLA-DR4 has been suggested for Mexican patients. Unfortunately, erythema dyschromicum perstans became a wastebasket term for the panoply of dermatological disorders that heal with prominent postinflammatory change in persons of color. It is now believed that most cases previously called erythema dyschromicum perstans are actually cases of lichen planus pigmentosus. Childhood cases may represent idiopathic eruptive macular pigmentation. True erythema dyschromicum perstans, if it exists, is quite rare, and largely restricted to certain geographic regions.

At the active border the characteristic histologic features of erythema dyschromicum perstans are those of a lichenoid dermatitis. In the centers of the lesions, the histologic changes are those of postinflammatory pigmentation. Therapeutic agents used for LP may benefit the acute inflammatory stage, but have limited effect on the pigmented lesions. Clofazimine, 100 mg/day for patients over 40 kg, and every other day for patients under 40 kg, has been reported to induce clearing in approximately 50%, but clofazimine pigment may complicate prolonged treatment. Dapsone has also been reported as effective. In some affected children, spontaneous improvement has occurred, leading some to suggest that no treatment is reasonable.

Idiopathic eruptive macular pigmentation

Although rarely reported, this condition is not rare. Young persons (mean age 11 years) in one study presented with asymptomatic widespread brown to gray macules of up to several centimeters in diameter on the neck, trunk, and proximal extremities. Lesions are not confluent and there is no history of preceding inflammation. Lesions may spontaneously involute. Some cases reported as erythema dyschromicum perstans in childhood may actually represent this entity.

Akagi A, et al: Linear hyperpigmentation with extensive epidermal apoptosis: a variant of linear lichen planus pigmentosus. J Am Acad Dermatol 2004; 50:S78.

Anbar T, et al: A clinical and epidemiological study of lichen planus among Egyptians of Al-Minya province. Dermatol Online 2005; 11:4.

Correa M, et al: HLA-DR association with the genetic susceptibility to develop ashy dermatosis in Mexican mestizo patients. J Am Acad Dermatol 2007; 56:(4):617.

Ince U: Lichen striatus in an adult patient treated with pimecrolimus. J Eur Acad Dermatol Venereol 2006; 20:360.

Jang KA, et al: Idiopathic eruptive macular pigmentation: report of 10 cases. J Am Acad Dermatol 2001; 44:351.

Jansen T, et al: Lichen planus actinicus treated with acitretin and topical corticosteroids. J Eur Acad Dermatol Venereol 2002; 16:171.

Kanwar AJ, et al: A study of 124 Indian patients with lichen planus pigmentosus. Clin Exp Dermatol 2003; 28:481.

Kashima A, et al: Two Japanese cases of lichen planus pigmentosus inversus. Int J Dermatol 2007; 46:740.

Kim G, Mikkilineni R: Lichen planus actinicus. Dermatol 2007; 13:13.

Torrelo A, et al: Erythema dyschromicum perstans in children: a report of 14 cases. J Eur Acad Dermatol Venereol 2005; 19:422.

Volz A, et al: Idiopathic eruptive macular pigmentation in a 7-year-old girl. Case report and discussion of differences from erythema dyschromicum perstans. Br J Dermatol 2007; 157:799.

Keratosis lichenoides chronica

This very rare dermatosis is characterized by its chronicity. In adults the disease begins in the late twenties. Typical lesions are papulonodular, hyperkeratotic, and covered with gray scales. These lesions favor the extremities and buttocks. Although initially discrete, the lesions frequently coalesce to

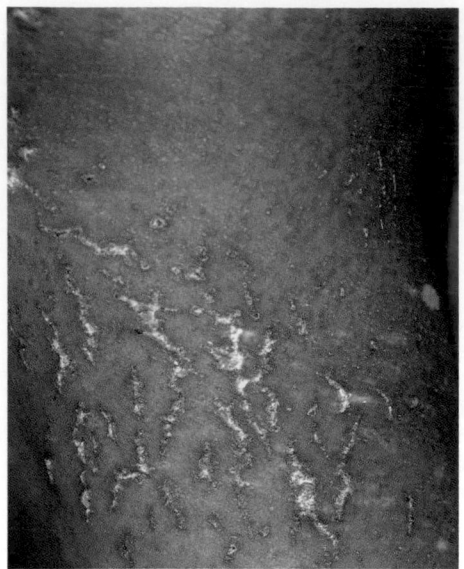

Fig. 12-12 Keratosis lichenoides chronica.

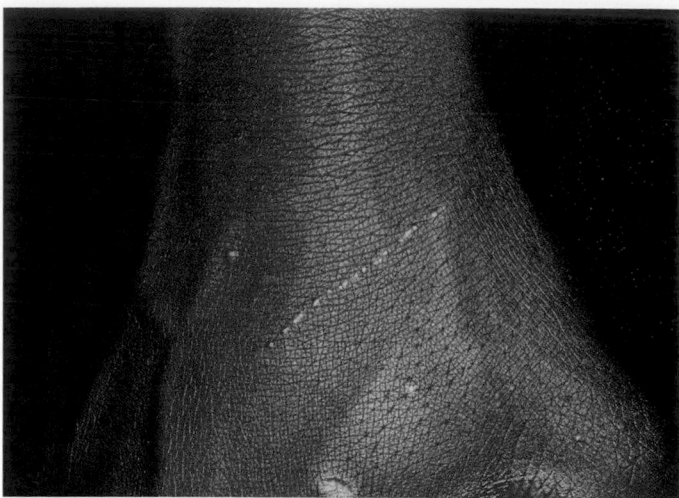

Fig. 12-13 Lichen nitidus, linear lesion from trauma.

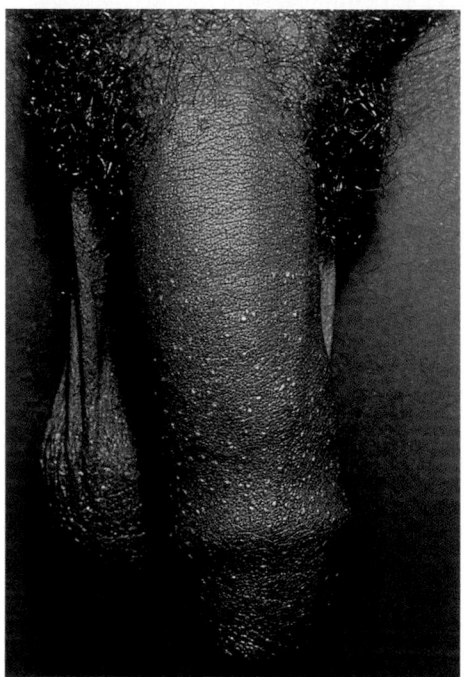

Fig. 12-14 Lichen nitidus, characteristic lesions of the penile shaft.

form linear and reticulate arrays of warty lichenoid lesions (Fig. 12-12). Lesions are infundibulocentric and acrosyringocentric. Keratotic plugs and prominent telangiectasia may be present. The palms and soles have discrete hyperkeratotic papules. There is an associated sharply marginated erythema, scaling, and telangiectasia of the face, superficially resembling seborrheic dermatitis or rosacea. Nail changes, including thickening of the nail plate, yellowing, longitudinal ridging, onycholysis, hyperkeratosis of the nailbed, paronychia, and warty lesions of the periungual areas, have been described. In addition, painful oral aphthae-like lesions often occur. Other findings include hoarseness due to vocal cord edema, and involvement of the eyelids (one-third of patients), conjunctiva, iris, or anterior chamber. Topical calcipotriol, PUVA, re-PUVA, bath PUVA, photodynamic therapy, and oral retinoids (isotretinoin and acitretin) may all prove beneficial. Keratosis lichenoides chronica rarely responds to topical or systemic steroids. Childhood cases are rare and differ from adult cases. They start in the first year of life, and have prominent facial purpura and erythema, especially on the cheeks. There are familial associations in more than half of childhood cases, suggesting an autosomal-recessive inheritance.

Histologically, there is irregular acanthosis or epidermal atrophy with hyperkeratosis and zones of parakeratosis. A lichenoid infiltrate, consisting primarily of lymphocytes, and vacuolar alteration at the basal cell layer, but concentrated around the infundibular and acrosyringia. Marked follicular plugging and plugging of the acrosyringia are characteristic.

Avermaete A, et al: Keratosis lichenoides chronica: characteristics and response to acitretin. Br J Dermatol 2001; 144:422.

Boer A: Keratosis lichenoides chronica: proposal of a concept. Am J Dermatopath 2006; 28:260.

Kunte C, et al: Keratosis lichenoides chronica: treatment with bath-PUVA. Acta Derm Venereol 2007; 87:182.

Lopez Navarro N, et al: Keratosis lichenoides chronica: response to photodynamic therapy. J Dermatologic Treatment 2008; 19:124.

Ruis-Maldonaldo R, et al: Keratosis lichenoides chronica in pediatric patients: a different disease. J Am Acad Dermatol 2007; 56:S1.

Lichen nitidus

Clinical features

Lichen nitidus (LN) is a chronic inflammatory disease characterized by minute, shiny, flat-topped, pale, exquisitely discrete, uniform papules, rarely larger than 1–2 mm. Children and young adults are primarily affected. Pruritus is usually minimal or absent, but may be more prominent in more generalized cases. Linear arrays of papules (Koebner phenomenon) are common, especially on the penis, forearms, and dorsal hands. Initially, lesions are localized and often remain limited to a few areas, chiefly the penis and lower abdomen, the inner surfaces of the thighs, and the flexor aspects of the wrists and dorsal hands/forearms (Figs 12-13 and 12-14). In other cases, the disease assumes a more widespread distribution, and the papules fuse into erythematous, finely scaly plaques. The reddish color varies with tints of yellow, brown, or violet. Unusual variants of LN include vesicular, hemorrhagic, linear, purpuric (resembling a pigmented purpuric dermatosis), and spinous follicular (resembling lichen spinulosus).

Palm and sole involvement may occur in LN, and the disease may be restricted to these areas. It presents with multiple, tiny, hyperkeratotic papules. The papules may coalesce to form diffuse hyperkeratotic plaques that fissure. The differentiation of LN from hyperkeratotic hand eczema and lichen planus of the palms is aided by the presence of a keratotic plug in the center of lesions of palmoplantar LN. Nail involvement with pitting; beaded, longitudinal ridging; and nailfold inflammation have been reported. Oral involvement, with gray–yellow papules or petechiae of the hard palate, is rare.

A variant of LN, termed actinic lichen nitidus, has been reported in dark-skinned patients from the Middle East and Indian subcontinent. Cases seen in African Americans have also been termed "pinpoint, papular polymorphous light eruption (PMLE)," or known by the older term "summer actinic lichenoid eruption." These cases all have lesions clinically and histologically identical to LN, which are limited to the sun-exposed areas of the dorsal hands, brachioradial area, and posterior neck. The LN histology may represent subacute or chronic lesions of pinpoint PMLE. Actinic LN/pinpoint papular PMLE usually responds to sun protection, with or without topical steroids.

The course of LN is slowly progressive, with a tendency for remission. The lesions may remain stationary for years but eventually they often disappear spontaneously and entirely. The cause of LN is unknown. Rare familial cases do occur. It is clinically and histologically distinct from lichen planus, and immunohistochemical studies also suggest they are distinct disorders. However, patients have been reported who have had both disorders, suggesting some common pathogenic basis. Both LP and LN have been reported as being secondary to hepatitis B immunization, and during treatment of hepatitis with interferon-α. There are also reports of patients with both LN and Crohn's disease, another condition with granulomatous inflammation. LN has a characteristic histologic appearance. Dermal papillae are widened and contain a dense infiltrate composed of lymphocytes, histiocytes, and melanophages. Multinucleate giant cells are often present, imparting a granulomatous appearance to the infiltrate. The epidermal rete ridges on either side of the papilla form a clawlike collarette. The overlying epidermis is attenuated, and there is usually vacuolar alteration of its basal layer. At times the infiltrate may extend down adjacent hair follicles and eccrine ducts, making distinction of LN from lichen scrofulosorum and lichen striatus difficult.

Because LN is usually asymptomatic, treatment is often not necessary. Topical application of high or superpotent topical corticosteroids or topical calcineurin inhibitors may suppress pruritus and lead to resolution of skin lesions. Narrow-band UVB and PUVA could be considered in more generalized and symptomatic cases. Anecdotal reports suggest therapeutic benefit from oral retinoids (etretinate and acitretin). As in lichen planus, refractory cases requiring aggressive therapy may respond to cyclosporine A.

Al Mutari N, et al: Generalized lichen nitidus. Ped Dermatol 2005; 22:158.

Bansal I, et al: Pinpoint papular variant of polymorphous light eruption: clinical and pathological correlation. Euro Acad Dermatol 2006; 20:406.

Dobbs CR, Murphy SJ: Lichen nitidus treated with topical tacrolimus. J Drugs Dermatol 2004; 3:683.

Fetil E, et al: Lichen nitidus after hepatitis B vaccine. Int Soc Dermatol 2004; 43:956.

Lernia V, et al: Lichen planus appearing subsequent to generalized lichen nitidus in a child. Ped Dermatol 2007; 24:453.

MacDonald AJ, et al: Lichen nitidus and lichen spinulosus or spinous follicular lichen nitidus. Clin Exp Dermatol 2005; 30:435.

Modi S, et al: Lichen nitidus actinicus: a distinct facial presentation in 3 pre-pubertal African-American girls. Dermatol Online J 2008; 14:10.

Park JH, et al: Treatment of generalized lichen nitidus with narrowband ultraviolet B. J Am Acad Dermatol 2006; 54:545.

Rallis E, et al: Generalized purpuric lichen nitidus: report of a case and review of the literature. Dermatol Online J 2007; 13:5.

Sanders S, et al: Periappendageal lichen nitidus: report of a case. J Cutan Pathol 2002; 29:125.

Scheinfeld NS, et al: Crohn's disease and lichen nitidus: a case report and comparison of common histopathologic features. Inflamm Bowel Dis 2001; 7:314.

Schelar M, et al: Generalized lichen nitidus with involvement of the palms following interferon alpha treatment. Dermatol 2007; 215:236.

Srivastava M, et al: Lassueur Graham Little Piccardi syndrome. Dermatol Online J 2007; 13:12.

Summey B, et al: Actinic lichen nitidus. Cutis 2008; 81:266.

Yanez S, Val-Bernal F: Purpuric generalized lichen nitidus: an unusual eruption simulating pigmented purpuric dermatosis. Dermatol 2004; 208:167.

Yoon TY, et al: Two cases of perforating lichen nitidus. J Dermatol 2006; 33:278.

Lichen striatus

Lichen striatus is a fairly common self-limited eruption that is seen primarily in young children (mean age 3 years). Girls are affected 2–3 times more frequently than boys. Lesions begin as small papules that are erythematous and slightly scaly (Fig. 12-15). In more darkly pigmented persons, hypopigmentation is prominent and may be purely macular. The 1–3 mm papules coalesce to form a band 1–3 cm wide, either continuous or interrupted, which over a few weeks progresses down the extremity or around the trunk, following lines of Blaschko. An extremity is more commonly involved, but trunk lesions, or lesions extending from the trunk on to an extremity, can also occur. About 10% of cases occur on the head. Multiple bands can uncommonly occur. Lesions are usually asymptomatic but pruritus may occur, especially in patients who are also atopic.

Nail involvement can occur if the process extends down the digit to the nail. Most commonly, the lichen striatus appears first on the skin, but the skin and nail abnormality may appear simultaneously. Uncommonly, only the nail may be involved for months, with later appearance of the band on the skin, or the nail may remain the sole area of involvement throughout the course of the disease. Nail-plate thinning, longitudinal ridging, splitting, and nailbed hyperkeratosis may be seen. Often only a part of the nail is involved. The histology of involved nails is identical to that of the skin lesions.

The active lesions of lichen striatus last for an average of 1 year, but may persist for up to 4 years. Eventually, all the lesions, including dystrophic nails, spontaneously resolve without scarring. Hypopigmentation may persist for several years. Hyperpigmentation is uncommon (<5%) and should suggest a diagnosis of linear lichen planus instead. Relapses can occur in up to 5% of cases, either in the same distribution or in a different anatomic region.

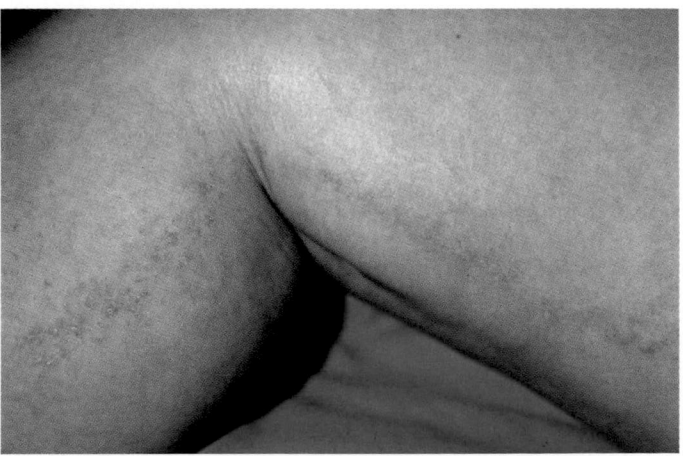

Fig. 12-15 Lichen striatus.

The histologic features of lichen striatus vary, partly reflecting the stage of evolution of the lesion. There may be a spongiotic dermatitis, but most frequently a lichenoid component is present. There is a bandlike infiltrate with necrotic keratinocytes at the dermoepidermal junction. Granulomatous inflammation may occasionally be present. Typically there is a dense lymphoid infiltrate around the eccrine sweat glands and ducts. This helps to distinguish lichen striatus from lichen planus.

Multiple reports exist of simultaneous cases in siblings. There is also a seasonal variation, with most cases occurring in the spring and summer. Epidemic outbreaks have been reported. These suggest a viral etiology or trigger. Trauma has also been reported to precipitate an outbreak of lichen striatus.

Adult cases of lichen striatus differ from those in childhood, being rarer and more papulovesicular, affecting multiple regions, resolving more rapidly (less than 2 months), and relapsing more frequently (up to one-third of cases). Histologically, they show more spongiotic and less lichenoid features. This has led some authors to call these cases "adult Blaschkitis" or "Grosshans–Marot disease." This splitting is probably not of any clinical utility.

Usually the diagnosis is straightforward in the setting of a young child, with the sudden onset of an eruption following the lines of Blaschko. The differential diagnosis could include linear lichen planus, linear psoriasis, inflammatory linear verrucous epidermal nevus, epidermal nevus, linear cutaneous lupus erythematosus, and verruca plana. Histologic evaluation will usually distinguish these entities, but is rarely required.

Treatment is usually not necessary. Parents may be reassured of the uniformly excellent prognosis. Topical steroids and topical tacrolimus or pimecrolimus may accelerate the resolution of lesions. In children with an acquired nail dystrophy of one or two digits, this diagnosis must be considered, and watchful waiting might be considered before biopsying the nail.

Campanati A, et al: Lichen striatus in adults and pimecrolimus: open, off-label clinical study. Int J Dermatol 2008; 47:732.

Hofer T: Lichen striatus in adults or adult blaschkitis. Dermatol 2003; 207:89.

Jo JH, et al: Early treatment of multiple and spreading lichen striatus with topical tacrolimus. J Am Acad Dermatol 2007; 57:904.

Karakas M, et al: Lichen striatus following HBV vaccination. J Dermatol 2005; 32:506.

Keegan B, et al: Pediatric blaschkitis: expanding the spectrum of childhood acquired Blaschko linear dermatoses. Ped Dermatol 2007; 24:621.

Leposavic R, et al: Onychodystrophy and subungual hyperkeratosis due to lichen striatus. Arch Dermatol 2002; 138:1099.

Patrizi A, et al: Lichen striatus: clinical and laboratory features of 115 children. Ped Dermatol 2004; 21:197.

Shepherd V, et al: Lichen striatus in an adult following trauma. Aus J Dermatol 2005; 46:25.

Sorgentini C, et al: Lichen striatus in an adult: successful treatment with tacrolimus. Br J Dermatol 2004; 150:770.

Taniguchi K, et al: Lichen striatus: description of 89 cases in children. Ped Dermatol 2004; 21:440.

Lichen sclerosus (lichen sclerosus et atrophicus)

Lichen sclerosus is a chronic disease of the skin and mucosa. The terms lichen sclerosus et atrophicus, kraurosis vulvae, and balanitis xerotica obliterans are synonymous but have been replaced by the single term lichen sclerosus (LS). LS can present from childhood to old age. Although it occurs in all races, whites appear to be preferentially affected. Both sexes are affected both before and after puberty, with females predominating at all ages. The prevalence is about 1.7% in the general female population.

The pathogenesis of LS is poorly understood. Autoimmune diseases (thyroid disease, vitiligo, alopecia areata, and pernicious anemia) occur in between one-fifth and one-third of women with LS, but are much less common in men. Psoriasis is increased in women with LS, reported to occur in 7.5–17% of patients. Autoantibodies to extracellular matrix protein (ECM) 1 are found in 80% of LS patients (as compared to 4% of controls and 7–10% of patients with other autoimmune diseases). The titer of the ECM 1 autoantibody correlates with the disease severity. The importance of this humoral autoimmunity in the pathogenesis of LS is currently unclear.

In females, there is a bimodal age distribution—prepubertal and postmenopausal. The initial lesions of LS are white, polygonal, flat-topped papules, plaques, or atrophic patches (Fig. 12-16). Lesions may be surrounded by an erythematous to violaceous halo. In atrophic lesions, the skin is smooth, slightly wrinkled, soft, and white (Fig. 12-17). Bullae, often hemorrhagic, telangiectasias, and fixed areas of purpura may occur on the patches. About 40% of women with LS are asymptomatic. However, when women referred to specialists are questioned, virtually 100% are symptomatic. Itching is frequently severe, especially in the anogenital area. In the genital area, fissuring and erosion may occur. This may result in dysuria, urethral and vaginal discharge, dyspareunia, and burning pain. Normal anatomic structures may be obliterated, with loss of the labia minora, clitoral hood, and urethral meatus. In women, this perineal involvement typically affects the

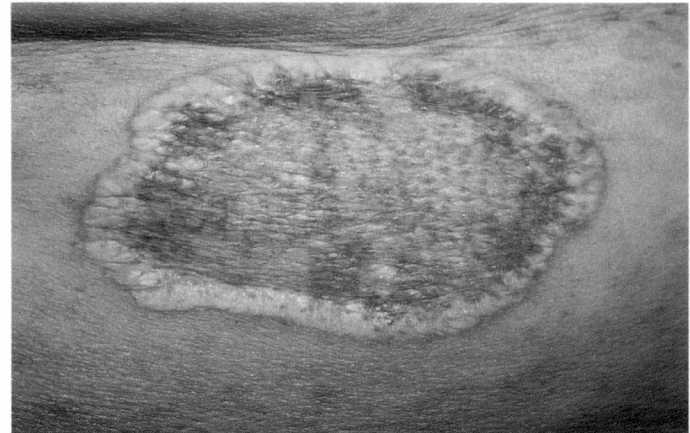

Fig. 12-16 Lichen sclerosus of the glabrous skin.

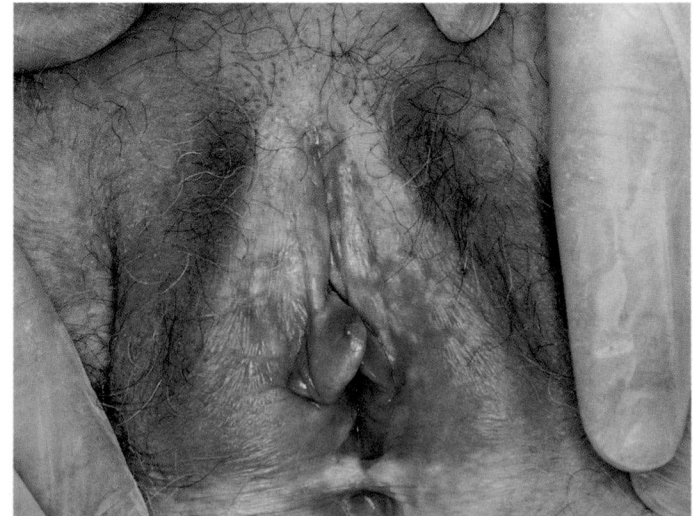

Fig. 12-17 Lichen sclerosus, white atrophic lesions with loss of normal tissue markings.

vulvar and perianal areas, giving a "figure-eight" or "hour-glass" appearance. Introital stenosis or fusion may occur. The vaginal and cervical mucosa are not involved by LS (in contrast to lichen planus). Prepubertal girls may also be affected and usually have vulvar and perianal lesions. Vulvar disease is associated with similar skin changes to those in adult women, and pruritus may be a prominent symptom. Perianal involvement may produce significant symptomatology of constipation, stool holding, and rectorrhagia due to rectal fissures. Infantile perineal protrusion refers to a pyramidal soft-tissue swelling covered by red or rose-colored skin along the median perineal raphe (the skin between the posterior fourchette and the anus). This occurs only in girls and appears to be a manifestation of LS in some prepubertal girls. Two-thirds of girls with LS have been evaluated for sexual abuse, largely due to the ecchymoses that accompany the lesions. If risk of sexual abuse is suspected, appropriate investigations must be performed.

There is clearly a relationship between the hormonal milieu and LS. Postmenopausal women are preferentially affected. Pregnancy leads to improvement, and often complete resolution. Oral contraceptive pill (OCP) use is common in premenopausal women with LS. These OCPs are often anti-androgenic. Stopping these agents and treating with standard topicals leads to significant improvement, suggesting that the anti-androgen OCPs may have accelerated the appearance of the LS. However, treatment of postmenopausal women with estrogen supplementation does not alter the incidence or course of their LS.

In males, lesions are atrophic and may be markedly hypopigmented or depigmented, resembling vitiligo. Lesions usually involve only the glans penis, but may extend on to the penile shaft and scrotum. If the glans is involved, hemorrhage is common, and shallow erosions may occur. LS of the glans does not usually lead to nonhealing erosions of the glans, but rather simply skin fragility. Phimosis and paraphimosis are common complications of LS in men (Fig. 12-18). Between 15% and 100% of circumcision specimens from prepubertal boys show features of LS. Sixty percent of acquired phimosis in boys and at least 10% in adult men are associated with LS. Most men with LS are uncircumcised. However, circumcision does not universally "cure" LS in boys or men, with at least 50% of men so treated continuing to have lesions of LS. Urethral meatal stenosis may occur and requires surgical correction. Perianal involvement by LS is much less common in men and boys.

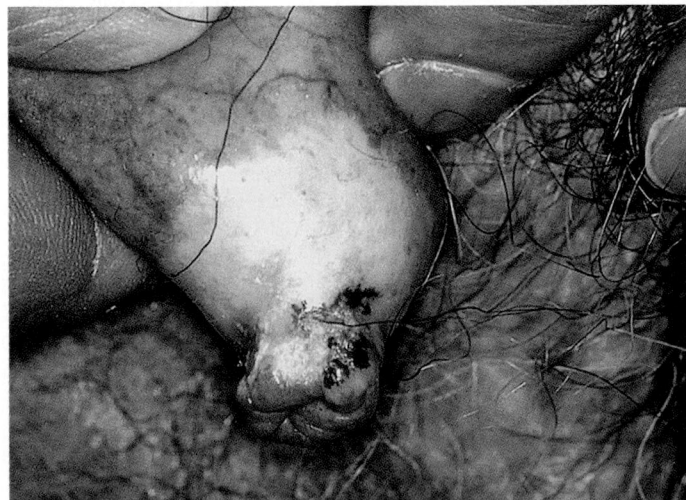

Fig. 12-18 Lichen sclerosus, phimosis; note the hemorrhagic macule. (Courtesy of Shyam Verma MD)

Extragenital lesions are most frequent on the upper back, chest, and breasts, and are usually asymptomatic. The tongue and oral mucosa may also be involved, either alone or with lesions elsewhere. Peristomal involvement around colostomy sites may occur. Patients having only extragenital lesions with histologic features of both LS and morphea have been reported. They may simultaneously have other cutaneous lesions of morphea or atrophoderma of Pasini and Pierini. These patients are best viewed as having morphea with overlying LS-like changes, rather than a form of LS. Rarely, in Europe, *Borrelia* has been reported to cause extragenital LS, and treatment with antibiotics has arrested the progression of the lesions.

Lichen sclerosus and cancer

Although the risk is not as high as was proposed early in this century, LS of the genitalia is a condition with increased risk for genital squamous cell carcinoma (SCC) in both women and men. The lifetime risk for women who are carefully followed appears to be 5% or less, but is clearly higher than for the general population. In one study, 14 of 23 (60%) anogenital SCCs in women arose on a background of LS. Human papillomavirus (HPV) appears to be associated with only about 15% of SCCs arising in women with LS. Hypertrophic vulvar lesions and age beyond 60 are clear risk factors for the development of SCC in women with LS. Such lesions and patients should be evaluated carefully. In men with LS the risk for genital SCC is less than in women with LS. However, between 44% and 55% of cases of penile SCC are associated with LS. Oncogenic HPV types do not appear to be associated with LS-associated penile cancer. The use of potent topical steroids and calcineurin inhibitors can be associated with activation of latent HPV infection and is of theoretical concern.

Histopathology

Early lesions are characterized by an interface dermatitis with vacuolar alteration of keratinocytes. With evolution the epidermis is thinned and the rete ridges are effaced. Compact orthokeratosis and follicular and eccrine plugging are present. The upper dermis is edematous, with the upper dermal collagen homogenized. Immediately beneath the altered papillary dermis there is a sparse bandlike and perivascular lymphoid infiltrate. In pruritic lesions, coexistent changes of lichen simplex chronicus may be seen, with acanthosis rather than atrophy of the epidermis.

Differential diagnosis

Extragenital LS must be differentiated from guttate morphea and lichen planus, especially of the atrophic type. Anogenital LS must be distinguished from genital lichen planus, lichen simplex chronicus, vulvar intraepithelial neoplasia (SCC in situ), and extramammary Paget's disease. The white color and atrophic surface are characteristic, and such areas are most fruitful if biopsied to confirm the diagnosis.

Treatment

The use of superpotent topical steroids has dramatically changed the management of anogenital LS. They are universally accepted as the treatment of choice for all forms of genital LS. Most patients will respond to once daily application of these agents and can subsequently be tapered to less frequent applications (once or twice a week) or to lower-strength steroids. In general, weekend application of an ultrapotent steroid is more effective than daily application of a mild steroid. Generally, the untreated lesions are atrophic, and pulsed weekend applications of a potent topical steroid treatment are associated with clinical and histologic reversal of the epidermal atrophy as the inflammatory process is controlled. Coexistent candidiasis may be present or appears with this treatment, and can be managed with topical or oral agents. Penile, vulvar, and prepubertal LS in girls have all been documented to respond to this form of treatment. Phimosis in young boys should be treated initially with potent topical steroids. The degree of symptomatic improvement far exceeds the objective improvement. The majority of patients have dramatic reduction in their itching and burning with topical clobetasol. However, the visible white, atrophic, scarred vulvar skin is often only minimally improved. It is unclear if aggressive topical therapy of LS reduces the risk of cancer development. Vulvar pain associated with LS may have a neuropathic component (as in vulvodynia), and treatment with tricyclic antidepressants (amitriptyline, for example), gabapentin, and duloxetine hydrochloride may be tried.

Topical tacrolimus 0.1% and 0.03% ointments and pimecrolimus 1% cream have also been demonstrated to be effective in genital LS. However, since superpotent steroids have proven so effective in genital LS, topical calcineurin inhibitors should be reserved for patients in whom topical steroids are ineffective or not tolerated. Close clinical follow-up is recommended, since the long-term risk of applying topical calcineurin inhibitors to skin predisposed to malignant degeneration is not known. Topical calcipotriol may also be of benefit. Topical testosterone was no more effective than emollient and in one trial was worse than emollients as maintenance therapy. It is no longer recommended. Hydroxychloroquine, calcitriol, topical 8% progesterone cream, topical calcipotriol, topical tretinoin, cyclosporine, and hydroxyurea can be considered in refractory cases. UVA-1 phototherapy led to moderate improvement in 3 out of 7 patients unresponsive to topical steroids. Some patients responded to topical corticosteroids following the UV treatment. Surgical treatments can be effective, starting with cryotherapy, which has been reported as helpful in three-quarters of patients with severe vulvar itch. Carbon dioxide ablation in male patients led to long-term remissions. Photodynamic therapy has brought significant improvement in multiple reports and can be considered in refractory cases. Extragenital LS is very difficult to treat. If superpotent topical steroids are ineffective, potassium p-aminobenzoic acid, PUVA, UVA-1, narrow-band UVB, calcipotriol, or antimalarials may be tried.

Alexiades Armenakas M, et al: Laser mediated photodynamic therapy of lichen sclerosus. J Drugs Dermatol 2004; 3:S25.

Assmann T, et al: Tacrolimus ointment for the treatment of vulvar lichen sclerosus. J Am Acad Dermatol 2003; 48:935.

Ayhan A, et al: Topical testosterone versus clobetasol for vulvar lichen sclerosus. Int J Gyne Obs 2007; 96:117.

Barbara E, et al: High prevalence of concomitant anogenital lichen sclerosus and extragenital psoriasis in adult women. Obs & Gyne 2008; 111:1143.

Baskan EB, et al: Open label trial of cyclosporine for vulvar lichen sclerosus. J Am Acad Dermatol 2007; 57:276.

Beattie PE, et al: UVA1 phototherapy for genital lichen sclerosus. Clin Exp Dermatol 2006; 31:343.

Birenbaum D, et al: High prevalence of thyroid disease in patients with lichen sclerosus. J Repro Med 2007; 52:28.

Bohm M, et al: Successful treatment of anogenital lichen sclerosus with topical tacrolimus. Arch Dermatol 2003; 139:922.

Boms S, et al: Pimecrolimus 1% cream for anogenital lichen sclerosus in childhood. BMC Dermatol 2004; 4:1471.

Bornstein J, et al: Clobetasol dipropionate 0.05% versus testosterone propionate 2% topical application for severe vulvar lichen sclerosus. Am J Obstet Gynecol 1998; 178:80.

Colbert R, et al: Progressive extragenital lichen sclerosus successfully treated with narrowband UV-B phototherapy. Arch Dermatol 2007; 143:19.

Cooper S, et al: The association of lichen sclerosus and erosive lichen planus of the vulva with autoimmune disease. Arch Dermatol 2008; 144:1432.

Dalmau J, et al: Psoralen UVA treatment for generalized prepubertal extragenital lichen sclerosus et atrophicus. J Am Acad Dermatol 2006; 55:S56.

Eisendle K, et al: Possible role of *Borrelia burgdorferi sensu lato* infection in lichen sclerosus. Arch Dermatol 2008; 144:591.

Goldstein A, et al: Pimecrolimus for the treatment of vulvar lichen sclerosus. J Repro Med 2004; 49:778.

Goldstein A, et al: Prevalence of vulvar lichen sclerosus in a general gynecology practice. J Repro Med 2005; 50:477.

Gunthert A, et al: Early onset vulvar lichen sclerosus in premenopausal women and oral contraceptives. Euro J Obs & Gyne 2008; 137:56.

Gupta S, et al: Treatment of genital lichen sclerosus with topical calcipotriol. Intl J STD & AIDS 2005; 16:772.

Hengge UR, et al: Multicentre, phase II trial on the safety and efficacy of topical tacrolimus ointment for the treatment of lichen sclerosus. Br J Dermatol 2006; 155:1021.

Hernandez-Machin B, et al: Infantile pyramidal protrusion localized at the vulva as a manifestation of lichen sclerosus et atrophicus. J Am Acad Dermatol 2007; 56:S49.

Jones R, et al: Clinically identifying women with vulvar lichen sclerosus at increased risk of squamous cell carcinoma. J Repro Med 2004; 49:808.

Khachemoune A, et al: Infantile perineal protrusion. J Am Acad Dermatol 2006; 54:1046.

Kreuter A, et al: Low-dose ultraviolet A1 phototherapy for extragenital lichen sclerosus: results of a preliminary study. J Am Acad Dermatol 2002; 46:251.

Maronn M, et al: Constipation as a feature of anogenital lichen sclerosus in children. Pediatr 2005; 115:e230.

Neill SM, et al: Guidelines for the management of lichen sclerosus. Br J Dermatol 2002; 147:640.

Oyama N, et al: Development of antigen-specific ELISA for circulating autoantibodies to extracellular matrix protein 1 in lichen sclerosus. J Clin Invest 2004; 113:1550.

Poindexter G, Morrell D: Anogenital pruritus: lichen sclerosus in children. Pediatr Annals 2007; 36:785.

Powell J, et al: High incidence of lichen sclerosus in patients with squamous cell carcinoma of the penis. Br J Dermatol 2001; 145:85.

Renaud Vilmer C: Effect of long term topical application of a potent steroid on the course of the disease. Arch Dermatol 2004; 140:709.

Romero A, et al: Treatment of recalcitrant erosive vulvar lichen sclerosus with photodynamic therapy. J Am Acad Dermatol 2007; 57:S46.

Simpkin S, et al: Clinical review of 202 patients with vulval lichen sclerosus: a possible association with psoriasis. Aus J Dermatol 2007; 48:28.

Stucket M, et al: The outcome after cryosurgery and intralesional steroid injection in vulvar lichen sclerosus corresponds to preoperative histopathological findings. Dermatol 2005; 210:218.

Thami GP, Kaur S: Genital lichen sclerosus, squamous cell carcinoma and circumcision. Br J Dermatol 2003; 148:1058.

Tomson N, Sterling JC: Hydroxycarbamide: a treatment for lichen sclerosus? Br J Dermatol 2007; 157:609.

Vincent MV, Mackinnon E: The response of clinical balanitis xerotica obliterans to the application of topical steroid-based creams. J Pediatr Sur 2005; 40:709.

Virgili A, et al: Open study of topical 0.025% tretinoin in the treatment of vulvar lichen sclerosus. J Reprod Med 1995; 40:614.

Windahl T: Is carbon dioxide laser treatment of lichen sclerosus effective in the long run? Scandin J Uro Nephro 2006; 40:208.

13 Acne

Acne vulgaris

Clinical features

Acne vulgaris is a chronic inflammatory disease of the pilo-sebaceous follicles, characterized by comedones, papules, pustules, nodules, and often scars. The comedo is the primary lesion of acne. It may be seen as a flat or slightly elevated papule with a dilated central opening filled with blackened keratin (open comedo or blackhead) (Fig. 13-1). Closed comedones (whiteheads) are usually 1 mm yellowish papules that may require stretching of the skin to visualize. Macrocomedones, which are uncommon, may reach 3–4 mm in size. The papules and pustules are 1–5 mm in size, and are caused by inflammation, so there is erythema and edema (Fig. 13-2). They may enlarge, become more nodular, and coalesce into plaques of several centimeters that are indurated or fluctuant, contain sinus tracts, and discharge serosanguinous or yellowish pus (Fig. 13-3).

Patients will typically have a variety of lesions in various states of formation and resolution. In light-skinned patients, lesions often resolve with a reddish-purple macule that is short-lived. In dark-skinned individuals, macular hyperpigmentation results and this may last several months (Fig. 13-4). Acne scars are heterogeneous in appearance. Morphologies include deep, narrow ice-pick scars seen most commonly on the temples and cheeks, canyon-type atrophic lesions on the face (Fig. 13-5), whitish-yellow papular scars on the trunk and chin, anetoderma-type scars on the trunk, and hypertrophic and keloidal elevated scars on the neck and trunk.

Acne affects primarily the face, neck, upper trunk (Fig. 13-6), and upper arms. On the face it occurs most frequently on the cheeks, and to a lesser degree on the nose, forehead, and chin. The ears may be involved, with large comedones in the concha, cysts in the lobes, and sometimes pre- and retro-auricular comedones and cysts. On the neck, especially in the nuchal area, large cystic lesions may predominate.

Acne typically begins at puberty and is often the first sign of increased sex hormone production. When acne begins at the age of 8–12 years, it is frequently comedonal in character, affecting primarily the forehead and cheeks. It may remain mild in its expression with only an occasional inflammatory papule. However, as hormone levels rise into the middle teenage years, more severe inflammatory pustules and nodules occur, with spread to other sites. Young men tend to have an oilier complexion and more severe widespread disease than young women. Women may experience a flare of their papulo-pustular lesions a week or so before menstruation. Acne may also begin in 20–35-year-old women who have not experienced teenage acne. This acne frequently manifests as papules, pustules, and deep painful persistent nodules on the jawline, chin, and upper neck.

Acne is primarily a disease of the adolescent, with 85% of all teenagers being affected to some degree. It occurs with

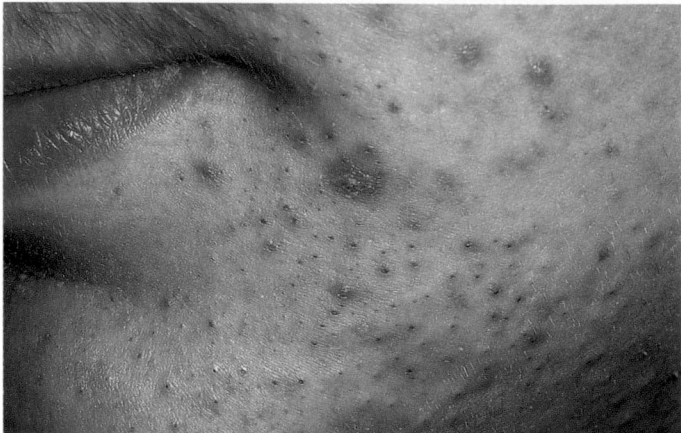

Fig. 13-1 Acne vulgaris, with comedones, on the chin.

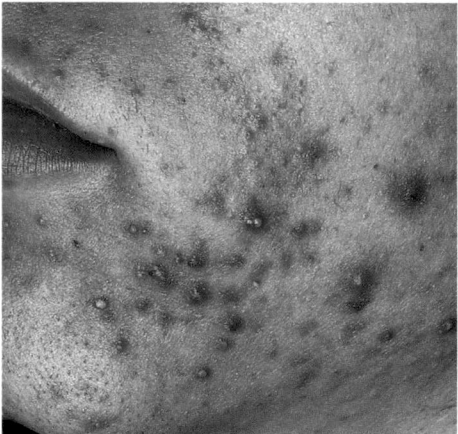

Fig. 13-2 Acne vulgaris, with papules and pustules, on the cheek.

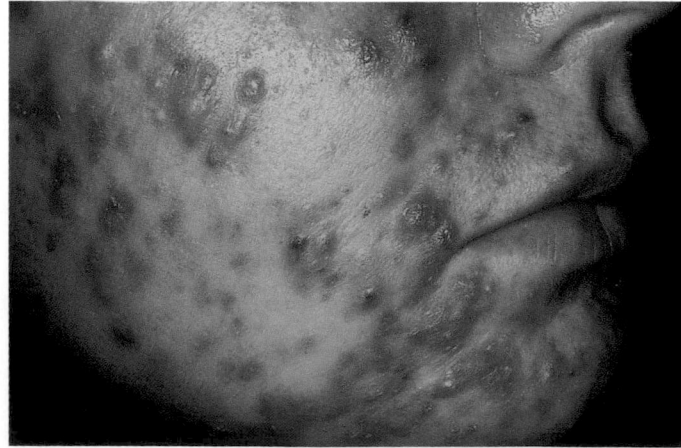

Fig. 13-3 Inflammatory acne with papules and nodules.

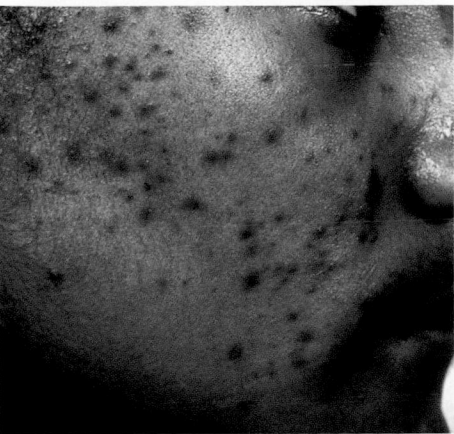

Fig. 13-4 Postinflammatory hyperpigmentation at sites of acne lesions.

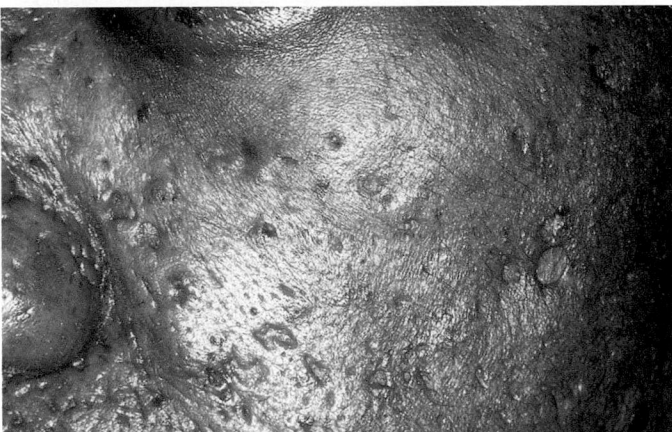

Fig. 13-5 Acne scarring on the cheek.

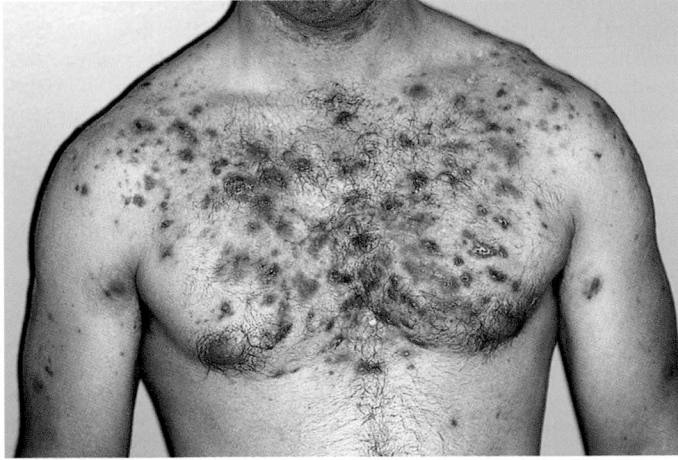

Fig. 13-6 Upper chest involvement with acne.

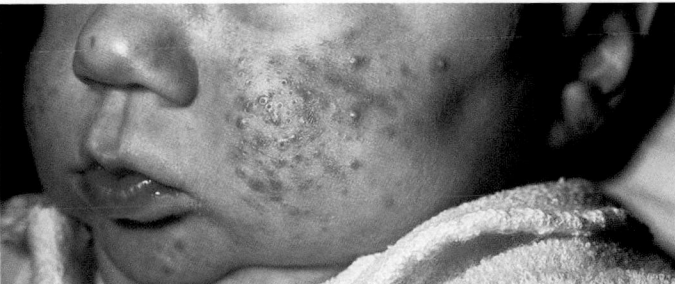

Fig. 13-7 Infantile acne.

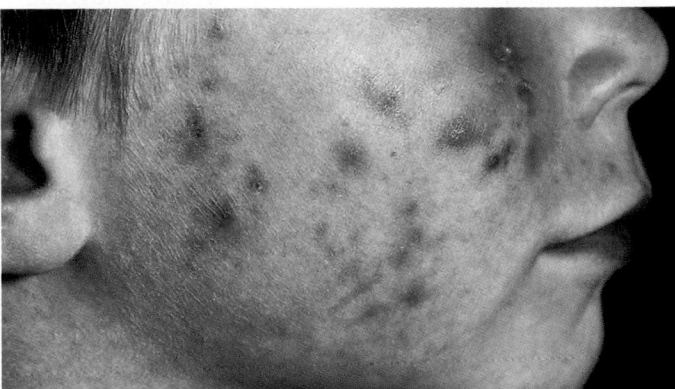

Fig. 13-8 Childhood acne.

greatest frequency between the ages of 15 and 18 in both sexes. Generally, involution of the disease occurs before age 25; however, great variability in age at onset and of resolution occurs. Around 12% of women and 3% of men will continue to have clinical acne until 44 years of age. A few will have inflammatory papules and nodules into late adulthood.

Neonatal acne is a common condition that develops a few days after birth, has a male sex preponderance, and is characterized by transient facial papules or pustules which usually clear spontaneously in a few days or weeks (Fig. 13-7). Infantile acne includes those cases that persist beyond the neonatal period or have an onset after the first 4 weeks of life. The acne process can extend into childhood, puberty, or adult life. In prolonged cases, topical benzoyl peroxide, erythromycin, or the retinoids may be effective. With more inflammatory disease, oral erythromycin, 125 mg twice a day, or trimethoprim, 100 mg twice a day, may be added to topical medications. Oral isotretinoin has been utilized in the infantile period and is effective. Childhood acne may evolve from persistent infantile acne or begin after age 2. It is uncommon and has a male predominance. Grouped comedones, papules, pustules, and nodules can occur alone or in any combination, usually limited to the face (Fig. 13-8). The duration is variable, from a few weeks to several years, and occasionally extends into more severe pubertal acne. Often there is a strong family history of moderately severe acne.

Pathogenesis

Acne vulgaris is exclusively a follicular disease, with the principle abnormality being comedo formation. It is produced by the impaction and distension of the follicles with a keratinous plug in the lower infundibulum. The keratinous plug is caused by hyperproliferation and abnormal differentiation of keratinocytes of unknown causes. Androgens, alterations in lipid composition, and an abnormal response to local cytokines are all hypothesized to be important. Androgen stimulation of the sebaceous glands is critical. Acne begins after sebum secretion increases and women with hyperandrogenic states often manifest acne, along with hirsutism and menstrual abnormalities. Treatment directed at reducing sebaceous secretion, such as isotretinoin, estrogens or antiandrogens, is effective in clearing acne.

As the retained cells block the follicular opening, the lower portion of the follicle is dilated by entrapped sebum. Disruption of the follicular epithelium permits discharge of the follicular contents into the dermis. The combination of keratin, sebum, and microorganisms, particularly *Propionibacterium acnes*, leads to the release of proinflammatory mediators and the accumulation of lymphocytes, neutrophils, and foreign body giant cells. This, in turn, causes the formation of inflammatory papules, pustules, and nodulocystic lesions.

Additional factors may exacerbate acne or, in a predisposed patient, cause the onset of acne. Comedogenic greasy or occlusive products may induce closed comedones and at times inflammatory lesions. Other types of cosmetics may initiate or worsen acne, but acne cosmetica is uncommon as most cosmetics are tested for comedogenicity.

Many types of mechanical or frictional forces can aggravate existing acne. A common problem is the overexuberant washing some patients feel may help rid them of their blackheads or oiliness. A key feature of mechanical or frictional acne is an unusual distribution of the acne lesions. Provocative factors include chin straps, violins, hats, collars, surgical tape, orthopedic casts, chairs, and seats. One acne patient who had laser hair removal developed flares of inflammatory lesions localized to the acne-prone sites after each laser session; the legs and abdomen were spared. All the above factors are likely to irritate the follicular epithelium and exacerbate the changes that lead to comedogenesis and follicular rupture. Prophylactic measures designed to interdict these various mechanical forces are beneficial.

In all women or children with acne the possibility of a hyperandrogenic state should be considered. In the former, the presence of irregular menses, hirsutism, or androgenetic alopecia increases the likelihood of finding clinically significant hyperandrogenism. Additionally, gynecologic endocrine evaluation may be indicated in women who have acne resistant to conventional therapy, who relapse quickly after a course of isotretinoin, or in whom there is a sudden onset of severe acne. Screening tests to exclude a virilizing tumor include serum dehydroepiandrosterone sulfate (DHEAS) and testosterone, obtained 2 weeks before the onset of menses. DHEAS levels may be very high in adrenal tumors (>800mcg/dl) or less dramatic in congenital adrenal hyperplasia (400–800mcgm/dl). Ovarian tumor is suggested by testosterone levels above 200 ng/dL. Many patients with late-onset congenital adrenal hyperplasia will have normal levels of DHEAS. Although 17-hydroxyprogesterone and adrenocorticotropic hormone (ACTH) stimulation tests have been used in this setting, the baseline 17-hydroxyprogesterone may be normal in some women with adult 21-hydroxylase deficiency, and ACTH stimulation may result in overdiagnosis of the syndrome. It is not clear that screening for adult-onset 21-hydroxylase deficiency improves patient outcome. Patients with polycystic ovarian syndrome (PCOS) may have a high serum testosterone level (150–200 ng/dL) or an increase in the luteinizing hormone (LH)/follicle stimulating hormone (FSH) ratio (>2–3), but recent American College of Obstetricians and Gynecologists (ACOG) guidelines suggest that laboratory and imaging studies are best used to exclude a virilizing tumor. The diagnosis of PCOS is made clinically by the presence of anovulation (fewer than nine periods per year or periods >40 days apart) and signs of hyperandrogenism, such as acne and hirsutism.

Acne neonatorum is explained by circulating maternal hormones, whereas acne extending or developing after the neonatal period may be a form of acne cosmetica, acne venenata, drug-induced acne, or part of an endocrinologic disorder. In the absence of any of these etiologies, qualitative or quantitative alterations of cutaneous androgen, metabolism, or increased end-organ sensitivity could be postulated as pathogenetic mechanisms for preadolescent acne.

Pathology

Comedones reveal a thinned epithelium and a dilated follicular canal filled with lamellar lipid-impregnated keratinous material. In pustular cases there are folliculocentric abscesses surrounded by a dense inflammatory exudate of lymphocytes and polymorphonuclear leukocytes. In addition to these findings, indolent nodular lesions frequently show plasma cells, foreign body giant cells, and proliferation of fibroblasts. Epithelial-lined sinus tracts may form.

Treatment

General principles

It is important to take a complete historical record of prior therapies, including all over-the-counter products. The dose, timing, combinations, side effects, and response to interventions should be obtained. Corticosteroids, anabolic steroids, neuroleptics, lithium, and cyclosporine may worsen acne. A family history of acne and, if present, its tendency to scarring should be noted. Women should be queried regularly about menstrual irregularities and hair growth in a male pattern, as well as use of cosmetics.

Failure of treatment may be because of drug interactions, coexisting conditions, or antibiotic resistance; however, the most common and important cause is lack of adherence to the treatment plan. Utilizing medications that are well tolerated, have convenient dosing regimens, and are cosmetically acceptable will help, but thorough patient education is essential. Explaining how lesions form, and the expected response to, and duration and possible side effects of treatment, and giving clear unambiguous instructions are key. Patients should be aware of the difference between active inflammatory lesions and the purplish-red or hyperpigmented macules of inactive resolved lesions. Topical application to the entire affected area rather than to specific lesions should be emphasized, and the fact that oral and topical medications should be used daily as the treatment is preventative in nature should be discussed.

A high glycemic diet may worsen acne, however the strength of its influence is unknown. The authors do not counsel patients to alter their diets. Scrubbing of the face increases irritation and may worsen acne. Use of only the prescribed medications and avoidance of potentially drying over-the-counter products, such as astringents, harsh cleansers, or antibacterial soaps, should be emphasized. Non-comedogenic cosmetics are recommended, and pressed powders and oil-based products should be avoided.

Medical therapy

Systemic and topical retinoids, systemic and topical antimicrobials, and systemic hormonal therapy are the main therapeutic classes of treatment available. Treatment guidelines are outlined in Box 13-1.

Topical treatment

As all topical treatments are preventative, use for 6–8 weeks is required to judge their efficacy. The entire acne-affected area is treated, not just the lesions, and long-term usage is the rule. In many patients, topical therapy may be effective as maintenance therapy after initial control is achieved with a combination of oral and topical treatment.

Topical retinoids It has long been appreciated that these agents are especially effective in promoting normal desquamation of the follicular epithelium; thus, they reduce comedones and inhibit the development of new lesions. Additionally, they have a marked anti-inflammatory effect, inhibiting the activity of leukocytes, the release of proinflammatory cytokines and other mediators, and the expression of transcription factors and toll-like receptors involved in immunomodulation. They also help penetration of other active agents. Thus, they should

Box 13-1 Acne treatment

Mild

1. Comedonal
   - Topical retinoid ± physical extraction (first line)
   - Alternate retinoid, salicylic acid, azelaic acid (second line)
2. Papular/pustular
   - Topical antimicrobial combination + topical retinoid, benzoyl peroxide wash if mild trunkal lesions (first line)
   - Alternate antimicrobials + alternate topical retinoids, azelaic acid, sodium sulfacetamide–sulfur, salicylic acid (second line)

Moderate

1. Papular/pustular
   - Oral antibiotic + topical retinoid + benzoyl peroxide (first line)
   - Alternate antibiotic, alternate topical retinoid, alternate benzoyl peroxide (second line)
   - In women, spironolactone + oral birth control pill + topical retinoids ± topical antibiotic and/or benzoyl peroxide
   - Isotretinoin if relapses quickly off oral antibiotics, does not clear, or scars

Severe

1. Nodular/conglobate
   - Isotretinoin
   - Oral antibiotic + topical retinoid + benzoyl peroxide
   - In women, spironolactone + oral birth control pill + topical retinoid ± topical or oral antibiotics and/or benzoyl peroxide

be utilized in nearly every patient with acne and are the preferred agents in maintenance therapy.

Tretinoin was the first of this group of agents to be used for acne. Popular forms of tretinoin are 0.025% and 0.05% in a cream base because these are less irritating than the gels and liquids. Its incorporation into microspheres and a polyolprepolymer also helps to limit irritation and make the product more stable in the presence of light and oxidizers. Tretinoin treatment may take 8–12 weeks before improvement occurs. When patients are tolerating the medication and are slow to respond, retinoic acid gel or solution may be utilized. Tretinoin should be applied at night and is in pregnancy category C.

Adapalene is a well-tolerated retinoid-like compound, which has efficacy equivalent to the lower concentrations of tretinoin. As it is light-stable, it may be applied in either the morning or the evening. It is in pregnancy category C. Tazarotene is comparatively strong in its action, but also relatively irritating. It should be applied once at night or every other night, and as it is in pregnancy category X, contraceptive counseling should be provided.

Initially utilizing retinoids on an every-other-night basis, or using a moisturizer with them, may lessen their irritancy. They are also particularly useful in patients with skin of color as they may lighten postinflammatory hyperpigmentation.

Benzoyl peroxide Benzoyl peroxide has a potent antibacterial effect. *P. acnes* resistance does not develop during use. Its concomitant use during treatment with antibiotics will limit the development of resistance, even if only given for short 2- to 7-day pulses. While it is most effective in inflammatory acne, some studies have shown it to be comedolytic also. The wash formulations may be utilized for mild trunkal acne when systemic therapies are not required.

Treatment is usually once or twice a day. Benzoyl peroxide may irritate the skin and produce peeling. Water-based formulations of lowest strength are least irritating. Application

lessened to once a day or every other day will also help limit this. Allergic contact dermatitis will rarely develop, suggested by the complaint of itch rather than stinging or burning. It is in pregnancy category C.

Topical antibacterials Topical clindamycin and erythromycin are available in a number of formulations. In general, they are well tolerated and are effective in mild to moderate inflammatory acne. These topical products are in pregnancy category B. Use of these topical antibiotics alone, however, is not recommended because of increasing antibiotic resistance. As mentioned above, concurrent therapy with benzoyl peroxide will limit this problem. Concomitant use with a topical retinoid will hasten the response and allow for more rapid discontinuance of the antibiotic. Dapsone is available topically in a gel formulation. Hemolytic anemia may occur and a discoloration of the skin is not uncommon when benzoyl peroxide is applied after topical dapsone. Additionally, concomitant oral use of trimethoprim/sulfamethoxazole will increase the systemic absorption of topical dapsone. It is in pregnancy category C.

Sulfur, sodium sulfacetamide, resorcin, and salicylic acid Although benzoyl peroxide, retinoids, and topical antibiotics have largely supplanted these older medications, sulfur, resorcin, and salicylic acid preparations are still useful and moderately helpful if the newer medications are not tolerated. They are frequently found in over-the-counter preparations. Sulfacetamide–sulfur combination products are mildly effective in both acne and rosacea. The latter should be avoided in patients with known hypersensitivity to sulfonamides.

Azelaic acid This dicarboxylic acid is remarkably free from adverse actions and has mild efficacy in both inflammatory and comedonal acne. It may help to lighten postinflammatory hyperpigmentation and is in pregnancy category B.

Combination topical therapy Several products are available which combine antibiotics such as clindamycin and benzoyl peroxide, or retinoids and either antibiotics or benzoyl peroxide. In general these medications increase adherence, as they require less frequent application of medication, and they may also limit irritation compared with the cumulative topical application of each product separately. However, they limit flexibility and may cause more irritation than a single product used alone.

Oral antibiotics

These agents are indicated for moderate to severe acne, in patients with inflammatory disease in whom topical combinations have failed or are not tolerated, for the treatment of chest, back, or shoulder acne, or in patients in whom absolute control is deemed essential, such as those who scar with each lesion or develop inflammatory hyperpigmentation. It generally takes 6–8 weeks to judge efficacy. Starting at a high dose and reducing it after control is preferred. Working to maintain control eventually with topical retinoids or retinoid–benzoyl peroxide combination therapy is ideal; however, keeping patients free of disease for 1–2 months before each decrease in dosage is best to prevent flaring. Most courses of oral therapy are of at least 3–6 months' duration.

There is concern that oral antibiotics may reduce the effectiveness of oral birth control pills. It is appropriate for this as yet unproved (except with rifampin, which is not used for acne) association to be discussed with patients and a second form of birth control offered.

Tetracycline Tetracycline is the safest and cheapest choice, and will give a positive response in many patients. It is usually given at an initial dose of 250–500 mg 1–4 times a day, with gradual reduction of the dose, depending on clinical response. It is best taken on an empty stomach, at least 30 min before meals and 2 h afterwards, which often limits dosage to twice a day. Calcium or iron in food supplements combines with tetracycline, reducing absorption by as much as half.

Vaginitis or perianal itching may result from tetracycline therapy in about 5% of patients, with *Candida albicans* usually present in the involved site. The only other common side effects are gastrointestinal symptoms such as nausea. To reduce the incidence of esophagitis, tetracyclines should not be taken at bedtime. Staining of growing teeth occurs, precluding its use in pregnant women and in children under the age of 9 or 10. Tetracycline should also be avoided when renal function is impaired.

Doxycycline The usual dose is 50–100 mg once or twice a day, depending on the disease severity. Photosensitivity reactions are not uncommon with this form of tetracycline and can be dramatic. Subantimicrobial-dose doxycycline, doxycycline hyclate 20 mg, may be given twice daily. The advantage of this is that the anti-inflammatory activity is being utilized but no antibiotic resistance results because of the low dose. A sustained-release 40 mg formulation is also available. These low-dose preparations appear to be of low efficacy, however.

Minocycline Minocycline is the most effective oral antibiotic in treating acne vulgaris. In patients whose *P. acnes* develops tetracycline resistance, minocycline is an alternative. The usual dose is 50–100 mg once or twice a day, depending on the severity of disease. Its absorption is less affected by milk and food than is that of tetracycline. Vertigo may occur and beginning therapy with a single dose in the evening may be prudent. An extended-release preparation is also available, which limits the vestibular side effects. Pigmentation in areas of inflammation, of oral tissues, in postacne osteoma or scars, in a photo-distributed pattern, on the shins, in the sclera, nailbed, ear cartilage, teeth, or in a generalized pattern may also be seen (Fig. 13-9). Additionally, lupus-like syndromes, a hypersensitivity syndrome (consisting of fever, hepatitis, and eosinophilia), serum sickness, pneumonitis, and hepatitis are uncommon but potentially serious adverse effects of minocycline.

Erythromycin For those who cannot take tetracyclines because of side effects or in pregnant women requiring oral antibiotic therapy, erythromycin may be considered. The efficacy is low. Side effects are mostly gastrointestinal upset; vaginal itching is a rare occurrence. The initial dose is 250–500 mg 2–4 times a day, reduced gradually after control is achieved. Erythromycin may increase blood levels of other drugs metabolized by the cytochrome P450 system.

Clindamycin Past experience has shown clindamycin to give an excellent response in the treatment of acne; however, the potential for the development of pseudomembranous colitis and the availability of retinoids has limited its use. The initial dose is 150 mg three times a day, reduced gradually as control is achieved.

Other antibiotics Sulfonamides are occasionally prescribed; however, the potential for severe drug eruptions limits their use. Trimethoprim–sulfamethoxazole (Bactrim, Septra), in double-strength doses twice a day initially, is effective in many cases unresponsive to other antibiotics. Trimethoprim alone, 300 mg twice a day, is also useful. Amoxicillin, in doses from 250 mg twice daily to 500 mg three times a day, is also an alternative and may be useful in pregnancy as it falls into pregnancy category B. Dapsone has been used in severe acne conglobata, but is rarely used today. Isotretinoin is favored.

Bacterial resistance *P. acnes* antimicrobial resistance has become a clinically relevant problem. Erythromycin and clindamycin resistance is widespread and usually presents simultaneously. Once *P. acnes* becomes resistant to tetracycline, it is also resistant to doxycycline, so if lack of efficacy due to prolonged oral therapy with one of them is suspected, a switch to minocycline is necessary. While concomitant use of benzoyl peroxide will help limit cutaneous drug resistance problems, it is now appreciated that *Staphylococcus aureus* in the nares, streptococci in the oral cavity, and enterobacteria in the gut may also become resistant, and close contacts, including treating dermatologists, may harbor such drug-resistant bacteria. Strategies to prevent antibiotic resistance include limiting the duration of treatment, stressing the importance of adherence to the treatment plan, restricting the use of antibiotics to inflammatory acne, encouraging retreatment with the same antibiotic unless it has lost its efficacy, avoiding the use of dissimilar oral and topical antibiotics at the same time, and using isotretinoin if unable to maintain clearance without oral antibacterial treatment.

Hormonal therapy

Hormonal interventions in women may be beneficial in the absence of abnormal laboratory tests. The work-up for the woman with signs of hyperandrogenism, such as acne, menstrual irregularities, hirsutism, or androgenetic alopecia, is presented above. Women with normal laboratory values often respond to hormonal therapy. Results take longer to be seen with these agents, with first evidence of improvement often not apparent for 3 months and continued improved response seen for at least 6 months. Particularly good candidates for hormonal treatment include women with PCOS, late-onset adrenal hyperplasia, or another identifiable endocrinologic condition; and women with late-onset acne, severe acne, acne that has not responded to other oral and topical therapies, or acne that has relapsed quickly after isotretinoin treatment. Women with acne primarily located on the lower face and neck, and deep-seated nodules that are painful and long-lasting, are often quite responsive to hormonal intervention (Fig. 13-10).

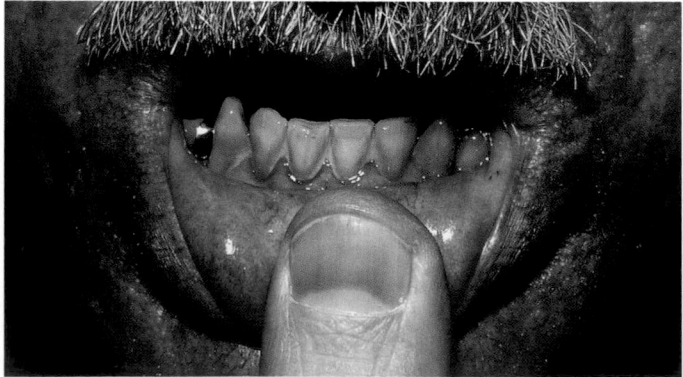

Fig. 13-9 Minocycline-induced blue pigmentation of the teeth and nails.

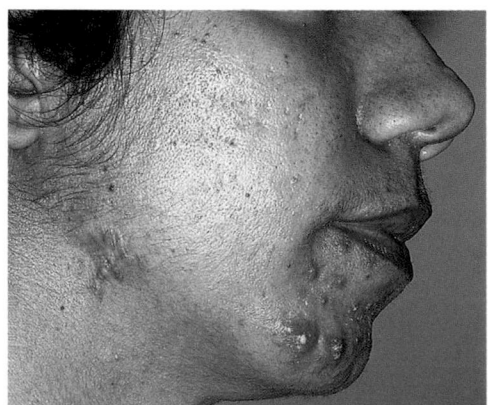

Fig. 13-10 Typical jawline lesions in an adult woman.

Oral contraceptives These agents block both adrenal and ovarian androgens. Ortho Tri-Cyclen, Estrostep, Alesse, Yasmin, and Yaz are examples of birth control pills that have beneficial effects on acne. Both the physician and the patient should be familiar with the adverse reactions associated with oral contraceptives, such as nausea, vomiting, abnormal menses, melasma, weight gain, breast tenderness, and rarely thrombophlebitis, pulmonary embolism, and hypertension.

Spironolactone As pregnancy while on antiandrogen treatment will result in feminization of a male fetus, spironolactone is usually prescribed in combination with oral contraceptives. It may be effective in doses from 25–200 mg/day. Most women will tolerate a starting dose of 50–100 mg/day. Most also tolerate 150 mg per day but many will have side effects at 200 mg per day. Side effects are dose-dependent and include breast tenderness, headache, dizziness, lightheadedness, fatigue, irregular menstrual periods, and diuresis. In a study by Shaw in patients treated with 50–100 mg/day, hyperkalemia was measurable, but in the absence of renal or cardiac disease was clinically insignificant. In his series, a third of patients cleared, a third had marked improvement, a quarter showed partial improvement, and 7% had no response. Spironolactone is often used with other topical or oral acne therapy. Several months of treatment are usually required to see benefit.

Dexamethasone Dexamethasone, in doses from 0.125 to 0.5 mg given once at night, reduces androgen excess and may alleviate cystic acne. Corticosteroids are effective in the treatment of adult-onset adrenal hyperplasia, but antiandrogens are also used increasingly in this setting.

Prednisone Although steroids may produce steroid acne, they are also effective anti-inflammatory agents in severe and intractable acne vulgaris. In severe cystic acne and acne conglobata, corticosteroid treatment is effective; however, side effects restrict its use. It is generally only given to patients with severe inflammatory acne during the first few weeks of treatment with isotretinoin, for initial reduction of inflammation, and to reduce isotretinoin-induced flares.

Other hormonal agents Finasteride, flutamide, estrogen, gonadotropin-releasing agonists, and metformin (by decreasing testosterone levels) have all been shown to have a beneficial effect on acne but due to side effects, expense, or other considerations are not commonly used.

Oral retinoid therapy

Isotretinoin This drug is approved only for severe cystic acne: however, it is useful in less severe forms of acne so as to prevent the need for continuous treatment and the repeated office visits that many patients require. It was a consensus of experts that oral isotretinoin treatment is warranted for severe acne, poorly responsive acne that improves by less than 50% after 6 months of therapy with combined oral and topical antibiotics, acne that relapses off oral treatment, scars, or acne that induces psychological distress. Additionally, other agreed indications were Gram-negative folliculitis, inflammatory rosacea, pyoderma faciale, acne fulminans, and hidradenitis suppurativa.

This retinoid is a reliable remedy in nearly all acne patients (Fig. 13-11). The dose is 0.5–1 mg/kg/day in one or two daily doses. For severe trunkal acne in patients who tolerate higher doses, treatment may be given in doses up to 2 mg/kg/day. In practice, most patients are started at a 20–40 mg dose so as to avoid an early flare, and then increased to 40–80 mg/day so as to limit side effects, which generally are dose-related. Doses as low as 0.1 mg/kg/day are very nearly as effective as the higher doses in clearing acne; the disadvantage is that they are less likely to produce a prolonged remission even after 20 weeks of treatment. To obtain the greatest chance of a prolonged remission, patients should receive 120–150 mg/kg over the treatment course. An easy way to calculate the total dose needed is to multiply the weight in kilograms by 3. The product is the total number of 40 mg capsules needed to reach the low end of the dosage spectrum.

The major advantage of isotretinoin is that it is the only acne therapy that is not open-ended (i.e. that leads to a remission, which may last many months or years). Approximately 40–60% of patients remain acne-free after a single course of isotretinoin. Approximately one-third of the relapsing patients will need only topical therapy, the others oral treatments. Many patients in the latter category prefer to be retreated with isotretinoin due to its reliable efficacy and ability to predict side effects, as they will be similar to those experienced in the first course. In Azoulay et al's study, fully 26% of isotretinoin-treated patients received a second course within a 2-year period.

Some subsets of patients tend to relapse more often. In patients under 16, 40% need a second course of isotretinoin

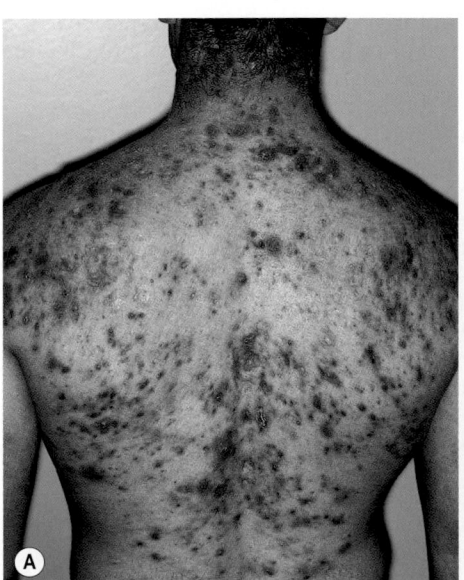
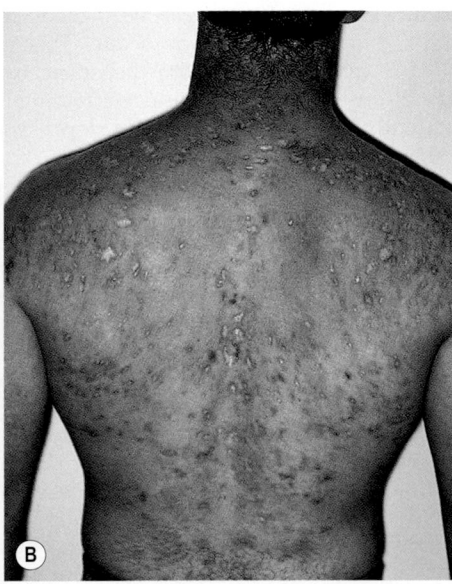

Fig. 13-11 A, Severe back acne before isotretinoin. B, Response to treatment.

within 1 year and 73% within 2 years. Adult women and patients with mild acne tend to relapse more often and more quickly than severely affected 17- to 22-year-olds. While patients' tolerance and response to repeated courses are similar to their experience with the first course, adult women who relapse may be better managed with hormonal therapies, and mild acne treated with standard therapy.

In adult acne patients, who frequently tolerate the side effects of isotretinoin less well, lower doses and/or intermittent therapy is possible. Goulden et al studied 80 adult acne patients whom they treated with 0.5 mg/kg/day for 1 week in every 4 over a period of 6 months. Acne resolved in 88% and 39% relapsed after 1 year. Seukeran and Cunliffe treated nine patients aged 56–75 years with 0.25 mg/kg/day for 6 months. All patients cleared and all but one remained clear 36 months later.

Patient education is critical in isotretinoin therapy. Its most serious adverse effect is the risk of severe damage to the fetus if it is given during pregnancy. Retinoid embryopathy is a well-defined syndrome characterized by craniofacial, cardiovascular, central nervous system, and thymus abnormalities. It is of the utmost importance that a woman of child-bearing potential follows closely the recommendations clearly outlined in extensive material provided by the manufacturer. The use of consent forms, contraception education, and unequivocal documentation of the absence of pregnancy through monthly laboratory testing are important components of a Food and Drug Administration (FDA)-mandated verification program designed to prevent pregnancy during treatment. Women should not become pregnant until off medication for at least 1 month. The drug is not mutagenic and there is no risk to a fetus conceived while the male partner is taking the drug.

Another major area of educational emphasis concerns the psychological effects of the medication. Reports of depression, psychosis, suicidal ideation, suicide, and attempted suicide have prompted numerous studies of the mental health of patients taking isotretinoin. While the usual outcome is an improvement of mood because of the clearance of the disease, and only one of the many large-scale population-based studies has found evidence of an elevated incidence of depression, there are a small number of patients who have developed depression and have positive dechallenge and rechallenge tests. Close monitoring for depression, fully educating the patient, and enlisting the help of a roommate or family member to look for changes in mood are all methods used to assess the psychological status of the patient on isotretinoin.

Inflammatory bowel disease (IBD) is a third concern. Patients with this condition have been successfully treated with isotretinoin without flaring, new onset of IBD in patients exposed to isotretinoin is of concern. The age of onset of IBD overlaps with the age at which acne will frequently be treated with isotretinoin and antibiotics. A review of Medwatch cases revealed 85 cases with new-onset IBD in isotretinoin users. Three cases improved off isotretinoin and then relapsed on re-exposure. Most did not improve or resolve with discontinuation of the medicine, with seven requiring surgery. Studies investigating a possible association of IBD and isotretinoin or tetracycline class antibiotics are ongoing. Some have reported significant associations, but results are either contradictory or are unverified.

Other side effects of isotretinoin are dose-dependent and generally not serious. Dry lips, skin, eyes, and oral and nasal mucosa occur in up to 90% of patients. These can be treated with moisturization. Dryness of the nasal mucosa leads to colonization by *S. aureus* in 80–90% of treated subjects. Skin abscesses, staphylococcal conjunctivitis, impetigo, facial cellulitis, and folliculitis may result. Such colonization may be avoided by the use of bacitracin ointment applied to the anterior nares twice a day during isotretinoin therapy. Arthralgias may occur but, like other side effects, do not require interruption of therapy unless severe. Monitoring of serum lipids is carried out, as some patients will develop hypertriglyceridemia. This may be controlled by avoidance of smoking and alcohol, and by following a diet that is low in fat. It should be realized that patients who develop this complication, and their families, are at risk for the development of the metabolic syndrome.

Liver function tests should be checked at regular intervals, depending on patient risk factors and the dose utilized.

Intralesional corticosteroids

Intralesional corticosteroids are especially effective in reducing inflammatory nodules. Kenalog-10 (triamcinolone acetonide 10 mg/mL) is best diluted with sterile normal saline solution to 2.5 mg/mL. Injecting less than 0.1 mL directly into the center of the nodule will help safeguard against atrophy and hypopigmentation.

Physical modalities

Local surgical treatment is helpful in bringing about quick resolution of the comedones, although many clinicians wait until after 2 or more months of topical retinoids to extract those that remain. The edge of the follicle is nicked with a No 11 scalpel blade and the contents of the comedo are expressed with a comedo extractor. Scarring is not produced by this procedure. Light electrode desiccation is an alternative. In isotretinoin-treated patients, macrocomedones present at weeks 10–15 may be expressed, since they tend to persist throughout therapy.

The use of photodynamic therapy and various forms of light, laser, or radiofrequency energy is under investigation. It is clear that there is an ability to destroy sebaceous glands or kill *P. acnes* with such interventions; however, the methods to deliver such treatments in an efficient, cost-effective, safe, relatively painfree, and practical manner are evolving. These treatments will be a welcome addition as they have the potential to provide care without the concerns associated with systemic drugs. More studies of larger patient populations with appropriate controls are needed to evaluate their place in the spectrum of acne treatments.

Complications

Even with the excellent treatment options available, scarring may occur. This may be quite prominent and often results from the cystic type of acne, although smaller lesions may produce scarring in some individuals. Pitted scars, widemouthed depressions, and keloids, primarily seen along the jawline and chest, are common types of scarring (Fig. 13-12). These may improve spontaneously over the course of a year or more. Many treatment options are available. Chemical peeling, ablative, nonablative, and vascular laser treatments, skin needling or rolling, dermabrasion, scar excision, subcision, punch grafts alone or followed by dermabrasion or laser smoothing, intralesional corticosteroids or fluorouracil, fractionated laser resurfacing, fat transfer, and the use of filler substances are among the procedures reported to be effective in improving the appearance.

Other complications from acne are prominent residual hyperpigmentation, especially in darker-skinned patients; pyogenic granuloma formation, which is more common in acne fulminans and in patients treated with high-dose isotretinoin; osteoma cutis, which consists of small, firm papules resulting from long-standing acne vulgaris; and solid facial

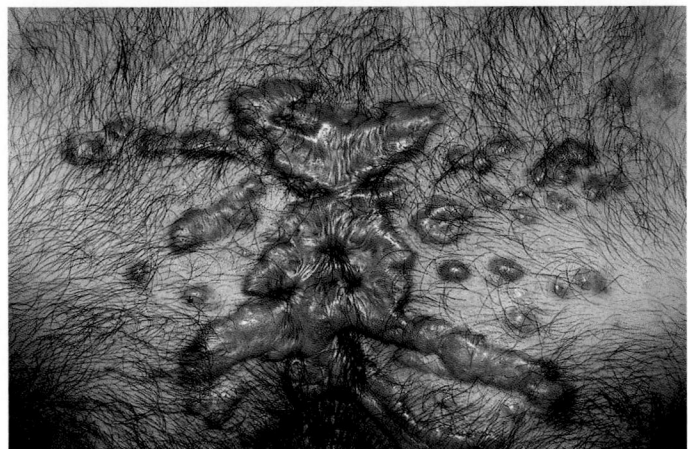

Fig. 13-12 Keloid of the chest secondary to acne.

edema. The latter is a persistent, firm facial swelling that is an uncommon, though distressing, result of acne vulgaris or acne rosacea. Both corticosteroids and isotretinoin have been reported to be effective treatments.

Arowojolu AO, et al: Combined oral contraceptive pills for treatment of acne. Cochrane Database Syst Rev 2007; 1:CD004425.

Autoniou C, et al: Clinical and therapeutic approach to childhood acne. Pediatr Dermatol 2009; 26:373.

Azoulay L, et al: Isotretinoin therapy and the incidence of acne relapse. Br J Dermatol 2007; 157:1240.

Azoulay L, et al: Isotretinoin and the risk of depression in patients with acne vulgaris. J Clin Psychiatry 2008; 69:S26.

Berard A, et al: Isotretinoin, pregnancies, abortions and birth defects. Br J Clin Pharmacol 2007; 63:196.

Bowe WP, et al: Diet and acne. J Am Acad Dermatol 2010; 63:124.

Bremmer JD, et al: Functional brain imaging alterations in acne patients treated with isotretinoin. Am J Psych 2005; 162:983.

Brown RJ, et al: Minocycline-induced drug hypersensitivity syndrome followed by multiple autoimmune sequelae. Arch Dermatol 2009; 145:63.

Chia CY, et al: Isotretinoin therapy and mood changes in adolescents with moderate to severe acne. Arch Dermatol 2005; 141:557.

Costello M, et al: Insulin-sensitising drugs versus the combined oral contraceptive pill for hirsutism, acne and risk of diabetes, cardiovascular disease, and endometrial cancer in polycystic ovary syndrome. Cochrane Database Syst Rev 2007; 1:CD005552.

Cunliffe WJ, Gollnick H: A clinical and therapeutic study of 29 patients with infantile acne. Br J Dermatol 2001; 145:463.

Ehrmann DA: Polycystic ovary syndrome. New Engl J Med 2005; 352:1223.

Frangos JE, et al: Acne and oral contraceptives. J Am Acad Dermatol 2008; 58:781.

Goldsmith LA, et al: American Academy of Dermatology Consensus Conference on the safe and optimal use of isotretinoin. J Am Acad Dermatol 2004; 50:900.

Gollnick H, et al: Management of acne. J Am Acad Dermatol 2003; 49:S1.

Goodman GJ, et al: The management of postacne scarring. Dermatol Surg 2007; 33:1175.

Goulden V, et al: Treatment of acne with intermittent isotretinoin. Br J Dermatol 1997; 137:106.

Hahm BJ, et al: Changes of psychiatric parameters and their relationships by oral isotretinoin in acne patients. J Dermatol 2009; 36:255.

Haider A, et al: Treatment of acne vulgaris. JAMA 2004; 292:726.

Hu S, et al: Fractional resurfacing for the treatment of atopic facial acne scars in Asian skin. Dermatol Surg 2009; 35:826.

Jacobs DG, et al: Suicide, depression, and isotretinoin. J Am Acad Dermatol 2001; 45:S168.

James WD: Clinical practice: acne. New Engl J Med 2005; 352:1463.

Katsambas A, et al: New and emerging treatments in dermatology: acne. Dermatol Ther 2008; 21:86.

Kim J, et al: Activation of Toll-like receptor 2 in acne triggers inflammatory cytokine responses. J Immunol 2002; 169:1535.

Lee AT, et al: Dermatologic manifestations of polycystic ovary syndrome. Am J Clin Dermatol 2007; 8:201.

Lee DH, et al: Comparison of a 585-nm pulsed dye laser and a 1064-nm Nd:YAG laser for the treatment of acne scars. J Am Acad Dermatol 2009; 60:801.

Levy R, et al: Effect of antibiotics on the oropharyngeal flora in patients with acne. Arch Dermatol 2003; 139:467.

Manolache L, et al: A case of solid facial oedema successfully treated with isotretinoin. J Eur Acad Dermatol Venereol 2009; 23:965.

Margolis D, et al: Potential association between the oral tetracycline class of antimicrobials used to treat acne and inflammatory bowel disease. Am J Gastroenterol 2010; (epub).

Norman RJ, et al: Polycystic ovary syndrome. Lancet 2007; 370:685.

Plewig G, Kligman AM: Acne and Rosacea, 3rd edn. New York: Springer, 2000.

Purdy S, et al: Acne. BMJ 2006; 333:949.

Railan D, et al: Laser treatment of acne, psoriasis, leukoderma and scars. Semin Cutan Med Surg 2009; 27:285.

Reddy D, et al: Possible association between isotretinoin and inflammatory bowel disease. Am J Gastroenterol 2006; 101:1569.

Rodonodi N, et al: High risk for hyperlipidemia and the metabolic syndrome after an episode of hypertriglyceridemia during 13-cis retinoic acid therapy for acne. Ann Intern Med 2002; 136:582.

Ross JI, et al: Antibiotic-resistant acne. Br J Dermatol 2003; 148:467.

Sakamoto FH, et al: Photodynamic therapy for acne vulgaris. J Am Acad Dermatol 2010; 63:195.

Seti TL, et al: Polycystic ovary syndrome. Am J Med 2007; 120:128.

Seukeran DC, Cunliffe WJ: Acne in the elderly. Br J Dermatol 1998; 139:99.

Shaw JC: Low-dose adjunctive spironolactone in the treatment of acne in a retrospective analysis of 85 consecutively treated patients. J Am Acad Dermatol 2000; 43:498.

Shaw JC, et al: Long-term safety of spironolactone in acne. J Cutan Med Surg 2002; 6:541.

Skidmore RA, et al: Effects of a subantimicrobial dose of doxycycline in the treatment of moderate acne. Arch Dermatol 2003; 139:459.

Strahan JE, et al: Cyclosporine-induced infantile nodulocystic acne. Arch Dermatol 2009; 145:797.

Strauss JS, et al: Guidelines of care for acne vulgaris management. J Am Acad Dermatol 2007; 56:651.

Taub AF: Procedural treatments for acne vulgaris. Dermatol Surg 2007; 33:1005.

Thiboutot D: Hormones and acne. Semin Cutan Med Surg 2001; 20:144.

Thiboutot D, et al: New insights into the management of acne. J Am Acad Dermatol 2009; 60:S1.

Torrelo A, et al: Severe acne infantum successfully treated with isotretinoin. Pediatr Dermatol 2005; 22:357.

Wysowaski DK, et al: An analysis of reports of depression and suicide in patients treated with isotretinoin. J Am Acad Dermatol 2001; 45:515.

Zaenglein AL, et al: Expert committee recommendations for acne management. Pediatrics 2006; 118:1188.

Acne conglobata

Cystic acne is the mildest form of acne conglobata (conglobate means shaped in a rounded mass or ball), an unusually severe type of acne. This form is characterized by numerous comedones (many of which are double or triple) and large abscesses with interconnecting sinuses, cysts, and grouped inflammatory nodules (Fig. 13-13). Suppuration is characteristic of acne conglobata. Pronounced scars remain after healing.

The cysts occur on the back, buttocks, chest, forehead, cheeks, anterior neck, and shoulders (Fig. 13-14). They contain a thick, yellowish, viscid, stringy, blood-tinged fluid. After incision and drainage of the cyst there is frequently a prompt refilling with the same type of material. These cysts are suggestive of the type found in hidradenitis suppurativa. Hidradenitis suppurativa and dissecting cellulitis of the scalp may be seen with acne conglobata, an association known as the follicular occlusion triad.

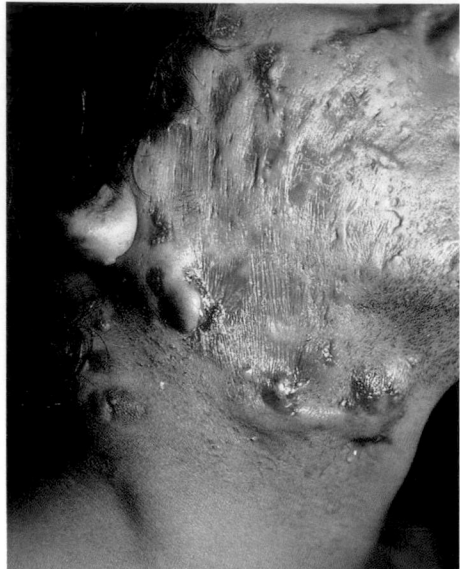

Fig. 13-13 Acne conglobata with fistula formation.

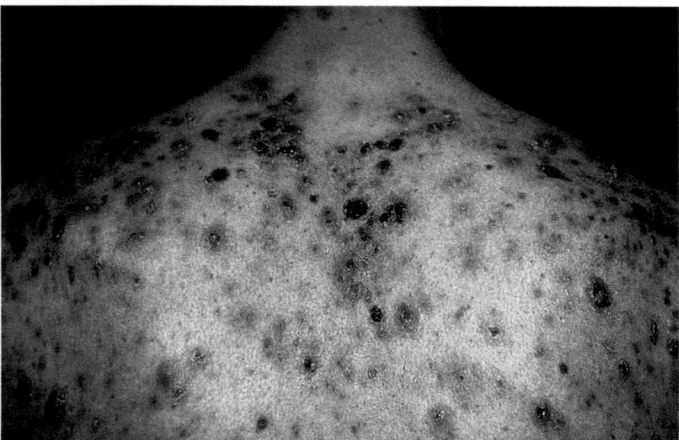

Fig. 13-14 Acne conglobata of the back.

This severe and painful disease occurs most frequently in young men around 16 years; it may extend and persist into adulthood and even into the fifth decade of life, especially over the posterior neck and back. Women are less frequently affected. Athletes and bodybuilders should be questioned about the use of anabolic steroids, which may induce such aggressive acne.

The therapy of choice in all but the earliest lesions is isotretinoin, 0.5–1 mg/kg/day to a total dose of 150 mg/kg, with a second course if resolution does not occur after a rest period of 2 months. Pretreatment with prednisone and low initial doses of isotretinoin, as described for acne fulminans, are recommended to avoid flaring of disease. CO_2 laser to open the sinus tracts and fractional laser to the scars is another method of therapy. Infliximab added to isotretinoin was a useful adjunct in one reported patient.

Gerber PA, et al: The dire consequences of doping. Lancet 2008; 372:656.
Hasegawa T, et al: Acne conglobata successfully treated by fractional laser after CO laser abrasion of cysts combined with topical tretinoin. J Dermatol 2009; 36:118.
Melnik B, et al: Abuse of anabolic-androgenic steroids and bodybuilding acne. J Dtsch Dermatol Ges 2007; 5:110.
Shirakawa M, et al: Treatment of acne conglobata with infliximab. J Am Acad Dermatol 2006; 55:344.

Acne fulminans

This rare form of extremely severe cystic acne occurs primarily in teenage boys. It is characterized by highly inflammatory nodules and plaques that undergo swift suppurative degeneration, leaving ragged ulcerations, mostly on the chest and back. The face is usually less severely involved. Fever and leukocytosis are common. Polyarthralgia and polymyalgia, destructive arthritis, and myopathy have been reported in association with it. Focal lytic bone lesions may be seen.

Prednisone, 40–60 mg, is necessary during the initial 4–6 weeks to calm the dramatic inflammatory response. After 4 weeks 10–20 mg of isotretinoin is added. This should be slowly increased to standard doses and continued for a full 120–150 mg/kg cumulative course. Large cysts may be opened and the contents expressed. Intralesional corticosteroids will aid their resolution. Infliximab may also be useful.

Iqbal M, et al: Acne fulminans with SAPHO syndrome treated with infliximab. J Am Acad Dermatol 2005; 52:S118.
Neely GM, et al: Acne fulminans. S D Med 2006; 59:387.
Seukeran DC, et al: The treatment of acne fulminans: a review of 25 cases. Br J Dermatol 1999; 141:307.

SAPHO syndrome

SAPHO syndrome is characterized by synovitis, acne, pustulosis, hyperostosis, and osteitis. Skin findings may include acne fulminans, acne conglobata, pustular psoriasis, hidradenitis suppurativa, dissecting cellulitis of the scalp, Sweet syndrome, Sneddon–Wilkinson disease, and palmoplantar pustulosis. The chest wall and mandible are the most common sites for musculoskeletal complaints. Bone changes of the anterior chest wall on nuclear scans are the most specific diagnostic findings. Acquired hyperostosis syndrome (AHYS) and, in a familial setting of a dominantly inherited disorder, pyogenic sterile arthritis, pyoderma gangrenosum, and acne (PAPA syndrome) both present with similar clinical scenerios. The latter is due to mutations in the CD2-binding protein on chromosome 15q. Systemic retinoids and infliximab have been successful in treating these patients. If isotretinoin is used, it should be initiated at a low dosage, such as 10 mg per day, in combination with prednisone for the first month to prevent flaring of the disease. Methotrexate, sulfasalazine, tumor necrosis factor (TNF) antagonists, and cyclosporine are other likely effective choices. Pamidronate is effective in treating the osteo-articular manifestations.

Colina M, et al: Sustained remission of SAPHO syndrome with pamidronate. Clin Exp Rheumatol 2009; 27:112.
Colina M, et al: Clinical and radiologic evolution of synovitis, acne, pustulosis, hyperostosis, and osteitis syndrome. Arthritis Rheum 2009; 61:813.
Galadari H, et al: Synovitis, acne, pustulosis, hyperostosis, and osteitis syndrome treated with a combination of isotretinoin and pamidronate. J Am Acad Dermatol 2009; 61:123.
Poindexter G, et al: Synovitis-acne-pustulosis-hyperostosis-osteitis syndrome. J Am Acad Dermatol 2008; 59(2Suppl 1):S53.
Sabugo F, et al: Infliximab can induce a prolonged clinical remission and a decrease in thyroid hormonal requirements in a patient with SAPHO syndrome and hypothyroidism. Clin Rhematol 2008; 27:533.
Tallon B, et al: Peculiarities of PAPA syndrome. Rheumatology (Oxford) 2006; 45:1140.

Other acne variants

Tropical acne

Tropical acne is unusually severe acne occurring in the tropics during the seasons when the weather is hot and humid.

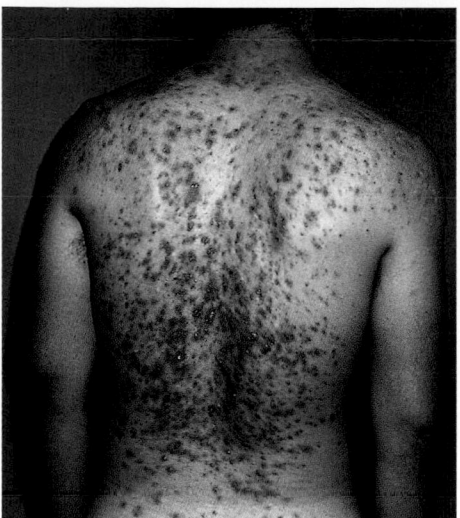

Fig. 13-15 Tropical acne.

Nodular, cystic, and pustular lesions occur chiefly on the back, buttocks, and thighs (Fig. 13-15). Characteristically, the face is spared. Conglobate abscesses occur often, especially on the back. Comedones are sparse. Acne tropicalis usually occurs in young adults who may have had acne vulgaris at an earlier age. This is especially true of those in the armed forces stationed in the tropics and carrying backpacks. Treatment is that for cystic acne, but acne tropicalis may persist until the patient moves to a cooler and less humid climate.

Acne aestivalis

Also known as Mallorca acne, this rare form of acne starts in the spring, progresses during the summer, and resolves completely in the fall. It affects almost exclusively women between the ages of 25 and 40. Dull red, dome-shaped, hard, small papules, usually not larger than 3–4 mm, develop on the cheeks and commonly extend on to the sides of the neck, chest, shoulders, and characteristically the upper arms. Comedones and pustules are notably absent or sparse. Acne aestivalis does not respond to antibiotics but benefits from application of retinoic acid.

Excoriated acne

Also known as picker's acne and acne excoriée des jeunes filles, excoriated acne is seen primarily in young women with a superficial type of acne in which the primary lesions are trivial or even nonexistent, but in which the compulsive neurotic habit of picking the face and squeezing minute comedones produces secondary lesions that crust and may leave scars. Often the lesion that is excoriated is minute, seen only in a magnifying mirror.

This condition may be a sign of depression or anxiety. It is an obsessive–compulsive symptom. If the patient admits to picking but being unable to stop this habit, improvement may follow support and acne therapy. However, most patients will require interventions with selective serotonin reuptake inhibitors, such as fluoxetine, paroxetine, or sertraline, behavior modification, or psychotherapy. Other pharmacologic treatments that have been successful in case reports include doxepin, clomipramine, naltrexone, pimozide, and olanzapine.

Arnold LM, et al: Psychogenic excoriation. CNS Drugs 2001; 15:351.
Brabek E, et al: Herpetic folliculitis and syringitis simulating acne excoriée. Arch Dermatol 2001; 37:97.

Hjorth N, et al: Acne aestivalis: Mallorca acne. Acta Dermatol Venereol 1972; 2:61.
Wells JM: Tropical acne—one hundred cases. J R Army Med Corps 1981; 127:55.

Acneiform eruptions

Acneiform eruptions are follicular eruptions characterized by papules and pustules resembling acne. Breaks in the epithelium and spillage of follicular contents into the dermis lead to the lesions. They are not necessarily confined to the usual sites of acne vulgaris, often have a sudden onset, are monomorphous, and usually appear in a patient well past adolescence. If secondary to a drug, an eruption begins within days of initiation of the medication, may be accompanied by fever and malaise, and resolves when the drug is stopped.

Acneiform eruptions may originate from skin exposure to various industrial chemicals, such as fumes generated in the manufacture of chlorine and its byproducts. These chlorinated hydrocarbons may cause chloracne, consisting of cysts, pustules, folliculitis, and comedones. The most potent acneiform-inducing agents are the polyhalogenated hydrocarbons, notably dioxin (2,3,7,8 tetrachlorobenzodioxin). Cutting and lubricating oils, crude coal tar applied to the skin for medicinal purposes, heavy tar distillates, coal tar pitch, and asbestos are known to cause acneiform eruptions. Acne venenata is another term applied to this process.

Acneiform eruptions are induced by medications such as iodides from radiopaque contrast media or potassium iodide, bromides in drugs such as propantheline bromide, testosterone, cyclosporine, antiepileptic medications, lithium, and systemic corticosteroids. When medium or high doses of corticosteroids are taken for as short a time as 3–5 days, a distinctive eruption may occur, known as steroid acne. It is a sudden outcropping of inflamed papules, most numerous on the upper trunk and arms (Fig. 13-16), but also seen on the face. The lesions typically present as papules rather than comedones; however, a histologic study confirmed they begin follicularly with microcomedone formation. Tretinoin (Retin-A), 0.05% cream applied once or twice a day, may clear the lesions within 1–3 months despite the continuation of high doses of corticosteroid. Oral antibiotics and other typical acne medications are also effective. Topical steroids, especially the fluorinated types or when applied under occlusion, may also induce an acneiform eruption. Topical tacrolimus and pimecrolimus may both induce a papulopustular eruption. Epidermal growth factor inhibitors, including monoclonal antibodies and tyrosine kinase inhibitors used in cancer therapy, produce a folliculitis in the majority of treated patients. Often oral minocycline and topical benzoyl peroxide are given prophylactically at the outset of the cancer therapy to prevent what may be a dose-limiting reaction. Finally, radiation therapy for malignancy can induce acne in the radiation port.

Agero AL, et al: Dermatologic side effects associated with the epidermal growth factor receptor inhibitors. J Am Acad Dermatol 2006; 55:657.
Antille C, et al: Induction of rosaceiform dermatitis during treatment of facial inflammatory dermatoses with tacrolimus ointment. Arch Dermatol 2004; 140:457.
El Sayed F, et al: Rosaceiform eruption to pimecrolimus. J Am Acad Dermatol 2006; 54:548.
Hengge UR, et al: Adverse effects of topical glucocorticoids. J Am Acad Dermatol 2006; 54:1.
Hu JC, et al: Cutaneous side effects of epidermal growth factor receptor inhibitors. J Am Acad Dermatol 2007; 56:317.
Li T, et al: Skin toxicities associated with epidermal growth factor receptor inhibitors. Target Oncol 2009; 4:107.
Melnik B, et al: Abuse of anabolic-androgenic steroids and bodybuilding acne. J Dtsch Dermatol Ges 2007; 5:110.

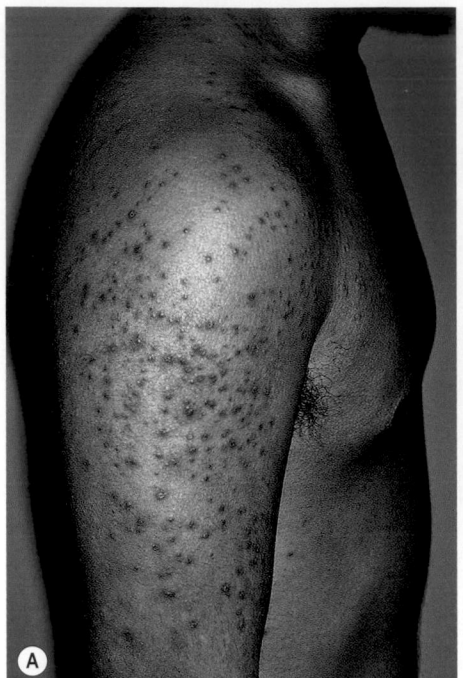
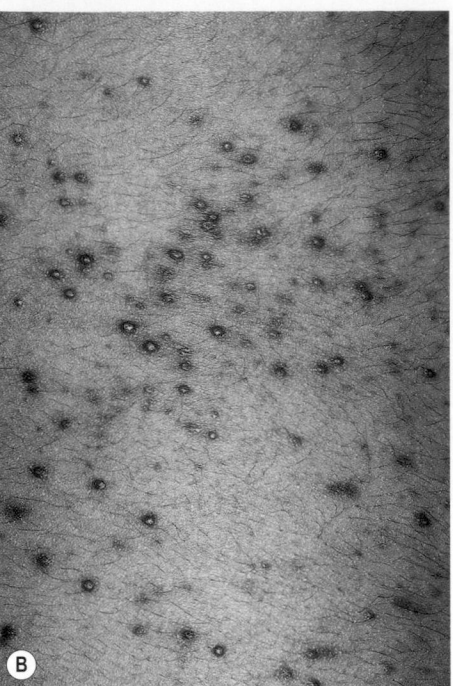

Fig. 13-16 A and B, Steroid acne. (Courtesy of Curt Samlaska, MD)

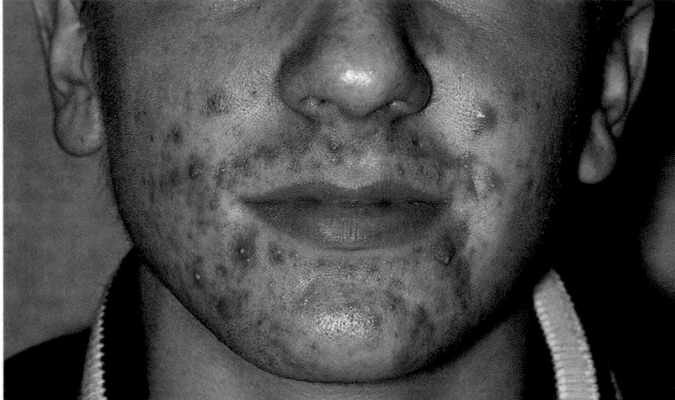

Fig. 13-17 Gram-negative folliculitis.

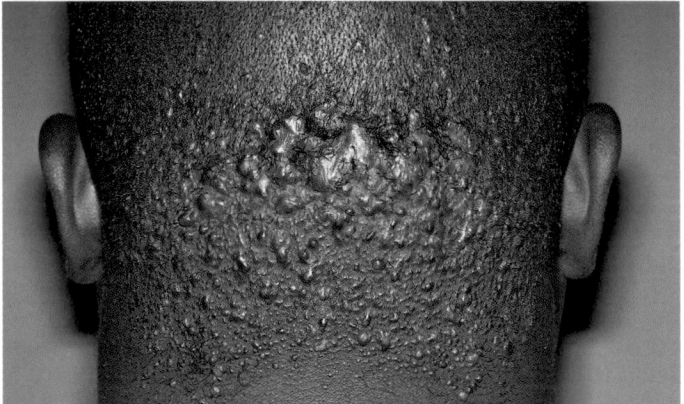

Fig. 13-18 Acne keloidalis nuchae.

Pelclova D, et al: Adverse health effects in humans exposed to 2,3,7,8-tetrachlorodibenzo-p-dioxin (TCDD). Rev Environ Health 2006; 21:119.
Plewig G, et al: Acneiform dermatoses. Dermatology 1998; 196:102.

Gram-negative folliculitis

Gram-negative folliculitis occurs in patients who have had moderately inflammatory acne for long periods and have been treated with long-term antibiotics, mainly tetracyclines. While on antibiotic treatment, patients develop either superficial pustules 3–6 mm in diameter flaring out from the anterior nares, or fluctuant, deep-seated nodules (Fig. 13-17). Culture of these lesions usually reveals a species of *Klebsiella, Escherichia coli, Enterobacter*, or, from the deep cystic lesions, *Proteus*.

With long-term, broad-spectrum antibiotic therapy the anterior nares may become colonized with these Gram-negative organisms. As the use of long-term antibiotic therapy declines, this disease has become less common.

Isotretinoin is very effective and is the treatment of choice in this disease. James and Leyden have shown that this treatment not only clears the acne component of the disease but also eliminates the colonization of the anterior nares with Gram-negative organisms. If isotretinoin cannot be tolerated or is contraindicated, amoxicillin or trimethoprim–sulfamethoxazole may be effective in suppressing the disease.

Boni R, et al: Treatment of Gram-negative folliculitis in patients with acne. Am J Clin Dermatol 2003; 4:273.
Neubert U, et al: Bacteriologic and immunologic aspects of Gram-negative folliculitis: a study of 46 patients. Int J Dermatol 1999; 38:270.

Acne keloidalis

Acne keloidalis is most frequently encountered in young adult Black, Hispanic, or Asian men who otherwise are in excellent health. It is not associated with acne vulgaris and is a primary cicatricial alopecia variant. It is a persistent folliculitis and perifolliculitis of the back of the neck that presents as inflammatory papules and pustules. Over time fibrosis ensues with coalescence of firm papules into keloidal plaques (Fig. 13-18). At times, sinus tract formation results.

Histologically, acne keloidalis is characterized by perifollicular, chronic (lymphocytic and plasmacytic) inflammation, most intense at the level of the isthmus and lower infundibulum of terminal hairs. There is lamellar fibroplasia, most marked at the level of the isthmus and, eventually, in the keloidal masses, the connective tissue becomes sclerotic, forming hypertrophic scars or keloids. Persistent free hairs in the dermis may be responsible for the prolonged inflammation and eventual scarring.

Topical therapy with potent steroid ointments or foams alone, or following tretinoin gel, twice a day is useful for the follicular papules. Oral antibiotics of the tetracycline group may be added and are helpful in suppressing the inflammatory response. Triamcinolone acetonide by intralesional injection, using Kenalog-10, into the inflammatory follicular lesions, and Kenalog-40 into the hypertrophic scars and keloids, is useful in reducing inflammation and fibrosis. Smaller lesions may be excised to a level below the hair follicle and closed. This may be followed by Kenalog-40 every 3 weeks. For larger lesions, deep excision or CO_2 laser ablation left to heal by primary intention may be necessary. Laser hair removal with the Nd:YAG laser may be utilized as a preventative measure.

Adegbidi H, et al: Keloid acne of the neck. Int J Dermatol 2005; 44(Suppl 1):49.

Bajaj V, et al: Surgical excision of acne keloidalis nuchae with secondary intention healing. Clin Exp Dermatol 2008; 33:53.

Ogunbiyi A, et al: Acne keloidalis in females. J Natl Med Assoc 2005; 97:1178.

Sperling LC, et al: Acne keloidalis is a form of primary scarring alopecia. Arch Dermatol 2000; 136:479.

Hidradenitis suppurativa

Clinical features

Hidradenitis suppurativa is a chronic disease characterized by recurrent abscess formation, primarily within the folded areas of skin that contain both terminal hairs and apocrine glands. The primary site of inflammation is not the gland but the terminal hair. Dissecting terminal folliculitis is a term Plewig uses to unify diseases primarily affecting the terminal hair follicle such as hidradenitis suppurativa, acne keloidalis nuchae, pilonidal sinus, and dissecting cellulitis of the scalp. The axilla is the most commonly affected site. Among other areas, the inguinal and submammary areas are favored in women (Figs 13-19 and 13-20), with the buttock, perianal, and atypical areas (such as retroauricular and trunk) more often affected in men, although any and all areas may be affected in either sex. It is a postpubertal process that affects women approximately four times more often than men.

The disease is characterized by the development of tender, red nodules, which at first are firm but soon become fluctuant and painful. Rupture of the lesion, suppuration, formation of sinus tracts, and extensive scarring are distinctive. As one area heals, recurrent lesions form, so that the course of the disease is protracted. It may eventually lead to the formation of honeycombed, fistulous tracts with chronic infection. The individual lesions contain a thick, viscous, mucoid, suppurative material. When a probe is used to explore the suppurating nodule, a burrowing sinus tract is usually detected that may extend for many centimeters, running horizontally just underneath the skin surface.

Disease severity varies and may be quantified by the Sartorius scale. This takes into account the number, type, and sites of lesions. Also to be considered is the impact on the quality of life that this chronic, recurrent, painful, odiferous, messy condition has. The majority of the approximately 1% of the population affected by this disease are mildly affected; however, severe debilitating disease is commonly observed. In this affected group, men outnumber women. Men more often have a history of acne and pilonidal cysts than women. Squamous cell carcinoma (after an average of 19 years of active disease), interstitial keratitis, spondyloarthropathy, urethral

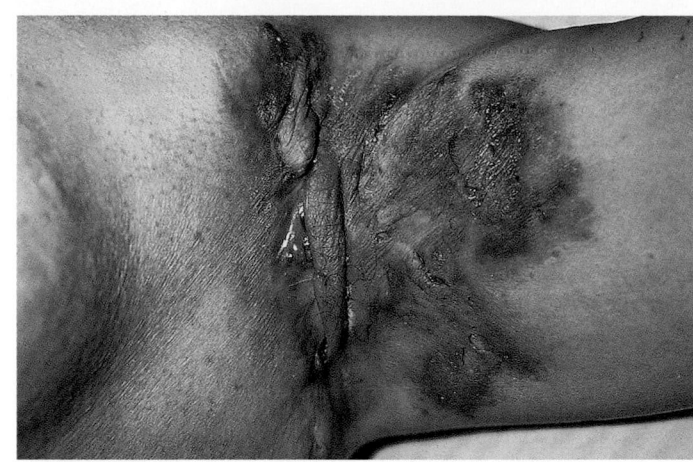

Fig. 13-19 Hidradentitis of the axilla.

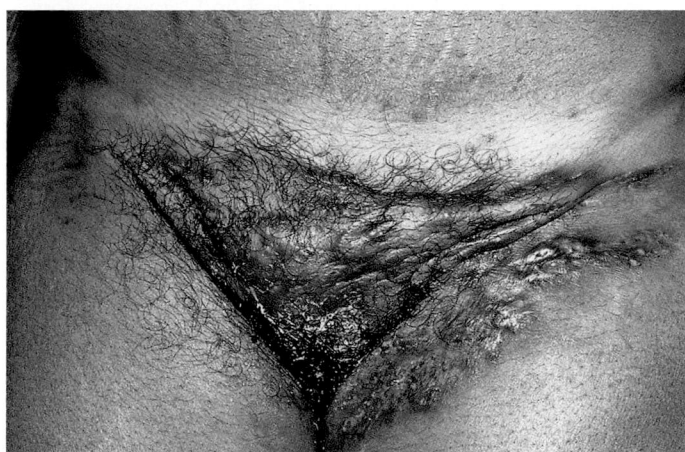

Fig. 13-20 Hidradentitis of the groin.

vesical and rectal fistulas, anemia, hypoproteinemia, and amyloidosis have been reported to complicate hidradenitis suppurativa, but are rare. Significant lymphedema of the penis and groin, along with alteration of the anatomy because of surgical intervention, often makes physical examination of these sites difficult. The risk of squamous cell carcinoma occurring as an ulceration or thickening in a skin crease, which can metastasize and cause death, requires attention to detail in this regard.

Etiology

Detailed histologic studies of hidradenitis suppurativa reveal that terminal follicle hyperkeratosis is followed by rupture of the follicular epithelium, and release of keratin, sebum, bacteria, and hairs into the dermis. The resulting inflammatory process engulfs the apocrine gland, and leads to rupture of the overlying skin, fibrosis, and sinus tract formation. Secondary bacterial infection with *Staphylococcus aureus, Streptococcus pyogenes,* and various Gram-negative organisms may occur. The initiating event is unknown. Associated findings of obesity, mechanical friction, smoking, immunologic dysfunction, and endocrinologic abnormalities such as diabetes and hyperandrogenism are seen in varying frequencies in different studies. Mechanical friction, often worsened by obesity, is an exacerbating factor, as is bacterial infection. There is an autosomal-dominantly inherited form of this disease. One study revealed that those with a positive family history tended to have less severe disease.

Differential diagnosis

Hidradenitis is to be differentiated from common furuncles, which are typically unilateral. Hidradenitis must also be differentiated from Bartholin abscess, scrofuloderma, actinomycosis, granuloma inguinale, and lymphogranuloma venereum.

Treatment

Despite the numerous forms of treatment available, a permanent cure is uncommon. The earliest lesions often heal quickly with intralesional steroid therapy, and this should be tried initially in combination with topical cleocin or oral tetracycline or minocycline. Topical daily cleansing with an antibacterial soap, chlorhexidine solution, or benzoyl peroxide wash is an important preventative measure. Additionally, laser hair removal, if performed, should be done in unaffected sites as a preventative therapy. Reduction of friction by wearing loose-fitting clothing and weight loss if needed, and avoidance of excessive sweating through the use of topical aluminum chloride or botulinum toxin A injections and heat avoidance may help. In cases with draining sinuses, culture of the pus may reveal *S. aureus* or Gram-negative organisms. The latter are usually cultured in chronic cases. Antibiotics should be selected based on sensitivities of the cultured organism. Useful systemic antibiotics include the tetracyclines, amoxicillin, sulfamethoxazole/trimethoprim DS, dapsone, clindamycin or antibiotic plus rifampin combination. Incision and drainage is strongly discouraged.

Isotretinoin is effective in some cases, but a remission seldom follows its use. In the largest study to date, Boer et al treated 68 patients with a mean dose of 0.56 mg/kg of isotretinoin for 4–6 months. Clearing was obtained in 23.5% and long-term remission was seen in 16.2%. Secondary infection with *S. aureus* often occurs. Infliximab, etanercept, and adalimumab may clear the condition during their use; however, response is variable. In women, spironolactone and oral birth control pills are often an excellent choice, and finasteride in men or postmenopausal women may also be a helpful adjuvant. Cyclosporine may work well in selected cases.

Photodynamic therapy and lasers have also been investigated to various degrees in hidradenitis. Methyl-aminolaevulinate or 5-aminolevulinic acid prior to blue or red light activation (photodynamic therapy) has had reports of success in some cases, but also anecdotal reports of lack of efficacy. It is inconvenient, costly, and often painful, and does not produce remission, so further studies are required before such treatment can be recommended. Neodymium-doped yttrium aluminum garnet laser treatment has been reported to be quite effective in a prospective, randomized controlled trial of 22 severely affected individuals. After a series of three monthly sessions resulted in significant improvement, Nd:YAG laser treatment holds real promise in the therapy of hidradenitis.

Chances of permanent cure are best when excision of the affected areas is done. Wide surgical excision, using intra-operative color-marking of sinus tracts, is most effective at limiting recurrence; however, it has moderate morbidity, especially in the groin and perianal areas. The recurrence rate is low in the axillary and perianal areas; however, the inguinal folds and especially the submammary sites more often recur so that excision of the latter site is uncommonly recommended. CO_2 laser may also destroy lesions and sinus tracts. The open areas may be closed or left to heal secondarily.

Alikhan A, et al: Hidradenitis suppurativa. J Am Acad Dermatol 2009; 60:539.

Blanco R, et al: Long-term successful adalimumab therapy in severe hidradenitis suppurativa. Arch Dermatol 2009; 145:580.
Boer J, et al: Long-term results of isotretinoin in the treatment of 68 patients with hidradenitis suppurativa. J Am Acad Dermatol 1999; 40:73.
Buimer MG, et al: Hidradenitis suppurativa. Br J Surg 2009; 96:350.
Canoui-Poitrine F, et al: Clinical characteristics of a series of 302 French patients with hidradenitis suppurativa, with an analysis of factors associated with disease severity. J Am Acad Dermatol 2009; 61:51.
Chandramohan K, et al: Squamous cell carcinoma arising from perianal lesion in a familial case of hidradenitis suppurativa. Int Wound J 2009; 6:141.
Joseph MA, et al: Hidradenitis suppurativa treated with finasteride. J Dermatolog Treat 2005; 18:75.
Kaur MR, et al: Hidradenitis suppurativa treated with dapsone. J Dermatolog Treat 2006; 17:211.
Kraft JN, et al: Hidradenitis suppurativa in 64 female patients: retrospective study comparing oral antibiotics and antiandrogen therapy. J Cutan Med Surg 2007; 11:125.
Lam J, et al: Hidradenitis suppurativa. Pediatr Dermatol 2007; 24:465.
Lee RA, et al: Hidradenitis suppurativa. Adv Dermatol 2007; 23:289.
Lee RA, et al: A prospective clinical trial of open-label etanercept for the treatment of hidradenitis suppurativa. J Am Acad Dermatol 2009; 60:565.
Madan V, et al: Outcomes of treatment of nine cases of recalcitrant severe hidradenitis suppurativa with carbon dioxide laser. Br J Dermatol 2008; 159:1309.
Mandal A, et al: Experience with different treatment modules in hidradenitis suppurativa. Surgeon 2005; 3:23.
Matusiak L, et al: Hidradenitis suppurativa and associated factors: still unsolved problems. J Am Acad Dermatol 2009; 61:362.
Mendoca CO, et al: Clindamycin and rifampicin combination therapy for hidradenitis suppurativa. Br J Dermatol 2006; 154:977.
Montes-Romero JA, et al: Amyloidosis secondary to hidradenitis suppurativa. Eur J Intern Med 2008; 19:e32.
Revuz JE, et al: Prevalence and factors associated with hidradenitis suppurativa: results from two case-control studies. J Am Acad Dermatol 2008; 59:596.
Rubin RJ, et al: Perianal hidradenitis suppurativa. Surg Clin North Am 1994; 74:1317.
Saraceno R, et al: Methyl aminolaevulinate photodynamic therapy for the treatment of hidradenitis suppurativa and pilonidal cysts. Photodermatol Photoimmunol Photomed 2009; 25:164.
Tierney E, et al: Randomized control trial for the treatment of hidradenitis suppurativa with a neodymium-doped yttrium aluminium garnet laser. Dermatol Surg 2009; 35:1.
Wolkenstein P, et al: Quality of life impairment in hidradenitis suppurativa. J Am Acad Dermatol 2007; 56:621.

Dissecting cellulitis of the scalp

Also known as perifolliculitis capitis abscedens et suffodiens, this is an uncommon chronic suppurative disease of the scalp characterized by numerous follicular and perifollicular inflammatory nodules. These nodules suppurate and undermine to form intercommunicating sinuses as long as 5 cm (Fig. 13-21). Scarring and alopecia ensue, although seropurulent drainage may last indefinitely. Adult black men are most commonly affected, and the vertex and occiput of the scalp are the sites of predilection.

The primary lesions are follicular and perifollicular erythematous papules which progress to abscesses. This disease is a variant of dissecting terminal hair folliculitis, along with hidradenitis suppurativa, acne keloidalis nuchae, and pilonidal sinus. Coagulase-positive *S. aureus* may be found in the lesions.

Treatment is generally unsuccessful unless the most vigorous procedures are followed. The combination of intralesional steroid injections and isotretinoin at a dose of 0.5–1.5 mg/kg/day for 6–12 months may be successful. Starting at a lower dose such as 10 mg per day for the first month or two may prevent a flare of the condition. The length of remission with isotretinoin is variable, but treatment may be repeated with similar results expected. Oral antibiotics such as the

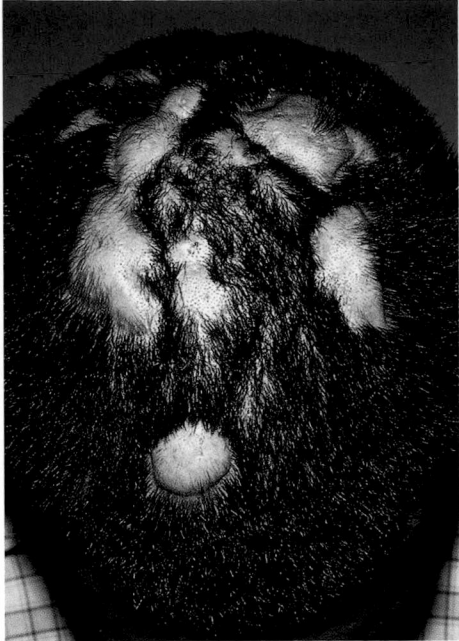

Fig. 13-21 Dissecting folliculitis. (Courtesy of Curt Samlaska, MD)

tetracyclines, trimethoprim–sulfamethoxazole, or the quinolones may produce good results. If *S. aureus* is cultured, the combination of oral rifampin and clindamycin has produced excellent results.

A surgical approach is at times necessary. Marsupialization or excision of sinus tracks may help limit inflammation. The Nd:YAG laser used with the intent to remove hair has led to long-term improvement.

Georgala S, et al: Dissecting cellulitis of the scalp treated with rifampicin and isotretinoin. Cutis 2008; 82:195.

Greenblatt DT, et al: Dissecting cellulitis of the scalp responding to oral quinolones. Clin Exp Dermatol 2008; 33:99.

Krasner BD, et al: Dissecting cellulitis treated with the long-pulsed Nd:YAG laser. Dermatol Surg 2006; 32:1039.

Sukhatme SV, et al: Refractory dissecting cellulitis of the scalp treated with adalimumab. J Drugs Dermatol 2008; 7:981.

Acne miliaris necrotica (acne varioliformis)

Acne miliaris necrotica consists of follicular vesicopustules, sometimes occurring as solitary lesions that are usually very itchy. They appear anywhere in the scalp or adjacent areas, rupture early, and dry up after a few days. In some patients, especially those who manipulate the lesions, *S. aureus* may be cultured. If they leave large scars, the term acne varioliformis is used; they are probably not separate diseases.

Treatment is with culture-directed antibiotics, or if the culture is negative, oral tetracycline or minocycline. Doxepin is helpful if patients manipulate their lesions.

Fisher DA: Acne necroticans and *Staphylococcus aureus*. J Am Acad Dermatol 1988; 18:1136.

Kossard S, et al: Necrotizing lymphocytic folliculitis: the early lesion of acne necrotica. J Am Acad Dermatol 1987; 16:1007.

Zirn JR, et al: Chronic acneiform eruption with crateriform scars. Arch Dermatol 1996; 132:1365.

Rosacea

Clinical features

Rosacea is characterized by a persistent erythema of the convex surfaces of the face, with the cheeks and nose most frequently

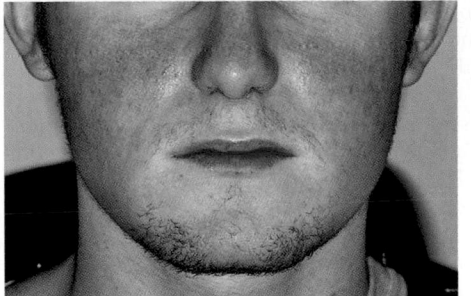

Fig. 13-22 Erythrotelangiectatic rosacea.

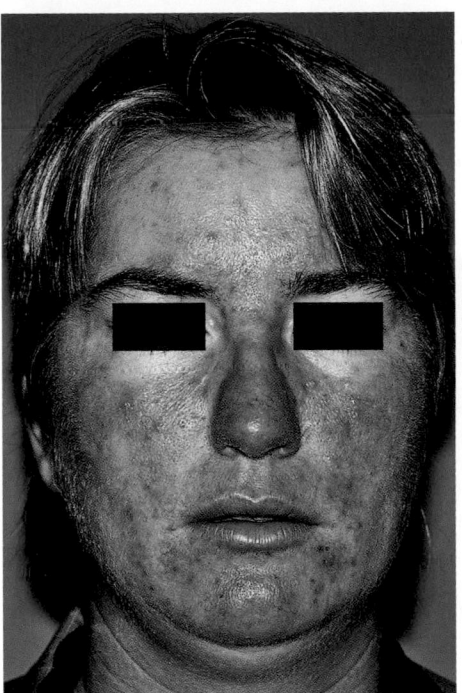

Fig. 13-23 Papulopustular rosacea. (Courtesy of Curt Samlaska, MD)

affected, followed by involvement of the brow and chin. There is a tendency to spare the periocular skin. Rosacea occurs most often in light-skinned women between the ages of 30 and 50; however, the severe type with phymatous changes occurs almost exclusively in men. Additional features commonly manifested include telangiectasia, flushing, erythematous papules and pustules. These tend to cluster in patterns, allowing for the identification of several subsets of patients, the importance of their recognition being that the therapeutic implications differ.

The erythrotelangiectatic type (Fig. 13-22) is characterized by a prominent history of a prolonged (over 10 min) flushing reaction to various stimuli, such as emotional stress, hot drinks, alcohol, spicy foods, exercise, cold or hot weather, or hot baths and showers. Often a burning or stinging sensation accompanies the flush, but sweating, lightheadedness, and palpitations do not. The skin is of fine texture, may have a roughness and scaling of the affected central facial sites, and is easily irritated. Over time a purplish suffusion and prominent telangiectasia may result.

The papulopustular subset of patients manifests a strikingly red central face accompanied by erythematous papules often surmounted by a pinpoint pustule (Fig. 13-23). The history of flushing is also present in most patients, but usually symptoms of irritancy are not prominent. The skin is of normal or at times slightly sebaceous quality and edema of the affected sites may be present. Such edema may dominate the clinical presentation, with the forehead, eyelids, and cheeks variably affected. This has been termed Morbihan's disease and is most likely to complicate the papulopustular and glandular types.

In the glandular type of rosacea, men with thick sebaceous skin predominate. The papules are edematous, the pustules are often 0.5–1.0 cm in size, and nodulocystic lesions may be present (Fig. 13-24). They tend to cluster in the central face, but in affected women the chin is favored. There is frequently a history of adolescent acne and typical scars may be seen. Flushing is less common, as is telangiectasia, but persistent edema may be problematic. It is in this subtype that rhinophyma (Fig. 13-25) most commonly occurs. Hypertrophic, hyperemic, large nodular masses are centered over the distal half of the nose. Rarely, such soft tissue overgrowth can affect the chin, ears, or forehead. Hugely dilated follicles contain long vermicular plugs of sebum and keratin. The histologic features are pilosebaceous gland hyperplasia with fibrosis, inflammation, and telangiectasia.

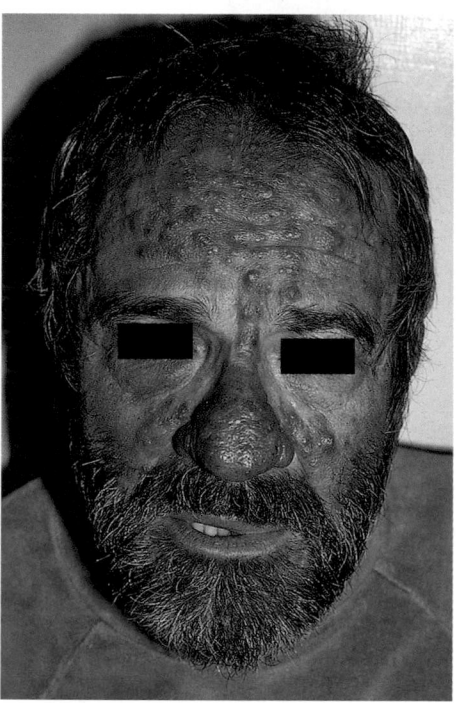

Fig. 13-24 Glandular rosacea.

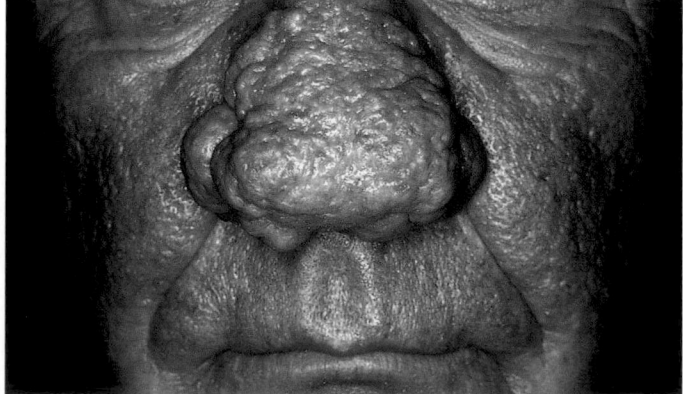

Fig. 13-25 Rhinophyma.

Etiology

The cause of rosacea remains unknown. Most patients have an abnormal vasomotor response to thermal and other stimuli, as described above. Additionally, chronic solar damage is an important contributor in producing damage to the dermal matrix and ground substance, especially in the erythrotelangiectatic subtype. Chronic vasodilatation, edema, and compromise of lymphatic drainage occur and lead to telangiectasia and fibrosis. Pilosebaceous unit abnormalities are not commonly felt to be part of the pathogenesis of this condition; however, some evidence points to abnormalities being present, especially in the glandular type of patient. It is to be expected that the pathogenic factors will vary among the subsets of patients. *Demodex* and *Helicobacter pylori* have been extensively investigated and do not appear to be central to the etiology of rosacea.

Other clinical considerations

Ocular findings

Blepharitis, recurrent chalazion, and conjunctivitis may be seen in all subsets of rosacea (Fig. 13-26). The eye itself may be affected, with keratitis, iritis, and episcleritis. An abnormal Schirmer test occurs in 40% of rosacea patients. Complaints are often of a gritty, stinging, itchy, or burning sensation in the eye. Light sensitivity and a foreign body sensation are also present at times. Ocular rosacea occurs equally in men and women. Such eye findings may occur before the skin disease. Since these findings have therapeutic implications and patients will not always complain of them to their dermatologist, these signs and symptoms should be actively sought when evaluating rosacea patients.

Extrafacial lesions

Flushing may involve the ears, lateral facial contours, neck, upper chest, and scalp. Papules and pustules may be present in persistent erythema of the scalp or the earlobes.

Topical steroid use

Long-term use of topical steroids on the face may result in persistent erythema, papules, and pustules. The sites involved correspond to the areas of application and are not necessarily limited to the central convexities. Treatment is discontinuance of the offending drug and institution of topical tacrolimus in combination with short-term minocycline. Topical tacrolimus itself has paradoxically been reported to induce a rosacea-like reaction, so coverage with minocycline while discontinuing topical steroids is necessary. Additionally, drinking alcohol after application of tacrolimus or pimecrolimus may induce

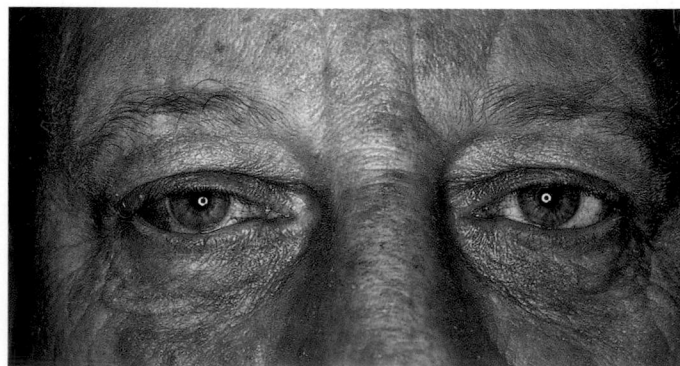

Fig. 13-26 Ocular rosacea.

flushing, which may be confused with new-onset flushing related to rosacea.

Perioral dermatitis

While this condition has been classified within the umbrella of rosacea variants, its distribution, signs, and symptoms vary such that it is included separately in this chapter.

Granulomatous lesions

Some patients with persistent facial erythema of the convexities will have, on biopsy of an erythematous papule, a granulomatous response closely resembling sarcoidosis or a necrotizing granuloma. Many experienced clinicians will accurately predict such findings from the clinical examination. Here the most important consideration is the fact that the response to treatment may be slower. When involvement of granulomatous facial papules includes the eyelids and upper lip, and is not associated with vascular manifestations, such as flushing, erythema, or telangiectasia, the term granulomatous facial dermatitis is preferred. This condition is discussed separately.

Differential diagnosis

The persistent erythema of the central face should be differentiated from that seen in polycythemia vera, carcinoid, mastocytosis, and connective tissue disease (lupus erythematosus, dermatomyositis, and mixed connective tissue disease). These conditions do not have associated papules and pustules, will manifest a variety of systemic symptoms and extrafacial signs, and specific laboratory markers are available to confirm clinical suspicions. Haber syndrome is a genodermatosis characterized by a rosacea-like facial dermatosis and multiple verrucous lesions on non-sun-exposed skin. Onset of the facial lesions is in the first two decades of life, in contrast to the later onset of rosacea. While rosacea may occur in human immunodeficiency virus (HIV) disease, a papulonodular eruption of the face that may simulate acne rosacea also occurs in patients with acquired immunodeficiency syndrome (AIDS). On expressing the contents of hair follicles with a comedo extractor, numerous *Demodex* mites are seen. In such cases, success with permethrin cream and lindane has been reported, and also lotions containing 5% benzoyl peroxide and 5% precipitated sulfur (Sulfoxyl) are helpful.

Treatment

Treatments are directed at specific findings manifested by rosacea patients. Since erythema, telangiectases, papules and pustules, phymas, flushing, ocular symptoms, and skin sensitivity are variably present in the three subsets of disease, the specific approach utilized will differ according to the factors present. Other treatments are useful in all patients.

General nonpharmacologic and nonsurgical interventions

Sunscreens are an important component of therapy for all patients. They should be applied each morning. Those containing physical blockers in a dimethicone or cyclomethicone vehicle are in general better tolerated, especially by the erythrotelangiectatic patients, than those with chemical agents. General avoidance of irritants such as astringents, peeling or acidic agents, and abrasive or exfoliant preparations is recommended. Cosmetic coverage of the erythema and telangiectases is best with a light green or yellow-tinted foundation set with powder.

If flushing is induced by specific trigger factors, their avoidance as much as possible is best. Soybe hypothesized that the central face is predisposed to rosacea as the edema and lack of movement of tissues with muscular movement may lead to lymphedema and inflammation. Circular massage for several minutes a day led to impressive improvement. This benign intervention may be considered and ought to be studied. Artificial tears and cleansing the lids with warm water two times daily will help ocular symptoms.

Topical therapy

Metronidazole, sodium sulfacetamide, sulfur cleansers and creams, and azelaic acid are approved for use in rosacea. They are the most commonly prescribed medications and are especially useful for the papulopustular patients and some patients with the erythrotelangiectatic type. Benzoyl peroxide and topical clindamycin, alone or in combination, are often quite beneficial and well tolerated by the glandular subset of patients. If oral antibiotics are needed, the topical products may be used to maintain remission after discontinuance of oral preparations.

Pimecrolimus or tacrolimus may also improve selected patients' erythema, especially those with an accompanying roughness or scaling of the skin surface. They help the irritated erythrotelangiectatic and at times the papulopustular patients, but are not effective in the glandular type, and tacrolimus in its ointment base may exacerbate the inflammatory component in these patients. They calm inflammation and abate symptoms, but require brief (no longer than 1 week) pretreatment with a potent topical steroid to be tolerated initially. The role of topical retinoids requires study. Many rosacea patients may tolerate a night-time application of tretinoin if cetaphil lotion is used immediately prior to use. Retinoids may help repair sun-damaged skin and normalize some of the abnormalities present. Topical application of a selective $\alpha 1$-adrenergic receptor agonist, oxymetazoline, helped one patient's flushing and redness, but this treatment requires more data before it can be recommended since rebound erythema is a concern.

Oral therapy

Oral antibiotics, particularly tetracycline 250–500 mg each morning, doxycycline 50–100 mg once or twice daily, or minocycline 50–100 mg once or twice a day, control more aggressive papular and pustular lesions, and aid in the treatment of ocular lesions. Subantimicrobial doxycycline is also available in a 40 mg extended-release formulation. It is only occasionally useful in the author's experience. Oral antibiotics should be discontinued once clearance of the inflammatory lesions is obtained; usually 2 or 3 months is necessary. The topical approved preparations above should be used as long-term maintenance after clearance with the oral medications, as disease will recur in most patients if all therapy is stopped. If significant ocular symptoms are present, oral antibiotics are an effective and convenient method of relieving both the skin and eye concerns. Isotretinoin given in lower doses than in acne vulgaris, and at times as a long-term suppressant, may be necessary for management of more resistant disease. It produces dramatic improvement even in cases resistant to other forms of therapy, but relapse often occurs in a few weeks or months. The authors rarely use oral metronidazole (side effects) or the macrolides (lack of efficacy) despite their reported utility in this condition.

Oral medications for reduction of flushing are uncommonly helpful. Occasionally an escalating dose of propranolol or clonidine is helpful in reducing symptomatic flushing, but most affected patients find the side effects occur before the beneficial effects are evident. One method is to start propranolol at 10 mg three times daily, and if no response is seen in 2 weeks, to increase the dose by 10 mg at one dose, then again every 2 weeks until either side effects require discontinuation or response occurs. Responses are mostly seen at a dose of 20–40 mg three times daily.

Surgical intervention

Surgical approaches to the reshaping of rhinophyma have included the use of a heated scalpel, electrocautery, dermabrasion, laser ablation, tangential excision combined with scissor sculpting, and radiofrequency electrosurgery. Often a combination of these approaches is used to obtain the best esthetic result. Lasers and light devices are useful for treating the erythema and telangiectases, but the cost is not covered by insurance and this limits their availability. In a comparative study the pulsed dye laser and intense pulse light device both significantly reduced erythema, telangiectasia, and patient-reported symptoms, and performed similarly well. Some vascular and CO_2 fractionated lasers may also help in dermal collagen remodeling and nonablative rejuvenation, such that the dermal matrix may be strengthened. For the patient incapacitated by flushing, burning, and stinging, endoscopic transthoracic sympathectomy may be considered, but this extreme measure should only rarely be considered, as serious complications may result.

An advocacy group that supports research and education in rosacea, the National Rosacea Society, is an excellent resource for patients.

Aloi F, et al: The clinicopathologic spectrum of rhinophyma. J Am Acad Dermatol 2000; 42:468.

Altinyazar HC, et al: Adapalene vs metronidazole gel for the treatment of rosacea. Int J Dermatol 2005; 44:252.

Antille C, et al: Induction of rosaceiform dermatitis during treatment of facial inflammatory dermatoses with tacrolimus ointment. Arch Dermatol 2004; 140:457.

Craige H, et al: Symptomatic treatment of idiopathic and rosacea-associated cutaneous flushing with propranolol. J Am Acad Dermatol 2005; 53:881.

Crawford GH, et al: Rosacea I. J Am Acad Dermatol 2004; 5:327.

Crawford KM, et al: Pimecrolimus for treatment of acne rosacea. Skin Med 2005; 4:147.

Elewski BE, et al: Rosacea. J Eur Acad Dermatol Venereol 2010; epub.

El Sayed F, et al: Rosaceiform eruption to pimecrolimus. J Am Acad Dermatol 2006; 54:548.

Garg G, et al: Clinical efficacy of tacrolimus in rosacea. J Eur Acad Dermatol Venereol 2009; 23:239.

Izikson L, et al: The flushing patient. J Am Acad Dermatol 2006; 55:193.

Karabulut AA, et al: A randomized, single-blind, placebo-controlled, split-face study with pimecrolimus cream 1% for papulopustular rosacea. J Eur Acad Dermatol Venereol 2008; 22:729.

Kilty S, et al: Surgical treatment of rhinophyma. J Otolaryngol Head Neck Surg 2008; 37:269.

Kroshinshky D, et al: Pediatric rosacea. Dermatol Ther 2006; 19:196.

Lee DH, et al: Pimecrolimus 1% cream for the treatment of steroid-induced rosacea. Br J Dermatol 2008; 158:1069.

Liu RH, et al: Azelaic acid in the treatment of papulopustular rosacea. Arch Dermatol 2006; 142:1047.

Neuhaus IM, et al: Comparative efficacy of nonpurpuragenic pulsed dye laser and intense pulsed light for erythematotelangiectatic rosacea. Dermatol Surg 2009; 35:920.

Ogunleye T, et al: Ethanol-induced flushing with topical pimecrolimus use. Dermatitis 2008; 19:E1.

Pelle MT, et al: Rosacea II. Therapy. J Am Acad Dermatol 2004; 51:499.

Powell FC: Clinical practice: rosacea. N Engl J Med 2005; 352:793.

Shanler SD, et al: Successful treatment of the erythema and flushing of rosacea using a topically applied selective alpha 1-adrenergic receptor agonist, oxymetazoline. Arch Dermatol 2007; 143:1369.

Stone DU, et al: Ocular rosacea. Curr Opin Ophthalmol 2004; 15:499.

van Zuuren E, et al: Interventions for rosacea. Cochrane Database Syst Rev 2005; 20:CD003262.

Van Zuuren EJ, et al: Systematic review of rosacea treatments. J Am Acad Dermatol 2007; 56:107.

Wilkin J, et al: Standard classification of rosacea: report of the National Rosacea Society Expert Committee on the Classification and Staging of Rosacea. J Am Acad Dermatol 2002; 46:584.

Yoon TY, et al: Pimecrolimus-induced rosacea-like demodicidosis. Int J Dermatol 2007; 46:1103.

Zhao YE, et al: Retrospective analysis of the association between Demodex infestation and rosacea. Arch Dermatol 2010; 146:896.

Pyoderma faciale

This uncommon eruptive facial disorder consists of a dramatically fulminant onset of superficial and deep abscesses, cystic lesions (Fig. 13-27), and sometimes sinus tracts. Edema and at times an intense reddish or cyanotic erythema accompany this pustular process. The lesions often contain greenish or yellowish purulent material. Older cysts contain an oily substance. The condition occurs mostly in postadolescent women. It is distinguished from acne by the absence of comedones, rapid onset, fulminating course, and absence of acne on the back and

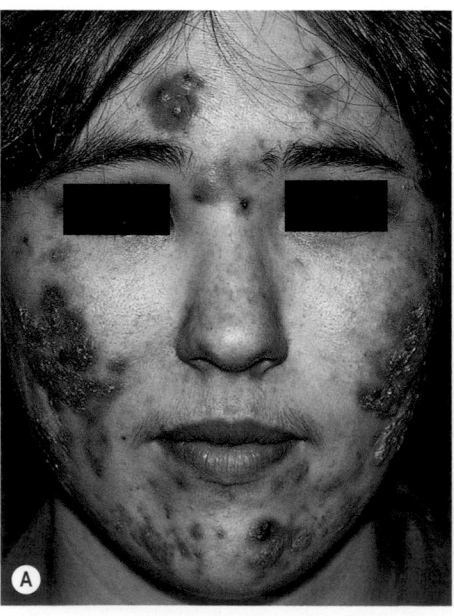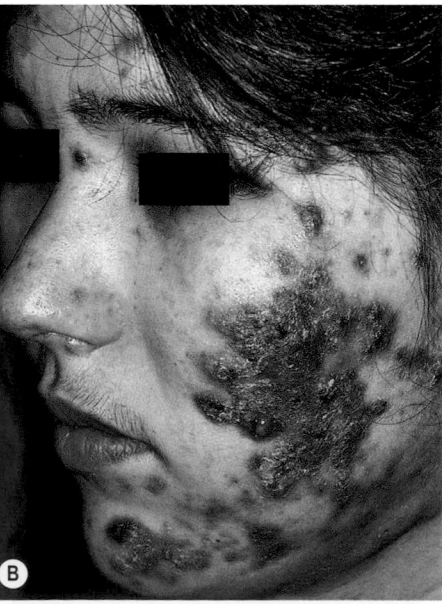

Fig. 13-27 A and B, Pyoderma faciale. (Courtesy of Curt Samlaska, MD)

chest. Pyoderma faciale is differentiated from rosacea by the inconsistent history of flushing, the absence of pre-existing erythema or telangiectases of the convex portions of the face, and by the large abscesses and nodules.

Treatment is similar to that of acne fulminans. Oral steroids are given for several weeks followed by the addition of isotretinoin, 10–20 mg, increasing to 0.5–1 mg/kg only after the acute inflammatory component is well under control. Steroids may usually be discontinued after several weeks of isotretinoin, but the latter should be given for a full 120–150 mg/kg total dose. As patients are predominately women of child-bearing age, pregnancy issues require full discussion. Indeed, four of Plewig et al's patients were pregnant and thus could not use isotretinoin.

Akhyani M, et al: The association of pyoderma faciale and erythema nodosum. Clin Exp Dermatol 2007; 32:275.
Crawford GH, et al: Pyoderma faciale. J Am Acad Dermatol 2005; 53:1106.
Fender AB, et al: Pyoderma faciale. Cutis 2008; 81:488.
Plewig G, et al: Pyoderma faciale. Arch Dermatol 1992; 128:1611.

Perioral dermatitis

This common perioral eruption consists of discrete papules and pustules on an erythematous and at times scaling base. It is a distinctive dermatitis confined symmetrically around the mouth, with a clear zone of some 5 mm between the vermilion border and the affected skin (Fig. 13-28). There is no itching; however, an uncomfortable burning sensation may be present. It occurs almost exclusively in women between the ages of 20 and 35. The use of fluorinated topical steroids is the most frequently identified cause. Exposure may be in the form of creams, ointments, or inhalers.

Treatment includes discontinuing topical steroids or protecting the skin from the inhaled product. Additionally, tetracycline, 250–500 mg once a day, or minocycline, 100 mg once or twice a day, will lead to control. Tacrolimus ointment 0.1% or pimecrolimus cream will prevent flaring after stopping steroid use. In those patients without steroid exposure, oral or topical antibiotics, and topical adapalene, azelaic acid, and metronidazole have been successful in clearing the eruption.

Periorbital dermatitis

Periorbital (periocular) dermatitis is a variant of perioral dermatitis occurring on the lower eyelids and skin adjacent to the upper and lower eyelids. Fluorinated topical steroids have been implicated as the cause. If intranasal inhaled steroids are used, a perinasal distribution may be seen. Prompt response to the same treatment employed in the perioral site is expected.

Chen AY, et al: Steroid-induced rosacealike dermatitis. Cutis 2009; 83:198.
Nguyen V, et al: Periorificial dermatitis in children and adolescents. J Am Acad Dermatol 2006; 55:781.
Poulos GA, et al: Perioral dermatitis associated with an inhaled corticosteroid. Arch Dermatol 2007; 142:1460.
Schwarz T, et al: A randomized, double-blind, vehicle-controlled study of 1% pimecrolimus cream in adult patients with perioral dermatitis. J Am Acad Dermatol 2008; 59:34.
Weber K, et al: Critical appraisal of reports on the treatment of perioral dermatitis. Dermatology 2005; 210:300.

Granulomatous facial dermatitis

Several dermatoses of the face characterized by granulomas are included in this category. Patients with persistent facial erythema involving one or more convex surfaces of the face will have lesions that show a granulomatous reaction histologically, and are included within rosacea. Some patients have no other stigmata of rosacea and their nosology is unclear. These other entities, which meet no other criteria for rosacea other than having pink papules on the face, are included here. Skowron et al have proposed the term FIGURE (facial idiopathic granulomas with regressive evolution).

Lupus miliaris disseminatus faciei

Firm, yellowish-brown or red, 1–3 mm, monomorphous, smooth-surfaced papules are present not only on the butterfly areas but also on the lateral areas, below the mandible, and periorificially (Fig. 13-29). The eyelid skin is characteristically involved. The discrete papules appear as yellowish-brown lesions on diascopy and as caseating epithelioid cell granulomas histologically. Patients usually lack a history of flushing, do not have persistent erythema or telangiectasia, have involvement of the eyelids, and heal with scarring, as opposed to rosacea patients. Long-term therapy with minocycline or isotretinoin may be used, often with gratifying results. Eventually, self-involution is expected but may take several years to occur.

Granulomatous perioral dermatitis in children

In otherwise healthy prepubertal children a profusion of grouped papules may develop on the perioral, periocular, and perinasal areas (Fig. 13-30). Eight of the initial 59 reported

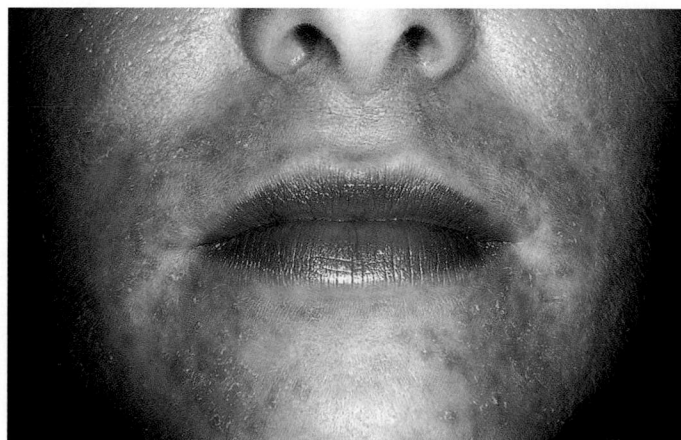

Fig. 13-28 Perioral dermatitis.

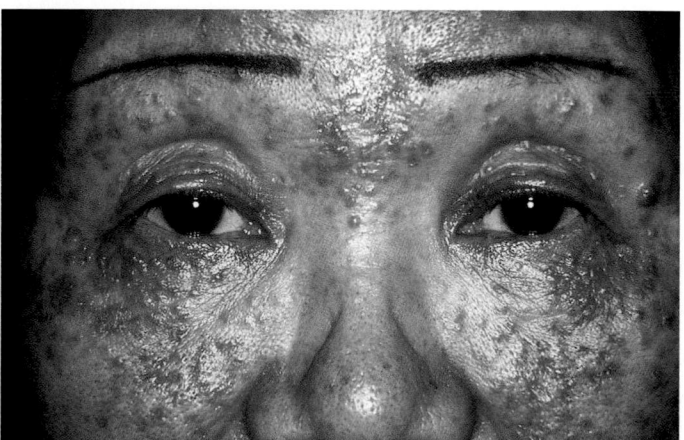

Fig. 13-29 Lupus miliaris.

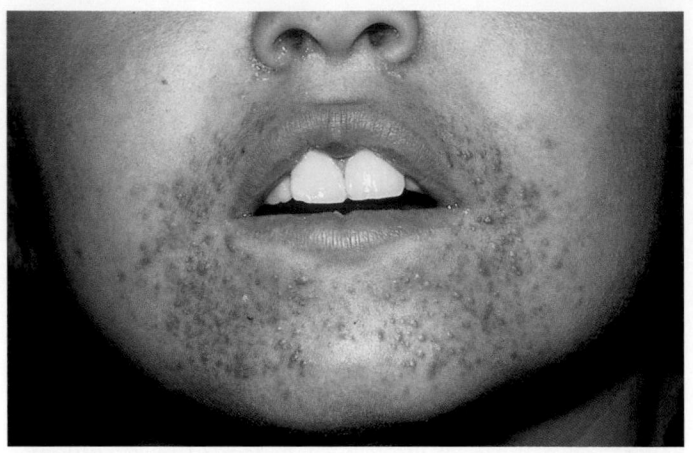

Fig. 13-30 Childhood granulomatous facial dermatitis.

cases have also had generalized lesions. Besides extremity and trunkal lesions, several of the girls have had dramatic lesions of the labia majora. Both sexes are affected equally. Children with skin of color (Afro-Caribbean, African American, and Asian) dominate the reports but white patients are also susceptible. Because the histologic appearance is granulomatous, sarcoidosis is often considered. Topical steroids, however, may worsen the condition and systemic involvement is not present. Topical metronidazole, erythromycin, sulfacetamide–sulfur combinations, and oral macrolide and tetracycline are usually effective.

Choi YL, et al: Case of childhood granulomatous periorificial dermatitis in a Korean boy treated by oral erythromycin. J Dermatol 2006; 33:806.
Lucas CR, et al: Granulomatous periorificial dermatitis. J Cutan Med Surg 2009; 13:115.
Misago N, et al: Childhood granulomatous periorificial dermatitis. J Eur Acad Dermatol 2005; 19:470.
Skowron F, et al: F.I.G.U.R.E.: facial idiopathic granulomas with regressive evolution. Dermatology 2000; 201:289.
Tarm K, et al: Granulomatous periorificial dermatitis. Cutis 2004; 73:399.
Urbatsch AJ, et al: Extrafacial and generalized granulomatous periorificial dermatitis. Arch Dermatol 2002; 138:1354.
Van de Scheur MR, et al: Lupus miliaris disseminatus faciei. Dermatology 2003; 206:120.

 Bonus images for this chapter can be found online at
http://www.expertconsult.com

Fig. 13-1 Minocycline-induced pigmentation at sites of inflammation in a patient with acne.
Fig. 13-2 Staphylococcal infection while on Accutane. (Courtesy of Curt Samlaska, MD)
Fig. 13-3 Acne conglobata.
Fig. 13-4 Rosacea.
Fig. 13-5 Steroid rosacea.

Bacterial Infections

14

Bacterial infections in the skin often have distinct morphologic characteristics that should alert the clinician to the fact that a potentially treatable and reversible condition exists. These cutaneous signs may be an indication of a generalized systemic process or simply an isolated superficial event.

Immunodeficiencies with low immunoglobulins, neutropenia, reduced neutrophil migration or killing, and disease caused by the human immunodeficiency virus (HIV) may be associated with severe or refractory pyogenic infections. Atopic dermatitis and syndromes with atopic-like dermatitis are also predisposed to bacterial infections.

The categorization of these infections will be first those diseases caused by Gram-positive bacteria, then those caused by Gram-negative bacteria, and finally several miscellaneous diseases caused by the rickettsiae, mycoplasmas, chlamydiae, and spirochetes.

Center for Communicable Diseases (CDC): STD treatment guidelines 2006. MMWR 2006; 55:1.

Fernandez-Obregon AC, et al: Current use of anti-infectives in dermatology. Expert Rev Anti Infect Ther 2005; 3:557.

Grice EA, et al: Topographical and temporal diversity of the human skin microbiome. Science 2009; 324:1190.

Hogan MT: Cutaneous infections associated with HIV/AIDS. Dermatol Clin 2006; 24:473.

Lupi O, et al: Tropical dermatology: bacterial tropical diseases. J Am Acad Dermatol 2006; 54:559.

May AK: Skin and soft tissue infections. Surg Clin North Am 2009; 89:403.

Nathwani D: New antibiotics for the management of complicated skin and soft tissue infections. Int J Antimicrob Agents 2009; 34(Suppl 1):S24.

Schauber J, et al: Antimicrobial peptides and the skin immune defense system. J Allergy Clin Immunol 2008; 122:261.

Schweiger ES, et al: Novel antibacterial agents for skin and skin structure infections. J Am Acad Dermatol 2004; 50:331.

Wu JJ, et al: Vaccines and immunotherapies for the prevention of infectious diseases having cutaneous manifestations. J Am Acad Dermatol 2004; 50:495.

INFECTIONS CAUSED BY GRAM-POSITIVE ORGANISMS

Staphylococcal infections

The skin lesions induced by this Gram-positive coccus appear usually as pustules, furuncles, or erosions with honey-colored crusts; however, bullae, widespread erythema and desquamation, or vegetating pyodermas may also be indicators of *Staphylococcus aureus* infection. Purulent purpura may indicate bacteremia or endocarditis caused by *S. aureus*, or, in immunocompromised patients, *S. epidermidis*. Two distinctive cutaneous lesions that occur with endocarditis are the Osler node and Janeway lesion or spot. The former is a painful, erythematous nodule with a pale center located on the fingertips. The latter is a nontender, angular hemorrhagic lesion of the palms (Fig. 14-1) and soles. These lesions are likely to be due to septic emboli.

S. aureus is a normal inhabitant of the anterior nares in 20–40% of adults, and also resides on the hands and perineum in smaller numbers of individuals. Nasal carriers are particularly prone to infections with this bacterium because of its continuous presence on the skin and nasal mucosa. Spread of infection in the hospital setting is frequently traced to the hands of a healthcare worker. Proper handwashing technique is essential in limiting this nosocomial complication. HIV-infected patients are at least twice as commonly nasal carriers, and they tend to harbor *S. aureus* in higher frequency and density at other sites of the body, thus predisposing them to skin and systemic infection.

Antibiotic resistance has become a clinically important consideration in many infections, but meticillin-resistant *S. aureus* (MRSA), which has been a nosocomial problem for years, is now a common community-acquired skin infection. MRSA infection may be suspected from a knowledge of local patterns of resistance, lack of response to initial meticillin-sensitive *S. aureus* (MSSA)-directed therapy, such as cefalexin, and factors predisposing to colonization and infection with this organism. Predisposing factors include age (older than 65), exposure to others with MRSA infection, prior antibiotic therapy, and recent hospitalization or chronic illness. In patients with risk factors, multiple drug resistance is likely and treatment with intravenous vancomycin or linezolid may be necessary. In community-acquired infection in patients without risk factors, clindamycin, trimethoprim–sulfamethoxazole (alone or combined with rifampin), minocycline, or oral linezolid will often be effective. Definitive antibiotic therapy may be tailored to the antibiotic susceptibility of the cultured organism.

Superficial pustular folliculitis (impetigo of Bockhart)

Bockhart impetigo is a superficial folliculitis with thin-walled pustules at the follicle orifices. Favorite locations are the extremities and scalp, although it is also seen on the face, especially periorally. These fragile, yellowish-white, domed pustules develop in crops and heal in a few days. *S. aureus* is the most frequent cause. The infection may secondarily arise in scratches, insect bites, or other skin injuries.

Sycosis vulgaris (sycosis barbae)

Sycosis vulgaris, formerly known as barber's itch, is a perifollicular, chronic, pustular staphylococcal infection of the bearded region (Fig. 14-2), characterized by the presence of inflammatory papules and pustules, and a tendency to recurrence. The disease begins with erythema and burning or itching, usually on the upper lip near the nose. In a day or two one or more pinhead-sized pustules, pierced by hairs, develop.

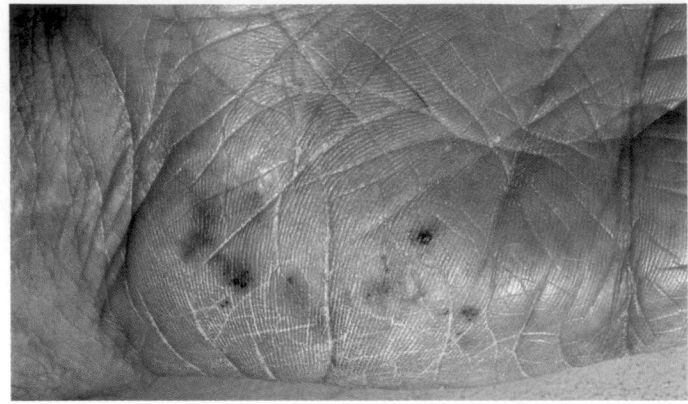

Fig. 14-1 Janeway lesion in subacute bacterial endocarditis.

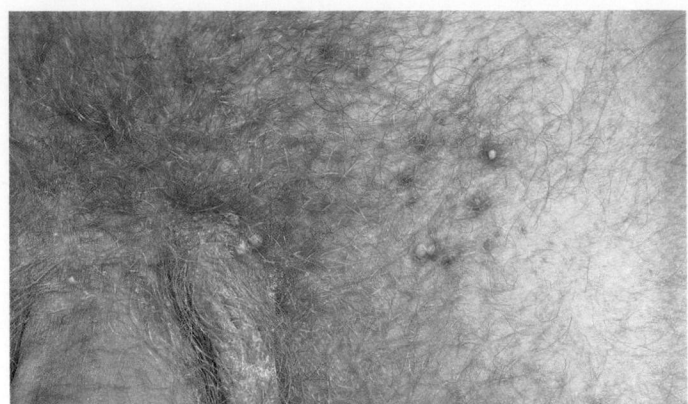

Fig. 14-3 Staphylococcal folliculitis.

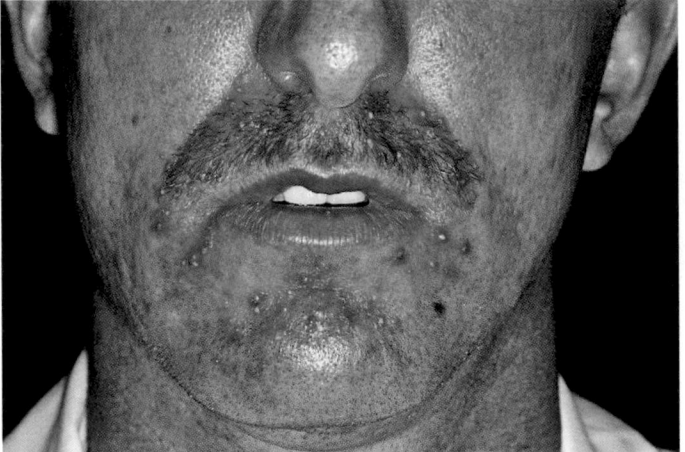

Fig. 14-2 Sycosis barbae.

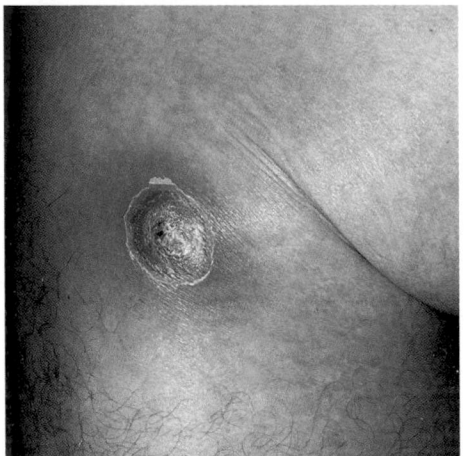

Fig. 14-4 Staphylococcal abscess.

These rupture after shaving or washing and leave an erythematous spot, which is later the site of a fresh crop of pustules. In this manner the infection persists and gradually spreads. At times the infection may extend deep into the follicles. A hairless, atrophic scar bordered by pustules and crusts may result. Marginal blepharitis with conjunctivitis is usually present in severe cases of sycosis.

Sycosis vulgaris is to be distinguished from tinea, acne vulgaris, pseudofolliculitis barbae, and herpetic sycosis. Tinea barbae rarely affects the upper lip, which is a common location for sycosis. In tinea barbae the involvement is usually in the submaxillary region or on the chin, and spores and hyphae are found in the hairs. Pseudofolliculitis barbae manifests torpid papules at the sites of ingrowing beard hairs in black men. In herpes simplex the duration is usually only a few days and even in persistent cases there are vesicles, which help to differentiate the disease from sycosis vulgaris.

Folliculitis

Staphylococcal folliculitis may affect other areas, such as the eyelashes, axillae, pubis, and thighs (Fig. 14-3). On the pubis it may be transmitted among sexual partners, and miniepidemics of folliculitis and furunculosis of the genital and gluteal areas may be considered a sexually transmitted disease (STD). Staphylococcal folliculitis has also been reported frequently among patients with acquired immunodeficiency syndrome (AIDS) and may be a cause of pruritus. An atypical, plaque-like form has been reported.

Treatment

Deep lesions of folliculitis represent small follicular abscesses and must be drained. Superficial pustules will rupture and drain spontaneously. Many patients will heal with drainage and topical therapy. Bactroban or retapamulin ointment and topical cleocin solution are effective topical agents. Skin surface staphylococcal carriage in abrasions and eczematous areas may be addressed with topical antibiotics as above, topical chlorhexidine, or bleach baths. The latter can be prepared by adding one half-cup of Clorox bleach to a tub of bathwater. If drainage and topical therapy fail or if there is accompanying soft-tissue infection, a first-generation cephalosporin, or a penicillinase-resistant penicillin such as dicloxacillin, is indicated, unless MRSA is suspected (see above). When the inflammation is acute, hot, wet soaks with Burow solution diluted 1 : 20 (Domeboro) are beneficial. An anhydrous formulation of aluminum chloride (Drysol, Xerac-AC) is effective when used once a night for chronic folliculitis, especially of the buttocks. Antibiotic ophthalmic ointments are used for blepharitis.

Furunculosis

A furuncle, or boil, is an acute, round, tender, circumscribed, perifollicular staphylococcal abscess that generally ends in central suppuration (Fig. 14-4). A carbuncle is merely two or more confluent furuncles, with separate heads.

The lesions begin in hair follicles, and often continue for a prolonged period by autoinoculation. Some lesions disappear

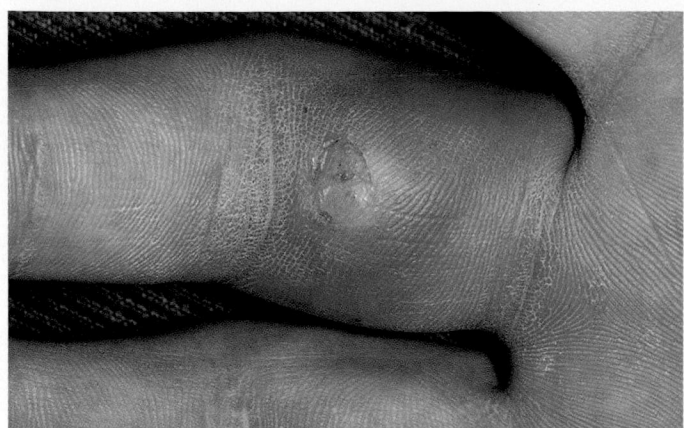

Fig. 14-5 Staphylococcal abscess in a diabetic patient.

before rupture, but most undergo central necrosis and rupture through the skin, discharging purulent, necrotic debris. Sites of predilection are the nape, axillae, and buttocks, but boils may occur anywhere.

The integrity of the skin surface may be impaired by irritation, pressure, friction, hyperhidrosis, dermatitis, dermatophytosis, or shaving, among other factors. Local barrier compromise predisposes to infection by providing a portal of entry for the ubiquitous *S. aureus*. The proximate cause is either contagion or autoinoculation from a carrier focus, usually in the nose or groin.

Certain systemic disorders may predispose to furunculosis: alcoholism; malnutrition; blood dyscrasias; disorders of neutrophil function; iatrogenic or other immunosuppression, including AIDS; and diabetes (Fig. 14-5). Patients with several of these diseases, as well as those receiving renal dialysis or under treatment with isotretinoin or acitretin, are often nasal carriers of *S. aureus*. Additionally, atopic dermatitis also predisposes to the *S. aureus* carrier state. This fact helps explain the observed increases in the incidence of infections in these diseases.

Hospital furunculosis

Epidemics of staphylococcal infections occur in hospitals. Marked resistance to antibacterial agents in these cases is commonplace. Attempts to control these outbreaks center on meticulous handwashing. In nurseries, a fall in neonatal colonization and infections with *S. aureus* and non-group A streptococci may be achieved by using a 4% solution of chlorhexidine for skin and umbilical cord care.

Treatment

Warm compresses and antibiotics taken internally may arrest early furuncles. A penicillinase-resistant penicillin or a first-generation cephalosporin should be given orally in a dose of 1–2 g/day according to the severity of the case. Meticillin-resistant and even vancomycin-resistant strains occur, as described above. In cases of staphylococcal infections that are unresponsive to these usual measures, antibiotic-resistant strains should be suspected and sensitivities checked. Bactroban applied to the anterior nares daily for 5 days and bleach baths may help prevent recurrence.

When the lesions are incipient and acutely inflamed, incision should be strictly avoided and moist heat employed. When the furuncle has become localized and shows definite fluctuation, incision with drainage is indicated. The cavity should be packed with iodoform or vaseline gauze. In these cases, oral antibiotics are not usually necessary.

In boils of the external auditory canal, upper lip, and nose, incision and drainage is generally only performed if antibiotic

therapy fails. In these latter circumstances, antibiotic ointment (Bactroban) should be applied, and antibiotics given internally. Warm saline-solution compresses should be applied liberally.

Chronic furunculosis

Despite treatment, recurrences of some boils may be anticipated. Usually no underlying disease is present to predispose to this; rather, autoinoculation and intrafamilial spread among colonized individuals are responsible.

One of the most important factors in prevention is to avoid autoinoculation. It is important to emphasize that the nasal carrier state predisposes to chronic furunculosis. The skin surface in the region of the furuncles may be a source of colonization, especially if there are cuts, excoriation, or eczematous changes. In addition, the hazard of contamination from the perianal and intertriginous areas is to be considered. In general, indications for elimination of the carriage state are recurrent infection, evidence of spread to others, or high-risk individuals in the household.

Routine precautions to be taken in attempting to break the cycle of recurrent furunculosis should be the daily use of a chlorhexidine wash, with special attention to the axillae, groin, and perianal area; laundering of bedding and clothing on a daily basis initially; the use of bleach baths; and frequent handwashing. Additionally, the application of Bactroban ointment twice a day to the nares of patients and family members every fourth week has been found to be effective. Rifampin, 600 mg/day, combined with dicloxacillin for MSSA or trimethoprim-sulfamethoxazole for MRSA, for 10 days, or low-dose (150 mg/day) clindamycin for 3 months are other options that are effective in eradicating the nasal carriage state. The use of bacitracin ointment inside the nares twice a day throughout the course of isotretinoin therapy eliminates, or markedly reduces, the risk of inducing nasal carriage of *S. aureus*, and hence staphylococcal infections.

Pyogenic paronychia

Paronychia is an inflammatory reaction involving the folds of the skin surrounding the fingernail. It is characterized by acute or chronic purulent, tender, and painful swellings of the tissues around the nail, caused by an abscess in the nailfold. When the infection becomes chronic, horizontal ridges appear at the base of the nail. With recurrent bouts new ridges appear.

The primary predisposing factor that is identifiable is separation of the eponychium from the nail plate. The separation is usually caused by trauma as a result of moisture-induced maceration of the nailfolds from frequent wetting of the hands. The relationship is close enough to justify treating chronic paronychia as work-related in bartenders, food servers, nurses, and others who often wet their hands. The moist grooves of the nail and nailfold become secondarily invaded by pyogenic cocci and yeasts. The causative bacteria are usually *S. aureus*, *Streptococcus pyogenes*, *Pseudomonas* species, *Proteus* species, or anaerobes. The pathogenic yeast is most frequently *Candida albicans*.

The bacteria usually cause acute abscess formation (*Staphylococcus*) (Fig. 14-6) or erythema and swelling (*Streptococcus*) (Fig. 14-7), and *C. albicans* most frequently causes a chronic swelling. If an abscess is suspected, applying light pressure with the index finger against the distal volar aspect of the affected digit will better demonstrate the extent of the collected pus by inducing a well-demarcated blanching. Smears of purulent material will help confirm the clinical impression. Myremecial warts may at times mimic

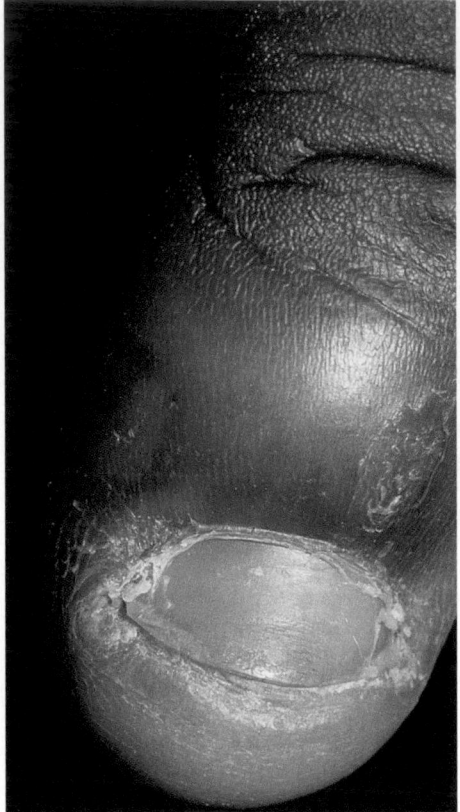

Fig. 14-6 Staphylococcal paronychia.

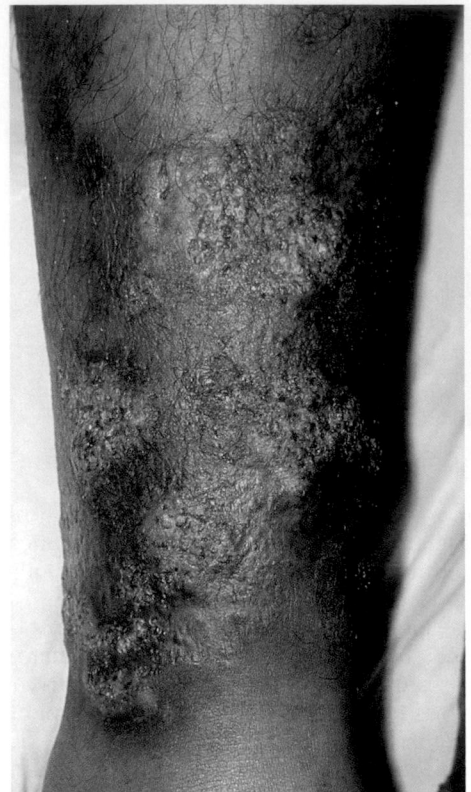

Fig. 14-8 Botryomycosis.

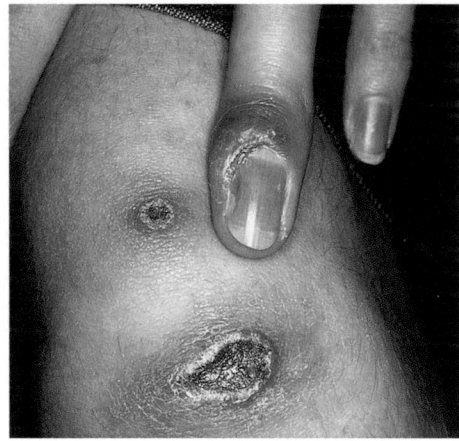

Fig. 14-7 Streptococcal paronychia and impetigo.

paronychia. Subungual black macules followed by edema, pain, and swelling have been reported to be a sign of osteomyelitis caused by *S. aureus* or *Streptococcus viridans*, in children with atopic dermatitis.

Treatment of pyogenic paronychia consists mostly of protection against trauma and concentrated efforts to keep the affected fingernails meticulously dry. Rubber or plastic gloves over cotton gloves should be used whenever the hand must be placed in water. Acutely inflamed pyogenic abscesses should be incised and drained. The abscess may often be opened by pushing the nailfold away from the nail plate. In acute suppurative paronychia, especially if stains show pyogenic cocci, a semisynthetic penicillin or a cephalosporin with excellent staphylococcal activity should be given orally. If these are ineffective, MRSA or a mixed anaerobic bacteria infection should be suspected. Augmentin for the latter or treatment dictated by the sensitivities of the cultured organism

will improve cure rates. Rarely, long-term antibiotic therapy may be required.

While *Candida* is the most frequently recovered organism in chronic paronychia, topical or oral antifungals lead to cure in only about 50% of cases. If topical steroids are used to decrease inflammation and allow for tissue repair, cure results more reliably (nearly 80% in one study). Often an antifungal liquid such as miconazole is combined with a topical corticosteroid cream or ointment.

Botryomycosis

Botryomycosis is an uncommon, chronic, indolent disorder characterized by nodular, crusted, purulent lesions (Fig. 14-8). Sinuses that discharge sulfur granules are present. These heal with atrophic scars. The granules most commonly yield *S. aureus* on culture, although cases caused by *Pseudomonas aeruginosa*, *Escherichia coli*, *Proteus*, *Bacteroides*, and *Streptococcus* have been reported. Botryomycosis occurs frequently in patients with altered immune function, such as those with neutrophilic defects. Other predisposing factors include diabetes, HIV infection, alcoholism, and Job syndrome. Appropriate antibiotics, surgical drainage, and surgical excision are methods used to treat botryomycosis.

Blastomycosis-like pyoderma

Large verrucous plaques with elevated borders and multiple pustules occur. Most patients have some underlying systemic or local host compromise. Bacteria such as *S. aureus*, *P. aeruginosa*, *Proteus*, *E. coli*, or streptococci may be isolated. Antibiotics appropriate for the organism isolated are curative; however, response may be delayed and prolonged therapy required. Acitretin may also be useful.

Pyomyositis

S. aureus abscess formation within the deep, large, striated muscles usually presents with fever and muscle pain. It is more common in the tropics, where it may affect adults but most commonly occurs in children. In temperate climates it occurs in children and patients with AIDS. The most frequent site in tropical disease is the thigh, while in HIV-infected patients the deltoid muscle is most often involved, followed closely by the quadriceps. Swelling and, occasionally, erythema or yellow or purplish discoloration are visible signs of pyomyositis, but these are late findings. Magnetic resonance imaging (MRI) with gadolinium injection will help delineate the extent of disease. Drainage of the abscess and appropriate systemic antibiotics are the recommended treatment.

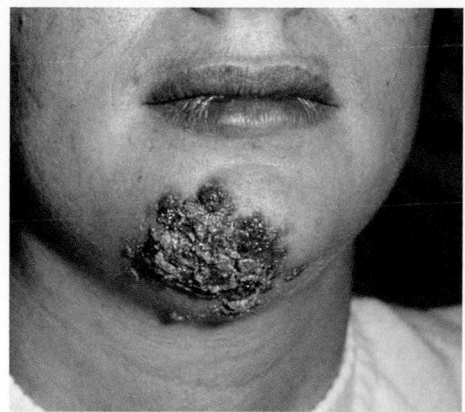

Fig. 14-9 Impetigo.

Impetigo contagiosa

Impetigo contagiosa is a staphylococcal, streptococcal, or combined infection characterized by discrete, thin-walled vesicles that rapidly become pustular and then rupture. Impetigo occurs most frequently on the exposed parts of the body: the face (Fig. 14-9), hands, neck, and extremities. Impetigo on the scalp is a frequent complication of pediculosis capitis.

The disease begins with 2 mm erythematous macules, which may shortly develop into vesicles or bullae. As soon as these lesions rupture, a thin, straw-colored, seropurulent discharge is noted. The exudate dries to form loosely stratified golden-yellow crusts, which accumulate layer upon layer until they are thick and friable.

The crusts can usually be removed readily, leaving a smooth, red, moist surface that soon collects droplets of fresh exudate again; these are spread to other parts of the body by fingers or towels. As the lesions spread peripherally and the skin clears centrally, large circles are formed by fusion of the spreading lesions to produce gyrate patterns. In streptococcal-induced impetigo, regional lymphadenopathy is common, but not serious.

Most studies find 50–70% of cases are due to *S. aureus*, with the remainder being due to either *S. pyogenes* or a combination of these two organisms. Streptococci may represent an early pathogen in the pathogenesis of impetigo, with staphylococci replacing streptococci as the lesion matures. Group B streptococci are associated with newborn impetigo and groups C and G are rarely isolated from impetigo, as opposed to the usual group A.

Impetigo occurs most frequently in early childhood (Fig. 14-10), although all ages may be affected. It occurs in the temperate zone, mostly during the summer in hot, humid weather. Common sources of infection for children are pets, dirty fingernails, and other children in schools, daycare centers, or crowded housing areas; for adults, common sources include infected children and self-inoculation from nasal or perineal carriage. Impetigo often complicates pediculosis capitis, scabies, herpes simplex, insect bites, poison ivy, eczema, and other exudative, pustular, or itching skin diseases.

Group A β-hemolytic streptococcal skin infections are sometimes followed by acute glomerulonephritis (AGN). Nephritogenic streptococci are generally associated with impetigo rather than with upper respiratory infections. There is no evidence that AGN occurs with staphylococcal impetigo. The important factor predisposing to AGN is the serotype of the streptococcus producing the impetigo. Type 49, 55, 57, and 60 strains and strain M-type 2 are related to nephritis.

The incidence of AGN with impetigo varies from about 2% to 5% (10–15% with nephritogenic strains of streptococcus) and occurs most frequently in childhood, generally under the age of 6. The prognosis in children is mostly excellent; however,

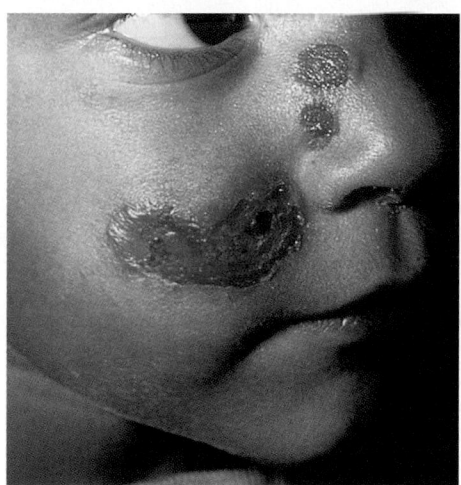

Fig. 14-10 Impetigo.

in adults the prognosis is not as good. Treatment, however early and however appropriate, is not believed to reduce the risk of occurrence of AGN.

The histopathology is that of an extremely superficial inflammation about the funnel-shaped upper portion of the pilo-sebaceous follicles. A subcorneal vesicopustule is formed, containing a few scattered cocci, together with debris of polymorphonuclear leukocytes and epidermal cells. In the dermis there is a mild inflammatory reaction—vascular dilation, edema, and infiltration of polymorphonuclear leukocytes.

Impetigo may simulate several diseases. The circinate patches are frequently mistaken for ringworm, but clinically are quite different. Impetigo is characterized by superficial, very weepy lesions covered by thick, bright yellow or orange crusts with loose edges, which do not resemble the scaling patches with peripheral erythema seen in tinea. Impetigo may be mistaken for *Toxicodendron* dermatitis, but it is more crusted and pustular, and more liable to involve the nostrils, corners of the mouth, and ears; it is not associated with the puffing of the eyelids, the linear lesions, or the itchiness that are so often present in dermatitis caused by poison ivy or oak. In varicella the lesions are small, widely distributed, discrete, umbilicated vesicles that are usually also present in the mouth, a site not involved by impetigo. In ecthyma the lesions are crusted ulcers, not erosions.

Treatment

Systemic antibiotics combined with topical therapy are advised. Because most cases are caused by *Staphylococcus*, a semisynthetic penicillin or a first-generation cephalosporin is recommended, unless MRSA is suspected, as detailed above. All treatment should be given for 7 days. It is necessary to soak off the crusts frequently, after which an antibacterial ointment should be applied. If the lesions are localized, especially if facial, and are present in an otherwise healthy child, topical therapy may be effective as the sole treatment.

Applying antibiotic ointment as a prophylactic to sites of skin trauma will prevent impetigo in high-risk children attending daycare centers. In one study infections were reduced by 47% with antibiotic ointment compared with 15% with a placebo. Additionally, if recurrent staphylococcal impetigo develops, a culture of the anterior nares may yield this organism. Such carrier states may be treated by application of mupirocin ointment to the anterior nares twice a day or a 10-day course of rifampin, 600 mg/day combined with dicloxacillin (for MSSA) or trimethoprim–sulfamethoxazole (for MRSA).

Bullous impetigo

This variety of impetigo occurs characteristically in newborn infants, though it may occur at any age. The neonatal type is highly contagious and is a threat in nurseries. In most cases the disease begins between the fourth and tenth days of life with the appearance of bullae, which may appear on any part of the body. Common early sites are the face and hands. Constitutional symptoms are at first absent, but later weakness and fever or a subnormal temperature may be present. Diarrhea with green stools frequently occurs. Bacteremia, pneumonia, or meningitis may develop rapidly, with fatal termination.

In warm climates particularly, adults may have bullous impetigo (Fig. 14-11), most often in the axillae or groins, or on the hands. Usually no scalp lesions are present. The lesions are strikingly large, fragile bullae, suggestive of pemphigus. When these rupture they leave circinate, weepy, or crusted lesions, and in this stage it may be called impetigo circinata. Children with bullous impetigo may give a history of an insect bite at the site of onset of lesions. The majority are caused by phage types 71 or 55 coagulase-positive *S. aureus* or a related group 2 phage type. Bullous impetigo may be an early manifestation of HIV infection.

Staphylococcal scalded skin syndrome

Staphylococcal scalded skin syndrome (SSSS) is a generalized, confluent, superficially exfoliative disease, occurring most commonly in neonates and young children. It was known in the past as Ritter's disease or dermatitis exfoliativa neonatorum. It has been reported to occur rarely in adults. When it does occur in an adult, usually either renal compromise or immunosuppression is a predisposing factor.

SSSS is a febrile, rapidly evolving, generalized, desquamative infectious disease, in which the skin exfoliates in sheets. It does not separate at the dermoepidermal junction, as in toxic (drug-induced) epidermal necrolysis (TEN), but within the granular layer. The lesions are thus much more superficial and less severe than in TEN, and healing is much more rapid. They also extend far beyond areas of actual staphylococcal infection, by action of the exfoliative exotoxins types A and B elaborated by the staphylococcus in remote sites. Usually the staphylococci are present at a distant focus, such as the pharynx, nose, ear, or conjunctiva. Septicemia or a cutaneous infection may also be the causative focus.

Its clinical manifestations begin abruptly with fever, skin tenderness, and erythema involving the neck, groins, and axillae (Fig. 14-12). There is sparing of the palms, soles, and mucous membranes. Nikolsky sign is positive. Generalized exfoliation follows within the next hours to days, with large sheets of epidermis separating.

Group 2 *S. aureus*, most commonly phage types 71 or 55, is the causative agent in most cases. If cultures are taken, they should be obtained from the mucous membranes because the skin erythema and desquamation are due to the distant effects of the exfoliative toxins, unlike the situation in bullous impetigo, where *S. aureus* is present in the lesions.

Rapid diagnosis can be made by examining frozen sections of a blister roof and observing that the full thickness of the epidermis is not necrotic as in TEN but rather is cleaved below the granular layer. The exfoliative toxins A, B, and D specifically cleave desmoglein 1, the antigenic target of autoantibodies in pemphigus foliaceus, thus accounting for the clinical and histologic similarity to pemphigus observed in SSSS and

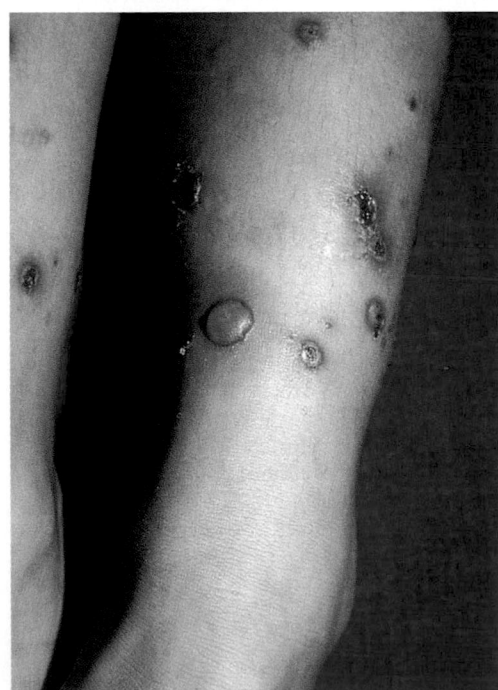

Fig. 14-11 Bullous impetigo.

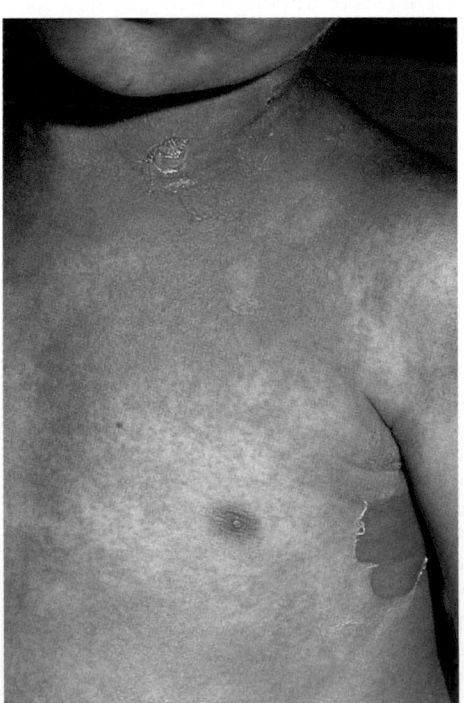

Fig. 14-12 Staphylococcal scalded skin syndrome.

bullous impetigo. Treatment of choice is a penicillinase-resistant penicillin such as dicloxacillin combined with fluid therapy and general supportive measures. If MRSA is cultured, and response is sluggish, antibiotics directed according to the susceptibilities of the recovered organism are needed. The prognosis is good in children; however, the mortality rate in adults can reach 60%.

Gram-positive toxic shock syndromes

Toxic shock syndrome (TSS) is an acute, febrile, multisystem illness, having as one of its major diagnostic criteria a widespread macular erythematous eruption. It is usually caused by toxin-producing strains of *S. aureus*, most of which were initially isolated from the cervical mucosa in menstruating young women. Now cases are most often due to infections in wounds, catheters, contraceptive diaphragms, or nasal packing. The mortality of these nonmenstrual cases is higher (up to 20%) compared with menstrual-related cases (under 5%), probably as a result of delayed diagnoses. Additionally, a very similar syndrome has been defined in which the cause is group A, or rarely group B, streptococci. This latter multiorgan disease has systemic components similar to classic staphylococcal TSS; however, the infection is usually a rapidly progressive, destructive soft-tissue infection such as necrotizing fasciitis. Those with an underlying chronic illness, recently recovered from varicella, or using nonsteroidal anti-inflammatory agents are predisposed. It has a case fatality rate of 30%. The streptococci are usually of M-types 1 and 3, with 80% of the isolates producing pyrogenic exotoxin A.

The Center for Communicable Diseases (CDC) case definition of staphylococcal TSS includes the following: a temperature of 38.9°C or higher, an erythematous eruption, desquamation of the palms and soles 1–2 weeks after onset (Fig. 14-13), hypotension, and involvement of three or more other systems—gastrointestinal (vomiting, diarrhea), muscular (myalgias, increased creatinine phosphokinase level), mucous membrane (hyperemia), renal (pyuria without infection or raised creatinine or blood urea nitrogen levels), hepatic (increased bilirubin, SGOT, or SGPT), hematologic (platelets <100000/mm³), or central nervous system (CNS) (disorientation). In addition, serologic tests for Rocky Mountain spotted fever, leptospirosis, and rubeola, and cultures of blood, urine, and cerebrospinal fluid should be negative. Procalcitonin, an indicator of severe bacterial infection may be a biologic marker for the toxic shock syndromes. Bulbar conjunctival hyperemia and palmar edema are two additional clinical clues. Streptococcal TSS is defined by isolation of group A β-hemolytic streptococci, hypotension, and two or more of the following: renal impairment, coagulopathy, hepatic involvement, acute respiratory distress syndrome, a generalized erythematous macular eruption that may desquamate, and soft tissue necrosis, myositis, or gangrene.

Around 90% of the early cases occurred in young women between the first and sixth days of a menstrual period. During the initial outbreak, the majority were using a superabsorbent tampon. Cases occur in women using contraceptive sponges, in patients with nasal packing after rhinoplasty, and in patients with staphylococcal infections of bone, lung, or soft tissue. The offending *S. aureus* strain produces one or more exotoxins.

Histologic findings are spongiosis and neutrophils scattered throughout the epidermis, individual necrotic keratinocytes, perivascular and interstitial infiltrates composed of lymphocytes and neutrophils, and edema of the papillary dermis. TSS must be differentiated from viral exanthems, Kawasaki's disease, scarlet fever, recurrent toxin-mediated perianal erythema, drug eruptions, Rocky Mountain spotted fever, systemic lupus erythematosus, TEN, and SSSS. In Kawasaki's

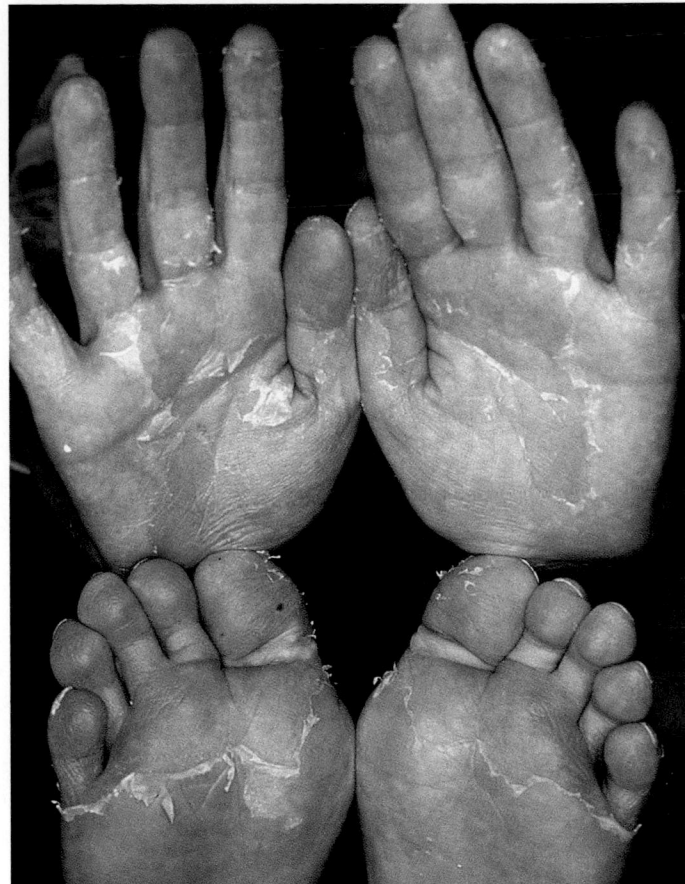

Fig. 14-13 Desquamation of the palms and soles.

disease, TSS toxin-producing staphylococcus has been recovered and streptococci that produce pyrogenic exotoxin B and C may be isolated; thus, some feel Kawasaki's disease is caused by toxin-secreting bacteria.

Treatment consists of systemic antibiotics such as nafcillin, 1–1.5 g intravenously every 4 h, vigorous fluid therapy to treat shock, and drainage of the *S. aureus*-infected site.

Antoniou T, et al: Prevalence of community-associated methicillin-resistant *Staphylococcus aureus* colonization in men who have sex with men. Int J STD AIDS 2009; 20:180.

Atanaskova N, et al: Innovative management of recurrent furunculosis. Dermatol Clin 2010; 28:479.

Bickels J, et al: Primary pyomyositis. J Bone Joint Surg 2002; 4:2277.

Brewer JD, et al: Staphylococcal scalded skin syndrome and toxic shock syndrome after tooth extraction. J Am Acad Dermatol 2008; 59:342.

Caum RS, et al: Skin and soft-tissue infections caused by methicillin-resistant *Staphylococcus aureus*. N Engl J Med 2007: 357:380.

Datta R, et al: Risk of infection and death due to methicillin-resistant *Staphylococcus aureus* in long-term carriers. Clin Infect Dis 2008; 47:176.

Dobson CM, et al: Adult staphylococcal scalded skin syndrome. Br J Dermatol 2003; 48:1068.

Durupt F, et al: Prevalence of *Staphylococcus aureus* toxins and nasal carriage in furunculosis and impetigo. Br J Dermatol 2007: 157:43.

Elliott DJ, et al: Empiric antimicrobial therapy for pediatric skin and soft-tissue infections in the era of methicillin-resistant *Staphylococcus aureus*. Pediatrics 2009; 123:e959.

Elston DM: Community-acquired methicillin-resistant *Staphylococcus aureus*. J Am Acad Dermatol 2007; 56:1.

Elston DM: How to handle a CA-MRSA outbreak. Dermatol Clin 2009; 27:43.

Gould FK, et al: Guidelines for the prophylaxis and treatment of methicillin-resistant *Staphylococcus aureus* infections in the United Kingdom. J Antimicrob Chemother 2009; 63:849.

Kato M, et al: Procalcitonin as a biomarker for toxic shock syndrome. Acta Derm Venereol 2010; 90:441.

Kazakova SV, et al: A clone of methicillin-resistant *Staphylococcus aureus* among professional football players. New Engl J Med 2005; 352:468.

Kil EH, et al: Methicillin-resistant *Staphyloccocus aureus*. Parts 1–4. Cutis 2008; 81:227, 247, 237, 343.

Kirkland EB, et al: Methicillin-resistant *Staphylococcus aureus* and athletes. J Am Acad Dermatol 2008; 59:494.

Koning S, et al: Interventions for impetigo. Cochrane Database Syst Rev 2004; 2:CDC 003261.

Koning S, et al: Efficacy and safety of retapamulin ointment as treatment of impetigo. Br J Dermatol 2008; 158:1077.

Lappin E, et al: Gram-positive toxic shock syndromes. Lancet Infect Dis 2009; 9:281.

Luelmo-Aguilar J, et al: Folliculitis. Am J Clin Dermatol 2004; 5:301.

Manfredi R, et al: Epidemiology and microbiology of cellulitis and bacterial soft tissue infection during HIV disease. J Cutan Pathol 2002; 29:168.

Marcinak JF, et al: Treatment of community-acquired methicillin-resistant *Staphylococcus aureus* in children. Curr Opin Infect Dis 2003; 16:265.

Mollering RC Jr: A 39-year-old man with a skin Infection. JAMA 2008; 299:79.

Occelli P, et al: Outbreak of staphylococcal bullous impetigo in a maternity ward linked to an asymptomatic health care worker. J Hosp Infect 2007; 67:264.

Patel GK, et al: Staphylococcal scalded skin syndrome. Am J Clin Dermatol 2003; 4:165.

Patrizi A, et al: Recurrent toxin-mediated perineal erythema. Arch Dermatol 2008; 144:239.

Rertveit S, et al: Impetigo in epidemic and nonepidemic phases. Br J Dermatol 2007; 157:100.

Rubenstein E, et al: Botryomycosis—like pyoderma in the genital region of a human immunodeficiency virus (HIV)—positive man successfully treated with dapsone. Int J Dermatol 2010; 49:842.

Scheinfeld NS: Is blistering distal dactylitis a variant of bullous impetigo? Clin Exp Dermatol 2007; 32:314.

Scheinpflug K, et al: Staphylococcal scalded skin syndrome in an adult patient with T-lymphoblastic non-Hodgkin's lymphoma. Oncologie 2008; 31:616.

Shapiro M, et al: Cutaneous microenvironment of HIV-seropositive and HIV-seronegative individuals, with special reference to *Staphylococcus aureus* colonization. J Clin Microbiol 2000; 38:3174.

Sica RS, et al: Prevalence of methicillin-resistant *Staphylococcus aureus* in the setting of dermatologic surgery. Dermatol Surg 2009; 35:420.

Stanley JR, et al: Pemphigus, bullous impetigo, and the staphylococcal scalded-skin syndrome. N Engl J Med 2006; 355:1800.

Suh L, et al: Methicillin-resistant *Staphylococcus aureus* colonization with atopic dermatitis. Pediatr Dermatol 2008; 25:528.

Templet JT, et al: Botryomycosis presenting as pruritic papules in an HIV-positive patient. Cutis 2007; 80:45.

Tosti A, et al: Topical steroids versus systemic antifungals in the treatment of chronic paronychia. J Am Acad Dermatol 2002; 47:73.

Turkmen A, et al: Digital pressure test for paronychia. Br Assoc Plast Surg 2004; 57:93.

Van Rijen M, et al: Mupirocin ointment for preventing *Staphylococcus aureus* infections in nasal carriers. Cochrane Database Syst Rev 2008; 4:CD006216.

Wollina U: Acute paronychia. J Eur Acad Dermatol Venereol 2001; 15:82.

Yang LP, et al: Spotlight on retapamulin in impetigo and other uncomplicated superficial skin infections. Am J Clin Dermatol 2008; 9:411.

Streptococcal skin infections

Ecthyma

Ecthyma is an ulcerative staphylococcal or streptococcal pyoderma, nearly always of the shins or dorsal feet. The disease begins with a vesicle or vesicopustule, which enlarges and in a few days becomes thickly crusted. When the crust is removed there is a superficial saucer-shaped ulcer with a raw base and elevated edges (Fig. 14-14). In urban areas these lesions are

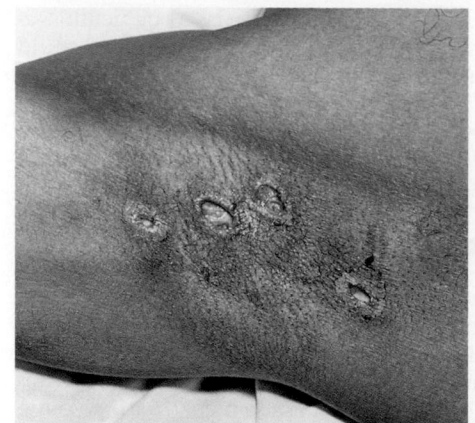

Fig. 14-14 Ecthyma.

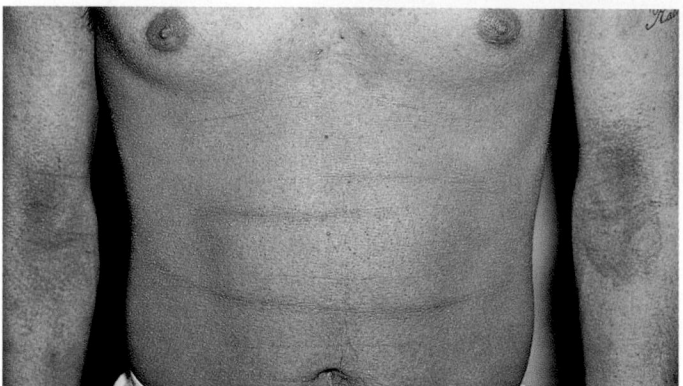

Fig. 14-15 Scarlet fever.

due to *S. aureus* and are seen in intravenous drug users and HIV-infected patients.

The lesions tend to heal after a few weeks, leaving scars, but rarely may proceed to gangrene when resistance is low. In fact, in a debilitated patient a focus of pyogenic infection elsewhere often precedes the onset of ecthyma in many cases. Local adenopathy may be present. Uncleanliness, malnutrition, and trauma are predisposing causes.

Treatment is cleansing with soap and water, followed by the application of mupirocin, retapamulin, or bacitracin ointment, twice a day. Oral dicloxacillin or a first-generation cephalosporin is also indicated, with adjustments made according to the cultured organism's susceptibilities.

Scarlet fever

Scarlet fever is a diffuse erythematous exanthem that occurs during the course of streptococcal pharyngitis. It affects primarily children, who develop the eruption 24–48 h after the onset of pharyngeal symptoms. The tonsils are red, edematous, and covered with exudate. The tongue has a white coating through which reddened, hypertrophied papillae project, giving the so-called white strawberry tongue appearance. By the fourth or fifth day the coating disappears, the tongue is bright red, and the red strawberry tongue remains.

The cutaneous eruption begins on the neck, then spreads to the trunk (Fig. 14-15) and finally the extremities. Within the widespread erythema are 1–2 mm papules, which give the skin a rough sandpaper quality. There is accentuation over the skinfolds, and a linear petechial eruption, called Pastia lines, is often present in the antecubital and axillary folds. There is facial flushing and circumoral pallor. A branny desquamation occurs as the eruption fades, with peeling of the palms and soles taking place about 2 weeks after the acute illness. The latter may be the only evidence that the disease has occurred.

The eruption is produced by erythrogenic exotoxin-producing group A streptococci. Cultures of the pharynx will recover this organism. Rarely, scarlet fever may be related to a surgical wound or burn infection with streptococci. An elevated antistreptolysin O titer may provide evidence of recent infection if cultures are not taken early. A condition known as staphylococcal scarlatina has been described that mimics scarlet fever; however, the strawberry tongue is not seen.

Penicillin, erythromycin, or dicloxacillin treatment is curative, and the prognosis is excellent.

Recurrent toxin-mediated perianal erythema

This recently described condition manifests as a perineal erysipelas-like erythema that resolves with desquamation. Strawberry tongue, erythema of the hands with desquamation, and a mild fever 1 or 2 days before the eruption are other signs. In some patients, a staphylococcal or streptococcal pharyngitis, impetigo, or perianal streptococcal dermatitis is present. There may be recurrences in individual patients. Streptococcal pyrogenic exotoxins A and B or toxic shock syndrome toxin 1 may be responsible for the skin findings.

Erysipelas

Also once known as St Anthony's fire and ignis sacer, erysipelas is an acute β-hemolytic group A streptococcal infection of the skin involving the superficial dermal lymphatics. Occasional cases caused by streptococci of group C or G are reported in adults. Group B streptococcus is often responsible in the newborn and may be the cause of abdominal or perineal erysipelas in postpartum women. It is characterized by local redness, heat, swelling, and a highly characteristic raised, indurated border (Fig. 14-16A). The onset is often preceded by prodromal symptoms of malaise for several hours, which may be accompanied by a severe constitutional reaction with chills, high fever, headache, vomiting, and joint pains. There is commonly a polymorphonuclear leukocytosis of 20 000/mm³ or more. However, many cases present solely as an erythematous lesion without associated systemic complaints.

The skin lesions may vary from transient hyperemia followed by slight desquamation to intense inflammation with vesicles or bullae. The eruption begins at any one point as an erythematous patch and spreads by peripheral extension. In the early stages the affected skin is scarlet, hot to the touch, branny, and swollen. A distinctive feature of the inflammation is the advancing edge of the patch. This is raised and sharply demarcated, and feels like a wall to the palpating finger. In some cases vesicles or bullae that contain seropurulent fluid occur and may result in local gangrene.

The legs and face are the most common sites affected. When on the face the inflammation generally begins on the cheek near the nose or in front of the lobe of the ear and spreads upward to the scalp, the hairline acting in some instances as a barrier against further extension. When on the legs, edema and bullous lesions are prominent features in many cases (Fig. 14-16B). Septicemia, deep cellulitis, or necrotizing fasciitis may occur as complications.

Predisposing causes are operative wounds, fissures (in the nares, in the auditory meatus, under the lobes of the ears, on the anus or penis, and between or under the toes, usually the little toe), abrasions or scratches, venous insufficiency, obesity, lymphedema, and chronic leg ulcers.

Recognition of the disease generally is not difficult. It may be confused with contact dermatitis from plants, drugs, or dyes, and with angioneurotic edema; however, with each of these, fever, pain, and tenderness are absent and itching is severe. A butterfly pattern on the face may mimic lupus erythematosus and ear involvement may suggest relapsing polychondritis.

Systemic penicillin is rapidly effective. Improvement in the general condition occurs in 24–48 h, but resolution of the cutaneous lesion may require several days. Vigorous treatment with antibiotics should be continued for at least 10 days. Locally, ice bags and cold compresses may be used. Leg involvement, especially when bullae are present, will more likely require hospitalization with intravenous antibiotics. The elderly, those with underlying immunocompromise, a longer duration of illness prior to presentation, and patients with leg ulcers will require longer inpatient stays.

Cellulitis

Cellulitis is a suppurative inflammation involving the subcutaneous tissue, caused most frequently by *S. pyogenes* or *S. aureus*. Usually, but not always, this follows some discernible

Fig. 14-16 Erysipelas.

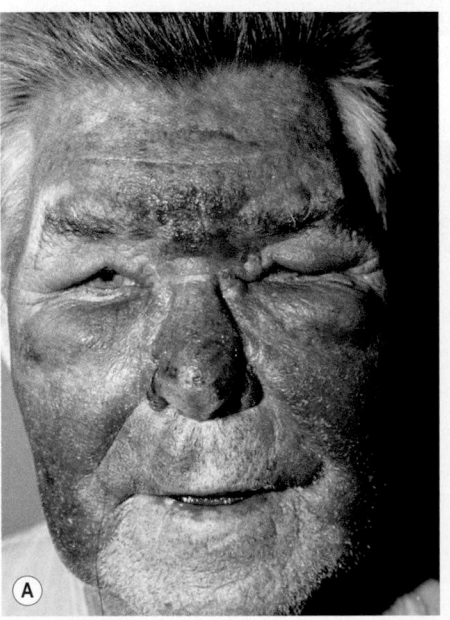

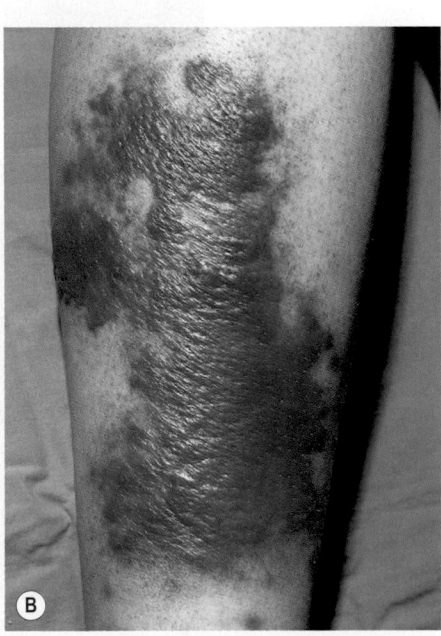

(A)

(B)

wound. On the leg tinea pedis is the most common portal of entry. Mild local erythema and tenderness, malaise, and chilly sensations, or a sudden chill and fever may be present at the onset. The erythema rapidly becomes intense and spreads (Fig. 14-17). The area becomes infiltrated and pits on pressure. Sometimes the central part becomes nodular and surmounted by a vesicle that ruptures and discharges pus and necrotic material. Streaks of lymphangitis may spread from the area to the neighboring lymph glands (Fig. 14-18). Gangrene, metastatic abscesses, and grave sepsis may follow. These complications are unusual in immunocompetent adults, but children and compromised adults are at higher risk.

Hook evaluated 50 patients with cellulitis prospectively by culture of the primary site of infection (when one was present), and also by aspiration of the advancing edge, by skin biopsy, and by blood culture. In 24 patients the primary site was identified and in 17 β-hemolytic streptococci were isolated, with *S. aureus* being present in 13. Kielhofner et al also evaluated needle aspirates in cellulitis. Of 87 patients, 33 were culture-positive. Of significance is the fact that 26 of 46 patients (57%) were positive if there was coexistent underlying disease, such as hematologic malignancy, diabetes mellitus, intravenous drug abuse, or cardiovascular disorders. *S. aureus* was present in 33% and group A streptococci in 27%. Other cultures were seldom positive and yielded no additional information.

Initial empiric therapy should cover both staphylococci and streptococci. Initial therapy will be guided as in the above staphylococcal discussion. MRSA should be considered, and treatment strategies chosen may depend on whether the infection was hospital- or community-acquired, as outlined above.

Chronic recurrent erysipelas, chronic lymphangitis

Erysipelas or cellulitis may be recurrent. Predisposing factors include alcoholism, diabetes, immunodeficiency, tinea pedis, venous stasis, lymphedema with or without lymphangiectasias, prosthetic surgery of the knee, a history of saphenous phlebectomy, lymphadenectomy, or irradiation. Chronic lymphedema is the end result of recurrent bouts of bacterial lymphangitis and obstruction of the major lymphatic channels of the skin. The final result is a permanent hypertrophic fibrosis to which the term elephantiasis nostras has been given. It must be differentiated from lymphangioma, acquired lymphangiectasia, and other causes such as neoplasms or filariasis.

During periods of active lymphangitis, antibiotics in large doses are beneficial and their use must be continued intermittently in smaller maintenance doses for long periods to achieve their full benefits. Compression therapy to decrease lymphedema will aid in the prevention of recurrence.

Necrotizing fasciitis

Necrotizing fasciitis is an acute necrotizing infection involving the fascia. It may follow surgery or perforating trauma, or may occur de novo. Within 24–48 h redness, pain, and edema quickly progress to central patches of dusky blue discoloration, with or without serosanguineous blisters (Fig. 14-19). Anesthesia of the involved skin is very characteristic. By the fourth or fifth day, these purple areas become gangrenous.

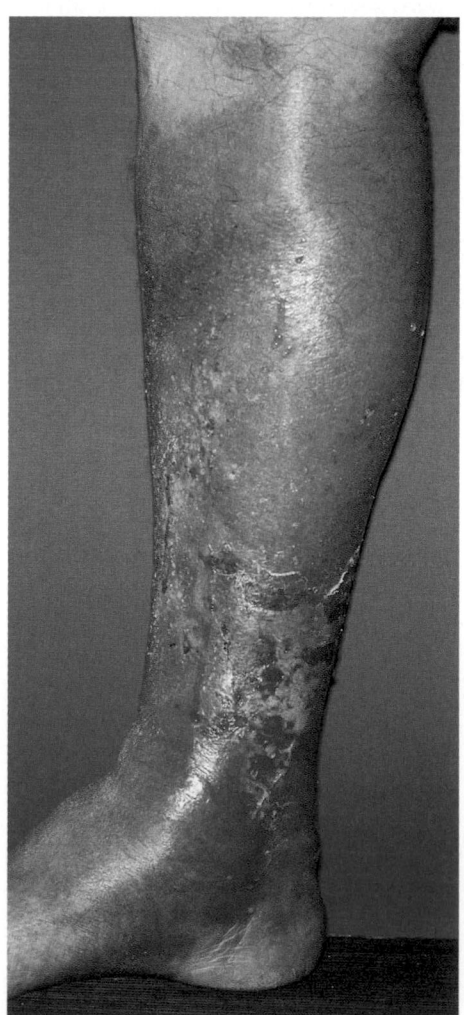

Fig. 14-17 Cellulitis.

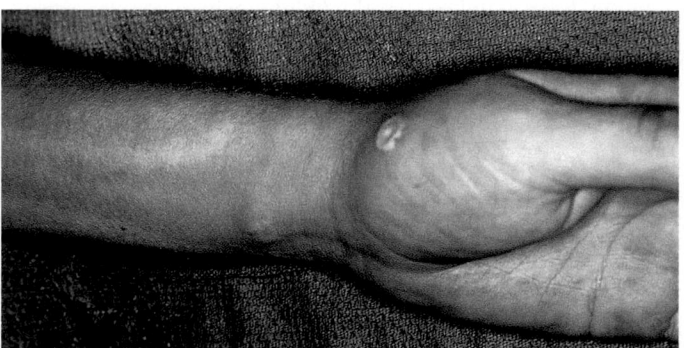

Fig. 14-18 Lymphangitis.

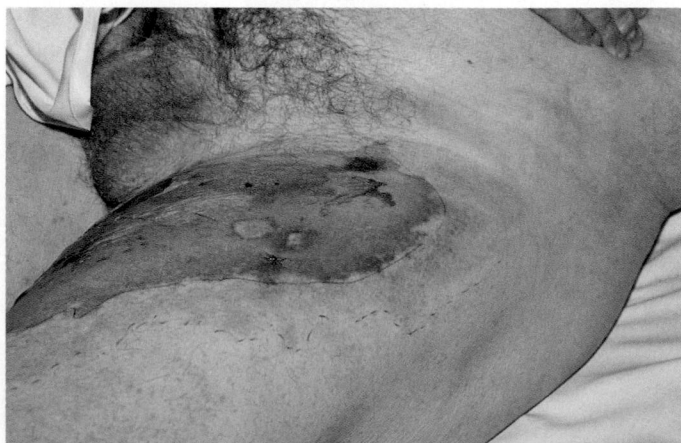

Fig. 14-19 Necrotizing fasciitis.

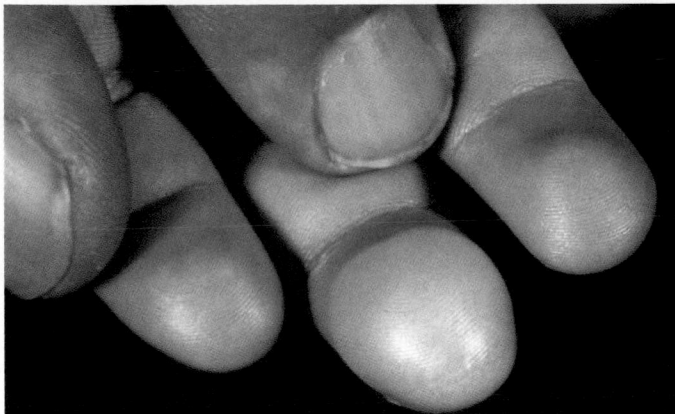

Fig. 14-20 Blistering dactylitis.

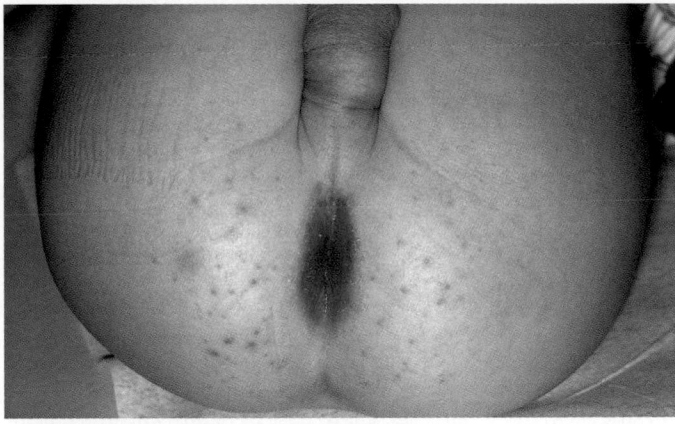

Fig. 14-21 Perianal dermatitis.

Many forms of virulent bacteria have been cultured from necrotizing fasciitis, including microaerophilic β-hemolytic streptococci, hemolytic staphylococcus, coliforms, enterococci, *Pseudomonas*, and *Bacteroides*. Both aerobic and anaerobic cultures should always be taken.

Early surgical debridement is an essential component of successful therapy. Signs and tests that can aid in delineating the extent of deep involvement include the presence of hypotension, an admission white blood cell count greater than 15.4 mm^3, serum sodium less than 135 mmol/L, and an MRI. It may be necessary to infiltrate the site with anesthetic, make a 2 cm incision down to the fascia, and probe with the finger. Lack of bleeding, a murky discharge, and lack of resistance to the probing finger are ominous signs. Treatment should include early surgical debridement, intravenously administered appropriate antibiotics, and supportive care. There may be a 20% mortality even in the best of circumstances. Poor prognostic factors are age over 50, underlying diabetes or atherosclerosis, delay of more than 7 days in diagnosis and surgical intervention, and infection on or near the trunk rather than the more commonly involved extremities. Neonatal necrotizing fasciitis most commonly occurs on the abdominal wall and has a higher mortality rate than in adults.

Blistering distal dactylitis

Blistering distal dactylitis is characterized by tense superficial blisters occurring on a tender erythematous base over the volar fat pad of the phalanx of a finger or thumb or occasionally a toe (Fig. 14-20). The typical patient is aged between 2 and 16. Group A β-hemolytic streptococcus or *S. aureus* is the most common cause. These organisms may be cultured from blister fluid and occasionally from clinically inapparent infections of the nasopharynx or conjunctiva.

Perineal dermatitis

Clinically, this entity presents most commonly as a superficial perianal, well-demarcated rim of erythema (Fig. 14-21); sometimes fissuring may also be seen. Pain or tenderness, especially prominent on defecation, may lead to fecal retention in affected patients, who are usually between ages 1 and 8. It may not resemble a cellulitis, but rather a dermatitis. It may also affect the vulval and penile tissues. Group A streptococci are most often the cause; however, *S. aureus* may be recovered rarely. As the vast majority of infections are due to streptococci, a systemic penicillin or erythromycin combined with a topical antiseptic or antibiotic is the treatment of choice. The duration should be 14–21 days, depending on clinical response. Post-

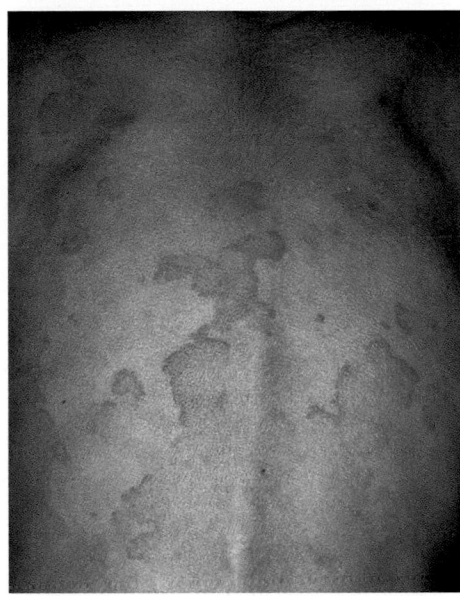

Fig. 14-22 Erythema marginatum.

treatment swabs and urinalysis to monitor for post-streptococcal glomerulonephritis are recommended.

Streptococcal intertrigo

Infants and young children may develop a fiery-red erythema and maceration in the neck, axillae, or inguinal folds. There are no satellite lesions. It may be painful and have a foul odor. Group A β-hemolytic streptococci are the cause, and topical antibiotics and oral penicillin combined with a low-potency topical steroid is curative.

Erythema marginatum

Delayed nonsuppurative sequelae of streptococcal infections include erythema nodosum, post-streptococcal glomerulonephritis, and rheumatic fever. While the latter only follows pharyngitis or tonsillitis, two skin signs are among the diagnostic criteria of rheumatic fever—erythema marginatum and subcutaneous nodules. The remaining major signs making up the revised Jones criteria are carditis, polyarthritis, and chorea. Erythema marginatum appears as a spreading patchy erythema that migrates peripherally and often forms polycyclic configurations (Fig. 14-22). It is evanescent, appearing for a few hours or days on the trunk or proximal extremities. Heat may make it more visible and successive crops may appear over several weeks. It is usually part of the early phase of the disease, coexisting with carditis but usually preceding the arthritis. Children younger than 5 are more likely to manifest the eruption than older patients. A skin biopsy will show a perivascular and interstitial polymorphonuclear leukocyte predominance. In contrast, the subcutaneous nodules occur over bony prominences and appear as a late manifestation. The lesions usually are asymptomatic and resolve spontaneously.

Group B streptococcal infection

Streptococcus agalactiae is the major cause of bacterial sepsis and meningitis in neonates. It may cause orbital cellulitis or facial erysipelas in these patients. Up to 25% of healthy adults harbor group B streptococcus in their genital or gastrointestinal tract. It has been reported to cause balanitis, toxic shock-like syndrome, cellulitis, perianal dermatitis, recurrent erysipelas, or blistering dactylitis in adults. Diabetes mellitus, neurologic impairment, cirrhosis, and peripheral vascular disease predispose patients to infection with this organism. In the postpartum period, abdominal or perineal erysipelas may be due to this organism.

Streptococcus iniae infections

Cellulitis of the hands may be caused by this fish pathogen. In Asian cuisine tilapia (also known as St Peter's fish or Hawaiian sunfish) is often purchased live from aquariums in retail stores. In cleaning the freshly killed fish before cooking, puncture wounds of the skin may be sustained from the dorsal fin, a fish bone, or a knife. Preparation of other raw seafood may also lead to this infection. Within 24 h fever, lymphangitis, and cellulitis without skin necrosis or bulla formation occur. Treatment with penicillin is curative.

Bachmeyer C, et al: Relapsing erysipelas of the buttock due to *Streptococcus agalactiae* in an immunocompetent woman. Clin Exp Dermatol 2009; 34:267.

Bellapianta JM, et al: Necrotizing fasciitis. J Am Acad Orthop Surg 2009; 17:174.

Bonnetblanc JM, et al: Erysipelas. Am J Clin Dermatol 2003; 4:157.

Buckland GT 3rd, et al: Persistent periorbital and facial lymphedema associated with group A beta-hemolytic streptococcal infection. Ophthal Plast Reconstr Surg 2007; 23:161.

Chong FY, et al: Blistering erysipelas. Singapore Med J 2008; 49:809.

Cox NH: Oedema as a risk factor for multiple episodes of cellulitis/erysipelas of the lower leg. Br J Dermatol 2006; 155:947.

Dahl PR, et al: Fulminant group A streptococcal necrotizing fasciitis. J Am Acad Dermatol 2002; 47:489.

Damstra RJ, et al: Erysipelas as a sign of subclinical primary lymphoedema. Br J Dermatol 2008; 158:1210.

Del Giudice P, et al: Severe relapsing erysipelas associated with chronic *Streptococcus agalactiae* vaginal cononization. Clin Infect Dis 2006; 43:1141.

Elston DM: Epidemiology and prevention of skin and soft tissue infections. Cutis 2004; 73:3.

Gabillot-Carre M, et al: Acute bacterial skin infections and cellulitis. Curr Opin Infect Dis 2007; 23:324.

Herbst R: Perineal streptococcal dermatitis/disease. Am J Clin Dermatol 2003; 4:555.

Honig PJ, et al: Streptococcal intertrigo. Pediatrics 2003; 112:1427.

Hook EW III: Acute cellulitis. Arch Dermatol 1987; 123:460.

Kielhofner MA, et al: Influence of underlying disease process on the utility of cellulitis needle aspirates. Arch Intern Med 1988; 148:2451.

Kilburn SA, et al: Interventions for cellulitis and erysipelas. Cochrane Database Syst Rev 2010; 6:CD004299.

Koh TH, et al: Streptococcal cellulitis following preparation of fresh raw seafood. Zoonoses Public Health 2009: 56:206.

Lau SK, et al: Invasive *Streptococcus iniae* infections outside North America. J Clin Microbiol 2003; 41:1004.

Leclerc S, et al: Recurrent erysipelas: 47 cases. Dermatology 2007; 214:52.

Lehane L, et al: Topically acquired bacterial zoonoses from fish. Med J Aust 2000; 173:256.

Manders SM, et al: Recurrent toxin-mediated perineal erythema. Arch Dermatol 1996; 132:57.

Martin JM, et al: Group A streptococcus. Semin Pediatr Infect Dis 2006; 17:140.

Mittal MK, et al: Group B streptococcal cellulitis in infancy. Pediatr Emerg Care 2007; 23:324.

Morris A: Cellulitis and erysipelas. Clin Evid 2006; 15:2207.

Neri I, et al: Streptococcal intertrigo. Pediatr Dermatol 2007; 24:577.

Olsen FJ, et al: Severe necrotizing fasciitis in an HIV-positive patient caused by methicillin-resistant *Staphylococcus aureus*. J Clin Microbiol 2008; 46:1144.

Patrizi A, et al: Recurrent toxin-mediated perineal erythema. Arch Dermatol 2008; 144:239.

Ravisha MS, et al: Rheumatic fever and rheumatic heart disease. Arch Med Res 2003; 34:382.

Reich HL, et al: Group B streptococcal toxic shock-like syndrome. Arch Dermatol 2004; 140:163.

Sarani B, et al: Necrotizing fasciitis. J Am Coll Surg 2009; 208:279.

Scheinfeld N: A review and report of blistering distal dactylitis due to *Staphylococcus aureus* in two HIV-positive men. Dermatol Online J 2007; 13:8.

Shimizu T, et al: Necrotizing fasciitis. Intern Med 2010; 49:1051.

Stevens DL, et al: Cellulitis and soft-tissue infections. Ann Intern Med 2009; 150:ITC11.

Sun JR, et al: Invasive infection with *Streptococcus iniae* in Taiwan. J Med Microbiol 2007; 56:1246.

Swartz MN: Cellulitis. N Engl J Med 2004; 350:904.

Tani LY, et al: Rheumatic fever in children younger than 5 years. Pediatrics 2003; 112:1065.

Wall DB, et al: A simple model to help distinguish necrotizing fasciitis from nonnecrotizing soft tissue infection. J Am Coll Surg 2000; 191:227.

Wasserzug O, et al: A cluster of ecthyma outbreaks caused by a single clone of invasive and highly infective *Streptococcus pyogenes*. Clin Infect Dis 2009; 48:1213.

Miscellaneous Gram-positive skin infections

Erysipeloid of Rosenbach

The most frequent form of erysipeloid is a purplish margined swelling on the hands. The first symptom is pain at the site of inoculation; this is followed by swelling and erythema. The most distinctive feature is the sharply marginated and often polygonal patches of bluish erythema (Fig. 14-23). The erythema slowly spreads to produce a sharply defined, slightly elevated zone that extends peripherally as the central portion

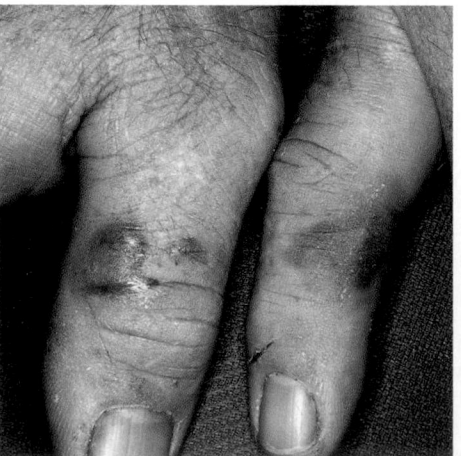

Fig. 14-23 Erysipeloid.

fades away. If the finger is involved, the swelling and tenseness make movement difficult. Vesicles frequently occur.

Another characteristic of the disease is its migratory nature; new purplish-red patches appear at nearby areas. If the infection originally involved one finger, eventually all of the fingers and the dorsum of the hand, palm, or both may become infected, the erythema appearing and disappearing; or extension may take place by continuity. The disease involutes without desquamation or suppuration.

A diffuse or generalized eruption in regions remote from the site of inoculation may occur, with fever and arthritic symptoms. Rarely, septicemia may eventuate in endocarditis, with prolonged fever and constitutional symptoms.

The infection is caused by *Erysipelothrix rhusiopathiae*. *E. rhusiopathiae* is present on dead matter of animal origin. Swine are more frequently infected than any other animal. A large percentage of healthy swine are carriers of the organism. Turkeys are also often infected and the disease may arise from handling contaminated dressed turkeys. It is also present in the slime of saltwater fish, on crabs, and on other shellfish.

The disease is widespread along the entire Atlantic seacoast among commercial fishermen who handle live fish, crabs, and shellfish. The infection also occurs among veterinarians and in the meat-packing industry, principally from handling pork products.

E. rhusiopathiae is a rod-shaped, nonmotile, Gram-positive organism that tends to form long-branching filaments. The organism is cultured best on media fortified with serum, at room temperature.

Treatment

The majority of the mild cases of erysipeloid run a self-limited course of about 3 weeks. In some patients, after a short period of apparent cure, the eruption reappears either in the same area or, more likely, in an adjacent previously uninvolved area. Penicillin, 1 g/day for 5–10 days, or ampicillin, 500 mg four times daily, is the best treatment for localized disease. If penicillin cannot be used, ciprofloxacin, clindamycin, or imipenem may be used. For systemic forms 12–20 million units/day of intravenous penicillin for up to 6 weeks may be necessary.

Varella JC, et al: Erysipeloid. Int J Dermatol 2005; 44:497.
Veraldi S, et al: Erysipeloid. Clin Exp Dermatol 2009; 34:859.

Pneumococcal cellulitis

Cellulitis may be caused by *Streptococcus pneumoniae*. Children present with facial or periorbital cellulitis, which may manifest a violaceous hue or bullae. Most patients under 36 months of age are previously healthy. Fever, leukocytosis, and septicemia are nearly universal. Response to treatment with penicillin or, in resistant cases, vancomycin is excellent. As most reported disease was caused by those strains included in the pneumococcal vaccine, this condition has become rare, as has occurred with *Haemophilus influenzae* cellulitis. Chronically ill or immunosuppressed adults also may develop pneumococcal cellulitis, or other soft tissue infections such as abscesses or pyomyositis. In patients with diabetes or substance abuse, extremity involvement is the rule, while in those with systemic lupus erythematosus, nephritic syndrome, hematologic disorders or HIV disease, the head, neck, and upper torso are typically affected. Skin involvement may also be seen as a surgical wound infection. Septicemia, tissue necrosis, and suppurative complications are frequent, so aggressive management with surgical drainage and intravenous antibiotics directed at the susceptibility of the cultured organism is vital.

Capdevilla O, et al: Bacteremic pneumococcal cellulitis compared with bacteremic cellulitis caused by *Staphylococcus aureus* and *Streptococcus pyogenes*. Eur J Clin Microbiol Infect Dis 2003; 22:337.
Garcia-Lechuz JM, et al: *Streptococcus pneumoniae* skin and soft tissue infections. Eur J Clin Microbiol Infect Dis 2007; 26:247.
Givner LB, et al: Pneumococcal cellulitis in children. Pediatrics 2000; 106:e61.

Anthrax

Cutaneous anthrax is uncommon in much of the world; human infection generally results from contact with infected animals or the handling of hides or other animal products from stock that has died from splenic fever. Cattlemen, woolsorters, tanners, butchers, and workers in the goat-hair industry are most liable to infection. Human-to-human transmission has occurred from contact with dressings from lesions. As the spores of *Bacillus anthracis* persist and may be aerosolized, it is a bioterrorism threat. In 2001 an outbreak of cutaneous disease resulted from powder-containing envelopes being sent through the mail.

Anthrax is an acute infectious disease characterized by a rapidly necrosing, painless eschar with suppurative regional adenitis. Three forms of the disease occur in humans: cutaneous, accounting for 95% of cases worldwide and nearly all US cases; inhalation, known as woolsorter's disease; and gastrointestinal, not yet reported in the US. The first clinical manifestation of the cutaneous form is an inflammatory papule, which begins about 3–7 days after inoculation, usually on an exposed site. The inflammation develops rapidly so that there is a bulla surrounded by intense edema and infiltration within another 24–36 h. It then ruptures spontaneously and a dark brown or black eschar is visible surrounded by vesicles situated on a red, hot, swollen, and indurated area. The lesion is neither tender nor painful. This is of diagnostic importance. Pustules are almost never present. The regional lymph glands become tender and enlarged, and frequently suppurate.

In severe cases the inflammatory signs increase; there is extensive edematous swelling and other bullae and necrotic lesions develop, accompanied by a high temperature and prostration, terminating in death in a few days or weeks. This may occur in up to 20% of untreated cases. In mild cases the constitutional symptoms are sometimes slight; the gangrenous skin sloughs and the resulting ulcer heals.

Internally, inhalation anthrax is manifested as a necrotizing, hemorrhagic mediastinal infection. Anthrax spores involve the alveoli, then the hilar and tracheobronchial nodes. Bacteremia followed by hemorrhagic meningitis is the usual sequence of events, almost always ending in death. Gastrointestinal anthrax results when spores are ingested and multiply in the intestinal submucosa. A necrotic ulcerative lesion in the terminal ileum or cecum may lead to hemorrhage.

The disease is produced by *Bacillus anthracis*, a large, square-ended, rod-shaped, Gram-positive organism, which occurs singly or in pairs in smears from the blood or in material from the local lesion, or in long chains on artificial media, where it tends to form spores. The bacillus possesses three virulence factors: a polyglutamate acid capsule inhibiting phagocytosis; an edema toxin, composed of edema factor and a transport protein termed protective antigen; and lethal toxin, composed of lethal factor plus protective antigen.

A biopsy should be obtained. This allows for immunohistochemical and polymerase chain reaction (PCR) studies, as well as routine histology and tissue Gram stain. Microscopically, there is loss of the epidermis at the site of the ulcer, with surrounding spongiosis and intraepidermal vesicles. Leukocytes are abundant in the epidermis. The dermis is edematous and infiltrated with abundant erythrocytes and neutrophils. Vasodilation is marked. The causative organisms are numerous and are easily seen, especially with Gram stain.

The diagnosis is made by demonstration of the causative agent in smears and cultures of the local material. Because aerobic nonpathogenic bacilli may be confused with *B. anthracis*, a specific γ-bacteriophage may be used to identify the organism. All virulent strains are pathogenic to mice. A four-fold rise in the enzyme-linked immunosorbent assay (ELISA) titer in paired serum specimens for antibodies against protective antigen or capsular antigens confirms the diagnosis. The characteristic gangrenous lesion, surrounded by vesiculation, intense swelling and redness, lack of pain, and the occupation of the victim are accessory factors. Staphylococcal carbuncle is the most easily confused entity, but here tenderness is prominent.

Early diagnosis and prompt treatment with ciprofloxacin, 500 mg, or doxycycline, 100 mg, both given twice a day for 60 days, are curative in the cutaneous form when there are no systemic symptoms, lesions are not on the head or neck and are without significant edema, and the patient is not a child under 2. In these latter conditions, more aggressive intravenous therapy is required, as outlined in the CDC management guidelines available at the CDC website. Asymptomatic exposed individuals should be given prophylactic treatment with a 6-week course of doxycycline or ciprofloxacin. A vaccine is available.

Carucci JA, et al: Cutaneous anthrax management algorithm. J Am Acad Dermatol 2002; 47:766.

Inglesby TV, et al: Anthrax as a biological weapon. JAMA 2002; 287:2236.

Kman NE, et al: Infectious agents of bioterrorism. Emerg Med Clin North Am 2008; 26:517.

McGovern TW, et al: Cutaneous manifestations of biologic warfare and related threat agents. Arch Dermatol 1999; 135:311.

Shadomy SV, et al: Anthrax. J Am Vet Med Assoc 2008; 233:63.

Swartz MN: Recognition and management of anthrax. N Engl J Med 2001; 345:1621.

Listeriosis

Listeria monocytogenes is a Gram-positive bacillus with rounded ends that may be isolated from soil, water, animals, and asymptomatic individuals. Human infection probably occurs via the gastrointestinal tract; however, in the majority of patients the portal of entry is unknown. Infections in humans usually produce meningitis or encephalitis with monocytosis. Risk factors include alcoholism, advanced age, pregnancy, and immunosuppression.

Cutaneous listeriosis is a rare disease. Veterinarians may contract cutaneous listeriosis from an aborting cow. The organism in the skin lesions is identical to that isolated from the fetus. The eruption consists of erythematous tender papules and pustules scattered over the hands and arms. There may be axillary lymphadenopathy, fever, malaise, and headache. Treatment with sulfonamides causes the disease to disappear within a few days.

Neonates are also at risk. Smith et al reported a newborn of an HIV-infected mother who died with a diffuse papular, petechial, and pustular eruption secondary to disseminated listeriosis. Listeria may cause a granulomatous disease of infants (granulomatosis infanta peptica). The endocarditis, meningitis, and encephalitis caused by *Listeria* may be accompanied by petechiae and papules in the skin.

Cases of listeriosis may easily be missed on bacteriologic examination, because the organism produces few colonies on original culture and may be dismissed as a streptococcus or as a contaminant diphtheroid because of the similarity in Gram-stained specimens. Serologic tests help to make the diagnosis.

L. monocytogenes is sensitive to most antibiotics. Ampicillin is the recommended antibiotic of choice, while trimethoprim–sulfamethoxazole is an effective alternate agent.

Cossart P, et al: *Listeria monocytogenes*, a unique model in infection biology. Microbes Infect 2008; 10:1041.

Gilchrist M: Cutaneous *Listeria* infection. Br J Hosp Med (Lond) 2009; 70:659.

Smith KJ, et al: Diffuse petechial pustular lesions in a newborn. Arch Dermatol 1994; 130:243.

Cutaneous diphtheria

The skin may become infected by the Klebs–Loeffler bacillus, *Corynebacterium diphtheriae,* in the form of ulcerations. The ulcer is punched out and has hard, rolled, elevated edges with a pale blue tinge (Fig. 14-24). Often the lesion is covered with a leathery, grayish membrane. Regional lymph nodes may be affected. Another type of skin involvement is that occurring in eczematous, impetiginous, vesicular, or pustular scratches, from which C. *diphtheriae* may be recovered. Postdiphtherial paralysis and potentially fatal cardiac complications may occur. These are mediated by a potent exotoxin, which stops protein production at the ribosome level.

Cutaneous diphtheria is common in tropical areas. Most of the cases occurring in the US are in nonimmunized migrant farm worker families and in elderly alcoholics. Travelers to developing countries may also import disease.

Treatment consists of intramuscular injections of diphtheria antitoxin, 20 000–40 000 U, after a conjunctival test has been performed to rule out hypersensitivity to horse serum. One drop of antitoxin diluted 1:10 is placed in one eye and a drop of saline in the other eye. If after 30 min there is no reaction, 20 000–40 000 U of antitoxin is given. Erythromycin, 2 g/day, is the drug of choice, unless large proportions of resistant organism are known in the area. In severe cases intravenous penicillin G, 600 000 U/day for 14 days, is indicated. Rifampin, 600 mg/day for 7 days, will eliminate the carrier state.

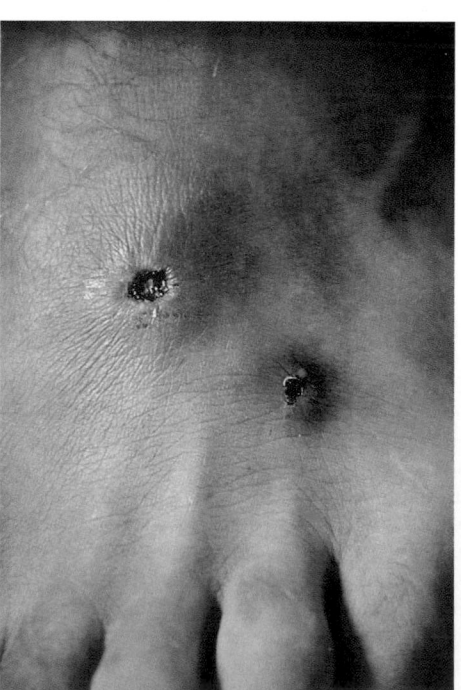

Fig. 14-24 Cutaneous diphtheria.

Connell TG, et al: Skin ulcers in a returned traveller. Lancet 2005; 365:726.
Lee PL, et al: Cutaneous diphtheroid infection and review of other cutaneous Gram-positive bacillus infections. Cutis 2007; 79:371.
Sing A, et al: Imported cutaneous diphtheria, Germany, 1997–2003. Emerg Infec Dis 2005; 11:343.
Vetrichevvel TP, et al: Cutaneous diphtheria masquerading as a sexually transmitted disease. Indian J Dermatol Venereol Leprol 2008; 74:187.

Corynebacterium jeikeium sepsis

Corynebacterium jeikeium colonizes the skin of healthy individuals, with the highest concentration being in the axillary and perineal areas. Hospitalized patients are more heavily colonized. Patients with granulocytopenia, indwelling catheters, prosthetic devices, exposure to multiple antibiotics, and valvular defects are at highest risk for the development of sepsis or endocarditis. A papular eruption, cellulitis, subcutaneous abscesses, tissue necrosis, hemorrhagic pustules, and palpable purpura may be seen on the skin. Vancomycin is the drug of choice. Mortality is over 30% in those with leukopenia, but only 5% if the marrow recovers. Hematopoietic growth factors should then be considered as adjunctive therapy in these patients.

Olson JM, et al: Cutaneous manifestations of *Corynebacterium jeikeium* sepsis. Int J Dermatol 2009; 48:886.

Desert sore

Also known as veldt sore, septic sore, diphtheric desert sore, and Barcoo rot, desert sore is an ulcerative disease that is endemic among bushmen and soldiers in Australia and Burma. The disease is characterized by the occurrence of grouped vesicles on the extremities, chiefly on the shins, knees, and backs of the hands. These rupture and form superficial indolent ulcers. The ulcers enlarge and may attain a diameter of 2 cm. The floor of the ulcer may be covered by a diphtheritic membrane. The original lesions may start as insect bites. Cultures show staphylococci, streptococci, and *Corynebacterium diphtheriae*. Treatment of the desert sore is with diphtheria antitoxin if *C. diphtheriae* is present. Antibiotic ointments are used topically, and oral penicillin or erythromycin is the treatment of choice.

Bailey H: Ulcers of the leg and their differential diagnosis. Dermatol Trop 1962; 1:45.

Tropical ulcer

Tropical ulcer is also known as tropical phagedena, Aden ulcer, Malabar ulcer, and jungle rot, as well as various native terms. It occurs on exposed parts of the body, chiefly the legs and arms, and frequently on pre-existing abrasions or sores, sometimes beginning from a mere scratch. As a rule, only one extremity is affected and usually there is a single lesion, although it is not uncommon to find multiple ulcers on both legs. Satellite lesions ordinarily occur as a result of autoinoculation.

The lesions begin with inflammatory papules that progress into vesicles and rupture with the formation of an ulcer. The ulcers vary in diameter and may, through coalescence, form extensive lesions. The lesions of some varieties are elevated or deeply depressed, and generally the edges are undermined and either smooth or ragged. At times the ulcers are covered by thick, dirty crusts or by whitish pseudomembranes. The edges are flat, without thickening, and around them there is a zone of inflammation characterized by redness, swelling, and some tenderness. Other than a slight itching, there is usually no distress.

The disease is most common in native laborers and in schoolchildren during the rainy season; it is probably caused in many instances by the bites of insects, filth, and pyogenic infection. Malnutrition appears to be a predisposing factor.

Tropical ulcer is a descriptive term used when more specific etiologic classification is not documented. If investigated microbiologically, anaerobic bacteria together with aerobes, some of them facultative anaerobes, are present in early lesions. The differential diagnosis includes a wide variety of conditions. The septic desert ulcer is superficial and shows *C. diphtheriae*. The gummatous ulcer is punched out, with a sinking floor. Other signs of syphilis are present, and the serologic test for syphilis is positive. The tuberculous ulcer is undermined and usually not found on the leg. The mycobacterium can be isolated from the lesion. The mycotic ulcer is noduloulcerative, with demonstrable fungi both by direct microscopic examination and by culture. The frambesia ulcer grows rapidly and yields *Treponema pertenue*. The Buruli ulcer shows abundant *Mycobacterium ulcerans* in biopsies. The leishmanial ulcer contains *Leishmania tropica*; it is not usually found on the leg. Carcinoma must be considered in any leg ulcer of long duration. A biopsy is indicated.

The arteriosclerotic ulcer is seen in older people at sites of frequent trauma; it is deep and penetrates through the deep fascia to expose tendons. The hypertensive ischemic ulcer is caused by thrombosis of the cutaneous arterioles. These painful ulcers are extremely shallow, usually bilateral, and seen most frequently on the mid- and lower parts of the leg. Varicosities are usually absent. The varicose or venous ulcer is shallow and has irregularly shaped edges. It is located typically on the lower half of the shins, mostly above and anterior to the medial malleolus along the course of the long saphenous vein.

The ulcers of blood dyscrasias are frequent in sickle cell anemia, in hereditary spherocytosis, Mediterranean anemia, and Felty syndrome. The diagnosis is aided by the fact that there is hypersplenism in each of these diseases. The ulcer of rheumatoid arthritis occurs frequently in patients who have abundant concomitant subcutaneous nodules. The ulcer of Kaposi sarcoma frequently occurs on the lower extremities and is accompanied by a purpuric discoloration of the skin and by other violaceous nodules that may occur anywhere on the body. In the tropics it is endemic among the South African Bantus.

Prevention of the disease is aided by protection from insect bites and from predisposing causes, such as debility, malnutrition, and filth. Topical and systemic antibiotic treatment is indicated in most patients.

Aribi M, et al: Tropical phagedenic ulcer. Eur J Dermatol 1999; 9:321.
MacDonald P: Tropical ulcers. J Wound Care 2003; 12:85.

Erythrasma

Erythrasma is characterized by sharply delineated, dry, brown, slightly scaling patches occurring in the intertriginous areas, especially the axillae, the genitocrural crease (Fig. 14-25), and the webs between the fourth and fifth toes and, less commonly, the third and fourth toes. There may also be patches in the intergluteal cleft, perianal skin, and inframammary area. Rarely, widespread eruptions with lamellated plaques occur.

The lesions are asymptomatic except in the groins, where there may be some itching and burning. Patients with extensive erythrasma have been found to have diabetes mellitus or other debilitating diseases.

Erythrasma is caused by the diphtheroid *Corynebacterium minutissimum*. This Gram-positive non-spore-forming

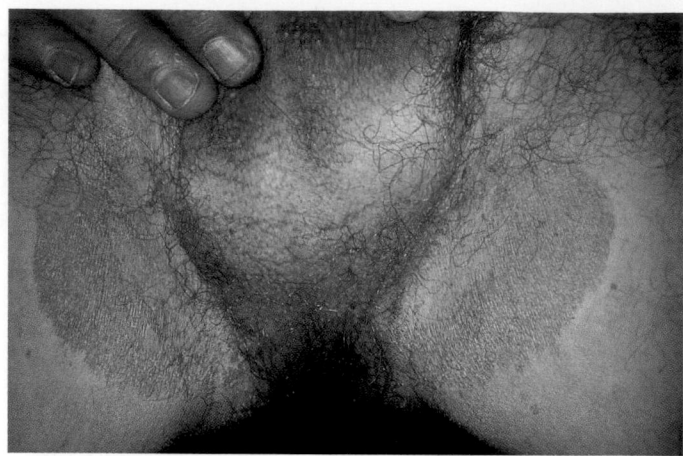

Fig. 14-25 Erythrasma.

rod-shaped organism may occasionally cause cutaneous granulomas or bacteremia in immunocompromised patients. Two other diseases caused by a *Corynebacterium*, pitted keratolysis and trichomycosis axillaris, may occur as a triad. In the differential diagnosis, tinea cruris caused by fungi, intertrigo, seborrheic dermatitis, inverse psoriasis, candidiasis, and lichen simplex chronicus must be considered.

The Wood's light is the diagnostic medium for erythrasma. The affected areas show a coral red fluorescence, which results from the presence of a porphyrin. Washing of the affected area before examination may eliminate the fluorescence. Topical erythromycin solution or topical clindamycin is easily applied and rapidly effective. Oral erythromycin, 250 mg four times a day for 1 week, tolnaftate solution, applied twice a day for 2–3 weeks, and topical miconazole are equally effective.

Rho N-K, et al: A corynebacterial triad. J Am Acad Dermatol 2008; 58:S57.
Santos-Juanes J, et al: Cutaneous granulomas caused by *Corynebacterium minutissimum* in an HIV-infected man. J Eur Acad Dermatol Venereol 2002; 16:643.

Arcanobacterium haemolyticum infection

This pleomorphic, nonmotile, non-spore-forming, β-hemolytic, Gram-positive bacillus causes pharyngitis and an exanthem in young adults. Acute pharyngitis in the 10- to 30-year-old age group is only due to group A streptococci 10–25% of the time. A proportion of the remainder will be caused by *Arcanobacterium haemolyticum*.

The exanthem is an erythematous morbilliform or scarlatiniform eruption involving the trunk and extremities. Although it usually spares the face, palms, and soles, atypical acral involvement has been reported. The general clinical presentation may include mild pharyngitis, severe diphtheria-like illness, or even septicemia.

Cultures for this organism should be done on 5% blood agar plates and observed for 48 h. The diagnostic features are enhanced by a 5–8% CO_2 atmosphere during incubation at 37°C. Routine pharyngeal specimens are done on sheep blood agar and will miss the growth of this organism because of its slow hemolytic rate and growth of normal throat flora. Treatment of choice is erythromycin, or in the case of severe infection, high-dose penicillin G.

Gaston DA, Zurowski SM: *Arcanobacterium haemolyticum* pharyngitis and exanthem. Arch Dermatol 1996; 132:61.
Mehta CL: *Arcanobacterium haemolyticum*. J Am Acad Dermatol 2003; 48:298.

Intertrigo

Intertrigo is a superficial inflammatory dermatitis occurring where two skin surfaces are in apposition. It is discussed here because of its clinical association with several diseases in this chapter. As a result of friction (skin rubbing skin), heat, and moisture, the affected fold becomes erythematous, macerated, and secondarily infected. There may be erosions, fissures, and exudation, with symptoms of burning and itching. Intertrigo is most frequently seen during hot and humid weather, chiefly in obese persons. Children and the elderly are also predisposed. This type of dermatitis may involve the retroauricular areas; the folds of the upper eyelids; the creases of the neck, axillae, and antecubital areas; finger webs; inframammary area; umbilicus; inguinal, perineal, and intergluteal areas; popliteal spaces; and toe webs.

As a result of the maceration, a secondary infection by bacteria or fungi is induced. The inframammary area in obese women is most frequently the site of intertriginous candidiasis. The groins are also frequently affected by fungal (yeast or dermatophyte) infection. Bacterial infection may be caused by streptococci, staphylococci, *Pseudomonas*, or *Corynebacteria*. Streptococcal intertrigo favors the neck, axillary, and inguinal folds of young children. There is a well-demarcated fiery-red, moist, shiny surface, a foul smell and an absence of satellite lesions.

In the differential diagnosis, seborrheic dermatitis typically involves the skinfolds. Intertriginous psoriasis and erythrasma are frequently overlooked, especially when the inguinal and intergluteal areas or fourth toe webs are involved, as in erythrasma. Fissured groin lesions may be a manifestation of Langerhans cell histiocytosis.

Treatment is directed toward the elimination of the maceration. Appropriate antibiotics or fungicides are applied locally. The apposing skin surfaces may be separated with gauze or other appropriate dressings. Botulinum toxin type A has been used to dry out areas predisposed to recurrent disease. Castellani paint is also useful, as is an antibacterial ointment. Low-potency topical corticosteroids and topical tacrolimus are helpful to reduce inflammation, but should always be used in conjunction with a topical antifungal or antimicrobial agent.

Chapman MS, et al: 0.1% tacrolimus ointment for the treatment of intertrigo. Arch Dermatol 2005; 141:787.
Honig PJ, et al: Streptococcal intertrigo. Pediatrics 2003; 112:1427.
Neri I, et al: Streptococcal intertrigo. Pediatr Dermatol 2007; 24:577.
Santiago-et-Sanchez-Mateos JL, et al: Botulinum toxin type A for the preventative treatment of intertrigo in a patient with Darier's disease and inguinal hyperhidrosis. Dermatol Surg 2008; 34:1733.

Pitted keratolysis

In this bacterial infection of the plantar stratum corneum the thick, weight-bearing portions of the soles become gradually covered with shallow asymptomatic discrete round pits 1–3 mm in diameter, some of which become confluent, forming furrows (Fig. 14-26). Men with very sweaty feet during hot, humid weather are most susceptible. Rarely, palmar lesions may occur. No discomfort is produced, though the lesions are often malodorous.

Most disease is caused by *Kytococcus sedentarius*. It produces two serine proteases which can degrade keratin. Clinical diagnosis is not difficult, based on its unique appearance. Histologic examination generally demonstrates keratin pits lined by small cocci as well as filamentous bacteria.

Topical erythromycin or clindamycin is curative. Miconazole or clotrimazole cream and Whitfield ointment are effective alternatives. Both 5% benzoyl peroxide gel and a 10–20%

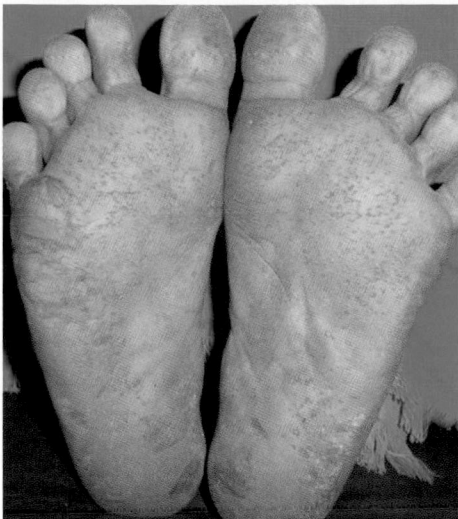

Fig. 14-26 Pitted keratolysis. (Courtesy of Shyam Verma, MD)

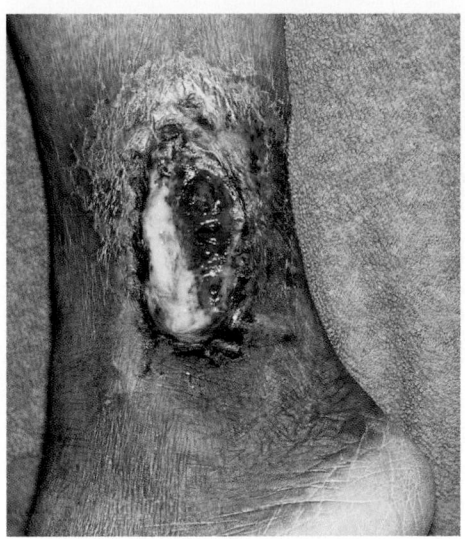

Fig. 14-27 Clostridial gas gangrene.

solution of aluminum chloride may be used. Botulinum toxin helps if there is associated hyperhidrosis.

Blaise G, et al: *Corynebacterium*-associated skin infections. Int J Dermatol 2008; 47:884.

Tamura BM, et al: Plantar hyperhidrosis and pitted keratolysis treated with botulinum toxin injection. Dermatol Surg 2004; 30:1510.

Walling HW: Primary hyperhidosis increases the risk of cutaneous infection. J Am Acad Dermatol 2009; 61:242.

Clostridial infections and gangrene of the skin (dermatitis gangrenosa)

Gangrene of the skin results from loss of the blood supply of a particular area and, in some instances, from bacterial invasion that promotes necrosis and sloughing of the skin. The various forms of bacterial infection causing gangrene will be discussed here. The infectious causes are often severe and acute in nature. These may involve deep tissues and MRI may delineate the depth of involvement. Vascular gangrene, purpura fulminans, and diabetic gangrene are covered in Chapter 35; vaccinia gangrenosa in Chapter 19; and necrotizing fasciitis earlier in this chapter.

Gas gangrene (clostridial myonecrosis)

Gas gangrene is the most severe form of infectious gangrene; it develops in deep lacerated wounds of muscle tissue (Fig. 14-27). The incubation period is only a few hours. Onset is usually sudden and is characterized by a chill, a rise in temperature, marked prostration, and severe local pain. Gas bubbles (chiefly hydrogen) produced by the infection cause crepitation when the area is palpated. A mousy odor is characteristic. A plain radiograph will demonstrate the air. Gas gangrene is caused by a variety of species of the genus *Clostridium*, most frequently *Clostridium perfringens*, *Clostridium oedematiens*, *Clostridium septicum*, *Clostridium difficile*, and *Clostridium haemolyticum*. These are thick, Gram-positive rods. *Clostridium* spores are resistant to skin sterilization chemicals; if injecting a site that is being soiled by stool incontinence, a mechanical wash prior to the sterile procedure, followed by an occlusive sterile dressing, is recommended.

A subacute variety occurs, which may be due to an anaerobic streptococcus (peptostreptococcus), *Bacteroides*, or *Prevotella*. This nonclostridial myositis may be clinically similar, but with delayed onset (several days). The purulent exudate has a foul odor, and Gram-positive cocci in chains are present. It is important to distinguish these two entities, since involved muscle may recover in nonclostridial myositis, and debridement may safely be limited to removal of grossly necrotic muscle. Infections with both clostridial and nonclostridial organisms such as *Streptococcus faecalis*, *Streptococcus anginosus*, *Proteus*, *E. coli*, *Bacteroides*, and *Klebsiella* species may also cause crepitant cellulitis, when the infection is limited to the subcutaneous tissue. Treatment of all clostridial infections is wide surgical debridement and intensive antibiotic therapy with intravenous penicillin G and clindamycin. Occasional cases of clindamycin-resistant *C. perfringens* are being reported. In such cases vancomycin may be an effective alternative. Hyperbaric oxygen therapy may be of value if immediately available. Infections in patients with cirrhosis and diabetes have a poorer prognosis.

Chronic undermining burrowing ulcers (Meleney gangrene)

This entity was first described by Meleney as postoperative progressive bacterial synergetic gangrene. It usually follows drainage of peritoneal abscess, lung abscess, or chronic empyema. After 1 or 2 weeks the wound markings or retention suture holes assume a carbunculoid appearance, finally differentiating into three skin zones: outer, bright red; middle, dusky purple; and inner, gangrenous with a central area of granulation tissue. The pain is excruciating. In Meleney postoperative progressive gangrene, the essential organism is a microaerophilic, non-hemolytic streptococcus (peptostreptococcus) in the spreading periphery of the lesion, associated with *S. aureus* or Enterobacteriaceae in the zone of gangrene. This disease is differentiated from ecthyma gangrenosum, which begins as vesicles rapidly progressing to pustulation and gangrenous ulceration in debilitated subjects, and is due to *P. aeruginosa*. Amebic infection with gangrene usually follows amebic abscess of the liver. The margins of the ulcer are raised and everted, and the granulations have the appearance of raw beef covered with shreds of necrotic material. Glairy pus can be expressed from the margins. Pyoderma gangrenosum occurs in a different setting, lacks the bacterial findings, and does not respond to antibiotic therapy. Fusospirochetal gangrene occurs following a human bite.

Wide excision and grafting are primary therapy. Antimicrobial agents, penicillin, and an aminoglycoside should be given as adjunctive therapy.

Fournier gangrene of the penis or scrotum

Fournier syndrome is a gangrenous infection of the penis, scrotum, or perineum, which may be due to infection with group A streptococci or a mixed infection with enteric bacilli and anaerobes. This is usually considered a form of necrotizing fasciitis, as it spreads along fascial planes. Peak incidence is between 20 and 50 years, but cases have been reported in children. Diabetes mellitus, obesity, poor personal hygiene, long-standing oral steroid therapy, and chronic alcoholism are predisposing factors. Culture for aerobic and anaerobic organisms should be carried out, and appropriate antibiotics started; surgical debridement and general support should be instituted.

Bhatnagar AM, et al: Fournier's gangrene. N Z Med J 2008; 121:46.

Campbell T, et al: Clinicopathologic challenge. Int J Dermatol 2008; 47:783.

Khanna N: Clindamycin-resistant *Clostridium perfringens* cellulitis. J Tissue Viability 2008; 17:95.

Ling I, et al: The crackling thigh. N Z Med J 2009; 122:81.

Majeski JA, et al: Necrotizing soft tissue infections. South Med J 2003; 96:900.

McHugh RC, et al: Clostridial sacroiliitis in a patient with fecal incontinence. Pain Phys 2008; 11:249.

Singh G, et al: Necrotising infections of soft tissues—a clinical profile. Eur J Surg 2002; 168:366.

Ullah S, et al: Fournier's gangrene. Surgeon 2009; 7:138.

Actinomycosis

Actinomyces are anaerobic, Gram-positive, filamentous bacteria. They colonize the mouth, colon, and urogenital track. Infections are seen most often in the cervicofacial area but also commonly on the abdominal region, thoracic area, or pelvis. Middle-aged men are affected most often. The lesions begin as firm nodules or plaques and develop draining sinuses. Grains or sulfur granules may be present in the exudate, just as in fungal mycetomas. In the cervicofacial region, the infection is known as lumpy jaw. The underlying bone may be involved with periostitis or osteomyelitis. Mandibular infection is seen four times as often as maxillary involvement (Fig. 14-28). The abdomen may be involved after a ruptured appendix or a gastrointestinal surgical procedure. Extension of the infection into the abdominal wall may produce draining sinuses on the abdominal skin. In the thoracic region, lung infection may spread to the thoracic wall.

Oropharyngeal actinomycosis is usually caused by *Actinomyces israelii* and *Actinomyces gerencseriae*. The condition is often clinically misdiagnosed as a malignancy, and it is the histological appearance of the characteristic granules that allows diagnosis. Sulfur granules consist of fine delicate branching filaments. Eosinophilic clubs composed of immunoglobulin are seen at the periphery of the granule (Splendore–Hoeppli's phenomenon). They resemble rays; hence the name, ray fungus (*Actinomyces*). Gram stain demonstrates long Gram-positive filaments.

The crushed granule is used for inoculating cultures containing brain–heart infusion blood agar, incubated under anaerobic conditions at 37°C. Culture is difficult; therefore direct microscopy is important.

Penicillin G in large doses, 10–20 MU/day for 1 month, followed by 4–6 g/day of oral penicillin for another 2 months, may produce successful and lasting results. Other effective medications have been ampicillin, erythromycin, tetracyclines, ceftriaxone, and clindamycin. Surgical incision, drainage, and excision of devitalized tissue are important.

Acevedo F, et al: Actinomycosis: a great pretender. Int J Infect Dis 2008; 12:358.

Garner JP, et al: Abdominal actinomycosis. Int J Surg 2007; 5:441.

Lancella A, et al: Two unusual presentations of cervicofacial actinomycosis and a review of the literature. Acta Otorhinolaryngol Ital 2008; 28:89.

Ozgediz D, et al: Abdominal actinomycosis after laparoscopic cholecystectomy. Surg Infect (Larchmt) 2009; 10:297.

Yi F, et al: Actinomycotic infection of the abdominal wall mimicking a malignant neoplasm. Sur Infect (Larchmt) 2008; 9:85.

Nocardiosis

Nocardiosis usually begins as a pulmonary infection from which dissemination occurs. Dissemination occurs most commonly in association with debilitating conditions, such as Hodgkin disease, periarteritis nodosa, leukemia, AIDS, organ transplants, or systemic lupus erythematosus. Skin involvement is seen in 10% of disseminated cases in the form of abscesses or vesiculopustular lesions (Fig. 14-29). Primary cutaneous disease also occurs in healthy individuals in the form of a draining abscess or lymphangitic nodules following a cutaneous injury.

Nocardia asteroides is usually responsible for the disseminated form of nocardiosis. *Nocardia brasiliensis* is the most common cause of primary cutaneous disease. A prick by a thorn or briar, other penetrating injury, or an insect bite or sting may be the inciting event.

Nocardia are Gram-positive, partially acid-fast, aerobic, filamentous bacteria. Some are branched, but filaments tend to be shorter and more fragmentary than those of *Actinomyces*. The surrounding red layer of immunoglobulin tends to be smooth rather than club-shaped. On Sabouraud dextrose agar, without antibacterial additives, there are creamy or

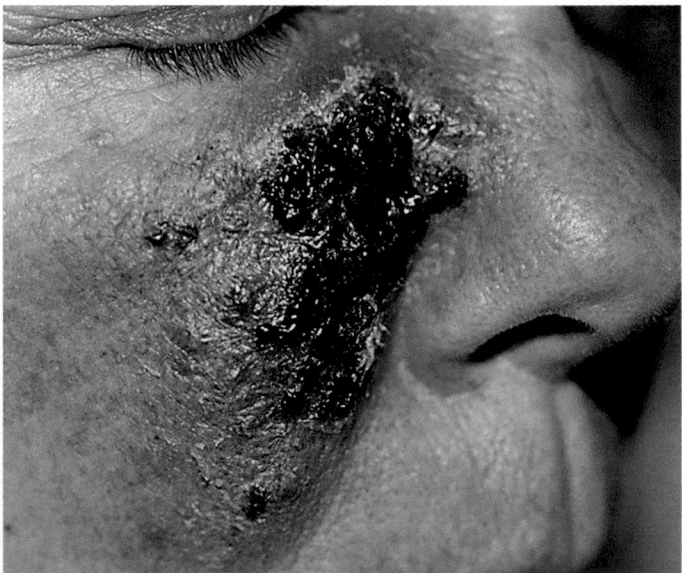

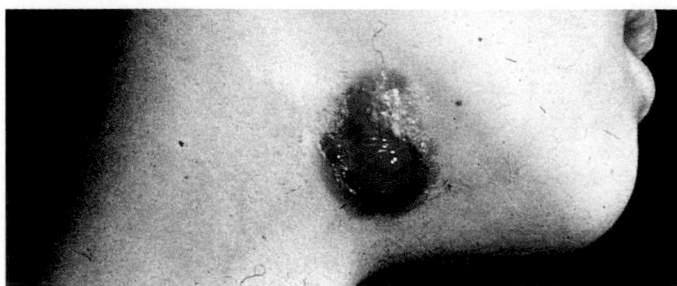

Fig. 14-28 Actinomycosis.

Fig. 14-29 Nocardiosis.

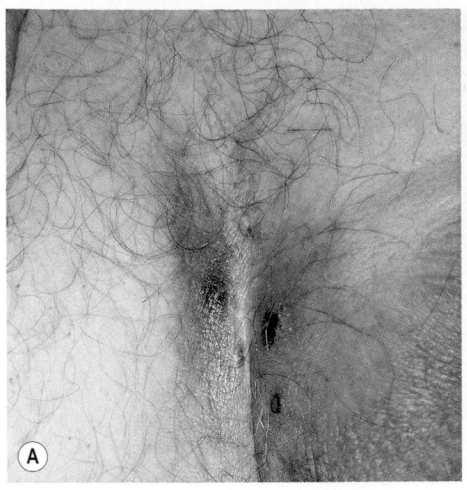
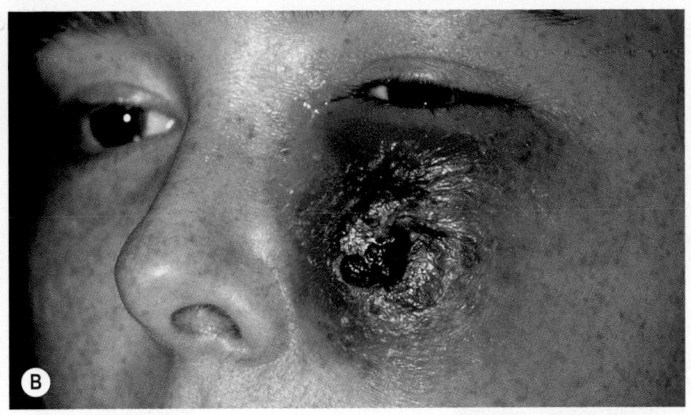

Fig. 14-30 A and B, Ecthyma gangrenosum.

moist, white colonies, which later become chalky and orange-colored.

Trimethoprim–sulfamethoxazole (Bactrim, Septra), four tablets twice a day for 6–12 weeks, is the drug of first choice. Minocycline for *N. asteroides* and augmentin for *N. brasiliensis* are alternatives. Amikacin has been used in combination with a variety of other antibiotics. Synergism has been observed with amikacin in combination with cefotaxime, imipenem, or sparfloxacin.

Bryant E, et al: Lymphocutaneous nocardiosis. Cutis 2010; 85:73.

Gosselink C, et al: Nocardiosis causing pedal actinomycetoma. J Foot Ankle Surg 2008; 47:457.

Saubolle MA, et al: Nocardiosis: review of clinical and laboratory experience. J Clin Microbiol 2003; 41:4497.

Smego RA Jr, et al: Lymphocutaneous syndrome. A review of non-sporothrix causes. Medicine (Baltimore) 1999; 78:38.

INFECTIONS CAUSED BY GRAM-NEGATIVE ORGANISMS

Pseudomonas infections

Ecthyma gangrenosum

In the gravely ill patient opalescent, tense vesicles or pustules are surrounded by narrow pink to violaceous halos. These lesions quickly become hemorrhagic and violaceous, and rupture to become round ulcers with necrotic black centers (Fig. 14-30). They are usually on the buttocks and extremities, and are often grouped closely together.

Ecthyma gangrenosum occurs in debilitated persons who may be suffering from leukemia, in the severely burned patient, in pancytopenia or neutropenia, or in patients with a functional neutrophilic defect, terminal carcinoma, or other severe chronic disease. Healthy infants may develop lesions in the perineal area after antibiotic therapy in conjunction with maceration of the diaper area.

The classic vesicle suggests the diagnosis. The contents of the vesicles or hemorrhagic pustules will show Gram-negative bacilli on Gram stain and cultures will be positive for *P. aeruginosa*. As this is usually a manifestation of sepsis, the blood culture will show *P. aeruginosa*. However, in healthy infants with diaper-area lesions, in patients with HIV infection, and in other occasional cases, early lesions may occur at a portal of entry, allowing for diagnosis and treatment before evolution into sepsis occurs.

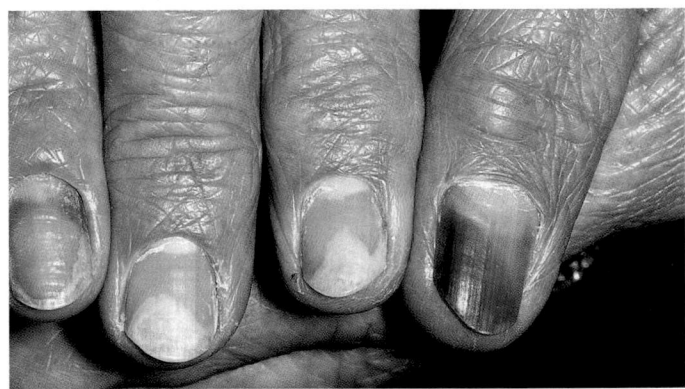

Fig. 14-31 Green nail syndrome complicating onycholysis.

Recommended treatment is the immediate institution of intravenous antipseudomonal penicillin. The addition of granulocyte–macrophage colony-stimulating factor to stimulate both proliferation and differentiation of myeloid precursors is an adjunct in a patient with myelodysplasia or treatment-induced neutropenia. Patients have a poorer prognosis if there are multiple lesions, if there is a delay in diagnosis and institution of appropriate therapy, and if neutropenia does not resolve by the end of a course of antibiotics. Instrumentation or catheterization increases the risk of this infection.

Other lesions are also seen with *Pseudomonas* septicemia. These may be sharply demarcated areas of cellulitis, macules, papules, plaques, and nodules, characteristically found on the trunk. *Pseudomonas mesophilica*, *Burkholderia cepacia*, *Citrobacter freundii*, and *Stenotrophomonas maltophilia* may also produce such skin lesions in immunocompromised individuals.

Several patients with AIDS have been reported who developed nodular skin lesions or abscesses secondary to *P. aeruginosa*. Generally, these patients are systemically ill; however, blood cultures are negative.

Green nail syndrome

Green nail syndrome is characterized by onycholysis of the distal portion of the nail and a striking greenish discoloration in the separated areas (Fig. 14-31). It is frequently associated with paronychia in persons whose hands are often in water. Overgrowth of *P. aeruginosa* accounts for the pigment. Soaking

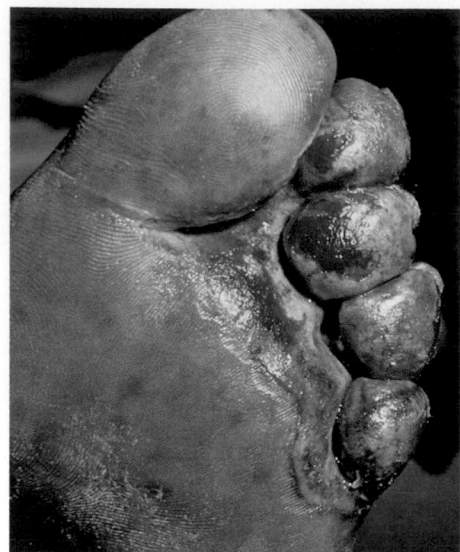

Fig. 14-32 Gram-negative toe web infection.

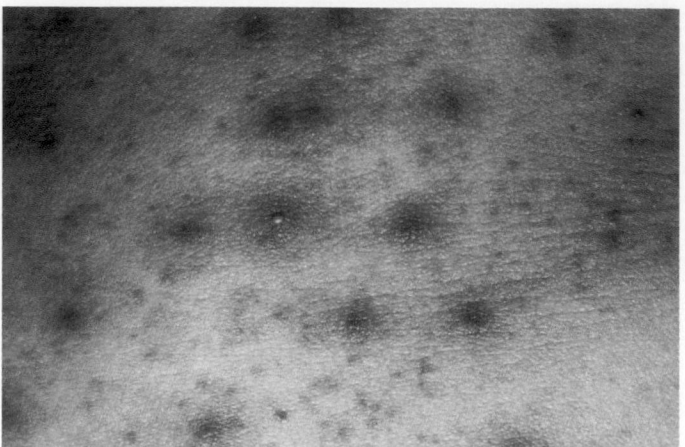

Fig. 14-33 Pseudomonas hot tub folliculitis.

the affected finger in a 1% acetic acid solution twice a day has been found to be helpful. Trimming the onycholytic nail plate followed by application of Neosporin solution twice a day is also effective. Green foot syndrome results from colonization of rubber sports shoes with *P. aeruginosa*. The organism produces pyoverdin, which stains the foot and toenails.

Gram-negative toe web infection

This type of infection often begins with dermatophytosis. Dermatophytosis may progress with increasing inflammation, maceration, and inflammation to dermatophytosis complex, where many types of Gram-negative organism may be recovered, but it is harder to culture dermatophytes. Finally, denudation with purulent or serous discharge and marked edema and erythema of the surrounding tissue may be seen (Fig. 14-32). Prolonged immersion may also cause hydration and maceration of the interdigital spaces, with overgrowth of Gram-negative organisms. *P. aeruginosa* is the most prominent among them, but commonly a mixture of other Gram-negative organisms, such as *E. coli* and *Proteus*, are present. Patients may suffer from red, painful nodules of the calf that do not drain, spontaneously involute, then reappear 1–2 weeks later. Culture of these subcutaneous abscesses will reveal *Pseudomonas* or other Gram-negatives, which are likely to originate in the macerated toe webs.

Early dermatophytosis, dermatophytosis simplex, may simply be treated with topical antifungals. However, once the scaling and peeling progress to white maceration, soggy scaling, bad odor, edema, and fissuring, treatment must also include topical antibiotics or acetic acid compresses. Drying of the interdigital spaces with a fan is a helpful adjunct. Full-blown Gram-negative toe web infection with widespread denudation and erythema, purulence, and edema requires systemic antibiotics. A third-generation cephalosporin or a fluoroquinolone is recommended.

Blastomycosis-like pyoderma

Large verrucous plaques with elevated borders and multiple pustules may occur as a chronic vegetating infection. Most patients have an underlying systemic or local host compromise. Bacteria such as *P. aeruginosa*, *S. aureus*, *Proteus*, *E. coli*, or streptococci may be isolated.

Pseudomonas aeruginosa folliculitis (hot tub folliculitis)

Pseudomonal folliculitis is characterized by pruritic follicular, maculopapular, vesicular, or pustular lesions occurring within 1–4 days after bathing in a hot tub, whirlpool, or public swimming pool (Fig. 14-33). As the water temperature rises, free chlorine levels fall, even though total chlorine levels appear adequate. This allows the bacteria to proliferate. Diving suits may become colonized and wearing them may result in *P. aeruginosa* folliculitis. Most lesions occur on the sides of the trunk, axillae, buttocks, and proximal extremities. The apocrine areas of the breasts and axilla are often involved. Associated complaints may include earache, sore throat, headache, fever, and malaise. Rarely, systemic infection may result; breast abscess and bacteremia have been reported. Large community outbreaks have occurred associated with public pools, and 27 employees of a cardboard manufacturing facility who were exposed to wet work developed *Pseudomonas* folliculitis of the extremities as an occupational disorder.

The folliculitis involutes usually within 7–14 days without therapy, although on occasion multiple prolonged recurrent episodes have been reported. In patients with fever, constitutional symptoms, or prolonged disease, a third-generation oral cephalosporin or a fluoroquinolone such as ciprofloxacin or ofloxacin may be useful. Preventive measures have been water filtration, automatic chlorination to maintain a free chlorine level of 1 ppm, maintenance of water at pH 7.2–7.8, and frequent changing of the water. Bromination of the water and ozone ionization are other options.

Pseudomonas hot-foot syndrome was reported in a group of 40 children who developed painful, erythematous plantar nodules or pustules after wading in a community pool whose floor was coated with abrasive grit. One biopsy showed neutrophilic eccrine hidradenitis and one dermal microabscesses. Most were treated symptomatically and resolution occurred within 2 weeks.

External otitis

Swelling, maceration, and pain may be present. In up to 70% of cases *P. aeruginosa* may be cultured. This is especially common in swimmers. Local applications of antipseudomonal and anti-inflammatory Cortisporin otic solution or suspension, or 2% acetic acid compresses with topical steroids, will help clear this infection. In patients with otorrhea or pus emanating from the canal, if the symptoms have been present for

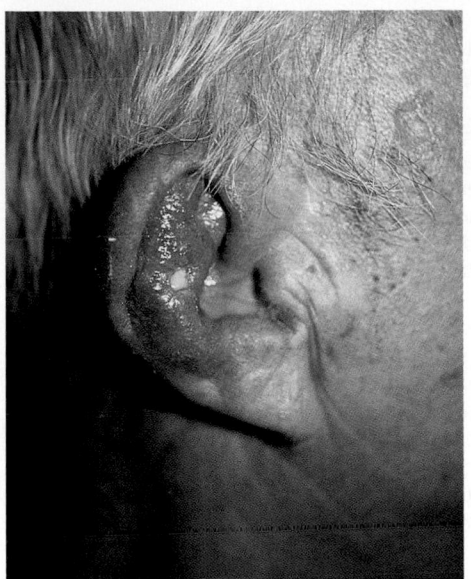

Fig. 14-34 *Pseudomonas* external otitis after shave biopsy.

a week or more, or if diabetes or an immunologic defect is present, cleansing of the canal, visualizing the tympanic membrane for perforation, and other precautions will be most readily handled by an otolaryngology consultation. Application of otic Domeboro solution after swimming will help prevent recurrence. Fungi such as *Candida* and *Aspergillus* are other causes. Antifungal solutions, such as ciclopiroxolamine solution, combined with steroid solutions are effective in otomycosis. There is also a threat of external otitis occurring after ear surgery (Fig. 14-34). If the patient is a swimmer or has diabetes, acetic acid compresses for a day or two before surgery may prevent this complication.

External otitis must be distinguished from allergic contact dermatitis due to neomycin in Cortisporin otic suspension. Allergic contact dermatitis produces severe pruritus, although tenderness may also be noted. Dermatitis may extend down the side of the cheek in a pattern suggesting drainage of the suspension.

A severe type, referred to as malignant external otitis, occurs in elderly patients with diabetes or in those immunocompromised with HIV infection, on chemotherapy, or living with organ transplants. The swelling, pain, and erythema are more pronounced, with purulence and a foul odor. Facial nerve palsy develops in 30% of cases, and cartilage necrosis may occur. This is a life-threatening infection in these older, compromised individuals, and requires swift institution and prolonged administration (4–6 weeks) of oral quinolone antibiotics.

Finally, commercial ear piercing of the upper ear cartilage may lead to infection with *Pseudomonas*, with resulting cosmetic deformity a reported complication.

Gram-negative folliculitis

Although this is usually due to Enterobacteriaceae, *Klebsiella, Escherichia, Proteus,* or *Serratia*, occasional cases caused by *Pseudomonas* have been seen. They differ from Gram-negative infection in patients with acne in that the site of *Pseudomonas* colonization is the external ear, and topical therapy alone to the face and ears is sufficient for cure. Finally, an outbreak of Gram-negative pustular dermatitis on the legs, arms, torso, and buttocks occurred in a group of college students who hosted a mud-wrestling social event.

Abdulhak AAB, et al: *Stenotrophomonas maltophilia* infections of intact skin. Diagn Microbiol Infec Dis 2009; 63:330.

Aste N, et al: Gram-negative bacterial toe web infection. J Am Acad Dermatol 2001; 45:537.

Aygencel G, et al: *Burkholderia cepacia* as a cause of ecthyma gangrenosum-like lesions. Infection 2008; 36:271.

Carfrae MJ, et al: Malignant otitis externa. Otolaryngol Clin North Am 2008; 41:537.

Cho SB, et al: Green nail syndrome associated with military footwear. Clin Exp Dermatol 2008; 33:791.

Fiorillo L, et al: The *Pseudomonas* hot-foot syndrome. N Engl J Med 2001; 345:335.

Goolamali SI, et al: Ecthyma gangrenosum. Clin Exp Dermatol 2009; 34:e180.

Handley RT, et al: Otitis externa. JAAPA 2009; 22:44.

Hewitt DJ, et al: Industrial *Pseudomonas* folliculitis. Am J Ind Med 2006; 49:895.

Kaya TI, et al: Blue underpants sign: a diagnostic clue for *Pseudomonas aeruginosa* intertrigo of the groin. J Am Acad Dermatol 2005: 53:869.

Keene WE, et al: Outbreak of *Pseudomonas aeruginosa* infections caused by commercial piercing of the upper ear cartilage. JAMA 2004; 291:981.

Nakai N, et al: Ecthyma gangrenosum without *Pseudomonas* septicemia in a kidney transplant patient. J Dermatol 2008; 35:585.

Neubert U, et al: Bacteriologic and immunologic aspects of Gram-negative folliculitis. Int J Dermatol 1999; 38:270.

Nieves D, et al: Smoldering Gram-negative cellulitis. J Am Acad Dermatol 1999; 41:319.

Osguthorpe JD, et al: Otitis externa. Am Fam Physician 2006; 74:1510.

Reich HL, et al: Nonpseudomonal ecthyma gangrenosum. J Am Acad Dermatol 2004; 50:S114.

Rubin Grandis J, et al: The changing face of malignant (necrotising) external otitis. Lancet Infect Dis 2004; 4:34.

Sawalka SS, et al: Blastomycosis-like pyoderma. Indian J Dermatol Venereol Leprol 2007; 73:117.

Zomorrodi A, et al: Ecthyma gangrenosum. Pediatr Infect Dis 2002; 21:1161.

Malacoplakia (malakoplakia)

This rare granuloma, originally reported only in the genitourinary tract of immunosuppressed renal transplant recipients, may also occur in the skin and subcutaneous tissues of other patients with deficient immune responsiveness such as is present in HIV infection. Patients are unable to resist infections with S. *aureus,* P. *aeruginosa,* and E. *coli*. There is defective intracellular digestion of the bacteria once they have been phagocytosed.

The granulomas may arise as masslike lesions or nodules, abscesses or ulcerations. They favor the perineum, but also affect the abdominal wall, thorax, extremities, and axilla. The tongue is also a site of appearance, usually presenting as a mass lesion.

Histologically, there are foamy eosinophilic Hansemann macrophages containing calcified, concentrically laminated, intracytoplasmic bodies called Michaelis–Gutmann bodies. Scattered immunoblasts, neutrophils, and lymphocytes are found in the dermis.

Successful treatment depends on the isolated organism; a fluoroquinolone such as ciprofloxacin or ofloxacin is usually useful.

Diapera MJ, et al: Malacoplakia of the tongue. Am J Otolaryngol 2009; 30:101.

Flann S, et al: Cutaneous malakoplakia in an abdominal skin fold. J Am Acad Dermatol 2010; 62:896.

Savant SR, et al: Cutaneous malakoplakia in an HIV-infected patient. Int J STD AIDS 2007; 18:435.

Haemophilus influenzae cellulitis

Haemophilus influenzae type B causes a distinctive bluish or purplish-red cellulitis of the face accompanied by fever in children younger than age 2. The condition is rarely seen in countries where the vaccination is available. It is given at 2, 4, and 6 months of age. The importance of recognizing the entity is related to the bacteremia that often accompanies the cellulitis. The bacteremia may lead to meningitis, orbital cellulitis, osteomyelitis, or pyarthrosis. Cultures of the blood and needle aspirates of the cellulitis should yield the organism. Cefotaxime or ceftriaxone is effective. In a family with children under the age of 4, the index case, both parents, and children at risk (unvaccinated) should be given rifampin to clear the nasal carriage state and prevent secondary cases.

Rimon A, et al: Periorbital cellulitis in the era of *Haemophilus influenzae* type B vaccine. J Pediatr Ophthalmol Strabismus 2008; 45:300.

Chancroid

Chancroid (soft chancre) is an infectious, ulcerative STD caused by the Gram-negative bacillus *Haemophilus ducreyi* (the Ducrey bacillus). One or more deep or superficial tender ulcers on the genitalia, and painful inguinal adenitis in 50%, which may suppurate, are characteristic of the disease. Men outnumber women manyfold.

Chancroid begins as an inflammatory macule or pustule 1–5 days—or rarely as long as 2 weeks—after intercourse. It generally appears on the distal penis or perianal area in men, or on the vulva, cervix, or perianal area in women. However, many cases of extragenital infection on the hands, eyelids, lips, or breasts have been reported. Autoinoculation frequently forms kissing lesions on the genitalia, and women are apt to have more numerous lesions.

The pustule ruptures early with the formation of a ragged ulcer that lacks the induration of a chancre, usually being soft with an indefinite inflammatory thickening. The ulcers appear punched out or have undermined irregular edges surrounded by mild hyperemia (Fig. 14-35). The base is covered with a purulent, dirty exudate. The ulcers bleed easily and are very tender.

A number of clinical variants have been described, including granuloma inguinale-like, giant ulcers, serpiginous ulcers, transient chancroid, and follicular and papular variants.

Only about half the cases of genital chancroid manifest inguinal adenitis. Suppuration of the bubo (inguinal lymph node) may occur despite early antibiotic therapy. The lymphadenitis of chancroid, mostly unilateral, is tender and may rupture spontaneously. Left untreated, the site of perforation of the broken-down bubo may assume the features of a soft chancre (chancrous bubo).

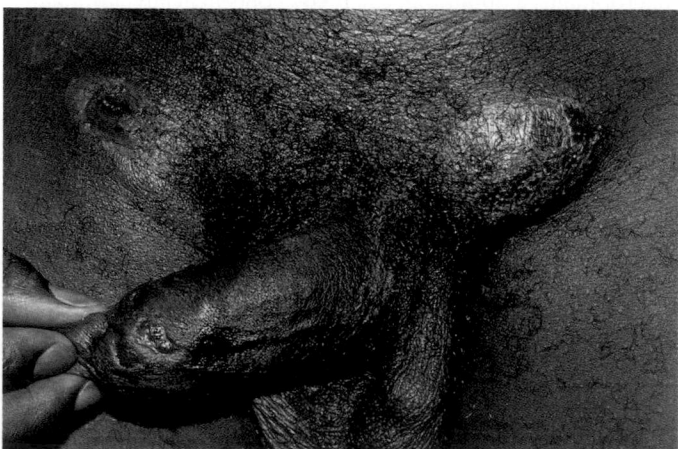

Fig. 14-35 Chancroid.

As a result of mixed infection, phagedenic and gangrenous features may develop. Chronic, painful, destructive ulcers, which begin on the prepuce or glans and spread by direct extension along the shaft of the penis, are present. They may sometimes attack the scrotum or pubes. The edges of the ulcer are likely to be elevated, firm, and undermined. The granulating base, which bleeds easily, is covered with a thick, purulent exudate and dirty, necrotic detritus. The neighboring skin may be edematous and dusky red, and the regional lymph glands may be swollen, although this is not necessarily a marked feature. There is severe mutilation as a result of sloughing, without any evidence of spontaneous healing.

This type of phagedena (spreading and sloughing ulceration) is a rare complication of chancre and chancroidal infections together with another secondary bacterial infection. Treatment is by the use of antibiotics locally and internally, directed against secondary bacteria, as well as the primary process. Multiple infections may be present, such as chancroid, syphilis, or granuloma inguinale.

On histologic investigation the ulcer may include a superficial necrotic zone with an infiltrate consisting of neutrophils, lymphocytes, and red blood cells. Deep to this, new vessel formation is present, with vascular proliferation. Deeper still is an infiltrate of lymphocytes and plasma cells. Ducrey bacilli may or may not be seen in the sections.

The definitive diagnosis of chancroid requires identification by culture. Solid-media culture techniques have made definitive diagnosis possible, and permit sensitivity testing; however, culture is unavailable in many settings and recovery is only about 80% successful. Specimens for culture should be taken from the purulent ulcer base and active border without extensive cleaning. They should be inoculated in the clinic, as transport systems have not been evaluated. The selective medium contains vancomycin, and cultures are done in a water-saturated environment with 1–5% CO_2, at a temperature of 33°C. Occasional outbreaks are due to vancomycin-sensitive strains. In these cases, culture will only be successful using vancomycin-free media.

Smears are only diagnostic in 50% of cases in the best hands. A probable diagnosis is made by a clinically compatible examination and negative testing for those conditions whose presentation may mimic chanchroid. Probably the disease for which chancroid is most frequently mistaken is herpes progenitalis. A history of recurrent grouped vesicles at the same site should help eliminate the chance of a misdiagnosis. Traumatic ulcerations should also be ruled out. These occur mostly along the frenulum or as multiple erosions on the prepuce. Adenopathy is absent and some degree of phimosis is present.

The clinical features that differentiate chancroid from syphilitic chancre are described in Chapter 18. However, the diagnosis of chancroid does not rule out syphilis. Either the lesion may already be a mixed sore or the subsequent development of syphilis should be anticipated, since the incubation period of the chancre is much longer than that of chancroid. Repeated darkfield examinations for *Treponema pallidum* are necessary, even in a sore where the diagnosis of chancroid has been established. Serologic tests for syphilis should be obtained initially, and monthly for the next 3 months, and serologic testing for HIV infection should also be done. Chancroidal genital ulcer disease facilitates the transmission of HIV infection. In HIV-infected patients, chanchroid may have a prolonged incubation period, the number of ulcers may be increased, extragenital sites are more frequently affected, antibiotic therapy fails more often, and healing is slower when it does occur. Complications such as penile amputation from a deep transverse ulcer may result.

Treatment

The treatment of choice for chancroid is azithromycin, 1 g orally in a single dose. Erythromycin, 500 mg four times a day for 7 days; ceftriaxone, 250 mg intramuscularly in a single dose; and ciprofloxacin, 500 mg orally twice a day for 3 days, are also recommended treatments. Ciprofloxacin should not be used in pregnant or lactating women, or in children younger than 17 years of age. Partners who have had sexual contact with the patient within the 10 days before the onset of symptoms should be treated with a recommended regimen.

Phimosis that does not subside following irrigation of the preputial cavity may have to be relieved by a dorsal slit. Circumcision should be deferred for at least 2 or 3 months. If frank pus is already present, repeated aspirations (not incisions) may be necessary.

Bong CT, et al: *Haemophilus ducreyi.* Microbes Infect 2002; 4:1141.
Mohammed TT, et al: Chancroid and HIV infection: a review. Int J Dermatol 2008; 47:1.
STD Guidelines 2006. MMWR 2006; 55:1.
Weiss HA: Male circumcision as a preventative measure against HIV and other sexually transmitted diseases. Curr Opin Infect Dis 2007; 20:66.

Granuloma inguinale (granuloma venereum, donovanosis)

Granuloma inguinale is a mildly contagious, chronic, granulomatous, locally destructive disease characterized by progressive, indolent, serpiginous ulcerations of the groins, pubes, genitalia, and anus.

The disease begins as single or multiple subcutaneous nodules, which erode through the skin to produce clean, sharply defined lesions, which are usually painless. More than 80% of cases demonstrate hypertrophic, vegetative granulation tissue, which is soft, has a beefy-red appearance, and bleeds readily (Fig. 14-36A). Approximately 10% of cases have ulcerative lesions with overhanging edges and a dry or moist floor (Fig. 14-36B). A membranous exudate may cover the floor of fine granulations, and the lesions are moderately painful. Occasional cases are misdiagnosed as carcinoma of the penis. The lesions enlarge by autoinoculation and peripheral extension with satellite lesions, and by gradual undermining of tissue at the advancing edge.

The genitalia are involved in 90% of cases, inguinal region in 10%, anal region in 5–10%, and distal sites in 1–5%. Lesions are limited to the genitalia in approximately 80% of cases and to the inguinal region in less than 5%. In men, the lesions most commonly occur on the prepuce or glans, and in women, lesions on the labia are most common.

The incubation period is unknown; it may vary between 8 and 80 days, with a 2- to 3-week period being most common.

Persisting sinuses and hypertrophic scars, devoid of pigment, are fairly characteristic of the disease. The regional lymph nodes are usually not enlarged. In later stages, as a result of cicatrization, the lymph channels are sometimes blocked and pseudoelephantiasis of the genitals (esthiomene) may occur. Mutilation of the genitals and destruction of deeper tissues are observed in some instances.

Dissemination from the inguinal region may be by hematogenous or lymphatic routes. There may be involvement of liver, other organs, eyes, face, lips, larynx, chest, and, rarely, bones. During childbearing the cervical lesions may extend to the internal genital organs. Squamous cell carcinoma may rarely supervene.

Granuloma inguinale is caused by the Gram-negative bacterium *Klebsiella granulomatis*. It is sexually transmitted in the majority of cases with the occurrence of conjugal infection in 12–52% of marital or steady sexual partners. Also, it is speculated that *K. granulomatis* is an intestinal inhabitant that leads to granuloma inguinale through auto-inoculation, or sexually through vaginal intercourse if the vagina is contaminated by enteric bacteria, or through rectal intercourse, heterosexual or homosexual. *K. granulomatis* probably requires direct inoculation through a break in the skin or mucosa to cause infection. Those affected are generally young adults.

On histologic investigation, in the center of the lesion, the epidermis is replaced by serum, fibrin, and polymorphonuclear leukocytes. At the periphery the epidermis demonstrates pseudoepitheliomatus hyperplasia. In the dermis there is a dense granulomatous infiltration composed chiefly of plasma cells and histiocytes, and scattered throughout are small abscesses containing polymorphonuclear leukocytes.

Characteristic pale-staining macrophages that have intracytoplasmic inclusion bodies are found. The parasitized histiocytes may measure 20 μm or more in diameter. The ovoid Donovan bodies measure 1–2 μm and may be visualized by using Giemsa or silver stains. The best method, however, is toluidine blue staining of semi-thin, plastic-embedded sections. Crushed smears of fresh biopsy material stained with Wright or Giemsa stain permit the demonstration of Donovan bodies and provide rapid diagnosis.

Granuloma inguinale may be confused with ulcerations of the groin caused by syphilis or carcinoma, but it is differentiated from these diseases by its long duration and slow course,

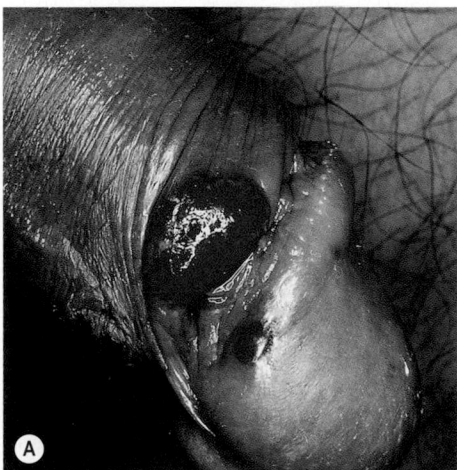
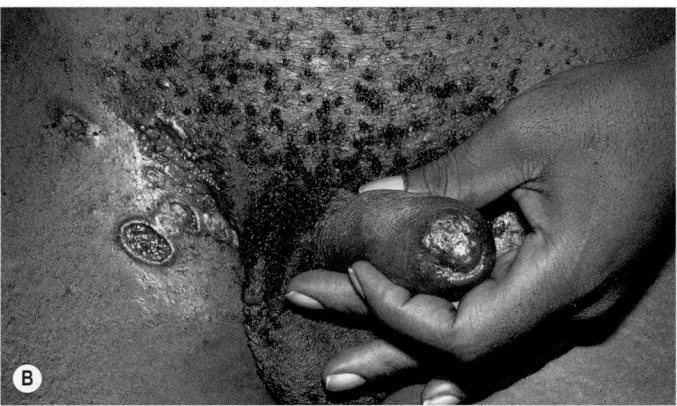

Fig. 14-36 Granuloma inguinale.

by the absence of lymphatic involvement, and, in the case of syphilis, by a negative test for syphilis and failure to respond to antisyphilitic treatment. It should not be overlooked that other venereal diseases, especially syphilis, often coexist with granuloma inguinale. Additionally, all patients presenting with STDs should be tested for HIV infection and their sexual partners evaluated. Lymphogranuloma venereum at an early stage would most likely be accompanied by inguinal adenitis. In later stages, when stasis, excoriations, and enlargement of the outer genitalia are common to granuloma inguinale and lymphogranuloma venereum, the absence of a positive lymphogranuloma venereum complement-fixation test and the presence of Donovan bodies in the lesions permit the diagnosis of granuloma inguinale.

Treatment

Trimethoprim–sulfamethoxazole, one double-strength tablet orally twice a day for a minimum of 3 weeks, or doxycycline, 100 mg orally twice a day for a minimum of 3 weeks, is the recommended regimen. Therapy should be continued until all lesions have healed completely. Alternative regimens are ciprofloxacin, 750 mg orally twice a day for a minimum of 3 weeks; erythromycin base, 500 mg orally four times a day for a minimum of 3 weeks, or azithromycin, 1 g orally once a week for at least 3 weeks, is also effective. The addition of an aminoglycoside (gentamicin), 1 mg/kg intravenously every 8 h, should be considered if lesions do no respond within the first few days and in HIV-infected patients.

Rosen T, et al: Antibiotic use in sexually transmissible diseases. Dermatol Clin 2009; 27:49.
STD Guidelines 2006. MMWR 2006; 55:1.
Velho PE, et al: Donovanosis. Braz J Infect Dis 2008; 12:521.

Gonococcal dermatitis

Primary gonococcal dermatitis is a rare infection that occurs after primary inoculation of the skin from an infected focus. It may present as grouped pustules on an erythematous base on the finger, simulating herpetic whitlow, with or without an ascending lymphangitis. Scalp abscesses in infants may occur secondary to direct fetal monitoring in mothers with gonorrhea. It may also cause an inflammation of the median raphe or a lymphangitis of the penis with or without accompanying urethritis. Treatment is the same as that of gonorrheal urethritis. A single oral dose of cefixime, 400 mg, is usually curative. Ceftriaxone is also effective as a 125 mg single intramuscular dose.

Gonococcemia

Gonococcemia is characterized by a hemorrhagic vesiculopustular eruption, bouts of fever, and arthralgia or actual arthritis of one or several joints. The skin lesions begin as tiny erythematous macules that evolve into vesicopustules on a deeply erythematous or hemorrhagic base or into purpuric macules that may be as much as 2 cm in diameter (Fig. 14-37). These purpuric lesions occur acrally, mostly on the palms and soles, and over joints. They are accompanied by fever, chills, malaise, migratory polyarthralgia, myalgia, and tenosynovitis. The vesicopustules are usually tender and sparse, and occur principally on the extremities. Involution of the lesions takes place in about 4 days.

Many patients are women with asymptomatic anogenital infections in whom dissemination occurs during pregnancy or menstruation. Liver function abnormalities, myocarditis, pericarditis, endocarditis, and meningitis may complicate this infection. In severe or recurrent cases complement deficiency,

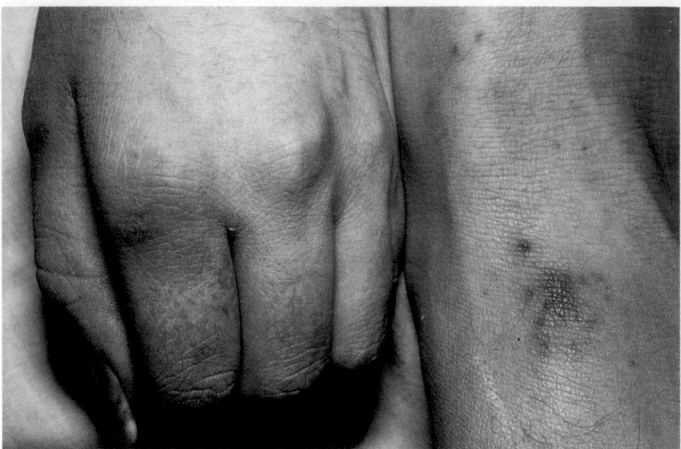

Fig. 14-37 Gonococcemia.

especially of the late (C5, C6, C7, or C8) components, should be investigated.

The causative organism is *Neisseria gonorrhoeae*. These organisms can at times be demonstrated in the early skin lesion histologically, by smears, and by cultures. Gonococci may be found in the blood, genitourinary tract, pharynx, joints, and skin.

The skin lesions of gonococcemia may be identical to those seen in meningococcemia, nongonococcal bacterial endocarditis, rheumatoid arthritis, the rickettsial diseases, systemic lupus erythematosus, periarteritis nodosa, Haverhill fever, and typhoid fever. Septic emboli with any Gram-negative organism or *Candida* classically manifest as hemorrhagic pustules.

The treatment of choice for disseminated gonococcal infection is ceftriaxone, 1 g/day intravenously or intramuscularly for 24–48 h after improvement begins. Then therapy may be switched to cefixime, 400 mg orally twice a day, for at least 1 week. Alternative initial drugs include cefotaxime, 1 g every 8 h, or ceftizoxime, 1 g every 8 h. Spectinomycin, 2 g intramuscularly every 12 h, may be used for persons allergic to β-lactam drugs.

If a cephalosporin is used, either doxycycline, 100 mg twice a day for 7 days, or azithromycin, 1 g as a single dose, should be given to treat coexisting chlamydial infection. Serologic testing for HIV infection should also be done, as well as screening for syphilis. Sex partners within 30 days for symptomatic infection and 60 days for asymptomatic infection should be referred for treatment.

Burgis JT, et al: Disseminated gonococcal infection in pregnancy presenting as meningitis and dermatitis. Obstet Gynecol 2006; 108:798.
Mahendran SM: Disseminated gonococcal infection presenting as cutaneous lesions in pregnancy. J Obstet Gynecol 2007; 27:617.
Mehrany K, et al: Disseminated gonococcemia. Int J Dermatol 2003; 42:208.
Rosen T, et al: Antibiotic use in sexually transmitted disease. Dermatol Clin 2009; 27:49.
STD Guidelines 2006. MMWR 2006; 55:1.

Meningococcemia

Acute meningococcemia presents with fever, chills, hypotension, and meningitis. Half to two-thirds of patients develop a petechial eruption, most frequently on the trunk and lower extremities, which may progress to ecchymoses, bullous hemorrhagic lesions, and ischemic necrosis (Fig. 14-38). Often acral petechiae are present, and petechiae may be noted on the eyelids. Angular infarctive lesions with an erythematous rim

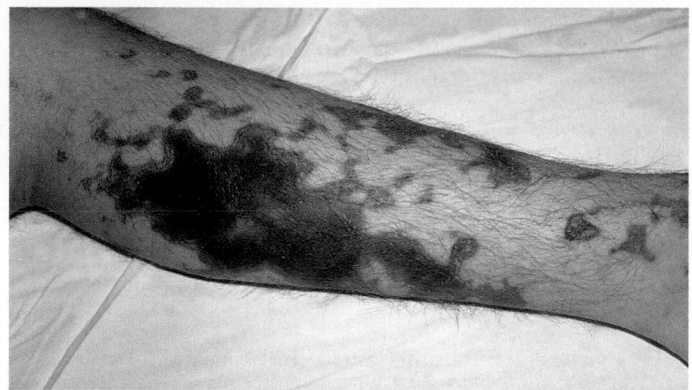

Fig. 14-38 Meningococcemia.

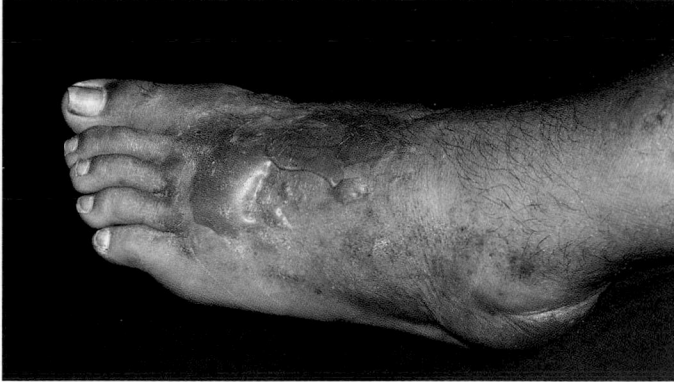

Fig. 14-39 *Vibrio vulnificus* infection. (Courtesy of Curt Samlaska, MD)

and gun-metal gray interior are characteristic of meningococcal sepsis. Occasionally, a transient, blanchable, morbilliform eruption is the only cutaneous finding. The oral and conjunctival mucous membranes may be affected.

Meningococcemia primarily affects young children, males more frequently than females. Patients with asplenia, immunoglobulin deficiencies, or inherited or acquired deficiencies of the terminal components of complement or properdin are predisposed to infection.

A rare variant is chronic meningococcemia. There are recurrent episodes of fever, arthralgias, and erythematous macules that may evolve into lesions with central hemorrhage. Acral hemorrhagic pustules, similar to those found in gonococcal sepsis, may be seen. Patients are generally young adults with fevers lasting 12 h interspersed with 1–4 days of well-being.

The disease is caused by the fastidious Gram-negative diplococcus *Neisseria meningitidis*. It has a polysaccharide capsule that is important in its virulence and serotyping. The human nasopharynx is the only known reservoir, with carriage rates in the general population estimated to be 5–10%.

Treatment is with penicillin G, 300 000 U/kg/day intravenously up to 24 MU/day for 10–14 days. Cefotaxime, ceftriaxone, chloramphenicol, and trimethoprim–sulfamethoxazole are alternatives. One dose of ciprofloxacin, 500 mg, is given after the initial course of antibiotics to clear nasal carriage. Household members and daycare and close school contacts should receive prophylactic therapy. Rifampin, 10 mg/kg every 12 h for 2 days, is an alternative for children. A polyvalent vaccine is effective against groups A, C, Y, and W-135, and is recommended for high-risk groups.

Ahlawat S, et al: Meningococcal meningitis outbreak control strategies. J Commun Dis 2000; 32:264.

Duggal S, et al: Recent outbreak of meningococcal meningitis: a microbiological study with brief review of the literature. J Commun Dis 2007; 39:209.

Milonovich LM: Meningococcemia. J Pediatr Health Care 2007; 21:75.

Ploysangam T, et al: Chronic meningococcemia in childhood. Pediatr Dermatol 1996; 13:483.

Vibrio vulnificus infection

Infection with *Vibrio vulnificus*, a Gram-negative rod of the non-cholera group of vibrios, may produce both a rapidly expanding cellulitis or a life-threatening septicemia in patients who have been exposed to the organism. This infection mainly occurs along the Atlantic seacoast. It may be acquired via the gastrointestinal tract, where, after being ingested with raw oysters or other seafood, the bacterium enters the bloodstream at the level of the duodenum. Pulmonary infection by the aspiration of seawater has been reported. Localized skin infection may result after exposure of an open wound to seawater.

Skin lesions characteristically begin within 24–48 h of exposure, with localized tenderness followed by erythema, edema, and indurated plaques. They occur in nearly 90% of patients and are most common on the lower extremities. A purplish discoloration develops centrally and then undergoes necrosis, forming hemorrhagic bullae or ulcers (Fig. 14-39). Other reported lesions include hemorrhagic bullae, pustules, petechiae, generalized macules or papules, and gangrene.

If the skin is invaded primarily, septicemia may not develop, but the lesions may be progressive and at times limb amputation may be necessary. With septicemia, cellulitic lesions are the result of seeding of the subcutaneous tissue during bacteremia. Patients with advanced liver disease are at particular risk for developing septicemia. Other predisposing disorders are immunosuppression, alcoholism, adrenal insufficiency, diabetes, renal failure, male sex, and iron-overload states. The virulence of the bacterium is related to the production of exotoxin and various other factors. The mortality in patients with septicemia is greater than 50%.

Treatment of this fulminant infection, which rapidly produces septic shock, includes antibiotics, surgical debridement, and appropriate resuscitative therapy. Doxycycline together with ceftazidime is the treatment of choice. In patients with preexisting hepatic dysfunction or immunocompromise and whose wounds are exposed to or acquired in saltwater, prophylactic antibiotic coverage with doxycycline, 100 mg every 12 h, and cleansing with 0.025% sodium hypochlorite solution may prevent progressive infection.

Borrenstein M, et al: Infections with *Vibrio vulnificus*. Dermatol Clin 2003; 21:245.

Kuo YL, et al: Necrotizing fasciitis caused by *Vibrio vulnificus*. Eur J Clin Microbiol Infect Dis 2007; 26:785.

Oliver JD: Wound infections caused by *Vibrio vulnificus* and other marine bacteria. Epidemiol Infect 2005; 133:383.

Patel VJ, et al: *Vibrio vulnificus* septicaemia and leg ulcer. J Am Acad Dermatol 2002; 46:S144.

Tsai YH, et al: Necrotizing soft-tissue infections and primary sepsis caused by *Vibrio vulnificus* and *Vibrio cholerae* non-01. J Truama 2009; 66:899.

Chromobacteriosis and *Aeromonas* infections

Chromobacteria are a genus of Gram-negative rods that produce various discolorations on gelatin broth. They have been shown to be common water and soil saprophytes of the southeastern US and Australia. Several types of cutaneous lesions are caused by chromobacteria, ranging from fluctuating abscesses and local cellulitis to anthrax-like carbuncular lesions with lymphangitis and fatal septicemia. *Chromobacterium violaceum*, the most common organism in this genus, produces a violet pigment. Patients with chronic granulomatous disease may be at particular risk. Systemic aminoglycosides are indicated.

A Gram-negative bacterium, *Aeromonas hydrophilia*, another typical soil and water saprophyte, may cause similar skin infections manifesting as cellulitis, pustules, furuncles, gas gangrene, or ecthyma gangrenosum-like lesions, after water-related trauma and abrasions. Folliculitis caused by *Aeromonas hydrophilia* may mimic *Pseudomonas folliculitis*. The treatment of choice is ciprofloxacin.

Julia Manresa M, et al: Aeromonas hydrophilia folliculitis associated with an inflatable swimming pool. Pediatr Dermatol 2009; 26:601.
Moore CC, et al: Successful treatment of an infant with *Chromobacterium violaceum* sepsis. Clin Infect Dis 2001; 32:E107.
Mulholland A, et al: A possible new cause of spa bath folliculitis: *Aeromonas hydrophilia*. Austral J Dermatol 2008; 49:39.
Tsai YH, et al: Necrotizing soft-tissue infections and sepsis caused by *Vibrio vulnificus* compared with those caused by *Aeromonas* species. J Bone Joint Surg Am 2007; 89:631.

Salmonellosis

Salmonellae are a genus of Gram-negative rods that exist in humans either in a carrier state or as a cause of active enteric or systemic infection. Most cases of typhoid fever caused by *Salmonella typhi* are acquired by ingestion of contaminated food or water. Pets such as lizards, snakes, and turtles carry *Salmonella* organisms and acquisition of the organism in petting zoos has also been reported. Poultry and poultry products are the most important sources and are believed to be the cause in about half of common-source epidemics. Hand washing and thorough cooking of meats are recommended preventative measures.

After an incubation period of 1–2 weeks, there is usually an acute onset of fever, chills, headache, constipation, and bronchitis. After 7–10 days of fever and diarrhea, skin lesions, rose-colored macules or papules ("rose spots") 2–5 mm in diameter, appear on the anterior trunk, between the umbilicus and nipples. They occur in crops, each group of 10–20 lesions lasting 3–4 days, the total duration of the exanthem being 2–3 weeks in untreated cases. Rose spots occur in 50–60% of cases. A more extensive erythematous eruption occurring early in the course, erythema typhosum, is rarely reported, as are erythema nodosum, urticaria, and ulcers or subcutaneous abscesses.

The diagnosis is confirmed by culturing the organism from blood, stool, skin, or bone marrow. If the organism is not grown on *Shigella–Salmonella* medium, or not analyzed correctly, it may be erroneously reported as a coliform. The preferred antibiotics are either ciprofloxacin or ceftriaxone.

Occasionally, *S. typhi* may cause skin lesions without systemic infection. Also, infection with non-typhoid *Salmonella*, such as *S. enterica*, may cause enteric fever with rose spots.

Coburn B, et al: Salmonella, the host and disease. Immunol Cell Biol 2007; 85:112.
Marzano AV, et al: Cutaneous infection caused by *Salmonella typhi*. J Eur Acad Dermatol Venereol 2003; 17:575.
Nishie H, et al: Non-typhoid *Salmonella* infection associated with rose spots. Br J Dermatol 1999; 140:558.

Shigellosis

Shigellae are small Gram-negative rods that cause bacillary dysentery, an acute diarrheal illness. Most cases are a result of person-to-person transmission; however, widespread epidemics have resulted from contaminated food and water. Small, blanchable, erythematous macules on the extremities, as well as petechial or morbilliform eruptions, may occur. Stoll reported a man who had sex with men who developed a 1 cm

furuncle on the dorsal penile shaft from which a pure culture of *Shigella flexneri* was grown. Shigellosis may then occur as a purely cutaneous form of STD. *Shigella* and *Salmonella* are among the organisms reported to induce the postdysenteric form of Reiter syndrome. Therapy with a fluoroquinolone is curative.

Carter JD, et al: Reactive arthritis. Rheum Dis Clin North Am 2009; 35:21.
Stoll DM: Cutaneous shigellosis. Arch Dermatol 1986; 122:22.

Helicobacter cellulitis

Fever, bacteremia, cellulitis, and arthritis may all be caused by *Helicobacter cinaedi* or *canis*. Generally, these manifestations occur in HIV-infected patients; however, malignancy, diabetes, and alcoholism are other predisposing conditions. Occasionally, *Helicobacter* has been reported to cause postsurgical wound infections and sepsis in otherwise healthy individuals. The cellulitis may be multifocal and recurrent, and have a distinctive red–brown or copper color with minimal warmth. Ciprofloxacin is generally effective.

Itamura T, et al: Helicobacter cinaedi cellulitis and bacteremia in immunocompetent hosts after orthopedic surgery. J Clin Microbiol 2007; 45:31.
Leemann C, et al: First case of bacteremia and multifocal cellulitis due to *Helicobacter canis* in an immunocompetent patient. J Clin Microbiol 2006; 44:4598.
Yoda K, et al: Isolation of *Helicobacter cinaedi* from a sepsis patient with cellulitis. Jpn J Infect Dis 2009; 62:169.

Rhinoscleroma

Rhinoscleroma is a chronic, inflammatory, granulomatous disease of the upper respiratory tract characterized by sclerosis, deformity, remission, and eventual debility. Death resulting from obstructive sequelae may occur. The infection is limited to the nose, pharynx, and adjacent structures.

The disease begins insidiously with nasal catarrh, increased nasal secretion, and subsequent crusting. Gradually, there ensues a nodular or rather diffuse sclerotic enlargement of the nose, upper lip, palate, or neighboring structures (Fig. 14-40). The nodules at first are small, hard, subepidermal, and freely movable, but they gradually fuse to form sclerotic plaques that adhere to the underlying parts. Ulceration is common. The lesions have a distinctive stony hardness, are insensitive, and are of a dusky purple or ivory color. Hyperpigmentation can be expected in dark-complexioned individuals.

In the more advanced stages of rhinoscleroma, the reactive growth produces extensive mutilation of the face and marked disfigurement. Complete obstruction of the nares, superficial erosions, and seropurulent exudation may occur.

A microorganism, *Klebsiella pneumoniae*, ssp. *rhinoscleromatis*, first isolated by von Frisch, is the causative agent. The rhinoscleroma bacillus is a Gram-negative rod, short, nonmotile, round at the ends, always encapsulated in a gelatinous capsule, and measuring 2–3 μm. It is found in the throats of scleroma patients only.

The disease occurs in both sexes, and is most common during the third and fourth decades of life. Although endemic in Austria and southern Russia, and occasionally found in Brazil, Argentina, Chile, Spain, Italy, Sweden, and the US, it is especially prevalent in El Salvador, where many workers in the dye industry have been affected. Rare familial cases have been reported; when this occurs, the condition may present in childhood.

In the primary stage of nasal catarrh, the histologic picture is that of a mild, nonspecific inflammation. When proliferation and tumefaction develop, the granulomatous tumor is made

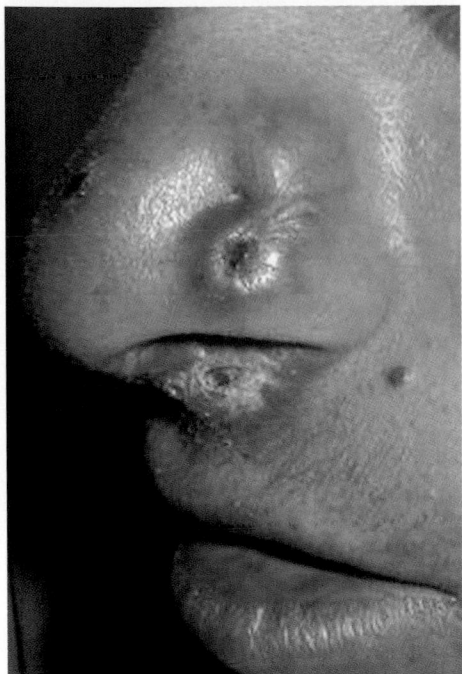

Fig. 14-40 Rhinoscleroma. (Courtesy of Jason Robbins, MD)

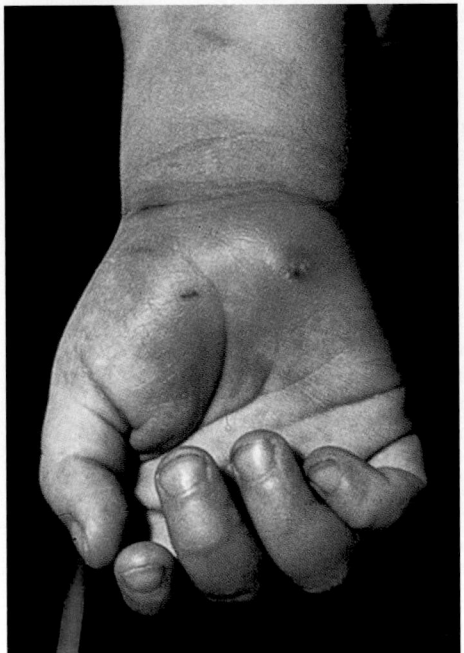

Fig. 14-41 *Pasteurella multocida* infection.

up largely of plasma cells, Mikulicz cells, an occasional hyaline degenerated plasma cell (Russell body), a few spindle cells, and fibrosis. The bacilli are found within foamy macrophages (Mikulicz cells). They are best visualized with the Warthin–Starry silver stain.

Rhinoscleroma has such distinctive features that its diagnosis should not be difficult. The diagnosis depends on bacteriologic, histopathologic, and serologic tests. Heat-killed antigen gives a positive complement-fixation reaction with scleroma patients' serum. Titers run as high as 1:1280. Clinically, it can be confused with syphilitic gumma, sarcoid, leishmaniasis, frambesia, keloid, lepra, hypertrophic forms of tuberculosis, and rhinosporidiosis.

Treatment

This disease is usually progressive and resistant to therapy; however, it may respond well to the fluoroquinolones, but therapy should be prolonged, lasting at least 3 or 4 months to try to limit the chance of relapse. Corticosteroids are useful in the acute phase. Surgical intervention or CO_2 laser treatments may be needed to prevent airway obstruction or to correct deformities.

Abalkhail A, et al: Rhinoscleroma. Singapore Med J 2007; 48:148.
Bhargava D, et al: Palatal presentation of scleroma. J Laryngol Otol 2001; 115:679.
De Pontual L, et al: Rhinoscleroma: a French national retrospective study of epidemiological and clinical features. Clin Infec Dis 2008; 47:1396.
Fernandez-Vozmediano JM, et al: Rhinoscleroma in three siblings. Pediatr Dermatol 2004; 21:134.

Pasteurellosis

Primary cutaneous (ulceroglandular) *Pasteurella hemolytica* infection may occur in patients with skin injury and exposure to this organism. *P. hemolytica* is a common pathogen of domestic animals, being associated with shipping fever in cattle and septicemia in lambs and newborn pigs. The lacerations become inflamed, lymphangitis and fever develop, and axillary lymph nodes become enlarged. Diagnosis is based on demonstration of the bacteria on culture of the lesions.

Pasteurella multocida is a small, nonmotile, Gram-negative, bipolar-staining bacterium. It is known to be part of the normal oral and nasal flora of cats and dogs, but may also be an animal pathogen. The most common type of human infection follows injuries from animal bites, principally cat and dog bites, but also cat scratches. Following animal trauma, erythema, swelling, pain, and tenderness develop within a few hours of the bite, with a gray-colored serous or sanguinopurulent drainage from the puncture wounds (Fig. 14-41). There may or may not be regional lymphadenopathy or evidence of systemic toxicity such as chills and fever. Septicemia may follow the local infection in rare cases, and tenosynovitis and osteomyelitis appear with some frequency. Though a Gram-negative bacillus, treatment is with systemic penicillin G in addition to careful cleansing and tetanus prophylaxis.

Chun ML, et al: Postoperative wound infection with *Pasteurella multocida* from a pet cat. Am J Obstet Gynecol 2003; 188:1115.
Luchansky M, et al: Cat bite in an old patient. Eur J Emerg Med 2003; 10:130.
Olshtain-Pops K, et al: *Pasteurella multocida* sepsis. IMAJ 2008; 10:648.

Dog and human bite pathogens

It is recommended that all cat bites and scratches, all sutured wounds of any animal source, and any other animal injuries of an unusual type or source be treated with antibiotics in addition to careful cleansing and tetanus prophylaxis. While *Pasteurella* species (*cunis* in dogs and *multocida* in cats) are usually present in bite site cultures, a complex mix of various other pathogens, such as streptococci, staphylococci, *Moraxella*, *Neisseria*, *Fusobacterium*, *Bacteroides*, and those individually discussed below, make the combination amoxicillin–clavulanate the best choice of initial therapy. Gatifloxacin and linezolid are other effective medications.

Capnocytophaga canimorsus, formerly referred to as DF-2, is a Gram-negative rod that is part of the normal oral flora of dogs and cats. It is associated with severe septicemia after dog bites. Patients who have undergone splenectomy are at particular risk. Alcoholism, chronic respiratory disease, and other medical conditions also predispose to infection; only one-quarter of patients were healthy before infection with

C. canimorsus. A characteristic finding is a necrotizing eschar at the site of the bite. Fever, nausea, and vomiting occur abruptly within 1–3 days, and the eschar develops soon thereafter. Disseminated intravascular coagulation and extensive dry gangrene may complicate the course. Sepsis after a dog bite is another hazard faced by splenectomized patients in addition to their particular problems with pneumococcus, *H. influenzae* group B, babesiosis, *N. meningitidis*, and group A streptococcus. *C. canimorsus* is difficult to identify by conventional cultures. Laboratory personnel need to be aware of the clinical suspicion of infection with this organism. A false-positive latex agglutination test for cryptococcal antigen in the spinal fluid may occur. Treatment is with intensive intravenous antibiotics. In less severely affected patients amoxicillin–clavulanate may be effective.

Eugonic fermenting bacteria (EF-4) and *Bergeyella zoohelcum* are other oral and nasal commensals in dogs; thus, most reports of human disease follow animal bites. *Eikenella corrodens*, a facultative Gram-negative bacillus, is a normal inhabitant of the human mouth. Most infections are caused by human bites or fist fights. Amoxicillin–clavulanate or penicillin G is effective.

Gaastra W, et al: *Capnocytophaga canimorsus*. Vet Microbiol 2009 (Epub 5 Feb).
Griego RD, et al: Dog, cat, and human bites. J Am Acad Dermatol 1995; 33:1019.
Grob JJ, et al: Extensive skin ulceration due to EF-4 bacterial infection in a patient with AIDS. Br J Dermatol 1989; 121:507.
Kravetz JD, et al: Cat-associated zoonoses. Arch Intern Med 2002; 162:1945.
Oehler RL, et al: Bite-related and septic syndromes caused by cats and dogs. Lancet Infect Dis 2009; 9:439.

Glanders

Once known as equinia, farcy, and malleus, glanders is a rare, usually fatal, infectious disease that occurs in humans by inoculation with *Burkholderia mallei*. It is encountered in those who handle horses, mules, or donkeys.

The distinctive skin lesion is an inflammatory papule or vesicle that arises at the site of inoculation, rapidly becomes nodular, pustular, and ulcerative, and forms an irregular excavation with undermined edges and a base covered with a purulent and sanguineous exudate. In a few days or weeks other nodules (called "farcy buds") develop along the lymphatics in the adjacent skin or subcutaneous tissues; subsequently, these break down. In the acute form, the skin involvement may be severe and accompanied by grave diarrhea. In the chronic form, there are few skin lesions and milder constitutional symptoms, but repeated cycles of healing and breakdown of nodules may occur for weeks.

The respiratory mucous membranes are especially susceptible to the disease. After accidental inhalation, first catarrhal symptoms are present and there may be epistaxis or a mucoid nasal discharge. The nasal discharge is a characteristic feature of the disease.

The diagnosis is established by finding the Gram-negative organism in this discharge or in the skin ulcers, and should be confirmed by serum agglutination. This organism has been fatal to many laboratory workers, and exposure in this setting is increasing, with *B. mallei* considered a bioterrorism threat.

Treatment is chiefly by immediate surgical excision of the inoculated lesions and antibiotics. Augmentin, doxycycline, or trimethoprim–sulfamethoxazole for up to 5 months' duration may be effective in disease limited to the skin, while parenteral ceftazidime can be used for severe or septic infection. Imipenem and doxycycline combination cured an infected laboratory worker.

Bovine farcy also occurs and is caused by *Nocardia farcinica*. Schiff et al reported a nonimmunocompromised patient with an infected facial laceration. Osteomyelitis complicated the course. Amikacin treatment after surgical debridement resulted in complete cure.

Dvorak GD, et al: Glanders. J Am Vet Med Assoc 2008; 233:570.
Schiff TA, et al: Cutaneous *Nocardia farcinica* infection in a nonimmunocompromised patient. Clin Infect Dis 1993; 16:756.
Srinivasan A, et al: Glanders in a military research microbiologist. N Engl J Med 2001; 345:256.
Whitlock GC, et al: Glanders. FEMS Microbiol Lett 2007; 277:115.

Melioidosis

Melioidosis (Whitmore's disease) is a specific infection caused by a glanders-like bacillus, *Burkholderia pseudomallei*. The disease has an acute pulmonary and septicemic form in which multiple miliary abscesses in the viscera occur, resulting in rapid death. Less often, it runs a chronic course, with subcutaneous abscesses and multiple sinuses of the soft tissues. Its clinical characteristics are similar to glanders, disseminated fungal infections, and tuberculosis. Severe urticaria and necrotizing fasciitis are uncommon complications.

Melioidosis is endemic in Southeast Asia and should be suspected in military personnel and travelers who have characteristic symptoms of a febrile illness and have been in that region. Recrudescence of disease after a long latency period may occur. Diagnosis is made from the recovery of the bacillus from the skin lesions or sputum, and by serologic tests.

Effective therapy is guided by the antibiotic sensitivity of the specific strain. For the acute septicemic phase, ceftazidime or imipenem is indicated. The majority of chronic cutaneous infections respond well to trimethoprim–sulfamethoxazole and doxycycline. Maintenance with this combination should continue for 20 weeks.

Cheng AC, et al: Melioidosis. Clin Microbiol Rev 2005; 18:383.
Gibney KB, et al: Cutaneous melioidosis in the tropical top end of Australia. Clin Infect Dis 2008; 47:603.
Tran D, et al: Cutaneous melioidosis. Clin Exp Dermatol 2002: 27:280.
Tzeng WT, et al: Recurrent cutaneous melioidosis treated with surgery and antibiotics. J Plast Reconstr Aesthet Surg 2009; 62:280.
White NJ, et al: Melioidosis. Lancet 2003; 361:1715.

Infections caused by *Bartonella*

Bartonella are aerobic, fastidious, Gram-negative bacilli. Several species cause human diseases, including *Bartonella henselae* (cat-scratch disease and bacillary angiomatosis), *Bartonella quintana* (trench fever and bacillary angiomatosis), *Bartonella bacilliformis* (verruga peruana and Oroya fever), and *Bartonella clarridgeiae* (a possible cause of cat-scratch disease). These agents are transmitted by arthropod vectors in some cases. Unique to this genus is the ability to cause vascular proliferation, as is seen in bacillary angiomatosis and verruga peruana. The bartonellae in affected tissue stain poorly with tissue Gram stain, and are usually identified in tissue using modified silver stains such as Warthin–Starry. They are difficult to culture, making tissue identification of characteristic bacilli an important diagnostic test. Electron microscopy and PCR can be used if routine staining is negative.

Cat-scratch disease

Cat-scratch disease is relatively common. About 22 000 cases are reported annually in the US, with between 60% and 90% of cases occurring in children and young adults. Cat-scratch disease is the most frequent cause of chronic lymphadenopathy in children and young adults.

B. henselae causes the vast majority of cases of cat-scratch disease. The infectious agent is transmitted from cat to cat by fleas, and from cats to humans by cat scratches or bites. Rarely, dog bites may transmit this infection. The organism can be found in the primary skin and conjunctival lesions, lymph nodes, and other affected tissues. In geographic areas where cat fleas are present, about 40% of cats are asymptomatically bacteremic with this organism.

The primary skin lesion appears within 3–5 days after the cat scratch, and may last for several weeks (Fig. 14-42). It is present in 50–90% of patients. The primary lesion is not crusted and lymphangitis does not extend from it. The primary lesion may resemble an insect bite but is not pruritic. It heals within a few weeks, usually with no scarring.

Lymphadenopathy, the hallmark of the disease, appears within a week or two after the primary lesions or between 10 and 50 days (average 17 days) after inoculation. Usually, the lymphadenopathy is regional and unilateral. Because most inoculations occur on the upper extremities, epitrochlear and axillary lymphadenopathy is most common (50%), followed by cervical (25%) or inguinal (18%). Generalized lymphadenopathy does not occur, but systemic symptoms such as fever, malaise, and anorexia may be present. Without treatment the adenopathy resolves over a few weeks to months, with spontaneous suppuration occurring in between 10% and 50% of cases. If the primary inoculation is in the conjunctiva, there is chronic granulomatous conjunctivitis and preauricular adenopathy—the so-called oculoglandular syndrome of Parinaud. Uncommonly, acute encephalopathy, osteolytic lesions, hepatic and splenic abscesses, hypercalcemia, and pulmonary manifestations have been reported. In addition, erythema nodosum and a diffuse exanthem may accompany cat-scratch disease.

Diagnosis is made largely on clinical features. The primary skin lesion or lymph node may be biopsied and the infectious agent identified. Involved lymph nodes and skin lesions demonstrate granulomatous inflammation with central "stellate" necrosis. A serologic test is available but is not reproducibly positive early in the disease, limiting its usefulness. Cat-scratch skin testing (Hanger and Rose test) can be used but is rarely required if the history and clinical features are characteristic. Other infectious and neoplastic causes of localized lymph-adenopathy, such as tularemia, sporotrichosis, atypical mycobacterial infection, and Hodgkin disease, may need to be excluded.

The vast majority of cases of cat-scratch disease resolve spontaneously without antibiotic therapy. Such therapy has not been demonstrated to shorten the duration of the disease in most typical cases. Fluctuant lymph nodes should be aspirated, not incised and drained. In patients with severe visceral disease, azithromycin, erythromycin, tetracycline or doxycycline is effective.

Trench fever

Trench fever is caused by *Bartonella quintana*, which is spread from person to person by the body louse. Urban cases of trench fever caused by this agent are now most commonly seen in homeless louse-infested persons.

Patients present with fever that initially lasts about a week, then recurs about every 5 days. Other symptoms are headache, neck, shin, and back pain. Endocarditis may occur. There are no skin lesions.

Treatment has not been studied systematically. Ceftriaxone for 7 days, followed by erythromycin or another macrolide for 2–4 months, is one effective regimen.

Bacillary angiomatosis

Bacillary angiomatosis describes a clinical condition characterized by vascular skin lesions resembling pyogenic granulomas (Fig. 14-43). Only two organisms have been proven to cause bacillary angiomatosis: *B. henselae* (the cause of cat-scratch disease) and *B. quintana* (the cause of trench fever). The skin lesions caused by these two agents are identical. If the bacillary angiomatosis is caused by *B. henselae*, there is usually a history of cat exposure, and the same *Bartonella* can also be isolated from the blood of the source cat. Bacillary angiomatosis caused by *B. quintana* is associated with homelessness and louse infestation. The incubation period is unknown but may be years.

Bacillary angiomatosis occurs primarily in the setting of immunosuppression, especially AIDS. The helper T-cell count is usually less than 50/mL. Other immunosuppressed patients,

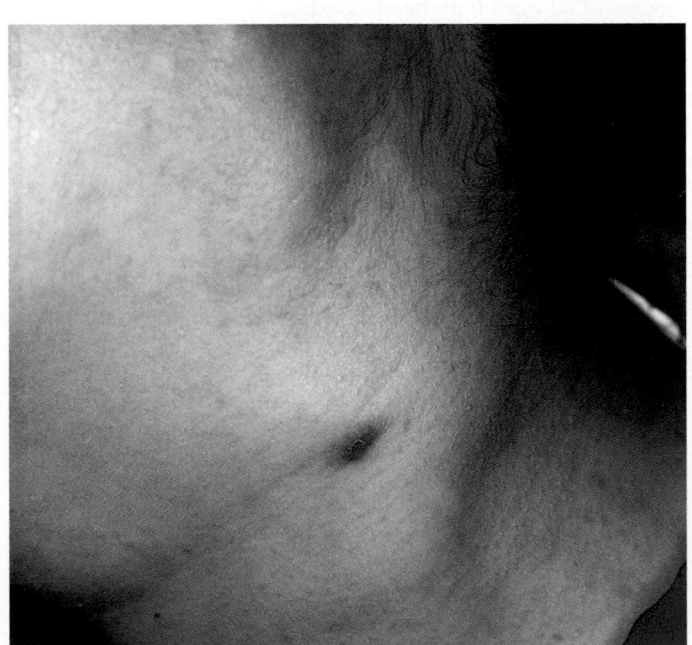

Fig. 14-42 Primary cat-scratch lesion with lymphadenopathy.

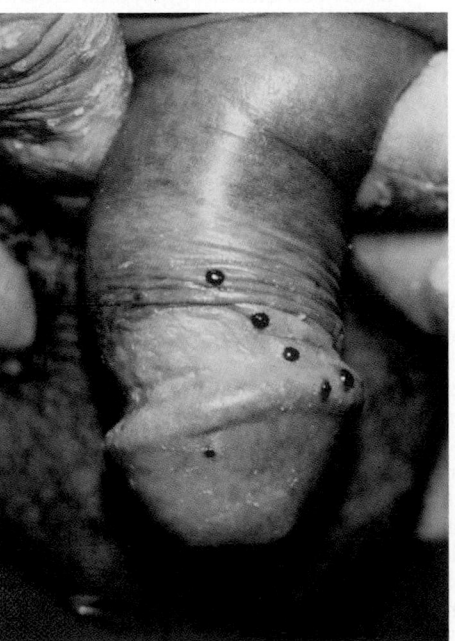

Fig. 14-43 Bacillary angiomatosis.

such as those with leukemia or transplants, may acquire the condition. Rarely, bacillary angiomatosis can occur in HIV-negative persons with no apparent immune impairment. In immunoincompetent hosts, the bacteria proliferate locally and are frequently blood-borne. The local proliferation of bacteria produces the angiogenic vascular endothelial growth factor (VEGF), leading to endothelial cell proliferation and the characteristic skin lesions. Immunocompetent hosts resist this bacterial proliferation, resulting in granulomatous and necrotic, rather than angiomatous, lesions.

Several different forms of cutaneous lesions occur. The most common form resembles pyogenic granuloma, which may exhibit a surrounding collarete of scale. Less commonly, subcutaneous masses, plaques, and ulcerations may occur. A single patient may exhibit several of these morphologies. Lesions are tender and bleed easily. Subcutaneous nodules are also tender and may be poorly marginated. Lesions may number from one to thousands, usually with the number gradually increasing over time if the patient is untreated.

In the setting of bacillary angiomatosis, the infection must be considered disseminated. Bacteremia is detected in about 50% of affected AIDS patients leading to involvement of many visceral sites, most frequently the lymph node, liver and spleen, and bone. Less commonly, pulmonary, gastrointestinal, muscle, oral, and brain lesions can occur. *B. henselae* is usually associated with lymph node and liver and spleen involvement, whereas *B. quintana* more often causes bone disease and subcutaneous masses. Visceral disease can be confirmed by appropriate radiologic or imaging studies. Bone lesions are typically lytic, resembling osteomyelitis. In the liver and spleen "peliosis" occurs. Liver function tests characteristically demonstrate a very elevated lactic dehydrogenase level, an elevated alkaline phosphatase level, slight elevation of the levels of hepatocellular enzymes, and a normal bilirubin level. Lesions on other epithelial surfaces, in muscle, and in lymph nodes are usually angiomatous.

Biopsies of bacillary angiomatosis skin lesions have the same low-power appearance as a pyogenic granuloma, with the proliferation of endothelial cells, forming normal small blood vessels. Bacillary angiomatosis is distinguished from pyogenic granuloma by the presence of neutrophils throughout the lesion, not just on the surface, as is seen in a pyogenic granuloma. The neutrophils are sometimes aggregated around granular material that stains slightly purple. This purple material represents clusters of organisms, which can at times be confirmed by modified silver stain such as the Steiner stain. Tissue Gram stain does not routinely stain the bacteria in bacillary angiomatosis lesions. Electron microscopy may identify bacteria in cases in which special stains are negative. Bacillary angiomatosis is easily distinguished histologically from Kaposi sarcoma. In patch or plaque lesions of Kaposi sarcoma the new blood vessels are abnormal in appearance, being angulated. Endothelial proliferation in Kaposi sarcoma is seen in the dermis around the eccrine units, follicular structures, and existing normal vessels. Nodular Kaposi sarcoma is a spindle cell tumor with slits rather than well-formed blood vessels. Neutrophils and purple granular material are not found in Kaposi sarcoma, but intracellular hyaline globules are present.

The natural history of bacillary angiomatosis is extremely variable. In most patients, however, either lesions remain stable or the size or number of lesions gradually increases over time. The initial lesions are usually the largest, and multiple satellite or disseminated smaller lesions occur, representing miliary spread. Untreated bacillary angiomatosis can be fatal, with patients dying of visceral disease or respiratory compromise from obstructing lesions.

The diagnosis of bacillary angiomatosis is virtually always made by identifying the infectious agent in affected tissue. The organisms can also be cultured from the lesions and the patient's blood. However, these organisms grow very slowly, so cultures may not be positive for more than 1 month. Thus, tissue and blood cultures are usually confirmatory in nature. Antibodies to *Bartonella* can be detected in most patients by an indirect fluorescence assay. Because of its limited availability and background positivity in the general population of cat owners, this test is not generally useful in establishing the diagnosis of bacillary angiomatosis.

Treatment

Bacillary angiomatosis is dramatically responsive to erythromycin, 500 mg four times a day, or doxycycline, 100 mg twice a day. Minocycline, tetracycline, clarithromycin, azithromycin, roxithromycin, and chloramphenicol may also be effective. Trimethoprim–sulfamethoxazole, ciprofloxacin, penicillins, and cephalosporins are not effective. Prophylactic regimens containing a macrolide antibiotic or rifampin prevent the development of bacillary angiomatosis. Treatment duration depends on the extent of visceral involvement. In cases with skin lesions or bacteremia only, at least 8 weeks of treatment are required. For liver and spleen involvement 3–6 months of treatment are recommended, and for bone disease, at least 6 months of treatment should be considered. Once treatment is begun, symptoms begin to resolve within hours to days. A Jarisch–Herxheimer reaction may occur with the first dose of antibiotic. If patients relapse after an apparently adequate course of treatment, chronic suppressive antibiotic therapy should be considered.

Oroya fever and verruga peruana

Oroya fever and verruga peruana represent two stages of the same infection. Oroya fever (Carrion's disease) is the acute febrile stage, and verruga peruana the chronic delayed stage. These conditions are limited to and endemic in Peru and a few neighboring countries in the Andes, and restricted to valleys between 500 and 3200 m above sea level. Both of these conditions are caused by *B. bacilliformis*, which is transmitted by a sandfly, usually *Lutzomyia verrucarum*. Humans represent the only known reservoir. Men represent about three-quarters of cases and all ages may be affected.

After an incubation period averaging 3 weeks, the acute infection, Oroya fever, develops. Symptomatology is highly variable. Some patients have very mild symptoms. Others may have high fevers, headache, and arthralgias. Severe hemolytic anemia can develop, sometimes with leukopenia, and thrombocytopenia. Untreated, the fatality rate is 40–88%, and with antibiotic treatment is still 8%. After the acute infection resolves, a latency period follows, lasting from weeks to months. The eruptive verruga peruana then occur. They are angiomatous, pyogenic granuloma-like lesions, virtually identical clinically and histologically to the lesions of bacillary angiomatosis (Fig. 14-44). They may be large and few in number (mular form), small and disseminated (miliary form), or nodular and deep. Visceral disease has not been found in verruga peruana, which is rarely fatal. Lesions usually heal spontaneously over several weeks to months without scarring. A lasting immunity results from infection.

The diagnosis of Oroya fever is made by identifying the bacteria within or attached to circulating erythrocytes using a Giemsa stain. Verruga peruana can be diagnosed by skin biopsy, showing the same features as bacillary angiomatosis, but with the organisms staining with Giemsa stain.

The antibiotic treatment of choice for Oroya fever is chloramphenicol, 2 g/day, since *Salmonella* coinfection is the most

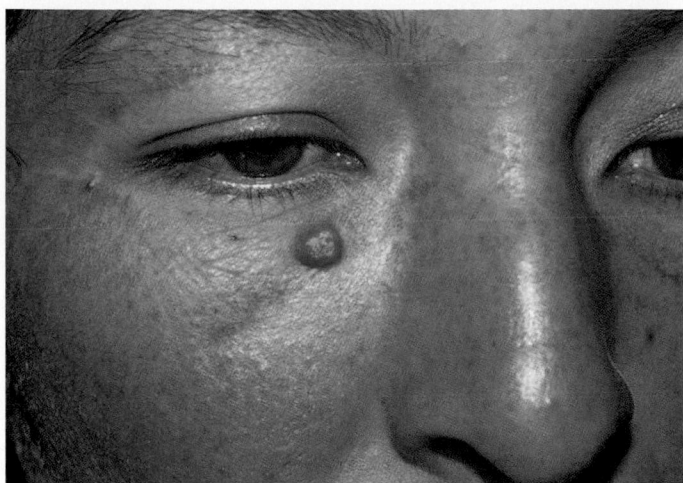

Fig. 14-44 Verruga peruana. (Courtesy of Francisco Bravo, MD)

frequent cause of death. Protection from sandfly bites is all-important.

Brouqui P, et al: Arthropod-borne diseases in homeless. Ann N Y Acad Sci 2006; 1078:223.
Chen TC, et al: Cat scratch disease from a domestic dog. J Formos Med Assoc 2007; 106:S65.
Florin TA, et al: Beyond cat scratch disease. Pediatrics 2008; 121:e1413.
Grilo N, et al: Cutaneous bacillary angiomatosis. S Afr Med J 2009; 99:220.
Guibal F, et al: High seroprevalence to *Bartonella quintana* in homeless patients with cutaneous parasitic infestations in downtown Paris. J Am Acad Dermatol 2001; 44:219.
Kempf VA, et al: Evidence of a leading role for VEGF in *Bartonella henselae*-induced endothelial proliferations. Cell Microbiol 2001; 3:623.
Maguina C, et al: Bartonellosis. Clin Dermatol 2009; 27:271.
Petersen K, et al: Bacillary angiomatosis in a patient with chronic lymphocytic leukemia. Infection 2008; 36:480.
Raoult D: From cat scratch disease to *Bartonella henselae* infection. CID 2007; 45:1541.

Plague

Plague normally involves an interaction among *Yersinia pestis*, wild rodents, and fleas parasitic on the rodents. Infection in humans with *Y. pestis* is accidental and usually presents as bubonic plague. Other clinical forms include pneumonic and septicemic plague.

In the milder form, the initial manifestations are general malaise, fever, and pain or tenderness in areas of regional lymph nodes, most often in the inguinal or axillary regions. In more severe infections, findings of toxicity, prostration, shock, and, occasionally, hemorrhagic phenomena prevail. Less common symptoms include abdominal pain, nausea, vomiting, constipation followed by diarrhea, generalized macular erythema, and petechiae. Rarely, vesicular and pustular skin lesions occur.

Plague is caused by *Y. pestis*, a pleomorphic, Gram-negative bacillus. The principal animal hosts involved have been rock squirrels, prairie dogs, chipmunks, marmots, skunks, deer mice, wood rats, rabbits, and hares. Transmission occurs through contact with infected rodent fleas or rodents, pneumonic spread, or infected exudates. *Xenopsylla cheopis* (Oriental rat flea) has traditionally been considered the vector in human outbreaks, but *Diamanus montanus*, *Thrassis bacchi*, and *Opisocrostis hirsutus* are species of fleas on wild animals responsible for spreading sylvatic plague in the US. Rodents carried home by dogs or cats are a potential source—and an important one in veterinarians—of infection. The bites,

scratches, or contact with other infectious material while handling infected cats are an increasing risk factor as residential development continues in areas of plague foci in the western US. In the US, 89% of cases since 1945 have occurred in the Rocky Mountain states.

Blood, bubo or parabubo aspirates, exudates, and sputum should be examined by smears stained with Gram stain or specific fluorescent antibody techniques, culture, and animal inoculation. A retrospective diagnosis can be made by serologic analysis.

The most effective drugs against *Y. pestis* are gentamicin and streptomycin; they should be given intravenously. Other effective drugs include chloramphenicol, the tetracyclines, and ciprofloxacin. Nearly all cases are fatal if not treated promptly.

Josko D: *Yersinia pestis*. Clin Lab Sci 2004; 17:25.
Lieberman JM: North American zoonoses. Pediatr Ann 2009; 38:193.
Meffert JJ: Biological warfare from a dermatologic perspective. Curr Allergy Asthma Rep 2003; 3:304.
Prentice MB, et al: Plague. Lancet 2007; 369:1196.

Rat-bite fever

This febrile, systemic illness is usually acquired by direct contact with rats or other small rodents, which carry the Gram-negative organisms *Spirillum minor* and *Streptobacillus moniliformis* among their oropharyngeal flora. *S. moniliformis* is the principal cause in the US. Crowded living conditions, homelessness, working with rats in medical research or in pet shops, or having one as a pet are predisposing factors in some infected patients. Although it usually follows a rat bite, infection may follow the bites of squirrels, cats, weasels, pigs, and a variety of other carnivores that feed on rats.

There are at least two distinct forms of rat-bite fever: "sodoku," caused by *S. minor*; and septicemia, caused by *S. moniliformis*, otherwise known as epidemic arthritic erythema or Haverhill fever. The latter usually follows the bite of a rat, but some cases have been caused by contaminated milk. The clinical manifestations of these two infections are similar in that both produce a systemic illness characterized by fever, rash, and constitutional symptoms. However, clinical differentiation is possible.

In the streptobacillary form, incubation is brief, usually lasting 10 days after the bite, when chills and fever occur. Within 2–4 more days the generalized morbilliform eruption appears and spreads to include the palms and soles. It may become petechial. Arthralgia is prominent, and pleural effusion may occur. Endocarditis, pneumonia, and septic infarcts often follow, and 10% of untreated cases may die from these causes.

Although infection with *S. minor* also begins abruptly with chills and fever, the incubation period is longer, ranging from 1 to 4 weeks. The bite site is often inflamed and may become ulcerated. Lymphangitis may be present. The eruption begins with erythematous macules on the abdomen, resembling rose spots, which enlarge, become purplish-red, and form extensive indurated plaques. Arthritis may rarely occur. Endocarditis, nephritis, meningitis, and hepatitis are potential complications. Around 6% of untreated patients die.

In both types of disease a leukocytosis of 15000–30000/mm^3 is present, sometimes with eosinophilia. A biologic false-positive venereal disease research laboratory (VDRL) test is found in 25–50% of cases. The course without treatment is generally from 1 to 2 weeks, though relapses may occur for months.

The diagnosis is confirmed by culturing the causative organism from the blood or joint aspirate, or demonstration of an antibody response in the streptobacillary form. *S. minor* is demonstrable by animal inoculation with the patient's blood, usually in the guinea pig or mouse. Their blood will show large numbers of organisms in Wright-stained smears. Demonstration of *S. minor* in a darkfield preparation of exudate from an infected site establishes the diagnosis.

Rat-bite fever must be differentiated from erysipelas, pyogenic cellulitis, viral exanthems, gonococcemia, meningococcemia, and Rocky Mountain spotted fever.

Prompt cauterization of bites by nitric acid may prevent the disease. Cleansing of the wound, tetanus prophylaxis, and 3 days of penicillin (2 g/day) are recommended for patients seen shortly after a bite. Both types respond readily to penicillin, tetracycline, or streptomycin therapy.

Cunningham BB, et al: Rat bite fever. J Am Acad Dermatol 1998; 38:330.
Gaastra W, et al: Rat bite fever. J Vet Microbiol 2009; 133:211.
Lieberman JM: North American zoonoses. Pediatr Ann 2009; 38:193.

Tularemia

Tularemia, also known as Ohara's disease or deer fly fever, is a febrile disease caused by *Francisella tularensis*, a short, nonmotile, non-spore-forming, Gram-negative coccobacillus. Tularemia is characterized by sudden onset, with chills, headache, and leukocytosis, after an incubation period of 2–7 days. Its clinical course is divided into several general types. The causative organism poses a bioterrorism threat.

The vast majority are the ulceroglandular type, which begins with a primary papule or nodule that rapidly ulcerates at the site of infection. This usually occurs through contact with tissues or body fluid of infected mammals, via an abrasion or scratch (Fig. 14-45), usually on the fingers, neck, or conjunctiva. The bites of a tick, *Dermacentor andersoni* or *Amblyomma americanum*, and of a deer fly, *Chrysops discalis*, also transmit this disease, and in such cases primary lesions are usually found on the legs or the perineum. The primary ulcer is tender, firm, indolent, and punched out, with a necrotic base that heals with scar formation in about 6 weeks. A lymphangitis spreads from the primary lesion; the regional lymph glands become swollen, painful, and inflamed, and tend to break down, forming subcutaneous suppurative nodules resembling those of sporotrichosis. The ulcers extend in a chain from the ulcer to the enlarged lymphatic glands.

The course of the ulceroglandular type is marked in the early stages by headache, anorexia, and vomiting, and by articular and muscular pains. The fever is at first continuous, varying between 102 and 104°F, and later shows morning remissions, then falls by lysis to normal. Other skin lesions are encountered in the course of the disease, which are in no way characteristic and are probably of a toxic nature. A macular, papular, vesicular, or petechial exanthem may occur. Erythema multiforme and erythema nodosum often occur. The clinical similarity of the primary ulcer of tularemia to a chancre of sporotrichosis is important in the differential diagnosis.

In the typhoidal type the site of inoculation is not known and there is no local sore or adenopathy. This form of the disease is characterized by persistent fever, malaise, gastrointestinal symptoms, and the presence of specific agglutinins in the blood serum after the first week.

Other uncommon types include an oculoglandular form, in which primary conjunctivitis is accompanied by enlargement of the regional lymph nodes; the pneumonic type, which occurs rarely in laboratory workers and is most severe; the oropharyngeal form, which may occur after ingestion of infected and inadequately cooked meat; and the glandular type, in which there is no primary lesion at the site of infection, but there is enlargement of regional lymph glands followed by generalized involvement. Several cases, mostly in children, have been acquired from cat bites, the cats having previously bitten infected rabbits.

The most frequent sources of human infection are the handling of wild rabbits and the bite of deer flies or ticks. Outbreaks of the disease occur chiefly at those times of the year when contact with these sources of infection is likely. No instance of the spread of the infection from person to person by contact has been reported. The disease occurs most often in the western and southern US, although cases have been reported in almost all parts of the US and in Japan. In Russia and other countries in the northern hemisphere it may be contracted from polluted water contaminated by infected rodent carcasses.

A definite diagnosis is made by staining smears obtained from the exudate with specific fluorescent antibody. *F. tularensis* can be cultured only on special media containing cystine glucose blood agar or other selective media. Routine culture media do not support growth. The bacilli can be identified by inoculating guinea pigs intraperitoneally with sputum or with bronchial or gastric washings, exudate from draining lymph nodes, or blood. The agglutination titer becomes positive in the majority of patients after 2 weeks of illness. A four-fold rise in titer is diagnostic; a single convalescent titer of 1:160 or greater is diagnostic of past or current infection. PCR is also successful in identifying the infectious agent.

The main histologic feature of tularemia is that of a granuloma; the tissue reaction consists primarily of a massing of endothelial cells and the formation of giant cells. Central necrosis and liquefaction occur, accompanied by polymorphonuclear leukocytic infiltration. Surrounding this is a tuberculoid granulomatous zone, and peripherally lymphocytes form a third zone. Small secondary lesions may develop. These pass through the same stages and tend to fuse with the primary one.

All butchers, hunters, cooks, and others who dress rabbits should wear protective gloves when doing so. Thorough cooking destroys the infection in a rabbit, thus rendering an infected animal harmless as food. Ticks should be removed promptly, and tick repellents may be of value for people with occupations that require frequent exposure to them.

Streptomycin, 1 g intramuscularly every 12 h for 10 days, is the treatment of choice. Obvious clinical improvement occurs after 48 h, although the fever may persist for as long as a week after treatment is begun. Gentamicin is also effective, but the tetracyclines are useful only if given in high doses for 15 days. In vitro testing and numerous case reports and small case series are documenting the excellent effects of the quinolones, especially ciprofloxacin, 500–750 mg twice a day for 10 days, or levofloxacin, 500 mg/day for 2 weeks.

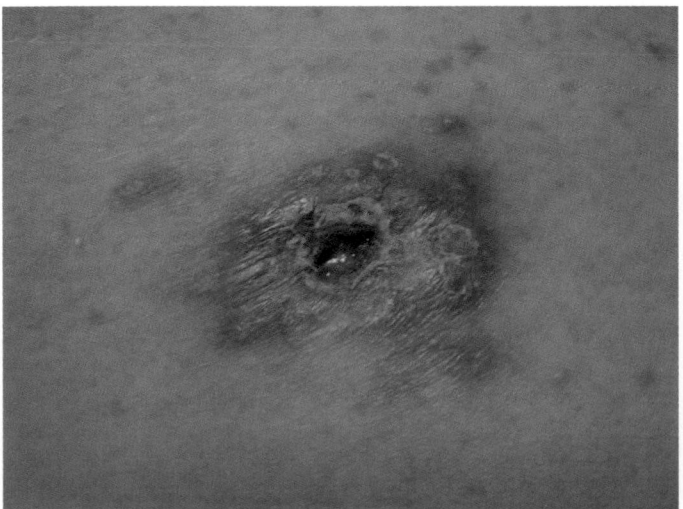

Fig. 14-45 Tularemia. (Courtesy of Steve Hess, MD)

Anonymous: Tularemia—Missouri, 2000–2007. MMWR 2009; 58:744.
Byington CL, et al: Tularemia with vesicular skin lesions may be mistaken for infection with herpes viruses. Clin Infect Dis 2008; 47:e4.
McGinley-Smith DE, et al: Dermatoses from ticks. J Am Acad Dermatol 2003; 49:363.
McGovern TW, et al: Cutaneous manifestations of biological warfare and related threat agents. Arch Dermatol 1999; 135:311.
Nigrovic LE, et al: Tularemia. Infect Dis Clin North Am 2008; 22:489.
Sjostedt A: Tularemia. Ann N Y Acad Sci 2007; 1105:1.

Brucellosis

Brucellosis is also known as undulant fever. Brucellae are Gram-negative rods that produce an acute febrile illness with headache, or at times an indolent chronic disease characterized by weakness, malaise, and low-grade fever. Brucellosis is acquired primarily by contact with infected animals or animal products. Primarily, workers in the meat-packing industry are at risk; however, veterinarians, pet owners, and travelers who consume unpasteurized milk or cheese may also acquire the disease.

Approximately 5–10% of patients develop skin lesions. The variety of cutaneous manifestations reported is large. Erythematous papules, diffuse erythema, abscesses, erysipelas-like lesions, leukocytoclastic vasculitis, thrombocytopenic purpura, Stevens–Johnson syndrome, and erythema nodosum-like lesions are some possible findings. Biopsy may reveal noncaseating granulomas.

Diagnosis is by culture of blood, bone marrow, or granulomas, and may be confirmed by a rising serum enzyme-linked immunosorbent assay (ELISA) or agglutination titer. PCR is available as well. Treatment is with doxycycline and streptomycin in combination for 6 weeks.

Franco MP, et al: Human brucellosis infection. Lancet Infect Dis 2007; 19:1.
Glynn MK, et al: Brucellosis. J Am Vet Med Assoc 2008; 233:900.
Metin A, et al: Cutaneous findings encountered in brucellosis and review of the literature. Int J Dermatol 2001; 40:434.
Pappas G, et al: Brucellosis. New Engl J Med 2005; 352:2325.

RICKETTSIAL DISEASES

Rickettsiae are obligate, intracellular, Gram-negative bacteria. The natural reservoirs of these organisms are the blood-sucking arthropods; when transmitted to humans through insect inoculation, the rickettsiae may produce disease. Most of the human diseases incurred are characterized by skin eruptions, fever, headache, malaise, and prostration. Diagnosis is usually made by indirect fluorescence antibody testing, which may be confirmed by Western blot or PCR; therapy is with doxycycline, 100 mg twice a day for 7 days. In addition to those diseases discussed in the following sections, Q fever, caused by *Coxiella burnetii*, is an acute, febrile illness from this general class that uncommonly has skin manifestations, but these are nonspecific and nondiagnostic in nature.

Typhus group

Louse-borne epidemic typhus, caused by *Rickettsia prowazekii*, mouse, cat, or rat flea-borne endemic typhus, caused by *Rickettsia typhi*, and scrub typhus, a mite-borne infection caused by *Rickettsia tsutsugamushi*, constitute this group.

Epidemic typhus

Humans contract epidemic typhus from an infestation by body lice (*Pediculus humanus* var. *corporis*), which harbor the rickettsiae. *R. prowazekii* is not transmitted transovarially, since it kills the louse 1–3 weeks after infection. For many years humans were the only known vector, but several cases of sporadic disease have been reported in which there was direct or indirect contact with the flying squirrel, and a reservoir apparently exists in this animal. While the louse feeds on the person's skin, it defecates. The organisms in the feces are scratched into the skin. Some 2 weeks after infection the prodromal symptoms of chills, fever, aches, and pains appear. After 5 days a pink macular eruption appears on the trunk and axillary folds and rapidly spreads to the rest of the body, but usually spares the face, palms, and soles. These macules may later become hemorrhagic, and gangrene of the fingers, toes, nose, and earlobes may occur. Mortality is 6–30% in epidemics, with the highest death and complication rates occurring in patients over the age of 60.

Serologic testing using immunofluorescent antibody (IFA) and Western blot for specificity becomes positive after the 8th–12th day of illness.

Doxycycline, 100 mg twice a day for 7 days, is curative. Prophylaxis is by vaccination and delousing; people who succumb are usually living under miserable sanitary conditions such as occur during war and following natural disasters. Vaccination is suggested only for special high-risk groups.

Brill–Zinsser disease may occur as a recrudescence of previous infection, with a similar but milder course of illness, which more closely resembles endemic typhus.

Endemic typhus

Endemic (murine) typhus is a natural infection of rats and mice by *R. typhi*, sporadically transmitted to humans by the rat flea, *Xenopsylla cheopis*. In south Texas, the disease is transmitted by the cat flea *Ctenocephalides felis*, with opposums as the natural reservoir of disease. It has the same skin manifestations as epidemic typhus (Fig. 14-46), but they are less severe, and gangrene does not supervene. Approximately 50% of patients with murine typhus had a skin eruption. Serologic testing using IFA and Western blot for specificity becomes positive in 50% of patients at 1 week and nearly all by 2 weeks. Fever and severe headache are suggestive early symptoms.

This disease occurs worldwide. In the US, the southeastern states and those bordering the Gulf of Mexico have been the most common sites of incidence. It most often occurs in urban settings, with peak incidence in the summer and fall.

Treatment is the same as that for louse-borne (epidemic) typhus.

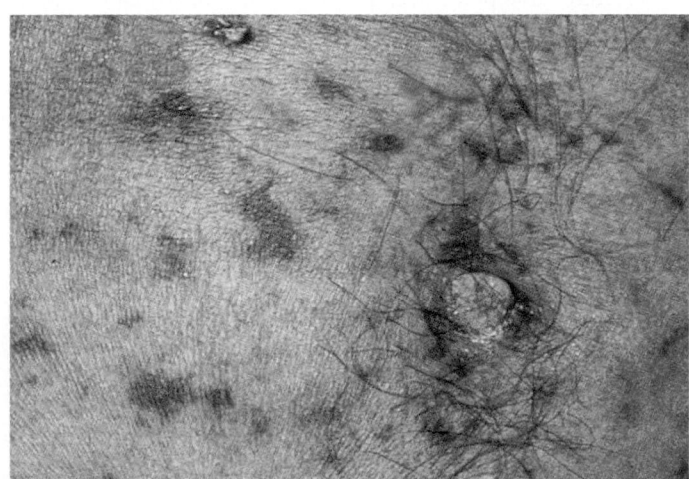

Fig. 14-46 Endemic typhus. (Courtesy of Richard DeVillez, MD)

Scrub typhus

Also known as tsutsugamushi fever, scrub typhus is characterized by fever, chills, intense headache, skin lesions, and pneumonitis. The primary lesion is an erythematous papule at the site of a mite bite, most commonly on the scrotum, groin, or ankle. It becomes indurated, and a multilocular vesicle rests on top of the papule. Eventually, a necrotic ulcer with eschar and surrounding indurated erythema develops and there is regional lymphadenopathy. Some 10 days after a mite bite, fever, chills, and prostration develop, and within 5 days thereafter pneumonitis and the skin eruption evolve. The erythematous macular eruption begins on the trunk, extends peripherally, and fades in a few days. Deafness and tinnitus occur in about one-fifth of untreated cases.

Scrub typhus is caused by *R. tsutsugamushi*. The vector is the trombiculid red mite (chigger), which infests wild rodents in scrub or secondary vegetation in transitional terrain between forests and clearings in Far Eastern countries such as Japan, Korea, Southeast Asia, and Australia.

Serologic diagnosis and treatment are as for other forms of rickettsias; however, in areas of the world where there is reduced susceptibility to tetracyclines, such as Thailand, rifampin is more reliable.

Spotted fever group

This group includes Rocky Mountain spotted fever, caused by *R. rickettsii*; Mediterranean (boutonneuse) fever, which when seen in Africa has been called Kenyan or South African tick-bite fever, caused by *Rickettsia conorii*; North Asian tick-borne rickettsiosis, caused by *Rickettsia sibirica*; Queensland tick typhus, caused by *Rickettsia australis*; African tick-bite fever, caused by *Rickettsia africae*; Flinders Island spotted fever, caused by *Rickettsia honei*; Yucatan spotted fever, caused by *Rickettsia felis* carried by the cat flea vector *Ctenocephalides felis*; Japanese spotted fever, caused by *Rickettsia japonica*; a spotted fever in the US caused by *Rickettsia parkeri*; and Russian vesicular rickettsiosis, caused by *Rickettsia akari*. Additionally, tick-borne lymphadenopathy (TIBOLA) and *Dermacentor*-borne necrosis–eschar–lymphadenopathy (DEBONEL) are linked to a disease transmitted by the *Dermacentor* tick; they have distinctive features. The tick usually attaches to the scalp, and will cause an eschar and sometimes alopecia. Adenopathy, fever, and a spotted eruption occur.

Only the first two types of spotted fever will be discussed in detail. They all are characterized by headache, fever, and a rash, the latter most frequently being a pink papular eruption, which may have petechiae, and in the case of African tick-bite fever, eschars. All are treated with doxycycline, 100 mg twice a day for 7 days. Most respond well and complications are minimal. Ticks are the vectors of all but the Yucatan spotted fever. Tick prevention strategies are outlined in Chapter 20.

Rocky Mountain spotted fever

One to 2 weeks after the tick bite, chills, fever, and weakness occur. An eruption appears, but unlike typhus it begins on the ankles, wrists, and forehead rather than on the trunk. The initial lesions are small, red macules, which blanch on pressure and rapidly become papular in untreated patients. Spread to the trunk occurs over 6–18 h, and the lesions become petechial and hemorrhagic over a period of 2–4 days (Fig. 14-47).

A vasculitis of the skin is the pathologic process, and *R. rickettsii* can be found in these initial macules by applying a fluorescent antibody technique to frozen sections. This is a very specific, but not very sensitive, method.

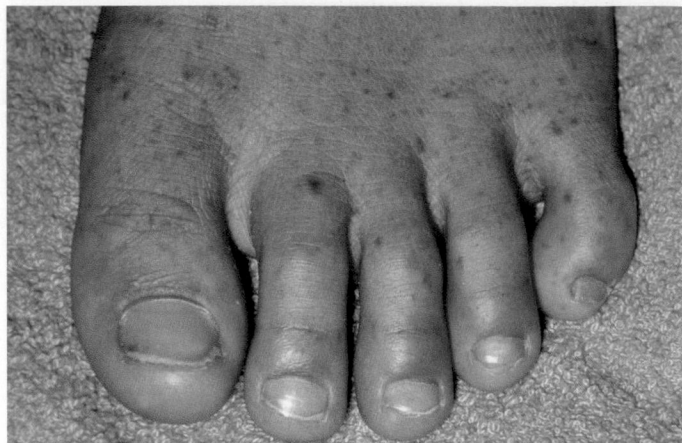

Fig. 14-47 Rocky Mountain spotted fever.

In the 10–20% of cases without a rash, the risk of a delay in diagnosis and a fatal outcome is greatest, with the case fatality rate rising precipitously if antibiotics are not initiated before the fifth day. An eschar will occasionally be present at the tick bite site and is a subtle clue to the diagnosis. In severe untreated cases a multisystem disorder appears, with renal, pulmonary, and central and peripheral nervous system abnormalities, and hepatomegaly most commonly found. Mortality in older persons approaches 60%; it is far lower in younger patients.

Ticks spread the causative organism, *R. rickettsii*. Principal offenders are the wood tick (*Dermacentor andersoni*), the dog tick (*D. variabilis* and *R. sanguineus* in Arizona), and the Lone Star tick (*Amblyomma americanum*).

Antibodies become positive in the second or third week of illness, too late to be of help when the decision to institute therapy is necessary. This decision is made by clinical considerations. A clue may be the recent illness of a pet dog, as *R. rickettsii* will cause symptomatic illness in infected dogs.

Treatment is with doxycycline, 100 mg twice a day for 7 days.

Mediterranean spotted fever

Boutonneuse fever, or Mediterranean fever, is an acute febrile disease endemic in southern Europe and northern Africa, and is the prototype of the spotted fever group of diseases. It affects children mostly and is characterized by a sudden onset with chills, high fever, headache, and lassitude. The tick bite produces a small, indurated papule known as tache noire, which becomes a necrotic ulcer (Fig. 14-48). The erythematous macular and papular eruption develops on the trunk (Fig. 14-49), palms, and soles.

The causative organism is *R. conorii*, transmitted by the dog tick, *Rhipicephalus sanguineus*.

As with all rickettsial diseases, the diagnosis is confirmed with serology and treatment is with doxycycline. Even without therapy the prognosis is good, and complications are rare.

Rickettsialpox

First recognized in New York in 1946, rickettsialpox has been found in other cities of the US and in Russia. It is an acute febrile disease characterized by the appearance of an initial lesion at the site of the mite bite about a week before the onset of the fever. This firm, 5–15 mm round or oval vesicle persists for 3–4 weeks and heals with a small pigmented scar. Regional lymphadenitis is present. The fever is remittent and lasts about

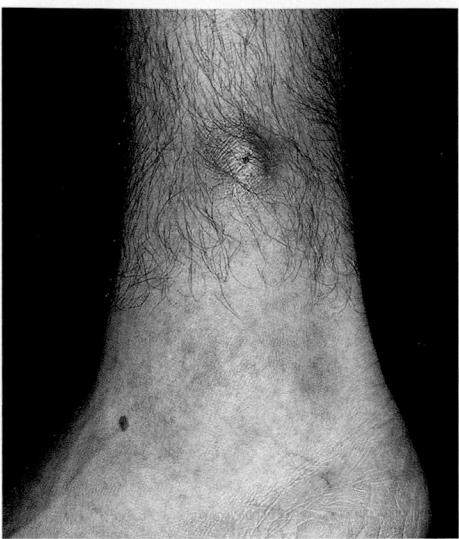

Fig. 14-48 Tache noire in boutonneuse fever.

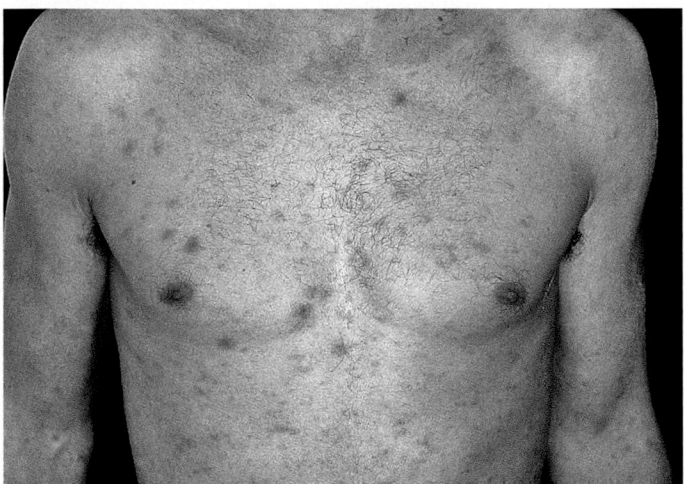

Fig. 14-49 Boutonneuse fever.

5 days. Chills, sweats, headache, and backache accompany the fever. A rash resembling varicella develops 3 or 4 days after the onset of fever. This secondary eruption is papulovesicular, numbers approximately 5–50 lesions, and is generalized in distribution. It fades in about 1 week.

The rodent mite, *Allodermanyssus* (*Liponyssoides*) *sanguineus*, transmits the causative organism, *Rickettsia akari*. The house mouse (*Mus musculus*) is the reservoir. All cases have occurred in neighborhoods infested by mice, on which the rodent mite has been found.

Diagnosis is confirmed by serologic testing. The disease is self-limited, and complete involution occurs in at most 2 weeks. Doxycycline is the agent of choice for treatment.

Bechah Y, et al: Epidemic typhus. Lancet Infect Dis 2008; 8:417.
Cazorla C, et al: Tick-borne diseases. Infect Dis Clin North Am 2008; 22:531.
Chen LF, et al: What's new in Rocky Mountain spotted fever? Infect Dis Clin North Am 2008; 22:515.
Civen R, et al: Murine typhus. Clin Infect Dis 2008; 46:913.
Cragun WC, et al: The expanding spectrum of eschar-associated rickettsioses in the United States. Arch Dermatol 2010; 146:641.
Dantas-Torres F: Rocky Mountain spotted fever. Lancet Infect Dis 2007; 7:724.
Demma LJ, et al: Rocky Mountain spotted fever from an unexpected tick vector in Arizona. New Engl J Med 2005; 353:587.
Elston DM: Tick bites and skin rashes. Curr Opin Infec Dis 2010; 23:132.

Koss T, et al: Increased detection of rickettsialpox in a New York City hospital following the anthrax outbreak of 2001. Arch Dermatol 2003; 139:1545.
Lutwick LI: Brill–Zinsser disease. Lancet 2001; 357:1198.
Nachega JB, et al: Travel-acquired scrub typhus. J Travel Med 2007; 14:352.
Panpanich R, et al: Antibiotics for treating scrub typhus. Cochrane Database Syst Rev 2002; 3:CD002150.
Paddock CD, et al: *Rickettsia parkeri*: a newly recognized cause of spotted fever rickettsiosis in the United States. Clin Infect Dis 2004; 38:805.
Rovery C, et al: Mediterranean spotted fever. Infect Dis Clin N Am 2008; 22:515.
Saini R, et al: Rickettsialpox: a report of three cases and a review of the literature. J Am Acad Dermatol 2004; 51:S65.
Schuster J, et al: African tick bite fever. J Dtsch Dermatol Ges 2008; 6:379.
Walker DH: Rickettsiae and rickettsial infections. Clin Infec Dis 2007; 45:S39.
Walker DH, et al: Emerging and re-emerging tick-transmitted rickettsial and ehrlichial infections. Med Clin North Am 2008; 92:1345.

Ehrlichiosis

These tick-borne organisms, which affect phagocytic cells, manifest as a febrile illness accompanied by headache and a rash. Human monocytic erhlichiosis (HME) is caused by *Ehrlichia chaffeensis*; human granulocytic anaplasmosis (HGA) by *Anaplasma phagocytophilia* groups; Sennetsu fever, a mononucleosis-type illness, by *Ehrlichia sennetsu*; and *Ehrlichia ewingii* also occasionally produces a similar symptomatic illness.

HME is transmitted by *Amblyomma americanum* or *Dermacentor variabilis*. It is most common in men between the ages of 30 and 60. The predominant regions reporting the disease are the south central, southeastern, and mid-Atlantic states. The same *Ixodes* ticks that transmit Lyme disease and babesiosis transmit HGA, and the infection occurs in the same geographic areas, the northeast and Pacific northwestern US. Coinfection with these agents occurs.

Skin eruptions are present in only about one-third of patients with HME and 10% of those with HGA. The lesions are usually present on the trunk and are nondiagnostic. A mottled or diffuse erythema, a fine petechial eruption, lower extremity vasculitis, and a macular, papular, vesicular, or urticarial morphology have all been seen. Acral edema with desquamation and petechiae of the palate may be present. Involvement of the kidneys, lungs, and CNS occurs in severe cases.

If the diagnosis is suspected, a complete blood count will usually show thrombocytopenia and leukopenia. The leukocytes should be inspected microscopically for intracytoplasmic microcolonies called morulae. They are seen more frequently in HGA than in HME. Indirect immunofluorescent antibodies and the PCR analysis are positive, but asymptomatic infection is frequent and seroprevalence rates are high in endemic areas. Culture of the organism is diagnostic. Doxycycline is the treatment of choice, 100 mg twice a day for 7 days. Severe life-threatening disease is usually seen in the immunosuppressed population.

Bakken JS, et al: Clinical diagnosis and treatment of human granulocytotropic anaplasmosis. Ann N Y Acad Sci 2006; 1078:236.
Ganguly S, et al: Tick-borne ehrlichiosis infection in human beings. J Vector Borne Dis 2008; 45:273.
Ismail N, et al: Human ehrlichiosis and anaplasmosis. Clin Lab Med 2010; 30:261.
McGinley-Smith DE, et al: Dermatoses from ticks. J Am Acad Dermatol 2003; 49:363.
Openshaw JJ, et al: Human ehrlichiosis. South J Med 2007; 100:769.

Leptospirosis

Leptospirosis is also known as Weil's disease, pretibial fever, and Fort Bragg fever. It is a systemic disease caused by many strains of the genus *Leptospira*. After an incubation period of 8–12 days, Weil's disease (icteric leptospirosis) starts with an abrupt onset of chills, followed by high fever, intense jaundice, petechiae, and purpura on both skin and mucous membranes, and renal disease, manifested by proteinuria, hematuria, and azotemia. Death may occur in 5–10% of cases, as a result of renal failure, vascular collapse, or hemorrhage. Leukocytosis of 15 000–30 000/mm³ and lymphocytosis in the spinal fluid are commonly present.

Pretibial fever ("Fort Bragg fever," anicteric leptospirosis) has an associated acute exanthematous infectious erythema, generally most marked on the shins. High fever, conjunctival suffusion, nausea, vomiting, and headache characterize the septicemic first stage. This lasts 3–7 days, followed by a 1–3-day absence of fever. During the second stage, when IgM antibody develops, headache is intense, fever returns, and ocular manifestations, such as conjunctival hemorrhage and suffusion, ocular pain, and photophobia, are prominent. At this time the eruption occurs. It consists of 1–5 cm erythematous patches or plaques that histologically show only edema and nonspecific perivascular infiltrate. The skin lesions resolve spontaneously after 4–7 days. There may be different clinical manifestations from identical strains of *Leptospira*.

Leptospira interrogans, serotype *icterohaemorrhagiae*, has been the most common cause of Weil's disease, whereas pretibial fever is most commonly associated with serotype *autumnalis*. Humans acquire both types accidentally from urine or tissues of infected animals, or indirectly from contaminated soil or from drinking or swimming in contaminated water. Travelers to the tropics who enjoy water sports are at risk. In the continental US, dogs and cats are the most common animal source; worldwide, rats are more often responsible. Leptospira enter the body through abraded or diseased skin, and the gastrointestinal or upper respiratory tract.

Leptospirosis may be diagnosed by finding the causative spirochetes in the blood by darkfield microscopy during the first week of illness, and by blood cultures, guinea pig inoculation, and the demonstration of rising antibodies during the second week of the disease. The microagglutination serologic test is the test of choice, but PCR and ELISA testing are also available.

Treatment with tetracyclines and penicillin shortens the disease duration if given early. Doxycycline, 100 mg/day for a week, is effective in mild disease; however, intravenous penicillin is necessary in severely affected patients. A dose of 200 mg once a week may help prevent infection while visiting a hyperendemic area.

Brett-Major DM, et al: Antibiotic prophylaxis for leptospirosis. Cochrane Database Syst Rev 2009: CD007342.
Buharti AR, et al: Leptospirosis. Lancet Infect Dis 2003; 3:757.
Guerra MA: Leptospirosis. J Am Vet Med Assoc 2009; 234:472.
Phraisuwan P, et al: Leptospirosis. Emerg Infect Dis 2002; 8:1455.

Borreliosis

Spirochetes of the genus *Borrelia* are the cause of Lyme disease. This multisystem infection first presents with skin findings and over the course of time multiple cutaneous signs may occur. These microorganisms are also the cause of relapsing fever, an acute illness characterized by paroxysms of fever. The more common type of relapsing fever is tick-borne, occasionally being reported in the US. A louse-borne type is endemic only in Ethiopia. The nonspecific macular or petechial eruption occurs near the end of the 3–5-day febrile crisis.

Lyme disease

Borrelia burgdorferi sensu lato species complex are responsible for inducing Lyme disease. These spirochetes are transmitted to humans by various members of the family of hard ticks, Ixodidae. Four genomic subspecies are recognized to be geographically prominent and cause varying skin and systemic disease manifestations. *Borrelia burgdorferi sensu stricto* causes Lyme disease in the northeast, midwest, and western US, and *Borrelia lonestari* causes disease in the southern US where the only skin finding is the diagnostic early manifestation, erythema migrans. *Borrelia lonestari* is the cause of STARI (Masters disease), a condition characterized by erythema migrans, headache, stiff neck, myalgia, and arthralgia. *Borrelia garinii* and *Borrelia afzelii* are present in Europe, with the former being the principle agent of Lyme neuroborreliosis and the latter associated with acrodermatitis chronica atrophicans, lymphocytoma, and, in some cases, morphea and lichen sclerosis et atrophicus. If it is not treated in the early stage, chronic arthritis and neurologic and cardiac complications frequently develop.

Diagnosing early Lyme disease depends on recognition of the skin eruption. Approximately 50% of patients recall a tick bite, which leaves a small red macule or papule at the site. The areas most often involved are the legs, groins, and axilla, with adults having lower-extremity lesions most often and children being more likely to manifest erythema migrans on the trunk. Between 3 and 32 (median 7) days after the bite, there is gradual expansion of the redness around the papule (Fig. 14-50A). The advancing border is usually slightly raised, warm, red to bluish-red, and free of any scale. Centrally, the site of the bite may clear, leaving only a ring of peripheral erythema, or it may remain red, becoming indurated, vesicular, or necrotic. In Europe, the large annular variety is most common, while in the US the lesions are usually homogenous or have a central redness. The annular erythema usually grows to a median diameter of 15 cm, but may range from 3 to 68 cm (Fig. 14-50B). It is accompanied by a burning sensation in half the patients; rarely is it pruritic or painful. Localized alopecia may result at the site of erythema migrans.

Between 25% and 50% of patients will develop multiple secondary annular lesions, similar in appearance to the primary lesion, but without indurated centers and generally of smaller size (Fig. 14-51). They spare the palms and soles. Their number ranges from 2 to 100. Without treatment, erythema migrans and the secondary lesions fade in a median of 28 days, although some may be present for months. Of untreated cases, 10% experience recurrences of erythema migrans over the following months. European cases of *Borrelia*-induced lymphocytoma occur early in general, from the time of erythema migrans until 10 months later. These are B-cell proliferations and present as red, indurated papules and plaques, which occur most commonly on the areola or earlobe.

Diffuse urticaria, malar erythema, and conjunctivitis may be present during this early period. Malaise, fever, fatigue, headaches, stiff neck, arthralgia, myalgia, lymphadenopathy, anorexia, and nausea and vomiting may accompany early signs and symptoms of infection. Usually the symptoms are of mild severity, mimicking a slight flu-like illness, except in patients coinfected with babesiosis, as is the case in approximately 10% of cases in southern New England. *Ehrlichia* coinfections may also occur, as the latter two diseases are also tick-transmitted infections.

Around 10% of untreated patients eventually develop a chronic arthritis of the knees, which in half of these leads to

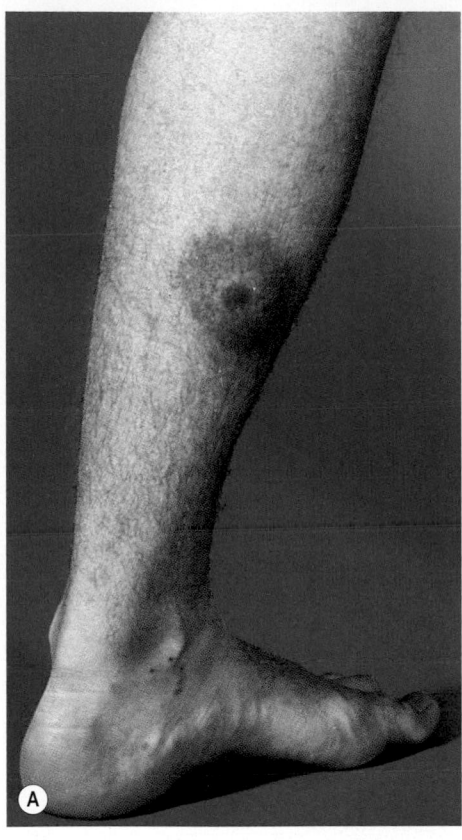

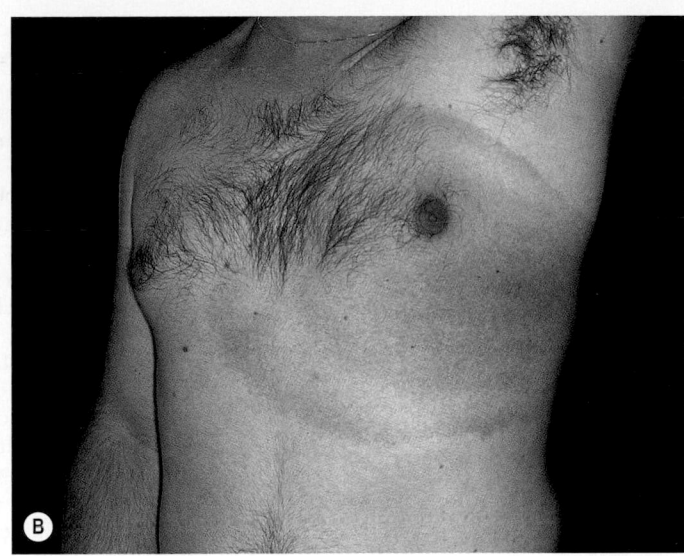

Fig. 14-50 A and B, Erythema migrans.

severe disability. Cardiac involvement occurs most often in young men, with fluctuating degrees of atrioventricular block or complete heart block occurring over a brief time (3 days to 6 weeks) early in the course of the illness. Neurologic findings include stiff neck, headache, meningitis, Bell palsy, and cranial and peripheral neuropathies, and are much more commonly manifested in European cases. Nonspecific findings include an elevated sedimentation rate in 50%, and an elevated IgM level, mild anemia, and elevated liver function tests in 20%.

Males and females are equally affected, and the age range most commonly affected is 20–50. Onset of illness is generally between May and November, with more than 80% of cases in the northern hemisphere identified in June, July, or August. In the US, tick transmission of Lyme disease is by *Ixodes scapularis* in the northeast and midwest, *Ixodes pacificus* is incriminated in the west, and in the south disease is transmitted by *Amblyomma americanum*. European cases are transmitted by the tick *Ixodes ricinus*.

The different subtypes of *Borrelia* present in Europe account for the fact that the clinical illness resulting from infection is somewhat different from that seen in the US. European erythema migrans occurs more often in females. It is less likely to have multiple lesions; untreated lesions last longer; there are more laboratory abnormalities in Lyme disease; the arthritis symptoms are prominent in the US but unusual in Europe; and the neurologic manifestations differ. In Europe, infection may lead to Bannwarth syndrome, which is characterized by focal, severe, radicular pains, lymphocytic meningitis, and cranial nerve paralysis. Acrodermatitis chronica atrophicans and some cases of morphea, atrophoderma of Pasini and Pierini, anetoderma, and lichen sclerosus et atrophicus are late cutaneous sequelae of *B. afzelii* or *B. garinii* infection in Europe. Some patients with morphea-type lesions may have histopathologic features of an interstitial granulomatous dermatitis with histiocytic pseudorosettes present.

Several cases of transplacental transmission of *Borrelia*, resulting in infant death, have been reported. However, studies of Lyme disease in pregnancy have generally failed to implicate an association with fetal malformations directly.

On histologic investigation there is a superficial and deep perivascular and interstitial mixed-cell infiltrate. Lymphocytes, plasma cells, and eosinophils may be seen, the latter especially prominent when the center of the lesion is biopsied. Warthin–Starry staining may reveal spirochetes in the upper dermis.

The clinical finding of erythema migrans is the most sensitive evidence of early infection. Serologic conversion in the US is as follows: 27% when symptoms present for fewer than 7 days, 41% with symptoms for 7–14 days, and 88% with symptoms longer than 2 weeks. For this reason the diagnosis is made through recognition of erythema migrans. While culture and PCR analysis is specific, it is not sensitive and is not available in most areas. Serologic testing is then the

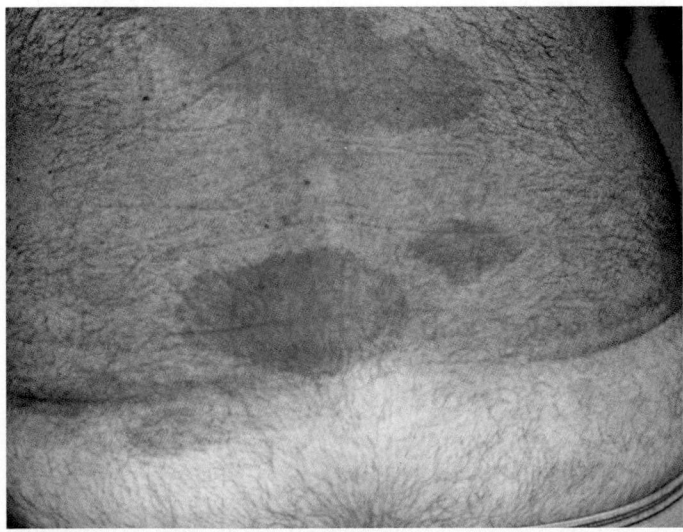

Fig. 14-51 Secondary lesions of erythema migrans.

confirmatory test. The screening examination is the ELISA. It is 89% sensitive and 72% specific, so when it is positive or indeterminate, a Western blot is used to confirm the result. False-positive tests occur in syphilis, pinta, yaws, leptospirosis, relapsing fever, infectious mononucleosis, and disease associated with autoantibody formation. The VDRL is negative in *B. burgdorferi* infection.

Treatment

The treatment of choice in adults is doxycycline, 100 mg twice a day for 10–30 days. Many authorities recommend at least 3 weeks of treatment. Amoxicillin, 500 mg twice a day for 21 days, or cefuroxime axetil, 500 mg twice a day for 21 days, is also effective. Doxycycline is also effective against *Ehrlichia* while the β-lactams are not. Children under age 9 should be treated with amoxicillin, 20 mg/kg/day in divided doses. Pregnant women with localized early Lyme disease should take amoxicillin; however, if disseminated disease is present, parenteral penicillin G or ceftriaxone is used. Immunodeficient patients may also benefit from intravenous penicillin or ceftriaxone, although the data are not robust for this recommendation.

More aggressive regimens are sometimes necessary for carditis and neurologic and arthritic involvement. For Bell palsy, first-degree heart block, and the first course of therapy for arthritis, treatment is a 28-day course of oral doxycycline or amoxicillin. For more severe manifestations in the CNS or heart and for resistant arthritis, parenteral dosing regimens are indicated.

Tick-control environmental measures and personal avoidance strategies are worthwhile when outdoor activities are planned in tick-infested areas. Inspecting for ticks after returning from outdoor activity is a good preventive measure. The tick needs to be attached for more than 24 h to transmit disease in the US. Nymphs are small; they may be hard to see. Beware of the freckle that moves. Prophylactic antibiotic therapy with one dose of 200 mg doxycycline after a known tick bite with a partially engorged *I. scapularis* in high-incidence areas is 87% effective. An effective vaccine was withdrawn from the market due to poor sales.

Acrodermatitis chronica atrophicans

Also known as primary diffuse atrophy, acrodermatitis chronica atrophicans (ACA) is characterized by the appearance on the extremities of diffuse reddish or bluish-red, paper-thin skin. The underlying blood vessels are easily seen through the epidermis. It occurs almost exclusively in Europe.

The disease begins on the backs of the hands and feet, then gradually spreads to involve the forearms, then the arms, and the lower extremities, knees and shins. Occasionally, even the trunk may become involved.

In the beginning the areas may be slightly edematous and scaly, but generally they are level with the skin and smooth. After several weeks to months the skin has a smooth, soft, thin, velvety feel and may easily be lifted into fine folds. It may have a peculiar pinkish gray color and a crumpled cigarette-paper appearance. Well-defined, smooth, edematous, bandlike thickenings develop and may extend from a finger to the elbow (ulnar bands) or develop in the skin over the shins. With progression of the disease, marked atrophy of the skin occurs.

Subcutaneous fibrous nodules may form, chiefly over the elbows, wrists, and knees. They may be single or multiple, and are firm and painless. Diffuse extensive calcification of the soft tissues may be revealed by radiographic examination. Xanthomatous tumors may occur in the skin. Hypertrophic osteoarthritis of the hands is frequently observed. Occasionally,

atrophy of the bones of the involved extremities is encountered. Ulcerations and carcinoma may supervene on the atrophic patches. The disease is slowly progressive but may remain stationary for long periods. Patches may change slightly from time to time, but complete involution never occurs.

ACA is a spirochetosis, a late sequel of infection with *Borrelia afzelii*. It is tick-transmitted by *Ixodes ricinus*. Nearly all patients with ACA have a positive test for antibodies to the spirochete, and Warthin–Starry stains demonstrate the organism in tissue in some cases. The organism has been cultured from skin lesions of ACA.

Histologically, there is marked atrophy of the epidermis and dermis without fibrosis. The elastic tissue is absent, and the cutaneous appendages are atrophic. In the dermis a bandlike lymphocytic infiltration is seen, which varies in abundance according to the stage of the disease. The epidermis is slightly hyperkeratotic and flattened, and beneath it there is a distinctive narrow zone of connective tissue in which the elastic tissue is intact.

Antibiotic therapy as for other forms of borreliosis cures most patients with ACA.

Aberer E: What should one do in case of a tick bite? Curr Probl Dermatol 2009; 37:155.

Dandache P, et al: Erythema migrans. Infect Dis Clin North Am 2008; 22:235.

Dworkin MS, et al: Tick-borne relapsing fever. Infect Dis Clin North Am 2008; 22:449.

Eisendle K, et al: The expanding spectrum of cutaneous borreliosis. G Ital Dermatol Venereol 2009; 144:157.

Feder HM Jr: Lyme disease in children. Infect Dis Clin North Am 2008; 22:315.

Grange F, et al: *Borrelia burgdorferi*-associated lymphocytoma cutis simulating a primary cutaneous large B-cell lymphoma. J Am Acad Dermatol 2002; 47:530.

Hengge UR, et al: Lyme borreliosis. Lancet Infect Dis 2003; 3:489.

Hubalek Z: Epidemiology of Lyme borreliosis. Curr Probl Dermatol 2009; 37:31.

Lipker D, et al: How accurate is a clinical diagnosis of ECM? Arch Dermatol 2004; 140:620.

Masters EJ, et al: STARI, or Masters disease. Infect Dis Clin N Am 2008; 22:361.

Moreno C, et al: Interstitial granulomatous dermatitis with histiocytic pseudorosettes? A new histopathologic pattern in cutaneous borreliosis. J Am Acad Dermatol 2003; 48:376.

Mullegger RR: Skin manifestations of Lyme borreliosis. Am J Clin Dermatol 2008; 9: 355.

Murray TS, et al: Lyme disease. Clin Lab Med 2010; 30:311.

Nowakowski J, et al: Long-term follow-up of patients with culture-confirmed Lyme disease. Am J Med 2003; 115:91.

Smetanick MT, et al: Acrodermatitis chronica atrophicans. Cutis 2010; 85:247.

Stanek G, et al: Lyme disease. Infect Dis Clin North Am 2008; 22:327.

Walsh CA, et al: Lyme disease in pregnancy. Obstet Gynecol Surv 2007; 62:41.

Mycoplasma

Mycoplasmas are distinct from true bacteria in that they lack a cell wall and differ from viruses in that they grow on cell-free media. *Mycoplasma pneumoniae* (Eaton agent) is an important cause of acute respiratory disease in children and young adults. It has been estimated that in the summer it may account for 50% of pneumonias.

Skin eruptions occur during the course of infection in approximately 25% of patients. The most frequently reported is Stevens–Johnson syndrome. Erythema nodosum and Gianotti–Crosti syndrome have been occasionally reported, as well as isolated mucositis without any or minimal skin lesions. Other exanthems include urticarial, vesicular, vesiculopustular, maculopapular, scarlatiniform, petechial, purpuric, and morbilliform lesions, distributed primarily on the trunk, arms, and legs. Ulcerative stomatitis and conjunctivitis may be present.

The diagnosis of *M. pneumoniae* infection is made in the acute situation by clinical means, but definitive diagnosis is made by enzyme immunoassay, PCR, or complement fixation techniques. Cold agglutinins with a titer of 1:128 or more are usually due to *M. pneumoniae* infection. Occasionally, acrocyanosis may occur secondary to cold agglutinin disease, which clears with antibiotic therapy.

Treatment is with either a macrolide (erythromycin, azithromycin, or clarithromycin) or doxycycline for 7 days.

Atkinson TP, et al: Epidemiology, clinical manifestations, pathogenesis and laboratory detection of *Mycoplasma pneumoniae* infections. FEMS Microbiol Rev 2008; 32:956.

Manoharan S, et al: Gianotti–Crosti syndrome in an adult following recent *Mycoplasma pneumoniae* infection. Australas J Dermatol 2005; 46:106.

Schalock PC, et al: *Mycoplasma pneumoniae*-induced cutaneous disease. Internat J Dermatol 2009; 48:673.

Chlamydial infections

Two species of chlamydia, *Chlamydia trachomatis* and *Chlamydia psittaci*, have been recognized. The two species share a major common antigen, and there are numerous serotypes within each species. In humans, *Chlamydia* causes trachoma, inclusion conjunctivitis, nongonococcal urethritis, cervicitis, epididymitis, proctitis, endometritis, salpingitis, pneumonia in the newborn, psittacosis (ornithosis), and lymphogranuloma venereum.

Lymphogranuloma venereum

Lymphogranuloma venereum (LGV) is an STD caused by microorganisms of the *Chlamydia trachomatis* group and characterized by suppurative inguinal adenitis with matted lymph nodes, inguinal bubo with secondary ulceration, and constitutional symptoms.

After an incubation period of 3–20 days, a primary lesion consisting of a 2–3 mm herpetiform vesicle or erosion develops on the glans penis, prepuce, or coronal sulcus, or at the meatus. In men who have sex with men the lesion may be in the rectum. In women it occurs on the vulva, vagina, or cervix. The lesion is painless and soon becomes a shallow ulceration. The initial symptom may be urethritis or proctitis. Extragenital primary infections of LGV are rare. An ulcerating lesion may appear at the site of infection on the fingers, lips, or tongue. In patients with HIV infection, a painful perianal ulcer may occur. Primary lesions heal in a few days.

About 2 weeks after the appearance of the primary lesion, enlargement of the regional lymph nodes occurs (Fig. 14-52). In one-third of cases, the lymphadenopathy is bilateral. In the rather characteristic inguinal adenitis of LGV in men, the nodes in a chain fuse together into a large mass. The color of the skin overlying the mass usually becomes violaceous, the swelling is tender, and the bubo may break down, forming multiple fistulous openings. Adenopathy above and below the Poupart ligament produces the characteristic, but not diagnostic, groove sign. Along with the local adenitis there may be systemic symptoms of malaise, joint pains, conjunctivitis, loss of appetite, weight loss, and fever, which may persist for several weeks. Cases with septic temperatures, enlarged liver and spleen, and even encephalitis have occasionally been observed.

Primary lesions of LGV are rarely observed in female patients; women also have a lower incidence of inguinal

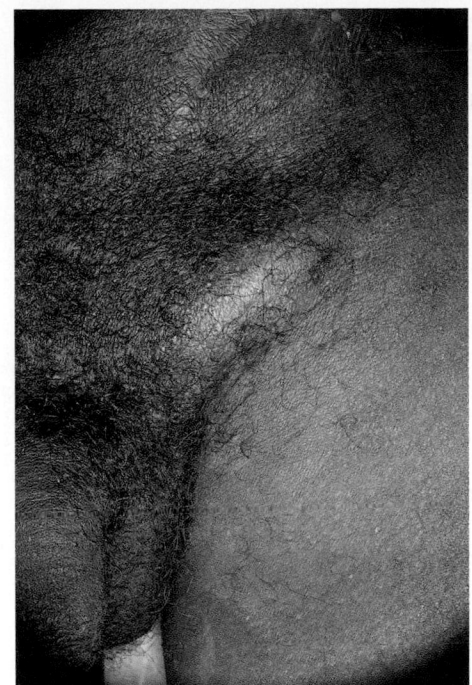

Fig. 14-52 Lymphogranuloma venereum.

buboes. Their bubo is typically pararectal in location. The diagnosis is recognized only much later when the patient presents with an increasingly pronounced inflammatory stricture, which may be annular or tubular, of the lower rectal wall. Because most of the lymph channels running from the vulva drain into the nodes around the lower part of the rectum, an inflammatory reaction in these nodes results in secondary involvement of the rectal wall. The iliac nodes may also be involved.

LGV may start in the rectum as proctitis, which may then progress to the formation of a stricture. The clinical hallmark is bloody, mucopurulent rectal discharge. The stricture can usually be felt with the examining finger 4–6 cm above the anus. Untreated rectal strictures in men and women may eventually require colostomy. With or without rectal strictures, women may in later stages of the disease show elephantiasis of the genitals with chronic ulcerations and scarring of the vulva (esthiomene). Such a reaction is rare in men.

Cutaneous eruptions take the form of erythema nodosum, erythema multiforme, photosensitivity, and scarlatiniform eruptions. Arthritis associated with LGV involves the finger, wrist, ankle, knee, or shoulder joints. Marked weight loss, pronounced secondary anemia, weakness, and mental depression are often encountered in the course of the anorectal syndrome. Colitis resulting from LGV is limited to the rectum and rectosigmoid structures. Perianal fistulas or sinuses are often seen in cases of anorectal LGV.

Among the various extragenital manifestations that occur are glossitis with regional adenitis, unilateral conjunctivitis with edema of the lids caused by lymphatic blockage with lymphadenopathy, acute meningitis, meningoencephalitis, and pneumonia.

The diagnosis by nucleic acid amplification tests identifies the organism in a wide variety of specimens including urine, urethral, rectal and ulcer swabs, bubo aspirates, and biopsy specimens. The complement fixation test is the most feasible and the simplest serologic test for detecting antibodies in resource-poor locales. These antibodies become detectable some 4 weeks after onset of illness. A titer of 1:64 is highly suggestive. Microhemagglutination inhibition assays are also available and not only confirm the diagnosis but also identify the strain. Three serotypes, designated L1, L2, and L3, are known for the LGV chlamydia. Characteristic surface antigens allow separation of the LGV chlamydias from the agents that cause trachoma, inclusion conjunctivitis, urethritis, and cervicitis, which also belong to the *C. trachomatis* group.

LGV occurs in all races and the highest incidence is found in the 20–40-year-old group. Asymptomatic female contacts who shed the organism from the cervix are an important reservoir of infection. The classic disease in men is uncommon in the US, whereas anorectal LGV is increasing in men who have sex with men.

The characteristic changes in the lymph nodes consist of an infectious granuloma with the formation of stellate abscesses. There is an outer zone of epithelioid cells with a central necrotic core composed of debris of lymphocytes, and leukocytes. In lesions of long duration, plasma cells may be present. Stellate abscess also occurs in cat-scratch disease, atypical mycobacterial infection, tularemia, and sporotrichosis.

As opposed to LGV, with chancroid a primary chancre or multiple chancroidal ulcers are present and may permit the demonstration of *H. ducreyi*. The skin lesions are characteristic and usually much larger and more persistent than the primary lesion of LGV. Donovan bodies are demonstrable in granuloma inguinale; however, inguinal adenitis is not characteristic. Esthiomene may also be seen in both diseases.

If the primary lesion of LGV is well developed, it may be confused with the primary lesion of syphilis. In any genital lesion, darkfield examination for *Treponema pallidum* is indicated if available. Syphilitic inguinal adenitis shows small, hard, nontender glands. It should be emphasized again that all venereal infections may be mixed infections and that observation for simultaneous or subsequent development of another venereal disease should be unrelenting. This includes serologic testing for HIV disease. Late stages of LGV esthiomene with ulcerating and cicatrizing lesions have to be differentiated from syphilis by search for spirochetes, the serologic tests for syphilis, and complement fixation tests.

Treatment

The recommended treatment is doxycycline, 100 mg twice a day for 3 weeks. An alternative is erythromycin, 500 mg four times a day for 21 days. Sexual partners within the prior 30 days should also be treated. The fluctuant nodules are aspirated from above through healthy adjacent normal skin to prevent rupture.

Bebear C, et al: Genital *Chlamydia trachomatis* infections. Clin Microbiol Infect 2009; 15:4.

Center for Communicable Diseases (CDC): STD treatment guidelines 2006. MMWR 2006; 55:1.

Kapoor S: Re-emergence of lymphogranuloma venereum. J Eur Acad Dermatol Venereol 2008; 22:409.

McLean CA, et al: Treatment of lymphogranuloma venereum. Clin Infect Dis 2007; 4 Suppl 3:S147.

Richardson D, et al: Lymphogranuloma venereum. Int J STD and AIDS 2007; 18:11.

White JA: Manifestations and mangement of lymphogranuloma venereum. Curr Opin Infect Dis 2009; 22:57.

Bonus images for this chapter can be found online at

http://www.expertconsult.com

Diseases Resulting from Fungi and Yeasts

15

SUPERFICIAL AND DEEP MYCOSES

An estimated 20–25% of the world's population has some form of fungal infection, usually an anthropophilic *Trichophyton* infection, making fungal infections the most common type of infection worldwide. Cutaneous infections are divided into superficial and deep mycoses. Most mycotic infections are superficial and are limited to the stratum corneum, hair, and nails. In contrast, most deep mycoses are evidence of disseminated infection, typically with a primary pulmonary focus. Although blastomycosis, histoplasmosis, and coccidioidomycosis generally present as skin lesions, they are almost always evidence of a systemic infection. There are a few deep mycoses that result from direct inoculation into the skin by a thorn or other foreign body. These include cutaneous lymphangitic sporotrichosis, primary cutaneous phaeohyphomycosis, and chromomycosis. Although phaeohyphomycosis generally begins as a skin infection, in immunosuppressed patients there is a great risk of dissemination and death. Even cutaneous sporotrichosis may occasionally disseminate. Although most cutaneous aspergillosis represents cutaneous embolization from a systemic (often a pulmonary) focus, in burn victims *Aspergillus* commonly colonizes the burn eschar. This colonization may often be treated with debridement alone. Deep incisional biopsies are required to determine if there has been invasion of viable tissue beneath the eschar. Evidence of viable tissue invasion suggests a likelihood of systemic dissemination and is usually an indication for systemic antifungal therapy.

The major fungi that cause only stratum corneum, hair, and nail infection are the dermatophytes. They are classified in three genera: *Microsporum*, *Trichophyton*, and *Epidermophyton*. Superficial fungal infections are divided into:

1. tinea capitis (ringworm of the scalp and kerion)
2. tinea barbae (ringworm of the beard)
3. tinea faciei
4. tinea corporis
5. tinea manus
6. tinea pedis
7. tinea cruris
8. onychomycosis (fungus infection of the nails).

Superficial mycoses are subdivided according to the causative dermatophyte. This is important because the antifungal agents vary somewhat in spectrum. For instance, higher doses of terbinafine are required to treat *Microsporum canis* infections than are needed to treat *Trichophyton* spp. The identity of the pathogen may also be important for pinning down a zoonotic reservoir of infection (a cat or dog for *M. canis* infections, cattle for *Trichophyton verrucosum*, and rats for granular zoophilic *Trichophyton mentagrophytes*).

Susceptibility and prevalence

Local and systemic immunosuppression may promote widespread tinea infection. Local immunosuppression is usually related to the use of a potent topical corticosteroid, but may also occur with use of a topical calcineurin inhibitor. A wide range of systemically immunocompromised states may result in severe forms of dermatophyte infection. These include primary immunodeficiency syndromes, acquired immunodeficiency syndrome (AIDS), connective tissue disease, and cancer chemotherapy. A defective cutaneous barrier, as in patients with ichthyosis, can also predispose to widespread tinea infection. Use of topical corticosteroids, occlusion, and shaving is associated with fungal folliculitis.

Genetic susceptibility to certain forms of fungal infection may be related to the types of keratin or degree or mix of cutaneous lipids produced. Surface antigens, such as the ABO system, may also be important, with patients with blood type A being somewhat more prone to chronic disease.

Data from the Icelandic population suggest a prevalence of symptomatic mycologically determined onychomycosis of 11.1%. The prevalence doubled with a history of cancer, psoriasis, tinea pedis interdigitalis, moccasin tinea pedis, parents with onychomycosis, children with onychomycosis, spouse with onychomycosis, regular swimming, and age over 50. Fungal disease accounts for 30–40% of all foot disease.

Many individuals will carry *Trichophyton rubrum* asymptomatically, and this tendency may be inherited in an autosomal-dominant fashion. When they are exposed to a hot humid climate or occlusive footwear, the disease often becomes symptomatic. Reported prevalence rates are therefore heavily affected by climate, footwear, and lifestyle.

Antifungal therapy

Topical agents provide safe, cost-effective therapy for limited superficial fungal infections. Available agents include clotrimazole, naftifine, miconazole, ciclopirox, econazole, oxiconazole, ketoconazole, sulconazole, tolnaftate, butenafine, and terbinafine. Clotrimazole, miconazole, tolnaftate and terbinafine are available without a prescription in the US.

When considering the use of an oral antifungal agent, factors include the type of infection, organism, spectrum, pharmacokinetic profile, safety, compliance, and cost. Griseofulvin has a long safety record, but requires much longer courses of therapy than newer agents. Topical antifungals remain very cost-effective for limited cutaneous disease.

Various classes of antifungal are in use. The imidazoles include clotrimazole, miconazole, econazole, sulconazole, oxiconazole, voriconazole, and ketoconazole. They work by inhibition of the cytochrome P450 14-α-demethylase, an essential enzyme in ergosterol synthesis. Nystatin is a polyene that works by irreversibly binding to ergosterol, an essential component of fungal cell membranes. Naftifine, terbinafine, and butenafine are allylamines, and their mode of action is inhibition of squalene epoxydation. The triazoles include itraconazole and fluconazole, which affect the cytochrome P450 system. As this system is responsible for the metabolism of numerous drugs, interactions can occur, some of which may be life-threatening.

For both itraconazole and griseofulvin, food increases absorption. For itraconazole and ketoconazole, antacids, H_2 antagonists and proton pump inhibitors lower absorption. Terbinafine is less active against *Candida* and *Microsporum* spp in vitro. In vivo, adequate doses can be effective against these organisms. Terbinafine has limited efficacy in the oral treatment of tinea versicolor but is effective topically. Although few drug interactions have been reported with terbinafine and the bioavailability is unchanged in food, hepatotoxicity, leukopenia, toxic epidermal necrolysis, and taste disturbances occur uncommonly. Ketoconazole has a wide spectrum against dermatophytes, yeasts, and some systemic mycoses. It has the potential for serious drug interactions and a higher incidence of hepatotoxicity than other available agents. The risk of liver toxicity with single doses is minimal, but for many indications, the drug has largely been replaced by fluconazole.

Fluconazole is mainly used to treat *Candida* infections, but has shown efficacy in the treatment of dermatophytoses both in daily and in weekly doses. Patients may have trouble remembering intermittent dosing schedules. In one study, daily dosing with terbinafine was rated by patients as more convenient than monthly pulsed dosing with itraconazole and was associated with higher overall satisfaction.

Both terbinafine and itraconazole have been shown to be effective and well tolerated in several studies of the treatment of tinea capitis and onychomycosis in children, but itraconazole has been associated with reports of heart failure.

Voriconazole has exceptional activity against a wide variety of yeasts, as well as many other fungal pathogens, but has been associated with photosensitivity, premature photoaging, actinic keratoses, squamous cell carcinoma, melanoma, and porphyria. Posaconazole has significant in vitro activity against *Candida* spp, although some resistance has been reported to this drug.

The echinocandins inhibit β-(1,3)-glucan synthesis, thus damaging fungal cell walls. They are active against most *Candida* spp and fungistatic against *Aspergillus* spp. They have limited activity against zygomycetes, *Cryptococcus neoformans* or *Fusarium* spp. Caspofungin was the first drug in this class to be marketed in the US for refractory invasive aspergillosis. Micafungin also belongs to this class of antifungal agent. Adverse events are uncommon but include phlebitis, fever, elevated liver enzymes, and mild hemolysis. The drugs must be given intravenously. Metabolism is mainly hepatic. In the setting of *Candida* sepsis, results are similar to those achieved with amphotericin B, with substantially lower toxicity. They may be used together with other antifungal agents in the treatment of life-threatening systemic fungal infections, such as disseminated aspergillosis refractory to other regimens. Screenings of members of sports teams can reduce the incidence of infection.

Cowen EW, et al: Chronic phototoxicity and aggressive squamous cell carcinoma of the skin in children and adults during treatment with voriconazole. J Am Acad Dermatol 2010; 62(1):31–37.

Havlickova B, et al: Epidemiological trends in skin mycoses worldwide. Mycoses 2008 Sep; 51(Suppl 4):2–15.

Petrikkos G, et al: Recent advances in antifungal chemotherapy. Int J Antimicrob Agents 2007 Aug; 30(2):108–117.

Sigurgeirsson B, et al: Risk factors associated with onychomycosis. J Eur Acad Dermatol Venereol 2004; 18:48.

THE SUPERFICIAL MYCOSES

Tinea capitis

Tinea capitis, also known as scalp ringworm, can be caused by all the pathogenic dermatophytes except for *Epidermophyton floccosum* and *Trichophyton concentricum*. In the US, most cases are caused by *Trichophyton tonsurans* (which has replaced *Microsporum audouinii* as the most common pathogen). Pet exposure is associated with tinea capitis caused by *M. canis*. Immigrant populations have a high incidence of tinea capitis with organisms common in their regions of origin. Among African and Arab immigrants, *Trichophyton soudanense*, *Trichophyton violaceum* and *M. audouinii* are particularly common.

Tinea capitis occurs mainly in children, although it may be seen at all ages. Boys have tinea capitis more frequently than girls; however, in epidemics caused by *T. tonsurans* there is often equal frequency in the sexes. African American children have a higher incidence of *T. tonsurans* infections than Anglo Americans. The infection is also common among Latin American children.

T. tonsurans produces black dot ringworm, as well as subtle seborrheic-like scaling and inflammatory kerion. Black dot tinea may also be caused by *T. violaceum*, an organism rarely seen in the US. Both of these organisms produce chains of large spores within the hair shaft (large spore endothrix) (Fig. 15-1). They do not produce fluorescence with a Wood's light.

The *M. canis* complex includes a group of organisms that produce small spores visible on the outside of the hair shaft (small spore ectothrix). These fungi fluoresce under Wood's light examination. The *M. canis* complex includes *M. canis*, *M. canis distortum*, *Microsporum ferrugineum*, and *M. audouinii*. *M. canis* infections begin as scaly, erythematous, papular eruptions with loose and broken-off hairs. The lesions commonly become highly inflammatory, although *M. audouinii* has less of a tendency to produce inflammatory lesions. Deep, tender, boggy plaques exuding pus are known as kerion celsii (Fig. 15-2). Kerion may be followed by scarring and permanent alopecia in the areas of inflammation and suppuration. Systemic steroids for a short period along with appropriate antifungal therapy will greatly diminish the inflammatory response and reduce the risk of scarring, and should be considered in the setting of highly inflammatory lesions.

Asymptomatic carriers of *T. tonsurans* are common, and represent a source of infection for classmates and siblings. Numerous studies have shown that 5–15% of urban children in western countries have positive scalp dermatophyte

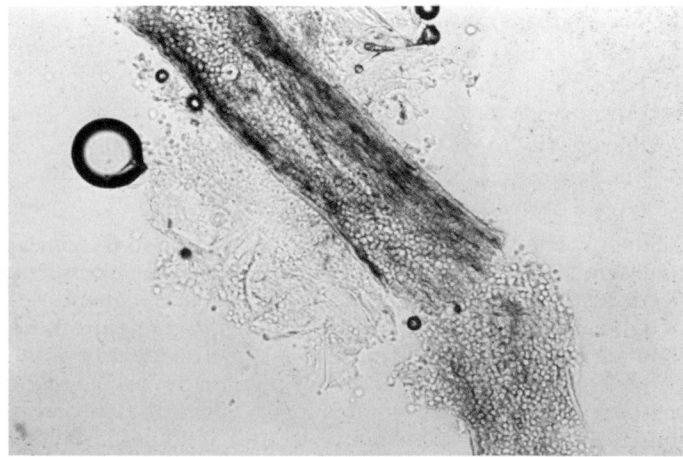

Fig. 15-1 Endothrix hair mount, note spores within the hair shaft.

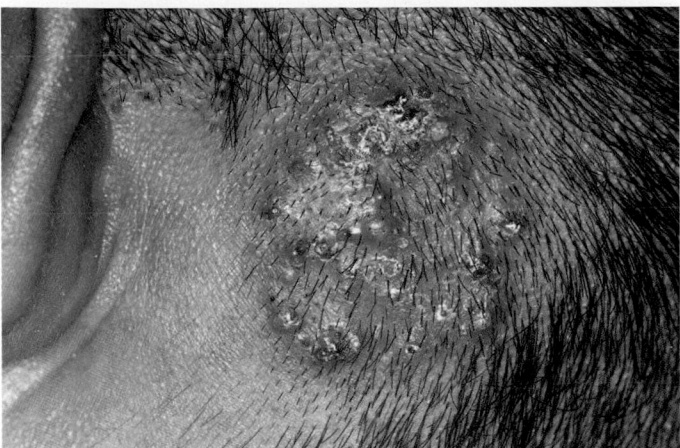

Fig. 15-2 Kerion.

cultures. In one study, 60% of children with a positive scalp culture were asymptomatic. All of these children were African American. The presence of scalp scaling and the use of a dandruff shampoo were associated with an increased likelihood of carrying a fungal organism. It is unlikely that dandruff shampoos predispose to tinea. More likely, they provide incomplete treatment of minimally symptomatic tinea that produces a subtle seborrheic scale.

The prevalence of various dermatophytes varies throughout the world. Where animal herding is an important part of the economy, zoonotic fungi account for a significant proportion of cases of tinea. In Asia, organisms vary significantly by region. In a study of 204 Iraqi schoolchildren with tinea capitis, *Trichophyton verrucosum* was the most common organism. Both *T. rubrum* and *T. mentagrophytes* var. *mentagrophytes* were more common than *T. tonsurans*. In south central Asia, *T. violaceum* is the most common dermatophytic species isolated, with *M. audouinii* a close second. Other common organisms include *Trichophyton schoenleinii*, *T. tonsurans*, *Microsporum gypseum*, *T. verrucosum*, and *T. mentagrophytes*. In east Asia, *T. violaceum* and *M. ferrugineum* are important pathogens. In Europe, African/Caribbean immigrants account for a large proportion of new patients with tinea capitis. Important pathogens include *T. tonsurans*, *M. audouinii* var. *langeronii*, *Trichophyton soudanense*, and *T. violaceum*. *Trichophyton megninii* is a rare cause of tinea capitis largely restricted to southwest Europe. In Africa, large-scale epidemics are associated with *T. soudanense*, *T. violaceum*, *T. schoenleinii* and *Microsporum* spp. In Australia, the predominantly white population experiences infections, mostly with *M. canis*, but *T. tonsurans* is now equal in prevalence in some areas of the continent.

Favus

Favus, which is very rare in the US, appears chiefly on the scalp but may affect the glabrous skin and nails. On the scalp, concave sulfur-yellow crusts form around loose, wiry hairs. Atrophic scarring ensues, leaving a smooth, glossy, thin, paper-white patch. On the glabrous skin the lesions are pinhead to 2 cm in diameter with cup-shaped crusts called scutulae, usually pierced by a hair as on the scalp. The scutulae have a distinctive mousy odor. When the nails are affected they become brittle, irregularly thickened, and crusted under the free margins.

Favus among the Bantus in South Africa is called, in Afrikaans, witkop (whitehead). It is also prevalent in the Middle East, southeastern Europe, and the countries bordering the Mediterranean Sea.

Pathogenesis and natural history

The incubation period of anthropophilic tinea capitis lasts 2–4 days, although the period is highly variable and asymptomatic carriers are common. The hyphae grow downward into the follicle, on the hair's surface, and the intrafollicular hyphae break up into chains of spores. There is a period of spread (4 days to 4 months) during which the lesions enlarge and new lesions appear. At about 3 weeks hairs break off a few millimeters above the skin surface. Within the hair, hyphae descend to the upper limit of the keratogenous zone and here form Adamson "fringe" on about the 12th day. No new lesions develop during the refractory period (4 months to several years). The clinical appearance is constant, with the host and parasite at equilibrium. This is followed by a period of involution in which the formation of spores gradually diminishes. Zoonotic fungal infections are commonly more highly inflammatory, but undergo similar phases of evolution.

Diagnosis

Wood's light

Ultraviolet (UV) light of 365 nm wavelength is obtained by passing the beam through a Wood's filter composed of nickel oxide-containing glass. This apparatus, commonly known as the Wood's light, is commonly used to demonstrate fungal fluorescence. Fluorescent-positive infections are caused by *M. audouinii*, *M. canis*, *M. ferrugineum*, *M. distortum*, and *T. schoenleinii*. In a dark room the skin under this light fluoresces faintly blue, and dandruff commonly is bright blue–white. Infected hair fluoresces bright green or yellow–green. The fluorescent substance is a pteridine. Large spore endothrix organisms (such as *T. tonsurans* and *T. violaceum*) and *T. verrucosum* (a cause of large spore ectothrix) do not fluoresce.

Laboratory examination

For demonstration of the fungus in a highly inflammatory plaque, two or three loose hairs are carefully removed with epilating forceps from the suspected areas. If fluorescence occurs, it is important to choose these hairs. Bear in mind that hairs infected with *T. tonsurans* do not fluoresce. In "black dot" ringworm or in patients with seborrheic scale, small broken fragments of infected hair will adhere to a moist gauze pad rubbed across the scalp. The hairs are placed on a slide and covered with a drop of a 10–20% KOH solution. Then a coverslip is applied, and the specimen is warmed until the hairs are macerated. Dimethyl sulfoxide (DMSO) can be added to the KOH solution in concentrations of up to 40%. This additive allows for rapid clearing of keratin without heating. Once the hairs have softened, they are compressed through the coverslip and examined first with a low-power objective and then with a high-power objective for detail. The patterns of endothrix and ectothrix involvement described above, together with local prevalence data, allow for identification of the organism.

Exact identification of the causative fungus is generally determined by culture, although molecular sequencing offers a more rapid alternative. For culture, several infected hairs are planted on Sabouraud dextrose agar, Sabouraud agar with chloramphenicol, Mycosel agar, or dermatophyte test medium (DTM). Cultures are best collected by rubbing the lesion vigorously with a moistened cotton swab or gauze pad, then streaking the cotton over the agar surface. On the first three media, a distinctive growth appears within 1–2 weeks. Most frequently, the diagnosis is made by the gross appearance of the culture growth, together with the microscopic appearance. In the case of *Trichophyton* spp, growth on different nutrient agars is often required to identify the organisms beyond genus. DTM not only contains antibiotics to reduce growth of contaminants but also contains a colored pH indicator to denote the alkali-producing dermatophytes. A few nonpathogenic saprophytes will also produce alkalinization and in the occasional case of onychomycosis of toenails caused by airborne molds, a culture medium containing an antibiotic may inhibit growth of the true pathogen.

T. tonsurans

This microorganism grows slowly in culture to produce a granular or powdery yellow to red, brown, or buff colony. Crater formation with radial grooves may be produced. Swollen microconidia may be seen regularly. Diagnosis is confirmed by the fact that cultures grow poorly or not at all without thiamine.

T. mentagrophytes

The colony is velvety, granular, or fluffy. It may be flat or furrowed, light buff, white, or sometimes pink. The back of the culture can vary from buff to dark red. Round microconidia borne laterally and in clusters confirm the diagnosis within 2 weeks. Spiral hyphae are sometimes prominent.

T. verrucosum

Growth is slow and cannot be observed well for at least 3 weeks. The colony is compact, glassy, velvety, heaped or furrowed, and usually white, but may be yellow or gray. The colony may crack the agar. Chlamydospores (round swellings along the hyphal structure) are present in early cultures, and microconidia may be seen.

M. audouinii

Culture typically shows a slowly growing, matted, velvety, light brown colony, the back of which is reddish brown to orange. The colony edge is generally striate, rather than smooth. Under the microscope a few large multiseptate macroconidia may be seen. Microconidia in a lateral position on the hyphae are clavate. Racquet mycelia, terminal chlamydospores, and pectinate hyphae are sometimes seen.

M. canis

The culture grossly shows profuse, cottony, aerial mycelia that are distinctly striate at the periphery, while sometimes tending to become powdery in the center. The color is buff to light brown. The back of the colony is lemon to orange–yellow. There are numerous spindle-shaped, thick-walled echinulate macroconidia. Clavate microconidia may be found, along with chlamydospores and pectinate bodies.

Differential diagnosis

Tinea capitis must be differentiated clinically from chronic staphylococcal folliculitis, pediculosis capitis, psoriasis, seborrheic dermatitis, secondary syphilis, trichotillomania, alopecia areata, lupus erythematosus, lichen planus, lichen simplex chronicus, and various inflammatory follicular conditions. The distinctive clinical features of tinea capitis are broken-off stumps of hairs, often in rounded patches in which there are crusts or pustules and few hairs. The broken-off hairs are loose and when examined are found to be surrounded by, or to contain, the fungus. Diffuse seborrheic scaling with hair loss is a common presentation of *T. tonsurans* infections.

In alopecia areata the affected patches are bald, and the skin is smooth and shiny without any signs of inflammation or scaling. Stumps of broken-off hairs are infrequently found, and no fungi are demonstrable. In seborrheic dermatitis the

involved areas are covered by fine, dry, or greasy scales. Hair may be lost, but the hairs are not broken. Atopic dermatitis is rarely associated with localized scalp involvement, and clinical examination frequently reveals more typical generalized findings. In psoriasis, well-demarcated, sometimes diffuse, areas of erythema and white or silver scaling are noted. Lichen simplex chronicus is frequently localized to the inferior margin of the occipital scalp. In trichotillomania, as in alopecia areata, inflammation and scaling are absent. Circumscribed lesions are very rare. Serologic testing, scalp biopsies, and immunofluorescent studies may be indicated if the alopecia of secondary syphilis or lupus erythematosus is a serious consideration. It should be noted that adult patients with lupus erythematosus are susceptible to tinea capitis, which may be photosensitive and difficult to distinguish from plaques of lupus without biopsy and KOH examinations.

Treatment

Numerous clinical trials exist that demonstrate the effectiveness of itraconazole, terbinafine, and fluconazole. Despite these studies, griseofulvin remains the most commonly used antifungal agent in children. It has a long safety record, and pediatricians and family practitioners are generally comfortable with the drug. A meta-analysis of published studies shows mean efficacy for griseofulvin treatment of about 68% for *Trichophyton* spp and 88% for *Microsporum*. For the ultramicronized form, doses start at 10 mg/kg/day. The tablets can be crushed and given with ice cream. Grifulvin V oral suspension is less readily absorbed. The dose is 20 mg/kg/day. Treatment should continue for 2–4 months, or for at least 2 weeks after negative laboratory examinations are obtained. Doses much higher than those reflected in drug labeling are commonly needed. For *Trichophyton* infections, terbinafine is commonly effective in doses of 3–6 mg/kg/day for 1–4 weeks. Alternate dosing schedules for terbinafine include one 250 mg tablet for patients over 40 kg, 125 mg (half of a 250 mg tablet) for those 20–40 kg, and 62.5 mg (one-quarter of a 250 mg tablet) for those under 20 kg. *Microsporum* infections require higher doses and longer courses of therapy with terbinafine. Itraconazole has been shown to be effective in doses of 5 mg/kg/day for 2–3 weeks, and fluconazole at doses of 6 mg/kg/day for 2–3 weeks. Reports of heart failure with itraconazole have limited its use.

Selenium sulfide shampoo or ketoconazole shampoo left on the scalp for 5 min three times a week can be used as adjunctive therapy to oral antifungal agents to reduce the shedding of fungal spores. Combs, brushes, and hats should be cleaned carefully and natural bristle brushes must be discarded.

Prognosis

Recurrence usually does not occur when adequate amounts of griseofulvin, fluconazole, or terbinafine have been taken, although exposure to infected persons, asymptomatic carriers, or contaminated fomites will increase the relapse rate. Without medication there is spontaneous clearing at about the age of 15, except with *T. tonsurans*, which often persists into adult life.

Dermatophytids

In cases of inflammatory tinea capitis, widespread "id" eruptions may appear concomitantly on the trunk and extremities. These are vesicular, lichenoid, papulosquamous, or pustular. They represent a systemic reaction to fungal antigens. Although they are commonly refractory to topical corticosteroids, they typically clear rapidly after treatment of the fungal infection.

The most common type of id reaction is seen on the hands and sides of the fingers when there is an acute fungus infection of the feet. These lesions are mostly vesicular and are extremely pruritic and even tender). Secondary bacterial infection may occur; however, fungus is not demonstrable in a true dermatophytid. The onset is at times accompanied by fever, anorexia, generalized adenopathy, spleen enlargement, and leukocytosis. Dermatophytid reactions due to inflammatory tinea capitis may occasionally present as widespread eruption, usually follicular, lichenoid, or papulosquamous. Rarely, the eruption may be morbilliform or scarlatiniform. The erysipelas-like dermatophytid is most commonly seen on the shin, where it appears as an elevated, sharply defined, erysipelas-like plaque about the size of the hand, usually with toe web tinea on the same side. This form of id reaction responds to systemic steroids and treatment of the tinea.

The histologic picture is characterized by spongiotic vesicles and a superficial, perivascular, predominantly lymphohistiocytic infiltrate. Eosinophils may be present. Diagnosis of a dermatophytid reaction is dependent on the demonstration of a fungus at some site remote from the suspect lesions of the dermatophytid, the absence of fungus in the id lesion, and involution of the lesion as the fungal infection subsides.

Tinea barbae

Ringworm of the beard, also known as tinea sycosis and barber's itch, is not a common disease. It occurs chiefly among those in agricultural pursuits, especially those in contact with farm animals. The involvement is mostly one-sided on the neck or face. Two clinical types are distinguished: deep, nodular, suppurative lesions; and superficial, crusted, partially bald patches with folliculitis (Fig. 15-3).

The deep type develops slowly and produces nodular thickenings and kerion-like swellings, usually caused by *T. mentagrophytes* or *T. verrucosum*. As a rule the swellings are confluent and form diffuse boggy infiltrations with abscesses. The overlying skin is inflamed, the hairs are loose or absent, and pus may be expressed through the remaining follicular openings. Generally, the lesions are limited to one part of the face or neck in men. The superficial crusted type is characterized by a less inflammatory pustular folliculitis, and may be associated with *T. violaceum* or *T. rubrum*. The affected hairs can sometimes be easily extracted. Rarely, *E. floccosum* may cause widespread verrucous lesions known as verrucous epidermophytosis.

Diagnosis

The clinical diagnosis is confirmed by the microscopic mounts of extracted hairs or a biopsy specimen. Culture can be performed on extracted hairs or tissue homogenates of biopsy specimens.

Differential diagnosis

The differential diagnosis includes staphylococcal folliculitis (sycosis vulgaris) and herpetic infections. Tinea barbae differs from sycosis vulgaris by usually sparing the upper lip, and by often being unilateral. In sycosis vulgaris the lesions are pustules and papules, pierced in the center by a hair, which is loose and easily extracted after suppuration has occurred. Herpetic infections usually demonstrate umbilicated vesicles. Tzanck preparations have a low diagnostic yield, but viral culture or direct fluorescent antibody is virtually always positive.

Treatment

As in tinea capitis, oral antifungal agents are required to cure tinea barbae. Topical agents are only helpful as adjunctive therapy. Oral agents are used in the same doses and for the same durations as in tinea capitis.

Tinea faciei

Fungal infection of the face is frequently misdiagnosed (Fig. 15-4). Typical annular rings are usually lacking and the lesions are exquisitely photosensitive. Frequently, a misdiagnosis of lupus erythematosus is made. Biopsies for direct immunofluorescence often demonstrate some reactants on sun-exposed skin, adding to the possible diagnostic confusion. Erythematous, slightly scaling, indistinct borders may be present at the periphery of the lesions, and are the best location for KOH examination. If topical corticosteroids have been used, fungal folliculitis is a frequent finding. A biopsy may be required to establish the diagnosis. A high index of suspicion is required, as fungal hyphae may be few in number or confined to hair follicles. The inflammatory pattern may be psoriasiform spongiotic or vacuolar interface. The latter pattern has the potential to perpetuate confusion with lupus erythematosus.

Usually the infection is caused by *T. rubrum*, *T. mentagrophytes*, or *M. canis*. Tinea faciei caused by *Microsporum nanum* has been described in hog farmers. If fungal folliculitis is present, oral medication is required. If no folliculitis is present, the infection generally responds well to topical therapy. Oral agents are appropriate for widespread infections.

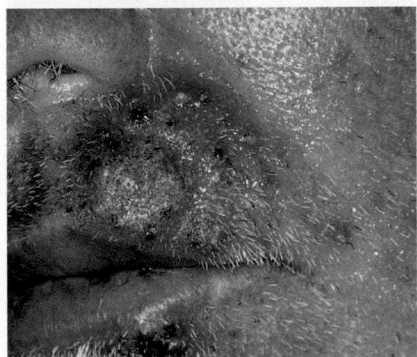

Fig. 15-3 Tinea barbae.

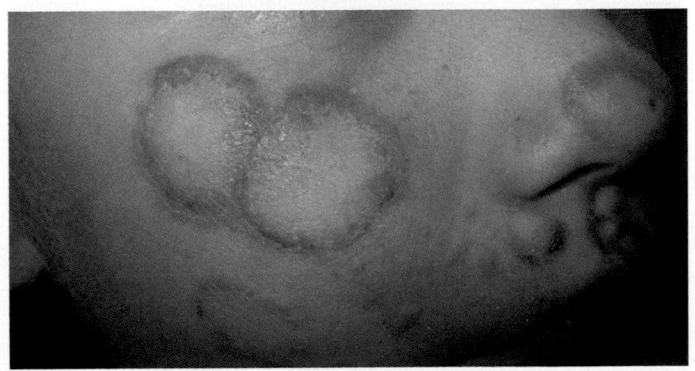

Fig. 15-4 Tinea faciei.

Tinea corporis (tinea circinata)

Tinea corporis includes all superficial dermatophyte infections of the skin other than those involving the scalp, beard, face, hands, feet, and groin. This form of ringworm is characterized by one or more circular, sharply circumscribed, slightly erythematous, dry, scaly, usually hypopigmented patches. An advancing scaling edge is usually prominent (Fig. 15-5). Progressive central clearing produces annular outlines that give them the name "ringworm." Lesions may widen to form rings many centimeters in diameter. In some cases concentric circles or polycyclic lesions form, making intricate patterns. Widespread tinea corporis may be the presenting sign of AIDS, or may be related to the use of a topical corticosteroid or calcineurin inhibitor.

In the US, *T. rubrum*, *M. canis*, and *T. mentagrophytes* are common causes, although infection can be caused by any of the dermatophytes. Multiple small lesions are commonly caused by exposure to a pet with *M. canis*. Other zoonotic fungi, such as granular zoophilic *T. mentagrophytes* related to Southeast Asian bamboo rats, can cause widespread epidemics of highly inflammatory tinea corporis.

Tinea gladiatorum is a common problem for wrestlers. In Pennsylvania, during the 1998–1999 wrestling season, about 85% of responding teams had at least one wrestler diagnosed with ringworm, despite the fact that 97% used preventive practices. One-third of these teams reported that a wrestler missed a match because of the infection. Opponents, equipment, and mats represent potential sources of infection.

Diagnosis

The diagnosis is relatively easily made by finding the fungus under the microscope in skin scrapings. In addition, skin scrapings can be cultured on a suitable medium. Growth of the fungus on culture medium is apparent within a week or two at most and, in most instances, is identifiable to the genus level by the gross and microscopic appearance of the culture. Biopsy of a chronic refractory dermatosis often reveals tinea incognito.

Other diseases that may closely resemble tinea corporis are pityriasis rosea, impetigo, nummular dermatitis, secondary and tertiary syphilids, seborrheic dermatitis, and psoriasis. These are distinguished by KOH examination and culture.

Treatment

Localized disease without fungal folliculitis may be treated with topical therapy. Sulconazole (Exelderm), oxiconazole (Oxistat), miconazole (Monistat cream or lotion, or Micatin cream), clotrimazole (Lotrimin or Mycelex cream), econazole (Spectazole), naftifine (Naftin), ketoconazole (Nizoral), ciclopirox olamine (Loprox), terbinafine (Lamisil), and butenafine (Mentax) are currently available and effective. Most treatment times are between 2 and 4 weeks with twice a day use. Econazole, ketoconazole, oxiconazole, and terbinafine may be used once a day. With terbinafine the course can be shortened to 1 week. Combination products with a potent corticosteroid (such as clotrimazole/betamethasone) frequently produce widespread tinea and fungal folliculitis. Their use should be discouraged.

Extensive disease or fungal folliculitis requires systemic antifungal treatment. When tinea corporis is caused by *T. tonsurans*, *T. mentagrophytes*, or *T. rubrum*, griseofulvin, terbinafine, itraconazole, and fluconazole are all effective. Shorter courses are possible with newer antifungals. Terbinafine therapy for *M. canis* typically requires higher doses and longer courses of therapy.

The ultra-micronized form of griseofulvin may be effective in doses from 500–1000 mg/day for 4–6 weeks. Approximately 10% of individuals will experience nausea or headache with griseofulvin. These symptoms commonly respond to a temporary reduction in dosage. Absorption of griseofulvin is improved when given with whole milk or ice cream. Effective blood levels in children occur at doses of 10–20 mg/kg/day, although higher doses are commonly needed. Terbinafine at 250 mg/day for 1–2 weeks; itraconazole, 200 mg/day for 1 week; and fluconazole, 150 mg once a week for 4 weeks, have been effective doses in adults.

Other forms of tinea corporis

Fungal folliculitis (Majocchi granuloma) and tinea incognito

Occasionally, a deep, pustular type of tinea circinata resembling a carbuncle or kerion is observed on the glabrous skin (Fig. 15-6). This type of lesion is a fungal folliculitis caused most often by *T. rubrum* or *T. mentagrophytes* infecting hairs at the site of involvement. It presents as a circumscribed, annular, raised, crusty, and boggy granuloma in which the follicles are distended with viscid purulent material. These occur most frequently on the shins or wrists. The lesions are often seen in areas of occlusion or shaving, or when a topical corticosteroid has been used. In immunosuppressed patients the lesions may be deep and nodular. Often, patients have been treated with a shot-gun approach, using both topical corticosteroids and

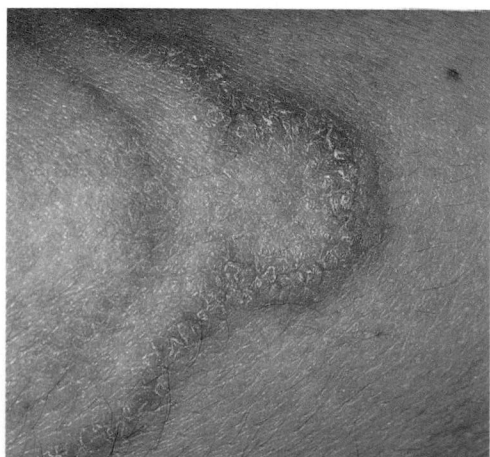

Fig. 15-5 Tinea corporis.

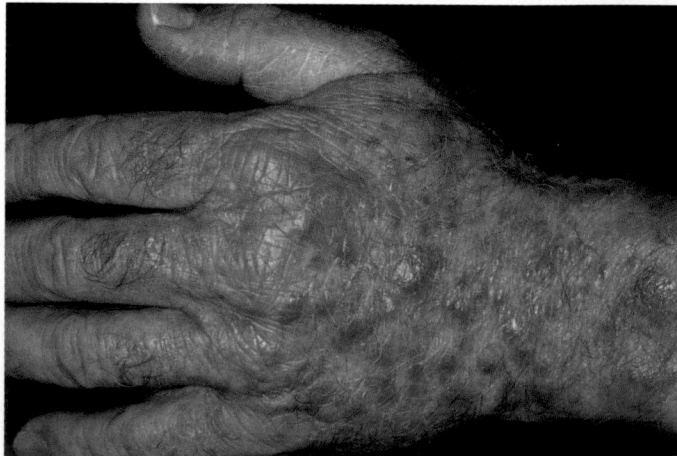

Fig. 15-6 Majocchi granuloma.

antifungal agents. If a topical antifungal has been used recently, KOH examination and culture may be negative. A biopsy may be required to establish the diagnosis. Oral therapy is necessary to cure the lesions.

Tinea incognito is a term applied to atypical clinical lesions of tinea, usually produced by treatment with a topical corticosteroid or occasionally a calcineurin inhibitor. The lesions are often widespread, and may lack an advancing raised scaly border. The diagnosis may be established by KOH examination or biopsy.

Tinea imbricata (Tokelau)

Tinea imbricata is a superficial fungal infection limited to southwest Polynesia, Melanesia, Southeast Asia, India, and Central America. It is characterized by concentric rings of scales forming extensive patches with polycyclic borders. Erythema is typically minimal. The eruption begins with one or several small, rounded macules on the trunk and arms. The small macular patch splits in the center and forms large, flaky scales attached at the periphery. As the resultant ring spreads peripherally, another brownish macule appears in the center and undergoes the process of splitting and peripheral extension. This is repeated over and over again. When fully developed, the eruption is characterized by concentrically arranged rings or parallel undulating lines of scales overlapping each other like shingles on a roof (imbrex means shingle).

The causative fungus is *T. concentricum*. Microscopically, the scrapings show interlacing, septate, mycelial filaments that branch dichotomously. Polyhedral spores are also present. Griseofulvin has been used, but the recurrence rate is high. In one study, terbinafine, 250 mg/day for 4 weeks, was effective in all of 43 patients. Itraconazole at a dose of 100 mg/day failed in 4 of 40 patients, but this may reflect the dose used in the study.

Tinea cruris

Tinea cruris, also known as jock itch and crotch itch, occurs most frequently in men on the upper and inner surfaces of the thighs, especially during the summer when the humidity is high. It begins as a small erythematous and scaling or vesicular and crusted patch that spreads peripherally and partly clears in the center (Fig. 15-7), so that the patch is characterized chiefly by its curved, well-defined border, particularly on its lower edge. The border may have vesicles, pustules, or papules. It may extend downward on the thighs and backward on the perineum or about the anus. The scrotum is rarely involved.

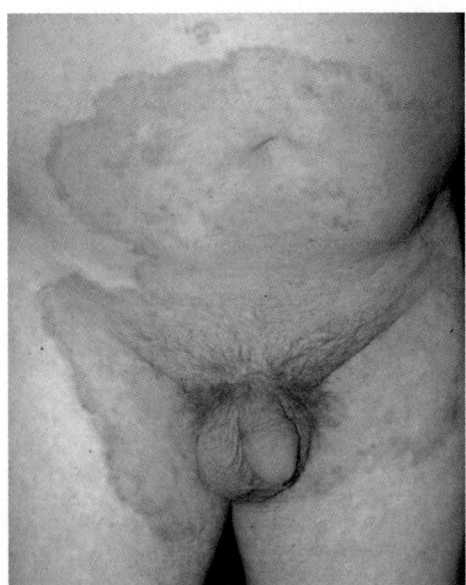

Fig. 15-7 Tinea cruris.

Etiology and differential diagnosis

Ringworm of the groin is usually caused by *T. rubrum*, *T. mentagrophytes*, or *E. floccosum*. Infection with *Candida albicans* may closely mimic tinea cruris, but is usually moister, more inflammatory, and associated with satellite macules. *Candida* often produces collarette scales and satellite pustules.

The crural region is also a common site for erythrasma, seborrheic dermatitis, pemphigus vegetans, and intertriginous psoriasis. Erythrasma often has a copper color, and is diagnosed by the Wood's light examination, which produces coral-red fluorescence. Seborrheic dermatitis generally involves the central chest and axillae in addition to the groin. Pemphigus vegetans produces macerated and eroded lesions. Diagnosis is established by biopsy and immunofluorescence. Inverse psoriasis may be associated with collarette scales, or with serpiginous arrays of pustules at the border of inflammatory lesions. When more typical lesions of psoriasis are lacking, a biopsy may be required to establish the diagnosis.

Treatment

The reduction of perspiration and enhancement of evaporation from the crural area are important prophylactic measures. The area should be kept as dry as possible by the wearing of loose underclothing and trousers. Plain talcum powder or antifungal powders are helpful. Specific topical and oral treatment is the same as that described earlier for tinea corporis.

Tinea of hands and feet

Dermatophytosis of the feet, long popularly called athlete's foot, is by far the most common fungal disease. *T. rubrum* causes the majority of infections, and there may be an autosomal-dominant predisposition to this form of infection. *T. rubrum* typically produces a relatively noninflammatory type of dermatophytosis characterized by a dull erythema and pronounced silvery scaling that may involve the entire sole and sides of the foot, giving a moccasin or sandal appearance. One hand may be involved. The eruption may also be limited to a small patch adjacent to a fungus-infected toenail, or to a patch between or under the toes. Sometimes an extensive, patchy, scaly eruption covers most of the trunk, buttocks, and extremities. Rarely, there is a patchy hyperkeratosis resembling verrucous epidermal nevus.

Generally, tinea infection of the hands is of the dry, scaly, and erythematous type that is suggestive of *T. rubrum* infection. Other areas are frequently affected at the same time, especially the combination of both feet and one hand (Fig. 15-8). Tinea pedis caused by anthropophilic *T. mentagrophytes* (*interdigitale*) presents with three distinct appearances. One is composed of multilocular bullae involving the thin skin of the plantar arch and along the sides of the feet and heel. The second presents with erythema and desquamation between the toes. The third is white superficial onychomycosis. In the human immunodeficiency virus (HIV)-positive population, this latter syndrome is usually caused by *T. rubrum*. Interdigital tinea must be distinguished from simple maceration caused by a closed web space. The latter does not respond to antifungal therapy. Interdigital tinea must also be distinguished from Gram-negative toe web infection. Diabetic patients develop interdigital fungal infections at a younger age than patients without diabetes.

T. mentagrophytes often produces acutely inflammatory multilocular bullae (Fig. 15-9). The burning and itching that accompany the formation of the vesicles may cause great discomfort, which is relieved by opening the tense vesicles. They contain a clear straw-colored tenacious fluid. Extensive or

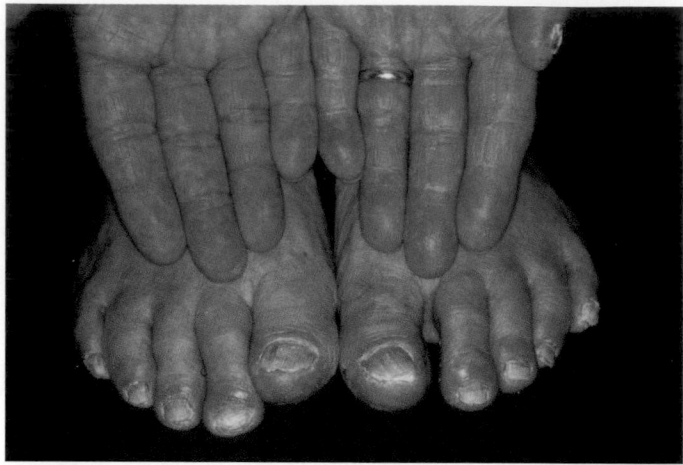

Fig. 15-8 One hand of "two foot, one hand" fungal infection.

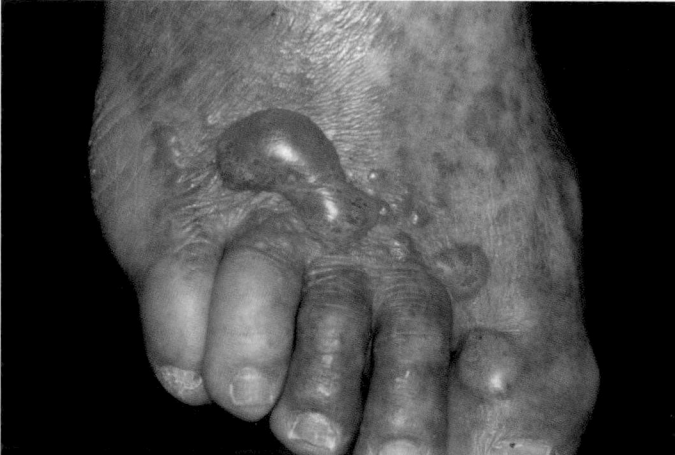

Fig. 15-9 Bullous tinea.

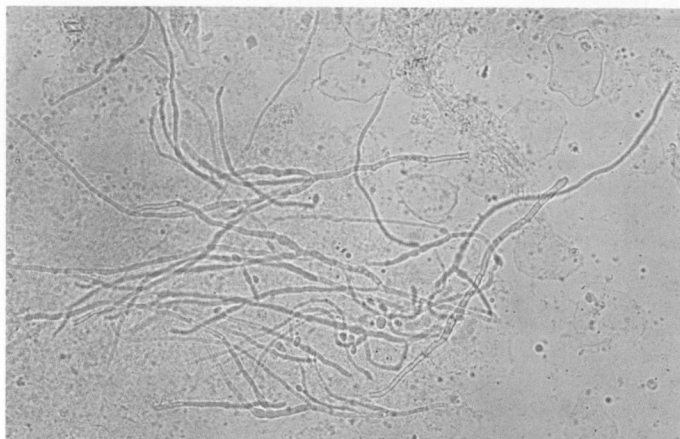

Fig. 15-10 Positive KOH examination.

acute eruptions on the soles may be incapacitating. The fissures between the toes, as well as the vesicles, may become secondarily infected with pyogenic cocci, which may lead to recurrent attacks of lymphangitis and inguinal adenitis. Gram-negative toe-web infections may also supervene. Hyperhidrosis is frequently present in this type of dermatophytosis. The sweat between the toes and on the soles has a high pH, and damp keratin is a good culture medium for the fungi.

Dermatophytid of the hands may be associated with inflammatory tinea of the feet and begins with the appearance of groups of minute, clear vesicles on the palms and fingers. The itching may be intense. As a rule, both hands are involved and the eruption tends to be symmetrical; however, there are cases in which only one hand is affected. The dorsa and sides of the feet may also be affected.

Diagnosis

Demonstration of the fungus by microscopic examination of the scrapings taken from the involved site establishes the diagnosis. Copious dry scale from the instep, heel, and sides of the foot can be gathered by scraping with the edge of a glass microscope slide. Bullae should be unroofed and either the entire roof mounted intact or scrapings made from the underside of the roof. A drop of a 10–20% solution of KOH is added to the material on the glass slide. A coverslip is placed over the specimen and pressed down firmly. Gentle heat is applied

until the scales are thoroughly macerated. The addition of 20–40% DMSO speeds clearing of keratin without the need for heating. A staining method using 100 mg of chlorazol black E dye in 10 mL of DMSO and adding it to a 5% aqueous solution of KOH can be helpful. Toluidine blue, 0.1%, can also be used on thin specimens, but contains no clearing agent to dissolve keratin.

The mycelia (Fig. 15-10) may be seen under low power, but better observation of both hyphae and spores is obtained by the use of 10X objective with the condenser cranked down or the light aperture closed by two-thirds. The lines of juncture of normal epidermal cells dissolve into a branching network that may easily be mistaken for fungus structures ("mosaic false hyphae"). This is the most common artifact misinterpreted as a positive KOH examination. Cotton and synthetic fibers from socks may also mimic hyphae.

Material may also be placed on Sabouraud dextrose agar, Sabouraud agar with chloramphenicol, Mycosel agar, or DTM. The last three agars inhibit growth of bacterial or saprophytic contaminants. The last two may inhibit some pathogenic nondermatophytes. The alkaline metabolites produced by growth of dermatophytes change the color of the pH indicator in DTM medium from yellow to red.

Prophylaxis

Hyperhidrosis is a predisposing factor for tinea infections. Because the disease often starts on the feet, the patient should be advised to dry the toes thoroughly after bathing. Dryness of the parts is essential if reinfection is to be avoided.

The use of a good antiseptic powder on the feet after bathing, particularly between the toes, is strongly advised for susceptible persons. Tolnaftate powder (Tinactin powder) or Zeasorb medicated powder is an excellent dusting powder for the feet. Plain talc, cornstarch, or rice powder may be dusted into socks and shoes to keep the feet dry. Periodic use of a topical antifungal agent may be required, especially when hot occlusive footwear is worn.

Treatment

Clotrimazole, miconazole, sulconazole, oxiconazole, ciclopirox, econazole, ketoconazole, naftifine, terbinafine, flutrimazol, bifonazole, and butenafine are effective topical antifungal agents. When there is significant maceration between the toes, the toes may be separated by foam or cotton inserts in the evening. Aluminum chloride 10% solution or aluminum acetate, 1 part to 20 parts of water, can be beneficial. Topical antibiotic ointments, such as gentamicin (Garamycin), which are effective against Gram-negative organisms, are helpful additions in some moist interdigital lesions. In the ulcerative type of Gram-negative toe-web infections, systemic antibiotic therapy is necessary. (See Chapter 14 for a discussion of Gram-negative toe-web infections.) Keratolytic agents containing salicylic acid, resorcinol, lactic acid, and urea may be useful in some cases, although all may lead to maceration if occluded.

Treatment of fungal infection of the skin of the feet and hands with griseofulvin in doses of 500–1000 mg/day can be effective. Dosage for children is 10–20 mg/kg/day. The period of therapy depends on the response of the lesions. Repeated KOH scrapings and cultures should be negative. Much shorter courses are possible with newer antifungal agents. Recommended adult dosing for terbinafine is 250 mg/day for 1–2 weeks; for itraconazole, 200 mg twice a day for 1 week; and for fluconazole, 150 mg once a week for 4 weeks. Abbreviated schedules and intermittent dosing with other agents may be possible, but require further study. In one small study, itraconazole was given in doses of 100 mg twice a day immediately after meals on 2 consecutive days. The regimen produced good to excellent responses in all patients within 14 days.

Onychomycosis (tinea unguium)

Onychomycosis is defined as the infection of the nail plate by fungus and represents up to 30% of diagnosed superficial fungal infections. *T. rubrum* accounts for most cases, but many fungi may be causative. Other etiologic agents include *E. floccosum* and various species of *Microsporum* and *Trichophyton* fungi. It may also be caused by yeasts and nondermatophytic molds.

There are four classic types of onychomycosis:

1. Distal subungual onychomycosis: primarily involves the distal nailbed and the hyponychium, with secondary involvement of the underside of the nail plate of fingernails and toenails (Fig. 15-11). It is usually caused by *T. rubrum*.
2. White superficial onychomycosis (leukonychia trichophytica): this is an invasion of the toenail plate on the surface of the nail. It is produced by *T. mentagrophytes*, species of *Cephalosporium* and *Aspergillus*, and *Fusarium oxysporum* fungi. In the HIV-positive population, it is commonly caused by *T. rubrum*.

3. Proximal subungual onychomycosis (Fig. 15-12): involves the nail plate mainly from the proximal nailfold, producing a specific clinical picture. It is produced by *T. rubrum* and *T. megninii*, and may be an indication of HIV infection.
4. *Candida* onychomycosis: produces destruction of the nail and massive nailbed hyperkeratosis. It is due to *C. albicans* and is seen in patients with chronic mucocutaneous candidiasis.

Onychomycosis caused by *T. rubrum* usually starts at the distal corner of the nail and involves the junction of the nail and its bed. A yellowish discoloration occurs, which spreads proximally as a streak in the nail. Later, subungual hyperkeratosis becomes prominent and spreads until the entire nail is affected. Gradually, the entire nail becomes brittle and separated from its bed as a result of the piling-up of subungual keratin. Fingernails and toenails present a similar appearance, and the skin of the soles is likely to be involved, with characteristic branny scaling and erythema.

Onychomycosis caused by *T. mentagrophytes* is usually superficial, and there is no paronychial inflammation. The infection generally begins with scaling of the nail under the overhanging cuticle and remains localized to a portion of the nail. In time, however, the entire nail plate may be involved. White superficial onychomycosis is the name given to one type of superficial nail infection caused by this fungus in which small, chalky white spots appear on or in the nail plate. They are so superficial that they may be easily shaved off. *T. violaceum*, *T. schoenleinii*, and *T. tonsurans* occasionally invade the nails, as does *Trichosporon beigelii*.

Scopulariopsis brevicaulis has been infrequently isolated from onychomycosis. Infection usually begins at the lateral edge of the nail, burrows beneath the plate, and produces large quantities of cheesy debris. *Nattrassia mangiferae* (*Hendersonula toruloidea*) and *Scytalidium hyalinum* have been reported to cause onychomycosis, as well as a moccasin-type tinea pedis. In addition to the more common features of onychomycosis, such as nail-plate thickening, opacification, and onycholysis, features of infection with these fungi include lateral nail invasion alone, paronychia, and transverse fracture of the proximal nail plate. When these agents are suspected, culture must be done with a medium that does not contain cycloheximide (found in Mycosel agar). Oral ketoconazole and griseofulvin are not effective in the treatment of these organisms.

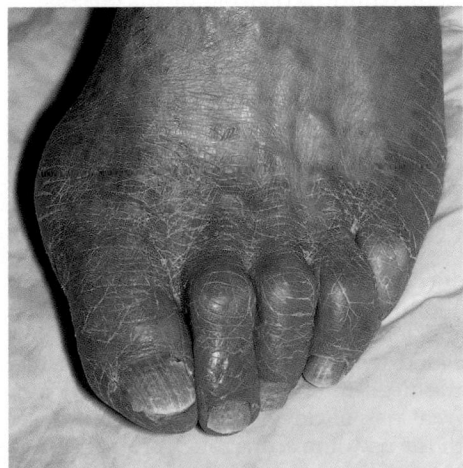

Fig. 15-11 Distal subungual onychomycosis and tinea pedis.

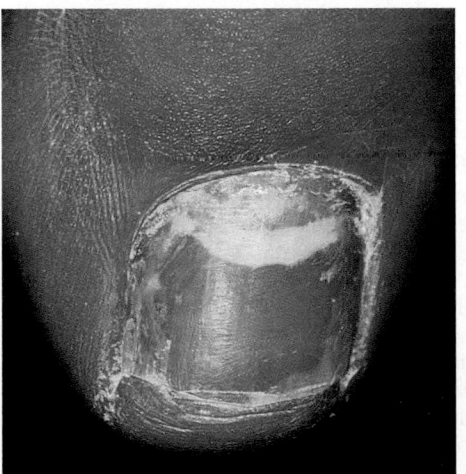

Fig. 15-12 White proximal subungual onychomycosis.

The pathogen is heavily influenced by heredity, geography, and footwear. In the US, most tinea pedis and onychomycosis are caused by *T. rubrum*. In a rural school in Mexico where most people wear nonocclusive leather sandals, *Trichosporon cutaneum*, *Candida* spp and *T. mentagrophytes* accounted for most infection. *T. rubrum* was not isolated in any patient. Cutaneous *Scytalidium* infections are common in patients from the tropics, especially the West Indies and Africa. They commonly carry the organism with them, even when they emigrate to more temperate climates.

Diagnosis

The demonstration of fungus is made by microscopic examination or by culture. The submitted clippings or curettings must include dystrophic subungual debris. Samples obtained via a drilling technique may have a higher yield than those obtained via a curettage. Immediate examination may be made if very thin shavings or curettings are taken from the diseased nailbed and examined with KOH solution. A variety of stains such as chlorazol black E can be added to improve sensitivity. Histologic examination, polymerase chain reaction (PCR), and calcofluor white microscopy and culture have also been used.

Histopathologic examination with periodic acid-Schiff (PAS) stain has been found to be 41–93% sensitive in various studies. It has proved more sensitive than either KOH or culture in several studies. In one study, in which histology was 85% sensitive, KOH dissolution and centrifugation combined with PAS was 57% sensitive, while calcofluor white fluorescent staining and chlorazol black E were each found to be 53% sensitive. Culture on Sabouraud agar with chloramphenicol and cycloheximide (Mycosel) agar was 32% sensitive. Other studies have shown the sensitivity of culture to be 30–70%. Combining KOH and culture has yielded sensitivities in the range of 80–85%.

Both office and central laboratories can be used to isolate fungi, but false-negative results are common in both settings. In one study, office DTM culture was positive in 102 of 184 patients (55%), while the central laboratory detected the infection in 78 of 184 (42%). The two tests were in agreement (both positive or both negative) in 114 of 184 patients (62%). In a similar study, DTM cultures were positive in 51% (n = 345), while central laboratory cultures were positive in 44% (n = 297). The two cultures were in agreement in 68% of cases. Dermatophytes accounted for about 90% of the confirmed infections in each study.

As no single method offers 100% sensitivity, a variety of methods are still in use. KOH has the advantage of being performed rapidly in the office. Histologic examination usually provides results within 24 h, while culture can take days to weeks. Identification of genus and species is only possible with culture.

Differential diagnosis

Dystrophic nails can be produced by psoriasis, lichen planus, eczema, and contact dermatitis, and may be clinically indistinguishable from fungal nails. Confirmatory tests to identify the fungus are mandatory in order to establish a diagnosis. Psoriasis may involve other nails with pitting, onycholysis, oil spots, and salmon patches, or by heaped-up subungual keratinization. Typical features of psoriasis may be present on other areas of skin. Lichen planus may produce rough nails or pterygium formation and may involve the oral mucosa or skin. Eczema and contact dermatitis affect the adjacent nailfold. Hyperkeratotic ("Norwegian") scabies can also produce dystrophic nails, but is associated with generalized hyperkeratosis.

Onychomycosis among psoriasis patients is reported with varying prevalence, but occurs roughly in the range of 22% compared to 13% for patients with other skin diseases. Onychomycosis occurs more frequently in men than in women with psoriasis.

Treatment

Many patients with onychomycosis are not symptomatic, and may not seek treatment. Patients with diabetes or peripheral neuropathy may be at higher risk for complications related to onychomycosis, and the benefits of treatment may be greater in this population. These factors, as well as cost and risk of recurrence, should be considered as part of the decision to treat onychomycosis.

The topical management of onychomycosis has improved with the introduction of ciclopirox and amorolfine nail lacquers. These agents are modestly effective at moderate cost. A lacquer containing encecalin extract of *Ageratina pichinchensis* also looks promising as a topical agent. Other topical agents are of little benefit, and no topical agent achieves the cure rates possible with oral therapy.

For disease involving fingernails, terbinafine is given in doses of 250 mg/day for 6–8 weeks. For toenails, the course of treatment is generally 12–16 weeks. Itraconazole is generally given as pulsed dosing, 200 mg twice a day for 1 week of each month, for 2 months when treating fingernails and for 3–4 months when treating toenails. Fluconazole, at doses of 150–300 mg once a week for 6–12 months, appears to be effective. Around 20% of patients will not respond to treatment. The presence of a dermatophytoma within the nail may be associated with a higher risk of failure. Dermatophytomas present as yellow streaks within the nail, and may respond to unroofing and curettage. Several studies have suggested that continuous therapy with terbinafine for 4 months is cost-effective when compared with other possible agents and regimens. Most clinical trials have been industry-sponsored and little independent research is available for review. For onychomycosis in children, terbinafine, itraconazole, and fluconazole have all been shown to be effective. Dosage depends on body weight, as indicated above. Duration of treatment is the same as for adults.

Treatment with systemic antifungals is very effective in onychomycosis caused by *Aspergillus* spp. *Scopulariopsis brevicaulis* and *Fusarium* spp infection is difficult to eradicate and treatment with both systemic antifungals and topical nail lacquers may be appropriate. Nail avulsion represents another option. *Candida* onychomycosis is always a sign of immunodepression. Systemic treatment with itraconazole or fluconazole is usually effective, but relapses are the rule. When treating *Candida* infections, combinations of topical and systemic treatment can be used for synergistic effect. The combination of topical amorolfine and oral itraconazole, which interferes with different steps of ergosterol synthesis, has been shown to exhibit substantial synergy in this setting. Combination treatment with topical amorolfine and two pulses of itraconazole may be as effective as three pulses of itraconazole, with lower cost.

The Food and Drug Administration (FDA) has issued a health advisory to announce serious risks associated with the use of itraconazole and terbinafine. The advisory states that both have been associated with serious liver problems resulting in liver failure, the need for transplantation, and death. There is a small but real risk of developing congestive heart failure associated with the use of itraconazole. Terbinafine has been associated with subacute cutaneous lupus erythematosus. Significant drug interactions may occur in patients on itraconazole who are also treated with drugs metabolized by the cytochrome P450 pathway. Interactions with terbinafine and the tricyclic antidepressant desipramine have been reported.

Itraconazole pulsed treatment has been shown to have a low incidence of liver function abnormalities (alanine aminotransferase [ALT], aspartate aminotransferase [AST], alkaline phosphatase, and total bilirubin). Product labeling recommends liver function tests for patients receiving continuous itraconazole for periods exceeding 1 month. Monitoring is required for the pulsed regimen if the patient has a history of hepatic disease, has abnormal baseline liver function tests, or development of signs or symptoms suggestive of liver dysfunction. Phenobarbital shows potential for the cytoprotection of hepatocytes to itraconazole- but not fluconazole-induced cytotoxicity in vitro, suggesting the possibility of regimens to reduce the risk of toxicity further.

Molds are sensitive to UV and visible light, and *T. rubrum* in culture has been shown to be susceptible to UV C radiation, photodynamic therapy (PDT), and psoralen with UVA (PUVA). For PDT with broad-band white light, the phthalocyanines and photofrin displayed a fungistatic effect, whereas porphyrins caused photodynamic killing of the dermatophyte. 5,10,15-Tris(4-methylpyridinium)-20-phenyl-(21H,23H)-porphine trichloride and deuteroporphyrin monomethylester showed superior results in vitro. Further study of various methods of phototherapy is warranted.

Ahmad SR, et al. Congestive heart failure associated with itraconazole. Lancet 2001; 357:1766.

Baran R, et al: Review of antifungal therapy and the severity index for assessing onychomycosis: part I. J Dermatolog Treat 2008; 19(2):72–81.

Baran R, et al: Review of antifungal therapy, part II: treatment rationale, including specific patient populations. J Dermatolog Treat 2008; 19(3):168–175.

Bell-Syer SE, et al: Oral treatments for fungal infections of the skin of the foot. Cochrane Database Syst Rev 2002; 2:CD003584.

Carrillo-Muñoz AJ, et al: Terbinafine susceptibility patterns for onychomycosis-causative dermatophytes and Scopulariopsis brevicaulis. Int J Antimicrob Agents 2008 Jun; 31(6):540–543.

Dai T, et al: Ultraviolet C inactivation of dermatophytes: implications for treatment of onychomycosis. Br J Dermatol 2008 Jun; 158(6):1239–1246.

Daniel CR 3rd, et al: Commentary: the illusory tinea unguium cure. J Am Acad Dermatol 2010 Mar; 62(3):415–417.

Das S, et al: Laboratory-based epidemiological study of superficial fungal infections. J Dermatol 2007 Apr; 34(4):248–253.

Elewski BE, et al: Terbinafine hydrochloride oral granules versus oral griseofulvin suspension in children with tinea capitis: results of two randomized, investigator-blinded, multicenter, international, controlled trials. J Am Acad Dermatol 2008 Jul; 59(1):41–54.

Gupta AK, et al: Meta-analysis: griseofulvin efficacy in the treatment of tinea capitis. J Drugs Dermatol 2008 Apr; 7(4):369–372.

Hirose N, et al: Management and follow-up survey of Trichophyton tonsurans infection in a university judo club. Mycoses 2008 May; 51(3):243–247.

Hivnor CM, et al: Terbinafine-induced subacute cutaneous lupus erythematosus. Cutis 2008 Feb; 81(2):156–157.

Kakourou T, et al: Guidelines for the management of tinea capitis in children. Pediatr Dermatol 2010 May; 27(3):226–228.

Kye YC: Successful treatment of tinea pedis with a topical agent containing isoconazole nitrate and diflucortolone valerate. Mycoses 2008 Sep; 51(Suppl 4):48–49.

Legge BS, et al: The incidence of tinea pedis in diabetic versus nondiabetic patients with interdigital macerations: a prospective study. J Am Podiatr Med Assoc 2008 Sep–Oct; 98(5):353–356.

Loo DS: Systemic antifungal agents: an update of established and new therapies. Adv Dermatol 2006; 22:101–124.

McPherson ME, et al: High prevalence of tinea capitis in newly arrived migrants at an English-language school, Melbourne, 2005. Med J Aust 2008 Jul 7; 189(1):13–16.

Seebacher C, et al: Tinea capitis: ringworm of the scalp. Mycoses 2007 May; 50(3):218–226.

Sharma R, et al: A virulent genotype of Microsporum canis is responsible for the majority of human infections. J Med Microbiol 2007 Oct; 56(Pt 10):1377–1385.

Shemer A, et al: Collection of fungi samples from nails: comparative study of curettage and drilling techniques. J Eur Acad Dermatol Venereol 2008 Feb; 22(2):182–185.

Shenoy MM, et al: Comparison of potassium hydroxide mount and mycological culture with histopathologic examination using periodic acid-Schiff staining of the nail clippings in the diagnosis of onychomycosis. Indian J Dermatol Venereol Leprol 2008 May–Jun; 74(3):226–229.

Smijs TG, et al: Morphological changes of the dermatophyte Trichophyton rubrum after photodynamic treatment: a scanning electron microscopy study. Med Mycol 2008 Jun; 46(4):315–325.

Watanabe D, et al: Successful treatment of toenail onychomycosis with photodynamic therapy. Arch Dermatol 2008 Jan; 144(1):19–21.

Zhang AY, et al: Advances in topical and systemic antifungals. Dermatol Clin 2007 Apr; 25(2):165–183, vi.

Candidiasis

Candidiasis is also known as candidosis or moniliasis. *C. albicans* is a common inhabitant of the human gastrointestinal and genitourinary tracts, and skin. Under the right conditions, it becomes a pathogen, causing lesions of the skin, nails, and mucous membranes. The intertriginous areas are frequently affected. Here warmth, moisture, and maceration of the skin permit the organism to thrive. The areas most often involved are the perianal and inguinal folds, abdominal creases, inframammary creases, interdigital areas, nailfolds, and axillae.

C. albicans is largely an opportunistic organism, acting as a pathogen in the presence of impaired immune response, or where local conditions favor growth. Warmth and moisture favor candidal growth. Reductions in competing flora during antibiotic therapy can also favor candidal growth. Higher skin pH favors candidal growth. Diapers, panty liners, and other occlusive products raise skin pH and may predispose to skin infections of *C. albicans*. A topical acidic buffer may be helpful as a preventive measure for recurrent *Candida*-induced skin rash.

Diagnosis

Under the microscope the KOH preparation may show spores and pseudohyphae. On Gram stain the yeast forms dense, Gram-positive, ovoid bodies, 2–5 μm in diameter. A combination of Gomori methenamine silver (GMS) and Congo red staining can be helpful in the differential diagnosis of fungal infections. *Blastomyces* and *Pityrosporum* are positive for both, while *Candida* and *Histoplasma* are GMS-positive and Congo red-negative.

Candida proliferates in both budding and mycelial forms in the stratum corneum or superficial mucosa. Budding yeast and pseudohyphae are easier to detect in histologic section with a PAS stain. Whereas dermatophyte hyphae tend to run parallel to the skin surface, *Candida* pseudohyphae have more of a tendency to vertical orientation.

In culture *C. albicans* should be differentiated from other forms of *Candida* that are only rarely pathogenic, such as *Candida krusei*, *Candida stellatoidea*, *Candida tropicalis*, *Candida pseudotropicalis*, and *Candida guilliermondii*. Culture on Sabouraud glucose agar shows a growth of creamy, grayish, moist colonies in about 4 days. In time the colonies form small, rootlike penetrations into the agar. Microscopic examination of the colony shows clusters of budding cells. When inoculated into cornmeal agar culture, thick-walled, round chlamydospores characteristic of *C. albicans* are produced.

Topical anticandidal agents

Most of the topical agents marketed for tinea are also effective for candidiasis. These include clotrimazole (Lotrimin, Mycelex), econazole (Spectazole), ketoconazole (Nizoral), miconazole (Monistat-Derm Lotion, Micatin), oxiconazole (Oxistat), sulconazole (Exelderm), naftifine (Naftin), terconazole, ciclopirox olamine (Loprox), butenafine (Mentax), terbinafine (Lamisil), nystatin, and topical amphotericin B lotion. Older agents such as gentian violet, Castellani paint, and boric acid are still sometimes used.

Other agents

Fluconazole has a remarkable safety record, even when used long-term in patients with *Candida* related to genodermatoses. Posaconazole, itraconazole, voriconazole, echinocandins, anidulafungin and amphotericin B are also used in various settings. Various flavonoid compounds, including apigenin and kaempferol, alkaloid ibogaine (an indole), and the protoberberine alkaloid berberine have been studied for their inhibitory effects. Kaempferol has shown a survival benefit in patients with systemic infections. Topical applications of each of these agents accelerated elimination from cutaneous sites of inoculation.

Oral candidiasis (thrush)

The mucous membrane of the mouth may be involved in healthy infants. In the newborn the infection may be acquired from contact with the vaginal tract of the mother. In older children and adults, thrush is commonly seen following antibiotic therapy. It may also be a sign of immunosuppression.

Grayish-white membranous plaques are found on the surface of the mucous membrane. The base of these plaques is moist, reddish, and macerated (Fig. 15-13). In its spread the angles of the mouth may become involved, and lesions in the intertriginous areas may occur, especially in marasmic infants. The diaper area is especially susceptible to this infection. Most of the intertriginous areas and even the exposed skin may be involved, with small pustules that quickly turn into macerated and erythematous scaling patches.

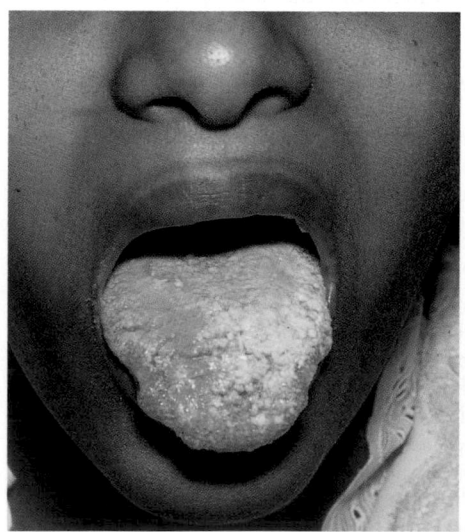

Fig. 15-13 Thrush.

In adults, the appearance may resemble that seen in children, or may be drier and more erythematous. Saliva inhibits the growth of *Candida*, and a dry mouth predisposes to candidal growth. Broad-spectrum antibiotics also predispose to candidiasis. The papillae of the tongue may appear atrophic, with the surface smooth, glazed, and bright red. Frequently the infection extends on to the angles of the mouth to form perlèche. This appearance is common in elderly, debilitated, and malnourished patients, and in patients with diabetes. It is often the first manifestation of AIDS, and is present in nearly all untreated patients with full-blown AIDS. The observation of oral "thrush" in an adult with no known predisposing factors warrants a search for other evidence of infection with HIV, such as lymphadenopathy, leukopenia, or HIV antibodies in the serum.

Various treatment options are available. Infants are commonly treated with oral nystatin suspension. An adult can let clotrimazole troches dissolve in the mouth. A single 150 mg dose of fluconazole is effective for many mucocutaneous infections in adults. In immunosuppressed patients, 200 mg/day is the starting dose, but much higher doses are often needed. Itraconazole, 200 mg/day for 5–10 days, can also be effective. Although terbinafine is commonly thought of as a dermatophyte drug, it can also be effective for *Candida* infections at doses of 250 mg/day.

Perlèche

Perlèche, or angular cheilitis, is characterized by maceration and transverse fissuring of the oral commissures. The earliest lesions are ill-defined, grayish-white, thickened areas with slight erythema of the mucous membrane at the oral commissure. When more fully developed, this thickening has a bluish-white or mother-of-pearl color and may be contiguous with a wedge-shaped erythematous scaling dermatitis of the skin portion of the commissure. Fissures, maceration, and crust formation ensue. Soft, pinhead-sized papules may appear. Involvement is usually bilateral. Perlèche is commonly related to *C. albicans*, but may also harbor coagulase-positive *S. aureus* and Gram-negative bacteria. Similar changes may occur in riboflavin deficiency or other nutritional deficiency.

Identical fissuring occurs at the mucocutaneous junction from drooling in persons with malocclusion caused by ill-fitting dentures and in the aged in whom atrophy of the alveolar ridges ("closing" the bite) has caused the upper lip to overhang the lower at the commissures. There is sometimes a vertical shortening of the lower third of the face.

If infection is due to *C. albicans*, anticandidal creams are effective, but the response is more rapid if they are used in combination with a mid-strength topical corticosteroid. If the perlèche is due to vertical shortening of the lower third of the face, dental or oral surgical intervention may be helpful. Injection of collagen into the depressed sulcus at the oral commissure can be beneficial.

Candidal vulvovaginitis

C. albicans is a common inhabitant of the vaginal tract. Overgrowth can cause severe pruritus, burning, and discharge. The labia may be erythematous, moist, and macerated, and the cervix hyperemic, swollen, and eroded, showing small vesicles on its surface. The vaginal discharge is not usually profuse and varies from watery, to thick and white or curdlike.

This type of infection may develop during pregnancy, in diabetes, or secondary to therapy with broad-spectrum antibiotics. Recurrent vulvovaginal candidiasis has also been associated with long-term tamoxifen treatment. Candidal balanitis may be present in an uncircumcised sexual partner. Diagnosis is established by the clinical symptoms and findings, as well as the demonstration of the fungus by KOH microscopic examination and culture.

Oral fluconazole, 150 mg given once, is easy and effective. In some patients with predisposing factors, longer courses of fluconazole, 100–200 mg/day, or itraconazole, 200 mg/day for 5–10 days, may be needed. Topical options include miconazole, nystatin, clotrimazole, and terconazole. Probiotic, anticandidal bacteria have also been advocated.

Candida glabrata vaginitis may be refractory to azole drugs and can be difficult to eradicate. Topical boric acid, amphotericin B, and flucytosine may be helpful in this setting.

Candidal intertrigo

The pruritic intertriginous eruptions caused by *C. albicans* may arise between the folds of the genitals; in groins or armpits; between the buttocks; under large, pendulous breasts; under overhanging abdominal folds; or in the umbilicus. The pink to red intertriginous moist patches are surrounded by a thin, overhanging fringe of somewhat macerated epidermis ("collarette" scale). Some eruptions in the inguinal region may resemble tinea cruris, but usually there is less scaliness and a greater tendency to fissuring. Persistent excoriation and subsequent lichenification and drying may, in the course of time, modify the original appearance. Often, tiny, superficial, white pustules are observed closely adjacent to the patches. When present, *Candida* can cause flares of inverse psoriasis, but there is no increase in the prevalence of *Candida* in the intertriginous areas of patients with either psoriasis or atopic dermatitis.

Topical anticandidal preparations are usually effective, but recurrence is common. Combinations of a topical anticandidal agent with a mid-strength corticosteroid may lead to more rapid relief. Castellani paint may also be helpful. Colorless Castellani paint is often preferred by patients.

Diaper candidiasis

The diagnosis of candidiasis may be suspected from the finding of involvement of the folds and occurrence of many small erythematous desquamating "satellite" or "daughter" lesions scattered along the edges of the larger macules (Fig. 15-14). Topical anticandidal agents are effective. They are sometimes compounded in zinc oxide ointment to act as a barrier against the irritating effect of urine. Recurrent diaper

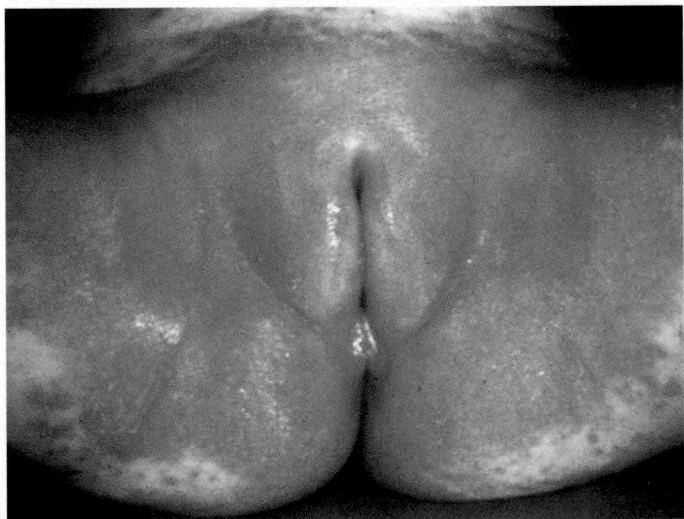

Fig. 15-14 Diaper candidiasis.

candidiasis may be associated with oral and gut colonization, and may respond to the addition of oral nystatin suspension.

Congenital cutaneous candidiasis

Premature rupture of membranes together with a birth canal infected with *C. albicans* may lead to congenital cutaneous candidiasis. The eruption is usually noted within a few hours of delivery. Erythematous macules progress to thin-walled pustules, which rupture, dry, and desquamate within a week or so. Lesions are usually widespread, involving the trunk, neck, and head, and at times the palms and soles, including the nailfolds. The oral cavity and diaper area are spared, in contrast to the usual type of acquired neonatal infection. The differential diagnosis includes other neonatal vesiculopustular disorders, such as listeriosis, syphilis, staphylococcal, and herpes infections, erythema toxicum neonatorum, transient neonatal pustular melanosis, miliaria rubra, drug eruption, and congenital icthyosiform erythroderma. If infection is suspected early, the amniotic fluid, placenta, and cord should be examined for evidence of infection.

Infants with candidiasis limited to the skin have favorable outcomes; however, systemic involvement may occur. Disseminated infection is suggested by evidence of respiratory distress or other laboratory or clinical signs of neonatal sepsis. Dissemination is more common in infants who weigh less than 1500 g. Treatment with broad-spectrum antibiotics and altered immune responsiveness can also predispose to dissemination. Infants with congenital cutaneous candidiasis and any of the above factors may be considered for systemic antifungal therapy.

Perianal candidiasis

C. albicans infection may present as pruritus ani. Perianal dermatitis with erythema, oozing, and maceration is present. Pruritus and burning can be extremely severe. Satellite lesions may be present, but their absence does not exclude candidiasis. *Candida* growth is also enhanced on abnormal tissue, such as extramammary Paget's disease. If the tissue does not return to normal after the candidiasis is treated, a biopsy may be warranted.

Candidal paronychia

Inflammation of the nailfold produces redness, edema, and tenderness of the proximal nailfolds, and gradual thickening and brownish discoloration of the nail plates. Usually the fingernails only are affected. Patients commonly have an atopic background.

While acute paronychia is usually staphylococcal in origin, chronic paronychia is commonly multifactorial in origin. Irritant dermatitis and candidiasis may play important roles. In one study, treatment with a topical corticosteroid was superior to treatment with an anticandidal agent. Avoidance of irritants and wet work is essential. Anticandidal agents may be of use in this setting, and may be used in combination with a topical corticosteroid.

Candidal paronychia is frequently seen in patients with diabetes, and one aspect of the treatment consists of bringing the diabetes under control. The avoidance of chronic exposure to moisture and irritants is also essential in these patients. If topical treatment fails, oral fluconazole once a week or itraconazole in pulsed dosing can be effective.

Repetitive contact urticaria or allergic contact dermatitis to foods and spices may mimic candidal paronychia. Patch and radioallergosorbent testing (RAST) may be of value.

Erosio interdigitalis blastomycetica

This form of candidiasis is seen as an oval-shaped area of macerated white skin on the web between and extending on to the sides of the fingers. Usually at the center of the lesion there are one or more fissures with raw, red bases; as the condition progresses the macerated skin peels off, leaving a painful, raw, denuded area surrounded by a collar of overhanging white epidermis. It is nearly always the third web, between the middle and ring fingers, that is affected. The moisture beneath the ring macerates the skin and predisposes to infection. The disease is also seen in patients with diabetes and those who do wet work.

Intertriginous lesions between the toes are similar. Usually the white, sodden epidermis is thick and does not peel off freely. On the feet it is the fourth interspace that is most often involved, but the areas are apt to be multiple. Clinically, this may be indistinguishable from tinea pedis. Diagnosis is made by culture. Lesions may respond to drying, topical anticandidal agents or applications of filter paper soaked with Castellani's paint.

Chronic mucocutaneous candidiasis

The term chronic mucocutaneous candidiasis designates a heterogeneous group of patients whose infection with *Candida* is chronic but limited to mucosal surfaces, skin, and nails. Onset is typically before age 6. Onset in adult life may herald the occurrence of thymoma. These cases may be either inherited or sporadic. Inherited types may be associated with endocrinopathy. Oral lesions are diffuse, and perlèche and lip fissures are common. The nails become thickened and dystrophic, with associated paronychia. Hyperkeratotic, hornlike, or granulomatous lesions are often seen (Figs 15-15 and 15-16).

Patients with mucocutaneous candidiasis have a selective defect in immunity that leaves them vulnerable to candidiasis. The underlying defect is unknown, and it is likely that this condition represents a group of disorders with a similar phenotype. Abnormalities of type 1 cytokine production in response to *Candida* have been reported. Specifically, there may be markedly impaired production of interleukin (IL)-12 and dramatically increased levels of IL-6 and IL-10. Reductions in natural killer (NK) cells have also been noted. In a five-generation Italian family with chronic mucocutaneous candidiasis affecting only the nails, low serum intercellular adhesion molecule 1 (ICAM-1) was noted. The defect was linked to a 19cM pericentromeric region on chromosome 11. Chronic mucocutaneous candidiasis with thyroid disease has been linked to chromosomes 2p.

Systemic fluconazole, itraconazole, or ketoconazole is necessary to control the disease. Courses are typically prolonged, repeated, and given at higher than the usual recommended dose. Patients with achlorhydria may have problems with absorption of itraconazole and ketoconazole. Cimetidine was reported to restore deficient cell-mediated immunity in four adults from one family, at a dose of 300 mg four times a day.

Systemic candidiasis

C. albicans is capable of causing disseminated disease and sepsis, invariably when host defenses are compromised. Those who are at high risk include patients with malignancies, especially leukemias and lymphomas, in which there may be impaired immune defenses; patients with AIDS; debilitated and malnourished patients; patients with transplants requiring immunosuppressive drugs for prolonged periods; patients receiving oral cortisone; patients who have had multiple surgical operations, especially cardiac surgery; patients with indwelling intravenous catheters; and intravenous drug abusers.

The initial sign of systemic candidiasis may be fever of unknown origin, pulmonary infiltration, gastrointestinal bleeding, endocarditis, renal failure, meningitis, osteomyelitis, endophthalmitis, peritonitis, proximal muscle weakness and tenderness, or a disseminated maculopapular exanthema. The cutaneous lesions begin as erythematous macules that may become papular, pustular, hemorrhagic, or ulcerative. Deep abscesses may occur. The trunk and extremities are the usual sites of involvement. Proximal muscle tenderness frequently accompanies the exanthema and may be a valuable clue to the correct diagnosis.

The demonstration of microorganisms or a positive culture will substantiate a diagnosis of candidiasis only if the microorganism is found in tissues or fluids ordinarily sterile for *Candida* and if the clinical picture is compatible. *Candida* colonization of endotracheal tubes used in supporting low-birth

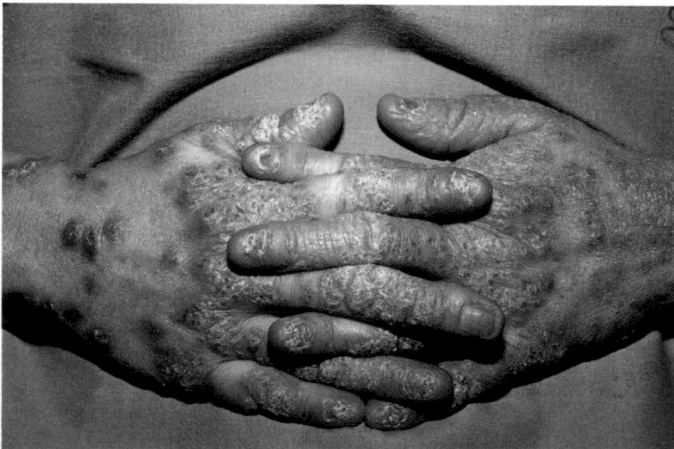

Fig. 15-15 Hand and nail involvement in chronic mucocutaneous candidiasis.

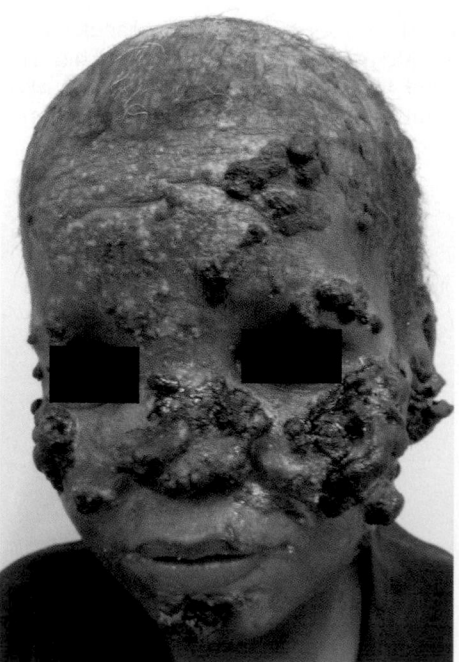

Fig. 15-16 Chronic mucocutaneous candidiasis. (Courtesy of Leslie Castelo-Soccio, MD)

weight neonates predisposes to systemic disease. If *Candida* is cultured within the first week of life, there is a high rate of systemic disease.

The mortality attributed to systemic candidosis has declined because of early empiric antifungal treatment and better prophylaxis. Data in children are similar to those in adults. Although amphotericin B remains the gold standard of treatment in systemic candidiasis, other safer options are available. Amphotericin B is now available in liposome-encapsulated forms, which appear to be less toxic. Fluconazole has been shown to be effective as prophylaxis of bone marrow transplantation, as well as in the treatment of oropharyngeal candidosis and candidemia in nonneutropenic patients. At high doses, it is sometimes used for *Candida* in neutropenic patients. Voriconazole is a new triazole antifungal that acts by inhibiting the synthesis of ergosterol in the fungal cell membrane. Posaconazole is a triazole active against *Candida*, although some problems with resistance have been reported. Caspofungin is an echinocandin antifungal that inhibits β-1,3-D-glucan synthesis in the cell wall. Micafungin and anidulafungin are echinocandins. The newer triazoles and echinocandins have broad spectrums and are effective against invasive *Aspergillus* and *Candida* infections. Voriconazole has produced liver abnormalities, rash, and visual disturbances, and these must be monitored during therapy. A meta-analysis of studies of *Candida* sepsis concluded that clinical efficacy was similar among the agents studied, but microbiological failure was more common with fluconazole than with amphotericin B or anidulafungin. Amphotericin B had a higher rate of adverse events than fluconazole or the echinocandins. Some data favor caspofungin or micafungin over anidulafungin in neutropenic patients. The anti-arrhythmic drug amiodarone has some fungicidal activity and low doses of amiodarone have been reported to produce a synergistic effect with fluconazole in fluconazole-resistant *C. albicans*. Despite advances in treatment, the mortality rates associated with systemic candidiasis remain high, with an overall mortality in the range of 30–50% and attributable mortality of approximately 30%.

Candidid

As in dermatophytosis, patients with candidiasis may develop secondary id reactions. They are much less common than the reactions seen with acute inflammatory dermatophytosis. The reactions, which have been reported to clear with treatment of candidal infection, are usually of the erythema annulare centrifugum or chronic urticaria type.

Antibiotic (iatrogenic) candidiasis

The use of oral antibiotics, such as the tetracyclines and their related products, may induce clinical candidiasis involving the mouth, gastrointestinal tract, or perianal area. In addition, vulvovaginitis may occur. It has been suggested that perhaps the bacterial flora in the gastrointestinal system are changed by suppression of some of the antibiotic-sensitive bacteria, thereby permitting other organisms such as *Candida* to flourish. Fluconazole, 150 mg once, will treat this adequately if antibiotic therapy is given for a limited time. For more prolonged courses of antibiotic therapy, the dose of fluconazole may have to be repeated, or a longer course of a topical agent may be used.

Arendse T, et al: *Candida* species: species distribution and antifungal susceptibility patterns. S Afr Med J 2008 Jun; 98(6):455–456.

Axelson GK, et al: Evaluation of the use of Congo red staining in the differential diagnosis of *Candida* vs. various other yeast-form fungal organisms. J Cutan Pathol 2008 Jan; 35(1):27–30.

Blyth CC, et al: Antifungal therapy in infants and children with proven, probable or suspected invasive fungal infections. Cochrane Database Syst Rev 2010; 2:CD006343.

Foureur N, et al: Prospective aetiological study of diaper dermatitis in the elderly. Br J Dermatol 2006 Nov; 155(5):941–946.

Gafter-Gvili A, et al: Treatment of invasive candidal infections: systematic review and meta-analysis. Mayo Clin Proc 2008 Sep; 83(9):1011–1021.

Hoyer LL, et al: *Candida* here, and *Candida* there, and *Candida* everywhere! Future Microbiol 2008 Jun; 3:271–273.

Lass-Flörl C: Invasive fungal infections in pediatric patients: a review focusing on antifungal therapy. Expert Rev Anti Infect Ther 2010; 8(2):127–135.

Leibovici V, et al: Prevalence of *Candida* on the tongue and intertriginous areas of psoriatic and atopic dermatitis patients. Mycoses 2008 Jan; 51(1):63–66.

Mansur AT, et al: Long-term use of fluconazole for verrucous plaques of cutaneous candidiasis in KID syndrome. Eur J Dermatol 2008 Jul–Aug; 18(4):469–470.

Marr KA: Fungal infections in oncology patients: update on epidemiology, prevention, and treatment. Curr Opin Oncol 2010; 22(2):138–142.

Rüping MJ, et al: Antifungal treatment strategies in high-risk patients. Mycoses 2008 Sep; 51(Suppl 2):46–51.

Sabol K, et al: Anidulafungin in the treatment of invasive fungal infections. Ther Clin Risk Manag 2008 Feb; 4(1):71–78.

Vazquez JA: Invasive fungal infections in the intensive care unit. Semin Respir Crit Care Med 2010; 31(1):79–86.

Yordanov M, et al: Inhibition of *Candida albicans* extracellular enzyme activity by selected natural substances and their application in *Candida* infection. Can J Microbiol 2008 Jun; 54(6):435–440.

Geotrichosis

Geotrichum candidum is an ascomycetous anamorph yeast-like fungus commonly found as part of the natural flora of milk. It is also found on fruit and tomatoes, and in soil. It is used commercially as a maturing agent for cheese. Individual strains may be more mold- or yeast-like. Substantial genetic polymorphism has been noted in this organism. Strains with a mold-like phenotype tend to have larger genomes than those with a yeast-like phenotype.

In immunosuppressed individuals, *G. candidum* or *Geotrichum capitatum* (*Blastoschizomyces capitatus*) may act as an opportunistic pathogen, causing disseminated or mucocutaneous geotrichosis. Mucocutaneous disease is characterized by erythema, pseudomembranes, and mucopurulent sputum similar to that seen in thrush. The intestinal, bronchial, and pulmonary forms are similar to candidal infection. *G. candidum* is commonly isolated as a saprophyte. If it is cultured repeatedly from diseased tissue, it should be assumed to be acting as a pathogen.

The diagnosis is made by the repeated demonstration of the organism by KOH microscopic examination and by its culture from sputum on Sabouraud dextrose agar. Direct examination shows branching septate mycelium and chains of rectangular cells. In culture there is a mealy growth at room temperature. The hyphae form rectangular arthrospores.

Treatment of mucocutaneous disease can be accomplished with oral nystatin or mycostatin suspension in some cases. For more severe or disseminated disease, liposomal amphotericin B, caspofungin, voriconazole, itraconazole, flucytosine, or combinations of these agents have been effective.

Etienne A, et al: Successful treatment of disseminated *Geotrichum capitatum* infection with a combination of caspofungin and voriconazole in an immunocompromised patient. Mycoses 2008 May; 51(3):270–272.

Hattori H, et al: A case of oral geotrichosis caused by *Geotrichum capitatum* in an old patient. Jpn J Infect Dis 2007 Sep; 60(5):300–301.

Pottier I, et al: Safety assessment of dairy microorganisms: *Geotrichum candidum*. Int J Food Microbiol 2008 Sep 1; 126(3):327–332.

Sfakianakis A, et al: Invasive cutaneous infection with *Geotrichum candidum*: sequential treatment with amphotericin B and voriconazole. Med Mycol 2007 Feb; 45(1):81–84.

Tinea nigra

Hortaea werneckii (formerly *Phaeoannellomyces werneckii*) is a black yeast-like hyphomycete that is widely distributed in hot, humid environments. The organism is common in the tropics. In the US, the infection is commonly seen along the Gulf coast. New taxonomic analysis has led some to classify *Cladosporium castellanii* as the etiological agent of tinea nigra in humans and confirmed that this fungus is the same as *Stenella araguata*.

Tinea nigra presents as one or several brown or black spots on the palms or soles. The lesions may be mistaken for nevi or melanoma. The pigment is confined to the stratum corneum and scrapes off easily. Dermoscopy has also been used to differentiate the lesions from melanocytic tumors. The fungus can easily be demonstrated by means of KOH or culture. In KOH preparations, the hyphae appear brown or golden in color. Young colonies are glossy, black, and yeast-like, but older colonies are filamentous and grayish. The pigment produced by the fungal hyphae is melanin. Culture will identify the organism, and PCR can be useful for rapid identification of *H. werneckii*.

Topical imidazoles and allylamines, such as clotrimazole, miconazole, ketoconazole, sulconazole, econazole, and terbinafine, have been reported as effective. Griseofulvin is not effective. Simply shaving away the superficial epidermis with a blade is frequently both diagnostic and curative.

Crous PW, et al: Delimiting *Cladosporium* from morphologically similar genera. Stud Mycol 2007; 58:33–56.
Kannan P, et al: Prevalence of dermatophytes and other fungal agents isolated from clinical samples. Indian J Med Microbiol 2006 Jul; 24(3):212–215.
Larangeira de Almeida H Jr, et al: Bilateral tinea nigra in a temperate climate. Dermatol Online J 2007 Jul 13; 13(3):25.
Rosen T, et al: Rapid treatment of tinea nigra palmaris with ciclopirox olamine gel, 0.77%. Skinmed 2006 Jul–Aug; 5(4):201–203.

Piedra (trichosporosis)

In black piedra, dark, pinhead to pebble-sized formations occur on the hairs of the scalp, brows, lashes, or beard. These nodules are distributed irregularly along the length of the shaft. White piedra is commonly caused by *T. beigelii* or *Trichosporon inkin*, and occurs more commonly in temperate climates. Based on molecular analysis, the taxon *T. beigelii* has been replaced by several species. A synergistic corynebacterial infection is often present in white piedra, as demonstrated by culture and electron microscopy. *T. beigelii* has also been implicated as a cause of onychomycosis. *T. inkin* is implicated as an etiologic agent of pubic white piedra. *Trichosporon asahii* causes white piedra and onychomycosis, and has been isolated from black piedra. *Trichosporon* spp can also cause disseminated disease in immunosuppressed patients, and *T. asahii* has produced disseminated cutaneous infections in immunocompetent hosts. In white piedra, patients present with yellow or beige-colored, soft, slimy sheaths coating the hair shafts (Fig. 15-17). The sheaths are composed of hyphae, arthrospores, and bacteria. The culture shows cream-colored, soft colonies composed of blastospores and septate hyphae, which fragment into arthrospores.

Black piedra, usually caused by *Piedraia hortai*, occurs mostly in the tropics, especially in South America and Asia. The node-like masses in KOH preparations show numerous oval asci containing 2–8 ascospores and mycelium. Cultures produce black colonies composed of hyphae and chlamydospores.

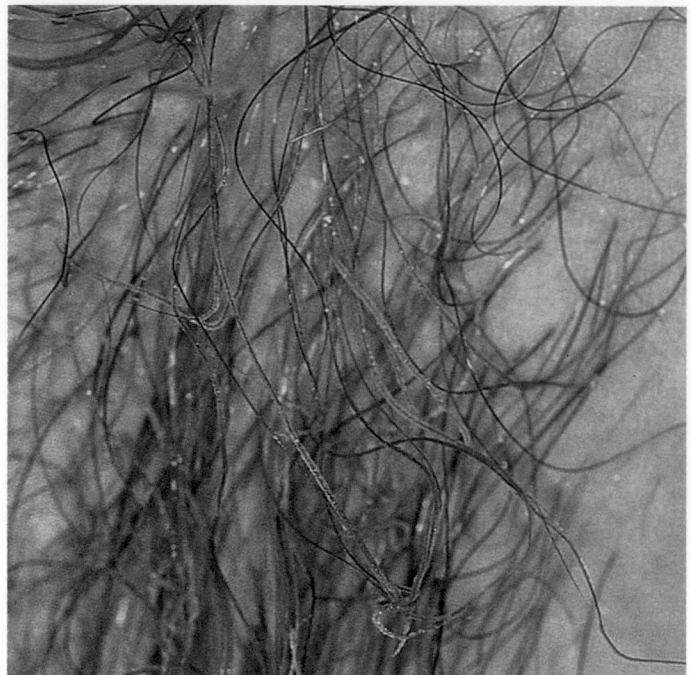

Fig. 15-17 White piedra.

Treatment may be accomplished by cutting or shaving the hair, but this may not be acceptable to the patient. Oral and topical terbinafine have been effective in black piedra. For white piedra, oral itraconazole, topical imidazoles, ciclopirox olamine, 2% selenium sulfide, 6% precipitated sulfur in petrolatum, chlorhexidine solutions, Castellani paint, zinc pyrithione, amphotericin B lotion, and 2–10% glutaraldehyde have all been used successfully. Unfortunately, the recurrence rate is high. Spontaneous remissions are sometimes observed.

Chagas-Neto TC, et al: Update on the genus *Trichosporon*. Mycopathologia 2008 Sep; 166(3):121–132.
David C, et al: Disseminated *Trichosporon inkin* and *Histoplasma capsulatum* in a patient with newly diagnosed AIDS. J Am Acad Dermatol 2008 Aug; 59(2 Suppl 1):S13–S15.
Kanitakis J, et al: Black piedra: report of a French case associated with *Trichosporon asahii*. Int J Dermatol 2006 Oct; 45(10):1258–1260.
Kiken DA, et al: White piedra in children. J Am Acad Dermatol 2006 Dec; 55(6):956–961.
Kim SH, et al: Chronic cutaneous disseminated *Trichosporon asahii* infection in a nonimmunocompromised patient. J Am Acad Dermatol 2008 Aug; 59(2 Suppl 1):S37–S39.
Pulvirenti N, et al: Superficial cutaneous *Trichosporon asahii* infection in an immunocompetent host. Int J Dermatol 2006 Dec; 45(12): 1428–1431.

Tinea versicolor (pityriasis versicolor)

Tinea versicolor is caused by *Malassezia furfur* and related fungi. The yeast phase of this organism is classified as *Pityrosporum orbiculare*. The genus includes 12 lipid-dependent species and a single non lipid-dependent species (*Malassezia pachydermatis*), that colonizes the skin and mucosal sites of healthy cats and dogs. These organisms are part of the normal follicular flora. They produce skin lesions when they grow in the hyphal phase. Tinea versicolor commonly presents as hypo- or hyperpigmented coalescing scaly macules on the trunk and upper arms (Fig. 15-18). Pink, atrophic, and trichrome variants exist and can produce striking clinical pictures. The eruption is more common during the summer months, and favors oily areas of skin. Sites of predilection are the sternal region and the sides of the chest, abdomen, back, pubis, neck, and intertriginous areas. Mild itching and

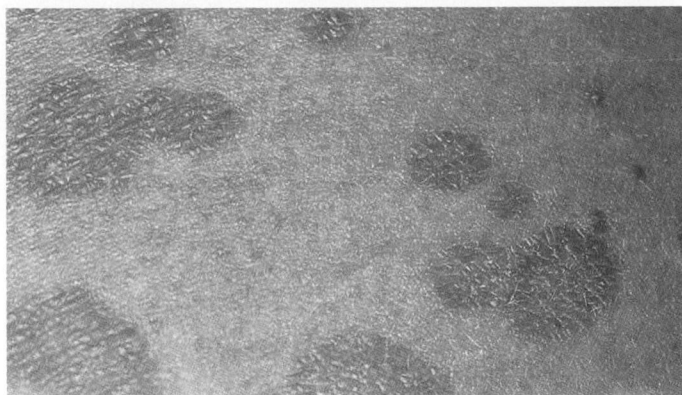

Fig. 15-18 Tinea versicolor.

inflammation about the patches may be present. In some instances many follicular papules are present. The face and scalp may be affected. Facial lesions occur fairly commonly in infants and immunocompromised patients. The disease may even occur on the scalp, palms, and soles. Penile lesions may occur as well, and the organism is commonly isolated from patients with balanoposthitis.

In hypopigmented tinea versicolor, abnormally small and poorly melanized melanosomes are produced, and are not transferred to keratinocytes properly. This becomes most conspicuous in dark-skinned people. This hypopigmentation may persist for weeks or months after the fungal disease is cured unless an effort is made to regain the lost pigmentation through UV exposure.

Diagnosis

The fungus is easily demonstrated in scrapings of the profuse scales that cover the lesions. Tape stripping of the lesions can also be performed. Microscopically, there are short, thick fungal hyphae and large numbers of variously sized spores. This combination of strands of mycelium and numerous spores is commonly referred to as "spaghetti and meatballs." The fungus can be highlighted by a variety of stains, including Parker blue–black ink (mixed 1:1 with 20% KOH) and 1% Chicago sky blue 6B with 8% KOH. Identification by culture requires lipid enrichment of the media, and is rarely done to establish the diagnosis. Wood's light examination accentuates pigment changes, and may demonstrate yellow–green fluorescence of the lesions in adjacent follicles.

Biopsy will demonstrate a thick basket-weave stratum corneum with hyphae and spores. In the atrophic variant, epidermal colonization with hyphae and spores is accompanied by effacement of the rete ridges, subepidermal fibroplasia, pigment incontinence, and elastolysis.

Differential diagnosis

Tinea versicolor must be differentiated from seborrheic dermatitis, pityriasis rosea, pityriasis rubra pilaris, pityriasis alba, Hansen's disease, syphilis, and vitiligo. In the atrophic variant, the lesions may suggest parapsoriasis, mycosis fungoides, anetoderma, lupus erythematosus, or steroid atrophy.

The diagnosis in all forms of tinea versicolor is generally easily established by KOH examination. In seborrheic dermatitis the patches have an erythematous yellowish tint and the scales are soft and greasy, whereas in tinea versicolor the scales are furfuraceous (fluffy). Macular syphilid consists of faint pink lesions, less than 1 cm in diameter, irregularly round or oval, which are distributed principally on the nape, sides of

the trunk, and flexor aspects of the extremities. They are slightly indurated with a peripheral scale, and may be copper-colored. There may be general adenopathy. Serologic tests are positive in this phase of syphilis, but prozone reactions may occur, and the serum may have to be diluted.

Treatment

Imidazoles, triazoles, selenium sulfide, ciclopirox olamine, zinc pyrithione, sulfur preparations, salicylic acid preparations, propylene glycol, and benzoyl peroxide have been used successfully as topical agents. Selenium sulfide lotion is very cost-effective and can be applied daily for a week, washed off after 10 min. It is also effective in a single overnight application. This can be repeated monthly as prophylaxis. The scalp can be shampooed monthly with selenium sulfide to reduce scalp colonization. Zinc pyrithione soap is also cost-effective and well tolerated for treatment and prophylaxis.

Ketoconazole, in 400 mg doses repeated at monthly intervals, is very effective. Oral itraconazole, 200 mg once a day for 7 days, is effective and can be followed by prophylactic treatment with itraconazole, 200 mg twice a day on 1 day a month. In a study of 50 patients, 400 mg single-dose itraconazole was shown to be equivalent to 200 mg/day itraconazole for 7 days. Fluconazole, 400 mg once, may also be effective, and can be repeated at monthly intervals. In a study of 128 patients, weekly dosing with two 150 mg capsules of fluconazole for 2 weeks was equivalent to weekly dosing of two 200 mg tablets of ketoconazole for 2 weeks. The effect of a single dose, not repeated in 2 weeks, was not assessed in this study, and may have proved just as effective. Although terbinafine has been shown to be ineffective via the oral route, it is effective topically. Twice a day applications are superior to once a day applications. Alternatively, 5-aminolevulinic acid photodynamic therapy has been reported as effective.

Patients should be informed that the hypo- and hyperpigmentation will take time to resolve and is not a sign of treatment failure. Relapse is likely if prophylactic doses are not given occasionally, but many options are available for prophylactic treatment. After initial therapy, patients may prefer weekly washing with a topical zinc pyrithione bar, single overnight applications of selenium sulfide, ketoconazole, econazole or bifonazole shampoo every 30–60 days, or monthly oral therapy.

Pityrosporum folliculitis

Pityrosporum folliculitis has been a controversial entity, but its prompt response to antifungal agents suggests that *Pityrosporum* yeast is indeed pathogenic. Criteria for diagnosis include characteristic morphology, demonstration of yellow–green Wood's light fluorescence of the papules or demonstration of *Pityrosporum* yeast in smears or biopsies, and prompt response to antifungal treatment. Lesions tend to be chronic, moderately itchy, dome-shaped, follicular papules and tiny pustules involving the upper back and adjacent areas. The face and scalp may be involved, and the lesions are sometimes found in association with either tinea versicolor or seborrheic dermatitis. *Pityrosporum* folliculitis is more common in organ or marrow transplant recipients. As *Pityrosporum* yeast is normally part of the follicular flora, alterations in flora may favour uncontrolled growth of the yeast. One such instance occurs when *Propionibacterium acnes* is suppressed by tetracycline therapy.

The eruption responds to oral fluconazole, 400 mg once; ketoconazole, 400 mg once; or itraconazole, 200 mg/day for 5–7 days. Topical therapy with 2.5% selenium sulfide applied overnight is also generally effective. Other treatments include 30–50% propylene glycol in water, and topical imidazole creams. Relapses are common, but prophylaxis may be successful with monthly applications of selenium sulfide or maintenance doses of topical econazole.

Alsterholm M, et al: Frequency of bacteria, *Candida* and *Malassezia* species in balanoposthitis. Acta Derm Venereol 2008; 88(4):331–336.

Cafarchia C, et al: The pathogenesis of *Malassezia* yeasts. Parassitologia 2008 Jun; 50(1–2):65–67.

Difonzo EM, et al: Skin diseases associated with *Malassezia* species in humans. Clinical features and diagnostic criteria. Parassitologia 2008 Jun; 50(1-2):69–71.

Faergemann J, et al: A double-blind, randomized, placebo-controlled, dose-finding study of oral pramiconazole in the treatment of pityriasis versicolor. J Am Acad Dermatol 2009; 61(6):971–976.

Galuppi R, et al: Epidemiology and variability of *Malassezia* spp. Parassitologia 2008 Jun; 50(1–2):73–76.

Guillot J, et al: The genus *Malassezia*: old facts and new concepts. Parassitologia 2008 Jun; 50(1–2):77–79.

Khaddar RK, et al: Penile shaft involvement in pityriasis versicolor. Acta Dermatovenerol Alp Panonica Adriat 2008 Jun; 17(2):86–89.

Kim YJ, et al: Successful treatment of pityriasis versicolor with 5-aminolevulinic acid photodynamic therapy. Arch Dermatol 2007 Sep; 143(9):1218–1220.

Lim SL, et al: New contrast stain for the rapid diagnosis of pityriasis versicolor. Arch Dermatol 2008 Aug; 144(8):1058–1059.

Wahab MA, et al: Single dose (400 mg) versus 7 day (200 mg) daily dose itraconazole in the treatment of tinea versicolor: a randomized clinical trial. Mymensingh Med J 2010; 19(1):72–76.

THE DEEP MYCOSES

Most deep cutaneous fungal infections are a manifestation of systemic infection from inhalation of aeorosolized fungus. When primary infection is introduced directly into the skin from puncture wounds, abrasions, or other trauma, a chancriform or verrucous lesion will form that may be accompanied by secondary lymphangitis. Chest radiographs should be taken when investigating patients with deep mycoses except for the classic inoculation types, such as sporotrichosis, mycetoma, chromoblastomycosis, and phaeohyphomycosis.

Coccidioidomycosis

Coccidioidomycosis is also known as coccidioidal granuloma, valley fever, and San Joaquin valley fever.

Primary pulmonary coccidioidomycosis

Inhalation of *Coccidioides immitis*, followed by an incubation period of 10 days to several weeks, produces a respiratory infection that may be mild, with only a low-grade fever resembling a flulike illness. Approximately 60% of infected persons are entirely asymptomatic. Severe symptoms of chills, high fever, night sweats, severe headache, backache, and malaise may ensue in a minority. A large percentage of patients show lung changes on roentgenographic examination. These include hilar adenopathy, peribronchial infiltration, or an infiltrate compatible with bronchopneumonia. At the time of onset a generalized maculopapular eruption may be present, which may be confused with a drug eruption, measles, or scarlet fever.

Within a few weeks the pulmonary symptoms subside. In about 30% of women and in 15% of men, allergic skin manifestations appear in the form of erythema nodosum over the shins and sometimes over the thighs, hips, and buttocks. These tender lesions may become confluent, gradually turn from purple to brown, and then disappear in about 3 weeks. Erythema nodosum is a favorable prognostic sign and occurs mostly in white individuals with transient self-limited disease.

Sometimes erythema multiforme may develop in a similar clinical setting.

Although valley fever is usually self-limited and patients recover spontaneously, a small percentage steadily progress into the chronic, progressive, disseminated form. The propensity for disseminated disease is several-fold higher in Hispanics and Native Americans, and many times higher for African Americans, Filipinos, and Vietnamese. In women, pregnancy may predispose to systemic disease. Infants, the elderly, persons with blood types B or AB, and immunosuppressed patients, including those with AIDS, are also at increased risk for severe disease.

Disseminated coccidioidomycosis (coccidioidal granuloma)

Dissemination occurs in less than 1% of infections, but its incidence is heavily influenced by the factors listed above. Target organs include the bones, joints, viscera, brain, meninges, and skin. A single organ or multiple organs may be involved.

Skin lesions occur in 15–20% of patients with disseminated disease. They may appear as verrucous nodules (Fig. 15-19), as pink papules resembling basal cell carcinoma, or as subcutaneous abscesses. The face is frequently involved. Some chronic lesions develop into plaques that resemble mycosis fungoides or North American blastomycosis. In patients with AIDS, umbilicated papules may mimic molluscum contagiosum. Umbilicated papules are more commonly associated with cryptococcosis, but can occur with a variety of fungi.

Primary cutaneous coccidioidomycosis

This form occurs rarely, and skin disease should be considered a manifestation of disseminated disease unless there is a definite history of inoculation or a colonized splinter is found in the lesion. Between 1 and 3 weeks following inoculation an

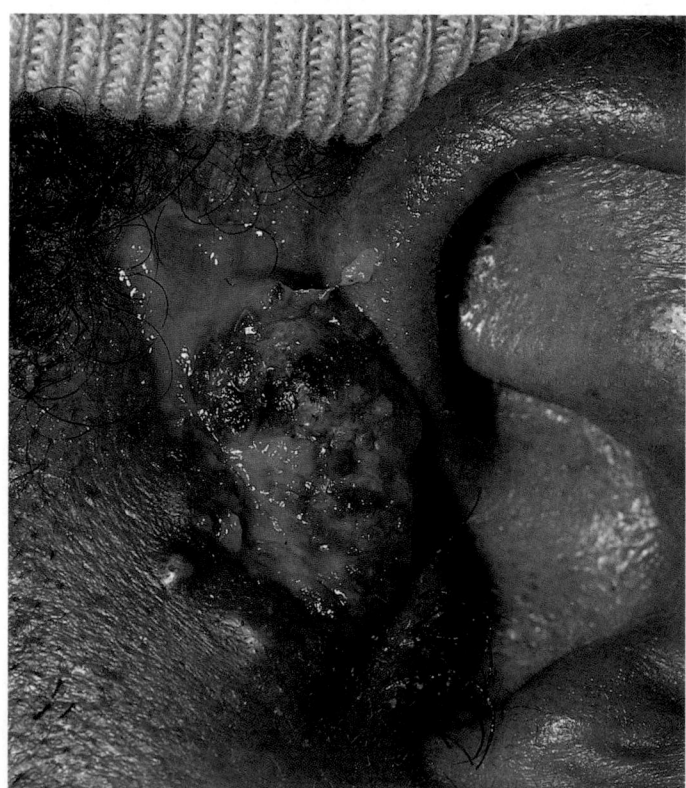

Fig. 15-19 Disseminated coccidioidomycosis. (Courtesy of Curt Samlaska, MD)

indurated nodule develops that may ulcerate. Later, nodules appear along the lymphatic vessels. Spontaneous recovery may result after several weeks, although most patients are treated with systemic agents.

Etiology and pathology

The causative organism, *C. immitis*, has been isolated from the soil and from vegetation. It is commonly found in the burrows of rodents, often at a depth of about 20 cm. Epidemics occur when the soil is disrupted to a depth of 20 cm or more. This can occur as a result of road work, laying of telephone or electric cable, dust storms, and earthquakes. A large outbreak occurred in 1994 in Ventura County, California, after the Northridge earthquake. Outbreaks occur sporadically in California and Arizona. Outbreaks in military personnel are often related to training in endemic areas.

C. immitis is dimorphous, reproducing brittle mycelia at room temperature, and spherules in tissue. Spherules are unencapsulated with a thick refractile wall and a granular interior. They measure 5–200 µm in diameter, but average 20 µm. Endosporulation can occur, and the organism can resemble *Rhinosporidium*. Compared to the latter organism, *Coccidioides* is typically much smaller and more uniform in size. It also lacks the small central nucleus that is uniformly present in non-sporulating *Rhinosporidium*.

Culture

Coccidioides is readily grown at room temperature, and is highly infectious. For this reason, culture of deep fungi should never be attempted in the office setting. Cultures should only be performed in laboratories with biocontainment hoods. The colonies appear on Sabouraud dextrose agar within 2–7 days as small, slightly raised disks penetrating the medium. Older cultures become covered with a dusty layer of aerial hyphae and assume a brownish color with age. In culture, spherical bodies throw out filaments of barrel-shaped arthrospores. Mycelia are branched and septate, 2–8 µm in diameter. PCR primers and a DNA hybridization probe test that targets organism-specific ribosomal RNA show promise for rapid identification.

Epidemiology

The disease principally occurs in limited areas in the western hemisphere. The original diagnosis was in a soldier from Argentina, where the disease is endemic in the Gran Chaco area. It is also endemic in northern Mexico, Venezuela, and the southwestern US (the lower Sonoran Life Zone). In highly endemic areas, most residents will have been infected, and new residents have a good chance of becoming infected within 6 months. Very few will develop disseminated disease, although the attack rate has recently increased in both California and Arizona.

Differential diagnosis

Clinically, it is extremely difficult to differentiate this disease from blastomycosis, which it closely resembles. Definite diagnosis depends on serologic testing and the demonstration of *C. immitis* microscopically, culturally, or by animal inoculation. Guinea pigs inoculated with *C. immitis* die from the systemic infection, whereas no evidence of infection is apparent after inoculation with *Blastomyces*. Intradermal testing with coccidioidin has largely been replaced by serologic testing. A positive reaction of the delayed tuberculin type develops early

and remains high in those who resist the disease well. A negative skin test occurs with dissemination.

Immunology

The first widely used skin test, coccidioidin, was developed in the 1940s. In the 1970s, spherulin was found to be more sensitive. Cross-reactions can occur with histoplasmin, blastomycin, and paracoccidioidin. In vitro tests of cellular immunity yield comparable results and skin testing has generally been replaced by serologic testing. Precipitin, latex agglutination, immunodiffusion, and complement fixation serologic tests have been developed. The precipitin, immunodiffusion, enzyme immunoassay (EIA), and latex agglutination tests are useful in very recent infection, since a maximum titer is reached in 1–2 weeks. They permit detection of coccidioidal IgM in early coccidioidomycosis. In later infections, the complement fixation test is useful. In primary coccidioidomycosis the titer is low, whereas in subsequent dissemination there is a rapid rise in titer. When the disease has disseminated, cerebrospinal, synovial, and peritoneal fluid can be tested for coccidioidal antibody. The *Coccidioides*-specific EIA detects antigenuria in about 70% of patients with coccidioidomycosis and is negative in more than 99% of controls without fungal infections. Cross-reactions with other systemic mycoses occur in 10.7% of patients. An isolated positive EIA IgM usually means disseminated disease.

Treatment

Amphotericin B is active against the organism, but less toxic drugs are now available. Fluconazole, at doses of 400–800 mg/day, is commonly used. Treatment must be continued for 12 months or longer. Many patients will require ongoing suppressive therapy. In patients infected with HIV, lifetime suppressive doses of 200 mg/day are advised and potent antiretroviral therapy is associated with improved outcomes. In coccidioidomycotic meningitis, fluconazole, 400–600 mg/day, is given indefinitely. Fluconazole and itraconazole have similar efficacies in the treatment of progressive nonmeningeal coccidioidomycosis. In meningeal disease itraconazole is not effective and amphotericin needs to be given intrathecally in addition to intravenously. Liposomal amphotericin is effective in animal models of meningeal disease without the need for intrathecal administration. Newer agents that have activity against *C. immitis* include voriconazole, caspofungin, and posaconazole. Voriconazole has been used successfully in meningeal disease. Azole resistance has been reported and should be suspected in patients with refractory disease.

Ampel NM: New perspectives on coccidioidomycosis. Proc Am Thorac Soc 2010 May; 7(3):181–185.

Durkin M, et al: Diagnosis of coccidioidomycosis with use of the *Coccidioides* antigen enzyme immunoassay. Clin Infect Dis 2008 Oct 15; 47(8):e69–e73.

Jewell K, et al: Genetic diversity among clinical *Coccidioides* spp. isolates in Arizona. Med Mycol 2008 Aug; 46(5):449–455 (Epub 2008 Mar 10).

Kriesel JD, et al: Persistent pulmonary infection with an azole-resistant *Coccidioides* species. Med Mycol 2008 Sep; 46(6):607–610.

Masannat FY, et al: Coccidioidomycosis in patients with HIV-1 infection in the era of potent antiretroviral therapy. Clin Infect Dis 2010; 50(1):1–7.

Montone KT, et al: In situ hybridization for Coccidioides immitis 5.8S ribosomal RNA sequences in formalin-fixed, paraffin-embedded pulmonary specimens using a locked nucleic acid probe: a rapid means for identification in tissue sections. Diagn Mol Pathol 2010 Jun; 19(2):99–104.

Noor O, et al: An unusual case of coccidioidomycosis presenting with skin lesions. Am J Dermatopathol 2008 Oct; 30(5):481–483.

Parish JM, et al: Coccidioidomycosis. Mayo Clin Proc 2008 Mar; 83(3):343–348.

Wheat LJ: Nonculture diagnostic methods for invasive fungal infections. Curr Infect Dis Rep 2007 Nov; 9(6):4654–4671.

Histoplasmosis

Histoplasmosis is caused by inhalation of airborne spores. It may be asymptomatic or cause limited lung disease. Dissemination to other organs, including the skin, occurs in about 1 in 2000 acute infections. Immunodeficiency, old age, and systemic corticosteroids predispose to widespread disease. Cases misdiagnosed as sarcoidosis and treated with corticosteroids have disseminated widely. In disseminated disease, mucous membranes are involved much more commonly than skin. Primary cutaneous disease is exceedingly rare.

Primary pulmonary histoplasmosis

Primary pulmonary histoplasmosis is usually a benign self-limited form of acute pneumonitis characterized by fever, malaise, night sweats, chest pain, cough, and hilar adenopathy. Resolution of the pneumonitis occurs rapidly, and the only residua may be calcifications in the lung and a positive skin test to histoplasmin. However, serious pneumonitis caused by histoplasmosis does occur. Such cases have been reported among cave workers in Mexico and travelers returning from Central America. A chronic pulmonary form may occur in patients with emphysema.

Approximately 10% of patients with acute symptomatic infection develop arthritis and erythema nodosum. During a large midwestern epidemic, about 4% of patients diagnosed with histoplasmosis presented with erythema nodosum. Erythema multiforme has also been described.

Progressive disseminated histoplasmosis

Most patients who develop this severe form are immunocompromised or taking systemic corticosteroids. Leukemia, lymphoma, lupus erythematosus, renal transplantation, or AIDS is a frequent predisposing disease. Cases have also been reported in patients receiving low-dose methotrexate for psoriasis. Approximately 20% have no identifiable risk factor.

The reticuloendothelial system, genitourinary tract, adrenals, gastrointestinal tract, adrenal glands, and heart may be involved. Ulcerations and granulomas of the oronasopharynx are the most common mucocutaneous lesions, occurring in about 20% of patients with disseminated disease (Fig. 15-20). Beginning as solid, indurated plaques, they ulcerate and become deepseated, painful, and secondarily infected. Perianal lesions may also occur.

Skin lesions are present in approximately 6% of patients with dissemination and may be more common in patients with

AIDS and in renal transplant recipients. Recently, cases have been reported in association with infliximab therapy. The morphologic patterns are nonspecific and protean, including umbilicated nodules, papules, plaques (Fig. 15-21), and ulcers. Cellulitis may also occur. Abscesses, pyoderma, pustules, and furuncles may be the first lesions on the skin. Demonstration of the organisms is readily made from histologic sections and cultures of the exudate. The most common manifestation in children is purpura. Usually it appears a few days before death and is probably caused by severe involvement of the reticuloendothelial system, with emaciation, chronic fever, and severe gastrointestinal symptoms.

In the HIV-positive population, dyspnea, a platelet count of <100 000 platelets/mm^3, and lactate dehydrogenase levels of more than two-fold the upper limit of the normal range are poor prognostic factors, and are independently associated with death during the first 30 days of antifungal treatment.

Primary cutaneous histoplasmosis

This rare entity is characterized by a chancre-type lesion with regional adenopathy. It has been reported on the penis.

African histoplasmosis

This type is caused by *Histoplasma duboisii*, now classified as a variant of *Histoplasma capsulatum*. Skin lesions are much more common and include superficial cutaneous granulomas, subcutaneous granulomas, and osteomyelitic lesions with secondary involvement of the skin (cold abscesses). In addition, papular, nodular, circinate, eczematoid, and psoriasiform lesions may be seen. The granulomas are dome-shaped nodules, painless but slightly pruritic. There may be skin and mucous membrane manifestations such as ulcerations of the nose, mouth, pharynx, genitals, and anus. These ulcers are chronic, superficial lesions with no induration or noticeable inflammatory reaction. Erythema nodosum occurs frequently. Emaciation and chronic fevers are common systemic signs.

Etiology and pathology

Histoplasmosis was first discovered in Panama by ST Darling in 1906. It is caused by *H. capsulatum*, a dimorphic fungus that exists as a soil saprophyte. The organism is frequently found in bat and bird feces.

In tissue there are 2–3 μm round bodies within the cytoplasm of large macrophages. A pseudocapsule surrounds each organism. The organisms bear a striking resemblance to those of leishmaniasis, but lack a kinetoplast and are distributed evenly throughout the cytoplasm, while leishmanial organisms often line up at the periphery of the cell like light bulbs on a movie

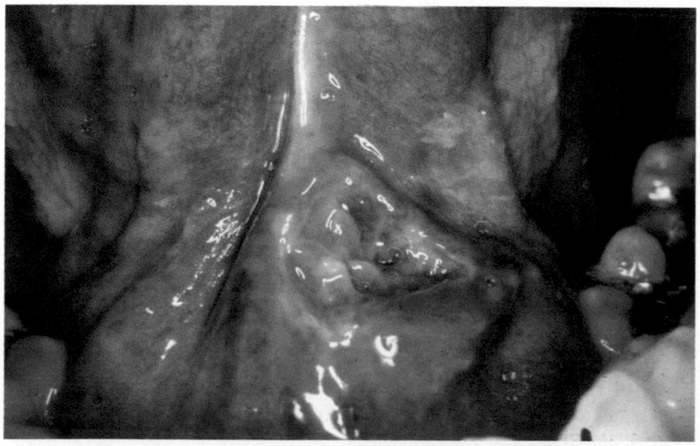

Fig. 15-20 Ulcer of disseminated histoplasmosis.

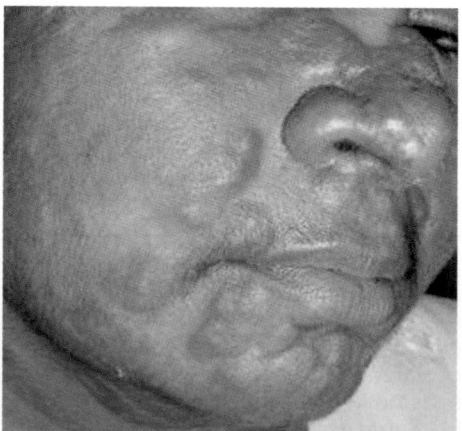

Fig. 15-21 Disseminated histoplasmosis. (Courtesy of Shyam Verma, MD)

marquee. Budding forms may rarely be present, and mycelial and pleomorphic budding forms are sometimes seen in cavitary pulmonary disease, endocardial disease, aortic plaques, or skin lesions. Morphologically, these forms resemble *Candida* more than typical intracellular *Histoplasma*. On direct examination the organism may be demonstrated in the peripheral blood, sputum, bronchial washings, spinal fluid, sternal marrow, lymph node touch smears, or ulcers when stained with Giemsa, PAS, or Gomori methenamine silver stains. In African histoplasmosis, the organisms are 10–13 μm in diameter and are typically found within multinucleated giant cells.

The mycelial phase may be demonstrated on Sabouraud dextrose agar, Mycosel medium, or brain–heart infusion agar to which blood has been added. A white, fluffy colony is found, with microconidia and echinulate macroconidia. One set of cultures should be inoculated at room temperature to demonstrate the mycelial phase and another at 37°C to produce the yeast phase. In disseminated disease the bone marrow is frequently involved. Blood, urine, and tissue from oral and skin lesions should also be cultured. PCR probes are available for rapid culture confirmation.

Epidemiology

Although histoplasmosis occurs throughout the world, it is most common in North America, especially in the central states of the US along the Mississippi River basin. Histoplasmosis is found frequently in river valley areas in the tropical and temperate zones. The Nile River valley seems to be one exception. Besides the Mississippi and Ohio river valleys, it has been found along the Potomac, Delaware, Hudson, and St Lawrence rivers. It has been reported in the major river valleys of South America, Central Africa, and Southeast Asia. The disease is heavily endemic in Puerto Rico and Nicaragua.

Transmission of the disease does not occur between individuals; instead, the infection is contracted from the soil by inhalation of the spores, especially in a dusty atmosphere. Feces of birds and bats contain the fungus. The spores have been demonstrated in the excreta of starlings, chickens, and bats. The disease may be contracted by persons who enter caves inhabited by bats or birds. Epidemics have been reported from exposure to silos, abandoned chicken houses, and storm cellars. Infected people throughout the world number in the many millions.

In an outbreak in Indianapolis in 1978, 488 clinically recognized cases occurred, and 55 had disseminated disease. The actual number infected was probably well over 100 000. Nineteen died, none of whom were under the age of 1. Fatal or disseminated infections occurred in 74% of immunosuppressed persons, compared with 6.5% of those without immunosuppression. Age over 54 was a worse prognostic factor than chronic lung disease in nonimmunosuppressed persons. Disseminated histoplasmosis is seen as an opportunistic infection in HIV-infected individuals, reflecting impaired cellular immune function.

Immunology

The best diagnostic test has been the urinary enzyme-linked immunosorbent assay (ELISA), but PCR assays are now available and demonstrate excellent sensitivity. Serologic testing for antibodies requires that the patient has normal immune responsiveness and is further limited by a high rate of false-positives and false-negatives, especially cross-reactions with blastomycosis. The complement fixation test, when positive at a titer of 1:32 or greater, indicates active or recent infection. Because of the limitations of serologic studies, culture remains the gold standard.

Treatment

Whereas minimal disease heals spontaneously in the majority of cases, moderate to severe disease requires therapy. Amphotericin B is the treatment of choice in severely ill patients and all immunocompromised patients. In patients infected with HIV a suppressive dose of 200 mg/day of itraconazole follows the intravenous amphotericin. Itraconazole, 200 mg/day for 9 months, may be given for moderate disease in immunocompetent patients. Most patients initially treated with amphotericin B respond quickly and can be switched to itraconazole.

Epifanio RN, et al: Disseminated histoplasmosis with oral manifestation. Spec Care Dentist 2007 Nov–Dec; 27(6):236–239.

Friedman A, et al: Sudden onset of verrucous plaques to the face and trunk: a case of cutaneous histoplasmosis in the setting of HIV. Dermatol Online J 2008 Feb 28; 14(2):19.

Galandiuk S, et al: Infliximab-induced disseminated histoplasmosis in a patient with Crohn's disease. Nat Clin Pract Gastroenterol Hepatol 2008 May; 5(5):283–287.

Kauffman CA: Diagnosis of histoplasmosis in immunosuppressed patients. Curr Opin Infect Dis 2008 Aug; 21(4):421–425.

Marques SA, et al: Histoplasmosis presenting as cellulitis 18 years after renal transplantation. Med Mycol 2008 Aug; 1:1–4.

Pfaller MA, et al: Epidemiology of invasive mycoses in North America. Crit Rev Microbiol 2010; 36(1):1–53.

Simon S, et al: Detection of *Histoplasma capsulatum* DNA in human samples by real-time polymerase chain reaction. Diagn Microbiol Infect Dis 2010 Mar; 66(3):268–273.

White J, et al: Oral histoplasmosis as the initial indication of HIV infection: a case report. SADJ 2007 Nov; 62(10):452, 454–455.

Winthrop KL, et al: Mycobacterial and other serious infections in patients receiving anti-tumor necrosis factor and other newly approved biologic therapies: case finding through the Emerging Infections Network. Clin Infect Dis 2008 Jun 1; 46(11):1738–1740.

Cryptococcosis

Cryptococcosis generally begins as a pulmonary infection and remains localized to the lung in 90% of cases. In the remaining 10% the organisms hematogenously disseminate to other organs, with the central nervous system (CNS) and the skin the two most common secondary sites. Patients in the latter group are usually immunocompromised or debilitated. The incidence of dissemination is much higher in patients with AIDS, occurring in up to 50% of this population.

Primary pulmonary cryptococcosis infection may be so mild that the symptoms of fever, cough, and pain may be absent. On the other hand, some cases may be severe enough to cause death. Radiographic studies will reveal disease at this stage.

When dissemination occurs, the organism has a special affinity for the CNS. It is the most common cause of mycotic meningitis. There may be restlessness, hallucinations, depression, severe headache, vertigo, nausea and vomiting, nuchal rigidity, epileptiform seizures, and symptoms of intraocular hypertension. Other organs, such as the liver, skin, spleen, myocardium, and skeletal system, as well as the lymph nodes, may be involved. Disseminated cryptococcosis can present in many organ systems; hepatitis, osteomyelitis, prostatitis, pyelonephritis, peritonitis, and skin involvement have all been reported as initial manifestations of disease. The incidence of skin involvement in cases of cryptococcosis is between 10% and 15%, although it is lower in the HIV-infected population. Cutaneous lesions may precede overt systemic disease by 2–8 months.

Skin infection with cryptococcosis occurs most frequently on the head and neck. A variety of morphologic lesions have been reported, including subcutaneous swellings, abscesses,

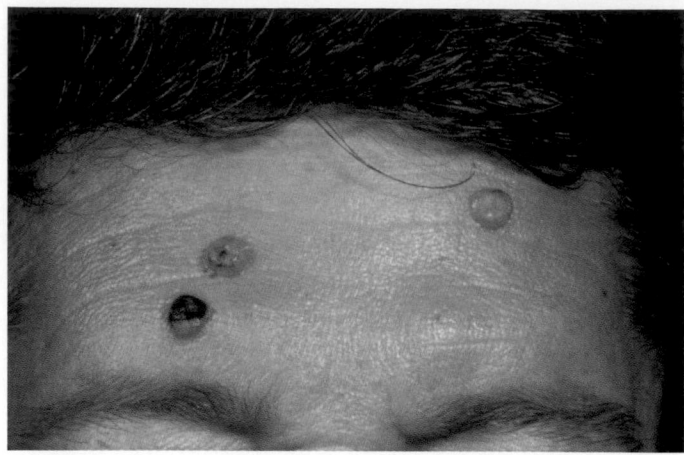

Fig. 15-22 Disseminated cryptococcosis.

blisters, tumorlike masses, molluscum contagiosum-like lesions, draining sinuses, ulcers, eczematous plaques, granulomas, papules, nodules, pustules, acneiform lesions, plaques, and cellulitis (Fig. 15-22). Presentation as an isolated penile plaque has been reported. Approximately 50% of patients with HIV will develop molluscum contagiosum-like lesions. In these patients there is often a central hemorrhagic crust. Lesions may first become evident in HIV-infected patients during highly active antiretroviral therapy (HAART). Solitary cutaneous lesions and indolent cellulitis may be the presenting signs of disseminated disease.

Primary inoculation cryptococcosis is a very rare disease. To establish the diagnosis, there should be a clear history of implantation or a foreign body found in association with the organism. Usually, primary inoculation disease presents as a solitary skin lesion on an exposed area, frequently in the form of a whitlow. Risk factors include outdoor activities and exposure to bird droppings. *Cryptococcus neoformans* serotype D is more commonly associated with primary cutaneous disease. Although primary cutaneous disease exists, for all practical purposes, identification of cryptococci in the skin indicates disseminated disease with a poor prognosis, and it requires a search for other sites of involvement.

Etiology and pathology

The causative organism is *C. neoformans*. It appears in tissue as a pleomorphic budding yeast. The organisms vary markedly in size and shape, in contrast to most other fungal organisms. The capsule is usually prominent, although it is inversely proportional to the extent of the granulomatous reaction. Generally, the capsule is easily identified in hematoxylin and eosin (H&E) sections, although mucicarmine, methylene blue or alcian blue staining can also be used. Usually, multiple yeast share a common capsule. *Cryptococcus* stains well with the Fontana–Masson stain for melanin.

Epidemiology

Cryptococcosis has a worldwide distribution and affects both humans and animals. The organism has been recovered from human skin, soil, dust, and pigeon droppings. The latter, when deposited on window ledges in large cities, are a source of infection. The patient with disseminated cryptococcosis usually has a concomitant debilitating disease, such as AIDS, cancer, leukemia, lymphoma, renal failure, hepatitis, alveolar proteinosis, severe diabetes mellitus, sarcoidosis, tuberculosis, or silicosis. Long-term oral prednisone or immunosuppressive therapy for chronic illnesses, such as renal transplantation,

sarcoidosis, or connective tissue disease, may also be a factor. Cases are being reported in association with anti-tumor necrosis factor (TNF)-α biologics. The portal of entry is the lung. Males outnumber females 2:1. Cryptococcosis is most frequent in persons aged 30–60 years.

Patients with AIDS are particularly at risk for disseminated disease. Cryptococcosis is the fourth leading cause of opportunistic infection and the second most common fungal opportunist, with 5–9% of patients manifesting symptomatic disease. Dissemination occurs in 50% of patients with AIDS; skin involvement is reported to be present in 6% of patients with AIDS.

Immunology

The latex slide agglutination test is sensitive and specific. It may give false-positives in the presence of rheumatoid factor. Direct microscopic examination and latex agglutination have been used with lesional skin scrapings to aid in rapid diagnosis. The complement fixation test for cryptococcal polysaccharide, the indirect fluorescence test, and the EIA for cryptococcal antigen detection are all helpful, but the last is capable of detecting the presence of antigen earlier and at a lower concentration than the other two tests.

Mycology

For direct examination, a drop of serum or exudate is placed on a slide and then covered with a coverslip. If examination shows yeast, one drop of 10% KOH can be added to half of the coverslip and one drop of India ink to the other half to demonstrate the capsule.

The organism produces a moist, shiny, white colony on Sabouraud dextrose agar. With aging the culture may turn to a cream and then a tan color. Subcultures from Sabouraud agar may be made on to cornmeal agar, and on to urea medium to aid in distinguishing the yeast from *Candida* and other yeasts. A commercially available DNA probe detection assay allows rapid culture confirmation.

Treatment

In seriously ill patients, amphotericin B intravenously initially, followed by fluconazole orally, is standard treatment. In less severely ill non-AIDS patients, fluconazole 400–600 mg/day for 8–10 weeks, may be effective. In non-AIDS meningitis, flucytosine is given in combination with amphotericin B, and in patients infected with HIV fluconazole is given indefinitely at a suppressive dose of 200 mg/day. In one study of AIDS patients suffering from cryptococcal meningitis, 600 mg/day of either fluconazole or itraconazole showed efficacy. The availability of voriconazole has expanded the number of options available. In disease refractory to other drugs, voriconazole has shown a response rate of 38.9%. Caspofungin has limited activity against cryptococcosis.

Allegue F, et al: Primary cutaneous cryptococcosis presenting as a whitlow. Acta Derm Venereol 2007; 87(5):443–444.

Calista D, et al: Cutaneous cryptococcosis of the penis. Dermatol Online J 2008 Jul 15; 14(7):9.

Chipungu GA, et al: Cutaneous cryptococcosis erroneously diagnosed as *Histoplasma capsulatum* infection. S Afr Med J 2008 Feb; 98(2):85–86.

Devirgiliis V, et al: Cutaneous cryptococcosis in a patient affected by chronic lymphocytic leukaemia: a case report. Int J Immunopathol Pharmacol 2008 Apr–Jun; 21(2):463–466.

Hoang JK, et al: Localized cutaneous *Cryptococcus albidus* infection in a 14-year-old boy on etanercept therapy. Pediatr Dermatol 2007 May–Jun; 24(3):285–288.

Jasch KC, et al: Pyoderma gangrenosum-like primary cutaneous cryptococcosis. Acta Derm Venereol 2008; 88(1):76–77.

Sing Y, et al: Cryptococcal inflammatory pseudotumors. Am J Surg Pathol 2007 Oct; 31(10):1521–1527.

Soon CW, et al: Primary cutaneous cryptococcosis in Hawai'i. Hawaii Med J 2007 Jan; 66(1):14–15.

Wilson ML, et al: Primary cutaneous cryptococcosis during therapy with methotrexate and adalimumab. J Drugs Dermatol 2008 Jan; 7(1):53–54.

Yao Z, et al: Management of cryptococcosis in non-HIV-related patients. Med Mycol 2005 May; 43(3):245–251.

North American blastomycosis

North American blastomycosis is also known as Gilchrist's disease, blastomycosis, and blastomycetic dermatitis.

Most cutaneous blastomycosis is the result of dissemination from a primary pulmonary focus. The lesions are chronic, slowly progressive, verrucous, and granulomatous, and are characterized by thick crusts, warty vegetations (Fig. 15-23), discharging sinuses, and pustules along the advancing edge. The lesions are often multiple and are located mostly on exposed skin. Papillomatous proliferation is most pronounced in lesions on the hands and feet, where the patches become very thick. There is a tendency for the patches to involute centrally and to form white scars while they spread peripherally. The crusts are thick and dirty gray or brown. Beneath them there are exuberant granulations covered with a seropurulent exudate, which oozes out of small sinuses that extend down to indolent subcutaneous abscesses. Lower-extremity nodules and plaques clinically and histologically suggestive of Sweet syndrome have also been described.

The primary infection is almost always in the upper or middle lobes of the lungs, and most cases never develop cutaneous dissemination. When dissemination does occur, the most common site is the skin, accounting for at least 80% of cases of disseminated disease. It also frequently disseminates to bone, especially the ribs and vertebrae. Other targets are the CNS, liver, spleen, and genitourinary system.

Cutaneous blastomycosis rarely occurs as a result of primary cutaneous inoculation. Such cases have a clear history of inoculation, and present with a small primary nodule and subsequent secondary nodules along the draining lymphatics, creating a picture similar to sporotrichosis. Healing takes place within several months.

Etiology and pathology

The fungus *Blastomyces dermatitidis* causes North American blastomycosis and was first described by Gilchrist in 1894. It is frequently found in soil and animal habitats. *B. dermatitidis* is a dimorphic fungus with a mycelial phase at room temperature and a yeast phase at 37°C. Direct microscopic examination of a KOH slide of the specimen should always be made, since culture of the fungus is difficult and the organism may be found in purulent exudates obtained from skin lesions. The specimen should be cultured by a qualified laboratory on Sabouraud dextrose agar, Mycosel, and brain–heart infusion agar to which blood has been added. Aerial mycelium will develop in 10–14 days, forming a white, cottony growth that turns tan with age. The structures are septate mycelia with characteristic conidia on the sides of hyphae. The conidia are 3–5 μm and variously shaped from round to oval forms. Culture at 37°C produces a slow-growing, wrinkled yeast with spherules, single budding cells, and some abortive hyphae. A DNA probe detection assay is commercially available for rapid culture confirmation.

Cutaneous blastomycosis usually demonstrates marked pseudoepitheliomatous hyperplasia of the epidermis with neutrophilic abscesses. Giant cells are frequently present in the dermal infiltrate. Organisms are typically few in number and are most commonly found within giant cells or intraepidermal abscesses. The organism is a thick-walled yeast, usually 5–7 μm in diameter, although giant forms have been reported in tissue. The organism lacks a capsule, but has a thick and distinctly asymmetrical refractile wall. Broad-based budding may occasionally be noted. Rarely, acute skin lesions may lack pseudoepitheliomatous hyperplasia and demonstrate a diffuse neutrophilic dermal infiltrate. They may present as cutaneous nodules, sometimes with a very localized distribution.

Primary cutaneous blastomycosis demonstrates a neutrophilic infiltrate with many budding cells of blastomycetes. In later lesions, a granulomatous infiltrate is found. The lymph nodes may show marked inflammatory changes, giant cells containing the organisms, lymphocytes, and plasma cells.

Lung involvement may show many changes that are suggestive of tuberculosis with tubercle formation. Purulent abscesses may occur in the lungs and bone. The abscesses may sometimes contain many organisms.

Epidemiology

North American blastomycosis is prevalent in the southeastern US and the Ohio and Mississippi river basins, reaching epidemic proportions in Kentucky and Mississippi; the latter has the highest prevalence of blastomycosis in North America. There is a male to female ratio of approximately 6:1, and most patients are over the age of 60. Often the cutaneous form occurs without a known history of pulmonary lesions.

Outdoor activity after periods of heavy rain is a risk factor for acute pulmonary disease. Beaver lodges are a common site for the fungus, and some reports have linked outbreaks of disease with outings near a beaver lodge. Blastomycosis has also been reported from the bite of a dog suffering from pulmonary blastomycosis. Transmission has been reported between men with prostatic involvement and their sexual partners.

Risk factors for symptomatic disease include pre-existing illness. In one study, one-quarter of patients with blastomycosis had underlying immunosuppression, and 22% had diabetes mellitus. In the south, African Americans have a higher incidence than whites and the mortality rate is also higher among African Americans.

Immunology

Serologic tests are performed by immunodiffusion or ELISA. Commercial antigen test kits are available for rapid diagnosis.

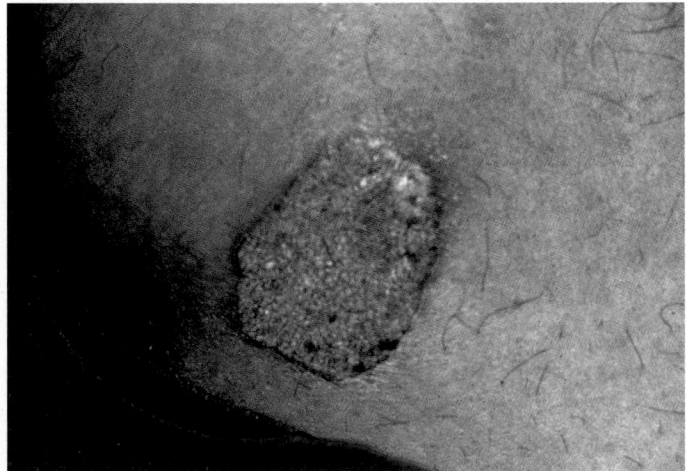

Fig. 15-23 North American blastomycosis.

Differential diagnosis

Blastomycosis may closely resemble halogenoderma, blastomycosis-like pyoderma, pemphigus vegetans, tuberculosis verrucosa cutis, syphilis, granuloma inguinale, drug eruptions, and trichophytic granuloma. The diagnosis is established by demonstration of the organism or serologic testing. The course of blastomycosis is more rapid and involvement is more extensive than in the verrucous type of tuberculosis. Vegetative lesions of tertiary syphilis are usually accompanied by other signs of the disease and have a predilection for the scalp and mucocutaneous junctions. Bromide and iodide eruptions are generally more acutely inflammatory, but may be indistinguishable from blastomycosis. Biopsy, drug history, and blood iodine or bromine levels may be required to distinguish the two.

Treatment

Itraconazole, at a dose of 200–400 mg/day for 6 months, is the treatment of choice. Amphotericin B, for a total dose of 1.5 g, may be required for very ill patients. Some data suggest that for those with life-threatening disease, initial treatment with a lipid formulation of amphotericin B should be followed by a prolonged course of oral voriconazole. Fluconazole, 400–800 mg/day for at least 6 months, is effective in 85% of patients with non-life-threatening disease. Voriconazole has also been used alone for patients with less serious disease.

Bariola JR, et al: Blastomycosis of the central nervous system: a multicenter review of diagnosis and treatment in the modern era. Clin Infect Dis 2010; 50(6):797–804.

Garvey K, et al: Chronic disseminated cutaneous blastomycosis in an 11-year-old, with a brief review of the literature. Pediatr Dermatol 2006 Nov–Dec; 23(6):541–545.

Kisso B, et al: Blastomycosis presenting as recurrent tender cutaneous nodules. S D Med 2006 Jun; 59(6):255–259.

Levy AL, et al: Verrucous nodules on the toes of a renal transplant recipient. Cutaneous blastomycosis. Arch Dermatol 2007 May; 143(5):653–658.

Mason AR, et al: Cutaneous blastomycosis: a diagnostic challenge. Int J Dermatol 2008 Aug; 47(8):824–830.

Patel AJ, et al: Diagnosis of blastomycosis in surgical pathology and cytopathology: correlation with microbiologic culture. Am J Surg Pathol 2010 Feb; 34(2):256–261.

South American blastomycosis

Mucocutaneous involvement in South American blastomycosis, also known as paracoccidioidal granuloma and paracoccidioidomycosis, is almost always a sign of disseminated disease, primarily in the lungs. Rare cases may arise from inoculation. In Brazil, the disease causes about 200 deaths per year.

The mucocutaneous type usually begins in the mouth, where small papules and ulcerations appear. Gingival lesions are most common, followed by lesions of the tongue and lips. With time, adjacent tissues are affected, and ultimately extensive ulcerations destroy the nose, lips, and face (Fig. 15-24). Skin lesions may show ulcerations, pseudoepeliomatous hyperplasia, and microabscesses. The lymphangitic type manifests itself by enlargement of the regional lymph nodes soon after the appearance of the initial lesions about the mouth. The adenopathy may extend to the supraclavicular and axillary regions. Nodes may become greatly enlarged and break down with ulcerations that secondarily involve the skin, causing severe pain and dysphagia with progressive cachexia and

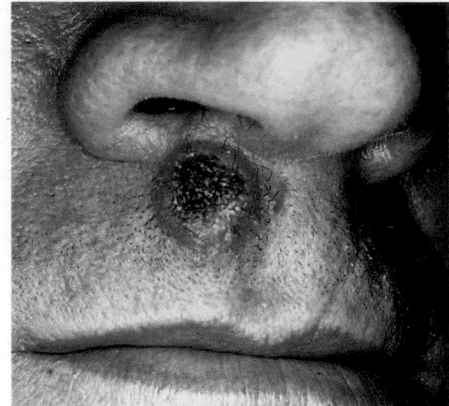

Fig. 15-24 Paracoccidioidomycosis. (Courtesy of Maria Silvia Negrao, MD)

death. Primary skin lesions are less common. The infection may closely simulate Hodgkin disease, especially when the suprahyoid, preauricular, or retroauricular groups of lymph nodes are involved.

There is a visceral type, caused by hematogenous spread of the disease to the liver, adrenal glands, spleen, intestines, and other organs. There is also a mixed type that has the combined symptomatology of the mucocutaneous, lymphangitic, and visceral types. The disease may either present as a rapidly progressive acute disease, or follow a subacute course, or occur as a chronic, slowly advancing form.

Etiology and pathology

Lutz first described South American blastomycosis in Brazil in 1908. It is caused by the fungus *Paracoccidioides brasiliensis*, a member of the phylum Ascomycota, order Onygenales, and family Onygenaceae.

Biopsies may demonstrate pseudoepeliomatous hyperplasia, abscess formation, or ulceration. A granulomatous inflammatory infiltrate is frequently present, consisting of lymphocytes, epithelioid cells, and Langerhans giant cells. The organism appears as a round cell, 10–60 μm in diameter, with a delicate wall. Multiple buds may be present, creating a resemblance to a mariner's wheel.

This chronic granulomatous disease is endemic in Brazil and also occurs in Argentina and Venezuela. Occasional cases have been reported in the US, Mexico, Central America, Europe, and Asia. Most of these patients have a travel history to endemic areas. The disease is generally found among laborers, mostly in men. Although the initial infection is usually respiratory, some individuals may become infected by picking their teeth with twigs or from chewing leaves. Armadillos may harbor the disease.

The fact that the disease is 15 times more common in men is of particular interest, since it has been shown that 17 β-estradiol inhibits transition from the mycelial to the tissue-invasive yeast form. *P. brasiliensis* can lodge in periodontal tissues and some cases start after extraction of teeth. Many cases have been reported in patients with AIDS, where the course is usually acute and severe.

Mycology

In culture the colony is cream-colored, compact, and powdery. Chlamydospores are round or oval. Elongate lateral conidia may be present.

Immunology

Complement fixation tests are positive in 97% of severe cases, and the titer rises as the disease becomes more severe. With improvement, the titer decreases. Immunodiffusion tests are commonly employed for diagnosis and post-therapy follow-up. The test is highly specific but only about 90% sensitive. IgG1 antibodies usually bind well. False-negative tests are commonly related to low-avidity IgG2 antibodies directed against fungal carbohydrate epitopes. Antibody responses to different antigens vary during the course of the disease. Sera from patients with severe acute or chronic disease recognized a greater number of antigens. Reactivity with BAT-exoAg persists after clinical recovery, and IgG reactivity against the 160 kD antigen is the most persistent marker of *P. brasiliensis* infection. The gp43 and gp70 antigen detection assay has improved detection of this organism.

Bronchoalveolar lavage fluid demonstrates low but detectable amounts of IL-6, TNF-α, and macrophage inflammatory protein (MIP)-1α produced by alveolar macrophages. Specific antibodies are mainly of the IgG2 isotype. MIP-1α selectively attracts CD8+ T cells. In skin lesions, Langerhans cells have short and irregular dendrites, and are decreased in number. FXIIIa-positive dendrocytes are increased in number and have prominent dendrites. The organism is frequently found within FXIIIa-positive dendrocytes. Melanin is present within the fungus and appears to contribute to virulence by reducing susceptibility to the host response as well as to pharmacologic agents.

Treatment

Itraconazole, 200 mg/day for 6 months, is the treatment of choice for most patients as it is well tolerated and shows an excellent response in 90%. Ketoconazole, 400 mg/day for 6–18 months, is equally effective, but not as well tolerated. Fluconazole, amphotericin B, and the sulfonamides also have activity against the yeast, although sulfa resistance has been reported. Many patients, especially those with AIDS, are given long-term suppressive therapy with a sulfa drug, so the emergence of resistance is of concern. In a randomized trial, itraconazole, ketoconazole, and sulfadiazine showed similar efficacy in the initial treatment of the disease. In vitro, terbinafine is highly active against isolates of *P. brasiliensis*, and may have a role as an alternate agent. Interferon (IFN)-γ and granulocyte–macrophage colony-stimulating factor enhance the antifungal effect of fluconazole in animal models. Ajoene (4,5,9-trithiadodeca-1,6,11-triene 9-oxide) is a naturally occurring compound that demonstrates activity against the organism. There has been considerable effort to design vaccines effective for prevention and to be used as adjuvant therapy.

Benard G: An overview of the immunopathology of human paracoccidioidomycosis. Mycopathologia 2008 Apr–May; 165(4–5):209–221.

de Almeida Soares CM, et al: A centennial: discovery of *Paracoccidioides brasiliensis*. Mycopathologia 2008 Apr–May; 165(4–5):179–181.

de Camargo ZP: Serology of paracoccidioidomycosis. Mycopathologia 2008 Apr–May; 165(4–5):289–302.

Maluf ML, et al: Antifungal activity of ajoene on experimental murine paracoccidioidomycosis. Rev Iberoam Micol 2008 Sep 30; 25(3):163–166.

Restrepo A, et al: Co-existence of integumentary lesions and lung x-ray abnormalities in patients with paracoccidioidomycosis (PCM). Am J Trop Med Hyg 2008 Aug; 79(2):159–163.

Taborda CP, et al: Melanin as a virulence factor of *Paracoccidioides brasiliensis* and other dimorphic pathogenic fungi: a minireview. Mycopathologia 2008 Apr–May; 165(4–5):331–339.

Travassos LR, et al: Attempts at a peptide vaccine against paracoccidioidomycosis, adjuvant to chemotherapy. Mycopathologia 2008 Apr–May; 165(4–5):341–352.

Sporotrichosis

Sporotrichosis usually occurs as a result of direct inoculation by a thorn, cat's claw, or other minor penetrating injury. The earliest manifestation may be a small nodule which may heal and disappear before the onset of other lesions. In the course of a few weeks nodules generally develop along the draining lymphatics (Fig. 15-25). These lesions are at first small, dusky red, painless, and firm. In time the overlying skin becomes adherent to them and may ulcerate. When the lesions occur on the face, the lymphatic drainage is radial, rather than linear, and secondary nodules occur as rosettes around the primary lesion.

Regional lymphangitic sporotrichosis is the common type, accounting for 75% of cases. Fixed cutaneous sporotrichosis is seen in 20% of cases and is characterized by a solitary ulcer, plaque, or crateriform nodule without regional lymphangitis (Fig. 15-26). It may also present as localized rosacea-like lesions

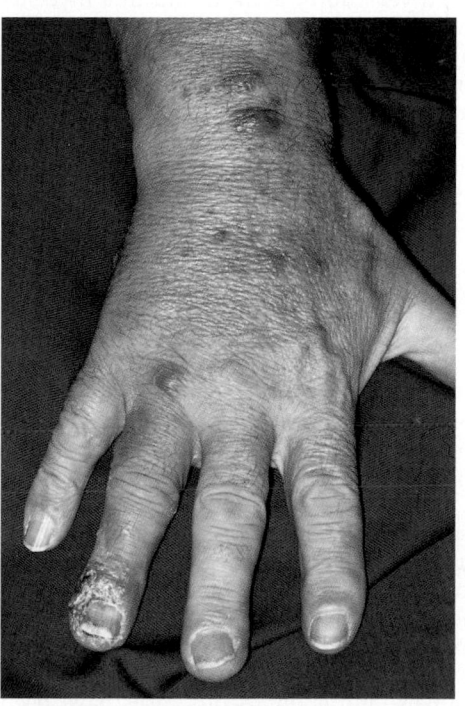

Fig. 15-25 Sporotrichosis.

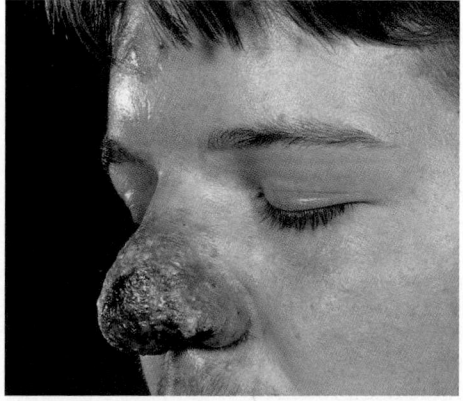

Fig. 15-26 Fixed cutaneous sporotrichosis.

of the face without regional lymphangitis. Increased host resistance, a smaller inoculum, facial location, and variations in strain pathogenicity have all been suggested as reasons for the fixed cutaneous form. The distribution in children is similar to that in adults.

Disseminated disease is the least common form. Factors that predispose to extracutaneous disease include oral prednisone therapy, other immunosuppressive drugs including TNF-α inhibitors, chronic alcoholism, diabetes mellitus, hematologic malignancies, and AIDS. Systemic invasion may produce cutaneous, pulmonary, gastrointestinal, articular, and brain lesions. Arthritis or bone involvement occurs in most cases. The cutaneous lesions are reddish, tender nodules, which soften, form cold abscesses, and eventually suppurate, leaving chronic ulcers or fistulas. These are usually around arthritic joints and the face and scalp, but may occur anywhere on the skin. At times only internal involvement is apparent.

Etiology and pathology

Sporotrichosis is caused by *Sporothrix schenckii*, a dimorphic fungus that grows in a yeast form at 37°C and in a mycelial form at room temperature. Cutaneous disease typically presents with palisading granulomatous dermatitis surrounding a stellate suppurative abscess. Organisms appear as cigar-shaped yeast in tissue, but are rare in North American cases. In Asian cases of sporotrichosis, the organisms are frequently more numerous. Asteroid bodies and mycelial elements are prevalent in regional lymphangitic sporotrichosis. PCR methods of detection have been developed.

Epidemiology

There seems to be no geographic limitation to the occurrence of sporotrichosis. Most often the primary invasion is seen as an occupational disease in gardeners, florists, and laborers following injuries by thorns, straw, or sphagnum moss. The pathogen commonly lives as a saprophyte on grasses, shrubs, and other plants. Carnations, rose bushes, barberry shrubs, and sphagnum moss are common sources. Infection may also be noted after insect stings. High humidity and high temperature favor infection. An epidemic of sporotrichosis among South African diamond miners was ascribed to inoculation of the organism by rubbing against the supporting wooden beams in the mines. Experimentally, it has been produced in many laboratory animals, and spontaneous cases have been observed in horses, mules, dogs, cats, mice, and rats. In cats, sporotrichosis commonly produces disseminated disease. The organism may be found on the claws, and transmitted to humans through cat scratches. Epidemics related to cat exposure have been documented.

Mycology

On Sabouraud agar a moist, white colony develops within 3–7 days. The surface becomes wrinkled and folded. Later the culture turns tan and, ultimately, black, as the organism is capable of producing melanin. In slide culture preparations the colony shows septate branching mycelia. Conidia are found in clusters or in sleevelike arrangements on delicate sterigmata. If the culture is grown at 37°C, grayish-yellow, velvety yeast-like colonies are produced. Cigar-shaped, round, oval, and budding cells, hyphae, and conidia may be seen microscopically.

Immunology

Culture extracts from *S. schenckii*, known as sporotrichins, will produce a delayed tuberculin-type reaction in persons who have had sporotrichosis. The test is fairly reliable, but only indicates previous exposure. Agglutination testing has been developed, but clinical diagnosis, biopsy, and culture remain the most common means of establishing a diagnosis.

Differential diagnosis

Demonstration by culture establishes the diagnosis, and it is important to differentiate sporotrichosis from other lymphangitic infections. Atypical mycobacteriosis (especially *Mycobacterium marinum*), leishmaniasis, and nocardiosis all produce lymphangitic spread. In contrast, tuberculosis, cat-scratch disease, tularemia, glanders, melioidosis, lymphogranuloma venereum, and anthrax produce ulceroglandular syndromes (an ulcer with regional lymphadenopathy rather than an ulcer with nodules along the lymphatic vessels).

Treatment

Itraconazole is effective at a dose of 100–200 mg/day for several months. Pulse dosing has also been used, with 400 mg/day for 1 week with a 3-week break, repeated until lesions are clear. Some data also suggest that terbinafine at a dose of 250 mg per day is effective, although the mean time for clearance in one study was in the order of 14 weeks. For cutaneous forms, potassium iodide, in doses of 2–6 g/day, remains an effective and inexpensive therapeutic option, and may be effective in cases where itraconazole therapy fails. Decades of experience demonstrate its effectiveness despite the absence of published high-level evidence. Iodide therapy usually requires 6–12 weeks of treatment. Generally, it is best to begin with five drops of the saturated solution in grapefruit or orange juice three times a day after meals. The drops can also be put in milk, but strong-flavored citrus juices are better at masking the taste. The dose should be gradually increased until 30–50 drops are taken three times a day. The drug is not suitable for pregnant women. Adverse effects of iodide therapy include nausea, vomiting, parotid swelling, acneiform rash, coryza, sneezing, swelling of the eyelids, hypothyroidism, a brassy taste, increased lacrimation and salivation, flares of psoriasis, and occasionally, depression. Most of the side effects can be controlled by stopping the drug for a few days and reinstituting therapy at a reduced dosage. Application of local hot compresses, hot packs, or a heating pad twice a day has been advocated as a useful adjunct, as *S. schenckii* is intolerant to temperatures above 38.5°C (101°F).

In adult disseminated cases, itraconazole, 300 mg twice a day for 6 months, followed by 200 mg twice a day, is the treatment of choice. In children, the drug is dosed based on weight and therapeutic response. The drug may have to be continued for many months. Amphotericin B, 0.5 mg/kg/day, is an alternative, but sensitivity to this is strain-dependent. *S. schenckii* is more sensitive to itraconazole than voriconazole, but the latter drug may also represent a therapeutic option.

Barros MB, et al: Endemic of zoonotic sporotrichosis: profile of cases in children. Pediatr Infect Dis J 2008 Mar; 27(3):246–250.

Bonifaz A, et al: Sporotrichosis in childhood: clinical and therapeutic experience in 25 patients. Pediatr Dermatol 2007 Jul–Aug; 24(4):369–372.

Bonifaz A, et al: Cutaneous sporotrichosis: intermittent treatment (pulses) with itraconazole. Eur J Dermatol 2008 Jan–Feb; 18(1):61–64.

Dinubile MJ: Nodular lymphangitis: a distinctive clinical entity with finite etiologies. Curr Infect Dis Rep 2008 Sep; 10(5):404–410.

Francesconi G, et al: Terbinafine (250 mg/day): an effective and safe treatment of cutaneous sporotrichosis. J Eur Acad Dermatol Venereol 2009 Nov; 23(11):1273–1276.

Fujii H, et al: A case of atypical sporotrichosis with multifocal cutaneous ulcers. Clin Exp Dermatol 2008 Mar; 33(2):135–138.

Hay RJ, et al: Outbreaks of sporotrichosis. Curr Opin Infect Dis 2008 Apr; 21(2):119–121.

Kauffman CA, et al: Clinical practice guidelines for the management of sporotrichosis: 2007 update by the Infectious Diseases Society of America. Clin Infect Dis 2007 Nov 15; 45(10):1255–1265.

Schubach A, et al: Epidemic sporotrichosis. Curr Opin Infect Dis 2008 Apr; 21(2):129–133.

Xavier MH, et al: Cat-transmitted cutaneous lymphatic sporotrichosis. Dermatol Online J 2008 Jul 15; 14(7):4.

Xue S, et al: Oral potassium iodide for the treatment of sporotrichosis. Cochrane Database Syst Rev 2009 Oct 7; (4):CD006136.

Chromoblastomycosis

Chromoblastomycosis usually affects one of the lower extremities (Fig. 15-27). It occurs as a result of direct inoculation of the organism into the skin. As a rule, lesions begin as a small, pink, scaly papule or warty growth on some part of the foot or lower leg, then slowly spread through direct extension and satellite lesions. With time, lesions develop a verrucous or nodular border and central atrophy and scarring. Small lesions may resemble common warts. Regional lymphadenitis may occur as a result of secondary bacterial infection, and a lymphangitic pattern of infection has been reported. In rare instances, the disease begins on an upper extremity or the face. Longitudinal melanonychia has been reported. Rarely, CNS involvement has been reported, both with and without associated skin lesions.

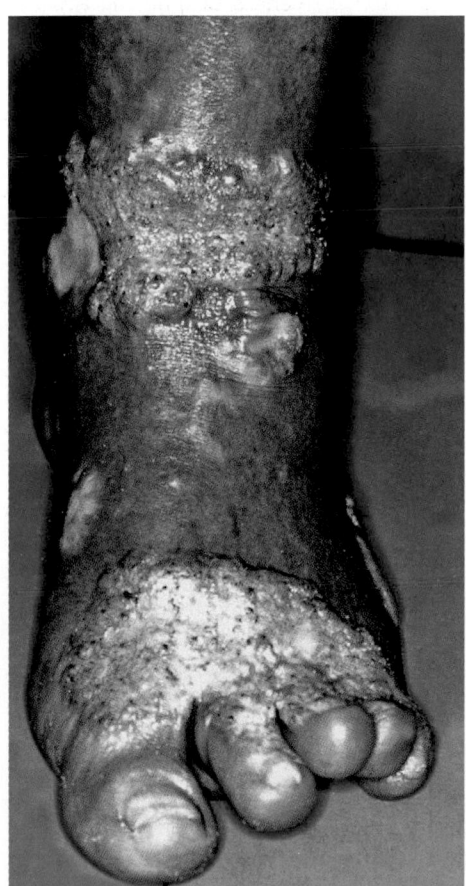

Fig. 15-27 Chromoblasiomycosis. (Courtesy of Maria Silvia Negrao, MD)

There is a 4:1 male predominance, and farmers account for almost 75% of patients with the disease. The disease is slowly progressive, and the average time between the appearance of lesions and diagnosis is almost 15 years. Lesions occur at sites of minor trauma. A thorn injury is remembered in about 16% of patients. Squamous cell carcinoma may occur in long-standing cases.

Etiology and pathology

Most cases are caused by one of five dematiaceous fungi. *Fonsecaea pedrosoi* is the most common cause, and accounts for 90% or more of the cases reported in South America. It has also been reported as the most common cause in other parts of the world. Other agents include *Phialophora verrucosa*, *Fonsecaea compacta*, *Cladosporium carrionii*, and *Rhinocladiella aquaspersa*. *Exophiala spinifera* and *Exophiala jeanselmei* have been reported in isolated cases. Patients may have more than one organism, and cutaneous lesions caused by both paracoccidioidomycosis and chromoblastomycosis have been reported in the same patient. Patients may also have chromoblastomycosis concurrently with mycetoma or invasive phaeohyphomycosis. CNS lesions have been associated with *Cladosporium trichoides* (*Xylohypha* or *Cladophialophora bantiana*), as well as other organisms to include *F. pedrosoi*. Most of the reported cases are really phaeohyphomycosis, rather than chromoblastomycosis, because the organism grows in the hyphal form.

Histopathologically, lesions are characterized by pseudoepitheliomatous hyperplasia with intraepidermal abscess, a dermal granulomatous reaction, and the presence of pigmented fungal sclerotic bodies. The fungi often appear in clusters that reproduce by equatorial septation, rather than by budding. The presence of sclerotic bodies (Medlar bodies, "copper pennies") rather than hyphae distinguishes the infection from invasive phaeohyphomycosis. The organisms are often seen in association with an embedded splinter. Medlar bodies are usually easily identified, but Ziehl–Neelsen and Wade–Fite stains have also been used to identify the pathogenic organisms, as has duplex PCR.

Staining for fungal antigens has demonstrated that they accumulate in macrophages and occasionally in factor XIIIa-positive dendrocytes or Langerhans cells. The immune response to the organism appears to affect the clinical and histologic presentation. Patients with verrucous plaques demonstrate a type T-helper 2 (Th2) immunologic response, while those with erythematous atrophic plaque have a type Th1 response. Immune stimulation with recombinant IL-12 or anti-IL-10 can restore an antigen-specific Th1-type response in monocytes from patients with severe disease.

Epidemiology

Chromoblastomycosis was first recognized in Brazil by Pedroso in 1911. Since then it has been found in other parts of South America and the Caribbean, Madagascar, South Asia, East Asia, the US, Russia, and many other countries. Barefooted farm workers bear the largest burden of infection. Trauma from wood products and soil exposure results in implantation of the organism, and dissemination is rare.

Mycology

The microorganisms produce black, slowly growing, heaped-up colonies. The genera differ according to the type of conidiophore produced. All produce melanin.

Treatment

Treatment is difficult, and the disease often affects those who can ill afford medication. In some series, only about 30% of patients were cured, although almost 60% improved. About 10% fail therapy outright, and recrudescence of the disease is noted in more than 40% of patients. Smaller lesions of chromoblastomycosis are best treated by surgical excision or cryotherapy. In one study of 22 patients, the number of cryosurgeries varied from 1 to 22, and treatment lasted for up to 126 months. Only three patients did not respond. If the lesions are extensive, itraconazole, 100 mg/day or more, is given for at least 18 months. Terbinafine, 500 mg/day for 6–12 months, has been effective in some patients. In refractory cases, itraconazole may be combined with cryotherapy, application of heat (local hyperthermia), or CO_2 laser vaporization. Alternate-week therapy with itraconazole and terbinafine has also been reported. Local hyperthermia alone has been reported as effective in some cases, and has been combined with CO_2 laser vaporization. Despite these options, some lesions remain resistant, and amputation may be unavoidable in some patients. Combination amphotericin B and itraconazole has been used in resistant cases, as has isolated limb infusion with melphalan and actinomycin D.

Damian DL, et al: Treatment of refractory chromomycosis by isolated limb infusion with melphalan and actinomycin D. J Cutan Med Surg 2006 Jan–Feb; 10(1):48–51.

de Andrade TS, et al: Rapid identification of *Fonsecaea* by duplex polymerase chain reaction in isolates from patients with chromoblastomycosis. Diagn Microbiol Infect Dis 2007 Mar; 57(3):267–272.

Garnica M, et al: Difficult mycoses of the skin: advances in the epidemiology and management of eumycetoma, phaeohyphomycosis and chromoblastomycosis. Curr Opin Infect Dis 2009 Dec; 22(6):559–563.

Lokuhetty MD, et al: Ziehl–Neelson and Wade–Fite stains to demonstrate medlar bodies of chromoblastomycosis. J Cutan Pathol 2007 Jan; 34(1):71–72.

López Martínez R, et al: Chromoblastomycosis. Clin Dermatol 2007 Mar–Apr; 25(2):188–194.

Muhammed K, et al: Lymphangitic chromoblastomycosis. Indian J Dermatol Venereol Leprol 2006 Nov–Dec; 72(6):443–445.

Paniz-Mondolfi AE, et al: Extensive chromoblastomycosis caused by *Fonsecaea pedrosoi* successfully treated with a combination of amphotericin B and itraconazole. Med Mycol 2008 Mar; 46(2):179–184.

Santos AL, et al: Biology and pathogenesis of *Fonsecaea pedrosoi*, the major etiologic agent of chromoblastomycosis. FEMS Microbiol Rev 2007 Sep; 31(5):570–591.

Sarti HM, et al: Longitudinal melanonychia secondary to chromoblastomycosis due to *Fonsecaea pedrosoi*. Int J Dermatol 2008 Jul; 47(7):764–765.

Sousa MG, et al: *Fonsecaea pedrosoi* infection induces differential modulation of costimulatory molecules and cytokines in monocytes from patients with severe and mild forms of chromoblastomycosis. J Leukoc Biol 2008 Sep; 84(3):864–870.

Phaeohyphomycosis

This heterogeneous group of mycotic infections is caused by dematiaceous fungi whose morphologic characteristics in tissue include hyphae, yeast-like cells, or a combination of these. This contrasts with chromomycosis, in which the organism forms round sclerotic bodies.

There are many types of clinical lesion caused by these organisms. Tinea nigra is an example of superficial infection. Alternariosis can also present as a superficial pigmented fungal infection in immunocompetent patients. Subcutaneous disease occurs most commonly as indolent abscesses at the site of minor trauma (so called "phaeomycotic cyst"). *E. jeanselmei* is the most common cause of this presentation in temperate

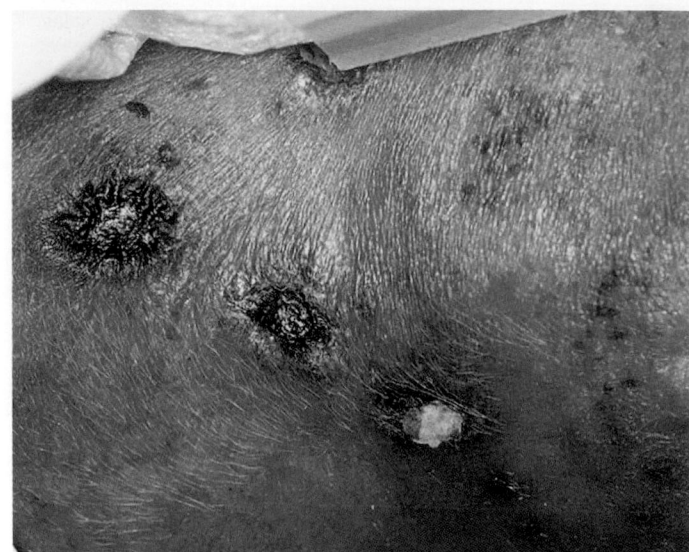

Fig. 15-28 Phaeohyphomycosis.

climates. Systemic phaeohyphomycosis is largely a disease of immunocompromised patients, although primary cerebral forms occur in immunocompetent patients. Localized forms occur primarily as a result of primary inoculation of the organism into the skin. Disseminated disease may also begin as a skin infection, although catheter sepsis is being recognized as a cause of disseminated infection. The lesions commonly appear as dry black leathery eschars with a scalloped erythematous edematous border (Fig. 15-28). *Bipolaris spicifera* is the most common cause of disseminated disease, although *Scedosporium prolificans* has been reported as the most common organism in some areas. The presence of melanin in the cell wall may be a virulence factor for these fungi. Eosinophilia is noted in about 10% of patients with disseminated disease. The disease often disseminates to many organs. Endocarditis is mostly reported on porcine valves. In some series, the mortality rate of disseminated disease is about 80%. More than a half of patients with primary CNS disease have no known underlying immunodeficiency. Mortality rates from CNS infections are high regardless of immune status.

Etiology and pathology

Many black molds are capable of causing phaeohyphomycosis. Among them are *Exophiala jeanselmei*, *Bipolaris spicifera*, *Alternaria* spp, *Dactylaria gallopava*, *Phialophora parasitica*, *Cladosporium sphaerospermum*, *Wangiella dermatitidis*, *Exserohilum rostratum*, *Cladophialophora bantiana*, *Wallemia sebi*, and *Chaetomium globosum*. Some fungi, such as *P. verrucosa*, can cause both phaeohyphomycosis and chromoblastomycosis. Some fungi, such as *E. jeanselmei*, may cause mycetoma (characterized by grain formation) in some patients, and phaeohyphomycosis or chromoblastomycosis in others.

All these organisms produce pigmented hyphae in tissue and culture, although the pigment may only be visible focally in some histologic sections. Melanin can be stained by the Fontana–Masson method, but many molds produce enough melanin to stain positive, and a positive stain should not be misinterpreted as proof of phaeohyphomycosis. Organisms as diverse as zygomycetes and dermatophytes can stain with the Fontana–Masson stain. When hyphae appear brown in tissue, there is little question as to the diagnosis, but when the organism appears hyaline in tissue, the presence of melanin staining must be interpreted in the context of the fungal morphology. Most organisms of phaeohyphomycosis produce thick refractile walls, and have prominent bubbly cytoplasm. This contrasts with the thin, delicate walls of organisms such as *Aspergillus*, *Fusarium*, and dermatophytes. Zygomycetes are aseptate, and usually appear hollow in tissue sections. Their thick refractile wall usually stains intensely red with H&E, contrasting with the pale wall of a phaeomycotic organism. Some organisms, like *Bipolaris*, produce round, dilated structures that resemble spores in tissue. The mix of round structures and hyphae is a helpful clue to the presence of a black mold in tissue.

Treatment

Phaeomycotic cysts are best treated with excision. Superficial phaeohyphomycosis may respond to topical antifungal agents and superficial debridement. For invasive and disseminated disease, surgical excision should generally be combined with antifungal therapy. Itraconazole has the best record of treating this group of infections, and doses of 400 mg/day or higher are commonly needed. Reproducible fungal sensitivity studies are now available through a few reference laboratories, but the process is slow, and patients with disseminated disease have little time to spare. Some organisms respond to amphotericin B or terbinafine. Combinations of terbinafine and triazoles have been successful clinically, and the combination of terbinafine and fluconazole has shown promise in vitro. For CNS disease, combinations of amphotericin B, flucytosine, and itraconazole may improve survival rates. Voriconazole has a broad spectrum of activity against these fungi, but clinical experience is limited. Complete excision of primary brain lesions may be prudent when possible. In widely disseminated disease, excision of lesions becomes impractical, but debulking of skin disease may be of some value.

Alternariosis

Alternaria is a genus of molds recognized as common plant pathogens but also as a cause of human infection. As a pigmented fungus, it is one of the emerging causes of phaeohyphomycosis. Most reported cases of invasive infection have occurred in immunocompromised patients, with the most frequent risk factors being solid organ transplantation and Cushing's syndrome. Cutaneous alternariosis usually presents as focal ulcerated papules and plaques or pigmented patches on exposed skin of the face, forearms and hands, or knees of immunocompetent patients. Topical corticosteroids may predispose to local infection. Localized disease in immunocompetent patients may respond to local debridement or wide surgical excision. Itraconazole has been successful, although resistance has also been reported. Terbinafine, posaconazole, voriconazole, ketoconazole, and intralesional miconazole have also been used successfully.

Guarro J, et al: Subcutaneous phaeohyphomycosis caused by *Wallemia sebi* in an immunocompetent host. J Clin Microbiol 2008 Mar; 46(3):1129–1131.

Martínez-González MC, et al: Three cases of cutaneous phaeohyphomycosis by *Exophiala jeanselmei*. Eur J Dermatol 2008 May–Jun;18(3):313–316.

Neoh CY, et al: Cutaneous phaeohyphomycosis due to *Cladophialophora bantiana* in an immunocompetent patient. Clin Exp Dermatol 2007 Sep; 32(5):539–540.

Pastor FJ, et al: *Alternaria* infections: laboratory diagnosis and relevant clinical features. Clin Microbiol Infect 2008 Aug; 14(8):734–746.

Podda L, et al: Breakthrough cutaneous alternariosis in a patient with acute lymphoblastic leukemia: clinical features and diagnostic issues. Leuk Lymphoma 2008 Jan; 49(1):154–155.

Qiu-Xia C, et al: Subcutaneous phaeohyphomycosis caused by *Cladosporium sphaerospermum*. Mycoses 2008 Jan; 51(1):79–80.

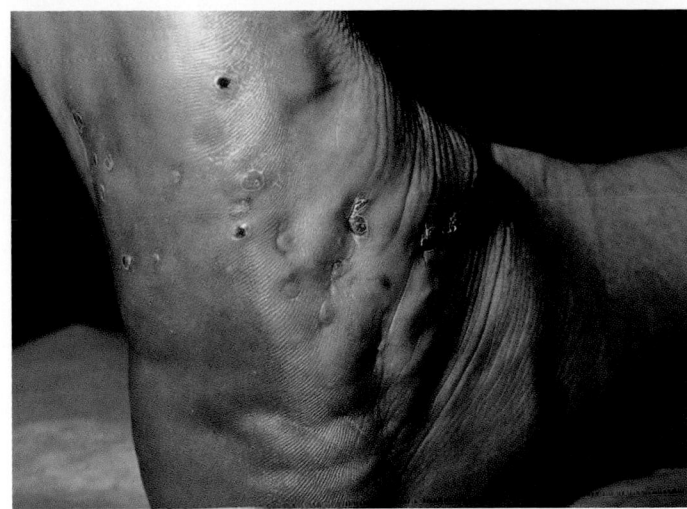

Fig. 15-29 Mycetoma.

Mycetoma

Mycetoma, also known as Madura foot and maduromycosis, is a chronic, granulomatous, subcutaneous, inflammatory disease caused by filamentous bacteria (actinomycetoma) or true fungi (eumycetoma). The organisms enter the skin by traumatic inoculation. Both forms of mycetoma present as progressive subcutaneous swelling with sinus tracts that discharge grains (Fig. 15-29).

The disease progresses slowly. Mycetomas generally begin on the instep or the toe webs. The lesion is commonly relatively painless, nontender, and firm. The overlying skin may be normal or attached to the underlying tumor. Mature lesions often have nodules and draining sinuses. Not only the skin and subcutaneous tissues, but also the underlying fascia and bone are involved. Other parts of the body, such as the hands, arms, chest, jaw, and buttocks, may be involved. Exposed sites are most common, and lesions in covered areas are nearly always actinomycetomas.

Etiology and pathology

Mycetoma is divided into actinomycetoma, produced by bacteria, and eumycetoma, produced by true fungi. Actinomycetomas are caused by *Nocardia*, *Actinomadura*, or *Actinomyces* spp. Eumycetomas are caused by true fungi, including pigmented fungi such as *Madurella* spp, and hyaline fungi such as *Pseudallescheria* and *Acremonium* (*Cephalosporium*). Organisms include *Pseudallescheria boydii* (which may occasionally disseminate as the anamorph or asexual form, *Scedosporium apiospermum*), *Madurella grisea*, *Madurella mycetomatis*, *Acremonium falciforme*, *Acremonium recifei*, *Leptosphaeria senegalensis*, *E. jeanselmei*, *Pyrenochaeta romeri*, and *Phialophora verrucosa*. Examples of actinomycetomas are those caused by *Nocardia asteroides*, *Nocardia brasiliensis*, *Nocardia caviae*, *Actinomadura madurae*, *Actinomadura pelletieri*, *Actinomyces israelii*, and *Streptomyces somaliensis*. *A. israelii* is the major cause of lumpy jaw, a form of mycetoma.

Almost all actinomycetomas produce light-colored grains, as do hyaline fungi. The list of light-grain organisms includes *A. israelii*, *A. madurae*, *Nocardia* spp, *S. somaliensis*, *P. boydii*, *Acremonium* spp, *Aspergillus nidulans*, *Fusarium* spp, and *Neotestudina rosatii*. Red grains are usually produced by *A. pelletieri*, although red pigment-producing colonies that differed from this organism (they were positive for casein hydrolysis and negative for nitrate reduction and hydrolysis tests of xanthine, hypoxanthine, and tyrosine) have been described and provisionally identified as *Actinomadura vinacea*. Pigmented fungi produce dark grains. These organisms include *M. grisea*, *M. mycetomatis*, *Curvularia geniculata*, *Helminthosporium speciferum*, *L. senegalensis*, *E. jeanselmei*, *P. verrucosa*, and *P. romeri*.

Histologic sections demonstrate stellate abscesses containing grains. Gram stain of an actinomycotic grain shows Gram-positive, thin filaments, 1–2 μm thick, embedded in a Gram-negative amorphous matrix. Club formation in the periphery of a grain may be seen. Special stains for demonstration of fungi, such as PAS and Gomori methenamine silver, will clearly show hyphae and other fungal structures within the grain. Hyphae of 2–5 μm in thickness suggest true fungal mycetoma.

Epidemiology

The mycetoma belt stretches between the latitudes of 15° south and 30° north. Relatively arid areas have higher rates of infection than humid areas. In the western hemisphere the incidence is highest in Mexico, followed by Venezuela and Argentina. In Africa it is found most frequently in Senegal, Sudan, and Somalia. Mycetomas are also reported in large numbers in India. Actinomycetomas outnumber eumycetomas by 3:1, which is a blessing as the former is much more responsive to therapy. The male to female ratio varies from 2:1 to 5:1.

Mycology

For true fungi (eumycetoma), cultures are made from the grains on Sabouraud dextrose agar containing 0.5% yeast extract and suitable antibiotics. Cultures should be incubated at 37°C and room temperature. For actinomycetes grains, culture should be made in brain–heart infusion agar, incubated aerobically and anaerobically at 37°C, and on Sabouraud dextrose agar with 0.5% yeast extract, incubated aerobically at 37°C and room temperature. The specimen for culture should be taken from a deep site, preferably from the base of a biopsy. Cultures should be processed by a reference laboratory and should not be grown in an office laboratory.

Diagnosis

Mycetoma may be diagnosed by keeping in mind a triad of signs, namely: tumefaction, sinuses, and granules. Pus gathered from a deep sinus will show the granules when examined with the microscope. The slide containing the specimen should have a drop of 10% NaOH added and a coverslip placed on top. A biopsy may be required. Radiographs will show the bone involvement and MRI images may show the "dot in a circle" sign, corresponding to grains.

Treatment

Actinomycetomas generally respond to antibiotic therapy, although advanced cases may also need surgery. In *A. israelii* infection, penicillin in large doses is curative. *N. asteroides* or *N. brasiliensis* is usually treated with sulfonamides. A combination of rifampicin and co-trimoxazole has also been used. Severe refractory disease may respond to imipenem.

Patients in the early stage of eumycetoma may be successfully treated by surgical removal of the area. In the more advanced stages, a combination of antifungal therapy and surgery may be successful. In some cases of eumycetoma, amputation will be necessary. Surgical excision combined

with itraconazole, 200 mg twice a day until clinically well, may be effective in cases caused by *P. boydii*. *P. boydii* is not generally responsive to amphotericin, although liposome-encapsulated forms may have an effect. In one study, 30 isolates of *P. boydii* were tested for activity of posaconazole, fluconazole, and itraconazole in a mouse model of disseminated disease. Posaconazole was as effective as fluconazole and more effective than itraconazole.

Ameen M, et al: Efficacy of imipenem therapy for *Nocardia* actinomycetomas refractory to sulfonamides. J Am Acad Dermatol 2010 Feb; 62(2):239–246.

Castro LG, et al: Clinical and mycologic findings and therapeutic outcome of 27 mycetoma patients from São Paulo, Brazil. Int J Dermatol 2008 Feb; 47(2):160–163.

Gosselink C, et al: Nocardiosis causing pedal actinomycetoma: a case report and review of the literature. J Foot Ankle Surg 2008 Sep–Oct; 47(5):457–462.

Joshi R: Treatment of actinomycetoma with combination of rifampicin and co-trimoxazole. Indian J Dermatol Venereol Leprol 2008 Mar–Apr; 74(2):166–168.

Liu A, et al: Actinomycetoma with negative culture: a therapeutic challenge. Dermatol Online J 2008 Apr 15; 14(4):5.

Severo LC, et al: Mycetoma caused by *Exophiala jeanselmei*. Report of a case successfully treated with itraconazole and review of the literature. Rev Iberoam Micol 1999 Mar; 16(1):57–59.

Keloidal blastomycosis (lobomycosis)

Keloidal blastomycosis was originally described by Jorge Lobo in 1931. Most cases have occurred in countries in Central and South America. One occurred in an aquarium attendant in Europe who cared for an infected dolphin. One occurred in an American who had walked under the pounding water of Angel Falls on a trip to South America. The disease has been identified in a significant proportion of dolphins inhabiting the Indian River Lagoon in Florida and estuarine waters near Charleston, SC. Low albumin levels and a defective immune response are found in infected dolphins, and infection is linked to fresh water effluents emptying into the bodies of water.

The disease may involve any part of the body and the lesions appear characteristically keloidal (Fig. 15-30). Fistulas may occur. The nodules gradually increase in size by invasion of the surrounding normal skin or through the superficial lymphatics. Long-standing cases may involve the regional lymph nodes. A common location is the ear, which may resemble the cauliflower ear of a boxer. Disseminated disease has also been described.

The fungus is probably acquired from water, soil, or vegetation in forested areas where the disease is prevalent. Agricultural laborers have been most frequently affected, but the sex distribution is almost equal.

The causative organism, *Lacazia loboi* (formerly *Loboa loboi* and *Paracoccidioides loboi*), is an obligate parasite. Culture has not been successful, but the organism can grow in mouse footpads. Histologically, the epidermis is atrophic. The organisms are thick-walled, refractile spherules, larger than those of *P. brasiliensis*. One or two buds may be seen, but never multiple budding as in *P. brasiliensis*. The organisms are typically numerous and appear in chains of spheres connected by short narrow tubes like a child's pop beads. The cellular infiltrate is composed of histiocytes, giant cells, and lymphocytes. In dolphin tissue, the organism appears significantly smaller than in human tissue. This may be a manifestation of the host response, or may indicate that the organism in the two hosts may not be identical. Isolation of the organism for study is accomplished via the proteolytic enzyme dispase followed by molecular analysis of 18S ribosomal sequences.

Surgical excision of the affected areas may be curative when the lesions are small, but recurrence is common. Complete

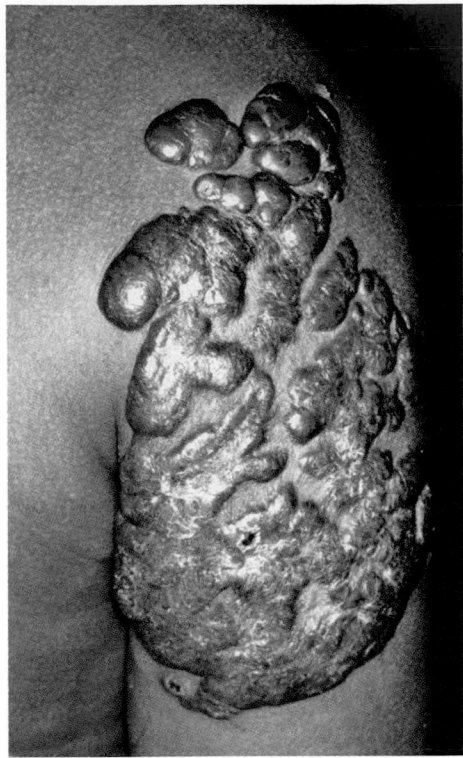

Fig. 15-30 Lobomycosis. (Courtesy of Maria Silvia Negrao, MD)

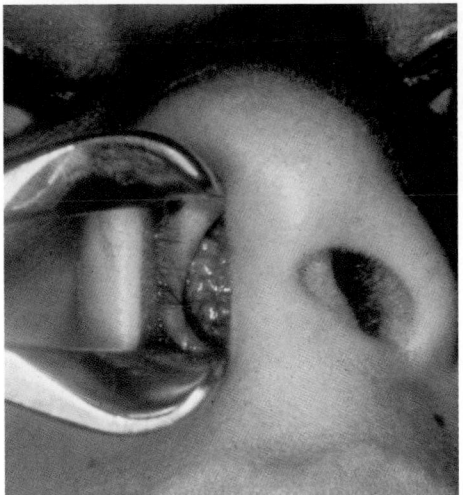

Fig. 15-31 Rhinosporidiosis.

resolution has been reported in a patient treated for 1 year with a combination of itraconazole, 100 mg/day, and clofazimine, 100 mg/day. Combination therapy with excision, itraconazole, and cryotherapy has also been reported.

Al-Daraji WI, et al: Lobomycosis in African patients. Br J Dermatol 2008 Jul; 159(1):234–236.

Carneiro FP, et al: Lobomycosis: diagnosis and management of relapsed and multifocal lesions. Diagn Microbiol Infect Dis 2009 Sep; 65(1):62–64.

Fonseca JJ: Lobomycosis. Int J Surg Pathol 2007 Jan; 15(1):62–63.

Paniz-Mondolfi AE, et al: Lobomycosis in Venezuela. Int J Dermatol 2007 Feb; 46(2):180–185.

Reif JS, et al: Evaluation and comparison of the health status of Atlantic bottlenose dolphins from the Indian River Lagoon, Florida, and Charleston, South Carolina. J Am Vet Med Assoc 2008 Jul 15; 233(2):299–307.

Talhari C, et al: Disseminated lobomycosis. Int J Dermatol 2008 Jun; 47(6):582–583.

Rhinosporidiosis

Rhinosporidiosis is a polypoid disease usually involving mucosal surfaces, especially the nasal mucosa (Fig. 15-31). Conjunctival, lacrimal, oral, and urethral tissues may also be involved, and genital lesions may resemble condylomata. The lesions begin as small papillomas and develop into pedunculated tumors with fissured and warty surfaces. Grayish-white flecks may be noted on the tissue, corresponding to transepithelial elimination of large sporangia. Bleeding occurs easily. Disseminated cutaneous lesions are rare. Conjunctival lesions begin as small, pinkish papillary nodules. Later they become larger, dark, and lobulated. Rectal and vaginal lesions have been reported. Like penile lesions, they may resemble condylomata or polyps. Widespread dissemination rarely occurs, and bone involvement has been described. The disease is endemic in Sri Lanka and India, but also occurs in parts of East Asia and in Latin America. It has been seen in the southern US, the UK, and Italy.

Rhinosporidium seeberi, an organism found in stagnant water, is the causative organism. It has been characterized as either a fungus or protist. The organisms appear as spherules 7–10 μm in diameter, which are contained within large cystic sporangia that may be as large as 300 μm in diameter. When the organism does not form endospores, it resembles *C. immitis* spherules, but differs by the regular presence of a central nucleus within each organism. The organisms are usually present within a polypoid structure. A granulomatous response is seen in about 50% of cases, and gigantic foreign body giant cells can rarely be noted filled with organisms.

Suppurative inflammation may be observed at the site of rupture of sporangia. Transepithelial elimination of sporangia is common. Destruction of the involved area by excision or electrosurgery is the most common method of treatment. Antifungal agents have been of little value. Culture of the organism is easiest when it is grown together with the cyanobacterium *Microcystis aeruginosa*. These are unicellular prokaryotic organisms found in pond water together with *R. seeberi*. The two organisms have also been shown to grow together in tissue, suggesting that rhinosporidiosis may represent a synergistic infection of the fungus and cyanobacterium. As drugs such as ciprofloxacin are active against *M. aeruginosa*, trials of antibiotic therapy may be of value.

Azad NS, et al: Rhinosporidiosis presenting as an urethral polyp. J Coll Physicians Surg Pak 2008 May; 18(5):314–315.

Echejoh GO, et al: Nasal rhinosporidiosis. J Natl Med Assoc 2008 Jun; 100(6):713–715.

Ghorpade A: Rhinosporidiosis: gigantic cells with engulfed sporangia of *Rhinosporidium seeberi* in the case of dermosporidiosis. Int J Dermatol 2008 Jul; 47(7):694–695.

Pandey N, et al: Oculosporidiosis. Indian J Ophthalmol 2008 Jan–Feb; 56(1):81.

Sudarshan V, et al: Rhinosporidiosis in Raipur, Chhattisgarh: a report of 462 cases. Indian J Pathol Microbiol 2007 Oct; 50(4):718–721.

Tolat SN, et al: Disseminated cutaneous rhinosporidiomas in an immunocompetent male. Indian J Dermatol Venereol Leprol 2007 Sep–Oct; 73(5):343–345.

Zygomycosis (phycomycosis)

There are a number of important pathogens in the class Zygomycetes. The two orders within this class that cause cutaneous infection most often are the Mucorales and Entomophthorales.

Entomophthoromycosis

Infections caused by the order Entomophthorales have been named entomophthoromycosis, rhinoentomophthoromycosis, conidiobolomycosis, or basidiobolomycosis. They occur usually in healthy individuals, and, unlike mucormycosis, often run an indolent course. The infections may be classified as cutaneous, subcutaneous, visceral, and disseminated.

Subcutaneous lesions occur in two basic types, each involving different anatomic sites. They occur either as well-circumscribed subcutaneous masses involving the nose, paranasal tissue, and upper lip, or as nodular, subcutaneous lesions located on the extremities, buttocks, and trunk.

Etiology

Conidiobolus coronatus typically causes the perinasal disease, whereas *Basidiobolus ranarum* causes the type of subcutaneous disease seen on the face.

Epidemiology

Occurrence is worldwide. It was first reported in Indonesia, where it is prevalent. Since then reports have come from Africa, Asia, and the Americas. Generally, infection occurs in a belt between 15° north and 15° south of the equator.

Diagnosis

Isolation and identification of the causative fungus are fundamental to the diagnosis. Culture on Sabouraud dextrose agar is made of nasal discharge, abscess fluid, or biopsy specimens. Biopsy specimens will show fibroblastic proliferation and an inflammatory reaction with lymphocytes, plasma cells, histiocytes, eosinophils, and giant cells. The organisms appear as broad hyphae that are generally aseptate and may be branched at right angles. The Splendore–Hoeppli phenomenon is common and appears as eosinophilic sleeves around the hyphae. Pythiosis, a primitive aquatic hyphal organism that acts as a zoonotic pathogen, may affect humans and has a similar appearance.

Treatment

Potassium iodide has been the drug of choice, although amphotericin B, co-trimoxazole, ketoconazole, itraconazole, and fluconazole have also been used successfully. Excision of small lesions is an alternative method of management, but the recurrence rate is significant. Rare human cases of pythiosis have responded to amphotericin B.

Mucormycosis

Mucormycosis refers to infections caused by the order Mucorales of the class Zygomycetes. They characteristically are acute, rapidly developing, and often fatal. In some series, the death rate is about 80%. Most infections occur in ketoacidotic diabetics, but leukemia, lymphoma, AIDS, iatrogenic immunosuppression, burns, chronic renal failure, and malnourishment all predispose to these infections. Infection has also been associated with methotrexate, prednisone, and infliximab therapy. Healthy individuals have been reported to develop these infections, and in contrast to mucocutaneous disease, 50% of patients with primary cutaneous zygomycosis are immunocompetent. Some have occurred after trauma or as a result of contaminated surgical dressings.

The five major clinical forms (rhinocerebral, pulmonary, cutaneous, gastrointestinal, and disseminated) all demonstrate vasculotropism of the organisms. This leads to infarction, gangrene, and the formation of black, necrotic, purulent debris. Ulceration, cellulitis, ecthyma gangrenosum-like lesions, and necrotic abscesses may occur. The infection may involve the skin through traumatic implantation or by hematogenous dissemination.

Etiology

The fungi that cause this infection are ubiquitous molds common in the soil, on decomposing plant and animal matter, and in the air. The pathogenic genera include *Rhizopus, Absidia, Mucor, Cunninghamella, Apophysomyces, Rhizomucor, Saksenaea, Mortierella,* and *Cokeromyces.*

Diagnosis

Tissue obtained by biopsy or curettage is examined microscopically and cultured. Prompt diagnosis is essential in this rapidly fatal infection. Histologically, the organism generally appears as eosinophilic, thick-walled hyphae that look hollow in cross-section. The organism is quite irregular in outline and right-angle branching is common. The organisms are highly vasculotropic and dissect along the media of muscular vessels, resulting in infarction of tissue.

Treatment

A combination of excision of affected tissue and antifungal therapy, usually with amphotericin B, is necessary in most cases. Very limited disease may be treated with excision alone, but this approach may be risky. Liposomal amphotericin B is more effective than conventional amphotericin B in animal models of infection. Clinical data also suggest the superiority of liposomal forms of amphotericin B. Arterial infusion of liposomal amphotericin B may be superior to intravenous therapy in some serious limb infections.

In both animal models and human disease, other antifungal agents have proved to be effective, but their effectiveness varies from one zygomycete to another. Itraconazole has been shown to be inactive against *Rhizopus microsporus* and *Rhizopus oryzae,* but partially active against *Absidia corymbifera.* Posaconazole has been shown to be inactive against *R. oryzae* but partially active against *A. corymbifera.* Posaconazole has activity against *R. microsporus,* and has been effective in some human infections. Breakthrough infections have been noted during posaconazole prophylaxis and some data suggest that liposomal amphotericin B is associated with better outcomes in the setting of established disease. Echinocandins have limited activity against zygomycetes, but FK463, a new echinocandin, and even caspofungin, have been used successfully. As these drugs have spotty coverage against zygomycetes, they are best used in combination with other agents, or when other agents have failed.

Mohs micrographic surgery has been used for margin control during excision of infected tissue. The speed of interpretation of each stage and the potential for tissue conservation are advantages of this method. Fungal stains, such as Gomori methenamine silver, have been used in this setting, but zygomycetes show variable staining with fungal stains. Often H&E is the optimal stain, and the organisms may stain avidly with a tissue Gram stain.

Gadadhar H, et al: Cutaneous mucormycosis complicating methotrexate, prednisone, and infliximab therapy. J Clin Rheumatol 2007 Dec; 13(6):361–362.

Ledgard JP, et al: Primary cutaneous zygomycosis in a burns patient: a review. J Burn Care Res 2008 Mar–Apr; 29(2):286–290.

Reddy IS, et al: Primary cutaneous mucormycosis (zygomycosis) caused by *Apophysomyces elegans.* Indian J Dermatol Venereol Leprol 2008 Jul–Aug; 74(4):367–370.

Rüping MJ, et al: Forty-one recent cases of invasive zygomycosis from a global clinical registry. J Antimicrob Chemother 2010; 65(2):296–302.

Simbli M, et al: Nosocomial post-traumatic cutaneous mucormycosis: a systematic review. Scand J Infect Dis 2008; 40(6–7):577–582.

Visser DH, et al: Diagnosis and treatment of cutaneous zygomycosis. Pediatr Infect Dis J 2007 Dec; 26(12):1165–1166.

Hyalohyphomycosis

The term hyalohyphomycosis contrasts with phaeohyphomycosis and refers to those opportunistic mycotic infections caused by nondematiaceous molds. Most of these organisms are septate, and, compared with black molds, most have delicate walls. Organisms include *Penicillium* and *Paecilomyces*. Disseminated infections with *Scedosporium apiospermum* (the asexual form of *Pseudallescheria boydii*) are also grouped in this category. Some authors use the term broadly to encompass infections with all light-colored molds, including *Fusarium*. Although *Aspergillus* is a light-colored mold that appears similar in tissue to other forms of hyalohyphomycosis, it is usually grouped separately, as organisms other than *Aspergillus* are more likely to cause wide dissemination and CNS disease in some reported series.

These organisms are ubiquitous; they occur as saprophytes in soil or water or on decomposing organic debris. They generally do not cause disease except in immunocompromised patients. *Fusarium solani* (keratomycosis) and *Fusarium oxysporum* (white superficial onychomycosis) are exceptions. Localized hyalohyphomycosis has also occurred in immunocompetent patients following traumatic implantation. There is no classic clinical morphology to the lesions, but keratotic masses, ulcerations, ecthyma gangrenosum-like lesions, erythematous nodules, dark eschars, and disseminated erythema have been described (Fig. 15-32).

Penicillium marneffei infection is an indicator of HIV disease, especially in Southeast Asia. This organism is dimorphic and appears in tissue as small intracellular organisms within histiocytes. The histologic similarity to histoplasmosis is striking.

Most of these infections are treated with a combination of excision and amphotericin B. Some organisms respond well to itraconazole alone or with an echinocandin.

Fusariosis

Fusarium has emerged as an important pathogen, especially in patients with hematologic malignancy, neutropenia, and T-cell immunodeficiency, particularly those with hematopoietic stem-cell transplants and graft versus host disease. Skin involvement is present in about 70% of patients, and the infection may sometimes begin in the skin and then disseminate. Many cases begin in the lungs or sinuses, then disseminate to the skin. Blood cultures are commonly positive, but skin biopsies provide the highest diagnostic yield. Contaminated hospital plumbing may be a source of fusariosis. *Fusarium* has been cultured from drains, water tanks, sink faucet aerators, and shower heads. Aerosolization of *Fusarium* spp by shower heads has been documented.

The mortality rate is high, but has improved with the availability of new antifungal agents. Neutropenia, a factor predicting mortality, must be controlled with colony-stimulating factors. Liposomal encapsulated amphotericin has good activity against *Fusarium*. Liposomal amphotericin B, together with terbinafine, has been effective for disseminated cutaneous *Fusarium proliferatum* infection. Voriconazole and posaconazole have also been used successfully. Posaconazole can raise calcineurin inhibitor levels in the blood, and these must be closely monitored during therapy. Some treatment failures may relate to unpredictable bioavailability. Pentamidine is active in vitro against many *Fusarium* spp. Some data suggest that IFN-γ plus granulocyte macrophage-colony stimulating factor may be helpful for refractory disseminated infection.

Aspergillosis

Aspergillosis is second only to candidiasis in frequency of opportunistic fungal disease in patients with leukemia and other hematologic neoplasia. Neutropenia remains the key risk factor for invasive aspergillosis in this population. Lymphocytes, especially NK cells, are also critical in host defense, and immunosuppressive agents create a risk of infection. Other risk factors include prolonged corticosteroid therapy, graft versus host disease, and cytomegalovirus infection. Solid organ transplant patients are also predisposed to *Aspergillus* infections. Pulmonary involvement is usually present in invasive disease, but skin lesions are present in only about 10% of cases. Biopsy of a skin lesion may establish the diagnosis when other studies have failed. Blood culture is an insensitive method of diagnosis. Serum antigenic assays are being developed, but suffer from limited sensitivity and specificity.

Aspergillus fumigatus is the most common cause of disseminated aspergillosis with cutaneous involvement. The organism grows on media without cycloheximide in 24 h or longer. In tissue, the organisms appear as slender hyphae with delicate walls and bubbly cytoplasm. The appearance is identical to that of *Fusarium*, except for the lack of vesicular swellings along hyphae. The hyphae in both are septate with 45° branching. Both tend to be vasculotropic and are associated with cutaneous necrosis. *Aspergillus flavus* rarely causes fungus balls in lung, but is a common cause of fungal sinusitis and skin lesions. *Aspergillus niger* is a rare cause of disseminated infection with skin lesions. In third-degree burns, *Aspergillus* commonly colonizes the eschar. Deep incisional biopsies are required to distinguish invasive disease from colonization.

Primary cutaneous aspergillosis

Primary cutaneous aspergillosis is a rare disease. Most cases occur at the site of intravenous cannulas in immunosuppressed patients. Hemorrhagic bullae and necrotic ulcers may be present (Fig. 15-33). *A. flavus* is most commonly associated with this form of infection. Patients must be treated aggressively, as the fungus may disseminate from the skin lesion.

Aspergillus is a frequent contaminant in cultures from thickened, friable, dystrophic nails, and various *Aspergillus* spp

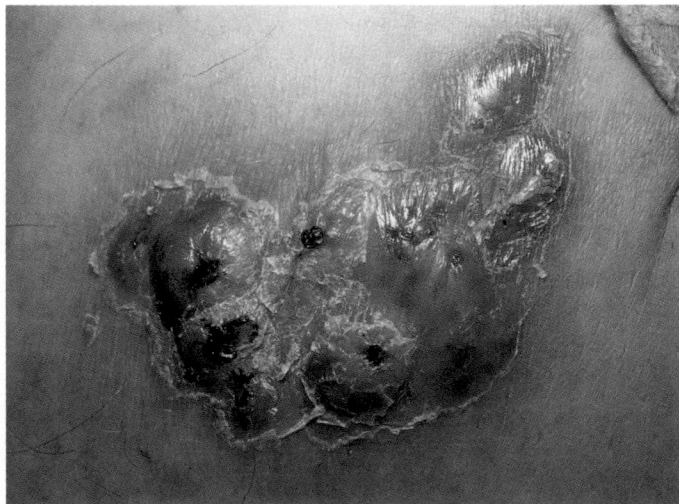

Fig. 15-32, Hyalohyphomycosis caused by *Paecilomyces*. (Courtesy of Dan Loo, MD)

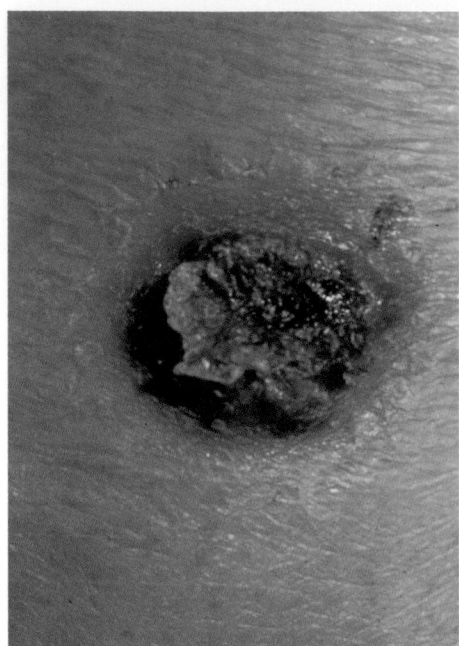

Fig. 15-33 Primary aspergillosis.

have been implicated as true etiologic agents of onychomycosis. Nail infection may respond to itraconazole.

Otomycosis

The ear canal may be infected by *A. fumigatus*, *A. flavus*, and *A. niger*. Pathogenic bacteria, especially *Pseudomonas aeruginosa*, are often found concurrently. The colonization may be benign, but malignant otitis may occasionally occur, especially in diabetic or iatrogenically immunosuppressed patients. Invasive disease must be treated with systemic agents.

Treatment

Amphotericin B has been the drug of choice in invasive aspergillosis, but triazoles have activity against the fungus. Voriconazole shows excellent activity against *Aspergillus* spp, including itraconazole- and amphotericin B-resistant strains of *A. fumigatus*. Some data suggest it is superior to amphotericin B, with lower overall toxicity, although visual disturbances, photosensitivity, skin cancer, and skin rash can be a problem with this drug. Voriconazole takes some time to achieve therapeutic levels, and the use of caspofungin in combination with voriconazole can provide coverage against *Aspergillus* infection during this period. Echinocandins are fungistatic against *Aspergillus* spp, but have also proved clinically useful.

Alexander BD, et al: Posaconazole as salvage therapy in patients with invasive fungal infections after solid organ transplant. Transplantation 2008 Sep 27; 86(6):791–796.
Gardner JM, et al: Chronic cutaneous fusariosis. Arch Dermatol 2005 Jun; 141(6):794–795.
Hedayati MT, et al: *Aspergillus flavus*: human pathogen, allergen and mycotoxin producer. Microbiology 2007 Jun; 153(Pt 6):1677–1692.
Ho DY, et al: Treating disseminated fusariosis: amphotericin B, voriconazole or both? Mycoses 2007 May; 50(3):227–231.
Lewis R, et al: Progressive fusariosis: unpredictable posaconazole bioavailability, and feasibility of recombinant interferon-gamma plus granulocyte macrophage-colony stimulating factor for refractory disseminated infection. Leuk Lymphoma 2008 Jan; 49(1):163–165.

Neuburger S, et al: Successful salvage treatment of disseminated cutaneous fusariosis with liposomal amphotericin B and terbinafine after allogeneic stem cell transplantation. Transpl Infect Dis 2008 Jul; 10(4):290–293.
Nucci M, et al: *Fusarium* infections in immunocompromised patients. Clin Microbiol Rev 2007 Oct; 20(4):695–704.
Pasqualotto AC: Differences in pathogenicity and clinical syndromes due to *Aspergillus fumigatus* and *Aspergillus flavus*. Med Mycol 2008 Jul; 25:1–10.
Pérez-Pérez L, et al: Ulcerous lesions disclosing cutaneous infection with *Fusarium solani*. Acta Derm Venereol 2007; 87(5):422–424.
Thomas A, et al: Clinical outcomes of lung-transplant recipients treated by voriconazole and caspofungin combination in aspergillosis. J Clin Pharm Ther 2010; 35(1):49–53.
Thomas LM, et al: Primary cutaneous aspergillosis in a patient with a solid organ transplant: case report and review of the literature. Cutis 2008 Feb; 81(2):127–130.
Thursky KA, et al: Recommendations for the treatment of established fungal infections. Intern Med J 2008 Jun; 38(6b):496–520.
Vennewald I, et al: Cutaneous infections due to opportunistic molds: uncommon presentations. Clin Dermatol 2005 Nov–Dec; 23(6):565–571.
Wiederhold NP, et al: Efficacy of posaconazole as treatment and prophylaxis against *Fusarium solani*. Antimicrob Agents Chemother 2010; 54(3):1055–1059.

DISEASE CAUSED BY ALGAE (PROTOTHECOSIS)

Protothecosis is caused by the *Prototheca* genus of saprophytic, achloric (nonpigmented) algae. These organisms reproduce asexually via internal septation or morulation. This reproductive method, along with the absence of glucosamine and muramic acid in the cell wall, separates the genus from the bacteria and fungi. Two *Prototheca* spp cause disease in humans, *Prototheca wickerhamii* and *Prototheca zopfii*. Stagnant water, tree slime, and soil appear to be the source of infection in most cases.

Skin lesions may present as verrucous lesions, ulcers, papulonodular lesions, or crusted papules with umbilication. Protothecosis of the olecranon bursa is usually seen in healthy individuals, but cutaneous infections have been most often reported in patients receiving immunosuppressive therapy and in those with renal failure, AIDS, hematologic malignancy, or diabetes mellitus. Neutropenia is not a common risk factor.

Prototheca spp are easily recognized in PAS-stained tissue specimens when the characteristic morulating cells are visible. These are more common in *P. wickerhamii*. The organism also appears with a single black nucleus and a slightly asymmetrical thick refractile wall. It grows on most routine mycologic media, but cycloheximide will suppress growth of *Prototheca* spp. Colonies on Sabouraud agar are smooth, creamy, and yeast-like. The use of fluorescent antibody reagents makes possible the rapid and reliable identification of *Prototheca* spp in culture and tissue.

Intravenous amphotericin B remains the most effective agent for *Prototheca* infections. Triazoles have been used, but appear to be less effective. Surgery, as well as topical amphotericin B and tetracycline, have been used for isolated cutaneous disease.

Dalmau J, et al: Treatment of protothecosis with voriconazole. J Am Acad Dermatol 2006 Nov; 55(5 Suppl):S122–S123.
Hightower KD, et al: Cutaneous protothecosis: a case report and review of the literature. Cutis 2007 Aug; 80(2):129–131.
Lass-Flörl C, et al: Human protothecosis. Clin Microbiol Rev 2007 Apr; 20(2):230–242.

Aspergillosis

16 Mycobacterial Diseases

Tuberculosis

No ideal classification scheme exists for cutaneous tuberculosis, but the system below is logical and takes into account the mechanism of disease acquisition. Unfortunately, unlike in Hansen's disease, these categories do not correlate perfectly to host immunity. There are four major categories of cutaneous tuberculosis:

1. Inoculation from an exogenous source (primary inoculation tuberculosis and tuberculosis verrucosa cutis).
2. Endogenous cutaneous spread contiguously or by autoinoculation (scrofuloderma, tuberculosis cutis orificialis).
3. Hematogenous spread to the skin (lupus vulgaris; acute miliary tuberculosis; tuberculosis ulcer, gumma, or abscess; tuberculous cellulitis). (Lupus vulgaris can also occur adjacent to lesions of scrofuloderma, suggesting that both hematogenous and local spread is capable of triggering this reaction pattern.)
4. Tuberculids (erythema induratum [Bazin disease], papulonecrotic tuberculid, and lichen scrofulosorum).

The finding of mycobacterial DNA by polymerase chain reaction (PCR) in tuberculids suggests that tuberculids also represent hematogenous dissemination of tuberculosis (TB), which is quickly controlled by the host, usually resulting in the absence of detectable organisms by culture and histologic methods. Miliary TB is the form with least effective host immunity. Tuberculous ulcer/abscess/cellulitis, and tuberculosis cutis orificialis are conditions of poor host immunity against *Mycobacterium tuberculosis*. Bacilli are prominent in these forms of cutaneous TB, and histologic and microbiologic confirmation is usually straightforward. This is fortunate, since cellular-based diagnostic modalities (purified protein derivative [PPD] and interferon-γ release assays [IGRA]) may be negative. Tuberculosis verrucosa cutis and lupus vulgaris are conditions of high host immunity to TB, and tuberculin skin tests and IGRA for TB will usually be positive. Scrofuloderma is usually associated with a positive PPD, and identification by culture and histologic methods is positive in only 20% and 40% respectively. In its initial stage primary inoculation TB will be multibacillary and culture-positive. As host immunity develops, the skin test becomes positive and the number of organisms on biopsy diminishes. The tuberculids also represent high host immune response manifestations of TB, and bacilli are rarely found.

Epidemiology

The increase in the numbers of cases of TB that started in the mid-1980s in the USA was associated with three phenomena: large numbers of immigrants from high-prevalence countries, the acquired immunodeficiency syndrome (AIDS)/human immunodeficiency virus (HIV) epidemic, and an increasing number of persons in congregative facilities (shelters for the homeless and prisons). Asians, African Americans, and Hispanics have the greatest risk for developing TB in the US. Aggressive diagnosis and treatment programs have led to a reduction in new cases of TB in the US. The infection rate in the US-born population of adults fell from 12.6% in 1970 to 2.5% in 2000. However, in the US, local pockets of TB are still found in regions of otherwise very low incidence. This is in part attributable to the persistently high infection rate in the foreign-born US population, whose infection rate has only fallen from 35.9% in 1970 to 21.3% in 1980.

In the developing world, TB is a tremendous health problem. Africa is home to 29% of all persons with TB worldwide. The incidence of TB in Africa doubled between 1990 and 2005, with new cases appearing at a rate of over 6/1000 in some countries. This has been driven largely by the HIV/AIDS epidemic. One-third or more of HIV-infected persons in Africa are also infected with *M. tuberculosis*. Latent TB is 100 times more likely to reactivate in persons with HIV infection, and HIV-infected persons are much more likely to acquire new tuberculous infection. In countries like India, while great progress has been made, TB is still very, very common, with 1.8 million new cases diagnosed every year, or 2 new cases per 1000 population per year. Infection rates are particularly high in India among healthcare workers; there are 17 new cases of TB for every 1000 medical residents per year.

TB has increasingly become resistant to first-line treatments. Strains of TB classified as multidrug-resistant (MDR-TB) are resistant to at least isoniazid and rifampin. Extensively drug-resistant TB (XDR-TB) is, in addition, resistant to any fluoroquinolone and at least one of the following: capreomycin, kanamycin, or amikacin. The emergence of these resistant strains of TB has made treatment more costly and more difficult. However, aggressive treatment protocols using multiple drugs for up to 2 years, and, when indicated, surgical techniques can cure up to 60% of even XDR-TB cases.

Cutaneous TB is an uncommon complication of tuberculous infection, with less than 2% of cases of TB having skin lesions, even in highly endemic areas. The types of cutaneous lesion that the patient will develop are dependent on multiple host factors:

1. Age: 25% of scrofuloderma cases and the majority of cases of lichen scrofulosorum occur in children.
2. Gender: women are 10 times more likely to develop erythema induratum, but men are 2–3 times more likely to have other forms of cutaneous TB.
3. Anatomic location: lupus vulgaris occurs on the face and extremities while TB verrucosa cutis occurs predominately on the sole and foot.
4. Nutritional status: tuberculous abscesses and scrofuloderma are associated with malnutrition.

The pattern of cutaneous TB has been changing over the last few decades, and is different in developed as opposed to developing nations. The average age of cases with cutaneous

TB has increased in developed countries, and tuberculids, especially erythema induratum, represent a larger proportion of cases. In Hong Kong, 85% of cases of cutaneous TB are tuberculids. This suggests that most cutaneous TB in adults will be found in patients infected in the distant past who are reactivating their disease, not recently infected persons. Cutaneous TB is uncommon in immunosuppressed hosts, since when they acquire new TB or reactivate their TB, it usually reactivates at a non-cutaneous site and is diagnosed before skin disease occurs. Miliary TB is the most commonly reported form of cutaneous TB in the setting of HIV. In areas of high TB endemicity in the developing world, true cutaneous TB is still common, and more than 50% of cases will occur before the age of 19. The likelihood of finding associated systemic TB is higher in children than adults. None the less, as opposed to all other forms of extrapulmonary TB, failing to find an underlying focus of TB in patients with cutaneous TB is not uncommon. Between 3% and 12% of cases of cutaneous TB will have an abnormal chest radiograph. Most commonly, TB of the lymph nodes will be found.

Tuberculin testing

The tuberculin skin test (TST) is designed to detect a memory cell-mediated immune response to *M. tuberculosis*. The test becomes positive between 2 and 10 weeks following infection and remains positive for many years, although it may wane with age. PPD preparations are currently used for testing in the US and Canada at a dose of 5 TU. The intradermal, or Mantoux, test is the standard, and it offers the highest degree of consistency and reliability. The test is read 48–72 h after intradermal injection. Induration measuring 5 mm or more is considered positive in HIV-infected patients, in those with risk factors for developing TB, in recent close contacts, or in those with chest x-ray findings consistent with healed TB. Because children are at increased risk of developing active TB after exposure, a 5 mm or larger reaction in contact investigations is considered positive. If the PPD measures more than 10 mm, it is considered positive in injection drug users, HIV-negative injection drug users, those born in foreign countries of high prevalence, mycobacteriology laboratory personnel, residents and employees in high-risk congregate facilities, and those with medical conditions that predispose to TB. If induration is more than 15 mm, it is positive in all others; 0–4 mm induration is negative. The lower the threshold for positivity for the TST, the less this represents true positivity (the higher number of false-positives). This is why a TST of less than 15 mm is considered positive only in patients at higher risk for having latent TB. Conversely, as the cutoff for true positivity is raised, the number of infected persons the TST detects will decrease (the number of false-negatives increases). A TST of over 6 mm will detect 89% of persons with latent TB, a TST of over 10 mm will detect 75%, and a TST of over 15 mm will detect only 47% of latently infected patients. At least 7% of patients with latent TB will have completely negative TSTs. Many intermediate TST responses may represent cross-reaction with atypical mycobacteria. Bacillus Calmette–Guérin (BCG) immunization leads to a positive tuberculin result in immunized children, but this reaction usually does not persist beyond 10 years. Repeated BCG immunization or BCG administration after the age of 2 years is more likely to result in a persistently positive TST on this basis. However, positive reactions in adults should not automatically be attributed to childhood BCG administration.

Reactivity to the tuberculin protein is impaired in certain conditions in which cellular immunity is impaired. Lymphoproliferative disorders, sarcoidosis, corticosteroids and immunosuppressive medications (including tumor necrosis factor [TNF]-inhibitors), severe protein deficiency, chronic renal failure, and numerous infectious illnesses, including HIV infection, are capable of diminishing tuberculin reactivity. In overwhelming TB (miliary disease), more than 50% of patients have a negative skin test before beginning therapy. A negative or doubtful reaction to a PPD preparation does not rule out TB infection, particularly in the face of suggestive symptoms and signs.

Until recently, the TST had been the gold standard to confirm the presence of infection with *M. tuberculosis*. TST has significant limitations, including low sensitivity in persons with compromised immune systems; negative tests in a substantial portion of persons with active TB (sensitivity only 77%); repeat visits to interpret; technical competence on the part of the person applying the test; booster effect of repeat testing creating potential false-positive results; and false-positive tests in persons with prior BCG vaccination. To overcome these obstacles, antigen-specific in vitro assays have been developed. They assay the amount of interferon (IFN)-γ released by peripheral blood T cells, and are called IGRAs (interferon-γ release assays). QuantiFERON-TB Gold, ELISpot^PLUS, and T-SPOT are three such tests. Results are variable with respect to the sensitivity and specificity of these assays, but they appear to be valuable in certain settings. They are no more sensitive or only slightly more sensitive than TST in detecting latent TB. However, they are considerably more specific in the BCG-vaccinated population, in whom the TST is only 60% specific whereas IGRAs are 93% specific. In addition, in persons with HIV and those receiving corticosteroids, IGRAs are much more likely to be positive than a TST in persons with *M. tuberculosis* infection. The clinical settings in which TSTs and IGRAs give either false-positive or false-negative values are different. If the TST is combined with an IGRA and the tests are concordant, false-negative results are 2% and false-positive tests only 1%. This suggests that the combination of a TST and an IGRA would be the optimal testing to assess for *M. tuberculosis* infection (latent or active). Either the two tests can be done simultaneously, or, if screening for latent TB in an otherwise immunologically normal person, the TST can be applied first, then an IGRA performed in all persons with a positive TST of more than 6 mm.

Appropriate screening prior to initiating anti-TNF therapy or immunosuppression in a dermatology patient would include the following:

1. Screen for active TB by history and physical examination (and chest x-ray where suspicion for TB is elevated).
2. Administer a TST and perhaps an IGRA.
3. Interpret the test results with caution in patients already on significant iatrogenic immunosuppressive or anti-TNF treatments.
4. Regularly monitor patients on anti-TNF agents for the development of TB with appropriate history, physical examination, and laboratory testing; and suspect and screen for TB if clinical symptoms may indicate infection.

BCG vaccination

BCG is a live attenuated strain of *Mycobacterium bovis* used in most parts of the world (except North America and Western Europe) to immunize infants. It enhances immunity to TB and is effective in reducing childhood TB, especially if given to neonates. Once the patient has been vaccinated, the tuberculin test becomes positive, and remains so for a period of less than 10 years (unless the person is BCG-immunized after age 2 or repeatedly immunized). In an adult who was vaccinated as a child in a foreign country with a high prevalence of TB and whose tuberculin test measures more than 10 mm, active TB should be assumed. The use of BCG instillation in the bladder for the treatment of bladder cancer has been associated with disseminated disease, usually pneumonitis, hepatitis, prostatitis, and abdominal aneurysms.

Dermatologic complications of BCG vaccination are rarely seen. Localized abscesses and regional suppurative adenitis occur at a rate of about 0.4 per 1000 vaccines. Excessive ulceration may occur if the BCG is inoculated too deeply. Scrofuloderma is rare. Disseminated infection is seen in between 1 and 4 cases per million infants vaccinated and is associated with a high mortality. Disseminated BCG develops only in the setting of immunodeficiency. Lupus vulgaris can occur rarely at the vaccination site, or at a distant site. It will respond to appropriate antituberculous treatment. Papular and papulonecrotic tuberculids, as well as erythema induratum, can occur following BCG immunization. They appear from 10 days to several months after vaccination. Treatment may not be necessary for the BCG-induced tuberculids, as they frequently heal in a few months with no treatment.

Inoculation cutaneous tuberculosis from an exogenous source

Primary inoculation tuberculosis (primary tuberculous complex, tuberculous chancre)

Primary inoculation TB develops at the site of inoculation of tubercle bacilli into a TB-free individual (Fig. 16-1). Regional lymphadenopathy usually occurs, completing the "complex." It occurs chiefly in children and affects the face or extremities. The inoculation can occur during tattooing, medical injections, nose-piercing, or external physical trauma. The earliest lesion, appearing 2–4 weeks after inoculation, is a painless brown–red papule, which develops into an indurated nodule or plaque that may ulcerate. This is the tuberculous chancre. Prominent regional lymphadenopathy appears 3–8 weeks after infection and, occasionally, cold, suppurative, and draining lesions may appear over involved lymph nodes. Primary tuberculous

complex occurs on the mucous membranes in about one-third of patients. Spontaneous healing usually occurs within a year or less, with the skin lesion healing first, then the lymph node, which is often persistently enlarged and calcified. Delayed suppuration of the affected lymph node, lupus vulgaris overlying the involved node, and occasionally dissemination may follow this form of cutaneous TB.

Histologically, there is a marked inflammatory response during the first 2 weeks, with many polymorphonuclear leukocytes and tubercle bacilli. During the next 2 weeks, the picture changes. Lymphocytes and epithelioid cells appear and replace the polymorphonuclear leukocytes. Distinct tubercles develop within 3 or 4 weeks of inoculation. Simultaneously, with the appearance of epithelioid cells, the number of tubercle bacilli decreases rapidly.

The differential diagnosis of primary inoculation TB extends over the spectrum of chancriform conditions of deep fungal or bacterial origin, such as sporotrichosis, blastomycosis, histoplasmosis, coccidioidomycosis, nocardiosis, syphilis, leishmaniasis, yaws, tularemia, and atypical mycobacterial disease. Pyogenic granuloma and cat-scratch disease must also be considered.

Paucibacillary cutaneous tuberculosis from an exogenous or endogenous source in persons with high immunity

Tuberculosis verrucosa cutis

Tuberculosis verrucosa cutis occurs from exogenous inoculation of bacilli into the skin of a previously sensitized person with strong immunity against *M. tuberculosis*. The tuberculin test is strongly positive. The prosecutor's wart resulting from inoculation during an autopsy is the prototype of tuberculosis verrucosa cutis.

Clinically, the lesion begins as a small papule, which becomes hyperkeratotic, resembling a wart. The lesion enlarges by peripheral expansion, with or without central clearing, sometimes reaching several centimeters or more in diameter (Fig. 16-2). Fissuring of the surface may occur, discharging purulent exudate. Lesions are almost always solitary, and regional adenopathy is usually present only if secondary bacterial infection occurs. Frequent locations for tuberculosis verrucosa cutis are on the dorsa of the fingers and hands in adults, and the ankles and buttocks in children.

The lesions are persistent, although usually superficial and limited in their extent. Local scarring, as seen in lupus vulgaris, can occur. Lesions may be separated by exudative or

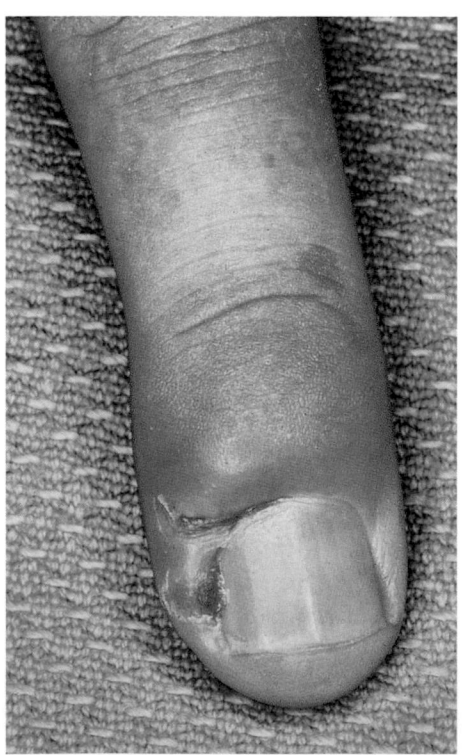

Fig. 16-1 Primary inoculation tuberculosis.

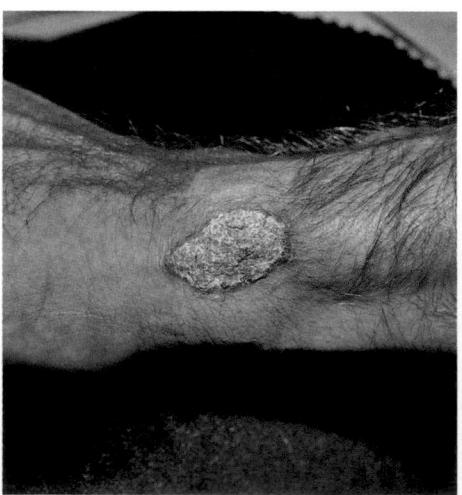

Fig. 16-2 Tuberculosis verrucosa cutis.

suppurative areas, but they seldom ulcerate and may heal spontaneously.

Histologically, there is pseudoepitheliomatous hyperplasia of the epidermis and hyperkeratosis. Suppurative and granulomatous inflammation is seen in the upper and mid-dermis, sometimes perforating through the epidermis. Caseation is rare. The number of acid-fast bacilli (AFB) is usually scant, and failure to find AFB should not be used to exclude the diagnosis. Culture will be positive in slightly more than 50% of cases.

Differential diagnosis Tuberculosis verrucosa cutis is differentiated only by culture from atypical mycobacteriosis caused by *Mycobacterium marinum*. It must also be distinguished from North American blastomycosis, chromoblastomycosis, verrucous epidermal nevus, hypertrophic lichen planus, halogenoderma, and verruca vulgaris.

Lupus vulgaris

Lupus vulgaris may appear at sites of inoculation, in scrofuloderma scars, or most commonly at distant sites from the initial infectious focus, probably by hematogenous dissemination. Approximately half of such cases will have evidence of TB elsewhere, so a complete evaluation is mandatory. Because lupus vulgaris is associated with moderately high immunity to TB, most patients will have a positive tuberculin test.

Lupus vulgaris typically is a single plaque composed of grouped red–brown papules, which, when blanched by diascopic pressure, have a pale brownish yellow or "apple-jelly" color. The papules (called lupomes) tend to heal slowly in one area and progress in another. They are minute, translucent, and embedded deeply and diffusely in the infiltrated dermis, expanding by the development of new papules at the periphery, which coalesce with the main plaque (Fig. 16-3). The plaques are slightly elevated. The disease is destructive (Fig. 16-4), frequently causes ulceration, and on involution leaves deforming scars as it slowly spreads peripherally over the years. Lupus vulgaris lesions of the head and neck can at times be associated with lymphangitis or lymphadenitis. If lesions involve the nose or the lobes of the ears, these structures are shrunken and scarred, as if nibbled away. Atrophy is prominent, and ectropion and eclabion may occur. The tip of the nose may be sharply pointed and beaklike, or the whole nose may be destroyed, and only the orifices and the posterior parts of the septum and turbinates visible. The upper lip, a site of predilection, may become diffusely swollen and thickened,

with fissures, adherent thin crusts, and ulcers. On the trunk and extremities, lesions may be annular or serpiginous, or may form gyrate patterns. On the hands and feet and around the genitals or buttocks, lesions may cause mutilation by destruction, scar formation, warty thickenings (Fig. 16-5), and elephantiasic enlargement.

An unusual form of lupus vulgaris may follow measles or another significant febrile illness. The window of immune deficiency caused by the acute illness results in dissemination of the TB hematogenously from a single focus of lupus vulgaris. Multiple erythematous papules in a generalized distribution appear a month or more after the illness. These lesions evolve to small papules and plaques clinically and histologically resembling lupus vulgaris. The TST is negative during the immediate period following the febrile illness, and then

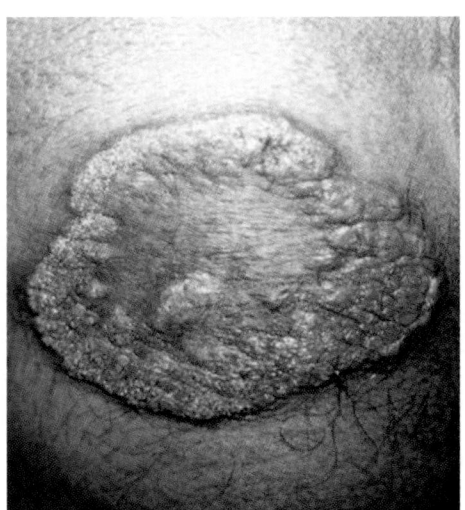

Fig. 16-4 Lupus vulgaris. (Courtesy of Shyam Verma, MD)

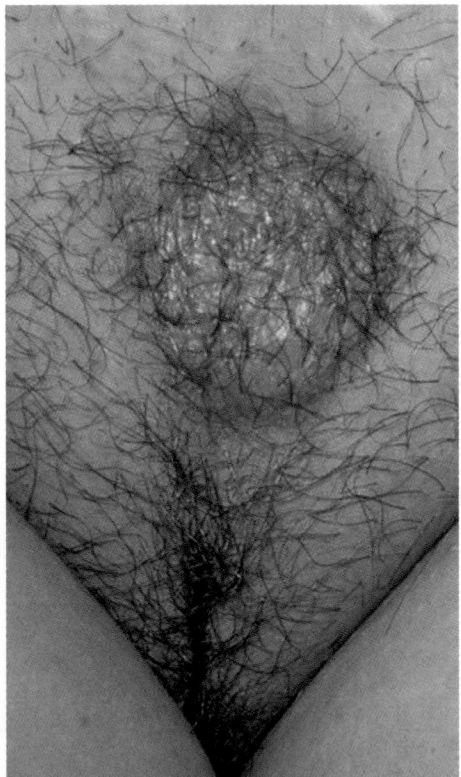

Fig. 16-5 Lupus vulgaris in the pubic area. (Courtesy of Shyam Verma, MD)

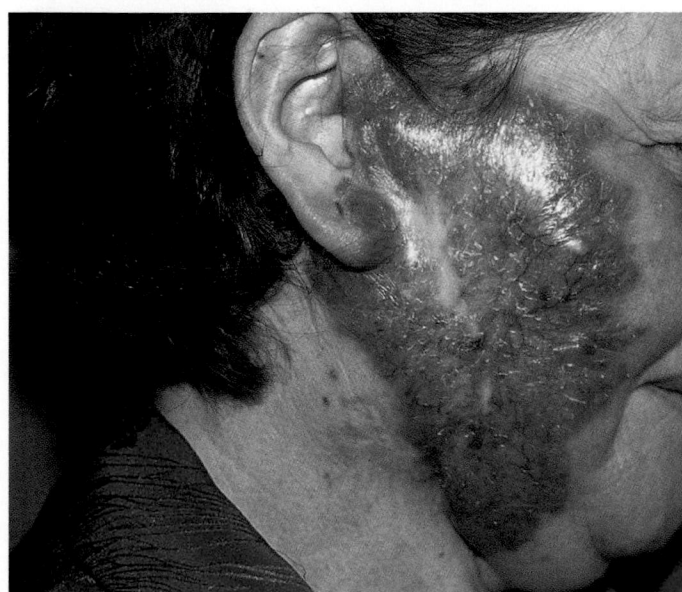

Fig. 16-3 Lupus vulgaris. (Courtesy of Dr Tavares-Bello, MD)

rapidly reverts to strongly positive. This is called "lupus vulgaris postexanthematicus."

While classically considered a scarring and atrophying process, lesions of the lips and ears may be quite hyperplastic. The lips may resemble cheilitis granulomatosis clinically and histologically. Uniform hyperplasia of the ear pinna and lobe may closely mimic "turkey ear," as described in sarcoidosis.

When the mucous membranes are involved, the lesions become papillomatous or ulcerative. They may appear as circumscribed, grayish, macerated, or granulating plaques. On the tongue, irregular, deep, painful fissures occur, sometimes associated with microglossia to the degree that nutrition is compromised.

The rate of progression of lupus vulgaris is slow, and a lesion may remain limited to a small area for several decades. The onset may be in childhood and persist throughout a lifetime. It may slowly spread, and new lesions may develop in other regions. In some instances, the lesions become papillomatous, vegetative, or thickly crusted, so that they have a rupioid appearance. Squamous cell carcinoma may develop in long-standing lesions.

Histologically, classic tubercles are the hallmark of lupus vulgaris. Caseation within the tubercles is seen in about half the cases and is rarely marked. Sarcoidosis may be simulated. The epidermis is affected secondarily, sometimes flattened and at other times hypertrophic. AFB are found in 10% or less of cases with standard acid-fast stains. PCR still lacks the sensitivity and specificity to diagnose paucibacillary forms of cutaneous TB reproducibly, and will be positive in about one-quarter of cases or less. Cultures of the skin lesions grow *M. tuberculosis* in about half the cases.

Colloid milia, acne vulgaris, sarcoidosis, or rosacea may simulate lupus vulgaris. Differentiation from tertiary syphilis, chronic discoid lupus erythematosus, Hansen's disease, systemic mycoses, and leishmaniasis may be more difficult, and biopsy and tissue cultures may be required.

Cutaneous tuberculosis from endogenous source by direct extension (scrofuloderma and periorificial TB)

Scrofuloderma is tuberculous involvement of the skin by direct extension from an underlying focus of infection. It occurs most frequently over the cervical lymph nodes but also may occur over bone or around joints if these are involved. Clinically, the lesions begin as subcutaneous masses, which enlarge to form nodules (Fig. 16-6). Suppuration occurs centrally. They may be erythematous or skin-colored, and usually the skin temperature is not increased over the mass. Lesions may drain, forming sinuses, or they may ulcerate with reddish granulation at the base (Fig. 16-7). Surgical procedures may incite lesions of scrofuloderma over joints or the abdominal cavity apparently by releasing the loculated focus and contaminating the track along which instruments are inserted. Scrofuloderma heals with characteristic cordlike scars, frequently allowing the diagnosis to be made many years later.

Perianal TB (tuberculosis fistulosa subcutanea) is characterized by a chronic anal fistula characteristically in men between 30 and 60 years of age. Involvement of the intestinal tract, especially the rectum, is present in most of these cases. Anal strictures and involvement of the scrotum may occur if disease is untreated.

Histologically, in scrofuloderma, the tuberculous process begins in the underlying lymph node or bone and extends through the deep dermis. Necrosis occurs with formation of a cavity filled with liquefied debris and polymorphonuclear leukocytes. At the periphery, more typical granulomatous

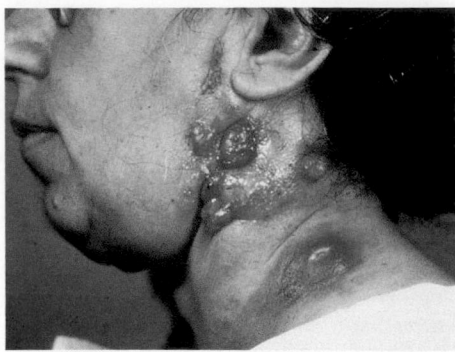

Fig. 16-6 Scrofuloderma. (Courtesy of James WD [ed]: Textbook, of Military Medicine, Office of the Surgeon General, United States Army, 1994)

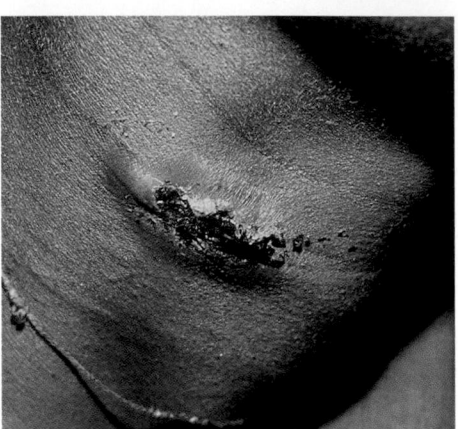

Fig. 16-7 Scrofuloderma.

inflammation is seen, along with AFB observed in slightly less than half of cases.

Scrofuloderma is to be differentiated from atypical mycobacterial infection, sporotrichosis, actinomycosis, coccidioidomycosis, and hidradenitis suppurativa. Lymphogranuloma venereum (LGV) favors the inguinal and perineal areas, and has positive serologic tests for LGV.

Tuberculosis cutis orificialis is a form of cutaneous TB that occurs at the mucocutaneous borders of the nose, mouth, anus, urinary meatus, and vagina, and on the mucous membrane of the mouth or tongue. It is caused by autoinoculation from underlying active visceral TB, particularly of the larynx, lungs, intestines, and genitourinary tract. It indicates failing resistance to the disease. Consequently, tuberculin positivity is variable but usually positive. Lesions ulcerate from the beginning and extend rapidly, with no tendency to spontaneous healing. The ulcers are usually soft and punched out, and have undermined edges.

Histologically, the ulcer base is usually composed largely of granulation tissue infiltrated with polymorphonuclear leukocytes. Deep and lateral to the ulcer, granulomatous inflammation may be found and AFB are numerous.

Cutaneous tuberculosis from hematogenous spread

Miliary (disseminated) tuberculosis

Miliary TB appears in the setting of fulminant TB of the lung or meninges. Generally, patients have other unmistakable signs of severe disseminated TB. It is most common in children but may occur in adults. Most reported instances of cutaneous TB seen in patients with AIDS are of this type. Miliary TB may also follow infectious illnesses that reduce immunity, especially measles. Because this represents uncontrolled hematogenous infection, the tuberculin test is negative. Lesions are generalized and may appear as erythematous macules or papules, pustules, subcutaneous nodules, and purpuric "vasculitic" lesions. Ulceration may occur, and the pain in the infarctive lesions may be substantial. The prognosis is guarded.

Skin biopsies show diffuse suppurative inflammation of the dermis or subcutis with predominantly polymorphonuclear leukocytes, at times forming abscesses. Caseating granulomas may be seen. AFB are abundant.

Metastatic tuberculous abscess, ulceration, or cellulitis

The hematogenous dissemination of mycobacteria from a primary focus may result in firm, nontender erythematous plaques (resembling cellulitis) or nodules. The nodules can evolve to form abscesses, ulcers, or draining sinus tracts. This form of cutaneous TB is usually seen in children, and most patients have decreased immunity from malnutrition, intercurrent infection, or an immunodeficiency state. Patients presenting with tuberculous skin ulcers may or may not have other foci of TB identified. Aerosolization of mycobacteria may occur during incision and drainage and during dressing changes, leading to secondary cases among surgical and nursing staff treating these ulcers. Histologically, abscess formation and numerous AFB are seen.

Sporotrichoid tuberculosis

While TB is usually felt to be spread either by direct extension or hematogenously, in about 3% of cases of cutaneous TB the lesions occur in a sporotrichoid pattern, suggesting lymphatic spread. Classically, this begins with a distal lesion, and new lesions appearing more proximally. Less commonly, a proximal lesion is present initially, and new lesions appear distally (retrograde lymphatic spread). The draining proximal lymph nodes may be enlarged. The individual lesions have the same morphology in any given patient, but different patients can have different morphologies. A string of lupus vulgaris-like lesions is most common. Less often, there is a string of deep nodules that may become fluctuant, drain to the surface, or ulcerate, forming linear scrofuloderma-like lesions. The draining lymph node may be enlarged (more often than in sporotrichoid atypical mycobacterial infection). The TST is positive. Underlying foci of systemic TB are often not found. Biopsy of the lesions (and affected lymph nodes) typically shows granulomatous inflammation, but AFB stains are usually negative. Culture may be positive.

This form of TB presents significant diagnostic problems, since sporotrichoid lesions would more commonly be a consequence of atypical mycobacteria or sporotrichosis. Since atypical mycobacteria, especially M. marinum, may result in a positive TST, confirming the diagnosis is difficult, even if AFB are found on biopsy. This is a clinical scenario in which the use of an IGRA to analyze the patient's immunological response specifically to M. tuberculosis, and PCR to speciate the infecting organism from the biopsy, can be very useful.

Tuberculous mastitis

Rarely, TB will present as subcutaneous nodules on the breast. The lesions can suppurate, forming abscesses, or break down, forming sinus tracts. While the condition favors women of child-bearing age, it can also affect men. Since it may closely resemble breast cancer, biopsies are frequently carried out. Abscesses may be incised and drained. The consequence of the ongoing inflammation, destroying the fat of the breast, and the surgical procedures can be a severely disfigured breast. An underlying focus of TB may at times be present in the underlying bone or at a distant site. TST is positive. Histology shows granulomatous inflammation with negative AFB stains. Culture is usually negative. This diagnosis should be considered in all patients with granulomatous mastitis from endemic areas of TB.

Tuberculids

Tuberculids are a group of skin eruptions associated with an underlying or silent focus of TB. They are diagnosed by their characteristic clinical features, histologic findings, a positive TST or IGRA, sometimes by the finding of TB at a distant site, and resolution of the eruption with antituberculous therapy. Tuberculids represent cutaneous lesions induced by hematogenous dissemination of tubercle bacilli to the skin. Lupus vulgaris may develop at the sites of tuberculids, and M. tuberculosis DNA may be found in tuberculid lesions by PCR. Tuberculids usually occur in persons with a strong immunity to TB (and thus having a positive PPD). This results in rapid destruction of the bacilli and autoinvolution of individual lesions in many cases. New lesions continue to appear, however, since hematogenous dissemination from the underlying focus continues. Tuberculids tend to be bilaterally symmetrical eruptions because they result from hematogenous dissemination.

Papulonecrotic tuberculid

Papulonecrotic tuberculid is usually an asymptomatic, chronic disorder, presenting in successive crops. Lesions are symmetrically distributed on the extensor extremities, especially on the tips of the elbows and on the knees; dorsal surfaces of the hands and feet; buttocks; face and ears; and glans penis. Lesions may favor pernio-prone sites and may be worse during winter months. Two-thirds of cases occur before the age of 30, and females are favored 3:1. Evidence of prior or active TB is found in between one-third and two-thirds of patients, especially in the lymph nodes. The TST is positive and may generate a necrotic reaction.

Typical lesions vary in size from 2 to 8 mm, and are firm, inflammatory papules that become pustular or necrotic. Lesions resolve slowly over several weeks, but occasional ulcers persist longer. Varioliform scarring follows the lesions. Crops recur over a course of months to years.

Papulonecrotic tuberculids may appear in association with other cutaneous manifestations of TB, particularly erythema induratum or scrofuloderma. Associated clinical phenomena have included tuberculous arteritis with gangrene in young adult Africans and the development of lupus vulgaris from lesions of papulonecrotic tuberculid. HIV-infected persons may develop papulonecrotic tuberculid.

Histologically, the epidermis is ulcerated in well-developed lesions. A palisaded collection of histiocytes surrounds an ovoid or wedge-shaped area of dermal necrosis. Well-formed tubercles are not seen, except in nonhealing lesions evolving into lupus vulgaris. Vascular changes are prominent, ranging from a mild lymphocytic vasculitis to fibrinoid necrosis and thrombotic occlusion of vessels. This is not a neutrophilic leukocytoclastic vasculitis, but rather a chronic granulomatous small-vessel vasculitis. Capillaries, venules, and arterioles may be involved. AFB stains are negative, but PCR may detect mycobacterial DNA in up to half of cases of papulonecrotic tuberculid.

Papulopustular secondary syphilis, pityriasis lichenoides et varioliformis acuta, Churg–Strauss granuloma, lymphomatoid papulosis, perforating granuloma annulare, perforating collagenosis, and necrotizing or septic vasculitis share clinical and histologic features with papulonecrotic tuberculid.

Lichen scrofulosorum

Also known as tuberculosis cutis lichenoides, lichen scrofulosorum consists of groups of indolent, minute, keratotic, discrete papules, scattered over the trunk. The lesions are 2–4 mm, follicular or parafollicular, and yellow–pink to reddish brown. They are firm and flat-topped, or surmounted by a tiny pustule or thin scale. The lesions are arranged in nummular or discoid groups, where they persist unchanged for months and cause no symptoms. They may slowly undergo spontaneous involution, followed at times by recurrences. Around 95% of cases of lichen scrofulosorum occur in children under the age of 20. Active TB at a distant site, usually the bones or lymph nodes, is present in about three-quarters of patients. The tuberculin test is always positive.

Histologically, lichen scrofulosorum shows noncaseating tuberculoid granulomas, situated just beneath the epidermis, between and surrounding hair follicles. Normally, tubercle bacilli are not seen in the pathologic specimens; nor can they be cultured from biopsy material.

Lichen nitidus, lichen planus, secondary syphilis, and sarcoidosis should be considered in the differential diagnosis.

Erythema induratum and vascular reactions due to tuberculosis (nodular tuberculid and nodular granulomatous phlebitis)

Erythema induratum (Bazin disease) is chronic and occurs predominantly (80%) in women of middle age. Lesions favor the posterior lower calf, which may also show acrocyanosis. Individual lesions are tender, erythematous or violaceous, 1–2 cm subcutaneous nodules (Fig. 16-8). Lesions resolve spontaneously, with or without ulceration, over several months and can heal with scarring. A clinically very similar condition called nodular granulomatous phlebitis is less common. It also affects women primarily and involves both the lower legs and thighs, usually along the course of the saphenous vein. Individual lesions evolve over weeks to months, but may recur for years in a seasonal pattern. They do not ulcerate or heal with scarring. The TST is positive. Idiopathic nodular vasculitis unassociated with TB may have identical clinical and histologic features, and this diagnosis is made when the PPD is negative.

The primary pathology occurs in the subcutaneous fat, which shows lobular panniculitis with fat necrosis. Granulomatous inflammation occurs in two-thirds of cases and is noncaseating. In addition, a granulomatous vasculitis of arterioles can be present in the fat and is the apparent cause of the fat necrosis. Biopsies of nodular granulomatous phlebitis show thrombosis of and granulomatous inflammation centered around veins in the deep dermis. AFB are not found on special stains or cultures of the biopsy. PCR may help to confirm these diagnoses; however, the positive PPD obviates the need for it. At times necrotizing vasculitis is present at the dermo-hypodermal junction. This reaction has been termed nodular tuberculid. The histology of nodular tuberculid may

be identical or very similar to polyarteritis nodosa. More rarely, small-vessel vasculitis (leukocytoclastic vasculitis) or Sweet-like lesions may be seen as a "reaction" to an underlying focus of TB.

Erythema induratum must be distinguished from erythema nodosum, nodular vasculitis, polyarteritis nodosa, tertiary syphilis, and other infectious and inflammatory panniculitides. Erythema nodosum is of relatively short duration and of rapid development, and chiefly affects the anterior rather than the posterior calves. It produces tender, painful, scarlet or contusiform nodules that appear simultaneously and do not ulcerate. Histology demonstrates a septal panniculitis. In erythema induratum the pain is less severe, and the lesions tend to evolve serially or in crops. A syphilitic gumma is usually unilateral and single, or may appear as a small, distinct group of lesions.

Diagnosis of cutaneous tuberculosis

Biopsy with acid-fast staining should be done when the history and physical examination suggest cutaneous TB. PCR testing is increasingly used to identify mycobacterial DNA in tissue specimens and other biologic samples. It may be positive when both stains and cultures are negative; however, in paucibacillary disease it is not reliably positive. Culture remains the gold standard and provides the means to determine antibiotic sensitivity and response to treatment.

Treatment

HIV testing is recommended for all patients diagnosed with TB, because they may require longer courses of therapy. In addition, every effort should be made to culture the organism for sensitivity testing, since MDR-TB is common in some communities. For all forms of cutaneous TB, multidrug chemotherapy is recommended. The recommendations of the local health clinics that manage other forms of TB should be followed. Three- or four-drug regimens are usually recommended for initial empiric treatment. Directly observed therapy is a strategy designed to ensure cure. Priority patients are those with prior treatment failure, pulmonary TB with a positive smear, HIV co-infection, current or prior drug use, drug-resistant disease, psychiatric illness, memory impairment, or prior nonadherence. Surgical excision is useful for the treatment of isolated lesions of lupus vulgaris and tuberculosis verrucosa cutis, and surgical intervention also may benefit some cases of scrofuloderma. Since in many cases of cutaneous TB, the organism has not been identified by either histology or culture, treatment is inherently empiric. Virtually all forms of cutaneous TB will have begun to respond to treatment by 6 weeks. Failure to respond within this timeframe should result in reconsideration of the diagnosis, assessment for compliance, and concern about drug resistance.

Almagro M, et al: Metastatic tuberculosis abscesses in an immunocompetent patient. Clin Exp Dermatol 2005; 30:247.

American Thoracic Society, CDC, and Infectious Diseases Society of America: Treatment of tuberculosis. MMWR 2003; 52:RR11.

Atasoy M, et al: Scrofuloderma following BCG vaccination. Ped Dermatol 2005; 22:179.

Bravo F, Eduardo G: Cutaneous tuberculosis. Clin Dermatol 2007; 25:173.

Caksen H, et al: Multiple metastatic tuberculous abscesses in a severely malnourished infant. Pediatr Dermatol 2002; 19:90

Casalini C, et al: Nodular lesion of the skin as primary cutaneous tuberculosis. J Travel Med 2003; 10:306.

Chee C, et al: Comparison of sensitivities of two commercial gamma interferon release assays for pulmonary tuberculosis. J Clin Microbiol 2008; 46:1935.

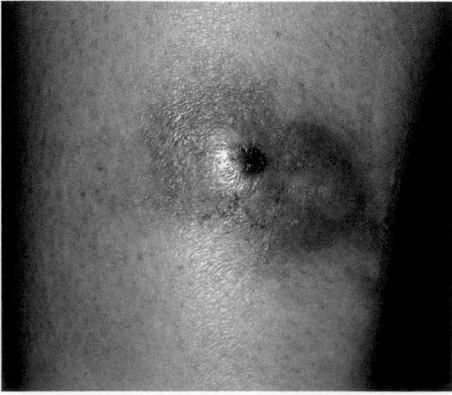

Fig. 16-8 Erythema induratum. (Courtesy of Curt Samlaska, MD)

Chintamani, et al: Port site tuberculosis following laparoscopic cholecystectomy. Trop Doctor 2005; 35:47.

Del Giudice P, et al: Unusual cutaneous manifestations of miliary tuberculosis. Clin Infect Dis 2000; 30:201.

Doherty S, et al: National psoriasis foundation consensus statement on screening for latent tuberculosis infection in patients with psoriasis treated with systemic and biologic agents. J Am Acad Dermatol 2008; 59:209.

Fernandez C, et al: Papulonecrotic tuberculid in a human immunodeficiency virus type-1 patient with multidrug-resistant tuberculosis. J Eur Acad Dermatol Venereol 2004; 18:369.

Foo C, Tan HH: A case of tuberculosis verrucosa cutis: undiagnosed for 44 years and resulting in fixed-flexion deformity of the arm. Clin Exp Dermatol 2005; 30:149.

Friedman PC, et al: Nodular tuberculid in a patient with HIV. J Am Acad Dermatol 2005; 53:S154.

Gandhi V, et al: Lichen scrofulosorum on the genitals: an unusual presentation. Int J Dermatol 2007; 46:548.

Ghorpade A: Lupus vulgaris over a tattoo mark: inoculation tuberculosis. J Eur Acad Dermatol Venereol 2003; 17:569.

Goktay F, et al: Detection of *Myobacterium tuberculosis* complex by line probe assay in a case with sporotrichoid skin lesions. Eur Dermatol Venereol 2007; 21:822.

Grabczysnka RC, Wilkinson JD: Nodular vasculitis: an indicator for ELISpot screening for tuberculosis. Clin Exp Dermatol 2007; 32:761.

Hamada M, et al: Epidemiology of cutaneous tuberculosis in Japan: a retrospective study from 1906 to 2002. Int J Dermatol 2004; 43:727.

High WA, et al: Cutaneous miliary tuberculosis in two patients with HIV infection. J Am Acad Dermatol 2004; 50:S110.

Ho CK, et al: Cutaneous tuberculosis in Hong Kong: an update. Hong Kong Med J 2006; 12:272.

Huang LH, et al: Disseminated cutaneous bacille Calmette–Guérin infection identified by polymerase chain reaction in a patient with X-linked severe combined immunodeficiency. Ped Dermatol 2006; 23:560.

Inoue T, et al: Erythema induratum of Bazin in an infant after bacille Calmette–Guérin vaccination. J Dermatol 2006; 33:268.

Jordaan HF, et al: Nodular tuberculid: a report of four patients. Ped Dermatol 2000; 17:183.

Kaur S, et al: Recalcitrant scrofuloderma due to rib tuberculosis. Ped Dermatol 2003; 20:309.

Kavala M, et al: Granulomatous cheilitis resulting from a tuberculide. Int J Dermatol 2004; 43:524.

Khan K, et al: Tuberculosis infection in the United States: national trends over three decades. Am J Respir Crit Care Med 2008; 177:455.

Khandpur S, Reddy BSN: Lupus vulgaris: unusual presentation over the face. J Eur Acad Dermatol Venereol 2003; 17:706.

Kumar B, et al: Childhood cutaneous tuberculosis. Int J Dermatol 2001; 40:26.

Lalvani A, Millington KA: Screening for tuberculosis infection prior to initiation of anti-TNF therapy. Autoimmun Rev 2008; 8:147.

Lee NH, et al: Tuberculous cellulitis. Clin Exp Dermatol 2000; 25:222.

Leon-Mateo A, et al: Perianal ulceration: a case of tuberculosis cutis orificialis. J Eur Acad Dermatol Venereol 2005; 19:364.

Lin CY, et al: Perianal tuberculosis during neutropenia: a rare case report and review of literature. Ann Hematol 2006; 85:547.

Makkar VR, et al: Lupus vulgaris postexanthematicus: a rare variant of lupus vulgaris with sarcoid-like histopathology. Clin Exp Dermatol 2005; 30:187.

McHugh A, et al: Nodular granulomatous phlebitis: a phlebitic tuberculid. Austral J Dermatol 2008; 49:220.

Menzies D, et al: Meta-analysis: new tests for the diagnosis of latent tuberculosis infection: areas of uncertainty and recommendation for research. Ann Intern Med 2007; 146:340.

Mitsuishi T, et al: Papulonecrotic tuberculid with spontaneous remission. J Dermatol 2006; 2:112.

Motswaledi HM, et al: Superficial thrombophlebitic tuberculide. Int J Dermatol 2006: 45:1337.

Motswaledi MH, Doman C: Lupus vulgaris with squamous cell carcinoma. J Cutan Pathol 2007; 34:939.

Muto J, et al: Papular tuberculides post-BCG vaccination: case report and review of the literature in Japan. Clin Exp Dermatol 2006; 31:611.

Ozkaya-Bayazit E, et al: Earlobe dermatitis. Arch Dermatol 2002; 138:1607.

Rai VM, et al: Tuberculous gluteal abscess coexisting with scrofuloderma and tubercular lymphadenitis. Dermatol Online J 2005; 11:14.

Rajagopala S, Agarwal R: Tuberculosis mastitis in men: case report and systematic review. Am J Med 2008; 121:539.

Ram R, et al: Isolated skin ulcers due to *Mycobacterium tuberculosis* in a renal allograft recipient. Nature Clin Prac Nephrol 2007; 3:688.

Raman M, et al: How soon does cutaneous tuberculosis respond to treatment? Int J Dermatol 2007; 73:243

Ramesh V, et al: A study of cutaneous tuberculosis in children. Pediatr Dermatol 1999; 16:264.

Ramesh V: Sporotrichoid cutaneous tuberculosis. Clin Exp Dermatol 2007; 32:680.

Safdar N, et al: An unintended consequence. N Engl J Med 2008; 358:1496.

Samuel A, et al: Bacillus Calmette–Guérin vaccine-induced lupus vulgaris in a child adopted from China. Ped Dermatol 2007; 24:E55.

Schoepfer AM, et al: Comparison of interferon gamma release assay versus tuberculin skin test for tuberculosis screening in inflammatory bowel disease. Am J Gastroenterol 2008; 103:1.

Singal A, et al: Lichen scrofulosorum: a prospective study of 39 patients. Int J Dermatol 2005; 44:489.

Singal A, et al: Multifocal scrofuloderma with disseminated tuberculosis in a severely malnourished child. Ped Dermatol 2005; 22:440.

Srivastava N, et al: Papulonecrotic tuberculid of the glans: worm-eaten appearance. Int J Dermatol 2007; 46:1324.

Torrelo A, et al: Lichen scrofulosorum. Pediatr Dermatol 2000; 17:373.

Umapathy KC, et al: Comprehensive findings on clinical, bacteriological, histopathological and therapeutic aspects of cutaneous tuberculosis. Trop Med Intl Health 2006; 11:1521.

Vashisht P, et al: Cutaneous tuberculosis in children and adolescents: a clinicohistological study. J Eur Acad Dermatol Venereol 2006; 21:40.

Welsh O, et al: Cutaneous tuberculosis confirmed by PCR in three patients with biopsy and culture negative for *Mycobacterium tuberculosis*. Int J Dermatol 2007; 46:734.

Williams C, et al: Turkey ear: a diagnosis or a physical sign? Br J Dermatol 2007; 157:816.

Winje BA, et al: Screening for tuberculosis infection among newly arrived asylum seekers: comparison of quantiFERON TB gold with tuberculin skin test. BioMed Infec Dis 2008; 8:65.

Wong HW, et al: Papular eruption on a tattoo: a case of primary inoculation tuberculosis. Aus J Dermatol 2005; 46:84.

Atypical mycobacteriosis

Many facultative pathogens and saprophytes, which are acid-fast mycobacteria but do not cause TB or Hansen's disease, are grouped under the designation "atypical" mycobacteria. They exist in a wide variety of natural sources, such as soil, water, and animals; most human disease is acquired from the environment. The number of cases of human infection with these organisms is increasing, or increasingly recognized. This is due to improved culture and identification techniques, and the increasingly large immunocompromised population.

Classification of mycobacteria

The old classification scheme based on identifying these organisms in the laboratory was:

- Group I: photochromogens (*Mycobacterium marinum*)
- Group II: scotochromogens
- Group III: nonchromogens (*M. avium intracellulare*, *Mycobacterium haemophilum*)
- Group IV: rapid growers.

M. marinum, *Mycobacterium ulcerans*, and *M. haemophilum* are now recognized as common pathogens in certain settings and geographic locations. Rapidly growing mycobacteria (RGM) of the *Mycobacterium fortuitum*, *chelonae*, and *abscessus* group are usually associated with previous surgery, injection, or trauma.

The number of new species of non-tuberculous mycobacteria has been growing dramatically, with now at least 90 known species. Many of these organisms do not cause infection and are simply commensals or saprophytes. They are found in water and soil, and their identification after contamination of clinical specimens has at times been responsible for pseudo-outbreaks of infection.

The clinical care of the patient with atypical mycobacterial infection depends on culturing and identifying the responsible agent from tissue specimens. The laboratory should be familiar with the special media, necessary incubation times and temperature, and identification characteristics of these organisms. Even with modern techniques, recovery of these organisms from infections is not universal. Granuloma formation may not occur in histological sections, and AFB stains may be negative. For this reason, if atypical mycobacterial infection is suspected, a biopsy should be carried out, part of which should be cultured at high and low temperatures and on special media, AFB stains of the tissue should be performed, and in selected cases PCR for specific species from fresh tissue or the paraffin fixed material should be considered. At times, a clinical diagnosis must be made and empiric therapy given.

Swimming pool granuloma (aquarium granuloma)

M. marinum is found in fresh and salt water, and can infect fish, often killing home aquarium fish. It grows optimally at 30°C. The vast majority of infections in the US and Europe are now associated with home aquariums. Fishermen, fish sellers, and persons involved in aquaculture are also at risk. Skin lesions favor males (60%). History of an injury preceding or simultaneous with exposure to contaminated water is usually present. Exposure can be indirect, such as contact with a bucket used to empty an aquarium. An indolent lesion usually starts about 3 weeks after exposure as a small papule or nodule located on the hands, knees, elbows, or feet (Fig. 16-9). It often has a keratotic or warty surface. A sporotrichoid pattern with a succession of nodules ascending the arm is common. Less commonly, ulcers and abscesses may be the presentation,

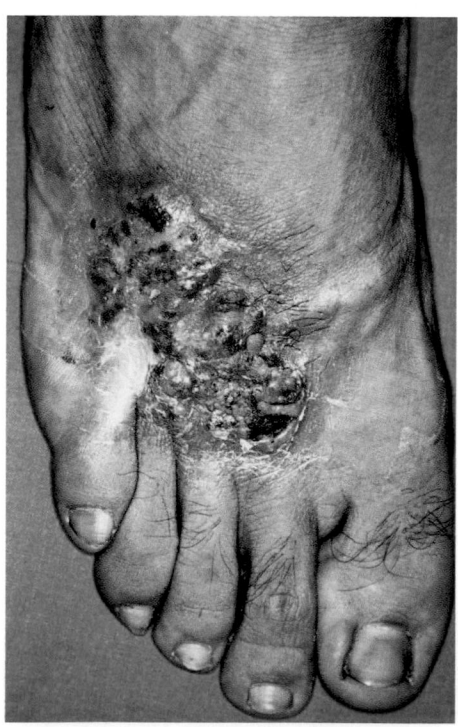

Fig. 16-9 Swimming pool granuloma.

especially in immunosuppressed hosts. Tenosynovitis, bursitis, arthritis, and even osteitis are the most frequent forms of deep structure involvement, with involvement of the tendon sheaths of the dorsal hands and less commonly the palms. This may limit range of motion and result in significant thickening and induration. Such cases may require surgical, as well as medical, management. The natural history is for slow progression, and lesions may be relatively indolent for years. Spontaneous resolution may occur in 10–20% of patients with skin lesions only after a period of many months. Immunosuppressed patients may develop widely disseminated lesions that are progressive.

Histopathologically, there is a suppurative and granulomatous reaction with overlying hyperkeratosis and acanthosis. Acid-fast organisms are found in only about 20% of cases. Tissue culture will be positive in about three-quarters of cases. The TST to *M. tuberculosis* usually becomes positive in those who have had *M. marinum* infection.

Treatment of the patient is determined by the extent of the infection and the immune status of the patient. Optimal treatment has not yet been established, and favorable outcome cannot be related to any specific antibiotic or antibiotic combination. Failure of every antibiotic used has been documented. Single-agent therapy is acceptable for immunocompetent patients with infections limited to skin and soft tissue only. Minocycline, 100 mg twice a day, seems to be the single best agent, with doxycycline, 100 mg twice a day, or clarithromycin, 500 mg twice a day, as alternatives. Some patients have failed on doxycycline but responded to minocycline. Combination treatment with minocycline plus clarithromycin, or rifampin, rifabutin, or amikacin added to minocycline and/or clarithromycin seems appropriate based on in vitro sensitivities of numerous isolates. Ethambutol and the quinolones have poor minimum inhibitory concentrations and their use is associated with treatment failure. The sensitivities of the organism isolated can be used in cases failing initial empiric treatment. Immunosuppressed hosts and persons with involvement of deep structures should receive combination treatment. For localized lesions in the immunocompetent host, treatment is recommended for at least 1–2 months after resolution of lesions, which is usually 3–4 months in total. More than 90% of such patients will be cured. Only about 75% of patients with deep structure infections will be cured with antibiotics, with or without supplemental surgery. In this situation treatment is often prolonged—many months to years. Photodynamic therapy has been effectively used in one case with a single lesion of the finger.

Buruli ulcer

Buruli ulcer is also known as Bairnsdale ulcer and Searl ulcer. This is the third most common type of mycobacterial skin infection in immunocompetent people. In Africa 75% of cases occur in children, and the elderly are disproportionately affected. In endemic areas in Australia, the elderly are seven times more likely to be infected. Lesions favor the extremities. The lesion begins as a solitary, hard, painless, subcutaneous nodule called the "preulcerative" stage. There can be significant local edema at this point. If untreated, some, but not all lesions ulcerate and expand by undermining the surrounding skin (Fig. 16-10). They may become very large, exposing muscle and tendon over a large portion of an affected extremity. Despite their appearance, the lesions are remarkably painless. Persons with hemoglobin SS or SC are as much as five times more likely to develop osteomyelitis from *M. ulcerans*. Histologically, there is extensive coagulative necrosis, little cellular infiltrate, and numerous clumps of AFB in the center of the area of necrosis.

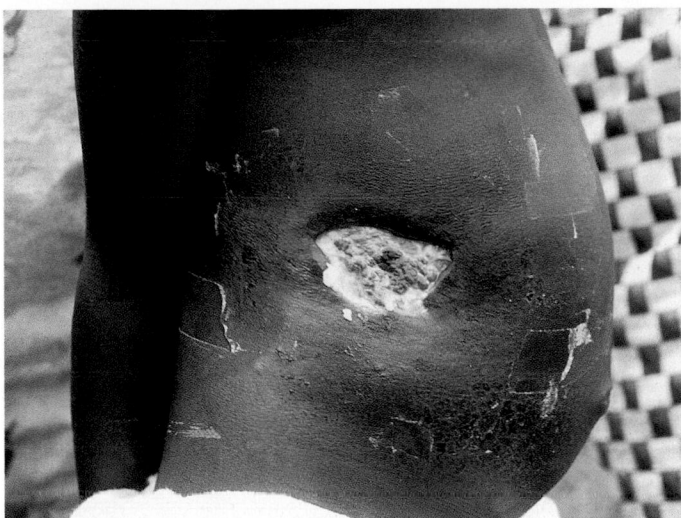

Fig. 16-10 Buruli ulcer.

M. ulcerans is the cause of Buruli ulcer. This organism occurs in Australia, numerous African nations (especially in West Africa), Asia, French Guyana, Peru, Suriname, Mexico, and Brazil.

The pathogenesis of this infection is now well worked out. *M. ulcerans* produces a toxin, mycolactone, responsible for the extensive necrosis and ulceration seen in these infections. In addition to having cellular toxicity, mycolactone is also locally immunosuppressive. Tissue necrosis creates a microaerophilic environment that favors the growth of *M. ulcerans*. Strains of *M. ulcerans* lacking mycolactone are not capable of producing disease. This toxin is also critical in maintaining the life cycle of the organism, as noted below.

M. ulcerans grows under a biofilm on aquatic plants. Snails and other water animals eat the contaminated plants, and carnivorous insects eat the plant-consuming molluscs. *M. ulcerans* moves from the gut of the carnivorous insects to their salivary glands. Only *M. ulcerans* spp producing mycolactone are capable of establishing a reservoir in the insect salivary gland. *M. ulcerans* is found in no other tissue in the biting insects, and produces no biofilm in the insect salivary gland. When these insects bite a human, they inoculate the mycobacteria into the host and begin the infection. Infection in the human is again associated with the production of the biofilm, which makes treatment difficult. This explains the association between infection and exposure to water, especially swampy water. Interestingly, being repeatedly bitten by these carnivorous insects results in the production of antibodies against the insect salivary contents. This "allergy" to the insect saliva is protective against *M. ulcerans* infection, explaining why persons working chronically in swampy water are at lower risk for infection than those visiting the area, and perhaps why children and the elderly are at greater risk for infection due to reduced production of these antibodies. In Australia, mosquito bites are associated with the development of *M. ulcerans* infection, and the bacteria can be isolated from trapped insects in areas of *M. ulcerans* epidemics. Whether the mosquitoes carry the infection by the same mechanism as the carnivorous water insects is unknown.

The diagnosis is often made clinically in areas of endemicity. AFB smears of the edge of ulcerative lesions or of aspirates from the center of preulcerative lesions, culture of the lesion, PCR, and histological examination are all available techniques to confirm the diagnosis. AFB stains are positive in up to 80% of lesions. Culture has a similar positivity rate. PCR may be slightly less sensitive. When AFB smears, culture, and PCR are all done on the same lesion, one test is positive in 94% of cases, two are positive in 83% of cases, and only 50% of cases yielded positive results by all three methods. Around 7% of cases will be negative with all three tests. In developed countries, excisional biopsies with AFB staining can be used, and will be positive in about 60% of cases. Preulcerative lesions give the highest culture results, since ulcerative lesions contain fewer organisms and are contaminated. AFB smears and PCR have similar sensitivity in preulcerative and ulcerative lesions. The organism is very stable in transport and has been cultured up to 26 weeks after sample collection if transported to the laboratory appropriately.

Treatment includes systemic antibiotics and surgery. Daily observed treatment for 8 weeks with streptomycin, 15 mg/kg intramuscularly, and rifampin, 10 mg/kg orally, is dramatically effective. The overall efficacy of this treatment regimen was 73% of patients, and 96% in lesions less than 10 cm in diameter (early lesions) without surgery. Healing is slow, with half of lesions healing by 24 weeks (with only 8 weeks of antibiotic treatment), and some requiring more than 9 months to heal. Clarithromycin, 7.5 mg/kg orally once daily, may be substituted for the last 4 weeks of streptomycin therapy with virtually equal efficacy. In larger lesions (over 15 cm) and in lesions failing antibiotic treatment alone, surgical excision with delayed grafting is the standard treatment offered. In a large series of more than 200 patients, all patients who completed the full course of antibiotics with or without surgery were cured—a success rate of 100% by 3 months after the antibiotics were completed. At 1-year follow-up, only 1.4% of patients had recurrences.

Severe scarring can occur as a consequence of untreated and large lesions, resulting in contracture deformities or amputations. If the periocular tissues are affected, enucleation of the eye may be required. Multiple metastatic skin lesions can occur. Bone lesions are uncommon and in three-quarters of the patients occur at a site distant from the primary Buruli ulcer. Rarely, death may result.

Other atypical mycobacterial infections

Mycobacterium haemophilum

M. haemophilum most commonly infects immunosuppressed patients with AIDS, organ transplants, or leukemia and lymphoma. The reservoir for the organism is unknown but felt to be water. Because *M. haemophilum* grows preferentially at 30–32°C, skin lesions, often at acral sites, predominate. Papules, plaques (at times cellulitis-like), and dermal or subcutaneous nodules are the primary lesions. These initial lesions break down in many cases, forming painful, draining ulcers. Septic arthritis, osteomyelitis, and pulmonary nodules may occur. *M. haemophilum* has specific growth requirements, and so isolation is not possible using routine laboratory culture techniques. If *M. haemophilum* infection is suspected, the laboratory should be notified in order that it can prepare the special media necessary to isolate it. *M. haemophilum* is sensitive to ciprofloxacin, clarithromycin, amikacin, rifampin, and rifabutin. It is resistant to ethambutol, isoniazid, and pyrazinamide. Treatment is for 1 year.

Rapid-growing mycobacterium

The organisms of the *M. fortuitum* group and *M. chelonae/abscessus* group usually cause subcutaneous abscesses or cellulitis. These organisms are frequently resistant to standard antituberculosis medications. Infections commonly occur after trauma in immunocompetent patients. Infections may follow a variety of cosmetic surgery procedures, skin

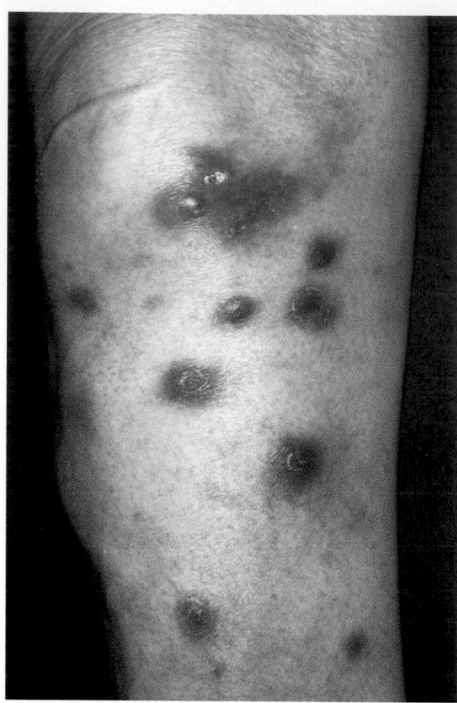

Fig. 16-11 Disseminated *Mycobacterium chelonae* infection.

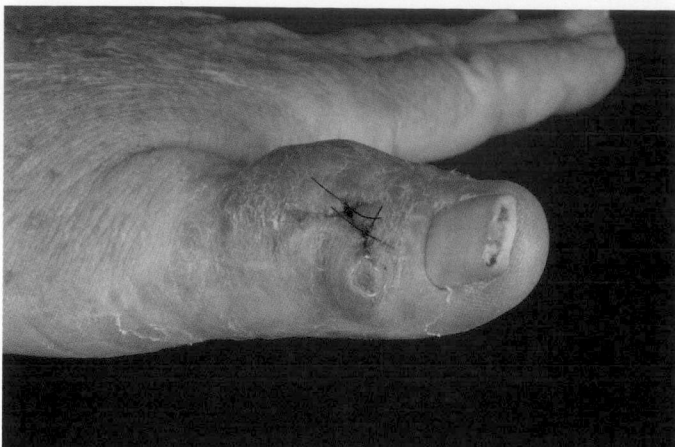

Fig. 16-12 *Mycobacterium avium–intracellulare* primary inoculation in a healthy woman.

piercings, catheterizations, or injections. Outbreaks of leg abscesses caused by *M. fortuitum* have been acquired in nail salon whirlpool foot baths. Most cases are restricted to the skin and start as small erythematous papules, many of which spontaneously heal. Others progress to large, fluctuant abscesses, which are quite painful and can ulcerate. Sporotrichoid or disseminated disease may occur in immunocompromised patients (Fig. 16-11), but proximal adenopathy is rarely found. Shaving of the legs prior to visiting the nail salon appears to be a risk factor for acquiring infection. In renal transplant cases, tender, nodular lesions of the legs are most common. Deep extension into bone underlying a chronic ulcer can occur. Since these infections on the skin are indolent and the organisms grow rapidly, waiting for susceptibilities can be considered. Treatment is determined by extent of disease and immune status of the patient. For *M. chelonae/abscessus* infections, clarithromycin, 500 mg twice a day for 6 or more months, is effective and well tolerated in many patients with disseminated cutaneous infection. Monotherapy may allow resistance to occur, but this rarely happens in immunocompetent patients with simple skin infections. In severe cases and in the setting of immunosuppression, combination treatment can be considered. Tobramycin, amikacin, linezolid, clarithromycin, and tigecycline have the highest percentage of susceptible isolates of *M. chelonae/abscessus*. The optimal regimen for treatment of *M. fortuitum* has not been defined, and combination treatment is often recommended. Amikacin plus cefoxitin or imipenem or a quinolone can be recommended for initial therapy. If only oral agents are to be used for skin-limited disease, clarithromycin, 500 mg twice daily, doxycycline, 100 mg twice daily, trimethoprim–sulfamethoxazole, 1 DS twice daily, or levofloxacin, 500–750 mg once daily, are acceptable agents. Surgical excision, debridement, and drainage may reduce duration of therapy.

Mycobacterium avium–intracellulare complex

This was an uncommon cause of skin infection before the AIDS epidemic. In patients with AIDS who develop disseminated *M. avium–intracellulare* complex infections, the skin may be involved by hematogenous dissemination and may present as nodules, ulcers, or pustules, or have a cellulitis-like appear-

ance. Immunocompromised children with chronic pulmonary infections are also at risk. Only occasional reports of immunocompetent patients with inoculation-type lesions have been reported (Fig. 16-12). Therapy for disseminated infection is undertaken with at least three agents, most commonly clarithromycin or azithromycin, ethambutol, and rifabutin. Adequate antiretroviral therapy should be assured in HIV-infected persons.

Mycobacterium kansasii

M. kansasii very rarely causes skin infection, usually following minor trauma. Three-quarters of cases occur in the setting of immunosuppression. Lesions can be papules, nodules, pustules, cellulitis, or sporotrichoid. Treatment is not standardized, but initial treatment with isoniazid, rifampin, and ethambutol until 12 months after clearing has been proposed. Azithromycin or clarithromycin can be added if necessary. However, individual cases have responded to single-agent therapy with minocycline or erythromycin. Surgical removal can be beneficial if practical. In immunosuppressed hosts, cutaneous lesions can occur via hematogenous dissemination, and a visceral source, especially pulmonary, should be sought.

Aubry A, et al: Sixty-three cases of *Mycobacterium marinum* infection. Arch Intern Med 2002; 162:1746.

Bartralot R, et al: Clinical patterns of cutaneous nontuberculous mycobacterial infections. Br J Dermatol 2005; 152:727.

Breathnach A, et al: Cutaneous *Mycobacterium kansasii* infection. Clin Infect Dis 1995; 20:812.

Brown-Elliott BA, et al: Newly described or emerging human species of nontuberculous mycobacteria. Infect Dis Clin North Am 2002; 16:187.

Chauty A, et al: Promising clinical efficacy of streptomycin–rifampin combination for treatment of Buruli ulcer (*Myobacterium ulcerans* disease). Antimicrob Agents and Chemothe 2007; 51:4029

Chaves A, et al: Primary cutaneous *Mycobacterium kansasii* infection in a child. Pediatr Dermatol 2001; 18:131.

Cummins D, et al: *Mycobacterium marinum* with different responses to second-generation tetracyclines. Int Journal of Derm 2005; 44:518.

Czelusta A, et al: Cutaneous *Mycobacerium kansasii* infection in a patient with systemic lupus erythematosus. J Am Acad Dermatol 1999; 40:359.

Dodiuk-Gad R, et al: Nontuberculous *Myobacterium* infections of the skin, a retrospective study of 25 cases. J Am Acad Dermatol 2007; 57:413.

Doedens R, et al: Transmission of *Mycobacterium marinum* from fish to a very young child. Pediatr Infec Dis J 2008; 27:81.

Fox LP, et al: *Mycobacterium abscessus* cellulitis and multifocal abscesses of the breasts in a transsexual from illicit intramammary injections of silicone. J Am Acad Dermatol 2004; 50:450.

Fujita N, et al: Levofloxacin alone efficiently treated a cutaneous *Mycobacterium fortuitum* infection. J Dermatol 2002; 29:452.

Ho MH, et al: A typical mycobacterial cutaneous infections in Hong Kong: 10-year retrospective study. Med J 2006; 12:21

Johnson PDR, et al: *Mycobacterium ulcerans* in mosquitoes captured during outbreak of Buruli ulcer, Southeastern Australia. Emerg Inf Dis 2007; 12:1653.

Kayal JD, et al: Sporotrichoid cutaneous *Mycobacterium avium* complex infection. J Am Acad Dermatol 2002; 47:S249.

Liao CH, et al: Skin and soft tissue infection caused by non-tuberculous mycobacteria. Intl J Tuberc Lung Dis 2007; 11:96.

Lin, JH, et al: Disseminated cutaneous *Mycobacterium haemophilum* infection with severe hypercalcaemia in a failed renal transplant recipient. Br J Dermatol 2003; 149:200.

Marsollier L, et al: Impact of *Mycobacterium ulcerans* biofilm on transmissibility to ecological niches and Buruli ulcer pathogenesis. PLoS Pathogens 2007; 3:0582.

Marsollier L, et al: Protection against *Mycobacterium ulcerans* lesion development by exposure to aquatic insect saliva. PLoS Med 2007; 4:0288.

Nackers F, et al: Association between haemoglobin variant S and C and *Mycobacterium ulcerans* disease (Buruli ulcer): a case-control study in Benin. Trop Med Int Health 2007; 12:511.

Nienhuis WA, et al: Antimicrobial treatment for early, limited *Mycobacterium ulcerans* infections. Lancet 2010; 375:664.

Paech V, et al: Remission of cutaneous *Mycobacterium haemophilum* infection as a result of antiretroviral therapy in an HIV-infected patient. Clin Infect Dis 2002; 34:1017.

Pang HN, et al: *Mycobacterium marinum* as a cause of chronic granulomatous tenosynovitis in the hand. J Infec 2007; 54:584.

Petrini B: *Mycobacterium abscessus:* an emerging rapid-growing potential pathogen. APMIS 2006; 114:319.

Quainoo ME, et al: Diagnosis of *Mycobacterium ulcerans* infection (Buruli ulcer) at a treatment centre in Ghana: a retrospective analysis of laboratory results of clinically diagnosed cases. Trop Med and Int Health 2008; 13:191.

Quek TYJ, et al: Risk of factors for *Mycobacterium ulcerans* infection, Southeastern Australia. Emerging Infec 2007; 13:1161.

Redbord KP, et al: Atypical *Mycobacterium* furunculosis occurring after pedicures. Am Acad Dermatolo 2005; 54:520.

Santin M, et al: *Mycobacterium kansasii* disease among patients infected with HIV type 1. Int J Tuberc Lung Dis 2003; 7:673.

Sniezek PJ, et al: Rapidly growing mycobacterial infections after pedicures. Arch Dermatol 2003; 139:629.

Streit M, et al: Disseminated *Mycobacterium marinum* infection with extensive cutaneous eruption and bacteremia in an immunocompromised patient. Eur J Dermatol 2006; 16:79.

Ucko M, Colorni A: *Myobacterium marimum* infection in fish and humans in Israel. J Clin Microbio 2005; 43:892.

Walsh D, et al: Buruli ulcer (*Myobacterium ulcerans* infection). Trans R Soc Trop Med Hyg 2008; 102:969.

Wiegell S, et al: *Myobacterium marinum* infection cured by photodynamic therapy. Am Med Assoc 2006; 142:1241.

Winthrop KL, et al: The clinical management and outcome of nail salon-acquired *Mycobacterium fortuitum* skin infection. Clin Infect Dis 2004; 38:38.

Bonus images for this chapter can be found online at
http://www.expertconsult.com

Fig. 16-1 Sporotrichoid atypical mycobacteriosis.

Fig. 16-2 Disseminated *Mycobacterium marinum* infection in systemic lupus erythematosus. (Courtesy of Curt Samlaska, MD)

Fig. 16-3 *Mycobacterium fortuitum* infection.

Fig. 16-4 *Mycobacterium avium-intracellulare* complex ulceration.

17 Hansen's Disease

Epidemiology

The World Health Organization (WHO) has committed itself to eliminating Hansen's disease as a public health problem. Elimination (not eradication) is considered as a prevalence of less than 1 case in 10 000 persons in any country. This target was globally met in 2000. The number of new cases of Hansen's disease declined from more than 750 000 in 2001 to 250 000 in 2007. As of 2008, three countries have yet to meet this elimination goal: Brazil, Nepal, and Timor-Leste. Hansen's disease is endemic in certain regions, with 95% of cases for the last two decades reported from 17 countries. Brazil, India, and Indonesia account for 76% of all cases worldwide Although 90% of cases diagnosed in the US are imported, Hansen's disease is endemic in the coastal southeastern US and in Hawaii. In the southeastern US cases may be related to exposure to armadillos, a natural host for the infectious agent.

It is believed that more than 90% of persons exposed to *Mycobacterium leprae* are able to resist infection. In endemic areas, 1.7–31% of the population is seropositive for antibodies to leprosy-specific antigens, suggesting widespread exposure to the bacillus. Around 17% of household contacts of multibacillary patients have *M. leprae* which is detectable by polymerase chain reaction (PCR) on skin swabs and 4% in nasal swabs. This clears after the multibacillary patient has been treated with multidrug therapy (MDT) for 2 months. Thus, it appears that while many persons can be transiently infected, they are able to resist overt clinical infection.

There appears to be a genetic basis for susceptibility to acquire Hansen's disease. Monozygotic twins have concordant disease in 60–85% of cases, and dizygotic twins in only 15–25%. Numerous genes have been identified as possibly conferring susceptibility to infection with *M. leprae*. Different genes have been identified in different populations, suggesting there may be multiple genetic causes of susceptibility to infection with *M. leprae*. Tight genetic linkage with the PARK2/PACRG regulatory region, HLA-DRB1, and lymphotoxin A (LTA+80) has been detected. *PARK2* is a gene involved in the development of Parkinson's disease, and LTA+80 is a low-production lymphotoxin A allele associated with malaria parasitemia.

In adults, cases in men outnumber those in women 1.5:1. Although Hansen's disease occurs at all ages, most cases appearing or acquired in endemic areas present before the age of 35. Patients exposed to armadillos present on average at age 50. The latency period between exposure and overt signs of disease is usually 5 years for paucibacillary cases, and an average of 10 years in multibacillary cases. Infected women are likely to present during or immediately after pregnancy.

The mode of transmission remains controversial. Except for cases associated with armadillo exposure, other cases of Hansen's disease are felt to be the only possible source of infection. Rarely, tatooing or other penetrating injury to the skin can be the route of infection. Multibacillary cases are much more infectious than paucibacillary cases, so the nature of the source case is the most important factor in transmission. Contact is associated with acquiring infection. Household contacts represent 28% of new Hansen's disease patients; they are at 8–10 times greater risk of acquiring disease if the household contact has lepromatous disease, as opposed to only 2–4 times if the contact has tuberculoid leprosy. In 80% of all new cases of Hansen's disease, there is a clear history of social contact with an untreated case of Hansen's disease. By PCR *M. leprae* can be detected on the intact skin by saline washings in up to 90% of multibacillary cases with a high bacterial load (bacterial index [BI] of over 3). Up to 70% of nasal swabs are similarly positive. While the swabs from the patients remain positive after 3 months of MDT, the household contacts swabs become negative, suggesting that the bacilli seen in patients are nonviable and that the risk of transmission is substantially reduced after the index patient is treated. Unfortunately, it may be possible that persons are infectious from their skin or nasal secretions with no clinical evidence of Hansen's disease (multibacillary patients who are not yet symptomatic and without identifiable skin lesions). This may make strategies relying on treatment of contacts of known Hansen's disease ineffective in eradicating the disease. In non-endemic areas transmission to contacts is very rare, a reassuring fact for the families of patients diagnosed in areas where Hansen's disease is uncommon. The last case of secondary transmission of Hansen's disease in the UK was in 1923!

The infectious agent

All cases of human and animal leprosy are caused by the same organism, *M. leprae*. This is a weakly acid-fast organism that has not been successfully cultured in vitro. It grows best at temperatures (30°C) below the core body temperature of humans. This explains the localization of Hansen's disease lesions to cooler areas of the body and the sparing of the midline and scalp. The organism may be cultivated in mouse footpads and most effectively in armadillos, whose lower body temperature is more optimal for growth of *M. leprae*. Phenolic glycolipid-1 (PGL-1) is a surface glycolipid unique to the leprosy bacillus. In infected tissues, the leprosy bacillus favors intracellular locations, within macrophages and nerves. The genome of the leprosy bacillus has been sequenced and compared to its close relative, the tuberculous bacillus. The genome of *M. leprae* contains only 50% functional genes, apparently the result of significant reductive evolution. Like other intracellular parasites, and in the absence of the ability to share DNA with other bacteria, *M. leprae* has lost many nonessential genes, including those involved in energy metabolism, making it dependent on the intracellular environment for essential nutrients. This may explain the extremely long generation time, 12–14 days, and the inability to culture *M. leprae* in vitro. All *M. leprae* isolates are very homogenous genetically and can be divided into only four genetic variants. These genetic variations are not correlated with virulence.

Diagnosis

A diagnosis of Hansen's disease must be considered in any patient with neurologic and cutaneous lesions. The diagnosis is frequently delayed in the developed world; clinicians do not readily think of Hansen's disease, since they may not have seen it before. In the US, this diagnostic delay averages 1½–2 years. In the UK, in over 80% of cases of Hansen's disease, the correct diagnosis was not suspected during the initial medical evaluations.

Hansen's disease is diagnosed, as with other infectious diseases, by identifying the infectious organism in affected tissue. Because the organism cannot be cultured, this may be very difficult. Skin biopsies from skin or nerve lesions, stained for the bacillus with Fite-Faraco stain, are usually performed in the developed world. In some Hansen's disease clinics, and in the developing world where disease is endemic, organisms are identified in slit smears of the skin. Smears are very specific, but 70% of all patients with Hansen's disease have negative smears. Smears are taken from lesions and cooler areas of the skin, such as the earlobes, elbows, and knees. If organisms are found on skin smears, the patient is said to be multibacillary. If the results of skin smears are negative (and there are five or fewer lesions), the patient is called paucibacillary.

Nerve involvement is detected by enlargement of peripheral nerves and lesional loss of sensation. Enlarged nerves are found in over 90% of patients with multibacillary Hansen's disease, and in 75–85% of patients with paucibacillary disease. About 70% of Hansen's disease lesions have reduced sensation, but lesional dysesthesia is not detected in patients with multibacillary disease, the most infectious form.

Serologic tests to detect antibodies against *M. leprae*-unique antigens (PGL-1) and PCR to detect small numbers of organisms in infected tissue have not improved diagnosis. They are universally positive in patients with multibacillary disease, in whom the diagnosis is not difficult. In paucibacillary patients these tests are often negative, and in endemic areas there is a high background rate of positivity of serologic tests. These tests are, therefore, of no real value in the diagnosis of patients with cutaneous Hansen's disease. In pure neural Hansen's disease, however, about 50% of patients are seropositive, and serologic testing might be of use in that setting. Seropositivity might also be used to identify persons in endemic areas at risk of developing Hansen's disease, and chemoprophylaxis could be directed at these persons. Also, seropositivity for antibodies to PGL-1 may be used as a surrogate field marker for high bacterial load (multibacillary status) and to identify those patients who might require longer therapy to cure their infection. Since PGL-1 antibody tests are best for detecting patients with poor cell-mediated immunity against *M. leprae* and who consequently have high humoral immunity against *M. leprae* and multibacillary disease, there is a need for a diagnostic test to identify those persons who have adequate cell-mediated immunity, but may be at risk of developing paucibacillary Hansen's disease. The lepromin skin test has not served this need, in contrast to tuberculin skin testing. Based on the technology of the T cell interferon (IFN)-γ production-based assays for *M. tuberculosis* infection, researchers have identified unique peptides of *M. leprae* and have developed a research IFN-γ release assay (IGRA). This was able to detect all paucibacillary cases in a Hansen's disease cohort. In addition, 13/14 household contacts of Hansen's disease patients were positive in this assay. Ideally, in endemic areas, both serological and cell-based assays could be used to detect all patients with Hansen's disease.

Classification

Hansen's disease may present with a broad spectrum of clinical diseases. The Ridley and Jopling scale classifies cases based on clinical, bacteriologic, immunologic, and histopathologic features (Table 17-1). In many exposed patients the infection apparently clears spontaneously and no clinical lesions develop. Patients who do develop clinical disease are broadly classified into two groups for the purposes of treatment and for trials that compare treatment strategies. Paucibacillary patients have few or no organisms in their lesions, and usually 3–5 lesions or fewer (for treatment purposes, the finding of acid-fast bacilli by stains or smears classifies a patient as having paucibacillary Hansen's disease). Multibacillary patients have multiple, symmetrical lesions, and organisms detectable by biopsy or smears. The individual's cell-mediated immune response to the organism determines the form Hansen's disease will take in the individual. If the cell-mediated immune response against *M. leprae* is strong, the number of organisms will be low (paucibacillary), and conversely if this response is inadequate, the number of organisms will be high (multibacillary).

The most common outcome after exposure is probably spontaneous cure. If skin disease does appear, the initial clinical lesion may be a single hypopigmented patch, perhaps with slight anesthesia. This is called indeterminate disease, since the course of the disease cannot be predicted at this stage. The lesion may clear spontaneously or may progress to any other form of Hansen's disease.

The spectrum of leprosy has two stable poles, the tuberculoid and lepromatous forms (see Table 17-1). These so-called

Table 17-1 Spectrum of host–parasite relationship in Hansen's disease

	High resistance		Unstable resistance		No resistance
	Tuberculoid (TT)	**Borderline Tuberculoid (BT)**	**Borderline (BB)**	**Borderline Lepromatous (BL)**	**Lepromatous (LL)**
Lesions	1–3	Few	Few or many asymmetrical	Many	Numerous and symmetrical
Smear for bacilli	0	1+	2+	3+	4+
Lepromin test	3+	2+	+	+	0
Histology	Epithelioid cells decreasing ⟶ Nerve destruction, sarcoid-like granuloma			Increasing histiocytes, foam cells, granuloma, xanthoma-like	

Adapted from Dr JH Petit.

polar forms do not change; the patient remains in one or the other form throughout the course of the disease. The polar tuberculoid form (called TT), the form of high cell-mediated immunity, is characterized by less than five lesions (often only one) and very few organisms (paucibacillary disease). The patients have strong cell-mediated immunity against the organism. The natural history of many TT leprosy patients is for spontaneous cure over several years. The polar lepromatous form (called LL) has very limited cell-mediated immunity against the organism, lesions are numerous, and they contain many organisms (multibacillary). Between these two poles is every possible degree of infection, forming the borderline spectrum. Cases near the tuberculoid pole are called borderline tuberculoid (BT), those near the lepromatous pole are called borderline lepromatous (BL), and those in the middle are called borderline borderline (BB). Borderline disease is characteristically unstable, and with time cases move from the TT to the LL pole, a process called downgrading.

Hansen's disease may involve only the nerves. This pure neural disease may be indeterminate, tuberculoid, or lepromatous (paucibacillary or multibacillary), and is so classified. In Nepal and India, pure neural Hansen's disease may represent as much as 5% of all new cases of Hansen's disease.

Early and indeterminate Hansen's disease

Usually, the onset of Hansen's disease is insidious. Prodromal symptoms are generally so slight that the disease is not recognized until the appearance of a cutaneous eruption. Actually, the first clinical manifestation in 90% of patients is numbness, and years may elapse before skin lesions or other signs are identified. The earliest sensory changes are loss of the senses of temperature and light touch, most often in the feet or hands. The inability to discriminate hot from cold may be lost before pinprick sensibility. Such dissociation of sensibility is especially suspicious. The distribution of these neural signs and their intensity will depend on the type of disease that is evolving.

Often the first lesion noted is a solitary, ill-defined, hypopigmented macule that merges into the surrounding normal skin. Less often, erythematous macules may be present. Such lesions are most likely to occur on the cheeks, upper arms, thighs, and buttocks. Examination reveals that sensory functions are either normal or minimally altered. Peripheral nerves are not enlarged, and plaques and nodules do not occur. Histologically, a variable lymphocytic infiltrate (without granulomas) is seen, sometimes with involvement of the cutaneous nerves. Usually, no bacilli, or only a few, are seen on biopsy of this indeterminate form. It is the classification, not the diagnosis, that is indeterminate. Few cases remain in this state; they evolve into lepromatous, tuberculoid, or borderline types, or (if cell-mediated immunity is good) often spontaneously resolve and never develop other signs or symptoms of Hansen's disease.

Tuberculoid leprosy

Tuberculoid lesions are solitary or few in number (five or less) and asymmetrically distributed. Lesions may be hypopigmented or erythematous, and are usually dry, scaly, and hairless (Fig. 17-1). The typical lesion of tuberculoid leprosy is the large, erythematous plaque with a sharply defined and elevated border that slopes down to a flattened atrophic center. This has been described as having the appearance of "a saucer right side up." Lesions may also be macular and hypopigmented or erythematous, resembling clinically indeterminate lesions. The presence of palpable induration and neurologic findings distinguishes indeterminate lesions from tuberculoid

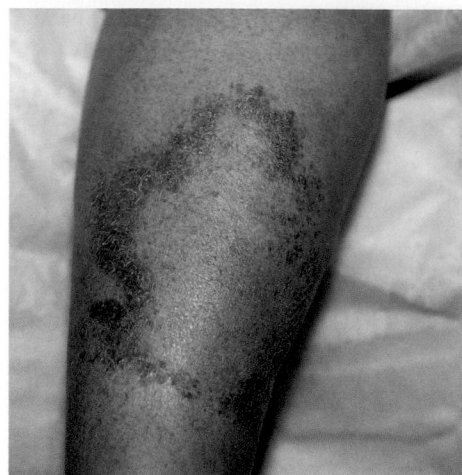

Fig. 17-1 Tuberculoid leprosy.

lesions clinically. The most common locations are the face, limbs, or trunk; the scalp, axillae, groin, and perineum are not involved.

A tuberculoid lesion is anesthetic or hypesthetic and anhidrotic, and superficial peripheral nerves serving or proximal to the lesion are enlarged, tender, or both. The greater auricular nerve and the superficial peroneal nerve may be visibly enlarged. Nerve involvement is early and prominent in tuberculoid leprosy, leading to characteristic changes in the muscle groups served. There may be atrophy of the interosseous muscles of the hand, with wasting of the thenar and hypothenar eminences, contracture of the fingers, paralysis of the facial muscles, and foot drop. Facial nerve damage dramatically increases the risk for ocular involvement and vision loss.

The evolution of the lesions is generally slow. There is often spontaneous remission of the lesions in about 3 years, or remission may result sooner with treatment. Spontaneous involution may leave pigmentary disturbances.

Borderline tuberculoid leprosy

Borderline tuberculoid lesions are similar to tuberculoid lesions, except that they are smaller and more numerous (Fig. 17-2). Satellite lesions around large macules or plaques are characteristic.

Borderline leprosy

In borderline leprosy, the skin lesions are numerous (but countable) and consist of red, irregularly shaped plaques. Small satellite lesions may surround larger plaques. Lesions are generalized but asymmetrical. The edges of lesions are not so well defined as the ones seen in the tuberculoid pole. Nerves may be thickened and tender, but anesthesia is only moderate in the lesions.

Borderline lepromatous leprosy

In borderline lepromatous leprosy, the lesions are symmetrical, numerous (too many to count), and may include macules, papules, plaques, and nodules. The number of small lepromatous lesions outnumbers the larger borderline-type lesions. Nerve involvement appears later; nerves are enlarged, tender, or both, and it is important to note that involvement is symmetrical. Sensation and sweating over individual lesions are normal. Patients usually do not show the features of full-blown lepromatous leprosy, such as madarosis (loss of the eyebrows), keratitis, nasal ulceration, and leonine facies.

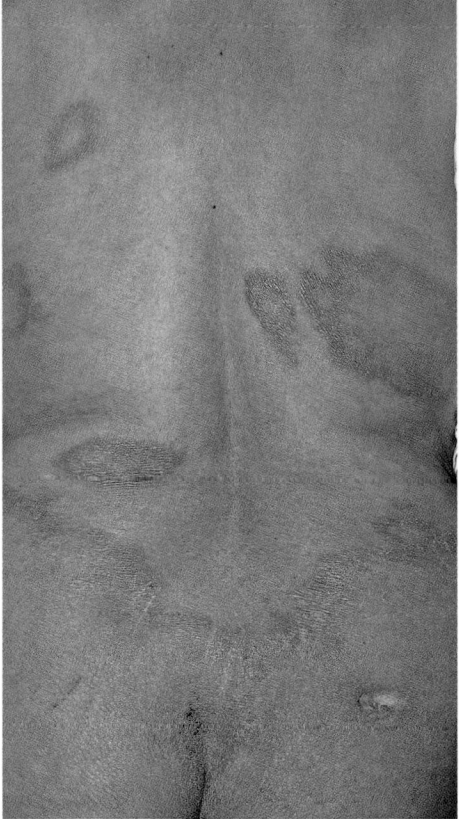

Fig. 17-2 Borderline tuberculoid leprosy.

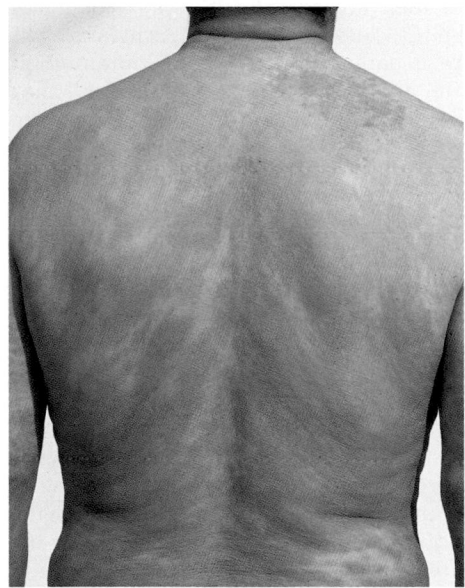

Fig. 17-3 Lepromatous leprosy.

Lepromatous leprosy

Lepromatous leprosy may begin as such or develop following indeterminate leprosy or from downgrading of borderline leprosy. The cutaneous lesions of lepromatous leprosy consist mainly of pale macules (Fig. 17-3) or diffuse infiltration of the skin. There is a tendency for the disease to become progressively worse without treatment. Lepromatous leprosy may be divided into a polar form (LL$_p$) and a subpolar form (LL$_s$); these forms may behave differently.

Macular lepromatous leprosy lesions are diffusely and symmetrically distributed over the body. Tuberculoid macules are

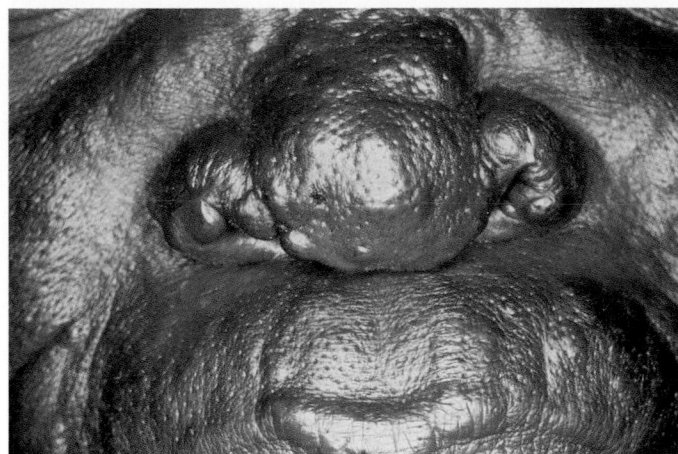

Fig. 17-4 Lepromatous leprosy.

large and few in number, whereas lepromatous macules are small and numerous. Lepromatous macules are ill defined, show no change in skin texture, and blend imperceptibly into the surrounding skin. There is little or no loss of sensation over the lesions, there is no nerve thickening, and there are no changes in sweating. A slow, progressive loss of hair takes place from the outer third of the eyebrows, then the eyelashes, and finally, the body; however, the scalp hair usually remains unchanged.

Lepromatous infiltrations may be divided into the diffuse, plaque, and nodular types (Fig. 17-4). The diffuse type is characterized by the development of a diffuse infiltration of the face, especially the forehead, madarosis, and a waxy and shiny appearance of the skin, sometimes described as a "varnished" appearance. Diffuse leprosy of Lucio is a striking form, uncommon except in western Mexico and certain other Latin American areas, where nearly one-third of lepromatous cases may be of this type. This form of lepromatous leprosy is characterized by diffuse lepromatous infiltration of the skin; localized lepromas do not form. A unique complication of this subtype is the reactional state referred to as Lucio's phenomenon (erythema necroticans).

The infiltrations may be manifested by the development of nodules called lepromas. The early nodules are ill defined and occur most often in acral parts: ears (Fig. 17-5), brows, nose, chin, elbows, hands, buttocks, or knees.

Nerve involvement invariably occurs in lepromatous leprosy, but develops very slowly. Like the skin lesions, nerve disease is bilaterally symmetrical, usually in a stocking-glove pattern. This is frequently misdiagnosed as diabetic neuropathy in the US if it is the presenting manifestation.

Histoid leprosy

Histoid leprosy is an uncommon form of multibacillary leprosy in which skin lesions appear as yellow–red, shiny, large papules and nodules in the dermis or subcutaneous tissue (Fig. 17-6). Lesions appear on a background of normal skin. They vary in size from 1 to 15 mm in diameter, and may appear anywhere on the body but favor the buttocks, lower back, face, and bony prominences. This pattern may appear de novo, but was mostly described in patients with resistance to dapsone.

Nerve involvement

Nerve involvement is characteristic and unique to Hansen's disease. This neural predilection or neurotropism is a histopathologic hallmark of Hansen's disease. Nerve

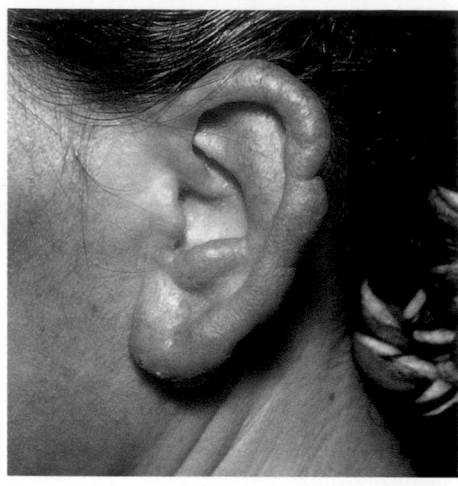

Fig. 17-5 Lepromatous leprosy, enlargement of the earlobe.

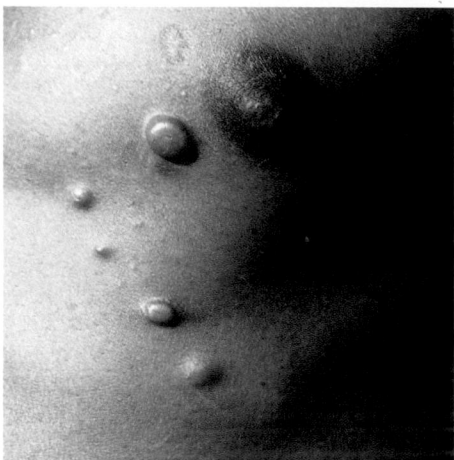

Fig. 17-6 Histoid leprosy.

(multibacillary). Nerve disease can be symptomatic or asymptomatic.

Leprosy bacilli may be delivered to the nerves via the perineural and endoneural blood vessels. Once the bacilli transgress the endothelial basal lamina and are in the endoneurium, they either enter resident macrophages or selectively enter Schwann cells. Damage to the nerves could then occur by several mechanisms:

1. obstruction of neural vessels
2. vasculitis of neural vessels
3. interference with the metabolism of the Schwann cell, making it unable to support the neuron
4. immunologic attack on endothelium or nerves
5. infiltration and proliferation of *M. leprae* in the closed and relatively nonexpandable endoneural and perineural spaces.

Different and multiple mechanisms may occur in different forms of Hansen's disease and in the same patient over time. The selective ability of *M. leprae* to enter Schwann cells is unique among bacteria. The *M. leprae*-unique PGL-1 phenolic glycolipid, expressed abundantly on the surface of leprosy bacilli, binds selectively to the α2 G module of laminin 2. This α2 chain is tissue-restricted and specifically expressed on peripheral nerve Schwann cells. The binding of *M. leprae* to laminin 2 places it in apposition to the Schwann cell basement membrane when laminin 2 binds to the dystroglycan complex on the Schwann cell membrane. These bound *M. leprae* are endocytosed into the Schwann cells, giving *M. leprae* selective access to the inside of Schwann cells. Other accessory binding molecules may facilitate the binding and endocytosis. The nerves become immunologic targets when they present *M. leprae* antigens on their surface in the context of major histocompatibility (MHC) class II molecules. Schwann cells and hence nerves are usually protected from immunologic attack mediated by the adaptive immune system since they rarely present MHC class II antigens on their surface. In Hansen's disease, expression of these immunologic molecules occurs on the surface of Schwann cells, making them potential targets for CD4+ cytotoxic T cells. This mechanism may be important in the nerve damage that occurs in type I (reversal) reactions.

The neural signs in Hansen's disease are dysesthesia, nerve enlargement, muscular weakness and wasting, and trophic changes. The lesions of the vasomotor nerves accompany the sensory disturbances or may precede them. Dysesthesia develops in a progressive manner. The first symptom is usually an inability to distinguish hot and cold. Subsequently, the perception of light touch is lost, then that of pain, and lastly the sense of deep touch. At times the sensory changes in large Hansen's disease lesions are not uniform because of the variation in the involvement of the individual neural filaments supplying the area. Therefore, the areas of dysesthesia may not conform to the distribution of any particular nerve, nor (except in lepromatous cases) are they symmetrical.

Nerve involvement affects chiefly (and is most easily observed in) the more superficial nerve trunks, such as the ulnar, median, radial, peroneal, posterior tibial, fifth and seventh cranial nerves, and especially the great auricular nerve. Beaded enlargements, nodules, or spindle-shaped swellings may be found, which at first may be tender. Neural abscesses may form. The ulnar nerve near the internal condyle of the humerus may be as thick as the little finger, round, and stiff, and often easily felt several centimeters above the elbow.

As a result of the nerve damage, areas of anesthesia, paralysis, and trophic disorders in the peripheral parts of the extremities gradually develop. Muscular paralysis and atrophy generally affect the small muscles of the hands and feet or

involvement is responsible for the clinical findings of anesthesia within lesions (paucibacillary and borderline leprosy), and of a progressive "stocking-glove" peripheral neuropathy (lepromatous leprosy). The neuropathy is termed "primary impairments" (WHO grade 1). Secondary (or visible) impairments (WHO grade 2) are a consequence of the neuropathy and include skin fissures, wounds, clawing of digits, contractures, shortening of digits, and blindness. Neural damage leads to deformities and in endemic regions results in Hansen's disease being a major cause of "limitations of activity" (formerly called disability) and "restrictions in social participation" (formerly termed handicap). Neuropathy is present in 1.3–3.5% of paucibacillary cases and 7.5–24% of multibacillary cases undergoing MDT. Secondary impairments occur in 33–56% of multibacillary cases. Neuropathy may progress, even after effective MDT, and secondary impairments may continue to appear for years as a consequence of the neuropathy. This requires patients with neuropathy to be constantly monitored, even though they are "cured" of their infection.

Nerve enlargement is rare in other skin diseases, so the finding of skin lesions with enlarged nerves should raise the possibility of Hansen's disease. Nerve involvement tends to occur with skin lesions, and the pattern of nerve involvement parallels the skin disease. Tuberculoid leprosy is characterized by asymmetrical nerve involvement localized to the skin lesions. Lepromatous nerve involvement is symmetrical and not associated with skin lesions. Nerve involvement without skin lesions, called pure neural leprosy, can occur and may be either tuberculoid (paucibacillary) or lepromatous

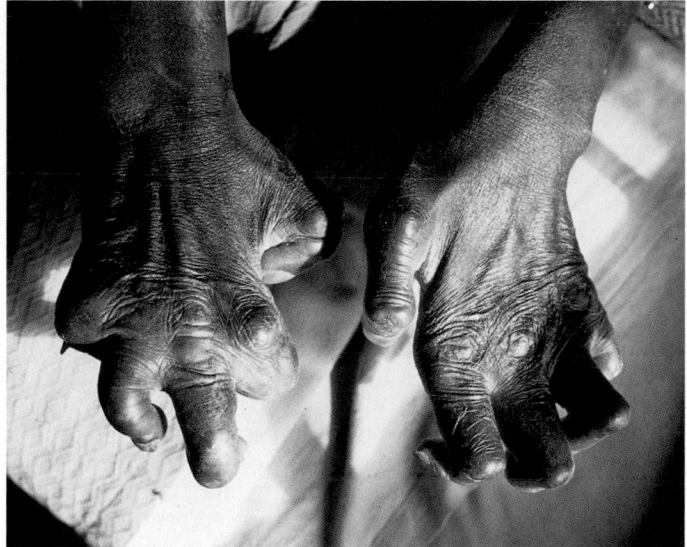

Fig. 17-7 Claw hand of Hansen's disease.

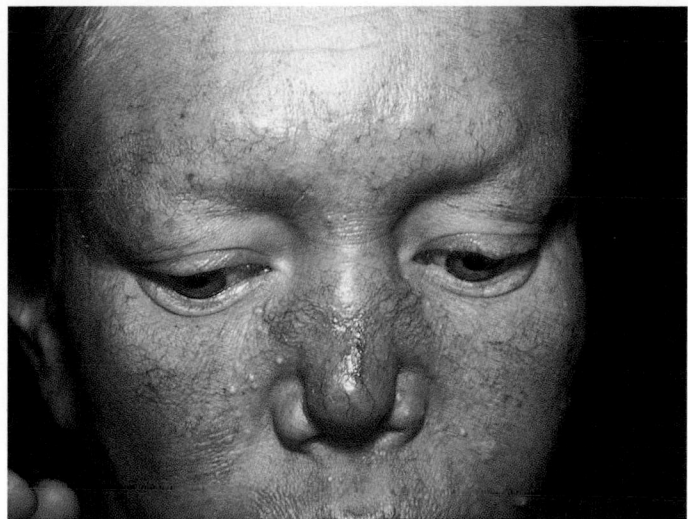

Fig. 17-8 Lepromatous leprosy with collapse of nasal bridge.

some of the facial muscles, producing weakness and progressive atrophy. Deeper motor nerves are only rarely involved. The fingers develop contractures, with the formation of a claw hand (Fig. 17-7), and, as the result of resorption of phalangeal bones, fingers and toes become shorter. Ptosis, ectropion, and a masklike appearance occur from damage to the fifth and seventh cranial nerves.

Subsequent to nerve damage ulceration, hyperkeratosis, bullae, alopecia, anhidrosis, and mal perforans pedis can develop. Trophic ulceration usually manifests as a perforating ulcer on the ball or heel of the foot.

Ocular involvement

Corneal erosions, exposure keratitis, and ulcerations may occur as a result of involvement of the seventh nerve. Specific changes may include corneal opacity, avascular keratitis, pannus formation, interstitial keratitis, and corneal lepromas. The corneal opacities enlarge and finally form visible white flecks called pearls. When (in borderline lepromatous or lepromatous cases only) the iris and the ciliary body become involved, miliary lepromata (iris pearls), nodular lepromata, chronic granulomatous iritis, and acute diffuse iridocyclitis may result. Of multibacillary patients, 2.8–4.6% are blind at diagnosis and 11% will have a potentially blinding process.

Mucous membrane involvement

The mucous membranes may also be affected, especially in the nose, mouth, and larynx. The nasal mucosa is most commonly involved, and lepromatous patients, if queried, frequently complain of chronic nasal congestion. By far the most common lesions in the nose are infiltrations and nodules. Perforation of the nasal septum may occur in advanced cases, with collapse of the nasal bridge (Fig. 17-8). Saddle-nose deformities and loss of the upper incisor teeth can occur.

Nodules occurring on the vocal cords will produce hoarseness.

Visceral involvement

In lepromatous leprosy, the body is diffusely involved and bacteremia occurs. Except for the gastrointestinal tract, lungs, and brain, virtually every organ can contain leprosy bacilli. The lymph nodes, bone marrow, liver, spleen, and testicles are most heavily infected. Visceral infection is restricted mostly to the reticuloendothelial system, which, despite extensive involvement, rarely produces symptoms or findings. Testicular atrophy, with resultant gynecomastia or premature osteoporosis, is an exception. Secondary amyloidosis with renal impairment may complicate multibacillary leprosy. Glomerulonephritis occurs in more than 5% and perhaps as many as 50% of Hansen's disease patients, and is not correlated with bacillary load or the presence of erythema nodosum leprosum.

Pregnancy and Hansen's disease

Hansen's disease may be complicated in several ways by pregnancy. As a state of relative immunosuppression, pregnancy may lead to an exacerbation or reactivation after apparent cure. In addition, pregnancy or, more commonly, the period immediately after delivery may be associated with the appearance of reactional states in patients with Hansen's disease. Pregnant patients with Hansen's disease cannot be given certain medications used to treat Hansen's disease, such as thalidomide, ofloxacin, and minocycline. MDT is tolerated by pregnant women if these restricted agents are avoided.

Human immunodeficiency virus (HIV) and Hansen's disease

HIV infection, while a cause of profound immunosuppression of the cell-mediated immune system, does not seem to have an adverse effect on the course of Hansen's disease. Patients are treated with the same agents and can be expected to have similar outcomes in general. Duration of treatment with MDT may need to be extended in patients with HIV infection. Treatment of HIV-infected patients with Hansen's disease using effective antiretroviral drugs may be associated with the appearance of reactional states (usually type I) as part of the immune reconstitution syndrome. This virtually always occurs in the first 6 months of antiviral therapy.

Pathogenesis

The patient's immune reaction to the leprosy bacillus is a critical element in determining the outcome of infection. Tuberculoid patients make well-formed granulomas that contain helper T cells, whereas lepromatous patients have poorly formed granulomas and suppressor T cells predominate. The cytokine profile in tuberculoid lesions is that of good cell-mediated immunity with IFN-γ and interleukin (IL)-2 being present. In lepromatous patients, these cytokines are reduced and IL-4, 5, and 10, cytokines that downregulate cell-mediated immunity and enhance suppressor function and antibody production, are prominent. Lepromatous leprosy thus represents a classic helper T-cell type 2 (Th2) response to *M. leprae*. Lepromatous patients have polyclonal hypergammaglobulinaemia and high antibody titers to *M. leprae* unique antigens, and may have false-positive syphilis serology, rheumatoid factor, and antinuclear antibodies. Although the cell-mediated immune response of lepromatous patients to *M. leprae* is reduced, these patients are not immune-suppressed for other infectious agents. Tuberculosis behaves normally in patients with lepromatous leprosy.

Histopathology

Ideally, biopsies should be performed from the active border of typical lesions and should extend into the subcutaneous tissue. Punch biopsies are usually adequate. Fite-Faraco stain is optimal for demonstrating *M. leprae*. Because the diagnosis of Hansen's disease is associated with significant social implications, evaluation must be complete, to include evaluation of multiple sections in paucibacillary cases, and consultation with a pathologist experienced in the diagnosis of Hansen's disease can be helpful if the diagnosis is suspected but organisms cannot be identified in the affected tissue, especially in paucibacillary disease and reactional states. PCR testing has not been very useful, as it is positive in only 50% of paucibacillary cases. The histologic features of Hansen's disease correlate with the clinical pattern of disease. Nerve involvement is characteristic of Hansen's disease, and histologic perineural and neural involvement should raise the possibility of Hansen's disease.

Tuberculoid leprosy

Dermal tuberculoid granulomas, consisting of groups of epithelioid cells with giant cells, are found in tuberculoid leprosy. The granulomas are elongated and generally run parallel to the surface, following neurovascular bundles. The epithelioid cells are not vacuolated or lipidized. The granulomas extend up to the epidermis, with no grenz zone. Lymphocytes are found at the periphery of the granulomas. Acid-fast bacilli are rare. The most important specific diagnostic feature, next to finding bacilli, is selective destruction of nerve trunks and the finding of perineural concentric fibrosis. An S-100 stain may demonstrate this selective neural destruction by demonstrating unrecognizable nerve remnants in the inflammatory foci. Bacilli are most frequently found in nerves, but the subepidermal zone and arrector pili muscles are other fruitful areas.

Borderline tuberculoid leprosy

The histopathology of the borderline tuberculoid type is similar to that seen in the tuberculoid variety, but epithelioid cells may show some vacuolation, bacilli are more abundant, and a grenz zone separates the inflammatory infiltrate from the overlying epidermis.

Borderline leprosy

In borderline leprosy, granulomas are less well organized, giant cells are not seen, the macrophages have some foamy cytoplasm, and organisms are abundant.

Borderline lepromatous leprosy

In borderline lepromatous lesions, foamy histiocytes, rather than epithelioid cells, make up the majority of the granuloma. Lymphocytes are still present and may be numerous in the granulomas, but are dispersed diffusely within them, not organized at the periphery. Perineural involvement with lymphocyte infiltration may be present. Organisms are abundant and may be found in clumps.

Lepromatous leprosy

In lepromatous leprosy, granulomas are composed primarily of bacilli- and lipid-laden histocytes. These are the so-called lepra cells or foam cells of Virchow. The infiltrate is localized in the dermis and may be purely perivascular or sheetlike and separated from the epidermis by a well-defined grenz zone. Acid-fast bacilli are typically abundant and appear as round clumps (globi). Pure polar lepromatous leprosy differs from the subpolar type primarily in the paucity of lymphocytes in the pure polar form.

Reactional states

Reactions are a characteristic and clinically important aspect of Hansen's disease. Around 50% of patients will experience a reaction after the institution of MDT. In addition to antibiotic therapy, intercurrent infections, vaccination, pregnancy, vitamin A, iodides, and bromide may trigger reactions. Reactions can be severe and are an important cause of permanent nerve damage in borderline patients. Reactional states are frequently abrupt in their appearance, as opposed to Hansen's disease itself, which changes slowly. It is therefore a common reason for patients to seek consultation. In addition, if the patient feels that the chemotherapy is triggering the reaction, he/she will tend to discontinue the treatment, leading to treatment failure.

Reactional states are divided into two forms, called type 1 and type 2 reactions. Type 1 reactions are caused by cell-mediated immune inflammation within existing skin lesions. They generally occur in patients with borderline leprosy (BT, BB, BL). Type 2 reactions are mediated by immune complexes and occur in lepromatous patients (BL, LL).

Type 1 reactions (reversal, lepra, and downgrading reactions)

Type 1 reactions represent an enhanced cell-mediated immune response to *M. leprae*, and commonly occur after treatment is initiated. If the reactions occur with antibiotic chemotherapy, they are called reversal reactions, and if they occur as borderline disease shifts toward the lepromatous pole (downgrading), they are called downgrading reactions. These two reaction types are clinically identical. Patients in all parts of the borderline spectrum may be affected by type 1 reactions, but these are most severe in patients with borderline lepromatous leprosy who have a large amount of *M. leprae* antigen and therefore have prolonged and repeated reactions during treatment.

Type 1 reactions clinically present with inflammation of existing lesions (Fig. 17-9). There are no systemic symptoms (such as fever, chills, and arthralgias). Lesions swell, become erythematous, and are sometimes tender, simulating cellulitis. In severe cases, ulceration can occur.

Patients may state that new lesions appeared with the reaction, but these probably represent subclinical lesions that were highlighted by the reaction. The major complication of type 1

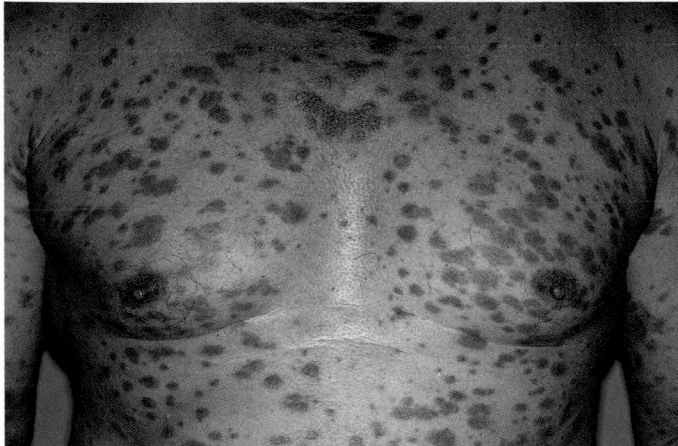

Fig. 17-9 Type I reaction. (Courtesy of Curt Samlaska, MD)

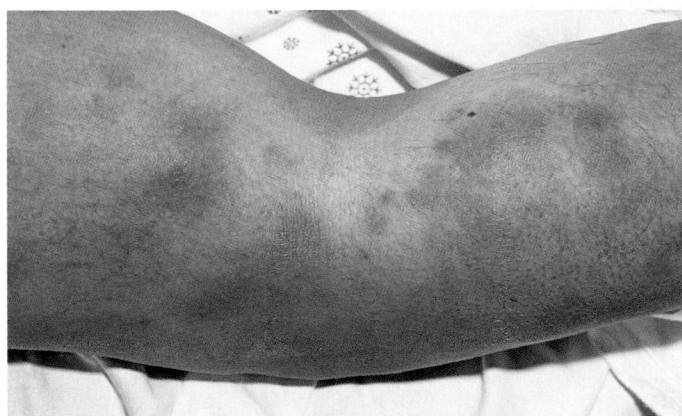

Fig. 17-10 Erythema nodosum leprosum.

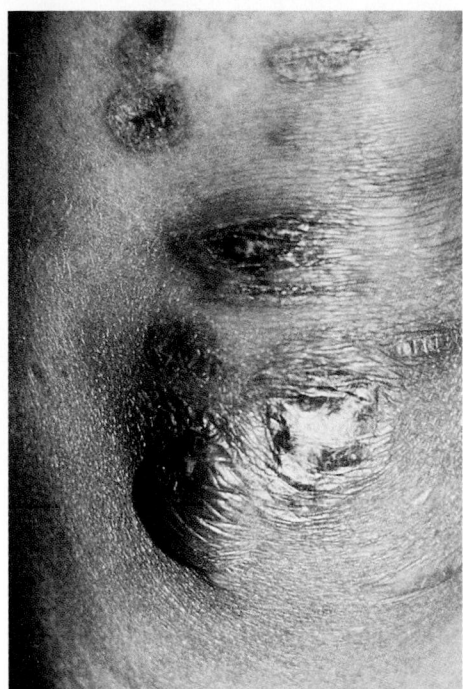

Fig. 17-11 Lucio's phenomenon, early bullous lesions.

ENL is a multisystem disease and can produce conjunctivitis, neuritis, keratitis, iritis, synovitis, nephritis, hepatosplenomegaly, orchitis, and lymphadenopathy. The intensity of the reaction may vary from mild to severe and it may last from a few days to weeks, months, or even years. Histologically, ENL demonstrates a leukocytoclastic vasculitis. Laboratory evaluation will reveal an elevated sedimentation rate, an elevated C-reactive protein, and a neutrophilia.

Lucio's phenomenon

Lucio's phenomenon is an uncommon and unusual reaction that occurs in patients with diffuse lepromatous leprosy of the "la bonita" type, most commonly found in western Mexico. Some consider it a subset of ENL, but it differs in that it lacks neutrophilia and systemic symptoms. It is not associated with institution of antibiotic treatment as is ENL, but it is commonly the reason for initial presentation in affected patients. Purpuric macules evolve to bullous lesions that rapidly ulcerate, especially below the knees (Fig. 17-11). They may be painful, but may also be relatively asymptomatic. Histologically, bacilli are numerous, and in addition to being in the dermis, are seen within blood vessel walls with thrombosis of mid-dermal vessels resulting in cutaneous infarction. Fever, splenomegaly, lymphadenopathy, glomerulonephritis, anemia, hypoalbuminemia, polyclonal gammopathy, and hypocalcemia can be associated. If the patient is diagnosed early, before significant metabolic and infectious complications occur, the outcome is favorable.

Treatment

Before 1982, dapsone monotherapy was the standard treatment for Hansen's disease, and while it was effective in many patients, primary and secondary dapsone-resistant cases occurred. In addition, multibacillary patients required lifelong treatment, which had inherent compliance problems. To circumvent these problems and shorten therapeutic courses, WHO proposed MDT. This has been very effective in treating active cases of Hansen's disease. The number of antibiotics

reactions is nerve damage. As the cell-mediated inflammation attacks *M. leprae* antigen, any infected tissue compartment can be damaged. Because bacilli are preferentially in nerves, neural symptoms and findings are often present. Reversal reaction occurring within a nerve may lead to sudden loss of nerve function and to permanent damage to that nerve. This makes type 1 reactions an emergency. In this setting, affected nerves are enlarged and tender. In other patients, the neuritis may be subacute or chronic and of limited acute symptomatology, but may still result in severe nerve damage. Histologically, skin lesions show perivascular and perineural edema and large numbers of lymphocytes. Severe reactions may demonstrate tissue necrosis. Bacilli are reduced.

Type 2 reactions (erythema nodosum leprosum)

Erythema nodosum leprosum (ENL) occurs in half of patients with borderline lepromatous or lepromatous leprosy, 90% of the time within a few years of institution of antibiotic treatment for Hansen's disease or during pregnancy. ENL is a circulating immune complex-mediated disease. As such, in contrast to type 1 reactions, it can result in multisystem involvement and is usually accompanied by systemic symptoms (fever, myalgias, arthralgias, anorexia). Skin lesions are characteristically erythematous, subcutaneous, and dermal nodules that are widely distributed (Fig. 17-10). They do not occur at the sites of existing skin lesions. Severe skin lesions can ulcerate. Unlike classic erythema nodosum, lesions are generalized and favor the extensor arms and medial thighs.

used and the duration of treatment are determined by the bacterial load the patient exhibits. This can be assessed by slit skin smear, where finding any bacilli classifies the patient as multibacillary. On skin biopsy the same criterion is used, i.e. finding any bacilli identifies the patient as multibacillary. The number of lesions constitutes the "field" classification system, and patients are classified as having 1 lesion, 2–5 lesions in one anatomic region (paucibacillary), or over 5 (multibacillary). This classification can result in undertreatment of patients with few lesions, but who are actually multibacillary. Three other reasons can result in undertreatment of patients:

1. failure or inability to do a skin biopsy
2. classifying patients with more than five lesions as "tuberculoid" and hence "paucibacillary"
3. failure to understand that, although the patient has histologic and clinical features of "tuberculoid" disease, organisms are identified on skin biopsy and hence he/she requires treatment for multibacillary disease.

All patients with more than five lesions and those with organisms identified on skin biopsy should be treated for multibacillary Hansen's disease. Failure may also result from noncompliance, drug resistance, relapse after apparent clinical and bacteriologic cure, and persistence. Persisters are viable organisms that, by mouse footpad testing, are sensitive to the antimicrobial agents given but persist in tissue despite bactericidal tissue levels in the patient. They are usually found in macrophages or nerves. These persisters correlate with relapse occurring 6–9 years following MDT. Since relapses may occur many years after MDT, where adequate healthcare resources exist, multibacillary patients should be followed annually to examine for evidence of relapse, reaction, or progression of neuropathy.

There are several different MDT recommendations, but only two are given here — those recommended by the Public Health Service for patients in the US and those recommended by WHO. Because dapsone resistance is less common in the US, and effective compliance programs can be developed to enhance monotherapy, dapsone monotherapy may still be considered after MDT in the US. For paucibacillary cases (no organisms found on skin smears or skin biopsy; five lesions or less; indeterminate and tuberculoid leprosy) in the US, the recommendation is 600 mg/day of rifampin and 100 mg/day of dapsone for 12 months. Paucibacillary patients who relapse with paucibacillary disease are treated with an appropriate regimen for multibacillary disease. In the US, multibacillary cases receive 100 mg/day of dapsone, 50 mg/day of clofazimine, and 600 mg/day of rifampin, or a standard WHO regimen (see below) for 2 years (Fig. 17-12). For multibacillary patients who refuse clofazimine, 100 mg of minocycline or 400 mg/day of ofloxacin may be substituted. Clarithromycin, 500 mg/day, may also be used in treatment regimens. Multibacillary relapses, whether the initial diagnosis was paucibacillary or multibacillary disease, should have a mouse footpad sensitivity study carried out, and be treated with an appropriate multidrug regimen for 2 years, followed by daily life-long dapsone or clofazimine, depending on sensitivity testing.

The WHO-recommended protocols are shorter and cheaper than those recommended in the US. There is concern that the reduction of MDT from 2 years to 1 year may lead to increased numbers of relapses, especially among patients with high bacillary loads (BI over 4 on skin smear). The WHO recommendation for paucibacillary disease (no bacilli on smears or biopsy; five or fewer lesions; indeterminate and tuberculoid patients) is 600 mg of rifampin under supervision once a month for 6 months and 100 mg/day of dapsone for 6 months, unsupervised, with completion of the treatment within 9 months. For

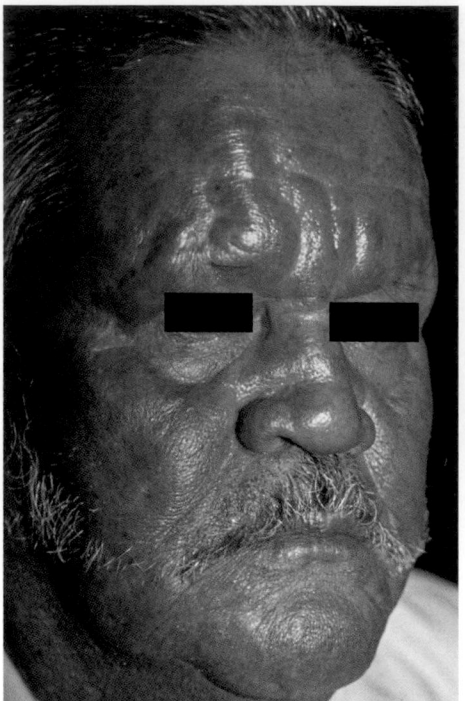

Fig. 17-12 Lepromatous leprosy with discoloration secondary to clofazimine.

single-lesion paucibacillary disease a single dose of 600 mg of rifampin, 400 mg of ofloxacin, and 100 mg of minocycline (ROM), all at one time, is given. This one-dose ROM treatment is less effective than the 6-month regimen for paucibacillary disease. Multibacillary patients (BT, BB, BL, and LL; more than five lesions; any bacilli seen on smears or biopsies) are treated with rifampin, 600 mg, and clofazimine, 300 mg, once a month under supervision, with dapsone, 100 mg/day, and clofazimine, 50 mg/day. Treatment is for 12 months. For patients intolerant of clofazimine, an alternative regimen is rifampin, 600 mg, ofloxacin, 400 mg, and minocycline, 100 mg, all once monthly for 24 doses. An alternative for the patient intolerant or resistant to rifampin or dapsone is clofazimine, 50 mg, ofloxacin, 400 mg, and minocycline, 100 mg, daily for 6 months, followed by 18 months of clofazimine, 50 mg daily, plus either ofloxacin, 400 mg/day, or minocycline, 100 mg/ day. At the end of treatment, visible skin lesions are often still present, especially with the WHO short-duration treatments. Paucibacillary lesions tend to clear 1–2 years after the 6-month treatment course. In the US, treatment could be continued until skin lesions are clear, even if the recommended duration of treatment has been passed. With short-duration MDT, it is very difficult to distinguish clinical relapse (failure of treatment) from late type 1 reactions causing skin lesions to reappear. Pathologic examination (biopsy) or an empiric trial of prednisone for several months may be considered in these cases.

There is significant disagreement regarding the effectiveness of the 1- or 2-year WHO-recommended MDT regimens. Relapse rates for multibacillary patients treated with MDT for 1 or 2 years have been reported to be as high as 7–20% overall, and 13–39% with BI of 4 or greater at diagnosis. Based on this information, patients with BL/LL disease with a BI of 4 or greater are at greatest risk for relapse, and should be treated beyond the 1-year recommended period, with treatment continued until smear negativity.

Adjunctive treatments

Once neurologic complications have occurred, patients with Hansen's disease should be offered occupational therapy. This should include training on how to avoid injury to insensitive skin of the hands and feet. Special shoes may be required. Ocular complications are frequent, and an ophthalmologist with specific skill in treating patients with Hansen's disease is an invaluable member of the treatment team.

Management of reactions

Even though reactions may appear after drug treatment is instituted, it is not advisable to discontinue or reduce anti-leprosy medication because of these. In mild reactions—those without neurologic complications or severe systemic symptoms or findings—treatment may be supportive. Bed rest and administration of aspirin or nonsteroidal anti-inflammatory agents may be used.

Type 1 reactions are usually managed with systemic corticosteroids. Prednisone is given orally, starting at a dose of 40–60 mg/day. Neuritis and eye lesions are urgent indications for systemic steroid therapy. Nerve abscesses may also need to be surgically drained immediately to preserve and recover nerve function. The corticosteroid dose and duration are determined by the clinical course of the reaction. Once the reaction is controlled, the prednisone may need to be tapered slowly—over months to years. The minimum dose required and alternate-day treatment should be used in corticosteroid courses of more than 1 month in duration. Clofazimine appears to have some activity against type 1 reactions and may be added to the treatment in doses of up to 300 mg/day if tolerated. Cyclosporine can be used if steroids fail or as a steroid-sparing agent. The starting dose would be 5–10 mg/kg. If during treatment the function of some nerves fails to improve while the function of others normalizes, the possibility of mechanical compression should be evaluated by surgical exploration. Transposition of the ulnar nerve does not seem to be more effective than immunosuppressive treatment for ulnar nerve dysfunction.

Thalidomide has been demonstrated to be uniquely effective against ENL and is the treatment of choice. Thalidomide is a potent teratogen and should not be given to women of child-bearing potential. The initial recommended dosage is up to 400 mg/day in patients weighing more than 50 kg. This dose is highly sedating in some patients, and patients may complain of central nervous system side effects, even at doses of 100 mg/day. For this reason, such a high dose should be used for only a brief period, or in milder cases treatment may be started at a much lower dose, such as 100–200 mg/day. In cases in which there is an acute episode of ENL, the drug may be discontinued after a few weeks to months. In chronic type 2 reactions, an attempt to discontinue the drug should be made every 6 months. Systemic corticosteroids are also effective in type 2 reactions, but long-term use may lead to complications. Clofazimine in higher doses (up to 300 mg/day) is effective in ENL, and may be used alone or to reduce corticosteroid or thalidomide doses. The combination of pentoxifylline, 400–800 mg twice a day, and clofazimine, 300 mg/day, can be used in ENL when thalidomide cannot be used or to avoid the use of systemic steroids to manage severe ENL. Pentoxifylline alone is inferior to steroids and thalidomide, but can be considered in milder cases. Tumor necrosis factor (TNF) inhibitors, specifically infliximab, have been reported to be effective in treating recurrent ENL.

Lucio's phenomenon is poorly responsive to both corticosteroids and thalidomide. Effective antimicrobial chemotherapy for lepromatous leprosy is the only recommended treatment, combined with wound management for leg ulcers.

Prevention

Because a defect in cell-mediated immunity is inherent in the development of Hansen's disease, vaccine therapies are being tested. Bacillus Calmette–Guérin (BCG) vaccination alone provides about 34–80% protection against infection. In the UK, BCG immunization is given to household contacts under the age of 12. Vaccines have been produced and are effective. It is unclear if they will be needed except in the areas of highest endemicity, as MDT has been effective in reducing the prevalence of disease. Since 80% of patients have contact with multibacillary patients, prevention depends on treating active multibacillary patients and examining exposed persons on an annual basis to detect early evidence of infection. Prophylactic antibiotic regimens have been used in such exposed patients and demonstrate a reduction in new Hansen's disease cases by more than 50% in the first 2 years. Interestingly, patients who had less contact with the source patient benefited more. In the UK, close contacts under the age of 12 whose source case was lepromatous are given rifampin, 15 mg/kg once a month for 6 months. Several trials of chemoprophylaxis in whole endemic regions (once-yearly MDT with single-dose rifampin, minocycline, and clofazimine) have shown early promise and may be useful in hyperendemic regions.

Alter A, et al: Leprosy as a genetic model for susceptibility to common infectious disease. Hum Genet 2008; 123:227.

Ang P, et al: Fatal Lucio's phenomenon in 2 patients with previously undiagnosed leprosy. J Am Acad Dermatol 2003; 48:958.

Batista M, et al: Leprosy reversal reaction as immune reconstitution inflammatory syndrome in patients with AIDS. Clin Infec Dis 2008; 46:56.

Britton W, Lockwood D: Leprosy. Lancet 2004; 363:1209.

Bruce S, et al: Armadillo exposure and Hansen's disease: an epidemiologic survey in southern Texas. J Am Acad Dermatol 2000; 43:223.

Eiglmeier K, et al: The decaying genome of Mycobactcrium leprae. Lepr Rev 2001; 72:387.

Faber WR, et al: Treatment of recurrent erythema nodosum leprosum with infliximab. N Engl J Med 2006; 17:355.

Fogagnolo L, et al: Vasculonecrotic reactions in leprosy. Braz J Infec Dis 2007; 3:378.

Gelber RH: Relapse rate in MB leprosy patients treated with 2 years of WHO-MDT is not low. Int J Lepr Other Mycobact Dis 2004; 72:493.

Geluk A, et al: Rational combination of peptides derived from different Mycobacterium leprae proteins improves sensitivity for immunodiagnosis of M. leprae infection. Clin Vaccine Immunol 2008; 15:522.

Ghorpade A: Inoculable leprosy. Int J Dermatol 2009; 48:1267.

Ho CK, Lo KK: Epidemiology of leprosy and response to treatment in Hong Kong. HK Med J 2006; 12:174.

Job CK, et al: Transmission of leprosy: a study of skin and nasal secretions of household contacts of leprosy patients using PCR. Am J Trop Med Hyg 2008; 78:518.

Klioze AM, Ramos-Caro FA: Visceral leprosy. Int J Dermatol 2000; 39:641.

Martiniuk F, et al: Leprosy as immune reconstitution inflammatory syndrome in HIV-positive persons. Emerg Infect Dis 2007; 13:9.

Menicucci LA, et al: Microscopic leprosy skin lesions in primary neuritic leprosy. J Am Acad Dermatol 2005; 52:648.

Moet FJ, et al: Effectiveness of single dose rifampicin in preventing leprosy in close contacts of patients with newly diagnosed leprosy: cluster randomised controlled trial. Br Med J 2008; 5:761.

Moschella S: An update on the diagnosis and treatment of leprosy. J Am Acad Dermatol 2004; 51:417.

Oskam L, et al: Serology: recent developments, strengths, limitations and prospects: a state of the art overview. Leprosy Rev 2003; 74:196.

Rambukkana A: Molecular basis for the peripheral nerve predilection of Mycobacterium leprae. Curr Opin Microbiol 2001; 4:21.

Scollard DM: Endothelial cells and the pathogenesis of lepromatous neuritis: insights from the armadillo model. Microbes Infect 2000; 2:1835.

Shegal V, et al: The imperatives of leprosy treatment in the pre- and post-global leprosy elimination era: appraisal of changing the scenario to current status. J Derm Treat 2008; 19:82.

Spierings E, et al: The role of Schwann cells, T cells and *Mycobacterium leprae* in the immunopathogenesis of nerve damage in leprosy. Leprosy Rev 2000; 71:S121.

Tourlaki A, et al: Necrotic erythema nodosum leprosum as the first manifestation of borderline lepromatous leprosy. Arch Dermatol 2008; 44:818.

Walker S, et al: Leprosy. Clin in Dermatol 2007; 25:165.

World Health Weekly Organization: Global leprosy situation, beginning of 2008. Wkly Epidemiol Rec 2008; 83:293.

Bonus images for this chapter can be found online at

http://www.expertconsult.com

Fig. 17-1 Borderline lepromatous leprosy.

Fig. 17-2 Lepromatous leprosy, multiple papules and nodules.

Fig. 17-3 Borderline tuberculoid leprosy.

Fig. 17-4 Borderline leprosy.

Fig. 17-5 Lepromatous leprosy, hyperpigmentation due to clofazimine.

Fig. 17-6 Type I reaction.

Fig. 17-7 Acral burns due to peripheral sensory neuropathy, lepromatous leprosy.

Syphilis, Yaws, Bejel, and Pinta   18

Syphilis

Syphilis, also known as lues, is a contagious, sexually transmitted disease caused by the spirochete *Treponema pallidum* subspecies *pallidum*. The only known host is the human. The spirochete enters through the skin or mucous membranes, on which the primary manifestations are seen. In congenital syphilis the treponeme crosses the placenta and infects the fetus. The risk of acquiring infection from sexual contact with an infected partner in the previous 30 days is between 16% and 30%. Syphilis results in multiple patterns of skin and visceral disease and is potentially life-long.

Syphilis, yaws, pinta, and endemic syphilis are closely related. Apparently, yaws first arose with humans in Africa and spread with human migrations to Europe and Asia. Endemic syphilis evolved from yaws and became endemic in the Middle East and the Balkans at some later date. Yaws moved with human migration to the New World and became endemic in South America. Syphilis, *T. pallidum pallidum*, may have originated in the New World from *T. pallidum pertenue*, the organism causing yaws (much as human immunodeficiency virus [HIV] evolved in Africa from simian immunodeficiency virus [SIV]). A tribe in Guyana with a spirochetal infection with features of both yaws and syphilis was identified. Sequencing the genome of this spirochete suggested that it was the ancestor of *T. pallidum pallidum*. This lends support to the theory that syphilis originated more recently in the New World and was brought back to Europe by sailors who went to the New World with Christopher Columbus. Exactly how and when it became primarily a venereally transmitted disease is unclear, but apparently this happened around the end of the 15th century.

T. pallidum is a delicate spiral spirochete that is actively motile. The number of spirals varies from 4 to 14 and the entire length is 5–20 μm. It can be demonstrated in preparations from fresh primary or secondary lesions by darkfield microscopy or by fluorescent antibody techniques. The motility is characteristic, consisting of three movements: a projection in the direction of the long axis, a rotation on its long axis, and a bending or twisting from side to side. The precise uniformity of the spiral coils is not distorted during these movements. Microscopic characteristics of *T. pallidum* cannot be distinguished from commensal oral treponemes, so darkfield examination of oral lesions is untrustworthy. Direct fluorescent antibody testing can be used for confirmation. The electron microscope shows the organism to have an axial filament with several fibrils, a protoplasmic cylinder, and a thin membranaceous envelope called the periplast.

The genome of *T. pallidum* has been sequenced and contains about one-quarter of the number of genes of most bacteria. It lacks significant metabolic capacity. It is very temperature-sensitive, with some enzymes working poorly at typical body temperature (perhaps explaining why fever therapy was effective). These two factors may contribute to the inability to culture the organism in vitro. *T. pallidum* is an effective pathogen, as it disseminates widely and rapidly after infection. It is in the bloodstream within hours of intratesticular injection and in numerous organs including the brain within 18 hours after inoculation. Once the organisms reach a tissue, they are able to persist for decades. In each tissue the number of organisms is very low, perhaps below a "critical antigenic mass." In addition, *T. pallidum* expresses very few antigenic targets on its surface (only about 1% as many as *Escherichia coli*). The outer membrane proteins of *T. pallidum* also undergo rapid mutation so that during an infection the host accumulates numerous subpopulations of organisms with different surface antigens. This low infection load, widespread dissemination, poor surface antigen expression, and rapid evolution of antigenically distinct subpopulations may allow the infection to persist despite the development by the host of antigen-specific antibodies and immune cells.

Syphilis remains a major health problem throughout the world. This is despite there having been a highly effective and economical treatment for more than 50 years. The story of the US and world epidemiology of syphilis illustrates a movement of infection from one population to another due to changing social conditions and behaviors. Just as the health systems respond to one epidemic, another appears. Using serologic testing, contact tracing, and penicillin treatment, the health departments in the US reduced the incidence of syphilis dramatically from the turn of the century through the mid-1950s. Then the incidence gradually increased through the next two decades and into the 1980s. In the early 1980s, half the cases of syphilis diagnosed were in men who have sex with men (MSM). Changes in sexual behavioral patterns among gay men in response to the acquired immunodeficiency syndrome (AIDS) epidemic reduced the number of these cases, but in the late 1980s syphilis again began to increase dramatically, associated with drug usage, especially crack cocaine. The incidence of syphilis increased disproportionately among socioeconomically disadvantaged minority populations, especially in major cities. Throughout the 1990s the rate of syphilis fell in the US, so that by 1999 the national rate of 2.6 cases in 100 000 was the lowest level ever recorded. In addition, half of new cases were concentrated in 28 counties, mainly in the southeastern US and in selected urban areas. With the advent of effective antiretroviral therapy for HIV, there was a change in sexual behavior in MSM, including those with HIV infection. Epidemics of syphilis in this group have now occurred in New York, Atlanta, Fort Lauderdale, Miami, Chicago, Houston, Los Angeles, and San Francisco. Similar epidemics have occurred in MSM in Europe. This epidemic is characterized by an older average age, anonymous sex partners (often met on the Internet), use of amphetamines and Viagra, being HIV-positive, and oral sex as the sole sexual exposure. In addition, there was a syphilis epidemic in Russia and the newly independent states starting in the late 1990s, with rates of syphilis 34 times that of Western Europe. There have also been outbreaks of syphilis in heterosexuals associated with commercial sex workers in the UK. Worldwide it is estimated that there are about 12 million persons infected annually with syphilis, 2 million of whom are pregnant women. The Centers for Disease Control (CDC) and the World Health Organization (WHO) have undertaken campaigns to eradicate syphilis. The shifting epidemiology of syphilis over the last 50 years suggests it will not be an easy task without an effective vaccine. Until that time reporting of all cases to public health departments for tracing and treatment of contacts, and widespread screening of persons at risk (including all pregnant women) should be continued.

Serologic tests

Serologic testing for infection with *T. pallidum*, as in tuberculosis, is undergoing changes that incorporate newer technologies into establishing the diagnosis. Currently, most testing in the US uses older technologies, while in the UK newer technologies have been adopted. Tests are considered either "treponemal" or "nontreponemal." Treponemal tests detect specific antitreponemal antibodies, via enzyme immunoassay (EIA) or *T. pallidum* particle assay (TPPA). These new treponemal tests have high rates of specificity and sensitivity exceeding 95%, even in patients with primary syphilis. Nontreponemal tests are based on the fact that serum of persons with syphilis aggregates a cardiolipin–cholesterol–lecithin antigen. This aggregation can be viewed directly in tubes or on cards or slides, or can be examined in an autoanalyzer. Because these tests use lipoidal antigens rather than *T. pallidum* or components of it, they are called nontreponemal antigen tests. The most widely used nontreponemal tests are the rapid plasma reagin (RPR) and venereal disease research laboratory (VDRL) tests. These nontreponemal tests are the standard tests used in the US, and become positive, as a rule, within 5–6 weeks of infection, shortly before the chancre heals. Tests are generally strongly positive throughout the secondary phase, except in rare patients with AIDS, whose response is less predictable, and usually become negative during therapy, especially if therapy is begun within the first year of infection. Results may also become negative after a few decades, even without treatment. EIA tests are available that detect both IgG- and IgM-specific antibodies against *T. pallidum*. The IgM becomes detectable 2–3 weeks after infection (around the time of the appearance of the chancre). The IgG test becomes positive at 4–5 weeks, so the IgM test is much more useful in diagnosing primary syphilis. The "treponemal" tests used in the US are the microhemagglutination assay for *T. pallidum* (MHA-TP) or the fluorescent treponemal antibody absorption (FTA-ABS) test. These specific treponemal tests are also positive earlier than the nontreponemal tests and may be used to confirm the diagnosis of primary syphilis in a patient with a negative RPR/VDRL. The EIA, TPPA, FTA-ABS and MHA-TP remain positive for life in the majority of patients, although in between 13% and 24% of patients these tests will become negative with treatment, regardless of stage and HIV status. The IgM EIA test, however, becomes negative following treatment in early syphilis, so that at 1 year, 92% of treated early syphilis patients are negative on the IgM EIA.

Since all these tests can have false-positives, although this is much less likely with the new EIA and TPPA tests, all positive results are confirmed by another test. In most US cities this involves screening the patient with a nontreponemal test, usually an RPR, and confirming all positives with a specific treponemal test, usually an MHA-TP. If a treponemal test, such as the TPPA or EIA, is used for initial screening, then the other specific treponemal test should be used to confirm the first test. A nontreponemal RPR/VDRL is also performed on all positives to determine the titer and monitor treatment

success. If the initial screening treponemal specific test is positive, but the nontreponemal test is negative, then a history of prior syphilis and treatment should be sought. If prior syphilis and adequate treatment can be documented and there is no evidence on examination of either primary or late syphilis, then the patient is followed and considered serofast following treatment. If the nontreponemal test is negative, but a second treponemal test is positive, and no prior history of syphilis and its treatment can be found, then the patient is considered to have late latent syphilis (less likely, recent infection) and is treated appropriately. He/she is considered noninfectious. If the two treponemal tests are discordant, one positive and the other negative, a third treponemal specific test can be ordered, or the case can be referred to a public health department for expert consultation. Since the nontreponemal tests are falsely negative in 25% or more of cases of primary syphilis and in up to 40% of cases of late syphilis, in these settings a specific treponemal test should also be performed as a screening test.

In resource-poor countries, serological testing for syphilis is largely unavailable since reagents require refrigeration or the tests require electrical equipment for processing. In Bangladesh and in some countries in sub-Saharan Africa and South America, more than 75% of women receive prenatal care, but only about 40% receive prenatal syphilis screening. Since syphilis is endemic in these regions, with infection rates in pregnant women exceeding 1%, millions of pregnant women with syphilis go undiagnosed, resulting in millions of cases of congenital syphilis. More than half a million babies die of congenital syphilis in sub-Saharan Africa every year. New rapid treponemal specific tests that can be used in these resource-poor countries have been developed. They cost only US$0.31–0.41 per test and await available funding to be put into use.

Nontreponemal tests are very valuable in following the efficacy of treatment in syphilis. By diluting the serum serially, the strength of the reaction can be stated in dilutions, the number given being the highest dilution giving a positive test result. In primary infection the titer may be only 1:2; in secondary syphilis it is regularly high, 1:32–1:256 or higher; in late syphilis, much lower as a rule, perhaps 1:4 or 1:8. The rise of titer in early infection is of great potential diagnostic value, as is the fall after proper treatment or the rise again if there is reinfection or relapse. Patients with very high antibody titers, as occur in secondary syphilis, may have a false-negative result when undiluted serum is tested. This "prozone" phenomenon will be overcome by diluting the serum.

Biologic false-positive test results

"Biologic false-positive" (BFP) is used to denote a positive serological test for syphilis in persons with no history or clinical evidence of syphilis. The term BFP is usually applied to the situation of a positive nontreponemal test and a negative treponemal test. Around 90% of BFP test results are of low titer (less than 1:8). Acute BFP reactions are defined as those that revert to negative in less than 6 months; those that persist for more than 6 months are categorized as chronic. Acute BFP reactions may result from vaccinations, infections (infectious mononucleosis, hepatitis, measles, typhoid, varicella, influenza, lymphogranuloma venereum, malaria), and pregnancy. Chronic BFP reactions are seen in connective tissue diseases, especially systemic lupus erythematosus (SLE) (44%), chronic liver disease, multiple blood transfusions/intravenous drug usage, and advancing age.

False-positive results to specific treponemal tests are less common but have been reported to occur in lupus erythematosus, drug-induced lupus, scleroderma, rheumatoid arthritis, smallpox vaccination, pregnancy, other related treponemal infections (see below), and genital herpes simplex infections.

A pattern of beaded fluorescence associated with FTA-ABS testing may be found in the sera of patients without treponemal disease who have SLE. The beading phenomenon, however, is not specific for SLE or even for connective tissue diseases.

Cutaneous syphilis

Chancre (primary stage)

The chancre is usually the first cutaneous lesion, appearing 18–21 days after infection. The typical incipient chancre is a small red papule or a crusted superficial erosion. In a few days to weeks it becomes a round or oval, indurated, slightly elevated papule, with an eroded but not ulcerated surface that exudes a serous fluid (Fig. 18-1). On palpation it has a cartilage-like consistency. The lesion is usually, but not invariably, painless. This is the uncomplicated or classic Hunterian chancre. The regional lymph nodes on one or both sides are usually enlarged, firm, and nontender, and do not suppurate. Adenopathy begins 1 or 2 weeks after the appearance of the chancre. The Hunterian chancre leaves no scar when it heals.

Chancres generally occur singly, although they may be multiple (Fig. 18-2); they vary in diameter from a few millimeters to several centimeters. In women the genital chancre is less often observed because of its location within the vagina or on the cervix. Extensive edema of the labia or cervix may occur. In men the chancre is commonly located in the coronal sulcus or on either side of the frenum. A chancre in the prepuce, being too hard to bend, will flip over all at once when the prepuce is drawn back, a phenomenon called a dory flop, from the resemblance to the movement of a broad-beamed skiff or dory as it is being turned upside down. Untreated, the chancre tends to heal spontaneously in 1–4 months. About the time of its disappearance, or usually a little before, constitutional symptoms and objective signs of generalized (secondary) syphilis occur.

Extragenital chancres may be larger than those on the genitalia. They affect the lips, tongue, tonsil, female breast, index finger, and, especially in MSM, the anus. The presenting complaints of an anal chancre include an anal sore or fissure and irritation or bleeding on defecation. Anal chancre must be ruled out in any anal fissure not at the 6 or 12 o'clock positions. When there is a secondary eruption, no visible chancre, and the glands below Poupart's ligament are markedly enlarged, anal chancre should be suspected.

Atypical chancres are common (Fig. 18-3). Simultaneous infection by a spirochete and another microbial agent may produce an atypical chancre. The mixed chancre caused by infection with *Haemophilus ducreyi* and *T. pallidum* will produce a lesion that runs a course different from either chancroid or primary syphilis alone. Such a sore begins a few days after exposure, since the incubation period for chancroid is short, and later the sore may transform into an indurated syphilitic lesion. A phagedenic chancre results from the combination of a syphilitic chancre and contaminating bacteria that may cause severe tissue destruction and result in scarring. Edema indurativum, or penile venereal edema, is marked solid edema of the labia or the prepuce and glans penis accompanying a chancre. Chancre redux is relapse of a chancre with insufficient treatment. It is accompanied by enlarged lymph nodes. Pseudochancre redux is a gumma occurring at the site of a

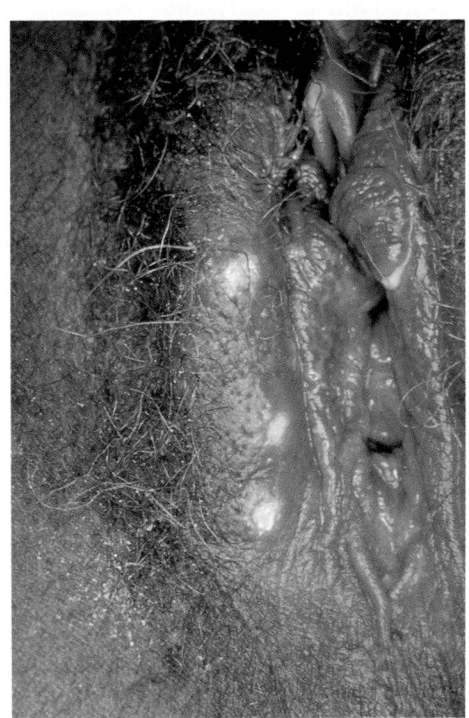

Fig. 18-2 Multiple chancres in a woman.

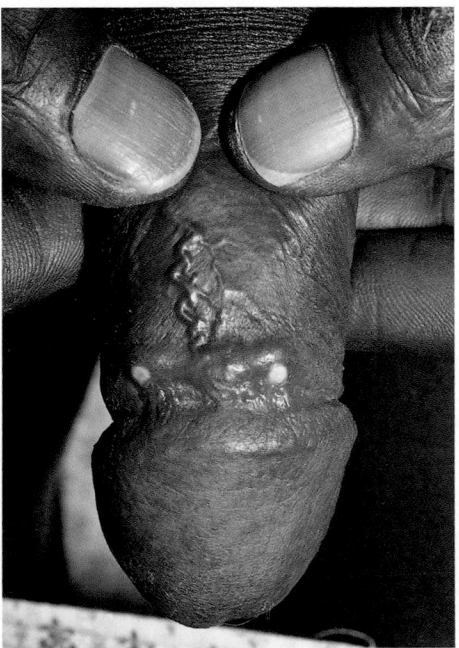

Fig. 18-3 Primary syphilis, atypical chancres, diagnosis confirmed by biopsy.

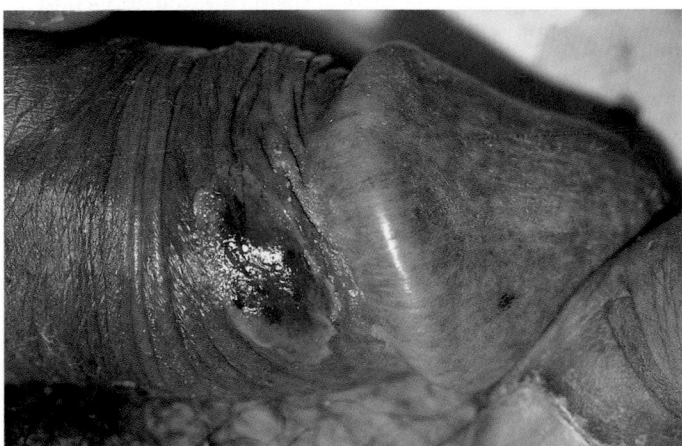

Fig. 18-1 Primary syphilis, chancre.

previous chancre. It is distinguished from relapsing chancre by the absence of lymphadenopathy and a negative darkfield examination. Syphilitic balanitis of Follmann may occur in the absence of a chancre. The lesions may be exudative, circinate, or erosive.

Histologic evaluation of a syphilitic chancre reveals an ulcer covered by neutrophils and fibrin. Subjacent there is a dense infiltrate of lymphocytes and plasma cells. Blood vessels are prominent with plump endothelial cells. Spirochetes are numerous in untreated chancres and can be demonstrated with an appropriate silver stain, such as the Warthin–Starry, Levaditi, or Steiner methods, or by immunoperoxidase staining. They are best found in the overlying epithelium or adjacent or overlying blood vessels in the upper dermis.

In a patient who presents with an acute genital ulceration, a darkfield examination should be performed if this investigation is available. The finding of typical *T. pallidum* in a sore on the cutaneous surface establishes a diagnosis of syphilis. *Treponema pertenue*, which causes yaws, and *Treponema carateum*, which causes pinta, are both indistinguishable morphologically from *T. pallidum*, but the diseases that they produce are usually easy to recognize. Commensal spirochetes of the oral mucosa are indistinguishable from *T. pallidum*, making oral darkfield examinations unreliable. If the darkfield examination results are negative, the examination should be repeated daily for several days, especially if the patient has been applying any topical antibacterial agents.

The lesion selected for examination is cleansed with water and dried. It is grasped firmly between the thumb and index finger and abraded sufficiently to cause clear or faintly blood-stained plasma to exude when squeezed. In the case of an eroded chancre, a few vigorous rubs with dry gauze are usually sufficient. If the lesion is made to bleed, it is necessary to wait until free bleeding has stopped to obtain satisfactory plasma. The surface of a clean coverslip is touched to the surface of the lesion so that plasma adheres. Then it is dropped on a slide and pressed down so that the plasma spreads out in as thin a film as possible. Immersion oil forms the interface between the condenser and slide and between the coverslip and objective. The specimen must be examined quickly, before the thin film of plasma dries.

An alternative to darkfield microscopy is the direct fluorescent antibody test (DFAT-TP) for the identification of *T. pallidum* in lesions. Serous exudate from a suspected lesion is collected as described above, placed on a slide, and allowed to dry. Many health departments will examine such specimens with fluorescent antibodies specific to *T. pallidum*. The method, unlike the darkfield examination, can be used for diagnosing oral lesions. Multiplex polymerase chain reaction (PCR) is also an accurate and reproducible method for diagnosing genital ulcerations. It has the advantage of being able to diagnose multiple infectious agents simultaneously. In genital ulcer disease outbreaks it should be made available.

The results of serologic tests for syphilis are positive in 75% (nontreponemal tests) to 90% (treponemal tests) of patients with primary syphilis; both these tests should be performed in every patient with suspected primary syphilis. The likelihood of positivity depends on the duration of infection. If the chancre has been present for several weeks, test results are usually positive.

A syphilitic chancre must be differentiated from chancroid. The chancre has an incubation period of 3 weeks; is usually a painless erosion, not an ulcer; has no surrounding inflammatory zone; and is round or oval. The edge is not undermined, and the surface is smooth and at the level of the skin. It has a dark, velvety red, lacquered appearance, is without an overlying membrane, and is cartilage-hard on palpation. Lymphadenopathy may be bilateral and is nontender and

nonsuppurative. Chancroid, on the other hand, has a short incubation period of 4–7 days; the ulcer is acutely inflamed, is extremely painful, and has a surrounding inflammatory zone. The ulcer edge is undermined and extends into the dermis. It is covered by a membrane, and is soft to the touch. Lymphadenopathy is usually unilateral and tender, and may suppurate. Chancroid lesions are usually multiple and extend into each other. Darkfield examination and cultures for chancroid confirm the diagnosis. However, since a combination of a syphilitic chancre and chancroid (mixed sores) is indistinguishable from chancroid alone, appropriate direct and serologic testing should be performed to investigate the presence of syphilis. Multiplex PCR allows for the simultaneous diagnosis of multiple infectious agents in genital ulcer diseases.

The primary lesion of granuloma inguinale begins as an indurated nodule that erodes to produce hypertrophic, vegetative granulation tissue. It is soft and beefy-red, and bleeds readily. A smear of clean granulation tissue from the lesion stained with Wright or Giemsa stain reveals Donovan bodies in the cytoplasm of macrophages.

The primary lesion of lymphogranuloma venereum (LGV) is usually a small, painless, transient papule or a superficial nonindurated ulcer. It most commonly occurs on the coronal sulcus, prepuce, or glans in men, or on the fourchette, vagina, or cervix in women. A primary genital lesion is noticed by about 30% of infected heterosexual men, but less frequently in women. Primary lesions are followed in 7–30 days by adenopathy of the regional lymph nodes. LGV is confirmed by serologic tests.

Herpes simplex begins with grouped vesicles, often accompanied or preceded by burning pain. After rupture of the vesicles, irregular, tender, soft erosions form.

Secondary syphilis

Cutaneous lesions

The skin manifestations of secondary syphilis have been called syphilids and occur in 80% or more of cases of secondary syphilis. The early eruptions are symmetrical, more or less generalized, superficial, nondestructive, exanthematic, transient, and macular; later they are maculopapular or papular eruptions, which are usually polymorphous, and less often scaly, pustular, or pigmented. The early manifestations are apt to be distributed over the face, shoulders, flanks, palms and soles, and anal or genital regions. The severity varies widely. The presence of lesions on the palms and soles is strongly suggestive. However, a generalized syphilid can spare the palms and soles. The individual lesions are generally less than 1 cm in diameter, except in the later secondary or relapsing secondary eruptions.

Macular eruptions The earliest form of macular secondary syphilis begins with the appearance of an exanthematic erythema 6–8 weeks after the development of the chancre, which may still be present. The syphilitic exanthem extends rapidly, so that it is usually pronounced a few days after onset. It may be evanescent, lasting only a few hours or days, or it may last several months, or partially recur after having disappeared. This macular eruption appears first on the sides of the trunk, about the navel, and on the inner surfaces of the extremities.

Individual lesions of macular secondary syphilis consist of round indistinct macules that are nonconfluent and may rarely be slightly elevated or urticarial. The color varies from a light pink or rose to brownish-red. The macular eruption may not be noticed on black skin and may be so faint that it is not recognized on other skin colors also. Pain, burning, and itching are usually absent, although pruritus may be present in 10–40% of cases. Simultaneous with the onset of the eruption there is a generalized shotty adenopathy most readily palpable in

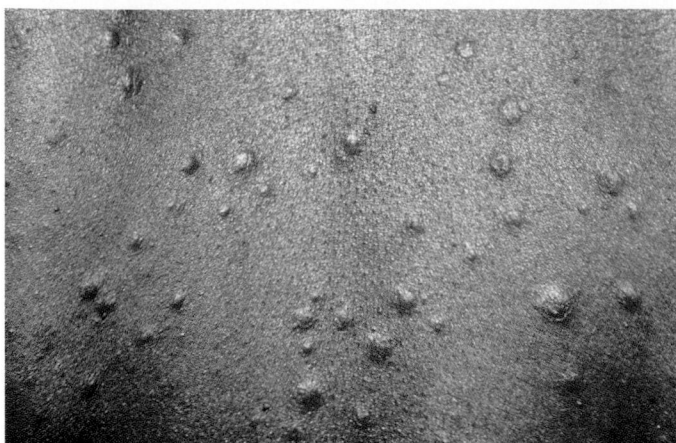

Fig. 18-4 Secondary syphilis.

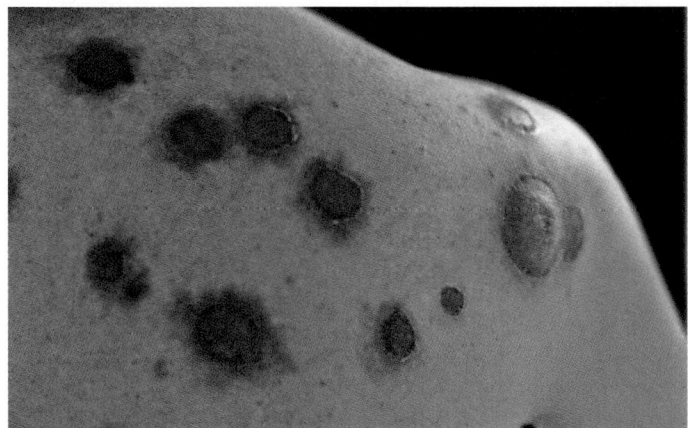

Fig. 18-5 Secondary syphilis, late, larger lesions.

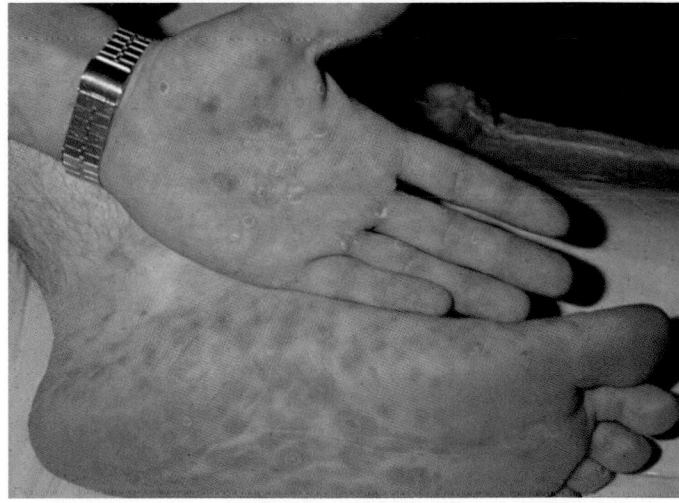

Fig. 18-6 Secondary syphilis, red flat-topped papules of the palms and soles.

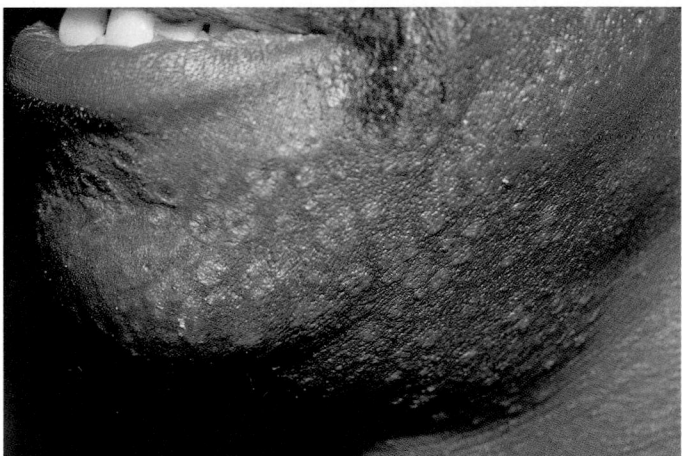

Fig. 18-7 Annular secondary syphilis.

the posterior cervical, axillary, and epitrochlear areas. Rarely, secondary syphilis may cause livedo reticularis. The macular eruption may disappear spontaneously after a few days or weeks without any residuum, or may result in postinflammatory hyperpigmentation. After a varying interval, macular syphilis may be followed by other eruptions.

Papular eruptions The papular types of eruption usually arise a little later than the macular. The fully developed lesions are of a raw ham or coppery shade, and round. While most frequently lesions are from 2 to 5 mm in diameter, nodules coalescing to large plaques can occur (Figs 18-4 and 18-5). They are often only slightly raised, but a deep, firm infiltration is palpable. The surface is smooth, sometimes shiny, and at other times covered with a thick, adherent scale. When this desquamates, it leaves a characteristic collarette of scales overhanging the border of the papule.

Papules are frequently distributed on the face and flexures of the arms and lower legs but are often distributed all over the trunk. Palmar and plantar involvement characteristically appears as indurated, yellowish-red spots (Fig. 18-6). Ollendorf's sign is present; the papule is exquisitely tender to the touch of a blunt probe. Healing lesions frequently leave hyperpigmented spots that, especially on the palms and soles, may persist for weeks or months. Split papules are hypertrophic, fissured papules that form in the creases of the alae nasi and at the oral commissures. These may persist for a long period. The papulosquamous syphilids, in which the adherent scales covering the lesions more or less dominate the picture, may produce a psoriasiform eruption. Follicular or lichenoid syphilids, which occur much less frequently, appear as minute

scale-capped papules. If they are at the ostia of hair follicles, they are likely to be conical; elsewhere on the skin, they are domed. Often they are grouped to form scaling plaques in which the minute coalescing papules are still discernible.

Like the other syphilids, papular eruptions tend to be disseminated but may also be localized, asymmetrical, configurate, hypertrophic, or confluent. The arrangement may be corymbose or in patches, rings, or serpiginous patterns.

The annular syphilid, like sarcoidosis (which it may mimic), is more common in blacks (Fig. 18-7). It is often located on the cheeks, especially close to the angle of the mouth. Here it may form annular, arcuate, or gyrate patterns of delicate, slightly raised, infiltrated, finely scaling ridges. These ridges are made up of minute, flat-topped papules, and the boundaries between ridges may be difficult to discern. An old term for annular syphilids was nickels and dimes.

The corymbose syphilid is another infrequent variant, usually occurring late in the secondary stage, in which a large central papule is surrounded by a group of minute satellite papules. The pustular syphilids are among the rarer manifestations of secondary syphilis. They occur widely scattered over the trunk and extremities, but they usually involve the face, especially the forehead. The pustule usually arises on a red, infiltrated base. Involution is usually slow, resulting in a small, rather persistent, crust-covered, superficial ulceration. Lesions in which the ulceration is deep are called ecthymatous. Closely related is the rupial syphilid, a lesion in which a relatively

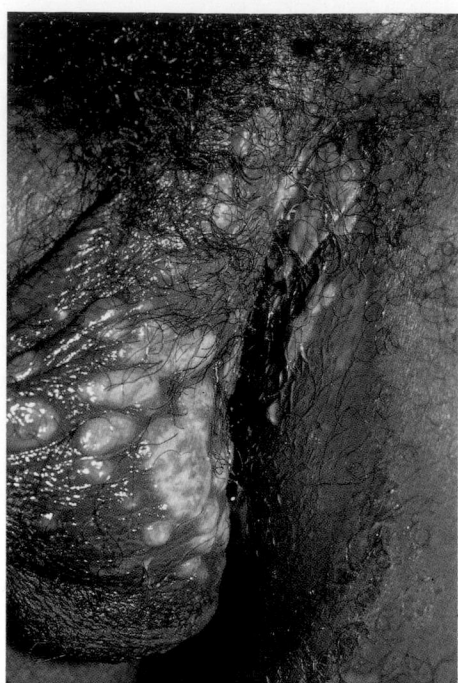

Fig. 18-8 Condylomata of the scrotum.

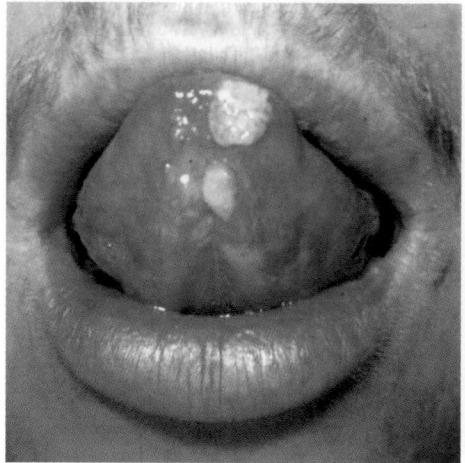

Fig. 18-9 Mucous patches of secondary syphilis.

superficial ulceration is covered with a pile of terraced crusts resembling an oyster shell. Lues maligna is a rare form of secondary syphilis with severe ulcerations, pustules, or rupioid lesions, accompanied by severe constitutional symptoms.

Condylomata lata are papular lesions, relatively broad and flat, located on folds of moist skin, especially about the genitalia and anus; they may become hypertrophic and, instead of infiltrating deeply, protrude above the surface, forming a soft, red, often mushroom-like mass 1–3 cm in diameter, usually with a smooth, moist, weeping, gray surface (Fig. 18-8). Condyloma lata may be lobulated but are not covered by the digitate elevations characteristic of venereal warts (condylomata acuminata).

Syphilitic alopecia is irregularly distributed so that the scalp has a moth-eaten appearance. It is unusual, occurring in about 5% of patients with secondary syphilis. Smooth circular areas of alopecia mimicking alopecia areata may occur in syphilis, and an ophiasis pattern may rarely be seen.

Mucous membrane lesions are present in one-third of patients with secondary syphilis; they may be the only manifestation of the infection. The most common mucosal lesion in the early phase is the syphilitic sore throat, a diffuse pharyngitis that may be associated with tonsillitis or laryngitis. Hoarseness and sometimes complete aphonia may be present. On the tongue, smooth, small or large, well-defined patches devoid of papillae may be seen (Fig. 18-9), most frequently on the dorsum near the median raphe. Ulcerations may occur on the tongue and lips during the late secondary period, at times resembling aphthae or major aphthae. A rare variant of syphilis is one presenting with oral and cutaneous erosions that histologically show the features of pemphigus vulgaris with a suprabasilar acantholytic blister and positive direct and indirect immunofluorescence finding of pemphigus as well.

Mucous patches are the most characteristic mucous membrane lesions of secondary syphilis. They are macerated, flat, grayish, rounded erosions covered by a delicate, soggy membrane. These highly infectious lesions are about 5 mm in diameter and teem with treponema. They occur on the tonsils, tongue, pharynx, gums, lips, and buccal areas, or on the genitalia, chiefly in women. In the latter they are most common on the labia minora, vaginal mucosa, and cervix. Such mucous erosions are transitory and change from week to week, or even from day to day.

Relapsing secondary syphilis

The early lesions of syphilis undergo involution either spontaneously or with treatment. Relapses occur in about 25% of untreated patients, 90% within the first year. Such relapses may take place at the site of previous lesions, on the skin or in the viscera. Recurrent eruptions tend to be more configurate or annular, larger, and asymmetrical.

Systemic involvement

The lymphatic system in secondary syphilis is characteristically involved. The lymph nodes most frequently affected are the inguinal, posterior cervical, postauricular, and epitrochlear. The nodes are shotty, firm, slightly enlarged, nontender, and discrete.

Acute glomerulonephritis, gastritis or gastric ulceration, proctitis, hepatitis, acute meningitis, unilateral sensorineural hearing loss, iritis, anterior uveitis, optic neuritis, Bell palsy, multiple pulmonary nodular infiltrates, periostitis, osteomyelitis, polyarthritis, and tenosynovitis may all be seen in secondary syphilis.

Histopathology

Macules of secondary syphilis feature superficial and deep perivascular infiltrates of lymphocytes, macrophages, and plasma cells without epidermal change, or accompanied by slight vacuolar change at the dermoepidermal junction.

Papules and plaques of secondary syphilis usually show dense superficial and deep infiltrates of lymphocytes, macrophages, and plasma cells. These cells are usually distributed in a bandlike pattern in the papillary dermis and cuffed around blood vessels, accompanied by psoriasiform epidermal hyperplasia and hyperkeratosis. Clusters of neutrophils are commonly present within the stratum corneum. The presence of numerous macrophages often gives the infiltrates a pallid appearance under scanning magnification. Vacuolar degeneration of keratinocytes is often present, giving the lesions a "psoriasiform and lichenoid" histologic pattern with slender elongated rete ridges. Plasma cells are said to be absent in 10–30% of cases. As lesions age, macrophages become more numerous, so that in late secondary lues, granulomatous foci are often present, mimicking sarcoidosis. Condylomata lata show spongiform pustules within areas of papillated epithelial hyperplasia and spirochetes are numerous. Spirochetes are most numerous within the epidermis and around superficial vessels. PCR and immunoperoxidase may identify *T. pallidum* infection when silver stains are negative.

Diagnosis and differential diagnosis

The nontreponemal serologic tests for syphilis are almost invariably strongly reactive in secondary syphilis. An exception occurs when very high titers of antibody are present, producing a false-negative result (prozone phenomenon). The true positivity of the serum is detected on dilutional testing. Identification of spirochetes by darkfield examination or histologic examination of affected tissues may be used to confirm the diagnosis, especially in patients who are seronegative.

Syphilis has long been known as the "great imitator," because the various cutaneous manifestations may simulate almost any cutaneous or systemic disease. Pityriasis rosea may be mistaken for secondary syphilis, especially since both begin on the trunk. The herald patch, the oval patches with a fine scale at the edge, patterned in the lines of skin cleavage, the absence of lymphadenopathy, and infrequent mucous membrane lesions help to distinguish pityriasis rosea from secondary syphilis. Drug eruptions may produce a similar picture; however, they tend to be scarlatiniform or morbilliform. Drug eruptions are often pruritic, whereas secondary syphilis usually is not. Lichen planus may resemble papular syphilid. The characteristic papule of lichen planus is flat-topped and polygonal, has Wickham's striae, and exhibits the Koebner phenomenon. Pruritus is severe in lichen planus, and less common and less severe in syphilis. Psoriasis may be distinguished from papulosquamous secondary syphilis by the presence of adenopathy, mucous patches, and alopecia in the latter. Sarcoidosis may produce lesions morphologically identical to secondary syphilis. Histologically, multisystem involvement, adenopathy, and granulomatous inflammation are common to both diseases. Serologic testing and biopsy specimens will distinguish these two disorders.

The differential diagnosis of mucous membrane lesions of secondary syphilis is of importance. Infectious mononucleosis may cause a biologic false-positive test for syphilis but is diagnosed by a high heterophile antibody titer. Geographic tongue may be confused with the desquamative patches of syphilis or with mucous patches. Lingua geographica occurs principally near the edges of the tongue in relatively large areas, which are often fused and have lobulated contours. It continues for several months or years and changes in extent and degree of involvement from day to day. Recurrent aphthous ulceration produces one or several painful ulcers, 1–3 mm in diameter, surrounded by hyperemic edges, with a grayish covering membrane, on nonkeratinized mucosal epithelium, especially in the gingival sulcus. A prolonged, recurrent history is characteristic. Syphilis of the lateral tongue may resemble oral hairy leukoplakia.

Latent syphilis

After the lesions of secondary syphilis have involuted, a latent period occurs. This may last for a few months or continue for the remainder of the infected person's life. Between 60% and 70% of untreated infected patients remain latently asymptomatic for life. During this latent period there are no clinical signs of syphilis, but the serologic tests for syphilis are reactive. During the early latent period infectivity persists; for at least 2 years a woman with early latent syphilis may infect her unborn child. For treatment purposes it is important to distinguish early latency (less than 1 year's duration) from late latency (of more than 1 year or unknown duration).

Late syphilis

For treatment purposes, late syphilis is defined by the CDC as infection of more than 1 year in duration, or by the WHO as more than 2 years in duration. Only about one-third of

patients with late syphilis will develop complications of their infection.

Tertiary cutaneous syphilis

Tertiary syphilids most often occur 3–5 years after infection. Around 16% of untreated patients will develop tertiary lesions of the skin, mucous membrane, bone, or joints. Skin lesions tend to be localized, to occur in groups, to be destructive, and to heal with scarring. Treponema are usually not found by silver stains or darkfield examination but may be demonstrated by PCR.

Two main types of tertiary syphilid are recognized, the nodular syphilid and the gumma, although the distinction is sometimes difficult to make. The nodular, noduloulcerative, or tubercular type consists of reddish-brown or copper-colored firm papules or nodules, 2 mm in diameter or larger. The individual lesions are usually covered with adherent scales or crusts (Fig. 18-10). The lesions tend to form rings and to undergo involution as new lesions develop just beyond them, so that characteristic circular or serpiginous patterns are produced. A distinctive and characteristic type is the kidney-shaped lesion. These frequently occur on the extensor surfaces of the arms and on the back. Individual lesions are composed of nodules in different stages of development so that it is common to find scars and pigmentation together with fresh and also ulcerated lesions. On the face the nodular eruption closely resembles lupus vulgaris. When the disease is untreated, the process may last for years, slowly marching across large areas of skin. The nodules may enlarge and eventually break down to form painless, rounded, smooth-bottomed ulcers, a few millimeters deep. These punched-out ulcers arise side by side and form serpiginous syphilitic ulcers, palm-sized in aggregate, enduring for many years (Fig. 18-11).

Gummas may occur as unilateral, isolated, single or disseminated lesions, or in serpiginous patterns resembling those of the nodular syphilid. They may be restricted to the skin or, originating in the deeper tissues, break down and secondarily involve the skin. The individual lesions, which begin as small nodules, slowly enlarge to several centimeters. Central necrosis is extensive and may lead to the formation of a deep

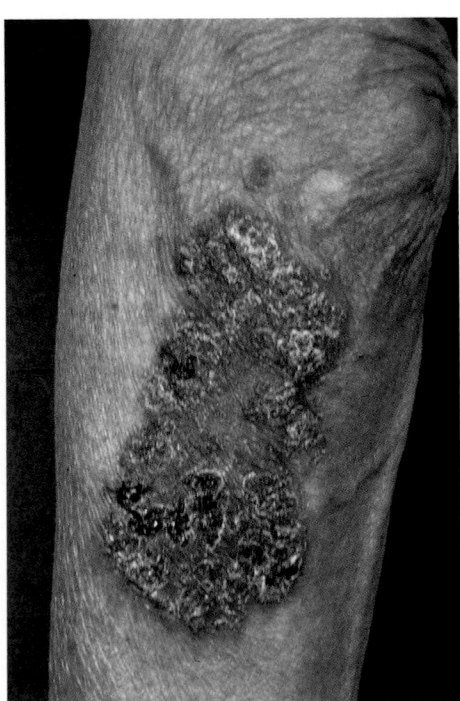

Fig. 18-10 Tertiary syphilis.

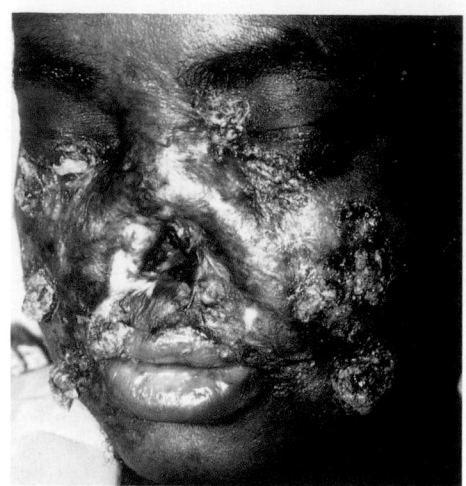

Fig. 18-11 Destruction of the central face in tertiary syphilis.

punched-out ulcer with steep sides and a gelatinous, necrotic base. Again, progression may take place in one area while healing proceeds in another. Perhaps the most frequent site of isolated gummas is the lower legs, where deep punched-out ulcers are formed, often in large infiltrated areas. On the lower extremities gummas are frequently mistaken for erythema induratum.

Lesions may be isolated to the mucous membranes, often the tongue, on which non-indurated punched-out ulcers occur. A superficial glossitis may cause irregular ulcers, atrophy of the papillae, and smooth, shiny scarring, a condition known as smooth atrophy. In interstitial glossitis there is an underlying induration. In the advanced stages, tertiary syphilis of the tongue may lead to a diffuse enlargement (macroglossia). Perforation of the hard palate from gummatous involvement is a characteristic tertiary manifestation. It generally occurs near the center of the hard palate. Destruction of the nasal septum may also occur.

Histologically, nodular lesions of late syphilis usually have changes that resemble those of secondary lesions, with the addition of tuberculoid granulomas containing varying numbers of multinucleate giant cells. The epidermis is often atrophic rather than hyperplastic. In gummas, there is necrosis within granulomas and fibrosis as lesions resolve. Spirochetes are scant.

For diagnosis of late syphilis clinicians rely heavily on specific treponemal tests. The nontreponemal tests, such as the VDRL and RPR, are positive in approximately 60% of cases. When there are mucous membrane lesions for which a diagnosis of carcinoma must also be considered, histologic examination is performed. Darkfield examination is not indicated, since it is always negative, but PCR of biopsy material may be positive. When not ulcerated, lesions of tertiary syphilis must be distinguished from malignant tumors, leukemids, and sarcoidosis. The ulcerated tertiary syphilids must be differentiated from other infections such as scrofuloderma, atypical mycobacterial infection, and deep fungal infections. Wegener's granulomatosis and ulcerated cutaneous malignancies must be considered Histology and appropriate cultures may be required.

Late osseous syphilis

Not infrequently, gummatous lesions involve the periosteum and the bone. Skeletal tertiary syphilis most commonly affects the head and face, and the tibia. Late manifestations of syphilis may produce periostitis, osteomyelitis, osteitis, and gummatous osteoarthritis. Osteocope (bone pain), most often at night, is a suggestive symptom.

Syphilitic joint lesions also occur, with the Charcot joint being the most prevalent manifestation. They are often associated with tabes dorsalis and occur most frequently in men. Although any joint may be involved, the knees and ankles are the most frequently affected. There is hydrops, then loss of the contours of the joint, hypermobility, and no pain. It is readily diagnosed by x-ray examination.

Neurosyphilis

Central nervous system (CNS) infection can occur at any stage of syphilis, even the primary stage. Most persons with CNS involvement have no symptoms. Finding cerebrospinal fluid (CSF) pleocytosis or a positive CSF VDRL has been used to confirm the diagnosis of CNS infection by *T. pallidum*. Unfortunately, a significant proportion of patients with CSF infection with *T. pallidum* will have a negative CSF-VDRL (46%) and non-diagnostic CSF pleocytosis (less than 20 white blood cells/μL) (33%). In patients with a negative CSF-VDRL but pleocytosis, an FTA can be performed on the CSF and is 100% sensitive but not specific for CNS syphilis. Combining this with flow cytometry to look for B cells in the CSF, which is 100% specific but only 40% sensitive, will allow the confirmation or exclusion of neurosyphilis in most cases with CSF pleocytosis. The likelihood of having CNS infection is ten-fold greater in persons with an RPR of greater than or equal to 1:32. Between 4% and 9% of persons with untreated syphilis will develop clinically symptomatic neurosyphilis, often during the first year or two of infection (while they have "early" syphilis). HIV-negative persons with negative CSF examinations have almost no risk of developing neurosyphilis; however, CSF evaluations are not routinely performed in asymptomatic persons with early syphilis, so identifying those at risk for symptomic neurosyphilis is problematic. Infection of the CNS by *T. pallidum* may also be strain-dependent, and eventually typing the infecting strain may predict those at highest risk for neurosyphilis.

Because infection of the CNS is common and the recommended treatments with benzathine penicillin do not reach treponemacidal levels in the CSF, there has been persistent concern regarding the failure to diagnose and treat asymptomatic neurosyphilis. It appears that, although treatment does not clear the spirochetes from the CSF, most non-HIV-infected persons are able to clear the CNS infection spontaneously. CSF evaluation is recommended in all patients with syphilis with any neurologic, auditory, or ophthalmic signs or symptoms, possibly resulting from syphilis, independent of stage or HIV status. In borderline cases, those with an RPR of greater than or equal to 1:32 should have CSF evaluation. All HIV-positive patients with RPR greater than or equal to 1:32 should be considered for immediate CSF evaluation, regardless of symptoms, especially if their CD4 count is 350 cells/μL or less. Patients with latent syphilis should have CSF evaluation if they are HIV-positive or fail initial therapy, or if therapy other than penicillin is planned for syphilis of more than 1 year in duration. Patients with tertiary syphilis should have CSF evaluation before treatment to exclude neurosyphilis. An appropriate fall in the serum RPR after treatment for neurosyphilis predicts clearing the CNS infection, so a repeat lumbar puncture following therapy is not required in HIV-negative or HIV-positive patients adequately treated for neurosyphilis.

Early neurosyphilis

Early neurosyphilis is mainly meningeal, occurring in the first year of infection. Meningeal neurosyphilis manifests as meningitis, with fever, headache, stiff neck, nausea, vomiting, cranial nerve disorders (loss of hearing, [often unilateral], facial weakness, photophobia, blurred vision), seizures, and delirium.

Meningovascular neurosyphilis

Meningovascular neurosyphilis most frequently occurs 4–7 years after infection. It is caused by thrombosis of vessels in the CNS and presents as in other CNS ischemic events. Hemiplegia, aphasia, hemianopsia, transverse myelitis, and progressive muscular atrophy may occur. Cranial nerve palsies may also occur, such as eighth nerve deafness and eye changes. The eyes may show fixed pupils, Argyll Robertson pupils, or anisocoria.

Late (parenchymatous) neurosyphilis

Parenchymatous neurosyphilis tends to occur more than 10 years after infection. There are two classic clinical patterns: tabes dorsalis and general paresis.

Tabes dorsalis is the degeneration of the dorsal roots of the spinal nerves and of the posterior columns of the spinal cord. The symptoms and signs are numerous. Gastric crisis with severe pain and vomiting is the most frequent symptom. Other symptoms are lancinating pains, urination difficulties, paresthesias (numbness, tingling, and burning), spinal ataxia, diplopia, strabismus, vertigo, and deafness. The signs that may be present are Argyll Robertson pupils, absent or reduced reflexes, Romberg sign, sensory loss (deep tendon tenderness, vibration, and position), atonic bladder, trophic changes, malum perforans pedis, Charcot joints, and optic atrophy.

Paresis has prodromal manifestations of headache, fatigability, and inability to concentrate. Later, personality changes occur, along with memory loss and apathy. Grandiose ideas, megalomania, delusions, hallucinations, and finally dementia may occur.

Late cardiovascular syphilis

Late cardiovascular syphilis occurs in about 10% of untreated patients. Aortitis is the basic lesion of cardiovascular syphilis, resulting in aortic insufficiency, coronary disease, and ultimately aortic aneurysm.

Congenital syphilis

Congenital syphilis has reappeared with heterosexual syphilis epidemics in the UK. In sub-Saharan Africa, where prenatal syphilis testing is not available, even for women with prenatal care, congenital syphilis is common. A total of 21% of all perinatal deaths in sub-Saharan Africa are due to congenital syphilis. Prenatal syphilis is acquired in utero from the mother, who usually has early syphilis. Infection through the placenta usually does not occur before the fourth month, so treatment of the mother within the first two trimesters will almost always prevent negative outcomes. If the mother has early syphilis and prenatal infection occurs soon after the fourth month, fetal death and miscarriage occur in about 40% of pregnancies. During the remainder of the pregnancy, infection is equally likely to produce characteristic developmental physical stigmata or, after the eighth month, active, infectious congenital syphilis. Forty percent of pregnancies in women with untreated early syphilis will result in a syphilitic infant. Infant mortality from congenital syphilis can be in excess of 10%. In utero infection of the fetus is rare when the pregnant mother has had syphilis for 2 or more years. Two-thirds of neonates with congenital syphilis are normal at birth, and only detected by serologic testing. Lesions occurring within the first 2 years of life are called early congenital syphilis and those developing thereafter are called late congenital syphilis. The clinical manifestations of these two syndromes are different.

Early congenital syphilis

Early congenital syphilis describes those cases presenting within the first 2 years of life. Cutaneous manifestations appear most commonly during the third week of life, but sometimes occur as late as 3 months after birth. Neonates born with findings of congenital syphilis are usually severely affected. They may be premature, and are often marasmic, fretful, and dehydrated. The face is pinched and drawn, resembling that of an old man or woman. Multisystem disease is characteristic.

Snuffles, a form of rhinitis, is the most frequent and often the first specific finding. The nose is blocked, often with blood-stained mucus, and a copious discharge of mucus runs down over the lips. The nasal obstruction often interferes with the child's nursing. In persistent and progressive cases, ulcerations develop that may involve the bones and ultimately cause perforation of the nasal septum or development of saddle nose, which are important stigmata later in the disease.

Cutaneous lesions of congenital syphilis resemble those of acquired secondary syphilis and occur in 30–60% of infants with syphilis. The early skin eruptions are usually morbilliform, and more rarely, purely papular. The lesions are at first a bright or violaceous red, later fading to a coppery color. The papules may become large and infiltrated; frequently scaling is pronounced. There is secondary pustule formation with crusting, especially in lesions that appear 1 or more years after birth. The eruption shows a marked predilection for the face, arms, buttocks, legs, palms, and soles.

Syphilitic pemphigus, a bullous eruption, usually on the palms and soles, is a relatively uncommon lesion. Lesions are present at birth or appear in the first week of life. They are teeming with spirochetes. The bullae quickly become purulent and rupture, leaving weeping erosions. They are found also on the eponychium, wrists, ankles, and, infrequently, other parts of the body. Even in the absence of bullous lesions, desquamation is common, often preceded by edema and erythema, especially on the palms and soles.

Various morphologies of cutaneous lesions occur on the face, perineum, and intertriginous areas. They are usually fissured lesions resembling mucous patches. In these sites radial scarring often results, leading to rhagades. Condylomata lata, large, moist, hypertrophic papules, are found about the anus and in other folds of the body. They are more common around the first year of life than in the newborn period. In the second or third year, recurrent secondary eruptions are likely to take the papulopustular form. Annular lesions similar to those in adults occur. Mucous patches in the mouth or on the vulva are seen infrequently.

Bone lesions occur in 70–80% of cases of early congenital syphilis. Epiphysitis is common and apparently causes pain on motion, leading to the infant's refusing to move (Parrot pseudoparalysis). Radiologic features of the bone lesions in congenital syphilis during the first 6 months after birth are quite characteristic, and x-ray films are an important part of the evaluation of a child suspected of having congenital syphilis. Bone lesions occur chiefly at the epiphyseal ends of the long bones. The changes may be classified as osteochondritis, osteomyelitis, and osteoperiostitis.

A general enlargement of the lymph nodes usually occurs, with enlargement of the spleen. Clinical evidence of involvement of the liver is common, manifested both by hepatomegaly and elevated liver function test results, and interstitial hepatitis is a frequent finding at autopsy. The nephrotic syndrome, and less commonly, acute glomerulonephritis have been reported in congenital syphilis.

Symptomatic or asymptomatic neurosyphilis, as demonstrated by a positive CSF serologic test, may be present. Eighty-six percent of infants with congenital syphilis diagnosed by clinical and laboratory findings born to mothers with untreated early syphilis will have CNS involvement, compared with only 8% of those with no clinical or laboratory findings. All infants with early congenital syphilis are treated as if they have neurosyphilis since it is very common, and CSF-VDRL may be negative, even in documented CNS infection. Clinical manifestations may not appear until the third to sixth month of life and are meningeal or meningovascular in origin. Meningitis, obstructive hydrocephalus, cranial nerve palsies, and cerebrovascular accidents may all occur.

Late congenital syphilis

Although no sharp line can be drawn between early and late congenital syphilis, children who appear normal at birth and develop the first signs of the disease after the age of 2 years show a different clinical picture. Lesions of late congenital syphilis are of two types: malformations of tissue affected at critical growth periods (stigmata) and persistent inflammatory foci.

Inflammatory late congenital syphilis

Lesions of the cornea, bones, and CNS are the most important. Interstitial keratitis, which begins with intense pericorneal inflammation and persists to characteristic diffuse clouding of the cornea without surface ulceration, occurs in 20–50% of cases of late congenital syphilis. If persistent, it leads to permanent partial or complete opacity of the cornea. Syphilitic interstitial keratitis must be differentiated from Cogan syndrome, consisting of nonsyphilitic interstitial keratitis, usually bilateral, associated with vestibuloauditory symptoms, such as deafness, tinnitus, vertigo, nystagmus, and ataxia. It is congenital.

Perisynovitis (Clutton joints), which affects the knees, leads to symmetrical, painless swelling. Gummas may also be found in any of the long bones or in the skull. Ulcerating gummas are frequently seen. They probably begin more often in the soft parts or in the underlying bone than in the skin itself, and when they occur in the nasal septum or palate, may lead to painless perforation.

The CNS lesions in late congenital syphilis are, as in late adult neurosyphilis, usually parenchymatous (tabes dorsalis or generalized paresis). Seizures are a frequent symptom in congenital cases.

Malformations (stigmata)

The destructive effects of syphilis in young children often leave scars or developmental defects called stigmata, which persist throughout life and enable a diagnosis to be made of congenital syphilis. Hutchinson emphasized the diagnostic importance of changes in the incisor teeth, opacities of the cornea, and eighth nerve deafness, which have since become known as the Hutchinson triad. Hutchinson's teeth, corneal scars, saber shins, rhagades of the lips, saddle nose, and mulberry molars are of diagnostic importance. (Fig. 18-12).

Hutchinson's teeth are a malformation of the central upper incisors that appear in the second or permanent teeth. The characteristic teeth are cylindrical rather than flattened, the cutting edge is narrower than the base, and in the center of the cutting edge a notch may develop (Fig. 18-13). The mulberry molar (usually the first molar, appearing about the age of 6 years) is a hyperplastic tooth, the flat occlusal surface of which is covered with a group of little knobs representing abortive cusps. Nasal chondritis in infancy results in flattening of the nasal bones, forming a so-called saddle nose. The unilateral thickening of the inner third of one clavicle (Higouménaki's sign) is a hyperostosis resulting from syphilitic osteitis in individuals who have had late congenital syphilis. The lesion appears typically on the right side in right-handed persons and on the left side in left-handed persons.

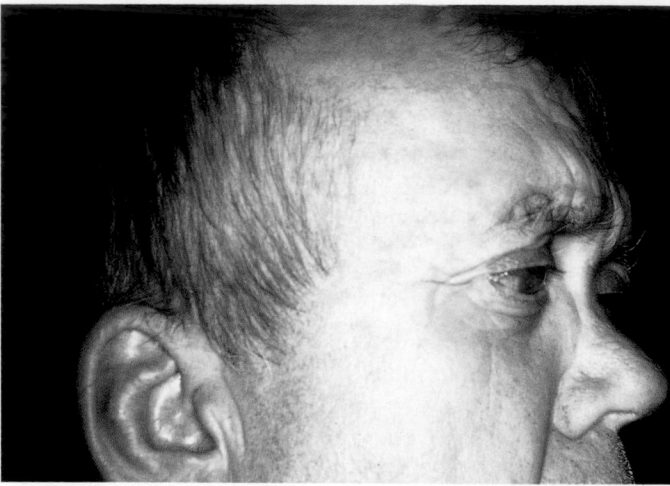

Fig. 18-12 Frontal bossing, interstitial keratitis and saddle nose in congenital syphilis.

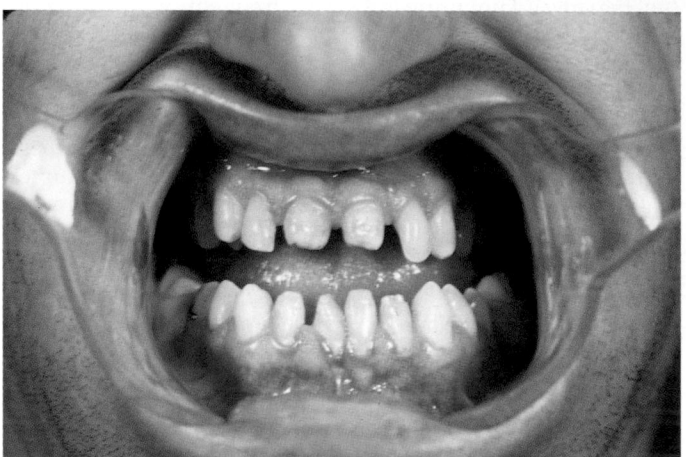

Fig. 18-13 Hutchinson's teeth.

Diagnosis

Infants of women who meet the following criteria should be evaluated for congenital syphilis:

1. maternal untreated syphilis, inadequate treatment, or no documentation of adequate treatment
2. treatment of maternal syphilis with erythromycin
3. treatment less than 1 month before delivery
4. inadequate maternal response to treatment
5. appropriate treatment before pregnancy, but insufficient serologic follow-up to document adequacy of therapy.

The results of serologic tests for syphilis for every woman delivering a baby must be known before the discharge of that baby from the hospital. Serologic testing of the mother and child at delivery are recommended. Evaluation of the children noted above might include:

1. a complete physical examination for findings of congenital syphilis
2. nontreponemal serology of the infant's serum (not cord blood)
3. CNS evaluation
4. pathologic evaluation of the placenta using specific antitreponemal antibody staining.

Treatment

Penicillin remains the drug of choice for treatment of all stages of syphilis. Erythromycin is not recommended for treatment of any stage or form of syphilis. HIV testing is recommended in all patients with syphilis. Treatment for HIV-infected patients is discussed later. Patients with primary, secondary, or early latent syphilis known to be of less than 1 year in duration can be treated with a single intramuscular injection of 2.4 MU of benzathine penicillin G. In nonpregnant, penicillin-allergic, HIV-negative patients, tetracycline, 500 mg orally four times a day, or doxycycline, 100 mg orally twice a day for 2 weeks, is recommended. Ceftriaxone, 1 g intramuscularly or intravenously for 8–10 days, is an acceptable alternative if the patient cannot tolerate the above options. Azithromycin and erythromycin can no longer be recommended as treatment for syphilis due to the widespread presence of resistance (over 75% in San Francisco). This is due to a mutation in the gene encoding a part of the ribosome responsible for the binding of macrolides. Close follow-up is recommended for all patients treated with non-penicillin-based regimens. These alternative agents are not recommended for persons with HIV infection and syphilis.

The recommended treatment of late or late latent syphilis of more than 1 year in duration in an HIV-negative patient is benzathine penicillin G 2.4 MU intramuscularly once a week for 3 weeks. In a penicillin-allergic, nonpregnant, HIV-negative patient, tetracycline, 500 mg orally four times a day, or doxycycline, 100 mg orally twice a day for 30 days, is recommended. CSF evaluation is recommended if neurologic or ophthalmologic findings are present, if there is evidence of active late (tertiary) syphilis, if treatment has previously failed, if the nontreponemal serum titer is 1:32 or higher, or if any regimen not based on penicillin is planned.

Recommended treatment regimens for neurosyphilis include penicillin G crystalline, 3–4 MU intravenously every 4 h for 10–14 days, or procaine penicillin, 2.4 MU/day intramuscularly, plus probenecid, 500 mg orally four times a day, both for 10–14 days. These regimens are shorter than those for treatment of late syphilis, so they may be followed by benzathine penicillin G, 2.4 MU intramuscularly, once a week for 3 weeks. Patients allergic to penicillin should have their allergy confirmed by skin testing. If allergy exists, desensitization and treatment with penicillin are recommended.

Treatment of congenital syphilis in the neonate is complex. Therapy should be undertaken in consultation with a pediatric infectious disease specialist. Management strategies can be found in the CDC *Guidelines for the Management of Sexually Transmitted Diseases*. Older children with congenital syphilis should have a CSF evaluation and be treated with aqueous crystalline penicillin G, 200000–300000 U/kg/day intravenously or intramuscularly (50 000 U every 4–6 h) for 10–14 days.

Pregnant women with syphilis should be treated with penicillin in doses appropriate for the stage of syphilis. A second dose of benzathine penicillin, 2.4 MU intramuscularly, may be administered 1 week after the initial dose in pregnant women with primary, secondary, or early latent syphilis. Sonographic evaluation of the fetus in the second half of pregnancy for signs of congenital infection may facilitate management and counseling. Expert consultation should be sought in cases where evidence of fetal syphilis is found, as fetal treatment failure is increased in this scenario. Follow-up quantitative serologic tests should be performed monthly until delivery. Pregnant women who are allergic to penicillin should be skin-tested and desensitized if test results are positive.

Jarisch–Herxheimer or Herxheimer reaction

A febrile reaction often occurs after the initial dose of antisyphilitic treatment, especially penicillin, is given. It occurs in about 60% of patients treated for seronegative primary syphilis, 90% of those with seropositive primary or secondary syphilis, and 30% of those with neurosyphilis. The reaction generally occurs 6–8 h after treatment and consists of shaking chills, fever, malaise, sore throat, myalgia, headache, tachycardia, and exacerbation of the inflammatory reaction at sites of localized spirochetal infection. A vesicular Herxheimer reaction can occur. A Herxheimer reaction in pregnancy may induce premature labor and fetal distress. Every effort should be made to avoid this complication. Early in pregnancy, women should rest and take acetaminophen for fever. Women treated after 20 weeks of pregnancy should seek obstetric evaluation if they experience fever, decreased fetal movement, or regular contractions within 24 h of treatment. An increase of inflammation in a vital structure may have serious consequences, as when there is an aneurysm of the aorta or iritis. When the CNS is involved, special importance is attached to avoiding the Herxheimer reaction, even though the paralyses that may result are often transitory. It is important to distinguish the Herxheimer reaction from a drug reaction to penicillin or other antibiotics. The reaction has also been described in other spirochetal diseases, such as leptospirosis and louse-borne relapsing fever.

Treatment of sex partners

Sexual partners of persons with syphilis should be identified. Persons who are exposed within 90 days of the diagnosis of primary, secondary, or early latent syphilis, even if seronegative, should be treated presumptively. If the exposure was longer than 90 days ago but follow-up is uncertain, presumptive treatment should be given. If the infectious source has a serologic titer of greater than 1:32, they should be presumed to have infectious early syphilis and sexual partners should be treated. At-risk partners are identified as those exposed within 3 months plus the duration of the primary lesions, for 6 months plus the duration of the secondary lesions, or 1 year for latent syphilis. Treatment of sexual partners is based on their clinical and serologic findings. If they are seronegative but had exposures as outlined above, treatment would be as for early syphilis, with benzathine penicillin, 2.4 MU intramuscularly as one dose.

Serologic testing after treatment

Before therapy and then regularly thereafter, quantitative VDRL or RPR testing should be performed on patients who are to be treated for syphilis to ensure appropriate response. For primary and secondary syphilis in an HIV-negative non-pregnant patient, testing is repeated every 3 months in the first year, every 6 months in the second year, and yearly thereafter. At least a four-fold decrease in titer would be expected 6 months after therapy, but 15% of patients with recommended treatment will not achieve this serologic response by 1 year. Patients with prior episodes of syphilis may respond more slowly. If response is inadequate, HIV testing (if HIV status is unknown) and CSF evaluation are recommended. For HIV-negative patients who fail to respond and who have a normal CSF evaluation, optimal management is unclear. Close follow-up must be assured. If it is decided to retreat the patient, 3-weekly injections of benzathine penicillin G, 2.4 MU, are recommended. A four-fold increase in serologic titer clearly indicates treatment failure or reinfection. These patients should have HIV testing and CSF analysis, with treatment determined by the results of these tests.

The serological response for patients with latent syphilis is slower, but a four-fold decrease in titer should be seen by 12–24 months. If no such response occurs, HIV testing and CSF evaluation are recommended. Patients treated for latent or late syphilis may be serofast, so that failure to observe a titer fall in these patients does not in itself indicate a need for retreatment. If the titer is less than 1:32, the possibility of a serofast state exists, and retreatment should be planned on an individual basis.

Seroreversion in specific treponemal tests can occur. By 36 months 24% of patients treated for early syphilis had a negative FTA-ABS and 13% a negative MHA-TP.

Syphilis and HIV disease

Syphilis and other genital ulcer diseases enhance the risk of transmission and acquisition of HIV. This may be due to the fact that early lesions of syphilis contain mononuclear cells with enhanced expression of CCR5, the coreceptor for HIV-1. HIV testing is recommended in all patients with syphilis.

Most HIV-infected patients with syphilis exhibit the classic clinical manifestations with appropriate serologic titers for that stage of disease. Response to treatment, both clinical and serologic in HIV-infected patients with syphilis, generally follow the clinical and serologic patterns seen in patients without coexisting HIV infection. In a large study that compared HIV-positive with HIV-negative patients with syphilis, the former were more likely to present with secondary syphilis (53% vs 33%) and were more likely to have a chancre that persisted when they had secondary syphilis (43% vs 15%). Unusual clinical manifestations of syphilis in HIV range from florid skin lesions to few atypical ones, but these are exceptions, not the rule. Since most HIV-infected patients in large urban areas in the US and Western Europe who acquire syphilis are men who have sex with men, chancres may be in atypical locations, such as the lips, tongue, or anus.

In general, the nontreponemal tests are of higher titer in HIV-infected persons. Rarely, the serologic response to infection may be impaired or delayed, and seronegative secondary syphilis has been reported. Biopsy of the skin lesions and histopathologic evaluation with silver stains will confirm the diagnosis of syphilis in such cases. This approach, along with darkfield examination of appropriate lesions, should be considered if the clinical eruption is characteristic of syphilis and the serologic tests yield negative results.

Neurosyphilis has been frequently reported in HIV-infected persons, even after appropriate therapy for early syphilis. Manifestations have been those of early neurosyphilis or meningeal or meningovascular syphilis. These have included headache, fever, hemiplegia, and cranial nerve deficits, especially deafness (cranial nerve VIII), decreased vision (cranial nerve II), and ocular palsies (cranial nerves III and VI). Whether HIV-infected persons are at increased risk for these complications or whether they occur more quickly is unknown. It is known that spirochetes are no more likely to remain in the CSF after treatment in HIV-infected persons than in HIV-negative persons. Whether the impaired host immunity allows these residual spirochetes to cause clinical relapse more frequently or more quickly in the setting of HIV is unknown.

HIV-infected patients who have primary or secondary syphilis, who are not allergic to penicillin, and who have no neurologic or psychiatric findings should be treated with benzathine penicillin G, 2.4 MU intramuscularly. The CDC recommendations are for one injectin, but allow that some experts recommend more treatment, up to 3 consecutive weeks of therapy. Patients who are allergic to penicillin should be desensitized and treated with penicillin. Following treatment, the patient should have serologic follow-up with quantitative nontreponemal tests at 3, 6, 9, 12, and 24 months. Failure of the titer to fall is an indication for re-evaluation, including lumbar puncture.

Because of the concerns about neurologic relapse in the setting of HIV disease, more careful CNS evaluation is advocated. Lumbar puncture is recommended in HIV-infected persons with latent syphilis (of any duration), late syphilis (even with a normal neurologic examination), and HIV-infected persons with any neurologic or psychiatric signs or symptoms. If the RPR is greater than or equal to 1:32 and the CD4 count is less than 350, neurosyphilis is more likely and lumbar puncture could be considered. Treatment in these patients will be determined by the result of their CSF evaluation. HIV-infected persons with primary and secondary syphilis should be counseled about their possible increased risk of CNS relapse.

Benzathine penicillin, 2.4 MU intramuscularly, should be used to treat all HIV-infected contacts of persons with syphilis who are at risk of acquiring infection.

Aquilina C, et al: Secondary syphilis simulating oral hairy leukoplakia. J Am Acad Dermatol 2003; 49:749.

Augenbraun MH: Treatment of syphilis 2001: nonpregnant adults. Clin Infect Dis 2002; 35:S187.

Battistella M, et al: Extensive nodular secondary syphilis with prozone phenomenon. Arch Dermatol 2008; 144:1078.

Bowring J, et al: Stroke in pregnancy associated with syphilis. Jpn Obstet Gynaecol Res 2008; 34:405.

Carlesimo M, et al: Isolated oral erosions: an unusual manifestation of secondary syphilis. Dermatol Online J 2008; 14:23.

Centers for Disease Control and Prevention: Syphilis testing algorithms using treponemal tests for initial screening—four laboratories, New York City, 2005–2006. MMWR 2008; 57:872.

Centers for Disease Control and Prevention: Sexually transmitted diseases treatment guidelines 2006. MMWR 2006; 55:1.

Cha JM, et al: Rectal syphilis mimicking rectal cancer. Yonsei Med J 2010; 51:276.

Chan SY, et al: Syphilis causing hearing loss. Int J STD & AIDS 2008; 19:721.

Cheng S, French P: Unilateral penile swelling: an unusual presentation of primary syphilis. Intl J STD & AIDS 2008; 19:640.

Chuck A, et al: Cost effectiveness of enzyme immunoassay and immunoblot testing for the diagnosis of syphilis. Int J STD & AIDS 2007; 19:393.

Crevel RV, et al: Syphilis presenting as isolated cervical lymphadenopathy: two related cases. J Infec 2009; 51:76.

Dorfman DH, et al: Congenital syphilis presenting in infants after the newborn period. N Engl J Med 1990; 323:1299.

Eccleston K, et al: Primary syphilis. Int J STD & AIDS 2008; 19:145.

Farnsworth N, Rosen T: Endemic treponematosis: review and update. Clin Dermatol 2006; 24:181.

Flynn TR, et al: A 37-year-old man with a lesion on the tongue. N Engl J Med 2010; 362:740.

Fowler VG, et al: Failure of benzathine penicillin in a case of seronegative secondary syphilis in a patient with acquired immunodeficiency syndrome: case report and review of the literature. Arch Dermatol 2001; 137:1374.

French P: Syphilis. Br Med J 2007; 334:143.

Harper K, et al: On the origin of the treponematoses: a phylogenetic approach. PLoS Neg Trop Dis 2008; 2:e148.

Hutchinson CM, et al: Altered clinical presentation of early syphilis in patients with human immunodeficiency virus infection. Ann Intern Med 1994; 121:94.

Jeans AR, et al: Sensorineural hearing loss due to secondary syphilis. Int J STD & AIDS 2008; 19:355.

Kenneth K, et al: Azithromycin resistance in *Treponema pallidum*. Curr Op Infec Dis 2008; 21:83.

Kent M, Romanelli F: Reexamining syphilis: an update on epidemiology, clinical manifestation and management. Ann Pharmaco 2008; 42:226.

LaFond R, Lukehart S: Biological basis for syphilis. Clin Microbio Rev 2006; 19:29.

Lee JY, Lee ES: Erythema multiforme-like lesions in syphilis. Br J Dermatol 2003; 149:658.

Lewis DA, Young H: Syphilis. Sex Transm Infect 2006; 82:iv13.

Malone JL, et al: Syphilis and neurosyphilis in a human immunodeficiency virus type-1 seropositive population: evidence for frequent serologic relapse after therapy. Am J Med 1995; 99:55.

Marra C: Déjà vu all over again: when to perform a lumbar puncture in HIV-infected patients with syphilis. Sex Trans Dis 2007; 34:145.

Marra C, et al: Alternative cerebrospinal fluid tests to diagnose neurosyphilis in HIV-infected individuals. Neurology 2004; 63:85.

Marra C, et al: Cerebrospinal fluid abnormalities in patients with syphilis: association with clinical and laboratory features. J Infec Dis 2004; 189:369.

Marra C, et al: Normalization of cerebrospinal fluid abnormalities after neurosyphilis therapy: does HIV status matter? Clin Infec Dis 2004; 38:1001.

Marra C, et al: Normalization of serum rapid plasma reagin titer predicts normalization of cerebrospinal fluid and clinical abnormalities after treatment of neurosyphilis. Clin Infec Dis 2008; 47:893.

Marra CM, et al: A pilot study evaluating ceftriaxone and penicillin G as treatment agents for neurosyphilis in human immunodeficiency virus-infected individuals. Clin Infect Dis 2000; 30:540.

McComb ME, et al: Secondary syphilis presenting as pseudolymphoma of the skin. J Am Acad Dermatol 2003; 49:S174.

McMillan A, Young H: Qualitative and quantitative aspects of the serological diagnosis of early syphilis. Int J STD & AIDS 2008; 19:620.

McMillan A, Young H: Reactivity in the venereal disease research laboratory test and the Mercia® IgM enzyme immunoassay after treatment of early syphilis. Int J STD & AIDS 2008; 19:689.

Mignogna MD, et al: Secondary syphilis mimicking pemphigus vulgaris. J Euro Acad Dermatol Venereol 2008; 23:479.

Monastirli A, et al: Lichen planus-like secondary syphilis in an 83-year-old woman. Clin Exp Dermatol 2008; 33:780.

Nessa K, et al: Field evaluation of simple rapid test in the diagnosis of syphilis. Int J STD & AIDS 2008; 19:316.

Parish JL: Treponemal infections in the pediatric population. Clin Dermatol 2000; 18:687.

Peeling RW, et al: Rapid tests for sexually transmitted infections (STIs): the way forward. Sex Transm Infec 2006; 82:v1.

Peterman T, et al: The changing epidemiology of syphilis. Sex Transm Dis 2005; 32:v1.

Pournavas CC, et al: Extensive annular verrucous late secondary syphilis. Br J Dermatol 2005; 152:1343.

Rosen T, et al: Vesicular Jarisch–Herxheimer reaction. Arch Dermatol 1989; 125:77.

Simms I, Broutet N: Congenital syphilis re-emerging. JDDG 2008; 6:269.

Sing A, et al: Characteristics of primary and late syphilis cases which were initially non-reactive with the rapid plasma reagin as the screening test. Int J STD & AIDS 2008; 19:464.

Stoner B: Current controversies in the management of adult syphilis. Clin Infec Dis 2007; 44:S130.

Tantalo L, et al: *Treponema pallidum* strain-specific differences in neuroinvasion and clinical phenotype in a rabbit model. J Infec Dis 2005; 191:75.

Thami GP, et al: The changing face of syphilis: from mimic to disguise. Arch Dermatol 2001; 137:1373.

Varela P, et al: Two recent cases of tertiary syphilis. Eur J Dermatol 1999; 9:300.

Veraldi S, et al: Multiple aphthoid syphilitic chancres of the oral cavity. Int J STD & AIDS 2008; 19:486.

Vural M, et al: A premature newborn with vesiculobullous skin lesions. Eur J Pediatr 2003; 162:197.

Wendel GD, et al: Treatment of syphilis in pregnancy and prevention of congenital syphilis. Clin Infect Dis 2002; 35:S200.

Workkowski K: Centers for Disease Control and Prevention: Sexually transmitted diseases treatment guidelines 2006. MMWR 2006; 55:R-11.

Yinnon AM: Serologic response to treatment of syphilis in patients with HIV infection. Arch Intern Med 1996; 156:321.

Nonvenereal treponematoses: yaws, endemic syphilis, and pinta

This group of diseases is called the endemic or nonvenereal treponematoses. They share many epidemiological and pathologic features. Like venereal syphilis, the clinical manifestations are divided into early and late stages. Early disease is considered infectious, and lasts for approximately 5 years. There are periods of latency. The histology is very similar in all the diseases, and similar to venereal syphilis. Cutaneous manifestations are prominent. The bones and mucosa may also be involved in some cases (except in pinta). The involvement of other organ systems and congenital disease is not seen. Children younger than 15 years are primarily affected. Person-to-person contact, or sharing of a drinking vessel, is the mode of transmission. The endemic treponematoses are closely related to poverty and a lack of available health services. They are described as occurring where the road ends. These diseases tend to occur in the tropics, especially yaws, and the wearing of few clothes and a hot, humid climate are associated with higher prevalence. In endemic areas, as hygiene improves, "attenuated" forms of yaws and endemic syphilis appear. A larger percentage of the population is latently infected, and secondary lesions are fewer in number, drier, and limited to moist skinfolds. Instead of several "crops" of eruptions lasting months to years, infected persons have only a single crop. Transmission is thus reduced, although a large percentage of the population may be infected. Yaws has been eradicated from many previously endemic areas so that the number of cases currently is less than 5% of what it was 50 years ago. Unfortunately, yaws is still focally endemic in Africa (especially among the pygmies), Indonesia, Timor Leste, Papua New Guinea, the Solomon Islands, and Vanuatu. The pockets of infection in the Amazon region may be vanishing.

Yaws (pian, frambesia, bouba)

Yaws is caused by *T. pallidum* subsp *pertenue*. It is transmitted nonsexually, by contact with infectious lesions. Yaws predominantly affects children younger than 15 years of age. The disease has a disabling course, affecting the skin, bones, and joints, and is divided into early (primary and secondary) and late (tertiary) disease.

Early yaws

A primary papule or group of papules appears at the site of inoculation after an incubation period of about 3 weeks (10 days to 3 months), during which there may be headache, malaise, and other mild constitutional symptoms. The initial lesion becomes crusted and larger (2–5 cm), and is known as the mother yaw (maman pian). The crusts are amber–yellow. They may be knocked off, forming an ulcer with a red, pulpy, granulated surface, but quickly reform, so that the typical yaws lesion is crusted. The lesion is not indurated. There may be some regional adenopathy.

Exposed parts are most frequently involved—the extremities, particularly the lower legs, feet, buttocks, and face—although the mother's breasts and trunk may be infected by her child. The lesion is practically always extragenital, and when genital, is a result of accidental contact rather than intercourse. After being present for about 3–6 months, the mother yaw spontaneously disappears, leaving slight atrophy and depigmentation.

Weeks or months after the primary lesion appears, secondary yaws develops. Secondary lesions resemble the mother yaw, but they are smaller and may appear around the primary lesions or in a generalized pattern. The secondary lesions may clear centrally and coalesce peripherally, forming annular lesions (ringworm yaws or tinea yaws) (Fig. 18-14). The palms and soles may be involved, resembling secondary syphilis. In some sites, especially around the body orifices and in the armpits, groins, and gluteal crease, condylomatous lesions may arise, resembling condyloma lata of secondary syphilis. In drier endemic regions and during drier seasons, lesions tend to be fewer, less papillomatous, and more scaly, and instead of being generalized, favor the folds of the axillae, groin, and oral cavity. Yaws in the dry seasons and regions closely resembles endemic syphilis. The palms and soles may develop thick, hyperkeratotic plaques that fissure. They are

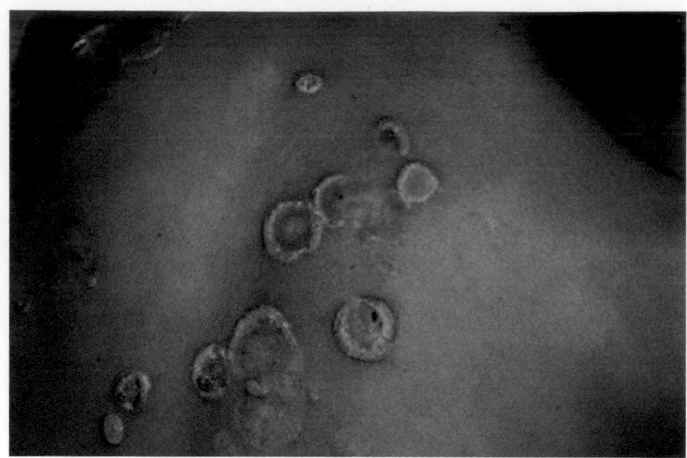

Fig. 18-14 Secondary lesions, yaws.

painful, resulting in a crablike gait (crab yaws). At times there is paronychia. Generalized lymphadenopathy, arthralgias, headaches, and malaise are common. With improved nutrition and hygiene, an "attenuated" form, with only scattered, flat, gray lesions in intertriginous areas, has been described.

In the course of a few weeks or months the secondary lesions may undergo spontaneous involution, leaving either no skin changes or hypopigmented macules that later become hyperpigmented. However, the eruption may persist for many months as a result of fresh recurrent outbreaks. The course is slower in adults than in children, in whom the secondary period rarely lasts longer than 6 months. During latency, skin lesions may relapse for as long as 5 years. Painful osteoperiostitis and polydactylitis may present in early yaws as fusiform swelling of the hands, feet, arms, and legs.

Late yaws

The disease usually terminates with the secondary stage, but in about 10% it progresses to the late stage, usually 5–10 years after initial infection. The typical late yaws skin lesions are gummas that present as indolent ulcers with clean-cut or undermined edges. They tend to fuse to form configurate and, occasionally, serpiginous patterns clinically indistinguishable from those of tertiary syphilis. On healing, these lesions scar, leading to contractures and deformities. Hyperkeratotic palmoplantar plaques and keratoderma frequently recur in the late stage.

Similar processes may occur in the skeletal system and other deep structures, leading to painful nodes on the bones, or destruction of the palate and nasal bone (gangosa). There may be periostitis, particularly of the tibia (saber shin, saber tibia), epiphysitis, chronic synovitis, and juxta-articular nodules. Goundou is a rare proliferative osteitis initially affecting the nasal aspects of the maxilla. Two large hard tumors form on the lateral aspects of the nose. These can significantly obstruct vision. The process may extend into other bones of the central face, affecting the palate and nose, and resulting in protrusion of the whole central face as a mass. Although yaws is classically felt to spare the eye and nervous system, abnormal CSF findings in early yaws and scattered reports of eye and neurologic findings in patients with late yaws suggest that yaws, like syphilis, has the potential to cause neurologic or ophthalmic sequelae, although very rarely.

Histopathology

Early yaws shows epidermal edema, acanthosis, papillomatosis, neutrophilic intraepidermal microabscesses, and a moderate to dense perivascular infiltrate of lymphocytes and plasma cells. Treponema are usually demonstrable in the primary and

secondary stages with the use of the same silver stains employed in diagnosing syphilis. Tertiary yaws shows features identical to the gumma of tertiary syphilis.

Diagnosis

The diagnosis should be suspected from the typical clinical appearance in a person living in an endemic region. The presence of keratoderma palmaris et plantaris in such a person is highly suggestive of yaws. Darkfield demonstration of spirochetes in the early lesions and a reactive VDRL or RPR test can be used to confirm primary and secondary yaws.

Endemic syphilis (bejel)

Bejel is a Bedouin term for this nonvenereal treponematosis, which occurs primarily in the seminomadic tribes who live in the arid regions of North Africa, Southwest Asia, and the eastern Mediterranean. The etiologic agent of bejel is *T. pallidum* subsp *endemicum*. It occurs primarily in childhood and is spread by skin contact or from mouth to mouth by kissing or use of contaminated drinking vessels. The skin, oral mucosa, and skeletal system are primarily involved.

Primary lesions are rare, probably occurring undetected in the oropharyngeal mucosa. The most common presentation is with secondary oral lesions resembling mucous patches. These are shallow, relatively painless ulcerations, occasionally accompanied by laryngitis. Split papules, angular cheilitis, condylomatous lesions of the moist folds of the axillae and groin, and a nonpruritic generalized papular eruption may be seen. Generalized lymphadenopathy is common. Osteoperiostitis of the long bones may occur, causing nocturnal leg pains.

Untreated secondary bejel heals in 6–9 months. The tertiary stage can occur between 6 months and several years after the early symptoms resolve. In the tertiary stage, leg pain (periosteitis) and gummatous ulcerations of the skin, nasopharynx, and bone occur. Gangosa (rhinopharyngitis mutilans) can result. Rarely reported neurologic sequelae seem to be restricted to the eye, including uveitis, choroiditis, chorioretinitis, and optic atrophy. As with yaws, with improved nutrition, an attenuated form of endemic syphilis occurs, often presenting with leg pain from periostitis. The diagnosis of bejel is confirmed by the same means as for venereal syphilis.

Pinta

Pinta is an infectious, nonvenereal, endemic treponematosis caused by *Treponema carateum*. The mode of transmission is unknown, but repeated, direct, lesion-to-skin contact is likely. Only skin lesions occur. By contrast with yaws and bejel, pinta affects persons of all ages, favoring those between 14 and 30 years. It was once prevalent in the forests and rural areas of Central and South America, and Cuba, but it is now rarely reported. The manifestations of pinta may be divided into primary, secondary (early), and tertiary (late) stages, but historically patients may describe continuous evolution from secondary dyspigmented lesions to the characteristic achromic lesions of tertiary pinta.

Primary stage

It is believed that the initial lesion appears 7–60 days after inoculation. The lesion begins as a tiny red papule that becomes an elevated, ill-defined, erythematous, infiltrated plaque up to 10–12.5 cm in diameter in the course of 2–3 months. Expansion of the primary lesion may occur by fusion with surrounding satellite macules or papules. Ultimately, it becomes impossible to distinguish the primary lesion from the secondary lesions. At no time is there erosion or ulceration such as occurs in the syphilitic chancre. Most initial lesions of pinta develop on the legs and other uncovered parts. The RPR and VDRL are nonreactive in the primary stage. Darkfield examination may be positive.

Secondary stage

The secondary stage appears from 5 months to 1 year or more after infection. It begins with small, scaling papules that may enlarge and coalesce, simulating psoriasis, ringworm, eczema, syphilis, or Hansen's disease. They are located mostly on the extremities and face, and frequently are somewhat circinate. Over time, the initially red to violaceous lesions show postinflammatory hyperpigmentation in shades of gray, blue, or brown, or hypopigmentation. Secondary lesions are classified as erythematous, desquamative, hypochromic, or hyperchromic. Multiple different morphologies may be present simultaneously, giving a very polymorphous appearance. Nontreponemal tests for syphilis are reactive in the secondary stage in about 60% of patients. Darkfield examination may show spirochetes.

Late dyschromic stage

Until the 1940s, the late pigmentary changes were the only recognized clinical manifestations of pinta. These have an insidious onset, usually in adolescents or young adults, of widespread depigmented macules resembling vitiligo. The lesions are located chiefly on the face, waistline, wrist flexures, and trochanteric region, although at times diffuse involvement occurs, so that large areas on the trunk and extremities are affected. The lesions are symmetrical in over one-third of patients. Hemipinta is a rare variety of the disease in which the pigmentary disturbances affect only half of the body. In the late dyschromic stage of pinta, the serologic test for syphilis is positive in nearly all patients.

Histopathology

Skin lesions in early pinta show moderate acanthosis; occasionally, lichenoid changes with basal layer vacuolization; and an upper dermal perivascular infiltrate of lymphocytes and plasma cells. Melanophages are prominent in the upper dermis. Spirochetes may be demonstrated in the epidermis by special stains in primary, secondary, and hyperpigmented lesions of tertiary pinta. In tertiary pinta the depigmented skin shows a loss of basal pigment, pigmentary incontinence, and virtually no dermal inflammatory infiltrate. Spirochetes are rarely found in depigmented tertiary lesions.

Treatment

The treatment of choice is benzathine penicillin G, 1.2–2.4 MU intramuscularly (0.6–1.2 MU for children under 10 years of age). In penicillin-allergic patients, tetracycline, 500 mg four times a day for adults (or erythromycin for children, 8–10 mg/kg four times a day for 15 days), is recommended. Penicillin-resistant yaws has been reported from New Guinea. In tertiary pinta, the blue color gradually disappears, as do the areas of partial depigmentation. The vitiliginous areas, if present for more than 5 years, are permanent. Eradication of these diseases is possible with persistent and effective treatment strategies. These include:

1. screening of the whole population in endemic areas
2. diagnosis of patients seen at health services and by community outreach
3. health education
4. improved hygiene (soap and water).

If more than 10% of the population is affected, the whole population is treated (mass treatment). If 5–10% of the population is affected, treat all active cases, all children under the age of 15, and all contacts (juvenile mass treatment). If under 5% of the population is infected, treat all active cases and all household and close personal contacts (selective mass treatment). Unfortunately, with the areas affected by the endemic treponematoses also struggling with epidemics of HIV, tuberculosis, and malaria, eradication programs have been largely discontinued.

Anselmi M, et al: Community participation eliminates yaws in Ecuador. Trop Med Int Health 2003; 8:634.

Mafart B: Goundou: a historical form of yaws. Lancet 2002; 360:1168.

Walker SL, Hay RJ: Yaws: a review of the last 50 years. Int J Dermatol 2000; 39:258.

Woltsche-Kuhr I, et al: Pinta in Austria (or Cuba). Arch Dermatol 1999; 135:685.

Bonus images for this chapter can be found online at http://www.expertconsult.com

19 Viral Diseases

Viruses are obligatory intracellular parasites. The structural components of a viral particle (virion) consist of a central core of nucleic acid, a protective protein coat (capsid), and (in certain groups of viruses only) an outermost membrane or envelope. The capsid of the simplest viruses is made up of many identical polypeptides (structural units) that fold and interact with one another to form morphologic units (capsomeres). The number of capsomeres is believed to be constant for each virus with cubic symmetry, and it is an important criterion in the classification of viruses. The protein coat determines serologic specificity, protects the nucleic acid from enzymatic degradation in biologic environments, controls host specificity, and increases the efficiency of infection. The outermost membrane of the enveloped viruses is essential for the attachment to, and penetration of, host cells. The envelope also contains important viral antigens.

Two main groups of viruses are distinguished: DNA and RNA. The DNA virus types are parvovirus, papovavirus, adenovirus, herpesvirus, and poxvirus. RNA viruses are picornavirus, togavirus, reovirus, coronavirus, orthomyxovirus, retrovirus, arenavirus, rhabdovirus, and paramyxovirus. Some viruses are distinguished by their mode of transmission: arthropod-borne viruses, respiratory viruses, fecal–oral or intestinal viruses, venereal viruses, and penetrating wound viruses.

Herpesvirus group

The herpesviruses are medium-sized viruses that contain double-stranded DNA and replicate in the cell nucleus. They are characterized by the ability to produce latent, but lifelong infection by infecting immunologically protected cells (immune cells and nerves). Intermittently, they have replicative episodes with amplification of the viral numbers in anatomic sites that are conducive to transmission from one host to the next (genital skin, orolabial region). The vast majority of infected persons remain asymptomatic. Viruses in this group are varicella zoster virus (VZV); herpes simplex virus (HSV)-1 and 2; cytomegalovirus (CMV); Epstein–Barr virus (EBV); human herpesviruses (HHV)-6, 7, and 8; *Herpesvirus simiae* (B virus); and other viruses of animals.

Herpes simplex

Infection with HSV is one of the most prevalent infections worldwide. HSV-1 infection, the cause of most cases of orolabial herpes, is more common than infection with HSV-2, the cause of most cases of genital herpes. Between 30% and 95% of adults (depending on the country and group tested) are seropositive for HSV-1. Seroprevalence for HSV-2 is lower, and it appears at the age of onset of sexual activity. In Scandinavia, the rate of infection with HSV-2 increases from 2% in 15-year-olds to 25% in 30-year-olds. About 2.4% of adults become infected annually with HSV-2 in their third decade of life. In the US about 25% of adults are infected with HSV-2. In sexually transmitted disease (STD) clinic patients, the infection rate is between 30% and 50%. In sub-Saharan Africa, infection rates are between 60% and 95%. Worldwide, the seroprevalence is higher in human immunodeficiency virus (HIV)-infected persons. Serologic data have demonstrated that many more people are infected than give a history of clinical disease. For HSV-1, about 50% of infected persons give a history of orolabial lesions. For HSV-2, 20% of infected persons are completely asymptomatic (latent infection), 20% have recurrent genital herpes they recognize, and 60% have clinical lesions that they do not recognize as genital herpes (subclinical or unrecognized infection). Most persons with HSV-2 infection are symptomatic, but the majority do not recognize that their symptoms are caused by HSV. All persons infected with HSV-1 and 2 infection are potentially infectious even if they have no clinical signs or symptoms.

HSV infections are classified as either "first episode" or "recurrent." Most patients have no lesions or findings when they are initially infected with an HSV. When the patient has his/her first clinical lesion, this is usually a recurrence. Since the initial clinical presentation is not associated with a new infection, the old terminology of "primary" infection has been abandoned. Instead, the initial clinical presentation is called a "first episode" and may represent a true primary infection or a recurrence. Persons with chronic or acute immunosuppression may have prolonged and atypical clinical courses.

Infections with HSV-1 or 2 are diagnosed by specific and nonspecific methods. The most common procedure used in the office is the Tzanck smear. It is nonspecific since both HSV and VZV infections result in the formation of multinucleate epidermal giant cells. The multiple nuclei are molded or fit together like pieces of a puzzle. Although the technique is rapid, its success depends heavily on the skill of the interpreter. The accuracy rate is between 60% and 90%, with a false-positive rate of 3–13%. The direct fluorescent antibody (DFA) test is more accurate and will identify virus type; results can be available in hours if a virology laboratory is nearby. Viral culture is very specific and relatively rapid (compared to serological tests), since HSV is stable in transport and grows readily and rapidly in culture. Results are often available in 48–72 h. However, the sensitivity may be as low as 25–50%, since nearby viral laboratories are not readily available to many practitioners. Polymerase chain reaction (PCR) is as specific as viral culture and can be performed on dried or fixed tissue. It is four times more sensitive than viral culture when compared head to head. Skin biopsies of lesions can detect viropathic changes caused by HSV, and with specific HSV antibodies, immunoperoxidase techniques can accurately diagnose infection. The accuracy of various tests is dependent on lesion morphology. Only acute, vesicular lesions are likely to be positive with Tzanck smears. Crusted, eroded, or ulcerative lesions are best diagnosed by viral culture, fluorescent antibody, histologic methods, or PCR.

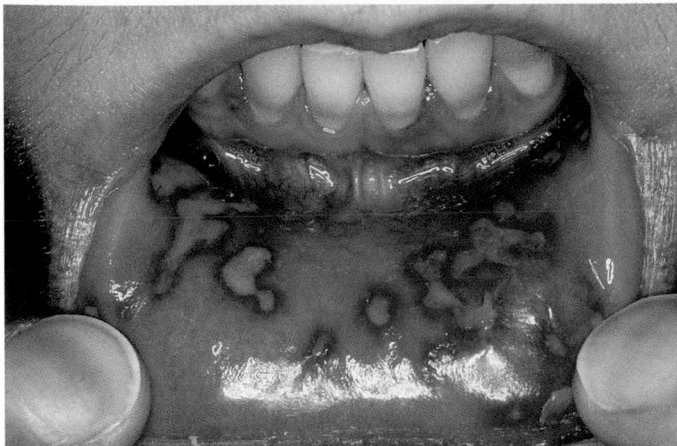

Fig. 19-1 Herpetic gingivostomatitis, extensive erosions of the oral mucosa.

Serologic tests are generally not used in determining whether a skin lesion is due to HSV infection. A positive serologic test indicates only that the individual is infected with that virus, not that the viral infection is the cause of the current lesion. Second-generation enzyme-linked immunosorbent assay (ELISA) tests and G protein-specific Western blot serologic tests can detect specific infection with HSV-1 and 2 but cannot determine the duration or source of that infection. In addition to determining the infection rate in various populations, serologic tests are most useful in evaluating couples in which only one partner gives a history of genital herpes (discordant couples), in couples at risk for neonatal herpes infection, and for possible HSV vaccination when it becomes available.

Orolabial herpes

Orolabial herpes is virtually always caused by HSV-1. In 1% or less of newly infected persons, herpetic gingivostomatitis develops, chiefly in children and young adults (Fig. 19-1). The onset is often accompanied by high fever, regional lymphadenopathy, and malaise. The herpetic lesions in the mouth are usually broken vesicles that appear as erosions or ulcers covered with a white membrane. The erosions may become widespread on the oral mucosa, tongue, and tonsils, and the gingiva margin is commonly eroded. Herpetic gingivostomatitis produces pain, foul breath, and dysphagia. In young children, dehydration may occur. It may cause pharyngitis, with ulcerative or exudative lesions of the posterior pharynx. The duration, untreated, is 1–2 weeks. If the initial episode of herpetic gingivostomatitis or herpes labialis is so severe that an intravenous delivery is required, acyclovir, 5 mg/kg three times a day, is recommended. Oral therapeutic options include acyclovir suspension, 15 mg/kg five times daily for 7 days, valacyclovir, 1 g twice daily for 7 days, or famciclovir, 500 mg twice daily for 7 days. This therapy reduces the duration of the illness by more than 50%.

The most frequent clinical manifestation of orolabial herpes is the "cold sore" or "fever blister." Recurrent HSV-1 is the cause 95% or more of the time, and typically presents as grouped blisters on an erythematous base. The lips near the vermilion are most frequently involved. Lesions may, however, occur wherever the virus was inoculated or proliferated during the initial episode (Fig. 19-2). Recurrences may be seen on the cheeks, eyelids, and earlobes. Oral recurrent HSV usually affects the keratinized surfaces of the hard palate and attached gingiva. Outbreaks are variable in severity, partly related to the trigger of the outbreak. Some outbreaks are small and resolve rapidly, while others may be severe, involving both the upper and lower lips (Fig. 19-3). In severe outbreaks, lip

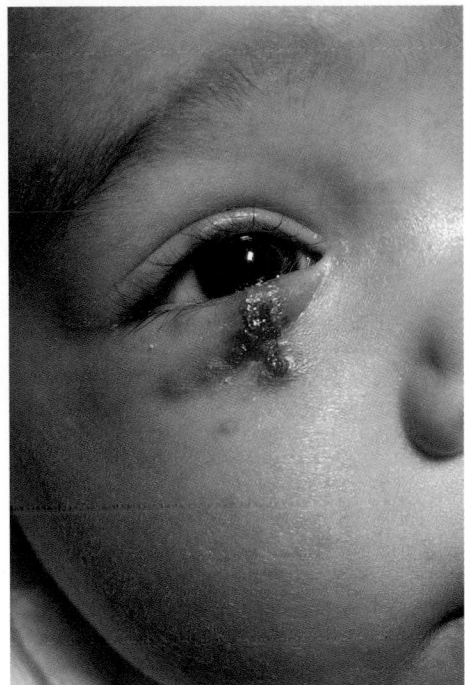

Fig. 19-2 HSV-1, eyelid infection from a "kiss" from an infected adult.

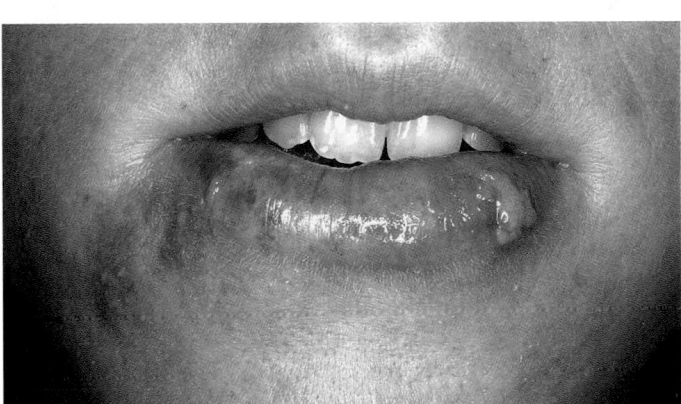

Fig. 19-3 Orolabial herpes simplex, severe outbreak triggered by a sunburn.

swelling is often present. Patient symptomatology is variable. A prodrome of up to 24 h of tingling, itching, or burning may precede the outbreak. Local discomfort, as well as headache, nasal congestion, or mild flu-like symptoms, may occur. Ultraviolet (UV) exposure, especially UVB, is a frequent trigger of recurrent orolabial HSV, and the severity of the outbreak may correlate with the intensity of the sun exposure. Surgical and dental procedures of the lips (or other areas previously affected with HSV) may trigger recurrences, and a history of prior HSV should be solicited in all patients in whom such procedures are recommended (see below).

In most patients recurrent orolabial herpes represents more of a nuisance than a disease. Because UVB radiation is a common trigger, use of a sunblock daily on the lips and facial skin may reduce recurrences. All topical therapies for the acute treatment of recurrent orolabial herpes have limited efficacy, reducing disease duration and pain by 1 day or less. Tetracaine cream, penciclovir cream, and acyclovir cream (not ointment) have some limited efficacy. Topical acyclovir ointment and docosanol cream provide minimal to no reduction in healing time or discomfort. The minimal benefit from these topical agents suggests that they should not be recommended when patients present to dermatologists for significant symptomatic orolabial herpes outbreaks. If oral therapy is contemplated for patients with severely symptomatic recurrences of orolabial HSV, it must be remembered that much higher doses of oral antivirals are required than for the treatment of genital herpes. Intermittent treatment with valacyclovir, 2 g twice a day for 1 day, or famciclovir, 1.5 g as a single dose, starting at the onset of the prodrome are simple and effective oral 1 day regimens. Since the patient's own inflammatory reaction against the virus contributes substantially to the severity of lesions of orolabial herpes simplex, topical therapy with a high-potency topical steroid (fluocinonide gel 0.05%, three times a day) in combination with an oral antiviral leads to more rapid reduction of pain, and reduces maximum lesion area and time to healing. In non-immunosuppressed patients, if episodic treatment for orolabial HSV is recommended and an oral agent is used, the addition of a high-potency topical steroid should be considered.

Although most patients with orolabial herpes simplex do not require treatment, certain medical and dental procedures may trigger outbreaks of HSV. If the cutaneous surface has been damaged by the surgical procedure (such as a dermabrasion, chemical peel, or laser resurfacing procedure), the surgical site can be infected by the virus and may result in prolonged healing and possible scarring. Prophylaxis is regularly used before such surgeries in patients with a history of orolabial herpes simplex. Famciclovir, 250 mg twice a day, and valacyclovir, 500 mg twice a day, are prophylactic options, to be begun 24 h before the procedure, or the morning of the procedure and continued for 14 days. Prophylaxis could also be considered before skiing or tropical vacations and extensive dental procedures at the same dosages.

Herpetic sycosis

Recurrent or initial herpes simplex infections (usually due to HSV-1) may primarily affect the hair follicle. The clinical appearance may vary from a few eroded follicular papules (resembling acne excoriée) to extensive lesions involving the whole beard area (Fig. 19-4). Close razor blade shaving imme-

diately prior to initial exposure or in the presence of an acute orolabial lesion may be associated with a more extensive eruption. The onset may be very acute (over days), or more subacute or chronic. Diagnostic clues include the tendency for erosions, a self-limited course of 2–3 weeks, and an appropriate risk behavior. The diagnosis may be confirmed by biopsy. Although the herpes infection is primarily in the follicle, surface cultures of eroded lesions will usually be positive in the first 5–7 days of the eruption.

Herpes gladiatorum

HSV-1 infection is highly contagious to susceptible persons who wrestle with an infected individual with an active lesion. One-third of susceptible wrestlers will become infected after a single match. In tournaments and wrestling camps, outbreaks can be epidemic, affecting up to 20% of all participants. Lesions usually occur on the lateral side of the neck, the side of the face, and the forearm, all areas in direct contact with the face of the infected wrestler (Fig. 19-5). Vesicles appear 4–11 days after exposure, often preceded by 24 h of malaise, sore throat, and fever. Ocular symptoms may occur. Lesions are frequently misdiagnosed as a bacterial folliculitis. Any wrestler with a confirmed history of orolabial herpes should be on suppressive antiviral therapy during all periods of training and competition. Rugby players, especially forwards who participate in scrums, are also at risk.

Herpetic whitlow

HSV infection may uncommonly occur on the fingers or periungually. Lesions begin with tenderness and erythema, usually of the lateral nailfold or on the palm. Deep-seated blisters develop 24–48 h after symptoms begin (Fig. 19-6). The blisters may be very small, requiring careful inspection to detect them. Deep-seated lesions that appear unilocular may be mistaken for a paronychia or other inflammatory process. Lesions may progress to erosions, or heal without ever impairing epidermal integrity due to the thick stratum corneum in this location. Herpetic whitlow may simulate a felon. Swelling of the affected hand is not uncommon. Lymphatic streaking

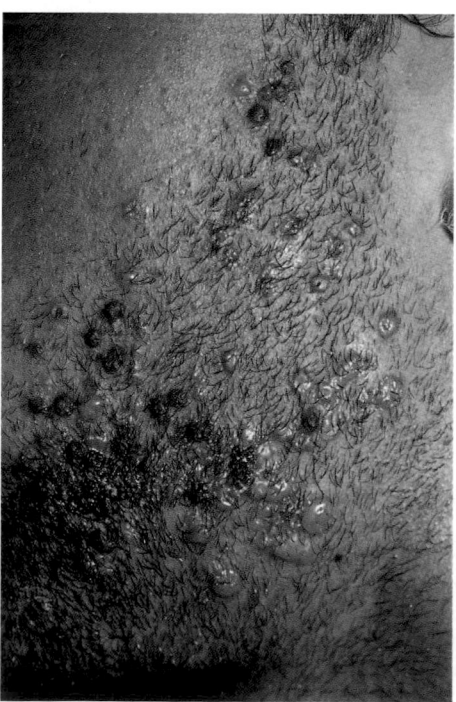

Fig. 19-4 Herpetic sycosis.

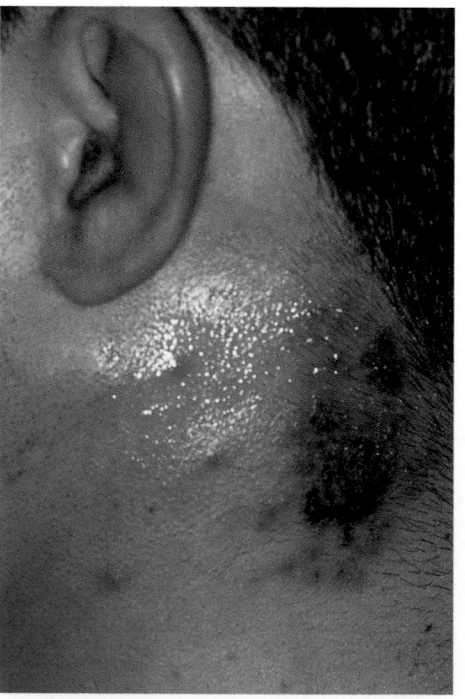

Fig. 19-5 Herpes gladiatorum, neck lesions of HSV-1.

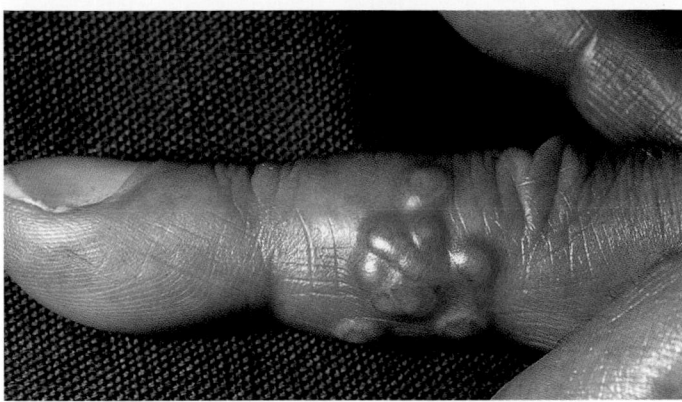

Fig. 19-6 Herpetic whitlow, classic grouped blisters.

and swelling of the epitrochlear or axillary lymph nodes may occur, mimicking a bacterial cellulitis. Repeated episodes of herpetic lymphangitis may lead to persistent lymphedema of the affected hand. Herpetic whitlow has become much less frequent among healthcare workers since the institution of universal precautions and glove use during contact with the oral mucosa. Currently, most cases are seen in persons with herpes elsewhere. Children may be infected while thumb sucking or nail biting during their initial herpes outbreak or by touching an infectious lesion of an adult. Herpetic whitlow is bimodal in distribution, with about 20% of cases occurring in children younger than 10 years old, and 55% of cases between the ages of 20 and 40. All cases in children are caused by HSV-1, but in adults up to three-quarters of cases are caused by HSV-2. Among adults, herpetic whitlow is twice as common in females. Herpetic whitlow in healthcare workers can be transmitted to patients. In patients whose oropharynx is exposed to the ungloved hands of healthcare workers with herpetic whitlow, 37% develop herpetic pharyngitis.

Herpetic keratoconjunctivitis

Herpes simplex infection of the eye is a common cause of blindness in the US. It occurs as a punctate or marginal keratitis, or as a dendritic corneal ulcer, which may cause disciform keratitis and leave scars that impair vision. Topical corticosteroids in this situation may induce perforation of the cornea. Vesicles may appear on the lids, and preauricular nodes may be enlarged and tender. Recurrences are common. Ocular symptoms in any person with an initial outbreak of HSV could represent ocular HSV, and an ophthalmological evaluation should be performed to exclude this possibility.

Genital herpes

Genital herpes infection is usually due to HSV-2, which causes 85% of initial infections and up to 98% of recurrent lesions. In the mid-1980s, the prevalence of genital herpes caused by HSV-1 began to increase because of changes in sexual habits and a falling prevalence of orolabial HSV-1 infection in developed nations, so that in some developed countries HSV-1 now causes up to 50% of anogenital herpes in women. HSV-1 in the genital area is much less likely to recur (only 20–50% of patients have a recurrence, and when a recurrence does occur, the average patient experiences only about one outbreak per year.

Genital herpes is spread by skin-to-skin contact, usually during sexual activity. The incubation period averages 5 days. Active lesions of HSV-2 contain live virus and are infectious. Persons with recurrent genital herpes shed virus asymptomatically between outbreaks (asymptomatic shedding). Even persons who are HSV-2-infected but have never had any clinical lesions or symptoms shed virus, so everyone who is HSV-2-infected is potentially infectious to a sexual partner. Asymptomatic shedding occurs simultaneously from several anatomic sites (penis, vagina, cervix, and rectum) and can occur through normally appearing intact skin and mucosae. In addition, persons with HSV-2 infection may have lesions they do not recognize as being caused by HSV (unrecognized outbreak) or have recurrent lesions that do not cause symptoms (subclinical outbreak). Most transmission of genital herpes occurs during subclinical or unrecognized outbreaks, or while the infected person is shedding asymptomatically.

The risk of transmission in monogamous couples, in which only one partner is infected, is about 5–10% annually, with women being at much greater risk than men for acquiring HSV-2 from their infected partner. Prior HSV-1 infection does not reduce the risk of being infected with HSV-2 but does make it more likely that initial infection will be asymptomatic. There is no strategy that absolutely prevents herpes transmission. All prevention strategies are more effective in reducing the risk of male-to-female transmission than female-to-male transmission. Condom use for all sexual exposures and avoiding sexual exposure when active lesions are present have been shown to be effective strategies, as has chronic suppressive therapy of the infected partner with valacyclovir, 500 mg/day.

The symptomatology during acquisition of infection with HSV-2 has a broad clinical spectrum from totally asymptomatic to severe genital ulcer disease (erosive vulvovaginitis or proctitis). Only 57% of new HSV-2 infections are symptomatic. Clinically, the majority of symptomatic initial herpes lesions are classic grouped blisters on an erythematous base. At times, the initial clinical episode is that of typical grouped blisters, but with a longer duration of 10–14 days. While uncommon and representing 1% or fewer of new infections, severe first-episode genital herpes can be a significant systemic illness. Grouped blisters and erosions appear in the vagina, in the rectum, or on the penis, with continued development of new blisters over 7–14 days. Lesions are bilaterally symmetrical and often extensive, and the inguinal lymph nodes can be enlarged bilaterally. Fever and flu-like symptoms may be present, but in women the major complaint is vaginal pain and dysuria (herpetic vulvovaginitis). The whole illness may last 3 weeks or more. If the inoculation occurs in the rectal area, severe proctitis may occur from extensive erosions in the anal canal and on the rectal mucosa. The initial clinical episode of genital herpes is treated with oral acyclovir, 200 mg five times a day or 400 mg three times a day; famciclovir, 250 mg three times a day; or valacyclovir, 1000 mg twice a day, all for 7–10 days. Since it is very difficult on clinical grounds to distinguish true initial (or primary) HSV-2 infection from a recurrence, all patients with their initial clinical episode receive the same therapy. Only serology can determine whether the person is totally HSV-naïve and suffering a true primary episode, is partially immune due to prior HSV-1 infection, or is already HSV-2-infected and their first clinical presentation is actually a recurrence. In fact, 25% of "initial" clinical episodes of genital herpes are actually recurrences.

Virtually all persons infected with HSV-2 will have recurrences, even if the initial infection was subclinical or asymptomatic. HSV-2 infection results in recurrences in the genital area six times more frequently than HSV-1. Twenty percent of persons with HSV-2 infection are truly asymptomatic, never having had either an initial lesion or recurrences. Twenty percent of patients have lesions they recognize as recurrent genital herpes and 60% have clinical lesions that are culture-positive for HSV-2, but are unrecognized by the patient as being caused by genital herpes. This large group of persons with subclinical or unrecognized genital herpes is infectious,

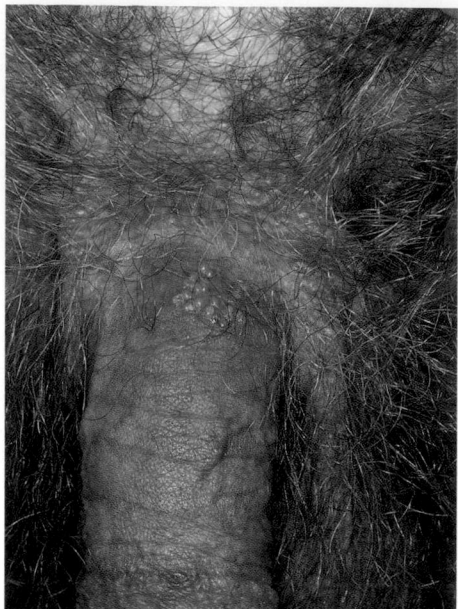

Fig. 19-7 Recurrent genital herpes.

at least intermittently, and represents one factor in the increasing number of new HSV-2 infections.

Typical recurrent genital herpes begins with a prodrome of burning, itching, or tingling. Usually within 24 h, red papules appear at the site, progress to blisters filled with clear fluid over 24 h, form erosions over the next 24–36 h, and heal in another 2–3 days (Fig. 19-7). The average total duration of a typical outbreak of genital herpes is 7 days. Lesions are usually grouped blisters, and the coalescent grouped erosions they evolve into characteristically have a scalloped border. Erosions or ulcerations from genital herpes are usually very tender and not indurated (as opposed to the chancre of primary syphilis). Lesions tend to recur in the same anatomic region, although not at exactly the same site (as opposed to a fixed drug eruption). Less classic clinical manifestations are tiny erosions or linear fissures on the genital skin. Lesions occur on the vulva, vagina, and cervical mucosa, as well as the penile and vulval skin. The upper buttock is a common site for recurrent genital herpes in both men and women. Intraurethral genital herpes may present with dysuria and a clear penile discharge, and is usually misdiagnosed as a more common, nongonococcal urethritis such as *Chlamydia* or *Ureaplasma*. Inguinal adenopathy may be present. Looking into the urethra and culturing any erosions will establish the diagnosis. Recurrent genital herpes heals without scarring unless the lesion is secondarily infected.

The natural history of untreated recurrent genital herpes is not well studied. Over the first several years of infection, the frequency of recurrences usually stays the same. Over longer periods (more than 3–5 years) the frequency of outbreaks decreases in at least two-thirds of patients treated with suppressive antiviral therapy.

Recurrent genital herpes is a problematic disease due to the social stigma associated with it. Because it is not curable, patients frequently demonstrate a significant emotional response when they are first diagnosed. These include anger (at the presumed source of the infection), depression, guilt, and the feeling they are not worthy. During the visit the healthcare worker should ask about a patient's feelings surrounding the diagnosis and any psychological complications that have occurred. This psychological component of genital herpes must be recognized, addressed directly with the patient,

and managed for the therapy of recurrent genital herpes to be successful.

Management of recurrent genital herpes should be individualized. A careful history, including a sexual history, should be obtained. Examination should include seeing the patient during an active recurrence, so that the infection can be confirmed. The diagnosis of recurrent genital herpes should not be made on clinical appearance alone because of the psychological impact of the diagnosis. The diagnosis is best confirmed by a viral culture or DFA examination, allowing for typing of the causative virus. If clinical lesions are not present, serology can determine if the patient is infected with HSV-2. If the patient is HSV-1-seropositive, but HSV-2-seronegative, the possibility of genital HSV-1 disease cannot be excluded.

Treatment depends on several factors, including the frequency of recurrences, severity of recurrences, infection status of the sexual partner, and psychological impact of the infection on the patient. For patients with few or mildly symptomatic recurrences, treatment is often not necessary. Counseling regarding transmission risk is required. In patients with severe but infrequent recurrences or in those who have severe psychological complications, intermittent therapy may be useful. To be effective, intermittent therapy must be initiated at the earliest sign of an outbreak. The patient must be given the medication before the recurrence, so treatment can be started by the patient when the first symptoms appear. Intermittent therapy only reduces the duration of the average recurrence by about 1 day. However, it is a powerful tool in the patient who is totally overwhelmed by each outbreak. The treatment of recurrent genital herpes is acyclovir, 200 mg five times a day or 800 mg twice a day, or famciclovir, 125 mg twice a day, all for 5 days. Shorter regimens that are equally effective include valacyclovir, 500 mg twice a day for 3 days; acyclovir, 800 mg three times a day for 2 days; or famciclovir, 1 g twice a day for one day.

For patients with frequent recurrences (more than 6–12 per year), suppressive therapy is more reasonable. Acyclovir, 400 mg twice a day, 200 mg three times a day, or 800 mg once a day, will suppress 85% of recurrences, and 20% of patients will be recurrence-free during suppressive therapy. Valacyclovir, 500 mg/day (or 1000 mg/day for persons with more than 10 recurrences per year), or famciclovir, 250 mg twice a day, are equally effective alternatives. Up to 5% of immunocompetent patients will have significant recurrences on these doses, and the dose of the antiviral may need to be increased. Chronic suppressive therapy reduces asymptomatic shedding by almost 95%. After 10 years of suppressive therapy a large number of patients can stop treatment with a substantial reduction in frequency of recurrences. Chronic suppressive therapy is very safe and laboratory monitoring is not required.

Intrauterine and neonatal herpes simplex

Neonatal herpes infection occurs in between 1 in 3000 and 1 in 20 000 live births, resulting in 1500–2200 cases of neonatal herpes annually in the US. Eighty-five percent of cases of neonatal herpes simplex infections occur at the time of delivery, 5% occur in utero with intact membranes, and 10–15% occur from nonmaternal sources after delivery. In utero infection may result in fetal anomalies, including skin lesions and scars, limb hypoplasia, microcephaly, microphthalmos, encephalitis, chorioretinitis, and intracerebral calcifications. It is either fatal or complicated by permanent neurologic sequelae.

Seventy percent of cases of neonatal herpes simplex are caused by HSV-2. Neonatal HSV-1 infections are usually acquired postnatally through contact with a person with orolabial disease, but can also occur intrapartum if the mother is genitally infected with HSV-1. The clinical spectrum of perinatally acquired neonatal herpes can be divided into three forms:

1. localized infection of the skin, eyes and/or mouth (SEM)
2. central nervous system (CNS) disease
3. disseminated disease (encephalitis, hepatitis, pneumonia, and coagulopathy).

The pattern of involvement at presentation is important prognostically. With treatment, localized disease (skin, eyes, or mouth) is rarely fatal, whereas brain or disseminated disease is fatal in 15–50% of neonates so affected. In treated neonates, long-term sequelae occur in 10% of neonates with localized disease. More than 50% of cases of CNS or disseminated neonatal herpes suffer neurologic disability.

In 68% of infected babies, skin vesicles are the presenting sign, and are a good source for virus recovery. However, 39% of neonates with disseminated disease, 32% with CNS disease, and 17% with SEM disease never develop vesicular skin lesions. Because the incubation period may be as long as 3 weeks, and averages about 1 week, skin lesions and symptoms may not appear until the child has been discharged from hospital.

The diagnosis of neonatal herpes is confirmed by viral culture or preferably immediate DFA staining of material from skin or ocular lesions. CNS involvement is detected by PCR of the cerebrospinal fluid (CSF). PCR of the CSF is negative in 24% of cases of neonatal CNS herpes infection, so empiric therapy pending other testing may be required. Neonatal herpes infections are treated with intravenous acyclovir, 60 mg/kg/day for 14 days for SEM disease, and 21 days for CNS and disseminated disease.

Seventy percent of mothers of infants with neonatal herpes simplex are asymptomatic at the time of delivery and have no history of genital herpes. Thus, extended history-taking is of no value in predicting which pregnancies may be complicated by neonatal herpes. The most important predictors of infection appear to be the nature of the mother's infection at delivery (first episode versus recurrent), and the presence of active lesions on the cervix, vagina, or vulvar area. The risk of infection for an infant delivered vaginally when the mother has active recurrent genital herpes infection is between 2% and 5%, whereas it is 26–56% if the maternal infection at delivery is a first episode. One strategy to prevent neonatal HSV would be to prevent transmission of HSV to at-risk women during pregnancy, eliminating initial HSV episodes during pregnancy. To accomplish this, pregnant women and their partners would be tested to identify discordant couples for HSV-1 and 2. If the woman is HSV-1-negative and the man is HSV-1-positive, orogenital contact during pregnancy should be avoided, and a condom should be used for all episodes of sexual contact. Valacyclovir suppression of the infected male could also be considered, but might have limited efficacy. If the woman is HSV-2-seronegative and her partner is HSV-2-seropositive, barrier protection for sexual contact during gestation is recommended, and valacyclovir suppression of the man could be considered. Abstinence from intercourse during the third trimester would also reduce the chances of an at-risk mother acquiring genital herpes that might first present perinatally. These strategies have not been tested and could not be guaranteed to prevent all cases of neonatal HSV. At a minimum, discordant couples should be made aware of the increased risk to the fetus that acquisition of HSV by the mother during pregnancy presents.

The appropriate management of pregnancies complicated by genital herpes is complex and there are still areas of controversy. Routine prenatal cultures are not recommended for women with recurrent genital herpes, as they do not predict shedding at the time of delivery. Such cultures may be of value

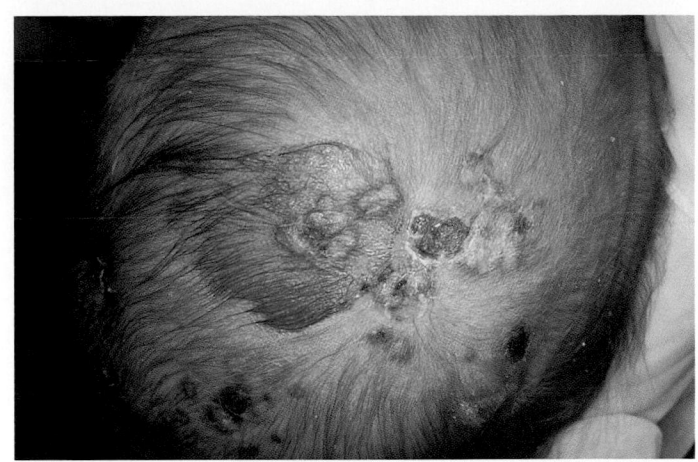

Fig. 19-8 Neonatal herpes, a scalp monitor was associated with infection of this neonate.

in women with primary genital herpes during pregnancy. Scalp electrodes should be avoided in deliveries where cervical shedding of HSV is possible, as they have been documented to increase the risk of infection of the newborn by up to seven-fold (Fig. 19-8). Vacuum-assisted delivery also increases the relative risk of neonatal transmission of HSV by between 2 and 27 times. Genital HSV-1 infection appears to be much more frequently transmitted intrapartum than HSV-2. The current recommendation is still to perform cesarean section in the setting of active genital lesions or prodromal symptoms. This will reduce the risk of transmission of HSV to the infant from 8% to 1% for women who are culture-positive from the cervix at time of delivery. However, this approach will not prevent all cases of neonatal herpes, is expensive, and has a high maternal morbidity (US$2.5 million to prevent each case of neonatal herpes, 1580 excess cesarian sections for every poor-outcome case of neonatal HSV prevented, and 0.57 maternal deaths for every neonatal death prevented.) Because the risk of neonatal herpes is much greater in mothers who experience their initial episode during pregnancy, antiviral treatment of all initial episodes of genital HSV in pregnancy is recommended (except in the first month of gestation where there may be an increased risk of spontaneous abortion). Standard acyclovir doses for initial episodes (acyclovir, 400 mg three times a day for 10 days) are recommended. This is especially true for all initial episodes in the third trimester. Chronic suppressive therapy with acyclovir has been used from 36 weeks' gestation to delivery in women with an initial episode of genital HSV during pregnancy to reduce outbreaks and prevent the need for cesarean section. This approach has been recommended by the American College of Obstetrics and Gynecology, and may also be considered for women with recurrent genital herpes.

The condition of extensive congenital erosions and vesicles healing with reticulate scarring may represent intrauterine neonatal herpes simplex (Fig. 19-9). The condition is rare since intrauterine HSV infection is rare and usually fatal. Probably only a few children survive to present later in life with the characteristic widespread reticulate scarring of the whole body. This may explain the associated CNS manifestations seen in many affected children. One of the authors (TB) has seen a child with this condition who developed infrequent widespread cutaneous blisters from which HSV could be cultured. Modern obstetric practices which screen for herpes in pregnant women and prophylactic treatment with acyclovir in the third trimester may prevent the condition, explaining the lack of recent cases.

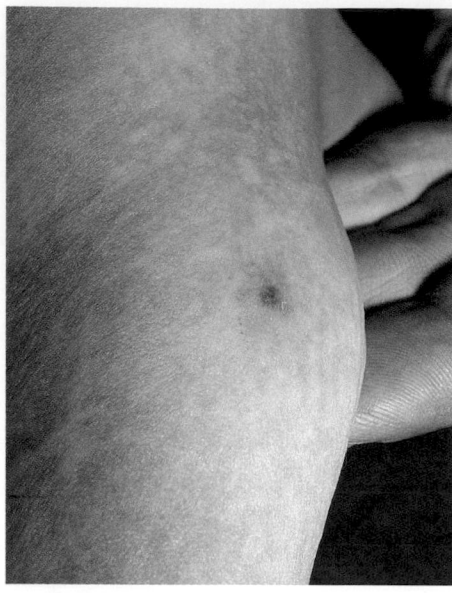

Fig. 19-9 Extensive congenital erosions and vesicles healing with reticulate scarring (the erosion on the arm was culture-positive for HSV-1).

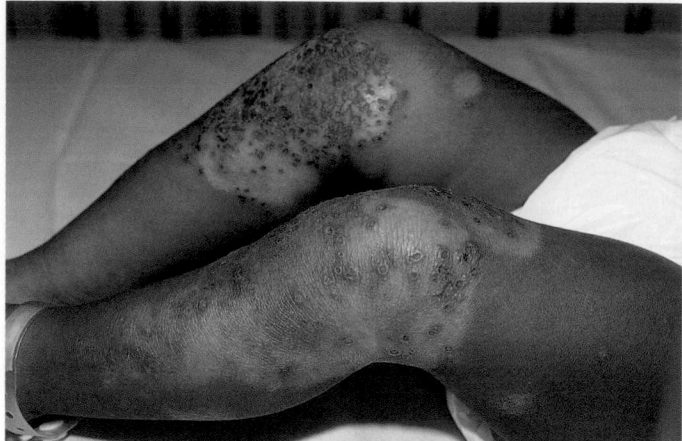

Fig. 19-10 Eczema herpeticum, sudden appearance of uniform erosions, accentuated in areas of active dermatitis.

Eczema herpeticum (Kaposi varicelliform eruption)

Infection with herpesvirus in patients with atopic dermatitis (AD) may result in spread of herpes simplex throughout the eczematous areas. This is called eczema herpeticum or Kaposi varicelliform eruption (KVE). In a large series the development of eczema herpeticum was associated with more severe atopic dermatitis, higher IgE levels, elevated eosinophil count, food and environmental allergies as defined by radioallergosorbent-testing (RAST), and onset of AD before age 5. Eczema herpeticum patients are also more likely to have *Staphylococcus aureus* and molluscum contagiosum infections. All these features identify AD patients who have significant Th2 shift of their immune system. The use of topical calcineurin inhibitors (TCIs) has been repeatedly associated with the development of eczema herpeticum. Bath or hot tub exposure has been reported as a risk factor for development of KVE. The Th2 shift of the immune system and the use of TCIs are both associated with a decrease in antimicrobial peptides in the epidermis, an important defense against cutaneous HSV infection. In addition, in Japan, polymorphisms in the *IL-18* gene are associated with eczema herpeticum complicating TCI treatment. The repair of the epidermal lipid barrier with physiologic lipid mixtures reverses some of the negative effects of the TCIs and may reduce the risk of eczema herpeticum.

In general, the term Kaposi varicelliform eruption is used for cases of disseminated cutaneous HSV associated with skin diseases other than atopic dermatitis. Cutaneous dissemination of HSV-1 or 2 may also occur in severe seborrheic dermatitis, scabies, Darier's disease, benign familial pemphigus, pemphigus (foliaceus or vulgaris), pemphigoid, cutaneous T-cell lymphoma, Wiskott–Aldrich syndrome, allergic and photoallergic contact dermatitis, and burns. In its severest form, hundreds of umbilicated vesicles may be present at the onset, with fever and regional adenopathy. Although the cutaneous eruption is alarming, the disease is often self-limited in healthy individuals. Much milder cases are considerably more common and probably go unrecognized and untreated. They present as a few superficial erosions or even small papules (Fig. 19-10). In patients with systemic immunosuppression in addition to an impaired barrier, such as patients with pemphigus and cutaneous T-cell lymphoma, KVE can be fatal, usually from *S. aureus* septicemia, but also from visceral dissemination of herpes simplex.

Psoriasis patients treated with immunosuppressives may suffer KVE as well, although this is less common. It usually occurs in the setting of worsening disease or erythroderma. Patients present with erosive lesions in the axilla and erosions of the psoriatic plaques. Lesions extend cephalad to caudad, and the development of large, ulcerated painful plaques can occur. The lesions are commonly co-infected with bacteria and yeast. Cultures positive for other pathogens do NOT exclude the diagnosis of KVE, and specific viral cultures, DFAs, and biopsies should be taken if the diagnosis of KVE is suspected. Given the limited toxicity of systemic antiviral therapy, treatment should be started immediately pending the return of laboratory confirmation. Depending on the severity of the disease, either intravenous or oral antiviral therapy should be given for KVE.

Immunocompromised patients

In patients with immunosuppression of the cell-mediated immune system by cytotoxic agents, corticosteroids, or congenital or acquired immunodeficiency, primary and recurrent cases of herpes simplex are more severe, more persistent, more symptomatic, and more resistant to therapy. In some settings (such as in bone marrow transplant recipients), the risk of severe reactivation is so high that prophylactic systemic antivirals are administered. In immunosuppressed patients, any erosive mucocutaneous lesion should be considered to be herpes simplex until proved otherwise, especially lesions in the genital and orolabial regions. Atypical morphologies are also seen.

Typically, lesions appear as erosions or crusts (Fig. 19-11). The early vesicular lesions may be transient or never seen. The three clinical hallmarks of herpes simplex infection are pain, an active vesicular border, and a scalloped periphery. Untreated erosive lesions may gradually expand, but they may also remain fixed and even become papular or vegetative, mimicking a wart or granulation tissue. In the oral mucosa numerous erosions may be seen, involving all surfaces (as opposed to only the hard, keratinized surfaces usually involved by recurrent oral herpes simplex in the immunocompetent host). The tongue may be affected with geometric fissures on the central dorsal surface (Fig. 19-12). Symptomatic stomatitis associated with cancer chemotherapy is at times caused or exacerbated by HSV infection. Herpetic whitlow presents as a painful paronychia that is initially vesicular and involves the lateral or proximal nailfolds. Untreated, it may lead to loss of the nail plate and ulceration of a large portion of the digit.

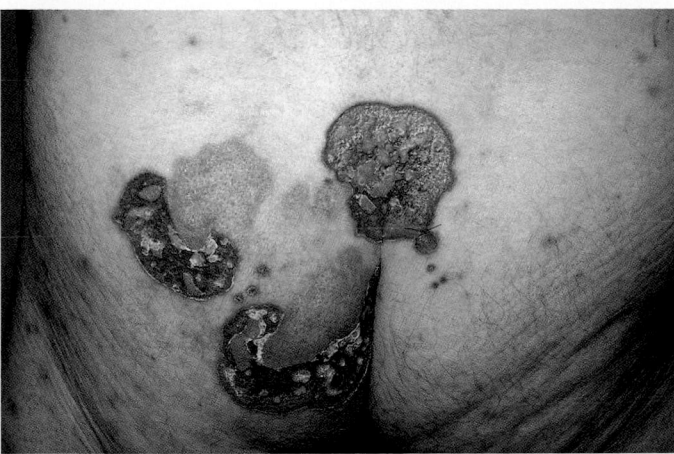

Fig. 19-11 Herpes simplex, HSV-2, infected areas spontaneously heal while new erosions appear.

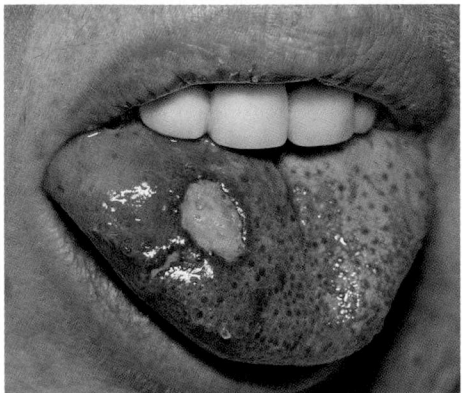

Fig. 19-12 Immunocompromised patient with tongue ulcer and fissures secondary to HSV.

Despite the frequent and severe skin infections caused by HSV in the immunosuppressed, visceral dissemination is unusual. Extension of oral HSV into the esophagus or trachea may develop spontaneously or as a complication of intubation through an infected oropharynx. Ocular involvement can occur from direct inoculation, and if lesions are present around the eye, careful ophthalmologic evaluation is required.

In an immunosuppressed host, since most lesions are ulcerative and not vesicular, Tzanck smears are of less value. Viral cultures taken from the ulcer margin are positive. DFA testing is specific and rapid, and is very useful in immunosuppressed hosts in whom therapeutic decisions need to be made expeditiously. At times, these tests are negative, but a skin biopsy will show typical herpetic changes in the epithelium adjacent to the ulceration. If an ulceration does not respond to treatment in 48 h and cultures are negative, a biopsy is recommended, as it may be the only technique that demonstrates the associated herpesvirus infection.

Therapy often can be instituted on clinical grounds pending confirmatory tests. Acyclovir, 400 mg orally three times a day; famciclovir, 500 mg twice a day; or valacyclovir, 1 g twice a day, all for a minimum of 5–10 days, is used. Therapy should continue until lesions are essentially healed. In severe infection, or in the hospitalized patient with moderate disease, intravenous acyclovir (5 mg/kg) can be given initially to control the disease. In patients with acquired immune deficiency syndrome (AIDS) and those with persistent immunosuppression, consideration should be given to chronic suppressive therapy with acyclovir, 400–800 mg twice or three times a day, or valacyclovir or famciclovir, both at a dose of 500 mg twice a day.

In the immunosuppressed host (but not in the immunocompetent host), long-duration treatment with acyclovir and its analogs, or treatment of large herpetic ulcerations, may be complicated by the development of acyclovir resistance. This resistance may be due to selection of acyclovir-resistant wild-type virus, which is present in large numbers on the surface of such large herpes lesions. In the immunocompetent host, these acyclovir-resistant mutants are few in number and eradicated by the host's immune system. The immunosuppressed host has much more HSV in their lesions, and in addition their own immune system is ineffective in killing the virus. These acyclovir-resistant viral strains may be difficult to culture and at times may only be identified by skin biopsy or PCR of the ulceration. Antiviral resistance is suspected if maximum oral doses of acyclovir, valacyclovir, or famciclovir do not lead to improvement. Intravenous acyclovir, except if given by constant infusion, will also invariably fail in such cases. Resistance to one drug is associated with resistance to all three of these drugs and is usually due to loss of the viral thymidine kinase. HSV isolates can be tested for sensitivity to acyclovir and some other antivirals. The standard treatment of acyclovir-resistant herpes simplex is intravenous foscarnet. In cases intolerant of or resistant to foscarnet, intravenous cidofovir may be used. Smaller lesions can sometimes be treated with topical trifluorothymidine (Viroptic) with or without topical or intralesional interferon (IFN)-α. Imiquimod may be of benefit in healing these lesions. Destruction of small lesions by desiccation followed by the above therapies may also be curative. If lesions recur, they may be acyclovir-sensitive or resistant, depending on the status of the virus in the dorsal root ganglion.

Histopathology

The vesicles of herpes simplex are intraepidermal. The affected epidermis and adjacent inflamed dermis are infiltrated with leukocytes and a serous exudate containing dissociated cells collects to form the vesicle. There is ballooning degeneration of the epidermal cells to produce acantholysis. The most characteristic feature is the presence of multinucleated giant cells which tend to mold together, forming a crude jigsaw puzzle appearance. The steel-gray color of the nucleus and peripheral condensation of the nucleoplasm may be clues to HSV infection, even if multinucleate cells are not seen. Immunoperoxidase stains can detect herpes simplex infection even in paraffin-fixed tissue, allowing the diagnosis to be absolutely confirmed from histologic material.

Differential diagnosis

Herpes labialis must most frequently be differentiated from impetigo. Herpetic lesions are composed of groups of tense, small vesicles, whereas in bullous impetigo the blisters are unilocular, occur at the periphery of a crust, and are flaccid. A mixed infection is not unusual and should especially be suspected in immunosuppressed hosts and when lesions are present in the typical herpetic regions around the mouth. Herpes zoster presents with clusters of lesions along a dermatome, but early on, if the number of zoster lesions is limited, it can be relatively indistinguishable from herpes simplex. In general, herpes zoster will be more painful and over 24 h will progress to involve more of the affected dermatome. DFA testing can rapidly make this distinction.

A genital herpes lesion, especially on the glans or corona, is easily mistaken for a syphilitic chancre or chancroid. Darkfield examination, multiplex PCR, and cultures for *Haemophilus ducreyi* on selective media will aid in making the diagnosis, as will diagnostic tests for HSV (Tzanck, culture, or DFA). Combined infections occur in up to 20% of cases, so finding a single pathogen may not complete the diagnostic evaluation.

Herpetic gingivostomatitis is often difficult to differentiate from aphthosis, streptococcal infections, diphtheria, coxsackievirus infections, and oral erythema multiforme. Aphthae have a tendency to occur mostly on the buccal and labial mucosae. They usually form shallow, grayish erosions, generally surrounded by a prominent ring of hyperemia. Aphthae commonly occur on nonattached mucosa while recurrent herpes of the oral cavity primarily affects the attached gingiva and palate.

Abudalu M, et al: Single-day, patient-initiated famciclovir therapy versus 3-day valacyclovir regime for recurrent genital herpes: a randomized, double blind, comparative trial. Clin Inf Dis 2008; 47:651.

Anderson B: The epidemiology and clinical analysis of several outbreaks of herpes gladiatorum. Med Sci Sports Exerc 2003; 35:1809.

Anzivino E, et al: Herpes simplex virus infection in pregnancy and in neonate: status of art of epidemiology, diagnosis, therapy and prevention. Vir J 2009; 6:40.

Ashley R: Performance and use of HSV type-specific serology test kits. Herpes 2002; 9:38.

Ban F, et al: Analysis of herpes simplex virus type 1 restriction fragment length polymorphism variants associated with herpes gladiatorum and Kaposi's varicelliform eruption in sumo wrestlers. J Gen Virol 2008; 89–2410.

Barlett BL: Famciclovir treatment options for patients with frequent outbreaks of recurrent genital herpes: the RELIEF trial. J Clin Virol 2008; 43:190.

Beck LA, et al: Phenotype of atopic dermatitis subjects with a history of eczema herpeticum. J Allergy Clin Immunol 2009; 124:260.

Beeson WH, Rachel JD: Valacyclovir prophylaxis for herpes simplex virus infection or infection recurrence following laser skin resurfacing. Dermatol Surg 2002; 28:331.

Bisaccia E, Scarborough D: Herpes simplex virus prophylaxis with famciclovir in patients undergoing aesthetic facial CO_2 laser resurfacing. Cutis 2003; 72:327.

Brabek E, et al: Herpetic folliculitis and syringitis simulating acne excoriée. Arch Dermatol 2001; 137:97.

Brown ZA, et al: Effect of serologic status and cesarean delivery on transmission rates of herpes simplex virus from mother to infant. JAMA 2003; 289:203.

Butler DF, et al: Acquired lymphedema of the hand due to herpes simplex virus type 2. Arch Dermatol 1999; 135:1125.

Carrasco DA, et al: Verrucous herpes of the scrotum in a human immunodeficiency virus-positive man: case report and review of the literature. J Eur Acad Dermatol Venereol 2002; 16:511.

Casper C, Wald A: Condom use and the prevention of genital herpes acquisition. Herpes 2002; 9:10.

Celum C, et al: Effect of aciclovir on HIV-1 acquisition in herpes simplex virus 2 seropositive women and men who have sex with men: a randomised, double-blind, placebo-controlled trial. Lancet 2008; 371:2109.

Cernik C, et al: The treatment of herpes simplex infections. Arch Intern Med 2008; 168:1137.

Chatis PA, et al: Successful treatment with foscarnet of an acyclovir-resistant mucocutaneous infection with herpes simplex virus in a patient with AIDS. N Engl J Med 1989; 320:279.

Chayavichitsilp P, et al: Herpes simplex. Ped in Rev 2009; 30:119.

Chosidow O, et al: Valacyclovir as a single dose during prodrome of herpes facialis: a pilot randomized double-blind clinical trial. Br J Dermatol 2003; 148:142.

Corey L, et al: Once-daily valacyclovir to reduce the risk of transmission of genital herpes. N Engl J Med 2004; 354:11.

Danielsen AG, et al: Chronic erosive herpes simplex virus infection of the penis in a human immunodeficiency virus-positive man, treated with imiquimod and famciclovir. Br J Dermatol 2002; 147:1020.

Enright AM, Prober CG: Neonatal herpes infection: diagnosis, treatment and prevention. Semin Neonatol 2002; 7:283.

Fatahzadeh M, Schwartz RA: Human herpes simplex virus infections: epidemiology, pathogenesis, symptomatology, diagnosis, and management. J Am Acad Dermatol 2007; 57:737.

Fife KH, et al: An international, randomized, double-blind, placebo-controlled study of valacyclovir for the suppression of herpes simplex virus type 2 genital herpes in newly diagnosed patients. Sex Transm Dis 2008; 35:668.

Gilbert J, et al: Topical imiquimod for acyclovir-unresponsive herpes simplex virus 2 infection. Arch Dermatol 2001; 137:1015.

Gilbert S, McBurney E: Use of valacyclovir for herpes simplex virus-1 (HSV-1) prophylaxis after facial resurfacing: a randomized clinical trial of dosing regimens. Dermatol Surg 2000; 26:50.

Grossman MC, et al: The Tzanck smear: can dermatologists accurately interpret it? J Am Acad Dermatol 1992; 27:403.

Gupta AK, et al: Extensive congenital erosions and vesicles healing with reticulate scarring. J Am Acad Dermatol 1987; 17:369.

Gupta R, et al: Genital herpes. Lancet 2007; 370:2127.

Howell MD, et al: Cathelicidin deficiency predisposes to eczema herpeticum. J Allergy Clin Immunol 2006; 117:836.

Husak R, et al: Pseudotumor of the tongue caused by herpes simplex virus type 2 in an HIV-1 infected immunosuppressed patient. Br J Dermatol 1998; 139:118.

Johansson AB, et al: Lower-limb hypoplasia due to intrauterine infection with herpes simplex virus type 2: possible confusion with intrauterine varicella-zoster syndrome. Clin Infect Dis 2004; 38:e57.

Jones CA, et al: Antiviral agents for treatment of herpes simplex virus infection in neonates. Cochrane Database Syst Rev 2009; 3:CD004206.

Hollier LM, et al: Third trimester antiviral prophylaxis for preventing maternal genital herpes simplex virus (HSV) recurrences and neonatal infection. Cochrane Database Syst Rev 2008; 1:CD004946.

Kaminester LH, et al: A double-blind, placebo-controlled study of topical tetracaine in the treatment of herpes labialis. J Am Acad Dermatol 1999; 41:996.

Kim M, et al: Topical calcineurin inhibitors compromise stratum corneum integrity, epidermal permeability and antimicrobial barrier function. Exp Dermatol 2009; Aug 23 (Epub ahead of print).

Kohelet D, et al: Herpes simplex virus infection after vacuum-assisted vaginally delivered infants of asymptomatic mothers. J Perinatol 2004; 24:147.

Kopp T, et al: Successful treatment of an acyclovir-resistant herpes simplex type 2 infection with cidofovir in an AIDS patient. Br J Dermatol 2002; 147:134.

Langenberg AGM, et al: A prospective study of new infections with herpes simplex virus type 1 and 2. N Engl J Med 1999; 341:1432.

Lanzafame M, et al: Unusual, rapidly growing ulcerative genital mass due to herpes simplex virus in a human immunodeficiency virus-infected woman. Br J Dermatol 2003; 149:193.

Lautenschlager S, Eichmann A: Urethritis: an underestimated clinical variant of genital herpes in men? J Am Acad Dermatol 2002; 46:307.

Lubbe J, et al: Adults with atopic dermatitis and herpes simplex and topical therapy with tacrolimus: what kind of prevention? Arch Dermatol 2003; 139:670.

McKeough MB, Spruance SL: Comparison of new topical treatments for herpes labialis: efficacy of penciclovir cream, acyclovir cream, and n-docosanol cream against experimental cutaneous herpes simplex virus type 1 infection. Arch Dermatol 2001; 137:1153.

Money D, et al: Genital herpes: gynaecological aspects. J Obstet Gynaecol 2008; 206:347.

Money D, et al: Guideline for the management of herpes simplex virus in pregnancy. J Obstet Gynaecol 2008; 208:518

Nahass GT, et al: Comparison of Tzanck smear, viral culture, and DNA diagnostic methods in detection of herpes simplex and varicella zoster infection. JAMA 1992; 268:2541.

Nikkels AF, Pierard GE: Chronic herpes simplex virus type I glossitis in an immunocompromised man. Br J Dermatol 1999; 140:343.

Osawa K, et al: Relationship between Kaposi's varicelliform eruption in Japanese patients with atopic dermatitis treated with tacrolimus ointment and genetic polymorphisms in the IL-19 gene promoter region. J Dermatol 2007; 34:531.

Paradisi A, et al: Kaposi's varicelliform eruption complicating allergic contact dermatitis. J Am Acad Dermatol 2006; 54:732.

Sacks SL: Efficacy of docosanol. J Am Acad Dermatol 2003; 49:558.

Santmyire-Rosenberger BR, et al: Psoriasis herpeticum: three cases of Kaposi's varicelliform eruption in psoriasis. J Am Acad Dermatol 2005; 53:52–56.

Segura S, et al: Eczema herpeticum during treatment of atopic dermatitis with 1% pimecrolimus cream. Acta Derm Venereol 2005; 85:524.

Sperling RS, et al: The effect of daily valacyclovir suppression on herpes simplex virus type 2 viral shedding in HSV-2 seropositive subjects without a history of genital herpes. Sex Transm Dis 2008; 35:286.

Spruance SL, et al: Single-dose, patient-initiated famciclovir: a randomized, double-blind, placebo-controlled trial for episodic treatment of herpes labialis. J Am Acad Dermatol 2006; 55:47.

Spruance SL, McKeough MB: Combination treatment with famciclovir and a topical corticosteroid gel versus famciclovir alone for experimental ultraviolet radiation-induced herpes simplex labialis: a pilot study. J Infect Dis 2000; 181:1906.

Stetson CL, et al: Herpetic whitlow during isotretinoin therapy. Int J Dermatol 2003; 42:496.

Wollenberg A, et al: Predisposing factors and clinical features of eczema herpeticum: a retrospective analysis of 100 cases. J Am Acad Dermatol 2003; 49:198.

Varicella

Varicella, commonly known as chickenpox, is the primary infection with the VZV. In temperate regions, 90% of cases occur in children younger than 10 years of age, with the highest age-specific incidence in children aged 1–4 years in unvaccinated children. More than 90% of adults in temperate countries have evidence of prior infection and are "immune" to varicella. In tropical countries, however, varicella tends to be a disease of teenagers, and only 60% of adults are "immune" serologically. The incubation period is 10–21 days (usually 14–15 days). Transmission is via the respiratory route and less commonly by direct contact with the lesions. A susceptible person may develop varicella following exposure to the lesions of herpes zoster. Infected persons are most infectious from 5 days before the appearance of the eruption, and most infectious 1–2 days prior to the appearance of the rash. Infectivity ceases 5–6 days after the eruption appears in most cases. There is an initial viral replication in the nasopharynx and conjunctiva, followed by infection of the reticuloendothelial system (liver spleen) between days 4 and 6. A secondary viremia occurs at days 11–20, resulting in infection of the epidermis and the appearance of the characteristic skin lesions. Low-grade fever, malaise, and headache are usually present but slight. The severity of the disease is age-dependent, with adults having more severe disease and a greater risk of visceral disease. In healthy children the death rate from varicella is 1.4 in 100 000 cases; in adults, 30.9 in 100 000 cases. Pregnant women have five times greater risk of an adverse outcome. As with most viral infections, immunosuppression may worsen the course of the disease. Lifelong immunity follows varicella and second episodes of "varicella" indicate either immunosuppression or another viral infection such as coxsackievirus.

Varicella is characterized by a vesicular eruption consisting of delicate "teardrop" vesicles on an erythematous base (Fig. 19-13). The eruption starts with faint macules that develop rapidly into vesicles within 24 h. Successive fresh crops of vesicles appear for a few days, mainly on the trunk, face, and oral mucosa. Initially, the exanthem may be limited to sun-exposed areas, the diaper area of infants, or sites of inflammation. The vesicles quickly become pustular and umbilicated, then crusted. Since the lesions appear in crops, lesions of various stages are present at the same time, a useful clue to the diagnosis. Lesions tend not to scar, but larger ones and those that become secondarily infected may heal with a characteristic round, depressed scar.

Secondary bacterial infection with *S. aureus* or a streptococcal organism is the most common complication of varicella (Fig. 19-14). Rarely, it may be complicated by osteomyelitis, other deep-seated infections, or septicemia. Other complications are rare. Pneumonia is uncommon in normal children but is seen in 1 in 400 adults with varicella. It may be bacterial or caused by the varicella, a difficult differential diagnosis. Cerebellar ataxia and encephalitis are the most common neurologic complications. Asymptomatic myocarditis and hepati-

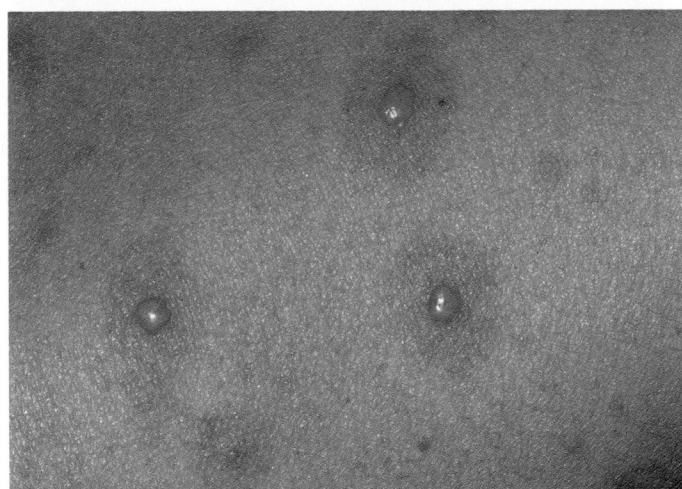

Fig. 19-13 Varicella.

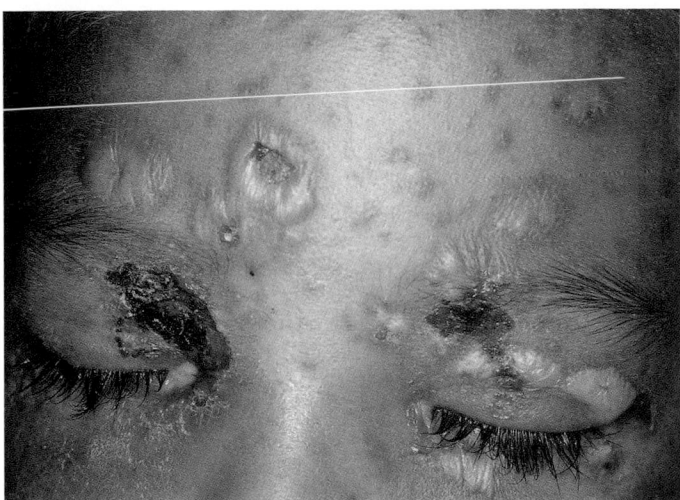

Fig. 19-14 Varicella with bullous impetigo as a complication.

tis are not uncommon in children with varicella, but these conditions are rarely significant and resolve spontaneously with no treatment. Reye syndrome, a syndrome of hepatitis and acute encephalopathy, is associated with the use of aspirin to treat the symptoms of varicella. Aspirin is absolutely contraindicated in patients with varicella. Any child with varicella and severe vomiting should be referred immediately to exclude Reye syndrome. Symptomatic thrombocytopenia is a rare manifestation of varicella, which can occur either with the exanthem or several weeks after. Purpura fulminans, a form of disseminated intravascular coagulation associated with low levels of protein C and S, may complicate varicella.

The diagnosis of varicella is easily made clinically. A Tzanck smear from a vesicle will usually show characteristic multinucleate giant cells. If needed, the most useful clinical test is a DFA test, which is rapid and will both confirm the infection and type the virus. Since the VZV grows poorly and slowly in the laboratory, viral culture is rarely indicated.

Treatment

Both immunocompetent children and adults with varicella benefit from acyclovir therapy if started early (within 24 h of the appearance of the eruption). Therapy does not appear to alter the development of adequate immunity to reinfection. Because the complications of varicella are infrequent in children, routine treatment is not recommended; therapeutic decisions are made on a case-by-case basis. Acyclovir therapy seems to benefit most secondary cases within a household, which tend to be more severe than the index case. In this setting, therapy can be instituted earlier. Therapy does not, however, return children to school sooner and the impact on parental work days missed is not known. The dose is 20 mg/kg (maximum 800 mg per dose) four times a day for 5 days. Aspirin and other salicylates should not be used as antipyretics in varicella because their use increases the risk of Reye syndrome. Topical antipruritic lotions, oatmeal baths, dressing the patient in light, cool clothing, and keeping the environment cool may all relieve some of the symptomatology. Children living in warm homes and kept very warm with clothing have anecdotally been observed to have more numerous skin lesions. Children with atopic dermatitis, Darier's disease, congenital ichthyosiform erythroderma, diabetes, cystic fibrosis, conditions requiring chronic salicylate or steroid therapy, and inborn errors of metabolism should be treated with acyclovir since they may suffer more complications or exacerbations of their underlying illness with varicella.

Varicella is more severe and complications are more common in adults. Between 5% and 14% of adults will have pulmonary involvement. Smokers and those with pre-existing lung disease (but not asthma) are at increased risk. The pneumonitis can progress rapidly and be fatal. Adults with varicella and at least one other risk factor should be evaluated with physical examination, pulse oximetry, and chest radiography. Antiviral treatment is recommended in all adolescents and adults (13 and older) with varicella. The dose is 800 mg four or five times a day for 5 days. Severe, fulminant cutaneous disease and visceral complications are treated with intravenous acyclovir, 10 mg/kg every 8 h, adjusted for creatinine clearance. If the patient is hospitalized for therapy, strict isolation is required. Patients with varicella should not be admitted to wards with immunocompromised hosts or on to pediatric wards, but rather are best placed on wards with healthy patients recovering from acute trauma.

Pregnant women and neonates

Maternal infection with the VZV during the first 20 weeks of gestation may result in a syndrome of congenital malformations (congenital varicella syndrome), as well as severe illness in the mother. In one study, 4 of 31 women with varicella in pregnancy developed varicella pneumonia. The risk for spontaneous abortion by 20 weeks is 3%; in an additional 0.7% of pregnancies, fetal death occurs after 20 weeks. The risk of preterm labor, as reported in various studies, has varied from no increase to a three-fold increase. Severe varicella and varicella pneumonia or disseminated disease in pregnancy should be treated with intravenous acyclovir. All varicella in pregnancy should be treated with oral acyclovir, 800 mg five times a day for 7 days (except perhaps during the first month, when a specialist should be consulted). In all women past 35 weeks of gestation or with increased risk of premature labor, admission and intravenous acyclovir, 10 mg/kg three times daily, should be recommended. The patient should be evaluated for pneumonia, renal function should be carefully monitored, and the patient should be switched to oral therapy once lesions stop appearing (usually in 48–72 hours).

Varicella zoster immune globulin (VZIG) should not be given once the pregnant woman has developed varicella. VZIG should be given for significant exposures (see below) within the first 72–96 h to ameliorate maternal varicella and prevent complications. Its use should be limited to seronegative women because of its cost and the high rate of asymptomatic infection in the US. The lack of a history of prior varicella is associated with seronegativity in only 20% or fewer of the US population.

Congenital varicella syndrome is characterized by a series of anomalies, including hypoplastic limbs (usually unilateral and lower extremity), cutaneous scars, and ocular and CNS disease. Female fetuses are affected more commonly than males. The overall risk for this syndrome is between 1% and 2% (the former figure from the largest series). The highest risk is from maternal varicella between weeks 13 and 20 when the risk is 2%. Infection of the fetus in utero may result in zoster occurring postnatally, often in the first 2 years of life. This occurs in about 1% of varicella-complicated pregnancies and the risk for this complication is greatest in varicella occurring in weeks 25–36 of gestation. The value of VZIG in preventing or modifying fetal complications of maternal varicella is unknown. In one study, however, of 97 patients with varicella in pregnancy who were treated with VZIG, none had complications of congenital varicella syndrome or infantile zoster, suggesting some efficacy for VZIG. Although apparently safe in pregnancy, acyclovir's efficacy in preventing fetal complications of maternal varicella is unknown.

If the mother develops varicella between 5 days before and 2 days after delivery, neonatal varicella can occur and be severe, as transplacental delivery of antivaricella antibody has been inadequate. These neonates develop varicella at 5–10 days of age. In such cases the administration of VZIG is warranted and acyclovir therapy intravenously should be considered.

Varicella vaccine

Live attenuated viral vaccine for varicella is a currently recommended childhood immunization. Two doses are now recommended, one between age 12 and 15 months and the second at 4–6 years. This double vaccination schedule is recommended since epidemics of varicella still occurred in children ages 9–11 in well-immunized communities, suggesting a waning of immunity by this age. Complications of varicella vaccination are uncommon. A mild skin eruption from which virus can usually not be isolated, occurring locally at the injection site within 2 days or generalized 1–3 weeks after immunization, occurs in 6% of children. Many of the breakthrough cases in vaccinated children are mild and many of the skin lesions were not vesicular (see modified varicella-like syndrome below). Prevention of severe varicella is virtually 100%, even when the vaccine is given within 36 h of exposure. Immunized children with no detectable antibody also have reduced severity of varicella after exposure. Secondary complications of varicella, including scarring, are virtually eliminated by vaccination.

Household exposure of immunosuppressed children to recently immunized siblings does not appear to pose a great risk. Children whose leukemia is in remission are also protected by the vaccine but may require three doses. Leukemic children still receiving chemotherapy have a complication rate from vaccination (usually a varicella-like eruption) approaching 50%. They may require acyclovir therapy. Unprotected close contacts developed varicella 15% of the time. In leukemic children, adequate immunization results in complete immunity in some and partial immunity in the rest, protecting them from severe varicella. Immunization also reduces the attack rate for zoster in leukemic children.

Modified varicella-like syndrome

Children immunized with live attenuated varicella vaccine may develop varicella of reduced severity on exposure to natural varicella. This has been called modified varicella-like syndrome (MVLS). The frequency of MVLS is between 0% and 2.7% per year and children with lower antibody titers are more likely to develop MVLS. The illness occurs an average of 15 days after exposure to varicella and consists primarily of macules and papules with relatively few vesicles. The average number of lesions is about 35–50, compared with natural varicella, which usually has about 300 lesions. The majority of patients are afebrile and the illness is mild, lasting fewer than 5 days on average.

Immunocompromised patients

Varicella cases can be extremely severe and even fatal in immunosuppressed patients, especially in individuals with impaired cell-mediated immunity. Before effective antiviral therapy nearly one-third of children with cancer developed complications of varicella and 7% died. In this setting, varicella pneumonia, hepatitis, and encephalitis are frequent. Prior varicella does not always protect the immunosuppressed host from multiple episodes. The skin lesions in the immunosuppressed host are usually identical to varicella in the healthy host; however, the number of lesions may be numerous (Fig. 19-15). In an immunosuppressed patient, the lesions more frequently become necrotic and ulceration may occur. Even if the lesions are few, the size of the lesion may be large (up to several centimeters) and necrosis of the full thickness of the dermis may occur. In HIV infection, varicella may be severe and fatal. Atypical cases of a few scattered lesions without a dermatomal distribution usually represent reactivation disease with dissemination. Chronic varicella may complicate HIV infection, resulting in ulcerative (ecthymatous) or hyperkeratotic (verrucous) lesions. These patterns of infection may be associated with acyclovir resistance.

The degree of immunosuppression likely to result in severe varicella has been a matter of debate. There are case reports of severe and even fatal varicella in otherwise healthy children given short courses of oral steroids or even using only inhaled steroids. In a case-control study, however, corticosteroid use did not appear to be a risk factor for the development of severe varicella. In the UK, any patient receiving or having received systemic steroids in the prior 3 months, regardless of dose, is considered at increased risk for severe varicella. Inhaled steroids are not considered an indication for prophylactic VZIG or antiviral treatment. A "high-risk" or significant exposure has been defined as:

1. household contact, i.e. living in the same house as a case of chickenpox or zoster
2. face-to-face contact with a case of chickenpox for at least 5 min
3. contact indoors with a case of chickenpox or herpes zoster for more than 1 h or, within a hospital setting, a case of chickenpox or herpes zoster in an adjacent bed or the same open ward.

Immunosuppressed children with no prior history of varicella and a high-risk exposure should be treated with VZIG as soon as possible after exposure (within 96 h). Pre-engraftment bone marrow transplant patients should be treated the same. VZIG treatment does not reduce the frequency of infection, but it does reduce the severity of infection and complications. The value of prophylactic antivirals is unknown. Parents of immunosuppressed children and their doctors should be aware that severe disease can occur and the parents counseled to return immediately after significant exposure or if varicella develops.

An unusual variant of recurrent varicella is seen in elderly patients with a history of varicella in childhood, who have a malignancy of the bone marrow and are on chemotherapy. They develop a mild illness with 10–40 widespread lesions and usually no systemic findings. This type of recurrent varicella tends to relapse. It is different from typical varicella, as all the lesions are in a single stage of development and for this reason could be easily confused with smallpox.

Ideally, management of varicella in the immunocompromised patient would involve prevention through the use of varicella vaccination before immunosuppression. Vaccination is safe if the person is more than 1 year from induction chemotherapy, chemotherapy is halted around the time of vaccination, and the lymphocyte count is higher than $700/mm^3$. Intravenous acyclovir at a dose of 10 mg/kg three times a day (or 500 mg/m^2 in children) is given as soon as the diagnosis of varicella is suspected. Intravenous therapy is continued until 2 days after all new vesicles have stopped. Oral antivirals are continued for a minimum of 10 days of treatment. VZIG is of no proven benefit once clinical disease has developed, but may be given if the patient has severe life-threatening disease and is not responding to intravenous acyclovir.

In HIV-infected adults, treatment is individualized. Persons with typical varicella should be evaluated for the presence of pneumonia or hepatitis. Valacyclovir, 1 g three times a day; famciclovir, 500 mg three times a day; or acyclovir, 800 mg every 4 h, may be used if no visceral complications are present. The former two agents may be preferable to acyclovir because of their enhanced oral bioavailability. Visceral disease mandates intravenous therapy. If the response to oral antiviral agents is not rapid, intravenous acyclovir therapy should be instituted. Antiviral treatment must be continued until all lesions are completely healed. Most cases of chronic or acyclovir-resistant VZV infection are associated with initial inadequate oral doses of acyclovir (either too short in duration, too low a dose, or in patients with gastrointestinal disease, in whom reduced gastrointestinal absorption may be associated with inadequate blood levels of acyclovir). Atypical disseminated cases must be treated aggressively until all lesions resolve. The diagnosis of acyclovir-resistant VZV infection may be difficult. Acyclovir-resistant VZV strains may be hard to culture and sensitivity testing is still not standardized or readily available for VZV. Acyclovir-resistant varicella is treated with foscarnet, and in cases failing that agent, cidofovir.

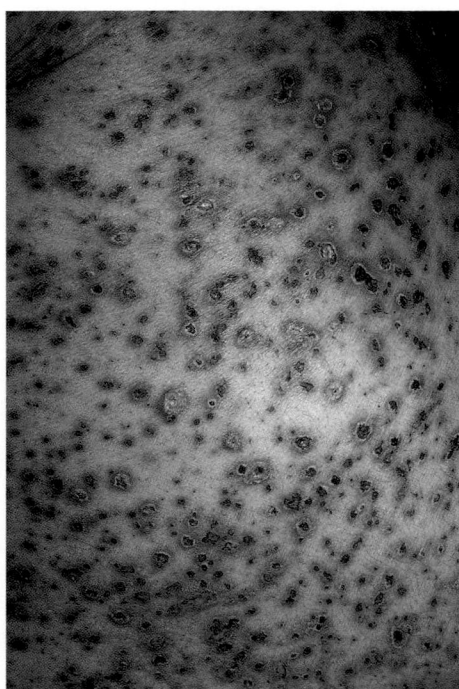

Fig. 19-15 Varicella in a patient with advanced Hodgkin disease.

Arvin AM: Antiviral therapy for varicella and herpes zoster. Semin Pediatr Infect Dis 2002; 13:12.

Asano Y: Clinicopathologic understanding and control of varicella-zoster virus infection. Vaccine 2008; 26:6487.

Clements DA: Modified varicella-like syndrome. Infect Dis Clin North Am 1996; 10:617.

Creed E, et al: Varicella zoster vaccines. Dermatolog Ther 2009; 22:143.

Enders G, et al: Consequences of varicella and herpes zoster in pregnancy: prospective study of 1739 cases. Lancet 1994; 343:1548.

Kasper WJ, et al: Fatal varicella after a single course of corticosteroids. Pediatr Infect Dis 1990; 9:729.

Marin M, et al: Varicella prevention in the United States: a review of successes and challenges. Pediatrics 2008; 122:e744.

Messner J, et al: Accentuated viral exanthems in areas of inflammation. J Am Acad Dermatol 1999; 40:345.

Mueller NH, et al: Varicella zoster virus infection: clinical features, molecular pathogenesis of disease, and latency. Neurol Clin 2008; 26:675.

Patel H, et al: Recent corticosteroid use and the risk of complicated varicella in otherwise immunocompetent children. Arch Pediatr Adolesc Med 1996; 150:409.

Santos-Juanes J, et al: Varicella complicated by group A streptococcal facial cellulitis. J Am Acad Dermatol 2001; 45:770.

Tunbridge AJ, et al: Chickenpox in adults: clinical management. J Infection 2008; 57:95.

Wu JJ, et al: Vaccines and immunotherapies for the prevention of infectious diseases having cutaneous manifestations. J Am Acad Dermatol 2004; 50:495.

Zampogna JC, Flowers FP: Persistent verrucous varicella as the initial manifestation of HIV infection. J Am Acad Dermatol 2001; 44:391.

Zoster (shingles, herpes zoster)

Zoster is caused by reactivation of VZV. Following primary infection or vaccination, VZV remains latent in the sensory dorsal root ganglion cells. The virus begins to replicate at some later time, traveling down the sensory nerve into the skin. Other than immunosuppression and age-related deficiency of cell-mediated immunity, the factors involved in reactivation are unknown.

The incidence of zoster increases with age. Below the age of 45, the annual incidence is less than 1 in 1000 persons. Among patients older than 75 years of age, the rate is more than four times greater. For white persons older than 80 years of age, the lifetime risk of developing zoster is 10–30%. Overall, about 1 in 3 unvaccinated persons will develop herpes zoster. For unknown reasons, being nonwhite reduces the risk for herpes zoster, with African Americans being four times less likely to develop zoster. Immunosuppression, especially hematologic malignancy and HIV infection, dramatically increases the risk for zoster. In HIV-infected persons the annual incidence is 30 in 1000 persons, or an annual risk of 3%. With the universal use of varicella vaccination and decrease in pediatric and adolescent varicella cases, older persons will no longer have periodic boosts of the anti-VZV immune activity. This could result in an increase in the incidence of zoster.

Herpes zoster classically occurs unilaterally within the distribution of a cranial or spinal sensory nerve, often with some overflow into the dermatomes above and below. The dermatomes most frequently affected are the thoracic (55%), cranial (20%, with the trigeminal nerve being the most common single nerve involved), lumbar (15%), and sacral (5%). The cutaneous eruption is frequently preceded by one to several days of pain in the affected area, although the pain may appear simultaneously or even following the skin eruption, or the eruption may be painless. The eruption initially presents as papules and plaques of erythema in the dermatome. Within hours the plaques develop blisters (Fig. 19-16). Lesions continue to appear for several days. The eruption may have few lesions or reach total confluence in the dermatome. Lesions may become hemorrhagic, necrotic, or bullous. Rarely, the

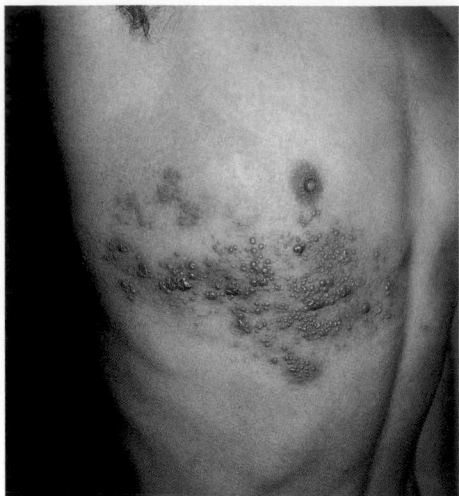

Fig. 19-16 Herpes zoster, classic dermatomal distribution.

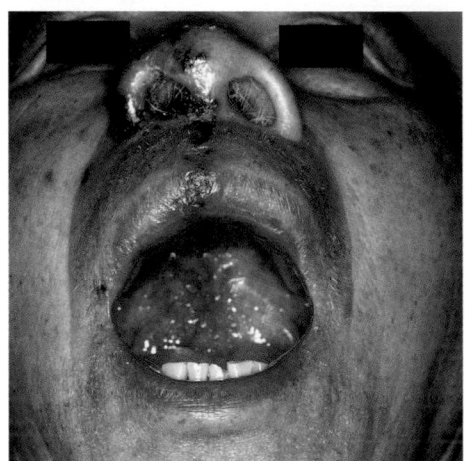

Fig. 19-17 Oral zoster.

patient may have pain, but no skin lesions (zoster sine herpete). There is a correlation with the pain severity and extent of the skin lesions, and elderly persons tend to have more severe pain. In patients under 30 years of age, the pain may be minimal. It is not uncommon for there to be scattered lesions outside the dermatome, usually fewer than 20. In the typical case, new vesicles appear for 1–5 days, become pustular, crust, and heal. The total duration of the eruption depends on three factors: patient age, severity of eruption, and presence of underlying immunosuppression. In younger patients, the total duration is 23 weeks, whereas in elderly patients, the cutaneous lesions of zoster may require 6 weeks or more to heal. Scarring is more common in elderly and immunosuppressed patients. Scarring also correlates with the severity of the initial eruption. Lesions may develop on the mucous membranes within the mouth in zoster of the maxillary (Fig. 19-17) or mandibular division of the facial nerve, or in the vagina in zoster in the S2 or S3 dermatome. Zoster may appear in recent surgical scars.

Zoster may rarely be seen in children under the age of 1 year. This can occur due to intrauterine exposure to VZV or due to exposure to VZV during the first few months of life. The maternal antibodies still present result in muted expression of varicella—subclinical or very mild disease. The immaturity of the infant's immune system results in poor immune response to the infection, allowing for early relapse in the form of zoster.

Disseminated herpes zoster

Disseminated herpes zoster is defined as more than 20 lesions outside the affected dermatome. It occurs chiefly in old or debilitated individuals, especially in patients with lymphoreticular malignancy or AIDS. Low levels of serum antibody against VZV are a highly significant risk factor in predicting dissemination of disease. The dermatomal lesions are sometimes hemorrhagic or gangrenous. The outlying vesicles or bullae, which are usually not grouped, resemble varicella and are often umbilicated and may be hemorrhagic. Visceral dissemination to the lungs and CNS may occur in the setting of disseminated zoster. Disseminated zoster requires careful evaluation and systemic antiviral therapy. This would initially be intravenous acyclovir, which may be changed to an oral antiviral agent once visceral involvement has been excluded and the patient has received at least 2–3 days of intravenous therapy.

Ophthalmic zoster

In herpes zoster ophthalmicus, the ophthalmic division of the fifth cranial nerve is involved. If the external division of the nasociliary branch is affected, with vesicles on the side and tip of the nose (Hutchinson's sign), the eye is involved 76% of the time, as compared with 34% when it is not involved (Fig. 19-18). Vesicles on the lid margin are virtually always associated with ocular involvement. In any case, the patient with ophthalmic zoster should be seen by an ophthalmologist. Systemic antiviral therapy should be started immediately, pending ophthalmologic evaluation. Ocular involvement is most commonly in the form of uveitis (92%) and keratitis (50%). Less common but more severe complications include glaucoma, optic neuritis, encephalitis, hemiplegia, and acute retinal necrosis. These complications are reduced from 50% of patients with herpes zoster ophthalmicus to 20–30% with effective antiviral therapy. Unlike the cutaneous lesions, ocular lesions of zoster and their complications tend to recur, sometimes as long as 10 years after the zoster episode.

Other complications

Motor nerve neuropathy occurs in about 3% of patients with zoster and is three times more common if zoster is associated with underlying malignancy. Seventy-five percent of cases

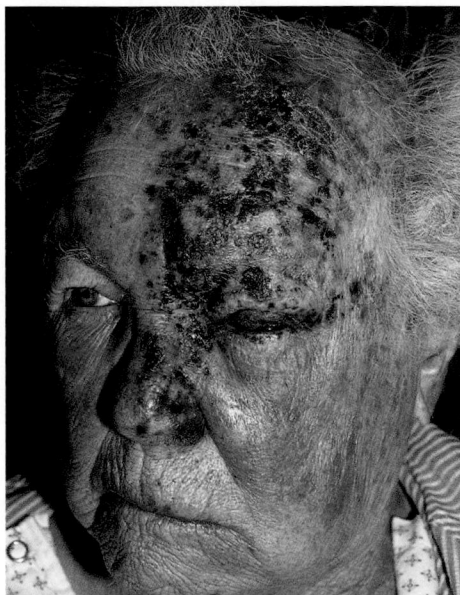

Fig. 19-18 Herpes zoster, involvement of the V1 dermatome.

slowly recover, leaving 25% with some residual motor deficit. If the sacral dermatome S3, or less often S2 or S4, is involved, urinary hesitancy or actual urinary retention may occur. Hematuria and pyuria may also be present. The prognosis is good for complete recovery. Similarly pseudo-obstruction, colonic spasm, dilatation, obstipation, constipation, and reduced anal sphincter tone can occur with thoracic (T6–T12), lumbar, or sacral zoster. Recovery is complete. Maxillary and mandibular alveolar bone necrosis may occur an average of 30 days after zoster of the maxillary or mandibular branches of the trigeminal nerve. Limited or widespread loss of teeth may result.

Ramsay Hunt syndrome results from involvement of the facial and auditory nerves by VSV. Herpetic inflammation of the geniculate ganglion is felt to be the cause of this syndrome. The presenting features include zoster of the external ear or tympanic membrane; herpes auricularis with ipsilateral facial paralysis; or herpes auricularis, facial paralysis, and auditory symptoms. Auditory symptoms include mild to severe tinnitus, deafness, vertigo, nausea and vomiting, and nystagmus.

Herpes zoster can be associated with delayed complications. Many of these are due to vasculopathies affecting the CNS or even peripheral arteries. Delayed contralateral hemiparesis, simulating stroke, is a rare but serious complication of herpes zoster that occurs weeks to months (mean 7 weeks) after an episode of zoster affecting the first branch of the trigeminal nerve. By direct extension along the intracranial branches of the trigeminal nerve, VZV gains access to the CNS and infects the cerebral arteries. Patients present with headache and hemiplegia. Arteriography is diagnostic, demonstrating thrombosis of the anterior or middle cerebral artery. This form of vasculopathy can also occur following varicella and may be the cause of up to one-third of ischemic strokes in children. The recognized vasculopathic complications of VZV have been expanded to include changes in mental status, aphasia, ataxia, hemisensory loss, and both hemianopia and monocular visual loss. Monocular vision loss can occur up to 6 months following zoster. Aneurysm, subarachnoid or cerebral hemorrhage, carotid dissection, and even peripheral vascular disease are other recognized forms of VZV vasculopathy. The vasculopathy may be multifocal and involve both large and small arteries. In more than one-third of cases VZV vasculopathy occurs without a rash. MRI is virtually always abnormal. The diagnosis is confirmed by VZV PCR and anti-VZV IgG antibody testing of the CSF. Since this is due to active viral replication in the vessels, the treatment is intravenous acyclovir, 10–15 mg/kg three times daily for a minimum of 14 days. In some patients, months of oral antivirals are given if symptoms are slow to resolve. A short burst of systemic steroids is sometimes also given.

Treatment

Middle-aged and elderly patients are urged to restrict their physical activities or even stay home in bed for a few days. Bed rest may be of paramount importance in the prevention of neuralgia. Younger patients may usually continue with their customary activities. Local applications of heat, as with an electric heating pad or a hot-water bottle, are recommended. Simple local application of gentle pressure with the hand or with an abdominal binder often gives great relief.

Antiviral therapy is the cornerstone in the management of herpes zoster. Since antiviral therapy does not reduce the rate of zoster-associated pain, clinicians may under-appreciate the tremendous benefit these antiviral drugs provide. The main benefit of therapy is in reduction of the duration and severity of zoster-associated pain. Therefore, treatment in immunocompetent patients is indicated for those at highest risk for persistent pain—those over 50 years of age. It is also recommended to treat all patients with painful or severe zoster, ophthalmic zoster, Ramsay Hunt syndrome, immunosuppression, cutaneous or visceral dissemination, and motor nerve involvement. In the most severe cases, especially in ophthalmic zoster and disseminated zoster, initial intravenous therapy may be considered. Therapy should be started as soon as the diagnosis is suspected, pending laboratory confirmation. It is preferable for treatment to be instituted within the first 3 or 4 days. In immunocompetent patients, the efficacy of starting treatment beyond this time is unknown. Treatment leads to more rapid resolution of the skin lesions and, most importantly, substantially decreases the duration of zoster-associated pain. Valacyclovir, 1000 mg, and famciclovir, 500 mg, may be given three times a day. These agents are as effective as or superior to acyclovir, 800 mg five times a day, probably because of better absorption and the fact that higher blood levels are achieved. They are as safe as acyclovir. If not contraindicated, they are preferred.

In the immunocompetent host, a total of 7 days of treatment has been shown to be as effective as 21 days of treatment. Valacyclovir and famciclovir must be dose-adjusted in patients with renal impairment. In an elderly patient, if the renal status is unknown, the newer agents may be started at twice-a-day dosing (which is almost as effective), pending evaluation of renal function, or acyclovir can be used. For patients with renal failure (creatinine clearance of less than 25 mL/min), acyclovir is preferable. In the setting of known or acquired renal failure, acyclovir neurotoxicity can occur from intravenous acyclovir or oral valacyclovir therapy. This can present in the acute setting as hallucinations, or with prolonged elevated blood levels, disorientation, dizziness, loss of decorum, incoherence, photophobia, difficulty speaking, delirium, confusion, agitation, and death delusion. Since acyclovir can reduce renal function, the patient's baseline renal function may have been normal, but high doses of acyclovir may have reduced renal function, leading to neurotoxic acyclovir levels.

In the immunosuppressed patient, an antiviral agent should always be given because of the increased risk of dissemination and zoster-associated complications. The doses are identical to those used in immunocompetent hosts. In immunosuppressed patients with ophthalmic zoster, disseminated zoster, or Ramsay Hunt syndrome, and in patients failing oral therapy, intravenous acyclovir should be used at a dose of 10 mg/kg three times a day, adjusted for renal function.

Since some of the pain during acute zoster (acute zoster neuritis) may have an inflammatory component, corticosteroids have been used during the acute episode. The use of corticosteroids in this setting is controversial. In selected older individuals, corticosteroid use is associated with better quality-of-life measures, reduction in time to uninterrupted sleep, quicker return to usual activities, and reduced analgesic use. A tapering dose of systemic steroids, starting at about 1 mg/kg and lasting 10–14 days, is adequate to achieve these benefits. Systemic steroids should not be used in immunosuppressed patients or when there is a contraindication to systemic steroid use. All factors being considered, the benefits of corticosteroid therapy during acute zoster appear to outweigh the risks in treatment-eligible patients. Reduction in postherpetic neuralgia by corticosteroids has never been documented despite multiple studies, but this is also true of antiviral therapy which reduces the severity and duration but not the prevalence of postherpetic neuralgia.

Zoster-associated pain (postherpetic neuralgia, PHN)

Pain is the most troublesome symptom of zoster. Eighty-four percent of patients over the age of 50 will have pain preceding the eruption and 89% will have pain with the eruption. Various terminologies are used to classify the pain. The simplest approach is to term all pain occurring immediately preceding or after zoster "zoster-associated pain" (ZAP). Another classification system separates acute pain (within the first 30 days), subacute pain (between 30 and 120 days), and chronic pain (lasting more than 120 days).

Two different mechanisms are proposed to cause ZAP: sensitization and deafferentation. Nociceptors (sensory nerves mediating pain) become sensitized following injury, resulting in ongoing discharge and hyperexcitability (peripheral sensitization). Prolonged discharge of the nociceptor enhances the dorsal horn neurons to afferent stimuli and expands the dorsal horn neuron's receptive field (central sensitization), leading to allodynia and hyperalgesia. In addition, neural destruction causes spontaneous activity in deafferented central neurons, generating constant pain. The spinal terminals of mechanoreceptors may contact receptors formerly occupied by C-fibers, leading to hyperalgesia and allodynia. The loss of function or death of dorsal horn neurons, which have an inhibitory effect on adjacent neurons, contributes to an increase in activity being transmitted up the spinal cord. The central sensitization is initially temporary (self-limited), but may become permanent.

The quality of the pain associated with herpes zoster varies, but three basic types have been described. There is the constant, monotonous, usually burning or deep, aching pain; the shooting, lancinating (neuritic) pain; and triggered pain. The latter is usually allodynia (pain with normal nonpainful stimuli such as light touch) or hyperalgesia (severe pain produced by a stimulus normally producing mild pain). The character and quality of acute zoster pain are identical to the pain that persists after the skin lesions have healed, although they be mediated by different mechanisms.

The rate of resolution of pain following herpes zoster is reported over a wide range. The following data are from a prospective study and do not represent selected patients, as are recruited in drug trials for herpes zoster. The tendency to have persistent pain is age-dependent, occurring for longer than 1 month in only 2% of persons under 40 years of age. Fifty percent of persons over 60 years of age and 75% of those over 70 years of age continue to have pain beyond 1 month. Although the natural history is for gradual improvement in persons over 70 years, 25% have some pain at 3 months and 10% have pain at 1 year. Severe pain lasting longer than 1 year is uncommon, but 8% of persons over 60 have mild pain and 2% still have moderate pain at 1 year.

ZAP, especially that of long duration, is very difficult to manage. Adequate medication should be provided to control the pain from the first visit. Once established, neuropathic pain is very difficult to control. Every effort should be made to prevent neuronal damage. In addition, chronic pain may lead to depression, complicating management of the pain. Patients with persistent moderate to severe pain may benefit from referral to a pain clinic. With this background, the importance of early and adequate antiviral therapy and pain control cannot be overemphasized.

Oral antiviral agents are recommended in all patients over 50 with pain in whom blisters are still present, even if they are not given within the first 96 h of the eruption. Oral analgesia should be maximized using acetaminophen, nonsteroidal anti-inflammatory drugs (NSAIDs), and opiate analgesia as required. Capsaicin applied topically every few hours may reduce pain, but the application itself may cause burning and the benefits are modest. Local anesthetics, such as 10% lidocaine in gel form, 5% lidocaine–prilocaine, or lidocaine patches (Lidoderm), may acutely reduce pain. These topical measures may provide some short-term analgesic effect, but do not appear to have any long-term benefit in reducing the severity or prevalence of ZAP. Sublesional anesthesia, epidural blocks, and sympathetic blocks with and without corticosteroids have been reported in large series, but rarely studied in a controlled manner. They provide acute relief of pain. Although the benefit of nerve blocks in preventing or treating persistent ZAP remains to be proven, they are a reasonable consideration in the acute setting if the patient is having very severe pain (unable to eat or sleep) and oral therapy has yet to be effective. They may also be used in patients who have failed the standard therapies listed below. A transcutaneous electrical nerve stimulation (TENS) unit may be beneficial for persistent neuralgia. Botulinum toxin, 100 U, spread out over the affected area in a checkerboard or fan-like pattern with 5 U per route, has dramatically improved PHN in four reported patients with thoracic zoster.

Despite this vast array of medication options, PHN is commonly difficult to treat for two reasons. The recommended medications are simply often not effective. Second, in the elderly who are most severely affected by PHN, these medications have significant and often intolerable side effects, limiting the dose one can prescribe. If multiple agents are combined to reduce the toxicity of any one agent, the side effects of these agents overlap (sedation, depression, constipation) and there may be drug–drug interactions, limiting combination treatment options.

Three classes of medication are used as standards to manage ZAP and PHN — tricyclic antidepressants, anti-seizure medications, and long-acting opiates. If opiate analgesia is required, it should be provided by a long-acting agent, and the duration of treatment should be limited and the patient transitioned to another class of agent. Constipation is a major side effect in the elderly. During painful zoster these patients ingest less fluid and fiber, enhancing the constipating effects of the opiates. Bulk laxatives should be recommended. Tramadol is an option for acute pain control, but drug interactions with the tricyclics must be monitored. The tricyclic antidepressants, such as amitriptyline (or nortriptyline) and desipramine, are well tested and documented as effective for the management of PHN. They are considered first-line agents in this condition. They are dosed at 25 mg/night (or 10 mg for those over the age of 65–70 years). The dose is increased by the same amount nightly until pain control is achieved or the maximum dose is reached. The ultimate dose is somewhere between 25 and 100 mg in a single nightly dose. The early use of amitriptyline was able to reduce the pain prevalence at 6 months, suggesting that early intervention is optimal. Venlafaxine (Effexor) may be used in patients who do not tolerate tricyclics. The starting dose is 25 mg/night and the dose is gradually titrated up as required. Gabapentin (Neurontin) and pregabalin (Lyrica) have been documented as aiding in the reduction of zoster-associated pain. The starting dose of gabapentin is usually 300 mg three times daily, escalating up to 3600 mg per day. Pregabalin has improved pharmacokinetics and is dosed at 300 mg or 600 mg daily, depending on renal function. There is better absorption and steadier blood levels. The anticonvulsants diphenylhydantoin, carbamazepine, and valproate; neuroleptics, such as chlorprothixene, and phenothiazines; and H_2-blockers, such as cimetidine, cannot be recommended, as they have been not been studied critically, many are poorly tolerated by the elderly, and some are associated with significant side effects. If the patient fails to respond to local measures, oral analgesics, including opiates, tricyclics, gabapentin, and venlafaxine, referral to a pain center is recommended.

Immunosuppressed patients

Patients with malignancy (especially Hodgkin disease and leukemia) are five times more likely to develop zoster than are their age-matched counterparts. Patients who also have a higher incidence of zoster include those with deficient immune systems, such as individuals who are immunosuppressed for organ transplantation or by connective tissue disease, or by the agents used to treat these conditions (especially corticosteroids, chemotherapeutic agents, cyclosporine, sirolimus and tacrolimus). Following stem cell transplantation for leukemia, up to 68% of patients will develop herpes zoster in the first 12 months (median 5 months). The cumulative incidence of VZV reactivation in this group may exceed 80% in the first 3 years. Although persons who are immunosuppressed have increased rates of zoster, screening for underlying malignancy, beyond a good history and physical examination, is not indicated in those with zoster. However, since zoster is 30 times more common in HIV-infected persons, the zoster patient under 50 years of age should be questioned about HIV risk factors. In pediatric patients with HIV infection and in other immunosuppressed children, zoster may rapidly follow primary varicella.

The clinical appearance of zoster in the immunosuppressed is usually identical to typical zoster, but the lesions may be more ulcerative and necrotic, and may scar more severely. Dermatomal zoster may appear, progress to involve the dermatome, and persist without resolution. Multidermatomal zoster is more common in the immunosuppressed. Visceral dissemination and fatal outcome are extremely rare in immunosuppressed patients (about 0.3%), but cutaneous dissemination is not uncommon, occurring in 12% of cancer patients, especially those with hematologic malignancies. Bone marrow transplant patients with zoster develop disseminated zoster 25% of the time, and visceral dissemination 10–15% of the time. Disseminated zoster may be associated with the syndrome of inappropriate antidiuretic hormone secretion (SIADH) and present with hyponatremia, abdominal pain, and ileus. This later presentation has been reported in stem cell transplant patients. Despite treatment with intravenous acyclovir, the SIADH can be fatal. In this setting the number of skin lesions may be small and the lesions resemble "papules" rather than vesicles. Mortality in patients with zoster who have undergone bone marrow transplantation is 5%. VZV IgG serostatus is determined before transplant and all seropositive patients receive prophylaxis with either acyclovir, 800 mg twice daily, or valacyclovir, 500 mg twice daily for 1 year or longer if the patient is on immunosuppressive therapy. In AIDS patients, ocular and neurologic complications of herpes zoster are increased. Immunosuppressed patients often have recurrences of zoster, up to 25% in patients with AIDS (Fig. 19-19).

Two atypical patterns of zoster have been described in AIDS patients: ecthymatous lesions, which are punched-out ulcerations with a central crust, and verrucous lesions (Fig. 19-20). These patterns were not reported before the AIDS epidemic. Atypical clinical patterns, especially the verrucous pattern, may correlate with acyclovir resistance.

Diagnosis

The same techniques used for the diagnosis of varicella are used to diagnose herpes zoster. The clinical appearance is often adequate to lead to suspicion of the diagnosis, and an in-office Tzanck smear can rapidly confirm the clinical suspicion. Zosteriform herpes simplex could also produce a positive result to a Tzanck smear, but the number of lesions is usually more limited and the degree of pain substantially less. Beyond Tzanck preparation, DFA testing is preferred to a viral culture, since it is rapid, types the virus, and has a higher yield than a culture will produce. When compared in documented VZV infections, Tzanck smear was 75% positive (with up to 10% false-positives and high variability, depending on the skill of

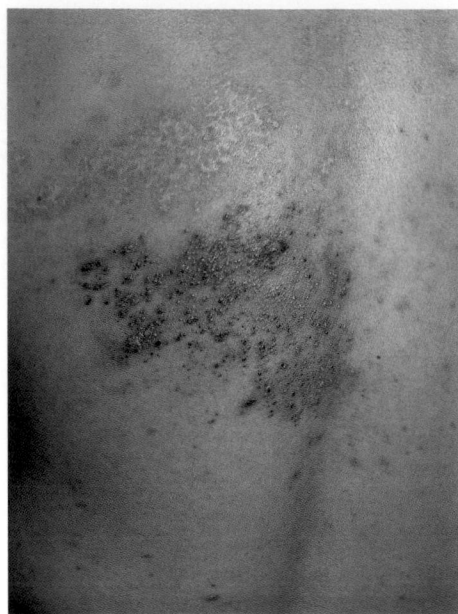

Fig. 19-19 Recurrent zoster in AIDS.

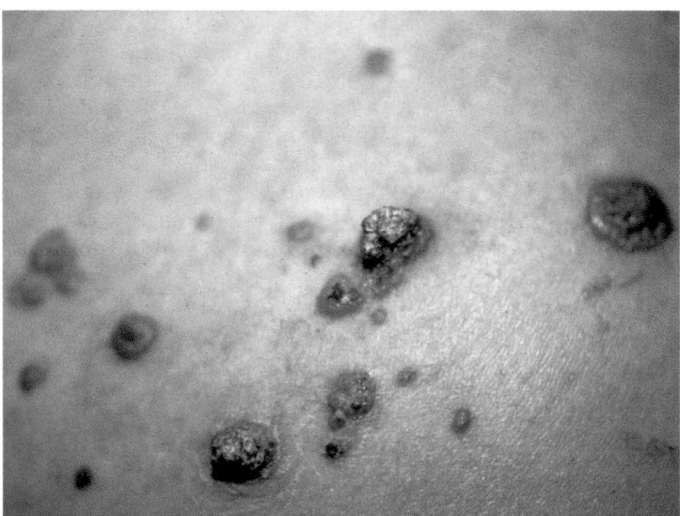

Fig. 19-20 Verrucous zoster in AIDS.

the examiner), and culture only 44% positive. PCR testing is 97% positive. In atypical lesions, biopsy may be necessary to demonstrate the typical herpesvirus cytopathic effects. Immunoperoxidase stain tests can then be performed on paraffin-fixed tissue to identify the VZV specifically. In cases in which acyclovir fails clinically, viral culture may be attempted and acyclovir sensitivity testing performed. It is not as standardized for VZV as it is for HSV and its availability is limited.

Histopathology

As in the case of herpes simplex, the vesicles in zoster are intraepidermal. Within and at the sides of the vesicle are found large, swollen cells called balloon cells, which are degenerated cells of the spinous layer. Acidophilic inclusion bodies similar to those seen in herpes simplex are present in the nuclei of the cells of the vesicle epithelium. Multinucleated keratinocytes, nuclear molding, and peripheral condensation of the nucleoplasm are characteristic and confirmatory of an infection with either HSV or VZV. In the vicinity of the vesicle there is marked intercellular and intracellular edema. In the upper part of the dermis, vascular dilatation, edema, and a perivascular infiltration of lymphocytes and polymorphonuclear leukocytes are present. Atypical lymphocytes may also be found. An underlying leukocytoclastic vasculitis is suggestive of VZV infection over HSV. Inflammatory and degenerative changes are also noted in the posterior root ganglia and in the dorsal nerve roots of the affected nerve. The lesions correspond to the areas of innervation of the affected nerve ganglion, with necrosis of the nerve cells.

Differential diagnosis

The distinctive clinical picture permits a diagnosis with little difficulty. A unilateral, painful eruption of grouped vesicles along a dermatome, with hyperesthesia and on occasion regional lymph node enlargement, is typical. Occasionally, segmental cutaneous paresthesias or pain may precede the eruption by 4 or 5 days. In such patients, prodromal symptoms are easily confused with the pain of angina pectoris, duodenal ulcer, biliary or renal colic, appendicitis, pleurodynia, or early glaucoma. The diagnosis becomes obvious once the cutaneous eruption appears. Herpes simplex and herpes zoster are confused if the lesions of HSV are linear (zosteriform HSV), or if the number of zoster lesions is small and localized to one site (not involving the whole dermatome). DFA testing or viral culture will distinguish them. DFA is generally preferred because it is rapid and sensitive.

Prevention of zoster

A vaccine using the same attenuated virus as in the varicella vaccination, but at much higher titers, has been licensed for the prevention of herpes zoster (Zostavax). It is recommended in all persons aged 60 years or older. This vaccination reduces the incidence of zoster by 50%. In addition, PHN was 67% lower in the vaccine recipients and the duration of ZAP was shortened. Burden of illness was also reduced. Those vaccinated between the ages of 60 and 69 had a greater reduction in zoster incidence than those over 70, but in both groups PHN and burden of illness were reduced similarly. Since it is a live virus vaccine, persons on antiviral medications must stop them 24 hours before immunization and not take them for 14 days following immunization. Immunosuppressed patients can be safely immunized following specific guidelines.

Inflammatory skin lesions following a zoster infection (isotopic response)

Following zoster, inflammatory skin lesions may rarely occur within the affected dermatome. Lesions usually appear within a month, or rarely, longer than 3 months, after the zoster. Clinically, the lesions are usually flat-topped or annular papules in the dermatome. Histologically, such papules most frequently demonstrate various patterns of granulomatous inflammation from typical granuloma annulare to sarcoidal reactions, or even granulomatous vasculitis (Fig. 19-21). Persistent viral genome has not been detected in these lesions, suggesting that continued antiviral therapy is not indicated. Persistent VZV glycoproteins may be the triggering antigens. Topical and intralesional therapy with corticosteroid medications is beneficial, but the natural history of these lesions is generally spontaneous resolution. Less commonly, other inflammatory skin diseases have been reported in areas of prior zoster, including lichen planus, lichen sclerosus, Kaposi sarcoma, graft versus host disease, morphea, and benign or even atypical lymphoid infiltrates. Leukemic infiltrates and lymphomas may affect zoster scars, as can metastatic carcinomas (inflammatory oncotaxis) or nonmelanoma skin cancers.

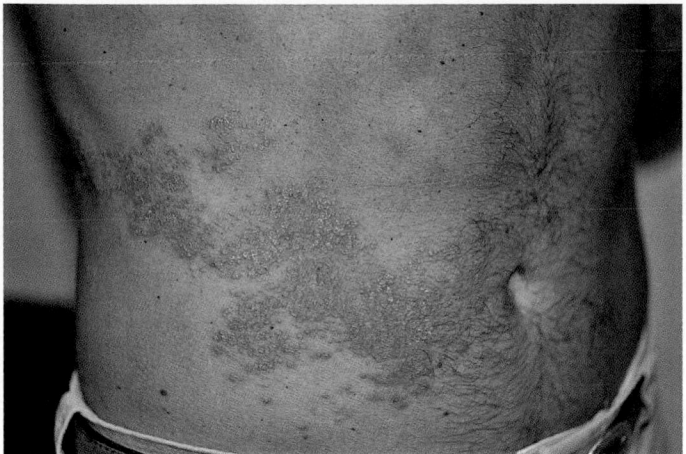

Fig. 19-21 Herpes zoster, dermatome previously affected by zoster developed a granulomatous dermatitis histologically consistent with granuloma annulare.

Arikawa J, et al: Mandibular alveolar bone necrosis after trigeminal herpes zoster. Int J Dermatol 2004; 43:136.

Asahi T, et al: Valacyclovir neurotoxicity: clinical experience and review of the literature. Eur J Neurol 2009; 16:457.

Au WY, et al: Disseminated zoster, hyponatraemia, severe abdominal pain and leukaemia relapse: recognition of a new clinical quartet after bone marrow transplantation. Br J Dermatol 2003; 149:862.

Betts RE: Vaccination strategies for the prevention of herpes zoster and postherpetic neuralgia. J Am Acad Dermatol 2007; 57:S143.

Chang SE: Subcutaneous granuloma annulare following herpes zoster. Int J Dermatol 2004; 43:298.

Chen PH, et al: Herpes zoster associated voiding dysfunction: a retrospective study and literature review. Arch Phys Med Rehab 2002; 83:1624.

Chiarello SE: Tumescent infiltration of corticosteroids, lidocaine, and epinephrine into dermatomes of acute herpetic pain or postherpetic neuralgia. Arch Dermatol 1998; 134:279.

Cohen JI: Strategies for zoster vaccination in immunocompromised patients. J Infect Dis 2008; 197:S237.

Gilden D, et al: Varicella zoster virus vasculopathies: diverse clinic manifestations, laboratory features, pathogenesis, and treatment. Lancet 2009; 8:731.

Harpaz R, et al: Prevention of herpes zoster. MMWR 2008; 57:1.

He L, et al: Corticosteroids for preventing postherpetic neuralgia. Cochrane Library 2009; 3.

Izu K, et al: Herpes zoster occurring as a solitary nodule on the index finger. Br J Dermatol 2004; 150:365.

Kurlan JG, et al: Herpes zoster in the first year of life following postnatal exposure to varicella-zoster virus. Arch Dermatol 2004; 140:1268.

Li Q, et al: Antiviral treatment for preventing postherpetic neuralgia. Cochrane Library 2009; 3.

Lui HS, et al: Botulinum toxin A relieved neuropathic pain in a case of post-herpetic neuralgia. Pain Med 2006; 7:89.

Mortada RA, et al: Unusual presentation of Ramsay Hunt syndrome in renal transplant patients: case report and literature review. Transpl Infec Dis 2009; 11:72–74.

Nikkels AF, et al: Atypical recurrent varicella in 4 patients with hemopathies. J Am Acad Dermatol 2003; 48:442.

Ruocco V, et al: Isotopic response after herpesvirus infection: an update. J Am Acad Dermatol 2002; 46:90.

Sadick NS, et al: Comparison of detection of varicella zoster virus by Tzanck smear, direct immunofluorescence with a monoclonal antibody, and virus isolation. J Am Acad Dermatol 1987; 17:64.

Sampathkumar P, et al: Herpes zoster (shingles) and postherpetic neuralgia. Mayo Clin Proc 2009; 84:274.

Sanli HE, et al: Granuloma annulare on herpes zoster scars in a Hodgkin's disease patient following autologous peripheral stem cell transplantation. J Eur Acad Dermatol Venereol 2006; 20:314.

Schmader K, et al: Racial differences in the occurrence of herpes zoster. J Infect Dis 1995; 171:701.

Schmader KE, Dworkin RH: Natural history and treatment of herpes zoster. J Pain 2008; 9:S3.

Song HJ, et al: Herpes zoster complicated by delayed intracranial haemorrhage. Clin Exper Dermatol 2008; 34:518.

Sotiriou E, et al: Severe post-herpetic neuralgia successfully treated with botulinum toxin A: three case reports. Acta Derm Venereol 2009; 89:214.

Styczynski J, et al: Management of HSV, VZV and EBV infections in patients with hematological malignancies and after SCT: guidelines from the Second European Conference on Infections in Leukemia. Bone Marrow Transp 2009; 43:757.

Tyring SK: Management of herpes zoster and postherpetic neuralgia. J Am Acad Dermatol 2007; 57:S136.

Uscategui T, et al: Antiviral therapy for Ramsay Hunt syndrome (herpes zoster oticus with facial palsy) in adults. Cochrane Library 2009; 3.

Watanabe T, et al: Papules on the nape: postherpetic granuloma annulare-like reaction (Wolf isotopic response). Arch Dermatol 2009; 145:589.

Weinberg JM: Herpes zoster: epidemiology, natural history, and common complications. J Am Acad Dermatol 2007; 57:S130.

Whitley RJ: A 70-year-old woman with shingles. Clin Crossroads 2009; 302:73.

Wu C, Raja S: An update on the treatment of postherpetic neuralgia. J of Pain 2008; 9:S19.

Epstein–Barr virus

Epstein–Barr virus (EBV) is a γ-herpesvirus. It infects human mucosal epithelial cells and B lymphocytes, and infection persists for the life of the host. EBV infection may be latent—not producing virions, but simply spread from mother cell to both daughter cells by copying the viral DNA with each host cell replication. Intermittently, infection may be productive, resulting in production and release of infectious virions. EBV infection may transit between latent and productive infection many times. The ability of EBV to maintain persistent infection is aided by the expression of the EBV nuclear antigen (EBNA)-1 viral gene product, which prevents cytotoxic T-lymphocyte response to the virus.

Initial infection with EBV occurs in childhood or early adulthood, so that by the early twenties, 95% of the population has been infected. The virus is shed into the saliva, so contact with oral secretions is the most common route of transmission. Primary infection may be asymptomatic or produce only a mild, nonspecific febrile illness, especially in younger children. In young adults, primary infection is more likely to be symptomatic and in 50% of cases produces a syndrome termed infectious mononucleosis. The incubation period is 3–7 weeks. Infectious mononucleosis is characterized by a constellation of findings: fever (up to 40°C), headache, lymphadenopathy, splenomegaly, and pharyngitis (sore throat).

Cutaneous and mucous membrane lesions are present in about 10% of patients with infectious mononucleosis; up to 70% of patients require hospitalization. Exanthems occur in 3–15% of children with infectious mononucleosis. Edema of the eyelids and a macular or morbilliform eruption are most common. The latter is usually on the trunk and upper extremities. Other less common eruptions are urticarial, vesicular, bullous, petechial, and purpuric types. The mucous membrane lesions consist of distinctive pinhead-sized petechiae, 5–20 in number, at the junction of the soft and hard palate (Forchheimer spots). Gianotti–Crosti syndrome (GCS) and the papular–purpuric glove and stocking syndrome are two specific viral exanthem patterns which may occur in the setting of asymptomatic primary EBV infection. EBV is now the leading cause of GCS worldwide. EBV reactivation has been uncommonly associated with drug-induced hypersensitivity syndrome (DRESS). EBV is also associated with enhanced insect bite reactions.

Painful genital ulcerations may precede the symptomatic phase of infectious mononucleosis, especially in premenarcheal girls. The ulcerations are up to 2 cm in diameter, single or multiple, and may be accompanied by marked swelling of the labia. Lesions last several weeks and heal spontaneously, often as the patient is developing symptoms of infectious mononucleosis. Transmission to patients via orogenital sex has been proposed, but the virus may also reach the vulvar mucosa hematogenously. EBV has been recovered by culture from these genital ulcerations. The lesions closely resemble herpetic ulcerations and fixed drug eruption, which must be considered in the differential diagnosis.

Laboratory evaluation in patients with infectious mononucleosis frequently shows an absolute lymphocytosis of greater than 50% and monocytosis with abnormally large lymphocytes. Atypical lymphocytes (Downey cells) usually represent at least 10% of the total leukocyte count. The white blood cell count ranges from 10 000 to 40 000/mm^3. Liver function tests may be elevated. Heterophile antibodies will be present in 95% or more of cases. In acute primary EBV infection the IgM antibodies to early antigen (EA) and viral capsid antigen (VCA) are found in high titer and fall during recovery. Antibodies to VCA and EBNA appear in the recovering phase and persist for years after primary infection. There is no specific therapy and in most cases no treatment is required. Acyclovir is not effective in altering the length or severity of infectious mononucleosis, although it is active against EBV in doses used for VZV. If patients have severe pharyngeal involvement with encroachment on the airway, 4 days of oral corticosteroid therapy (40–60 mg/day prednisone) is useful to induce a prompt reduction in pharyngeal swelling. Most patients recover completely.

Patients with mononucleosis treated with ampicillin, amoxicillin, or other semisynthetic penicillins commonly develop a generalized, pruritic, erythematous to copper-colored macular exanthem on the 7th–10th day of therapy. The eruption starts on the pressure points and extensor surfaces, generalizes, and becomes confluent. The eruption lasts about 1 week and resolves with desquamation. The eruption often does not recur when these medications are given after the acute mononucleosis has resolved.

Oral hairy leukoplakia (OHL) is a distinctive condition strongly associated with HIV. It appears as poorly demarcated, corrugated white plaques seen on the lateral aspects of the tongue (Fig. 19-22). Lesions on the other areas of the oral mucosa are simply white plaques without the typical corrugations. OHL can be distinguished from thrush by the fact that OHL cannot be removed by firm scraping with a tongue blade.

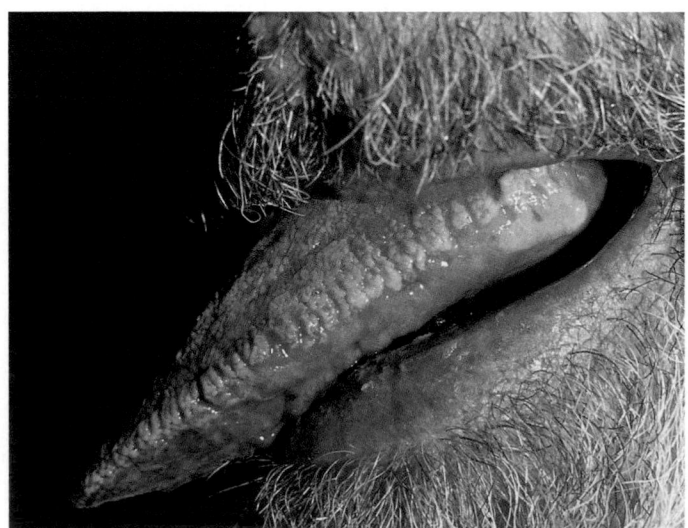

Fig. 19-22 Oral hairy leukoplakia.

More than one-third of patients with AIDS have OHL, but is not restricted to patients with HIV infection; it also occurs in other immunosuppressed hosts, especially renal and bone marrow transplant recipients, and those using inhaled steroids for chronic obstructive pulmonary disease. OHL can be a part of the immune reconstitution inflammatory syndrome (IRIS). EBV does not establish infection in the basal cell layer of the oral epithelium but is maintained by repeated direct infection of the epithelium by EBV in the oral cavity; it is not reactivation of EBV at the site. Only chronically immunosuppressed patients continuously shed EBV in their oral secretions; hence the restriction of OHL to immunosuppressed hosts. In normal persons a similar morphologic and histologic picture can be seen (pseudo-OHL), but EBV is not found in these patients' lesions. Thus, the finding of OHL warrants HIV testing. If results are negative, special histologic studies searching for EBV in the OHL biopsy should be performed. If EBV is found, a work-up for immunosuppression is recommended.

OHL is usually asymptomatic and requires no treatment. If treatment is requested in immunosuppressed hosts, podophyllin, applied for 30 s–1 min to the lesions once each month, is easiest. Tretinoin gel, applied topically twice a day, or oral acyclovir, 400 mg five times a day, is also effective. Lesions recur when treatment is discontinued.

In immunosuppressed and immunocompetent hosts, EBV may be responsible for benign and malignant disorders, some of which can be fatal. These include Kikuchi's histocytic necrotizing lymphadenitis, hydroa vacciniforme of the severe type, plasmablastic lymphoma, post-transplant lymphoproliferative disorder, Burkitt lymphoma, and nasopharyngeal carcinoma.

Cytomegalic inclusion disease

Congenital cytomegalovirus (CMV) infection, as documented by CMV excretion, is found in 1% of newborns. Ninety percent of these babies are asymptomatic. Clinical manifestations in infants may include jaundice, hepatosplenomegaly, cerebral calcifications, chorioretinitis, microcephaly, mental retardation, and deafness. Cutaneous manifestations may result from thrombocytopenia, with resultant petechiae, purpura, and ecchymoses. Purpuric lesions, which may be macular, papular, or nodular, may show extramedullary hematopoiesis (dermal erythropoiesis), producing the "blueberry muffin baby." A generalized vesicular eruption may very rarely occur. Most symptomatic cases occur within the first 2 months of life. Neonatal disease is more severe and sequelae are more frequent in neonates born of mothers with primary rather than recurrent CMV disease in pregnancy.

Between 50 and 80% of immunocompetent adults and up to 100% of HIV-infected men who have sex with men (MSM) are infected with CMV. Infection in adults may be acquired by exposure to infected children, sexual transmission, and transfusion of CMV-infected blood. Symptomatic primary infection in adults is unusual and is identical to infectious mononucleosis caused by EBV. An urticarial or morbilliform eruption or erythema nodosum may occur in primary CMV infection in immunocompetent adults. Ampicillin and amoxicillin administration will often result in a morbilliform eruption in acute CMV infection, similar to that seen in acute EBV infection.

CMV infection is very common in AIDS patients, most frequently causing retinitis (20% of patients), colitis (15%), cholangitis, encephalitis, polyradiculomyopathy, and adrenalitis. It occurs in the setting of very advanced HIV infection (usually with CD4 counts below 50) and has become much less common in the era of highly active antiretroviral therapy (HAART).

CMV infection in tissues is usually identified by the histologic finding of a typical CMV cytopathic effect. In a very small percentage of AIDS patients with CMV infection, skin lesions may occur that contain such cytopathic changes. In most cases CMV is found in association with another infectious process and the treatment of that other infection will lead to resolution of the CMV in the skin without treatment of the CMV. This is especially true of perianal HSV ulcerations. CMV may even be found in totally normal skin in CMV-viremic AIDS patients, suggesting that finding the CMV cytopathic effect is alone insufficient to imply a causal relationship of the CMV to any cutaneous lesion. Only in the case of perianal and oral ulcerations has the pathogenic role of CMV been documented. In unusual cases of very painful perianal ulcerations, only CMV infection is found histologically. The CMV cytopathic changes may be noted in the nerves at the base of these ulcerations, suggesting that CMV neuritis may be producing the severe pain that characterizes these cases. The diagnosis of CMV ulceration is one of exclusion. CMV cytopathic changes must be seen in the lesion and cultures, and histologic evidence of any other infectious agent must be negative. In these cases, clinically suggested by their location (perianal or oral) and painful nature, specific treatment with ganciclovir, foscarnet, or cidofovir will lead to healing of the ulceration and dramatic resolution of the pain.

Agaba PA, et al: Presentation and survival of patients with AIDS-related Kaposi's sarcoma in Jos, Nigeria. Int J STD AIDS 2009; 29:410.

Castelnuovo B, et al: Cause-specific mortality and the contribution of immune reconstitution inflammatory syndrome in the first 3 years after antiretroviral therapy initiation in an urban African cohort. Clin Infect Dis 2009; 49:965.

Crum-Cianflone N, et al: Cutaneous malignancies among HIV-infected persons. Arch Intern Med 2009; 169:1130.

Dal Maso L: Pattern of cancer risk in persons with AIDS in Italy in the HAART era. Brit J Cancer 2009; 100:840.

Dauden E, et al: Mucocutaneous presence of cytomegalovirus associated with human immunodeficiency virus infection. Arch Dermatol 2001; 137:443.

Hancox JG, et al: Perineal ulcers in an infant: an unusual presentation of postnatal cytomegalovirus infection. J Am Acad Dermatol 2006; 54:536.

Hudson LB, Perlman SE: Necrotizing genital ulcerations in a premenarcheal female with mononucleosis. Obstet Gynecol 1998; 92:642.

Jagannathan P, et al: Life-threatening immune reconstitution inflammatory syndrome after pneumocystis pneumonia: a cautionary case series. AIDS 2009; 23:13.

Lehloenya R, Meintjes G: Dermatologic manifestations of the immune reconstitution inflammatory syndrome. Dermatol Clin 2006; 24:549.

Mani D, et al: A retrospective analysis of AIDS-associated Kaposi's sarcoma in patients with undetectable HIV viral loads and CD4 counts greater than 300 cells/mm³. J Int Assoc Physicians AIDS Care 2009; 8:279.

Maurer T, et al: HIV-associated Kaposi's sarcoma with a high CD4 count and a low viral load. N Engl J Med 2007; 357:13.

Mendoza N: Mucocutaneous manifestations of Epstein–Barr virus infection. Am J Clin Dermatol 2008; 9:295.

Meyerle JH, Turiansky GW: Perianal ulcer in a patient with AIDS—diagnosis. Arch Dermatol 2004; 104:877.

Moodley M, et al: Vulval cytomegalovirus coexisting with herpes simplex virus in a patient with human immunodeficiency virus infection. Int J Obstet Gynaecol 2003; 110:1123.

Piperi E, et al: Oral hairy leukoplakia in HIV-negative patients: report of 10 Cases. Int J Surg Pathol 2008; Nov 25 (Epub ahead of print).

Ramdial PK, et al: Cytomegalovirus neuritis in perineal ulcers. J Cutan Pathol 2002; 29:439.

Ramirez-Amador VA, et al: Identification of oral candidosis, hairy leukoplakia and recurrent oral ulcers as distinct cases of immune reconstitution inflammatory syndrome. Int J STD AIDS 2009; 20:250.

Weiss DA, et al: Condyloma overgrowth caused by immune reconstitution inflammatory syndrome. Urology 2009 Jul 16 (Epub ahead of print).

Human herpesviruses-6 and 7

Infection with HHV-6 is almost universal in adults, with seropositivity in the 80–85% range in the US, and seroprevalence almost 100% in children. There are intermittent periods of viral reactivation throughout life; persistent infection occurs in several organs, particularly in the CNS. Acute seroconversion to HHV-6 and to HHV-7 each appears to be responsible for about one-third of roseola cases, and in the remaining third neither is found. HHV-6 infection occurs earlier than HHV-7, and second episodes of roseola in HHV-6-seropositive children may be caused by HHV-7. Primary infection with HHV-6 is associated with roseola only 9% of the time, and 18% of children with seroconversion have a rash. Primary infection may occur with only fever and no rash, or rash without fever. Other common findings include otitis media, diarrhea, and bulging fontanelles, sometimes with findings of meningoencephalitis. Uncommonly, hepatitis, intussusception, and even fatal multisystem disease may occur. In adults, acute HHV-6 infection resembles acute mononucleosis. Viral recovery is reduced in patients receiving acyclovir therapy, but ganciclovir is the recommended agent for treatment of severe disease associated with HHV-6. HHV-6 and 7 may be the etiologic agents responsible for pityriasis rosea.

As with other herpesviruses, the pattern of disease in HHV-6 may be different in immunosuppressed hosts. Chronic macular or papular generalized exanthems have been reported in two patients, one following bone marrow transplantation for severe combined immunodeficiency and one with acute leukemia who was undergoing chemotherapy. In the latter patient, the eruption cleared with recovery of the bone marrow.

Roseola infantum (exanthem subitum, sixth disease)

Roseola infantum is a common cause of sudden, unexplained high fever in young children between 6 and 36 months of age. Prodromal fever is usually high and convulsions and lymphadenopathy may accompany it. Suddenly, on about the fourth day, the fever drops. Coincident with the drop in temperature, a morbilliform erythema consisting of rose-colored discrete macules appears on the neck, trunk, and buttocks, and sometimes on the face and extremities. Often there is a blanched halo around the lesions. The eruption may also be papular or, rarely, even vesicular. The mucous membranes are spared. Complete resolution of the eruption occurs in 1–2 days. A case of spontaneously healing, generalized eruptive histiocytosis has been reported following exanthem subitum.

Human herpesvirus-8

HHV-8, a γ-herpesvirus, is most closely related to EBV and *Herpesvirus saimiri*. It has been found in virtually all patients with Kaposi sarcoma, including those who have AIDS (Fig. 19-23), in African cases; in elderly men from the Mediterranean basin; and in transplant patients. In addition, the seropositivity rate (infection rate) for this virus correlates with the prevalence of Kaposi sarcoma in a given population.

The background seroprevalence rate in North America and Northern Europe is near zero. Seroprevalence is highest in Kaposi sarcoma-endemic areas in sub-Saharan Africa (50–100%). In the general population in Italy, the seroprevalence is 10–15%, being 6–10% in children under age 16 and 22% after age 50. In south central Italy and Sardinia, seroprevalence rates are higher, being in the 20–25% range for the general population. In Italy, high rates of HHV-8 seropositivity are also seen in HIV-infected gay men (up to 60%), in female prostitutes (40%), and in heterosexual men who have had sex with prostitutes (40%). Infection with HHV-8 precedes and

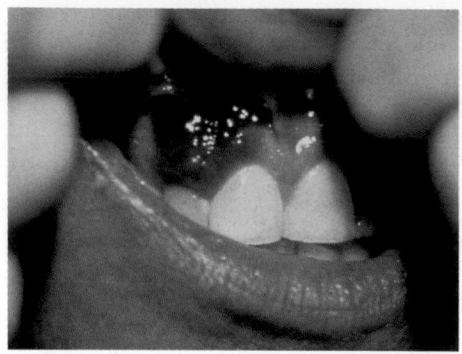

Fig. 19-23 Oral Kaposi sarcoma in AIDS associated with HHV-8.

predicts subsequent development of Kaposi sarcoma in HIV-infected men. In addition to Kaposi sarcoma lesions, HHV-8 can be found in saliva and in circulating blood cells in HHV-8-infected patients. HHV-8 is also found in the semen of up to 20% of patients with Kaposi sarcoma. Heterosexual partners of patients with classic Kaposi sarcoma have high rates of HHV-8 seropositivity (over 40%). These epidemiologic features all strongly support sexual transmission as an important mechanism of the spread of HHV-8. The finding of a significant number of infections in prepubertal children, however, suggests that nonsexual methods of transmission also exist. HHV-8 seroprevalence rates in heterosexual intravenous drug users and persons with HIV infection acquired via blood transfusion are not increased above the general population, suggesting that HHV-8 is poorly transmitted by blood and blood products.

HHV-8 is present in a rare type of B-cell lymphoma called body cavity-based B-cell lymphoma or primary effusion lymphoma (PEL), which presents with pleural, pericardial, and peritoneal malignant effusions. Rarely, this form of lymphoma may be associated with skin lesions, which histologically are CD30+ anaplastic large cell lymphoma. HHV-8 is also found in all cases of Castleman's disease associated with HIV infection and 10–50% of cases in HIV-negative persons. Exanthems and cutaneous nodules may accompany multicentric Castleman's disease, and HHV-8 has been identified in the skin lesions of one such patient.

Cattani P, et al: Age-specific seroprevalence of human herpesvirus 8 in Mediterranean regions. Clin Microbiol Infect 2003; 9:274.
Drago F: Pityriasis rosea: an update with critical appraisal of its possible herpesviral etiology. J Am Acad Dermatol 2008; 61:303.
Schwartz RA, et al: Kaposi sarcoma: a continuing conundrum. J Am Acad Dermatol 2008; 59:179.
Tamiya H, et al: Generalized eruptive histiocytoma with rapid progression and resolution following exanthema subitum. Clin Exper Dermatol 2005; 30:294.
Torigoe S, et al: Clinical manifestations associated with HHV-7 infection. Arch Dis Child 1995; 72:518.
Wyplosz A, et al: Initial human herpesvirus-8 rash and multicentric Castleman disease. Clin Infect Dis 2008: 47:684.
Yoshida M, et al: Exanthem subitum (roseola infantum) with vesicular lesions. Br J Dermatol 1995; 132:614.

B virus

B virus (*Herpesvirus simiae*) is endemic in Asiatic Old World monkeys (macaques) and may infect other monkeys housed in close quarters with infected monkeys. In macaques the disease is a recurrent vesicular eruption analogous to HSV in humans, with virus shed from conjunctiva, oral mucosa, and the urogenital area. Humans become infected after being bitten, scratched, or contaminated by an animal shedding B virus. Usually, patients are animal handlers or researchers.

Rare cases of respiratory or human-to-human contact spread have been reported. Within a few days of the bite, vesicles, erythema, necrosis, or edema appear at the site of inoculation. Regional lymph nodes are enlarged and tender. Fever is typically present. In a substantial number of human infections, rapid progression to neurologic disease occurs. This is initially manifested by peripheral nerve involvement (dysesthesia, paresthesia), then progresses to spinal cord involvement (myelitis and ascending paralysis with hyporeflexia), and finally to brain disease (decreased consciousness, seizures, and respiratory depression). Fifteen of 22 reported cases have died, and all survivors of encephalitis suffered severe neurologic sequelae. Treatment with acyclovir or ganciclovir has been successful in some cases, but other patients similarly treated have died. Because *H. simiae* infection may recur after a period of latency, lifetime surveillance is required. The Centers for Disease Control (CDC) have issued guidelines to protect workers from B virus infection.

Benson PM, et al: B virus (*Herpesvirus simiae*) and human infection. Arch Dermatol 1989; 125:1247.
Centers for Disease Control and Prevention: Fatal cercopithecine herpesvirus 1 (B virus) infection following a mucocutaneous exposure and interim recommendations for worker protection. MMWR 1998; 47:1073.
Ostrowski SR, et al: B-virus from pet macaque monkeys: an emerging threat in the United States? Emerg Infect Dis 1998; 4:117.

Infectious hepatitis

Hepatitis B virus

Hepatitis B virus (HBV) is a double-stranded DNA virus that is spread by blood and blood products, and sexually in Europe and the Western Hemisphere. In Africa and Asia, infection often occurs perinatally. HBV is the primary cause of hepatocellular carcinoma and may also cause liver failure and cirrhosis. Acute infection with HBV is associated with anorexia, nausea, right upper quadrant pain, and malaise. Between 20 and 30% of persons with acute HBV infection have a serum sickness-like illness with urticaria, arthralgias, and, occasionally, arthritis, glomerulonephritis, or vasculitis. These symptoms appear 1–6 weeks before the onset of clinically apparent liver disease. Immune complexes containing hepatitis B surface antigen and hypocomplementemia occur in the serum and in joint fluid. The process spontaneously resolves as antigen is cleared from the blood.

Hepatitis B is also associated with polyarteritis nodosa (PAN) in 7–8% of cases. This usually occurs within the first 6 months of infection, even during the acute phase, but may occur as long as 12 years after infection. Unlike the urticarial reaction, which is usually associated eventually with the development of clinical hepatitis, HBV infection associated with PAN may be silent.

A highly effective vaccine is available to prevent HBV infection. It is recommended as a part of standard childhood immunizations and all healthcare workers should be immunized. IFN-α and lamivudine may be used to treat active HBV infection, although following therapy, HBV viremia may recur.

Hepatitis C virus

Hepatitis C virus (HCV) is a single-stranded RNA virus that causes most cases of non-A, non-B viral hepatitis. Now that a serologic test is available to screen blood products for HCV infection, the vast majority of new cases of HCV infection are parenterally transmitted via intravenous drug usage. Sexual transmission, as compared to HBV, is uncommon (less than

1% transmission/year of exposure). Maternal to infant spread occurs in 5% of cases. Only about one-third of patients are symptomatic during acute infection. Between 55% and 85% of patients will have chronic infections. Although in most cases patients have minimal symptoms for the first one to two decades of infection, cirrhosis and liver failure, as well as hepatocellular carcinoma, are common sequelae. Chronic HCV infection is associated with various skin disorders, either by direct effect or as a consequence of the associated hepatic damage.

Cutaneous necrotizing vasculitis, which is usually associated with a circulating mixed cryoglobulin, occurs in approximately 1% of patients with chronic HCV infection. In 84% of cases of type II cryoglobulinemia, HCV infection is present. The most common clinical presentation is palpable purpura of the lower extremities (90% of cases). Livedo reticularis, urticaria, and subcutaneous nodules showing a granulomatous vasculitis may also occur. Arthropathy, glomerulonephritis, and neuropathy frequently accompany the skin eruption. Leg ulcers can occur in 10–20%. Histologically, in all cases a leukocytoclastic vasculitis is seen. In some cases, the vasculitis may involve small arteries, giving a histologic pattern similar to that seen in PAN. In various studies 5–20% of patients with PAN were HCV-positive, suggesting that both HBV and HCV can cause PAN. The presence of anti-HCV antibodies should not be used as the sole diagnostic test in persons with PAN, as PAN may cause a false-positive ELISA test for HCV. Rheumatoid factor, a type II cryoglobulin, and hypocomplementemia are found in up to 80% of cases. HCV-infected patients with mixed cryoglobulinemia are 35 times more likely to develop non-Hodgkin lymphoma, usually of the B-cell type.

Patients with porphyria cutanea tarda (PCT) often have hepatocellular abnormalities. Depending on the prevalence of HCV infection in the population studied, between 10 and 95% of sporadic (not familial) PCT cases are HCV-associated. Treatment of the HCV infection with IFN may lead to improvement of the PCT.

HCV infection has been associated with lichen planus. The likelihood of identifying HCV infection in a patient with lichen planus is greatest in geographic regions with high rates of HCV infection. Patients with mucosal ulcerative lichen planus are also more likely to be HCV-infected. Serologic testing in a patient should be considered if the patient has HCV risk factors or abnormal liver function tests, or is from a geographic region or population in which HCV infection is common. HCV may also be associated with cutaneous B-cell lymphoma, xerostomia (but not typical Sjögren syndrome), possibly erythema multiforme, and autoimmune thyroid disease. Approximately 15% of patients with HCV infection have pruritus. Pruritus virtually always is associated with advanced liver disease and abnormal liver function tests. Patients with pruritus and normal liver function tests and no history of hepatitis will rarely be found to be infected with HCV.

Necrolytic acral erythema is an uncommon condition uniquely associated with HCV infection. It resembles the "deficiency" dermatoses, except that it has an acral distribution. The clinical lesions are painful or pruritic, keratotic, well-defined plaques with raised red scaly borders, or diffuse hyperkeratosis (Fig. 19-24). Erosion and flaccid blisters may occur, contributing to the discomfort. The dorsal feet (less commonly, the dorsal hands), as well as the lower extremities, may be involved. Histologically, there is necrosis of the superficial portion of the epidermis, along with hyperkeratosis, loss of the granular cell layer, and parakeratosis. Intraepidermal spongiotic foci are present, which may be macroscopic at times, the cleavage plane being between the necrotic and viable epidermis. Zinc, essential fatty acid, and glucagon levels are normal, but the patients may be hypoalbuminemic

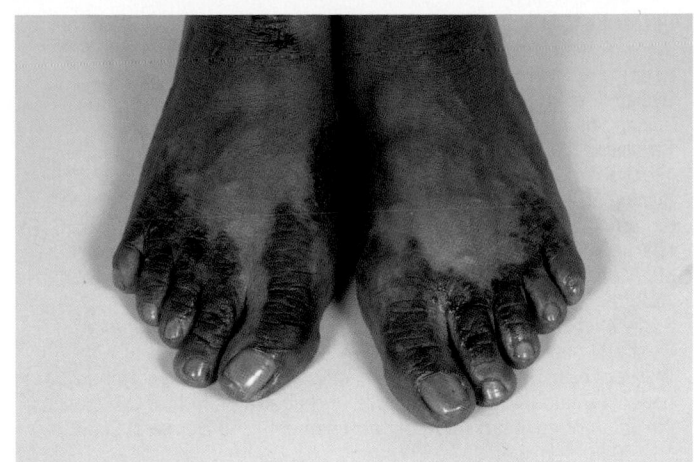

Fig. 19-24 Necrolytic acral erythema.

and have low serum amino acids due to their liver disease. Treatment of the associated HCV infection with IFN and ribavirin, or IFN plus zinc, has resulted in resolution. Hyperalimentation was also partially effective in some patients, as was amino acid supplementation with zinc.

A combination of IFN-α and ribavirin is used to treat patients with chronic HCV infection, with sustained responses (negative HCV in the blood at 12 months) in slightly over 50% of patients. Complications caused by the presence of the virus in the blood, such as vasculitis, improve with such treatment. The response of other associated conditions, such as lichen planus and PCT, is variable. Combined IFN and ribavirin therapy may be complicated by an eczematous eruption with pruritus in about 8% of patients and severe pruritus in about 1%. Eczema typically affects the distal extremities, dorsal hands, face, neck, and less commonly the trunk, axillae, and buttocks. The eruption may be photodistributed and photoexacerbated. These eczematous eruptions typically begin 2–4 months after treatment is begun. In affected patients, prior treatment with IFN alone was usually not associated with an eczematous eruption. Histologically, the eruptions show a spongiotic dermatitis. The eruption resolves completely if treatment is stopped for 2–3 weeks, but will recur when treatment is restarted. Aggressive therapy with antihistamines, emollients, and potent topical steroids will usually control the eczema, allowing uninterrupted continuation of treatment. The severity of the pruritus in these cases may relate to the tendency of liver disease to cause itch and the frequent psychiatric side effects of HCV and IFN (depression, anxiety), which may reduce itch threshold. Patients receiving IFN-α for HCV infection may develop cosmetically unsightly granulomatous nodules at filler injection sites.

Bonkovsky HL, Mehta S: Hepatitis C: a review and update. J Am Acad Dermatol 2001; 44:159.

Brandt O, et al: Gianotti–Crosti syndrome. J Am Acad Dermatol 2006; 54:136.

Cacoub P, Saadoun D: Hepatitis C virus infection induced vasculitis. Clin Rev Allerg Immunol 2008; 35:30.

Carbone M, et al: Course of oral lichen planus: a retrospective study of 808 northern Italian patients. Oral Dis 2009; 15:235.

Charles ED, et al: Hepatitis C virus-induced cryoglobulinemia. Kidney Int 2009; 76:818.

Cribier B, et al: Systematic cutaneous examination in hepatitis C virus infected patients. Acta Dermatol Venereol 1998; 78:355.

Cribier B, et al: Should patients with pruritus be tested for hepatitis C virus infection? A case-controlled study. Br J Dermatol 2000; 142:1249.

Dereure O, et al: Diffuse inflammatory lesions in patients treated with interferon alfa and ribavirin for hepatitis C: a series of 20 patients. Br J Dermatol 2002; 147:1142.

Descamps V, et al: Facial cosmetic filler injections as possible target for systemic sarcoidosis in patients treated with interferon for chronic hepatitis C: two cases. Dermatol 2008; 217:81.

Duman V, et al: Recurrent erythema multiforme and chronic hepatitis C: efficacy of interferon alpha. Br J Dermatol 2000; 142:1248.

Fernandes SS, et al: Erythema induratum and chronic hepatitis C infection. J Clin Virol 2009; 44:333.

Hivnor CM, et al: Necrolytic acral erythema: response to combination therapy with interferon and ribavirin. J Am Acad Dermatol 2004; 50:S121.

Khanna VJ, et al: Necrolytic acral erythema associated with hepatitis C: effective treatment with interferon alfa and zinc. Arch Dermatol 2000; 136:755.

Sovfir N, et al: Hepatitis C virus infection in cutaneous PAN. Arch Dermatol 1999; 135:1001.

Vazquez-Lopez F, et al: Eczema-like lesions and disruption of therapy in patients treated with interferon-alfa and ribavirin for chronic hepatitis C: the value of an interdisciplinary assessment. Br J Dermatol 2004; 150:1028.

Gianotti–Crosti syndrome (papular acrodermatitis of childhood, papulovesicular acrolocated syndrome)

Gianotti–Crosti syndrome (GCS) is a characteristic viral exanthem. It was initially associated with the early anicteric phase of HBV infection. With universal HBV immunization, HBV is now a rare cause of GCS. EBV is now the most common cause of GCS worldwide. Other implicated infectious agents have included adenovirus, CMV, enteroviruses (coxsackie A16, B4, and B5), vaccinia virus, rotavirus, hepatitis A and C, respiratory syncytial virus, parainfluenza virus, parvovirus B19, rubella virus, HHV-6, streptococcus, and *Mycobacterium avium* infection. Immunizations against poliovirus, diphtheria, pertussis, Japanese encephalitis, influenza, and hepatitis B and measles (together) have also caused this syndrome. The clinical features of GCS are identical, independent of the cause:

- The condition typically affects children between 6 months and 14 years of age (median age 2 years, 90% of cases occurring before the age of 4), and may rarely be seen in adults (women only). Chuh proposed diagnostic criteria involving the following positive clinical features:
  1. monomorphous flat-topped, pink-brown, papules or papulovesicles of 1–10 mm in diameter (Figs 19-25 and 19-26)
  2. any three or all four sites involved—face, buttocks, forearms, and extensor legs
  3. symmetry
  4. duration of at least 10 days.
- Negative clinical features:
  1. extensive truncal lesions
  2. scaly lesions.

The lesions develop over a few days but last longer than most viral exanthems (more than 10 days and up to many weeks). Lesion numbers may vary from a few to a generalized eruption coalescing to form plaques covering the face, trunk, and upper extremities. Early in the course of the eruption, the lesions will demonstrate a Koebner phenomenon. Pruritus is variable and the mucous membranes are spared, except when inflamed by the associated infectious agent. Depending on the cause, the lymph nodes, mainly inguinal and axillary, are moderately enlarged for 2–3 months. No treatment appears to shorten the course of the disease, which is self-limited.

Brandt O, et al: Gianotti–Crosti syndrome. J Am Acad Dermatol 2006; 54:136.

Dikici B, et al: A case of Gianotti–Crosti syndrome with HBV infection. Adv Med Sci 2008; 53:338.

Fastenberg M, Morrell DS: Acral papules: Gianotti–Crosti syndrome. Pediatr Ann 2007; 36:800.

Gumus P, et al: Gianotti–Crosti syndrome as the only manifestation of primary Epstein–Barr virus infection: a case report. Turk J Pediatr 2008; 50:302.

Karakas M, et al: Gianotti–Crosti syndrome in a child following hepatitis B virus vaccination. J Dermatol 2007; 34:117.

Kolivras A, Andre J: Gianotti–Crosti syndrome following hepatitis A vaccination. Pediatr Dermatol 2008; 25:650.

Monastirli A, et al: Gianotti–Crosti syndrome after hepatitis A vaccination. Acta Derm Venereol 2007; 87:174.

Xia Y, et al: Pruritic acral rash in a child: Gianotti–Crosti syndrome. Am Fam Physician 2008; 78:103.

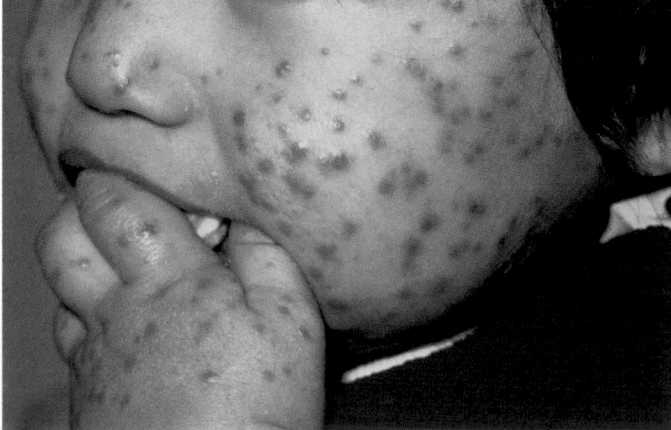

Fig. 19-25 Gianotti–Crosti syndrome.

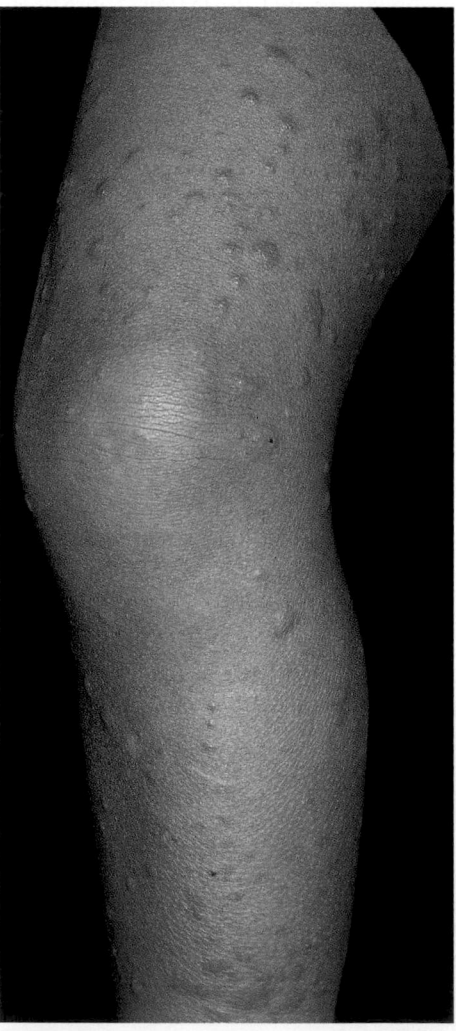

Fig. 19-26 Papules on the leg, Gianotti–Crosti syndrome. (Courtesy of Curt Samlaska, MD)

Poxvirus group

The poxviruses are DNA viruses of a high molecular weight. The viruses are 200–300 nm in diameter, and hence can be seen in routine histologic material. The orthopoxviruses include variola, vaccinia, monkeypox, cowpox, buffalopox, and Cantagalo and Aracatuba. The parapoxviruses are primarily zoonotic, and include orf, paravaccinia, bovine papular stomatitis, deerpox, and sealpox. Tanapox is the sole yatapoxvirus to cause human disease.

Variola major (smallpox)

Smallpox was eradicated worldwide in 1977. It continues to be of interest to dermatologists as it is a potential biologic warfare agent. Variola is spread via the respiratory route, with 37–88% of unvaccinated contacts becoming infected. The incubation period for smallpox is 7–17 days (average 10–12 days). The prodromal phase consists of 2–3 days of high fever (over 40°C), severe headache, and backache. The fever subsides and an exanthem covers the tongue, mouth, and oropharynx. This is followed in 1 day by the appearance of skin lesions. The skin lesions are distributed in a centrifugal pattern, the face, arms, and legs being more heavily involved than the trunk. Lesions appear first on the palms and soles, and feel like firm "BBs" under the skin. Beginning as erythematous macules (days 1–2), the lesions all in synchrony become 2–3 mm papules (days 2–4) and evolve to 2–5 mm vesicles (days 4–7) and 4–6 mm pustules (days 5–15). The pustules umbilicate, collapse, and form crusts beginning in the second week. The total evolution averages 2 weeks. Lesions on the palms and soles persist the longest. The crusts separate after about 1 more week, leaving scars (Fig. 19-27), which are permanent in 65–80% of the survivors. Patients are infectious from the onset of the exanthem through the first 7–10 days of the eruption. A variety of complications occur, including pneumonitis, blindness due to viral keratitis or secondary infection (1% of patients), encephalitis (less than 1% of patients), arthritis (2% of children), and osteitis. Immunity is lifelong. The mortality rate was 5–40% in undeveloped countries (and at a time prior to current intensive care and antiviral management).

Six clinical patterns of smallpox have been described. Variola major, or "ordinary smallpox," had a case fatality rate of 30%.

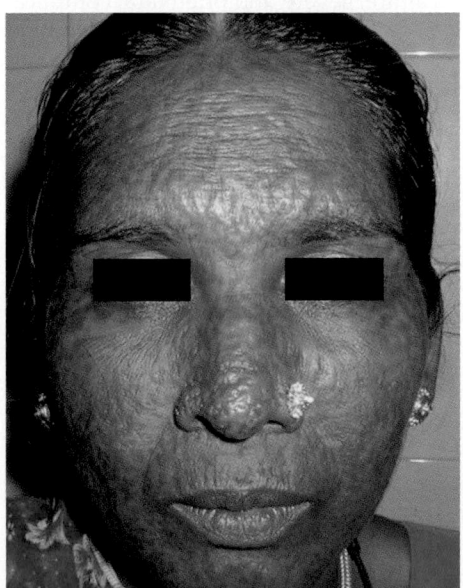

Fig. 19-27 Smallpox scars. (Courtesy of Shyam Verma, MD)

Modified variola represents a small percentage of unvaccinated patients and about 25% of vaccinated persons. The lesions are fewer, smaller, and more superficial, and evolve more rapidly. Fatalities were rare. Flat lesions occur in about 7% of persons, and evolve slowly and coalesce. Ninety-seven percent of unvaccinated persons with flat variola died. Hemorrhagic smallpox occurred in a small percentage of patients, resembles a purpuric eruption or vasculitis, and was universally fatal within a week. This variant is very hard to diagnose without a biopsy, but is highly infectious. Variola sine eruption describes infection in patients who develop flu-like symptoms but no skin lesions. They do not appear to be infectious. Variola minor appears to be a subtype of variola that is milder and resulted in death in less than 1% of patients.

Diagnosis is made by electron microscopy, viral culture, and PCR. Special laboratories, usually associated with the City and State Health Departments in the US, have the capacity to process these specimens and confirm the diagnosis. The differential diagnosis is primarily varicella, especially of the more severe form seen in adults. In varicella the prodrome lasts for 1–2 days; fever begins with the onset of the eruption (not preceding it by 1–3 days, as in variola); the eruption is concentrated on the torso (not centrifugally); individual lesions of different stages are present; and individual lesions evolve from vesicles to crust within 24 h. The diagnostic test of choice in this setting would be a Tzanck smear or DFA, which can rapidly confirm the diagnosis of varicella.

Treatment of smallpox includes strict isolation and protection of healthcare workers. Only vaccinated persons should treat the patient, and any of those exposed should immediately be vaccinated, as this modifies the disease. Cidofovir may be indicated, as it modifies infections by other orthopox viruses.

Breman JG, Henderson DA: Diagnosis and management of smallpox. N Engl J Med 2002; 346:1300.

Vaccinia

The vaccinia virus has been propagated in laboratories for immunization against smallpox. There are multiple strains used in vaccines and the rates of complications vary somewhat, depending on the strain used. New vaccines have been developed, but were not used during the mass immunizations that took place between 2002 and 2004, so their adverse reaction profiles are poorly understood. The available antiviral agents with activity against vaccinia are limited. If a case of vaccinia is encountered, the State Health Department or CDC should be contacted immediately for optimal management.

Vaccination

Vaccination is inoculation of live vaccinia virus into the epidermis and upper dermis by the multiple puncture technique. Between 3 and 5 days after inoculation, a papule forms, which becomes vesicular at days 5–8, then pustular, reaching a maximum size at days 8–10. The pustule dries from the center outward, revealing the pathognomonic umbilicated pustule, and forms a scab that separates 14–21 days after vaccination, resulting in a pitted scar. Formation by days 6–8 of a papule, vesicle, ulcer, or crusted lesion, surrounded by a rim of erythema and induration, is termed a "major reaction" or "take." The rim of erythema averages 3.5–4 cm in diameter in new vaccinees and peaks on days 9–11. Repeat vaccinees have reactions of a similar time course, but the maximum diameter of the erythema is only 1–2 cm. Reactions that do not match this description are considered equivocal and such persons cannot be considered immune. Revaccination should be considered. A large vaccination reaction, or "robust take," is the development of a plaque of erythema and induration of greater than 10 cm at the site of inoculation. This occurs in 10% of initial vaccines. It peaks at days 8–10 and resolves without treatment within 72 h. Cellulitis secondary to vaccination occurs in days 1–5 after vaccination or after several weeks, and progresses without treatment. Management should be expectant, but a bacterial culture may be taken. Since vaccinated patients may have fever at days 8–10 following vaccination, this is not helpful in separating cellulitis from a "robust take." Rarely, patients will develop lesions at the site of vaccination an average of 2 months following vaccination. The nature of these lesions is unknown, but they have not been identified as containing live virus and are self-limited.

Vaccination involves the inoculation of a live virus. Complications result from an abnormal response to the vaccination by the host or from inadvertent transmission to another person. Persons with defective cutaneous or systemic immunity are at particular risk for adverse outcomes from vaccination. Since some complications may be fatal, extremely careful steps must be taken to avoid complications.

Inadvertent inoculation and autoinoculation

Inadvertent inoculation of vaccinia may occur by transmission of virus via hands or fomites from the vaccination site to another skin area or the eye, or to another person. Accidental autoinoculation occurs in about 1 in 1000 vaccinees. Autoinoculation most commonly occurs around the eyes and elsewhere on the face, but the groin and other sites may be involved (Fig. 19-28). These lesions evolve in parallel with the primary vaccination site and, except for ocular lesions, cause no sequelae, except scarring at times. Any evidence of ocular inflammation in a recently vaccinated individual could represent ocular vaccinia infection and requires immediate ophthalmologic evaluation. Transmission to others (secondary transfer) is rare if the vaccination site is kept covered until it heals (7.4 in 100 000 primary vaccinees). It usually occurs within a household or through intimate contact. Serial transmission can occur among male sports partners. Correct bandaging of the vaccination site using foam or occlusive dressings and not gauze bandages, and treating the inoculation site with povidone iodine ointment beginning at 7 days after immuniza-

tion both can reduce viral shedding and might reduce autoinoculation and secondary cases.

Generalized vaccinia

Between 6 and 9 days after vaccination, a generalized vaccinia eruption may occur, in about 81 per 1 million new vaccinees or 32 per 1 million repeat vaccinees. The lesions are papulovesicles that become pustules and involute in 3 weeks, although successive crops may occur within that time. Generalized vaccinia may be accompanied by fever, but patients do not appear ill. Lesions may be generalized or limited to one anatomic region, and can number from a few to hundreds. They can be confused with multiple site autoinoculation, as well as erythema multiforme. The diagnosis is confirmed by biopsy, viral culture, or PCR. Generalized vaccinia is self-limited and does not require treatment in the immunocompetent host. In the setting of underlying immunodeficiency, early intervention with vaccinia immune globulin (VIG) may be beneficial.

Eczema vaccinatum

Eczema vaccinatum is analogous to eczema herpeticum, representing vaccinia virus infection superimposed on a chronic dermatitis, especially atopic dermatitis. Patients with Darier's disease, Netherton, and other disorders of cornification may also be at risk. Since patients with atopic dermatitis or any past history of atopic dermatitis should not be vaccinated, most cases of eczema vaccinatum represent secondary transfer to an at-risk individual from a recent vaccinee, usually a family member. The vesicles appear suddenly, mostly in areas of active dermatitis. The lesions are sometimes umbilicated and appear in crops, resembling smallpox or chickenpox. The onset is sudden and fresh vesicles appear for several days. Scarring is common. Often there is cervical adenopathy and fever, and affected persons are systemically ill (as opposed to those with generalized vaccinia). Secondary bacterial infection can complicate eczema vaccinatum. The mortality rate for eczema vaccinatum is 30–40% if untreated. VIG reduces mortality to 7%. Multiple doses of VIG and perhaps treatment with effective antivirals may be required. One case occurred during the recent mass vaccination of the US military.

Progressive vaccinia (vaccinia necrosum, vaccinia gangrenosum)

Progressive vaccinia is a rare, severe and often fatal complication of vaccination that occurs in persons who are immunodeficient. Most cases occur when infants with undiagnosed immunodeficiency are immunized. The initial vaccination site continues to progress and fails to heal after more than 15 days. The vaccination site is characterized by a painless but progressive necrosis and ulceration (Fig. 19-29), with or without metastatic lesions to distant sites (skin, bones, viscera). No inflammation is present at the sites of infection, even histologically. Inflammation may indicate secondary bacterial infection. Untreated progressive vaccinia is virtually always fatal. Progressive vaccinia is diagnosed by skin biopsy, viral culture, or PCR. VIG should be given, and antiviral antibiotics should be considered.

Cutaneous immunologic complications

A spectrum of erythematous eruptions occurs following vaccination. These eruptions are more common than generalized vaccinia, with which they are often confused. Cases of Stevens–Johnson syndrome following vaccination have been seen in the past, primarily in children, but apparently are rare in adult vaccinees (no cases among more than 30 000 civilian adult vaccinees).

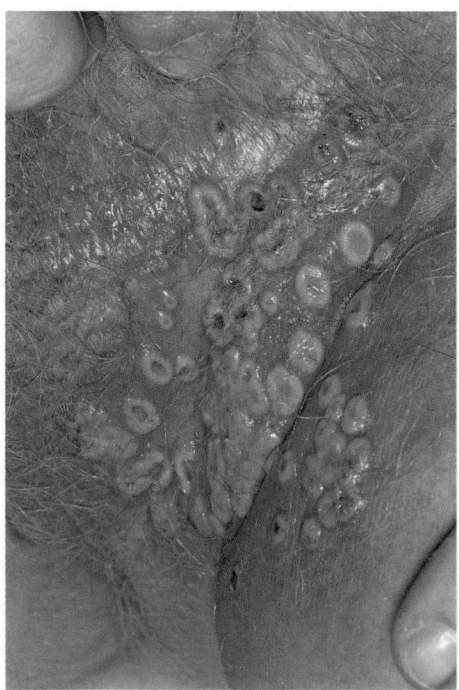

Fig. 19-28 Vaccinia, typical reaction at about 1 week.

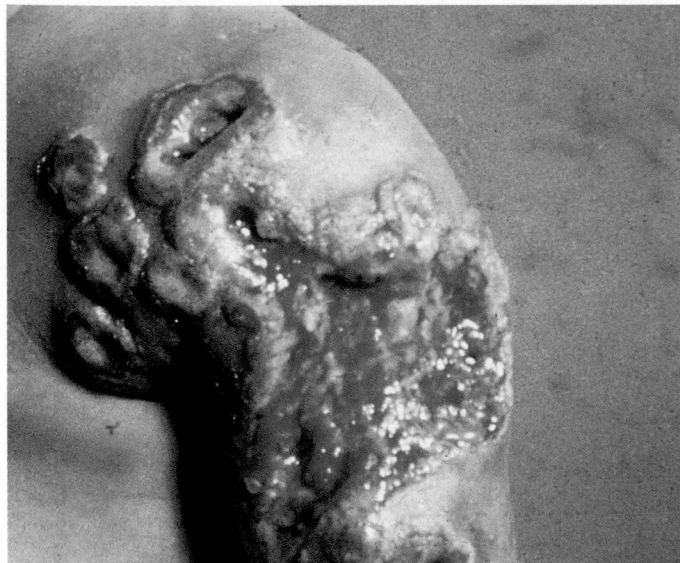

Fig. 19-29 Vaccinia, disseminated.

Benign hypersensitivity reactions to vaccinia

About 0.08% of vaccinees will develop a diffuse cutaneous eruption during the second week after vaccination, around the peak of the immunization site reaction. These have been classified as exanthematous (by far the most common), urticarial, and erythema multiforme-like (the most rare). A follicular eruption has also been reported (see below). All these reaction patterns evolve over 1–2 days, and resolve over days. Patients may have mild symptoms but are afebrile. At times, the eruption may evolve from around the inoculation site and generalize. This had been called "roseola vaccinia" in the past. Primary vaccinees are more likely to develop these reactions. Histology is non-specific, showing features of a viral exanthem (a mild spongiotic dermatitis). These reactions are distinguished from generalized vaccinia by a later onset (end of second week as opposed to days 6–9 after vaccination), prominent erythema, lack of vesicles and pustules, and negative laboratory testing for vaccinia virus. The eruptions described as erythema multiforme-like lack mucosal involvement and blistering, and more closely resemble urticaria multiforme (see Chapter 7). They are distinguished from erythema multiforme/Stevens–Johnson syndrome by the absence of atypical purpuric or typical targetoid lesions, lack of mucosal involvement, and histologic evaluation.

Post-vaccination follicular eruption

A generalized variant of this eruption occurred in 2.7% of new vaccinees and a localized variant in 7.4% during a trial of Aventis Pasteur smallpox vaccine. In the second week, 9–11 days following vaccination, multiple follicular, erythematous papules appeared, primarily on the face, trunk, and proximal extremities. Lesions were mildly pruritic. Over several days the lesions evolved to pustules, which resolved without scarring. Lesions were simultaneously at different stages of development. The number of lesions was usually limited and rarely exceeded 50. Lesions spontaneously resolved over a few days. Histologic evaluation revealed a suppurative folliculitis. No virus was detected in the lesions by PCR or viral culture.

Other skin lesions at vaccination scars

Melanomas, basal cell carcinomas, and squamous cell carcinomas have all occurred in vaccination scars. Benign lesions with a tendency to occur in scars, such as dermatofibromas, sarcoidosis, and granuloma annulare, also can occur in vaccination scars.

Bessinger GT, et al: Benign hypersensitivity reactions to smallpox vaccine. Int J Dermatol 2007; 4:460.

Centers for Disease Control and Prevention: Update on adverse events following civilian smallpox vaccination—United States, 2003. Arch Dermatol 2003; 139:1091.

Centers for Disease Control and Prevention: Secondary and tertiary transfer of vaccinia virus among U.S. military personnel—United States and worldwide, 2002–2004. Arch Dermatol 2004; 140:629.

Cono J, et al: Smallpox vaccination and adverse reactions. MMWR 2003; 52:1.

Curry JL, et al: Occurrence of a basal cell carcinoma and dermatofibroma in a smallpox vaccination scar. Dermatol Surg 2008; 34:132.

Fulginitis VA: Risks of smallpox vaccination. JAMA 2003; 290:1452.

Hammarlund E, et al: Traditional smallpox vaccination with reduced risk of inadvertent contact spread by administration of povidone iodine ointment. Vaccine 2008; 26:430.

Hivnor C, James W: Autoinoculation vaccinia. J Am Acad Dermatol 2003; 50:139.

Kaiser J: A tame virus runs amok. Science 2007; 316:1418.

Kroger A, et al: Dermatological lesions near the smallpox vaccination site after scab detachment. Clin Infec Dis 2008; 46:S227.

Lederman E, et al: Eczema vaccinatum resulting from the transmission of vaccinia virus from a smallpox vaccinee: an investigation of potential fomites in the home environment. Vaccine 2009; 27:375.

Lewis FS, Norton SA: Analysis of cases reported as generalized vaccinia during the US military smallpox vaccination program, December 2002 to December 2004. J Am Acad Dermatol 2006; 55:23.

Simpson EL, et al: Cutaneous responses to vaccinia in individuals with previous smallpox vaccination. J Am Acad Dermatol 2007; 57:442.

Talbot TR, et al: Focal and generalized folliculitis following smallpox vaccination among vaccinia-naïve recipients. JAMA 2003; 289:3290.

Talbot TR, et al: Optimal bandaging of smallpox vaccination sites to decrease the potential for secondary vaccinia transmission without impairing lesion healing. Infec Cont Hosp Epidemiol 2006; 27:1184.

Vora S, et al: Severe eczema vaccinatum in a household contact of a smallpox vaccinee. Clin Infec Dis 2008; 46:1555.

Waibel KH, Walsh DW: Smallpox vaccination site complications. Int J Dermatol 2006; 45:684.

Waibel KH, Walsh DW: Smallpox vaccination site reactions: two cases of exaggerated scarring and a brief review. Int J Dermatol 2006; 45:764.

Walling HW, et al: Squamous cell carcinoma in situ in a smallpox vaccination scar. Int J Dermatol 2008; 47:599.

Human monkeypox

Human monkeypox is a rare, sporadic zoonosis that occurs in remote areas of the tropical rainforests in central and western Africa. Monkeypox virus is an orthopoxvirus. The main vector for monkeypox is wild African rodents and monkeys. Humans and anteaters are accidental hosts. Direct contact with an infected animal or person appears to be required to acquire the infection. In Africa, more than 90% of cases occur in children under 15 years of age, in whom the fatality rate is 11%. The secondary attack rate in African households is 10%. A recent outbreak of 81 cases of monkeypox occurred in the US. Prairie dogs became infected when housed with infected African rodents. Persons who purchased the prairie dogs become infected, most commonly via bites or scratches, or through areas of damaged skin. The pattern of monkeypox seen in the US cases was different from that of African cases, since transmission was felt to be by inoculation, and many of the affected persons were previously immunized with vaccinia. Primary skin lesions occurred at sites of inoculation and limited spread occurred thereafter, with the appearance of 1–50 additional satellite and disseminated lesions over several days. Patients often had fever, respiratory symptoms, and characteristic lymphadenopathy (67%). About one-quarter required hospitalization, and only two children had serious clinical illness, one with encephalitis and one with severe oropharyngeal lesions.

In Africa, the disease is clinically similar to smallpox, with an incubation period of 10–14 days. Patients develop headache (100%); fever, sweats, and chills (82%); and lymphadenopathy (90%). Lymphadenopathy is not a feature of smallpox. The prodrome lasts 2 days, followed by the appearance of 2–5 mm papules. The lesions spread centrifugally and progress from papules to vesicles, then pustules all in a 14–21-day period. In 80% of cases, the lesions are largely monomorphic, but are more pleomorphic than smallpox. The distribution is generalized and the buccal mucosa can be affected. Lesions resolve with hemorrhagic crusts. The disease is self-limited. It is less severe in persons previously vaccinated against smallpox.

Buffalopoxvirus

Buffalopoxvirus is a subspecies of vaccinia virus and is endemic in buffalo herders in India. Lesions occur on the hands and arms of animal handlers and resemble a milder form of cowpox. Family members may be affected and children have developed lesions resembling eczema vaccinatum.

Zoonotic poxvirus infections

While these infections are uncommon, increasing numbers are being reported due to the popularity of exotic pets and travel to endemic areas. They continue to represent, in the case of orf, an important disease in animal husbandry. The diagnosis of zoonotic poxvirus infection is usually by epidemiologic history, clinical features, and electron microscopy, which can separate the various poxvirus genera. Laboratory culture is slow and PCR analysis of the viral DNA allows for speciation. Rarely is antiviral therapy indicated, as most diseases are self-limited. Cidofovir, and in some cases ribavirin and adefovir dipivoxil, would be anticipated to have activity against this group of viruses.

Cowpox

Cowpox is an orthopoxvirus related to smallpox and vaccinia, which is geographically restricted to the UK, Europe, Russia, and adjacent states. It is largely a zoonosis that rarely affects cattle. The domestic cat is the usual source of human infection, but the animal reservoirs are apparently small wild rodents (mice and voles) and human infection from contact with such rodents has been confirmed. Most cases occur in the late summer and in fall.

The incubation period is about 7 days. There is then an abrupt onset of fever, malaise, headache, and muscle pain. Lesions are usually solitary (72%), with co-primaries in 25%. Lesions occur on the hands and fingers in half the cases and the face in another third. Secondary lesions are uncommon and generalized disease is rare, usually occurring in patients with atopic dermatitis. The lesion progresses from a macule through a vesicular stage, then a pustule that becomes blue–purple and hemorrhagic. A hard, painful, 1–3 cm indurated eschar develops after 2–3 weeks and may resemble cutaneous anthrax. In anthrax, however, the eschar forms by day 6. Lesions are always painful and there is local lymphadenopathy, which is usually tender. The amount of surrounding edema and induration is much more marked than in orf. Patients are systemically ill until the eschar stage. Healing usually takes 6–8 weeks. Scarring is common.

Farmyard pox

Because closely related parapoxviruses of sheep and cattle cause similar disease in humans, orf and milker's nodules have been collectively called farmyard pox. The epidemiologic features are discussed separately, but the clinical and histologic features, which are identical, are discussed jointly. The diagnosis of these infections is based on taking an accurate history, and can virtually always be confirmed by routine histologic evaluation. The presence of a homologue gene of vascular endothelial growth factor (VEGF) may explain the vascular nature of lesions produced by parapoxviruses.

Milker's nodules/bovine papular stomatitis/pseudocowpox

These infections cause worldwide occupational disease of milkers or veterinarians, most commonly transmitted directly from the udders (milker's nodules) or muzzles (bovine papular stomatitis) of infected cows. Lesions are usually solitary or only a few in number, and are confined to the hands or forearms (Fig. 19-30). Numerous lesions have been reported in healing first- and second-degree burns in milker's nodules. These cases occurred on farms with infected cattle, but the patients had not had direct contact with the cattle, suggesting indirect viral transmission. It is unclear whether milker's nodules and bovine papular stomatitis are caused by one or two species of parapoxvirus.

Orf

Also known as ecthyma contagiosum, contagious pustular dermatosis, sheep pox, and infectious labial dermatitis, orf is a common disease in goat- and sheep-farming regions throughout the world (Fig. 19-31). Direct transmission from active

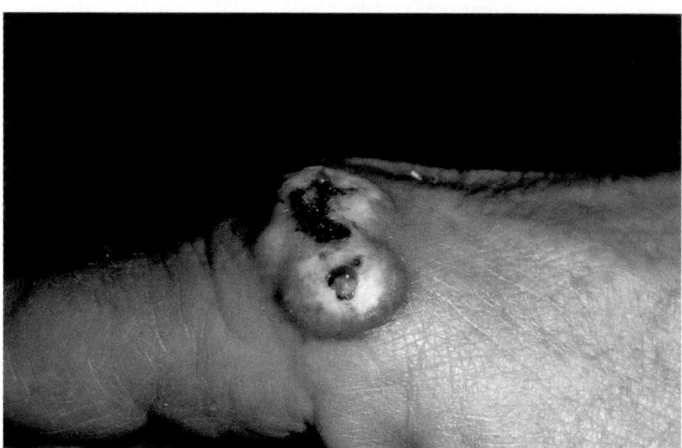

Fig. 19-30 Milker's nodule.

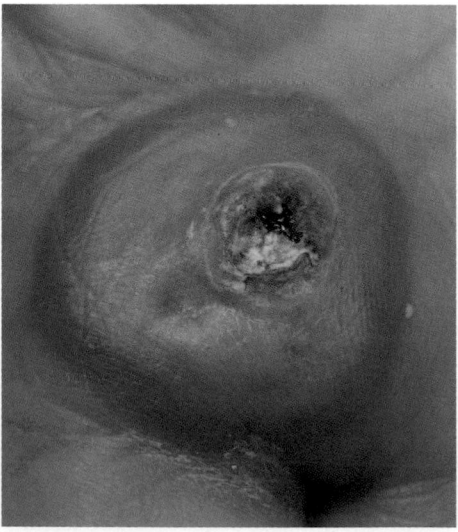

Fig. 19-31 Orf.

lesions on lambs is most common, but infection from fomites is also frequent, since the virus is resistant to heat and dryness. Autoinoculation to the genital area can occur, but human-to-human transmission is rare.

Clinical features

The incubation period for farmyard pox is about 1 week. Lesions are usually solitary and occur on the hands, fingers, or face. Lesions evolve through six stages:

1. A papule forms, which then becomes a target lesion with a red center surrounded successively with a white ring and then a red halo.
2. In the acute stage, a red, weeping nodule not unlike pyogenic granuloma appears.
3. In a hairy area, temporary alopecia ensues.
4. In the regenerative stage, the lesion becomes dry with black dots on the surface.
5. The nodule then becomes papillomatous.
6. The nodule finally flattens to form a dry crust, eventually healing.

Lesions are usually about 1 cm in diameter, except in immunosuppressed patients, in whom giant lesions may occur. Spontaneous resolution occurs in about 6 weeks, leaving minimal scarring. Mild swelling, fever, pain, and lymphadenitis may accompany the lesions, but these symptoms are milder than those seen in cowpox. Orf may be associated with an erythema multiforme-like eruption in about 5% of cases. Treatment is supportive, although shave excision may accelerate healing.

Histologic features

Histologic features correlate with the clinical stage. Nodules show a characteristic pseudoepitheliomatous hyperplasia covered by a parakeratotic crust. Keratinocytes always demonstrate viropathic changes of nuclear vacuolization and cytoplasmic 3–5 μm eosinophilic inclusions surrounded by a pale halo. The papillary dermis is markedly edematous. The dermal infiltrate, which is dense and extends from the interface to the deep dermis, consists of lymphocytes, histiocytes, neutrophils, and eosinophils. Massive capillary proliferation and dilation are present in the upper dermis.

Sealpox

Sealpox, caused by a parapoxvirus, closely resembles orf and has been described in seal handlers who have been bitten by infected harbor or grey seals. Up to 40% of seals in Europe and North America are serologically positive for the virus, suggesting infection is common.

Human tanapox

Tanapox infection is a yatapoxvirus infection endemic to equatorial Africa. It is spread from its natural hosts, nonhuman primates, through minor trauma. Human-to-human transmission is rare. Tanapox infection is manifested by mild fever of abrupt onset lasting 3–4 days, followed by the appearance of one or two pock lesions. Lesions are firm and cheesy, resembling cysts. The disease is self-limited and smallpox vaccination would not be expected to be protective. Rare cases have been imported into Europe and the US.

Parapoxvirus infections from wildlife

Smith et al reported two patients with solitary lesions on the fingers, one following direct inoculation while cleaning a deer and another at the site of a cut sustained on a camping trip in an area with wild deer. Lesions were present for more than 2 months before biopsy. Histologically, there was marked hyperkeratosis, parakeratosis, and pseudoepitheliomatous

hyperplasia. The midepidermal cells showed vacuolization with pyknotic nuclei. The dermis had prominent vascular proliferation. Viral particles were identified by electron microscopy in the keratinocytes. These may represent cases of red deer pox, caused by a distinct species of parapoxvirus. Reindeer poxvirus may cause similar disease.

Buttner M, Rziha HJ: Parapoxviruses: from the lesion to the viral genome. J Vet Med 2002; 49:7.

Centers for Disease Control: Update: multistate outbreak of monkeypox—Illinois, Indiana, Kansas, Missouri, Ohio, and Wisconsin, 2003. Arch Dermatol 2003; 139:1229.

Clark C, et al: Human smallpox resulting from a seal bite. Br J Dermatol 2005; 152:791.

De Clercq E: Cidofovir in the therapy and short-term prophylaxis of poxvirus infections. Trends Pharmacol Sci 2002; 23:456.

Dhar AD, et al: Tanapox infection in a college student. N Engl J Med 2004; 350:361.

Di Giulio DB, Eckburg PB: Human monkeypox: an emerging zoonosis. Lancet 2004; 4:15.

Di Giulio DB, Eckburg PB: Human monkeypox. Lancet 2004; 4:199.

Earl PL, et al: Immunogenicity of a highly attenuated MVA smallpox vaccine and protection against monkeypox. Nature 2004; 428:182.

Frey SE, Belshe RB: Poxvirus zoonoses: putting pocks into context. N Engl J Med 2004; 350:324.

Hawranek T, et al: Feline orthopoxvirus infection transmitted from cat to human. J Am Acad Dermatol 2003; 49:513.

Hönlinger B, et al: Generalized cowpox infection probably transmitted from a rat. Br J Dermatol 2005; 153:451.

Lewis-Jones S: Zoonotic poxvirus infections in humans. Curr Opin Infect Dis 2004; 17:81.

Nitsche A, et al: Viremia in human cowpox virus infection. J Clin Virol 2007; 40:160.

Quenelle DC, et al: Cutaneous infections of mice with vaccinia or cowpox viruses and efficacy of cidofovir. Antiviral Res 2004; 63:33.

Reed KD, et al: The detection of monkeypox in humans in the Western hemisphere. N Engl J Med 2004; 350:342.

Sale, TA, et al: Monkeypox: an epidemiologic and clinical comparison of African and US disease. J Am Acad Dermatol 2006; 55:478.

Smith KJ, et al: Parapoxvirus infections acquired after exposure to wildlife. Arch Dermatol 1991; 127:79.

Trindade GS, et al: Zoonotic vaccinia virus: clinical and immunological characteristics in a naturally infected patient. Clin Inf Dis 2009; 48:e37.

Wienecke R, et al: Cowpox virus infection in an 11-year-old girl. J Am Acad Dermatol 2000; 42:892.

Molluscum contagiosum

Molluscum contagiosum is caused by up to four closely related types of poxvirus, MCV-1 to 4 and their variants. Although the proportion of infection caused by the various types varies geographically, throughout the world MCV-1 infections are most common. In small children virtually all infections are caused by MCV-1. There is no difference in the anatomic region of isolation with regard to infecting type (as opposed to HSV, for example). In patients infected with HIV, however, MCV-2 causes the majority of infections (60%), suggesting that HIV infection-associated molluscum does not represent recrudescence of childhood molluscum.

Infection with MCV is worldwide. Three groups are primarily affected: young children, sexually active adults, and immunosuppressed persons, especially those with HIV infection. Molluscum is most easily transmitted by direct skin-to-skin contact, especially if the skin is wet. Swimming pools have been associated with infection.

In all forms of infection, the lesions are relatively similar. Individual lesions are smooth-surfaced, firm, dome-shaped, pearly papules, averaging 3–5 mm in diameter (Fig. 19-32). "Giant" lesions may be up to 1.5 cm in diameter. A central umbilication is characteristic. Irritated lesions may become crusted and even pustular, simulating secondary bacterial infection. This may precede spontaneous resolution. Lesions

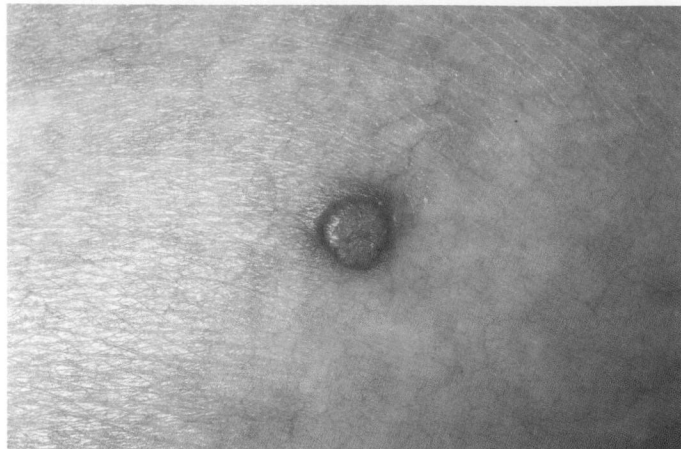

Fig. 19-32 Molluscum contagiosum.

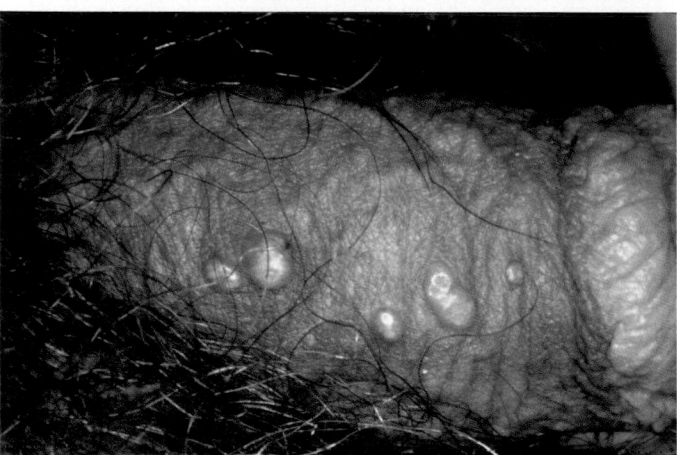

Fig. 19-33 Molluscum contagiosum of the penis.

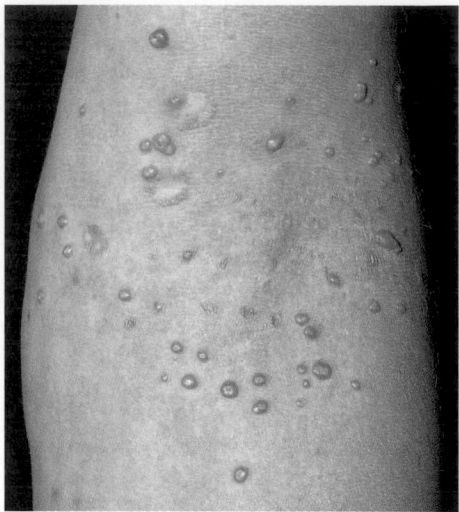

Fig. 19-34 Molluscum contagiosum, child with atopic dermatitis.

that rupture into the dermis may elicit a marked suppurative inflammatory reaction that resembles an abscess.

The clinical pattern depends on the risk group affected. In young children the lesions are usually generalized and number from a few to more than 100. Dermatitis surrounding a lesion usually heralds the resolution of that lesion. Lesions tend to be on the face, trunk, and extremities. Genital lesions occurring as part of a wider distribution occur in 10% of childhood cases. When molluscum is restricted to the genital area in a child, the possibility of sexual abuse must be considered.

In adults, molluscum is sexually transmitted and other STDs may coexist. There are usually fewer than 20 lesions; these favor the lower abdomen, upper thighs, and the penile shaft in men (Fig. 19-33). Mucosal involvement is very uncommon.

Immunosuppression, either systemic T-cell immunosuppression (usually HIV, but also sarcoidosis and malignancies) or abnormal cutaneous immunity (as in atopic dermatitis or topical steroid use), predisposes the individual to infection. In atopic dermatitis, lesions tend to be confined to dermatitic skin (Fig. 19-34).

Secondary infection may occur. In addition, in about 10% of lesions, a surrounding eczematous reaction is present (molluscum dermatitis). Rarely, erythema annulare centrifugum may be associated. Lesions on the eyelid margin or conjunctiva may be associated with a conjunctivitis or keratitis. Rarely, the molluscum lesions may present as a cutaneous horn (molluscum contagiosum cornuatum).

Between 10 and 30% of AIDS patients not receiving antiretroviral therapy have molluscum contagiosum. Virtually all

HIV-infected patients with molluscum contagiosum already have an AIDS diagnosis and a helper T-cell count of less than 100. In untreated HIV disease, lesions favor the face (especially the cheeks, neck, and eyelids) and genitalia. They may be few or numerous, forming confluent plaques. Giant lesions are not uncommon and may be confused with a basal cell carcinoma. Involvement of the oral and genital mucosa may occur, virtually always indicative of advanced AIDS (helper T-cell count less than 50). Facial disfigurement with numerous lesions can occur.

Molluscum contagiosum has a characteristic histopathology. Lesions primarily affect the follicular epithelium. The lesion is acanthotic and cup-shaped. In the cytoplasm of the prickle cells, numerous small eosinophilic and later basophilic inclusion bodies, called molluscum bodies or Henderson–Paterson bodies, are formed. Eventually, their bulk compresses the nucleus to the side of the cell. In the fully developed lesion each lobule empties into a central crater. Inflammatory changes are slight or absent. Characteristic brick-shaped poxvirus particles are seen on electron microscopy in the epidermis. Latent infection has not been found, except in untreated AIDS patients, in whom even normal-appearing skin may contain viral particles. Molluscum contagiosum virus contains an *IL-18* binding protein gene it apparently acquired from humans. This blocks the host's initial effective Th1 immune response against the virus by reducing local IFN-γ production.

The diagnosis is easily established in most instances because of the distinctive central umbilication of the dome-shaped lesion. This may be enhanced by light cryotherapy that leaves the umbilication appearing clear against a white (frozen) background. For confirmation, express the pasty core of a lesion, squash it between two microscope slides (or a slide and a cover glass) and stain it with Wright, Giemsa, or Gram stains. Firm compression between the slides is required.

Treatment is determined by the clinical setting. In young immunocompetent children, especially those with numerous lesions, the most practical course may be not to treat or to use only topical tretinoin. Aggressive treatment may be emotionally traumatic and can cause scarring. Spontaneous resolution is virtually a certainty in this setting, avoiding these sequelae. Individual lesions last 2–4 months each; the duration of infection is about 2 years. Continuous application of surgical tape to each lesion daily after bathing for 16 weeks led to cure in 90% of children so treated. Topical cantharidin, applied for 4–6 h to approximately 20 lesions per setting, led to resolution in 90% of patients and 8% of patients improved. This therapy is well tolerated, has a very high satisfaction rate for patients and their parents, and has rare complications. If lesions are limited and the child is cooperative, nicking the lesions with a blade to express the core (with or without the use of a comedo extractor), light cryotherapy, application of trichloroacetic acid (35–100%), or removal by curettage are all alternatives. The application of EMLA cream for 1 h before any painful treatments has made the management of molluscum in children much easier. Topical 5% sodium nitrite with 5% salicylic acid cures about 75% of patients. No controlled trials have confirmed the efficacy of imiquimod and it cannot be recommended for the treatment of molluscum.

In adults with genital molluscum, removal by cryotherapy or curettage is very effective. Neither imiquimod nor podophyllotoxin has been demonstrated to be effective. In fact, the failure of these agents to improve "genital warts" suggests the diagnosis of genital molluscum contagiosum. Sexual partners should be examined; screening for other coexistent STDs is mandatory.

In patients with atopic dermatitis, application of EMLA followed by curettage or cryotherapy is most practical. Caustic chemicals should not be used on atopic skin. Topical steroid application to the area should be reduced to the minimum strength possible. A brief course of antibiotic therapy should be considered after initial treatment, since dermatitic skin is frequently colonized with *S. aureus*.

In immunosuppressed patients, especially those with AIDS, management of molluscum can be very difficult. Aggressive treatment of the HIV infection with HAART, if it leads to improvement of the helper T-cell count, is predictably associated with a dramatic resolution of the lesions. This response is delayed 6–8 months from the institution of the treatment. Molluscum occurs frequently in the beard area, so shaving with a blade razor should be discontinued to prevent its spread. If lesions are few, curettage or core removal with a blade and comedo extractor is most effective. EMLA application may permit treatment without local anesthesia. Cantharone or 100% trichloroacetic acid may be applied to individual lesions. Temporary dyspigmentation and slight surface irregularities may occur. Cryotherapy may be effective but must be used with caution in persons of pigment. When lesions are numerous or confluent, treatment of the whole affected area may be required because of the possibility of latent infection. Trichloroacetic acid peels above 35% concentration (medium depth) or daily applications of 5-fluorouracil (5-FU) to the point of skin erosion may eradicate lesions, at least temporarily. At times, removal by curette is required. In patients with HIV infection, continuous application of tretinoin cream once nightly at the highest concentration tolerated seems to reduce the rate of appearance of new lesions. Topical 1–3% cidofovir application and systemic infusion of this agent have been reported to lead to dramatic resolution of molluscum in patients with AIDS.

Au WY, et al: Fulminant molluscum contagiosum infection and concomitant leukaemia cutis after bone marrow transplantation for chronic myeloid leukaemia. Br J Dermatol 2000; 143:1097.

Charteris DG, et al: Ophthalmic molluscum contagiosum. Br J Ophthalmol 1995; 79:476.

Diven DG: An overview of poxviruses. J Am Acad Dermatol 2001; 44:1.

Fornatora ML, et al: Intraoral molluscum contagiosum: a report of a case and a review of the literature. Oral Surg Oral Med Oral Pathol Oral Radiol Endod 2001; 92:318.

Meadows KP, et al: Resolution of recalcitrant molluscum contagiosum in HIV-infected patients treated with cidofovir. Arch Dermatol 1997; 133:987.

Silverberg NB, et al: Childhood molluscum contagiosum: experience with cantharidin therapy in 300 patients. J Am Acad Dermatol 2000; 43:503.

Toro JR, et al: Topical cidofovir: a novel treatment for recalcitrant molluscum contagiosum in children infected with human immunodeficiency virus 1. Arch Dermatol 2000; 136:983.

Watanabe T, et al: Antibodies to molluscum contagiosum virus in the general population and susceptible patients. Arch Dermatol 2000; 136:1518.

Xiang Y, Moss B: Molluscum contagiosum virus interleukin-18 (IL-18) binding protein is secreted as a full-length form that binds cell surface glycosaminoglycans through the C-terminal tail and a furin-cleaved form with only IL-18 binding domain. J Virol 2003; 77:2623.

Picornavirus group

Picornavirus designates viruses that were originally called enteroviruses (polioviruses, coxsackieviruses, and echoviruses), plus the rhinoviruses. The picornaviruses are small, single-stranded RNA, icosahedral viruses varying in size from 24 to 30 nm. Only the coxsackieviruses, echoviruses, and enterovirus types 70 and 71 are significant causes of skin disease.

Enterovirus infections

Person-to-person transmission occurs by the intestinal–oral route and, less commonly, the oral–oral or respiratory routes. Enteroviruses are identified by type-specific antigens. The type-specific antibodies appear in the blood about 1 week after infection has occurred and attain their maximum titer in 3 weeks. Viral cultures obtained from the rectum, pharynx, eye, and nose may isolate the infecting agent. Usually, the diagnosis is by clinical characteristics, and except in specific clinical settings, the causative virus is not identified. Enteroviral infections most frequently occur in children between the ages of 6 months and 6 years.

Many nonspecific exanthems and exanthems that occur during the summer and early fall are caused by coxsackievirus or echovirus. The exanthems are most typically diffuse macular or morbilliform erythemas, which sometimes also contain vesicular lesions, or petechial or purpuric areas. Echovirus 9 has caused an eruption resembling acute meningococcemia. Each type of exanthem has been associated with many subtypes of coxsackievirus or echovirus (one exanthem, many possible viral causes). Echovirus 9, the most prevalent enterovirus, causes a morbilliform exanthem, initially on the face and neck, then the trunk and extremities. Only occasionally is there an eruption on the palms and soles. Small red or white lesions on the soft palate may occur. The most common specific eruptions due to enteroviruses are hand-foot-and-mouth disease, herpangina, and roseola-like illnesses. Rare reported presentations of enterovirus infection include a unilateral vesicular eruption simulating herpes zoster, caused by echovirus 6; a fatal dermatomyositis-like illness in a patient with hypogammaglobulinemia, caused by echovirus 24; and a widespread vesicular eruption in atopic dermatitis that simulated Kaposi varicelliform eruption, caused by coxsackievirus A-16. Pleconaril and other new antienteroviral agents may be useful in severe enteroviral infections.

While the cutaneous eruptions due to these viruses are quite benign, infections with enterovirus 71 can be quite severe, with the development of brainstem encephalitis and fatal neurogenic pulmonary edema, as well as ascending flaccid paralysis resembling poliomyelitis. Epidemics with severe disease have been reported in Bulgaria, Hungary, Hong Kong, Japan, Australia, Malaysia, Singapore, and Taiwan; the latter had the worst epidemic, affecting more than 1 million people with 78 deaths in 1998.

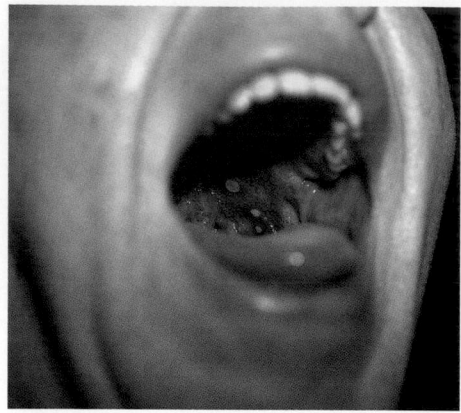

Fig. 19-35 Herpangina.

Herpangina

Herpangina, a disease of children worldwide, is caused by multiple types of coxsackievirus (most frequently A8, A10, and A16), echoviruses, and enterovirus 71. In the severe outbreaks in Taiwan, 10% of the fatal cases had herpangina. It begins with acute onset of fever, headache, sore throat, dysphagia, anorexia, and sometimes, stiff neck. The most significant finding, which is present in all cases, is of one or more yellowish-white, slightly raised 2 mm vesicles in the throat, usually surrounded by an intense areola (Fig. 19-35). The lesions are found most frequently on the anterior faucial pillars, tonsils, uvula, or soft palate. Only one or two lesions might appear during the course of the illness or the entire visible pharynx may be studded with them. The lesions often occur in small clusters and later coalesce. Usually, the individual or coalescent vesicles ulcerate, leaving a shallow, punched-out, grayish-yellow crater 2–4 mm in diameter. The lesions disappear in 5–10 days. Treatment is supportive, consisting of topical anesthetics.

Herpangina is differentiated from aphthosis and primary herpetic gingivostomatitis by the location of the lesions in the posterior oropharynx and by isolation of an enterovirus. Coxsackievirus A10 causes acute lymphonodular pharyngitis, a variant of herpangina, characterized by discrete yellow–white papules in the same distribution as herpangina.

Hand-foot-and-mouth disease

Hand-foot-and-mouth disease (HFMD) is usually a mild illness. It primarily affects children from 2 to 10, but exposed adults may also develop disease. Infection begins with a fever and sore mouth. In 90% of cases oral lesions develop; these consist of small (4–8 mm), rapidly ulcerating vesicles surrounded by a red areola on the buccal mucosa, tongue, soft palate, and gingiva. Lesions on the hands and feet are asymptomatic red papules that quickly become small, gray, 3–7 mm vesicles surrounded by a red halo. They are often oval, linear, or crescentic, and run parallel to the skin lines on the fingers and toes (Fig. 19-36). They are distributed sparsely on the dorsa of the fingers and toes, and more frequently on the palms and soles. Especially in children who wear diapers, vesicles and erythematous, edematous papules may occur on the buttocks (Fig. 19-37). The infection is usually mild and seldom lasts more than a week. Treatment is supportive, with the use of oral topical anesthetics. Onychomadesis may follow enteroviral infection and HFMD, about 1 month after the acute viral syndrome.

HFMD is most frequently caused by coxsackievirus A16 and less commonly by other coxsackie viruses (A5, A7, A9, A10, B1, B3, and B5), as well as enterovirus 71. In the severe Taiwanese enterovirus 71 outbreak, 80% of cases with CNS

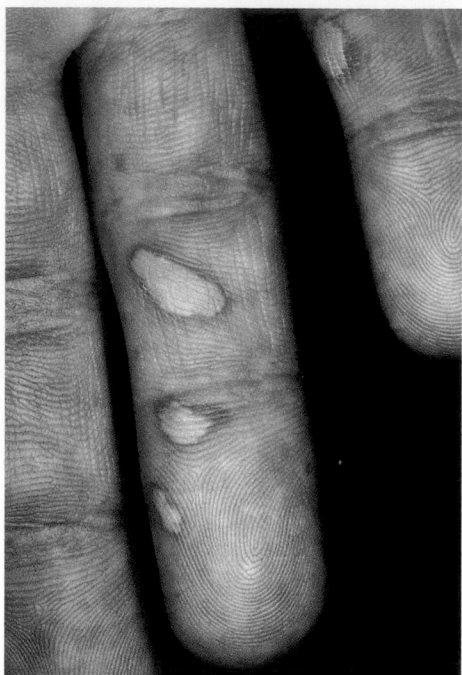

Fig. 19-36 Hand-foot-and-mouth disease. (Courtesy of James Fitzpatrick, MD)

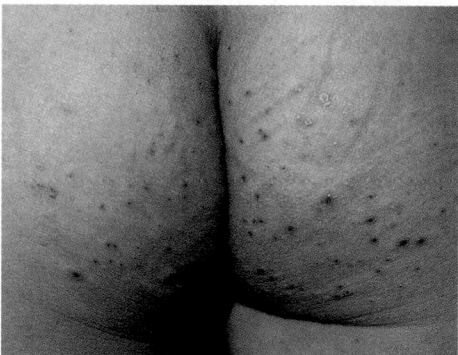

Fig. 19-37 Hand-foot-and-mouth disease.

disease had HFMD. No cases of HFMD associated with CNS disease were due to coxsackie A16, so the rapid discrimination of viral types may be vital in outbreaks of HFMD. The virus may be recovered from the skin vesicles. Histopathologic findings are those of an intraepidermal blister formed by vacuolar and reticular degeneration of keratinocytes similar to other viral blisters. Inclusion bodies and multinucleated giant cells are absent. HFMD is distinguished from herpangina by the distribution of the oral lesions and the presence of skin lesions. It is differentiated from erythema multiforme minor by the skin lesions, which are oval and gray, as opposed to targetoid, as in erythema multiforme. HFMD usually requires no treatment. Although the coxsackieviruses lack thymidine kinase, acyclovir has anecdotally been reported to hasten resolution of the eruption in two reports.

Boston exanthem disease

The so-called Boston exanthem disease occurred as an epidemic in Boston and was caused by echovirus 16, a now uncommon cause of viral exanthems. The eruption consisted of sparsely scattered, pale red macules and papules. In severe cases, the lesions were morbilliform and even vesicular. The eruption was chiefly on the face, chest, and back, and in some cases on the extremities. On the soft palate and tonsils, small ulcerations like those of herpangina were noted. There was little or no adenopathy. The incubation period was 3–8 days.

Eruptive pseudoangiomatosis

Eruptive pseudoangiomatosis has been described in two clusters—in the Mediterranean region and in South Korea. It favors the summer months in both regions. The disorder is characterized by the sudden appearance of 2–4 mm blanchable red papules that resemble angiomas. In children, it is usually associated with a viral syndrome, but most affected adults have no viral symptoms. In adults, females outnumber males 2:1. The red papules blanch on pressure and are often surrounded by a 1–2 mm pale halo. Lesions often number about 10, but may be much more numerous. Most lesions appear on the exposed surfaces of the face and extremities, but the trunk may also be affected. In children, lesions are short-lived, virtually always resolving within 10 days. Lesions may last slightly longer in adults. Annual recrudescences may occur. Epidemics have been described in adults, and even healthcare workers caring for patients with eruptive pseudo-angiomatosis have developed lesions. Histologically, dilated upper dermal vessels, but not increased numbers of blood vessels, with prominent endothelial cells are seen. Echoviruses 25 and 32 had been implicated in the initial reports. The occurrence in young children and the presence of miniepidemic outbreaks suggest an infectious trigger. This disorder closely resembles "erythema punctatum Higuchi," which is very common in Japan and known to be caused by *Culex pipiens pallens* bites. It appears that mosquito bites, viral infection, or enhanced insect bite reaction due to intercurrent viral infection are possible pathogenic causes of eruptive pseudoangiomatosis.

Chang LY: Enterovirus 71 in Taiwan. Pediatr Neonatol 2008; 49:103.

Chang LY, et al: Transmission and clinical features of enterovirus 71 infections in household contacts in Taiwan. JAMA 2004; 291:222.

Faulkner CF, et al: Hand, foot and mouth disease in an immunocompromised adult treated with acyclovir. Australas J Dermatol 2003; 44:203.

Jin SP, et al: Eruptive pseudo-angiomatosis lesions are associated with intravascular neutrophils and do not harbour Epstein–Barr virus. J Eur Acad Dermatol Venereol 2010; 24:163–167.

Lui Z, et al: Coxsackievirus-induced myocarditis: new trends in treatment. Expert Rev Anti Infect Ther 2005; 3:641.

Messner J, et al: Accentuated viral exanthems in areas of inflammation. J Am Acad Dermatol 1999; 40:345.

Patel S, Chamlin SL: A 4-year-old girl with abnormal fingernails. Pediat Ann 2006; 35:431.

Salazar A, et al: Onychomadesis outbreak in Valencia, Spain, June 2008. Euro Surveill 2008; 13:7.

Steiner I, et al: Viral encephalitis: a review of diagnostic methods and guidelines for management. Eur J Neurol 2005; 12:331.

Venturi C, et al: Eruptive pseudoangiomatosis in adults: a community outbreak. Arch Dermatol 2004; 140:757.

Paramyxovirus group

The paramyxoviruses are RNA viruses that range in size from 100 to 300 nm. In this group, the viral diseases of dermatologic interest are measles (rubeola) and German measles (rubella). Other viruses of this group are mumps virus, parainfluenza virus, Newcastle disease virus, and respiratory syncytial virus.

Measles

Measles is a highly infectious and potentially fatal viral infection. Highly effective two-dose vaccines are available, and when countries reach a rate of 95% vaccination, measles elimination has been achieved. However, measles remains a major health problem in many nations, including developed ones who provide immunizations to their populations. More than 12 000 cases of measles occurred in Europe in the 2-year period covering 2006–7. This epidemic is ongoing and has spurred an elimination program. Numerous hospitalizations and even deaths from measles are still occurring in these developed nations. The majority of cases are in unvaccinated persons, supporting the concept that vaccination (specifically two doses) is protective, and that these measles epidemics and deaths are preventable. Low vaccination levels exist in these countries for many reasons, some philosophical and some socioeconomic. Since the children in unvaccinated groups may share common schools, camps, and social networks, they provide a prime breeding ground for epidemics. Some developed European and Asian countries (notably Japan, with 200 000 cases annually) have not been able to achieve high immunization levels, meaning that their populations are still at risk. The lack of "herd" immunity in these nations leaves at particular risk those infants and susceptible children who cannot be immunized due to other medical conditions. In addition, the introduction of a case of measles can lead to an outbreak since many unprotected children can propagate the spread of the virus. Although cases of measles continue to be imported into the US, the high immunization rate has prevented such outbreaks. Countries with low immunization rates also serve as the source of nonendemic cases in countries with high immunization rates. In Africa and Southeast Asia, multiple socioeconomic factors have resulted in lack of immunization. Dermatologists and pediatricians in the Americas need to be alert for cases of measles when seeing persons from these countries or unvaccinated persons from the Americas who have traveled to nations known to have ongoing measles outbreaks.

Also known as rubeola and morbilli, measles was a worldwide disease that most commonly affected children under 15 months of age. In the current epidemics, however, older children and frequently adolescents are the age group primarily affected. Measles is spread by respiratory droplets and has an incubation period of 9–12 days.

The prodrome consists of fever, malaise, conjunctivitis, and prominent upper respiratory symptoms (nasal congestion, sneezing, coryza, and cough). After 1–7 days, the exanthem appears, usually as macular or morbilliform lesions on the anterior scalp line and behind the ears. Lesions begin as discrete erythematous papules that gradually coalesce. The rash spreads quickly over the face (Fig. 19-38), then by the second or third day (unlike the more rapid spread of rubella) extends down the trunk to the extremities. By the third day, the whole body is involved. Lesions are most prominent and confluent in the initially involved areas and may be more discrete on the extremities. Purpura may be present, especially on the extremities, and should not be confused with "black measles," a rare, disseminated intravascular coagulation-like complication of measles. Koplik spots, which are pathognomonic, appear during the prodrome (Fig. 19-39). They appear first on the buccal mucosa nearest to the lower molars as 1 mm white papules on an erythematous base. They may spread to involve other areas of the buccal mucosa and pharynx. After 6–7 days the exanthem clears, with simultaneous subsidence of the fever.

Complications include otitis media, pneumonia, encephalitis, and thrombocytopenic purpura. Encephalitis, although rare (less than 1% of cases), can be fatal. Infection in pregnant patients is associated with fetal death. Complications and fatalities are more common in children who are undernourished or have T-cell deficiencies. In HIV-infected children, the exanthem may be less prominent.

Modified measles occurs in a partially immune host as a result of prior infection, persistent maternal antibodies, or

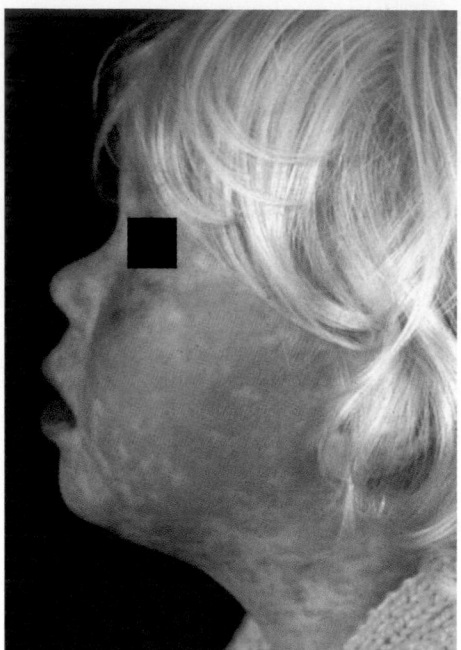

Fig. 19-38 Measles.

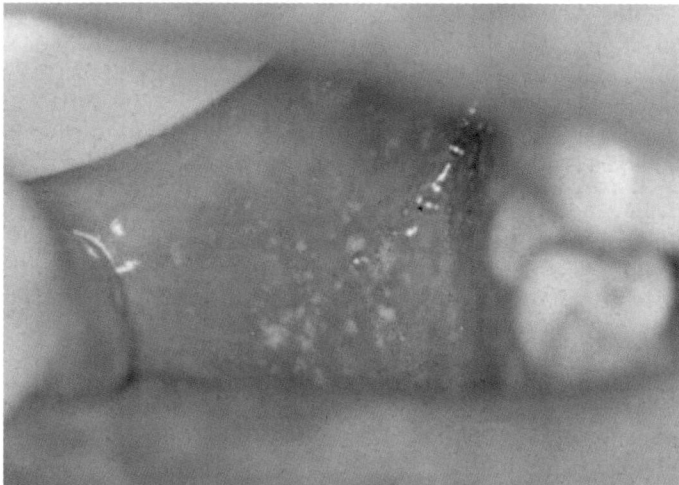

Fig. 19-39 Koplik spots.

immunization, and is a milder disease. Patients may have only fever, or fever and a rash. The course is shorter, the exanthem is less confluent, and Koplik spots may be absent. It is difficult to differentiate it from other viral exanthems.

A diagnosis of measles is established by the presence of a high fever, Koplik spots, the characteristic conjunctivitis, upper respiratory symptoms, and typical exanthem. Lymphopenia is common, with a decreased white blood cell count. Biopsies of skin lesions may show syncytial keratinocytic giant cells, similar to those seen in respiratory secretions. Laboratory confirmation can be with acute and convalescent serologic tests. Identification of virus-specific IgM (5 days after the rash is present) is highly suggestive of infection in an unimmunized individual. Too early a serum IgM assay may lead to a false-negative result and the test should be repeated. Virus isolation is also possible, but can be costly and technically challenging. The combination of IgM serological testing and virus isolation is the current gold standard. Immunofluorescence techniques can identify virus from clinical material. New PCR-based technologies can rapidly detect the measles virus genome in urine, oropharyngeal secretions, and blood, and are highly useful in modified and previously

vaccinated patients. Rubella, scarlet fever, secondary syphilis, enterovirus infections, and drug eruptions are in the differential diagnosis. Administration of high doses of vitamin A will reduce the morbidity and mortality of hospitalized children with measles. Two doses of retinyl palmitate, 200 000 IU 24 h apart, are recommended for all children 6–24 months of age, immunodeficient children, children with malnutrition or evidence of vitamin A deficiency, and recent immigrants from areas of high measles mortality. Otherwise, treatment is symptomatic, with bed rest, analgesics, and antipyretics.

Live virus vaccination is recommended at 12 months, with a booster prior to entering school (4–5 years). A faint maculopapular exanthem may occur 7–10 days after immunization. Prophylaxis should be offered to exposed susceptible persons. It must be provided within the first few days following exposure, so identification of susceptible persons is critical. Vaccination can be effective if given within 3 days of exposure and normal immune globulin at a dose of 0.25 mL/kg up to 6 days after contact. In an Australian outbreak, these strategies prevented 80% of possible secondary cases.

Rubella

Rubella, commonly known as German measles, is caused by a togavirus and probably spreads by respiratory secretions. The incubation period is 12–23 days (usually 15–21). Live virus vaccination is highly effective, providing lifelong immunity.

There is a prodrome of 1–5 days consisting of fever, malaise, sore throat, eye pain, headache, red eyes, runny nose, and adenopathy. Pain on lateral and upward eye movement is characteristic. The exanthem begins on the face and progresses caudad, covering the entire body in 24 h and resolving by the third day. The lesions are typically pale pink, morbilliform macules, smaller than those of rubeola. The eruption may resemble roseola or erythema infectiosum. An exanthem of pinhead-sized red macules or petechiae on the soft palate and uvula (Forchheimer's sign) may be seen. Posterior cervical, suboccipital, and postauricular lymphadenitis occurs in more than half of cases. Rubella is in general a much milder disease than rubeola. Arthritis and arthralgias are common complications, especially in adult women. These last a month or longer. The diagnosis is confirmed by finding rubella-specific IgM in oral fluids or the serum. This IgM develops rapidly, but 50% of sera drawn on the first day of the rash are negative. The virus is rapidly cleared from the blood, being absent by day 2 of the rash. However, the virus is found in oral secretions for 5–7 days after the rash has appeared. PCR-based techniques to identify virus in oral secretions may detect infection more effectively in earlier samples. The combination of PCR-based virus detection tests and identification of rubella virus-specific IgM will result in rapid confirmation of most cases of rubella within the first few days of appearance of disease symptoms.

Congenital rubella syndrome

Infants born to mothers who have had rubella during the first trimester of pregnancy may have congenital cataracts, cardiac defects, and deafness. Numerous other manifestations, such as glaucoma, microcephaly, and various visceral abnormalities, may emerge. Among the cutaneous expressions are thrombocytopenic purpura; hyperpigmentation of the navel, forehead, and cheeks; bluish-red, infiltrated, 2–8 mm lesions ("blueberry muffin" type), which represent dermal erythropoiesis; chronic urticaria; and reticulated erythema of the face and extremities.

Abernathy E, et al: Confirmation of rubella within 4 days of rash onset: comparison of rubella virus RNA detection in oral fluid with immunoglobulin M detection in serum or oral fluid. J Clin Microbiol 2009; 47:182.

Armstrong N, O'Donnell N: Anniversary of rubella epidemic. Lancet 2004; 354:328.

Centers for Disease Control and Prevention: Recommendations from an ad hoc meeting of the WHO Measles and Rubella Laboratory Network (LabNet) on use of alternative diagnostic samples for measles and rubella surveillance. MMWR 2009; 57:657.

Dobson R: Measles outbreak in Wales will get worse, officials predict. BMJ 2009; 338:1412.

Gomi H, Hiroshi T: Why is measles still endemic in Japan? Lancet 2004; 364:328.

Hussey GD, et al: A randomized, controlled trial of vitamin A in children with severe measles. N Engl J Med 1990; 323:160.

Kaneko M: Rubella outbreak on Tokunoshima Island in 2004: serological and epidemiological analysis of pregnant women with rubella. J Obstet Gynaecol Res 2006; 32:461.

Lowther SA, et al: Population immunity to measles virus and the effect of HIV-1 infection after a mass measles vaccination campaign in Lusaka, Zambia: a cross-sectional survey. Lancet 2009; 373:1025.

Masuno K, Sibuya K: Measles elimination: lack of progress in the Western Pacific region. Lancet 2009; 373:1008.

Muscat M, et al: Measles in Europe: an epidemiological assessment. Lancet 2009; 373:383.

Nagai M, et al: Modified adult measles in outbreaks in Japan, 2007–2008. J Med Virol 2009; 81:1094.

Nakayama T: Laboratory diagnosis of measles and rubella infection. Vaccine 2009; 27:3228.

Parent du Châtelet I, et al: Measles resurgence in France in 2008, a preliminary report. Euro Surveill 2009; 14(pii):19118.

Pena-Rey I, et al: Measles risk groups in Spain: implications for the European measles-elimination target. Vaccine 2009; 27:3927.

Sheppeard V, et al: The effectiveness of prophylaxis for measles contacts in NSW. NSW Public Health Bull 2009; 20:81.

Wichmann O, et al: Further efforts needed to achieve measles elimination in Germany: results in an outbreak investigation. Bull World Health Organ 2009; 87:108.

Asymmetric periflexural exanthem of childhood (APEC)

This clinical syndrome, also known as unilateral laterothoracic exanthem, occurs primarily in the late winter and early spring, and appears to be most common in Europe. It affects girls more often than boys (1.2–2:1). It occurs in children 8 months to 10 years of age, but most cases are between 2 and 3 years of age. Multiple cases have been reported in adults from Europe and China. Its cause is unknown, but a viral origin has been proposed, since it occurs in young children and is seasonal, and secondary cases in families have been reported. No reproducible viral etiology has been implicated; however, at least three cases attributed to parvovirus B19 have been reported. Clinically, two-thirds to three-quarters of affected children have symptoms of a mild upper respiratory or gastrointestinal infection, usually preceding the eruption. The lesions are usually discrete 1 mm erythematous papules that coalesce to poorly marginated morbilliform plaques. Pruritus is usually present, but mild. Lesions begin unilaterally close to a flexural area, usually the axilla (75% of cases). Spread is centrifugal, with new lesions appearing on the adjacent trunk and proximal extremity. Normal skin may intervene between lesions. The contralateral side is involved in 70% of cases after 5–15 days, but the asymmetrical nature is maintained throughout the illness. Lymphadenopathy of the nodes on the initially affected side occurs in about 70% of cases. The syndrome lasts 2–6 weeks on average, but may last more than 2 months, and resolves spontaneously. Topical steroids and oral antibiotics are of no benefit, but oral antihistamines may help associated pruritus. Histologically, a mild to moderate lymphocytic (CD8+ T-cell) infiltrate surrounds and involves the eccrine ducts but not the secretory coils. There may be an accompanying interface dermatitis of the upper eccrine duct and adjacent epidermis.

Chan PKS, et al: Asymmetric periflexural exanthema in an adult. Clin Exp Dermatol 2004; 29:311.

Gelmetti C, Caputo R: Asymmetric periflexural exanthema of childhood: who are you? J Eur Acad Dermatol Venereol 2001; 15:293.

Guimera-Martin-Neda G, et al: Asymmetric periflexural exanthem of childhood: report of two cases with parvovirus B19. J Eur Acad Dermatol Venereol 2006; 20:461.

Parvovirus group

Parvovirus B19 is the most common agent in this erythrovirus genus to cause human disease. Infection is worldwide, occurring in 50% of persons by age 15. The vast majority of elderly adults are seropositive. Infections are more common in the spring in temperate climates. Epidemics in communities occur about every 6 years. The virus is spread via the respiratory route and infection rates are very high within households. Most infections are asymptomatic. The propensity for parvovirus B19 to affect the bone marrow is reflected by the presence of thrombocytopenia or leukopenias during the acute infection. Parvovirus B19 is the prototype for the concept, "One virus, many exanthems." Erythema infectiosum and papular purpuric gloves and socks syndrome are both strongly associated with parvovirus B19 infection. Parvovirus B19 may also play a role in some cases of Gianotti–Crosti syndrome and APEC. Other known complications of this viral infection include arthropathy (especially in middle-aged females), aplastic crisis in hereditary spherocytosis and sickle cell disease, and chronic anemia in immunosuppressed patients. Infection of a pregnant woman leads to transplacental infection in 30% of cases and a fetal loss rate of 5–9%. Acute viral myocarditis and pericarditis are frequently secondary to parvovirus B19 infection.

Erythema infectiosum (fifth disease)

Erythema infectiosum is a worldwide benign infectious exanthem that occurs in epidemics in the late winter and early spring. In normal hosts (but not immunosuppressed or sickle-cell patients in crisis), viral shedding has stopped by the time the exanthem appears, making isolation unnecessary. The incubation period is 4–14 days (average 7 days). Uncommonly, a mild prodrome of headache, runny nose, and low-grade fever may precede the rash by 1 or 2 days.

Erythema infectiosum has three phases. It begins abruptly with an asymptomatic erythema of the cheeks, referred to as slapped cheek. The erythema is typically diffuse and macular, but tiny translucent papules may be present. It is most intense beneath the eyes and may extend over the cheeks in a butterfly-wing pattern. The perioral area, lids, and chin are usually unaffected. After 1–4 days the second phase begins, consisting of discrete erythematous macules and papules on the proximal extremities and later the trunk. This evolves into a reticulate or lacy pattern (Fig. 19.40). These two phases typically last 5–9 days. A characteristic third phase is the recurring stage. The eruption is markedly reduced or invisible, only to recur after the patient is exposed to heat (especially when bathing) or sunlight, or in response to crying or exercise. About 7% of children with erythema infectiosum have arthralgias, whereas 80% of adults have joint involvement. Necrotizing lymphadenitis may also occur in the cervical, epitrochlear, supraclavicular, and intra-abdominal lymph nodes. Children with aplastic crisis due to parvovirus B19 usually do not have a rash. However, even healthy children can develop significant bone marrow complications, albeit transient and self-limited.

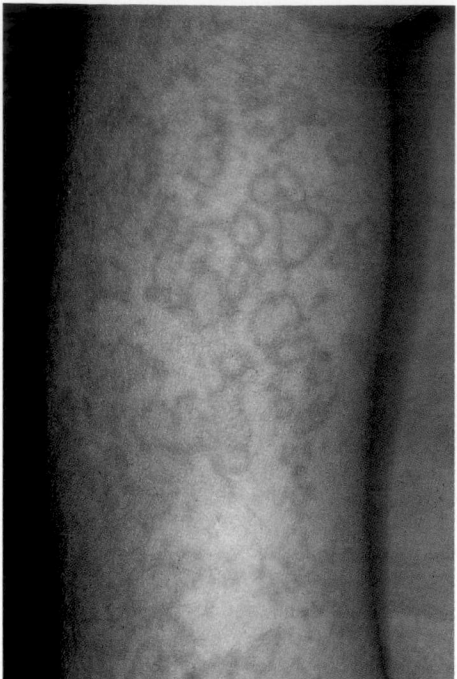

Fig. 19-40 Erythema infectiosum.

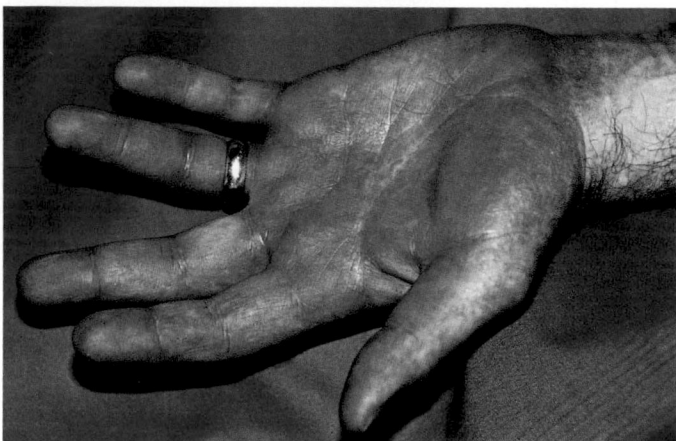

Fig. 19-41 Purpuric socks syndrome.

Papular purpuric gloves and socks syndrome

This syndrome, which is less common than erythema infectiosum, occurs primarily in teenagers and young adults. Pruritus, edema, and erythema of the hands and feet appear, and a fever is present. The lesions are sharply cut off at the wrists and ankles (Fig. 19-41). Over a few days they become purpuric. There is a mild erythema of the cheeks, elbows, knees, and groin folds. Lesions in the groin may become purpuric. Oral erosions, shallow ulcerations, aphthous ulcers on the labial mucosa, erythema of the pharynx, Koplik spots, or petechial lesions may be seen on the buccal or labial mucosa. The lips may be red and swollen. Vulvar edema and erythema accompanied by dysuria may be seen. An unusual variant is a unilateral petechial and erythematous eruption of the axilla. The acral erythema may rarely move proximally along lymphatics, simulating a lymphangitis. Transient lymphocytopenia, a drop in platelet count, and elevation of liver function tests may be seen. The syndrome resolves within 2 weeks. Evidence of seroconversion for parvovirus B19 has been found in most reported patients. Histologically, there is a dermal infiltrate of CD30+ T lymphocytes surrounding the upper dermal vessels.

There is an interface component and prominent extravasation of red blood cells in petechial lesions. Parvovirus B19 antigen has been found in the endothelial cells, sweat glands and ducts, and epidermis in three patients. In HIV-infected patients who develop papular purpuric gloves and socks syndrome (PPGSS), the eruption is more persistent (lasting 3 weeks to 4 months) and is associated with anemia.

Not all cases of PPGSS are caused by parvovirus B19. In adults, it may be associated with HBV infection. In children the syndrome occurs at an average age of 23 months. The eruption lasts an average of 5 weeks. In children CMV and EBV are the most common documented causes in Taiwan, where this syndrome appears to be very common in the last quarter of the year.

Other skin findings attributed to parvovirus B19

In some cases the exanthem of parvovirus B19 affects primarily the flexural areas, especially the groin. This may present as APEC (see above), petechiae in the groin, or an erythema studded with pustules in the groin and to a lesser degree in the axillae, resembling baboon syndrome. The petechial eruption of PPGSS may also involve the perioral area and has been termed the "acropetechial syndrome." An outbreak in Kerala, India, described 50 children mostly under the age of 2 years, who presented with high fever and a diffuse, intensely erythematous, tender skin eruption. The children were very irritable and cried when held. The skin was markedly swollen. Whole-body edema was present. The acute exanthem was followed by diffuse desquamation. There were no secondary cases. IgM for parvovirus B19 was detected in 15 of 24 cases tested. This was termed "red baby syndrome" by the authors. Infection with parvovirus B19 may trigger a hemophagocytic (or macrophage activation) syndrome. This presents with progressive cytopenias, liver dysfunction, coagulopathy, high ferritin, and hemophagocytosis. Numerous nonspecific eruptions have been described with hemophagocytic syndrome, including nodules, ulcers, purpura, and panniculitis. The diagnostic hemophagocytic cells may occasionally be identified in skin biopsies. Infection with parvovirus B19 may lead to cutaneous necrosis in persons with a hypercoagulable state, such as paroxysmal nocturnal hemoglobinuria.

Alfadley A, et al: Papular-purpuric "gloves and socks" syndrome in a mother and daughter. J Am Acad Dermatol 2003; 48:941.

Butler GJ, et al: Parvovirus B19 infection presenting as "bathing trunk" erythema with pustules. Australas J Dermatol 2006; 47:286.

Cholez C, et al: Cutaneous necrosis during paroxysmal nocturnal haemoglobinuria: role of parvovirus B19? J Eur Acad Dermatol Venereol 2005; 19:380.

Dyrsen ME, et al: Parvovirus B19-associated catastrophic endothelialitis with a Degos-like presentation. J Cutan Pathol 2008; 35:20.

Fruhauf J, et al: Bullous papular-purpuric gloves and socks syndrome in a 42-year-old female: molecular detection of parvovirus B19 DNA in lesional skin. J Am Acad Dermatol 2008; 60:691.

Ghigliotti G, et al: Papular-purpuric gloves and socks syndrome in HIV-positive patients. J Am Acad Dermatol 2000; 43:916.

Hsieh MY, Huang PH: The juvenile variant of papular-purpuric gloves and socks syndrome and its association with viral infections. Br J Dermatol 2004; 151:201.

Johnson LB, et al: Parvovirus B19 infection presenting with necrotizing lymphadenitis. Am J Med 2003; 114:340.

Kellermayer R, et al: Clinical presentation of parvovirus B19 infection in children with aplastic crisis. Pediatr Infect Dis J 2003; 22:1100.

McNeeley M, et al: Generalized petechial eruption induced by parvovirus B19 infection. J Am Acad Dermatol 2005; 52:S109.

Messina MF, et al: Purpuric gloves and socks syndrome caused by parvovirus B19 infection. Pediatr Infect Dis J 2003; 22:755.

Nicolay N, Cotter S: Clinical and epidemiological aspects of parvovirus B19 infections in Ireland, January 1996–June 2008. Euro Surveill 2009; 14(pii):19249.

Sakai H, et al: Hemophagocytic syndrome presenting with a facial erythema in a patient with systemic lupus erythematosus. J Am Acad Dermatol 2007; 57:S111.

Sasidharan CK, et al: Red baby syndrome: a new disease due to parvovirus B-19 observed in Kerala. Indian J Pediatr 2009; 76:309.

Seishima M, et al: Acute heart failure associated with human parvovirus B19 infection. Clin Exper Dermatol 2008; 33:588.

Sklavounou-Andrikopoulou A, et al: Oral manifestations of papular-purpuric "gloves and socks" syndrome due to parvovirus B19 infection: the first case presented in Greece and review of the literature. Oral Dis 2004; 10:118.

Yamada Y, et al: Human parvovirus B19 infection showing follicular purpuric papules with a baboon syndrome-like distribution. Br J Dermatol 2004; 150:770.

Young NS, Brown KE: Parvovirus B19. N Engl J Med 2004; 350:586.

Arbovirus group (togaviridae)

The arboviruses comprise the numerous arthropod-borne RNA viruses. These viruses multiply in vertebrates, as well as in arthropods. The vertebrates usually act as reservoirs and the arthropods as vectors of the various diseases.

West Nile fever

West Nile virus (WNV) is a flavivirus that is endemic in East Africa. It first appeared in eastern North America in 1999 and reached California by 2004. It is primarily an infection of the crow family (crows, ravens, magpies, and bluejays). It is spread by *Culex* mosquitoes. Approximately 80% of infected persons will have no symptoms. After an incubation period of 3–15 days, a febrile illness of sudden onset occurs. Headache, myalgia, arthralgia, conjunctivitis, pharyngitis, cough, adenopathy, abdominal pain, hepatitis, pancreatitis, and myocarditis are recognized clinical manifestations. The primary complications, however, are neurologic disease, including seizures (10% of symptomatic adults), ascending flaccid paralysis (like poliomyelitis), ataxia, meningitis, encephalitis, myelitis, cranial neuropathies, optic neuritis, and reduced level of consciousness. A significant percentage of affected persons are left with permanent neurologic sequelae. About 20% of hospitalized patients will have an exanthem. It is nonpruritic and composed of 50–100 erythematous, ill-defined macules 0.5–1 cm in diameter, primarily on the trunk and proximal extremities. It lasts 5–7 days and resolves without scaling.

Sandfly fever

Sandfly fever is also known as phlebotomus fever and pappataci fever. The vector, *Phlebotomus papatasii*, is found in the Mediterranean area (Sicilian, Naples, and Toscana virus), Russia, China, and India. While Sicilian and Naples sandfly fever viral infections disappeared or dramatically decreased with mosquito eradication programs, Toscana virus infection is still common. While most infected persons are asymptomatic, 80% of aseptic meningitis cases in the summer in endemic areas are due to this agent. Small pruritic papules appear on the skin after the sandfly bite and persist for 5 days. After an incubation period of another 5 days, fever, headache, malaise, nausea, conjunctival injection, stiff neck, and abdominal pains suddenly develop. The skin manifestations consist of a scarlatiniform eruption on the face and neck. Recovery is slow, with recurring bouts of fever. No specific treatment is available.

Dengue

More than 100 million cases of dengue occur annually worldwide, and the global prevalence is growing. In European hospitals evaluating patients with fever following trips to the tropics, dengue is the most common febrile illness in travelers returning from Southeast Asia who develop a fever within 1 month of the trip. It is transmitted by *Aedes* mosquitoes, which have adapted well to living around humans in urban environments. It affects primarily tropical regions where temperatures rarely drop below 20°C, favoring the reproduction of the mosquito vector. While Southeast Asia and the Western Pacific are most severely affected, India, Cuba, and the tropical Americas also have numerous cases. Persons of African ancestry appear to be at much decreased risk of developing dengue.

Dengue fever begins 2–15 days after the infectious mosquito bite. The clinical features are characteristic and consist of the sudden onset of high fevers accompanied by myalgias, headache, retro-orbital pain, and severe backache (breakbone fever). Common associated laboratory findings include elevated liver function tests (to about 3 times normal, on average), thrombocytopenia (platelet count below 100 000 in 50% of cases), and a leukopenia. These are present during the acute illness and help to suggest dengue as the correct diagnosis. About 50% of patients will develop a characteristic skin eruption. In 90% of patients, the eruption begins between days 3 and 5 of the illness, often as the fever defervesces. The skin eruption occurs in less than 10% of patients prior to the onset of fever. The eruption is most commonly generalized (50%), or involves only the extremities (30%) or the trunk (20%). Lesions are macular or morbilliform, and are usually confluent, characteristically sparing small islands of normal skin—"islands of white in a sea of red" (Fig. 19-42). Facial flushing may be prominent. The rash is either asymptomatic or mildly pruritic. Petechiae may be present, but the finding of cutaneous hemorrhage should raise the suspicion of dengue hemorrhagic fever/dengue shock syndrome (DHF/DSS; see below). Complete recovery occurs in 7–10 days. Biopsy of the exanthem shows minimal findings and is of no value in predicting the severity of the patient's condition, or in identifying DHF/DSS.

There are four serotypes of dengue. Following infection with one serotype, the individual is resistant to reinfection with that serotype. However, if that person becomes infected with another serotype, he/she is at risk of developing severe complications from the second episode of dengue. The patient's antidengue antibodies are incapable of preventing infection by or replication of the new dengue virus type. However, they do trigger increased viral phagocytosis by mononuclear cells and

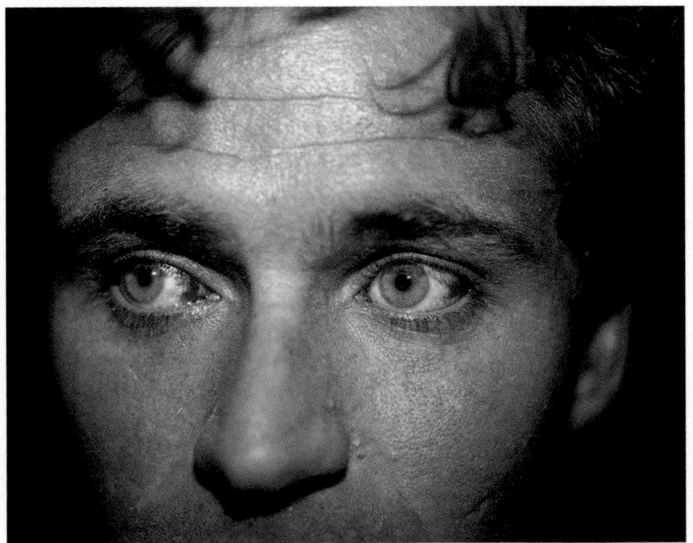

Fig. 19-42 Dengue.

amplified cytokine production. The syndrome that results is characterized by hemorrhage (dengue hemorrhagic fever/ DHF), at times with extensive plasma leakage (dengue shock syndrome/DSS). The fatality rate for DSS may be as high as 40%. DHF/DSS have been clearly defined by the World Health Organization (WHO). Persons with sickle-cell disease are at particular risk of developing DSS and death. DHF grade I presents with findings of dengue with thrombocytopenia, and a positive tourniquet test. Scrotal edema may be present. DHF grade II is DHF grade I plus spontaneous bleeding, most commonly into the skin, conjunctiva (20%), and oral cavity. DSS is grade II DHF plus circulatory failure (hypotension) and agitation. DSS may progress to grade IV, which is grade III plus profound shock (a blood pressure of 0). Only one-third of patients with DHF/DSS will have skin lesions, so their absence does not exclude the diagnosis.

The diagnosis of dengue is made by detection of dengue-specific IgM in the sera by ELISA, by acute and convalescent serologies demonstrating seroconversion. Some laboratories can detect viral RNA in acute serum samples. Given the theoretical risk of increasing DHF/DSS cases by immunizing persons against a single dengue virus type if they were to be exposed to another type, a quadrivalent vaccine would seem prudent. It has not been developed, so travelers' only preventive strategy is to avoid mosquito bites. In children, dengue fever and Kawasaki disease have occurred simultaneously. Since these two syndromes may be nearly identical in their presentation, this differential diagnosis can be extremely difficult. When both diagnoses have been made simultaneously, it was because there was persistent fever (beyond 1 week), a reactive thrombocytosis following the initial thrombocytopenia, and in some cases the development of characteristic cardiac lesions.

Alphavirus

In Finland, Sindbis virus infection is transmitted by the *Culiseta* mosquito. An eruption of multiple, erythematous, 2–4 mm papules with a surrounding halo is associated with fever and prominent arthralgias. The eruption and symptoms resolve over a few weeks. Histologically, the skin lesions show a perivascular lymphocytic infiltrate with large atypical cells, simulating lymphomatoid papulosis. CD30 does not stain the large cells, however, allowing their distinction.

Chikungunya virus is transmitted by the *Aedes* mosquito. Chikungunya is from the Makonde language of sub-Saharan Africa and means "that which bends up," describing the characteristic stooped posture due to the joint symptoms of the disease. It is endemic in Africa, India, Sri Lanka, Southeast Asia, the Philippines, Hong Kong, and the islands of the Indian Ocean. The incubation period is 2–7 days. The patient presents with the abrupt onset of high fever. Significant joint symptoms are characteristic and occur in 40% of infections. Most typically, there is swelling and pain in the small joints of the hands and feet. The joint symptoms may persist for weeks to months, with about 50% still having some symptoms at 6 months. Patients may develop neuropathic acral findings, including Raynaud, erythromelalgia, or severe acral coldness, as late sequelae. Headache occurs in 70% of patients, and nausea and vomiting in 60%. Lymphopenia, thrombocytopenia, and elevated liver function tests can be observed in the first week of the illness. While generally a nonfatal and self-limited illness, severe complications can occur, resulting in death in about 1 in 1000 infected persons.

About one-half to three-quarters or more of patients with Chikungunya virus infection develop a rash. It is pruritic in 20–50% of the patients. The most common and characteristic exanthem is described as morbilliform, and most frequently affects the arms, upper trunk, and face. It can be confluent and islands of sparing can be seen. It appears by the second day of the fever in more than half of patients, and in another 20% on the third or fourth day; only about one-fifth develop the eruption after the fifth day of the illness. Ecchymoses may appear during the acute illness. Aphthous-like ulcerations can occur in the oral, penoscrotal, and less commonly the axillary regions. These may be preceded by intense erythema and pain in the affected area. Following acute Chikungunya infection, hyperpigmentation of the skin may occur.

A bullous eruption may occur in acute Chikungunya virus infection. Ninety percent of those with a bullous eruption are under 1 year of age, and most of the severe bullous eruption cases occur in children under the age of 6 months. Seventeen percent of children develop a vesiculobullous component to their eruption, compared to only 3% of adults. There is an initial exanthem, followed in hours or days by flaccid or tense nonhemorrhagic blisters that rupture easily. Nikolsky's sign is positive. The genitalia, palms, and soles are spared. There is a close resemblance to toxic epidermal necrolysis (TEN) and up to 80% of the total body surface area may become denuded. High titers of virus are recovered from blister fluid (in excess of what is present in blood). Biopsy demonstrates an intraepidermal blister with acantholytic cells free-floating in the blister cavity. These patients are managed like burn patients and most recover. Skin grafting is usually not required.

The diagnosis of Chikungunya virus infection is made by detecting virus-specific IgM in the serum. Confirmation is with seroconversion over the next several months, with development of virus-specific IgG. PCR-based methods may detect viral genome in the blisters or serum during the acute illness.

It may be quite difficult to differentiate dengue fever from Chikungunya fever, since they are both endemic in the same geographic regions, and their clinical symptoms and laboratory findings are quite similar. Arthralgias occur in a significant percentage of patients with Chikungunya virus infection (approaching 100% of those with a rash), and are rare in patients with dengue. Neutropenia is seen in 80% of dengue patients and only 10% of Chikungunya patients. A positive tourniquet test does not distinguish these two infections, but thrombocytopenia is more common in dengue (85+%) as compared with Chikungunya (35%).

Bandyopadhyay D, et al: Mucocutaneous features of Chikungunya fever: a study from an outbreak in west Bengal, India. Int J Dermatol 2008; 47:1148.

Borgherini G, et al: Outbreak of Chikungunya on Reunion Island: early clinical and laboratory features in 157 adult patients. Clin Infec Dis 2007; 44:1401.

Bottieau E, et al: Fever after a stay in the tropics. Medicine 2007; 86:18.

Chen TC, et al: Dengue hemorrhagic fever complicated with acute idiopathic scrotal edema and polyneuropathy. Am J Trop Med Hyg 2008; 78:8.

de la C, Sierra B, et al: Race: a risk factor for dengue hemorrhagic fever. Arch Virol 2007; 152:533.

Del Giudice P, et al: Skin manifestations of West Nile virus infection. Dermatol 2005; 211:348.

Dionisio D, et al: Epidemiological, clinical and laboratory aspects of sandfly fever. Curr Opin Infect Dis 2003; 16:383.

Gonzalez D, et al: Classical dengue hemorrhagic fever resulting from two dengue infections spaced 20 years or more apart: Havana, dengue 3 epidemic, 2001–2002. Int J Infect Dis 2005; 5:280.

Hochedez P, et al: Chikungunya infection in travelers. Emer Inf Dis 2006; 12:1565.

Hochedez P, et al: Management of travelers with fever and exanthema, notably dengue and Chikungunya infections. Am J Trop Med Hyg 2008; 87:710.

Inanadar AC, et al: Cutaneous manifestations of Chikungunya fever: observations made during a recent outbreak in South India. Int J Dermatol 2008; 45:154.

Itoda I, et al: Clinical features of 62 imported cases of dengue fever in Japan. Am J Trop Med Hyg 2006; 75:470.

Lupi O, Tyring SK: Tropical dermatology: viral tropical diseases. J Am Acad Dermatol 2003; 49:979.

Martyn-Simmons CL, et al: A florid skin rash in a returning traveller. Clin Exp Dermatol 2007; 32:779.

Nicoletti L, et al: Chikungunya and dengue viruses in travelers. Emer Infec Dis 2008; 14:177.

Pistone T, et al: Cluster of Chikungunya virus infection in travelers returning from Senegal, 2006. J Trav Med 2009; 16:286.

Radakovic-Fijan S, et al: Dengue hemorrhagic fever in a British travel guide. J Am Acad Dermatol 2002; 46:430.

Rajapakse S, et al: Atypical manifestation of Chikungunya infection. Trans R Soc Trop Med Hyg 2009; Aug 26 (Epub ahead of print).

Robin S, et al: Severe bullous skin lesions associated with Chikungunya virus infection in small infants. Eur J Pediatr 2009 Aug 19 (Epub ahead of print).

Saadiah S, et al: Skin histopathology and immunopathology are not of prognostic value in dengue haemorrhagic fever. Br J Dermatol 2008; 158:836.

Simon R, et al: An emerging rheumatism among travelers returned from Indian Ocean islands: report of 47 cases. Medicine 2007; 86: 123.

Singh S, et al: Dengue fever and Kawasaki disease: a clinical dilemma: Rheumatol Int 2009; 29:717.

Solignat M, et al: Replication cycle of Chikungunya: a re-emerging arbovirus. Virology 2009; Sep 2 (Epub ahead of print).

Solomon T: Flavivirus encephalitis. N Engl J Med 2004; 351:370.

Thomas EA, et al: Cutaneous manifestations of dengue viral infection in Punjab (north India). Int J Dermatol 2007; 46:715.

Valassina M, et al: A Mediterranean arbovirus: the Toscana virus. J Neurovirol 2003; 9:577.

Papovavirus group

Papovaviruses are double-stranded, naked DNA viruses characterized as slow-growing. They replicate inside the nucleus. Because they contain no envelope, they are resistant to drying, freezing, and solvents. In addition to the human papillomaviruses (HPVs), which cause warts, papillomaviruses of rabbits and cattle, polyomaviruses of mice, and vacuolating viruses of monkeys are some of the other viruses in this group.

Warts (verruca)

There are more than 100 types of HPV. The genome of HPV consists of early genes (*E1*, *E2*, *E4*, *E5*, *E6*, and *E7*), two late genes (*L1* and *L2*), and in between an upstream regulatory region (URR). *L1* and *L2* code for the major and minor capsid proteins. A new HPV type is defined when there is less than 90% DNA homology with any other known type in the *L1* and *E6* genes. Viruses with 90–98% homologies are classified as subtypes. The gene sequences from HPVs throughout the world are similar. Most HPV types cause specific types of warts and favor certain anatomic locations, such as plantar warts, common warts, genital warts, and so on. Some wart types, e.g. HPV-27, may be found in several different locations. A large proportion of the HPV types rarely cause warts and appear to be pathogenic only in immunosuppressed patients or those with epidermodysplasia verruciformis. However, many persons may carry or be latently infected with these rare wart types, explaining the uniformity of gene sequence and clinical presentation all over the world. In the setting of immunosuppression, HPV types may cause warty lesions of a different clinical morphology than they would cause in an immunocompetent host.

Infection with HPV may be clinical, subclinical, or latent. Clinical lesions are visible by gross inspection. Subclinical lesions may be seen only by aided examination (e.g. the use of acetic acid soaking). Latent infection describes the presence of HPV or viral genome in apparently normal skin. Latent infection is thought to be common, especially in genital warts, and explains in part the failure of destructive methods to eradicate warts.

HPV infection is very common, as most people will experience infection during their lifetime. In schoolchildren in Australia, 22% were found to have nongenital cutaneous warts, with 16% having common warts, 6% having plantar warts, and 2% having flat (plane) warts. In the UK, the prevalence has been reported at between 4% and 5%. The peak age for cutaneous warts is in the teenage and early adult years, when infection rates reach 25% in some studies. White persons have visible cutaneous warts twice as frequently as other ethnicities. Genital warts begin to appear with sexual activity, and infection rates, including latent infection, exceed 50% in sexually active populations in many parts of the world.

HPVs have coexisted with humans for many millennia, and humans are their primary host and reservoir. HPVs have been successful pathogens of human because they evade the human immune response. This is primarily by avoiding expressing antigens on the surface of keratinocytes until the keratinocytes are above the level of the antigen-presenting cells in the epidermis. They also reduce Langerhans cells in the vicinity of infection. Through *E6* and *E7*, HPV reduces local production of key immune reactants such as TLR9 and IL-8, muting the local immune response. HPVs thus live in equilibrium with their human hosts through a combination of immune evasion and programmed immune suppression (tolerance).

Management of warts is based on their clinical appearance, their location, and the immune status of the patient. In general, warts of all types are more common and more difficult to treat in persons with suppressed immune systems. Except in WHIM syndrome (warts, hypogammaglobulinemia, infection, and myelokathexis), syndromes of reduced immunoglobulin production or B-cell function are not associated with increased HPV infection. However, situations where cell-mediated immunity is suppressed are associated with high rates of clinical HPV infection and HPV-induced neoplasias. The common clinical scenarios are iatrogenic medications (as in organ transplant recipients), viral infections that damage T cells (such as HIV), and congenital syndromes of T-cell immunodeficiency. WILD syndrome is the association of primary lymphedema, disseminated warts and anogenital dysplasia with depressed cell-mediated immunity. HPV 57 is present in the skin warts and multiple warts types are found in the genital lesions (HPV types 6, 51, 52, 61, 84). Because warts in some settings are important cofactors in cancer, histologic evaluation of warty lesions in these situations may be important.

Verruca vulgaris

Common warts are a significant cause of concern and frustration on the part of the patient (Figs 19-43 and 19-44). Social

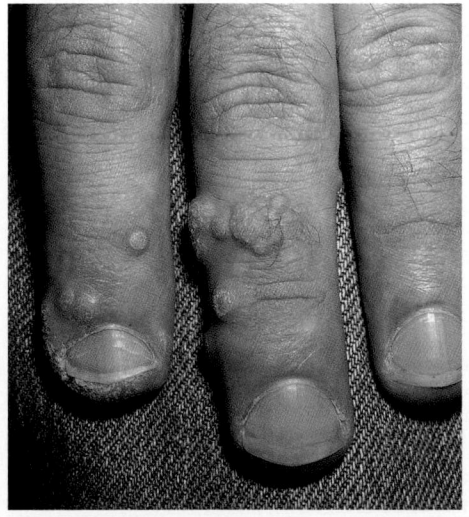

Fig. 19-43 Verruca vulgaris.

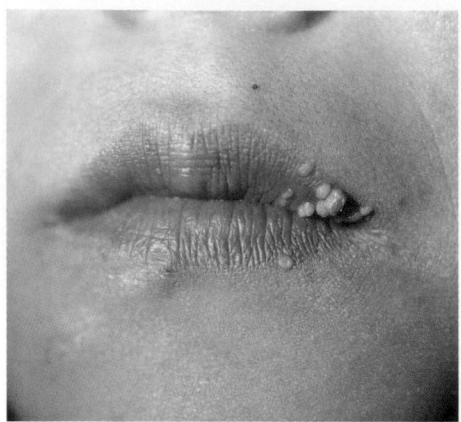

Fig. 19-44 Verruca, nail biter with periungual warts.

activities can be affected, lesions can be uncomfortable or bleed, and treatment is often painful and frustratingly ineffective. HPV-1, 2, 4, 27, 57, and 63 cause common warts. Common warts occur largely between the ages of 5 and 20, and only 15% occur after the age of 35. Frequent immersion of hands in water is a risk factor for common warts. Meat handlers (butchers), fish handlers, and other abattoir workers have a high incidence of common warts of the hands. The prevalence reaches 50% in those persons with direct contact with meat. Warts in butchers are caused by HPV-2 and 4, and up to 27% of hand warts from butchers are due to HPV-7. HPV-7 is very rarely found in warts in the general population (less than 0.3%), and in butchers it is found only on the hands where there is direct contact with meat. The source of HPV-7 is unknown, but HPV-7 is not bovine papillomavirus and does not come from the slaughtered animals. HPV-57 has been reported to cause dystrophy of all 10 fingernails, with marked subungual hyperkeratosis and destruction of the nail plate without periungual involvement.

The natural history of common warts is for them to resolve spontaneously. Reported clearance rates in children are 23% at 2 months, 30% at 3 months, 65–78% at 2 years, and 90% over 5 years. Common warts are usually located on the hands; they favor the fingers and palms. Periungual warts are more common in nail biters and may be confluent, involving the proximal and lateral nailfolds. Fissuring may lead to bleeding and tenderness. Lesions range in size from pinpoint to more than 1 cm, most averaging about 5 mm. They grow in size for weeks to months and usually present as elevated, rounded papules with a rough, grayish surface, which is so characteristic that it has given us the word verrucous, used to describe lesions with similar surface character (e.g. seborrheic keratosis). In some instances, a single wart (mother wart) appears and grows slowly for a long time, and then suddenly many new warts erupt. On the surface of the wart, tiny black dots may be visible, representing thrombosed, dilated capillaries. Trimming the surface keratin makes the capillaries more prominent and may be used as an aid in diagnosis. Warts do not have dermatoglyphics (fingerprint folds), as opposed to calluses, in which these lines are accentuated.

Common warts may occur anywhere on the skin, apparently spreading from the hands by autoinoculation. In nail biters, warts may be seen on the lips and tongue, usually in the middle half, and uncommonly in the commissures. Digitate or filiform warts tend to occur on the face and scalp, and present as single or multiple spikes stuck on the surface of the skin.

Pigmented warts

Pigmented warts have commonly been reported in Japan. They appear on the hands or feet, and resemble common warts

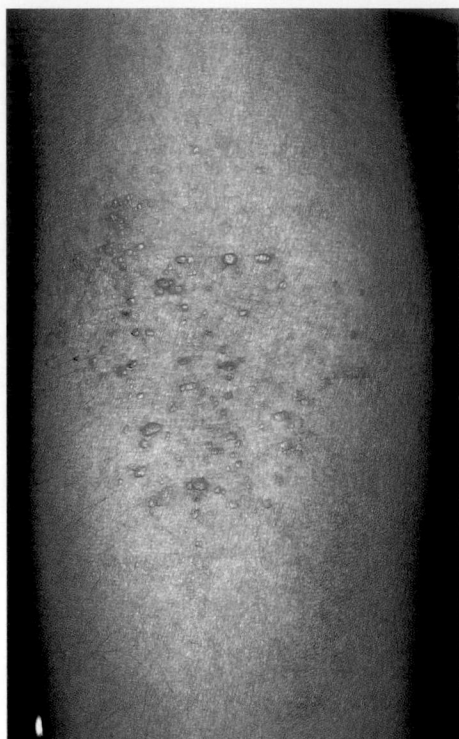

Fig. 19-45 Verruca plana, atopic dermatitis infected with numerous flat warts.

or plantar warts, except for their hyperpigmentation. They are caused by HPV-4, 65, and 60. The pigmentation is due to melanocytes in the basal cell layer of the HPV-infected tissue, which contain large amounts of melanin. This is proposed to be caused by "melanocyte blockade" or the inability of the melanocytes to transfer melanin to the HPV-infected cells.

Flat warts (verruca plana)

HPV-3, 10, 28, and 41 most often cause flat warts. Children and young adults are primarily affected. Sun exposure appears to be a risk factor for acquiring flat warts. They are common on swimmers and on the sun-exposed surfaces of the face and lower legs. Flat warts present most typically as 2–4 mm flat-topped papules that are slightly erythematous or brown on pale skin and hyperpigmented on darker skin. They are generally multiple and are grouped on the face, neck, dorsa of the hands, wrists, elbows, or knees (Fig. 19-45). The forehead, cheeks, and nose, and particularly the area around the mouth and the backs of the hands are the favorite locations. In men who shave their beards and in women who shave their legs, numerous flat warts may develop as a result of autoinoculation. A useful finding is the tendency for the warts to Koebnerize, forming linear, slightly raised, papular lesions. Hyperpigmented lesions occur, and when scarcely elevated, may be confused with lentigines or ephelides. Plaque-like lesions may be confused with verrucous nevus, lichen planus, and molluscum contagiosum. When lesions occur only on the central face and are erythematous, they can be easily confused with papular acne vulgaris. Of all clinical HPV infections, flat warts have the highest rate of spontaneous remission.

Plantar warts (verruca plantaris)

HPV-1, 2, 4, 27, and 57 cause plantar warts. These warts generally appear at pressure points on the ball of the foot, especially over the mid-metatarsal area. They may, however, be anywhere on the sole. Frequently, there are several lesions on one foot. Sometimes they are grouped or several contiguous warts

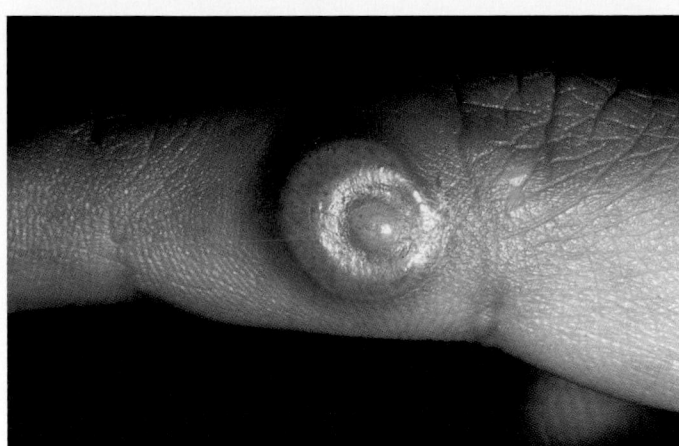

Fig. 19-46 Myrmecia.

fuse so that they appear as one. Such a plaque is known as a mosaic wart. The soft, pulpy cores are surrounded by a firm, horny ring. Over the surface of the plantar wart, most clearly if the top is shaved off, multiple small black points may be seen that represent dilated capillary loops within elongated dermal papillae. Plantar warts may be confused with corns or calluses, but have a soft central core and black or bleeding points when pared down, features that calluses do not have.

The myrmecia type of verruca occurs as smooth-surfaced, deep, often inflamed and tender papules or plaques, mostly on the palms or soles, but also beside or beneath the nails, or, less often, on the pulp of the digits (Fig. 19-46). They are distinctively dome-shaped and much bulkier beneath the surface than they appear. Myrmecia are caused by HPV-1. They can be mistaken for a paronychia or digital mucinous cyst.

HPV-60 causes a peculiar type of plantar wart called a ridged wart because of the persistence of the dermatoglyphics across the surface of the lesion. Typically, the warts are slightly elevated, skin-colored, 3–5 mm papules. They occur on non-weight-bearing areas and lack the typical features of plantar warts. HPV-60 also causes plantar verrucous cysts, 1.5–2 cm, epithelium-lined cysts on the plantar surface. These cysts tend to occur on weight-bearing areas, suggesting that HPV-infected epidermis is implanted into the dermis, forming the cyst. It is common to see ridged warts near plantar verrucous cysts.

Histologic features

Typical nongenital warts rarely require histologic confirmation. A biopsy may be useful in several settings, however. Histology can be used to distinguish warts from corns and other keratotic lesions that they resemble. This is enhanced by immunoperoxidase staining for HPV capsid antigen. Cytologic atypia and extension into the dermis suggest the diagnosis of an HPV-induced squamous cell carcinoma. There is a correlation between HPV type and the histologic features of the wart, allowing identification of the HPV types that cause specific lesions, a useful feature in the diagnosis of epidermodysplasia verruciformis, for example.

Treatment

The form of therapy used depends on the type of wart being treated, age of the patient, and previous therapies used and their success or failure. With any treatment modality at least 2 or 3 months of sustained management by that method is considered a reasonable therapeutic trial. Do not abandon any treatment too quickly. Since many nongenital warts will spontaneously regress, the treatment algorithm should allow for nonaggressive options and the patient should be offered the option of no treatment. Indications for treatment are pain, interference with function, social embarrassment, and risk of malignancy. Aims of therapy are:

1. to remove the wart
2. not to produce scarring
3. to induce lifelong immunity to prevent recurrence.

There are very few controlled studies on the treatment of cutaneous warts, so the evidence for all forms of treatment except cryotherapy is fair to poor.

Flat warts

Flat warts frequently undergo spontaneous remission, so therapy should be as mild as possible and potentially scarring therapies should be avoided. If lesions are few, light cryotherapy is a reasonable consideration. Topical salicylic acid products can also be used. Treatment with topical tretinoin once or twice a day, in the highest concentration tolerated to produce mild erythema of the warts without frank dermatitis, can be effective over several months. Tazarotene cream or gel may also be effective. Imiquimod 5% cream used up to once a day can be effective. If the warts fail to react initially to the imiquimod, tretinoin may be used in conjunction. Should this fail, 5-FU cream 5%, applied twice a day, may be very effective. Anthralin, although staining, could be similarly used for its irritant effect. For refractory lesions, laser therapy in very low fluences or photodynamic therapy might be considered before electrodesiccation because of the reduced risk of scarring. Ranitidine, 300 mg twice a day, cleared 56% of refractory flat warts in one study. Cimetidine alone or with levamisole may be considered. Topical immunotherapy with dinitrochlorobenzene (DNCB), squaric acid, or dyphencyprone, or intralesional Candida antigen injections, can be used on limited areas of flat warts. The induced dermatitis requires careful dose monitoring when treating facial lesions.

Common warts

Treatments for common warts involve two basic approaches: destruction of the wart and induction of local immune reactions (immunotherapy). Destructive methods are most commonly used as initial therapy by most practitioners. Cryotherapy is a reasonable first-line therapy for most common warts. The wart should be frozen adequately to produce a blister after 1 or 2 days. This correlates with a thaw time of 30–45 s for most common warts. A sustained 10 s freeze with a spray gun was found to be more effective than simply freezing to obtain a 2–3 mm halo around the wart. Aggressive cryotherapy can produce significant blistering and may be complicated by significant postprocedural pain for several days. Berth-Jones et al found that a single freeze–thaw cycle was as effective as two cycles. The ideal frequency of treatment is every 2 or 3 weeks, just as the old blister peels off. A spray device, while more costly, is quicker, and cannot spread infectious diseases (especially viral hepatitis) from one patient to the next. Children may be frightened by such a device, so a cotton-tipped swab is an option for them. Cryotherapy can be effective for periungual warts. Damage to the matrix is unusual or rare, since periungual warts usually affect the lateral nailfolds, not the proximal one. Complications of cryotherapy include hypopigmentation, uncommonly scarring, and rarely, damage to the digital nerve from freezing too deeply on the side of the digit. Patients with Fanconi anemia, cryoglobulinemia, poor peripheral circulation, and Raynaud may develop severe blisters when cryotherapy is used to treat their warts. Doughnut warts, with central clearing and an annular recurrence, may complicate cryotherapy.

Products containing salicylic acid with or without lactic acid are effective patient-applied treatments; these have an efficacy comparable to that of cryotherapy. After the wart-affected area is soaked in water for 5–10 min, the topical medication is applied, allowed to dry, and covered with a strip bandage for 24 h. This is repeated daily. The superficial keratinous debris may be removed by scraping with a table knife, pumice stone, or emery board.

A small amount of cantharone (0.7% cantharidin) is applied to the wart, allowed to dry, and covered for 24 h. A blister, similar to that produced by cryotherapy, develops in 24–72 h. These blisters may be as painful as or more painful than those following cryotherapy. Treatment is repeated every 2–3 weeks. Perhaps more than any other method, there is a tendency for cantharidin to produce doughnut warts, a round wart with a central clear zone at the site of the original wart. None the less, this agent is a very useful adjunct in the management of difficult-to-treat verrucas.

Simple occlusion with a relatively impermeable tape can be effective in eradicating warts. The key appears to be to keep the wart occluded as much of the time as possible. Duct tape, moleskin, or transparent tape (Blenderm) is a practical option. Fenestrated and semipermeable dressings have not been studied and may not be effective. This is a good initial option for children and others unwilling to have other forms of treatment. Unfortunately, in adults, the efficacy of duct tape for common warts is very low. Two months of treatment resolved common warts in only 20% of patients, and 75% of "resolved" warts recurred.

Bleomycin has high efficacy and is an important treatment for recalcitrant common warts. It is used at a concentration of 1 U/mL, which is injected into and immediately beneath the wart until it blanches. The multiple puncture technique of Shelley—delivering the medication into the wart by multiple punctures of the wart with a needle through a drop of bleomycin—may also be used, as may an air jet injector. For small warts (less than 5 mm), 0.1 mL is used; 0.2 mL is used for larger warts. The injection is painful enough to require local anesthesia in some patients. Pain can occur for up to 1 week. The wart becomes black, and the black eschar separates in 2–4 weeks. Treatment may be repeated every 3 weeks, but it is unusual for common warts to require more than one or two treatments. Scarring is rare. Response rates vary by location, but average 90% with two treatments for most common, nonplantar warts, even periungual ones. Treatment of finger warts with bleomycin may uncommonly be complicated by localized Raynaud phenomenon of treated fingers. Bleomycin treatment of digital warts may rarely result in digital necrosis and permanent nail dystrophy, so extreme caution should be used in treating warts around the nailfolds. Lymphangitis/cellulitis is a rare complication. In a patient receiving a total of 14 U for plantar warts, flagellate urticaria followed by characteristic bleomycin flagellate hyperpigmentation occurred.

Surgical ablation of warts can be effective treatment, but even complete destruction of a wart and the surrounding skin does not guarantee that the wart will not recur. Surgical methods should be reserved for warts that are refractory to more conservative approaches. Pulsed dye laser therapy appears to have similar efficacy to cryotherapy. With pulsed dye laser therapy less plume is produced than with CO_2 laser therapy. Depending on the fluences used, the treatment can be performed in two-thirds of patients without anesthesia, although some pain occurs. The energy setting is dependent on the particular device being used. The energy may be as low as 7 J/cm^2 for thinner lesions and up to 15 J/cm^2 for more hyperkeratotic ones. A short pulse duration (0.45 ms) is most effective. A 5 or 7 mm spot size is used and treatment is extended 2 mm beyond the visible wart. Immediately after treatment, the skin has a gray–black discoloration, which

evolves to an eschar over 10–14 days. Treatment is repeated every 2–4 weeks and up to five treatments may be required. In immunocompetent patients, response rates for refractory warts range from 70% to 90%. CO_2 laser destruction requires local anesthesia, causes scarring, and may lead to nail dystrophy. Its efficacy is between 56% and 81% in refractory warts. A potentially infectious plume is produced. Frequency-doubled Nd:YAG and 532 nm KTP lasers are also reported to be effective, but there is less evidence for their use. Photodynamic therapy with aminolevulinic acid 20%, using broad-band sources with variable intensities, produces a clearance rate of 40–75% for recalcitrant warts. Several treatments at 3 weekly intervals may be required. Significant pain can occur during treatment and lasts for up to 24 h, which limits its use in children.

Oral cimetidine, 30–40 mg/kg/day, has been anecdotally reported to lead to resolution of common warts, perhaps because of its immunomodulatory effects. When used as a single agent, however, in both children and adults, the efficacy is low (30%), comparable with a placebo. It may be beneficial as an adjunct to other methods, however, or for treatment of refractory warts. Oral zinc sulfate at a dose of 10 mg/kg, to a maximum of 600 mg per day, has been reported to clear 80% of warts in children and young adults in Iran. No recurrences were observed at 6 months. If other groups find this therapy efficacious, it might become a useful agent in wart therapy. There appear to be limited side effects. Heat treatment, either localized to the wart and delivered by radiofrequency or by application to the affected part by soaking it in a hot bath, has been reported to be effective. Treatment for 15 min at 43–50°C (107.6–122°F) to as short as 30 s at higher temperatures has been used. Extreme caution must be exercised to avoid scalding. Oral administration of acitretin or isotretinoin may also be used in refractory cases. Hypnotic suggestion and hypnoanalysis for warts have been reviewed by Shenefelt.

Immunotherapy with topical and intralesional agents has become a mainstay of wart therapy. The hope is that not only will the wart be eradicated, but the immune reaction induced in the wart may also lead to widespread and permanent immunity against warts. The commonly used agents are topical DNCB, squaric acid dibutyl ester, and diphencyprone, as well as intralesional Candida or mumps antigen. Patients may be initially sensitized at a distant site (usually the inner upper arm) with the topical agents, or the agent may be applied initially to the warts directly. Two treatment approaches are used and their efficacies have not been compared. Some practitioners apply topical agents in the office in higher concentrations (2–5%), but only every 2 weeks or so. Others give their patients take-home prescriptions to use on a daily basis, albeit at lower concentrations to start with (0.2–0.5%). In most cases the agents are dissolved in acetone. The treated wart should be kept covered for 24 h after application. If the reaction is overly severe, the strength of the application may be reduced. Wart tenderness may indicate the need to reduce treatment concentration. Warts may begin to resolve within a week or two, but on average, 2–3 months of treatment or more are required. For intralesional Candida antigen, treatments are repeated every 3–4 weeks. Overall cure rates for all three topical sensitizers and for intralesional antigen injection is 60–80%. Side effects of treatment include local pruritus, local pain, and a mild eczematous dermatitis. Intralesional Candida injections may be associated with IFN-mediated side effects such as swelling, fever, shaking chills, and a feeling of having "flu." This begins 6–8 hours after the treatment and resolves over 24–28 hours. Patients should be advised of these possible side effects. Most patients have no limitation of activities or function with topical immunotherapy. Scarring has not been reported.

The efficacy of imiquimod for common warts appears to be significantly less than cryotherapy or topical immunotherapy and it is considerably more expensive. The routine use of imiquimod in the treatment of common or plantar warts cannot be recommended. Topical cidofovir has been used in desperate situations, compounded in a 1–5% concentration applied directly to the wart on a daily basis. Local irritation and erosion may occur.

Plantar warts

In general, plantar warts are more refractory to any form of treatment than are common warts. Initial treatment usually involves daily application of salicylic acid in liquid, film, or plaster form after soaking. In failures, cryotherapy or cantharidin application may be attempted, alone or in combination. A second freeze–thaw cycle is beneficial when treating plantar warts with cryotherapy. Bleomycin injections, laser therapy, or topical immunotherapy, as discussed above, may be used in refractory cases. Surgical destruction with cautery or blunt dissection should be reserved for failures with nonscarring techniques, since a plantar scar may be persistently painful. CO_2 laser may also result in plantar scars. Photodynamic therapy may be effective in some cases. The optimum photosensitizing agent and light source are unknown.

Genital warts (external genital warts, EGW)

Genital warts are the most common STD. Among sexually active young adults in the US and Europe, infection rates as high as 50% in some cohorts have been found using sensitive PCR techniques. It is estimated that the lifetime risk for infection in sexually active young adults may be as high as 80%. The number of new cases of genital wart infection diagnosed in the US yearly may approach 1 million. In the vast majority of couples in whom one has evidence of HPV infection, the partner will be found to be concordantly infected. The risk of transmission is not known, however. A large portion of genital HPV infection is either subclinical or latent. Unfortunately, the infectivity of subclinical and latent infection is unknown. Subclinical and latent infection is probably responsible for most "recurrences" following treatment of genital warts. Since the methodology for determining HPV infection in males is less accurate and since women suffer the major complication of HPV infection—cervical cancer, virtually all data on HPV infection rates and epidemiology are derived from studies of women.

Genital HPV infection is closely linked with cancer of the cervix, glans penis, anus, vulvovaginal area, and periungual skin. Cancer occurs when there is integration of the HPV genome into the host DNA. In high-risk genital HPV types, E6 and E7 gene products bind to and inactivate p53 and retinoblastoma protein (pRb), respectively. This is felt to be important in relation to their ability to cause cancer. In most persons, genital HPV infection appears to be transient, lasting about 1–2 years, and results in no sequelae. In a small proportion (about 2% of immunocompetent persons), infection persists and in a small proportion of persons with persistent HPV infection cancer may develop (Fig. 19-47). Certain cofactors, such as the HPV type causing the infection, location of infection, cigarette smoking, uncircumcised status, and immunosuppressed status, are associated with progression to cancer. The transition zones of the cervix and anus are at highest risk for the development of cancer.

More than 30 HPV types are associated with genital warts. Patients are commonly infected with multiple HPV types. The HPV types producing genital infection are divided into two broad categories—those that produce benign lesions, or low-risk types (at least 12 types); and those associated with cancer, the so-called high-risk or oncogenic types (at least 15 types).

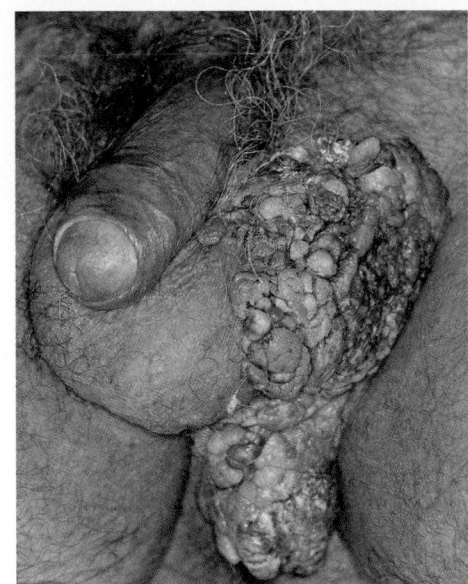

Fig. 19-47 Squamous cell carcinoma in persistent HPV infection.

The most common low-risk genital HPV types are HPV-6 and 11, and most HPV-induced genital dysplasias are caused by HPV-16 and 18. There is a strong correlation between the HPV type and the clinical appearance of HPV-induced genital lesions. Virtually all condylomata acuminata are caused by "benign" HPV-6 and 11. High-risk HPV-16 and 18 produce flat or sessile, often hyperpigmented lesions. For this reason, biopsy and HPV typing of EGW is rarely necessary.

Genital HPV infection is strongly associated with sexual intercourse. Female virgins rarely harbor HPV (about 1%). For women, insertive vaginal intercourse is strongly associated with acquiring genital HPV infection, with 50% of women testing positive for genital HPV within 5 years of the time of first sexual intercourse. However, sexual contact does not need to be penile–vaginal, as the risk of acquiring genital HPV infection was 10% in women who had nonpenetrative sexual exposure as compared to 1% of women who had no such exposure. Infection may occur at the introitus and then be spread to other sites by self-inoculation. Women who have sex with women may have genital HPV infection and still require regular gynecologic evaluations. Condom use may be partly, but not completely, protective for acquisition of genital HPV infection. In men the risk of genital HPV infection is associated with being uncircumcised, having had sex before age 17, having had more than six lifetime sexual partners, and having had sex with professional sex workers.

Condylomata acuminata

Condylomata on the skin surface appear as lobulated papules that average 2–5 mm in size, but they may range from microscopic to several centimeters in diameter and height. Lesions are frequently multifocal. Numerous genital warts may appear during pregnancy. Condylomata acuminata occur in men anywhere on the penis (Fig. 19-48) or about the anus. Scrotal condylomata occur in only 1% of immunocompetent male patients with warts (Fig. 19-49). Intraurethral condylomata may present with terminal hematuria, altered urinary stream, or urethral bleeding. In women, lesions appear on the mucosal surfaces of the vulva or cervix, on the perineum, or about the anus. Cauliflower-like masses may develop in moist, occluded areas such as the perianal skin, vulva, and inguinal folds. As a result of accumulation of purulent material in the clefts, these may be malodorous. Their color is generally gray, pale yellow, or pink. When perianal lesions occur, a prior history

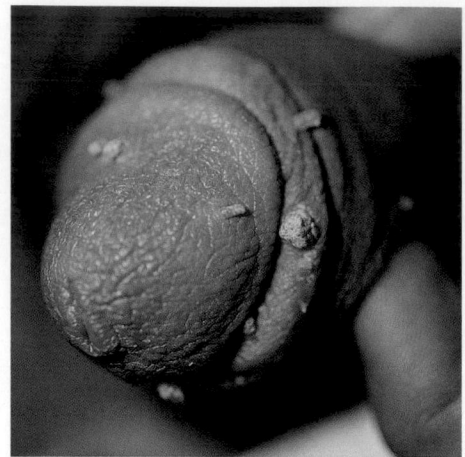

Fig. 19-48 Genital warts, keratotic type.

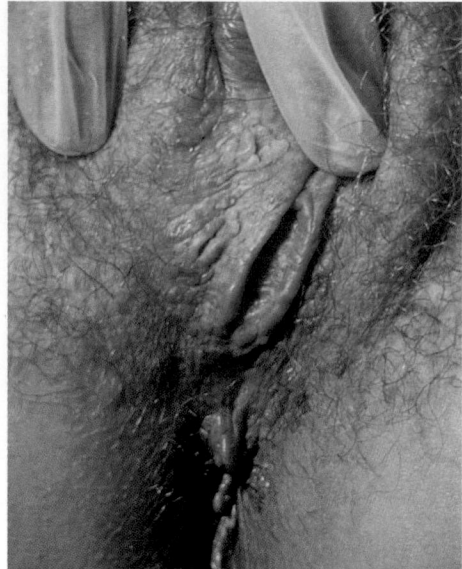

Fig. 19-50 Genital warts, bowenoid papulosis.

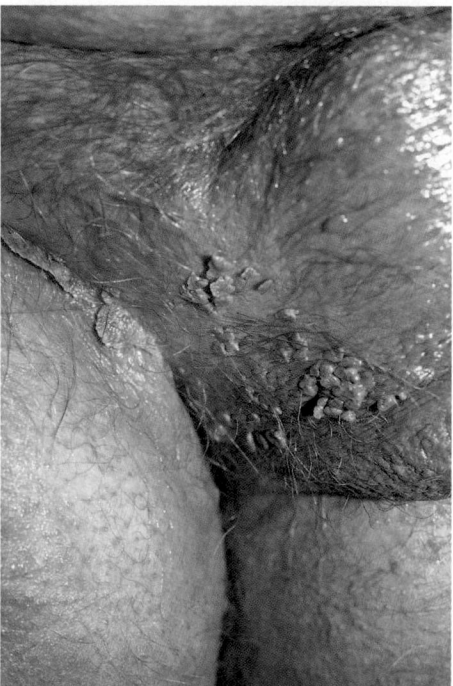

Fig. 19-49 Genital warts, condylomata acuminata.

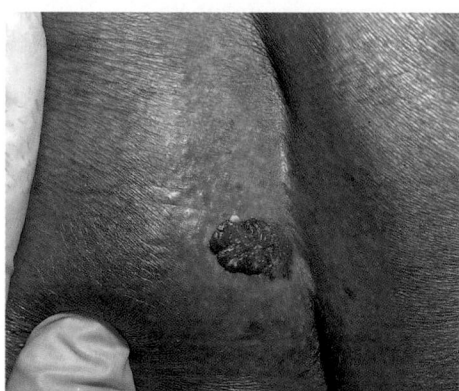

Fig. 19-51 Genital Bowen's disease.

of receptive anal intercourse will usually predict whether intra-anal warts are present and will help to determine the need for anoscopy. Immunosuppressed individuals and those with known high-risk HPV types should have routine anal pap smears to detect malignant change.

Genital warts are sexually transmitted and other STDs may be found in patients with genital warts. A complete history should be taken and the patient screened for other STDs as appropriate. Women with EGW should have a routine cervical cytologic screening to detect cervical dysplasia.

Bowenoid papulosis and HPV-induced genital dysplasias

Bowenoid papulosis is characterized by flat, often hyperpigmented papules a few millimeters to several centimeters in diameter. These occur singly or, more often, may be found in multiples on the penis, near the vulva, or perianally (Fig. 19-50). At times, similar lesions are seen outside the genital area in the absence of genital bowenoid papulosis. They occur most commonly on the neck or face and are more common in men. They contain HPV-16, 18, or other high-risk HPV types. Histologically, bowenoid papulosis demonstrates abnormal

epithelial maturation and cellular atypia closely resembling Bowen's disease. It is usually caused by HPV-16. On the glabrous external genitalia, bowenoid papulosis usually behaves similarly to other EGWs, but may progress to squamous cell carcinoma (SCC). On the glans penis of an uncircumcised male, and on the cervical, vaginal, or rectal mucosa, progression to invasive SCC is more likely (Fig. 19-51). Female partners of men with bowenoid papulosis and women with bowenoid papulosis have an increased risk of cervical dysplasia.

Giant condyloma acuminatum (Buschke–Lowenstein tumor)

Giant condyloma acuminatum is a rare, aggressive, wart-like growth that is a verrucous carcinoma. Unlike other HPV-induced genital carcinomas, this tumor is usually caused by HPV-6. It occurs most often on the glans or prepuce of an uncircumcised male; less often, it may occur on perianal skin or the vulva. Despite its bland histologic picture, it may invade deeply, and uncommonly it may metastasize to regional lymph nodes. Treatment is by complete surgical excision. Recurrence after radiation therapy may be associated with a more aggressive course.

Diagnosis

Even in women with confirmed cervical HPV infection, serologic tests are positive in only 50%, making serologic diagnosis of HPV infection of no use to the practicing clinician. HPV cannot be cultured. HPV typing via in situ hybridization or

PCR is useful in managing HPV infection of the cervix and in some cases of prepubertal HPV infection, but not in the management of EGW. Virtually all condylomata can be diagnosed by inspection. Bright lighting and magnification should be used when examining for genital HPV infection. Flat, sessile, and pigmented lesions are suggestive of bowenoid papulosis and may require a biopsy. Subclinical and latent infections are no longer sought or investigated because they are very common and there is no management strategy known to eradicate these forms of HPV infection. Soaking with acetic acid is not generally necessary, but may be helpful to detect early lesions under the foreskin. In patients with multiple recurrences, acetic acid soaking may determine the extent of infection, helping to define the area for application of topical therapies. The procedure is performed by soaking the external genitalia in men and the vagina and cervix in women with 3–5% acetic acid for up to 10 min. Genital warts turn white (acetowhitening), making them easily identifiable. Any process that alters the epidermal barrier will be acetowhite, however (dermatitis, for example), so only typical acetowhite lesions should be treated as warts. In atypical cases, a 2-week trial is attempted with a 1% hydrocortisone preparation plus a topical anticandidal imidazole cream. If the acetowhitening persists, a biopsy is performed and histologic evidence of HPV infection sought. Immunoperoxidase or in situ hybridization methods may aid in evaluation. PCR should probably not be performed on such biopsied specimens, except possibly in childhood cases. The high background rate of latent infection (up to 50%) makes interpretation of a positive PCR impossible. In contrast, chromogenic in situ hybridization clearing demonstrates the localization of positive nuclei within the lesion.

Treatment

Because no effective virus-specific agent exists for the treatment of genital warts, their recurrence is frequent. Treatment is not proven to reduce transmission to sexual partners or to prevent progression to dysplasia or cancer. Specifically, the treatment of male sexual partners of women with genital warts does not reduce the recurrence rate of warts in these women. Therefore, the goals of treatment must first be discussed with the patient, and perhaps with his/her sexual partner. Observation represents an acceptable option for some patients with typical condylomata acuminata. In some patients, only wart-free periods are achieved. As genital warts may cause discomfort, genital pruritus, malodor, bleeding, and substantial emotional distress, treatment is indicated if the patient desires it. Bleeding genital warts may increase the sexual transmission of HIV and hepatitis B and C. Bowenoid papulosis may be treated as discussed below when it occurs on the external genitalia. Lesions with atypical histology (squamous intraepithelial lesion) on mucosal surfaces and periungually are special cases and treatment must be associated with histologic confirmation of eradication in cases where topical methods are used.

The treatment chosen is in part dictated by the size of the warts and their location. The number of EGWs at the time of initial evaluation is strongly predictive of wart clearance. Patients with four or fewer EGWs will be clear with three or fewer treatments, whereas only 50% of patients with ten or more EGWs will be clear after three treatments. Only 1% of patients with 1–4 EGWs will still have lesions after eight treatments, but 20% of patients with ten or more EGWs will still have lesions after eight treatments. A more effective or aggressive treatment approach might be considered in patients with high numbers of EGWs.

Podophyllin is more effective in treating warts on occluded or moist surfaces, such as on the mucosa or under the prepuce.

It is available as a crude extract, usually in 25% concentration in tincture of benzoin. It is applied weekly by the physician and can be washed off 4–8 h later by the patient, depending on the severity of the reaction. After six consecutive weekly treatments, approximately 40% of patients are free of warts and 17% are free of warts at 3 months after treatment. Purified podophyllotoxin 0.5% solution or gel is applied by the patient twice a day for 3 consecutive days of each week in 4- to 6-week treatment cycles. Efficacy approaches 60% for typical condylomata and side effects are fewer than with standard, physician-applied podophyllin preparations. Therefore, whenever possible, podophyllotoxin should be used instead of classic podophyllin solutions.

Imiquimod, an immune response modifier that induces IFN locally at the site of application, has an efficacy similar to cryotherapy (about 50%) and yields a low recurrence rate (22%). It is available in a 250 mg sachet containing a 5% cream formulation. One sachet can cover up to 350 cm² when applied appropriately, allowing for several treatments with a single sachet if the treatment area is limited. It is more effective than podophyllotoxin in treating women with EGW, but only equally or slightly less effective in men, especially for warts on the penile shaft. Imiquimod is less effective than cryotherapy in the treatment of EGW. Therapeutic response to imiquimod is slow, requiring 10 or more weeks in some patients to see any effect. It is patient-applied, once a day for 3 alternate days per week (usually Monday, Wednesday, and Friday). Treatment results in mild to moderate irritation (less than with podophyllin or cryotherapy in men, but with a similar side-effect profile in women). Rare complications include flaring of psoriasis and psoriatic arthritis, vitiligo-like hypopigmentation, and the production of a local neuropathy. Imiquimod should be used cautiously in persons with psoriasis. Neuropathy is associated with application of excessive amounts, occlusion of the medication, and application to an eroded mucosa.

Imiquimod may be used to treat penile condyloma in circumcised and uncircumcised men, anal and perianal condyloma, and vulvar condyloma. It may be used as the initial treatment or in cases in which recurrence has been frequent after other forms of treatment were attempted. Several trials have demonstrated that the use of imiquimod following electrosurgical destruction of warts results in a significant reduction in recurrences (20% vs 65% in one study and 8% vs 25% in another). While the percentage of recurrences differed significantly in these studies, the imiquimod-treated patients in both studies had a 3–4-fold reduction in wart recurrence. The use of imiquimod following surgical destruction of condyloma should be considered in all immunocompetent patients, especially those who have had recurrence after a previous surgical procedure. It is unclear whether the imiquimod should be started before the surgical procedure or after healing of the surgical procedure. The duration of continued imiquimod therapy after ablation is also unknown, but since most recurrences occur during the first 3–6 months, 3 months of therapy would be reasonable. Application of imiquimod three times weekly following surgery may be more effective than use only twice weekly, although these two approaches have not been compared head to head. Suppositories containing about 5 mg of imiquimod appear to reduce the risk of recurrence of anal condyloma in immunocompetent men after surgical ablation of extensive anal disease. Imiquimod has been effective in the treatment of bowenoid papulosis in scattered case reports.

The topical application of green tea extract containing sinecatechins (Polyphenon E or Veregen) can be effective in treating EGW. A 15% ointment applied three times daily leads to EGW clearance in 60% of women and 45% of men. The average time to complete clearance is 16 weeks. Erythema and erosions at the application site occur in 50% of patients.

Bichloroacetic or trichloroacetic acid (TCA) 35–85% can be applied to condylomata weekly or biweekly. TCA is safe for use in pregnant patients. When compared with cryotherapy, TCA has the same or lower efficacy and causes more ulcerations and pain. It is not generally recommended for EGW, as other available treatments are more effective and cause less morbidity.

Cryotherapy with liquid nitrogen is more effective than podophyllin and imiquimod, approaching 70–80% resolution during treatment and 55% 3 months after treatment. One or two freeze–thaw cycles are applied to each wart every 1–3 weeks. A zone of 2 mm beyond the lesion is frozen. Cryotherapy is effective in dry as well as moist areas. Perianal lesions are more difficult to eradicate than other genital sites and two freeze–thaw cycles are recommended in this location. Cryotherapy is safe to use in pregnant patients. EMLA cream with or without subsequent lidocaine infiltration may be beneficial in reducing the pain of cryotherapy. The addition of podophyllin to cryotherapy does not result in statistically better results after 2 months of therapy and cannot be recommended as standard treatment.

Electrofulguration or electrocauterization with or without snip removal of the condyloma is more effective than TCA, cryotherapy, imiquimod, or podophyllin. Wart clearance during therapy is nearly 95% and wart cure at 3 months exceeds 70%. Local anesthesia is required and scarring may occur. Surgical removal is ideal for large exophytic warts that might require multiple treatments with other methods. It has high acceptance in patients who have had recurrences from other methods because results are immediate and cure rates higher.

The use of CO_2 laser in the treatment of genital warts has not been demonstrated to be more effective than simpler surgical methods. Although visible warts are eradicated by the laser, HPV DNA can still be detected at the previous site of the wart. The CO_2 laser has the advantage of being bloodless, but it is costlier and requires more technical skill on the part of the surgeon to avoid complications. It should be reserved for treatment of extensive lesions in which more cost-effective methods have been attempted and failed. Adjunctive photodynamic therapy does not prevent recurrence of EGW after CO_2 laser ablation. When compared to CO_2 laser ablation of EGWs, ALA-PDT demonstrated higher efficacy, fewer recurrences, and was less painful. ALA-PDT response rate is about 75%.

Any surgical method that generates a smoke plume is potentially infectious to the surgeon. HPV DNA is detected in the plumes generated during CO_2 laser or electrocoagulation treatment of genital warts. The laser-generated plume results in longer-duration HPV aerosol contamination and wider spread of detectable HPV DNA. If these methods of wart treatment are used, an approved face mask should be worn, a smoke evacuator should be operated at the surgical site during the procedure to remove the plume, and decontamination of the equipment after the surgery should be carried out.

5-FU 5% cream applied twice a day may be effective, especially in the treatment of flat, hyperpigmented lesions, such as those in bowenoid papulosis. Care must be taken to avoid application to the scrotum, as scrotal skin is prone to painful erosions. Twice-a-day instillation of 5-FU into the urethra can be used to treat intraurethral condylomata. The cone from a tube of Xylocaine jelly will fit on to the thread of the 5-FU tube, or the cream may be instilled with a syringe. It is typically left in place for 1 h before the patient voids. Care should be taken that drips of urine containing the medication do not contact the scrotum. 5-FU may also be used to treat intravaginal warts by instillation in the vagina, but is often associated with severe irritation. Intermittent therapy (twice a week for 10 weeks) is better tolerated than daily therapy. 5-FU is not commonly recommended for the treatment of typical EGWs because other methods of treatment are available.

The efficacy of systemic and intralesional IFN-α therapy has been found to be relatively low in eradicating genital warts. Intralesional therapy eradicates 40–60% of warts and systemic IFN treatment will eradicate warts in only about 20% of patients. IFN treatment of genital warts in patients with AIDS has even lower efficacy rates. Response rates to IFN have never reached the levels achieved with electrosurgical methods. Because of the high cost, frequent side effects, and low efficacy associated with IFN therapy, the CDC no longer recommends the use of IFN for the treatment of genital warts.

Human papillomavirus vaccination

HPV virus-like particles (VLPs) composed of spontaneous assembling L1 molecules have been used to develop a polyvalent vaccine against HPV 6, 11, 16, and 18. This vaccine is highly effective and is now approved in more than 100 countries for the immunization of prepubertal girls. In older women (age 24–45) the vaccine is also effective and may be given as a "catch-up" vaccine in women with no evidence of prior genital HPV infection with these HPV types. The protection was type-specific and did not prevent squamous intraepithelial lesions from other HPV types. Since HPV-16 and 18 are the primary HPV types associated with cervical cancer, it is hoped that the rate of cancers induced by these high-risk genital HPV types can be reduced by vaccination.

Genital warts in children

Children can acquire genital warts through vertical transmission perinatally, and through digital inoculation or autoinoculation, fomite or social nonsexual contact, and sexual abuse. HPV typing has demonstrated that most warts in the genital area of children are "genital" HPV types, and most children with genital warts have family members with a genital HPV infection.

HPV typing can be performed; however, the presence of genital types of HPV does not prove abuse and a finding of a nongenital HPV type does not exclude the possibility of sexual abuse. In children younger than 1 year of age, vertical transmission is possible and is probably the most common means of acquisition. The risk for sexual abuse is highest in children older than 3 years of age. When abuse is suspected, children should be referred to child protection services if the practitioner is not skilled in evaluating children for sexual abuse. Children between 1 and 3 years of age are primarily nonverbal and are difficult to evaluate. Management of such patients is on a case-by-case basis. Other STDs should be screened for in children who have a genital HPV infection. Usually, the management of children with anogenital warts (Fig. 19-52) requires a multidisciplinary team that should include a pediatrician. Genital warts in children often spontaneously resolve (75%), so nonintervention may be a reasonable consideration. Genital warts in children usually respond quickly to topical therapy, such as podophyllotoxin, imiquimod, or light cryotherapy. In refractory cases, surgical removal or electrocautery may be used. The use of a topical anesthetic is recommended before treatment.

Recurrent respiratory (laryngeal) papillomatosis

HPV-associated papillomas may occur throughout the respiratory tract, from the nose to the lungs. Recurrent respiratory papillomatosis has a bimodal distribution—in children under 5, and after the age of 15. Affected young children are born to mothers with genital condylomata and they present with hoarseness. The HPV types found in these lesions, HPV-6 and 11, are the types seen in genital condylomata. Treatment is with CO_2 laser surgery and IFN. Carcinoma that is often fatal

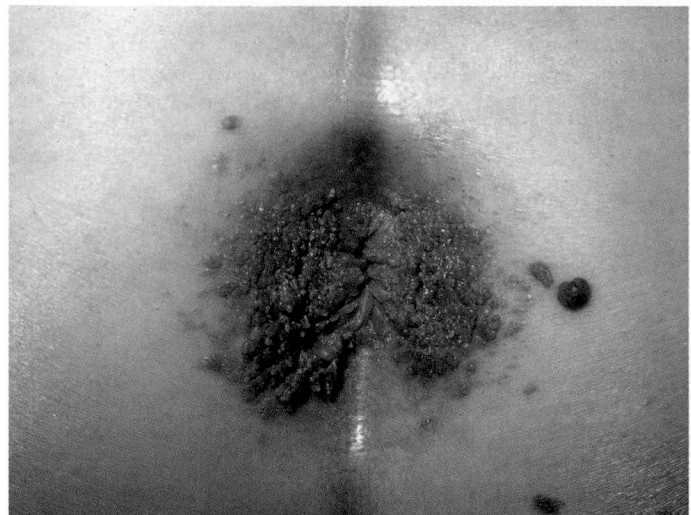

Fig. 19-52 Perianal warts in an 18-month-old child.

develops in 14% of patients, even in young children. The incidence of carcinoma is higher in those treated with radiation therapy.

Heck's disease

Small white to pinkish papules occur diffusely in the oral cavity in this disease, also known as focal epithelial hyperplasia. It occurs most commonly in Native Americans, in Greenland, and in Turkey. HPV-13, 24, and 32 have been associated. Lesions may spontaneously resolve. Treatment options include cryosurgery, CO_2 laser, electrosurgery, and topical (β), intralesional, and systemic IFN.

Epidermodysplasia verruciformis

Epidermodysplasia verruciformis (EV) is a rare, inherited disorder characterized by widespread HPV infection and cutaneous SCCs. Virtually always, it is inherited as an autosomal-recessive trait, although one well-documented kindred demonstrates an X-linked inheritance. About 10% of EV patients are products of consanguineous marriages. HPV types associated with this syndrome include those infecting normal hosts, such as HPV-3 and 10, as well as many "unique" HPV types. These HPV types, now numbering 19, are called EV HPVs and include HPV-5, 8, 9, 12, 14, 15, 17, 19 through 25, and 36 through 38. The genetic mutations causing EV are found in two closely linked genes, *EVER1* and *EVER2*. Seventy-five percent of all EV cases worldwide have homozygous invalidating mutations in one of these two genes. The *EVER* genes are transmembrane channel-like genes, so *EVER1* is also *TMC-6* and *EVER2* is also *TMC-8*. The functions of these genes and how they cause this syndrome are unknown.

The condition presents in childhood and continues throughout life. Skin lesions include flat wart-like lesions of the dorsal hands, extremities, face, and neck. They appear in childhood or young adulthood, apparently earlier in sunnier climates. The characteristic lesions are flatter than typical flat warts and may be quite abundant, growing to confluence (Fig. 19-53). Typical HPV 3- and 10-induced flat warts may be admixed. In addition, on the trunk are lesions that are red, tan, or brown patches/plaques or hypopigmented, very slightly scaly plaques resembling tinea versicolor. Plaques on the elbows may resemble psoriasis. Seborrheic keratosis-like lesions may also be seen on the forehead, neck, and trunk. Common warts are reported to be uncommon in some EV cohorts. In other EV patients, typical common warts of the hands and feet may be

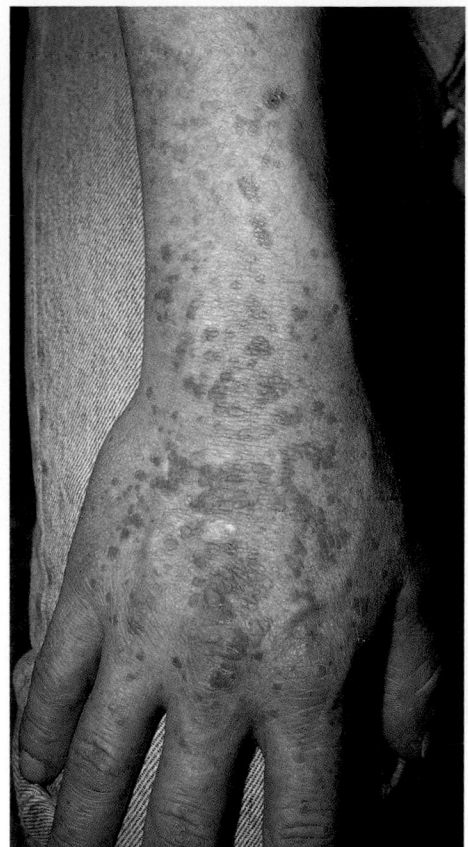

Fig. 19-53 Epidermodysplasia verruciformis.

present also. Some patients with extensive (more than 100) common and plantar warts that never resolve and simply grow to confluence have been called "generalized verrucosis." These patients do not develop skin cancers and live into adulthood. There are reports of patients with generalized verrucosis who also are infected with EV HPV types, suggesting a common pathogenesis. The genetic basis of generalized verrucosis is unknown.

The histologic features of an EV-specific HPV infection are very characteristic. The cells of the upper epidermis have a clear, smoky, or light-blue pale cytoplasm and a central pyknotic nucleus.

SCCs develop in about one-third of EV patients, an average of 24 years after the appearance of the characteristic EV skin lesions. Most often, skin cancers appear on sun-exposed surfaces, but they can appear on any part of the body. They begin to appear at the age of 20–40, again earlier in patients living in regions with high sun exposure. Skin cancers are less common in African patients, suggesting a protective effect of skin pigmentation. HPV-5, 8, and 47 are found in more than 90% of EV skin cancers. The SCCs may appear de novo, but usually appear on the background of numerous actinic keratoses and lesions of Bowen's disease (Fig. 19-54). Surgical treatment is recommended. Radiation therapy is contraindicated. If skin grafting is required, the grafts should be taken from sun-protected skin, such as the buttocks or inner upper arm.

Aside from surgical intervention for skin cancer, treatment for EV consists largely of preventive measures. Strict sun avoidance and protection should be started as soon as the syndrome is diagnosed. An approach similar to that for children with xeroderma pigmentosa could be instituted. ALA-PDT, topical 5-FU, imiquimod, cimetidine, systemic interferons, and oral retinoids may all have a place in managing patients with EV.

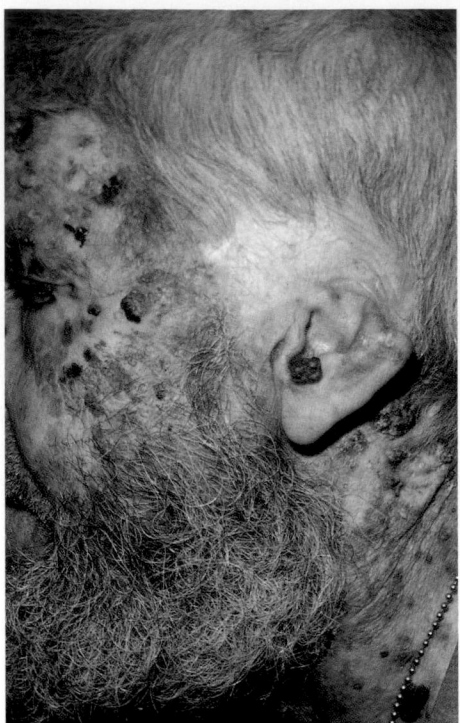

Fig. 19-54 Multiple SCCs in epidermodysplasia verruciformis.

The mechanism by which cancer occurs in patients with EV is unclear. HPV-5 proteins do not bind to p53 or pRb. The p53 mutations present in the SCCs of patients with EV are characteristic of those induced by UVB, confirming the close association of UV exposure and the development of cancer in patients with EV. EV HPV DNA has been reported to be found in a large percentage (35%) of the general population in very low copy number. EV HPV DNA is reported to be present on the skin in up to 80% of patients with psoriasis. EV HPV is not universally present in the skin cancers of EV patients, but is usually present in the precancerous lesions (AKs and SCC in situ). This suggests that EV HPV may be required only in early phases of carcinogenesis and therefore may not be found in well-developed SCCs.

Infection with EV HPV types has been reported in the immunosuppressed, especially those with HIV. Typical flat scaly lesions resembling tinea versicolor are most common. SCC has not been reported in these patients.

Immunosuppressed patients

Patients with defects in their cell-mediated immunity may have an increased frequency of HPV infection. Predisposing conditions include organ transplantation, immunosuppressive medications, congenital immunodeficiency diseases, lymphoma, and HIV infection.

Organ transplant recipients begin to develop warts soon after transplantation and by 5 years up to 90% of transplant patients have warts. Initially, these are common and plantar warts, but later numerous flat warts appear, particularly in sun-exposed areas. Depending on the background level of UV radiation, the lifetime risk for cutaneous carcinomas may exceed 40%. Skin cancers begin to appear 4 years or more after transplantation, occur in sun-exposed sites, and are more common in persons with skin types I and II. The duration and intensity of immunosuppression appear more important in causing the skin cancers than are the specific immunosuppressive agents used. The use of Voriconazole as prophylaxis or treatment for aspergillus infection may lead to accelerated development of skin cancers, especially squamous cell carci-

nomas and melanoma. Malignant lesions may resemble Bowen's disease, keratoacanthomas, SCCs, or warts. Genital warts are also increased and, especially in women, genital dysplasias are more frequent. The presence of keratotic lesions of any type on the skin is a strong predictor for the development of nonmelanoma skin cancer (NMSC) in organ transplant patients. The skin of organ transplant patients should be examined closely, and once skin cancers begin to appear, regular dermatologic examinations should be performed. It is especially important in immunosuppressed patients to monitor the genital and anal areas regularly for changing lesions and to have a low threshold for performing a biopsy.

In HIV disease, common, plantar, flat, oral and genital warts are all very common. Warty keratoses at the angle of the mouth, often bilateral, are a characteristic, and perhaps unique, manifestation of HPV infection in patients with AIDS. The warts are caused predominantly by HPV-2, 27, and 57. HPV-7 can be found in cutaneous, oral, and perioral warts in non-butchers with HIV infection. HPV-6 may be found in common warts. Genital warts are increased 15-fold among HIV-infected women. Fifty percent or more of HIV-infected MSM have evidence of anal HPV infection. Genital neoplasia associated with HPV-16 and 18 occurs much more frequently in HIV-infected women and MSM. Uncommonly, HIV-infected patients develop HPV 5- and 8-induced EV-like lesions. Although nongenital skin cancers are also common in some fair-skinned HIV-infected patients, HPV has not been demonstrated in the nongenital SCCs of these patients. With HAART therapy, warts may disappear. Paradoxically, increased rates of genital and oral warts are seen in HIV-infected persons with adequate control of their HIV infection. The likelihood of clearance of common warts in persons with HIV is related to the nadir of their helper T-cell count. HIV-infected persons whose helper T-cell count never falls below 200 are more likely to have sustained remission of their warts.

The treatment of warts in immunosuppressed hosts is very difficult. Although standard methods are used, their efficacy may be reduced. Imiquimod has low efficacy in this setting, but can be attempted. The addition of a second modality (podophyllin, 5% 5-FU, or surgery) to the imiquimod treatment may lead to improvement. Topical cidofovir (in concentrations from 1% to 5%) and intralesional cidofovir (7.5 mg/mL) have been effective in refractory anogenital and common warts in immunodeficient patients. Topical cidofovir is very expensive, is irritating, and can cause skin erosion and ulceration. Addition of sirolimus to the immunosuppressive regimen may be associated with decrease in the number of warts in organ transplant patients. Oral retinoids can be effective in reducing the rate of appearance of SCCs in organ transplant patients. In organ transplant patients with widespread actinic damage and many precancerous lesions, photodynamic therapy can be considered.

Abess A, et al: Flagellate hyperpigmentation following intralesional bleomycin treatment of verruca plantaris. Arch Dermatol 2003; 139:337.

Ahmed I, et al: Liquid nitrogen cryotherapy of common warts: cryospray vs. cotton wool bud. Br J Dermatol 2001; 144:1006.

Ashida M, et al: Protean manifestations of human papillomavirus type 60 infection on the extremities. Br J Dermatol 2002; 146:885.

Baron JM, et al: HPV 18-induced pigmented bowenoid papulosis of the neck. J Am Acad Dermatol 1999; 40:633.

Benson E: Imiquimod: potential risk of an immunostimulant. Australas J Dermatol 2004; 45:123.

Bleeker MCG, et al: Penile lesions and human papillomavirus in male sexual partners of women with cervical intraepithelial neoplasia. J Am Acad Dermatol 2002; 47:351.

Bonnez W: A comment on "Butcher's warts: dermatological heritage or testable misinformation?" Arch Dermatol 2002; 138:411.

Bouwes Bavinck JN, et al: Keratotic skin lesions and other risk factors are associated with skin cancer in organ-transplant recipients: a case-control study in the Netherlands, United Kingdom, Germany, France, and Italy. J Invest Dermatol 2007; 127:1647.

Brown T, et al: Vitiligo-like hypopigmentation associated with imiquimod treatment of genital warts. J Am Acad Dermatol 2005; 52:715.

Carrasco D, et al: Treatment of anogenital warts with imiquimod 5% cream followed by surgical excision of residual lesions. J Am Acad Dermatol 2002; 47:S212.

Castellsague X, et al: Male circumcision, penile human papillomavirus infection, and cervical cancer in female partners. N Engl J Med 2002; 346:1105.

Chen K, et al: Comparative study of photodynamic therapy vs CO_2 laser vaporization in treatment of condylomata acuminata, a randomized clinical trial. Br J Dermatol 2007; 156:516.

Chen S, et al: New therapies from old medicines. Nat Biotech 2008; 26:1077.

Ciconte A, et al: Warts are not merely blemishes on the skin: a study on the morbidity associated with having viral cutaneous warts. Australas J Dermatol 2003; 44:169.

Connolly M, et al: Cryotherapy of viral warts: a sustained 10-s freeze is more effective than the traditional method. Br J Dermatol 2001; 145:554.

Cowen EW, et al: Chronic phototoxicity and aggressive squamous cell carcinoma of the skin in children and adults during treatment with voriconazole. J Am Acad Dermatol 2010; 62:31.

Descamps V, et al: Topical cidofovir for bowenoid papulosis in an HIV-infected patient. Br J Dermatol 2001; 144:642.

Dharancy S, et al: Conversion to sirolimus: a useful strategy for recalcitrant cutaneous viral warts in liver transplant recipients. Liver Transp 2006; 12:1883.

Dicle O, et al: Choice of immunosuppressants and the risk of warts in renal transplant recipients. Acta Derm Venereol 2008; 88:294.

Durani BK, Jappe U: Successful treatment of facial plane warts with imiquimod. Br J Dermatol 2002; 147:1018.

Frazer IH: Interaction of human papillomaviruses with the host immune system: a well evolved relationship. Virol 2009; 384:410.

Garden JM, et al: Viral disease transmitted by laser-generated plume (Aerosol). Arch Dermatol 2002; 138:1303.

Gewirtzman A, et al: Epidermodysplasia verruciformis and human papilloma virus. Curr Opin Infect Dis 2008; 21:141.

Gibbs S: Topical immunotherapy with contact sensitizers for viral warts. Br J Dermatol 2002; 146:705.

Gibbs S, Harvey I: Topical treatments for cutaneous warts. Cochrane Database Syst Rev 2006; 19:3:CD001781.

Godfrey JC, et al: Successful treatment of bowenoid papulosis in a 9-year-old girl with vertically acquired human immunodeficiency virus. Pediatrics 2003; 112:e73.

Gross G, et al: A randomized, double-blind, four-arm parallel-group, placebo-controlled phase II/III study to investigate the clinical efficacy of two galenic formulations of Polyphenon® E in the treatment of external genital warts. J Eur Acad Dermatol Venereol 2007; 21:1404.

Guill CK, et al: Asymptomatic labial papules in a teenager. Arch Dermatol 2002; 138:1509.

Gul U, et al: Clinical aspects of epidermodysplasia verruciformis and review of the literature. Int J Dermatol 2007; 46:1069.

Hancox JG, et al: Hemorrhagic bullae after cryosurgery in a patient with hemophilia A. Dermatol Surg 2003; 29:1084.

Hivnor C, et al: Intravenous cidofovir for recalcitrant verruca vulgaris in the setting of HIV. Arch Dermatol 2004; 140:13.

Horn TD, et al: Intralesional immunotherapy of warts with mumps, candida and Trichophyton skin test antigens: a single-blinded, randomized and controlled trial. Arch Dermatol 2005; 141:589.

Hu E, Goldie S: The economic burden of noncervical human papillomavirus disease in the United States. Am J Obstet Gynecol 2008; 198:500.e1.

Jones JM, et al: A new and effective delivery system of bleomycin for the treatment of recalcitrant warts. J Am Acad Dermatol 2004; 50:P414.

Karaman G, et al: Ranitidine therapy for recalcitrant warts in adults: a preliminary study. J Eur Acad Dermatol Venereol 2001; 15:486.

Kaspari M, et al: Application of imiquimod by suppositories (anal tampons) efficiently prevents recurrences after ablation of anal canal condyloma. Br J Dermatol 2002; 147:757.

Kennedy CM, Boardman LA: New approaches to external genital warts and vulvar intraepithelial neoplasia. Clin Obstet Gynecol 2008; 51:518.

Kreuter A, et al: A human papillomavirus-associated disease with disseminated warts, depressed cell-mediated immunity, primary lymphedema and anogenital dysplasia. Arch Dermatol 2008; 144(3):366.

Lazarczyk M, et al: The EVER proteins as a natural barrier against papillomaviruses: a new insight into the pathogenesis of human papillomavirus infections. Microbiol Mol Biol Rev 2009; 73:348.

Lee SH, et al: Plantar warts of defined aetiology in adults and unresponsiveness to low dose cimetidine. Australas J Dermatol 2001; 42:220.

Longstaff E, von Krogh G: Condyloma eradication: self-therapy with 0.15–10.5% podophyllotoxin versus 20–25% podophyllin preparations: an integrated safety assessment. Regul Toxicol Pharmacol 2001; 33:117.

Loo WJ, Holt PJA: Bowenoid papulosis successfully treated with imiquimod. J Eur Acad Dermatol Venereol 2003; 17:363.

Majewski S, Jablonska S: Human papillomavirus type 7 and butcher's warts. Arch Dermatol 2001; 137:1655.

Majewski S, Jablonska S: Do epidermodysplasia verruciformis human papillomaviruses contribute to malignant and benign epidermal proliferations? Arch Dermatol 2002; 138:649.

Majewski S, et al: Imiquimod is highly effective for extensive, hyperproliferative condyloma in children. Pediatr Dermatol 2003; 20:440.

Mammas IN, et al: Human papilloma virus (HPV) infection in children and adolescents. Eur J Pediatr 2009; 168:267.

Martinelli C, et al: Resolution of recurrent perianal condylomata acuminata by topical cidofovir in patients with HIV infection. J Eur Acad Dermatol Venereol 2001; 15:568.

McCown H, et al: Global nail dystrophy associated with human papillomavirus type 57 infection. Br J Dermatol 1999; 141:731.

Micali G, et al: Treatment of cutaneous warts with squaric acid dibutylester: a decade of experience. Arch Dermatol 2000; 136:557.

Miller D, et al: Melanoma associated with long-term voriconazole therapy. Arch Dermatol 2010; 146(3):300.

Mizuki D, et al: Successful treatment of topical photodynamic therapy using 5-aminolevulinic acid for plane warts. Br J Dermatol 2003; 149:1087.

Moresi JM, et al: Treatment of anogenital warts in children with topical 0.05% podofilox gel and 5% imiquimod cream. Pediatr Dermatol 2001; 18:448.

Munoz G, et al: Safety, immunogenicity, and efficacy of quadrivalent human papillomavirus (types 6, 11, 16, 18) recombinant vaccine in women aged 24–45 years: a randomised, double-blind trial. Lancet 2009; 373:1949.

Nucci V, et al: Condyloma acuminatum of the tongue treated with photodynamic therapy. Clin Infec Dis 2009; 48:1330.

Orth G: Genetics of epidermodysplasia verruciformis: insights into host defense against papillomaviruses. Sem in Immunol 2006; 18:362.

Paraskevas KI, et al: Surgical management of giant condyloma acuminatum (Buschke–Lowenstein tumor) of the perianal region. Dermatol Surg 2007; 33:638.

Parsad D, et al: Cimetidine and levamisole versus cimetidine alone for recalcitrant warts in children. Pediatr Dermatol 2001; 18:349.

Pehoushek J, Smithe KJ: Imiquimod and 5% fluorouracil therapy for anal and perianal squamous cell carcinoma in situ in an HIV-1-positive man. Arch Dermatol 2001; 137:14.

Peterson CL, et al: Hand warts successfully treated with topical 5-aminolevulinic acid and intense pulsed light. Eur J Dermatol 2008; 18:207.

Petrow W, et al: Successful topical immunotherapy of bowenoid papulosis with imiquimod. Br J Dermatol 2001; 145:1022.

Robson KJ, et al: Pulsed-dye laser versus conventional therapy in the treatment of warts: a prospective randomized trial. J Am Acad Dermatol 2000; 43:275.

Rogers HD, et al: Acquired epidermodysplasia verruciformis. J Amer Acad Dermatol 2009; 60:315.

Schiffman M, Kjaer SK: Chapter 2: natural history of anogenital human papillomavirus infection and neoplasia. J Natl Cancer Inst Monogr 2003; 31:14.

Shenefelt PD: Biofeedback, cognitive-behavioral methods, and hypnosis in dermatology: is it all in your mind? Dermatol Ther 2003; 16:114.

Sherrard J, Riddell L: Comparison of the effectiveness of commonly used clinic-based treatments for external genital warts. Int J STD AIDS 2007; 18:365.

Shofer H, et al: Randomized, comparative trial on the sustained efficacy of topical imiquimod 5% cream versus conventional ablative methods in external anogenital warts. Eur J Dermatol 2006; 16:642.

Stefanaki C, et al: Comparison of cryotherapy to imiquimod 5% in the treatment of anogenital warts. Int J STD AIDS 2008; 19:441.

Steinhoff M, et al: Successful topical treatment of focal epithelial hyperplasia (Heck's disease) with interferon-β. Br J Dermatol 2001; 144:1067.

Sterling JC, et al: Guidelines for the management of cutaneous warts. Br J Dermatol 2001; 144:4.

Stockfleth E, et al: Topical Polyphenon E® in the treatment of external genital and perianal warts: a randomized controlled trial. Br J Dermatol 2008; 158:1329.

Szeimies RM, et al: Adjuvant photodynamic therapy does not prevent recurrence of condylomata acuminata after carbon dioxide laser ablation: a phase III, prospective, randomized, bicentric, double-blind study. Dermatol Surg 2009; 35:757.

Turnbull JR, et al: Regression of multiple viral warts in human immunodeficiency virus-infected patient treated by triple antiretroviral therapy. Br J Dermatol 2002; 146:330.

Vanhooteghem O, et al: Raynaud phenomenon after treatment of verruca vulgaris of the sole with intralesional injection of bleomycin. Pediatr Dermatol 2001; 18:249.

Wang YS, et al: Photodynamic therapy with 20% aminolevulinic acid for the treatment of recalcitrant viral warts in an Asian population. Int J Dermatol 2007; 46:1180.

Winer R, et al: Duct tape for the treatment of common warts in adults. Arch Dermatol 2007; 143:309.

Winer RL, et al: Genital human papillomavirus infection: incidence and risk factors in a cohort of female university students. Am J Epidemiol 2003; 157:218.

Wu JK, et al: Psoriasis induced by topical imiquimod. Australas J Dermatol 2004; 45:47.

Wulf HS, et al: Topical photodynamic therapy for prevention of new skin lesions in renal transplant recipients. Acta Derm Venereol 2006; 86:25.

Yaghoobi R, et al: Evaluation of oral zinc sulfate effect on recalcitrant multiple viral warts: a randomized placebo-controlled clinical trial. J Am Acad Dermatol 2009; 60:706.

Yanagi T, et al: Epidermodysplasia verruciformis and generalized verrucosis: the same disease? Clin Exper Dermatol 2006; 31:390.

Viral-associated trichodysplasia (cyclosporine-induced folliculodystrophy)

Organ transplant recipients on immunosuppressive regimens rarely develop a characteristic eruption of erythematous 1–3 mm facial papules. The midface, glabella, and chin are primarily affected. Lesions are numerous, may reach confluence, and can cause nasal distortion similar to that seen in rosacea and sarcoidosis (Fig. 19-55). Some papules have a central, keratotic white excrescence. Alopecia of the eyebrows and eyelashes may occur, but the scalp is spared. Histology is characteristic, showing massively distended, bulbous follicles with expansion of the inner root sheath cells containing numerous trichohyaline granules. Abrupt inner root sheath-type cornification is present. No hair shafts (or hair cortex) are present in the affected follicles. Electron microscopy demonstrates numerous viral particles about 40 nm in size with features suggestive of a papovavirus. Topical cidofovir 3% cream slowly improved one patient.

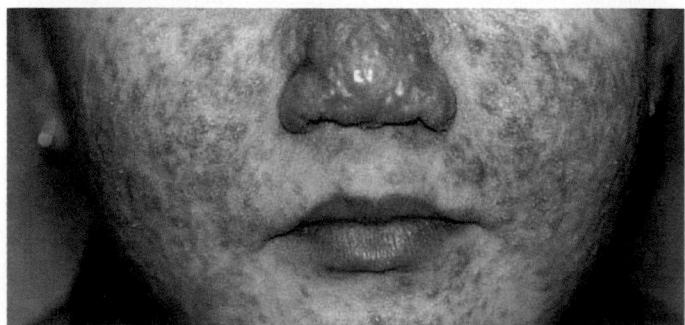

Fig. 19-55 Trichodysplasia. (Courtesy of Len Sperling, MD)

Chastain MA, Millikan LE: Pilomatrix dysplasia in an immunosuppressed patient. J Am Acad Dermatol 2000; 43:118.

Heaphy MR, et al: Cyclosporine-induced folliculodystrophy. J Am Acad Dermatol 2004; 50:310.

Sperling LC, et al: Viral-associated trichodysplasia in patients who are immunocompromised. J Am Acad Dermatol 2004; 50:318.

Retroviruses

These oncoviruses are unique in that they contain RNA, which is converted by a virally coded reverse transcriptase to DNA in the host cell. The target cell population is primarily CD4+ lymphocytes (primarily helper T cells), but also, in some cases, macrophages. For this reason they are called human T-lymphotropic viruses (HTLV). Transmission may be by sexual intercourse, blood products/intravenous drug use, and from mother to child during childbirth and breastfeeding. There is often a very long "latent" period from the time of infection until presentation with clinical disease.

Human T-lymphotropic virus-1

HTLV-1 is endemic in Japan, the Caribbean, South America (Brazil, Peru, Columbia), sub-Saharan Africa, Romania, among Australian Aborigines, and in the southeastern US. In endemic areas, infection rates may be quite high, with only a small percentage of infected patients ever developing clinical disease (estimated at about 3%). HTLV-1 is spread primarily by mother-to-infant transmission during breastfeeding, but also can be transmitted sexually (primarily male to female) or via blood transfusion or intravenous drug use. HTLV-1 uses the GLUT glucose transporter to enter cells. HTLV-1 is responsible for several clinical syndromes. About 1% of persons who are infected will develop adult T-cell leukemia-lymphoma (ATL), with more HTLV-1-infected persons in Japan developing ATL than in other populations. Infection in childhood through breastfeeding seems to be a risk factor for developing ATL. HTLV-1-associated myelopathy or tropical spastic paraparesis (HAM/TSP) is a less common degenerative neurologic syndrome.

There are four forms of ATL: smoldering, chronic, acute, and lymphomatous, usually progressing in that order. A primary cutaneous tumoral variant of ATL has been proposed. ATL is characterized by lymphadenopathy, hepatosplenomegaly, hypercalcemia, and skin lesions. Skin lesions in ATL include erythematous papules or nodules (Fig. 19-56). Prurigo may be a prodrome to the development of ATL. Histologically, the cutaneous infiltrates are pleomorphic, atypical lymphocytes

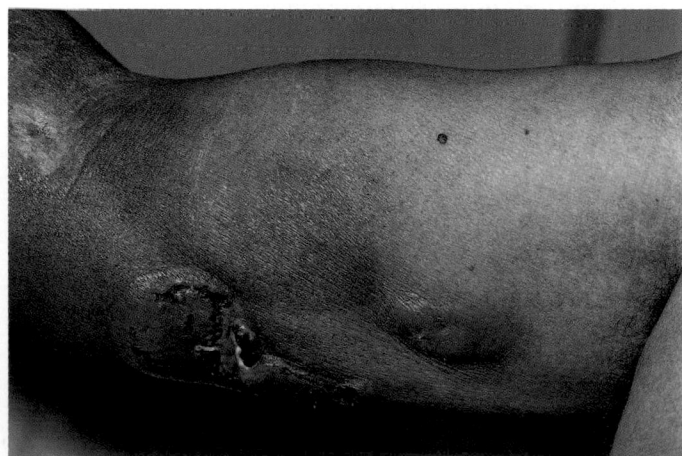

Fig. 19-56 HTLV-1-associated adult T-cell leukemia-lymphoma.

with characteristic "flower cells" representing HTLV-1-infected lymphocytes. Epidermotropism may be present, mimicking mycosis fungoides.

HTLV-1-infected patients often have an abnormal skin examination. If they are seropositive but asymptomatic, dermatophytosis (34%), seborrheic dermatitis (6%), and xerosis/acquired icthyosis (7%) are most commonly found. Vitiligo is also associated. Xerosis occurs in 82% of patients with HAM/TSP, seborrheic dermatitis in 33%, candidiasis and palmar erythema in 15%, and chronic eczema/photosensitivity in up to 20%. Biopsies from the areas of chronic eczema/photosensitivity may show features of ATL in up to 25% of these patients (smoldering ATL). Areas of positive biopsies are described as "atrophic." Scabies is seen in 2% of asymptomatic HTLV-1-infected patients and in 5% of those with HAM/TSP. The scabies may be of the hyperkeratotic (crusted) type and the finding of this pattern of scabies in a person from an HTLV-1 endemic region should trigger serologic testing for HTLV-1. The spectrum of skin disease seen in symptomatic HTLV-1-infected patients is remarkably similar to that seen in HIV-infected patients with CNS disease (xerosis/eczema, seborrheic dermatitis, and scabies).

"Infective dermatitis" occurs in children and less commonly in adults infected with HTLV-1. It is much rarer in Japan than other HTLV-1 endemic countries. Infective dermatitis is diagnosed by major and minor criteria, as delineated by La Grenade et al. Clinically, the children present at an early age (on average, about 7 years) with a chronic eczema of the scalp, axilla, groin, external auditory canal, retroauricular area, eyelid margins, paranasal areas, and neck. Exudation and crusting are the hallmarks of the skin lesions. Pruritus is mild. Clinically, infective dermatitis resembles a cross between infected atopic dermatitis and infected seborrheic dermatitis. There is a chronic nasal discharge. Cultures from the skin and nares are positive for *S. aureus* or β-hemolytic streptococcus, and the condition responds rapidly to antibiotics and topical steroids. Infective dermatitis is relapsing and recurrent. Skin biopsies show a nonspecific dermatitis; however, close examination may show atypical CD4+ cells infiltrating the epidermis, at times simulating ATL or cutaneous T-cell lymphoma. Up to one-third of patients with infective dermatitis have comorbidities, including pneumonitis, corneal opacities, and lymphocytosis with atypical lymphocytes. Careful neurological examination of children with infective dermatitis will often reveal abnormal neurological findings (weakness, lumbar pain, dysesthesias, and urinary disturbances).

Bittencourt AL, et al: Adult-onset infective dermatitis associated with HTLV-1: clinical and immunopathological aspects of two cases. Eur J Dermatol 2006; 16:62.

Bittencourt AL, et al: Manifestations of the human T-cell lymphotropic virus type 1 infection in childhood and adolescence. J Pediatria (Rio J) 2006; 82:411.

Goncalves DU, et al: Dermatologic lesions in asymptomatic blood donors seropositive for human T-cell lymphotrophic virus type-1. Am J Trop Med Hyg 2003; 68:562.

Kendall EA, et al: Early neurologic abnormalities associated with human T-cell lymphotropic virus type-1 infection in a cohort of Peruvian children. J Pediatr 2009; Jul 21 (Epub ahead of print).

La Grenade L, et al: Clinical, pathologic, and immunologic features of human T-lymphotrophic virus type 1-associated infective dermatitis in children. Arch Dermatol 1998; 134:439.

Lenzi MER, et al: Dermatological findings of human T-lymphotrophic virus type 1 (HTVL-1)-associated myelopathy/tropical spastic paraparesis. Clin Infect Dis 2003; 36:507.

Maragno L, et al: Human T-cell lymphotropic virus type 1 infective dermatitis emerging in adulthood. Int J Dermatol 2009; 48:723.

Verdonck K, et al: Human T-lymphotropic virus 1: recent knowledge about an ancient infection. Lancet 2007; 7:266.

Yamaguchi T, et al: Clinicopathological features of cutaneous lesions of adult T-cell leukaemia/lymphoma. Br J Dermatol 2005; 152:76.

Human immunodeficiency virus

Human immunodeficiency virus (HIV) infects human helper T cells, leading to a progressive immunodeficiency disease. In its end stages it is called acquired immunodeficiency syndrome (AIDS). Cutaneous manifestations are prominent, affecting up to 90% of HIV-infected persons. Many patients have multiple skin lesions of different kinds. The skin lesions or combinations of skin conditions are so unique that the diagnosis of HIV infection or AIDS can often be suspected from the skin examination alone. The skin findings can be classified into three broad categories: infections, inflammatory dermatoses, and neoplasms. The skin conditions also tend to appear at a specific stage in the progression of HIV disease, making them useful markers of the stage of HIV disease.

The natural history of HIV infection in the vast majority of patients is a gradual loss of helper T cells. The rate of this decline is variable, with some patients progressing rapidly and others very slowly or not at all (long-term nonprogressors). Soon after infection there is a seroconversion syndrome called primary HIV infection, or acute infection (group I). Patients recover from this syndrome and enter a relatively long latent period (asymptomatic infection or group II), which averages about 10 years. During this period patients may have persistent generalized lymphadenopathy (group III). When symptoms begin to appear they are often nonspecific and include fever, weight loss, chronic diarrhea, and mucocutaneous disease (group IV A). Helper T-cell counts in group II, III, and IV A patients usually range from 200 to 500. The skin findings at this stage (originally called AIDS-related complex [ARC]) include seborrheic dermatitis, psoriasis, Reiter syndrome, atopic dermatitis, herpes zoster, acne rosacea, oral hairy leukoplakia, onychomycosis, warts, recurrent *S. aureus* folliculitis, and mucocutaneous candidiasis.

Once the helper T-cell count is 200 or less, the patient is defined as having AIDS. In this stage of HIV disease, the skin lesions are more characteristic of immunodeficiency and include characteristic opportunistic infections: chronic herpes simplex, molluscum contagiosum, bartonellosis (bacillary angiomatosis), systemic fungal infections (cryptococcosis, histoplasmosis, coccidioidomycosis, and penicilliosis), and mycobacterial infection. Paradoxically, patients at this stage also have hyper-reactive skin and, frequently, inflammatory, often pruritic skin diseases. These skin conditions include eosinophilic folliculitis, granuloma annulare, drug reactions, enhanced reactions to insect bites, and photodermatitis.

When the T-cell count falls below 50, the patient is often said to have "advanced AIDS." These patients may have very unusual presentations of their opportunistic infections, including multicentric, refractory molluscum contagiosum; chronic herpes simplex; chronic cutaneous varicella zoster infection; cutaneous acanthamebiasis, cutaneous atypical mycobacterial infections (including *Mycobacterium avium* complex and *Mycobacterium haemophilum*), and crusted scabies. Treatment of their infections is often very difficult because of the significant chronic immunosuppression.

It is now clear that HIV itself is the cause of the loss of helper T cells and that effective treatment of HIV infection may halt or reverse the natural history of HIV disease. There are numerous antiretroviral agents and they are usually used in combinations called "cocktails." This combination treatment is called highly active antiretroviral therapy (HAART). A significant percentage of HIV-infected patients respond to HAART and may show dramatic improvement of their HIV disease. HIV disappears from the blood and helper T-cell counts rise. As expected, in patients who respond to HAART, opportunistic infections no longer occur, and subsequently mortality decreases. This is also true of cutaneous infectious conditions.

HIV-associated psoriasis usually improves substantially, especially if the patient did not have psoriasis prior to HIV infection.

HAART is typically associated with resolution of all forms of HIV-related cutaneous complications. However, some conditions may initially appear or be exacerbated by the sudden improvement of the immune status that occurs with eradication of HIV viremia and with increase in helper T-cell counts. This complex of manifestations has been termed the "immune reconstitution" or "immune restoration" syndrome (IRIS). IRIS occurs in between 15% and 25% of HIV-infected persons started on HAART. Persons with an opportunistic infection (OI), specifically cryptococcosis, tuberculosis, or *Pneumocystis* pneumonia, may be at higher risk if HAART is started as the OI is being treated. This marked inflammatory syndrome can be severe, and in resource-poor countries 5% of AIDS-related deaths in treated patients can be attributed to IRIS during the first year of HAART therapy. Half of IRIS-related conditions are dermatological. Three forms of IRIS occur:

1. A hidden OI is unmasked as the reconstituted immune system attacks the hidden pathogen. The presentation may be atypical. The appearance of cutaneous mycobacterial infections with HAART is an example.
2. In the setting of a documented OI, when HAART is started, the patient has worsening of the infection with new findings. This is not treatment failure, but enhanced immune response to the pathogen. This typically occurs with tuberculosis or cryptococcosis.
3. The development of new disorders is seen, infectious or inflammatory, or enhanced inflammatory responses around malignancies, especially Kaposi sarcoma. Eosinophilic folliculitis, acne flares, drug eruptions, Reiter's syndrome, lupus erythematosus, alopecia universalis, at times HPV infections (especially oral and genital), increased outbreaks of genital and orolabial herpes simplex, or molluscum contagiosum, herpes zoster, cytomegalovirus ulcerations, type I reactions in Hansen's disease, cutaneous mycobacterial and fungal infections, leishmaniasis, tattoo and foreign body granulomas, and sarcoidosis can be part of IRIS in the skin.

Primary HIV infection (acute seroconversion syndrome)

Several weeks after infection with HIV, an acute illness develops in a large proportion of individuals. The clinical syndrome is much like EBV infection, with fever, sore throat, cervical adenopathy, a rash, and oral, genital, and rectal ulceration. The skin eruption can be polymorphous (Figs 19-57 and 19-58). Most characteristic is a papular eruption of discrete, slightly scaly, oval lesions of the upper trunk. The lesions have a superficial resemblance to pityriasis rosea, but the peripheral scale is not prominent, and there is focal hemorrhage in the lesions. A Gianotti–Crosti-like papular eruption may also occur. Purpuric lesions along the margins of the palms and soles, as seen in immune complex disease, have been reported. The mucosal erosions resemble aphthae but are larger and can affect all parts of the mouth, pharynx, esophagus, and anal mucosa. Dysphagia may be prominent. The helper T-cell count falls abruptly during seroconversion. The level of immune impairment may be adequate to allow oral candidiasis or even *Pneumocystis jirovecii* (formerly *carinii*) pneumonia to develop. The diagnosis should be suspected in any at-risk individual with the correct constellation of symptoms. A direct measurement of HIV viral load will confirm the diagnosis. Combination antiviral therapy is instituted immediately.

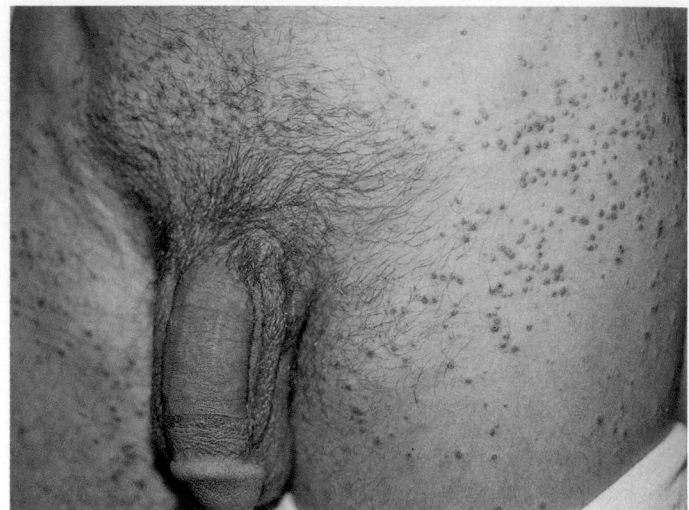

Fig. 19-57 Primary HIV infection.

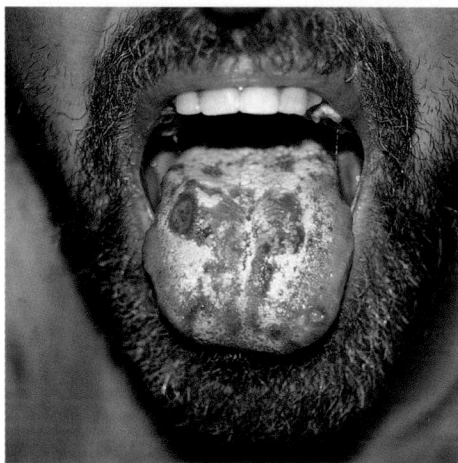

Fig. 19-58 Primary HIV infection. (Courtesy of Ginat Mirowski, MD)

HIV-associated pruritus

From early in the HIV epidemic, it was clear that pruritus was a marker of HIV infection throughout the world, occurring in up to 30% of patients. Pruritus is usually not caused by HIV disease itself but is related to inflammatory dermatoses associated with the disease. "Papular pruritic eruption" is not a specific disease, but a wastebasket diagnosis used to encompass patients with many forms of HIV-associated pruritus. Worldwide, it most commonly represents enhanced insect bite reactions. These pruritic eruptions are best subdivided into follicular and nonfollicular eruptions. The relative prevalence of these two patterns of pruritic eruptions is geographically distinct. In tropical and semitropical regions where biting insects are prominent, nonfollicular eruptions are most common, and probably represent insect bite hypersensitivity. In temperate regions, follicular pruritic eruptions are more common.

Eosinophilic folliculitis (EF) is the most common pruritic follicular eruption. It is seen in patients with a helper T-cell count of about 200. Clinically, it presents with urticarial follicular papules on the upper trunk, face, scalp, and neck (Fig. 19-59). Pustular lesions are uncommon; pustules are usually smaller than in bacterial folliculitis and represent end-stage lesions. They are uncommonly seen, since the pruritus is so severe that they are excoriated before the lesion evolves to this degree. Ninety percent of lesions occur above the nipple line on the anterior trunk, and lesions typically extend down the midline of the back to the lumbar spine. The disease waxes

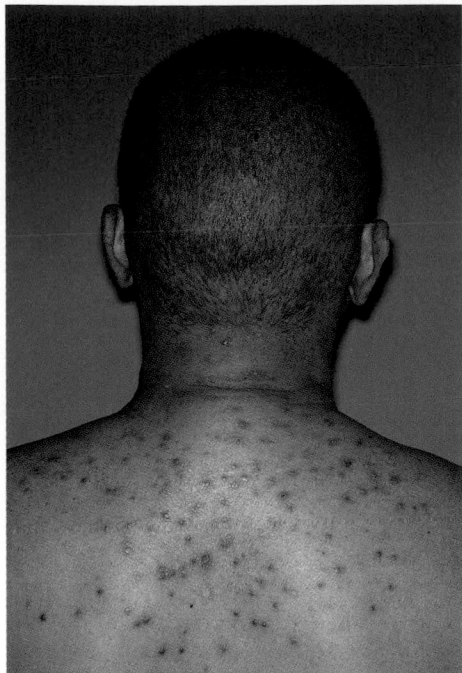

Fig. 19-59 Eosinophilic folliculitis. (Courtesy of Curt Samlaska, MD)

and wanes in severity and may spontaneously clear, only to flare unpredictably. A peripheral eosinophilia may be present and the serum IgE level may be elevated, suggesting this is a disorder mediated by T-helper 2 cells. Histologically, an infiltrate of mononuclear cells and eosinophils is seen around the upper portion of the hair follicle at the level of the sebaceous gland. As lesions evolve, eosinophils and lymphocytes enter the follicular structure and the sebaceous glands. Pustules are formed late and represent aggregates of eosinophils in the uppermost part of the follicle.

Initial treatment of eosinophilic folliculitis is topical steroids and antihistamines. If the patient fails to respond, phototherapy (UVB or PUVA) or itraconazole, 200 mg twice a day, may be effective. In some patients repeated applications of permethrin (every other night for up to 6 weeks) may be of benefit. This latter therapy is directed at *Demodex* mites, which may be the antigenic trigger of this condition. Isotretinoin is also effective, often after a few months, in a dose of about 0.5–1 mg/kg/day. HAART may lead to a flare of EF, but usually leads eventually to its resolution. Staphylococcal folliculitis, which may be severely pruritic in patients with HIV disease, and *Pityrosporum* folliculitis should be included in the differential diagnosis. These are excluded by bacterial culture and skin biopsy, respectively.

The other pruritic dermatoses that are not follicular can be divided into the primarily papular eruptions and the eczematous ones. The papular eruptions include scabies, insect bites, transient acantholytic dermatosis, granuloma annulare, and prurigo nodularis. The eczematous dermatoses include atopic-like dermatitis, seborrheic dermatitis, nummular eczema, xerotic eczema, photodermatitis, and drug eruptions. Patients may have multiple eruptions simultaneously, making differential diagnosis difficult. A skin biopsy from a representative lesion of every morphologic type on the patient may elucidate the true diagnosis. Treatment is determined by the diagnosis and is similar to treatment in persons without HIV infection with these same dermatoses. Special considerations in AIDS patients include the use of topical therapy plus ivermectin for crusted scabies and thalidomide for prurigo nodularis and photodermatitis. Both of these systemic agents are very effective if used appropriately.

HIV-associated neoplasia

Neoplasia is prominent in HIV infection and in some cases is highly suggestive of HIV infection. Kaposi sarcoma is an example. Other common neoplasms seen in patients with HIV infection include superficial basal cell carcinomas (BCCs) of the trunk, SCCs in sun-exposed areas, genital HPV-induced SCC, and extranodal B- and T-cell lymphomas. Lipomas, angiolipomas, and dermatofibromas may occur in association with HAART therapy. In the case of lipomas, their appearance is usually related to the peripheral fat loss that occurs with some HIV treatment regimens and with HIV disease itself.

Nonmelanoma skin cancers (NMSC) are very common in HIV-infected persons. HAART does not protect against the development of NMSC in HIV. The rate of development of BCC and SCC is not increased in persons with HIV infection. BCCs usually occur as superficial multicentric lesions on the trunk in fair-skinned males in their twenties to fifties. The ratio of BCC to SCC is not reversed in HIV disease, as it is in organ transplant recipients. BCCs behave in the same manner as they do in the immunocompetent host and standard management is usually adequate.

Actinically induced SCCs are also quite common and present in the standard manner as nodules, keratotic papules, or ulcerations. In most cases, their behavior is relatively benign and standard management is adequate. Removal of SCCs in sun-exposed areas by curettage and desiccation in patients with HIV infection is associated with an unacceptably high recurrence rate of about 15%. Complete excision is therefore recommended. The use of imiquimod to treat SCC in situ in the setting of HIV infection should be considered experimental, and if it is undertaken, very close follow-up is recommended. In a small subset of patients with AIDS, actinic SCCs can be very aggressive—they may double in size over weeks and may metastasize to regional lymph nodes or viscerally, leading to the death of the patient.

Genital SCCs, including cervical, vaginal, anal, penile, and nailbed SCC, all occur in patients with HIV infection. These neoplasms are increased in frequency, and the progression from HPV infection to neoplasia appears to be accelerated. This is analogous to the situation in organ transplant and other immunosuppressed patients. It appears that these cancers are associated with primarily "high-risk" HPV types.

For the dermatologist, there are three important manifestations of high-risk genital HPV infection in patients with HIV. Most common is perianal dysplasia, seen most frequently in MSM with a history of receptive anal intercourse. Dysplasia in this area may present as velvety white or hyperpigmented plaques involving the whole anal area and extending into the anal canal. These lesions may erode or ulcerate. Histology will demonstrate SCC in situ. The risk of progression of the lesions to anal SCC is unknown but is estimated to be at least 10 times higher than the rate of cervical cancer in women in the general population. The management of such lesions is unclear, but regular follow-up is clearly indicated and any masses in the anal canal should be immediately referred for biopsy. At some centers pap smear equivalents are performed. Imiquimod has been used as an adjunct in the management of genital warts and HPV-associated genital in situ dysplasias (not genital SCC). While it may be of benefit in patients with reconstituted immune systems on HAART, especially in combination with surgical ablation, the response rate is much lower than in immunocompetent patients. In the only placebo-controlled trial, done before standard HAART was available, imiquimod was no more effective than placebo in clearing genital warts in HIV infection (11% of genital warts cleared). Small case series of patients on HAART suggest clearance rates of about 30–50%.

The vulvar and penile skin may develop flat white or hyperpigmented macules from a few millimeters to several centimeters in diameter. These show SCC in situ and are analogous to bowenoid papulosis in the immunocompetent host. Rare cases of progression to SCC have occurred. Such lesions are best managed conservatively as warts and watched closely. Lesions of the penis and vulva, not at a transition zone or on mucosal surfaces, have a low risk of progressing to invasive SCC. Lesions of the glans penis that are red and fixed should be biopsied. If the changes of SCC in situ are found, these should be managed aggressively as SCC in situ. Topical 5-FU and superficial radiation therapy are effective. Close clinical follow-up is indicated. Periungual SCC has also been seen in patients with HIV infection. Any persistent keratotic or hyperpigmented lesion in the periungual area must be carefully evaluated. Management is surgical excision.

Extranodal B-cell and, less commonly, T-cell lymphomas are associated with the advanced immunosuppression of AIDS. The B-cell lymphomas and some of the T-cell lymphomas present as violaceous or plum-colored papules, nodules, or tumors. Once the diagnosis is established by biopsy, systemic chemotherapy is required. EBV is found in some cases. HAART is both protective against the development of non-Hodgkin lymphoma (NHL) and Hodgkin disease in HIV and substantially improves prognosis of HIV-infected patients with NHL. Mycosis fungoides can also be seen in patients with HIV infection, often in patients who have not yet developed AIDS. It presents with pruritic patches or plaques and may progress to tumor stage. EBV is not found in these cases. CD8+ pseudolymphoma is also seen in patients with untreated HIV infection, and may resolve with HAART.

Malignant melanoma (MM) is occasionally seen in persons with HIV infection. The rate of MM is up to four times higher in HIV-infected persons. These patients demonstrate the same risk factors as do other melanoma patients—multiple nevi, fair skin type, and prior intermittent intense sun exposure. HIV-infected patients with melanoma in the era prior to HAART had a significantly shorter disease-free survival and a reduced overall survival. Many fair-skinned patients infected with HIV complain of the new onset of atypical moles (analogous to organ transplant patients). Whether these confer an increased risk of melanoma is unknown.

AIDS and Kaposi sarcoma

Kaposi sarcoma (KS) was, along with *Pneumocystis* pneumonia, the harbinger of the AIDS epidemic. Many MSM and bisexual men presented with this tumor in the early 1980s, with a prevalence of up to 25% in some cohorts. HHV-8, a γ-herpesvirus, has been identified in these lesions. The clinical features of KS in patients with AIDS are different than those seen in elderly men who do not have AIDS. Patients with AIDS present with symmetrical widespread lesions, often numerous. Lesions begin as macules that may progress to tumors or nodules (Fig. 19-60). Any mucocutaneous surface may be involved, but areas of predilection include the hard palate, face, trunk, penis, and lower legs and soles. Visceral disease may be present and progressive. Edema may accompany lower leg lesions, and if it is significant, it is often associated with lymph node involvement in the inguinal area.

A diagnosis of KS is established by skin biopsy, which should be taken from the center of the most infiltrated plaque. Excessive bleeding is not usually a problem. Early macular lesions show atypical, angulated, ectatic vessels in the upper dermis associated with an inflammatory infiltrate containing plasma cells. Plaque lesions show aggregates of small vessels and endothelial cells in the upper dermis and surrounding adnexal structures. Nodules and tumors show the classic pattern of a spindle cell neoplasm with prominent extravasation of red blood cells.

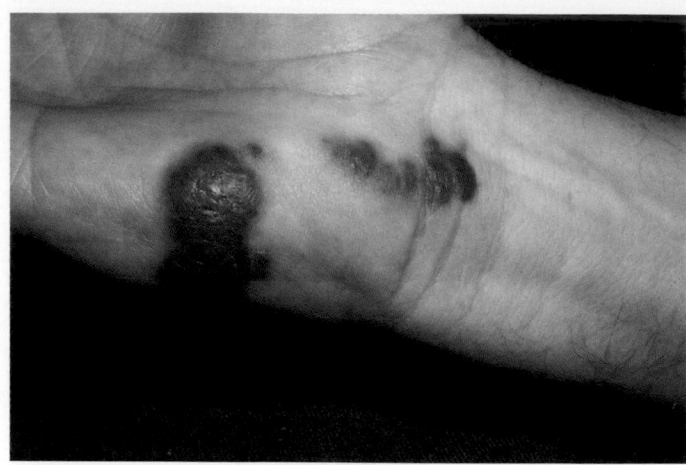

Fig. 19-60 Kaposi sarcoma in AIDS.

HAART has reduced the incidence of KS in HIV-infected patients by 10-fold. However, KS remains an important complication of HIV infection for two reasons:

1. HIV-associated KS is still common in sub-Saharan Africa. With HAART therapy, survival in Africa for HIV-infected persons over 1 year is nearly 100%, if they do not have KS. In patients with HIV disease and KS, however, survival is only 77%. This is due to the lack of effective cytotoxic therapy for KS in Africa. HIV-KS is more common in women than men in some clinics in Africa.

2. While HAART has substantially reduced the prevalence of KS in HIV disease in the developed world, HAART has not eliminated the disease. In fact, there remains a fairly substantial proportion of primarily gay men with HIV disease who also have KS (up to 13% of some cohorts). Twenty percent or more of these AIDS-KS patients have well-controlled HIV disease with long-term undetectable viral load and CD4 counts above 300. These patients have an overall good prognosis, but still may require cytotoxic or radiation therapy to control their KS. Patients with AIDS-KS and lower CD4 counts and detectable viral loads are more likely to have visceral disease. Up to one-third of these AIDS-KS patients died despite HAART and chemotherapy, suggesting that AIDS-KS in the setting of poor HIV control is a bad prognostic finding.

The treatment of AIDS-associated KS depends on the extent and aggressiveness of the disease. Effective HAART after about 6 months is associated with involution of KS lesions in 50% of patients. This should be the initial management in most patients with mild to moderate disease (fewer than 50 lesions, and fewer than 10 new lesions/month) who are not receiving anti-HIV treatment. Intralesional vinblastine, 0.2–0.4 mg/mL, can be infiltrated into lesions (as for a hypertrophic scar) and they will involute over several weeks. Hyperpigmentation usually remains. Cryotherapy is also effective but will leave postinflammatory hypopigmentation in pigmented persons. Persistent individual lesions and lesions of the soles and penis respond well to local irradiation therapy (one single treatment of 80 Gy or fractionated treatments to 150 Gy). For patients with moderate disease (more than 10 lesions, or mucosal or visceral involvement), HAART alone may not be adequate in controlling KS, and liposomal doxorubicin may need to be added to their treatment. For patients with symptomatic visceral disease, aggressive skin disease, marked edema, and pulmonary disease, systemic chemotherapy is indicated. Options include IFN-α, vinca alkaloids, bleomycin, and liposomal doxorubicin as first-line therapies, and taxol for treatment failures.

Agaba PA, et al: Presentation and survival of patients with AIDS-related Kaposi's sarcoma in Jos, Nigeria. Int J STD AIDS 2009; 29:410.

Aggarwal M, Rein J: Acute human immunodeficiency virus syndrome in an adolescent. Pediatrics 2003; 112:e323.

Alberici F, et al: Ivermectin alone or in combination with benzyl benzoate in the treatment of human immunodeficiency virus-associated scabies. Br J Dermatol 2000; 142:969.

Alonso N, et al: Prevalence of skin disease in HIV-positive pregnant women. Int J Dermatol 2003; 42:521.

Bonnet F, et al: Malignancy-related causes of death in human immunodeficiency virus-infected patients in the era of highly active antiretroviral therapy. Cancer 2004; 101:317.

Castelnuovo B, et al: Cause-specific mortality and the contribution of immune reconstitution inflammatory syndrome in the first 3 years after antiretroviral therapy initiation in an urban African cohort. Clin Infect Dis 2009; 49:965.

Crum-Cianflone N, et al: Cutaneous malignancies among HIV-infected persons. Arch Intern Med 2009; 169:1130.

Cusini M, et al: 5% Imiquimod cream for external anogenital warts in HIV-infected patients under HAART therapy. Int J STD AIDS 2004; 15:17.

Dal Maso L: Pattern of cancer risk in persons with AIDS in Italy in the HAART era. Brit J Cancer 2009; 100:840.

Dank JP, Colven R: Protease inhibitor-associated angiolipomatosis. J Am Acad Dermatol 2000; 42:129.

Diaz-Arrastia C, et al: Clinical and molecular responses in high-grade intraepithelial neoplasia treated with topical imiquimod 5%. Clin Cancer Res 2001; 7:3031.

Farrant P, Higgins E: A granulomatous response to tribal medicine as a feature of the immune reconstitution syndrome. Clin Exp Dermatol 2004; 29:366.

Fearfield LA, et al: Cutaneous squamous cell carcinoma with zosteriform metastases in a human immunodeficiency virus-infected patient. Br J Dermatol 2000; 142:573.

Gilson RJC, et al: A randomized, controlled, safety study using imiquimod for the topical treatment of anogenital warts in HIV-infected patients. AIDS 1999; 13:2397.

Hayes BB, et al: Eosinophilic folliculitis in 2 HIV-positive women. Arch Dermatol 2004; 140:463.

Husak R, et al: Refractory human papillomavirus-associated oral warts treated topically with 1–3% cidofovir solutions in human immunodeficiency virus type 1-infected patients. Br J Dermatol 2005; 153:382.

Jagannathan P, et al: Life-threatening immune reconstitution inflammatory syndrome after pneumocystis pneumonia: a cautionary case series. AIDS 2009; 23:13.

Kanitakis J, et al: Cutaneous leiomyomas (piloleiomyomas) in adult patients with human immunodeficiency virus infection. Br J Dermatol 2000; 143:1338.

Kerschmann RL, et al: Cutaneous presentations of lymphoma in HIV disease. Arch Dermatol 1995; 131:1281.

Kreuter A, et al: Treatment of anal intraepithelial neoplasia in patients with acquired HIV with imiquimod 5% cream. J Am Acad Dermatol 2004; 50:980.

Kreuter A, et al: Clinical spectrum and virologic characteristics of anal intraepithelial neoplasia in HIV infection. J Am Acad Dermatol 2005; 52:603.

Lehloenya R, Meintjes G: Dermatologic manifestations of the immune reconstitution inflammatory syndrome. Dermatol Clin 2006; 24:549.

Mani D, et al: A retrospective analysis of AIDS-associated Kaposi's sarcoma in patients with undetectable HIV viral loads and CD4 counts greater than 300 cells/mm³. J Int Assoc Physicians AIDS Care 2009; 8:279.

Martin-Carbonero L, et al: Pegylated liposomal doxorubicin plus highly active antiretroviral therapy versus highly active antiretroviral therapy alone in HIV patients with Kaposi's sarcoma. AIDS 2004; 18:1737.

Massad LS, et al: Effect of antiretroviral therapy on the incidence of genital warts and vulvar neoplasia among women with the human immunodeficiency virus. Am J Obstet Gynecol 2004; 190:1241.

Maurer T, et al: HIV-associated Kaposi's sarcoma with a high CD4 count and a low viral load. N Engl J Med 2007; 357:13.

Moussa R, et al: Buschke–Loewenstein lesion: another possible manifestation of immune restoration inflammatory syndrome? AIDS 2004; 18:1221.

Nguyen P, et al: Aggressive squamous cell carcinomas in persons infected with the human immunodeficiency virus. Arch Dermatol 2002; 138:758.

Rodrigues LKE, et al: Altered clinical course of malignant melanoma in HIV-positive patients. Arch Dermatol 2002; 138:765.

Rodwell GEL, Berger TG: Pruritus and cutaneous inflammatory conditions in HIV disease. Clin Dermatol 2000; 18:479.

Schartz NEC, et al: Regression of CD8+ pseudolymphoma after HIV antiviral triple therapy. J Am Acad Dermatol 2003; 49:139.

Seoane Reula E, et al: Role of antiretroviral therapies in mucocutaneous manifestations in HIV-infected children over a period of two decades. Br J Dermatol 2005; 153:382.

Trevenzoli M, et al: Sarcoidosis and HIV infection: a case report and a review of the literature. Postgrad Med J 2003; 79:535.

Wananukul S, et al: Mucocutaneous findings in pediatric AIDS related to degree of immunosuppression. Pediatr Dermatol 2003; 20:289.

Ward HA, et al: Cutaneous manifestation of antiretroviral therapy. J Am Acad Dermatol 2002; 46:284.

Weiss DA, et al: Condyloma overgrowth caused by immune reconstitution inflammatory syndrome. Urology 2009; Jul 16 (Epub ahead of print).

Yeni PG, et al: Treatment for adult HIV infection: 2004 Recommendations of the International AIDS Society—USA Panel. JAMA 2004; 292:251.

Bonus images for this chapter can be found online at http://www.expertconsult.com

20 Parasitic Infestations, Stings, and Bites

The major groups of animals responsible for bites, stings, and parasitic infections in humans belong to the phyla Arthropoda, Chordata, Cnidaria (formerly Coelenterata), Nemathelminthes, Platyhelminthes, Annelida, and Protozoa. Vector-borne disease continues to be a major worldwide public health threat. Mosquito-borne diseases, such as malaria, West Nile fever, and equine encephalitis, present risks for the resident population as well as travelers. Tick-borne diseases include Lyme disease, Rocky Mountain spotted fever, ehrlichiosis, tick-borne relapsing fever, tularemia, babesiosis, and Colorado tick fever. Children and those who work outdoors are at higher risk for contracting arthropod-borne diseases. Protection of children is complicated by the potential toxicity of agents used as repellents. This chapter will review parasitic diseases and the major causes of bites and stings, as well as strategies for prevention.

Alexander JO: Arthropods and human skin. Berlin: Springer, 1984.
de la Fuente J, et al: Overview: ticks as vectors of pathogens that cause disease in humans and animals. Front Biosci 2008; 13:6938–6946.
Goddard J: Arthropods of medical importance. Boca Raton: CRC, 2003.
Larkin JM: Ticks and tick-related illness. Med Health R I 2008; 91(7):209–211.
Stollery N: Infestations. Practitioner 2008; 252(1705):48, 50, 52–53.

PHYLUM PROTOZOA

The protozoa are one-celled organisms, divided into classes according to the nature of their locomotion. Class Sarcodina organisms move by temporary projections of cytoplasm (pseudopods); class Mastigophora by means of one or more flagella; and class Ciliata by short, hairlike projections of cytoplasm (cilia). Class Sporozoa have no special organs of locomotion.

Class Sarcodina

Amebiasis cutis

Entamoeba histolytica is an intestinal parasite transmitted by the fecal–oral route or by sexual contact. Cutaneous ulcers usually result from extension of an underlying amebic abscess; the most common sites are the trunk, abdomen, buttocks, genitalia, or perineum. Those on the abdomen may result from hepatic abscesses. Penile lesions are usually sexually acquired. Most lesions begin as deep abscesses that rupture and form ulcerations with distinct, raised, cordlike edges, and an erythematous halo approximately 2 cm wide. The base is covered with necrotic tissue and hemopurulent pus containing amebae. These lesions are from a few centimeters to 20 cm wide. Without treatment, slow progression of the ulcer occurs in an increasingly debilitated patient until death ensues. Patients may also present with fistulae, fissures, polypoid warty lesions, or nodules. Deep lesions are more likely to be associated with visceral lesions.

The sole manifestation of early amebiasis may be chronic urticaria. An estimated 10 million invasive cases occur annually, most of them in the tropics. Infection may be asymptomatic, or bloody diarrhea and hepatic abscesses may be present. In the US, the disease occurs chiefly in institutionalized patients, world travelers, recent immigrants, migrant workers, and men who have sex with men (MSM).

The histologic findings are those of a necrotic ulceration with many lymphocytes, neutrophils, plasma cells, and eosinophils. *E. histolytica* is found in the tissue, within blood and lymph vessels. The organism measures 50–60 μm in diameter, and has basophilic cytoplasm and a single eccentric nucleus with a central karyosome.

The organism is frequently demonstrable in fresh material from the base of the ulcer by direct smear. Culture of the protozoa confirms the diagnosis. Indirect hemagglutination test results remain elevated for years after the initial onset of invasive disease, whereas the results of gel diffusion precipitation tests and counterimmunoelectrophoresis become negative at 6 months. This property can be used to test for recurrent or active disease in persons coming from endemic areas.

When the perianal or perineal areas are involved, granuloma inguinale, lymphogranuloma venereum, deep mycosis, and syphilis must be considered. In chronic urticaria, fresh stool examinations by a trained technician are necessary.

The treatment of choice is metronidazole (Flagyl), 750 mg orally three times a day for 10 days. Abscesses may require surgical drainage.

Other ameba

Amebas of the genera *Acanthamoeba* and *Balamuthia* may also cause skin lesions in infected hosts. These organisms are ubiquitous in the environment and are found in soil, water, and air. Granulomatous amebic encephalitis is the most common manifestation of infection with these amebas. In the case of *Acanthamoeba*, invasive infections are nearly always in immunocompromised individuals, including those with acquired immunodeficiency syndrome (AIDS) and organ transplant patients, although *Acanthamoeba* can also involve the cornea in those who use homemade contact lens solution. Disseminated lesions present as pink or violaceous nodules that then enlarge, suppurate, and form ulcers with a necrotic eschar (Fig. 20-1). Other findings include fever, nasal congestion or discharge, epistaxis, cough, headaches, lethargy, altered mental status, and seizures. In patients infected with *Acanthamoeba* who have disease of the central nervous system (CNS), death is nearly universal within days to weeks. The organisms are visible on skin biopsy and culture is definitive. In patients without CNS involvement, the mortality rate is 75%, with successfully treated cases often managed with a

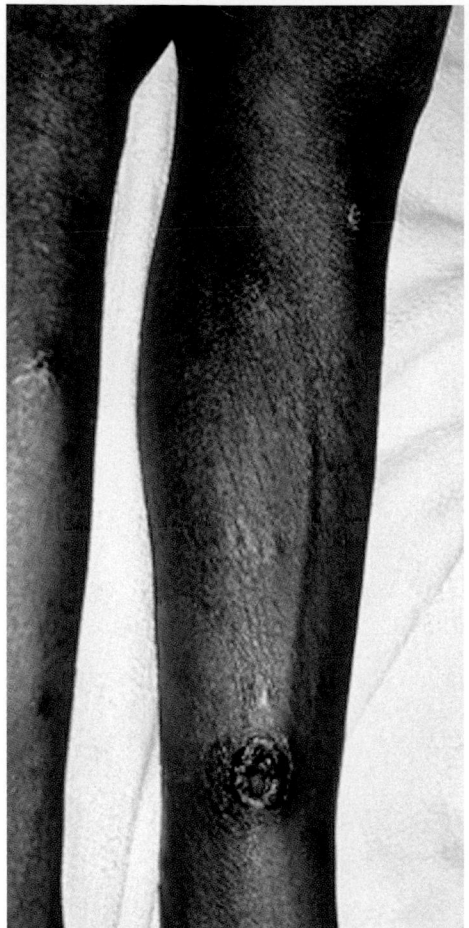

Fig. 20-1 Disseminated acanthameba in HIV disease.

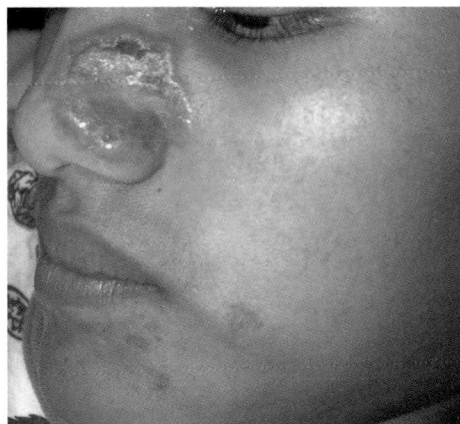

Fig. 20-2 *Balamuthia* infection. (Courtesy of Paco Bravo, MD)

combination of 5-fluorocytosine and sulfadiazine. In patients infected with *Balamuthia mandrillaris*, involvement of the central face is typical and pentamidine is favored for treatment (Fig. 20-2). Chlorhexidine topically and surgical debridement are local adjunctive measures that may prove beneficial.

Al-Daraji WI, et al: Primary cutaneous amebiasis with a fatal outcome. Am J Dermatopathol 2008; 30(4):398–400.

Kenner BM, et al: Cutaneous amebiasis in a child and review of the literature. Pediatr Dermatol 2006; 23(3):231–234.

Khan NA: Acanthamoeba: biology and increasing importance in human health. FEMS Microbiol Rev 2006; 30(4):564–595.

Verma GK, et al: Amoebiasis cutis: clinical suspicion is the key to early diagnosis. Australas J Dermatol 2010 Feb; 51(1):52–55.

Class Mastigophora

Organisms belonging to this class are known as flagellates. Many have an undulating membrane with flagella along their crest.

Trichomoniasis

Trichomonas vulvovaginitis is a common cause of vaginal pruritus, with burning and a frothy leukorrhea. The vaginal mucosa appears bright red from inflammation and may be mottled with pseudomembranous patches. The male urethra may also harbor the organism; in the male it causes urethritis and prostatitis. Occasionally, men may develop balanoposthitis. Erosive lesions on the glans and penis or abscesses of the median raphe may occur. Neonates may acquire the infection during passage through the birth canal, but they require treatment only if symptomatic or if colonization lasts more than 4 weeks. As this is otherwise nearly exclusively a sexually transmitted disorder (STD), *Trichomonas* vulvovaginitis in a child should prompt suspicion of sexual abuse.

Trichomoniasis is caused by *Trichomonas vaginalis*, a colorless pyriform flagellate 5–15 µm long. *T. vaginalis* is demonstrated in smears from affected areas. Testing by direct immunofluorescence is sensitive and specific, and PCR analysis is now available.

Metronidazole, 2 g in a single oral dose, is the treatment of choice. Alternatively, 500 mg twice a day for 7 days may be given. Patients should be warned not to drink alcohol for 24 h after the last dose because of the disulfiram-type effects of this medication. Male sex partners should also be treated. The use of metronidazole is contraindicated in pregnant women, and clotrimazole, applied intravaginally at a dosage of 100 mg a night for 2 weeks, may be used instead.

Bellanger AP, et al: Two unusual occurrences of trichomoniasis: rapid species identification by PCR. J Clin Microbiol 2008; 46(9):3159–3161.

Francis SC, et al: Prevalence of rectal *Trichomonas vaginalis* and *Mycoplasma genitalium* in male patients at the San Francisco STD clinic, 2005–2006. Sex Transm Dis 2008; 35(9):797–800.

Pavithran K: Trichomonal abscess of the median raphe of the penis. Int J Dermatol 1993; 32:820.

Leishmaniasis

Cutaneous leishmaniasis, American mucocutaneous leishmaniasis, and visceral leishmaniasis (kala-azar), which includes infantile leishmaniasis and post-kala-azar dermal leishmaniasis, are all caused by morphologically indistinguishable protozoa of the family Trypanosomidae, called *Leishmania* (pronounced leesh-may-nea). The clinical features of these diseases differ and they have, in general, different geographic distributions. The reason for the variable clinical manifestations may reside with the diversity of the organism, the immune status of the patient, and the genetic ability to initiate effective cell-mediated immune response to the specific infecting organism. It is known that the antigen-specific T-cell responses, which lead to the production of interferon (IFN) and interleukin (IL)-12, are important for healing of the lesions and the induction of lifelong, species-specific immunity to reinfection that results after natural infection. Both CD4 and CD8+ lymphocytes appear to be active in the immune response. IL-10-producing natural regulatory T cells may play a role in the downregulation of infection-induced immunity.

Cutaneous leishmaniasis

There are several types of lesion. All tend to occur on exposed parts, as all are transmitted by the sandfly. Old World leishmaniasis manifests mainly in the skin and has also been called Baghdad boil, Oriental sore, leishmaniasis tropica, Biskra button, Delhi boil, Aleppo boil, Kandahar sore, and Lahore sore. Mild visceral disease may occur. Skin lesions of New World infection have been termed uta, pian bois, and bay sore or chiclero ulcer.

Clinical features

In Old World leishmaniasis, lesions may present in two distinct types. One is the moist or rural type, a slowly growing, indurated, livid, indolent papule (Fig. 20-3), which enlarges in a few months to form a nodule that may ulcerate in a few weeks to form an ulcer as large as 5 cm in diameter. Spontaneous healing usually takes place within 6 months, leaving a characteristic scar. This type is contracted from rodent reservoirs such as gerbils via the sandfly vector. The incubation period is relatively short—1–4 weeks. The dry or urban type has a longer incubation period (2–8 months or longer), develops much more slowly, and heals more slowly than the rural type.

Rarely, after the initial or "mother" lesion is healed, at the borders of the healed area, a few soft red papules may appear that are covered with whitish scales and have the "apple jelly" characteristics of granulomatous diseases such as lupus vulgaris. These spread peripherally on a common erythematous base and are the lupoid type. This is also known as leishmaniasis recidivans and occurs most commonly with the urban type of disease, caused by *Leishmania tropica*. New World disease may also induce purely cutaneous lesions, of varied morphology. The primary papule may become nodular, verrucous, furuncular, or ulcerated, with an infiltrated red border (Fig. 20-4). Subcutaneous peripheral nodules, which eventually ulcerate, may signal extension of the disease. A linear or radial lymphangitic (sporotrichoid) pattern may occur with lymphadenopathy, and the nodes may rarely yield organisms. Facial lesions may coalesce and resemble erysipelas. Recidivans lesions are unusual in the New World form of disease. In Yucatan and Guatemala, a subtype of New World disease exists: the chiclero ulcer. The most frequent site of infection is the ear (Fig. 20-5). The lesions ulcerate and occur most frequently in workers who harvest chicle for chewing gum in forests, where there is high humidity. This form is a more chronic ulcer that may persist for years, destroying the ear cartilage and leading to deformity. The etiologic agent is *Leishmania mexicana* and the sandfly vector, *Lutzomyia flaviscutellata*.

Uta is a term used by Peruvians for leishmaniasis occurring in mountainous territory at 1200–1800 m above sea level. The ulcerating lesions are found on exposed sites and mucosal lesions do not occur.

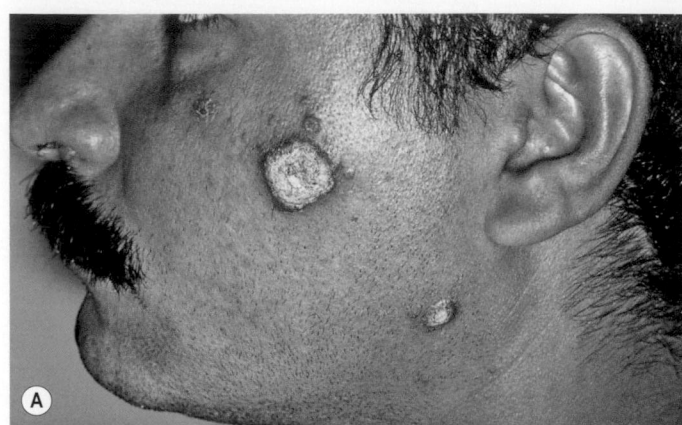
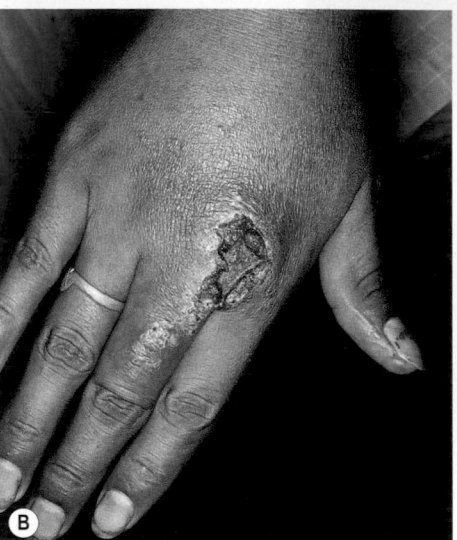

Fig. 20-4 A and B, New World leishmaniasis.

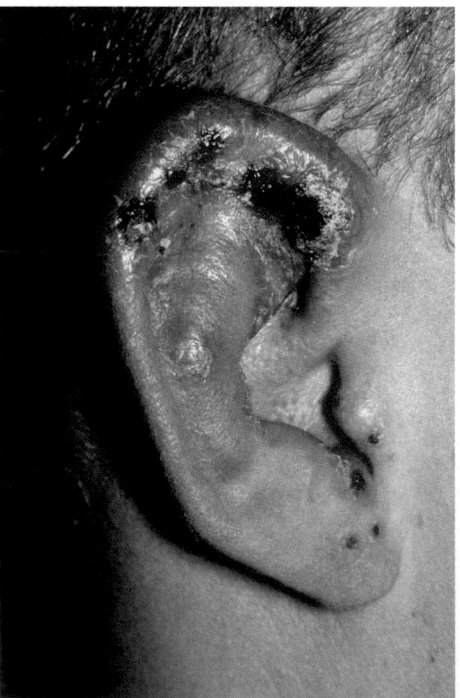

Fig. 20-5 Chiclero ulcer in leishmaniasis.

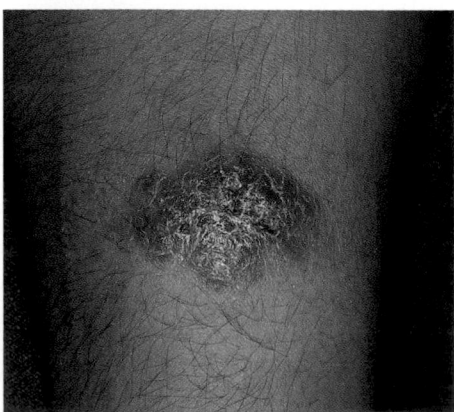

Fig. 20-3 Old World leishmaniasis.

Disseminated cutaneous leishmaniasis may be seen in both New and Old World disease. Multiple nonulcerated papules and plaques, chiefly on exposed surfaces, characterize this type. The disease begins with a single ulcer, nodule, or plaque from which satellite lesions may develop and disseminate to cover the entire body. The disease is progressive and treatment is usually ineffective. It is characterized by anergy to the organism. This type of leishmaniasis must be differentiated from lepromatous leprosy, xanthoma tuberosum, paracoccidioidal granuloma, Lobo's disease, and malignant lymphoma.

Etiologic factors

L. tropica, *Leishmania major*, *Leishmania aethiopica*, and *Leishmania infantum*, the cause of Mediterranean visceral leishmaniasis, may cause cutaneous leishmaniasis. Purely cutaneous leishmaniasis is also caused by several species present in the New World. *L. mexicana* does not induce mucosal disease. *Leishmania braziliensis guyanensis* produces cutaneous disease, as does *Leishmania braziliensis braziliensis* and *Leishmania braziliensis panamensis*; however, the latter two may also result in mucocutaneous disease.

Epidemiology

Cutaneous leishmaniasis is endemic in Asia Minor and to a lesser extent in many countries around the Mediterranean. Iran and Saudi Arabia have a high occurrence rate. In endemic areas, deliberate inoculation on the thigh is sometimes practiced so that scarring on the face—a frequent site for Oriental sore—may be avoided. Purely cutaneous lesions may also be found in the Americas. In the US, leishmaniasis is largely restricted to South Texas, although rare reports of human cutaneous disease have occurred as far north as Pennsylvania, and visceral leishmaniasis in immunosuppressed humans is being recognized as an emerging infection in areas not previously thought to be endemic for the disease.

Pathogenesis

The organism has an alternate life in vertebrates and in insect hosts. Man and other mammals, such as dogs and rodents, are the natural reservoir hosts. The vector hosts are *Phlebotomus* sandflies for the Old World type and *Phlebotomus perniciosus* and *Lutzomyia* sandflies for New World cutaneous leishmaniasis. After the insect has fed on blood, the flagellates (leptomonad, promastigote) develop in the gut in 8–20 days, after which migration occurs into the mouth parts; from here transmission into humans occurs by a bite. In humans, the flagella are lost and a leishmanial form (amastigote) is assumed.

Histopathology

An ulcer with a heavy infiltrate of histiocytes, lymphocytes, plasma cells, and polymorphonuclear leukocytes is seen. The parasitized histiocytes form tuberculoid granulomas in the dermis. Pseudoepitheliomatous hyperplasia may occur in the edges of the ulcer. Numerous organisms are present (mostly in histiocytes), which are nonencapsulated and contain a nucleus and a paranucleus. Wright, Giemsa, and monoclonal antibody staining may be helpful in identifying the organisms. The organisms are seen within histiocytes and often line up at the periphery of a vacuole like the bulbs surrounding a movie marquee. Polymerase chain reaction (PCR) primers are available for a variety of species. PCR is more sensitive than microscopy, but less sensitive than culture.

Diagnosis

In endemic areas, the diagnosis is not difficult. In other localities, cutaneous leishmaniasis may be confused with syphilis, yaws, lupus vulgaris, and pyogenic granulomas. The diagnosis is established by demonstration of the organism in smears. A punch biopsy specimen from the active edge of the ulcer is ideal for culture. It can be placed in Nicolle–Novy–MacNeal (NNN) medium and shipped at room temperature. Parasites can also be cultured from tissue fluid. A hypodermic needle is inserted into the normal skin and to the edge of the ulcer base. The needle is rotated to work loose some material and serum, which is then aspirated. A culture on NNN medium at 22–35°C (71.6–95°F) is recommended to demonstrate the leptomonads. As expected, PCR is the most sensitive diagnostic test for cutaneous leishmaniasis.

Treatment

Spontaneous healing of primary cutaneous lesions occurs, usually within 12–18 months, shorter for Old World disease. Reasons to treat a self-limited infection include avoiding disfiguring scars in exposed areas, notably the face; avoiding secondary infection; controlling disease in the population; and failure of spontaneous healing. In the diffuse cutaneous and recidivans types, the disease may persist for 20–40 years if not treated.

In areas in which localized cutaneous leishmaniasis is not complicated by recidivans or sporotrichoid forms, or by mucocutaneous disease, treatment with such topical modalities as paromomycin sulfate 15% plus methylbenzethonium chloride 12%, ketoconazole cream under occlusion, cryotherapy, local heat, photodynamic therapy, and laser ablation, or with intralesional sodium stibogluconate antimony or emetine hydrochloride may be effective and safe.

In the setting of Old World cutaneous leishmaniasis, some data suggest that intramuscular meglumine antimoniate in combination with intralesional meglumine antimoniate may be superior to intralesional therapy alone. A meta-analysis of studies of Old World cutaneous leishmaniasis concluded that pentamidine was similar in efficacy to pentavalent antimonials and both were superior to the other agents studied. Since then, a Pakistani study concluded that itraconazole was more effective and more economical, and had fewer side effects than meglumine antimoniate in both wet and dry types of cutaneous leishmaniasis. It should be noted that the number of patients was relatively small, and other studies have been disappointing. Oral fluconazole and zinc sulfate have been used to treat *L. major*. A similar meta-analysis of studies of New World cutaneous leishmaniasis concluded that meglumine might be the best agent in its class. Azithromycin has been used in New World disease, but is inferior to antimonials. Perilesional injections of IFN-γ have also been reported to be effective but are expensive.

In patients who are immunosuppressed or who acquire infection in areas where mucocutaneous disease may occur, systemic therapy is recommended. As with topical treatment, many alternatives have been reported to be effective. Sodium antimony gluconate (sodium stibogluconate) solution is given intramuscularly or intravenously, 20 mg/kg/day in two divided doses for 28 days. It can be obtained from the Centers for Disease Control (CDC) Drug Service (Atlanta, GA 30333). Repeated courses may be given. Antimony n-methyl glutamine (Glucantime) is used more often in Central and South America because of its local availability.

Other systemic medications reported to be effective include fluconazole, 200 mg per day for 6 weeks, ketoconazole, dapsone, rifampicin, and allopurinol. Some of these have not been subjected to controlled clinical trials, as is true of most topical treatments. The recidivans and disseminated cutaneous types may require prolonged courses or adjuvant IFN therapy. Amphotericin B may be used in antimony-resistant disease. Lipid formulations of amphotericin B are highly effective in short courses but are expensive. Liposomal amphotericin B may be especially helpful for *L. braziliensis* and *L. guyanensis* infections. Intramuscular pentamidine is also used for *L. guyanensis* cutaneous leishmaniasis, because this infection is resistant to systemic antimony. Miltefosine is being used for cutaneous disease in Colombia and Bolivia. It may prove to be the treatment of choice for diffuse cutaneous leishmaniasis and post-kala-azar dermal leishmaniasis. It is less toxic than most other available agents and its use is likely to increase in all forms of leishmaniasis, but some studies have shown it to be ineffective in *L. major* and *L. braziliensis* infections. Control depends chiefly on the success of antifly measures taken by health authorities and personal protection with protective clothing, screening, and repellents. Vaccines are being investigated but are not available.

Mucocutaneous leishmaniasis (leishmaniasis americana, espundia)

Clinical features

The initial infection, which occurs at the site of the fly bite, is a cutaneous ulcer. Secondary lesions on the mucosa usually occur at some time during the next 5 years (Fig. 20-6). The earliest mucosal lesion is usually hyperemia of the nasal septum with subsequent ulceration, which progresses to invade the septum and later the paranasal fossae. Perforation of the septum eventually takes place. For some time the nose remains unchanged externally, despite the internal destruction. At first, only a dry crust is observed, or a bright red infiltration or vegetation on the nasal septum, with symptoms of obstruction and small hemorrhages. Despite the mutilating and destructive character of leishmaniasis, it never involves the nasal bones. When the septum is destroyed, the nasal bridge and tip of the nose collapse, giving the appearance of a parrot beak, camel nose, or tapir nose.

It is important to recall that the four great chronic infections (syphilis, tuberculosis, Hansen's disease, and leishmaniasis) have a predilection for the nose. The ulcer may extend to the lips (Fig. 20-7) and continue to advance to the pharynx, attacking the soft palate, uvula, tonsils, gingiva, and tongue. The eventual mutilation is called espundia. Two perpendicular grooves at the union of the osseous palate and soft tissues, in the midst of the vegetative infiltration of the entire pharynx, are called the palate cross of espundia.

Only in exceptional cases does American leishmaniasis invade the genital or ocular mucous membranes. The frequency of mucous membrane involvement is variable. In Yucatan and Guatemala, it is an exception; in other countries, such as Brazil, it may occur in 80% of cases.

Etiologic factors

Mucocutaneous leishmaniasis is caused by *L. braziliensis braziliensis* and *L. braziliensis panamensis*. Leishmania has two forms: the nonflagellated form or leishmania, which is found in the tissues of humans and animals susceptible to the inoculation of the parasite; and the flagellated form or leptomonad, which is found in the digestive tract of the vector insect (*Lutzomyia* in mucocutaneous disease) and in cultures. The typical morphology of leishmania, as found in vertebrates, is round or oval, usually with one extremity more rounded than the other, measuring 2–4 μm × 1.5–2.5 μm, with cytoplasm, nucleus, and blepharoplast or kinetoplast.

Epidemiology

Mucocutaneous leishmaniasis is predominantly a rural and jungle disease. It most often occurs in damp and forested regions. The disease can be contracted at any time of the year, but the risk is highest just after the rainy season. All ages and races, and both sexes are equally affected. Epidemics parallel the El Niño cycle.

Histopathology

In the ulcerous type, marked irregular acanthosis and sometimes pseudoepitheliomatous hyperplasia can be found. The dermis shows a dense infiltration of histiocytes, lymphocytes, and plasma cells. In new lesions some neutrophils are observed. Large Langhans giant cells or typical tubercles are occasionally seen. Numerous organisms are present (mostly in histiocytes), which are nonencapsulated and contain a nucleus and a paranucleus. Wright, Giemsa, and monoclonal antibody staining may be helpful in identifying the organisms. In patients with granulomatous infiltrates containing intracellular parasites within histiocytes, leishmaniasis is one of several diseases to be considered, including rhinoscleroma, histoplasmosis, granuloma inguinale, Chagas' disease, *Penicillium marneffei* infection, and toxoplasmosis. Touch smears stained with Giemsa

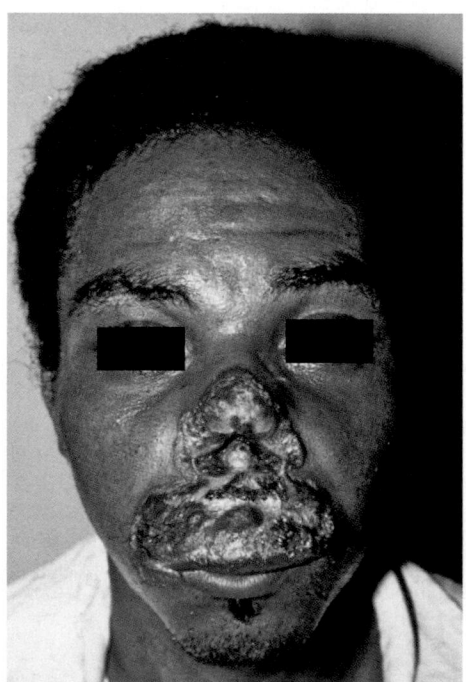

Fig. 20-7 Severe destructive mucocutaneous leishmaniasis. (Courtesy of Debra Kalter, MD)

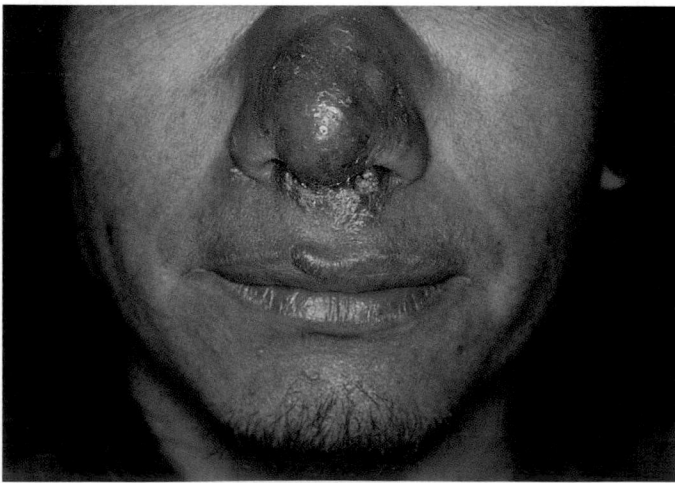

Fig. 20-6 Mucocutaneous leishmaniasis.

are helpful in many cases of cutaneous and mucocutaneous leishmaniasis.

Laboratory findings

Leishmania is demonstrated in the cutaneous and mucous membrane lesions by direct smears or cultures. In biopsy material stained with Wright stain, intracellular and extracellular organisms are seen with typical morphology of two chromatic structures: nucleus and parabasal body. In later mucosal lesions the scarcity of parasites makes identification difficult. The culture is done on NNN medium for leptomonads.

Prophylaxis

Although it is impractical to eliminate the insect vector, it is still the only valid measure for the control of this prevalent disease. Effective vaccines are not available.

Treatment

Treatment is the same as described for cutaneous leishmaniasis, except that antimony resistance is common in mucocutaneous disease. Combination therapy using antimonials with drugs such as rifampin or azithromycin, or adding immunomodulators such as IFN-γ, IL-2, or imiquimod may result in cure. Amphotericin B treatment may be necessary.

Visceral leishmaniasis (kala-azar, dumdum fever)

Clinical features

The earliest lesion is the cutaneous nodule or leishmanioma, which occurs at the site of the initial sandfly inoculation. Kala-azar, meaning "black fever," acquired its name because of the patchy macular darkening of the skin caused by deposits of melanin that develop in the later course of the disease. These patches are most marked over the forehead and temples, periorally, and on the mid-abdomen.

The primary target for the parasites is the reticuloendothelial system; the spleen, liver, bone marrow, and lymph nodes are attacked. The incubation period is 1–4 months. An intermittent fever, with temperatures ranging from 39° to 40°C (102–104°F), ushers in the disease. There are hepatosplenomegaly, agranulocytosis, anemia, and thrombocytopenia. Chills, fever, emaciation, weight loss, weakness, epistaxis, and purpura develop as the disease progresses. Susceptibility to secondary infection may produce pulmonary and gastrointestinal infection, ulcerations in the mouth (cancrum oris), and noma. Death occurs about 2 years from onset in untreated individuals.

Most infections are subclinical or asymptomatic. In patients with AIDS, papular and nodular skin lesions may occur. Dermatofibroma-type or Kaposi sarcoma-like brown to purple nodules are most commonly reported, although random biopsies of normal skin will reveal organisms; therefore, clinical correlation is necessary to attribute skin findings to Leishmania specifically.

Etiologic factors

L. donovani spp. donovani, infantum, and chagasi cause visceral leishmaniasis and are parasites of rodents, canines, and humans. They are nonflagellate oval organisms some 3 mm in diameter, known as Leishman–Donovan bodies. In the sandfly it is a leptomonad form with flagella.

Epidemiology

L.d. donovani causes visceral leishmaniasis in India, with the major reservoir being humans and the vector being Phlebotomus argentipes. L.d. infantum occurs in China, Africa, the Near East and Middle East, and the Mediterranean littoral, where the major reservoirs are dogs, and Phlebotomus perniciosus and Phlebotomus ariasi are the vectors of the Mediterranean type. American visceral leishmaniasis is caused by L. donovani chagasi and is transmitted by the sandfly Lutzomyia longipalpis. American visceral leishmaniasis principally affects domestic dogs, although explosive outbreaks of the human infection occur sporadically, when the number of L. longipalpis builds up to a high level in the presence of infected dogs. Canine visceral infections with L. infantum have been reported in foxhounds in various parts of the United States and Canada.

Diagnosis

Leishman–Donovan bodies may be present in the blood in individuals with kala-azar of India. Specimens for examination, in descending order of utility, include spleen pulp, sternal marrow, liver tissue, and exudate from lymph nodes. Culturing on NNN medium may also reveal the organisms.

Treatment

General supportive measures are essential. Pentavalent antimony has long been the drug of choice. In areas of drug resistance, amphotericin B is usually effective, but it is expensive and toxic, and requires intravenous administration. Miltefosine is an oral alkyl-phosphocholine analog that has proven as effective as amphotericin B in some trials. It is often used to treat visceral disease in India and Ethiopia. Mixed infections involving both Leishmania and Trypanosoma cruzi are becoming increasingly common in Central and South America because of overlapping endemic areas. Amiodarone has been used as an unconventional antiparasitic drug in this setting in addition to standard therapy.

Post-kala-azar dermal leishmaniasis

In kala-azar, the leishmanoid (amastigote) forms may be widely distributed throughout apparently normal skin. During and after recovery from the disease, a special form of dermal leishmaniasis known as post-kala-azar dermal leishmaniasis appears. This condition appears during or shortly after treatment in the African form, but its appearance may be delayed up to 10 years after treatment in the Indian form. It follows the treatment of visceral leishmaniasis in 50% of Sudanese patients and 5–10% of those seen in India. There are two constituents of the eruption: a macular, depigmented eruption found mainly on the face, arms, and upper part of the trunk; and a warty, papular eruption in which amastigotes can be found. Because it may persist for up to 20 years, these patients may act as a chronic reservoir of infection. This condition closely resembles Hansen's disease. High concentrations of IL-10 in the blood of visceral leishmaniasis patients predict those who will be affected by post-kala-azar dermal leishmaniaisis. Miltefosine may become the drug of choice.

Viscerotropic leishmaniasis

Twelve soldiers developed systemic infection with L. tropica while fighting in Operation Desert Storm in Saudi Arabia. None had symptoms of kala-azar, but most had fever, fatigue, malaise, cough, diarrhea, or abdominal pain. None had cutaneous disease. Diagnostic tests yielded positive results on bone marrow aspiration; lymph node involvement was also documented. Treatment with sodium stibogluconate led to improvement.

Ameen M: Cutaneous leishmaniasis: therapeutic strategies and future directions. Expert Opin Pharmacother 2007; 8(16):2689–2699.

Bari AU, et al: Many faces of cutaneous leishmaniasis. Indian J Dermatol Venereol Leprol 2008; 74(1):23–27.

Berman JJ: Treatment of leishmaniasis with miltefosine: 2008 status. Expert Opin Drug Metab Toxicol 2008; 4(9):1209–1216.

Clem A: A current perspective on leishmaniasis. J Glob Infect Dis 2010 May; 2(2):124–126.

González U, et al: Designing and reporting clinical trials on treatments for cutaneous leishmaniasis. Clin Infect Dis 2010 Aug 15; 51(4):409–419.

Kassi M, et al: Vector control in cutaneous leishmaniasis of the Old World: a review of literature. Dermatol Online J 2008; 14(6):1.

Krolewiecki AJ, et al: A randomized clinical trial comparing oral azithromycin and meglumine antimoniate for the treatment of American cutaneous leishmaniasis caused by *Leishmania (Viannia) braziliensis*. Am J Trop Med Hyg 2007; 77(4):640–646.

Minodier P, et al: Cutaneous leishmaniasis treatment. Travel Med Infect Dis 2007; 5(3):150–158.

Monsel G, et al: Recent developments in dermatological syndromes in returning travelers. Curr Opin Infect Dis 2008; 21(5):495–499.

Mosleh IM, et al: Efficacy of a weekly cryotherapy regimen to treat *Leishmania major* cutaneous leishmaniasis. J Am Acad Dermatol 2008 Apr; 58(4):617–624.

Nilforoushzadeh MA, et al: Successful treatment of lupoid cutaneous leishmaniasis with Glucantime and topical trichloroacetic acid (a case report). Korean J Parasitol 2008; 46(3):175–177.

Okwor I, et al: Persistent parasites and immunologic memory in cutaneous leishmaniasis: implications for vaccine designs and vaccination strategies. Immunol Res 2008; 41(2):123–136.

Paniz-Mondolfi AE, et al: Concurrent Chagas' disease and borderline disseminated cutaneous leishmaniasis: the role of amiodarone as an antitrypanosomatidae drug. Ther Clin Risk Manag 2008; 4(3):659–663.

Ramesh V, et al: Oral miltefosine in the treatment of post-kala-azar dermal leishmaniasis. Clin Exp Dermatol 2008; 33(1):103–105.

Ready PD: Leishmaniasis emergence and climate change. Rev Sci Tech 2008; 27(2):399–412.

Reithinger R, et al: Cutaneous leishmaniasis. Lancet Infect Dis 2007; 7(9):581–596.

Saleem K, et al: Comparison of oral itraconazole and intramuscular meglumine antimoniate in the treatment of cutaneous leishmaniasis. J Coll Physicians Surg Pak 2007; 17(12):713–716.

Shahbazi F, et al: Evaluation of PCR assay in diagnosis and identification of cutaneous leishmaniasis: a comparison with the parasitological methods. Parasitol Res 2008; 103(5):1159–1162.

Tripathi P, et al: Immune response to leishmania: paradox rather than paradigm. FEMS Immunol Med Microbiol 2007; 51(2):229–242.

Tuon FF, et al: Treatment of New World cutaneous leishmaniasis—a systematic review with a meta-analysis. Int J Dermatol 2008; 47(2):109–124.

van der Meide WF, et al: Treatment assessment by monitoring parasite load in skin biopsies from patients with cutaneous leishmaniasis, using quantitative nucleic acid sequence-based amplification. Clin Exp Dermatol 2008; 33(4):394–399.

Vélez I, et al: Efficacy of miltefosine for the treatment of American cutaneous leishmaniasis. Am J Trop Med Hyg 2010 Aug; 83(2):351–356.

Wright NA, et al: Cutaneous leishmaniasis in Texas: a northern spread of endemic areas. J Am Acad Dermatol 2008; 58(4):650–652.

Zeegelaar JE, et al: Imported tropical infectious ulcers in travelers. Am J Clin Dermatol 2008; 9(4):219–232.

Ziaei H, et al: Distribution frequency of pathogenic bacteria isolated from cutaneous leishmaniasis lesions. Korean J Parasitol 2008; 46(3):191–193.

Human trypanosomiasis

Three species of trypanosome are pathogenic to humans: *Trypanosoma gambiense* and *Trypanosoma rhodesiense* in Africa, and *Trypanosoma cruzi* in America. The skin manifestations are usually observed in the earlier stages of the disease as evanescent erythema, erythema multiforme, and edema, especially angioedema.

In the early stage of African trypanosomiasis, a trypanosome chancre may occur at the site of a tsetse fly bite. Then erythema with circumscribed swellings of angioedema, enlargement of the lymph nodes, fever, malaise, headache, and joint pains ensue. In the West African (Gambian) form, the illness is chronic, lasting several years, with progressive deterioration,

whereas the East African (Rhodesian) form is an acute illness, with a stormy, fatal course of weeks to months. The Rhodesian form is more often associated with cutaneous signs. Annular or deep erythema nodosum-like lesions are frequent manifestations (Fig. 20-8). Lymphadenopathy is generalized, but frequently there is a pronounced enlargement of the posterior cervical group (Winterbottom's sign).

In American trypanosomiasis (Chagas' disease), similar changes take place in the skin. The reduviid bug (kissing bug, assassin bug) (Fig. 20-9) usually bites at night, frequently at mucocutaneous junctions, where the bug's infected feces are deposited when it feeds. The unsuspecting sleeping person rubs the feces into the bite and becomes infected. If the bite of the infected bug occurs near the eye, Romana's sign develops; this consists of unilateral conjunctivitis and edema of the eyelids, with an ulceration or chagoma in the area. The bite of a "kissing bug" becomes markedly swollen and red, whether trypanosomes are involved or not. Acute Chagas' disease is usually a mild illness consisting of fever, malaise, edema of the face and lower extremities, and generalized lymphadenopathy. Skin lesions occurring in this phase include nodules at the site of inoculation, disseminated nodules, or morbilliform and urticarial lesions. In chronic Chagas' disease, which occurs in 10–30% of infected persons years to decades later, the heart (myocarditis, arrhythmias, thromboembolism, and cardiac failure) and the gastrointestinal system (megaesophagus and megacolon) are the most commonly involved organs. During the remaining infected but asymptomatic indeterminate phase, patients may transmit the disease through transfusion. When such patients become immunosuppressed

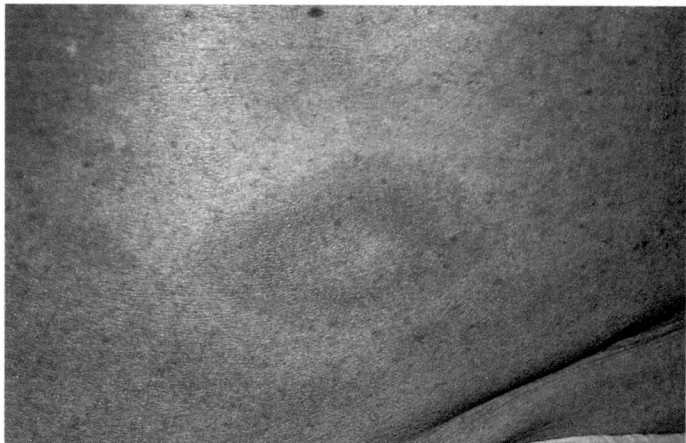

Fig. 20-8 African trypanosomiasis.

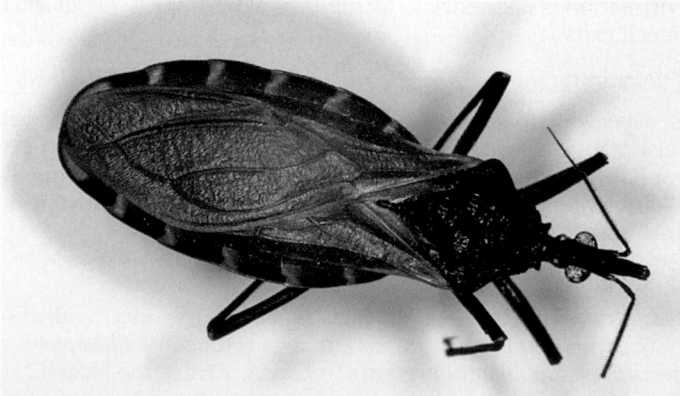

Fig. 20-9 Triatome reduviid bug.

(with AIDS or organ transplantation), reactivation skin lesions may occur.

Rhodesian trypanosomiasis is endemic among the cattle-raising tribes of East Africa, with the savannah habitat of the vectors determining its geographic distribution. Wild game and livestock are reservoir hosts, in addition to humans. The tsetse fly, *Glossina morsitans*, is the principal vector.

For Gambian trypanosomiasis, humans are the only vertebrate host and the palpalis group of tsetse flies is the invertebrate host. These flies are found close to the water, and their fastidious biologic requirements restrict their distribution, and thus that of the disease. Incidence is seasonal, with humidity and temperature being determining factors. The highest incidence is in males aged 20–40 years in tropical areas of West and Central Africa.

Chagas' disease is prevalent in Central and South America from the US to Argentina and Chile; the highest incidence is in Venezuela, Brazil, Uruguay, Paraguay, and Argentina. Approximately 29% of all male deaths in the 29–44-year-old age group in Brazil are ascribed to Chagas' disease.

Before CNS involvement has occurred in the Rhodesian form, suramin, a complex, non-metal-containing, organic compound, is the treatment of choice. When the CNS is involved, melarsoprol is the drug of choice. Pentamidine isethionate is the drug of choice for the Gambian disease. Eflornithine appears to be a good alternative to melarsoprol for second-stage West African trypanosomiasis. For American trypanosomiasis, treatment is of limited efficacy. Nifurtimox and benznidazole clear the parasitemia and reduce the severity of the acute illness. There is a high incidence of adverse effects, however. Although benznidazole reduces parasite load during the acute phase, it does not prevent chronic cardiac lesions. Ruthenium complexation improves bioavailability of benznidazole and has the potential to improve outcomes. Conservative treatment is the typical approach to the patient with congestive heart failure from Chagas myocarditis, but recent data suggest that clomipramine, a tricyclic antidepressant that inhibits *Trypanosoma cruzi*'s trypanothione reductase, improves the course of cardiac disease in animal models. Gastrointestinal complications may be treated surgically.

Bazán PC, et al: Chemotherapy of chronic indeterminate Chagas disease: a novel approach to treatment. Parasitol Res 2008; 103(3):663–669.

de Souza W: Trypanosomiasis and leishmaniasis "recent development in the chemotherapy of infectious diseases caused by parasitic protozoa". Curr Pharm Des 2008; 14(9):821.

LaForgia MP, et al: Cutaneous manifestations of reactivation of Chagas' disease in a renal transplant patient. Arch Dermatol 2003; 139:104.

McGovern TW, et al: Cutaneous manifestations of African trypanosomiasis. Arch Dermatol 1995; 131:1178.

Class Sporozoa

Toxoplasmosis

Toxoplasmosis is a zoonosis caused by a parasitic protozoan, *Toxoplasma gondii*. Infection may be either congenital or acquired. Congenital infection occurs from placental transmission. Abortion or stillbirth may result. However, a full-term child delivered to an infected mother may have a triad of hydrocephalus, chorioretinitis, and cerebral calcification. In addition, there may be hepatosplenomegaly and jaundice. Skin changes in toxoplasmosis are rare and clinically nonspecific.

In congenital toxoplasmosis, macular and hemorrhagic eruptions predominate. Blueberry muffin lesions, reflecting dermatoerythropoiesis, may be seen. Occasionally, abnormal hair growth and exfoliative dermatitis have also been observed. The differential diagnosis of congenital toxoplasmosis is the TORCH syndrome (toxoplasmosis, rubella, cytomegalovirus, and herpes simplex). In acquired toxoplasmosis, early skin manifestations consist of cutaneous and subcutaneous nodules, and macular, papular, and hemorrhagic eruptions. These may be followed by scarlatiniform desquamation, eruptions mimicking roseola, erythema multiforme, dermatomyositis or lichen planus, as well as exfoliative dermatitis. As a rule, the exanthem is accompanied by high fever and general malaise.

Diagnosis of acquired toxoplasmosis is of special importance to three groups of adults: healthy pregnant women concerned about recent exposure; adults with lymphadenopathy, fever, and myalgia, who might have some other serious disease, such as lymphoma; and immunocompromised persons, such as patients with AIDS, in whom toxoplasmosis might be fatal. It is the most common cause of focal encephalitis in patients with AIDS and this may be accompanied by a widespread papular eruption.

T. gondii is a crescent-shaped, oval, or round protozoan that can infect any mammalian or avian cell. The disease is often acquired through contact with animals, particularly cats. Reservoirs of infection have been reported in dogs, cats, cattle, sheep, pigs, rabbits, rats, pigeons, and chickens. The two major routes of transmission of *T. gondii* in humans are oral and congenital. Meats consumed by humans may contain tissue cysts, thus serving as a source of infection when eaten raw or undercooked. There is no evidence of direct human-to-human transmission, other than from mother to fetus.

The diagnosis cannot be made on clinical grounds alone. It may be established by isolation of *T. gondii*; demonstration of the protozoa in tissue sections, smears, or body fluids by Wright or Giemsa stain; characteristic lymph node histology; and serologic methods. In the setting of bone marrow transplantation, the organism has caused interface dermatitis, creating the potential for misdiagnosis as graft versus host disease.

A combination of pyrimethamine (Daraprim) and sulfadiazine acts synergistically and forms an effective treatment. Dosages and total treatment time vary according to the age and immunologic competence of the infected patient.

Sra KK, et al: Treatment of protozoan infections. Dermatol Ther 2004; 17(6):513–516.

Vidal CI, et al: Cutaneous toxoplasmosis histologically mimicking graft-versus-host disease. Am J Dermatopathol 2008; 30(5):492–493.

PHYLUM CNIDARIA

The cnidarians include the jellyfish, hydroids, Portuguese man-of-war, corals, and sea anemones. These are all radial marine animals, living mostly in ocean water. When a swimmer's skin contacts these organisms, they release a toxin through small spicules.

Portuguese man-of-war dermatitis

Stings by the Portuguese man-of-war (*Physalia physalis* in the Atlantic, or the much smaller *Physalia utriculus* or "bluebottle" in the Pacific) are characterized by linear lesions that are erythematous, urticarial, and even hemorrhagic. The forearms, sides of the trunk, thighs, and feet are common sites of involvement. The usual local manifestation is sharp, stinging, and intense pain. Internally, there may be severe dyspnea, prostration, nausea, abdominal cramps, lacrimation, and muscular pains. Death may occur if the areas stung are large in relation to the patient's size.

The fluid of the nematocysts contains toxin that is carried into the victim through barbs along the tentacle. The venom is a neurotoxic poison that can produce marked cardiac changes. Each Portuguese man-of-war is a colony of symbiotic organisms consisting of a blue to red float or pneumatophore with a gas gland, several gastrozooids measuring 1–20 mm, reproductive polyps, and the fishing tentacles bearing the nematocysts from which the barbs are ejected. The hydroid is found most frequently along the southeastern Florida coastline and in the Gulf of Mexico, and on windward coasts throughout the mid-Pacific and South Pacific. Safe Sea, a barrier cream, has been reported as being effective at preventing jellyfish stings off the coast of Florida, but studies of barrier creams in general have been mixed.

Jellyfish dermatitis

This produces lesions similar to those of the Portuguese man-of-war, except that the lesions are not so linear (Fig. 20-10). Immediate allergic reactions occur infrequently as urticaria, angioedema, or anaphylaxis. Delayed and persistent lesions also rarely occur.

The Australian sea wasp, *Chironex fleckeri*, which is colorless and transparent, is the most dangerous of all, with a sting that is often fatal. Another sea wasp, *Carybdea marsupialis*, much less dangerous, occurs in the Caribbean. *Rhopilema nomadica*, common in the Mediterranean, has been reported to cause severe delayed dermatitis.

Seabather's eruption is an acute dermatitis that begins a few hours after bathing in the waters along the coast of the Atlantic. It affects covered areas of the body as cnidarian larvae become entrapped under the bathing suit and the nematocyst releases its toxin because of external pressure. Thus, the buttocks and waist are affected primarily, with the breast also involved in women (Fig. 20-11). Erythematous macules and papules appear and may develop into pustules or vesicles. Urticarial plaques are also present in a smaller number of patients. Crops of new lesions may occur for up to 72 h, and the eruption persists for 10–14 days on average. It is quite pruritic.

Outbreaks in Florida are usually caused by larvae of the thimble jellyfish, *Linuche unguiculata*, which patients report as "black dots" in the water or their bathing suits. The larvae of the sea anemone, *Edwardstella lineata*, caused one epidemic of seabather's eruption in Long Island, New York. This organism also has nematocysts; thus, the mechanism of the eruption is the same as with the jellyfish-induced eruption. It is likely that different cnidarian envenomations in different waters produce a similar clinical picture. Other reports focus on spring plants, dinoflagellates, protozoans, or crustaceans as potential causes. Since trapping of cnidarian larvae with their nematocysts or other toxic or irritant substances under the bathing suit

accounts for this eruption, seabathers who take off their bathing suit and shower soon after leaving the water may limit it.

Hydroid, sea anemone, and coral dermatitis

Patients contacting the small marine hydroid, *Halecium*, may develop a dermatitis. The organism grows as a 1 cm-thick coat of moss on the submerged portions of vessels or pilings. Sea anemones (Fig. 20-12) produce reactions similar to those from jellyfish and hydroids. Coral cuts (Fig. 20-13) are injuries caused by the exoskeleton of the corals, *Milleporina*. They have a reputation for becoming inflamed and infected, and for delayed healing. The combination of implantation of fragments of coral skeleton and infection (since the cuts occur most commonly on the feet) probably accounts almost entirely for these symptoms. Detoxification as soon as possible after the injury is advisable for all these types of sting or cut.

Treatment of stings and cuts

Hot water immersion may be an effective remedy for many stings, but scald injuries must be avoided. Undischarged

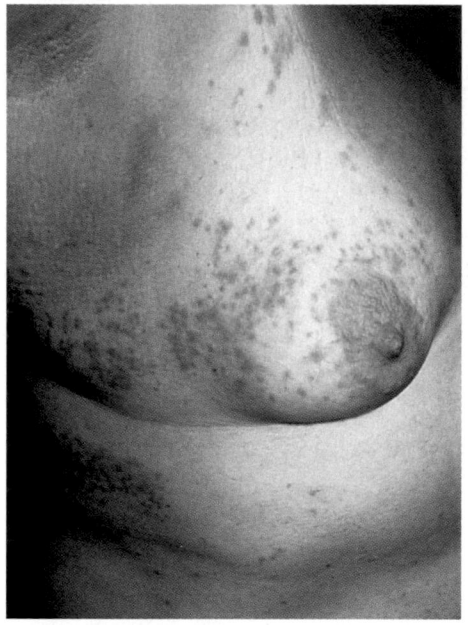

Fig. 20-11 Seabather's eruption.

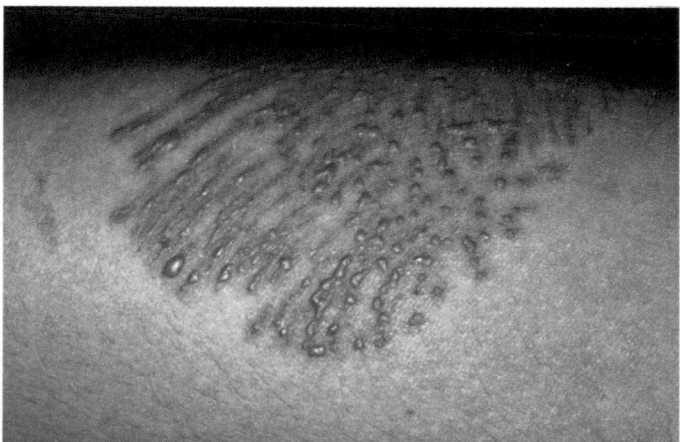

Fig. 20-10 Jellyfish sting. (Courtesy of Anthony Slagel, MD)

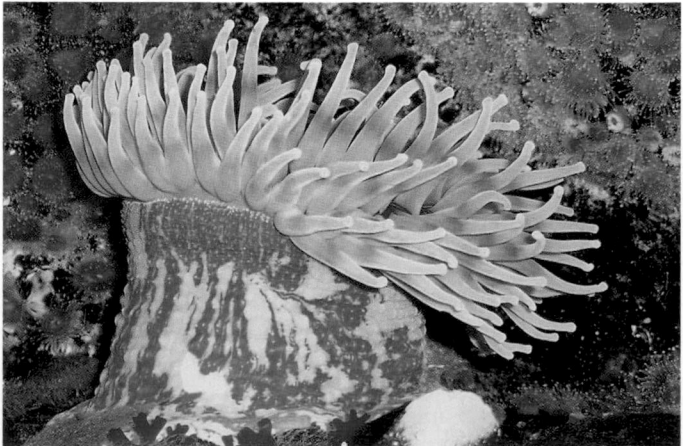

Fig. 20-12 Sea anemone.

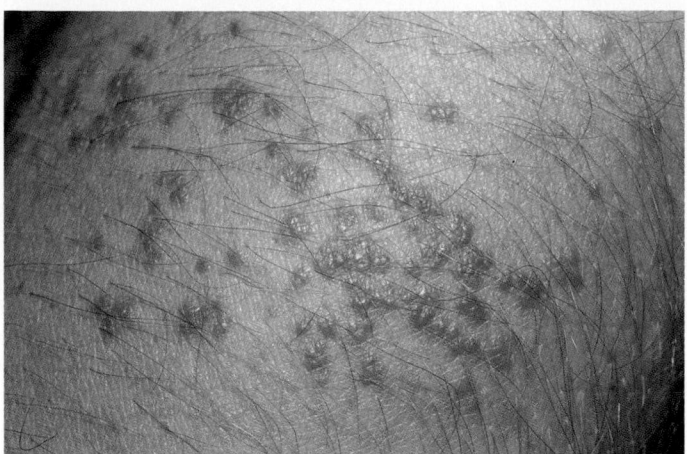

Fig. 20-13 Coral cuts. (Courtesy of Curt Samlaska, MD)

nematocytes may be removed with sea water, but never with fresh water, as this may cause them to discharge. Pacific *Chironex* (box jellyfish) nematocytes should always be inactivated with 5% acetic acid (vinegar) when it is available, but Pacific *Physalia* (bluebottle) nematocytes may discharge on contact with vinegar. Large visible tentacles may be removed with forceps in a double-gloved hand. Remaining nematocysts may be removed by applying a layer of shaving cream and shaving the area gently. Meat tenderizer may cause tissue damage and has been shown to be no better than placebo in some studies.

Pressure dressings and abrasion will worsen the envenomation. Topical anesthetics or steroids may be applied after decontamination. Systemic reactions may occur through either large amounts of venom or a previously sensitizing exposure from which anaphylaxis may result, and systemic treatment with epinephrine, antihistamines, or corticosteroids may be needed. Specific antivenin is available for the box jellyfish, *Chironex fleckeri*. This should be administered intravenously to limit myonecrosis. $MgSO_4$ may also be of value in the setting of box jellyfish envenomation. Recurrent jellyfish reactions have shown partial responses to tacrolimus ointment 0.1%.

Sponges and bristleworms

Sponges have horny spicules of silicon dioxide and calcium carbonate. Some sponges produce dermal irritants, such as halitoxin and okadaic acid, and others may be colonized by Cnidaria. Allergic or irritant reactions may result. Bristleworms may also produce stinging. All of these may be treated by first using adhesive tape to remove the spicules, then applying vinegar soaks, as described above, and finally, applying topical corticosteroid agents.

Sea urchin injuries

Puncture wounds inflicted by the brittle, fragile spines of sea urchins, mainly of genus *Diadema* or *Echinothrix*, are stained blue–black by the black spines and may contain fragments of the spines. The spines consist of calcium carbonate crystals, which most commonly induce an irritant reaction with pain and inflammation of several days' duration. Foreign-body or sarcoid-like granulomas may develop, as may a vesicular hypersensitivity reaction, 10 days after exposure. Injuries by spines of the genus *Tripneustes* have been reported to cause fatal envenomation, but this genus is not found on US coasts.

Starfish also have thorny spines that can sting and burn if they are stepped on or handled. Several different types of stinging fish also produce puncture wounds. Stingrays, scorpionfish, stonefish, catfish, and weaverfish may cause such envenomations.

These wounds should be immersed in nonscalding water (45°C [113°F]) for 30–90 min or until the pain subsides. Calcified fragments may be visible on x-ray evaluation, with fluoroscopy guiding extraction of spines, especially on the hands and feet. Sea urchin spines have been effectively removed using the erbium:YAG laser. Debridement and possibly antibiotic therapy for deep puncture wounds of the hands and feet are recommended. There is a specific antivenin for stonefish stings.

Seaweed dermatitis

Although this is caused by a marine alga and not by an animal, it deserves mention with other problems associated with swimming or wading. The dermatitis occurs 3–8 h after the individual emerges from the ocean. The distribution is in parts covered by a bathing suit: scrotum, penis, perineum, and perianal area. The dermatitis is caused by a marine plant, *Lyngbya majuscula* Gomont. It has been observed only in bathers swimming off the windward shore of Oahu, Hawaii. Seabather's eruption, clamdigger's itch, and swimmer's itch must be differentiated from seaweed dermatitis caused by marine algae. Prophylaxis is achieved by refraining from swimming in waters that are turbid with such algae. Swimmers should shower within 5 min of swimming. Active treatment in severe cases is the same as for acute burns.

Dogger Bank itch

Dogger Bank itch is an eczematous dermatitis caused by the sea chervil, *Alcyonidium hirsutum*, a seaweed-like animal colony. These sea mosses or sea mats are found on the Dogger Bank, an immense shelflike elevation under the North Sea between Scotland and Denmark.

Boulware DR: A randomized, controlled field trial for the prevention of jellyfish stings with a topical sting inhibitor. J Travel Med 2006; 13(3):166–171.

Burroughs R, et al: Aquatic antagonists: sea urchin dermatitis. Cutis 2005; 76(1):18–20.

Burnett JW: Lack of efficacy of a combination sunblock and "jellyfish sting inhibitor" topical preparation against *Physalia* sting. Dermatitis 2005; 16(3):151.

Elston DM: Aquatic antagonists: sea anemone dermatitis. Cutis 2006; 78(1):31–32.

Elston DM: Aquatic antagonists: sponge dermatitis. Cutis 2007; 80(4):279–280.

Haddad V Jr, et al: Tropical dermatology: marine and aquatic dermatology. J Am Acad Dermatol 2009 Nov; 61(5):733–735.

Rallis E, et al: Recurrent dermatitis after solitary envenomation by jellyfish partially responded to tacrolimus ointment 0.1%. J Eur Acad Dermatol Venereol 2007; 21(9):1287–1288.

Yoder JS, et al: Surveillance for waterborne disease and outbreaks associated with recreational water use and other aquatic facility-associated health events—United States, 2005–2006. MMWR Surveill Summ 2008; 57(9):1–29.

PHYLUM PLATYHELMINTHES

Phylum Platyhelminthes includes the flatworms, of which two classes, trematodes and cestodes, are parasitic to humans. The trematodes, or blood flukes, parasitize human skin or internal organs. The cestodes are segmented, ribbon-shaped flatworms that inhabit the intestinal tract as adults and involve the subcutaneous tissue, heart, muscle, and eye in the larval form. This is encased in a sac that eventually becomes calcified.

Class Trematoda

Schistosome cercarial dermatitis

Cercarial dermatitis is a severely pruritic, widespread, papular dermatitis caused by cercariae of schistosomes for which humans are not hosts (the usual animal hosts are waterfowl and rodents, such as muskrats).

The eggs in the excreta of these animals, when deposited in water, hatch into swimming miracidia. These enter a snail, where further development occurs. From the snail, the free-swimming cercariae emerge to invade human skin on accidental contact. The swimming, colorless, multicellular organisms are a little less than a millimeter long. Exposure to cercariae occurs when a person swims or, more often, wades in water containing them. They attack by burrowing into the skin, where they die. The species that causes this eruption cannot enter the bloodstream or deeper tissues.

After coming out of the water, the bather begins to itch and a transient erythematous eruption appears, but after a few hours, the eruption subsides, together with the itching. Then, after a quiescent period of 10–15 h, the symptoms recur, and erythematous macules and papules develop throughout the exposed parts that were in the water (Fig. 20-14). After several days the dermatitis heals spontaneously. There are two types: the freshwater swimmer's itch, and the saltwater marine dermatitis or clam digger's itch. It is not communicable.

Various genera and species of organism have been reported from various locations worldwide. An outbreak of cercarial dermatitis was reported from Delaware in 1991 in which the avian schistosome, *Microbilharzia variglandis*, was implicated as the causative organism. *Schistosoma spindale* cercaria caused a recent epidemic in southern Thailand.

Thoroughly washing, then drying with a towel after exposure can prevent the disease. Rubbing with alcohol is an additional preventive measure advocated by some. Snail populations can be controlled or waterfowl may be treated with medicated feedcorn to destroy the adult schistosomes and prevent outbreaks of swimmer's itch.

Visceral schistosomiasis (bilharziasis)

The cutaneous manifestation of schistosomiasis may begin with mild itching and a papular dermatitis of the feet and other parts after swimming in polluted streams containing cercariae. The types of schistosome causing this disease can penetrate into the bloodstream and eventually inhabit the venous system, draining the urinary bladder (*Schistosoma haematobium*) or the intestines (*Schistosoma mansoni* or *Schistosoma japonicum*). After an asymptomatic incubation period, there may be a sudden illness with fever and chills, pneumonitis, and eosinophilia. Petechial hemorrhages may occur.

Cutaneous schistosomal granulomas most frequently involve the genitalia, perineum, and buttocks. The eggs of *S. haematobium* or *S. mansoni* (Fig. 20-15) usually cause these bilharziomas. Vegetating, soft, cauliflower-shaped masses, fistulous tracts, and extensive hard masses occur; these are riddled by sinuses that exude a seropurulent discharge with a characteristic odor. Phagedenic ulcerations and pseudoelephantiasis of the scrotum, penis, or labia are sometimes encountered. Histologically, the nodules contain bilharzial ova undergoing degeneration, with calcification and a surrounding cellular reaction of histiocytes, eosinophils, and occasional giant cells. In some cases, eventual malignant changes have been noted in chronic lesions. Animal studies have shown a moderate Th1 response to parasite antigens in most tissues, but a strong Th2 response that propagates fibrogenesis within the liver. Infrequently, ectopic or extragenital lesions may occur, mainly on the trunk. This is a papular eruption tending to group in plaques and become darkly pigmented and scaly. A severe urticarial eruption known as urticarial fever or Katayama fever is frequently present along with an *S. japonicum* infection; it occurs with the beginning of oviposition, 4–8 weeks after infection. This condition occurs mainly in China, Japan, and the Philippines. In addition to the urticaria, fever, malaise, abdominal cramps, arthritis, and liver and spleen involvement are seen. This is felt to be a serum sickness-like reaction.

Preventive measures include reducing infection sources, preventing contamination by human excreta of snail-bearing waters, control of snail hosts, and avoiding exposure to cercaria-infested waters. Prophylactic measures are constantly sought to control one of the world's worst parasitic diseases, but as yet none has been found to be practical. For both *S. haematobium* and *S. mansoni*, praziquantel (Biltricide), 40 mg/kg orally for each of two treatments in 1 day, is the treatment of choice. *S. japonicum* treatment requires 60 mg/kg in three doses in 1 day. Schistosomicides exhibit toxicity for the host as well as for the parasite, and the risk of undesirable side effects may be enhanced by concomitant cardiac, renal, or hepatosplenic disease.

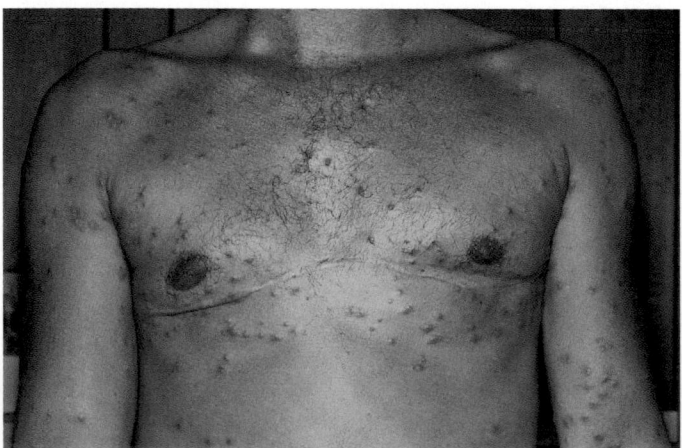

Fig. 20-14 Swimmer's itch.

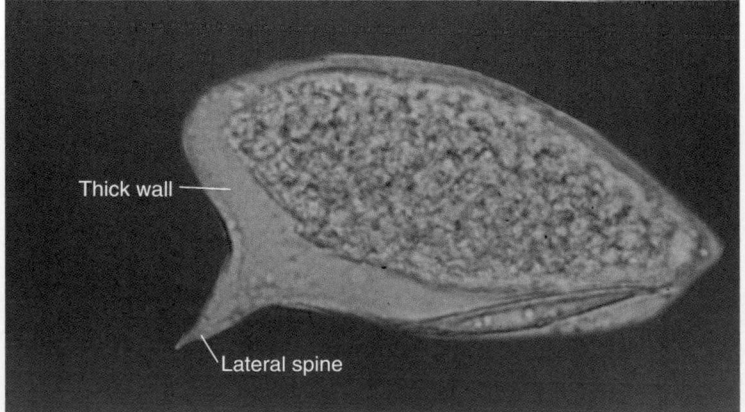

Fig. 20-15 Ova of *S. Mansoni* are characterized by a thick chitinous wall and a lateral spine.

Elston DM: *Schistosoma japonicum.* Cutis 2004; 73:299.

Salvana EM, et al: Schistosomiasis in travelers and immigrants. Curr Infect Dis Rep 2008; 10(1):42–49.

Wilson MS, et al: Immunopathology of schistosomiasis. Immunol Cell Biol 2007; 85(2):148–154.

Cysticercosis cutis

The natural intermediate host of the pork tapeworm, *Taenia solium*, is the pig, but under some circumstances humans act in this role. The larval stage of *T. solium* is *Cysticercus cellulosae*. Infection takes place by the ingestion of food contaminated with the eggs, or by reverse peristalsis of eggs or proglottides from the intestine to the stomach. Here the eggs hatch, freeing the oncospheres. These enter the general circulation and form cysts in various parts of the body, such as striated muscles, brain, eye, heart, and lung.

In the subcutaneous tissues, the lesions are usually painless nodules that contain cysticerci. They are more or less stationary, usually numerous, and often calcified, and are therefore demonstrable radiographically. Pain and ulceration may accompany the lesions. The disease is most prevalent in countries in which pigs feed on human feces. It may be confused with gumma, lipoma, and epithelioma. A positive diagnosis is established solely by incision and examination of the interior of the calcified tumor, where the parasite will be found. Fine needle aspiration has also been used to establish the diagnosis.

Albendazole or praziquantel is effective; however, the status of the CNS, spinal, and ocular involvement needs to be thoroughly assessed prior to treatment. The length of therapy and use of concomitant corticosteroids depend upon the location of the cysts. None of the regimens clears the calcified parasites, however, which need to be surgically removed.

Handa U, et al: Fine needle aspiration in the diagnosis of subcutaneous cysticercosis. Diagn Cytopathol 2008; 36(3):183–187.

Uthida-Tanaka AM, et al: Subcutaneous and cerebral cysticercosis. J Am Acad Dermatol 2004; 50(2 Suppl):S14–S17.

Sparganosis

Sparganosis is caused by the larva of the tapeworm *Spirometra*. The adult tapeworm lives in the intestines of dogs and cats. This is a rare tissue infection occurring in two forms. Application sparganosis occurs when an ulcer or infected eye is poulticed with the flesh of an infected intermediate host (such poultices are frequently used in the Orient). The larvae become encased in small nodules in the infected tissue. Ingestion sparganosis occurs when humans ingest inadequately cooked meat, such as snake or frog, or when a person drinks water that is contaminated with *Cyclops*, which is infected with plerocercoid larvae. One or two slightly pruritic or painful nodules may form in the subcutaneous tissue or on the trunk, breast, genitalia, or extremities. Cerebral disease may also occur. Diagnosis is usually made via excision of the nodule, although noninvasive imaging has also been used.

Humans are the accidental intermediate host of the *Sparganum*, which is the alternative name for the plerocercoid larva. Treatment is surgical removal or ethanol injection of the infected nodules (Fig. 20-16). This may be difficult because of the swelling and extensive vascularity.

Kim SH, et al: Scrotal sparganosis: with an emphasis on ultrasonographic findings. Urology 2008; 71(2):351.e11–12.

Moon HG, et al: Breast sparganosis presenting as a breast mass with vague migrating pain. J Am Coll Surg 2008; 207(2):292.

Sarukawa S, et al: Case of subcutaneous sparganosis: use of imaging in definitive preoperative diagnosis. J Dermatol 2007; 34(9):654–657.

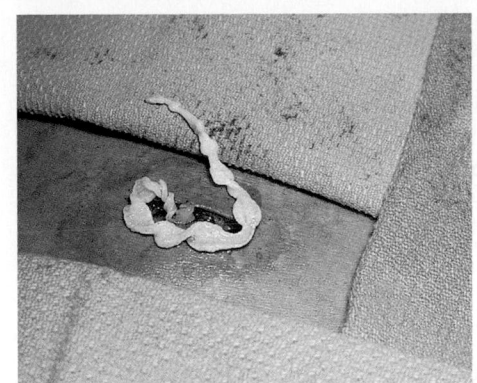

Fig. 20-16 Sparganosis.

Echinococcosis

Echinococcosis is also known as hydatid disease. In humans, infection is produced by the ova reaching the mouth from the hands, in food, or from containers soiled by ova-contaminated feces from an infected dog. This leads to *Echinococcus granulosus* infestation of the liver and the lungs. Soft, fluctuating, semitranslucent, cystic tumors may occur in the skin, sometimes in the supraumbilical area as fistulas from underlying liver involvement. These tumors become fibrotic or calcified after the death of the larva. Eosinophilia, intractable urticaria and pruritus, and even acute generalized exanthematous pustulosis may be present. Such reactive findings may be present as skin manifestations of many of the helminthic infections, including other types of tapeworm. The treatment is excision, with care being taken to avoid rupturing the cyst. Albendazole combined with percutaneous drainage may also be used. *Hymenolepis nana* is a cosmopolitan dwarf tapeworm endemic in the tropics, which may cause a treatment-resistant pruritic papular eruption associated with eosinophilia. Stool specimens for ova and parasites are definitive and praziquantel is curative.

Baldi A, et al: Echinococcal cysts with primary cutaneous localization. Br J Dermatol 2002; 147:807.

Cannistraci C, et al: Acute generalized exanthematous pustulosis in cystic echinococcosis. Br J Dermatol 2003; 148:1245.

Di Lernia V, et al: Skin eruption associated with *Hymenolepis nana* infection. Int J Dermatol 2004; 43:357.

PHYLUM ANNELIDA

Leeches

Leeches, of the class Hirudinea, are of marine, freshwater, or terrestrial types. After attaching to the skin, they secrete an anticoagulant, hirudin, and then engorge themselves with blood. Local symptoms at the site of the bite may include bullae, hemorrhage, pruritus, whealing, necrosis, or ulceration. Allergic reactions, including anaphylaxis, may result. Leeches may be removed by applying salt, alcohol, or vinegar, or by use of a match flame. Bleeding may then be stopped by direct pressure or by applying a styptic pencil to the site.

Leeches may be used medicinally to salvage tissue flaps that are threatened by venous congestion. However, *Aeromonas* infection, anetoderma, and pseudolymphoma may be complications of their attachment.

Abdelgabar AM, et al: The return of the leech. Int J Clin Pract 2003; 57:103.

Haycox CL, et al: Indications and complications of medicinal leech therapy. J Am Acad Dermatol 1995; 33:1053.

Ouderkirk JP, et al: *Aeromonas* meningitis complicating medicinal leech therapy. Clin Infect Dis 2004; 38:e36.

PHYLUM NEMATHELMINTHES

Phylum Nemathelminthes includes the roundworms, both free-living and parasitic forms. Multiplication is usually outside the host. Both the larval and adult stages may infect humans.

Class Nematoda

Enterobiasis (pinworm infection, seatworm infection, oxyuriasis)

The chief symptom of pinworm infestation, which occurs most frequently in children, is nocturnal pruritus ani. There is intense itching accompanied by excoriations of the anus, perineum, and pubic area. The vagina may become infested with the gravid pinworms. A pruritic papular dermatosis of the trunk and extremities may be observed infrequently. Restlessness, insomnia, enuresis, and irritability are but a few of the many symptoms ascribed to this exceedingly common infestation.

Oxyuriasis is caused by the roundworm *Enterobius vermicularis*, which may infest the small intestines, cecum, and large intestine of humans. The worms, especially gravid ones, migrate toward the rectum and at night emerge to the perianal and perineal regions to deposit thousands of ova; then the worm dries and dies outside the intestine. These ova are then carried back to the mouth of the host on the hands. The larvae hatch in the duodenum and migrate into the jejunum and ileum, where they reach maturity. Fertilization occurs in the cecum, thus completing the life cycle.

Humans are the only known host of the pinworm, which probably has the widest distribution of all the helminths. Infection occurs from hand-to-mouth transmission, often from handling soiled clothes, bedsheets, and other household articles. Ova under the fingernails are a common source of auto-infection. Ova may also be airborne and collect in dust that may be on furniture and the floor. Investigation may show that all members of the family of an affected person also harbor the infection. It is common in orphanages and mental institutions, and among people living in communal groups.

Rarely is it feasible to identify a dead pinworm in the stool. Diagnosis is best made by demonstration of ova in smears taken from the anal region early in the morning before the patient bathes or defecates. Such smears may be obtained with a small eye curette and placed on a glass slide with a drop of saline solution. It is also possible to use Scotch tape, looping the tape sticky-side out over a tongue depressor and then pressing it several times against the perianal region. The tape is then smoothed out on a glass slide. A drop of a solution containing iodine in xylol may be placed on the slide before the tape is applied to facilitate detection of any ova. These tests should be repeated on 3 consecutive days to rule out infection. Ova may be detected under the fingernails of the infected person.

Albendazole, 400 mg, mebendazole, 100 mg, or pyrantel pamoate, 11 mg/kg (maximum 1 g) given once and repeated in 2 weeks, is effective. Personal hygiene and cleanliness at home are important. Fingernails should be cut short and scrubbed frequently; they should be thoroughly cleaned on arising, before each meal, and after using the toilet. Sheets, underwear, towels, pajamas, and other clothing of the affected person should be laundered thoroughly and separately.

Elston DM: *Enterobius vermicularis* (pinworms, threadworms). Cutis 2003; 71:268.

Jacobson CC, et al: Parasitic infestations. J Am Acad Dermatol 2007; 56(6):1026–1043.

Hookworm disease (ground itch, uncinariasis, ancylostomiasis, necatoriasis)

The earliest skin lesions (ground itch) are erythematous macules and papules, which in a few hours become vesicles. These itchy lesions usually occur on the soles, toe webs, and ankles; they may be scattered or in groups. The content of the vesicles rapidly becomes purulent. These lesions are produced by invasion of the skin by the *Ancylostoma* or *Necator* larvae, and precede the generalized symptoms of the disease by 2 or 3 months. The cutaneous lesions last less than 2 weeks before the larvae continue their human life cycle. There may be as high as 40% eosinophilia around the fifth day of infection.

The onset of the constitutional disease is insidious and is accompanied by progressive iron-deficiency anemia and debility. During the course of the disease urticaria often occurs. The skin ultimately becomes dry and pale or yellowish.

Hookworm is a specific communicable disease caused by *Ancylostoma duodenale* or *Necator americanus*. In the soil, under propitious circumstances, they attain the stage of infective larvae in 5–7 days. When they come into accidental contact with bare feet, these tiny larvae (which can scarcely be seen with a small pocket lens) penetrate the skin and reach the capillaries. They are carried in the circulation to the lungs, where they pass through the capillary walls into the bronchi. They move up the trachea to the pharynx and, after being swallowed, eventually reach their habitat in the small intestine. Here they bury their heads in the mucosa and begin their sexual life.

Hookworm is prevalent in most tropical and subtropical countries, and is often endemic in swampy and sandy localities in temperate zones. In these latter regions the larvae are killed off each winter, but the soil is again contaminated from human sources the following summer. *N. americanus* prevails in the western hemisphere, Central and South Africa, South Asia, Australia, and the Pacific islands.

The defecation habits of infected individuals in endemic areas are largely responsible for its widespread distribution, as is the use of human feces for fertilization in many parts of the world. In addition, the climate is usually such that people go barefoot because of the heat or because they cannot afford shoes. Infection is thereby facilitated, especially through the toes.

Finding the eggs in the feces of a suspected individual establishes the diagnosis. The ova appear in the feces about 5 weeks after the onset of infection. The eggs may be found in direct fecal films if the infection is heavy, but in light infections it may be necessary to resort to zinc sulfate centrifugal flotation or other concentration methods. Mixed infections frequently occur.

Albendazole, 400 mg once, or mebendazole, 100 mg twice a day for 3 days or 500 mg once, or pyrantel pamoate, 11 mg/kg (maximum 1 g) each day for 3 days, is effective. Prophylaxis is largely a community problem and depends on preventing fecal contamination of the soil. This is best attained by proper sanitary disposal of feces, protecting individuals from exposure by educating them about sanitary procedures, and mass treatment through public health methods.

Nematode dermatitis

Miller et al described a patient who developed a persistent widespread folliculitis caused by *Ancylostoma caninum*. It was apparently acquired by his lying in grass contaminated by the droppings of his pet dogs and cats. A biopsy revealed hookworm larvae within the hair follicle. Oral thiabendazole was curative.

Creeping eruption (larva migrans)

Creeping eruption is a term applied to twisting, winding linear skin lesions produced by the burrowing of larvae. People who go barefoot on the beach, children playing in sandboxes, carpenters and plumbers working under homes, and gardeners are often victims. The most common areas involved are the feet, buttocks, genitals, and hands.

Slight local itching and the appearance of papules at the sites of infection characterize the onset. Intermittent stinging pain occurs, and thin, red, tortuous lines are formed in the skin. The larval migrations begin 4 days after inoculation and progress at the rate of about 2 cm/day. However, they may remain quiescent for several days or even months before beginning to migrate. The linear lesions are often interrupted by papules that mark the sites of resting larvae (Fig. 20-17). As the eruption advances, the old parts tend to fade, but sometimes there are purulent manifestations caused by secondary infection; erosions and excoriations caused by scratching frequently occur. If the progress of the disease is not interrupted by treatment, the larvae usually die in 2–8 weeks, with resolution of the eruption, although rarely it has been reported to persist for up to 1 year. At times, the larvae are removed from the skin by the fingernails in scratching. Eosinophilia may be present.

Loeffler syndrome, consisting of a patchy infiltrate of the lungs and eosinophilia as high as 50% in the blood and 90% in the sputum, may complicate creeping eruption.

The majority of cases in the US occur along the southeast coast and are caused by penetration by the larvae of a cat and dog hookworm, *Ancylostoma braziliense*. It is acquired from body contact with damp sand or earth that has been contaminated by the excreta of dogs and cats. The larvae of *A. caninum*, which also infests the dog and the cat, rarely produce a similar dermatitis. The diagnosis is typically made clinically, although biopsy may sometimes demonstrate the organism and even dermoscopy has been used.

Ivermectin, 200 µg/kg, generally given as a single 12 mg dose and repeated the next day, or albendazole, 400 mg/day for 3 days, is an effective treatment. Criteria for successful therapy are relief of symptoms and cessation of tract extension, which usually occurs within a week. Topical thiabendazole, compounded as a 10% suspension or a 15% cream used four times a day, will result in marked relief from pruritus in 3 days, and the tracts become inactive in 1 week. Topical metronidazole has also been reported to be effective.

Another condition, not to be confused with this helminthic disease, which also is called creeping eruption (or sandworm, as it is known in South Africa, particularly in Natal and Zululand), is caused by a small mite about 300 µm long that tunnels into the superficial layers of the epidermis.

Gnathostomiasis

Migratory, intermittent, erythematous, urticarial plaques characterize human gnathostomiasis. Each episode of painless swelling lasts from 7–10 days and recurs every 2–6 weeks. Movement of the underlying parasite may be as much as 1 cm/h. The total duration of the illness may be 10 years. Histopathologic examination of the skin swelling will demonstrate eosinophilic panniculitis. The clinical manifestation has been called larva migrans profundus.

The nematode *Gnathostoma dolorosi* or *spinigerum* is the cause; most cases occur in Asia or South America. Eating raw flesh from the second intermediate host, most commonly freshwater fish, in such preparations as sashimi and ceviche, allows humans to become the definitive host. Eating raw squid or snake is another less common exposure. As the larval cyst in the flesh is digested, it becomes motile and penetrates the gastric mucosa, usually within 24–48 h of ingestion. Symptoms then occur as migration of the parasite continues. Surgical removal is the treatment of choice, if the parasite can be located. This may be combined with albendazole, 400 mg/day or twice a day for 21 days, or ivermectin, 200 µg/kg/day for 2 days.

Creeping eruption in several reports from Japan has been found to be caused by a newly recognized causative parasite of the nematode superfamily Spiruroidea. Eating raw squid was associated with the onset of long, narrow lesions that were pruritic, linear, and migratory. Surgical removal is necessary; chemotherapy has been largely unsuccessful. Data regarding ivermectin are mixed.

Larva currens

Intestinal infections with *Strongyloides stercoralis* may be associated with a perianal larva migrans syndrome, called larva currens, because of the rapidity of larval migration (currens means "running" or "racing"). Larva currens is an autoinfection caused by penetration of the perianal skin by infectious larvae as they are excreted in the feces. An urticarial band is the prominent primary lesion of cutaneous strongyloidiasis. Strongyloidiasis, like the creeping eruption secondary to it, is often a chronic disease; infections may persist for more than 40 years. Approximately one-third of patients infected are asymptomatic.

Signs and symptoms of systemic strongyloidiasis include abdominal pain, diarrhea, constipation, nausea, vomiting,

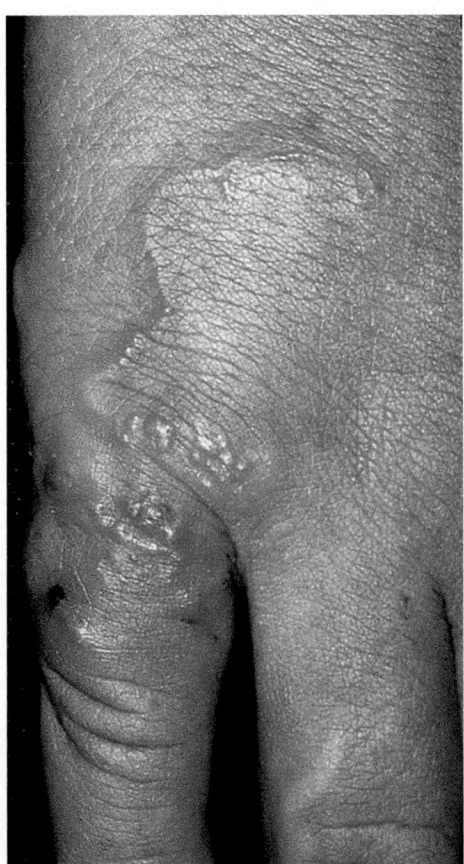

Fig. 20-17 Cutaneous larva migrans.

pneumonitis, urticaria, eosinophilic folliculitis, and a peripheral eosinophilia. The skin lesions originate within 30 cm of the anus and characteristically extend as much as 10 cm/day.

Fatal cases of hyperinfection occur in immunocompromised patients. In such patients the parasite load increases dramatically and can produce a fulminant illness. Widespread petechiae and purpura are helpful diagnostic signs of disseminated infection and chronic urticaria is a possible presenting sign. Periumbilical ecchymoses may appear as if they were caused by a thumbprint.

Administration of ivermectin, 200 µg/kg/day for 2 days, or thiabendazole 50 mg/kg/day in two doses (maximum 3 g/day) for 2 days, is the treatment of choice. Immunosuppressed hosts may be treated with thiabendazole, 25 mg/kg twice a day for 7–10 days.

There are free-living strongyloides known as *Pelodera* that can produce a creeping eruption also. Jones et al reported a case of widespread follicular, erythematous, dome-shaped papules and pustules that began within 24 h of working under a house. This eruption persisted for 1 month before presentation. Scraping the lesions revealed live and dead larvae of the free-living soil nematode, *Pelodera strongyloides*. Treatment with oral thiabendazole led to resolution.

Bussaratid V, et al: Efficacy of ivermectin treatment of cutaneous gnathostomiasis evaluated by placebo-controlled trial. Southeast Asian J Trop Med Public Health 2006; 37(3):433–440.

Fox LM: Ivermectin: uses and impact 20 years on. Curr Opin Infect Dis 2006; 19(6):588–593.

Heukelbach J, et al: Epidemiological and clinical characteristics of hookworm-related cutaneous larva migrans. Lancet Infect Dis 2008; 8(5):302–309.

Hochedez P, et al: Hookworm-related cutaneous larva migrans. J Travel Med 2007; 14(5):326–333.

Hotez PJ, et al: Hookworm infection. New Engl J Med 2004; 351:299.

Zalaudek I, et al: Entodermoscopy: a new tool for diagnosing skin infections and infestations. Dermatology 2008; 216(1):14–23.

Dracunculiasis (Guinea worm disease, dracontiasis, medina worm)

Guinea worm disease is now limited to remote villages in several sub-Saharan African countries. It is caused by *Dracunculus medinensis* and is contracted through drinking water that has been contaminated with infected water fleas in which *Dracunculus* is parasitic. In the stomach, the larvae penetrate into the mesentery, where they mature sexually in 10 weeks. Then the female worm burrows to the cutaneous surface to deposit her larvae and thus causes the specific skin manifestations. As the worm approaches the surface, it may be felt as a cordlike thickening and forms an indurated cutaneous papule. The papule may vesiculate and a painful ulcer develops, usually on the leg. The worm is often visible. When the parasite comes in contact with water, the worm rapidly discharges its larvae, which are ingested by water fleas (*Cyclops*), contaminating the water.

The cutaneous lesion is usually on the lower leg, but it may occur on the genitalia, buttocks, or arms (Fig. 20-18). In addition to the ulcers on the skin, there may be urticaria, gastrointestinal upsets, eosinophilia, and fever.

The disease may be prevented by boiling drinking water, providing safe drinking water through boreholes, or filtering the water through mesh fibers. Native treatment consists of gradually extracting the worm a little each day, with care not to rupture it; in the event of such an accident, the larvae escape into the tissues and produce fulminating inflammation. Surgical removal is the treatment of choice. Metronidazole, 500 mg/day, resolves the local inflammation and permits easier removal of the worm. Immersion in warm water pro-

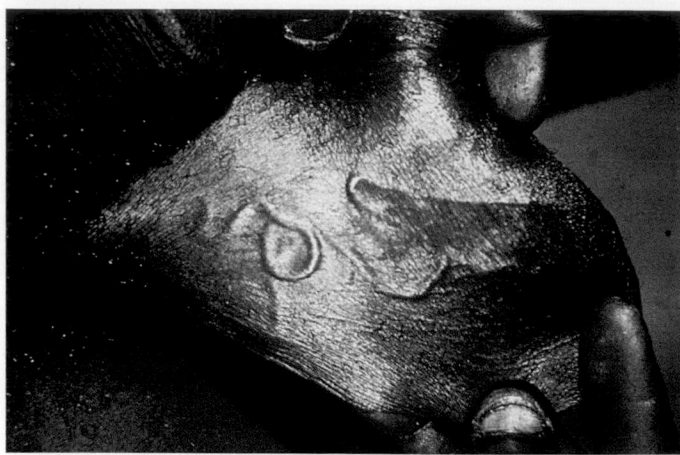

Fig. 20-18 Dracunculiasis.

motes emergence of the worm. Global eradication is within our grasp, and Guinea worm disease may become a historical footnote.

Bristol N: Donald R Hopkins: eradicating Guinea worm disease. Lancet 2008; 371(9624):1571.

Hopkins DR, et al: Dracunculiasis, onchocerciasis, schistosomiasis, and trachoma. Ann N Y Acad Sci 2008; 1136:45–52.

Filariasis

Elephantiasis tropica (elephantiasis arabum)

Filariasis is a widespread tropical disorder caused by infestation with filarial worms of *Wuchereria bancrofti*, *Brugia malayi*, or *Brugia timori* species. It is characterized by lymphedema, with resulting hypertrophy of the skin and subcutaneous tissues, and by enlargement and deformity of the affected parts, usually the legs, scrotum, or labia majora. The disease occurs more frequently in young men than in women.

The onset of elephantiasis is characterized by recurrent attacks of acute lymphangitis in the affected part, associated with chills and fever (elephantoid fever) that last for several days to several weeks. These episodes recur over several months to years. After each attack the swelling subsides only partially, and as recrudescences supervene, thickening and hypertrophy become increasingly pronounced. The overlying epidermis becomes stretched, thin, and shiny, and over the course of years, leathery, insensitive, and verrucous or papillomatous from secondary pyogenic infection. There may be a dozen or more attacks in a year.

In addition to involvement of the legs and scrotum, the scalp, vulva, penis, female breasts, and arms are at times affected, either alone or in association with the other regions. The manifestations vary according to the part involved. When the legs are attacked, both are usually affected in a somewhat symmetrical manner, the principal changes occurring on the posterior aspects above the ankles and on the dorsa of the feet. At first, the thickening may be slight and associated with edema that pits on pressure. Later, the parts become massive and pachydermatous, the thickened integument hanging in apposing folds, between which there is a fetid exudate (Fig. 20-19).

When the scrotum is affected, it gradually reaches an enormous size and the penis becomes hidden in it. The skin, which at first is glazed, is later coarse and verrucous, or, in far-advanced cases, ulcerated or gangrenous. Resistant urticaria may occur. Filarial orchitis and hydrocele are common. A testicle may enlarge rapidly to the size of an apple and be extremely painful. The swelling may subside within a few days, or the enlargement may be permanent. As a result of obstruction and dilation of the thoracic duct or some of its lower abdominal tributaries into the urinary tract, chyle appears in the urine, which assumes a milky appearance. Lobulated swellings of the inguinal and axillary glands, called varicose glands, are caused by obstructive varix and dilatation of the lymphatic vessels.

Filaria are transmitted person to person by the bites of a variety of mosquitoes of the *Culex*, *Aedes*, and *Anopheles* species. The adult worms are threadlike, cylindrical, and creamy white. The females are 4–10 cm long. Microfilarial embryos may be seen coiled each in its own membrane near the posterior tip. Fully grown, sheathed microfilariae are 130–320 μm long. The adult worms live in the lymphatic system, where they produce microfilariae. These either remain in the lymphatic vessels or enter the peripheral bloodstream. An intermediate host is necessary for the further development of the parasite.

It is important to realize that infestation by the filaria is often asymptomatic, and elephantiasis usually occurs only if hundreds of thousands of mosquito bites are suffered over a period of years, with episodes of intercurrent streptococcal lymphangitis. Filariasis was endemic in the considerable Samoan population of Hawaii for half a century, and only one case of elephantiasis has occurred among this group.

Search for the microfilariae should be made on fresh cover-slip films of blood (collected at night), urine, or other body fluid, and examined with a low-power objective lens. Calcified adult worms may be demonstrated on x-ray examination, and ultrasound can detect adult worms. At times, adult filariae are found in abscesses or in material taken for pathologic examination. Specific serologic tests and a simple card test for filarial antigen are available. The prognosis in regard to life is good, but living becomes burdensome unless the condition is alleviated.

Diethylcarbamazine, in increasing doses over a 14-day period, is the treatment of choice. This regimen clears microfilariae but not adult worms. A single dose of ivermectin may also be effective. Doxycycline kills the intracellular symbiotic bacteria, *Wolbachia*. This leads to long-term sterility of adult female worms. It is being studied to determine its place in the treatment of both bancroftian filariasis and onchocerciasis. A worldwide effort to eliminate these diseases is under way. Surgical operations have been devised to remove the edematous subcutaneous tissue from the scrotum and breast. Prophylactic measures consist of appropriate mosquito control. Diethylcarbamazine has been effective in mass prophylaxis and if a trip of over 1 month is planned to areas with endemic *W. bancrofti* and extensive exposure to mosquitoes is likely, taking 500 mg/day for 2 days each month is recommended.

Palumbo E: Filariasis: diagnosis, treatment and prevention. Acta Biomed 2008; 79(2):106–109.

Shenoy RK: Clinical and pathological aspects of filarial lymphedema and its management. Korean J Parasitol 2008; 46(3):119–125.

Loiasis (loa loa, Calabar swelling, tropical swelling, fugitive swelling)

Infection with *Loa loa* is often asymptomatic. In infected persons, the parasite develops slowly and there may even be an interval of as much as 3 years between infection and the appearance of symptoms, although the usual interval is 1 year. The first sign is often painful, localized, subcutaneous, nonpitting edema called Calabar or fugitive swelling (Fig. 20-20A). These are one or more slightly inflamed, edematous, transient swellings, usually about the size of a hen's egg. They usually last a few days and then subside, although recurrent swellings at the same site may eventually lead to a permanent cystlike protuberance. These swellings may result from hypersensitivity to the adult worm or to materials elaborated by it.

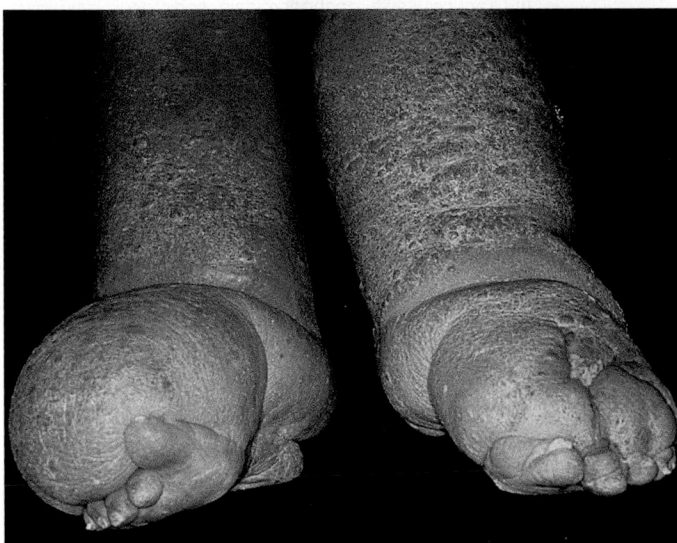

Fig. 20-19 Filarial elephantiasis.

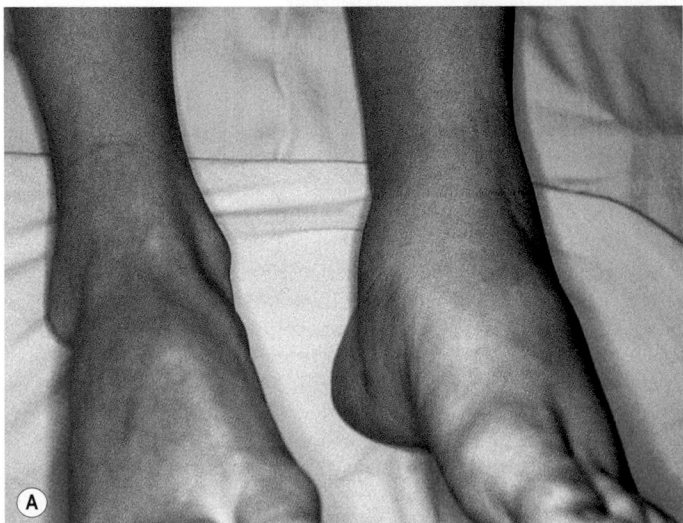

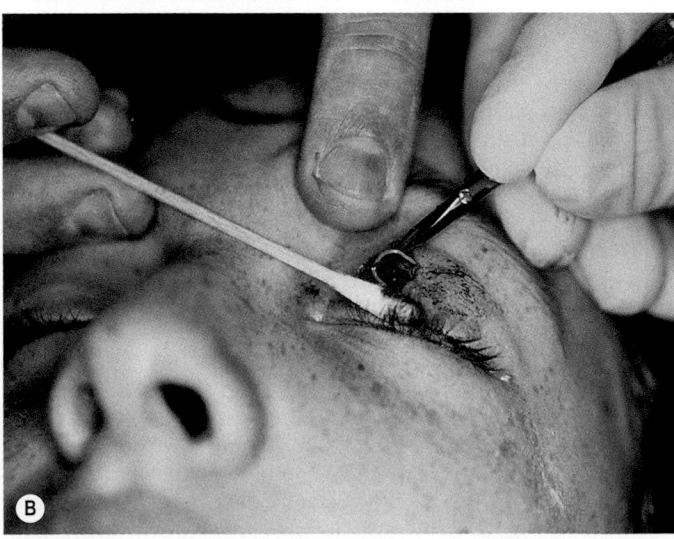

Fig. 20-20 A and B, Loiasis. (Courtesy of Curt Samlaska, MD)

Eosinophilia may be as high as 90% and often is between 60% and 80%.

The filariae may be noticed subcutaneously in the fingers, breasts, eyelids, or submucosally under the conjunctivae. The worm may be in the anterior chamber of the eye, the myocardium, or other sites. It has a predilection for loose tissues such as the eye region, the frenum of the tongue, and the genitalia. The wanderings of the adult parasite may be noticed because of a tingling and creeping sensation. The death of the filaria in the skin may lead to the formation of fluctuant cystic lesions.

Loiasis is widely distributed in West and Central Africa, where it is transmitted by the mango fly, *Chrysops dimidia* or *Chrysops silacea*. This fly bites only in the daytime. Humans are the only important reservoir for the parasite. The observation of the worm under the conjunctiva, Calabar swellings, and eosinophilia establish the diagnosis. Demonstration of the characteristic microfilariae in the blood during the day is possible in only some 20% of patients. Specific serologic tests are available, and luciferase immunoprecipitation systems can provide rapid diagnostic results with improved sensitivity and specificity compared with enzyme-linked immunosorbent assays (ELISA).

Removal of the adult parasite whenever it comes to the surface of the skin is mandatory (Fig. 20-20B). This must be done quickly by seizing the worm with forceps and placing a suture under it before cutting down to it. Worms that are not securely and rapidly grasped may escape into the deeper tissues.

Diethylcarbamazine kills both adults and microfilariae, and is given in increasing doses for 21 days. In regions in which onchocerciasis and loiasis are both endemic and ivermectin is used in a community-based elimination strategy for onchocerciasis, simultaneously infected patients with a high *Loa loa* load have a greater risk of serious side effects. If ivermectin treatment of these patients is undertaken, proper monitoring and appropriate supportive treatment should be available in anticipation of this risk. Diethylcarbamazine is an effective chemopreventive, using 300 mg/week in temporary residents of regions of Africa where *Loa loa* is endemic.

Burbelo PD, et al: Rapid, novel, specific, high-throughput assay for diagnosis of *Loa loa* infection. J Clin Microbiol 2008; 46(7):2298–2304.
Nam JN, et al: Surgical management of conjunctival loiasis. Ophthal Plast Reconstr Surg 2008; 24(4):316–317.
Padgett JJ, et al: Loiasis: African eye worm. Trans R Soc Trop Med Hyg 2008; 102(10):983–989.

Onchocerciasis

The skin lesions are characterized by pruritus, dermatitis, and onchocercomas. The dermatitis is variable in its appearance and probably relates to chronicity of infection, age of the patients, geographic area in which it was acquired, and relative immune responsiveness. Early in the course of the infection an itchy papular dermatitis may occur, and in visitors who acquire the infection this may be localized to one extremity (Fig. 20-21). In Central America, papules may appear only on the head and neck area. This unusual localization of insect bite-appearing papules with excoriations may lead to the diagnosis in travelers returning to their home countries. In Central America, another manifestation of the acute phase is acute swelling of the face with erythema and itching, known as erisipela de la costa. In Zaire and Central America, an acute urticarial eruption is seen. The inflammation, which is accompanied by hyperpigmentation, is known as mal morado.

As time passes, the dermatitis becomes chronic and remains papular; however, thickening, lichenification, and depigmentation occur (Fig. 20-22). Later, atrophy may supervene. When the depigmentation is spotted, it is known as leopard skin;

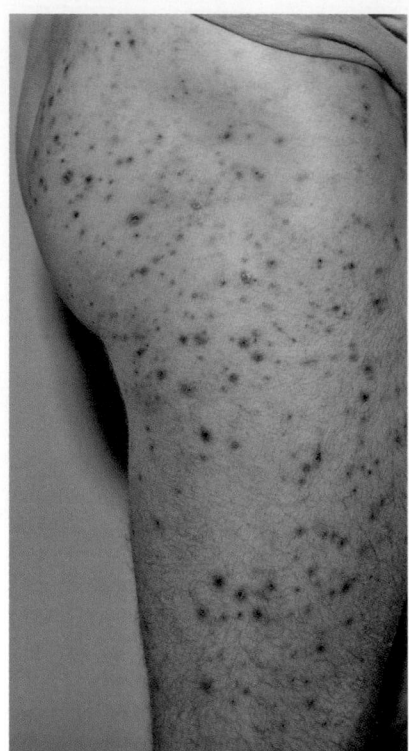

Fig. 20-21 Early onchocerciasis.

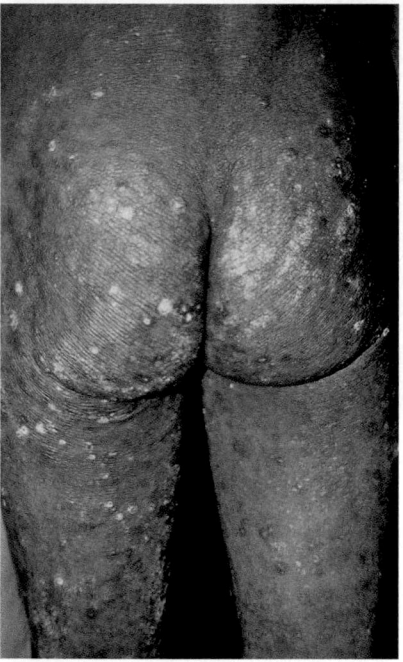

Fig. 20-22 Onchocerciasis. (Courtesy of Debra Kalter, MD)

when the skin is thickened, it is called elephant skin. When local edema and thickened, wrinkled, dry dermatitic changes predominate, it is sometimes called lizard skin.

In Saudi Arabia, Yemen, and East Africa, a localized type of onchocerciasis exists called sowda, which is Arabic for "black." It is characterized by localized, pruritic, asymmetrical, usually darkly pigmented, chronic lichenified dermatitis of one leg or one body region. It is also known as the chronic hyperreactive type, and an association with antidefensin antibodies suggests a reason for this enhanced reactivity against the parasite.

After a time, firm subcutaneous nodules, pea-sized or larger, develop on various sites of the body. These nodules are onchocercomas containing myriad microfilariae. These occur

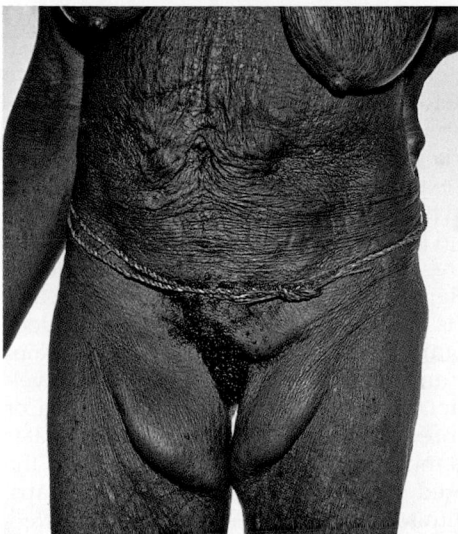

Fig. 20-23 Onchocerciasis.

in crops, are frequently painful, and their site varies. In parts of Africa, where natives are wholly or nearly unclothed, the lesions occur on the trunk, axillae, groin, and perineum. In Central and South America, the head, especially the scalp, is the usual site of involvement.

Firm, nontender lymphadenopathy is a common finding in patients with chronically infected onchocerciasis. "Hanging groin" describes the loose, atrophic skin sack that contains these large inguinal nodes (Fig. 20-23).

In about 5% of affected persons, serious eye lesions arise late in the disease, gradually leading to blindness.

Onchocerciasis is caused by *Onchocerca volvulus*, which is transmitted to humans by the bite of the black fly of the genus *Simulium*. It breeds in fast-flowing streams. When the black fly bites, it introduces larvae into the wound. The larvae reach adulthood in the subdermal connective tissue in about 1 year. Then millions of the progeny migrate back into the dermis and the aqueous humor of the eye.

Onchocerciasis occurs in Africa on the west coast, in the Sahara, Sudan, and the Victoria Nile division, where it is known as river blindness. In Central and South America, this disease is to be found in Guatemala, Brazil, Venezuela, and southern Mexico.

The presence of eosinophilia, skin lesions, and onchocercomas with ocular lesions is highly suggestive in endemic areas. Frequently, the microfilariae may be found in skin shavings or dermal lymph, even when no nodules are detectable. The scapular area is the favorite site for procuring specimens for examination by means of a skin snip. This is performed in the field or office by lifting the skin with an inserted needle and then clipping off a small, superficial portion of the skin with a sharp knife or scissors. The specimen is laid in a drop of normal saline solution on a slide, covered with a coverslip, and examined under the microscope. The filariae wriggle out at the edges of the skin slice.

Specific serologic and PCR-based diagnostic tests from blood and skin biopsies are available. Other filarial parasites can be detected in similar systems. When patients suspected of having onchocerciasis were given a single oral dose of 50 mg of diethylcarbamazine, a reaction consisting of edema, itching, fever, arthralgias, and an exacerbation of pruritus was described as a positive Mazzotti test reaction, which supported the diagnosis of onchocerciasis. The reaction may be related to *Wolbachia* organisms within the worms.

Onchocercomas may be surgically excised whenever feasible. Ivermectin as a single oral dose of 150 µg/kg is the drug of choice. Skin microfilaria counts remain low at the end of 6 months' observation. Ivermectin should be repeated every 6 months to suppress the dermal and ocular microfilarial counts. More frequent dosing does not appear to reduce microfilarial counts further.

Doxycycline kills the intracellular symbiotic bacteria, *Wolbachia*. It is being tested for long-term effects and determination of its place in the treatment of onchocerciasis and bancroftian filariasis. If there is eye involvement, prednisone, 1 mg/kg, should be started several days before treatment with ivermectin. Moxidectin and emodepside also appear promising as alternative drugs. There are community-based treatment protocols that have the objective of eliminating onchocerciasis from endemic areas. Severe reactions may occur in patients simultaneously infected with *Loa loa*.

Bottomley C, et al: Rates of microfilarial production by *Onchocerca volvulus* are not cumulatively reduced by multiple ivermectin treatments. Parasitology 2008; Oct 3:1–11

Boussinesq M: Onchocerciasis control: biological research is still needed. Parasite 2008; 15(3):510–514.

Haddad D: The NGDO Co-ordination Group for Onchocerciasis Control. Ann Trop Med Parasitol 2008; 102(Suppl 1):35–38.

Thylefors B: The Mectizan Donation Program (MDP). Ann Trop Med Parasitol 2008; 102(Suppl 1):39–44.

Trichinosis

Ingestion of *Trichinella spiralis* larva-containing cysts in inadequately cooked pork, bear, or walrus meat may cause trichinosis. It usually causes a puffy edema of the eyelids, redness of the conjunctivae, and sometimes urticaria or angioedema associated with hyperpyrexia, headache, erythema, gastrointestinal symptoms, muscle pains, and neurologic signs and symptoms. Ten percent of patients develop a bilateral, asymptomatic hand swelling that is especially prominent over the digits, and erythema along the perimeters of the palms and volar surfaces of the digits, which progresses to desquamation. In 20% of cases a nonspecific macular or petechial eruption occurs and splinter hemorrhages are occasionally present. Eosinophilia is not constant, but may be as high as 80%. In the average patient, eosinophilia begins about 1 week after infection and attains its height by the fourth week.

The immunofluorescence antibody test has the greatest value in establishing early diagnosis. The bentonite flocculation test, ELISA, and other serologic tests are limited by their inability to detect infection until the third or fourth week.

Diagnosis is confirmed by a muscle biopsy that demonstrates larvae of *Trichinella spiralis* in striated muscle. Unfortunately, trichinae cannot usually be demonstrated unless eosinophilic vasculitis and granulomas have been described on biopsy. A 2 mm-thick slice of the muscle biopsy may be compressed between two glass slides to demonstrate the cysts.

The condition is treated with albendazole, 400 mg twice a day for 14 days. Corticosteroidal agents are effective as a means of controlling the often severe symptoms and should be given at doses of 40–60 mg/day.

Li CK, et al: Inflammatory response during the muscle phase of *Trichinella spiralis* and *T. pseudospiralis* infections. Parasitol Res 2001; 87(9):708–714.

Renner R, et al: Chronic urticaria and angioedema with concomitant eosinophilic vasculitis due to *Trichinella* infection. Acta Derm Venereol 2008; 88(1):78–79.

Pneumocystosis

Pneumocystis jirovecii (formerly *carinii*) has features characteristic of both protozoa and fungi. It is an opportunistic infection, occurring primarily as a pulmonary infection in AIDS patients. Extrapulmonary involvement is uncommon and usually occurs in the reticuloendothelial system. Skin findings may occur. At least half of reported cases are of nodular growths in the auditory canal, with the remainder having nonspecific pink to skin-colored papules and nodules that may ulcerate. On biopsy, the dermis contains foamy material within which Giemsa-positive organisms are identified. Cutaneous botryomycosis caused by combined *Staphylococcus aureus* and *Pneumocystis jirovecii* has been reported in the setting of HIV infection. A 3-week course of trimethoprim–sulfamethoxazole combination is the treatment of choice. In combined infections, all pathogens require treatment.

Anuradha SA, et al: Extrapulmonary *Pneumocystis carinii* infection in an AIDS patient: a case report. Acta Cytol 2007; 51(4):599–601.

Saadat P, et al: Botryomycosis caused by *Staphylococcus aureus* and *Pneumocystis carinii* in a patient with acquired immunodeficiency disease. Clin Exp Dermatol 2008; 33(3):266–269.

PHYLUM ARTHROPODA

This phylum contains more species than all the other phyla put together. The following classes are of dermatologic significance: Myriapoda, Insecta, and Arachnida. Mosquitoes, flies, ticks, and fleas transmit diseases throughout the world. Bites and stings are always prevalent, but increase dramatically after natural disasters such as hurricanes and flooding.

Prevention of arthropod-related disease

Mosquitoes remain the most important vectors of arthropod-borne disease, and mosquito control programs are an essential component of the public health efforts of many states. Insect repellents are effective in preventing disease transmission and are especially important during travel to areas where vector-borne disease is endemic. Most are based on DEET (N,N-diethyl-3-methylbenzamide, previously called N,N-diethyl-m-toluamide). DEET has been tested against a wide range of arthropods, including mosquitoes, sandflies, ticks, and chiggers. The American Academy of Pediatrics recommends concentrations of 30% or less in products intended for use in children. As this represents a major market share for these products, many formulations that comply with the recommendation are available. Some evidence suggests that children do not have a higher incidence of adverse reactions when compared to adults, but even in adults there have been occasional reports of neurotoxicity. High concentrations of DEET can also produce erythema and irritation or bullous eruptions. Extended-release products reduce the need for repeated application, and appear to minimize the risk of complications. Overall, DEET has a good safety record in widespread use. Picaridin (KBR 3023) is a piperidine-derived repellent ingredient that is also effective against a range of arthropods. In some studies, it has been shown to be less irritating than DEET while providing comparable efficacy. The best studies for the evaluation of repellents are field trials that involve a range of arthropods. Arm box studies are still performed, but must be interpreted with caution. In a well-designed arm box study, soybean oil (Bite Blocker for Kids) performed reasonably well, and was second only to DEET in efficacy. Citronella did not perform well, and citronella candles have little documented efficacy. In contrast, neem oil is an effective mosquito repellent that is used in many areas of the world that are endemic for malaria. Geraniol candles demonstrate some efficacy, but only in the area immediately surrounding the candles. Repellency drops significantly at a distance of even 2 m. Candles with geraniol are twice as effective as those with linalool and five times as effective as those with citronella. IR3535 (ethyl butyl acetyl aminopropionate) in a variety of formulations has also demonstrated good efficacy against mosquitoes. Complete protection times in field trials ranged from 7.1 to 10.3 hours.

Travelers to malaria-endemic areas should follow CDC guidelines for malaria prophylaxis. They should also avoid night-time outdoor exposure and use protective measures such as repellents and bed netting. The anopheline mosquitoes that carry malaria tend to bite at night, so bed nets and screens are important measures. Mosquitoes that carry dengue mostly bite during the day. Repellents play a greater role in protection against dengue, as it is more difficult to limit daytime outdoor activity. Mosquito control programs depend largely on drainage of stagnant water and spraying of breeding areas. In developing countries, water barrels may be stocked with fish or turtles to consume mosquito larvae. Both can soil the water and the relative risks must be evaluated. In some studies, the risk has clearly favored stocking the barrel. Mosquito traps, including the Mosquito Magnet, have been shown to be effective for the control of mosquitoes in limited areas. Generally, mosquitoes fly upwind to bite, and downwind to return to their resting area. Mosquito traps must be positioned between the breeding and resting areas, and the area to be protected. Mosquito traps commonly use CO_2, heat, and chemical attractants. Some *Culex* mosquitoes are repelled by octenol, and the manufacturer may provide guidelines for areas where the attractant should not be used.

Prevention of disease from ticks and chiggers

Tick-borne diseases include rickettsial fevers, ehrlichiosis, Lyme disease, babesiosis, relapsing fever, and tularemia. Most require a sustained tick attachment of more than 24 h for effective transmission, and frequent tick checks with prompt removal of ticks is an important strategy for the prevention of tick-borne illness. Unfortunately, tick inspections frequently fail to identify the tick in time for prompt removal. Some data suggest that adult ticks are found and removed only 60% of the time within 36 h of attachment. Nymphal ticks are even more difficult to detect, and may be removed in as few as 10% of patients within the first 24 h. Because of this, repellents and acaricides remain critical for preventing tick-borne illness. Permethrin has cidal activity against a wide range of arthropods. Some North African *Hyalomma* ticks are resistant to permethrin, and may exhibit a paradoxical pheromone-like attachment response when exposed to the agent, but permethrin performs very well with other species of tick, as well as mosquitoes and chiggers. It can be used to treat clothing, sleeping bags, mosquito netting, and tents. Permethrin-treated clothing, used in conjunction with a repellent, provides exceptional protection against bites in most areas of the world. Permethrin has a good record of safety, although there is a report of congenital leukemia with 11q23/*MLL* rearrangement in a preterm female infant whose mother had abused permethrin because of a pathologic fear of spiders. Permethrin can induce cleavage of the *MLL* gene in cell culture, providing a plausible link between the agent and the leukemia. It should be emphasized that permethrin in this case was not used according to the manufacturer's instructions, and the theoretical risk of carcinogenicity should be weighed against the very real risk of death from arthropod-borne disease. Cardiac glycosides have also been used topically as acaricides and have performed well in limited studies.

Ixodes scapularis is the major North American vector for Lyme disease, human granulocytic ehrlichiosis, and human babesiosis. A Lyme vaccine was marketed in the US, but proved to be a commercial failure and was voluntarily withdrawn from the market. Prevention of Lyme disease now centers on prevention of tick attachments and on prompt tick removal. Back yards and recreational areas adjacent to wooded areas have higher rates of tick infestation. Tick numbers can be reduced by deer fencing, removal of leaf debris, application of an acaricide, and the creation of border beds with wood chip mulch or gravel. Bait boxes and deer feeding stations have been devised that are capable of delivering a topical acaricide while the animal feeds. Parasitic wasps control tick numbers in nature, but wasp populations may fluctuate, and investment in wasp control may be a risky venture compared with other forms of tick control. Other natural forms of tick control have been investigated, as they have the potential to become self-sustaining in the environment, at least for a period of time. Fungi and nematodes show some promise. In southern states, fire ants control tick populations by eating tick eggs.

Prevention of flea-borne illness

Fleas are important vectors of plague and endemic typhus. They may also be vectors of cat-scratch disease. Lufenuron is a maturation inhibitor that prevents fleas from breeding. It is commonly used in oral and injectable forms for the prevention of flea infestation in cats and dogs. Fipronil is used topically for the prevention of flea and tick infestation. Other agents in use include imidacloprid, selamectin, and nitenpyram. House sprays often include pyrethroids or pyriproxyfen. Powdered boric acid may be helpful for the treatment of infested carpets or floor boards. A knowledgeable veterinarian and an exterminator should be consulted.

Anon: Picardin—a new insect repellent. Med Lett Drugs Ther 2005; 47:46.

Borkhardt A, et al: Congenital leukaemia after heavy abuse of permethrin during pregnancy. Arch Dis Child Fetal Neonatal Ed 2003; 88:F436.

Carroll SP: Prolonged efficacy of IR3535 repellents against mosquitoes and blacklegged ticks in North America. J Med Entomol 2008; 45(4):706–714.

Corazza M, et al: Allergic contact dermatitis due to an insect repellent: double sensitization to picaridin and methyl glucose dioleate. Acta Derm Venereol 2005; 85:264.

Diaz JH: The impact of hurricanes and flooding disasters on hymenopterid-inflicted injuries. Am J Disaster Med 2007; 2(5):257–269.

Fradin MS, et al: Comparative efficacy of insect repellents against mosquito bites. N Engl J Med 2002; 347:13.

Müller GC, et al: Indoor protection against mosquito and sand fly bites: a comparison between citronella, linalool, and geraniol candles. J Am Mosq Control Assoc 2008; 24(1):150–153.

Müller GC, et al: Ability of essential oil candles to repel biting insects in high and low biting pressure environments. J Am Mosq Control Assoc 2008; 24(1):154–160.

Trongtokit Y, et al: Comparative repellency of 38 essential oils against mosquito bites. Phytother Res 2005; 19:303.

Class Myriapoda

Morphologically and genetically, the class Myriapoda is distinct from other groups of arthropod. This group contains the centipedes and millipedes. Both are capable of producing significant skin manifestations.

Centipede bites (Chilopoda)

Centipede bites are manifested by paired hemorrhagic marks that form a chevron shape caused by the large paired mouthparts (Fig. 20-24). The bite is surrounded by an erythematous swelling (Fig. 20-25) that may progress into a brawny edema or lymphangitis. Locally, there may be intense itching and pain, often associated with toxic constitutional symptoms. Most centipede bites run a benign self-limited course, and treatment is only supportive. Children are often bitten when

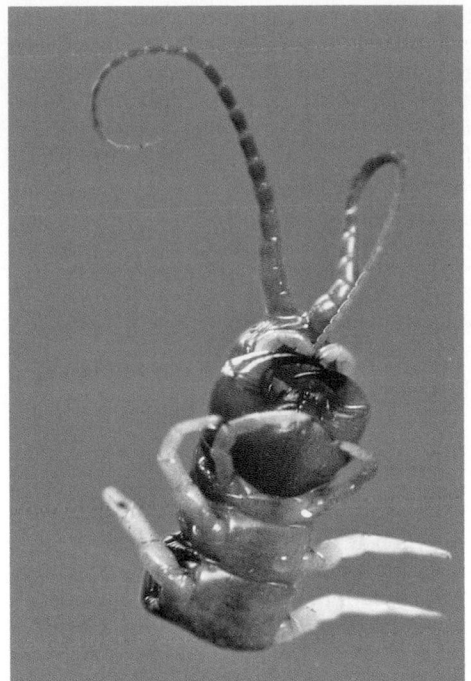

Fig. 20-24 Centipede.

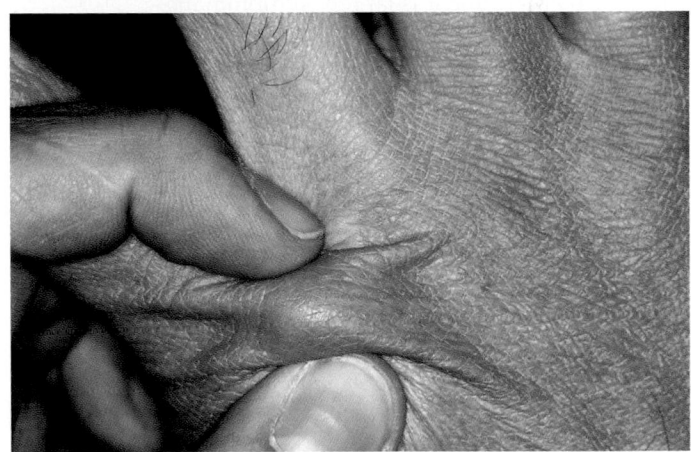

Fig. 20-25 Centipede bite.

they try to handle centipedes. As some species of *Scolopendra* in the western US will attain a length of 15–20 cm, the child may describe it as a snake. Recognition of the characteristic chevron shape is important to avoid inappropriate treatment with snake antivenin. In the eastern US, the common house centipede, *Scutigera coleoptrata*, does not bite humans. *Scolopendra subspinipes*, in Hawaii, inflicts a painful bite. As exotic species appear more commonly at pet stores and swap meets, envenomation by them will become more common.

In some tropical and subtropical areas, centipede bites account for about 17% of all envenomations (compared to the 45% caused by snakes and 20% by scorpions). Most bites occur at home and involve an upper extremity. Local pain and edema occur in up to 96% of patients, depending on the species involved. Treatment is largely symptomatic. Rest, ice, and elevation may be sufficient, but topical or intralesional anesthetics may be required in some cases. Tetanus immunization should be considered if the patient has not been immunized within the past 10 years. Centipede bites can result in Wells syndrome, requiring topical or intralesional corticosteroids. Rarely, bites may produce more serious toxic responses, including rhabdomyolysis, myocardial ischemia, proteinuria, and acute renal failure. These have been reported following the bite of *Scolopendra heros*, the giant desert centipede. Although centipedes have sometimes been found in association with corpses, injuries from the centipede tend to be postmortem and are rarely the cause of death. Ingestion of centipedes by children is usually associated with transient, self-limited toxic manifestations.

Guerrero AP: Centipede bites in Hawai'i: a brief case report and review of the literature. Hawaii Med J 2007; 66(5):125–127.
Hasan S, et al: Proteinuria associated with centipede bite. Pediatr Nephrol 2005; 20(4):550–551.
Malta MB, et al: Toxic activities of Brazilian centipede venoms. Toxicon 2008; 52(2):255–263.
Yildiz A, et al: Acute myocardial infarction in a young man caused by centipede sting. Emerg Med J 2006; 23(4):e30.

Millipede burns (Diplopoda)

Some millipedes secrete a toxic liquid that causes a brownish pigmentation or burn when it comes into contact with skin. Burns may progress to intense erythema and vesiculation. Millipedes may be found in laundry hung out to dry, and millipede burns in children have been misinterpreted as signs of child abuse. Recognition of the characteristic curved shape of the burn can be helpful in preventing misdiagnosis. Some millipedes can squirt their venom and ocular burns are reported. Washing off the toxin as soon as possible will limit the toxic effects. Other treatment is largely symptomatic.

Diplopods (Fig. 20-26) have evolved a complex array of chemicals for self-defense. Some primates take advantage of these chemicals. Two millipede compounds, 2-methyl-1,4-benzoquinone and 2-methoxy-3-methyl-1,4-benzoquinone, demonstrate a repellent effect against *Aedes aegypti* mosquitoes. Tufted and white-faced capuchin monkeys anoint themselves with the secretions to ward off mosquitoes. Effective commercial repellents are available for human use and millipede juice is not recommended.

Dar NR, et al: Millipede burn at an unusual site mimicking child abuse in an 8-year-old girl. Clin Pediatr (Phila) 2008; 47(5):490–492.
Hendrickson RG: Millipede exposure. Clin Toxicol (Phila) 2005; 43(3):211–212.

Class Insecta

Order Lepidoptera

Order Lepidoptera includes butterflies, moths, and their larval forms, caterpillars. Severe systemic reactions have occurred as the result of ingestion of some caterpillars, and with some species the sting alone can produce severe toxicity. *Lonomia achelous*, found in Latin America, can cause a fatal bleeding diathesis. The Spanish pine caterpillar, *Thaumetopoea pityocampa*, causes both dermatitis and anaphylactoid symptoms. Pine caterpillars are also an important cause of systemic reactions in China and Israel. The tussock moth, *Orgyia pseudotsugata*, causes respiratory symptoms in forestry workers in Oregon.

Caterpillar dermatitis

Irritation is produced by contact of the hairs with the skin. Toxins in the hairs can produce severe pain, local pruritic erythematous macules, and wheals, depending on the species. If the hairs get into the clothing, widespread persistent dermatitis may result. Not only the caterpillars, but also their egg covers and cocoons commonly contain stinging hairs. In the US the most common caterpillars of medical importance are the brown-tail moth caterpillar (*Nygmia phoeorrhoea*), puss caterpillar (*Megalopyge opercularis*) (Figs 20-27 and 20-28), saddleback caterpillar (*Sibine stimulae*) (Fig. 20-29), io moth caterpillar (*Automeris io*), crinkled flannel moth caterpillar (*Megalopyge crispata*), Oklahoma puss caterpillar (*Lagoa crispata*), Douglas fir tussock moth caterpillar(*Orgyia pseudotsugata*), buck moth caterpillar (*Hemileuca maia*), and flannel moth caterpillar (*Norape cretata*). The hairs of the European processionary caterpillar (*Thaumetopoea processionea*) are especially dangerous to the eyes, but ophthalmia nodosa

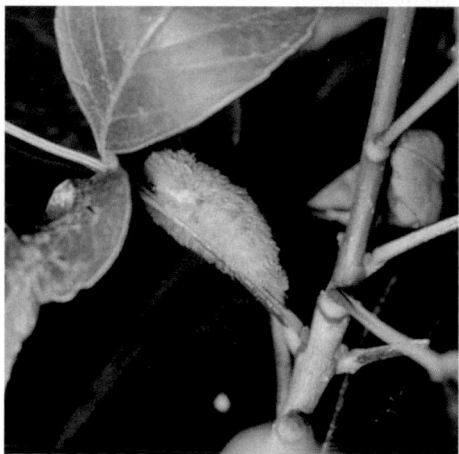
Fig. 20-27 Puss caterpillar.

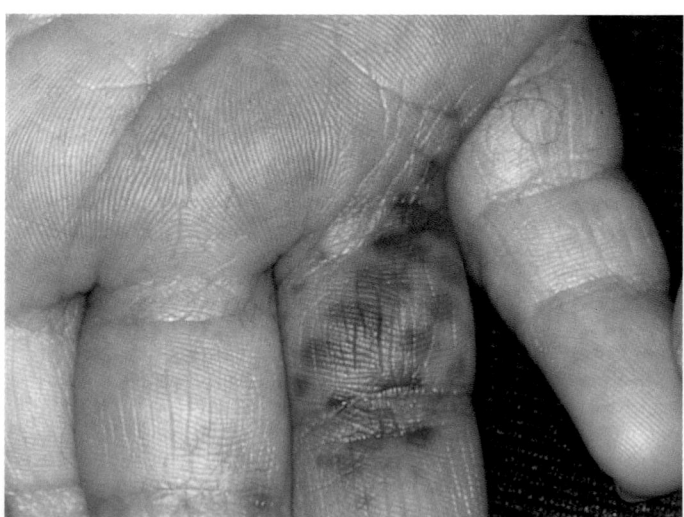
Fig. 20-28 Characteristic railroad track purpura of a puss caterpillar sting.

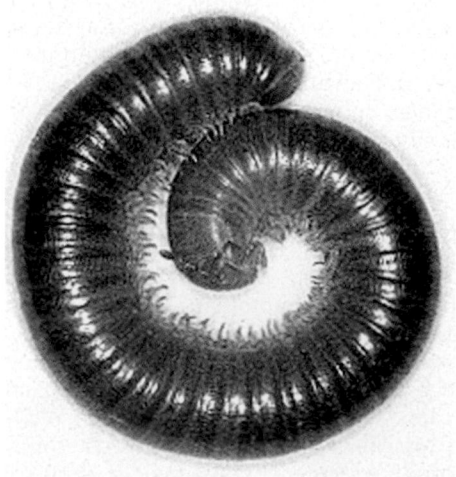
Fig. 20-26 Millipede.

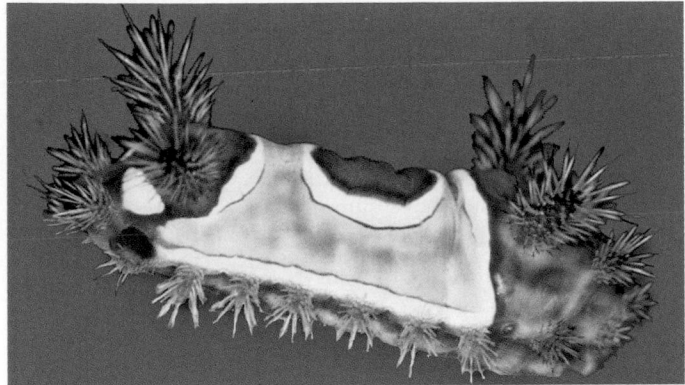

Fig. 20-29 Saddleback caterpillar.

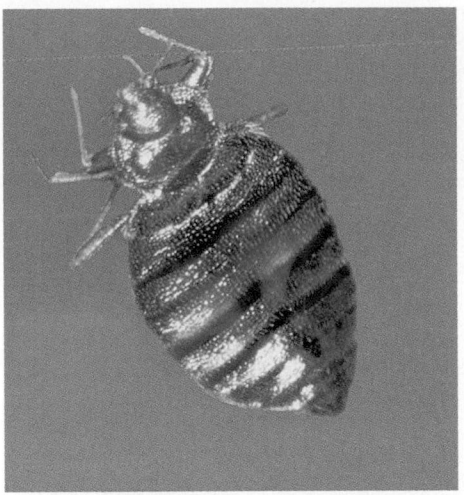

Fig. 20-30 Bedbug.

(a papular reaction to embedded hairs) can be seen with a wide variety of caterpillars and moths. Airborne processionary caterpillar hairs have caused large epidemics of caterpillar dermatitis.

Moth dermatitis

Moth dermatitis may be initiated by the hairs of the brown-tail moth (*Euproctis chrysorrhoea*), goat moth (*Cossus cossus*), puss moth (*Dicranura vinula*), gypsy moth (*Lymantria dispar*), and Douglas fir tussock moth (*Hemenocampa pseudotsugata*). In Latin America, the moths of the genus *Hylesia* are most frequently the cause of moth dermatitis. Severe conjunctivitis and pruritus are the first signs, and may persist for weeks aboard ships that have docked in ports where the moth is common. Caripito itch is named after Caripito, Venezuela, a port city where the moth is found. Korean yellow moth dermatitis is caused by *Euproctis flava* Bremer.

Topical applications of various analgesics, antibiotics, and oral antihistaminics are of little help. Topical or oral corticosteroids are sometimes helpful, as is scrubbing and tape stripping of skin. Contaminated clothing may need to be discarded if dermatitis persists after the clothing is washed.

Hossler EW: Caterpillars and moths: Part I. Dermatologic manifestations of encounters with Lepidoptera. J Am Acad Dermatol 2010 Jan; 62(1):1–10.

Hossler EW: Caterpillars and moths: Part II. Dermatologic manifestations of encounters with Lepidoptera. J Am Acad Dermatol 2010 Jan; 62(1):13–28.

Iserhard CA, et al: Occurrence of lepidopterism caused by the moth *Hylesia nigricans* (Berg) (Lepidoptera: Saturniidae) in Rio Grande do Sul state, Brazil. Neotrop Entomol 2007; 36(4):612–615.

Redd JT, et al: Outbreak of lepidopterism at a boy scout camp. J Am Acad Dermatol 2007; 56(6):952–955.

Order Hemiptera

The true bugs belong to the order Hemiptera. The order includes bedbugs, water bugs, chinch bugs, stink bugs, squash bugs, and reduviid bugs (kissing bugs, assassin bugs). The latter are vectors of South American trypanosomiasis. In most true bugs, the wings are half sclerotic and half membranous, and typically overlap. In bedbugs, the wings are vestigial.

Cimicosis (bedbug bites)

Bedbugs have flat oval bodies and retroverted mouthparts used for taking blood meals (Fig. 20-30). *Cimex lectularius* is the most common species in temperate climates, and *Cimex hemipterus* in tropical climates. Both are reddish brown and about the size of a tick. *C. hemipterus* is somewhat longer than *C. lectularius*. They breed through a process referred to as traumatic insemination, where the male punctures the female and deposits sperm into her body cavity. Bedbugs hide in

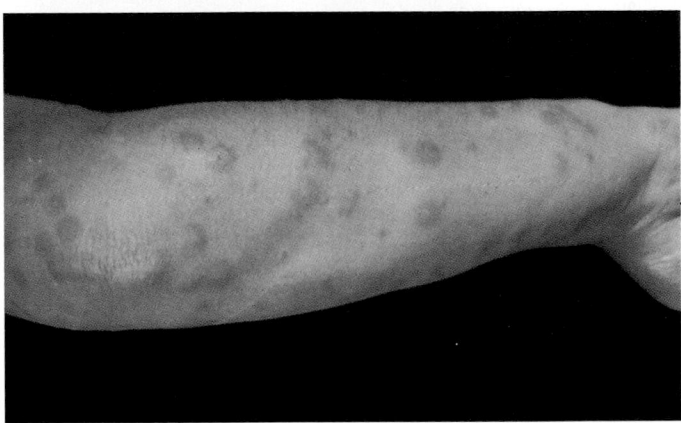

Fig. 20-31 Bedbug bites.

cracks and crevices, then descend to feed while the victim sleeps. It is common for bedbugs to inflict a series of bites in a row ("breakfast, lunch, and dinner"). Bites may mimic urticaria, and patients with papular urticaria commonly have antibodies to bedbug antigens. Bullous and urticarial reactions occur (Fig. 20-31). The incidence is rising in the US, and in some refugee camps, almost 90% of residents suffer from bedbug bites. Bedbugs are suspected vectors for Chagas' disease and hepatitis B, although data are sparse.

Bedbugs often infest bats and birds, and these hosts may be responsible for infestation in houses. Management of the infestation may require elimination of bird nests and bat roosts. Cracks and crevices should be eliminated, and the area treated with an insecticide such as dichlorvos or permethrin. As most insecticides have poor residual effect on mud bricks, wood, and fabric, frequent retreatment may be necessary. Microencapsulation of insecticides enhances persistence. Permethrin-impregnated bednets have been shown to be effective against bedbugs in tropical climates.

Abdel-Naser MB, et al: Patients with papular urticaria have IgG antibodies to bedbug (*Cimex lectularius*) antigens. Parasitol Res 2006; 98(6):550–556.

Anderson AL, et al: Bedbug infestations in the news: a picture of an emerging public health problem in the United States. J Environ Health 2008; 70(9):24–27, 52–53.

Scarupa MD, et al: Bedbug bites masquerading as urticaria. J Allergy Clin Immunol 2006; 117(6):1508–1509.

Reduviid bites

Triatome reduviid bugs (kissing bugs, assassin bugs, conenose bugs) descend on their victims while they sleep, and feed on

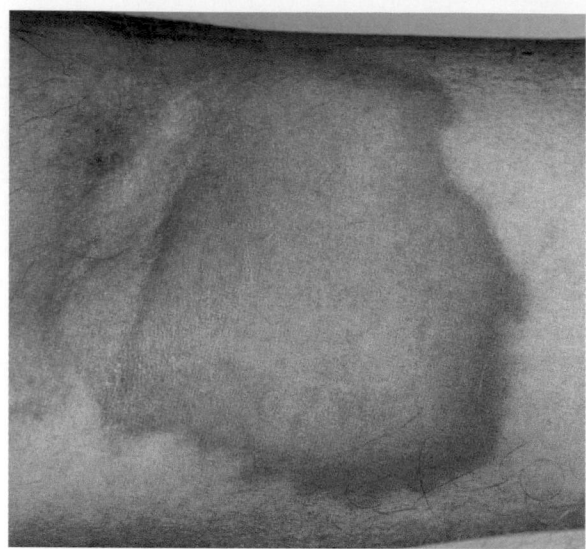

Fig. 20-32 Triatome bite.

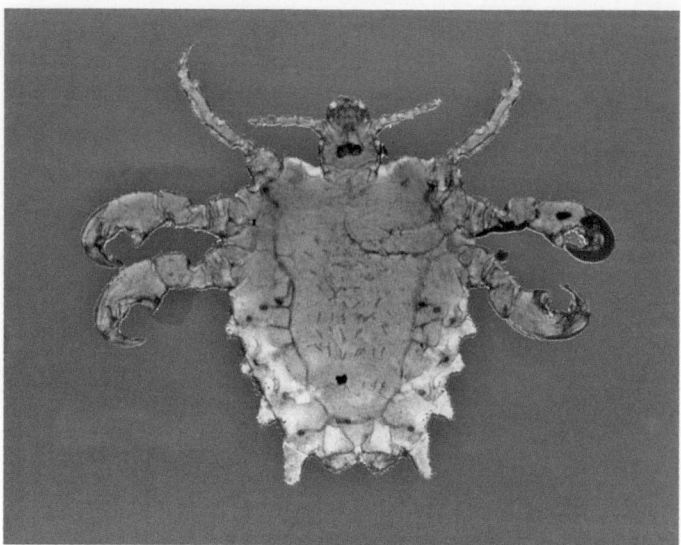

Fig. 20-33 Crab louse.

an exposed area of skin. The bite is typically painless, although the bugs are capable of producing a more painful defensive bite. Swelling and itching occur within hours of the bite (Fig. 20-32). Many Latin American species have a pronounced gastrocolic reflex and defecate when they feed. Romana's sign is unilateral eye swelling after a night-time encounter with a triatome bug. *Trypanosoma cruzi* is transmitted by the feces and rubbed into the bite. American trypanosomiasis can produce heart failure and megacolon. Triatome bugs infest thatch, cracks, and crevices, and infestation is associated with poor housing conditions. In nonendemic areas, bites are sporadic, and are often followed by a red swelling suggestive of cellulitis. Anaphylaxis has also occurred. *Arilus cristatus*, the wheal bug, is widely distributed and has an extremely painful defensive bite but it is not known to carry disease.

Elston DM: What's eating you? Wheel bug (Reduviidae: *Arilus cristatus*). Cutis 1998; 61:189.

Elston DM, et al: What's eating you? Triatome reduviids. Cutis 1999; 63:63.

Order Anoplura

Pediculosis

Three varieties of these flattened, wingless insects infest humans: *Pediculus humanus* var. *capitis* (the head louse), *P. humanus* var. *corporis* (the body louse), and *Phthirus pubis* (the pubic or crab louse) (Fig. 20-33). Rarely, zoonotic lice or louse-like psocids will cause infestation.

Pediculosis capitis

Pediculosis capitis is more common in children, but occurs in adults also. Patients present with intense pruritus of the scalp, and often have posterior cervical lymphadenopathy. Excoriations and small specks of louse dung are noted on the scalp, and secondary impetigo is common. Lice may be identified, especially when combing the hair. Nits may be present throughout the scalp, but are most common in the retroauricular region. Generally, only those ova close to the scalp are viable, and nits noted along the distal hair shaft are empty egg cases. In very humid climates, however, viable ova may be present along the entire length of the hair shaft. Peripilar keratin (hair) casts are remnants of the inner root sheath that encircle hair shafts. They may be mistaken for nits. While nits are firmly cemented to the hair, casts move freely along the

hair shaft. Headlice readily survive immersion in water, but remain fixed to scalp hairs. There is no evidence that swimming pools contribute to the spread of head lice.

Effective therapeutic agents must kill or remove both lice and ova. Ulesfia (containing benzyl alcohol) is the first non-neurotoxic FDA-approved treatment for lice and represents a significant advancement. Permethrin is the most widely used pediculicide in the US. It is available as an over-the-counter 1% cream rinse (Nix) and a 5% prescription cream (Elimite) that is marketed for the treatment of scabies. The 1% cream rinse must be applied after shampooing and drying the hair completely. Applying to dry hair lessens dilution of the medication. Product labeling states the medication should be applied for 10 min, then rinsed off, but longer applications may be required. Shampooing should not take place for 24 h afterward. Permethrin has a favorable safety profile, although congenital leukemia has been reported, as noted above, and the use of insecticidal shampoos is statistically associated with leukemia. Other reported side effects have included acute onset of stuttering in a toddler. Pyrethrins, combined with piperonyl butoxide (RID, A-200, R+C shampoo), are sold over the counter. Malathion 0.5% lotion (Ovide) is marketed as a prescription product in the US. The efficacy is partly dependent upon the vehicle, and the product is flammable and can be irritating to the eyes. As it has not been widely used in the US, resistance has not emerged. Lindane is also marketed as a prescription product. The efficacy is somewhat lower, and the product has potential neurotoxicity if abused and is not available in all areas. Carbaryl is used in many parts of the world, but not in the US. Because of the potential toxicity associated with chemical pediculicides, the future belongs to asphyxiating agents such as those that contain benzyl alcohol or dimeticone. Cure rates with dimeticone are significantly higher than those with permethrin in some studies. Other agents that asphyxiate or desiccate contain isopropyl myristate 50%.

Nit combing is an important adjunct to treatment, but is impractical as a primary method of therapy. Metal combs are more effective than plastic combs. Acidic cream rinses make the hair easier to comb but do not dissolve nit cement, which is similar in composition to amyloid. Various "natural" remedies are marketed that contain coconut oil, anise oil, and ylang ylang oil, but these agents are potential contact allergens, and there are few data regarding their safety and efficacy. Some data support the efficacy of tea tree oil, which is more potent than lavender or lemon oil. Some published data also support combination lotions containing 5% lavender, peppermint, and eucalyptus oils, or 10% eucalyptus and peppermint oils in various combinations of water and alcohol. The addition of 10% 1-dodecanol improves efficacy.

Aliphatic alcohols show promise as pediculicides, and crotamiton (Eurax), an antiscabietic agent, has some efficacy in the treatment of pediculosis. As no treatment is reliably ovicidal, retreatment in a week is reasonable for all patients. Resistance to pediculicides is an emerging problem in many parts of the world. The emergence of resistance to an agent is related to the frequency with which that agent is used. Knockdown resistance (KDR) is a common mechanism of resistance that manifests as lack of immobilization of the lice. Responsible gene mutations (*T929I* and *L932F*) have been identified and can be used to screen for KDR. In countries like the US, where permethrin is used commonly, permethrin-resistant lice have emerged. Cross-resistance among pyrethroids is typical. In the UK, resistance to malathion has been reported and multidrug-resistant lice have been identified. KDR results in slower killing of lice, but may be overcome to some degree by longer applications. Monooxygenase-based resistance to pyrethrins may be overcome by synergism with piperonyl butoxide. Sequential use of pediculicides may be useful in overcoming resistance, and systemic agents may play some role. Trimethoprim–sulfamethoxazole has been used as an off-label oral agent, although more recent data suggest it is ineffective. Shaving the head will cure head lice, but has poor patient acceptance in most cultures. Simple public health measures are also of value when epidemics of louse infestation occur in schools. Hats, scarves, and jackets should be stored separately under each child's desk. Louse education and inspections by the school nurse facilitate targeted treatment of infested individuals.

Pediculosis corporis

Pediculosis corporis (pediculosis vestimenti, "vagabond's disease") is caused by body lice that lay their eggs in the seams of clothing (Fig. 20-34). The parasite obtains its nourishment by descending to the skin and taking a blood meal. Generalized itching is accompanied by erythematous, blue and copper-colored macules, wheals, and lichenification. Secondary impetigo and furunculosis are common.

Body louse infestation is differentiated from scabies by the lack of involvement of the hands and feet, although infestation by both lice and scabies is common, and a given patient may suffer from lice, scabies, and flea infestation.

Lice may live in clothing for 1 month without a blood meal. If discarding the clothing is feasible, this is best. Destruction of body lice can also be accomplished by laundering the cloth-

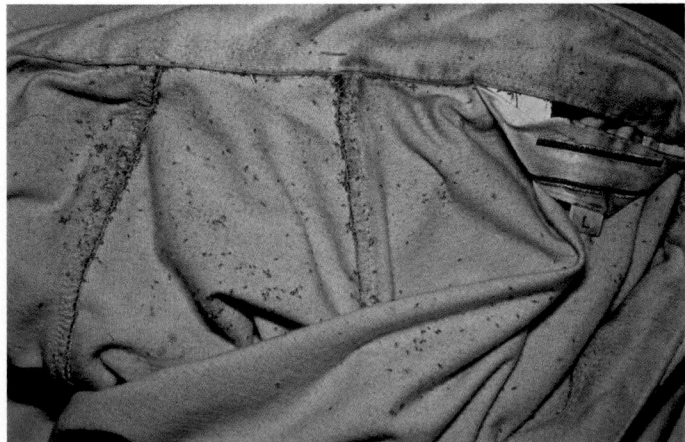

Fig. 20-34 Body lice in seams of clothing.

ing and bedding. Clothing placed in a dryer for 30 min at 65°C (149°F) is reliably disinfected. Pressing clothing with an iron, especially the seams, is also effective. Permethrin spray or 1% malathion powder can be used to treat clothing and reduce the risk of reinfestation.

Body lice are vectors for relapsing fever, trench fever, and epidemic typhus. These diseases are most prevalent among refugee populations. The trench fever organism is also an important cause of endocarditis among the homeless.

Pediculosis pubis (crabs)

Phthirus pubis, the crab louse, is found in the pubic region, as well as hairy areas of the legs, abdomen, chest, axillae, and arms. Pubic lice may also infest the eyelashes and scalp. The lice spread through close physical contact, and are commonly transmitted sexually. A diagnosis of pediculosis pubis should initiate a search for other STDs, including HIV. Contaminated bedding is also a source of infestation. Pubic louse nits are attached to the hairs at an acute angle. Other than the presence of lice and nits in the hair, the signs and symptoms are similar to those of body louse infestation.

Occasionally, blue or slate-colored macules occur in association with pediculosis pubis. These macules, called maculae ceruleae, are located chiefly on the sides of the trunk and on the inner aspects of the thighs. They are probably caused by altered blood pigments.

Treatment of pediculosis pubis is similar to that for head lice. The affected person's sexual contacts should be treated simultaneously. For eyelash involvement, a thick coating of petrolatum can be applied twice daily for 8 days, followed by mechanical removal of any remaining nits. Fluorescein and 4% pilocarpine gel are also effective. Clothing and fomites should be washed and dried by machine, or laundered and ironed.

Badiaga S, et al: The effect of a single dose of oral ivermectin on pruritus in the homeless. J Antimicrob Chemother 2008; 62(2):404–409.

Burgess IF, et al: Randomised, controlled, assessor blind trial comparing 4% dimeticone lotion with 0.5% malathion liquid for head louse infestation. PLoS ONE 2007; 2(11):e1127.

Elston DM: Drug-resistant lice. Arch Dermatol 2003; 139:1061.

Elston DM: Treating pediculosis—those nit-picking details. Pediatr Dermatol 2007; 24(4):415–416.

Galiczynski EM Jr, et al: What's eating you? Pubic lice (*Phthirus pubis*). Cutis 2008; 81(2):109–114.

Gonzalez Audino P, et al: Effectiveness of lotions based on essential oils from aromatic plants against permethrin resistant *Pediculus humanus capitis*. Arch Dermatol Res 2007; 299(8):389–392.

Hammond K, et al: Topical pyrethrin toxicity leading to acute-onset stuttering in a toddler. Am J Ther 2008; 15(4):323–324.

Heukelbach J, et al: A highly efficacious pediculicide based on dimeticone: randomized observer blinded comparative trial. BMC Infect Dis 2008; 8:115.

Kaul N, et al: North American efficacy and safety of a novel pediculicide rinse, isopropyl myristate 50% (Resultz). J Cutan Med Surg 2007; 11(5):161–167.

Mikhail M, et al: What's eating you? Body lice (*Pediculus humanus* var *corporis*). Cutis 2007; 80(5):397–398.

Oliveira FA, et al: High in vitro efficacy of Nyda L, a pediculicide containing dimeticone. J Eur Acad Dermatol Venereol 2007; 21(10):1325–1329.

Pinckney J 2nd, et al: Phthiriasis palpebrarum: a common culprit with uncommon presentation. Dermatol Online J 2008; 14(4):7.

Raoult D, et al: Molecular identification of lice from pre-Columbian mummies. J Infect Dis 2008; 197(4):535–543.

Speare R, et al: Comparative efficacy of two nit combs in removing head lice (*Pediculus humanus* var. *capitis*) and their eggs. Int J Dermatol 2007; 46(12):1275–1278.

Toloza AC, et al: Interspecific hybridization of eucalyptus as a potential tool to improve the bioactivity of essential oils against permethrin-resistant head lice from Argentina. Bioresour Technol 2008; 99(15):7341–7347.

Williamson EM, et al: An investigation and comparison of the bioactivity of selected essential oils on human lice and house dust mites. Fitoterapia 2007; 78(7–8):521–525.

Order Diptera

Order Diptera includes the two-winged biting flies and mosquitoes. Adult dipterids bite and spread disease, while larvae parasitize humans in the form of myiasis. Medically important families of flies include the Tabanidae (horsefly, deerfly, gadfly), which inflict extremely painful bites, and the Muscidae (housefly, stablefly, and tsetse fly). Tsetse fly bites transmit African trypanosomiasis. Simulidae include the black fly (buffalo gnat, turkey gnat), the vector of onchocerciasis. These flies are dark-colored and "hunchbacked." They may produce extremely painful bites that may be associated with fever, chills, and lymphadenitis. Black flies are seasonal annoyances in the northern US and Canada.

Psychodidae sandflies (Diptera: Phlebotominae) are small, hairy-winged flies that transmit leishmaniasis, sandfly fever, and verruga peruana. Sandfly fever viruses are a problem in Africa, the Mediterranean basin, and Central Asia, and are carried by *Phlebotomus* flies. *Lutzomyia* flies are common in Latin America and south Texas.

Culicidae, or mosquitoes, are vectors of many important diseases, such as filariasis, malaria, dengue, and yellow fever. Their bites may cause severe urticarial reactions. Ceratopogonidae, the biting midges or gnats, fly in swarms and produce erythematous, edematous lesions at the site of their bite.

Mosquito bites

Moisture, warmth, CO_2, estrogens, and lactic acid in sweat attract mosquitoes. Drinking alcohol also stimulates mosquito attraction. Mosquito bites are a common cause of papular urticaria. More severe local reactions are seen in young children, individuals with immunodeficiency, and those with new exposure to indigenous mosquitoes. Both necrotizing fasciitis and the hemophagocytic syndrome have been reported following mosquito bites, and exaggerated hypersensitivity reactions to mosquito bites are noted in a wide variety of Epstein–Barr virus (EBV)-associated lymphoproliferative disorders, especially natural killer (NK) cell proliferations. Mosquito bites may play a key role in reactivation of latent EBV infection. Effective repellents are mostly DEET- or picaridin-based. Effective mosquito traps are available, but electronic mosquito repellents appear to be of no value.

Enayati AA, et al: Electronic mosquito repellents for preventing mosquito bites and malaria infection. Cochrane Database Syst Rev 2007 Apr 18; (2):CD005434.

Moore SJ, et al: Are mosquitoes diverted from repellent-using individuals to non-users? Results of a field study in Bolivia. Trop Med Int Health 2007; 12(4):532–539.

Peng Z, et al: Advances in mosquito allergy. Curr Opin Allergy Clin Immunol 2007; 7(4):350–354.

Wang Q, et al: Comparison of the mosquito saliva-capture enzyme-linked immunosorbent assay and the unicap test in the diagnosis of mosquito allergy. Ann Allergy Asthma Immunol 2007; 99(2):199–200.

Ked itch

The sheep ked (*Melophagus ovinus*) feeds by thrusting its sharp mouth parts into the skin and sucking blood. Occasionally, it attacks woolsorters and sheepherders, causing pruritic, often hemorrhagic papules, nearly always with a central punctum. Deer keds attack humans in a similar way. The papules are very persistent and may last for up to 12 months. Favorite locations are the hips and the abdomen.

Myiasis

Myiasis is the infestation of human tissue by fly larvae. Forms of infestation include wound myiasis, furuncular myiasis, plaque myiasis, creeping dermal myiasis, and body cavity myiasis. Wound myiasis occurs when flies lay their eggs in an open wound. Furuncular myiasis often involves a mosquito vector that carries the fly egg. Plaque myiasis typically involves many maggots and occurs after flies lay their eggs on clothing. Creeping myiasis develops when the larvae of the *Gasterophilus* fly wander intradermally. The most common species are *Gasterophilus nasalis* and *Gasterophilus intestinalis*. An itching pink papule develops, followed by a tortuous line that extends by 1–30 cm a day. Body cavity myiasis may involve the orbit, nasal cavity, gastrointestinal tract, or urogenital system.

The human botfly, *Dermatobia hominis*, is a common cause of furuncular myiasis (Fig. 20-35) in the neotropical regions of the New World. The female glues its eggs to the body of a mosquito, stablefly, or tick. When the unwitting vector punctures the skin by biting, the larva emerges from the egg and enters the skin through the puncture wound. Over a period of several days, a painful furuncle develops in which the larva is present. Other larvae that frequently cause furuncular lesions in North America are the common cattle grub (*Hypoderma lineatum*), rabbit botfly (*Cuterebra cuniculi*), and *Wohlfahrtia vigil*. This last fly can penetrate infant skin, but not adult skin. Thus, nearly all reported cases have occurred in infants. The New World screw worm, *Cochliomyia hominivorax*, often involves the head and neck region. Larvae of Calliphoridae flies, especially *Phaenicia sericata*, the green blowfly, cause wound myiasis. Other blowflies, flesh flies (Sarcophagidae), and humpbacked flies (Phoridae) are less common causes of wound myiasis. In tropical Africa the Tumbu fly (*Cordylobia anthropophaga*) deposits her eggs on the ground or on clothing. The young maggots penetrate the skin and often form a plaque with many furuncular-appearing lesions. *Cordylobia ruandae* and *Cordylobia rodhaini* are less frequent causes of plaque myiasis.

Removal of the maggots of furuncular myiasis can be accomplished by injection of a local anesthetic into the skin, which causes the larva to bulge outward. The opening of the furuncle can also be occluded with hair gel, surgical lubricant, lard, petrolatum, or bacon, causing the larva to migrate outward. Successful treatment with ivermectin has also been reported.

Caissie R, et al: Cutaneous myiasis: diagnosis, treatment, and prevention. J Oral Maxillofac Surg 2008; 66(3):560–568.

de Souza Barbosa T, et al: Oral infection by *Diptera* larvae in children: a case report. Int J Dermatol 2008; 47(7):696–699.

McGraw TA, et al: Cutaneous myiasis. J Am Acad Dermatol 2008; 58(6):907–926.

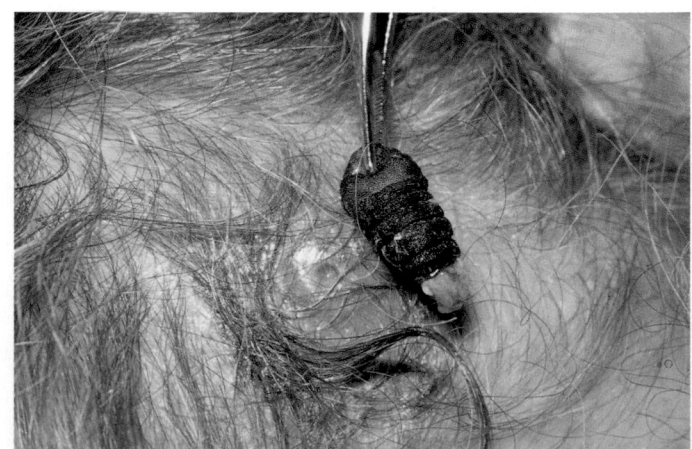

Fig. 20-35 Myiasis.

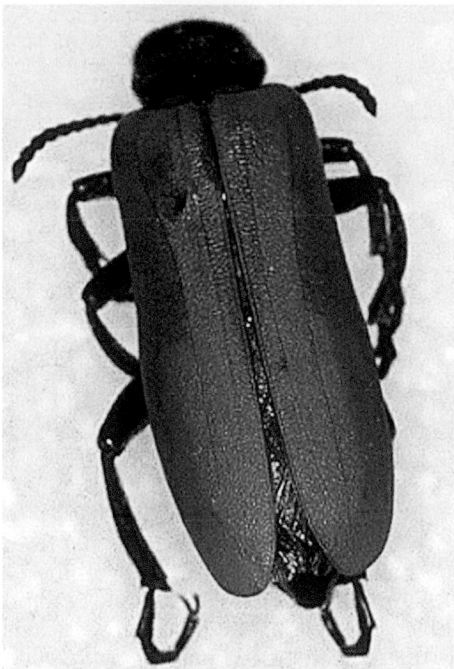

Fig. 20-36 Blister beetle.

Order Coleoptera

Blister beetle dermatitis

Blister beetle (Fig. 20-36) dermatitis occurs after contact with several groups of beetle. The Meloidae and Oedemeridae families produce injury to the skin by releasing a vesicating agent, cantharidin. Members of the family Staphylinidae (genus *Paederus*) contain a different vesicant, pederin. None of the beetles bites or stings; rather, they exude their blistering fluid if they are brushed against, pressed, or crushed on the skin. Many blister beetles are attracted at night by fluorescent lighting.

Slight burning and tingling of the skin occur within minutes, followed by the formation of bullae, often arranged in a linear fashion. "Kissing lesions" are observed when the blister beetle's excretion is deposited in the flexures of the elbows or other folds. Ingestion of beetles or cantharidin results in poisoning, presenting with hematuria and abdominal pain. In many tropical and subtropical habitats, rove beetles (genus *Paederus*) produce a patchy or linear erythematous vesicular eruption (Fig. 20-37). In parts of South America, it is known as podo. It occurs frequently during the rainy season and appears predominantly on the neck and exposed parts. Lymphadenopathy and fever are common. In the American southwest, outbreaks of rove beetle dermatitis have followed unusually rainy periods. In southeastern Australia, corneal erosions are caused by small Corylophidae beetles (*Orthoperus* spp).

Treatment consists of drainage of the bullae and application of cold wet compresses and topical antibiotic preparations. Early cleansing with acetone, ether, soap, or alcohol may be helpful to remove cantharidin.

Other beetles

Papulovesicular and urticarial dermatitis is caused by the common carpet beetle (Dermestidae: *Anthrenus scrophulariae*). The eruption involves the chest, neck, and forearms. The larvae inhabit warm houses throughout the winter months. They are reddish brown, fusiform, about 6 mm long, and covered by hairs. A generalized pruritic eruption has been attributed to the larvae of the carpet beetle, *Anthrenus verbasci*. Bombardier beetles of the family Carabidae (subfamily Brachininae) can cause skin burns with a deep yellow–brown color. Chemicals released when these beetles are crushed include acids, phenols, hydrocarbons, and quinines. When the beetle is threatened, chemical reactions produce an explosive spray of boiling hot benzoquinones from the tip of the abdomen. Dermestidae (skin beetles) and Cleridae (bone beetles) infest exposed human remains and are useful in estimating the postmortem interval. Rare cases of allergic angioedema have been reported after exposure to ladybugs.

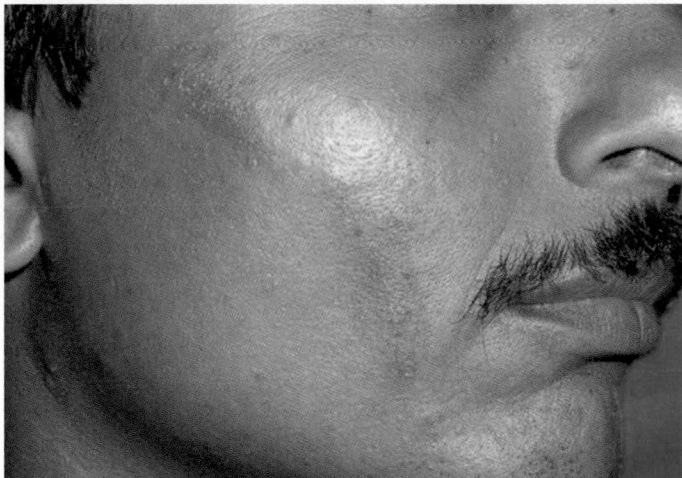

Fig. 20-37 *Paederus* dermatitis. (Courtesy of Shyam Verma, MD)

Elston DM: What's eating you? Blister beetles. Cutis 2004; 74(5):285–286.

Gnanaraj P, et al: An outbreak of *Paederus* dermatitis in a suburban hospital in South India: a report of 123 cases and review of literature. J Am Acad Dermatol 2007; 57(2):297–300.

Padhi T, et al: Clinicoepidemiological profile of 590 cases of beetle dermatitis in western Orissa. Indian J Dermatol Venereol Leprol 2007; 73(5):333–335.

Order Hymenoptera

Hymenopterids include bees, wasps, hornets, and ants. Stings by any of these may manifest the characteristic clinical and histologic features of eosinophilic cellulitis (Wells syndrome), complete with flame figures.

Bees and wasps

Yellowjackets are the principal cause of allergic reaction to insect stings, because they nest in the ground or in walls and are disturbed by outdoor activity, such as gardening or lawn mowing. Bees are generally docile and sting only when provoked, although Africanized bees display aggressive behavior. The allergens in vespid venom are phospholipase, hyaluronidase, and a protein known as antigen 5. Bee venom contains histamine, mellitin, hyaluronidase, a high molecular weight substance with acid phosphatase activity, and phospholipase A. The barbed ovipositor of the honeybee is torn out of the bee and remains in the skin after stinging. The bumble bee, wasp, and hornet are able to withdraw their stinger.

The reaction to these stings ranges from pain and mild local edema to exaggerated reactions that may last for days. Serum sickness, characterized by fever, urticaria, and joint pain, may occur 7–10 days after the sting. Severe anaphylactic shock and death may occur within minutes of the sting. Most hypersensitivity reactions have been shown to be mediated by specific IgE antibodies. Anaphylaxis to vespids may also be the presenting symptom of mastocytosis, with no demonstrable specific IgE against wasp venom. Granuloma annulare and subcutaneous granulomatous reactions have been reported. Contact allergy to propolis is common among beekeepers.

Treatment of local reactions consists of immediate application of ice packs or topical anesthetics. Chronic reaction sites may be injected with triamcinolone suspension diluted to 5 mg/mL with 2% lidocaine. Oral prednisone may be required for severe local reactions.

For severe systemic reactions, 0.3 mL of epinephrine (1:1000 aqueous solution) is injected intramuscularly. This may need to be repeated after 10 min. Susceptible persons should carry a source of injectable epinephrine. Corticosteroids and epinephrine may be required for several days following severe reactions. Hyposensitization by means of venom immunotherapy can reduce the risk of anaphylaxis in people at risk. Those at risk should be evaluated by an allergist. Rush desensitization regimens exist and ultra-rush sublingual immunotherapy looks promising.

Ants

The sting of most ants is painful, but that of the fire ants (*Solenopsis invicta*, *Solenopsis geminata*, or *Solenopsis richteri*) is especially painful. Fire ants are vicious and will produce many burning, painful stings within seconds if their mound is disturbed. The sting causes intense pain and whealing. Later, an intensely pruritic sterile pustule develops at the site (Fig. 20-38). Anaphylaxis, seizures, and mononeuropathy have been reported. The sting of harvester ants and soldier ants may produce similar reactions. Treatment options are similar to those for vespid stings.

Bilò BM, et al: Advances in hymenoptera venom immunotherapy. Curr Opin Allergy Clin Immunol 2007; 7(6):567–573.
Hafner T, et al: Long-term efficacy of venom immunotherapy. Ann Allergy Asthma Immunol 2008; 100(2):162–165.
Lewis FS, et al: What's eating you? Bees, part 1: characteristics, reactions, and management. Cutis 2007; 79(6):439–444.
Lewis FS, et al: What's eating you? Bees, part 2: venom immunotherapy and mastocytosis. Cutis 2007; 80(1):33–37.
Münstedt K, et al: Contact allergy to propolis in beekeepers. Allergol Immunopathol (Madr) 2007; 35(3):95–100.
Patriarca G, et al: Sublingual desensitization in patients with wasp venom allergy: preliminary results. Int J Immunopathol Pharmacol 2008; 21(3):669–678.
Takayama K, et al: Papular granuloma annulare with subcutaneous granulomatous reaction induced by a bee sting. Acta Derm Venereol 2008; 88(5):519–520.

Yanagawa Y, et al: Cutaneous hemorrhage or necrosis findings after *Vespa mandarinia* (wasp) stings may predict the occurrence of multiple organ injury: a case report and review of literature. Clin Toxicol (Phila) 2007; 45(7):803–807.

Order Siphonaptera

Fleas are wingless, with highly developed legs for jumping. They are blood-sucking parasites, infesting most warm-blooded animals. Fleas are important vectors of plague, endemic typhus, brucellosis, melioidosis, and erysipeloid.

Pulicosis (flea bites)

The species of flea that most commonly attack humans are the cat flea (*Ctenocephalides felis*) (Fig. 20-39), human flea (*Pulex irritans*), dog flea (*Ctenocephalides canis*), and oriental rat flea (*Xenopsylla cheopis*) (Fig. 20-40). The stick-tight flea (*Echidnophaga gallinacea*), mouse flea (*Leptopsylla segnis*), and chicken flea (*Ceratophyllus gallinae*) are sometimes implicated.

Fleas are small, brown insects about 2.5 mm long, flat from side to side, with long hind legs. They slip into clothing or jump actively when disturbed. They bite about the legs and waist and may be troublesome in houses where there are dogs or cats. The lesions are often grouped and may be arranged in zigzag lines. Hypersensitivity reactions may appear as papular urticaria, nodules, or bullae. Camphor and menthol preparations, topical corticosteroids, and topical anesthetics can be of benefit.

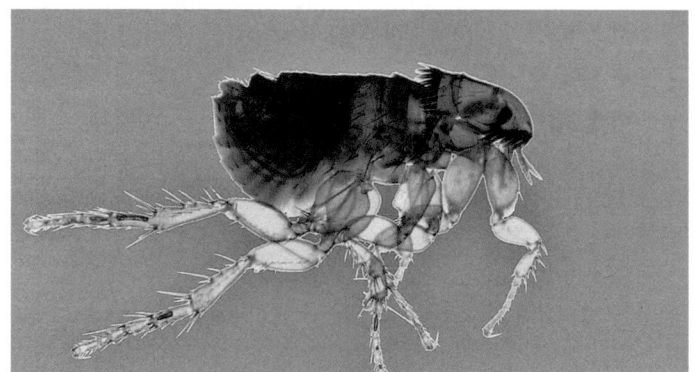

Fig. 20-39 Cat flea.

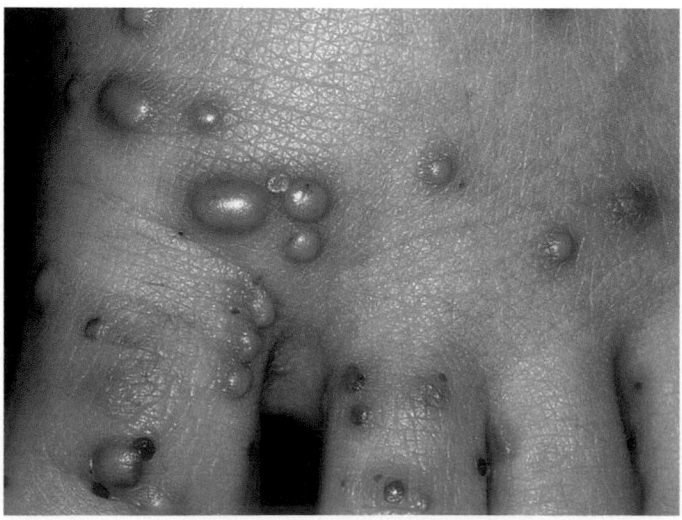

Fig. 20-38 Sterile pustules at the site of fire ant stings.

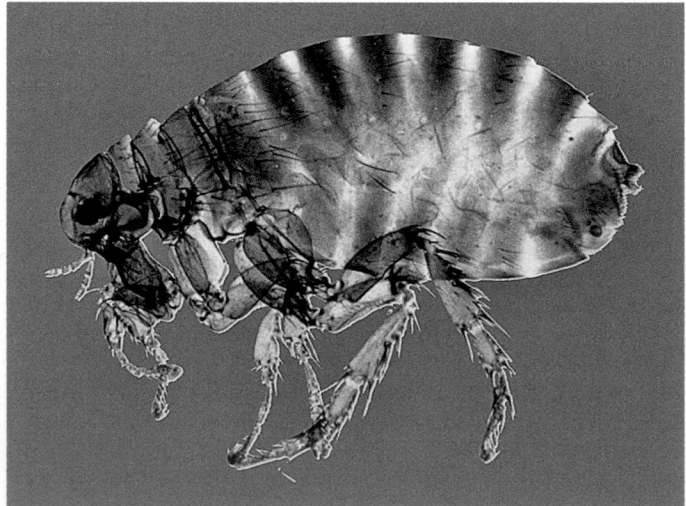

Fig. 20-40 Oriental rat flea.

Vectors of disease

Xenopsylla cheopis and *Xenopsylla braziliensis* are vectors of plague and endemic typhus. The cat flea (*Ctenocephalides felis*) is the vector for *Rickettsia felis* (a cause of endemic typhus). Plague and tularemia are transmitted by the squirrel flea, *Diamanus montanus*. Several species of flea are intermediate hosts of the dog tapeworm and rat tapeworm, which may be an incidental parasite of humans.

Tungiasis

Tunga penetrans is also known as nigua, the chigoe, sand flea, or jigger. It is a reddish-brown flea about 1 mm long. It resides in the Caribbean, equatorial Africa, Central and South America, India, and Pakistan. It was first reported in crewmen who sailed with Christopher Columbus.

The impregnated female chigoe burrows into the skin, often adjacent to a toenail, where she may be seen with the aid of dermoscopy. The eggs develop and drop to the ground. These eggs develop into larvae, which form cocoons from which the insects emerge in about 10 days. Skin lesions are pruritic swellings the size of a small pea (Fig. 20-41). These may occur on the ankles, feet, and soles, as well as the anogenital areas. The lesions become extremely painful and secondarily infected. Wearing open shoes and the presence of pigs in the area are risk factors for disease.

Curettage or excision of the burrows is recommended. Topical ivermectin, metrifonate, or thiabendazole can be used, and oral thiabendazole, 25 mg/kg/day, has been effective in heavily infested patients. Antibiotics should be used for the secondary infection and tetanus prophylaxis should be given. These lesions can be prevented by the wearing of shoes. Infested ground and buildings may be disinfected by the use of insecticides and growth inhibitors.

Cabrera R, et al: Tungiasis: eggs seen with dermoscopy. Br J Dermatol 2008; 158(3):635–636.

Ugbomoiko US, et al: Risk factors for tungiasis in Nigeria: identification of targets for effective intervention. PLoS Negl Trop Dis 2007; 1(3):e87.

Veraldi S, et al: Imported tungiasis: a report of 19 cases and review of the literature. Int J Dermatol 2007; 46(10):1061–1066.

Zalaudek I, et al: Entodermoscopy: a new tool for diagnosing skin infections and infestations. Dermatology 2008; 216(1):14–23.

Class Arachnida

Arachnida includes the ticks, mites, spiders, and scorpions. Adult and nymph stages of arachnids have four pairs of legs, while larval forms have six legs. Their bodies consist of cephalothorax and abdomen, in contrast to insects, which have three body segments.

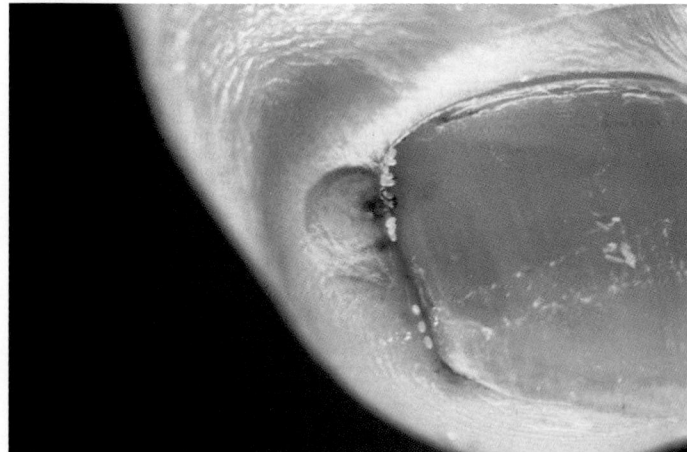

Fig. 20-41 Tungiasis.

Order Acarina

Tick bite

Several varieties of the family Ixodidae (hard ticks) and Argasidae (soft ticks) will attack human skin, but only hard ticks remain attached. In the US, *Ornithodoros hermsi*, *Ornithodoros turicata*, and *Ornithodoros parkeri* transmit tick-borne relapsing fever. The wood tick (*Dermacentor andersoni*) is an important disease vector in western states. It carries Rocky Mountain spotted fever, tularemia, ehrlichiosis, and Colorado tick fever. The dog tick (*Dermacentor variabilis*) (Fig. 20-42) is prevalent in the eastern states, and is the most common vector of Rocky Mountain spotted fever. It also carries tularemia. *Dermacentor marginatus* transmits tick-borne lymphadenopathy in Spain. The brown dog tick (*Rhipicephalus sanguineus*) is a vector of Rocky Mountain spotted fever, tularemia, and boutonneuse fever. The lone star tick (*Amblyomma americanum*) (Fig. 20-43) carries Rocky Mountain spotted fever, tularemia, and human monocytic ehrlichiosis. *Ixodes ricinus* in Europe and *Ixodes scapularis* and *Ixodes pacificus* in the US transmit *Borrelia burgdorferi*, the cause of Lyme disease. *Ixodes* ticks also transmit human granulocytic ehrlichiosis and babesiosis. The risk of disease transmission increases with the duration of tick attachment. Unfortunately, ticks commonly attach in areas where they are not noticed, allowing them to engorge and transmit disease.

The female hard tick attaches itself to the skin by sticking its proboscis into the flesh to suck blood from the superficial vessels. The insertion of the hypostome is generally unnoticed by the subject. The attached tick may be mistaken by the patient for a new mole (Fig. 20-44). The parasite slowly becomes engorged and then falls off. During this time, which may last for 7–12 days, the patient may suffer from fever, chills, headache, abdominal pain, and vomiting. This is called tick bite pyrexia. Removal of the engorged tick causes a subsidence of the general symptoms in 12–36 h.

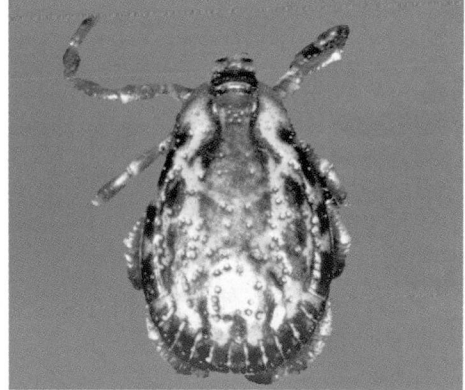

Fig. 20-42 *Dermacentor variabilis*.

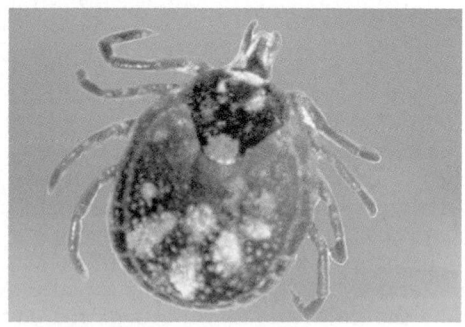

Fig. 20-43 Lone star tick.

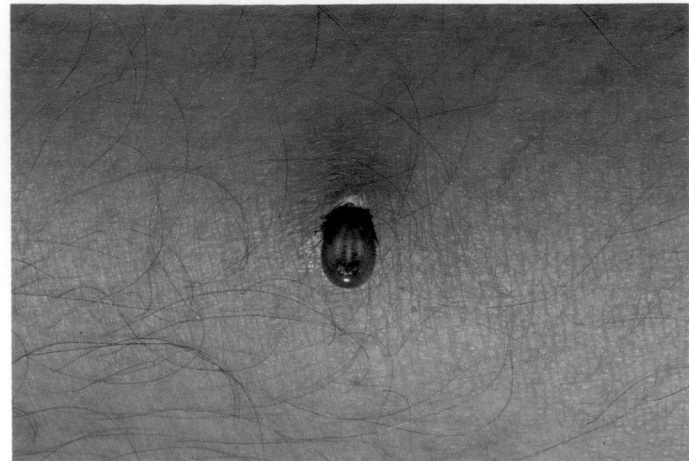

Fig. 20-44 Tick attached to skin.

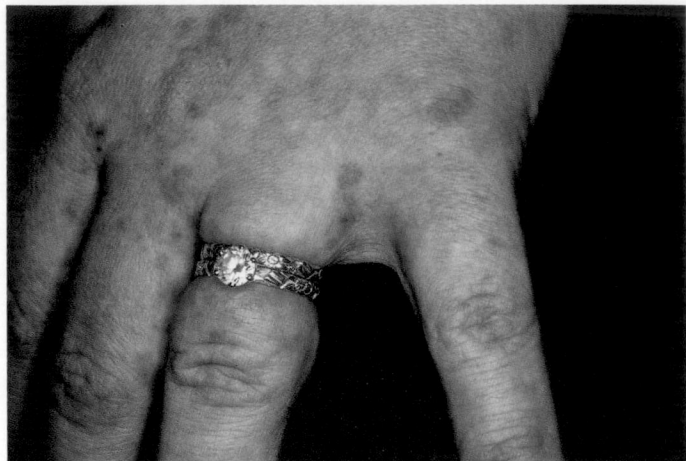

Fig. 20-45 Scabies.

The bites may be followed by small, severely pruritic, fibrous nodules (tick bite granulomas) that persist for months, or by pruritic circinate and arciform localized erythemas that may continue for months. Tick bite-induced alopecia has been reported.

Histologically, bite reactions demonstrate wedge-shaped necrosis with a neutrophilic infiltrate and vascular thrombosis or hemorrhage. Chronic bite reactions often have atypical CD30+ lymphocytes and eosinophils. Pseudolymphomas and immunocytomas may occur.

Tick paralysis

Tick paralysis most commonly affects children, and carries a mortality rate of about 10%. Flaccid paralysis begins in the legs, then the arms, and finally the neck, resembling Landry–Guillain–Barré syndrome. Bulbar paralysis, dysarthria, dysphagia, and death from respiratory failure may occur. Prompt recovery occurs if the tick is found and removed before the terminal stage. *Dermacentor* ticks in North America and *Ixodes* ticks in Australia are the most important causes of tick paralysis. As *Dermacentor* ticks commonly attach to the scalp, they may go unnoticed.

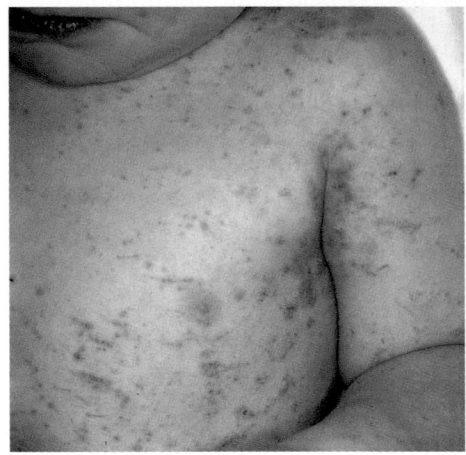

Fig. 20-46 Scabies.

Castelli E, et al: Local reactions to tick bites. Am J Dermatopathol 2008; 30(3):241–248.

Dworkin MS, et al: Tick-borne relapsing fever. Infect Dis Clin North Am 2008; 22(3):449–468.

Edlow JA, et al: Tick paralysis. Infect Dis Clin North Am 2008; 22(3):397–413.

Gunduz A, et al: Tick attachment sites. Wilderness Environ Med 2008; 19(1):4–6.

Larkin JM: Ticks and tick-related illness. Med Health R I 2008; 91(7):209–211.

Porta FS, et al: Tick-borne lymphadenopathy: a new infectious disease in children. Pediatr Infect Dis J 2008; 27(7):618–622.

Mites

Scabies

Sarcoptes scabiei, the itch mite, is an oval, ventrally flattened mite with dorsal spines. The fertilized female burrows into the stratum corneum and deposits her eggs. Scabies is characterized by pruritic papular lesions, excoriations, and burrows. Sites of predilection include the finger webs (Fig. 20-45), wrists, axillae (Fig. 20-46), areolae, umbilicus, lower abdomen, genitals (Fig. 20-47), and buttocks (Fig. 20-48). An imaginary circle intersecting the main sites of involvement—axillae, elbow flexures, wrists and hands, and crotch—has long been called the circle of Hebra. In adults, the scalp and face are usually spared, but in infants lesions are commonly present over the entire cutaneous surface. The burrows appear as slightly elevated, grayish, tortuous lines in the skin. A vesicle or pustule containing the mite may be noted at the end of the burrow, especially in infants and children. To identify burrows quickly, a drop of India ink or gentian violet can be applied to the infested area, then removed with alcohol. Thin threadlike burrows retain the ink.

The eruption varies considerably, depending on the length of infestation, previous sensitization, and previous treatment. It also varies with climate and the host's immunologic status. Lichenification, impetigo, and furunculosis may be present. Bullous lesions may contain many eosinophils, resembling bullous pemphigoid. Positive immunofluorescent findings may also be noted. Scabies may also resemble Langerhans cell histiocytosis clinically and histologically. Misdiagnosis has led to systemic treatment with toxic agents.

Dull red nodules may appear during active scabies; these are 3–5 mm in diameter, may or may not itch, and persist on the scrotum penis (Fig. 20-49), and vulva. Intralesional steroids, tar, or excision are methods of treatment for this troublesome condition, termed nodular scabies. Histologically, the lesions may suggest lymphoma.

Crusted scabies (Norwegian or hyperkeratotic scabies) is found in immunocompromised or debilitated patients, including those with neurologic disorders, Down syndrome, organ transplants, graft versus host disease, adult T-cell leukemia, Hansen's disease, or AIDS. In these patients, the infestation assumes a heavily scaling and crusted appearance. Crusts and scales teem with mites, and there is involvement of the face

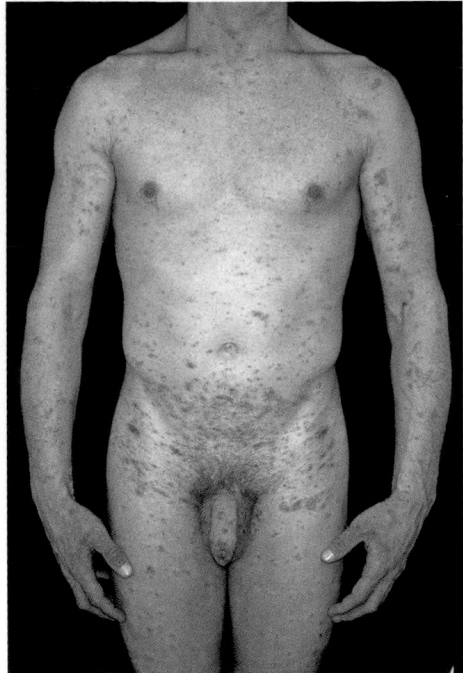

Fig. 20-47 Scabies.

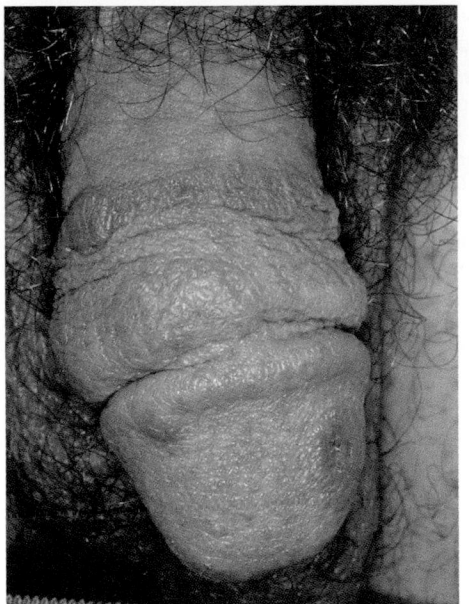

Fig. 20-49 Scabies.

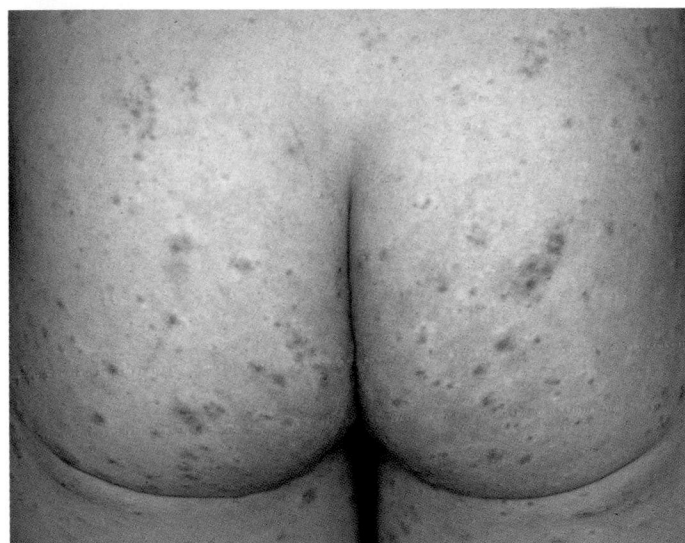

Fig. 20-48 Scabies.

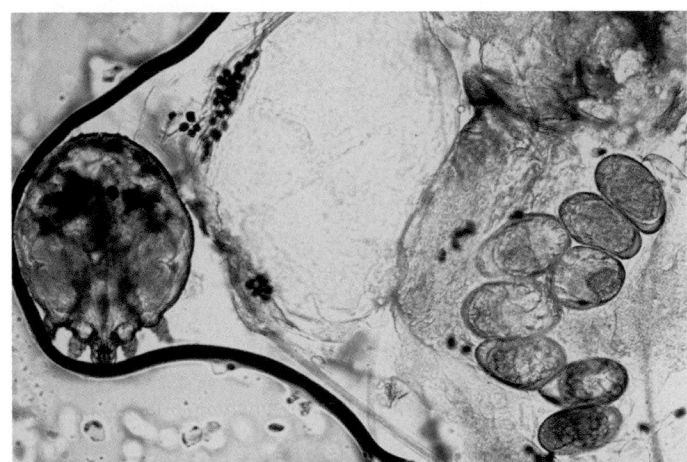

Fig. 20-50 Scabies mite, ova, and feces.

and especially the scalp. Itching may be slight. Psoriasis-like scaling is noted around and under the nails. The tips of the fingers are swollen and crusted; the nails are distorted. Severe fissuring and scaling of the genitalia and buttocks may be present. Pressure-bearing areas are the sites of predilection for the heavy keratotic lesions, in which the mites may abound.

Scabies is usually contracted by close personal contact, although it may also be transmitted by contaminated linens and clothing. Screening for other STDs is appropriate. Sensitization begins about 2–4 weeks after onset of infection. During this time the parasites may be on the skin and may burrow into it without causing pruritus or discomfort. Severe itching begins with sensitization of the host. In reinfections, itching begins within days and the reaction may be clinically more intense. The itching is most intense at night, whereas during the daytime the pruritus is tolerable but persistent. The eruption does not involve the face or scalp in adults. In women, itching of the nipples associated with a generalized pruritic papular eruption is characteristic; in men, itchy papules on the

scrotum and penis are equally typical. When more than one member of the family has pruritus, suspicion of scabies should be aroused. Whenever possible, though, it is advisable to identify the mite, as a diagnosis of scabies usually requires treatment of close physical contacts in addition to the patient. Because scabies cannot always be excluded by examination, treatment on presumption of scabies is sometimes necessary.

Positive diagnosis is made only by the demonstration of the mite under the microscope (Fig. 20-50). A burrow is sought and the position of the mite is determined. A surgical blade or sterile needle is used to remove the parasite. A drop of mineral or immersion oil can be placed on a lesion and gently scraped away with the epidermis beneath it. The majority of mites are found on the hands and wrists, less frequently (in decreasing order) at the elbows, genitalia, buttocks, and axillae. Children have often gathered mites and ova under the nails when scratching. A blunt curette can be used to gather material from under the nails for examination. Non-invasive techniques include dermoscopy and digital photography.

Permethrin 5% cream (Elimite) is the most widely used and most effective medication for scabies. It is a synthetic pyrethroid that is lethal to mites and has low toxicity for humans, although some concern has been raised about the association between topical insecticides and lymphoma.

Lindane (γ-benzene hexachloride) is also effective, with a low incidence of adverse effects when used properly. Because of the availability of less toxic agents, lindane is rarely used as a first-line agent. In much of the world, benzyl benzoate and 10% precipitated sulfur in white petrolatum are used to treat scabies. The scabicide should be thoroughly rubbed into the skin from the neck to the feet, with particular attention given to the creases, perianal areas, umbilicus, and free nail edge and folds. It is washed off 8–10 h later. Clothing and bed linen are changed and laundered thoroughly. Crotamiton (Eurax) has a lower cure rate than other available agents. When used, it should be applied on five successive nights and washed off 24 h after the last use.

Ivermectin has been used to control onchocerciasis since 1987, and is marketed in the US for the treatment of strongyloidiasis. Numerous publications attest to its efficacy in treating scabies. It is supplied as 3 and 6 mg pills, and is usually given at a dose of 200 µg/kg. Although an oral treatment is very convenient, it may not be any more effective than topical therapy. In the crusted type, it should be used in conjunction with a topical agent. It may need to be repeated two or three times at intervals of 1–2 weeks. The drug appears to have a good margin of safety, although neurotoxicity may be possible.

Individuals in close contact with the patient should be treated. Scabies in long-term healthcare institutions is an increasing problem. Delays in treating close contacts may result in large numbers requiring treatment.

Animal scabies Zoonotic scabies and scab mites may affect humans who come in close contact with the animal. The reaction resembles scabies, but typically runs a self-limited course. Burrows are usually absent.

Other mite diseases

***Demodex* mites** *Demodex folliculorum* is a vermiform mite that inhabits the pilosebaceous units of the nose, forehead, chin, and scalp. The mite has a flattened head, four pairs of short, peglike legs, and an elongated abdomen. *Demodex brevis* is shorter, and is more commonly found on the trunk.

In dogs, the lesions of demodectic mange contain numerous mites. In humans, there are convincing reports of demodectic blepharitis, demodectic folliculitis, demodectic abscess, and demodectic alopecia that respond to eradication of the mites. Some rosacea-like lesions may also be caused by *Demodex*. Treatment of the eruptions in which *Demodex* has been implicated consists of applying permethrin, sulfur, lindane, benzyl benzoate, or benzoyl peroxide. Oral ivermectin and metronidazole have also been used.

***Cheyletiella* dermatitis** *Cheyletiella yasguri*, *Cheyletiella blakei* (Fig. 20-51), and *Cheyletiella parasitovorax* are three species of nonburrowing mite that are parasitic on dogs, cats, and rabbits, respectively, where they present as "walking dandruff." They may bite humans when there is close contact with the animals, producing an itchy dermatitis resembling scabies or immu-

nobullous disease. The mites are similar in diameter to *S. scabiei*, but are elongated and have prominent anterior hooked palps. They may be found by brushing the animal's hair over a dark piece of paper. The brushings can be placed in alcohol, where the scales and hair sink while the mites float. The pet should be treated by a qualified veterinarian.

Chigger bite The trombiculid mites are known as chiggers, mower's mites, or red bugs. In North America, *Trombicula* (*Eutrombicula*) *alfreddugesi* attacks humans and animals. In Europe, the harvest mite, *Neotrombicula autumnalis*, is a common nuisance. Attacks occur chiefly during the summer and fall, when individuals have more frequent contact with mite-infested grass and bushes. The lesions occur chiefly on the legs (Fig. 20-52), and at the belt line and other sites at which clothing causes constriction. Penile lesions are common in males. Lesions generally consist of severely pruritic hemorrhagic puncta surrounded by red swellings. On the ankles, intensely pruritic, grouped, excoriated papules are noted. Several varieties of trombiculid mite in East Asia and the South Pacific are vectors of scrub typhus (tsutsugamushi fever).

Gamasoidosis Persons in contact with canaries, pigeons, and poultry are prone to develop gamasoidosis. The dermatosis occurs chiefly on the hands and arms, where the bite produces inflammatory, itchy papules. Any area on the body may be attacked and common additional sites are the groin, areolae, umbilicus, face, and scalp. The mites may wander from birds' nests as soon as the young birds begin to fly, and they may infest terrace cushions and furniture. In large metropolitan areas, especially where pigeons tend to gather, it is not unusual to see pigeons roosting on window ledges. Through the open windows or even through air conditioners, the pigeon mites attack humans and cause urticarial and papular eruptions. The tropical fowl mite (*Ornithonyssus bursa*), widely prevalent in wild birds in both continental US and Hawaii, may do this as well.

Two genera of mite, *Ornithonyssus* and *Dermanyssus*, commonly infest birds. *O. bursa* and *Ornithonyssus sylvarium* are the two common species of feather mite. *Dermanyssus gallinae*, the red or chicken mite, is also a common parasite of birds. *Dermanyssus* mites may carry *Erysipelothrix rhusiopathiae*. *D. gallinae* tends to leave the bird during the day and hide in cracks and crevices, and therefore can be killed without direct treatment of the bird. Thorough spraying of the surroundings with an agent such as malathion is effective. Mites of the *Ornithonyssus* group require treatment of the birds themselves. In pet stores, bird mites may be transmitted to rodents with human disease related to contact with a gerbil or hamster.

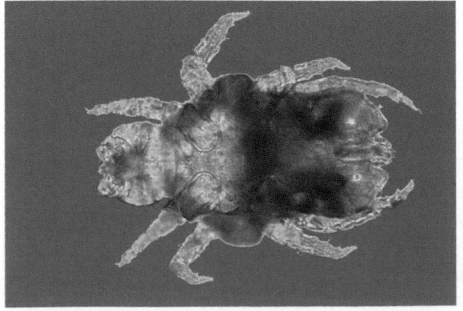

Fig. 20-51 *Cheyletiella blakei.*

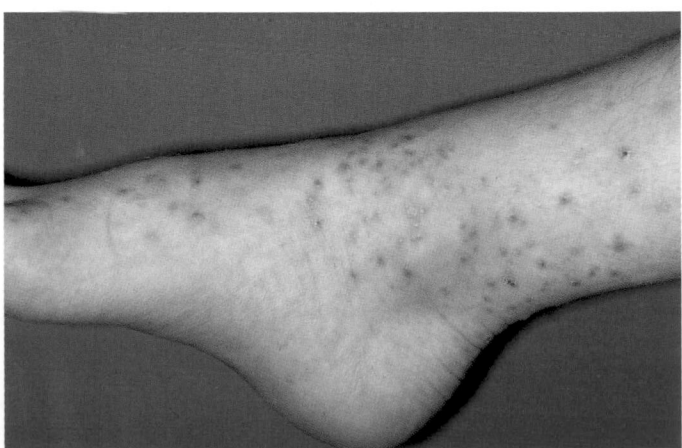

Fig. 20-52 Chigger bites.

Grocer's itch This is a pruritic dermatitis of the forearms, with occasional inflammatory and urticarial papules on the trunk. It results from the handling of figs, dates, and prunes, when it is caused by *Carpoglyphus passularum*, or from exposure to the cheese mite (*Glyciphagus domesticus*). This must be distinguished from grocer's eczema, which is caused by sensitization to flour, sugar, cinnamon, chocolate, and similar items.

Grain itch Grain itch is also known as straw itch, barley itch, mattress itch, and prairie itch. Causative mites include *Pyemotes tritici*, *Pyemotes ventricosus*, *Cheyletus malaccensis*, and *Tyrophagus putrescentiae* (the copra itch mite). Those chiefly affected are harvesters of wheat, hay, barley, oats, and other cereals, or farm hands and packers who have contact with straw. Grain itch has a typical lesion consisting of an urticarial papule on which there is a small vesicle. There is intense pruritus, with lesions occurring predominantly on the trunk. Frequently, there is a central hemorrhagic punctum in the beginning that rapidly turns into an ecchymosis with hemosiderin pigmentation.

Other mite-related dermatitis *Dermatophagoides pteronyssinus* and *Dermatophagoides farinae* are dust mites implicated in atopic diseases. *Lepidoglyphus destructor* is the hay mite. There have been outbreaks of *Pyemotes boylei* bites in homes fumigated for termites. Although mites do not appear capable of survival when forced to share an environment with termites, they thrive in locations in which there are termite carcasses. Vanillism is a dermatitis caused by *Acarus siro* and occurs in workers handling vanilla pods. Copra itch occurs on persons handling copra who are subject to *Tyrophagus longior* mite bites. Coolie itch is found in tea plantations in India and is caused by *Rhizoglyphus parasiticus*. It causes sore feet. Rat mite itch, caused by *Ornithonyssus bacoti*, the tropical rat mite, may result in an intensely pruritic dermatitis. This papulovesicular urticarial eruption is seen in workers in stores, factories, warehouse, and stockyards. The rat mite may transmit endemic typhus, rickettsial pox, equine encephalitis, tularemia, plague, and relapsing fever. Feather pillow dermatitis is a pruritic papular dermatitis traced to the Psoroptid carpet mite, *Dermatophagoides scheremetewskyi*, which may infest feather pillows. Finally, the house mouse mite, *Allodermanyssus* (*Liponyssoides*) *sanguineus*, is the vector of *Rickettsia akari*, the causative organism of rickettsialpox.

Levitt JO: Digital photography in the diagnosis of scabies. J Am Acad Dermatol 2008; 59(3):530.

Mumcuoglu KY, et al: Treatment of scabies infestations. Parasite 2008; 15(3):248–251.

Neynaber S, et al: Diagnosis of scabies with dermoscopy. CMAJ 2008; 178(12):1540–1541.

Strong M, et al: Interventions for treating scabies. Cochrane Database Syst Rev 2007; 3:CD000320.

Tjioe M, et al: Scabies outbreaks in nursing homes for the elderly: recognition, treatment options and control of reinfestation. Drugs Aging 2008; 25(4):299–306.

Wolf R, et al: Treatment of scabies and pediculosis: Facts and controversies. Clin Dermatol 2010 September–October; 28(5):511–518.

Yoon TY, et al: Pimecrolimus-induced rosacea-like demodicidosis. Int J Dermatol 2007; 46(10):1103–1105.

Order Scorpionidae

Scorpion sting

Scorpions (Fig. 20-53) are different from other arachnids in that they have an elongated abdomen ending in a stinger. They also have a cephalothorax, four pairs of legs, pincers, and mouth pincers. Two poison glands in the back of the abdomen empty into the stinger. Scorpions are found all over the world, especially in the tropics. They are nocturnal and hide during

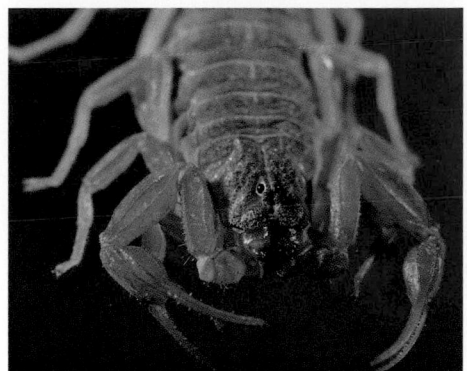

Fig. 20-53 Common *Centruroides* scorpion.

the daytime under table tops, and in closets, shoes, and folded blankets. Ground scorpions may burrow into gravel and children's sandboxes. Buthid scorpions include the most venomous species of medical importance. Important scorpions include *Tityus serrulatus*, found in Brazil, *Buthotus tamulus*, found in India, *Leiurus quinquestriatus* and *Androctonus crassicauda*, found in North Africa and southwest Asia, and *Centruroides suffusus*, found in Mexico. *Centruroides exilicauda* and *C. sculpturatus* are the most toxic scorpions in the United States. *Vaejovis* scorpions in the southeastern United States have been reported to cause "brown recluse-like" dermonecrotic reactions.

Scorpions sting only by accident or in self-defense. The venom causes pain, paresthesia, and variable swelling at the site of the sting. The sting of the Egyptian scorpion (*L. quinquestriatus*) has a mortality rate of 50% in children. The neurotoxic venom may produce numbness at the sting site, laryngeal edema, profuse sweating and salivation, cyanosis, nausea, and paresthesia of the tongue. There is little or no visible change at the site of the sting. Death may occur from cardiac or respiratory failure, especially in children. Renal and hepatic toxicity may also occur.

Treatment depends on the species and toxic symptoms. Antiarrhythmics, antiadrenergic agents, vasodilators, and calcium channel-blockers may be required. Antivenin is available for many species of scorpion.

Krkic-Dautovic S, et al: Acute renal insufficiency and toxic hepatitis following scorpions sting. Med Arh 2007; 61(2):123–124.

Ranu Alpay N, et al: Unusual presentations of scorpion envenomation. Hum Exp Toxicol 2008; 27(1):81–85.

Order Arachnidae

Arachnidism

Spiders are prevalent throughout the world. Most are beneficial to humans, as they trap many insects, but a few species are dangerous to humans. Many spider venoms are not well characterized, and in most cases of envenomation, the responsible spider is never identified. The Brazilian armed spider (*Phoneutria nigriventer*) is well characterized. Its venom contains neurotoxins that may be fatal in children. Various reactions to spider bites have been reported, including dermonecrotic reactions, systemic toxicity, and acute generalized exanthematous pustulosis.

Latrodectism

The various species of *Latrodectus* have similar toxins and cause similar reactions in humans. The black widow spider, *Latrodectus mactans*, is of chief concern in the continental US. It may also be found in the Caribbean. Black widows are web-building spiders, and are commonly found in woodpiles and

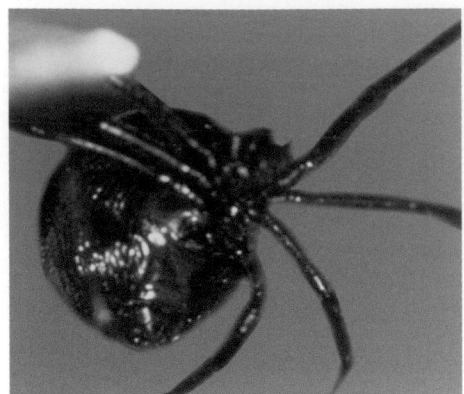

Fig. 20-54 Black widow.

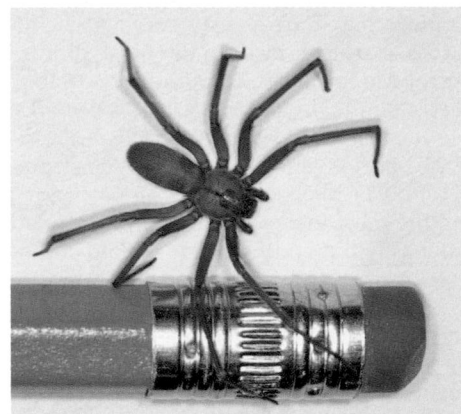

Fig. 20-55 Brown recluse spider.

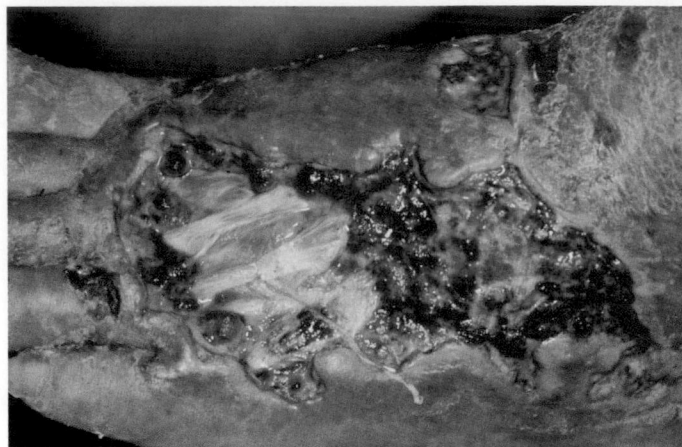

Fig. 20-56 Brown recluse spider bite.

The incidence of brown recluse bites is grossly overestimated. *Loxosceles rufescens*, *Loxosceles deserta*, and *Loxosceles arizonica* cause lesser degrees of skin necrosis. *Loxosceles laeta* occurs throughout Latin America and produces changes similar to those of *L. reclusa*. The venom contains a phospholipase enzyme, sphingomyelinase D, which is the major toxin. Hyaluronidase contributes to a gravity-dependent spread of the necrotic lesions.

In the localized type of reaction, known as necrotic cutaneous loxoscelism, extensive local necrosis develops (Fig. 20-56). A painful severe edematous reaction occurs within the first 8 h, with development of a bulla with surrounding zones of erythema and ischemia. In about a week the central portion becomes dark, demarcated, and gangrenous. Systemic loxoscelism is rare, but may be associated with minor-appearing bite reactions. Systemic toxic symptoms are associated with disseminated intravascular coagulation.

Treatment

Treatment consists of rest, ice, and elevation. Tetanus toxoid should be given if the patient has not received the immunization within 10 years. Some data suggest a trend towards better outcome with injections of intralesional triamcinolone, and there are anecdotal reports of sparing of necrosis in the injected site, while the areas above and below the injection site show necrosis. Antibiotics and conservative debridement may be needed for necrotic wounds. Dapsone has been used, but some studies show that it is no better than placebo, and it may be toxic, especially in the setting of venom-induced hemolysis. Colchicine has also been disappointing in animal models, but tetracyclines show some promise and deserve further study.

Funnel web spiders

Funnel web spiders include *Tegenaria agrestis* (the hobo spider or aggressive house spider of the Pacific Northwest) and *Atrax robustus* (the Sydney funnel web spider of Australia). Australian funnel web spiders are dangerous, but antivenin is available.

Tarantulas (Lycosidae: Theraphosidae)

Tarantulas are large, hairy hunting spiders. American species have urticating hairs that produce cutaneous wheal and flare reactions and embed in the cornea, causing ophthalmia nodosa.

under outhouse seats. Their venom may be less potent than that of related brown widow spiders, but they inject more of it. *Latrodectus curacaviensis* is native to South America, and Australia and New Zealand have related red-back spiders (*Latrodectus mactans hasselti*). *Latrodectus indistinctus* is found in Africa, and the brown widow, *Latrodectus geometricus*, is native to southern Africa and Madagascar.

The female *Latrodectus mactans* (Fig. 20-54) spider is 13 mm long and shiny black, with a red hourglass-shaped marking on its abdomen. The legs are long, with a spread of up to 4 cm. The black widow spider is not aggressive, and bites only when disturbed. Severe pain usually develops within a few minutes and spreads throughout the extremities and trunk. Within a few hours there may be chills, vomiting, violent cramps, delirium or partial paralysis, spasms, and abdominal rigidity. The abdominal pains are frequently most severe and may be mistaken for appendicitis, colic, or food poisoning. Toxic morbilliform erythema may occur. Myocarditis has also been reported.

Antivenin is indicated for severe symptoms of envenomation. Benzodiazepines reduce the associated tetany.

Loxoscelism

The brown recluse spider (*Loxosceles reclusa*) (Fig. 20-55) is the major cause of necrotic arachnidism in the US. It is most common in the lower Midwest and Southwest. This reclusive spider may be identified by a dark, violin-shaped marking over the cephalothorax and three sets of eyes, rather than the usual four. It is light brown and about 1 cm long, with a small body and long delicate legs. It is found in storage closets, basements, and cupboards, and among clothing. Outdoors it has been found in woodpiles, in grass, on rocky bluffs, and in barns. It stings in self-defense and is not an aggressive spider.

Davidovici BB, et al: Acute generalized exanthematous pustulosis following a spider bite: report of 3 cases. J Am Acad Dermatol 2006 Sep;55(3):525–529.

Isbister GK, et al: A randomised controlled trial of intramuscular vs. intravenous antivenom for latrodectism—the RAVE study. QJM 2008; 101(7):557–565.

King LE Jr: Common ground? Tetracyclines, matrix metalloproteinases, pustular dermatoses, and loxoscelism. J Invest Dermatol 2007; 127(6):1284–1286.

McGlasson DL, et al: Cutaneous and systemic effects of varying doses of brown recluse spider venom in a rabbit model. Clin Lab Sci 2007; 20(2):99–105.

Sari I, et al: Myocarditis after black widow spider envenomation. Am J Emerg Med 2008; 26(5):630.e1–3.

Swanson DL, et al: Loxoscelism. Clin Dermatol 2006; 24(3):213–221.

Vetter RS, et al: Of spiders and zebras: publication of inadequately documented loxoscelism case reports. J Am Acad Dermatol 2007; 56(6):1063–1064.

PHYLUM CHORDATA

Stingray injury

The two stingray families (Dasyatidae and Myliobatidae) are among the most venomous fish known to humans. Attacks generally occur as a result of an unwary victim stepping on a partially buried stingray. A puncture-type wound occurs about the ankles or feet, and later ulcerates. Sharp, shooting pain develops immediately, with edema and cyanosis. Symptoms of shock may occur.

Persons wading in shallow, muddy waters where stingrays may be found should shuffle their feet through the mud to frighten the fish away. Successful treatment is usually attained by immersing the injured part in hot water for 30–60 min. The water should be as hot as can be tolerated, since the venom is detoxified by heat. Meperidine hydrochloride administered intravenously or intramuscularly may be necessary. If the ulcer remains unhealed after 8 weeks, excision is indicated.

Snake bite

Venomous snake bites are a serious problem in some parts of the world. In the US the rattlesnake, cottonmouth moccasin, copperhead, and coral snake are the venomous snakes most frequently encountered. Patients are usually young men, with 98% of bites on the extremities, most often the hands or arms. In Europe, 39% of envenomations from exotic pets are snake bites from rattlesnakes, cobras, mambas, or other venomous snakes. Nearly 30 enzymes are found in snake venom, most of which are hydrolases. Snake venom has effects on the cardiovascular, hematologic, respiratory, and nervous systems. Severe envenomation may mimic brain death, with loss of other brainstem reflexes. Local effects at the bite site include the rapid onset of swelling, erythema, and ecchymosis. In more severe reactions, bullae and lymphangitis may appear. Fang marks are often visible and pain is common, except with Mojave rattlesnake bites. Antivenin is used in severe envenomation, and antitetanus measures are indicated. In the eastern United States, copperheads inflict most snake bites, followed by rattlesnakes and cottonmouths. Most of these children can be managed conservatively, although Crotalidae antivenin, antibiotics, and fasciotomy may be needed.

Lizard bite

Heloderma suspectum (the Gila monster) is found chiefly in Arizona and New Mexico. Another venomous lizard is the beaded lizard of southwestern Mexico (*Heloderma horridum*). Bites from these poisonous lizards may cause paralysis, dyspnea, and convulsions. Systemic toxicity usually resolves spontaneously with supportive care within 1 or 2 days. Death is rare. There is no antivenin.

Campbell BT, et al: Pediatric snakebites: lessons learned from 114 cases. J Pediatr Surg 2008; 43(7):1338–1341.

Langley RL: Animal bites and stings reported by United States poison control centers, 2001–2005. Wilderness Environ Med 2008; 19(1):7–14.

Schaper A, et al: Bites and stings by exotic pets in Europe: an 11 year analysis of 404 cases from Northeastern Germany and Southeastern France. Clin Toxicol (Phila) 2009; 47(1):39–43.

Bonus images for this chapter can be found online at http://www.expertconsult.com

Fig. 20-1 Leishmaniasis recidivans.
Fig. 20-2 New World leishmaniasis.
Fig. 20-3 Disseminated cutaneous leishmaniasis.
Fig. 20-4 Mucocutaneous leishmaniasis. (Courtesy of James Fitzpatrick, MD)
Fig. 20-5 Coral cuts. (Courtesy of Curt Samlaska, MD)
Fig. 20-6 Cutaneous larva migrans.
Fig. 20-7 Dracunculosis.
Fig. 20-8 Filarial elephantiasis.
Fig. 20-9 Trichinosis.
Fig. 20-10 Bedbug.
Fig. 20-11 Bedbug.
Fig. 20-12 Human flea.
Fig. 20-13 Stick-tight flea.
Fig. 20-14 *Rhipicephalus* tick, engorged female.
Fig. 20-15 Snake bite.

21 Chronic Blistering Dermatoses

In noninherited chronic blistering (vesicular or bullous) dermatoses, the cause of blistering is usually an autoimmune reaction, and the pattern of immunofluorescence is critical in establishing the diagnosis. Usually, antibodies are bound in perilesional skin, while lesional skin often fails to demonstrate deposits. Lower-extremity skin should be avoided if possible, as it may be prone to false-negative reactions.

Salt-split skin preparations are useful in determining the site of deposition of the autoantibodies. A 1M solution of NaCl predictably splits skin at the level of the lamina lucida. Localization of immune deposits to the roof or floor of this split is diagnostically useful. The identification of n-serrated and u-serrated patterns of immunoglobulin deposition provides the same information and may make salt-split skin immunofluorescence unnecessary. An n-serrated pattern (Fig. 21-1) corresponds to a split above the basal lamina, while a u-serrated pattern (Fig. 21-2) corresponds to a sub-lamina densa split. The patterns are best seen in areas where the basement membrane zone curves. Immunoprecipitation, enzyme-linked immunosorbent assay (ELISA), and immunoblotting have helped to define the molecular targets of the autoantibodies and have revolutionized testing for immunobullous diseases. Data vary concerning the sensitivity and specificity of these tests. In the setting of bullous pemphigoid, ELISA can produce apparent false-positives at rates of 7% or higher, based on non-NC16a antibodies, as well as on anti-BP 180 antibodies that bind to the pathogenic NC16a domain but do not produce clinical disease and are not associated with positive indirect immunofluorescent findings.

Transient acantholytic dermatosis (Grover's disease) is an idiopathic nonimmune vesiculobullous disease that may mimic the histologic patterns of immunobullous disease, but shows no specific findings on direct immunofluorescence (DIF). Specific dermatoses of pregnancy are discussed under the differential diagnosis of herpes gestationis.

The outlook for immunobullous diseases has improved since the introduction of rituximab, intravenous immunoglobulins, and less toxic immunosuppressive regimens. Oral and ocular involvement often requires a multidisciplinary approach.

Elchahal S, et al: Ocular manifestations of blistering diseases. Immunol Allergy Clin North Am 2008 Feb; 28(1):119–136.
Fine JD: Prevalence of autoantibodies to bullous pemphigoid antigens within the normal population. Arch Dermatol 2010 Jan; 146(1):74–75.
Gaines E, et al: Development of outcome measures for autoimmune dermatoses. Arch Dermatol Res 2008 Jan; 300(1):3–9.
Hertl M, et al: Recommendations for the use of rituximab (anti-CD20 antibody) in the treatment of autoimmune bullous skin diseases. J Dtsch Dermatol Ges 2008 May; 6(5):366–373.
Lo Russo L, et al: Diagnostic pathways and clinical significance of desquamative gingivitis. J Periodontol 2008 Jan; 79(1):4–24.
Mihai S, et al: Immunopathology and molecular diagnosis of autoimmune bullous diseases. J Cell Mol Med 2007 May–Jun; 11(3):462–481.
Schmidt E, et al: Rituximab in autoimmune bullous diseases: mixed responses and adverse effects. Br J Dermatol 2007 Feb; 156(2):352–356.
Segura S, et al: High-dose intravenous immunoglobulins for the treatment of autoimmune mucocutaneous blistering diseases: evaluation of its use in 19 cases. J Am Acad Dermatol 2007 Jun; 56(6):960–967.
Wieland CN, et al: Anti-bullous pemphigoid 180 and 230 antibodies in a sample of unaffected subjects. Arch Dermatol 2010 Jan; 146(1):21–25.

Pemphigus vulgaris

Clinical features

Pemphigus vulgaris (PV) is characterized by mucosal erosions and by thin-walled, relatively flaccid, easily ruptured bullae that appear on apparently normal skin and mucous membranes or on erythematous bases. The fluid in the bulla is clear at first but may become hemorrhagic or even seropurulent. The bullae rupture to form erosions. The denuded areas soon become partially or totally covered with crusts that have little or no tendency to heal. When they finally heal, lesions often leave hyperpigmented patches but no scarring.

PV usually appears first in the mouth (Fig. 21-3) (60% of cases) or at the site of a burn, radiation therapy, or other skin injury. Other common sites include the groin, scalp, face, neck, axillae, and genitals. The Nikolsky sign is present (intact epidermis shearing away from the underlying dermis, leaving a moist surface). The sign is elicited by slight pressure, twisting, or rubbing. The "bulla-spread phenomenon" (Asboe–Hansen sign) is elicited by pressure on an intact bulla, gently forcing the fluid to spread under the adjacent skin.

Short-lived bullae quickly rupture to involve most of the mucosa with painful erosions. The lesions extend on to the lips and form heavy, fissured crusts on the vermilion. Involvement of the throat produces hoarseness and difficulty in swallowing. The mouth odor is offensive. The esophagus may be involved, and sloughing of its entire lining in the form of a cast (esophagitis dissecans superficialis) may occur, even when the cutaneous disease appears to be well controlled. The conjunctiva, nasal mucosa, vagina, penis, and anus may also be involved. Chronic lesions may involve the face, scalp, or flexures. Widespread cutaneous disease (Fig. 21-4) may cause death through sepsis or fluid and electrolyte imbalance.

The diagnosis is made by histology, immunofluorescence pattern of perilesional skin or plucked hairs, indirect immunofluorescence (IIF) testing of serum, or ELISA testing for anti-desmoglein (Dsg)1 and Dsg3 autoantibodies. As in other autoimmune diseases, specific antibodies may be present in relatives of patients with pemphigus who do not manifest any signs of disease.

Epidemiology

PV occurs with equal frequency in men and women, usually in their fifth and sixth decades. It is rare in young persons. The

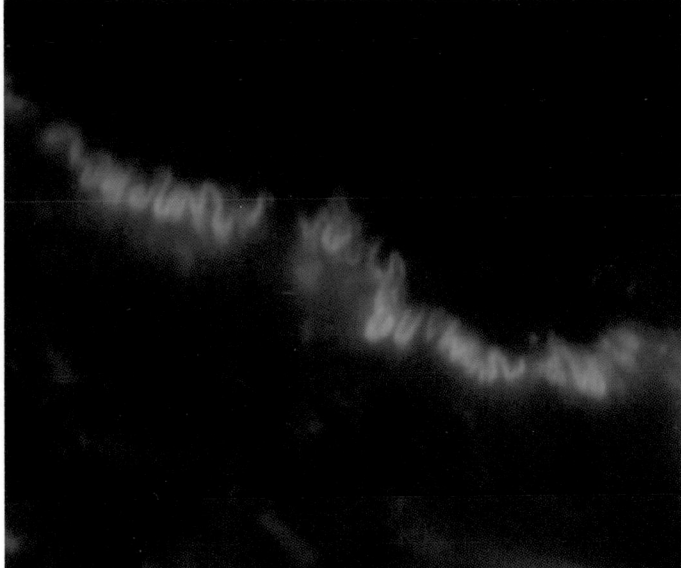

Fig. 21-1 N-serrated immunofluorescent pattern.

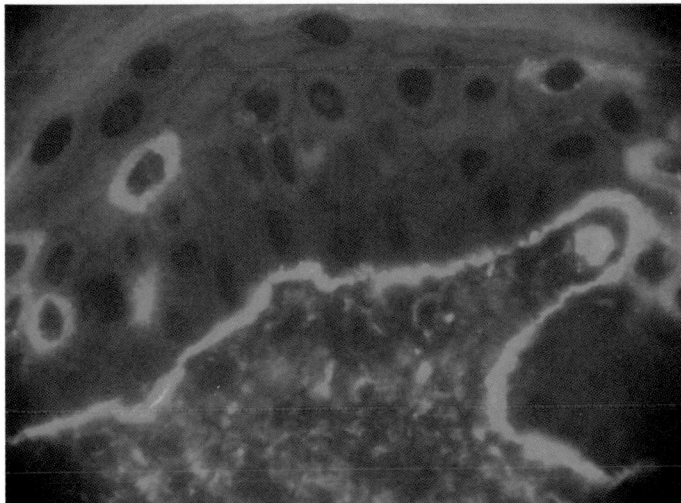

Fig. 21-2 U-serrated immunofluorescent pattern.

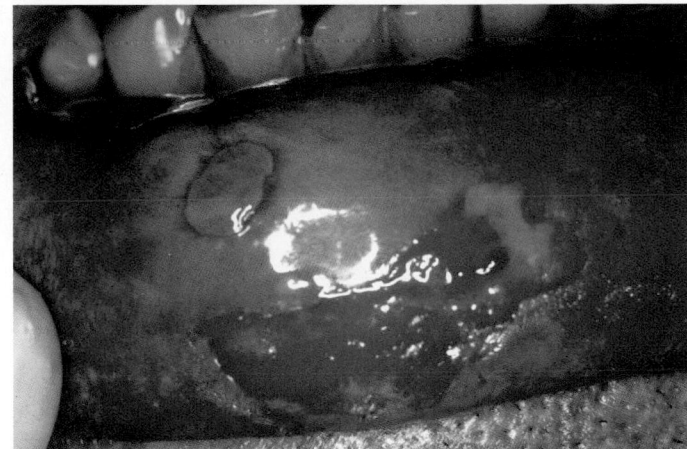

Fig. 21-3 Pemphigus vulgaris of the oral mucosa.

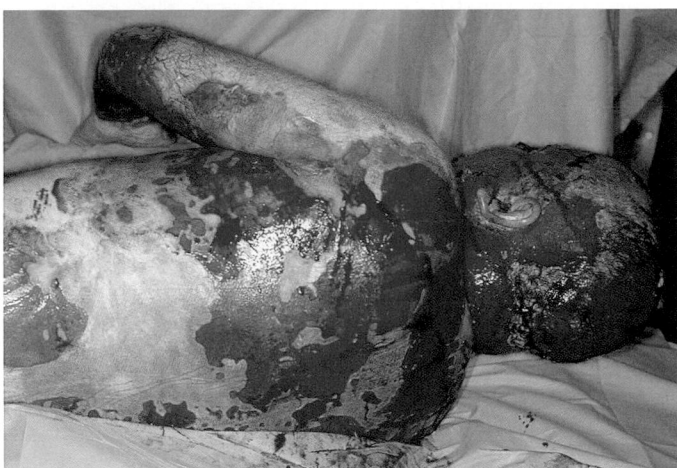

Fig. 21-4 Pemphigus vulgaris.

condition occurs more often in Jewish people and those of Mediterranean descent.

Etiologic factors

Antibodies in PV are most commonly directed against Dsg3. The presence of antibodies to both Dsg1 and Dsg3 correlates with mucocutaneous disease. If autoantibodies are only directed against Dsg3, mucosal lesions predominate. Both humoral and cellular autoimmunity are important in the pathogenesis of skin lesions. Antibody alone can produce acantholysis, without complement or inflammatory cells. Both IgG1 and IgG4 autoantibodies to Dsg3 occur in patients with pemphigus, but some data suggest that the IgG4 antibodies are pathogenic. Plasminogen activator is associated with antibody-mediated acantholysis. Involved T cells are usually CD4 cells that secrete a T-helper 2 (Th2)-like cytokine profile, although Th1 cells may also be involved in antibody production in chronic disease. IgG is found in both involved and clinically normal skin. C3 deposits are heavier in acantholytic areas. DIF may remain positive for years after clinical remission, and conversion to negative predicts sustained remission

after withdrawal of therapy. Pemphigus may be associated with myasthenia gravis and thymoma.

The PV antigen (130 kD transmembrane desmosomal glycoprotein) shows homology with the cadherin family of calcium-dependent cell adhesion molecules. With IIF, circulating antibodies can be demonstrated in 80–90% of patients. Circulating intercellular antibodies may also be present in patients with thermal or actinic burns, and in patients with drug eruptions. These antibodies are not directed against Dsg3. They do not bind to the epidermis in vivo and are often directed against ABO blood-group antigens.

Penicillamine treatment of rheumatoid arthritis has induced pemphigus, most often of the foliaceous type. Nearly all the reported cases have had a positive DIF and more than half have had a positive IIF. Penicillamine and captopril may induce acantholysis in organ explant cultures in the absence of autoantibody. The doses responsible for induction of disease have ranged from 250 to 1500 mg/day, and the drugs were taken for an average of 13 months before the onset of pemphigus. A long list of drugs, including captopril, enalapril, penicillin, thiopronine, interleukin (IL)-2, nifedipine, piroxicam, and rifampicin, has also been reported to induce pemphigus. Many of these contain either a sulfhydryl or an amide group. Only 10–15% of patients with drug-induced pemphigus have had oral lesions. Most disease resolves when the medication is discontinued, but some cases have persisted for many months.

Many studies have indicated a genetic predisposition to pemphigus and an association with other autoimmune diseases. Statistical analysis shows a skewed distribution of various human leukocyte antigens (HLA). Most patients are of HLA phenotype DR4 or DR6. In addition, an HLA-DQ restriction fragment has been identified in many patients with pemphigus. HLA-G is associated with pemphigus in Jewish patients. Thus, there may be a genetically inherited susceptibility to the disease. Additionally, a predisposition to develop other autoimmune diseases may occur in relatives of pemphigus patients.

Histopathology

The characteristic findings consist of suprabasilar acantholysis with intraepidermal blister formation. Acantholytic cells are round and show no intercellular bridges. Regeneration of the epidermis occurs, and may cause the split to appear to be higher as cells regenerate beneath the cleft. At least some areas typically still demonstrate the characteristic tombstone row of basal keratinocytes underneath the bulla. An early intact bulla shows the most characteristic histology. Asboe–Hansen modification of the Nikolsky test may be used to extend the bulla beyond its original margin to where secondary regenerative changes have not taken place.

In early disease, spongiosis with eosinophils may be noted in the epidermis, in the absence of acantholysis. In the setting of immunobullous disease, spongiosis with eosinophils is more likely to represent pemphigoid than pemphigus, and immunofluorescent findings readily distinguish the two.

DIF demonstrates a "chicken wire" pattern of intercellular IgG in perilesional skin or plucked hairs. C3 may also be present. The staining is uniform, not granular. IIF shows a similar pattern of staining. Prozone reactions occur, so the serum should be tested at a wide range of dilutions. Positive tests may be confirmed with ELISA for the antibody.

Treatment

Large-scale, prospective, double-blinded studies are few, and the management of PV is based largely on smaller open trials and clinical experience. A survey of 24 very experienced clinicians showed that half used prednisone in doses of 1 mg/kg/day, while half used higher doses. Adjuvant steroid-sparing agents were commonly employed, with almost half of the respondents reporting the use of azathioprine. Because of its tolerability and simpler dosing schedule, mycophenolate mofetil is commonly used in place of azathioprine. Other agents used less commonly include cyclophosphamide and methotrexate. Almost 40% of the clinicians aimed to replace prednisone with a steroid-sparing agent, while others were content to continue a low dose of prednisone. The survey suggests that, even among the world's experts, there is significant variation in how this difficult disease is managed. Rituximab and intravenous immunoglobulin therapy have produced dramatic responses in some patients with refractory disease, and some authorities now consider rituximab appropriate first-line therapy for patients with severe disease.

Most agents used to treat the disease are immunosuppressive, although the mechanism of action may not merely be suppression of T cells and antibody production. Methylprednisolone can directly block pemphigus antibody-induced acantholysis. It also upregulates expression of the genes encoding Dsg3 and periplakin, increases measurable levels of E-cadherin, Dsg1, and Dsg3, and interferes with phosphorylation of these adhesion molecules. Many of these effects antagonize those of pemphigus antibodies.

Topical treatment

The skin lesions are extremely painful in advanced cases. When there are extensive raw surfaces, prolonged daily baths are helpful in removing the thickened crusts and reducing the foul odor. Silver sulfadiazine (Silvadene) 1%, widely used for local therapy of burns, is an effective topical antimicrobial agent, suitable for treatment of limited disease. Silver nitrate-impregnated cotton batting, manufactured for burn units, can be used in more extensive disease. Very localized areas can be treated with silver nitrate-impregnated dressings such as Acticoat 7 or Aquacell Ag. Painful ulcerations of the lips and mouth may benefit from topical application of a mixture of equal parts of Maalox and elixir of diphenhydramine hydrochloride (Benadryl) or viscous xylocaine, especially before meals. The various commercial antiseptic mouthwashes are helpful in alleviating discomfort and malodor. Potent topical corticosteroids and topical tacrolimus have been successful in some patients with limited disease.

Systemic therapy

A common method of treatment for severe disease would be to begin with doses of prednisone adequate to control the disease. High doses of prednisone (100–150 mg) are sometimes needed, but prolonged high doses are associated with significant morbidity and mortality, so adjuvant therapy should be started early. During the early phase of therapy, if prednisone at 1 mg/kg/day proves inadequate, the drug is commonly increased to a split dose of 1 mg/kg twice a day. As the course of corticosteroid therapy is commonly longer than initially anticipated, it is good practice to begin vitamin D, calcium, weight-bearing exercise, and bisphosphonate therapy early in the course of treatment. Commonly used agents include alendronate, 70 mg/wk; risedronate, 35 mg/wk or 150 mg/mo; ibandronate, 150 mg/mo; teriparatide, 20 µg/d; or zoledronic acid, 5 mg infusion yearly.

Mycophenolate mofetil is commonly chosen as a steroid-sparing agent, at a dose of 1–1.5 g twice a day. Gastrointestinal intolerance is the most common side effect, and blood counts must be monitored. If the disease does not respond, either plasmapheresis or intravenous immunoglobulin (IVIG) is added to the regimen. Azathioprine is less expensive than mycophenolate mofetil, and is commonly used as an alternative when cost is an overriding issue. It is best dosed based on measurement of the patient's thiopurine methyltransferase (TPMT) level. The majority of patients metabolize the drug quickly, and may be underdosed if TPMT is not measured. Patients with high levels of the enzyme may require 2.5–3 mg/kg/day. Patients with mid-range levels are treated with 1–2.5 mg/kg/day. Patients who are deficient in the enzyme may be treated with very low doses or with a different agent. Allopurinol interferes with metabolism of the drug and increased serum levels may lead to toxicity. Patients with refractory disease may be treated with rituximab, intravenous immunoglobulins, or cyclophosphamide, either alone or in conjunction with plasmapheresis. Plasmapheresis alone is followed by rebound of antibody production, but the rebounding clone of plasma cells is sensitized to the effects of cytotoxic agents. Both daily cyclophosphamide dosing and pulse dosing schedules can be used alone or in combination with dexamethasone. Pulse dosing is usually given with mesna rescue and is associated with less bladder toxicity. Both dosing schedules should be planned early in the day with vigorous hydration to minimize the risk of bladder toxicity. Blood counts must be monitored closely. Other risks of therapy with high doses of corticosteroids and immunosuppressants include diabetes, infection, hypertension, and cardiorespiratory disease. All of these risks must be monitored, and all patients must receive gentle wound care and fluid and electrolyte management. In patients who cannot tolerate cyclophosphamide, chlorambucil has been used, but is associated with a greater risk of hematologic malignancy. Immunoadsorption represents a novel approach to therapy that could replace plasmapheresis. In addition to the use of IVIG as an adjuvant to conventional therapy, it has also been given as monotherapy. Onset of action is fairly rapid and may be seen within 1–2 weeks. There is a trend towards using rituximab early in the course of treatment if patients have significant disease.

The sooner the diagnosis is established and the sooner treatment is given, the more favorable the prognosis. The therapeutic effects are estimated by the number of new lesions per day and the rate of healing of new lesions. In patients with and Dsg3 antibodies, mucosal disease may still be active when cutaneous disease appears to be in remission. Pemphigus antibody titers can be performed on esophageal substrate, watching for a fall in titer. If, after 4–8 weeks of treatment, new blister formation is not suppressed, prednisone dosage may be increased to 150 mg/day. Dosage adjustments are, of course, made more frequently and aggressively in severe, progressive disease. Dividing the daily dose will usually result in greater efficacy but will also result in greater adrenal suppression. Additionally, intravenous pulse therapy with megadose corticosteroids (Solu-medrol), at a dose of 1 g/day over a period of 2–3 h, repeated daily for 5 days, may be employed for cases that are unresponsive to oral doses. Untreated disease is commonly fatal, but the clinician should remember that, in treated patients, side effects of therapy are the most common cause of death. Adjuvant therapy to decrease steroid dependence has reduced mortality.

Medication is continued until clinical disease is suppressed and pemphigus antibody disappears from the serum. Once the antibody is no longer present, a DIF test is repeated. A negative DIF is predictive of sustained remission after withdrawal of therapy.

Immunosuppressant therapy alone has been reported as a successful treatment of early stable PV. If a contraindication to the use of corticosteroids exists or only limited disease is present, these may be used as single agents. In general, however, combined treatment with corticosteroids is superior in gaining early control of the disease. Dexamethasone–cyclophosphamide therapy was studied in 32 patients with PV. Monthly pulses consisted of intravenous dexamethasone, 136 mg, for 3 consecutive days monthly, with intravenous cyclophosphamide, 500 mg, on the second day. Daily oral cyclophosphamide, 50 mg, and oral tapered courses of oral corticosteroids were given in the intervals between the pulses. All patients responded. Partial remissions were noted after 2–8 pulses. From 8 to 32 pulses were required to achieve complete remission. The duration of pulsed therapy correlated with both the disease severity and the time to achieve remission. Oral cyclophosphamide was successful in 17 of 20 patients who had failed therapy with prednisone and an antimetabolite. The median time to achieve complete remission was 8.5 months, and the median duration of treatment was 17 months. Plasmapheresis was used in nine patients. Hematuria developed in five patients and infections were noted in six. One patient developed bladder cancer 15 years after therapy.

Intramuscular or oral gold is no longer commonly used. Gold is less effective than immunosuppressive therapy, but its advantages include lack of carcinogenicity and infertility. A minimum of 6 months is required to judge the effectiveness of gold therapy. Infliximab or rituximab, an anti-CD20 monoclonal antibody, has been used successfully in several cases of refractory disease, but may be associated with serious infections and progressive multifocal leukoencephalopathy. Extracorporeal photochemotherapy has been used in a few patients, and dapsone may have some value as a steroid-sparing agent. Nicotinamide and tetracycline can be tried in patients with milder disease. In one study, it was successful in 2 of 6 patients. In another study, it was only successful in 1 of 10 patients. Data on the effectiveness of cyclosporine have been mixed. Etanercept has been used successfully in some patients.

Pemphigus vegetans

Pemphigus vegetans may present as localized plaques in the scalp or in two classic forms, the Neumann type (which generally begins and ends as typical pemphigus) and the Hallopeau type (which usually remains localized). Both types show pseudoepitheliomatous hyperplasia, and the Hallopeau type is characterized by eosinophil microabscesses within the epidermis.

Pemphigus vegetans may begin with flaccid bullae that become erosions and form fungating vegetations or papillomatous proliferations, especially in body folds or on the scalp. The tongue often shows cerebriform morphologic features early in the course of the disease. At times there is a tendency for the lesions to coalesce to form large patches or to arrange themselves into groups or figurate patterns.

The laboratory findings, etiologic factors, epidemiology, pathogenesis, and treatment of pemphigus vegetans are the same as those for pemphigus vulgaris. Captopril-induced pemphigus vegetans has been reported.

Pemphigus vegetans must be differentiated from other conditions characterized by pseudoepitheliomatous hyperplasia and microabscesses, including halogenoderma, chromoblastomycosis, blastomycosis, granuloma inguinale, blastomycosis-like pyoderma, condyloma lata, and amebic granulomas. The Hallopeau type is distinguished by the presence of eosinophils, and both types by immunofluorescent findings.

Allen KJ, et al: The efficacy and safety of rituximab in refractory pemphigus: a review of case reports. J Drugs Dermatol 2007 Sep; 6(9):883–889.

Aoyama Y, et al: Severe pemphigus vulgaris: successful combination therapy of plasmapheresis followed by intravenous high-dose immunoglobulin to prevent rebound increase in pathogenic IgG. Eur J Dermatol 2008 Sep–Oct; 18(5):557–560.

Chams-Davatchi C, et al: Randomized controlled open-label trial of four treatment regimens for pemphigus vulgaris. J Am Acad Dermatol 2007 Oct; 57(4):622–628.

Cianchini G, et al: Treatment of severe pemphigus with rituximab: report of 12 cases and a review of the literature. Arch Dermatol 2007 Aug; 143(8):1033–1038.

Czernik A, et al: Kinetics of response to conventional treatment in patients with pemphigus vulgaris. Arch Dermatol 2008 May; 144(5):682–683.

Daneshpazhooh M, et al: Thyroid autoimmunity and pemphigus vulgaris: is there a significant association? J Am Acad Dermatol 2010 Feb; 62(2):349–351.

Firooz A, et al: Role of thiopurine methyltransferase activity in the safety and efficacy of azathioprine in the treatment of pemphigus vulgaris. Arch Dermatol 2008 Sep; 144(9):1143–1147.

Günther C, et al: Successful therapy of pemphigus vulgaris with immunoadsorption using the TheraSorb adsorber. J Dtsch Dermatol Ges 2008 Aug; 6(8):661–663.

Hashimoto T: Treatment strategies for pemphigus vulgaris in Japan. Expert Opin Pharmacother 2008 Jun; 9(9):1519–1530.

Ishii N, et al: A clinical study of patients with pemphigus vulgaris and pemphigus foliaceous: an 11-year retrospective study (1996–2006). Clin Exp Dermatol 2008 Aug; 33(5):641–643.

Kitajima Y, et al: A perspective of pemphigus from bedside and laboratory-bench. Clin Rev Allergy Immunol 2007 Oct; 33(1–2):57–66.

Knudson RM, et al: The management of mucous membrane pemphigoid and pemphigus. Dermatol Ther 2010 May–Jun; 23(3):268–280.

Lehman JS, et al: Do safe and effective treatment options exist for patients with active pemphigus vulgaris who plan conception and pregnancy? Arch Dermatol 2008 Jun; 144(6):783–785.

Mao X, et al: Seeking approval: present and future therapies for pemphigus vulgaris. Curr Opin Investig Drugs 2008 May; 9(5):497–504.

Martin LK, et al: Interventions for pemphigus vulgaris and pemphigus foliaceus. Cochrane Database Syst Rev 2009 21; (1):CD006263.

Mignogna MD, et al: Adjuvant high-dose intravenous immunoglobulin therapy can be easily and safely introduced as an alternative treatment in patients with severe pemphigus vulgaris: a retrospective preliminary study. Am J Clin Dermatol 2008; 9(5):323–331.

Saraceno R, et al: Therapeutic options in an immunocompromised patient with pemphigus vulgaris: potential interest of plasmapheresis and extracorporeal photochemotherapy. Eur J Dermatol 2008 May–Jun; 18(3):354–356.

Shimanovich I, et al: Treatment of severe pemphigus with protein A immunoadsorption, rituximab and intravenous immunoglobulins. Br J Dermatol 2008 Feb; 158(2):382–388.

Sorce M, et al: Rituximab in refractory pemphigus vulgaris. Dermatol Ther 2008 Jul; 21(Suppl 1):S6–S9.

Stirling L, et al: Evidence-based pemphigus treatment? J Invest Dermatol 2010 Aug; 130(8):1963.

Valikhani M, et al: Impact of smoking on pemphigus. Int J Dermatol 2008 Jun; 47(6):567–570.

Werth VP, et al: Multicenter randomized, double-blind, placebo-controlled, clinical trial of dapsone as a glucocorticoid-sparing agent in maintenance-phase pemphigus vulgaris. Arch Dermatol 2008 Jan; 144(1):25–32.

Zivanovic D, et al: Dexamethasone-cyclophosphamide pulse therapy in pemphigus: a review of 72 cases. Am J Clin Dermatol 2010; 11(2):123–129.

Pemphigus foliaceus

Pemphigus foliaceus (PF) is characterized by flaccid bullae and localized or generalized exfoliation. Antibodies target Dsg1. Lesions start as small, flaccid bullae that rupture almost as they appear, leading to crusting. Below each crust is a moist surface with a tendency to bleed. A Nikolsky sign may be easily elicited by rubbing the skin (Fig. 21-5). After a time, the exfoliative characteristics predominate, with few bullae (Fig. 21-6). Adherent scale crusts may resemble corn flakes. A variant of pemphigus that has clinical features suggestive of dermatitis herpetiformis but has immunologic features of pemphigus has been called herpetiform pemphigus. Most of these patients represent a clinical variant of PF, with the remainder being PV patients. A few have also demonstrated desmocollin antibodies.

The Nikolsky sign is present in PF. Oral lesions are rarely seen, and then only as superficial erosive stomatitis. This may be because Dsg3, present throughout the epithelium, is unaltered in PF and provides enough adherence to maintain clinical integrity. Several patients have been described whose clinical picture shifted from PF to PV or vice versa, with an accompanying change in antibody profile.

Most patients with PF are not severely ill. They complain of burning, pain, and pruritus. The lesions may persist for many years without affecting general health. PF occurs mostly in adults between 40 and 50 years of age, but has also been reported in children. The sexes are affected equally. Prevalence of PF in people of Jewish heritage is much less than with PV. The drugs listed under PV more commonly induce PF.

The principal histologic finding consists of acantholysis in the upper epidermis, usually in the granular layer. The stratum corneum may be missing entirely, or separated from the underlying epidermis. Individual elongated acantholytic cells are noted above the epidermis or clinging to the underside of the stratum corneum.

DIF demonstrates intercellular IgG throughout the epidermis, although the deposits may be somewhat more prominent in the upper epidermis. IIF is positive in most patients, although prozone reactions occur and a wide range of dilutions should be tested. A sensitive and specific ELISA for detecting antibodies to Dsg1 is now available to confirm positive IIF results. Patients with a distinct clinical picture of PF or PV may have a mix of antibodies. Western blot has shown Dsg1 in roughly 86% of PF patients and 25% of PV patients. ELISA has shown anti-Dsg1 antibodies in up to 71% of PF patients and in 62% of PV patients. In one study, antibodies to Dsg3 were detected in 19 of 276 patients with PF and fogo selvagem who had only cutaneous disease. The antibody was capable of producing disease in laboratory animals, suggesting it was pathogenic in the PF patients. Therefore, ELISA studies must always be interpreted in the context of clinical, histologic, and immunofluorescence findings. In PV, Dsg3 mediates mucosal disease and cutaneous disease is associated with antibodies to Dsg1. A shift to predominantly Dsg1 antibodies has accompanied a clinical shift from PV to PF. Patients have also shifted from a pemphigus to a pemphigoid phenotype.

Dsg1, the antigen in PF, was first identified by immunoprecipitation consisting of polypeptides of molecular weight 260, 160, and 85 kD. The 260 kD molecule is a complex of the 160 and 85 kD polypeptides. The PF antibody binds to a 160 kD glycoprotein extracted from normal epidermis. This glycoprotein is identical to Dsg1. The 85 kD glycoprotein is plakoglobulin, a desmosomal and adherens junction-associated molecule. Desmogleins are cadherin-type adhesion molecules found in desmosomes. The N-terminal extracellular domain of Dsg1

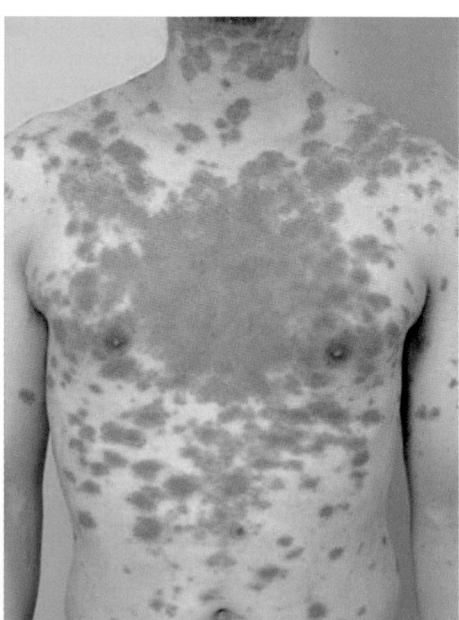

Fig. 21-6 Pemphigus foliaceus.

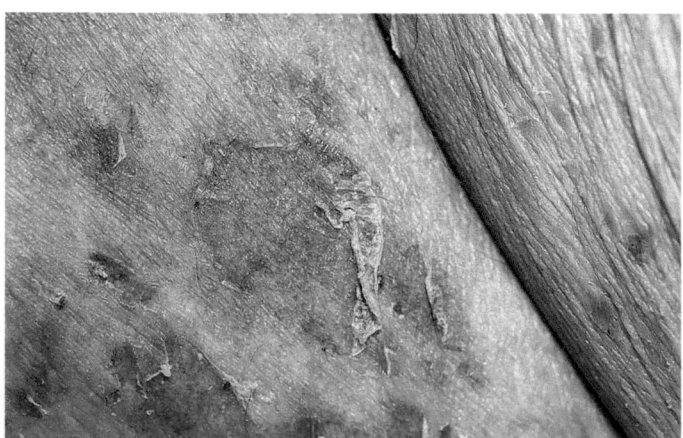

Fig. 21-5 Pemphigus foliaceus.

contains the dominant autoimmune epitopes in both PF and PV. Antibodies include both IgG1 and IgG4 subclasses. IgG4 antibodies appear to be pathogenic in most patients. In a subset of patients, IgG1 autoantibodies are pathogenic. E-cadherin autoantibodies often cross-react with Dsg1.

Treatment

Treatment is similar to that for PV and the two diseases often require similarly aggressive treatment. In fact, many clinical trials include patients with both diseases. PF patients are generally less ill and may not need oral corticosteroid therapy. Dapsone and hydroxychloroquine may be useful, either alone in mild cases or to reduce the steroid dose level. Very mild disease may be treated with topical corticosteroids or topical calcineurin inhibitors. Nicotinamide and tetracycline may be more effective than in PV. Azathioprine, mycophenolate mofetil, or cyclophosphamide may be needed, just as in PV. Rituximab, IVIG, and immunoablative high-dose cyclophosphamide without stem cell rescue have been used for refractory disease. Etanercept has been used and immunoadsorption with tryptophan-linked polyvinyl alcohol adsorbers or adsorption with plant lectins, such as wheat germ agglutinin, has been effective and holds promise as adjuvant therapy.

Endemic pemphigus (fogo selvagem)

Endemic pemphigus is found in tropical regions, mostly in certain interior areas of Brazil. Fifteen percent of cases are familial. The disease is common in children, adolescents, and young adults, with about one-third of cases occurring before the age of 20 and two-thirds by the age of 40. The initial lesions may be flaccid bullae, but later lesions are eczematoid, psoriasiform, impetiginous, or seborrheic in appearance. The midfacial areas may be involved. Melanoderma and verrucous vegetative lesions are not unusual, and exfoliative dermatitis may occur. The mucous membranes are not often involved. The Nikolsky sign is present. The disease is often seen in those with arthropod exposure, and may be initiated by an infectious agent, possibly carried by mosquitoes or black flies. Histologically and immunohistologically, fogo selvagem is identical to PF. Peripheral blood mononuclear cells from patients produce more IL-1β than those from healthy controls. A strong Th2 bias is also observed. IgM anti-Dsg1 antibodies are common in fogo selvagem, but not in other forms of pemphigus.

A distinct subset has been described in a rural area in northeastern Colombia. This subset differs from previously described forms of endemic pemphigus, and shares some immunoreactivity with paraneoplastic pemphigus. It is not, however, associated with malignant tumors. Clinically, the disease resembles Senear–Usher syndrome. A systemic form may affect internal organs and has a poorer prognosis. All patients appear to have antibodies to Dsg1. In addition, many sera react with desmoplakin I, envoplakin, and periplakin. A few Brazilian sera also react with plakins. None of the Colombian patients' sera reacted with Dsg3, but about half of Brazilian patients' sera reacted with Dsg3. This area of Colombia is a mining region and the population is exposed to high environmental levels of mercuric sulfides and selenides; these compounds have been found in the skin of patients with the disease.

Pemphigus erythematosus (Senear–Usher syndrome)

In Senear–Usher syndrome, the early lesions are circumscribed patches of erythema and crusting that clinically resemble lupus erythematosus and are immunopathologically positive for the lupus band in 80% of patients. The lesions are erythematous and thickly crusted, bullous, or even hyperkeratotic. These are usually localized on the nose, cheeks, and ears, sites frequently affected by lupus erythematosus. In addition, crusting and impetiginous lesions appear amid bullae on the scalp, chest, and extremities. In most patients, the disease runs an indolent course.

The histopathology is that of pemphigus foliaceus. DIF shows IgG and complement localized in both intercellular and basement membrane sites. At the dermoepidermal junction, the deposits are continuous and granular, as in lupus. In the epidermis, they resemble those of pemphigus. The antinuclear antibody is present in low titer in 30% of patients. Patients have demonstrated anti-Dsg1 but not anti-Dsg3 autoantibodies. Additional autoantibodies may be directed against bullous pemphigoid antigen 1 (BP230) and periplakin.

Patients often respond to low doses of prednisone, and may respond well to topical steroids and sunscreens. Immunosuppressants may be needed in severe cases.

Cohen SN, et al: Equal efficacy of topical tacrolimus and clobetasone butyrate in pemphigus foliaceus. Int J Dermatol 2006 Nov; 45(11):1379.

Dasher D, et al: Pemphigus foliaceus. Curr Dir Autoimmun 2008; 10:182–194.

Diaz LA, et al: The IgM anti-desmoglein 1 response distinguishes Brazilian pemphigus foliaceus (fogo selvagem) from other forms of pemphigus. J Invest Dermatol 2008 Mar; 128(3):667–675.

Gubinelli E, et al: Pemphigus foliaceus treated with etanercept. J Am Acad Dermatol 2006 Dec; 55(6):1107–1108.

Kim NH, et al: Antibody response in endemic pemphigus foliaceus. J Invest Dermatol 2008 Mar; 128(3):498.

Maeda JY, et al: Changes in the autoimmune blistering response: a clinical and immunopathological shift from pemphigus foliaceus to bullous pemphigoid. Clin Exp Dermatol 2006 Sep; 31(5):653–655.

Mutasim DF: Autoimmune bullous dermatoses in the elderly: an update on pathophysiology, diagnosis and management. Drugs Aging 2010; 27(1):1–19.

Rocha-Alvarez R, et al: Endemic pemphigus vulgaris. Arch Dermatol 2007 Jul; 143(7):895–899.

Serrão VV, et al: Successful treatment of recalcitrant pemphigus foliaceus with rituximab. J Eur Acad Dermatol Venereol 2008 Jun; 22(6):768–770.

Zaraa I, et al: Pemphigus vulgaris and pemphigus foliaceus: similar prognosis? Int J Dermatol 2007 Sep; 46(9):923–926.

Paraneoplastic pemphigus

In 1990, Anhalt et al described five patients with underlying neoplasms who presented with painful mucosal ulcerations and polymorphous skin lesions, which progressed to blistering eruptions on their trunk and extremities. Most patients described since then have had associated neoplasms or Castleman's disease. The mucosal lesions of paraneoplastic pemphigus (PNP) may appear lichenoid or more commonly may resemble Stevens–Johnson syndrome, with crusting of the lips. The skin lesions may appear as erythematous macules, lichenoid lesions, erythema multiforme-like lesions, flaccid bullae, and erosions typical of pemphigus, or with tense, more deep-set bullae.

Histologically, the lesions demonstrate epidermal acantholysis, suprabasal cleft formation, dyskeratotic keratinocytes, and vacuolar change of the basal epidermis. Biopsies that demonstrate both acantholysis and lichenoid change or individual cell necrosis should raise the suspicion of PNP.

It should be noted that all forms of pemphigus may be paraneoplastic; however, the specific disease dubbed "paraneoplastic pemphigus" has a characteristic clinical appearance as well as diagnostic immunologic findings, but is not universally associated with a neoplasm. DIF reveals IgG and C3 deposition in the intercellular spaces of the epithelium. IIF shows a similar pattern in a wide range of stratified squamous epithelium and transitional epithelium (such as rat bladder). About 25% of cases will be negative and some erythema multiforme may be falsely positive. Immunoprecipitation is the definitive test. It reveals a complex immune response with autoantibodies directed against four high molecular weight keratinocyte proteins. Antibody targets include desmoplakin 1 (250 kD), envoplakin (210 kD), the major plaque protein of hemidesmosomes BPAg1 (230 kD), and periplakin (190 kD). Many cases also recognize an additional antigen at 170 kD. Finally, antibodies to Dsg3 and Dsg1 are frequently present on ELISA. ELISA has also been used to detect anti-envoplakin and anti-periplakin autoantibodies. On DIF, some cases also demonstrate a linear or granular IgG and/or C3 at the basement membrane zone. Detection of the characteristic immunologic pattern may be delayed and tests should be repeated if the index of suspicion is high.

Whereas the dominant epitopes in PV reside in N-terminal regions of Dsg3, epitopes on Dsg3 in PNP are distributed more broadly through the extracellular domain. The N-terminal domains are still recognized more frequently than the C-terminal domains. IgG subclasses in PNP are IgG1- and IgG2-dominant, contrasting with the IgG4 dominance in PV. There is a significant association in PNP with HLA-DRB1*03 allele (61.5% of those studied). In one study, 8 of 9 fatal PNP cases had distinctive cell surface antibodies detected in a beaded pattern by complement indirect immunofluorescent (CIIF) tests on monkey esophagus. Three long-term survivors with PNP lacked this pattern, suggesting the test may have prognostic value.

A wide variety of both benign and malignant tumors are seen in these patients, and some have no identifiable neoplasm. The most common associations are non-Hodgkin lymphoma, chronic lymphocytic leukemia, Castleman tumor, sarcoma, and thymoma. Most reported patients die from their tumor. Others have died from bronchiolitis obliterans.

Therapy for the bullous dermatoses with prednisone and/or immunosuppressive agents should be balanced with treatment of the tumor. Immunoablative high-dose cyclophosphamide without stem-cell rescue, cyclosporine A, plasmapheresis, immunoapheresis, and rituximab have been successful in some cases. Even with treatment, the death rate remains higher than for other immunobullous diseases.

Bennett DD, et al: Delayed detection of autoantibodies in paraneoplastic pemphigus. J Am Acad Dermatol 2007 Dec; 57(6):1094–1095.

Park GT, et al: Paraneoplastic pemphigus without an underlying neoplasm. Br J Dermatol 2007 Mar; 156(3):563–566.

Peterson JD, et al: Effectiveness and side effects of anti-CD20 therapy for autoantibody-mediated blistering skin diseases: a comprehensive survey of 71 consecutive patients from the initial use to 2007. Ther Clin Risk Manag 2009; 5(1):1–7.

Zhu X, et al: Paraneoplastic pemphigus. J Dermatol 2007 Aug; 34(8):503–511.

Intraepidermal neutrophilic IgA dermatosis

In 1985, Huff et al reported the case of an elderly man having a chronic bullous dermatosis with unique histologic and immunopathologic findings. Clinically, there were generalized flaccid bullae, which rapidly ruptured and crusted. There was no scarring when the dermatosis healed. No mucosal lesions were present, and the distal extremities, face, and neck were spared. Neither grouping nor symmetry was present. Histologic findings consisted of neutrophilic exocytosis, and in some areas neutrophils were arranged in a linear fashion at the dermoepidermal junction. Later, intraepidermal abscesses were formed; no acantholysis was present. DIF repeatedly

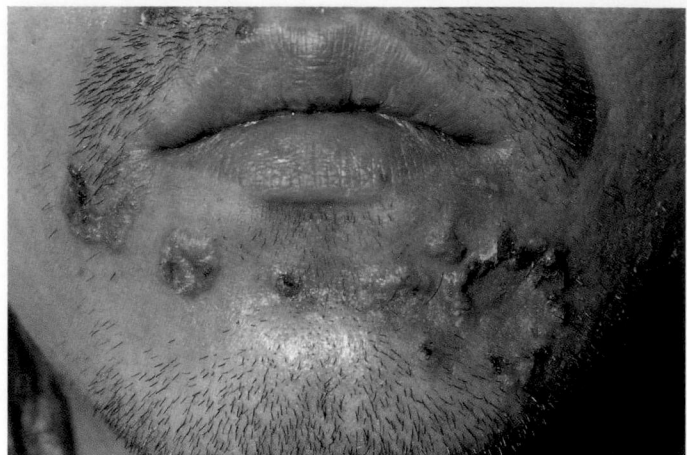

Fig. 21-7 Intraepidermal neutrophilic IgA dermatosis.

showed an intercellular deposition of IgA within the epidermis, with minimal staining of the basal layer. No circulating antibodies were found.

Since this report, many additional patients with intraepidermal IgA deposition have been described. They have been classified as belonging to two subsets, one closely mimicking pemphigus and the second simulating subcorneal pustular dermatosis (SPD). The former starts with vesicles that become pustular within a few days, enlarge peripherally, and rupture in the center, then forming a crust (Fig. 21-7). Continued peripheral vesiculation may lead to a flower-like appearance. The head, neck, and trunk are frequent sites of involvement. In some patients, the condition is induced by ultraviolet (UV) A light. The second subset presents much like Sneddon–Wilkinson disease, with serpiginous and annular pustules. Some cases have been induced by granulocyte–macrophage colony stimulating factor. Some patients have had associated malignancies.

Histologically, intraepidermal bullae with neutrophils, some eosinophils, and acantholysis are seen. DIF shows intraepidermal IgA deposition, usually throughout the epidermis, and IIF may reveal circulating autoantibody that binds to the same location. There is evidence that the IgA specificity in individual cases may be directed at either Dsg1 or Dsg3. Some patients have concurrent IgG intercellular antibodies directed at Dsg1, and some have a monoclonal IgA gammopathy. The antigen in SPD-type IgA pemphigus is desmocollin, a type of desmosomal cadherin. Some patients have a circulating IgA monoclonal gammopathy. It should be noted that IgA antibodies to desmogleins 1 and 3 may occur in pemphigus vulgaris, pemphigus foliaceus, and paraneoplastic pemphigus. Individual patients may express both anti-desmocollin 1 and anti-Dsg1 antibodies.

Therapy with topical corticosteroids may be effective in mild cases. Dapsone is often effective, and may be so even at doses as low as 25 mg/day. Oral corticosteroids may be necessary, and some resistant cases have required immunosuppressive agents and plasmapheresis. Colchicine, acitretin, adalimumab, mycophenolate mofetil, and isotretinoin have been effective in some patients.

Bliziotis I, et al: Regression of subcorneal pustular dermatosis type of IgA pemphigus lesions with azithromycin. J Infect 2005; 51:E31.

Düker I, et al: Subcorneal pustular dermatosis-type IgA pemphigus with autoantibodies to desmocollins 1, 2, and 3. Arch Dermatol 2009; 145(10):1159–1162.

Howell SM, et al: Rapid response of IgA pemphigus of the subcorneal pustular dermatosis subtype to treatment with adalimumab and mycophenolate mofetil. J Am Acad Dermatol 2005; 53:541.

Kopp T, et al: IgA pemphigus—occurrence of anti-desmocollin 1 and anti-desmoglein 1 antibody reactivity in an individual patient. J Dtsch Dermatol Ges 2006 Dec; 4(12):1045–1050.

Mentink LF, et al: Coexistence of IgA antibodies to desmogleins 1 and 3 in pemphigus vulgaris, pemphigus foliaceus and paraneoplastic pemphigus. Br J Dermatol 2007 Apr; 156(4):635–641.

Patrício P, et al: Autoimmune bullous dermatoses: a review. Ann N Y Acad Sci 2009; 1173:203–210.

Petropoulou H, et al: Immunoglobulin A pemphigus associated with immunoglobulin A gammopathy and lung cancer. J Dermatol 2008 Jun; 35(6):341–345.

Bullous pemphigoid

Clinical features

Bullous pemphigoid (BP) was described by Lever in 1953. Clinically, it is characterized by large, tense, subepidermal bullae with a predilection for the groin, axillae, trunk, thighs (Fig. 21 8), and flexor surfaces of the forearms. Key features distinguishing BP from other immunobullous diseases include subepidermal separation at the dermoepidermal junction, an inflammatory cell infiltrate that tends to be rich in eosinophils, and antibodies directed against two hemidesmosomal antigens, BP230 and BP180. Antibody detection rates vary by method and many normal patients will gave positive serologic tests but negative IIF.

After the bullae rupture, large denuded areas are seen, but the bullae and denuded areas do not tend to increase in size as they do in PV. Instead, the denuded areas show a tendency to heal spontaneously. In addition to the bullae, there often are erythematous patches and urticarial plaques (Fig. 21-9), with a tendency to central clearing. These patches and plaques may be present without bullae early in the course of the disease.

Later, bullae often occur on an urticarial base. Sometimes, targetoid lesions are present.

BP may begin at a localized site, frequently on the shins. The disease may also be limited to areas of radiation therapy, burns, or plaques of psoriasis. It may remain localized throughout the course of the disease or eventuate in generalized pemphigoid. Cases of the localized disease in which a vesicular eruption is limited to the palms or soles (dyshidrosiform pemphigoid) are occasionally observed. Young girls may present with localized vulvar erosions and ulcers that resemble the signs of child abuse (Fig. 21-10). These localized varieties have been shown to have circulating IgG antibody, which immunoprecipitates the 230 kD BP antigen.

Many other variants of BP have been described. A vesicular variant manifested by tense, small, occasionally grouped blisters, is termed vesicular pemphigoid. Other patients, mostly women, have papules and nodules of the scalp and extremities, with sparing of the mucous membranes, in a pattern resembling prurigo nodularis (pemphigoid nodularis). Cases resembling pemphigus vegetans, but with IgG and C3 at the basement membrane zone, are occasionally observed (pemphigoid vegetans). Erythroderma may be present (erythrodermic pemphigoid) or there may be no bullae at all (nonbullous variant). The latter type may present as generalized pruritus, pruritic eczema, or urticarial eruptions with peripheral eosinophilia. Overall, incidence of oral involvement is about 20%, but involvement of the pharynx, larynx, nasal mucosa, vulva, urethra, and eye is rare.

BP occurs most frequently in the elderly. The age of onset averages 65–75 years. It also occurs in young children, however, with clinical and pathologic findings similar to those in adults. Many of these cases begin with hand and foot bullae (Fig. 21-11). Facial involvement may be somewhat more common in children. In children, the course of disease is usually under 1 year, with most cases lasting 5 months or less.

In patients with lichen planus, a bullous eruption similar to BP may develop. This condition, called lichen planus pemphigoides, is sometimes related to the 230 kD antigen, the 180 kD antigen, or a unique 200 kD subepidermal antigen. A nonscarring eruption, with acute onset, widespread erosions, and severe mucous membrane involvement resembling toxic

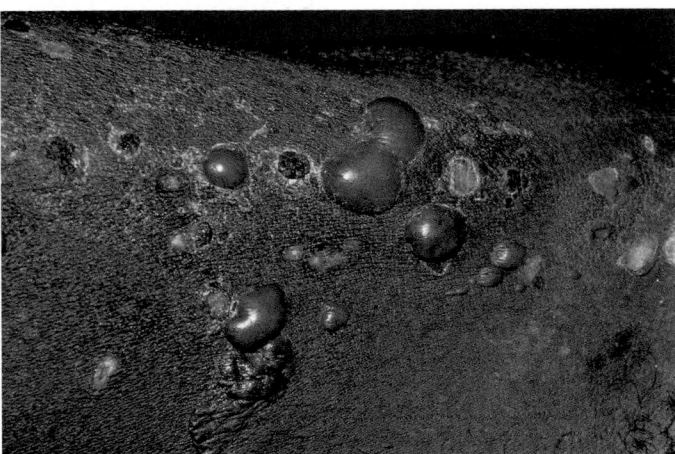

Fig. 21-8 Bullous pemphigoid.

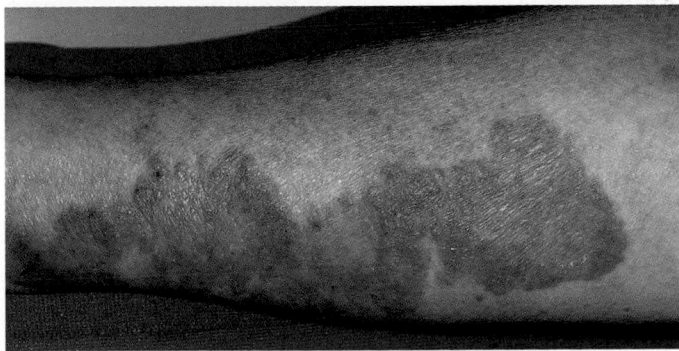

Fig. 21-9 Urticarial bullous pemphigoid.

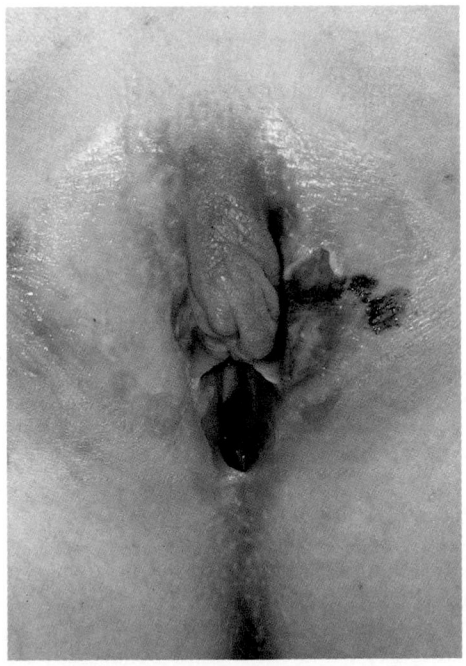

Fig. 21-10 Vulvar pemphigoid.

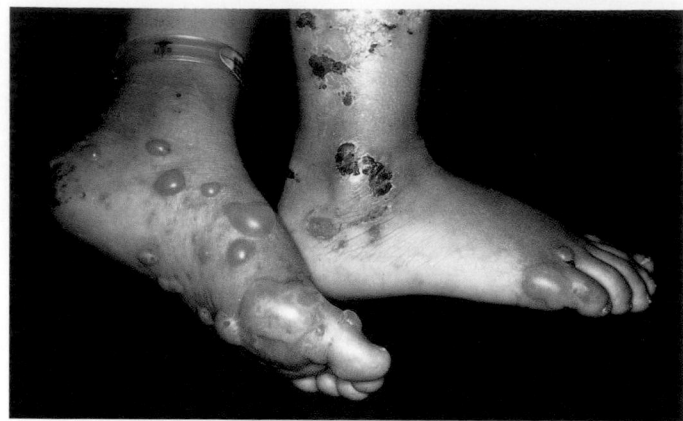

Fig. 21-11 Childhood bullous pemphigoid.

epidermal necrolysis or PV, has been referred to as anti-p105 pemphigoid. Linear IgG and C3 are noted at the basement membrane zone. The 105 kD antigen is found in the lower portion of the lamina lucida.

Etiologic factors

Circulating basement membrane zone antibodies of the IgG class are present in approximately 70% of patients with BP. In most instances, the antibodies fix complement in vitro, in contrast to pemphigus antibodies, which fail to do so. Complement is activated by both the classic and alternate pathways. No close correlation exists between the titer of antibodies and clinical disease activity.

Passive transfer mouse models suggest that subepidermal blistering is initiated by anti-BP180 antibodies. Blister formation involves complement activation, mast cells, and neutrophils. Basement membrane zone damage is caused by proteinases and reactive oxygen species released by the infiltrating neutrophils.

The site of IgG binding has been localized to the lamina lucida, with accentuation near hemidesmosomes. BP antigen 1 (BPAg1) is synthesized by the keratinocyte and is an intracytoplasmic hemidesmosomal plaque protein of molecular weight 230 kD with disulfide-linked chains. The second BP antigen (the 180 kD BPAg2) is a transmembrane protein with a long C-terminal collagenous domain that projects into the extracellular region below the hemidesmosome. The antibody to BPAg2 is the primary pathogenic factor. The noncollagenous (NC) 16A domain harbors the major epitopes of autoantibodies in BP. A predominance of the IgG4 subclass has been observed in several studies. In addition to this humoral response, infiltrating T-helper lymphocytes with a mixed Th1/Th2 cytokine profile may play a role in blister formation. Peripheral blood eosinophilia is present in 50% of pemphigoid patients.

BP has occasionally been reported to be associated with other diseases, such as diabetes mellitus, rheumatoid arthritis, PF, dermatomyositis, ulcerative colitis, myasthenia gravis, and thymoma. Drugs have been reported to induce BP; these include penicillamine, furosemide, captopril, penicillin, sulfasalazine, nalidixic acid, and enalapril.

Histopathology

The histologic changes are characterized by subepidermal bullae, by the absence of acantholysis, and by a superficial dermal infiltrate containing many eosinophils. The amount of inflammatory infiltrate varies, and individual bullae may be "infiltrate-poor" or "infiltrate-rich." Often the infiltrate contains many eosinophils, although neutrophil-predominant cases exist. Spongiosis with eosinophils occurs more frequently than in pemphigus. Urticarial lesions often demonstrate eosinophils lined up along the dermoepidermal junction.

Atypical presentations are fairly common. In one study of 23 new cases of BP, only 7 of 22 biopsy specimens showed subepidermal blister formation, and only 12 of these had a predominance of eosinophils in the blister cavity. In 23% of patients, the biopsy was not particularly suggestive of BP. DIF, IIF, immunoblot analysis, and ELISA are critical in establishing the diagnosis in such cases.

DIF is a more sensitive test than IIF, just as in pemphigus. In a positive test, continuous linear (tubular or toothpaste pattern) immunofluorescence is seen along the basement membrane zone. IgG and/or C3 are best found in perilesional skin. False-negative tests are somewhat more common on the lower extremities. A positive DIF test is found in nearly 100% of patients, with C3 most commonly present and IgG present in about 80% of cases. IgA and IgM are occasionally present.

About 20% of patients have negative staining for IgG on DIF, even though C3 is present. In some of these patients, IgG may be present at subthreshold levels that cannot be detected. Also, the major subclass, IgG4, shows limited reactivity with most commercial antihuman IgG conjugates. Double sandwich antibody immunofluorescence methods have been developed that offer greater sensitivity for IgG4 antibodies.

All histologic features present in BP may also be seen in epidermolysis bullosa acquisita (EBA); therefore, immunofluorescence testing on salt-split skin is sometimes performed to differentiate EBA from BP. Salt-split skin may be replaced by assessment of u-serrated (EBA) and n-serrated (BP) immunoglobuin patterns in DIF specimens and by serologic testing. C3 deposition is nearly always present in BP, whereas it may be absent in EBA. Type IV collagen mapping in BP localizes to the base of the blister. In EBA it stains the roof.

Bullous scabies can also mimic both the histology and DIF findings of BP.

Treatment

Relatively few controlled trials have been performed, and many recommendations are based on experience and consensus of opinion. A Cochrane Library search strategy identified seven randomized controlled trials through 2003. A total of 634 patients were enrolled in the trials. One comparing prednisolone, 0.75 mg/kg/day, with prednisolone, 1.25 mg/kg/day, found no statistical difference between the two. The same was true of a trial comparing methylprednisolone with prednisolone. Higher doses of prednisolone were associated with more severe side effects in these studies. Two trials confirmed that adjuvant therapy with azathioprine or plasma exchange could reduce the required steroid dose. Another trial failed to confirm the superiority of combination treatment (with either azathioprine or plasma exchange) over steroid alone, and one trial found no statistically significant difference between prednisolone and a combination of tetracycline and niacinamide. The steroid-treated group had more side effects. Another study compared ultrapotent topical corticosteroid treatment (clobetasol propionate cream 40 g/day) with oral prednisone (0.5–1 mg/kg/day). In those with severe disease, the 1 year survival rate was better in the topical corticosteroid group (76% vs 58%). Disease control at 3 weeks was also better in the topical steroid group (99% vs 91%). Side effects were common in both groups, but more common in the prednisone group (29% vs 54%). Among those with moderate disease, there were no significant differences between the two groups.

Even in those with fairly extensive disease, topical corticosteroid treatment should be attempted. Prednisone has long been the standard approach, but the complication rate must be weighed carefully, especially in those with severe disease. Oral therapy with tetracycline, 500 mg four times a day, combined with niacinamide, 500 mg three times a day, is effective in some cases. It should be noted that occasional patients with BP may respond to tetracycline alone or nicotinamide alone. Rituximab has proved effective in adults and has been used in infancy. Dapsone is also effective in some patients. Immunosuppressive therapy may still be necessary in resistant cases, either in combination with systemic or topical steroids, or as sole therapy. Azathioprine and mycophenolate mofetil demonstrate similar efficacy when used as steroid-sparing agents, and cumulative corticosteroid doses are similar. Mycophenolate mofetil is more expensive, but is easier to dose and is associated with less toxicity. Methotrexate, cyclophosphamide, chlorambucil, IVIG, and cyclosporine have also proved effective in some patients, and some data suggest that outcomes are better with methotrexate than with prednisone. Low-dose oral methotrexate has been shown to induce apoptosis of tissue eosinophils in patients with bullous pemphigoid. The effectiveness of intravenous IVIG is improved by the addition of an immunosuppressive agent. In exceptionally severe cases, pulse therapy with methylprednisolone, 15 mg/kg in 16 mL of bacteriostatic water over a period of 30–60 min/day for three doses, can be rapidly effective. Some patients may also respond to dapsone or sulfapyridine. These agents tend to be more effective in neutrophil-rich pemphigoid. Oral erythromycin and topical macrolactams have proved effective in some patients.

Double-filtration plasmapheresis (DFPP) may be more effective than conventional plasma exchange, possibly because it removes pathogenic cytokines. DFPP reduces a variety of cytokines, including IL-8, tumor necrosis factor (TNF)-α, and IL-2. IVIG produces faster clearance of antibody titers, and may be helpful in inducing and maintaining remission.

Course and prognosis

BP is usually self-limited over a 5–6-year period. This period is generally a year or less in children. Relapse occurs in 10–15% of patients once therapy is discontinued. The presence of circulating anti-BP180 antibodies, but not anti-BP230, is associated with a statistically increased chance of death in the first year after diagnosis. Other risk factors for death during the first year include greater age, higher daily steroid dosage at discharge, low serum albumin, and erythrocyte sedimentation rate greater than 30 mm/h. Much of the morbidity and mortality now relate to side effects of drug therapy, but with improvements in treatment, pemphigoid patients have similar mortality to age-matched controls. While IIF titers do not always correlate with disease activity, ELISA measurements of BP180NC16a show better correlation. The presence of IgE autoantibodies to BP180 correlate with a more severe course.

Beissert S, et al: A comparison of oral methylprednisolone plus azathioprine or mycophenolate mofetil for the treatment of bullous pemphigoid. Arch Dermatol 2007 Dec; 143(12):1536–1542.

Czernik A, et al: Improvement of intravenous immunoglobulin therapy for bullous pemphigoid by adding immunosuppressive agents: marked improvement in depletion of circulating autoantibodies. Arch Dermatol 2008 May; 144(5):658–661.

Dahlman-Ghozlan K, et al: Low-dose oral methotrexate induces apoptosis of tissue eosinophils in bullous pemphigoid. Acta Derm Venereol 2008; 88(3):219–222.

Feng S, et al: Serum levels of autoantibodies to BP180 correlate with disease activity in patients with bullous pemphigoid. Int J Dermatol 2008 Mar; 47(3):225–228.

Fine JD: Prevalence of autoantibodies to bullous pemphigoid antigens within the normal population. Arch Dermatol 2010; 146(1):74–75.

Iwata Y, et al: Correlation of IgE autoantibody to BP180 with a severe form of bullous pemphigoid. Arch Dermatol 2008 Jan; 144(1):41–48.

Joly P, et al: A comparison of oral and topical corticosteroids in patients with bullous pemphigoid. N Engl J Med 2002; 346:321.

Kasperkiewicz M, et al: The pathophysiology of bullous pemphigoid. Clin Rev Allergy Immunol 2007 Oct; 33(1–2):67–77.

Khumalo N, et al: Interventions for bullous pemphigoid. Cochrane Database Syst Rev 2005; 20:CD002292.

Kjellman P, et al: A retrospective analysis of patients with bullous pemphigoid treated with methotrexate. Arch Dermatol 2008 May; 144(5):612–616.

Leuci S, et al: Serological studies in bullous pemphigoid: a literature review of antibody titers at presentation and in clinical remission. Acta Derm Venereol 2010; 90(2):115–121.

Liu A, et al: A quick and simple serum test to differentiate bullous pemphigoid, epidermolysis bullosa acquisita, and anti-epiligrin cicatricial pemphigoid. Dermatol Online J 2008 Jul 15; 14(7):3.

Olasz EB, et al: Bullous pemphigoid and related subepidermal autoimmune blistering diseases. Curr Dir Autoimmun 2008; 10:141–166.

Parker SR, et al: Mortality of bullous pemphigoid: an evaluation of 223 patients and comparison with the mortality in the general population in the United States. J Am Acad Dermatol 2008 Oct; 59(4):582–588.

Schulze J, et al: Severe bullous pemphigoid in an infant—successful treatment with rituximab. Pediatr Dermatol 2008 Jul–Aug; 25(4):462–465.

Veien NK: Bullous pemphigoid masquerading as recurrent vesicular hand eczema. Acta Derm Venereol 2010; 90(1):4–5.

Wieland CN, et al: Anti-bullous pemphigoid 180 and 230 antibodies in a sample of unaffected subjects. Arch Dermatol 2010; 146(1):21–25.

Pemphigoid gestationis (herpes gestationis)

Clinical features

Pemphigoid gestationis (PG) is an autoimmune, inflammatory, bullous disease with onset during pregnancy or during the postpartum period. It occurs in approximately 1 in 50 000 pregnancies. The onset is usually during the second trimester, with urticarial plaques and papules developing around the umbilicus and extremities. Targetoid lesions may be present (Fig. 21-12). As the disease progresses, lesions may spread over the abdomen, back, chest, and extremities, including the palms and soles. The face, scalp, and oral mucosa are usually spared. Within the infiltrated erythematous plaques, tense vesicles and bullae erupt, often in an annular or polycyclic configuration. Pruritus is severe and may be paroxysmal. The disease will often flare shortly after delivery and then remit spontaneously, usually within 3 months. There is no scarring, except that caused by excoriations or secondary infections. Recurrences with subsequent pregnancies are common, and

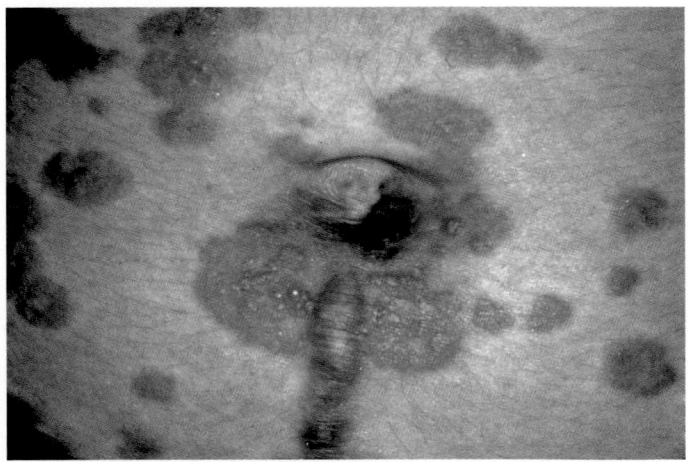

Fig. 21-12 Pemphigoid gestationis.

the disease may be provoked by subsequent menstrual periods or oral contraceptives. A number of cases of persistent disease have been reported.

Most study data suggest that fetal loss is not statistically increased, although infants are often born prematurely and are small for gestational age. In fewer than 5% of cases, infants manifest the disease in the form of urticarial lesions or bullae. The lesions are usually limited, and clear spontaneously without the need for therapy. Neonatal convulsions have been reported.

Etiologic factors

PG is an autoimmune, antibody-mediated disease. A complement-fixing IgG antibody is present in the serum, and is deposited in the lamina lucida. The antigen, transmembrane collagen XVII, is a component of fetal membranes and promotes migration of placental cytotrophoblastic cells. The antigenic epitopes are usually restricted to the N-terminal portion of the extracellular domain of BP180 (BPAg2). The antigenic N-terminal portion of MCW-1 is located in the noncollagenous domain (NC16A) of BP180. Other antigens are located nearby, and four major PG epitopes are clustered within a 22 amino acid region of the BP180 ectodomain. ELISA-based assays correlate antibody levels to disease activity. Both IgG1 and IgG3 subtypes have been noted, but a more recent study found IgG4 to be the predominant subtype, just as in BP.

Studies have documented an increased frequency of HLA-DR3, DR4, and C4 null alleles in patients with PG. A woman may have antibodies directed against her husband's HLA antigens. Black women rarely manifest PG, possibly related to the low incidence of HLA-DR4 in American black persons (Fig. 21-13). There is an increased frequency of Graves' disease in PG patients.

Pathogenesis

Pathogenesis is similar to that of BP. However, hormonal factors influence the disease manifestation. In addition to being seen in pregnant patients, menstruating women, and those taking oral contraceptives, the disease may occur in association with hydatidiform mole and choriocarcinoma. The IgG antibodies bind to the lamina lucida and fix complement. Activated eosinophils, neutrophils, and T cells with a predominant Th2 phenotype are involved in blister formation. Evidence of fetal microchimerism is lacking.

Patients with chronic PG tend to be older and multigravid, with a history of PG during previous pregnancies. They often

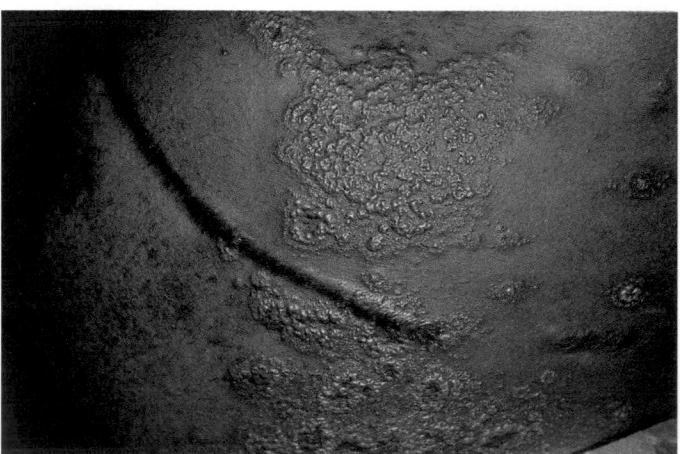

Fig. 21-13 Pemphigoid gestationis.

have widespread cutaneous and mucosal involvement. The IgG1 subclass is commonly present. Antibodies to a C-terminal portion of BP180 have been noted in a patient with chronic PG. This same region is targeted in patients with cicatricial pemphigoid and some with BP.

Histopathology

A subepidermal bulla with eosinophils and some neutrophils is usually present. In the urticarial stage, eosinophils may line up along the dermoepidermal junction, as in urticarial BP. Civatte bodies may be present. On DIF, all patients have C3 deposited in a linear pattern at the dermoepidermal junction. Approximately 25–40% also have detectable IgG. On conventional IIF testing, approximately 25% of patients have a circulating IgG anti-basement zone antibody, but in nearly 75% the PG factor, a complement-fixing IgG antibody, can be demonstrated by complement-enhanced immunofluorescence. Immunoelectron microscopy has demonstrated that the blister occurs at the level of the lamina lucida, with deposition of C3 and IgG at this site, exactly as in BP.

Differential diagnosis

The main diagnosis to be considered is pruritic urticarial papules and plaques of pregnancy (PUPPP). The differential diagnosis also includes erythema multiforme, drug reactions, and bullous scabies. Acrodermatitis enteropathica has also been reported to flare as a bullous eruption with each pregnancy. Biopsy, immunofluorescence findings, and clinical course establish the diagnosis.

Treatment

The use of potent topical steroids may be adequate in some milder cases of PG. Prednisone, in an oral dose of about 40 mg/day, is usually effective in the remainder of cases. The dose is tapered to the lowest effective amount given on alternate days. Pyridoxine has been reported to be effective in some cases. Persistent PG after delivery has been treated with various tetracyclines, together with nicotinamide. A few severe cases have required treatment with rituximab, cyclophosphamide, dapsone, methotrexate, IVIG, or plasmapheresis.

Other pregnancy-related dermatoses

Intrahepatic cholestasis of pregnancy (prurigo gravidarum)

This pregnancy-related disease has no primary skin lesions, and is usually manifested only as severe generalized pruritus and jaundice. Secondary excoriations may be present. It is caused by cholestasis, occurs late in pregnancy, resolves after delivery, and recurs with subsequent pregnancies. There is an increased incidence of fetal complications. It has been estimated to occur in 0.5% of 3192 pregnancies. Both ursodeoxycholic acid and S-adenosyl-l-methionine improve pruritus, but the former is more effective with regard to improving liver function. Delivery at 37 weeks is associated with better outcomes.

Polymorphic eruption of pregnancy

Some investigators have proposed grouping all the pruritic inflammatory dermatoses of pregnancy into the designation

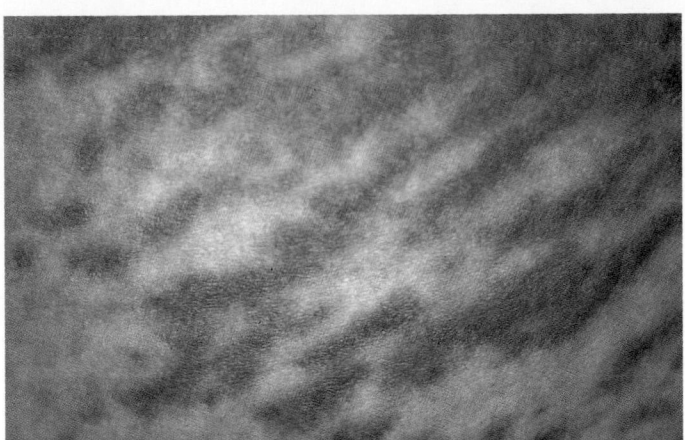

Fig. 21-14 Pruritic urticarial papules and plaques of pregnancy.

polymorphic eruption of pregnancy. This argument has some merit, as many of the pruritic eruptions of pregnancy are nonspecific or variable manifestations of PUPPP, and there are no consistent hormonal or immunopathogenetic factors that reliably separate them. These eruptions occur in approximately 1 in 120–240 pregnancies. They are more common with male fetuses and multiple gestation pregnancies.

Pruritic urticarial papules and plaques of pregnancy

Lawley et al first reported seven patients under the name pruritic urticarial papules and plaques of pregnancy (PUPPP) in 1979. This eruption is characterized by erythematous papules and plaques that begin as 1 or 2 mm lesions within the abdominal striae (Fig. 21-14). They then spread over the course of a few days to involve the abdomen, buttocks, thighs, and in some cases the arms and legs. The upper chest, face, and mucous membranes are generally spared. The lesions coalesce to form urticarial plaques, sometimes in figurate patterns, and occasionally spongiotic vesicles are present. Intense pruritus is characteristic. In contrast to PG, postpartum onset or exacerbation is uncommon. Fetal and maternal outcomes are not affected by this eruption, and only rarely do newborns manifest transient lesions of PUPPP.

This eruption occurs in primigravidas 75% of the time, and rarely recurs with subsequent pregnancies. It begins late in the third trimester and resolves with delivery. Many studies have investigated the relationship of maternal weight gain to the development of this dermatosis. Patients with PUPPP average more weight gain and greater abdominal distension than those without the disease. It is more common in those carrying twins or triplets.

Histologic findings consist of a perivascular lymphohistiocytic infiltrate in the upper and mid-dermis, with a variable number of eosinophils and dermal edema. The epidermis is usually normal, although focal spongiosis, parakeratosis, or scales or crust may be present. The results of a DIF test are negative or nonspecific.

Usually, potent topical steroids are required to control the eruption. A few patients require prednisone. The disease remits after delivery.

Papular dermatitis of pregnancy

Papular dermatitis of pregnancy is a controversial entity. It is defined as a pruritic, generalized eruption of 3–5 mm erythematous papules, each surmounted by a small, firm, central crust. The lesions may erupt at any time during pregnancy and usually resolve with delivery. Marked elevation of the 24 h urinary chorionic gonadotropin has been cited as a marker for the condition.

Administration of systemic corticosteroids is reportedly effective in controlling the eruption. The condition may recur in subsequent pregnancies. The high incidence of fetal deaths reported by Spangler is now felt to have been overstated.

Prurigo gestationis (Besnier)

This eruption consists of pruritic, excoriated papules of the proximal limbs and upper trunk; these occur most often between the 20th and 34th weeks of gestation. It clears in the postpartum period and usually does not recur.

Therapy with potent topical steroidal agents is recommended. No adverse effects on maternal or fetal health are seen. This eruption may simply be an expression of atopic dermatitis in pregnancy.

Pruritic folliculitis of pregnancy

Several authors have reported on pruritic folliculitis in gravid women, with small follicular pustules scattered widely over the trunk appearing during the second or third trimester and resolving by 2 or 3 weeks after delivery. Acute folliculitis and focal spongiosis with exocytosis of polymorphonuclear leukocytes are present on biopsy, and DIF results are negative. This condition may be a type of hormonally induced acne.

Linear IgM dermatosis of pregnancy

In 1988, Alcalay et al described a woman who developed small, red, follicular papules and pustules that, on immunofluorescence testing, showed linear deposits of IgM. This finding is common in a wide variety of dermatoses, and is nonspecific.

Impetigo herpetiformis

Impetigo herpetiformis is a form of severe pustular psoriasis occurring in pregnancy. It consists of an acute, usually febrile onset of grouped pustules on an erythematous base, which begins in the groin, axillae, and neck. There is a high peripheral white blood cell count, and hypocalcemia may be present. The histopathology is that of pustular psoriasis. The condition resolves with delivery, but recurrences with subsequent pregnancies may be expected. Fetal death is not uncommon, and results from placental insufficiency. Treatment is with systemic corticosteroids, in the range of 40–60 mg/day of oral prednisone. The condition is discussed in more detail in Chapter 10.

Al-Fouzan AW, et al: Herpes gestationis (pemphigoid gestationis). Clin Dermatol 2006 Mar–Apr; 24(2):109–112.

Ambros-Rudolph CM, et al: The specific dermatoses of pregnancy revisited and reclassified: results of a retrospective two-center study on 505 pregnant patients. J Am Acad Dermatol 2006 Mar; 54(3):395–404.

Aoyama Y, et al: Herpes gestationis in a mother and newborn: immunoclinical perspectives based on a weekly follow-up of the enzyme-linked immunosorbent assay index of a bullous pemphigoid antigen noncollagenous domain. Arch Dermatol 2007 Sep; 143(9):1168–1172.

Cianchini G, et al: Severe persistent pemphigoid gestationis: long-term remission with rituximab. Br J Dermatol 2007 Aug; 157(2):388–389.

D'Alessio MC, et al: No evidence for fetal microchimerism in the skin of patients with pemphigoid gestationis. Eur J Dermatol 2010; 20(1):122–123.

Huilaja L, et al: Pemphigoid gestationis autoantigen, transmembrane collagen XVII, promotes the migration of cytotrophoblastic cells of placenta and is a structural component of fetal membranes. Matrix Biol 2008 Apr; 27(3):190–200.

Lee RH, et al: Pregnancy outcomes during an era of aggressive management for intrahepatic cholestasis of pregnancy. Am J Perinatol 2008 Jun; 25(6):341–345.

Okumus N, et al: A case report of neonatal convulsions due to maternal herpes gestationis. J Child Neurol 2007 Apr; 22(4):488–491.

Patton T, et al: IgG4 as the predominant IgG subclass in pemphigoides gestationis. J Cutan Pathol 2006 Apr; 33(4):299–302.

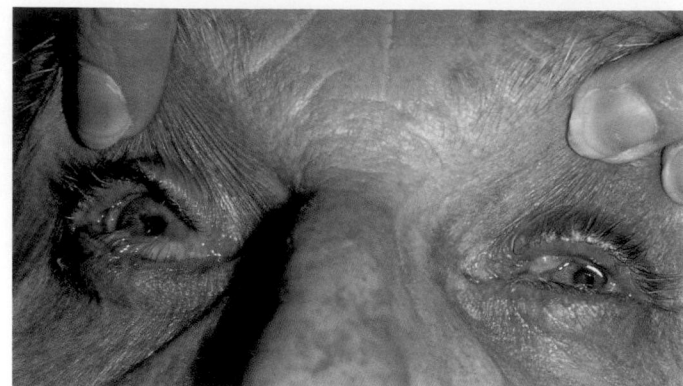

Fig. 21-15 Cicatricial pemphigoid.

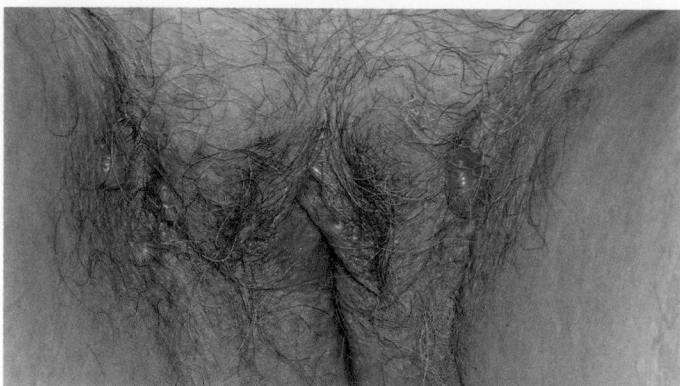

Fig. 21-16 Anti-laminin cicatricial pemphigoid with inguinal involvement. Blisters began at the same time colonic cancer was diagnosed.

Petropoulou H, et al: Polymorphic eruption of pregnancy. Int J Dermatol 2006 Jun; 45(6):642–648.

Regnier S, et al: A case-control study of polymorphic eruption of pregnancy. J Am Acad Dermatol 2008 Jan; 58(1):63–67.

Rodrigues Cdos S, et al: Persistent herpes gestationis treated with high-dose intravenous immunoglobulin. Acta Derm Venereol 2007; 87(2):184–186.

Roncaglia N, et al: A randomised controlled trial of ursodeoxycholic acid and S-adenosyl-l-methionine in the treatment of gestational cholestasis. Br J Obstet Gynaecol 2004; 111:17.

Cicatricial pemphigoid (benign mucosal pemphigoid)

In 1953, Lever suggested the designation benign mucosal pemphigoid for what had previously been called ocular pemphigus, cicatricial pemphigoid, or essential shrinkage of the conjunctiva. Because of its scarring nature, the designation cicatricial pemphigoid (CP) has gained predominance. The term encompasses a group of immunologically distinct immunobullous diseases with scarring.

Clinical features

CP usually occurs in older women, with a female to male ratio of approximately 2:1. The condition is characterized by evanescent vesicles that rupture quickly, leaving behind erosions and ulcers. In most patients, they primarily occur on the mucous membranes, especially the conjunctiva (Fig. 21-15) and oral mucosa. Oral lesions occur in approximately 90% of cases and conjunctival lesions in 66%. The oral mucosa may be the only affected site for years. Desquamative gingivitis, diffuse erythema of the marginal and attached mucosa associated with mucosal desquamation and pain, is often the presenting sign. The mucosa readily peels away in response to pressure from a cotton-tipped applicator or stream of air from a dental air hose. The gingivae are almost always involved, and the lingual surfaces less regularly. The palate, tongue, and tonsillar pillars may be involved.

The disorder is chronic. In ocular cases, it leads to scarring and progressive shrinkage of the ocular mucous membranes. Blindness may result. It is usually bilateral and associated with redness and flaccid vesicles on the conjunctiva, xerosis, and fibrous adhesions (symblepharon). Entropion, trichiasis, and corneal opacities develop, and ultimately, the adhesions attach both lids to the eyeball and narrow the palpebral fissure. Scarring may also develop in the pharynx, esophagus, larynx, and anogenital mucosa. Esophageal stricture may occur, and deafness has been reported.

Cutaneous lesions are seen in approximately 25% of patients. These begin as tense bullae, similar to those in BP. The bullae may occur on the face, scalp, neck, inguinal region (Fig. 21-16), or extremities. Generalized lesions may also occur. Some of these patients will have circulating antibodies targeted against the classic BP antigens, and should be classified as mucosal-predominant BP. Some have secondary antibodies against other antigens. Some patients have EBA, as the IgG autoantibody was found to target type VII collagen. Vegetating intertriginous lesions have been dubbed CP vegetans.

In Brunsting–Perry pemphigoid there are no mucosal lesions, but one or several circumscribed erythematous patches develop, on which recurrent crops of blisters appear. Ultimately, atrophic scarring results. Generally, the areas of involvement are confined to the head and neck. The average age at onset is 58, with a 2:1 male to female ratio. In contrast to BP, CP shows little tendency for remission. Although the disease is chronic and produces significant morbidity, the patient's general health is usually not jeopardized.

Etiologic factors

Circulating autoantibodies target the hemidesmosomal protein BP180, but the target epitopes differ from those usually targeted in BP. While most BP patients react with the noncollagenous domain (NC16a) on the extracellular N-terminal portion of BP180, most CP antibodies target C-terminal domains. Fluorescence typically is found on the epidermal side of 1 M NaCl split skin.

Although patients share a similar phenotype, CP is a heterogeneous group of autoimmune subepidermal blistering diseases. Although most patients' autoantibodies target BP180, others target laminin 5 (antiepiligrin cicatricial pemphigoid) or the β4 subunit of α6 β4 integrin. Some patients with a CP phenotype have antibodies to multiple epitopes, including the β4 subunit, BP180, and BP230. Other subsets of patients targeting unique basement membrane zone antigens will likely be identified.

A sensitive ELISA test for laminin 5 antibodies has made it easier to identify this subset of patients. Among those whose antibodies target laminin 5 (antiepiligrin CP), most exhibit antibodies to the α subunit, especially the G domains of the α3 subunit. Antibodies may also target the β3 and γ2 subunits. Other patients have been found to have autoantibodies that react with both laminin 6 and laminin 5, prompting the proposed designation of antilaminin cicatricial pemphigoid (Fig. 21-17). In antilaminin cicatricial pemphigoid, IgG anti-basement membrane zone autoantibodies bind to the dermal side of 1 M NaCl split skin. There is an increased relative risk

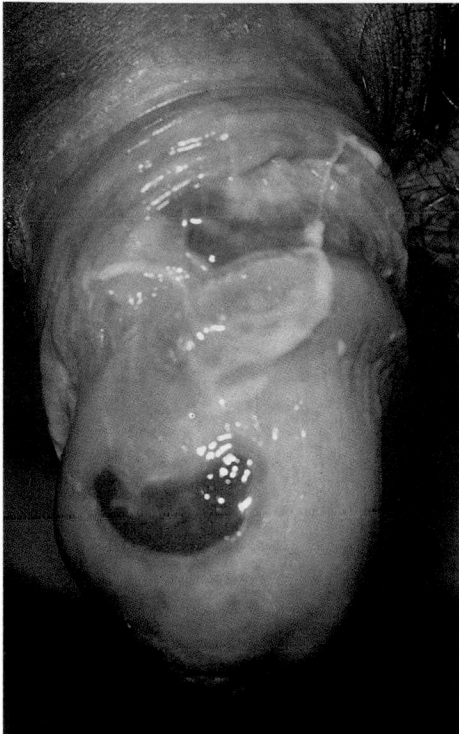

Fig. 21-17 Antilaminin cicatricial pemphigoid.

for solid cancers (mostly adenocarcinomas) in these patients. Tumors are commonly found during the first year of the disease. Like other forms of CP, the disease rarely remits spontaneously. In contrast to the increased tumor risk in antilaminin 5 CP, some data suggest that patients with antibodies to the β4 integrin subunit have a decreased risk of cancer.

Histopathology

The histologic findings are identical to those of bullous pemphigoid, except that fibrosis and scarring may be present in the upper dermis. Basement membrane separation occurs in the lamina lucida or below the lamina densa, depending on the targeted antibody. The inflammatory infiltrate is variable.

DIF testing of perilesional skin or mucosa reveals C3 and IgG at the lamina lucida in 80–95% of patients. The basement membrane zone of mucosal glands stains as well. IgA may be found occasionally. A circulating antibody to the basement membrane zone is found by IIF in about 20% of cases. Immunoelectron microscopy shows that lamina lucida antibodies bind at a deeper level than with BP. Most IIF-positive cases show IgG binding to the epidermal side of salt-split skin, although combined staining and dermal staining may be present in different subtypes, as noted above. Laser scanning confocal microscopy using fluorescein isothiocyanate-conjugated anti-human IgG antibody has been employed to determine the localization of IgG at the basement membrane zone, and may be of value in patients with negative IIF. "Knockout" skin substrates and fluorescent overlay antigen mapping have also been used to differentiate between anti-epiligrin CP and EBA.

Treatment

A review of studies using the Cochrane criteria found two small randomized controlled trials, both in patients with severe eye involvement. In one, 6 months of cyclophosphamide was superior to prednisone. In the second trial, 20 of 20 patients responded well to 3 months of cyclophosphamide, while only 14 of 20 responded to dapsone. Based on these limited data, and other uncontrolled trials, the reviewers concluded that severe ocular CP responds best to cyclophosphamide combined with corticosteroids, and that mild to moderate disease may respond to dapsone. Mycophenolate mofetil has also been used effectively.

In mild cases, oral hygiene, topical steroids, intralesional triamcinolone, or topical steroids occluded under vinyl inserts may be effective for desquamative gingivitis and other oral, genital, or cutaneous disease. Cream and gel formulations may be used, or the steroid may be compounded in Orabase. Topical sucralfate suspension may decrease the pain and healing time of the oral and genital ulcers. Cyclosporine washes have some efficacy but are too expensive for general use. Other topical calcineurin inhibitors have been used effectively. There have been reports of efficacy of thalidomide, tetracycline combined with niacinamide, dapsone, IVIG, etanercept, systemic corticosteroids, and immunosuppressive drugs.

Bruch-Gerharz D, et al: Mucous membrane pemphigoid: clinical aspects, immunopathological features and therapy. Eur J Dermatol 2007 May–Jun; 17(3):191 200.

Calabresi V, et al: Oral pemphigoid autoantibodies preferentially target BP180 ectodomain. Clin Immunol 2007 Feb; 122(2):207–213.

Canizares MJ, et al: Successful treatment of mucous membrane pemphigoid with etanercept in 3 patients. Arch Dermatol 2006 Nov; 142(11):1457–1461.

Daniel E, et al: Mycophenolate mofetil for ocular inflammation. Am J Ophthalmol 2010; 149(3):423–432.e1–2.

Galdos M, Etxebarría J: Intravenous immunoglobulin therapy for refractory ocular cicatricial pemphigoid: case report. Cornea 2008 Sep; 27(8):967–969.

Hingorani M, et al: Ocular cicatricial pemphigoid. Curr Opin Allergy Clin Immunol 2006 Oct; 6(5):373–378.

Kennedy JS, et al: Recalcitrant cicatricial pemphigoid treated with the anti-TNF-alpha agent etanercept. J Drugs Dermatol 2010; 9(1):68–70.

Letko E, et al: Relative risk for cancer in mucous membrane pemphigoid associated with antibodies to the beta4 integrin subunit. Clin Exp Dermatol 2007 Nov; 32(6):637–641.

Pujari SS, et al: Cyclophosphamide for ocular inflammatory diseases. Ophthalmology 2010; 117(2):356–365.

Sadler E, et al: A widening perspective regarding the relationship between anti-epiligrin cicatricial pemphigoid and cancer. J Dermatol Sci 2007 Jul; 47(1):1–7.

Woźniak K, et al: Cicatricial pemphigoid vegetans. Int J Dermatol 2007 Mar; 46(3):299–302.

Epidermolysis bullosa acquisita

Criteria for epidermolysis bullosa acquisita (EBA) were proposed in 1971 by Roenigk, and included:

1. clinical lesions of dystrophic epidermolysis bullosa, including increased skin fragility, trauma-induced blistering with erosions, atrophic scarring, milia over extensor surfaces (Fig. 21-18), and nail dystrophy
2. adult onset
3. lack of a family history of epidermolysis bullosa
4. exclusion of all other bullous diseases, such as porphyria cutanea tarda, pemphigoid, pemphigus, dermatitis herpetiformis, and bullous drug eruption.

In 1981, Roenigk et al extended these criteria to include:

5. IgG at the basement membrane zone by DIF
6. the demonstration of blister formation beneath the basal lamina
7. deposition of IgG beneath the basal lamina.

Since then, the clinical spectrum of this disease has expanded, with evidence that some patients have histologic findings

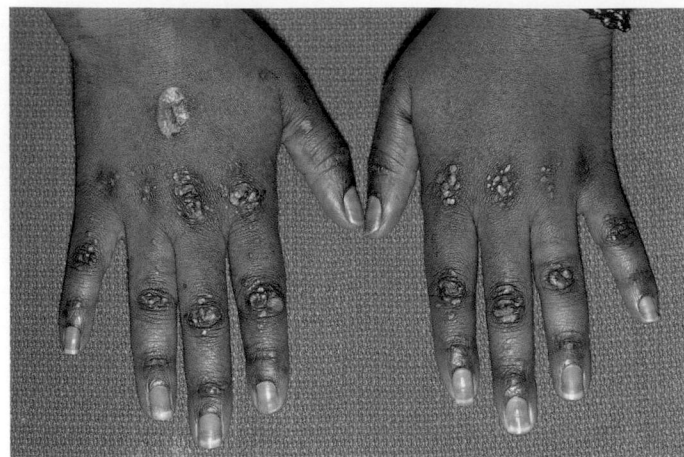

Fig. 21-18 Epidermolysis bullosa acquisita.

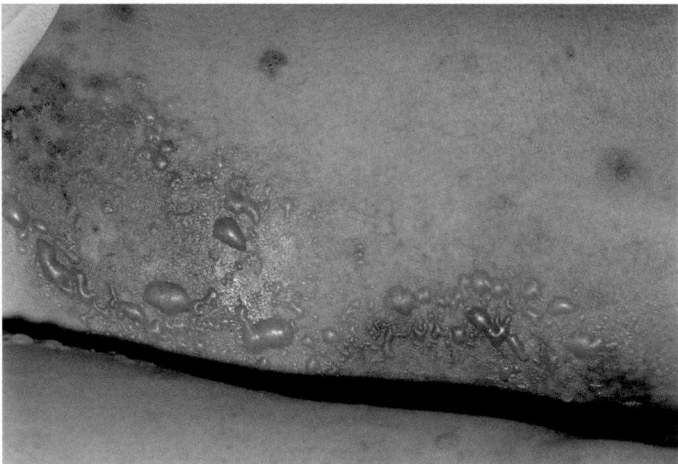

Fig. 21-19 Inflammatory epidermolysis bullosa acquisita.

identical to BP, but show positive immunofluorescence on the floor of salt-split skin. The antibodies have been found to target type VII collagen, a major component of anchoring fibrils. The target is the same as that in bullous lupus erythematosus. In some patients, it has been shown that autoantibodies bind to the NC-1 domain of collagen VII within the lamina densa. IIF studies reveal circulating anti-basement membrane zone antibodies in approximately half of cases. The antibodies are directed against multiple epitopes on the N-terminal noncollagenous domain of type VII collagen, in particular a region that demonstrates homology with cartilage matrix protein. The neonatal Fc receptor plays a regulatory role in immunoglobulin G homeostasis, maintaining antibody levels and promoting tissue injury in experimental EBA. It may represent a potential therapeutic target.

The noninflammatory clinical presentation of EBA is the most commonly recognized type. The association of EBA with many systemic diseases, such as myeloma, granulomatous colitis, diabetes, lymphoma, leukemia, amyloidosis, hepatitis C infection, and carcinoma, is well established. In rare instances, cases of this noninflammatory subset may mimic either BP or CP. When the onset is in childhood, hereditary dystrophic epidermolysis bullosa may be considered.

In 1982, Gammon described patients with generalized inflammatory bullous disease that resembled BP clinically (Fig. 21-19), but with immunologic and ultrastructural features of EBA. Many of these patients have associated diabetes mellitus, are HLA-DR2-positive, and progress to the trauma-induced scarring type of EBA in the long term. Approximately

5–10% of patients referred to medical centers as having BP may actually have EBA.

EBA patients usually have a predominance of neutrophils over eosinophils, although this is variable. On IIF, EBA patients are more likely to have linear IgG without concomitant C3 deposition than are patients with BP. Immunofluorescence on salt-split skin allows differentiation of the majority of cases without the need to resort to immunoblot techniques or immunoelectron microscopy. By DIF testing of the patient's salt-split skin biopsy, EBA will manifest IgG deposition only on the dermal side of the split, whereas the majority of BP patients will have IgG bound only to the epidermal side or to both sides. As demonstrated by IIF, the same results apply in the majority of cases. As noted above, some patients with BP have antibodies that target sub-lamina densa antigen. Absolute differentiation of these diseases is obtained by immunoelectron microscopy or immunoblot findings. In EBA, immunoblotting identifies 290 kD and 145 kD proteins, corresponding to type VII collagen. Blistering appears to be T cell-dependent.

Because bullous systemic lupus erythematosus (SLE) and EBA share anti-basement membrane zone antibodies of identical specificity, and there is clinical and histologic overlap as well, this differential diagnosis may be difficult. The following features help to identify EBA: skin fragility, predilection for traumatized areas, and healing with scars and milia. In SLE, sun-exposed skin is involved by preference, and the patient has a diagnosis of SLE established by American College of Rheumatology criteria; in bullous SLE there is usually a dramatic response to dapsone. In addition to the cases of bullous SLE that show linear IgG staining below the lamina densa with circulating IgG autoantibodies to the 290 kD and 145 kD antigens, some patients will show granular staining of IgG at the basement membrane zone without circulating IgG. EBA-like eruptions are rarely seen as a result of penicillamine therapy.

Purely IgA-mediated EBA has been described. The patients resemble linear IgA dermatosis or inflammatory IgG-mediated EBA. Only a minority demonstrate milia or scarring.

Treatment

A review of the literature using Cochrane criteria failed to identify any randomized controlled trials. The disease is often resistant to therapy, but good responses have been reported in some patients treated with systemic steroids alone or in combination with azathioprine or dapsone. Other agents reported to be effective include rituximab, mycophenolate mofetil, IVIG, cyclosporine, colchicine, plasmapheresis, photopheresis, infliximab, and the humanized murine monoclonal anti-Tac antibody, daclizumab. Extracorporeal photochemotherapy has been effective in a few patients with refractory disease. Supportive therapy, including control of infection, careful wound management, and maintenance of good nutrition, should be emphasized.

Chen M, et al: The cartilage matrix protein subdomain of type VII collagen is pathogenic for epidermolysis bullosa acquisita. Am J Pathol 2007 Jun; 170(6):2009–2018.

Remington J, et al: Autoimmunity to type VII collagen: epidermolysis bullosa acquisita. Curr Dir Autoimmun 2008; 10:195–205.

Sadler E, et al: Treatment-resistant classical epidermolysis bullosa acquisita responding to rituximab. Br J Dermatol 2007 Aug; 157(2):417–419.

Sesarman A, et al: Neonatal Fc receptor deficiency protects from tissue injury in experimental epidermolysis bullosa acquisita. J Mol Med 2008 Aug; 86(8):951–959.

Shook BA, et al: Epidermolysis bullosa acquisita occurring in 2 patients with hepatitis C. J Am Acad Dermatol 2006 May; 54(5):888–891.

Sitaru AG, et al: T cells are required for the production of blister-inducing autoantibodies in experimental epidermolysis bullosa acquisita. J Immunol 2010; 184(3):1596–1603.

Stein JA, et al: Epidermolysis bullosa acquisita. Dermatol Online J 2007 Jan 27; 13(1):15.

Wallet-Faber N, et al: Epidermolysis bullosa acquisita following bullous pemphigoid, successfully treated with the anti-CD20 monoclonal antibody rituximab. Dermatology 2007; 215(3):252–255.

Dermatitis herpetiformis (Duhring disease)

Clinical features

Dermatitis herpetiformis (DH) is a chronic, relapsing, severely pruritic disease characterized by grouped, symmetrical lesions on extensor surfaces, the scalp, nuchal area, and buttocks. As the lesions are severely pruritic, they generally present as excoriations. The eruption usually occurs on an erythematous base and may be papular, papulovesicular, vesiculobullous (Fig. 21-20), bullous, or urticarial. Linear petechial lesions may be noted on the volar surfaces of the fingers, as well as the palms. Pigmented spots alone over the lumbosacral region should arouse suspicion of DH. The mucous membranes are involved in rare cases, mostly when bullae are numerous. Laryngeal lesions may manifest as hoarseness. Itching and burning are usually intense, and their paroxysmal quality provokes scratching to the point of bleeding and, at times, scarring. Spontaneous remissions lasting as long as a week and terminating abruptly with a new crop of lesions are a characteristic feature of the disease. Perimenstrual flares may occur.

Between 77 and 90% of patients with DH and IgA deposits in the skin are HLA-B8-positive, a similar frequency to that observed in gluten-sensitive enteropathy (GSE). HLA antigens DR3 and DQw2 are also increased in frequency. Black and Asian patients are uncommon and some studies indicate that this may be because of HLA differences. These HLA markers are associated with other autoimmune diseases and indicate patients who appear to have an overactive immune response to common antigens and may clear immune complexes slowly. DH is more common in those with affected family members.

DH in childhood is usually similar to the adult type, has identical histologic and immunofluorescent findings, and has a high incidence of HLA-B8 and DR3 and abnormal jejunal biopsies. Palmar blisters and brown, hemorrhagic, purpuric macules may be more common than in adults. Treatment with sulfones results in prompt response, as in adults.

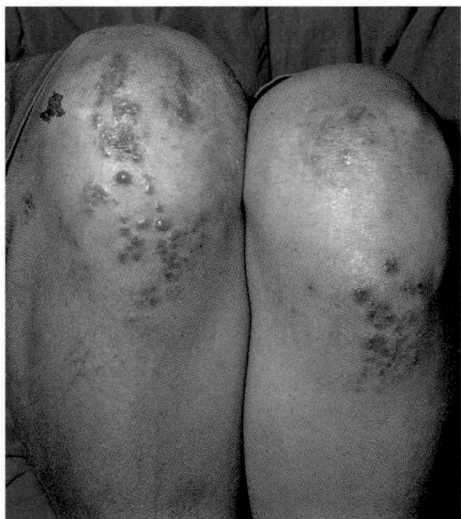

Fig. 21-20 Dermatitis herpetiformis.

Gluten, a protein found in cereals except for rice and corn, provokes flares of the disease. Villous atrophy of the jejunum and inflammation of the small bowel occur. IgA is bound to the skin, and this apparently activates complement, primarily via the alternate pathway. Oral iodides will cause a flare of the disease. Patch tests with 50% potassium iodide in petrolatum produce a bulla in uncontrolled DH, but only exceptionally in patients controlled by a gluten-free diet or by sulfone therapy.

Associated disease

Thyroid disorders are increased in incidence in patients with DH. Neurologic disease, including ataxia, may occur. An increased incidence of malignancy, especially small bowel lymphoma, has also been remarked upon in some studies, although others have noted this increase with celiac disease but not DH. In fact, the incidence of breast cancer may be lower in those with DH than in the general population.

Enteropathy

Between 70 and 100% of patients with DH have abnormalities in the jejunal mucosa, but most are asymptomatic. If given a high-gluten diet, virtually all patients with DH develop findings indistinguishable from celiac disease, and DH affects approximately 25% of patients presenting with celiac disease.

The dapsone requirement in DH is usually decreased after 3–6 months of a gluten-free diet. The majority of patients who adhere to a strict gluten-free diet can eventually stop their medication or significantly reduce the dosage. A gluten-free diet is not easy to follow, but may decrease the incidence of intestinal lymphoma.

Diagnosis

The distinction from linear IgA bullous dermatosis is often clinically impossible. Other conditions considered in the differential diagnosis at times are BP, bullous erythema multiforme, scabies, contact dermatitis, atopic dermatitis, nummular eczema, neurotic excoriations, insect bites, and chronic bullous disease of childhood. The finding of IgA in a granular pattern at the dermoepidermal junction with accentuation in the dermal papillae is specific for DH.

Autoantibodies

Circulating IgA antibodies against the smooth muscle cell endomysium (anti-endomysial antibodies) are present in 70% of DH patients, in nearly all patients with active celiac disease, and almost never in other conditions. Tissue transglutaminase (TTG) is the major autoantigen in GSE. IgA antibodies directed at TTG2 are common in patients with DH or celiac disease, but epidermal transglutaminase (TTG3) appears to be the most important antigen. Dietary exposure to gliadin proteins in wheat and related proteins from barley and rye induce flares of the disease. These proteins are high-affinity substrates for TTG. The two are often tightly bound, which may explain why an antibody response is generated against both gliadin and TTG. Gliadins can also be found in rice, corn, and oats, but these proteins are poor substrates for TTG. Some data suggest that a diet with moderate quantities of oats can be tolerated in patients with controlled DH or GSE.

Epidemiology

This disease has an equal male to female incidence. The average age of onset is between 20 and 40 years. It does occur with some frequency in children. Black and Asian persons are rarely affected.

Histopathology

The initial changes are first noted at the tips of the dermal papillae, where edema, focal fibrin, and neutrophilic micro-abscesses are seen. The cellular infiltrate contains many neutrophils, but may also include a few eosinophils. A subepidermal separation is noted histologically. Ultrastructurally, the split may begin in the lamina lucida. In a study of 24 cases of confirmed DH, 37.5% had nonspecific findings on hematoxylin and eosin (H&E) staining, including a lymphocytic infiltrate, ectatic capillaries, and fibrosis in the dermal papillae. Because of the potential for nonspecific biopsy findings, DIF studies are essential. Histologic differentiation of linear IgA bullous dermatosis from DH is extremely difficult unless DIF is performed.

DIF of noninvolved perilesional skin reveals deposits of IgA alone or together with C3 arranged in a granular pattern at the dermoepidermal junction. The granules may be vertically elongated, giving a "picket-fence" appearance. The deposits are typically accentuated in the dermal papillae. IgM and IgG deposits are occasionally observed in association with IgA. Deposits may be focal, so that multiple biopsies may be needed, and the deposits of antibody are more often seen in previously involved skin or normal-appearing skin adjacent to involved skin. IgA is observed by immunoelectron microscopy, either alone or in conjunction with C3, IgG, or IgM as clumps in the upper dermis. A fibrillar staining pattern exists when the immune deposits lie along dermal microfibrils. A few patients will have negative DIF despite typical clinical findings and evidence of anti-endomysial antibodies. IIF is rarely positive.

Treatment

The drugs chiefly used are dapsone and sulfapyridine. The most effective sulfone is diaminodiphenylsulfone (dapsone). The dose varies between 50 and 300 mg/day, usually starting with 100 mg/day and increasing gradually to an effective level or until side effects occur. Once a favorable response is attained, the dosage is decreased to the minimum that does not permit recurrence of signs and symptoms. When dapsone is discontinued abruptly, large bullae similar to those seen in BP frequently occur. Hemolytic anemia, leukopenia, methemoglobinemia, agranulocytosis, or peripheral neuropathy may occur with dapsone. Acute hemolytic anemia (which may be severe) occurs in patients with glucose-6-phosphate dehydrogenase (G6PD) deficiency, therefore a G6PD level should be measured before therapy. In those whose ethnic background makes G6PD deficiency unlikely, some authorities begin dapsone at a low starting dose (25 mg/day) and watch the patient closely for dark urine. The patient should be warned to report by telephone any incident of red or brown urine or blue nailbeds or lips. A blood count should be done weekly for 4 weeks, bimonthly for the next 3 months, and every 2–6 months thereafter. Liver function tests should be monitored bimonthly for the first 4 months, then checked with the hematologic studies every 4–6 months.

Agranulocytosis is rare. It typically occurs 1–3 months after initiation of drug therapy, and presents with sore throat, aphthae, or evidence of infection. The risk of agranulocytosis is higher in older individuals (>60 years) and non-white persons. The incidence varies with the disease. It is rarely seen in patients with Hansen's disease, but patients with DH have a 25- to 33-fold increased risk.

Sulfapyridine can also be used to treat the disease. After a test dose of 0.5 g of sulfapyridine, one tablet (0.5 g) is given four times a day. The dose is then increased if necessary, or reduced if possible. Usually, 1–4 g/day is required for good control. The drug is less water-soluble than dapsone, and patients should remain hydrated. Sulfasalazine, 500 mg three times a day, increased to 1.5 g three times a day as tolerated, may also be used, since sulfapyridine is a metabolic product. Gastrointestinal intolerance may limit the dosage. In rare patients, it is necessary to find alternatives to the sulfone drugs. Tetracycline/nicotinamide and colchicine have controlled individual patients.

Gluten-free diet

Patients must strictly avoid wheat, barley, and rye. Moderate amounts of oats may be tolerated. In Canada, standards for growing, processing, testing, and labeling of pure, uncontaminated oats have allowed adults to consume up to 70 g (roughly one-half to three-quarters of a cup) of oats and children to consume up to 25 g (one-quarter of a cup) daily without flares of disease. Corn and rice are generally well tolerated, corresponding to the poor binding of their gliadin proteins to TTG. Exacerbation of disease related to corn starch has been reported. If a gluten-free diet is followed strictly, the patient will almost certainly be able to take less medication or stop it altogether. Some evidence suggests that this may decrease the incidence of associated malignancy; however, it is a very difficult diet to follow. The diet will help to achieve a remission. Once a prolonged remission has been obtained, some gluten may be tolerated in a subset of patients. In one study, 38 patients who had followed a gluten-free diet for a mean of 8 years reintroduced gluten to their diets. Thirty-one experienced recurrence within an average of 2 months, but seven remained in remission for a mean follow-up of 12 years. IgA deposits did not recur in their skin. This report suggests that clinical and histologic remission can be maintained in some patients with DH despite the reintroduction of dietary gluten. For most patients, however, a gluten-free diet remains an important aspect of disease management. Support may be obtained from the American Celiac Society/Dietary Support Coalition, Annette Bentley, President, 59 Crystal Avenue, West Orange, NJ 07052-3570, 973-325-8837 (voice), 973-669-8808 (fax). A list of celiac societies can be found at http://www.nowheat.com/grfx/nowheat/primer/celisoc.htm or http://www.enabling.org/ia/celiac/groups/groupsus.html. A commercial website with a search engine can be found at http://www.celiac.com. Another commercial source for products can be found at http://www.glutenfreemall.com. A Google search using the terms "celiac society" or "gluten-free diet" is a good starting point for patients with the disease who want more information about the diet and commercially available products.

Al-Niaimi F, et al: Dermatitis herpetiformis exacerbated by cornstarch. J Am Acad Dermatol 2010; 62(3):510–511.

Beutner EH, et al: Methods for diagnosing dermatitis herpetiformis. J Am Acad Dermatol 2006 Dec; 55(6):1112–1113.

Haboubi NY, et al: Coeliac disease and oats: a systematic review. Postgrad Med J 2006 Oct; 82(972):672–678.

Helsing P, et al: Dermatitis herpetiformis presenting as ataxia in a child. Acta Derm Venereol 2007; 87(2):163–165.

Hull CM, et al: Elevation of IgA anti-epidermal transglutaminase antibodies in dermatitis herpetiformis. Br J Dermatol 2008 Jul; 159(1):120–124.

Lewis NR, et al: No increase in risk of fracture, malignancy or mortality in dermatitis herpetiformis: a cohort study. Aliment Pharmacol Ther 2008 Jun 1; 27(11):1140–1147.

Nino M, et al: A long-term gluten-free diet as an alternative treatment in severe forms of dermatitis herpetiformis. J Dermatolog Treat 2007; 18(1):10–12.

Rashid M, et al: Consumption of pure oats by individuals with celiac disease: a position statement by the Canadian Celiac Association. Can J Gastroenterol 2007 Oct; 21(10):649–651.

Templet JT, et al: Childhood dermatitis herpetiformis: a case report and review of the literature. Cutis 2007 Dec; 80(6):473–476.

Van L, et al: Dermatitis herpetiformis: potential for confusion with linear IgA bullous dermatosis on direct immunofluorescence. Dermatol Online J 2008 Jan 15; 14(1):21.

Viljamaa M, et al: Malignancies and mortality in patients with coeliac disease and dermatitis herpetiformis: 30-year population-based study. Dig Liver Dis 2006 Jun; 38(6):374–380.

Linear IgA bullous dermatosis

Linear IgA bullous dermatosis (LAD) is characterized by sub-epidermal blisters, a neutrophilic infiltrate, and a circulating IgA anti-basement membrane zone antibody with linear basement membrane zone deposits on DIF. Like CP, linear IgA disease is really a group of diseases with a similar immunofluorescent pattern.

Adult linear IgA disease

This acquired, autoimmune blistering disease may present with a clinical pattern of vesicles indistinguishable from DH, or with vesicles and bullae having a BP-like appearance. There may be urticarial lesions, and bullae may occur on an urticarial base, as in BP (Fig. 21-21). Unusual variants include morbilliform, prurigo-like, and eczematous presentation. Mucous membrane involvement may occur in up to 50% of cases. In some patients, oral and conjunctival lesions dominate the presentation, and scarring may occur, as in CP. In the majority of patients, there is no association with enteropathy or with HLA-B8. The disease tends to remit after several years in approximately 60% of patients. IgA is commonly directed against a 97 kD antigen in the lamina lucida. Some patients demonstrate both IgA and IgG antibodies to BP180, and IgA to LAD285. IgA and IgG reactivity has been found to all three portions of the BP180 ectodomain. In some patients, the strongest reactivity is to the C-terminal portion of BP180 (the major antigenic area in CP). This may explain cases of clinical overlap with CP. Antigenic targets for LAD are expressed by both keratinocytes and fibroblasts.

Linear IgA dermatosis commonly occurs as a drug-induced disease. In drug-induced disease, the eruption is self-limited,

there is less mucosal involvement, and there is usually no detectable circulating autoantibody. The IgA may be deposited in the sub-basal lamina area. Implicated drugs include vancomycin, lithium, amiodarone, carbamazepine, captopril, penicillin, amoxicillin, moxifloxacin, PUVA, furosemide, oxaprozin, IL-2, interferon (IFN)-α, phenytoin, diclofenac, statins, tea tree oil, angiotensin receptor antagonists, and glibenclamide. The antigen identified may be the 97 kD antigen, the 230 kD BP antigen, or the 180 kD BP antigen.

Some cases have been associated with internal malignancy, paraproteinemia, or infection. Sporadic reports have linked single cases with dermatomyositis, rheumatoid arthritis, acquired hemophilia, and multiple sclerosis, although these may be fortuitous associations.

Biopsies commonly demonstrate papillary dermal microabscess with neutrophils. As in DH, eosinophils may be present. Subepidermal bullae commonly contain a mixture of neutrophils and eosinophils. On DIF, a homogeneous linear (tubular or toothpaste) pattern of IgA is present at the basement membrane zone (Fig. 21-22). Some cases will have both linear IgA and IgG in combination at the basement membrane zone. A lack of C3 may be a clue that both immunoglobulins recognize the 97 kD antigen.

By IIF, only a minority will have circulating IgA autoantibody with anti-basement membrane specificity, and this is usually present in low titer. On salt-split skin, deposition may occur on the roof or base, or a combination of the two. This correlates with the fact that, on immunoelectron microscopy, deposition of the autoantibody may be present in the lamina lucida, below the lamina densa, or both. Some patients with sub-lamina densa deposits have EBA.

In drug-induced disease, the drug must be stopped. Many cases resolve quickly, but some require drug therapy with a corticosteroid or dapsone. Idiopathic disease generally responds to dapsone in doses similar to that described for DH. Other cases require topical or systemic steroids in addition, or as sole treatment. A combination of tetracycline, 2 g/day, and nicotinamide, 1.5 g/day, may be effective. Other patients have responded to mycophenolate mofetil, IVIG, colchicine, trimethoprim–sulfamethoxazole, or erythromycin. The rare patients with associated GSE may respond to a gluten-free diet.

Childhood linear IgA disease (chronic bullous disease of childhood)

Chronic bullous disease of childhood (CBDC) is an acquired, self-limited bullous disease that may begin by the time the

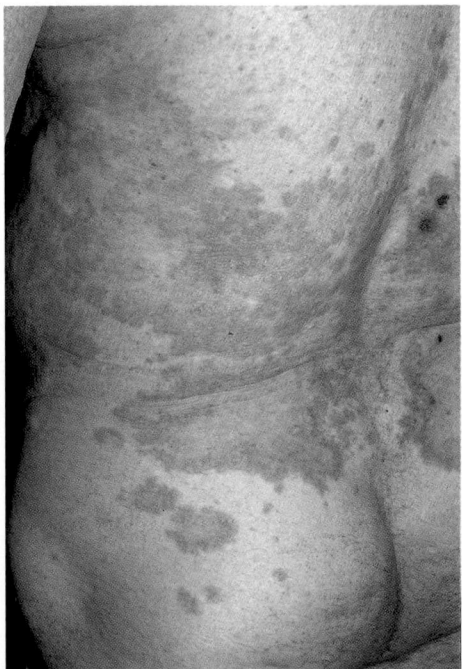

Fig. 21-21 Adult linear IgA disease.

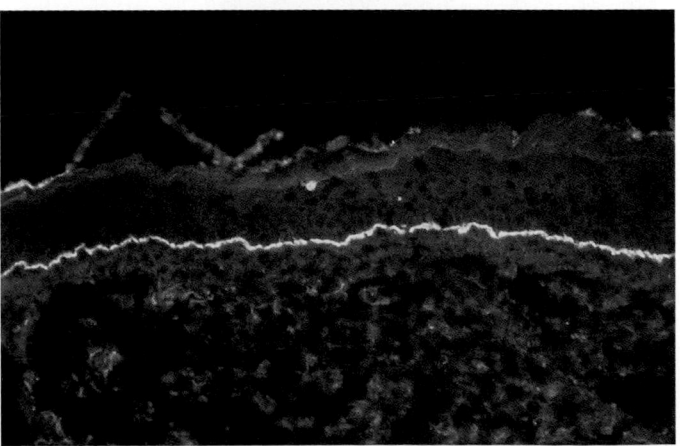

Fig. 21-22 Direct immunofluorescence of linear IgA disease.

patient is aged 2 or 3 and usually remits by age 13 (Fig. 21-23). The average age of onset is 5 years. Bullae develop on either erythematous or normal-appearing skin, preferentially involving the lower trunk, buttocks, genitalia, and thighs. Perioral and scalp lesions are common, and oral mucous membrane lesions may occur in up to 75% of patients. Bullae are often arranged in rosettes or an annular array, the so-called string of pearls configuration. Tense individual bullae similar to those present in BP are also seen. Pruritus is often severe.

The prime histologic finding is the presence of a subepidermal bulla filled with neutrophils. Eosinophils may be present, and in some cases they predominate. DIF reveals a linear deposition of IgA at the basement membrane zone identical to that seen in the adult forms of the disease. IIF is positive for circulating IgA anti-basement membrane zone antibodies in approximately 50% of cases, usually in low titer. In contrast to adults with LAD, children demonstrate an increased frequency of B8, DR3, and DQ2, and may be homozygous for these antigens. As in the adult disease, immunoelectron microscopy and immunomapping studies may demonstrate immune deposits within the lamina lucida, below the lamina densa, or both. Also as in adult disease, some children have both IgG and IgA deposits. GSE is rare, but IgA nephropathy may occur. Childhood linear IgA disease has occurred in conjunction with Crohn's disease.

Many patients' antibodies target the 97 kD peptide. Some children with sub-basal lamina deposits target type VII collagen and have EBA. Patients with only IgA or with both IgG and IgA circulating autoantibodies may target BP230 or BP180. Individual patients may have a combination of IgA against the 97 kD peptide, and IgG against BP230 and BP180. Collagen XVII/BP180 is a transmembrane protein with a soluble 120 kD ectodomain. In linear IgA dermatosis and CBDC, IgA targets the soluble ectodomain more efficiently than the full-length protein. Some sera target the Col15 domain.

The untreated disease runs a variable course, with eventual spontaneous resolution by adolescence being common. Treatment with either dapsone or sulfapyridine is usually successful. Occasional cases respond to topical steroids alone, and systemic steroids are sometimes necessary. Other patients have responded to mycophenolate mofetil, colchicine, topical calcineurin inhibitors, or dicloxacillin.

Billet SE, et al: A morbilliform variant of vancomycin-induced linear IgA bullous dermatosis. Arch Dermatol 2008 Jun; 144(6):774–778.

Farrant P, et al: Is erythromycin an effective treatment for chronic bullous disease of childhood? A national survey of members of the British Society for Paediatric Dermatology. Pediatr Dermatol 2008 Jul–Aug; 25(4):479–482.

Kharfi M, et al: Linear IgA bullous dermatosis: the more frequent bullous dermatosis of children. Dermatol Online J 2010; 16(1):2.

Navi D, et al: Drug-induced linear IgA bullous dermatosis. Dermatol Online J 2006 Sep 8; 12(5):12.

Peterson JD, et al: Linear IgA bullous dermatosis responsive to trimethoprim–sulfamethoxazole. Clin Exp Dermatol 2007 Nov; 32(6):756–758.

Rositto AE, et al: Linear IgA disease of childhood developing IgA nephropathy. Pediatr Dermatol 2008 May–Jun; 25(3):339–340.

Transient acantholytic dermatosis (Grover's disease)

In 1970, Grover described a new dermatosis that occurred predominantly in persons over 50 years of age and consisted of a sparse eruption of limited duration. The lesions were fragile vesicles that rapidly turned into crusted and keratotic erosions. He termed the condition transient acantholytic dermatosis (TAD). Since then, the majority of cases have been found to persist or recur, and the term persistent and recurrent acantholytic dermatosis may be a more accurate description of the disorder. The distribution is predominantly limited to the chest or shoulder girdle area and upper abdomen, and there is a strong male predominance (Fig. 21-24). The condition often appears or flares during periods of heat, sweating, or hospitalization. Many patients are asymptomatic and the condition may be an incidental finding on examination. Other patients complain of pruritus. Asteatotic eczema occurs five times as often among patients with TAD as in controls. The disorder has been described in the setting of a variety of malignancies, but may be associated with the hospitalization or type B symptoms rather than the malignancy itself. TAD has been reported with cetuximab. Patients on strict bed rest appear to have a higher incidence of the disease. The clinical differential diagnosis includes Galli–Galli disease, an acantholytic variant of Dowling–Degos disease that may resemble TAD clinically.

There are five histologic types resembling Darier's disease, PV, PF, benign familial pemphigus, or spongiotic dermatitis. The Darier type predominates. Often two or more types can

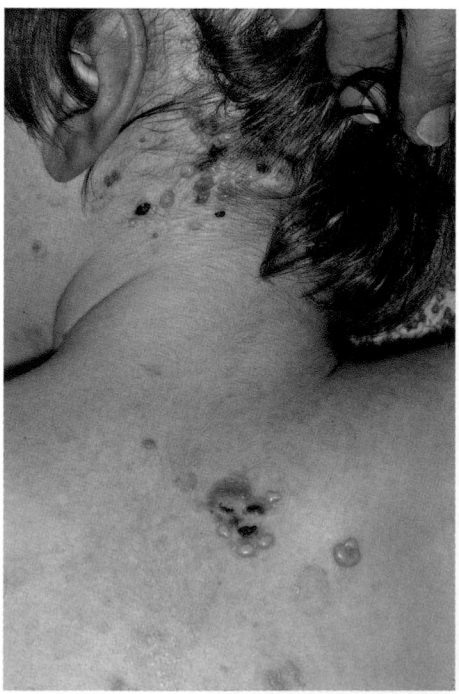

Fig. 21-23 Chronic bullous disease of childhood.

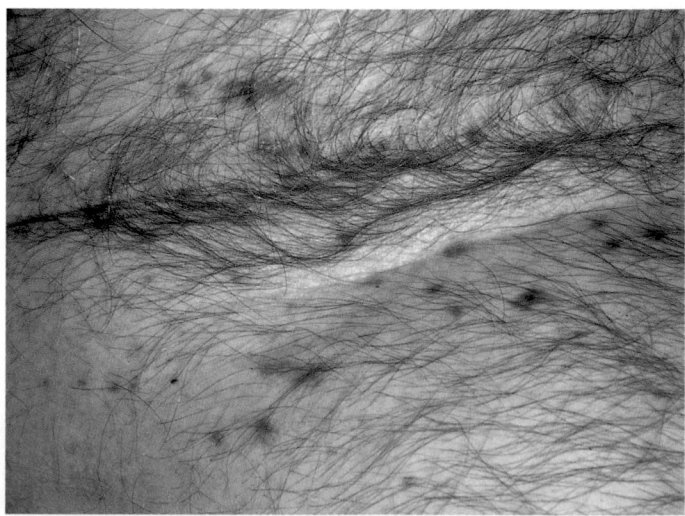

Fig. 21-24 Transient acantholytic dermatosis.

be found in a single biopsy specimen. DIF studies yield negative or nonspecific results. Although heat and sweating are significant risk factors, only a minority of cases are associated with acrosyringia histologically.

About 50% of patients respond to topical steroids. Control of fevers, hospital discharge, and avoidance of sun and sweating often result in improvement. Sustained remission has been described after a course of systemic corticosteroids. Topical antibiotics, isotretinoin, and dapsone have been successful in some patients. PUVA has been reported to result in an initial flare followed by slow clearance, and UVB therapy may produce clearing in some patients. Rituximab has produced clearing of TAD in patients being treated for lymphoma.

Gilchrist H, et al: Galli–Galli disease: a case report with review of the literature. J Am Acad Dermatol 2008 Feb; 58(2):299–302.

Ishibashi M, et al: Remission of transient acantholytic dermatosis after the treatment with rituximab for follicular lymphoma. Clin Exp Dermatol 2008 Mar; 33(2):206–207.

Julliard KN, et al: Antibiotic ointment in the treatment of Grover disease. Cutis 2007 Jul; 80(1):72–74.

Tscharner GG, et al: Grover's disease induced by cetuximab. Dermatology 2006; 213(1):37–39.

Bonus images for this chapter can be found online at http://www.expertconsult.com

22 Nutritional Diseases

A nutritional disease is caused either by insufficiency or, less often, by excess of one or more dietary essentials. Nutritional diseases are particularly common in underdeveloped tropical countries. Infants and children are particularly at risk for deficiency states, especially malnutrition. Frequently, patients have features of several of these disorders if their diets have been generally restricted. An intertriginous or acral eruption, a seborrheic dermatitis-like facial eruption, atrophic glossitis, and alopecia are common features of many nutritional deficiencies. This occurs because these nutrients are essential to overlapping metabolic pathways of fatty acid metabolism, resulting in abnormal arachidonic acid metabolism and abnormal differentiation of the epidermis. The abnormal epidermal differentiation results in impaired epidermal lipid and intercellular junction production and defective barrier function. Impaired disposal of free radicals may also occur. The histologic findings in many types of nutritional dermatosis are also similar.

In developed countries, alcoholism is the main cause of nutritional diseases. Nutritional diseases should also be suspected in postoperative patients; psychiatric patients, including those with anorexia nervosa and bulimia; patients on unusual diets; patients with surgical or inflammatory bowel dysfunction, especially Crohn's disease; and patients with severe oral erosive disease (such as pemphigus) which prevents eating. Bowel bypass surgery may result in nutritional deficiency. Cystic fibrosis may be accompanied by nutritional deficiency dermatitis. In the pediatric setting, nutritional deficiency may also occur because of parental ignorance of the nutritional requirements of their infants. The diagnosis of nutritional deficiency is often missed since physicians fail to take adequate dietary histories. The edema of protein malnutrition may mask the problem, as malnourished children may gain weight through edema, staying on the growth curve. The dermatitis produced by elevated glucagon levels from islet cell tumors of the pancreas (necrolytic migratory erythema) and a similar dermatosis seen in hepatitis C infection and other forms of hepatic insufficiency (necrolytic acral erythema and pseudoglucagonoma) probably also represent nutritional deficiency dermatoses. Deficiency states caused by inborn errors of metabolism are discussed in Chapter 26. In most cases the clinical findings and socioeconomic scenario are adequate to lead to suspicion of a specific deficiency state, and replacement therapy can confirm the diagnosis. Laboratory testing may be costly and inaccurate in some deficiency states, and patients with poor nutrition are often deficient in many nutrients simultaneously. Testing is indicated to confirm the diagnosis of zinc deficiency, in essential fatty acid deficiency, and in evaluating for possible glucagonoma syndrome.

Vitamin A

Hypovitaminosis A (phrynoderma)

Vitamin A is a fat-soluble vitamin found as retinyl esters in milk, fish oil, liver, and eggs, and as carotenoids in plants. Vitamin A deficiency is common in children in the developing world. It is rare in developed countries, where it is most commonly associated with diseases of fat malabsorption, such as bowel bypass surgery for obesity, pancreatic insufficiency, Crohn's disease, celiac disease, cystic fibrosis, and liver disease. Vitamin A is required for the normal keratinization of many mucosal surfaces. When it is deficient, the resultant abnormal keratinization leads to increased mortality from inflammatory disease of the gut and lung—diarrhea and pneumonia (especially in rubeola). Vitamin A supplementation of 200 000 IU/day for 2 days is recommended for children with rubeola.

While phrynoderma had classically been ascribed to and felt to be specific for vitamin A deficiency, in fact it is most frequently found as a disorder of multiple deficiencies, including vitamins A, B, C, E, and essential fatty acids. Replacing all these deficiencies leads to rapid improvement. Correcting only the B vitamin deficiency leads to more rapid improvement than replacing the vitamin A. This explains cases in which the cutaneous findings of phrynoderma were found without the classic eye findings of vitamin A deficiency. The skin eruption, termed phrynoderma, or "toadskin," resembles keratosis pilaris. It consists of keratotic papules of various sizes, distributed over the extremities and shoulders, surrounding and arising from the pilosebaceous follicles. Individual lesions are firm, pigmented papules containing a central intrafollicular keratotic plug, which projects from the follicle as a horny spine and leaves a pit when expressed. Lesions are of two sizes: 1–2 mm papules closely resembling keratosis pilaris, and the more diagnostic large 2–6 mm crateriform papules filled with a central keratotic plug. These later lesions may simulate a perforating disorder. The eruption of small lesions usually begins on the anterolateral aspect of the thighs or the posterolateral aspect of the upper arms. It then spreads to the extensor surfaces of both the upper and lower extremities, shoulders, abdomen, back, and buttocks, and finally reaches the face and posterior aspect of the neck. The hands and feet are not involved and only occasionally are there lesions on the midline of the trunk or in the axillary and anogenital areas. On the face, the eruption resembles acne because of the presence of many large comedones, but it differs from acne in respect of dryness of the skin. The large dome-shaped nodules are on the elbows and knees. They have a surrounding red or brown rim. The whole skin displays dryness, fine scaling, and hyperpigmentation. Hair casts may also be seen. Vitamin A deficiency can at times mimic vitamin C deficiency, since both conditions cause follicular hyperkeratosis, and bleeding and gingival disease can be a feature of vitamin A deficiency as well as scurvy. The histological findings of "deficiency dermatitis" which are common to many deficiency states (zinc, essential fatty acids, amino acids, glucagonoma, cystic fibrosis) are not features of either vitamin A or vitamin C deficiency.

In vitamin A deficiency, eye findings are prominent and often pathognomonic. These include night blindness, an inability to see bright light, xerophthalmia, xerosis corneae, and keratomalacia. The earliest finding is delayed adaptation to the dark (nyctalopia). Sometimes there are circumscribed areas of xerosis of the conjunctiva lateral to the cornea, occasionally forming well-defined white spots (Bitot spots). These are triangular, with the apex toward the canthus. Vitamin A deficiency is a major cause of blindness in children in the developing world.

The histologic findings of vitamin A deficiency are hyperkeratosis, horny plugs in the upper portion of the hair follicle, coiled hairs in the upper part of the follicle, severe atrophy of the sebaceous glands, and squamous metaplasia of the secretory cells of the eccrine sweat glands. If the follicles rupture, perifollicular granulomatous inflammation is found.

The diagnosis of vitamin A toxicity is confirmed by determination of the serum retinol level. The treatment is oral vitamin A, 100 000 IU/day for 2–3 days, followed by the recommended dietary requirement. Serum retinol levels are monitored to determine adequacy of supplementation and to avoid vitamin A toxicity.

Hypervitaminosis A

Because the skin findings of hypervitaminosis A are similar to the side effects of synthetic retinoid therapy, they are well recognized by most dermatologists. Children are at greater risk for toxicity than adults. Excess megavitamin ingestion may be the cause. In adults, as little as 25 000 IU/day may lead to toxicity, especially in persons with hepatic compromise from alcoholic, viral, or medication-induced hepatitis. Dialysis patients also are at increased risk, as vitamin A is not removed by dialysis. Standard hyperalimentation solutions contain significant amounts of vitamin A, and in burn victims with renal compromise, vitamin A toxicity can occur. If the patient is taking a synthetic retinoid, all vitamin A supplementation should be stopped.

Most cases of chronic hypervitaminosis A have been reported in children. There is loss of hair and coarseness of the remaining hair, loss of the eyebrows, exfoliative cheilitis, generalized exfoliation and pigmentation of the skin, and clubbing of the fingers. Moderate widespread itching may occur. Hepatomegaly, splenomegaly, hypochromic anemia, depressed serum proteins, and elevated liver function tests may be found. Bone growth may be retarded by premature closure of the epiphyses in children. Pseudotumor cerebri with papilledema may occur very early, before any other signs appear. In infants this may present as a bulging fontanelle.

In adults, the early signs are dryness of the lips and anorexia. These may be followed by joint and bone pains, follicular hyperkeratosis, branny desquamation of the skin, fissuring of the corners of the mouth and nostrils, dryness and loss of scalp hair and eyebrows, and dystrophy of the nails. Fatigue, myalgia, depression, anorexia, headache (from pseudotumor cerebri), strabismus, and weight loss commonly occur. Liver disease may be progressive and may lead to cirrhosis with chronic toxicity. Hypercalcemia commonly occurs in dialysis patients. Retinoids are teratogens, and birth defects may occur with excess vitamin A supplementation during pregnancy.

Bak H, Ahn SK: Pseudoglucagonoma syndrome in a patient with malnutrition. Arch Dermatol 2005; 141:914.

Bhalla K, et al: Hypercalcemia caused by iatrogenic hypervitaminosis A. J Am Diet Assoc 2005; 105:119.

Bremner NA, et al: Vitamin A toxicity in burns patients on long-term enteral feed. Burns 2007; 22:266.

Cheruvattath R, et al: Vitamin A toxicity: when one a day doesn't keep the doctor away. Liver Trans 2006; 12:1888.

Girard C, et al: Vitamin A deficiency phrynoderma associated with chronic giardiasis. Ped Derm 2006; 23:346.

Hivnor CM, et al: Necrolytic acral erythema: response to combination therapy with interferon and ribavirin. J Am Acad Dermatol 2004; 50:S121.

Khanna VJ, et al: Necrolytic acral erythema associated with hepatitis C. Arch Dermatol 2000; 136:755.

Maronn M, et al: Phrynoderma: a manifestation of vitamin A deficiency? … the rest of the story. Ped Derm 2005; 22:60.

Park YM, et al: Recurrent annular erythematous scaly patches. Arch Dermatol 2002; 138:405.

Smith KE, Fenske NA: Cutaneous manifestations of alcohol abuse. J Am Acad Dermatol 2000; 43:1.

Vitamin D

Although active vitamin D is produced in the skin, deficiency of vitamin D has no skin manifestations, except for alopecia. The elderly have decreased vitamin D cutaneous photosynthesis by reason of decreased sun exposure and poor intake of vitamin D, both of which predispose them to osteomalacia. Aggressive photoprotection may also reduce vitamin D levels. Patients with cutaneous lupus and other photosensitive diseases who are counseled to avoid the sun and use high sun protection factor (SPF) sunscreens are at particular risk. Other patients at risk include those who are debilitated with limited sun exposure; those taking anticonvulsants; those with fat malabsorption; and HIV-infected patients (especially dark-skinned patients living in northern climes). Vitamin D_3 supplementation of 400–800 IU per day should be recommended in all these groups of patients. Dermatologists who have patients at risk should also consider measuring vitamin D blood levels.

Cusak C, et al: Photoprotective behaviour and sunscreen use: impact on vitamin D levels in cutaneous lupus erythematosus. Photoderm Photoimmun Photomed 2008; 24:260.

Van den Bout-Van den Beukel CJ, et al: Vitamin D deficiency among HIV type 1-infected individuals in the Netherlands: effects of antiretroviral therapy. AIDS Res Hum Retroviruses 2008: 24:1375.

Vitamin K deficiency

Dietary deficiency of vitamin K, a fat-soluble vitamin, usually does not occur in adults because it is synthesized by bacteria in the large intestine. However, deficiency may occur in adults because of malabsorption caused by biliary disease, malabsorption syndromes, cystic fibrosis, or anorexia nervosa. Liver disease of all causes produces deficiency. Drugs such as coumarin, salicylates, cholestyramine, and perhaps the cephalosporins may induce a deficiency state. Newborns of mothers taking coumarin or phenytoin, or premature infants with an uncolonized intestine can be vitamin K-deficient. The result is a decrease in the vitamin K-dependent clotting factors II, VII, IX, and X. The cutaneous manifestations that result are purpura, hemorrhage, and ecchymosis. Treatment is 5–10 mg/day of intramuscular vitamin K for several days. In acute crises, fresh frozen plasma is used.

Humphries JE: Skin necrosis due to vitamin K deficiency. Am J Med 1993; 95:453.

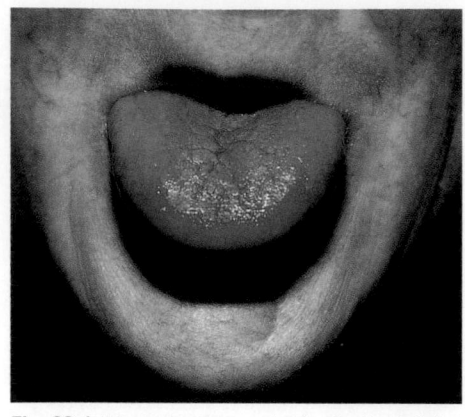

Fig. 22-1 Magenta tongue in riboflavin deficiency.

Soundararajan R, et al: Skin necrosis and protein C deficiency associated with vitamin K depletion in a patient with renal failure. Am J Med 1992; 93:467.

Vitamin B₁ deficiency

Vitamin B₁ (thiamine) deficiency results in beriberi. The skin manifestations are limited to edema and red burning tongue. Peripheral neuropathy is common, and congestive heart failure may develop.

Shenovy VV, et al: Congestive cardiac failure and anemia in a 15-year-old boy. J Postgrad Med 2000; 51:225.

Tran HA: A 74-year-old woman with increasing dyspnea. Arch Pathol Lab Med 2006; 130:e8.

Tsujino T, et al: Loop diuretic precipitated beriberi in a patient after pancreaticoduodenectomy: a case report. Am J Med Sci 2007; 334:407.

Vitamin B₂ deficiency

Vitamin B₂ (riboflavin) deficiency is seen most often in alcoholic patients; however, phototherapy for neonatal icterus, acute boric acid ingestion, hypothyroidism, and chlorpromazine use have been reported to cause it also. The classic findings are the oral–ocular–genital syndrome. The lips are prominently affected with angular cheilitis (perlèche) and cheilosis. The tongue is atrophic and magenta in colour (Fig. 22-1). A seborrheic-like dermatitis with follicular keratosis around the nares primarily affects the face. Genital dermatitis is worse in men than it is in women who have riboflavin deficiency. There is a confluent dermatitis of the scrotum, sparing the midline, with extension on to the thighs. In its mildest form it is slightly "irritating" and pruritic, especially when sweating. As the deficiency progresses, the scrotum goes through a mild acute dry phase with erythema and slight scale to a severe chronic dry phase with confluent red papules that spread to involve the perianal area and inner thighs, accompanied by fissuring and pain. Balanitis and phimosis may occur, requiring circumcision. In severe deficiency the entire scrotum becomes wet with increasing pain and fissuring. The final stage is accompanied by massive swelling so that the scrotum may reach the size of a football. Photophobia and blepharitis angularis occur. The response to 5 mg/day of riboflavin is dramatic.

Roe DA: Riboflavin deficiency. Semin Dermatol 1991; 10:293.

Vitamin B₆

Pyridoxine deficiency

Pyridoxine (vitamin B₆) deficiency may occur in cases of uremia and cirrhosis, as well as with the use of certain phar-

macologic agents. Skin changes include a seborrheic dermatitis-like eruption, atrophic glossitis with ulceration, angular cheilitis, conjunctivitis, and intertrigo. Occasionally, a pellagra-like eruption may occur. Neurologic symptoms include somnolence, confusion, and neuropathy.

Pyridoxine excess

Friedman et al reported a patient who ingested large doses of pyridoxine and developed a subepidermal vesicular dermatosis and sensory peripheral neuropathy. The bullous dermatosis resembled epidermolysis bullosa acquisita.

Friedman MA, et al: Subepidermal vesicular dermatosis and sensory peripheral neuropathy caused by pyridoxine abuse. J Am Acad Dermatol 1986; 14:915.

Vitamin B₁₂ deficiency

Vitamin B₁₂ (cyanocobalamin) is absorbed through the distal ileum after binding to gastric intrinsic factor in an acid pH. Deficiency is caused mainly by gastrointestinal abnormalities, such as a deficiency of intrinsic factor, achlorhydria (including that induced by medications), ileal diseases, and malabsorption syndromes resulting from pancreatic disease or sprue. Aggressive treatment for the eradication of *Helicobacter pylori* may cause B₁₂ deficiency, as can metformin administration and long-term antacid ingestion. Food-cobalamin malabsorption is a syndrome in which the body is unable to release vitamin B₁₂ from food or intestinal transport proteins especially with accompanying achlorhydria. These patients have adequate dietary vitamin B₁₂, but often have atrophic gastritis. A Schilling test will be normal. Congenital lack of transcobalamin II can also produce B₁₂ deficiency. Because of the large body stores in adults, deficiency occurs 3–6 years after gastrointestinal abnormalities.

Glossitis, hyperpigmentation, and canities are the main dermatologic manifestations. The tongue is bright red, sore, and atrophic. Linear atrophic lesions may be an early sign. The hyperpigmentation is generalized, but it is more commonly accentuated in exposed areas, such as the face and hands, and in the palmar creases and flexures, resembling Addison's disease. The nails may be pigmented. Premature gray hair may occur paradoxically. Megaloblastic anemia is often present. Weakness, paresthesias, numbness, ataxia, and other neurologic findings occur.

Parenteral replacement with intramuscular injections, 1 mg/week for 1 month, then 1 mg/month, leads to a reversal of the pigmentary changes in the skin, nails, mucous membranes, and hair. Mega-dose oral replacement of 1–2 mg per day may replace body stores by simple diffusion, independent of intrinsic factor. Neurologic defects may or may not improve with replacement.

Folic acid deficiency

Diffuse hyperpigmentation, glossitis, cheilitis, and megaloblastic anemia, identical to vitamin B₁₂ deficiency, occur in folic acid deficiency. Low folic acid is associated with neural tube defects which are more common in light-skinned people, suggesting an association between ultraviolet (UV) exposure and reduction in folic acid.

Dali-Youcef N, Andres E: An update on cobalamin deficiency in adults. Q J Med 2009; 102–117.

Der-Petrossian M, et al: Photodegradation of folic acid during extracorporeal photopheresis. Br J Dermatol 2007; 156:117.

Downham TF, et al: Hyperpigmentation and folate deficiency. Arch Dermatol 1976; 112:562.

Graella J, et al: Glossitis with linear lesions: an early sign of vitamin B₁₂ deficiency. J Am Acad Dermatol 2009; 60:498.
Lee HJ, Jo DY: A smooth, shiny tongue. N Engl J Med 2009; 360:e8.

Scurvy

Scurvy, or vitamin C deficiency, is the deficiency disease most commonly diagnosed by dermatologists, since cutaneous manifestations are early and prominent features. Elderly male alcoholics and psychiatric patients on restrictive diets are most commonly affected. Dialysis patients are also at risk. Smoking is a risk factor for low vitamin C levels. In the UK up to 25% of men and 16% of women in the low-income population had vitamin C levels in the deficient range.

The four Hs are characteristic of scurvy: hemorrhagic signs, hyperkeratosis of the hair follicles, hypochondriasis, and hematologic abnormalities. Perifollicular petechiae are the characteristic finding (Fig. 22-2). In addition, ecchymoses of various sizes, especially on the lower extremities, are common. These may be associated with tender nodules (subcutaneous and intramuscular hemorrhage) and subperiosteal hemorrhage, leading to pseudoparalysis in children. Woody edema may be present, simulating cellulitis. Subungual, subconjunctival, intramuscular, periosteal, and intra-articular hemorrhage may also occur. The referring diagnosis is often vasculitis.

Another characteristic finding is keratotic plugging of the hair follicles, chiefly on the anterior forearms, abdomen, and posterior thighs. The hair shafts are curled in follicles capped by keratotic plugs. This distinctive finding has been named "corkscrew hairs" (Fig. 22-3).

Hemorrhagic gingivitis occurs adjacent to teeth and presents as swelling and bleeding of the gums (Fig. 22-4). The teeth are loose and the breath is foul. Gingival disease may be absent, or may be the sole sign of scurvy. Edentulous areas do not develop gingivitis, and those with good oral hygiene have less prominent gingival involvement. Epistaxis, delayed wound healing, and depression may also occur. Frequently, anemia is present and may be the result of blood loss or associated deficiencies of other nutrients such as folate.

The diagnosis of scurvy is usually made on clinical grounds and confirmed by a positive response to vitamin C supplementation. A biopsy will exclude vasculitis and demonstrate follicular hyperkeratosis, coiled hairs, and perifollicular hemorrhage in the absence of inflammation. Serum ascorbic acid levels may be confirmatory in unusual cases. Treatment is with ascorbic acid, 1000 mg/day for a few days to 1 week, and a maintenance dose of 100 mg/day should be considered.

Arron ST, et al: Scurvy: a presenting sign of psychosis. J Am Acad Dermatol 2007; 57:S8
Chartler TK, et al: Palpable purpura in an elderly man. Arch Dermatol 2003; 139:1363.
Christopher K, et al: Early scurvy complicating anorexia nervosa. South Med J 2002; 95:1065.
Duggan CP, et al: Case 23-2007: a 9-year-old boy with bone pain, rash, and gingival hypertrophy. N Engl J Med 2009; 357:392.
Edge JC, Callen J: Scurvy masquerading as cellulitis. J Am Acad Dermatol 2004; 50:P170.
Frey JL, Shehan JM: Unknown: lower extremity papules associated with easy bruising. DOJ 2008; 14:19.
Li R, et al: Gingival hypertrophy: a solitary manifestation of scurvy. Am J Otolaryng 2008; 29:426.
Mosdol A, et al: Estimated prevalence and predictors of vitamin C deficiency within UK's low-income population. J Pub Health 2008; 30:456.
Ragunatha S, et al: Diffuse nonscarring alopecia of scalp: an indicator of early infantile scurvy? Pediatr Dermatol 2008; 25:644.
Singer R, et al: High prevalence of ascorbate deficiency in an Australian peritoneal dialysis population. Nephrology 2008; 13:17.
Walters RW, et al: Scurvy with manifestations limited to a previously injured extremity. J Am Acad Dermatol 2007; 57:S48.

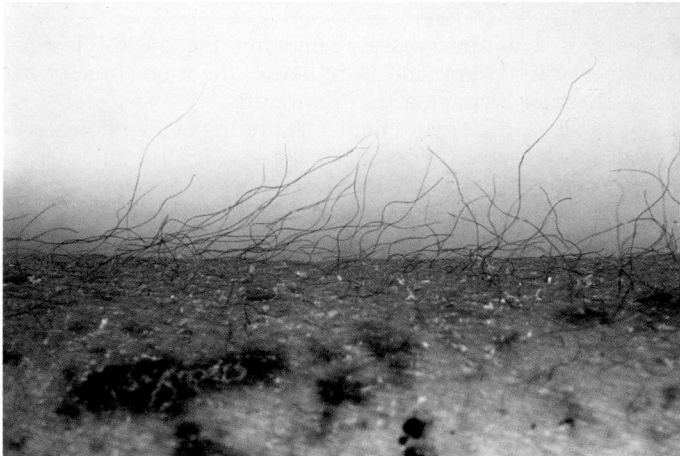

Fig. 22-3 Corkscrew hairs in scurvy.

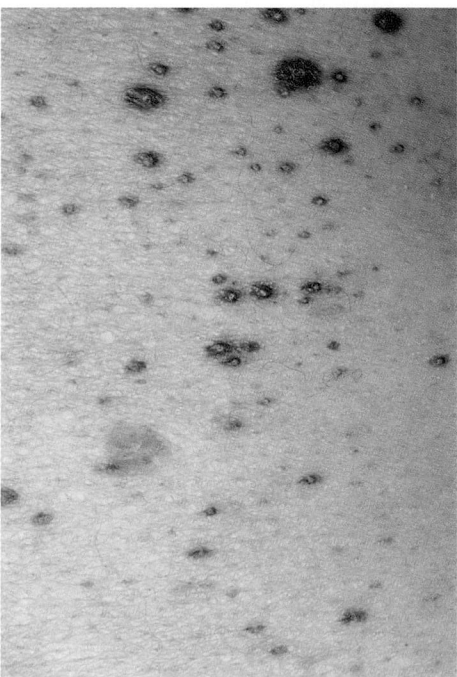

Fig. 22-2 Scurvy, perifollicular hemorrhage and follicular hyperkeratosis.

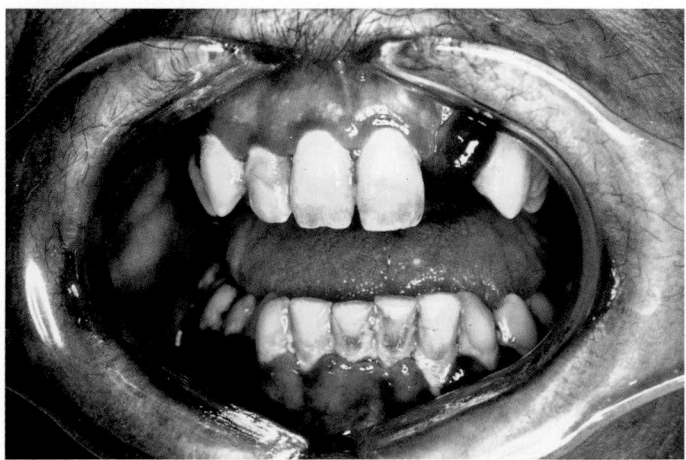

Fig. 22-4 Scurvy, gingivitis.

Niacin deficiency (pellagra)

Pellagra usually results from a deficiency of nicotinic acid (niacin, vitamin B₃) or its precursor amino acid, tryptophan. It is associated classically with a diet almost entirely composed of corn, millet, or sorghum. It can occur within 60 days of dietary niacin deficiency. Other vitamin deficiencies (especially pyridoxine) or malnutrition, which interfere with the conversion of tryptophan to niacin, often coexist. In developed countries, most cases of pellagra occur in alcoholics. Other possible causes of pellagra are:

* carcinoid tumors, which divert tryptophan to serotonin
* Hartnup disease (impaired absorption of tryptophan)
* gastrointestinal disorders, e.g. Crohn and gastrointestinal surgery
* prolonged intravenous supplementation
* psychiatric disease, including anorexia nervosa
* restrictive diets in adult patients with atopic dermatitis concerned about "food allergy."

Pellagra can also be induced by medications, most commonly isoniazid, azathioprine (and its metabolite 6-mercaptopurine), 5-fluorouracil, ethionamide, protionamide, and pyrazinamide. These medications may induce pellagra by interfering with niacin biosynthesis. The anticonvulsants, including hydantoins, phenobarbital, and carbamazepine, may rarely produce pellagra in a dose-dependent fashion.

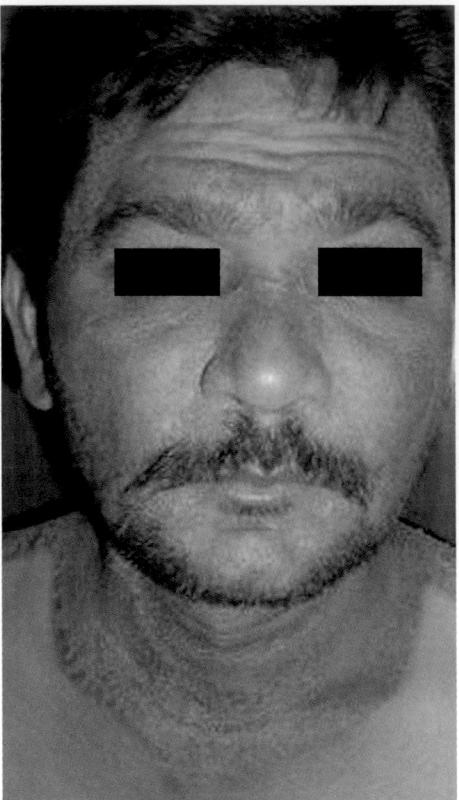

Fig. 22-5 Pellagra. (Courtesy of Shyam Verma, MD)

Clinical features

Pellagra is a chronic disease affecting the gastrointestinal tract, nervous system, and skin; hence, the mnemonic of the 3 Ds—diarrhea, dementia, and dermatitis.

The most characteristic cutaneous finding is the photosensitive eruption, which worsens in the spring and summer. It occurs symmetrically on the face, neck, and upper chest (Casal necklace; Fig. 22-5); extensor arms; and backs of the hands. Initially, there is erythema and swelling after sun exposure, accompanied by itching and burning or pain. In severe cases, the eruption may be vesicular or bullous (wet pellagra). When compared with normal sunburn, the pellagrous skin takes about four times longer to recover from the acute phototoxic injury. After several phototoxic events, thickening, scaling, and hyperpigmentation of the affected skin occurs. The skin has a copper or mahogany hue. In protracted cases, the skin ultimately becomes dry, smooth, paper-thin, and glassy with a parchment-like consistency. Scarring rarely occurs.

The nose is fairly characteristic. There is dull erythema of the bridge of the nose, with fine, yellow, powdery scales over the follicular orifices (sulfur flakes). The eruption resembles seborrheic dermatitis, except for its location. Plugs of inspissated sebum may project from dilated orifices on the nose, giving it a rough appearance.

At the onset, there is weakness, loss of appetite, abdominal pain, diarrhea, mental depression, and photosensitivity. Skin lesions may be the earliest sign, with phototoxicity being the presenting symptom in some cases. Neurologic and gastrointestinal symptoms can occur without skin changes. Delusions of parasitosis have been reported in pellagra. In the later stages of the disease, the neurologic symptoms may predominate. Apathy, depression, muscle weakness, paresthesias, headaches, and attacks of dizziness or falling are typical findings. Hallucinations, psychosis, seizures, dementia, neurologic degeneration, and coma may develop. The disease is progressive and can be fatal if untreated.

Pathology

Histologically, the findings in the skin vary according to the stage of the disease. The most characteristic finding is pallor and vacuolar changes of the keratinocytes in a band in the upper layers of the stratum malpighii, just below the granular cell layer, which may be attenuated. If marked, a cleft may form in the upper epidermis, correlating with the blistering seen in wet pellagra.

Diagnosis and treatment

If the characteristic skin findings are present, the diagnosis is not difficult clinically. Dietary treatment to correct the malnutrition is essential. Animal proteins, eggs, milk, and vegetables are beneficial. Supplementation with nicotinamide, 100 mg three times a day for several weeks, should be given. Fluid and electrolyte loss from diarrhea should be replaced, and in patients with gastrointestinal symptoms, possibly interfering with absorption, initial intravenous supplementation should be considered. Within 24 h of niacin therapy is begun, the skin lesions begin to resolve, confirming the diagnosis. Alcoholism must be treated if present, and the factors that may have led to pellagra must be corrected.

Ashourian N, Mousdicas N: Pellagra-like dermatitis. N Engl J Med 2009; 345:1614.

Bell HK, et al: Cutaneous manifestations of the malignant carcinoid syndrome. Br J Dermatol 2005; 152:71.

Cho S, et al: Wet pellagra. Int J Dermatol 2001; 40:543.

Jarrett P, et al: Pellagra, azathioprine, and inflammatory bowel disease. Clin Exp Dermatol 1997; 22:44.

Karthikeyan K, Thappa DM: Pellagra and skin. Int J Dermatol 2002; 41:476.

Kleyn CE: Cutaneous manifestations of the malignant carcinoid syndrome. J Am Acad Dermatol 2004; 50:P437.

Ladoyanni E, et al: Pellagra occurring in a patient with atopic dermatitis and food allergy. JEADV 2006; 21:394.

Lyon VB, Fairley JA: Anticonvulsant-induced pellagra. J Am Acad Dermatol 2002; 46:597.

MacDonald A, Forsyth A: Nutritional deficiencies and the skin. Clin Exper Dermatol 2005; 30:388.

Prakah R, et al: Rapid resolution of delusional parasitosis in pellagra with niacin augmentation therapy. Gen Hosp Psych 2008; 30:581.

Rabindranath D, et al: A rash imposition from a lifestyle omission: a case report of pellagra. Ulster Med J 2006; 75:92.

Stevens HP, et al: Pellagra secondary to 5-fluorouracil. Br J Dermatol 1993; 128:578.

Biotin deficiency

Biotin is universally available and is produced by intestinal bacteria. Therefore, deficiency is rare but can occur in patients with a short gut or malabsorption. Sometimes it occurs in individuals taking antibiotics or receiving parenteral nutrition. Ingestion of avidin, found in raw egg white, may bind biotin, leading to deficiency. The three autosomal-recessive syndromes holocarboxylase synthetase deficiency (multiple carboxylase deficiency), biotinidase deficiency, and the very rare syndrome of inability to transport biotin into cells all have similar clinical features, referred to as "multiple carboxylase deficiency." The holocarboxylase deficiency presents earlier and is termed the "neonatal" form, whereas the biotinidase deficiency may present later and is termed the "juvenile" form. Clinical presentation is variable, with some patients manifesting only certain features.

The skin and nervous system are primarily affected. A dermatitis similar to that found in cases of zinc deficiency and essential fatty acid deficiency is seen. It is periorificial and characterized by patchy, red, eroded lesions on the face and groin. *Candida* is regularly present on the lesions. Alopecia, sometimes total, including loss of the eyebrows and eyelashes, can occur. Conjunctivitis may be present. Neurologic findings are prominent. In adults, these include depression, lethargy, hallucinations, and limb paresthesias. In infants, neurologic findings include hypotonia, lethargy, a withdrawn behavior, ataxia, seizures, deafness, and developmental delay. The diagnosis of the inherited forms is made by detecting organic aminoaciduria of 3-hydroxyisovaleric acid. Measurement of serum biotinidase can distinguish biotinidase deficiency from holocarboxylase deficiency. Treatment consists of 10 mg of biotin/day, but depending on the severity of the enzyme mutation, higher doses may be required. Skin lesions resolve rapidly, but the neurologic damage may be permanent; hence, the importance of early diagnosis. One report suggested that valproic acid treatment in children, especially at doses of 40 mg/kg/day or higher, may lead to partial biotinidase deficiency, and that the skin lesions (seborrheic dermatitis-like rash and alopecia) improved with biotin supplementation at 10 mg/day.

Fleischman MH, et al: Case report and review of congenital biotinidase deficiency. J Am Acad Dermatol 2004; 50:P513.

Hove JLK, et al: Management of a patient with holocarboxylase synthetase deficiency. Mol Genet Metab 2008; 95:201.

Mardach R, et al: Biotin dependency due to a defect in biotin transport. J Clin Invest 2002; 109:1617.

Perez-Monjaras A, et al: Impaired biotinidase activity disrupts holocarboxylase synthetase expression in late onset multiple carboxylase deficiency. J Biol Chem 2008; 283:34150.

Rathi N, Rathi M: Biotinidase deficiency with hypertonia as unusual feature. Indian Pediatr 2009; 46:65.

Santer R, et al: Partial response to biotin therapy in a patient with holocarboxylase synthetase deficiency: clinical, biochemical, and molecular genetic aspects. Mol Genet Metab 2003; 79:160.

Schulpis KH, et al: Low serum biotinidase activity in children with valproic acid monotherapy. Epilepsia 2001; 42:1359.

Zinc deficiency

Zinc deficiency may be an inherited abnormality, acrodermatitis enteropathica, or it may be acquired. Acrodermatitis enteropathica is an autosomal-recessive, inherited disorder due to mutations in the *SLC39A4* gene that encodes the zinc transporter ZIP4. Acquired cases are termed acquired acrodermatitis enteropathica or acrodermatitis enteropathica-like syndrome. Premature infants are at particular risk because of inadequate body zinc stores, suboptimal absorption, and high zinc requirements. Normally, human breast milk has adequate zinc, and weaning classically precipitates clinical zinc deficiency in premature infants and in infants with acrodermatitis enteropathica. However, clinical zinc deficiency may occur in full-term and premature infants still breastfeeding. This is due to either low maternal breast milk zinc levels or a higher zinc requirement by the infant than the breast milk can provide (even though the zinc level in the breast milk is normal). A rare syndrome of congenital myopathy, recurrent diarrhea, microcephaly, and deafness has been associated with a neonatal bullous eruption characteristic of nutritional deficiency. These children have required very high doses of zinc supplementation.

Parenteral nutrition without adequate zinc content may lead to zinc deficiency. Acquired zinc deficiency also occurs in alcoholics as a result of poor nutritional intake and increased urinary excretion; as a complication of malabsorption, inflammatory bowel disease, or gastrointestinal surgery; and, occasionally, in cases of anorexia nervosa and acquired immunodeficiency syndrome (AIDS). Patients with severe erosive oral disease, such as pemphigus or graft versus host disease, may develop zinc deficiency due to malnourishment. Zinc requirements increase during metabolic stress, so symptomatic deficiency may present during infections, after trauma or surgery, with malignancy, during pregnancy, and with renal disease. Diets containing mainly cereal grains are high in phytate, which binds zinc, and have caused endemic zinc deficiency in certain areas of the Middle East and North Africa.

The dermatitis found in all forms of zinc deficiency is pustular and bullous, with an acral and periorificial distribution (Fig. 22-6). On the face, in the groin, and in other flexors there

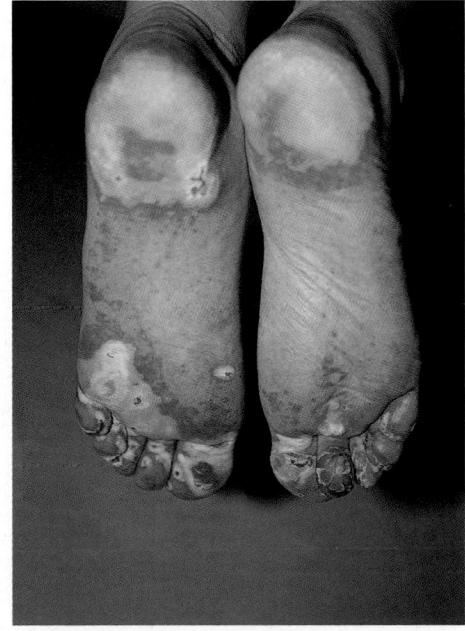

Fig. 22-6 Zinc deficiency, acquired in a patient who had severe nausea following a gastric bypass procedure and was unable to eat.

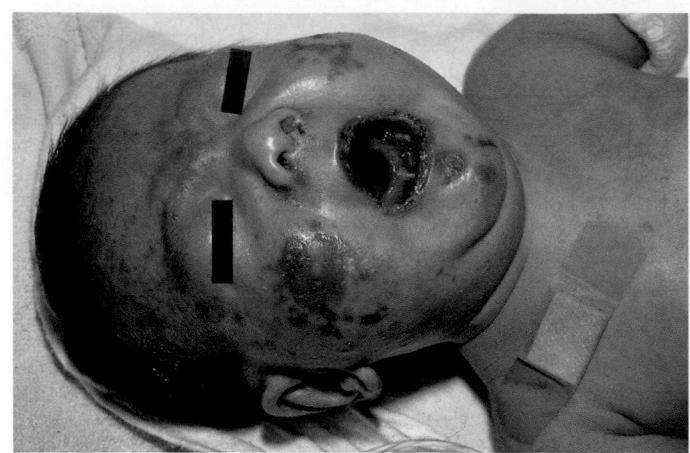

Fig. 22-7 Acrodermatitis enteropathica.

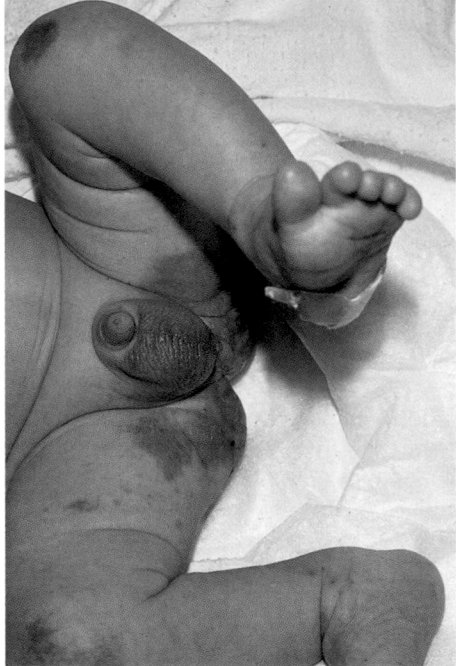

Fig. 22-8 Acrodermatitis enteropathica.

is a patchy, red, dry scaling with exudation and crusting. Angular cheilitis and stomatitis may be present (Fig. 22-7). The periungual areas are erythematous and scaling, and sometimes have superficial, flaccid pustules. Nail dystrophy may result, with thinning of the nails and accentuated longitudinal ridges. Chronic lesions may be more psoriasiform. Generalized alopecia may occur.

Diarrhea is present in most cases. Growth retardation, ophthalmic findings, impaired wound healing, and central nervous system manifestations occur. Patients are particularly irritable and emotionally labile.

The histopathologies of acquired and hereditary zinc deficiency are identical. There is vacuolation of the keratinocytes of the upper stratum malpighii. These areas of vacuolation may become confluent, forming a subcorneal bulla. In larger lesions, there may be total epidermal necrosis with subepidermal blister formation. Neutrophils are typically present. In the late stages of acrodermatitis enteropathica, this characteristic upper epidermal pallor is frequently absent, and the biopsy demonstrates only a psoriasiform dermatitis.

The diagnosis of zinc deficiency should be suspected in at-risk individuals with acral or periorificial dermatitis. In par-

ticular, chronic diaper rash with diarrhea in an infant should lead to evaluation for zinc deficiency (Fig. 22-8). The diagnosis can be confirmed by low serum zinc levels. A low serum alkaline phosphatase, a zinc-dependent enzyme, may be a valuable adjunctive test where the serum zinc level is normal or near normal. In some patients, even if the zinc level is in the normal range, a trial of zinc supplementation should be considered if the skin lesions are characteristic. Replacement is with zinc sulfate, 1–2 mg/kg/day (50 mg of elemental zinc per 220 mg zinc sulfate tablet). In acquired cases, transient treatment and addressing the underlying condition are adequate. In cases of acrodermatitis enteropathica, supplementation is 3 mg/kg/day and should be lifelong. Overzealous zinc supplementation should be avoided, as it may lead to low serum copper levels.

Alhaj E, et al: Diffuse alopecia in a child due to dietary zinc deficiency. Skinmed 2007; 6:199.

Bodemer AA, Lloyd R: Acrodermatitis enteropathica vs. acquired zinc deficiency. J Am Acad Dermatol 2004; 50:P174.

Chue CD, et al: An acrodermatitis enteropathica-like eruption secondary to acquired zinc deficiency in an exclusively breast-fed premature infant. Int J Dermatol 2008; 46:372.

Dinulos JGH, Zembowicz A: Case 32-2008: a 10-year-old girl with recurrent oral lesions and cutaneous bullae. N Engl J Med 2008; 359:1718

Fernandez-Torres R, et al: Facial crusted lesions and acral splitting. Am J Med 2008; 121:e7.

Hall MJ, et al: Recalcitrant psoriasiform rash. Pediatr Dermatol 2002; 19:180.

Inamadar AC, Palit A: Acrodermatitis enteropathica with depigmented skin lesions simulating vitiligo. Pediatr Dermatol 2007; 24:668.

Jensen SL, et al: Bullous lesions in acrodermatitis enteropathica delaying diagnosis of zinc deficiency: a report of two cases and review of the literature. J Cutan Pathol 2008; 35:1.

Kienast A, et al: Zinc-deficiency dermatitis in breast-fed infants. Eur J Pediatr 2007; 166:189.

Kim YJ, et al: Acrodermatitis enteropathica-like eruption associated with combined nutritional deficiency. J Korean Med Sci 2005; 20:908.

Levy J, et al: Congenital myopathy, recurrent secretory diarrhea, bullous eruption of skin, microcephaly, and deafness: a new genetic syndrome? Am J Med Genetics 2003; 116A:20.

Maverakis E, et al: Acrodermatitis enteropathica. DOJ 2007; 13:11.

Maverakis E, et al: Acrodermatitis enteropathica and an overview of zinc metabolism. J Am Acad Dermatol 2007; 56:116.

Perafan-Riveros C, et al: Acrodermatitis enteropathica: case report and review of the literature. Pediatr Dermatol 2002; 19:426.

Sanchez JE, et al: Acquired acrodermatitis enteropathica: case report of an atypical presentation. J Cutan Pathol 2007; 34:490.

Suchithra N, et al: Acrodermatitis enteropathica-like skin eruption in a case of short bowel syndrome following jejuno-transverse colon anastomosis. DOJ 2007; 13:20.

Tran KT, et al: Acquired acrodermatitis enteropathica caused by anorexia nervosa. J Am Acad Dermatol 2005; 53:361.

Essential fatty acid deficiency

Essential fatty acid (EFA) deficiency may develop in multiple settings: low-birth weight infants; cystic fibrosis; gastrointestinal abnormalities, including inflammatory bowel disease and intestinal surgery; and prolonged parenteral nutrition without EFA supplementation. The resulting dermatitis is similar to that seen in zinc and biotin deficiency, although characteristically more widespread, but with less periorificial involvement and mucous membrane and nail changes. There is a generalized xerosis, since EFAs constitute up to one-quarter of the fatty acids of the stratum corneum and are required for normal epidermal barrier function. Widespread erythema and an intertriginous weeping eruption are seen. The hair becomes lighter in color, and diffuse alopecia is present. Poor wound healing, growth failure, and increased risk of infection may occur. There is a decrease in linoleic acid and an increase in palmitoleic and oleic acids. A ratio of eicosatrienoic acid to arachidonic acid of more than 0.4 is diagnostic of EFA deficiency. Intravenous lipid therapy with Intralipid 10% reverses the process. In patients who develop pancreatitis from the fat emulsion infusion, topical safflower oil emulsion or soybean oil applications may be considered as a stopgap measure, waiting for the pancreatitis to improve. Topical treatment does not maintain liver and tissue stores.

The nutrient deficiency eruption seen in children with cystic fibrosis has been termed "CF nutrient deficiency dermatitis" or CFNDD. It shares features of acrodermatitis enteropathica, kwashiorkor, and EFA deficiency. It presents at 2 weeks to 6 months of age with erythematous papules that may be annular. The diaper area and perioral/periorbital regions are initially affected. It spreads to the extremities and progresses to widespread plaques. Laboratory abnormalities include anemia, hypoalbuminemia, elevated liver function tests, including an elevated alkaline phosphatase, low or normal zinc, low vitamin E, and at times EFA deficiency. Biopsy shows a psoriasiform dermatitis, but the upper dermal pallor may be absent. Treatment of CFNDD is general enhancement of the child's nutrition, addressing zinc, protein, and EFA deficiencies as well as other nutritional deficiencies. Zinc therapy alone does not improve CFNDD.

Bernstein ML, et al: Cutaneous manifestations of cystic fibrosis. Pediatr Dermatol 2008; 25:150.

Marcason W: Can cutaneous application of vegetable oil prevent an essential fatty acid deficiency? J Am Diet Assoc 2007; 107:1262.

Sacks GS, et al: Failure of topical vegetable oils to prevent essential fatty acid deficiency in a critically ill patient receiving long-term parenteral nutrition. J Parenter Enteral Nutr 1994; 18:274.

Iron deficiency

Iron deficiency is common, especially among actively menstruating women, and particularly if they have little red meat in their diets and have not made an effort to replace their losses with other foods. Mucocutaneous findings include koilonychia, glossitis, angular cheilitis, pruritus, and telogen effluvium diffuse hair loss. Plummer–Vinson syndrome is the combination of microcytic anemia, dysphagia, and glossitis, seen almost entirely in middle-aged women. The lips are thin and the opening of the mouth is small and inelastic, so that there is a rather characteristic appearance. Smooth atrophy of the tongue is pronounced. Koilonychia is present in 40–50% of patients, and alopecia may be present. An esophageal web in the postcricoid area may occur, presenting as difficulty swallowing, or the feeling that food is stuck in the throat. The diagnosis is confirmed by measuring the serum iron level. Treatment consists of iron sulfate supplementation, 325 mg three times a day.

Cockayne SE, Thomas SE: Scratching and fasting: a study of pruritus and anorexia nervosa. Br J Dermatol 1999; 141:747.

Rushton DH, et al: Is there really no clear association between low serum ferritin and chronic diffuse telogen hair loss? Br J Dermatol 2003; 148:1270.

Selenium deficiency

Selenium deficiency occurs in patients on parenteral nutrition, in areas where soil selenium content is poor, and in low-birth weight infants. Manifestations in children include hypopigmentation of the skin and hair (pseudoalbinism). Leukonychia and Terry-like nails have been reported. Cardiomyopathy, muscle pain, and weakness with elevated muscle enzymes are the major features. Treatment consists of 3 µg/kg/day of selenium.

Vinton NE, et al: Macrocytosis and pseudoalbinism: manifestations of selenium deficiency. J Pediatr 1987; 111:711.

Protein–energy malnutrition

Protein–energy malnutrition is a spectrum of related disease including marasmus, kwashiorkor, and marasmic kwashiorkor. These conditions are endemic in the developing world. Marasmus represents prolonged deficiency of protein and calories, and is diagnosed in children who are below 60% of their ideal body weight without edema or hypoproteinemia. Kwashiorkor occurs with protein deficiency but a relatively adequate caloric intake. It is diagnosed in children between 60% and 80% of their ideal body weight with edema or hypoproteinemia. Marasmic kwashiorkor shows features of both conditions and is diagnosed in children who are less than 60% of their ideal body weight with features of edema or hypoproteinemia.

These conditions are rare in developed countries, but occasionally, kwashiorkor may occur as a result of severe dietary restrictions instituted to improve infantile atopic dermatitis. In the US this may occur when rice beverage, which lacks protein, is substituted for cow's milk and soy in the diets of infants surviving largely on bottle feedings. Most cases, therefore, are in infants younger than 1 year of age.

Marasmus

In cases of marasmus, the skin is dry, wrinkled, and loose because of marked loss of subcutaneous fat. The "monkey facies," caused by loss of the buccal fat pad, is characteristic. In contrast to kwashiorkor, there is no edema or dermatosis.

Kwashiorkor

Kwashiorkor produces hair and skin changes, edema, impaired growth, and the characteristic potbelly. In cases diagnosed in the US due to dietary restriction or social chaos, edema has masked growth failure, resulting in the diagnosis of malnutrition being delayed. The hair and skin changes are usually striking. Africans call the victims of kwashiorkor "red children." The hair is hypopigmented, varying in color from a reddish-yellow to gray or even white. The hair is dry and lusterless; curly hair becomes soft and straight; and marked scaling (crackled hair) is seen. Especially striking is the flag sign, affecting long, normally dark hair. The hair grown during periods of poor nutrition is pale, so that alternating bands of pale and dark hair can be seen along a single strand, indicating alternating periods of good and poor nutrition. The nails are soft and thin.

The skin lesions are hypopigmented on dark skin and erythematous or purple on fair skin. Lesions first appear in areas of friction or pressure: the flexures, groin, buttocks, and elbows. Hyperpigmented patches occur with slightly raised edges. As they progress, they resemble old, dark, deteriorating enamel paint with peeling or desquamation. This has been described variously as "crazy pavement," "crackled skin," "mosaic skin," "enamel paint," and "flaky paint" (Fig. 22-9). In severe cases, the peeling leaves pale, ulcerated, hypopigmented areas with hyperpigmented borders.

Buno IJ, et al: The enamel paint sign in the dermatologic diagnosis of early-onset kwashiorkor. Arch Dermatol 1998; 134:107.

Heath ML, Sidbury R: Cutaneous manifestations of nutritional deficiency. Curr Op in Pediatr 2006; 18:417.

Kuhl J, et al: Skin signs as the presenting manifestation of severe nutritional deficiency: report of 2 cases. Arch Dermatol 2004; 140:521.

Liu T, et al: Kwashiorkor in the United States. Arch Dermatol 2001; 137:630.

McKenzie CA, et al: Childhood malnutrition is associated with a reduction in the total melanin content of scalp hair. Br J Nutr 2007; 98:159.

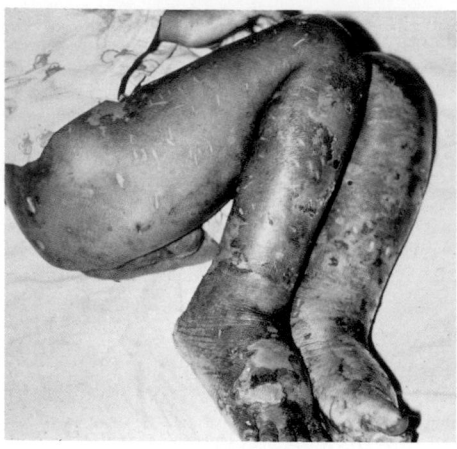

Fig. 22-9 Flaky paint sign, kwashiorkor.

Carotenemia and lycopenemia

Excessive ingestion of fruits and vegetables containing large amounts of β-carotene and lycopene can result in a yellowish discoloration of the skin, which is especially prominent on the palms, soles, and central face (areas of high sweat gland density). The sclerae are spared. Infants are most commonly affected, perhaps since pureeing fruits and vegetables makes these pigments more available for absorption. Carotenemia may also result from excess ingestion of β-carotene nutritional supplements and can be seen in hypothyroidism and anorexia nervosa.

Sale TA, et al: Carotenemia associated with increased consumption of green beans. J Am Acad Dermatol 2004; 50:P153.

Sivaramakrishnan VK, et al: Carotenemia in infancy and its association with prevalent feeding practices. Pediatr Derm 2006; 23:571.

Yuko T, et al: A case of carotenemia associated with ingestion of nutrient supplements. J Dermatol 2006: 2:132.

Bonus images for this chapter can be found online at

http://www.expertconsult.com

Diseases of Subcutaneous Fat

23

An inflammatory disorder that is primarily localized in the subcutaneous fat is termed a panniculitis. This group of disorders may be challenging for both the clinician and the dermatopathologist. Clinically, in all forms of panniculitis, lesions present as subcutaneous nodules. Histopathologically, the subcutaneous fat is a rather homogenous tissue and inflammatory processes may show considerable overlap. One way of classifying panniculitis is to separate erythema nodosum (EN), as the prototypical septal panniculitis, from those processes that primarily involve the fat lobules—the lobular panniculitides. Some lobular panniculitides are due to vasculitis (such as polyarteritis nodosa), and are discussed in other chapters. The remaining lobular panniculitides are categorized by their pathogenesis. Weber–Christian disease, Rothmann–Makai disease, lipomembranous or membranocystic panniculitis, and eosinophilic panniculitis are reaction patterns, and are not specific entities. Neutrophilic panniculitis may be infectious or may represent a variant of Sweet syndrome with primary involvement of the panniculus.

Given the depth of lesions in the panniculus, the choice of biopsy is critical in establishing the diagnosis. An incisional or excisional biopsy, narrow at the skin surface and wider in the panniculus, is the optimal procedure. An alternative double-punch method, using a 6–8 mm punch first, followed by a 4–6 mm punch at the depth of the first punch, may be considered, but is less ideal. Panniculitis is an area of dermatopathology where the skill of the dermatopathologist is critical in establishing good clinicopathologic correlation. If the biopsy report from an adequate biopsy specimen does not match the clinical findings, repeat the biopsy, or ask for a second opinion on the original specimen.

Requena L: Normal subcutaneous fat, necrosis of adipocytes and classification of the panniculitides. Semin Cutan Med Surg 2007 Jun; 26(2):66–70.

Septal panniculitis (acute and chronic erythema nodosum)

EN is the most common inflammatory panniculitis. It occurs in two forms: acute, which is common, and chronic, which is rare. Acute EN may occur at any age and in both sexes, but most cases occur in young adult women (female to male ratio, 3–6:1). The eruption consists of bilateral, symmetrical, deep, tender nodules and plaques 1–10 cm in diameter. Usually there are up to 10 lesions, but in severe cases many more may be found. Initially, the skin over the nodules is red, smooth, slightly elevated, and shiny (Fig. 23-1). The most common location is the pretibial area and lateral shins.

In general, the lesions should be primarily on the anterior rather than posterior calf. Lesions may also be seen on the upper legs, extensor arms, neck, and rarely the face. The onset is acute, and frequently associated with malaise, leg edema, and arthritis or arthralgia (usually of the ankles, knees, or

wrists). Fever, headache, episcleritis, conjunctivitis, and various gastrointestinal complaints may also be present. Over a few days, the lesions flatten, leaving a purple or blue–green color resembling a deep bruise (erythema contusiforme). Ulceration does not occur, and the lesions resolve without atrophy or scarring. The natural history is for the nodules to last a few days or weeks, appearing in crops, and then slowly involute. EN is much less common in children than adults, and affects boys and girls equally.

Acute EN is a reactive process. It is commonly associated with a streptococcal infection and in children this is by far the most common precipitant. Tuberculosis remains an important cause in areas where tuberculosis is endemic. Intestinal infection with *Yersinia*, *Salmonella*, or *Shigella* may precipitate EN. Other infectious causes include systemic fungal infections (coccidioidomycosis, histoplasmosis, sporotrichosis, and blastomycosis) and toxoplasmosis. EN-like lesions have been described in other infectious diseases such as *Helicobacter* septicemia, brucellosis, psittacosis, and cat-scratch disease. Since these organisms are fastidious, it has not always been possible to exclude the possibility that the EN-like lesions seen in these diseases actually represent septic foci in the panniculus. Sarcoidosis may present with fever, cough, joint pains, hilar adenopathy, and EN. This symptom complex, known as Löfgren syndrome, is especially common in Scandinavian, Irish, and Puerto Rican women. It generally responds well to therapy and runs a self-limited course. EN is frequently seen in patients with inflammatory bowel disease, more commonly Crohn's than ulcerative colitis. In this setting, it is not associated with overall disease severity, but is strongly associated with female sex, eye and joint involvement, and isolated colonic involvement. EN has been rarely reported in association with various hematologic malignancies, but this is less common than Sweet syndrome or pyoderma gangrenosum.

Drugs may also induce EN. The bromides, iodides, and sulfonamides were once the most frequent causative agents. Currently, oral contraceptives and hormone replacement therapy are the most common medications inducing EN. This association, the predominance in young women, and the occurrence of EN in pregnancy suggest that estrogens may predispose to the development of EN. Echinacea herbal therapy can also induce EN. While infliximab has been used to treat EN associated with Crohn disease, it has also produced EN upon multiple challenges in the setting of ankylosing spondylitis.

EN-like lesions have been described in Behçet syndrome and Sweet syndrome, and probably represent these inflammatory processes occurring in the fat, rather than the coexistence of two disorders. Histologically, the subcutaneous lesions of Behçet syndrome show features different from EN—a lobular or mixed lobular and septal pattern, and most importantly, a vasculitis which may be lymphocytic or leukocytoclastic, or may involve a small arteriole. This vasculitis is proposed to be

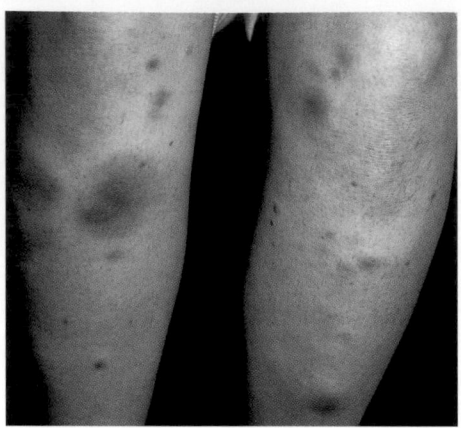

Fig. 23-1 Erythema nodosum, erythematous tender nodules on the anterior shins.

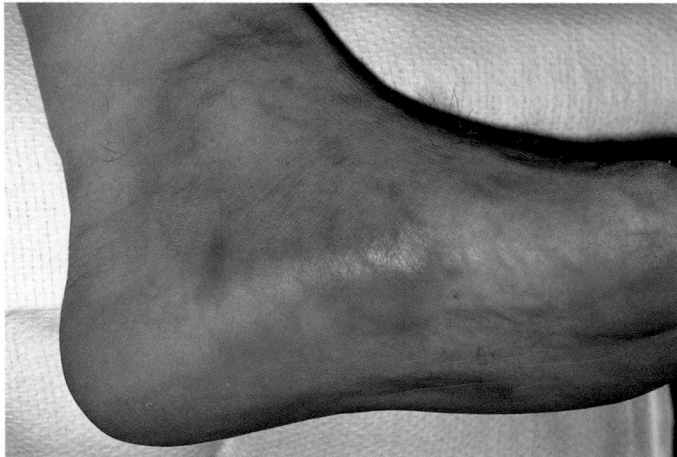

Fig. 23-2 Chronic erythema nodosum.

the primary event producing the subcutaneous lesions in Behçet syndrome.

A more chronic variant of EN, called chronic EN, EN migrans, or subacute migratory panniculitis of Vilanova and Piñol, is well described. This form of septal panniculitis is much less common than acute EN. It is distinguished from acute EN by the following features:

1. Lesions tend to occur in older women.
2. Lesions are unilateral or asymmetrical if bilateral (Fig. 23-2).
3. Lesions are not associated with systemic symptoms except arthralgias.
4. Lesions are painless or less tender than acute EN lesions.
5. Lesions are not associated with underlying diseases.
6. Lesions begin as a single lesion that tends to resolve, but migrates centrifugally, forming annular plaques of subcutaneous nodules with central clearing.
7. Lesions have a prolonged course of months to years.

In the differential diagnosis of EN, other forms of panniculitis must be considered. Erythema induratum (EI) usually affects primarily the posterior calves alone and runs a more chronic course, with the possibility of ulceration and scarring. Syphilitic gummas, as well as the nodules of sporotrichosis, are, as a rule, unilateral. Subcutaneous fat necrosis associated with pancreatitis and nodular vasculitis may also occur on the shins, but associated clinical features and/or histologic features will allow the differentiation to be made. Subacute infectious processes, such as *Helicobacter* cellulitis and atypical mycobacterial infection, may closely mimic EN. In most cases,

the classic picture of the acute onset of symmetrical, red, tender nodules on the anterior shins of a young woman will allow the diagnosis of EN to be easily made without a biopsy. However, if the case is atypical or does not evolve typically, a biopsy should be performed. In cases where the diagnosis of EN has been made in error, either the clinical features were atypical and a biopsy was not performed or was inadequate (punch biopsy), or the biopsy was misinterpreted by the pathologist.

EN is a septal panniculitis; the inflammatory infiltrate principally involves the connective tissue septa between fat lobules throughout the evolution of the lesion. The infiltrate may be composed of either neutrophils (early) or lymphocytes and other mononuclear cells (later), or a mixture, depending on the stage at which the lesion is biopsied. In older lesions histiocytes and multinucleate giant cells may predominate. Fat lobules are only secondarily affected by the inflammation, but some foamy histiocytes may be seen in the evolution of the lesions. Meischer radial granulomas, aggregates of histiocytes around stellate clefts, are characteristic but not diagnostic of EN. Leukocytoclastic vasculitis is not a histologic feature of EN. In chronic EN septal fibrosis and septal granulomas composed of epithelioid histiocytes are seen.

The management of EN involves three components: identifying the trigger; rest and elevation of the affected extremities; and specific anti-inflammatory medications. Since streptococcus is a common trigger, throat culture and ASO titer are indicated. A complete history of any preceding illness will often lead to clues. Preceding diarrhea might suggest *Yersinia* infection, for example. A travel and exposure history is especially important when considering endemic fungal infections. Four percent of patients with histoplasmosis present with EN, so in endemic areas this cause should be excluded. Early treatment of the infectious cause does not appear to shorten the duration of the EN, although EN triggered by infections tends to last longer if the infection is more chronic—streptococcal-induced EN will tend to last for a shorter period than tuberculosis-triggered EN. Bed rest is of great value and may be all that is required in mild cases. In children this is especially true. Gentle support hose are also helpful. Curtailing vigorous exercise during the acute attacks will shorten the course, and restriction of physical activities might prevent exacerbations and recurrences. Aspirin and nonsteroidal anti-inflammatory drugs (NSAIDs) such as indomethacin are often helpful. Potassium iodide is a safe and effective treatment. As a supersaturated solution, five drops three times a day, increased by one drop per dose per day up to 30 drops three times a day, is one easy-to-remember dose schedule. As a tablet, the dose is one 300 mg tablet three times a day. Induction of hypothyroidism by prolonged iodide therapy should be watched for. Once controlled, the therapy is gradually reduced over 2–3 weeks. Intralesional corticosteroid injections will control persistent lesions. Systemic steroids will result in rapid resolution of lesions, if not contraindicated by the underlying precipitating cause. In acute lesions, colchicine is often rapidly effective at a dose of 0.6 mg twice a day. For chronic EN, saturated solution of potassium iodide (SSKI) is often effective. In refractory cases, antimalarials may be tried.

The prognosis in acute EN is usually good, the attack running its course in 3–6 weeks. Recurrences do occur, especially if the underlying condition or infection is still present, or if physical activity is resumed too quickly. Chronic or atypical lesions should suggest an alternative diagnosis and require a biopsy.

Farhi D, et al: Significance of erythema nodosum and pyoderma gangrenosum in inflammatory bowel diseases: a cohort study of 2402 patients. Medicine (Baltimore) 2008 Sep; 87(5):281–293.

Patel RR, et al: Erythema nodosum in association with newly diagnosed hairy cell leukemia and group C streptococcus infection. Am J Dermatopathol 2008 Apr; 30(2):160–162.

Requena L, et al: Erythema nodosum. Dermatol Clin 2008 Oct; 26(4):425–438.

Rosen T, et al: Erythema nodosum associated with infliximab therapy. Dermatol Online J 2008 Apr 15; 14(4):3.

LOBULAR PANNICULITIS

Vessel-based lobular panniculitis

Inflammation or thrombosis of blood vessels may lead to fat necrosis due to ischemia. This can occur in primary forms of vasculitis, such as polyarteritis nodosa and Churg–Strauss syndrome, in metabolic disorders such as oxalosis and calciphylaxis, with atheromatous emboli, with heparin and coumarin necrosis, and with various coagulopathies. These entities are discussed in other chapters.

Nodular vasculitis

Clinically and histologically, nodular vasculitis is identical to EI. The two differ only by the presence of tuberculosis as a precipitating factor in EI. Nodular vasculitis presents as tender, subcutaneous nodules on the calves of middle-aged, thick-legged women (Fig. 23-3). Venous insufficiency may be present. Lesions are bilateral and less red and tender than EN; they often ulcerate, drain oily liquid, and recur over years.

The early lesions may show a suppurative vasculopathy, proposed by various authors to be an arteritis, a venulitis, or both. In some cases, no vasculitis is found, and (despite the name) the presence of a vasculitis is not required to establish the diagnosis of nodular vasculitis. Nodular vasculitis results in substantial lobular necrosis of adipocytes with suppuration. Necrosis of the lobule results in loss of the lipocyte membrane and pooling of lipid into variably sized round aggregates. As lesions evolve, the fat becomes increasingly necrotic, forming microcysts, and the disease progresses to the point where it may perforate through the epidermis, forming ulceration. Granulomatous inflammation appears adjacent to areas of fat necrosis, and eventually lesions resolve with fibrosis.

Non-tuberculous nodular vasculitis must be distinguished from EI. Because clinical and pathologic features are identical, the differentiation is made by searching for tuberculous infection in the patient, by applying a tuberculin skin test. If this is positive, the appropriate diagnosis is EI. Polymerase chain reaction (PCR) of the affected tissue may reveal the DNA of *Mycobacterium tuberculosis* in 50–70% of cases of EI. As a tuberculid, EI is a manifestation of cellular immunity to tuberculosis, and the purified protein derivative (PPD) test will always be positive. PCR of the tissue is not recommended in cases which are tuberculin skin test-negative. Gamma release assays are a sensitive method for diagnosis of tuberculosis and have proved helpful in the setting of EI. It should be noted that even in areas where tuberculosis is prevalent, EI is rare, representing only 1% of cutaneous manifestations of tuberculosis in one study. When present, EI may signal serious genitourinary involvement, including tuberculous epididymo-orchitis. Magro and coworkers proposed the name acute infectious id panniculitis for sterile neutrophil-dominant lobular panniculitis in response to non-tuberculous infectious organisms.

EI requires antibiotic therapy for the underlying tuberculosis. Treatment of nodular vasculitis is usually SSKI, as outlined for EN. This is effective in about half of cases. In the others, trials of colchicine, antimalarials, NSAIDs, mycophenolate mofetil, and systemic steroids may be attempted. Support stockings, elevation, and treatment of associated venous insufficiency may also improve nodular vasculitis.

Angus J, et al: Usefulness of the QuantiFERON test in the confirmation of latent tuberculosis in association with erythema induratum. Br J Dermatol 2007 Dec; 157(6):1293–1294.

Larsen S, et al: Extraintestinal manifestations of inflammatory bowel disease: epidemiology, diagnosis, and management. Ann Med 2010 Mar; 42(2):97–114.

Magro CM, et al: Acute infectious id panniculitis/panniculitic bacterid: a distinctive form of neutrophilic lobular panniculitis. J Cutan Pathol 2008 Oct; 35(10):941–946.

Mascaró JM Jr, et al: Erythema induratum of Bazin. Dermatol Clin 2008 Oct; 26(4):439–445.

Ramdial PK, et al: Tuberculids as sentinel lesions of tuberculous epididymo-orchitis. J Cutan Pathol 2007 Nov; 34(11):830–836.

Taverna JA, et al: Case reports: nodular vasculitis responsive to mycophenolate mofetil. J Drugs Dermatol 2006 Nov–Dec; 5(10):992–993.

Terranova M, et al: Clinical and epidemiological study of cutaneous tuberculosis in Northern Ethiopia. Dermatology 2008; 217(1): 89–93.

Sclerosing panniculitis (hypodermitis sclerodermiformis, lipodermatosclerosis, stasis panniculitis)

Sclerosing panniculitis occurs primarily on the medial lower third of the lower legs of women older than 40 (Fig. 23-4), with an above average body mass index. It may be bilateral. If not bilateral, the left leg only is affected, or the process is more severe on the left leg. If the right leg is primarily affected, deep venous thrombosis currently or in the past or a venous injury to the right leg must be considered. Typically, there is marked woody induration in a stocking distribution resulting in calves that resemble inverted champagne bottles. This induration results from fibrosis in the subcutaneous fat which may occur without the primary inflammatory panniculitis ever being clinically observed. It occurs multifocally and microscopically throughout the affected area. This pattern was called hypodermitis sclerodermiformis. When the areas of fat necrosis are larger, they present as erythematous, tender, subcutaneous

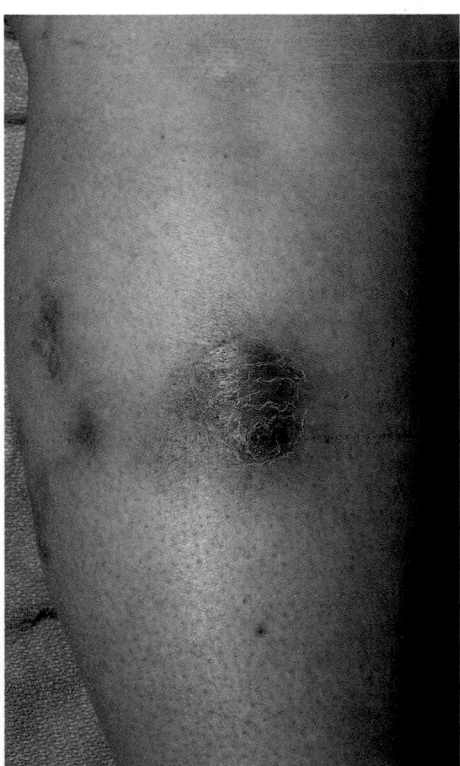

Fig. 23-3 Nodular vasculitis.

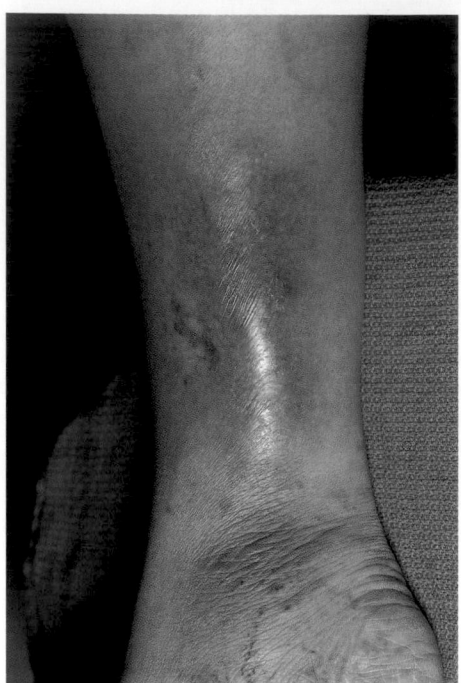

Fig. 23-4 Lipodermatosclerosis.

nodules or plaques. This is designated sclerosing panniculitis.

It is now recognized that these are two aspects of the same disease with a common pathogenesis—venous insufficiency. These patients may have venous varicosities, superficial thrombophlebitis, deep venous thrombosis, or several of these conditions. Even when venous disease is not clinically evident, evaluation of the venous system of the lower leg will frequently reveal insufficiency. Laboratory evaluation may reveal a genetic mutation in the fibrinolytic system resulting in increased thrombosis in these patients. Venous insufficiency results in hypoxia, necrosis of fat, inflammation, and eventual fibrosis. If hypoxemia is present from other causes such as pulmonary disease, sclerosing panniculitis may be more severe. Angiosarcoma has been reported as a rare complication in the setting of postphlebitic lipodermatosclerosis.

The histologic features of sclerosing panniculitis are characteristic, but not all features may be seen on every biopsy, since the histologic features change over time within the lesion. The overlying dermis frequently shows changes of stasis with nodular proliferation of thick-walled vessels, hemosiderin deposition, fibrosis, and atrophy. In early lesions there is ischemic necrosis in the center of the fat lobules manifested as "ghost cells"—pale cell walls with no nuclei. There is a sparse lymphocytic infiltrate in the fat septa. As the lesions evolve, the septa are thickened and fibrosed, and there is a mixed inflammatory infiltrate of lymphocytes, plasma cells, and macrophages. Foamy histiocytes are present around the areas of fat necrosis. Fat microcysts are characteristic (but not diagnostic) and appear as small cysts with feathery eosinophilic remnants of adipocytes lining the cyst cavity and resembling frost on a window, so-called lipomembranous fat necrosis. In later lesions these microcysts collapse and are replaced by fibrosis. Despite these characteristic features, biopsy should be avoided in these patients. Biopsies heal poorly and may lead to chronic leg ulcers. The diagnosis can usually be made clinically, and non-invasive techniques such as magnetic resonance imaging (MRI) have been used in an effort to avoid poorly healing wounds related to a biopsy. If a biopsy must be performed, it should be from the most proximal edge of involvement.

This diagnosis can be clinically confirmed if a careful vascular evaluation is performed. The location on the lower medial calf is unusual for EN. Most other panniculitides favor the posterior mid-calf. The gradual progression from the ankles proximally is characteristic of sclerosing panniculitis and not other forms of lobular panniculitis.

The treatment of sclerosing panniculitis may be difficult. Fibrotic areas may be irreversible. Graded compression stockings and elevation, standard treatments for venous insufficiency, are most effective in this condition. Application of pressure dressings, such as an Unna boot, can produce dramatic, if temporary, improvement. Greater compression—Unna boot with Coban and a foam buttress (bolster material to apply extra pressure to the red inflamed area) or the Profore boot—can be beneficial. Unfortunately, some patients cannot tolerate compression because of the pain of the lesions. Intralesional triamcinolone has been used, but is most effective when used in conjunction with compression. Pentoxiphylline, in doses of 400–800 mg three times a day, is useful, especially in cases not responding to compression and elevation alone, or in patients who are initially intolerant of compression dressings. Apparently by enhancing the fibrinolytic capacity of affected patients, stanozolol, 2–5 mg, or oxandrolone, 10 mg twice a day, may benefit some patients. It is rarely required if appropriate pressure dressings are applied and the patient is able to take full doses of pentoxiphylline. Stanozolol and oxandrolone may be virilizing for women and should be avoided if possible in women of childbearing potential. Stanozolol may induce hepatitis. Surgical treatment of varicosities and incompetent perforators may result in dramatic improvement in some patients.

Campbell LB, et al: Intralesional triamcinolone in the management of lipodermatosclerosis. J Am Acad Dermatol 2006 Jul; 55(1):166–168.
Chan CC, et al: Magnetic resonance imaging as a diagnostic tool for extensive lipodermatosclerosis. J Am Acad Dermatol 2008 Mar; 58(3):525–527.
Heymann WR: Lipodermatosclerosis. J Am Acad Dermatol 2009; 60(6):1022–1023.
Jowett AJ, et al: Angiosarcoma in an area of lipodermatosclerosis. Ann R Coll Surg Engl 2008 Jul; 90(5):W15–16.
Parnaby CN, et al: An overview of the surgical aspects of lower limb venous disease. Scott Med J 2009; 54(1):30–35.
Segura S, et al: Lipomembranous fat necrosis of the subcutaneous tissue. Dermatol Clin 2008 Oct; 26(4):509–517.
Vesić S, et al: Acute lipodermatosclerosis: an open clinical trial of stanozolol in patients unable to sustain compression therapy. Dermatol Online J 2008 Feb 28; 14(2):1.

Physical panniculitis

This category includes processes in the fat that occur from physical factors. Some are characterized by the presence of needle-like clefts—sclerema neonatorum, subcutaneous fat necrosis, and post-steroid panniculitis. Infants and children are most frequently affected, and in all these disorders metabolic differences in fat are apparently important pathogenically. Hypothermia or cold is frequently associated in some forms (cold panniculitis, sclerema, and subcutaneous fat necrosis). It may be difficult in some cases to separate mild cases of sclerema neonatorum clearly from subcutaneous fat necrosis, or differentiate cold panniculitis from subcutaneous fat necrosis of the newborn if the lesions are at sites of cold exposure. This is not surprising, since they may be pathogenically related. In general, cold panniculitis refers to localized cases where there is a history of local cold exposure, sclerema to cases presenting in severely ill children soon after birth with a poor prognosis, and subcutaneous fat necrosis (the most common variant) to cases with more limited lesions occurring in the first 6 weeks of life, sometimes with associated hypercalcemia. Traumatic fat necrosis occurs from damage to the subcutaneous fat resulting from trauma. All these conditions are treated supportively, and in all except sclerema neonatorum, spontaneous and complete recovery is expected.

Sclerema neonatorum

Sclerema neonatorum is the most severe and the rarest disorder in this group. It affects premature neonates who are gravely ill for other reasons or have experienced profound hypothermia. Affected neonates usually die, unless the underlying diseases can be reversed. In the first few days of life, the skin begins to harden, usually initially on the buttocks or lower extremities, and rapidly spreads to involve the whole body. The skin on the palms, soles, and genitalia is spared. The skin becomes dry, livid, cold, rigid, and board-like, so that the mobility of the parts is limited. The skin in the involved areas cannot be picked up. The skin of the entire body may appear half-frozen and is yellowish-white. Visceral fat may also be involved. Therapy is mostly supportive, but some data suggest exchange transfusion may improve survival.

Histologically, adipocytes are enlarged and filled with needle-like clefts in a radial array. Affected fat cells undergo necrosis. There is sparse inflammation, and histiocytes containing needle-like clefts are rare, possibly because most children die before granulomas can form.

Subcutaneous fat necrosis of the newborn

Subcutaneous fat necrosis of the newborn (SFN) occurs during the first 4 weeks of life (half in the first week) in term or post-term infants. A history of fetal distress, birth asphyxia, and meconium aspiration is common. Maternal cocaine use, severe neonatal anemia, thrombocytopenia, septicemia, and hypothermia have also been associated with SFN following delivery by emergency cesarian section and speaks against trauma as playing a role in SFN. Painful, firm to rubbery, erythematous nodules appear, usually on the upper back, buttocks, cheeks, or proximal extremities (Fig. 23-5). Lesions may fuse to form plaques and resolve spontaneously within 3 months with no scarring. In general, the infants remain well; however, hypoglycemia, thrombocytopenia, hypertriglyceridemia, lactic acidosis, and potentially life-threatening hypercalcemia may occur. Some degree of hypercalcemia occurred in more than 50% of recently reported cases, and in 4 of 11 consecutive cases seen at one institution. The hypercalcemia may appear weeks to months after the appearance and resolution of the skin lesions. Periodic serial serum calcium determinations for the first 3–4 months of life have been recommended. The pathogenesis of the hypercalcemia in SFN may be due to elevated prostaglandin E levels or inappropriately high levels of 1,25-hydroxyvitamin D. The mechanism of hypercalcemia in SFN has been postulated to be similar to that seen in other granulomatous conditions, such as sarcoidosis. Hypercalcemia may result in failure to thrive, irritability, apathy, hypotonia, seizures, and renal failure. The hypercalcemia is treated with hyperhydration, calcium-wasting diuretics (furosemide), and formulas low in calcium and vitamin D. Systemic steroids, calcitonin, and bisphosphonates may also be effective, when other methods fail to reduce the hypercalcemia.

Histologically, subcutaneous fat necrosis is a lobular panniculitis, with granular necrosis of adipocytes. Needle-shaped clefts are arranged radially within histiocytes, and multinucleate foamy histiocytes are present. Degranulating eosinophils may be present. Lesions may resolve with calcification and fibrosis. Fine-needle aspiration and touch preparations have confirmed this diagnosis, and characteristic ultrasound and MRI findings have been reported.

Cold panniculitis

Infants and young children are particularly predisposed to cold panniculitis. It has been described in children who suck on ice or popsicles (popsicle panniculitis), in the scrotum of prepubertal males (Fig. 23-6), and in infants treated for supraventricular tachycardia with the application of cold packs to the face. Most infants reported as affected have been black. Lesions occur within a few days of the cold application and appear as slightly erythematous, nontender, firm subcutaneous nodules. Equestrian panniculitis on the upper outer thighs of women riding horses in the cold appears to represent a form of perniosis rather than true panniculitis (see Chapter 3).

The typical patient with fat necrosis of the scrotum is a prepubertal (9–14-year-old) boy, who is heavy-set or even obese, with scrotal swelling, usually bilateral, associated with mild to moderate pain. The gait is often guarded and broad-based. There is a lack of systemic complaints and no symptoms related to voiding. The scrotal masses are bilateral and symmetrical in most cases. However, the lesions may be unilateral and there may be more than two. The masses are firm and tender, and do not transmit light. The overlying scrotal skin will be normal or red. Cryptorchidism is not unusual. The most common location of the lesions is near the perineum, consistent with the area of greatest concentration of scrotal fat

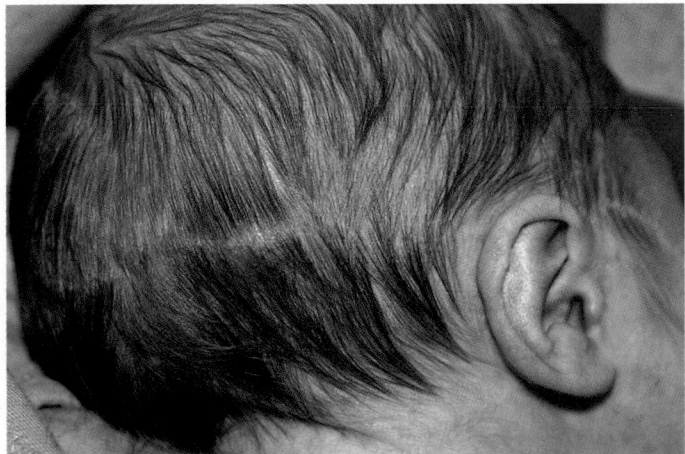

Fig. 23-5 Subcutaneous fat necrosis.

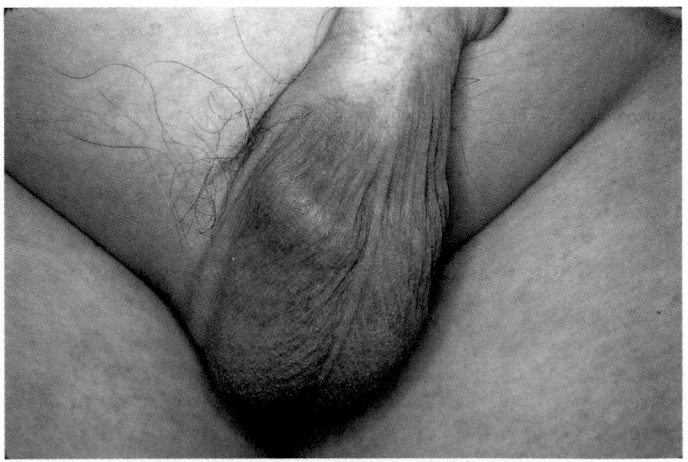

Fig. 23-6 Cold panniculitis.

in children. The adult scrotum lacks this fatty tissue. Without treatment lesions resolve over several days to weeks.

Histologically, there is necrosis of adipocytes within lobules of the upper subcutaneous fat adjacent to the lower dermis. A mixed inflammatory infiltrate of lymphocytes, neutrophils, and foam cells is present, and microcysts sometimes occur. This histology is not specific and the diagnosis relies largely on obtaining a history of cold exposure.

Alos N, et al: Pamidronate: treatment for severe hypercalcemia in neonatal subcutaneous fat necrosis. Horm Res 2006; 65(6):289–294.

Aucharaz KS, et al: Treatment of hypercalcaemia in subcutaneous fat necrosis is controversial. Horm Res 2007; 68(1):31.

Borgia F, et al: Subcutaneous fat necrosis of the newborn: be aware of hypercalcaemia. J Paediatr Child Health 2006 May; 42(5):316–318.

Isaiah JH, et al: Subcutaneous fat necrosis of the newborn and lactic acidosis. Pediatr Dermatol 2007 Jul–Aug; 24(4):435–436.

Lund JJ, et al: The utility of a touch preparation in the diagnosis of fluctuant subcutaneous fat necrosis of the newborn. Pediatr Dermatol 2009; 26(2):241–243.

Mahé E, et al: Subcutaneous fat necrosis of the newborn: a systematic evaluation of risk factors, clinical manifestations, complications and outcome of 16 children. Br J Dermatol 2007 Apr; 156(4):709–715.

Navarini-Meury S, et al: Sclerema neonatorum after therapeutic whole-body hypothermia. Arch Dis Child Fetal Neonatal Ed 2007 Jul; 92(4):F307.

Quesada-Cortés A, et al: Cold panniculitis. Dermatol Clin 2008 Oct; 26(4):485–489.

Tajirian A, et al: Subcutaneous fat necrosis of the newborn with eosinophilic granules. J Cutan Pathol 2007 Jul; 34(7):588–590.

Torrelo A, et al: Panniculitis in children. Dermatol Clin 2008 Oct; 26(4):491–500.

Vasireddy S, et al: MRI and US findings of subcutaneous fat necrosis of the newborn. Pediatr Radiol 2009; 39(1):73–76.

Zaulyanov LL, et al: Subcutaneous fat necrosis of the newborn and hyperferritinemia. Pediatr Dermatol 2007 Jan–Feb; 24(1):93.

Zeb A, et al: Sclerema neonatorum: a review of nomenclature, clinical presentation, histological features, differential diagnoses and management. J Perinatol 2008 Jul; 28(7):453–460.

Post-steroid panniculitis

This rare form of panniculitis occurs predominately in children treated acutely with high doses of systemic corticosteroids during rapid corticosteroid withdrawal. Substantial weight gain has usually occurred during the corticosteroid therapy. Firm subcutaneous nodules begin to appear within a month of tapering the corticosteroids. Areas of abundant subcutaneous fat are favored—the cheeks, trunk, and proximal extremities. Most cases resolve spontaneously within weeks, but if severe, the steroids must be reinstituted and tapered more slowly.

Histologically, the changes are identical to those seen in subcutaneous fat necrosis of the newborn. There is a lobular panniculitis with necrosis of adipocytes and needle-shaped clefts in both adipocytes and histiocytes. Foamy histiocytes are also present.

Silverman RA, et al: Poststeroid panniculitis. Pediatr Dermatol 1992; 5:92.

Traumatic panniculitis

Accidental trauma to the skin may induce necrosis of the fat. This is most common on the trunk and breasts of women. The prior history of trauma is frequently not recalled. Lesions present like a lipoma, as a firm, mobile subcutaneous mass (formerly reported as mobile encapsulated lipoma). Airbag injury may induce fat necrosis. The term myospherulosis (spherulocytosis) has been used to describe subcutaneous cystic lesions induced by trauma with hemorrhage into areas of high lipid content. Long-acting antibiotics formulated in oil

bases were associated with myospherulosis. The structures resemble the sporangia of rhinosporidiosis, but represent degenerated red blood cells rather than true fungal organisms. Accidental trauma to the upper anterolateral thigh from a desk or chair may result in semicircular bands of atrophy of fat called lipoatrophia semicircularis.

Histologically, there is a granulomatous lobular panniculitis with foamy histiocytes, membranous fat necrosis, and microcysts. Lesions heal with fibrosis of the septa. In myospherulosis, large round structures containing many smaller round eosinophilic bodies are noted. These represent degenerated erythrocytes.

Moreno A, et al: Traumatic panniculitis. Dermatol Clin 2008 Oct; 26(4):481–483.

Factitial panniculitis

Self-induced panniculitis is rarely reported, but it is not uncommon. It may be induced by the injection of organic materials, povidone, feces, saliva, vaginal fluid, and oils. In many cases, ulceration will occur. Factitial trauma may also induce a panniculitis. Medical personnel are at risk because they have ready access to syringes and needles. Pointed, detailed questioning of the patient may identify inconsistencies in the history, or the underlying cause for the behavior (e.g. attention-seeking, revenge, malingering).

The clinician must have a high index of suspicion in cases in which the clinical pattern is not characteristic of a known form of panniculitis. Inspection of early lesions for tell-tale healing injection sites may help confirm the diagnosis. A biopsy is often required. Culture may demonstrate a consistent pattern of fecal, oral, or vaginal flora. Biopsy demonstrates an acute lobular panniculitis with fat necrosis and a neutrophilic infiltrate. Careful evaluation of the biopsy material with polarization may identify foreign material. When the suspicion is high and no foreign material can be seen in the tissue, special evaluation by incineration and mass spectroscopy may identify the injected substance. Electron microscopy with x-ray emission spectrography can identify inorganic substances. Radiographs may demonstrate fractured needles or foreign bodies.

Sanmartín O, et al: Factitial panniculitis. Dermatol Clin 2008 Oct; 26(4):519–527.

Sclerosing lipogranuloma

Sclerosing lipogranuloma describes the granulomatous and fibrotic reaction that occurs in the panniculus from the injection of silicone or mineral oils. Topical application of an antibacterial ointment to an open wound can rarely result in the formation of lipogranuloma. In most cases the injections are intentional and cosmetic. The time from injection to onset of symptoms may be months to more than 10 years.

Lesions are usually localized to the penis, scrotum, breasts, nose, and buttocks, often after an attempt to augment the area by injection. The overlying skin is hyperpigmented and erythematous. Lesions are frequently diagnosed initially as cellulitis. On palpation, the skin is indurated and cannot be picked up between the fingers. The subcutaneous tissue is indurated, thickened, and lumpy. In some cases, there will be focal ulceration. The injected material will frequently migrate locally, extending beyond the sites of implantation. In some cases it is carried to other tissues, specifically the lymphoreticular system and lungs. Hepatosplenomegaly and pulmonary fibrosis may occur.

Histologically, the panniculus is replaced by the injected material, which is in various-sized vacuoles, giving the affected tissue a "Swiss cheese" appearance. Because the material is usually washed out during the tissue processing, the material itself is not seen, only the spaces it occupied in the tissue in vivo. The vacuoles are surrounded by histiocytes, many of which have ingested the material, giving their cytoplasm a vacuolated appearance. Fibrosis may be prominent. Frozen section can be used to demonstrate the lipid.

Jung SE, et al: Sclerosing lipogranuloma of the scrotum: sonographic findings and pathologic correlation. J Ultrasound Med 2007 Sep; 26(9):1231–1233.
Nyirády P, et al: Treatment and outcome of vaseline-induced sclerosing lipogranuloma of the penis. Urology 2008 Jun; 71(6):1132–1137.

ENZYME-RELATED PANNICULITIS

This category includes panniculitis induced by enzymes that damage fat (pancreatic panniculitis) and panniculitis caused by the absence of an enzyme critical in preventing tissue inflammation after injury (α1-antitrypsin).

Pancreatic panniculitis (subcutaneous fat necrosis)

Subcutaneous fat necrosis is most commonly associated with pancreatitis or pancreatic carcinoma, and more rarely with anatomic pancreatic abnormalities, pseudocysts, hypertriglyceridemia in association with nephrotic syndrome, or drug-induced pancreatitis. Men outnumber women 2:1 in cases of pancreatitis and 7:1 in cases of pancreatic carcinoma. In cases associated with pancreatic carcinoma, acinar cell carcinoma is most common. Even metastatic pancreatic carcinoma with no residual tumor in the pancreas may induce the syndrome. In 40% of cases, the skin lesions are the first symptom of the underlying pancreatic pathology and therefore represent an important clue to the diagnosis.

Skin lesions appear as tender or painless erythematous subcutaneous nodules from 1 to 5 cm in diameter (Fig. 23-7). The lower leg is the most common location, being affected in more than 90% of cases. Subcutaneous fat elsewhere may also be affected, except rarely on the head and neck. The number of lesions is usually fewer than 10 but may reach the hundreds.

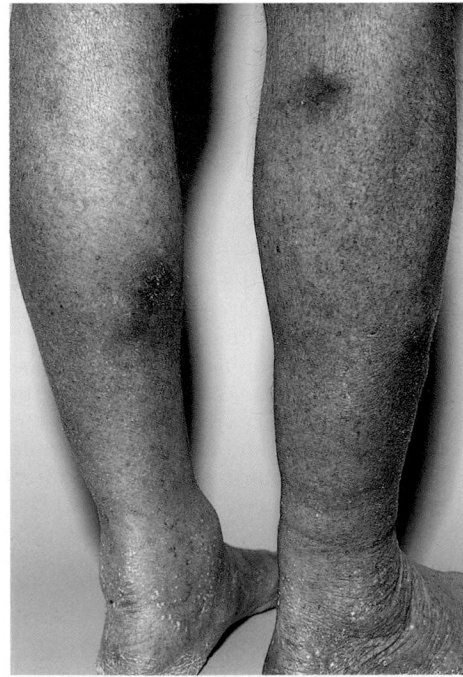

Fig. 23-7 Pancreatic fat necrosis.

In most cases the lesions involve, leaving an atrophic scar. If the fat necrosis is severe, however, the lesion develops into a sterile abscess that may break down, draining a thick, brown, oily material.

Pancreatic panniculitis is frequently accompanied by a constellation of findings related to fat necrosis in other organs. Importantly, abdominal symptoms may be completely absent. Arthritis is found in 54–88% of cases, and may be monoarticular, oligoarticular, and rarely polyarticular. The arthritis may be intermittent, migratory, or persistent, and is usually in joints adjacent to the lesions of panniculitis. Examination of the joint fluid reveals the presence of free fatty acids, suggesting it is due to fat necrosis adjacent to the joint space. Other findings are medullary fat necrosis of bone, polyserositis, and pulmonary infiltrates or embolism.

Laboratory evaluation is useful in establishing the diagnosis. In most patients the amylase or lipase, or both, are elevated. In many cases, however, one of the tests may be normal and the other abnormal, so both tests must be performed. Sixty percent of patients with pancreatic carcinoma and subcutaneous fat necrosis will have a peripheral eosinophilia.

The histologic features of pancreatic panniculitis are diagnostic. They include focal areas of fat necrosis with anucleate "ghost cells"; finely stippled basophilic material, representing calcium, within the residual rim of the necrotic cells and at the periphery of the affected foci; and a dense inflammatory polymorphous infiltrate at the periphery of the affected fat. The affected necrotic areas are relatively acellular. Several reports have suggested that the early features are those of a septal panniculitis, resembling EN. This may have represented sampling error but does indicate that if the initial sample is not diagnostic, another, perhaps more adequate, sample of a more advanced lesion should be considered.

The necrosis of fat at all affected sites is at least in part due to the release of fat-digesting enzymes, lipases, from the affected pancreatic tissue. These lipases spread hematogenously to the affected sites.

EN represents the primary differential consideration, since pancreatic panniculitis may not have abdominal symptoms, also favors the lower legs, and may be accompanied by joint symptoms. The distinction can be made by skin biopsy, serum amylase, and lipase determinations, and especially if eosinophilia is present, a search for a pancreatic neoplasm.

Treatment revolves mainly around treating the cause of the pancreatitis. Obstruction or stenosis of ducts should be repaired, pseudocysts drained, and in the case of pancreatic carcinoma, octreotide administered, if necessary.

Bogart MM, et al: Pancreatic panniculitis associated with acinic cell adenocarcinoma: a case report and review of the literature. Cutis 2007 Oct; 80(4):289–294.
García-Romero D, et al: Pancreatic panniculitis. Dermatol Clin 2008 Oct; 26(4):465–470.
Lee WS, et al: Fatal pancreatic panniculitis associated with acute pancreatitis: a case report. J Korean Med Sci 2007 Oct; 22(5):914–917.
Madarasingha NP, et al: Pancreatic panniculitis: a rare form of panniculitis. Dermatol Online J 2009; 15(3):17.
Suwattee P, et al: Pancreatic panniculitis in a 4-year-old child with nephrotic syndrome. Pediatr Dermatol 2007 Nov–Dec; 24(6):659–660.

Alpha1-antitrypsin deficiency panniculitis

Alpha1-antitrypsin is the most abundant antiprotease in circulation and a potent and irreversible inactivator of neutrophil elastase. Heterozygous deficiency of this enzyme occurs in 1 in 50 persons and homozygous deficiency in 1 in 2500 persons of European descent. Emphysema and liver disease are the most common manifestations of deficiency. A small percentage of patients with homozygous deficiency and the PiZZ or PiSZ phenotypes will develop panniculitis.

The panniculitis usually appears between the ages of 20 and 40 but can occur in childhood. Both sexes are equally affected. Lesions appear after relatively minor trauma and present as painful nodules on the extremities or trunk. They may spontaneously drain an oily, brown liquid. Multiple draining sinus tracts can occur, with lesions coalescing into large draining plaques.

The histologic findings in this form of panniculitis are dependent on the stage of the lesion. Early lesions show neutrophils splaying the collagen of the reticular dermis and subcutaneous septae. More fully evolved lesions show dissolution of the septae, with islands of normal fat "floating" in the spaces that represented the destroyed septae. This later finding is considered diagnostic by some. Elastic tissue stains may reveal decreased elastic tissue in the affected areas.

The clinical and histologic differential diagnosis is factitial panniculitis. This is not surprising since trauma produces both lesions, and in the case of the enzyme deficiency, the inflammation-produced enzymes are simply not inactivated, leading to more pronounced lesions than would be expected from that degree of trauma.

Replacement of the deficient enzyme will lead to resolution of the skin lesions, but is costly. Dapsone and doxycycline can also be therapeutic apparently by their ability to reduce neutrophil chemotaxis. Colchicine can be attempted if dapsone is not tolerated. These agents can reduce the requirement for enzyme replacement and should be considered as maintenance treatment in previously affected patients. Systemic steroids may exacerbate the panniculitis. Liver transplantation leads to normal levels of the enzyme and resolution of the panniculitis. Gene therapy and stem cell therapy appear promising.

Stoller JK, et al: Primary care diagnosis of alpha-1 antitrypsin deficiency: issues and opportunities. Cleve Clin J Med 2007 Dec; 74(12):869–874.

Valverde R, et al: Alpha-1-antitrypsin deficiency panniculitis. Dermatol Clin 2008 Oct; 26(4):447–451.

Wood AM, et al: Alpha one antitrypsin deficiency: from gene to treatment. Respiration 2007; 74(5):481–492.

Cytophagic histiocytic panniculitis

Cytophagic histiocytic panniculitis (CHP) is a multisystem disease characterized by widespread erythematous, painful, subcutaneous nodules, which may occasionally become ecchymotic or break down and form crusted ulcerations. There is a progressive febrile illness, with hepatosplenomegaly, pancytopenia, hypertriglyceridemia, and liver dysfunction. These result from the proliferation of benign-appearing histiocytes, which have a marked phagocytic capacity and extensively involve the reticuloendothelial system. Some patients progress to a terminal phase characterized by profound cytopenia, liver failure, and a terminal hemorrhagic diathesis.

CHP represents a spectrum of disease that occurs in children and adults. Some cases are triggered by viral infections (Epstein–Barr virus [EBV], human immunodeficiency virus [HIV]), and others represent subcutaneous B- or T-cell lymphomas. The benign cases are reportedly EBV-negative and the lymphoma-associated cases are EBV-positive.

Histologically, there is infiltration of the lobules of subcutaneous fat by histiocytes and inflammatory cells (primarily helper T cells), with fat necrosis and hemorrhage. The characteristic cell is a "bean bag" cell: a histiocyte stuffed with phagocytized red blood cells, lymphocytes, neutrophils, platelets, or fragments of these cells. These "bean bag" cells are not diagnostic of CHP and can be seen uncommonly in other panniculitides, especially lupus profundus. The presence of atypical lymphocytes or the detection of a clonal B- or T-cell proliferation supports the diagnosis of subcutaneous lymphoma in cases of CHP.

The treatment of CHP is difficult. If malignancy cannot be detected, cyclosporine has been effective in many cases, and combined treatment with high-dose corticosteroids, cyclosporine, and anakinra has been reported. If malignancy is detected, aggressive chemotherapy and perhaps bone marrow transplantation may be considered.

Behrens EM, et al: Interleukin 1 receptor antagonist to treat cytophagic histiocytic panniculitis with secondary hemophagocytic lymphohistiocytosis. J Rheumatol 2006 Oct; 33(10):2081–2084.

MISCELLANEOUS FORMS OF PANNICULITIS

Gouty panniculitis

Uric acid crystals may deposit initially in the subcutaneous fat, leading to lesions resembling other forms of panniculitis. Histologically, there is a lobular panniculitis with necrosis of adipocytes and infiltration of polymorphonuclear leukocytes. Feathery needle-like crystals in sheaves are present.

Dahiya A, et al: Gouty panniculitis in a healthy male. J Am Acad Dermatol 2007 Aug; 57(2 Suppl):S52–S54.

Lipodystrophy (lipoatrophy)

The lipodystrophies are conditions in which there is markedly reduced subcutaneous fat. They can be generalized (total), partial, or localized, and may be congenital or acquired. In the congenital types, women are more commonly and severely affected. Hypertriglyceridemia and diabetes mellitus with insulin resistance occur in many of the congenital and acquired forms of lipodystrophy. These syndromes were quite rare until the 1990s. With the advent of combination antiviral therapy for HIV infection (highly active antiretroviral therapy [HAART]), acquired lipodystrophy has become very common in geographic regions where HIV infection is prevalent. In addition, localized fat loss can be a consequence of therapeutic injections into the fat.

Congenital lipodystrophies

Congenital generalized lipodystrophy

Congenital generalized liposystrophy, also known as Berardinelli–Seip syndrome, is a rare autosomal-recessive condition. From birth there is an extreme paucity of fat in the subcutaneous tissue and other adipose tissues, giving affected persons a generalized muscular appearance. The mechanical fat of the palms, soles, joints, orbits, and scalp is not affected in some types of this syndrome. The children have a voracious appetite. They have increased height and height velocity, advanced bone age, muscular hypertrophy, and a masculine habitus. This habitus plus enlargement of the genitalia in infancy (clitoromegaly) can lead to the misdiagnosis of precocious puberty. Scalp hair is abundant and curly, and there is generalized hypertrichosis and hyperhidrosis. The abdomen is protuberant and the liver and spleen are enlarged. The overall appearance is acromegalic (Fig. 23-8) due to enlargement of the mandible, hands, and feet. Acanthosis nigricans is invariably present and often generalized. Hyperinsulinemia, insulin resistance, and diabetes appear often around puberty. The diabetes mellitus resists insulin and oral hypoglycemic therapy, but ketoacidosis does not occur. Hypertriglyceridemia occurs and can produce eruptive xanthomas; pancreatitis; and

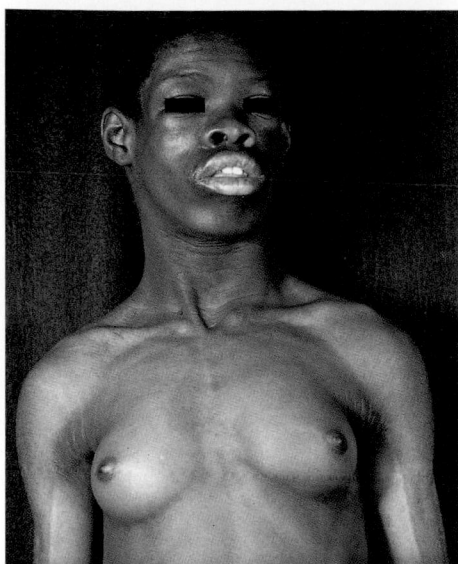

Fig. 23-8 Congenital generalized lipodystrophy.

fatty liver, which may eventuate in cirrhosis. Hypertrophic cardiomyopathy and mild mental retardation may occur. Lifespan is shortened, with patients frequently dying in young adulthood from complications of diabetes, or liver or heart disease. Mutations in three genes, *1-acylglycerol 3-phosphate-O-acyltransferase 2* (*AGPAT2*), *Berardinelli–Seip congenital lipodystrophy 2* (*BSCL2*), and *Caveolin-1* (*CAV1*), cause different subtypes of this disorder. A novel subtype with preservation of bone marrow fat, congenital muscular weakness, and cervical spine instability has also been described. Serum leptin and adiponectin levels are extremely low in various types. If leptin levels are low, leptin replacement decreases serum triglycerides and improves hyperglycemia. Twenty percent of patients with congenital generalized lipodystrophy do not have mutations in these two genes, suggesting there are other genetic causes.

Familial partial lipodystrophy

Familial partial lipodystrophy is a heterogenous autosomal-dominant group of disorders with distinct phenotypes. The most common variant is the Dunnigan type. Patients are normal at birth, but at around the time of puberty there is gradual loss of subcutaneous tissue from the arms and legs, and variably from the chest and anterior abdomen. Fat gain occurs in the face, neck, and intra-abdominally, resulting in a cushingoid appearance. Diabetes mellitus, hypertriglyceridemia, and atherosclerosis occur more frequently in female patients. The hypertriglyceridemia may result in pancreatitis and fatty liver, but cirrhosis has not been reported. The genetic defect in the Dunnigan variant of partial lipodystrophy is in the gene encoding lamins A and C (*LMNA*). Lamins are intermediate filaments integral to the nuclear envelope. The site of the mutation determines the phenotype expressed. Myopathy, muscular dystrophy, cardiomyopathy, and conducting system disturbances can occur in a minority of patients.

A second characterized form of familial partial lipodystrophy is related to mutations in the *PPAR-γ* gene. This rare syndrome is associated with marked loss of subcutaneous tissue of the forearms and calves, and less prominently on the upper arms and thighs. The trunk is spared and there is no excess fat on the neck. Diabetes mellitus, hypertriglyceridemia, hypertension, and hirsutism also occur. Other forms of familial partial lipodystrophy not associated with the above two mutations have been described, suggesting additional genetic causes of this syndrome.

Mandibuloacral dysplasia is an extremely rare autosomal-recessive condition with hypoplasia of the mandible and clavicle, acro-osteolysis, joint contractures, mottled cutaneous pigmentation, skin atrophy, alopecia, a bird-like facies, and dental anomalies. Two distinct patterns of lipodystrophy occur. Type A is characterized by loss of subcutaneous fat from the arms and legs, but normal to excess fat of the face and neck. Type B has a more generalized lipodystrophy. Hyperinsulinemia, insulin resistance, diabetes mellitus, and hyperlipidemia occur in some patients. Mutations in the *LMNA* gene have been reported in type A patients. Mutations in the zinc metalloproteinase (ZMPSTE24), which is involved in the processing of prelamin A, have also been responsible for mandibuloacral dysplasia. Autosomal-recessive neonatal progeroid syndrome is characterized by near total absence of fat from birth, with sparing of the sacral and gluteal areas.

Acquired lipodystrophy

Most cases are related to antiretroviral therapy, and severity may be related to genetic variations in resistin. Lipodystrophy occurs in up to 80% of HIV-infected patients, most of whom are being treated with combination anti-HIV therapy (HAART). The fat of the face, especially the buccal fat pads, buttocks, and limbs, is lost. There is increased fat deposition in other areas, especially the neck, upper back (buffalo hump), and intra-abdominally. It is related to non-nucleoside reverse transcriptase inhibitors which also inhibit the γDNA polymerase of mitochondria, leading to adipocyte apoptosis. As with the other acquired and inherited forms of lipodystrophy, patients may suffer from hypertriglyceridemia, hypercholesterolemia, and insulin resistance, especially if a protease inhibitor is a part of their treatment. Metformin therapy, at a dose of 500–850 mg twice a day, combined with exercise reduces the body mass index and waist circumference, as well as insulin resistance, but the trend has been towards treatment with thiazolidinediones. Antiretroviral-associated lipoatrophy slowly improves with prolonged rosiglitazone. Growth hormone reduces visceral fat, but the effects are short-lived. Various injectables may provide cosmetic improvement.

There are several idiopathic forms of acquired lipodystrophy. Although they appear later in life, are not inherited, and no genetic mutation has yet been described as being causal, they closely resemble the genetically determined diseases. Acquired lipodystrophy can be partial or generalized. In addition, hyperinsulinemia, hyperlipidemia, and diabetes mellitus may occur in patients with acquired lipodystrophy. Management involves controlling the hyperinsulinemia and its complications.

Acquired partial lipodystrophy (Barraquer–Simons syndrome)

Until HAART-associated lipodystrophy appeared, this was the most common form of lipodystrophy. Females outnumber males 4:1. It presents in the first and second decades. This progressive fat disorder is characterized by a diffuse and progressive loss of the subcutaneous fat that usually begins in the face and scalp, and progresses downward as far as the iliac crests, sparing the lower extremities. The upper half of the body looks emaciated and the cheeks sink in (Fig. 23-9A). There is an apparent, and sometimes real, adiposity of the buttocks, thighs, and legs, especially in affected women (Fig. 23-9B). The onset is insidious, with no discomfort or inflammation in the areas of fat loss. A few patients have developed other autoimmune diseases, including systemic lupus erythematosus and juvenile dermatomyositis.

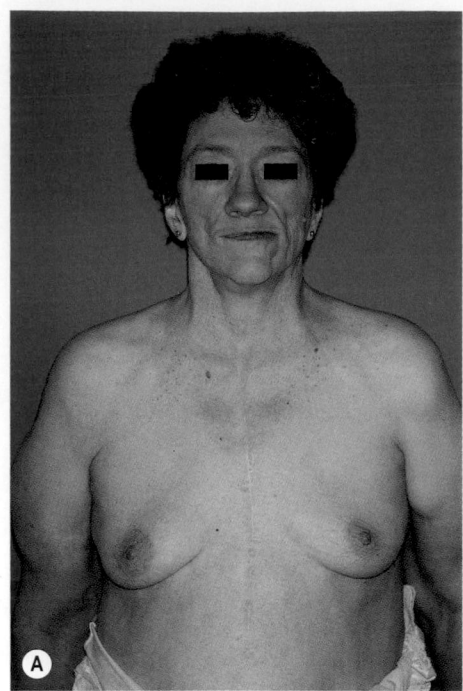
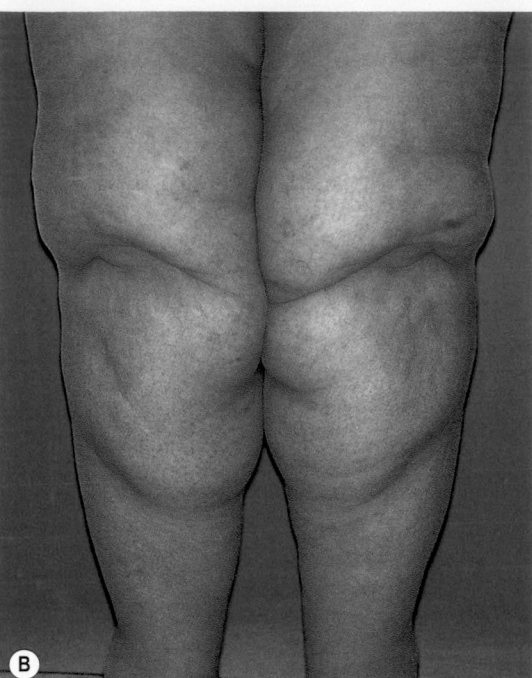

Fig. 23-9 Partial lipodystrophy, acquired. A, Face. B, hypertrophy of subcutaneous fat on the lower half of the body.

Downregulation of *PPAR-γ* and adiponectin, with impairment of mitochondrial gene expression, has been reported. Histologically, the skin is normal except for the absence of fat. Most patients with this form of lipodystrophy have reduced levels of C3 resulting from the presence of a circulating polyclonal IgG called "C3 nephritic factor." Proteinuria caused by membranoproliferative glomerulonephritis occurs in about 20% of patients, appearing about 8 years after the onset of the lipodystrophy. C3 nephritic factor stabilizes C3b,Bb (C3 convertase), leading to unopposed activation of the alternative complement system and excessive consumption of C3.

Acquired generalized lipodystrophy

This rare form of lipodystrophy appears during childhood or adolescence. Females outnumber males 3:1. The fat loss affects large areas of the body, particularly the face, arms, and legs. Mechanical fat of the palms and soles may be lost, but ocular and bone marrow fat are spared. Acanthosis nigricans is present. Hepatic steatosis and voracious appetite may be present. Cirrhosis occurs in about 20% of patients due to hepatitic steatosis or autoimmune hepatitis. Diabetes mellitus and hypertriglyceridemia may occur.

About 25% of patients will have a preceding inflammatory panniculitis at the onset of the syndrome. These patients tend to have less severe manifestations. Another 25% of patients with acquired generalized lipodystrophy have an associated connective tissue disease, especially juvenile dermatomyositis. Half of the patients give no history of panniculitis and have no connective tissue disease. One case has been associated with an abnormality of chromosome 10.

Centrifugal abdominal lipodystrophy

Most cases of "lipodystrophia centrifugalis abdominalis infantilis," as described by Imamura et al, have been reported from a single region of Japan. The cause is unknown. It is almost invariably a disease of childhood; 90% of cases begin at age 3. Girls outnumber boys 2:1. It is characterized by depression of the skin caused by loss of fat in the groin (80% of cases) or axilla (20% of cases). The atrophic area slowly enlarges centrifugally for 3–8 years in most cases, often stopping with the onset of

puberty. In 80% of cases the depressed area was surrounded by a discrete, erythematous border with scale. One-third of patients have multiple lesions and regional lymph nodes are enlarged in 65% of cases. The affected children are otherwise well. When the lesion stops expanding, the erythematous rim and lymphadenopathy disappear. After the progression stops, the skin returns to normal within a year or two.

Lipoatrophia annularis (Ferreira–Marques)

Lipoatrophia annularis primarily affects women and usually involves the upper extremity. The lipoatrophy may be preceded by erythema, a bracelet-shaped swelling, and tenderness of the entire extremity. This is followed by loss of subcutaneous fat so that the arm is divided into two parts by a depressed, atrophic, bracelet-like constriction. The depressed band is usually about 1 cm wide and up to 2 cm in depth. Arthralgias and pain of the affected extremity precede and accompany the process. The band persists for up to 20 years. The histology shows atrophy of the subcutaneous fat. The cause is unknown.

Localized lipodystrophy

Six months to 2 years after the initiation of insulin injections, localized atrophy of fat may develop at the sites, more frequently in children and women than in men. It may be a manifestation of connective tissue disease. This dystrophic change may resolve if patients are switched to human insulin. Much less often, insulin injections may result in lipohypertrophy. Rarely, injections of other medications may result in lipoatrophy.

Brown TT: Approach to the human immunodeficiency virus-infected patient with lipodystrophy. J Clin Endocrinol Metab 2008 Aug; 93(8):2937–2945.

Carey D, et al: Restorative interventions for HIV facial lipoatrophy. AIDS Rev 2008 Apr–Jun; 10(2):116–124.

Guallar JP, et al: Impaired expression of mitochondrial and adipogenic genes in adipose tissue from a patient with acquired partial lipodystrophy (Barraquer–Simons syndrome): a case report. J Med Case Reports 2008 Aug 27; 2:284.

Guaraldi G, et al: Lipodystrophy and quality of life of HIV-infected persons. AIDS Rev 2008 Jul–Sep; 10(3):152–161.

Herranz P, et al: Lipodystrophy syndromes. Dermatol Clin 2008 Oct; 26(4):569–578.

Macallan DC, et al: Treatment of altered body composition in HIV-associated lipodystrophy: comparison of rosiglitazone, pravastatin, and recombinant human growth hormone. HIV Clin Trials 2008 Jul–Aug; 9(4):254–268.

Marque M, et al: Lipoatrophic connective tissue panniculitis. Pediatr Dermatol 2010; 27(1):53–57.

Ranade K, et al: Genetic analysis implicates resistin in HIV lipodystrophy. AIDS 2008 Aug 20; 22(13):1561–1568.

Serrão VV, et al: Localized abdominal idiopathic lipodystrophy. Dermatol Online J 2008 Jul 15; 14(7):15.

Bonus images for this chapter can be found online at

http://www.expertconsult.com

Lipodystrophy

24 Endocrine Diseases

The skin interacts with the endocrine system in many ways. Some of these are discussed in this chapter.

Al Niaimi F, et al: Endocrinology and the skin. Br J Hosp Med (Lond) 2008; 69:510.

Jabbour S: Cutaneous manifestations of endocrine disorders. Am J Clin Dermatol 2003; 4:315.

Schneider JB, et al: Cutaneous manifestations of endocrine-metabolic disease and nutritional deficiency in the elderly. Dermatol Clin 2004; 22:23.

Acromegaly

Excess growth hormone in prepubertal children leads to gigantism, whereas once the epiphyseal growth plates close, such excess leads to acromegaly. In acromegaly, changes in the soft tissues and bones form a characteristic syndrome. In association with the well-known changes in the facial features caused by gigantic hypertrophy of the chin, nose, and supraorbital ridges, there is thickening, reddening, and wrinkling of the forehead, and exaggeration of the nasolabial grooves. The lips and tongue are thick. Cutis verticis gyrata is present in approximately 30% of patients. The hands and feet enlarge (Fig. 24-1), and there is gradual growth of the fingertips until they resemble drumsticks. There is diffuse hypertrophy of the skin, which is at least partly due to deposition of colloidal iron-positive material in the papillae and reticular dermis. This increased skin thickness can be demonstrated in lateral radiographs of the heel, with reversal toward normal after treatment. Skin thickness does not correlate well with growth hormone levels at the time of diagnosis. Skin tags are often present and the skin has an oily feel. Hypertrichosis, hyperpigmentation, and hyperhidrosis occur in many patients. The viscera also enlarge and patients may develop a variety of rheumatologic, cardiovascular, metabolic and respiratory complications.

The clinical changes may suggest the leonine facies of Hansen's disease, as well as Paget's disease, myxedema, and pachydermoperiostosis. Acromegaloid facial appearance syndrome is an inherited condition where only the facial changes are present, and no abnormality of growth hormone exists. Pseudoacromegaly is an acquired condition that may be seen in patients with severe insulin-resistant diabetes, which appears to be a fibroblast defect, or in patients on long-term minoxidil.

The cause of acromegaly is hypersecretion of growth hormone by the pituitary, usually because of an adenoma of the gland. Rare cases of ectopic growth hormone-releasing hormone producing tumors of the lung and pancreas have been reported. The peak age of diagnosis is in the forties. Measurement of serum insulin-like growth factor (somatomedin C), and of serum growth hormone after a glucose load, and magnetic resonance imaging (MRI) of the pituitary are diagnostic tests. It may occur as one of the manifestations of Carney complex, McCune–Albright syndrome, or multiple endocrine neoplasia-1.

The currently preferred treatment is a combination of transsphenoidal microsurgical excision of the tumor followed by medical therapy for residual disease. Octreotide and lanreotide are potent, long-acting inhibitors of growth hormone (somatostatin analogs) that are given as once-a-month or biweekly intramuscular depot injections. Fatigue, paresthesias, and headaches improve rapidly. With continuous treatment, soft-tissue swelling and facial coarsening improve as growth hormone levels decline in almost all patients. After 18–24 months of therapy 50% of patients will completely normalize, with the exception of hyperhidrosis, which persists in most patients. The dopamine agonist bromocriptine suppresses growth hormone secretion and is used as an adjuvant medical therapy in some cases. The growth hormone receptor antagonist pegvisomant is another medical option to normalize growth hormone secretion. Radiation is generally reserved for recalcitrant cases.

Al-Bedaia M, et al: Acromegaly presenting as cutis verticis gyrata. Int J Dermatol 2008; 47:164.

Ben-Shlomo A, et al: Skin manifestations in acromegaly. Clin Dermatol 2006; 24:256.

Davidovici BB, et al: Cutaneous manifestations of pituitary gland diseases. Clin Dermatol 2008; 26:288.

Nguyen KH, et al: Pseudoacromegaly induced by the long-term use of minoxidil. J Am Acad Dermatol 2003; 48:962.

Yaqub A, et al: Insulin-mediated pseudoacromegaly. W V Med J 2008; 1104:12.

Zen PR, et al: Acromegaloid facial appearance and hypertrichosis. Clin Dysmorphol 2004; 13:49.

Cushing syndrome

Chronic excess of glucocorticoids leads to a wide variety of signs and symptoms. Among the most prominent features of this syndrome is central obesity, affecting the face, neck, trunk, and markedly the abdomen, but sparing the limbs. There is classically deposition of fat over the upper back, referred to as a buffalo hump. This may be treated with liposuction. The face becomes moon-shaped, being wide and round. The peak age of onset is in the twenties and thirties.

The striking and distressing skin changes include hypertrichosis, dryness, acne, susceptibility to superficial dermatophyte and *Pityrosporon* infections, a plethora over the cheeks, anterior neck, and V of the chest, and the characteristic purplish, atrophic striae which may involve the abdomen (Fig. 24-2), buttocks, back, breasts, upper arms, and thighs. Skin fragility and thinning occur such that easy bruising and a cigarette paper-type wrinkling are present. The skin may easily pull off when adhesive tape is removed (Liddle's sign). The thinning of the skin can be demonstrated and measured in lateral radiographs of the heels. There is reversal with treatment. Women, who are affected four times more frequently than men in noniatrogenic cases, develop facial lanugo hypertrichosis, with thinning of the scalp hair. Occasionally, there may be livedo reticularis, purpura, ecchymosis, or brownish pigmentation. Poikiloderma-like changes have been observed. Opportunistic fungal infections occur; these may be with organisms that are not normally pathogenic, or may be uncommon presentations of common infections.

There is usually hypertension and marked generalized arteriosclerosis, with progressive weakness, prostration, and pains in the back, limbs, and abdomen; also kyphosis of the dorsal spine occurs, accentuating the buffalo appearance. Osteoporosis occurs and there is generally a loss of libido. In 20% of patients a disturbance in carbohydrate metabolism develops, with hyperglycemia, glycosuria, and diabetes mellitus.

These varied symptoms indicate a marked and widespread disturbance caused by the hyperactive adrenal cortex. When microadenomas of the pituitary produce these clinical findings, it is referred to as Cushing's disease. This accounts for only 10% of patients. Between 40% and 60% of additional cases are due to increased adrenocorticotropic hormone (ACTH) production by the pituitary, but no adenoma is identified. Adrenal adenomas and carcinomas, and ectopic production of

ACTH by other tumors, account for the remainder of cases of noniatrogenic Cushing syndrome. Iatrogenic Cushing syndrome is usually secondary to systemic administration of corticosteroids; however, absorption from topically applied steroids may occur, especially in children. Primary pigmented nodular adrenocortical disease leading to Cushing syndrome occurs in 30% of patients with Carney complex. With alcohol abuse the clinical findings of Cushing syndrome may be mimicked, producing the pseudo-Cushing syndrome.

A rapid screening test for Cushing syndrome consists of oral administration of 1 mg of dexamethasone at 11 pm, followed at 8 am by a fluorometric determination of plasma cortisol. A cortisol level below 3 µg/dL essentially rules out Cushing syndrome, except for the iatrogenic variety, in which there is adrenocortical hypoplasia, and the serum cortisol level is very low even without dexamethasone suppression. If this test is positive, it must be confirmed by doing a 24 h urinary free cortisol test. A value of at least three times the upper limit of normal is 95–100% sensitive and specific. A serum ACTH is then obtained to determine if the source is the adrenals, or a pituitary or ectopic tumor (low, normal or high, and very high, respectively). Treatment is primarily surgical removal of the tumor; however, radiation, chemotherapy, or medication that blocks steroid synthesis is occasionally employed.

Arnaldi G, et al: Diagnosis and complications of Cushing's syndrome. J Clin Endocrinol Metab 2003; 88:593.
Davidovici BB, et al: Cutaneous manifestations of pituitary gland diseases. Clin Dermatol 2008; 26:288.
Kim S, et al: Erysipeloid sporotrichosis in a woman with Cushing's disease. J Am Acad Dermatol 1999; 40:272.
Lionakis MS, et al: Glucocorticoids and invasive fungal infections. Lancet 2003; 362:1828.
Shibli-Rahhal A, et al: Cushing's syndrome. Clin Dermatol 2006; 24:260.
Vaughan ED Jr: Diseases of the adrenal gland. Med Clin North Am 2004; 88:443.

Addison's disease

Adrenal insufficiency is manifested in the skin primarily by hyperpigmentation (Fig. 24-3). It is diffuse but most prominently observed in sun-exposed areas and sites exposed to recurrent trauma or pressure. The axillae, perineum, and nipples are also affected. Palmar crease darkening in patients of lighter skin type, scar hyperpigmentation, and darkening of nevi, mucous membranes, hair, and nails may all be seen. An eruptive onset of multiple new nevi may be an early sign of Addison's disease. Occasionally, pigmentation may not occur; this is referred to as white Addison's disease. Decreased axillary and pubic hair is seen in women, as their androgen

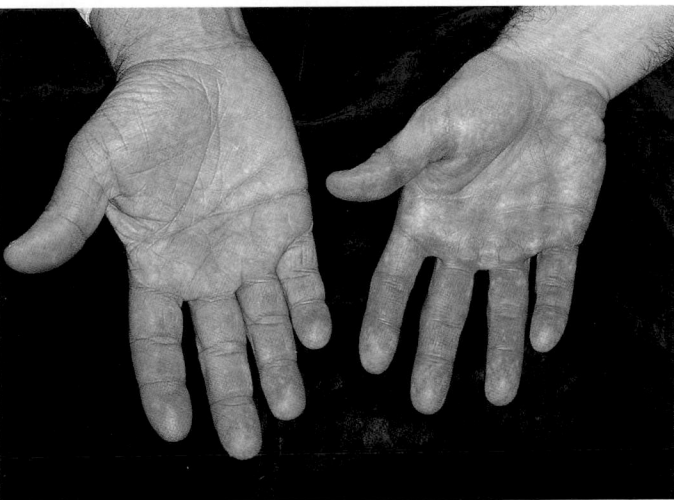

Fig. 24-1 Acromegaly. Patient with acromegaly on the left compared to normal-sized hand on the right.

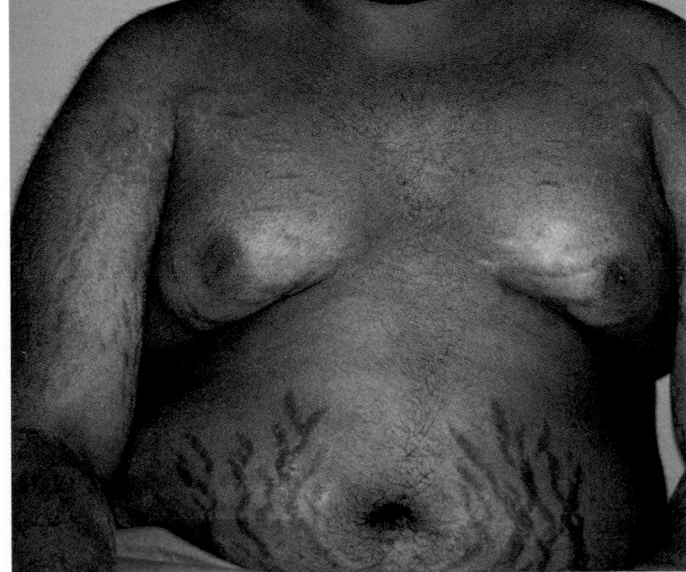

Fig. 24-2 Cushing syndrome.

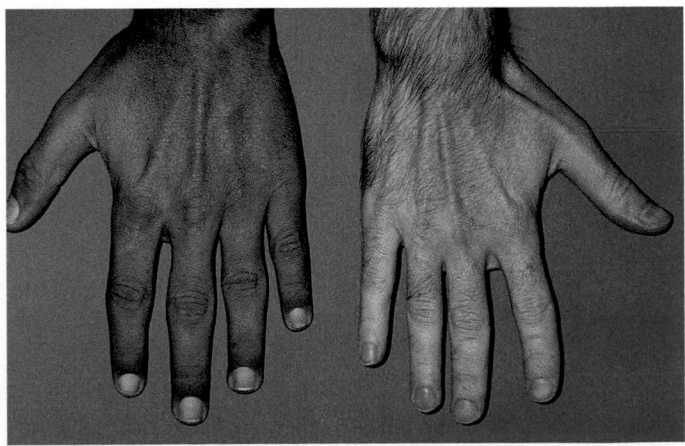

Fig. 24-3 Hyperpigmentation in Addison's disease.

production primarily occurs in the adrenals. Fibrosis and calcification of the pinnae of the ears are rare complications.

Systemic signs such as weight loss, nausea, vomiting, diarrhea, weakness, fatigue, and hypotension add specificity to the cutaneous abnormalities. Addison's disease is usually the result of autoantibody destruction of adrenocortical tissue; however, infection, hemorrhage, or infiltration may be the cause of adrenal insufficiency. In young boys suspected of having Addison's disease, adrenoleukodystrophy must be considered. Hyperpigmentation may precede neurologic signs, so very-long-chain fatty acid levels should be determined. Addison's disease may be part of polyglandular autoimmune syndromes I and II, in which various combinations of hypoparathyroidism, chronic candidiasis, vitiligo or autoimmune thyroiditis, and diabetes may occur.

Diagnosis is made by obtaining a serum cortisol, followed by stimulation with cosyntropin. Failure to see an elevation above 20 μg/dL in 1 h is diagnostic. Plasma ACTH is elevated in primary insufficiency but normal to low in patients with secondary adrenal insufficiency, where the damage is in the hypothalamic/pituitary axis. The adrenals should be imaged with computed tomography (CT) to exclude infiltration or infection. Treatment is the replacement of the glucocorticoids and mineralocorticoids.

Burk CJ, et al: Addison's disease, diffuse skin and mucosal hyperpigmentation with subtle "flu-like" symptoms. Pediatr Dermatol 2008; 25:215.

Kendereski A, et al: White Addison's disease. J Endocrinol Invest 1999; 22:395.

Nieman LK, et al: Addison's disease. Clin Dermatol 2006; 24:276.

Prat C, et al: Longitudinal melanonychia as the first sign of Addison's disease. J Am Acad Dermatol 2008; 58:522.

Shah SS, et al: Addisonian pigmentation of the oral mucosa. Cutis 2005; 76:97.

Panhypopituitarism and growth hormone deficiency

Pituitary failure results in many changes in the skin, hair, and nails as a result of the absence of pituitary hormone action on these sites. Pale, thin, dry skin is seen. Hypohidrosis is present. Diffuse loss of body hair occurs, with axillary, pubic, and head hair being especially thin. The nails are thin, fragile, and opaque, and grow slowly. Compromise of the pituitary is usually caused by a pituitary tumor, although infiltration, infection, trauma, hemorrhage or hypothalamic tumors may be the etiology. Thyroid hormone, glucocorticoids, sex steroids, and growth hormones are low and require replacement. A pituitary MRI will screen for tumors or infiltrative processes.

Davidovici BB, et al: Cutaneous manifestations of pituitary gland diseases. Clin Dermatol 2008; 26:288.

Smith JC: Hormone replacement therapy in hypopituitarism. Expert Opin Pharmacother 2004; 5:1023.

Androgen-dependent syndromes

The androgen-dependent syndromes are caused by the excessive production of adrenal or gonadal androgens by adrenal adenomas, carcinoma, or hyperplasia, Leydig cell tumors in men, and arrhenoblastomas and polycystic ovarian syndrome (PCOS) in women. The latter is defined as the association of biochemical or clinical androgenism with chronic anovulation without specific underlying disease of the adrenal or pituitary glands.

The cutaneous signs of excessive androgen in women include acne, hirsutism, temporal balding and androgen-induced patterned scalp hair loss, seborrhea, enlargement of the clitoris, and decreased breast size. Hyperpigmentation of the skin, areolae, genitalia, palmar creases, and buccal mucosa

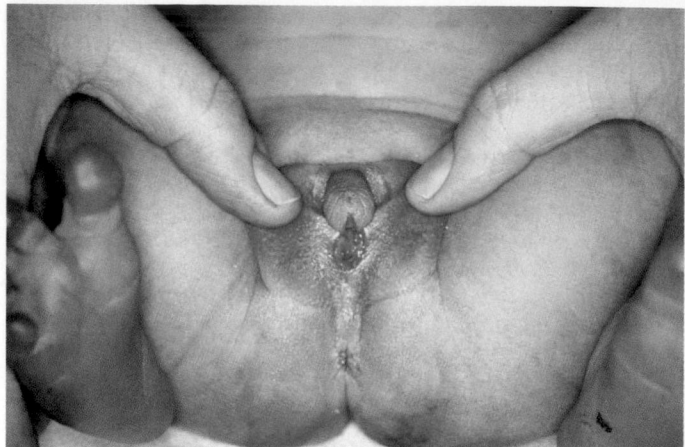

Fig. 24-4 Adrenogenital syndrome.

develops in some patients. Acanthosis nigricans is common in PCOS, reflecting insulin resistance. Diabetes mellitus, cardiovascular complications, and sleep apnea are associated comorbidities of PCOS. The association of endometrial cancer is suggested but remains unproven in women. Females may also develop a deepening voice, increased muscle mass, galactorrhea, and irregular or absent periods.

In the congenital adrenogenital syndrome, excess androgen is produced by an inherited defect in any of the five enzymatic steps required to convert cholesterol to cortisol. The formation of inadequate amounts of cortisol stimulates the pituitary to secrete excessive ACTH, which leads to excess androgen production. In boys, precocious puberty results. In girls, masculinization occurs, with the prominent cutaneous signs of excess androgen production (Fig. 24-4). Among these may be childhood acne. It may begin before age 9 and manifest as primarily comedonal lesions in the central face associated with advanced bone age. Many children with this presentation of acne, however, reveal no abnormality. Accelerated bone growth with early closure of the epiphyseal plates results in short stature. Early appearance of pubic and axillary hair is also seen.

Testing includes serum total testosterone and dehydroepiandrosterone sulfate (DHEA-S). If the total testosterone is greater than 200 ng/dL, ovarian imaging is indicated to assess for an ovarian tumor. If DHEA-S is 2–3 times the upper limit, an adrenal mass should be suspected and a CT scan of the adrenals is needed. In congenital adrenal hyperplasia, testing should include levels of cortisol, aldosterone, and precursor hormones, and in some cases Cortrosyn stimulation tests. Nonclassic adrenal hyperplasia is most commonly related to 21-hydroxylase deficiency, and may present as PCOS. It is best diagnosed by a corticotropin-stimulated 17-hydroxyprogesterone (17-HP) level greater than 10 ng/mL (30.3 nmol/L). The diagnosis can be confirmed by genotyping of the *CYP21* gene. The baseline 17-HP level has been used as a screening test. Although the sensitivity and specificity of the test have been challenged, levels of 17-HP lower than 2 ng/mL (6.0 nmol/L) have a fairly good negative predictive value, and those greater than 4 ng/mL (12.0 nmol/L) have a fairly good positive predictive value. The question remains whether treatment with corticosteroid replacement results in better outcomes than empiric antiandrogen therapy.

Treatment of the cutaneous signs of androgen excess is successful with an oral contraceptive and often also an androgen-blocking agent such as cyproterone acetate, flutamide, and finasteride. Spironolactone, which competes for the androgen cytosol receptors, has proved useful as a systemic antiandrogen in the treatment of hirsutism and acne. Laser hair removal and standard acne therapy are also effective. Adrenal–androgenic female pattern alopecia may improve with topical minoxidil or spironolactone. Metformin is commonly employed to improve insulin responsiveness. Chorionic villous biopsy may identify homozygous adrenogenital female fetuses and allow for dexamethasone therapy to prevent intrauterine virilization of the external genitalia.

Azziz R, et al: The Androgen Excess and PCOS Society criteria for the polycystic ovary syndrome. Fertil Steril 2009; 91:456.

Dewailly D: Nonclassic 21-hydroxylase deficiency. Semin Reprod Med 2002; 20:243.

Heymann WR: Hyperandrogenism and the skin. J Am Acad Dermatol 2004; 50:937.

Lee AT, et al: Dermatologic manifestations of polycystic ovary syndrome. Am J Clin Dermatol 2007; 8:201.

Martin KA, et al: Evaluation and treatment of hirsutism in premenopausal women. J Clin Endocrinol Metab 2008; 93:105.

Nisenblat V, et al: Androgens and polycystic ovary syndrome. Curr Opin Endocrinol Diabetes Obes 2009; 16:224–231.

Speiser PW, et al: Congenital adrenal hyperplasia. N Engl J Med 2003; 349:776.

Hypothyroidism

Hypothyroidism is a deficiency of circulating thyroid hormone, or rarely peripheral resistance to hormonal action. Deficiency may be caused by iodine deficiency, late-stage Hashimoto autoimmune thyroiditis, or pituitary or hypothalamic disease causing central hypothyroidism, or it may be iatrogenic secondary to surgery, radioactive iodine treatment, or drug therapy with lithium, interferon, or bexarotene. It may also complicate anticonvulsant and minocycline hypersensitivity syndromes, appearing approximately 2 months after the eruption has resolved. The condition produces various clinical manifestations, depending on when in life it occurs and on its severity. Middle-aged women are the most commonly affected adults. Patients with Turner and Down syndrome are predisposed to hypothyroidism and the production of thyroid autoantibodies. There are a wide array of immunologic conditions associated with Hashimoto thyroiditis such as autoimmune polyglandular syndrome types II and III, vitiligo, connective tissue disease, and autoimmune urticaria.

An autosomal-recessive variant of ectodermal dysplasia reported as ANOTHER (alopecia, nail dystrophy, ophthalmic complications, thyroid dysfunction, hypohidrosis, ephelides and enteropathy, and respiratory tract infections) syndrome has been described.

Cretinism

Thyroid deficiency in fetal life produces the characteristic picture of cretinism at birth and in the next few months of life. Depending on the degree of thyroid deficiency, a wide variety of signs and symptoms may be evident. The main consequence of extreme thyroid deficiency is cretinism and its attendant mental retardation, but much more prevalent are lesser degrees of intellectual and neurologic deficits seen in areas where iodized salt is still not routinely available.

The person with cretinism has cool, dry, pasty white to yellowish skin. Disturbances in the amount, texture, and distribution of the hair with patchy alopecia are common. Pigmentation is less than normal after exposure to sunlight. Sweating is greatly diminished. The lips are pale, thick, and protuberant. The tongue is usually enlarged, and there is delayed dentition. Wide-set eyes, a broad, flat nose, and periorbital puffiness characterize the face. A protuberant abdomen with umbilical hernia; acral swelling; coarse, dry, brittle nails; a clavicular fat pad; and hypothermia with cutis marmorata are also seen.

Myxedema

When lack of secretion of thyroid hormone is severe, myxedema is produced. The skin becomes rough and dry, and in severe cases of primary myxedema, ichthyosis vulgaris may be simulated. The facial skin is puffy; the expression is often dull and flat; macroglossia, swollen lips, and a broad nose are present; and chronic periorbital infiltration secondary to deposits of mucopolysaccharides frequently develops (Fig. 24-5A). Such infiltrate can lead to a cutis verticis gyrata appearance of the scalp. Carotenemia may cause a yellow tint in the skin that is especially prominent on the palms and soles. Diffuse hair loss is common, and the outer third of the

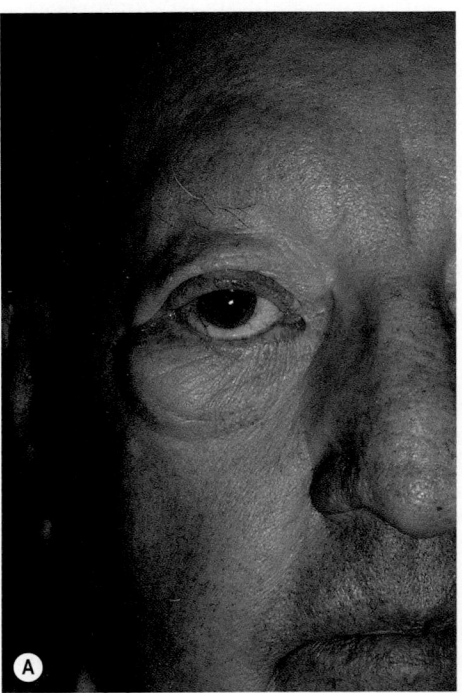

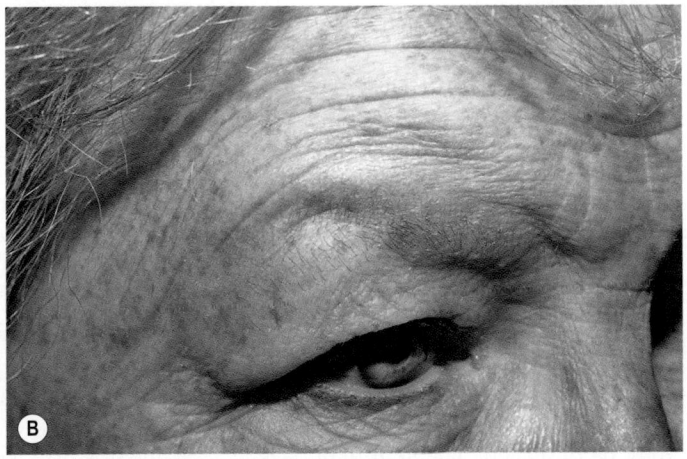

Fig. 24-5 A, Periorbital infiltration with mucopolysaccharides. B, Loss of lateral eyebrow.

eyebrows is shed (Fig. 24-5B). The hair becomes coarse and brittle. The free edges of the nails break easily, and onycholysis may occur.

Mild hypothyroidism

Lesser degrees of deficiency are common and far less easily diagnosed. Coldness of hands and feet in the absence of vascular disease, sensitivity to cool weather, lack of sweating, tendency to put on weight, need for extra sleep, drowsiness in the daytime, and constipation all suggest possible hypothyroidism and the need for appropriate tests. Palmoplantar keratoderma may be a sign of hypothyroidism and will resolve after thyroid replacement is given.

Diagnosis and treatment

An increased thyroid-stimulating hormone (TSH) test is the best diagnostic test for primary hypothyroidism. T3 and T4 are low. In Hashimoto thyroiditis, the most common cause of hypothyroidism in the US, thyroid peroxidase antibodies are present in 95% of patients and antithyroglobulin antibodies in 65%. In those with positive antibodies but normal thyroid function, hypothyroidism will develop at a rate of 5% per year. Thyroid hormone replacement will reverse the skin findings of hypothyroidism.

Ai J, et al: Autoimmune thyroid disease: etiology, pathogenesis, and dermatologic manifestations. J Am Acad Dermatol 2003; 48:641.

Brown RJ, et al: Minocycline-induced drug hypersensitivity syndrome followed by multiple autoimmune sequelae. Arch Dermatol 2009; 145:63.

Burman KD, et al: Dermatologic aspects of thyroid disease. Clin Dermatol 2006; 24:247.

Doshi DN, et al: Cutaneous manifestations of thyroid disease. Clin Dermatol 2008; 26:283.

Dunn JT: Endemic goiter and cretinism. J Pediatr Endocrinol Metab 2001; 14(Suppl 6):1469.

Gratton CEH, et al: Chronic urticaria. J Am Acad Dermatol 2002; 46:645.

Miller JJ, et al: Palmoplantar keratoderma associated with hypothyroidism. Br J Dermatol 1998; 139:741.

Nakatsui T, et al: Onycholysis and thyroid disease. J Cutan Med Surg 1998; 3:40.

Hyperthyroidism

Excessive quantities of circulating thyroid hormone may be caused by Graves' thyroiditis (diffuse toxic goiter), a multinodular toxic goiter (Plummer's disease) or a single toxic thyroid nodule, early Hashimoto autoimmune thyroiditis, a TSH-secreting pituitary adenoma, pituitary resistance to thyroid hormone, metastatic thyroid cancer, or excessive human chorionic gonadatropin. The most common etiology is Graves' disease, which accounts for about 55% of cases; it is mediated by thyroid-stimulating antibodies that bind to the TSH receptor, mimic the effects of TSH, and induce hyperthyroidism. There are many skin changes common to all forms of hyperthyroidism. The cutaneous surface is warm, moist, and smooth-textured. Palmar erythema or facial flushing may be seen. The hair is thin and has a downy texture, and nonscarring diffuse alopecia may be observed. The skin may darken to produce a bronzed appearance or melanoderma; sometimes melasma of the cheeks is seen. Nail changes are present in approximately 5% of patients with Plummer nails, a concave contour of the plate with distal onycholysis being characteristic. Hyperhidrosis may be noted.

Graves' disease has a female to male ratio of 7:1, and the peak age at onset is 20–30 years. It is the most common cause of noniatrogenic hyperthyroidism. Ophthalmopathy, pretibial

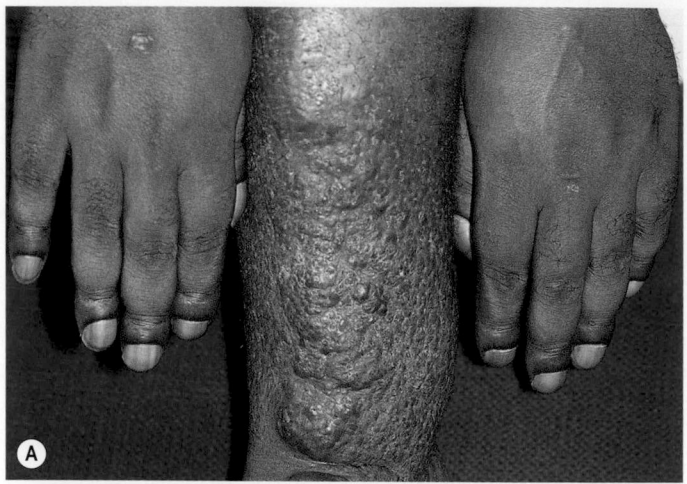

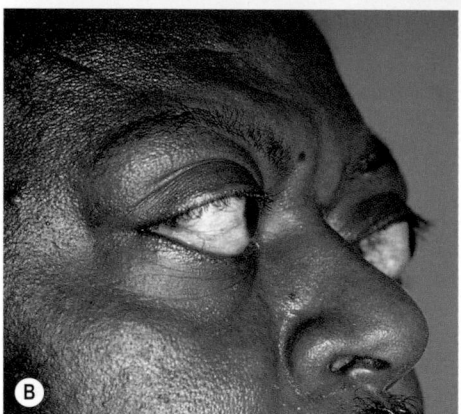

Fig. 24-6 A, Thyroid acropachy and pretibial myxoedema. B, Exophthalmos.

myxedema, and thyroid acropachy are findings nearly always limited to Graves patients (Fig. 24-6). Thyroid acropachy, seen in approximately 0.1–1% of Graves patients, is characterized by digital clubbing, soft-tissue swelling of the hands and feet, and diaphyseal proliferation of the periosteum in acral and distal long bones (tibia, fibula, ulna, and radius). It usually occurs after treatment of hyperthyroidism and is frequently associated with exophthalmos and pretibial myxedema. It may, however, occasionally precede the thyrotoxicosis and has been recognized in euthyroid and hypothyroid patients. It can be confused clinically with acromegaly, pachydermoperiostosis, pulmonary osteoarthropathy, or osteoperiostitis, but the radiologic findings are pathognomonic.

Pretibial myxedema, consisting of bilateral, localized, cutaneous accumulations of glycosaminoglycans, occurs in 4% of patients who have or have had Graves' disease. The morphology may vary from a nonpitting infiltration to nodules, plaques, and even an elephantiasic form where the skin is thickened, firm, and hyperpigmented from just below the knees to the feet. It may also uncommonly occur during the course of Hashimoto thyroiditis and primary hypothyroidism. Patients with pretibial myxedema regularly have associated ophthalmopathy and occasionally have thyroid acropachy. While it is not usually clinically apparent, approximately half of patients with Graves' disease have mucopolysaccharide deposition in the preradial area of the extensor aspects of the forearms. Lesions of the shoulder, hands, thigh, and scalp have been reported.

Improvement in the plaques of pretibial myxedema has resulted from intralesional injections of triamcinolone acetonide and with high-potency topical steroids under occlusion. Systemic steroids are usually not helpful. Compression stockings or complete decongestive physiotherapy, and a combination of manual lymphatic drainage, bandaging, and exercise, are useful and safe. Improvement with intravenous immunoglobulin of the skin, eye, and immunologic parameters has been reported in small series of patients. Pentoxifylline, octreotide, plasmapheresis, and cytotoxic drugs have all been reported to help in small numbers of patients, but negative reports also exist.

Vitiligo is present in 7% of patients with Graves' disease and occurs with an increased frequency in Hashimoto thyroiditis. Urticaria may be seen in patients with thyroid autoantibodies and may clear with the administration of thyroid hormone, even in euthyroid patients. A wide range of other autoimmune disorders may be seen in patients with Graves or Hashimoto autoimmune thyroiditis.

The TSH level is low in all patients except those with a TSH-secreting pituitary adenoma. Free T3 and T4 are elevated. Anti-TSH antibodies are present in nearly all Graves patients. A 24 h radioiodine scan will also help define the etiology. Treatment is with radioactive iodine or antithyroid drugs such as methimazole or propylthiouracil.

Ai J, et al: Autoimmune thyroid disease: etiology, pathogenesis, and dermatologic manifestations. J Am Acad Dermatol 2003; 48:641.

Anderson CK, et al: Triad of exophthalmos, pretibial myxedema, and acropachy in a patient with Graves' disease. J Am Acad Dermatol 2003; 48:970.

Artantas S, et al: Skin findings in thyroid diseases. Eur J Intern Med 2009; 20:158.

Doutre MS: Chronic urticaria and thyroid auto-immunity. Clin Rev Allergy Immunol 2006; 30:31.

Heymann W (ed): Thyroid Disorders with Cutaneous Manifestations. Heidelberg: Springer, 2008.

Mota A, et al: Thyroid acropachy. J Clin Rheumatol 2007; 13:360.

Pineda AM, et al: Oral pentoxifylline and topical clobetasol propionate ointment in the treatment of pretibial myxoedema, with concomitant improvement of Graves' ophthalmopathy. J Eur Acad Dermatol Venereol 2007, 21:1441.

Hypoparathyroidism

Varied changes in the skin and its appendages may be evident in this condition of parathyroid hormone (PTH) deficiency. Most pronounced is faulty dentition when hypoparathyroidism is present during development of the permanent teeth. The skin is dry and scaly. A diffuse scantiness of the hair and complete absence of axillary and pubic hair may be found. The nails are brittle and malformed. Onycholysis with fungal infection may be present. Of patients with idiopathic hypoparathyroidism, 15% develop mucocutaneous candidiasis. Hypoparathyroidism is the most frequent endocrine abnormality present in patients with the APECED (autoimmune polyendocrinopathy, candidiasis, ectodermal dystrophy) syndrome. In autoimmune polyendocrinopathy syndrome type I, hypoparathyroidism is present in association with Addison's disease and chronic candidiasis. Hypoparathyroidism may additionally occur in DiGeorge syndrome, or with parathyroid infiltration or their inadvertent surgical removal during thyroid surgery. Hypoparathyroidism with resultant hypocalcemia may trigger bouts of impetigo herpetiformis or pustular psoriasis.

Pseudohypoparathyroidism (PH) is an autosomal-dominant or X-linked inherited disorder characterized by end-organ unresponsiveness to PTH. The PTH and phosphorus levels are high, whereas the serum calcium is low. The typical clinical findings include short stature; obesity; round face; prominent forehead; low nasal bridge; attached earlobes; short neck; short, wide nails; delayed dentition; mental deficiency; amenorrhea; blue sclera; and cataracts. Brachycephaly, microcephaly, and shortened metacarpals or metatarsals, especially of

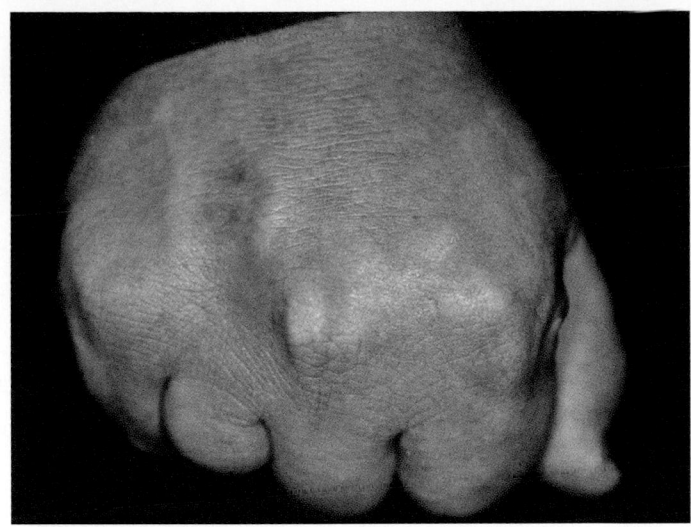

Fig. 24-7 Albright's sign in pseudohypoparathyroidism.

the fourth and fifth digits, occur because of premature epiphyseal closure. The latter results in short, stubby fingers and toes, with dimpling over the metacarpophalangeal joints (Albright's sign) (Fig. 24-7). Subcutaneous calcification and ossification occur commonly in this disorder, as they may in pseudopseudohypoparathyroidism (PPH), which has the same phenotype, but patients have normal serum and calcium levels. PH and PPH are two types of Albright hereditary osteodystrophy. In PH type 1a there is a defect in a G protein that couples receptors for several hormones to adenylate cyclase. This causes a generalized resistance to agents acting through the cAMP pathway and explains the frequent association of hypothyroidism and hypogonadism.

Betterle C, et al: Update on autoimmune polyendocrine syndromes (APS). Acta Biomed Ateneo Parmense 2003; 74:9.

Erbegci Z, et al: A case of recurrent impetigo herpetiformis with a positive family history. Int J Clin Pract 2000; 54:619.

Levine MA, et al: Genetic basis for resistance to parathyroid hormone. Horm Res 2003; 60(Suppl 3):87.

Shimizu T, et al: Massive calcification in pseudohypoparathyroidism. N Engl J Med 2003; 349:464.

Hyperparathyroidism

Whereas PTH regulates calcium levels, calcinosis cutis may develop from excess PTH. This can occur when the serum calcium/phosphorus product is greater than 65 mg/dL. This may manifest as large subcutaneous nodules or white, often linearly arranged, papules centered about joints. Additionally, calciphylaxis, while most common in the setting of secondary hyperparathyroidism and renal failure, may be seen occasionally in primary hyperparathyroidism.

Multiple endocrine neoplasia (MEN) type I is characterized by tumors of the parathyroids, endocrine pancreas, anterior pituitary, thyroid, and adrenal glands. The most commonly observed abnormality is hypercalcemia from hypersecreting tumors of the parathyroid glands. This autosomal-dominantly inherited disease usually presents in the fourth decade of life with clinical symptoms related to hypersecretion of hormone. Patients may also manifest multiple angiofibromas, collagenomas, café-au-lait macules, lipomas, confetti-like hypopigmentation, and gingival macules. The angiofibromas are smaller and less numerous than those present in tuberous sclerosis. Tumors in both MEN I and tuberous sclerosis apparently arise because of abnormalities within a tumor suppressor gene. The *MEN I* gene, which is present on chromosome 11, has a protein product termed menin whose function is yet to be delineated.

Additionally, approximately 20–40% of cases of sporadic parathyroid adenomas have been linked to overexpression of cyclin D1, a key regulator of the cell cycle.

Arnold A, et al: Molecular pathogenesis of primary hyperparathyroidism. J Bone Miner Res 2002; 17(Suppl 2):N30.

Mirza I, et al: An unusual presentation of calciphylaxis due to primary hyperparathyroidism. Arch Pathol Lab Med 2001; 125:1351.

Vidal A, et al: Cutaneous lesions associated to multiple endocrine neoplasia syndrome type 1. J Eur Acad Dermatol Venereol 2008, 22:835.

Xia Y, et al: Rapidly growing collagenomas in multiple endocrine neoplasia type 1. J Am Acad Dermatol 2007; 56:877.

Acanthosis nigricans

Acanthosis nigricans (AN) is characterized by hyperpigmentation and velvet-textured plaques, which are symmetrically distributed. The regions affected may be the face, neck, axillae (Fig. 24-8), external genitals, groin, inner aspects of the thighs, flexor and extensor surface of the elbows and knees, dorsal joints of the hands, umbilicus, and anus. With extensive involvement, lesions can be found on the areolae, conjunctiva, lips, and buccal mucosa, and around the umbilicus. Rarely, the involvement may be almost universal. The color of the patches is grayish, brownish, or black. The palms or soles may show thickening of the palmar skin with exaggeration of the dermatoglyphs. In severe cases a rugose hypertrophy occurs and can be a sign of malignancy. Small, papillomatous, non-pigmented lesions and pigmented macules may occasionally be found in the mucous membranes of the mouth, pharynx, and vagina. Acrochordons are a frequent accompaniment in the axillae and groin. There is a clear predisposition for certain racial groups to manifest AN, with Native Americans most commonly affected, followed by African Americans and Hispanics, all above the rates in Caucasians. This is obesity-independent.

Type I: acanthosis nigricans associated with malignancy

The rare type of AN may either precede (18%), accompany (60%), or follow (22%) the onset of the internal cancer. It is generally the most striking type clinically, both from the standpoint of extent of involvement and the pronounced nature of the lesions (Fig. 24-9). Most cases are associated with adenocarcinoma, especially of the gastrointestinal tract (60% stomach), lung, and breast, or less often the gallbladder, pancreas, esophagus, liver, prostate, kidney, colon, rectum, uterus, and ovaries. Other types of cancer and lymphoma may be seen also. A few cases have been observed in childhood, but most begin after puberty or in adulthood. This type should be highly suspected if widespread lesions develop in a nonobese male aged over 40.

Tripe palms (acanthosis palmaris) are characterized by thickened, velvety palms with pronounced dermatoglyphics; 95% occur in patients with cancer and 77% are seen with AN (Fig. 24-10). In 40% of these cases, tripe palms are the presenting sign of an undiagnosed malignancy. If only the palms are involved, lung cancer is most common, whereas in tripe palms associated with AN, gastric cancer is most frequent.

Type II: familial acanthosis nigricans

This exceedingly rare type is present at birth or may develop during childhood. It is commonly accentuated at puberty. It is not associated with an internal cancer and is inherited in an autosomal-dominant manner.

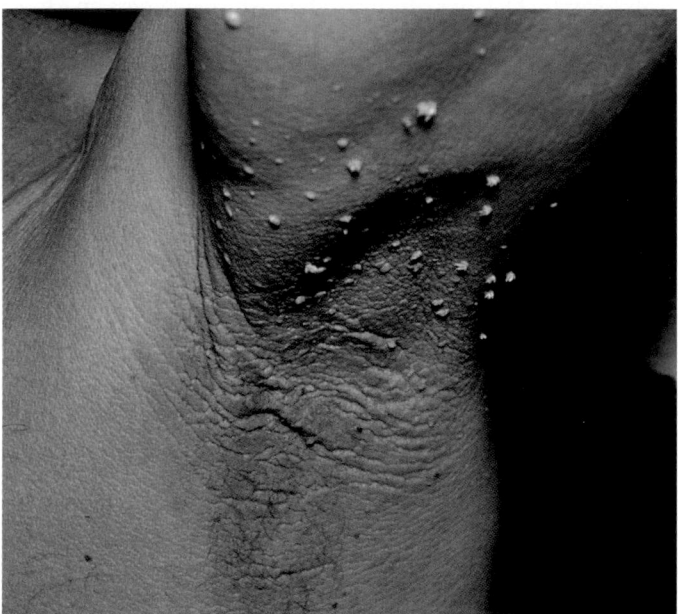

Fig. 24-8 Acanthosis nigricans.

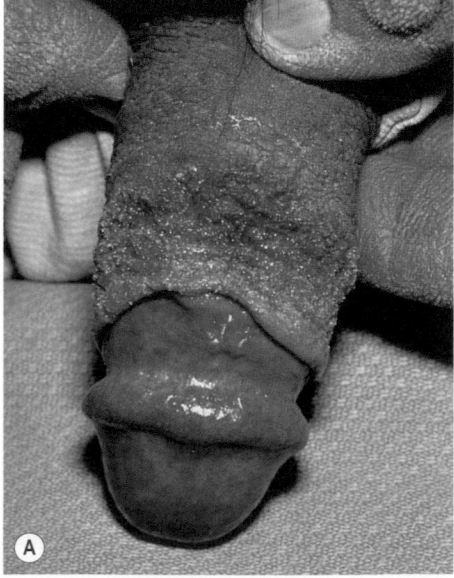

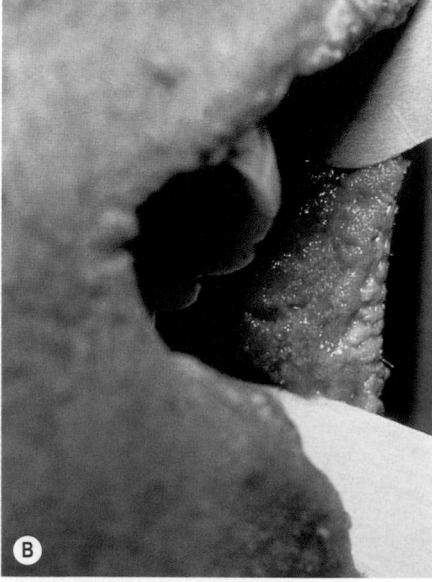

Fig. 24-9 A and B, Extensive acanthosis nigricans in a patient with stomach cancer.

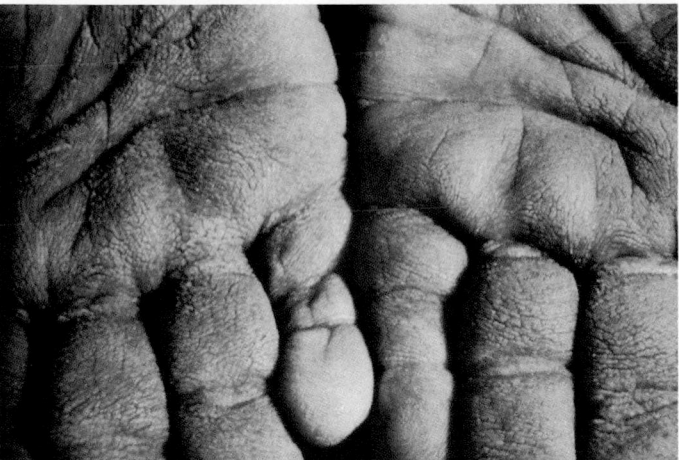

Fig. 24-10 Tripe palms.

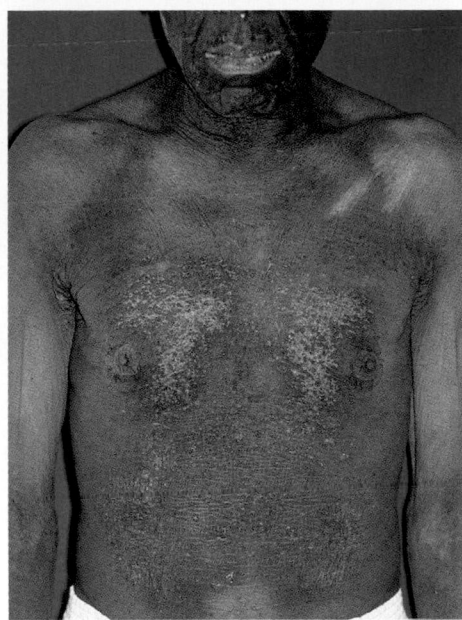

Fig. 24-11 Diffuse acanthosis nigricans in type B syndrome.

Type III: acanthosis nigricans associated with insulin-resistant states and syndromes

Type III is the most common variety of AN. It presents as a grayish, velvety thickening of the skin of the sides of the neck, axillae, and groins. It occurs in obese persons with or without endocrine disorders. It also occurs in acromegaly and gigantism, pseudoacromegaly, polycystic ovary syndrome, Cushing syndrome, diabetes mellitus, MORFAN syndrome (mental retardation, overgrowth, remarkable face, and AN), Addison's disease, Prader–Willi syndrome, Alström syndrome, ataxia-telangiectasia, hyperandrogenic states, hypogonadal syndromes, and the various well-recognized insulin-resistant states, including lipoatrophic diabetes, leprechaunism, pinealoma (Rabson–Mendenhall syndrome), acral hypertrophy syndrome; type A syndrome, where there is a defect in insulin-receptor, postreceptor pathways, or a lamin A mutation and type B syndrome, where autoantibodies to the insulin receptor are present. Whereas both type A and type B syndromes occur most commonly in black females, type A predominates in young children with hyperandrogenic manifestations. Many of the conditions associated with insulin resistance and AN manifest as hyperandrogenism and have been dubbed the HAIR-AN syndrome. In one group of women with hirsutism, obesity, and hyperandrogenism, vulvar AN was present in all patients, with other sites less frequently involved. Type B syndrome is seen in middle-aged patients with autoimmune disease (Fig. 24-11). Most, if not all, patients with this type of acanthosis nigricans may have either clinical or subclinical insulin resistance, and patients should have a glucose and insulin level drawn simultaneously. In adults a glucose to insulin ratio of less than 4.5 is abnormal, while in prepubertal children less than 7 is abnormal. Fasting glucose and lipoprotein profile, hemoglobin A1c, body weight, blood pressure, and an alanine aminotransferase (ALT) test for evaluation for fatty liver are other investigations that are useful in assessing patients with suspected insulin-resistant states.

Acanthosis nigricans may occur in fibroblast growth factor receptor defect syndromes such as Beare–Stevenson cutis gyrata syndrome, Crouzon syndrome, severe achondroplasia with developmental delay and AN (SADDAN), and thanatophoric dysplasia. Finally, other associated syndromes also manifest AN, including Bloom syndrome, Costello syndrome, Wilson's disease, benign encephalopathy, Hirschowitz syndrome, Capozucca syndrome, Down syndrome, Hermansky–Pudlack syndrome, Kabuki syndrome, hypothyroidism, Rud syndrome, and primary biliary cirrhosis. Drugs known to induce AN are nicotinic acid, niacinamide, somatotrophin, testosterone, triazinate, diethylstilbestrol, oral contraceptives, insulin, protease inhibitors, and glucocorticoids. Approximately 10% of renal transplant patients have AN.

The histopathology shows papillomatosis without thickening of the malpighian layer. Acanthosis was applied here to indicate the clinical bristly thickening of the skin and not as a histologic term. Hyperkeratosis and slight hyperpigmentation of the basal layer is present in most cases; it appears, however, that the clinically observed hyperpigmentation is due to hyperkeratosis and clinical thickening rather than to melanin.

The differential diagnosis includes intertriginous granular parakeratosis and several disorders of reticulated hyperpigmentation, including confluent and reticulated papillomatosis (Gougerot–Carteaud syndrome), Dowling–Degos' disease, Haber syndrome, and acropigmentatio reticularis of Kitamura. Granular parakeratosis presents as erythematous to brownish hyperkeratotic papules and plaques of the intertriginous regions. It is most often seen in middle-aged women in the axillae; however, the inguinal folds and submamamary areas may be involved. Histology reveals a thickened stratum corneum, severe compact parakeratosis with retention of keratohyalin granules, and vascular proliferation and ectasia. The cause is likely to be an irritant response to rubbing or to antiperspirants or deodorants. Dowling–Degos' disease is a familial nevoid anomaly with delayed onset in adult life. There is progressive, brown–black hyperpigmentation of flexures with associated soft fibromas and follicular hyperkeratoses. Pitted acneiform scars occur periorally.

Treatment of the type associated with malignancy consists of finding and removing the causal tumor. Early recognition and treatment may be life-saving. The type occurring with obesity usually improves with weight loss. If there is associated endocrinopathy, it must be treated as well. One patient with lipodystrophic diabetes improved during dietary supplementation with fish oil. Etretinate, metformin, tretinoin, calcipotriol, urea, salicyclic acid, CO_2 laser ablation, and long-pulsed alexandrite laser therapy have been reported as successful treatments in individual cases.

Ezra N, et al: Unilateral pruritic axillary rash: axillary granular parakeratosis. Arch Dermatol 2008; 144:1651.
Garcia Hidalgo L: Dermatological complications of obesity. Am J Clin Dermatol 2002; 3:497.

Hermanns-Lê T, et al: Acanthosis nigricans associated with insulin resistance. Am J Clin Dermatol 2004; 5:199.

Higgins SP, et al: Acanthosis nigricans: a practical approach to evaluation and management. Dermatol Online J 2008; 15:2.

Lee AT, et al: Dermatologic manifestations of polycystic ovary syndrome. Am J Clin Dermatol 2007; 8:201.

Malek R, et al: Treatment of type B insulin resistance. J Clin Endocrinol Metab 2010; 95:3641.

McGinness J, et al: Malignant acanthosis nigricans and tripe palms associated with pancreatic adenocarcinoma. Cutis 2006; 78:37.

Pentenero M, et al: Oral acanthosis nigricans, tripe palms and sign of Leser–Trelat in a patient with gastric adenocarcinoma. Int J Dermatol 2004; 43:530.

Rosenbach A, et al: Treatment of acanthosis nigricans of the axillae using a long-pulsed (5-msec) alexandrite laser. Dermatol Surg 2004; 30:1158.

Scheinfeld N: Confluent and reticulated papillomatosis. Am J Clin Dermatol 2006; 7:305.

Scheinfeld NS, et al: Granular parakeratosis. J Am Acad Dermatol 2005; 52:863.

Sinha S, et al: Juvenile acanthosis nigricans. J Am Acad Dermatol 2007; 57:502.

Bonus images for this chapter can be found online at

http://www.expertconsult.com

Fig. 24-1 Acromegaly.

Fig. 24-2 Pretibial myxedema. (Courtesy of Lawrence Lieblich, MD)

Fig. 24-3 Obesity-related acanthosis nigricans.

Abnormalities of Dermal Fibrous and Elastic Tissue

25

Collagen

Many types of collagen have been identified in tissues of vertebrates (Table 25-1). There are four families of collagens. Fibrillar collagens (types I, II, III, V, and XI) form fibrils that are among the most abundant proteins in the body. Type I collagen accounts for 60–90% of the dry weight of skin, ligaments, and demineralized bone. Type III collagen is abundant in fetal skin and blood vessels. It comprises 35% of the collagen in normal adult skin, but up to 40% in inflamed skin in the setting of contact dermatitis. Basement membrane-associated collagen is made up of types IV and VII. Fiber-associated collagens (types VIII, IX, and XIV) are found on the surface of type I and II collagens, and are believed to serve as flexible spacers among fibrils. Fibril-associated collagens with interrupted triple helices (FACITs) do not form fibrils themselves but are found attached to the surfaces of pre-existing fibrils of the fibril-forming collagens. FACITs are composed of types IX, XII, XIV, XVI, XIX, XX and XXI. Network-forming collagens are sheets formed from types VIII and X. Studies on types XV, XVII, and XIX demonstrate their widespread presence in basement membranes, particularly vascular endothelium, which may represent a new subgroup of collagens associated with angiogenic and pathologic processes. Type XVII collagen is also known as BP180, and contains the target antigens for several immunobullous diseases. Type VII collagen contains the target antigens for bullous lupus and epidermolysis bullosa acquisita. Type II collagen contains the target antigens for relapsing polychondritis.

The regulation of collagen synthesis and degradation is complex. Dermal fibrosis is largely related to increases in type I collagen mediated by proα1 and proα2 collagen genes. Transforming growth factor-β (TGF-β) results in increased type I procollagen synthesis. Angiotensin II type 1 receptor stimulation increases collagen production and inhibits collagen degradation, whereas type 2 receptor stimulation exerts the reverse effects.

Czarny-Ratajczak M, et al: Collagens, the basic proteins of the human body. J Appl Genet 2000; 41:317.

Elastosis perforans serpiginosa

In 1953, Lutz described a chronic papular keratotic eruption in an arciform shape located on the sides of the nape of the neck (Fig. 25-1). The papules range from 2 to 5 mm in diameter, and are grouped in a serpiginous or horseshoe-shaped arrangement. Although the lesions typically occur on the neck, other sites may be involved, such as the upper arms, face, lower extremities, and rarely the trunk. Disseminated lesions may occur in Down syndrome. Elastosis perforans serpiginosa (EPS) is most common in young adults. Men outnumber women 4:1. The disease runs a variable course with spontane-

ous resolution often occurring from 6 months to 5 years after onset. Often, atrophic scarring remains.

Approximately one-third of cases occur in patients with associated diseases, the most frequent concomitant disorder being Down syndrome. Approximately 1% of patients with Down syndrome have EPS, and the lesions are likely to be more extensive and persistent than in other patients. Progressive vaso-occlusive disease with stroke has been reported. Ehlers–Danlos syndrome, osteogenesis imperfecta, Marfan syndrome, Rothmund–Thomson syndrome, acrogeria, systemic sclerosis, morphea, XYY syndrome, and renal disease have also been associated with EPS. Reports of EPS associated with pseudoxanthoma elasticum have occurred with penicillamine. Evaluation for associated disease should be driven by associated signs and symptoms.

The distinctive histopathologic changes consist of elongated, tortuous channels in the epidermis into which eosinophilic elastic fibers perforate. The fibers are extruded from the dermis. There is degeneration and alteration of the elastic tissue in the adjacent papillary dermis with an accompanying inflammatory response. In penicillamine-associated disease, the fibers may have an irregular (bramble-bush) contour when examined with electron microscopy.

Treatment is difficult, but individual lesions may resolve following liquid nitrogen cryotherapy. Some cases have responded to CO_2, Er:YAG, or pulsed dye laser therapy. Topical retinoids have been reported to be of benefit.

Espinosa PS, et al: Elastosis perforans serpiginosa, Down syndrome, and moyamoya disease. Pediatr Neurol 2008 Apr; 38(4):287–288.
Lewis KG, et al: Acquired disorders of elastic tissue: part I. Increased elastic tissue and solar elastotic syndromes. J Am Acad Dermatol 2004; 51:1.
Suneja T, et al: Elastosis perforans serpiginosa. Skinmed 2007 Sep–Oct; 6(5):255–256.
Vearrier D, et al: What is standard of care in the evaluation of elastosis perforans serpiginosa? A survey of pediatric dermatologists. Pediatr Dermatol 2006 May–Jun; 23(3):219–224.

Reactive perforating collagenosis

In 1967, Mehregan reported a rare, familial, nonpruritic skin disorder characterized by papules that grow to a diameter of 4–6 mm and develop a central area of umbilication in which keratinous material is lodged. The discrete papules may be numerous and involve sites of frequent trauma such as the backs of the hands, forearms, elbows, and knees. The lesion reaches a maximum size of about 6 mm in 4 weeks and then regresses spontaneously in 6–8 weeks. The lesions are broader than those of EPS and a broad crust containing collagen fibers is extruded centrally. Koebnerization is often observed. Young children are most frequently affected. Most reports support an autosomal-recessive mode of inheritance; however, a family in which it appeared to be inherited by autosomal dominance has been reported. Acquired reactive perforating collagenosis is

Table 25-1 Collagen types

Collagen type	Gene*	Chromosome	Tissue distribution
I	COL1A1–2	17q21.3–q22	Skin, bone, tendon
I-trimer			Tumors, cell cultures, skin, liver
II	COL2A1	7q21.3–q22	Cartilage, vitreous
III	COL3A1	12q13–q14	Fetal skin, blood vessels, intestines
IV	COL4A1–6	13q34, 2q35–q37, Xq22	Basement membranes
V	COL5A1–3	9q34.2–q34.3	Ubiquitous
VI	COL6A1–3	21q22.3, 2q37	Aortic intima, placenta
VII	COL7A1	3p21	Amnion, anchoring fibrils
VIII	COL8A1–2	3q12–q13.1, 1p32.3–p34.3	Endothelial cell cultures
IX	COL9A1–3	6q12–q14, 1p32	Cartilage, type II collagen tissue
X	COL10A1	6q12–q22	Cartilage
XI	COL11A1–2, COL2A1	1p21	Cartilage, skin
XII	COL12A1	6	Skin, cartilage, cornea, limbal
XIII	COL13A1	10q22	Ubiquitous
XIV	COL14A1	8q23	Ubiquitous, fetal hair follicles, basement membranes
XV	COL15A1	9q21–22	Skin hemidesmosomes, kidney, liver, spleen
XVI	COL16A1	1p34–35	Ubiquitous
XVII	COL17A1	10q24.3	Skin hemidesmosomes (BP180)
XVIII	COL18A1	21q22.3	Ubiquitous, basement membranes
XIX	COL19A1	6q12–q14	Ubiquitous, basement membranes
XX	COL20A1		Corneal epithelium, embryonic skin, sternal cartilage, and tendon
XXI	COL21A1	6p11.2–12.3	Blood vessel walls
XXII	COL22A1	8q24.2	Tissue junctions such as BMZ of anagen hair follicle
XXIII			Rat prostate carcinoma cells
XXIV			Fetal cornea and bone
XXV			Precursor to Alzheimer amyloid plaque component
XXVI			Testis and ovary
XXVII			Chondrocytes, developing tissues including stomach, lung, gonad, skin, cochlea, and teeth

*A dash denotes a series of genes, i.e. COL14A1–2 means COL14A1 and COL14A2.

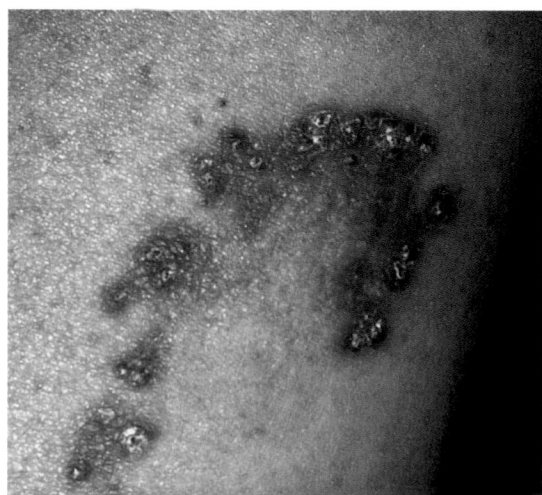

Fig. 25-1 Elastosis perforans serpiginosa.

discussed in Chapter 33 within the section on acquired perforating dermatosis.

No specific treatment is typically indicated, since the lesions involve spontaneously. Topical retinoids may be helpful in patients who require treatment.

Kumar V, et al: Familial reactive perforating collagenosis. J Dermatol 1998; 25:54.

Ramesh V, et al: Familial reactive perforating collagenosis: a clinical, histopathological study of 10 cases. J Eur Acad Dermatol Venereol 2007 Jul; 21(6):766–770.

Pseudoxanthoma elasticum

Pseudoxanthoma elasticum (PXE) is an inherited disorder involving the connective tissue of the skin, eye, and cardiovascular system. Many cases appear to be sporadic. In familial cases, both a recessive and a dominant inheritance pattern have been reported, with the recessive form apparently more common. The skin changes generally present as small,

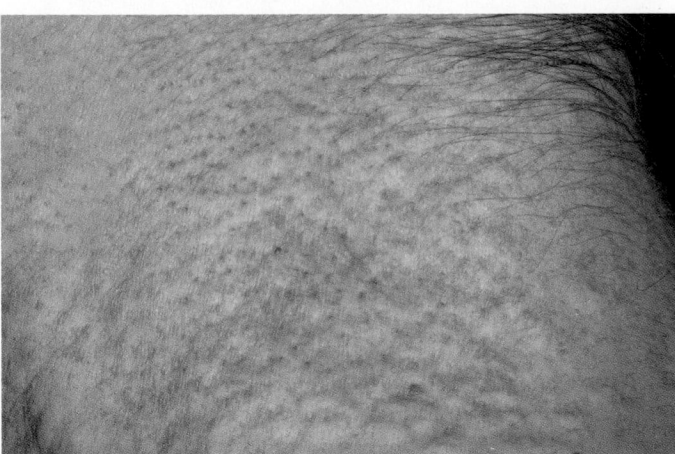

Fig. 25-2 Pseudoxanthoma elasticum.

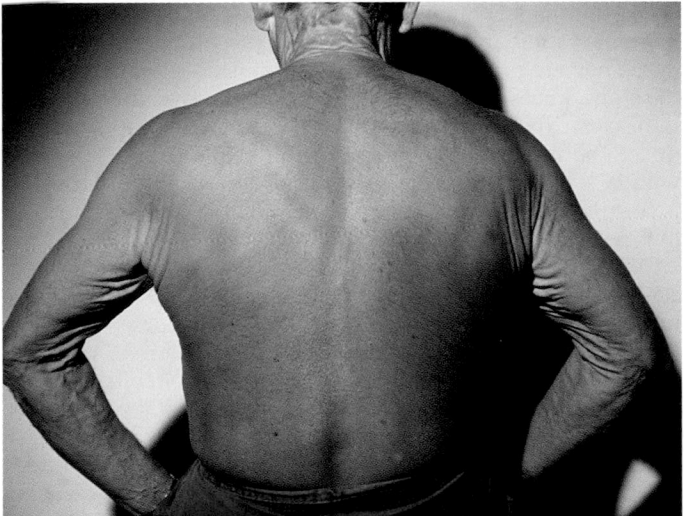

Fig. 25-3 Pseudoxanthoma elasticum.

On fundoscopic examination a reddish-brown band is evident around the optic disk, from which glistening streaks extend. With fluorescent photography early fluorescence of the angioid streaks and macular lesions is noted. In addition, there may be hemorrhages and exudates. Progressive loss of vision often starts after minor trauma to the eye. Drusen-like spots are commonly present, and show increased autofluorescence, unlike age-related drusen.

Vascular involvement commonly leads to hemorrhage. These vascular events are caused by the degeneration of the elastic fibers in the vascular media. Gastric hemorrhage occurs in 10% of patients, and viewed by gastroscopy diffuse rather than focal bleeding is common. Epistaxis occurs frequently, but hematuria is rare. PXE affects the elastic tissue of the cardiac valves, myocardium, and pericardium. In one study, mitral valve prolapse was found in 71% of 14 patients examined. Hypertension occurs in many patients older than age 30. Any patient with hypertension at a young age should be examined for stigmata of PXE. Leg cramps and intermittent claudication occur prematurely, and peripheral pulses are diminished or absent. Calcification of peripheral arteries is seen in many patients over age 30 and may be detected by radiograph. Accelerated coronary artery disease can occur, especially in association with hypertension. Extensive cutaneous calcification, and renal and testicular stones may occur.

Mutations in the *ABCC6* gene on the short arm of chromosome 16 have been implicated in the pathogenesis of PXE. *ABCC6* encodes an adenosine triphosphate (ATP)-binding cassette transporter and multidrug resistance protein. Although the most prominent manifestations of the disease are in the skin, eye, gut, and heart, mineralization of elastic fibers can be found in many organs.

Histologically, elastic fibers are fragmented and mineralized with calcium. They stain gray–blue with hematoxylin and eosin (H&E), and are twisted, curled, and broken, suggesting "raveled wool." Blind biopsies of scars or axillary skin in patients with a family history of PXE or with angioid streaks may sometimes show early changes of PXE. Calcium stains are helpful in identifying early disease.

The differential diagnosis includes PXE-like papillary dermal elastolysis, perforating calcific elastosis, and cutis laxa. Patients with PXE-like papillary dermal elastolysis may have cobble-stoned, yellow papules on the neck, similar to PXE, but lack any retinal or vascular alterations and the typical fragmentation of elastic fibers with calcium deposition on histology. Penicillamine may induce similar clinical and histologic features in patients with Wilson's disease or homocystinuria.

No definitive therapy is available to treat the skin disease. Some data suggest that patients benefit from limiting dietary calcium and phosphorus to the minimal daily requirement. Intravitreal bevacizumab has been used to treat choroidal neovascularization.

Finger RP, et al: Intravitreal bevacizumab for choroidal neovascularisation associated with pseudoxanthoma elasticum. Br J Ophthalmol 2008 Apr; 92(4):483–487.

Goede J, et al: Testicular microlithiasis in a 2-year-old boy with pseudoxanthoma elasticum. J Ultrasound Med 2008 Oct; 27(10):1503–1505.

Plomp AS, et al: ABCC6 mutations in pseudoxanthoma elasticum: an update including eight novel ones. Mol Vis 2008 Jan 24; 14:118–124.

Plomp AS, et al: Proposal for updating the pseudoxanthoma elasticum classification system and a review of the clinical findings. Am J Med Genet A 2010 Apr; 152A(4):1049–1058.

circumscribed, yellow to cream-colored papules on the sides of the neck and flexures, giving the skin a "plucked chicken skin" appearance (Fig. 25-2). Lax, redundant folds of skin may be present (Fig. 25-3). Nuchal comedones and milia en plaque may also be seen. Characteristic exaggerated nasolabial folds and mental creases are common. Mental creases appearing in patients under the age of 30 years are highly suggestive of PXE. In addition, the inguinal, periumbilical, and periauricular skin, as well as the mucosa of the soft palate, inner lip, stomach, rectum, and vagina, may be involved.

The characteristic retinal change is the angioid streak, which is the result of breaks in Bruch's elastic membrane. PXE can be demonstrated in more than half of patients with angioid streaks, and 85% of PXE patients will have retinal findings. The angioid streaks appear earlier than the skin changes, so that most cases are discovered by ophthalmologists. Angioid streaks may be the only sign of the disease for years. In such patients biopsies of the midportions of old scars may be diagnostic of PXE. The association of the skin lesions with angioid streaks is called Grönblad–Strandberg syndrome. Angioid streaks may also be seen in Ehlers–Danlos syndrome, Paget's disease of bone, diabetes, hemochromatosis, hemolytic anemia, hypercalcinosis, solar elastosis, neurofibromatosis, Sturge–Weber syndrome, tuberous sclerosis, myopia, sickle-cell anemia, trauma, lead poisoning, hyperphosphatemia, pituitary disorders, and intracranial disorders. PXE, Paget's disease of the bone, and sickle-cell disease account for the vast majority of patients with angioid streaks.

Perforating calcific elastosis

Also known as periumbilical perforating PXE and localized acquired cutaneous PXE, perforating calcific elastosis is an acquired, localized cutaneous disorder, most frequently found in obese, multiparous, middle-aged women. Lax, well-circumscribed, reticulated, or cobble-stoned plaques occur in the periumbilical region with keratotic surface papules. It is a distinct disorder that shares some features of PXE. As in PXE there may be calcific elastosis in the mid-dermis; however, hereditary PXE rarely causes perforating channels. None of the systemic features of PXE occurs in perforating calcific elastosis.

It is suggested that repeated trauma of pregnancy, obesity, and/or abdominal surgery promotes elastic fiber degeneration, resulting in localized disease. PXE can cause periumbilical lesions, and in the absence of documented perforation, evaluations to exclude PXE should be performed. There is no effective therapy.

Lopes LC, et al: Perforating calcific elastosis. J Eur Acad Dermatol Venereol 2003; 17:206.

Ehlers–Danlos syndromes

Ehlers–Danlos syndromes (EDSs), also known as cutis hyperelastica, India rubber skin, and elastic skin, are a group of genetically distinct connective tissue disorders characterized by excessive stretchability and fragility of the skin (Fig. 25-4), with hyperextensibility of the joints (Fig. 25-5) and a tendency toward easy scar formation and formation of fibrous or calcified pseudotumors. Atrophic scarring on the distal fingers and wide atrophic "fish-mouth" scars are typical. Patients demonstrate reduced thickness of the dermis, as determined by high-

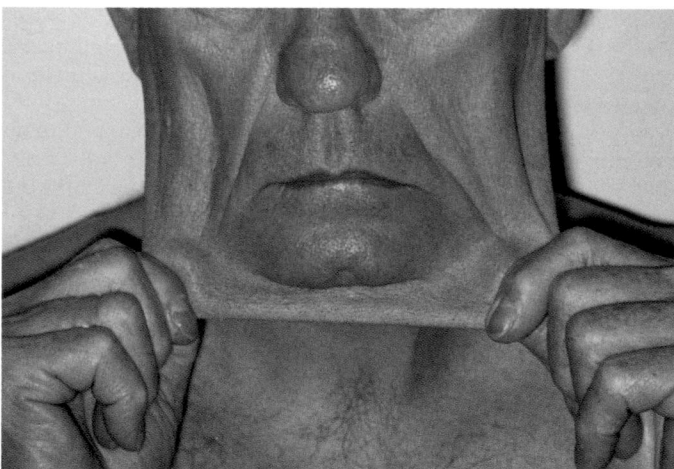

Fig. 25-4 Ehlers–Danlos syndrome.

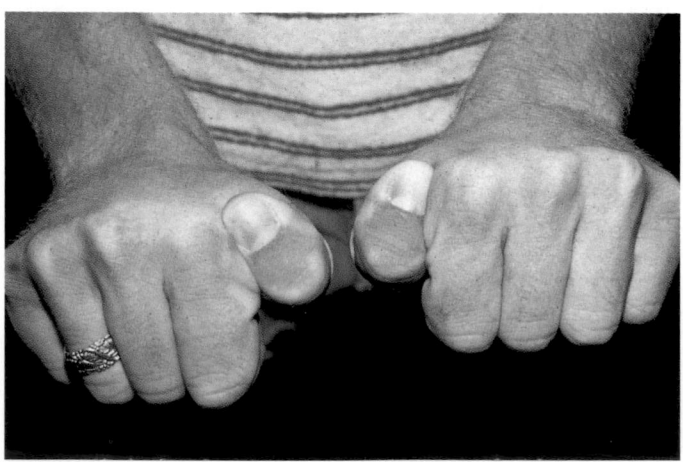

Fig. 25-5 Hyperextensible joints, Ehlers–Danlos syndrome.

resolution 20 MHz ultrasound. The reduction in thickness is most marked on the chest and distal lower leg. Rare oral manifestations have been reported, including supernumerary teeth and odontogenic keratocysts.

Classically, EDS has been divided into 10 numeric types, the salient features of which are listed in Table 25-2. Type IX EDS, an allelic variant of Menkes' disease, is now reclassified as the occipital horn syndrome and is identical to X-linked cutis laxa. It is related to mutations in an X-linked gene, *ATP7A*. Types I, II, III, V, VII, and VIII EDS have hyperextensible skin. In these patients, the integument may be stretched out like a rubber band and snaps back with equal resilience. This rubbery skin is most pronounced on the elbows, neck, and sides of the abdomen. The skin is velvety in appearance and feels like wet chamois cloth. Minor trauma may produce a gaping "fish-mouth" wound with large hematomas underneath. The subcutaneous calcifications are 2–8 mm oval nodules, mostly on the legs. Two types of nodule occur in patients with EDS. Molluscoid pseudotumors are soft, fleshy nodules seen in easily traumatized areas such as the ulnar forearms and shins. Spheroids are hard subcutaneous nodules that become calcified. They are probably the result of fat necrosis. Trauma over the shins, knees, hands, and elbows produces cigarette-paper-thin scars. Approximately 50% of these patients can touch the tip of the nose with their tongue (Gorlin's sign), compared with 10% of persons without the disorder. Aortic root dilation is seen in up to 20% of patients with EDS. It is more common in types I and II than in type III.

Patients with type IV EDS have thin, translucent skin, characteristic facial features, and vascular fragility. They are prone to arterial rupture and often have extensive bruising. Perforations of the intestines and uterus may occur. Atlantoaxial subluxation has been noted. Protein analysis of collagen III in cultured fibroblasts usually shows a defect. Some type IV patients demonstrate no abnormalities of collagen III, although a mutation in the *COL3A1* gene is identified. Type V patients have clinical features that are similar to the gravis/mitis form. Patients with type VI EDS may have microcornea, retinal detachment, and glaucoma, as well as scoliosis. In normal individuals, the ratio of hydroxylysylpyridinoline (HP) to lysylpyridinoline (LP) in urine is about 10:1. In patients with type VI EDS, the HP/LP ratio is reduced, ranging from 1:3 to 1:7. The spondylocheirodysplastic form is autosomal-recessive and caused by mutations in the zinc transporter gene, *SLC39A13*. This form includes hyperelastic, bruisable skin, joint hypermobility, contractures, protuberant eyes, bluish sclerae, short stature, finely wrinkled palms, thenar atrophy, and tapered digits. Skeletal dysplasia includes platyspondyly, osteopenia, and widened metaphyses. The urinary HP/LP ratio is approximately 1.

In type VIIA and VIIB EDS there is marked joint hypermobility and moderate cutaneous elasticity. Joint dislocations of the large joints, such as the hips, are common. Type VIIC EDS, the autosomal-recessive form, is referred to as dermatosparaxis. Patients with this type have severe skin fragility and sagging, redundant skin. Type VIII EDS manifests as periodontitis as well as easy bruising. Reductions of collagen type III alone or together with a reduction in collagen type I have been reported. When type IX EDS was redefined as a variant of Menkes syndrome, old-type X EDS was reclassified by some authors as new type IX. It is characterized by hypermobile joints, easy bruising, fish-mouth scars, mitral valve prolapse, and platelets resistant to aggregation with collagen and adenosine diphosphate (ADP) reagents. A qualitative deficiency of fibronectin was the suggested cause, although never confirmed. Since the deletion of old-type IX, old-type XI has been reclassified by some as new-type X, or the familial joint hypermobility syndrome.

Table 25-2 Features of Ehlers–Danlos syndromes

Ehlers-Danlos type	Gene	Inheritance*	Molecular abnormality	Clinical features
I	COL5A1–2†	AD	Type V collagen	Gravis type: joint laxity, skin hyperextensibility
II	COL5A1–2	AD	Type V collagen	Mitis type: same as EDS 1 but less severe
III	TNXB haploid	AD	Unknown	Hypermobility
IV	COL3A1	AD AR	Type III procollagen	Thin skin, bruising, ruptured blood vessels and viscera
V			Unknown	Skin hyperextensibility, easy bruising
VI	LH1, PLOD	AR	Lysyl hydroxylase deficiency	Severe eye defects and scoliosis
VIIA, VIIB	COL1A1–2	AD	Type I procollagen	Arthrochalasis, subluxations, moderate skin stretchability
VIIC		AR	Procollagen peptidase deficiency	Dermatosparaxis, severe stretchability, redundant skin
VIII	Heterogenous, only some map to chromosome 12p13	AD	Unknown	Same as EDS types I and II, periodontitis
Old-type IX, reclassified as a variant of Menkes' disease/occipital horn syndrome	ATP7A	X-linked	Lysyl oxidase	Abnormal facies, skeletal abnormalities including occipital horns, chronic diarrhea, and genitourinary abnormalities
X (new-type IX)		AR	Fibronectin	Bruising
Old-type XI (new-type X)			Familial joint hypermobility syndrome	Relationship to EDS unclear
Spondylocheirodysplastic	SLC39A13	AR		Hyperelastic, bruisable skin, joint hypermobility, contractures, tapered digits, skeletal dysplasia

*AD, autosomal-dominant; AR, autosomal-recessive.
†COL5A1–2 means COL5A1 and COL5A2 genes.

Because of the discovery of new types and confusion concerning the numbered types, an alternate classification scheme has been proposed that groups EDS by associated signs and symptoms, as well as known genetic mutations. This new classification combines numeric types I and II because they share the same mutations (Box 25.1).

Histology

Collagen fibers may appear fine. Factor XIIIa-positive dermal dendrocytes may be markedly reduced in the adventitial dermis and almost absent in the reticular dermis.

Treatment

Patients must be counseled to avoid trauma. Intestinal perforations in EDS type IV have been managed with porcine small intestinal submucosa grafts. Matrix metalloproteinase inhibitors produce changes in connective tissue, and are being evaluated as possible therapeutic agents.

Callewaert B, et al: Ehlers–Danlos syndromes and Marfan syndrome. Best Pract Res Clin Rheumatol 2008 Mar; 22(1):165–189.
Ferreira O Jr, et al: Odontogenic keratocyst and multiple supernumerary teeth in a patient with Ehlers–Danlos syndrome: a case report and review of the literature. Quintessence Int 2008 Mar; 39(3):251–256.
Giunta C, et al: Spondylocheiro dysplastic form of the Ehlers–Danlos syndrome: an autosomal-recessive entity caused by mutations in the zinc transporter gene SLC39A13. Am J Hum Genet 2008 Jun; 82(6):1290–1305.
Mataix J, et al: Periodontal Ehlers–Danlos syndrome associated with type III and I collagen deficiencies. Br J Dermatol 2008 Apr; 158(4):825–830.
Parapia LA, et al: Ehlers–Danlos syndrome: a historical review. Br J Haematol 2008 Apr; 141(1):32–35.
Walsh CA, et al: Ehlers–Danlos syndrome in pregnancy. Fetal Diagn Ther 2008; 24(1):79 (Epub 2008 May 27).

Marfan syndrome

Marfan syndrome is an autosomal-dominant disorder of connective tissue caused by mutations in the gene encoding fibrillin-1. It is one of the more common inherited diseases, with estimated incidence rates of 1 in 10000 in the US. Among the important abnormalities are tall stature, loose-jointedness, a dolichocephalic skull, high-arched palate, arachnodactyly (Fig. 25-6), pigeon breast, pes planus, poor muscle tone, and large, deformed ears. The aorta, chordae tendineae, and aortic and mitral valves are often involved. Ascending aortic aneurysm and mitral valve prolapse are commonly seen. Ectopia lentis, extensive striae over the hips and shoulders, dental anomalies, and, rarely, elastosis perforans serpiginosa have

Box 25-1 New classification for Ehlers–Danlos syndrome (EDS)

1. Classic type (gravis—EDS type I, and mitis II)*
2. Hypermobility type (hypermobile—EDS III)
3. Vascular types (arterial-ecchymotic—EDS type IV, Qatarian EDS)†
4. Kyphoscoliosis type (ocular-scoliotic—EDS type VI)
5. Arthrochalasia type (arthrochalasis multiplex congenita—EDS type VIIA and VIIB)
6. Dermatosparaxis type (human dermatosparaxis—EDS type VIIC)
7. Miscellaneous forms (X-linked—EDS type V, periodontitis; EDS type VIII, fibronectin-deficient EDS; EDS type X, familial hypermobility syndrome [formerly EDS type XI]; progeroid EDS; and unspecified forms). Some progeroid EDS is related to galactosyltransferase I deficiency.

*Mutations in the genes for collagen α1(V) chain (COL5A1), collagen α2(V) chain (COL5A2), tenascin-X (TNX), and collagen α1(I) chain (COL1A1) have been characterized in patients with classical EDS. All are autosomal-dominant, except the tenascin-X-related type, which is autosomal-recessive.

†A distinct vascular type of EDS was described in an extended family in Qatar. Features of the syndrome include skin hyperextensibility, joint hypermobility, tortuous systemic arteries, epicanthic folds, flat saggy cheeks, elongated facies, micrognathia, hernias, an elongated aortic arch, aortic aneurysms, bifid pulmonary artery, pulmonic stenosis, hypotonia, and arterial rupture. Linkage to the major loci of other types of EDS was excluded.

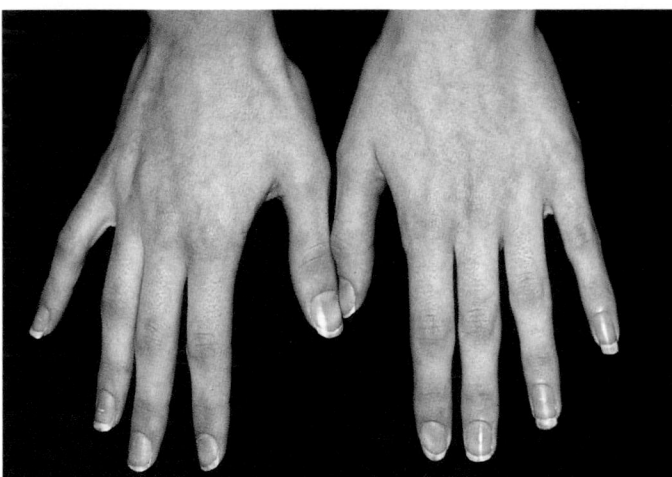

Fig. 25-6 Marfan syndrome.

been reported. Several cases document the occasional occurrence of spontaneous pneumothorax and congenital lung abnormalities.

Marfan syndrome is caused by a gene defect localized to chromosome 15 and producing abnormal elastic tissue in fibrillin 1 (aorta adventitia, the suspending ligaments of the lens, skin) and fibrillin 2 (elastin orientation in cartilage, aortic media, bronchi, and all tissues rich in elastin). Gene defects include substitutions, deletions, duplication missense, frameshift, splice site, and nonsense mutations. Ectopia lentis is more common in patients whose mutations involve a cysteine substitution in the gene for fibrillin 1, and less prevalent in those with premature termination mutations. Death may result from aortic root aneurysm rupture or dissection. Echocardiography is helpful for early detection of cardiovascular involvement. Surgical intervention may be required for aneurysms of the aortic root or for aortic dissection. Long-term

administration of propranolol may significantly reduce the rate of aortic dilatation, as may angiotensin II blockade. Long-term doxycycline may be helpful to inhibit matrix metalloproteinases. Some evidence suggests it may be more effective than atenolol in preventing progression of thoracic aortic aneurysms. Antisense ribozymes are promising for gene therapy.

Brooke BS, et al: Angiotensin II blockade and aortic-root dilation in Marfan's syndrome. N Engl J Med 2008 Jun 26; 358(26):2787–2795.
Chung AW, et al: Long-term doxycycline is more effective than atenolol to prevent thoracic aortic aneurysm in Marfan syndrome through the inhibition of matrix metalloproteinase-2 and -9. Circ Res 2008 Apr 25; 102(8):e73–85.
Frydman M: The Marfan syndrome. Isr Med Assoc J 2008 Mar; 10(3):175–178.
Pyeritz RE: Marfan syndrome and related disorders. Ann Thorac Surg 2008 Jul; 86(1):335–336.
Raanani E, et al: The multidisciplinary approach to the Marfan patient. Isr Med Assoc J 2008 Mar; 10(3):171–174.
Singh P, et al: Pregnancy outcome with Marfan's syndrome and aortic root replacement. J Obstet Gynaecol 2008 Feb; 28(2):226–228.

Homocystinuria

Homocystinuria, an inborn error in the metabolism of methionine, is characterized by the presence of homocysteine in the urine and deficiency of the enzyme cystathionine synthetase or methylenetetrahydrofolate reductase. Cystathionine β-synthase is a heme-containing enzyme that catalyzes pyridoxal 5'-phosphate-dependent conversion of serine and homocysteine to cystathionine. Over 130 gene mutations have been described. The defect results in increased levels of homocysteine and methionine, and decreased levels of cysteine. The incidence of the disorder varies from 1 in 344 000 worldwide to 1 in 65 000 in Ireland where the disorder is more common. Among the signs of homocystinuria are ectopia lentis, genu valgum, kyphoscoliosis, pigeon breast deformity, and frequent fractures. Generalized osteoporosis, arterial and venous thrombosis, and mental retardation are features of homocystinuria not found in Marfan syndrome. Half of all patients will have a serious vascular event before the age of 30, and 25% experience a serious event before the age of 16. The facial skin has a characteristic flush, especially on the malar areas, and the color has a tendency to become violaceous when the patient is reclining. Elsewhere the skin is blotchy red, suggestive of livedo reticularis. The hair is typically fine, sparse, and blond, and the teeth are irregularly aligned. Downward dislocation of the lens, as opposed to the upward displacement seen in Marfan syndrome, is a prominent feature. Treatment with pyridoxine, folic acid, and vitamin B_{12} produces variable results. A methionine-restricted, cysteine-supplemented diet is generally recommended. Unfortunately, some methionine-free baby formulas contain significant amounts of homocysteine and should be reformulated. Betaine supplementation has been shown to be effective. Wheat flour is rich in betaine, but the amounts ingested are smaller than those needed to treat the disease. It has been recommended that methionine-free formulas be supplemented with 150 mg/dL of betaine. Alfalfa and bean sprouts contain ample homocysteine, and excessive amounts should be avoided. Other vegetables do not contain large amounts of homocysteine. Vitamin C ameliorates endothelial dysfunction, and the effect appears to be independent of homocysteine concentration. Some of the beneficial effects of folate are also independent of homocysteine lowering. In an animal model of homocystinuria, 5-methyltetrahydrofolate decreased mortality, but folic acid did not.

Cattaneo M: Hyperhomocysteinemia and venous thromboembolism. Semin Thromb Hemost 2006 Oct; 32(7):716–723.

Lee PJ, et al: A rationale for cystine supplementation in severe homocystinuria. J Inherit Metab Dis 2007 Feb; 30(1):35–38.

Li D, et al: Mefolinate (5-methyltetrahydrofolate), but not folic acid, decreases mortality in an animal model of severe methylenetetrahydrofolate reductase deficiency. J Inherit Metab Dis 2008 Jun; 31(3):403–411.

McCully KS: Homocysteine, vitamins, and vascular disease prevention. Am J Clin Nutr 2007 Nov; 86(5):1563S–1568S.

Cutis laxa (generalized elastolysis)

Cutis laxa, also known as dermatomegaly, dermatolysis, chalazoderma, and pachydermatocele, is characterized by inelastic loose, redundant skin. Around the eyelids, cheeks, and neck the drooping skin produces a bloodhound-like facies. Usually the entire integument is involved. The shoulder girdle skin may look like that of a St Bernard dog. The abdomen is frequently the site of large, pendulous folds. There are two well-described genetic forms of cutis laxa, the autosomal-dominant and autosomal-recessive types. The dominant form is primarily a cutaneous, cosmetic form, with a good prognosis. The recessive form is more common, and is associated with significant internal involvement, including hernias, diverticula, pulmonary emphysema, cor pulmonale, aortic aneurysm, dental caries, large fontanelles, and osteoporosis. Pulmonary emphysema, cor pulmonale, and right-sided heart failure are often seen already in infancy. Frameshift and splicing mutations in the elastin gene have been reported in autosomal-dominant disease. Both homozygous and heterozygous missense mutations in the *fibulin-5* gene have been reported in some patients with the disease, especially in families with the recessive form. *Fibulin-4* mutations may cause autosomal recessive cutis laxa associated with emphysema, vascular tortuosity, ascending aortic aneurysm, inguinal and diaphragmatic hernia, joint laxity, and pectus excavatum. X-linked recessive cutis laxa is now known as the occipital horn syndrome (formerly type IX EDS). It is caused by a mutation in the copper-binding ion transporting ATPase, ATP7A, and is allelic to another X-linked disorder, Menkes' disease. Nonfamilial cases (Fig. 25-7) have been associated with urticaria, lupus erythematosus, glomerulonephritis, plasma cell dyscrasias, and systemic amyloidosis. These acquired cases may have a preceding inflammatory phase with large numbers of interstitial neutrophils, eosinophils, or macrophages engulfing elastic fibers. Isolated acral disease has been associated with myeloma and rheumatoid arthritis.

The Costello syndrome is characterized by increased prenatal growth, postnatal growth retardation, coarse facies, loose skin that resembles cutis laxa, cardiomyopathy, and gregarious personality. Patients are predisposed to abdominal and pelvic rhabdomyosarcoma in childhood. The disorder appears to be inherited as an autosomal-dominant trait. The de Barsy syndrome is associated with severe cutis laxa, mental and growth retardation, joint laxity, ocular abnormalities, and skeletal disease.

Mid-dermal elastolysis is an acquired, noninherited condition that usually affects young women. Wide areas of skin demonstrate atrophic wrinkling. Histologically, elastic tissue is absent from the mid-dermis. Many cases appear to be induced or aggravated by ultraviolet light exposure.

Claus S, et al: A p.C217R mutation in fibulin-5 from cutis laxa patients is associated with incomplete extracellular matrix formation in a skin equivalent model. J Invest Dermatol 2008 Jun; 128(6):1442–1450.

Graul-Neumann LM, et al: Highly variable cutis laxa resulting from a dominant splicing mutation of the elastin gene. Am J Med Genet A 2008 Apr 15; 146A(8):977–983.

Hucthagowder V, et al: Fibulin-4: a novel gene for an autosomal recessive cutis laxa syndrome. Am J Hum Genet 2006 Jun; 78(6):1075–1080.

Blepharochalasis

In blepharochalasis the eyelid skin becomes lax and falls in redundant folds over the lid margins. The condition may affect young adults, where a preceding inflammatory phase presents with episodes of lid swelling. Most cases are bilateral, but unilateral involvement may occur. Rarely, elastolysis of the earlobes may accompany blepharochalasis. It is generally sporadic, but a dominantly inherited form has been described. Biopsy shows lack of elastic fibers, and abundant IgA deposits have been demonstrated in some cases, possibly binding to fibulin and fibronectin. Sequelae include excess thin skin, fat herniation, lacrimal gland prolapse, ptosis, blepharophimosis, pseudoepicanthic fold, proptosis, conjunctival injection and cysts, entropion, and ectropion.

Ascher syndrome consists of progressive enlargement of the upper lip and blepharochalasis. The minor salivary glands of the affected areas are inflamed, resulting in superfluous folds of mucosa, giving the appearance of a double lip. There is a superficial resemblance to angioedema. Treatment is by surgical correction.

Huemer GM, et al: Unilateral blepharochalasis. Br J Plast Surg 2003; 56:293.

Schaeppi H, et al: Unilateral blepharochalasis with IgA-deposits. Hautarzt 2002; 53:613.

Anetoderma (macular atrophy)

Anetoderma is characterized by localized loss of elastic tissue resulting in herniation of subcutaneous tissue. The lesions protrude from the skin (Fig. 25-8), and on palpation have less resistance than the surrounding skin, producing the "button hole" sign identical to a neurofibroma. The surface skin may be slightly shiny, white, and crinkly. The usual locations are the trunk, especially on the shoulders, upper arms, and thighs. The intervening skin is normal.

Up to half of cases have an accompanying abnormality, such as lupus, antiphospholipid antibodies, Graves' disease, scleroderma, hypocomplementemia, hypergammaglobulinemia, autoimmune hemolysis, and infection with the human immunodeficiency virus (HIV). Screening for antiphospholipid antibodies is of particular importance, as they may produce a prothrombotic state, and some patients fulfill criteria for the antiphospholipid syndrome. The antibodies may be detected as anticardiolipin antibodies, anti-β2-glycoprotein-I antibodies, or a lupus anticoagulant. Patients may experience recurrent fetal loss, recurrent strokes, or recurrent deep vein thrombosis. Some cases of anetoderma may be related to

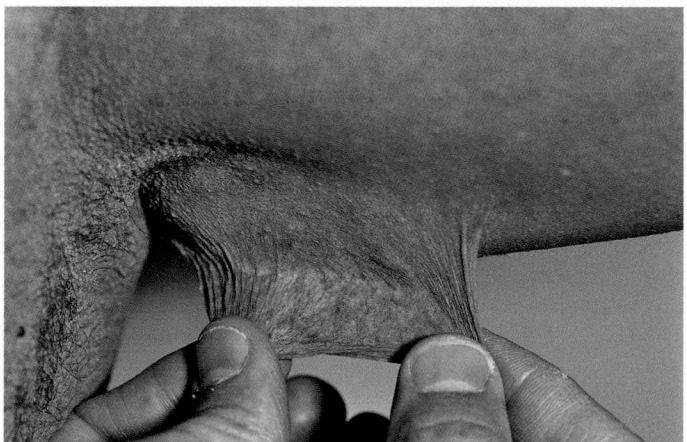

Fig. 25-7 Acquired cutis laxa.

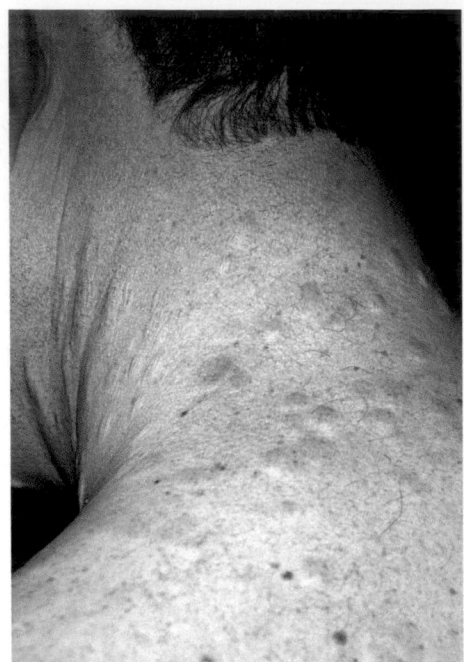

Fig. 25-8 Anetoderma.

Fig. 25-9 Linear focal elastosis on the lower back of an elderly man.

borreliosis. Rare familial cases have been noted. Secondary anetoderma may be related to previous lesions of acne, secondary syphilis, measles, lupus erythematosus, Hansen's disease, sarcoidosis, tuberous xanthoma, varicella, granuloma annulare, mastocytosis, and lymphoreticular malignancy.

Anetoderma of prematurity (congenital anetoderma) occurs in premature infants and may be related to pressure, adhesives, or changes in flow of ions or water under monitor leads. Intrauterine borreliosis has also been implicated.

Histologically, a loss of elastic tissue is noted with special stains. In the late stage, the skin looks normal in H&E sections. In the acute stage, a neutrophilic, lymphoid, or granulomatous response may be noted.

Hodak E, et al: Primary anetoderma and antiphospholipid antibodies: review of the literature. Clin Rev Allergy Immunol 2007 Apr; 32(2):162–166.

Ishida Y, et al: Coexistence of disseminated primary anetoderma and generalized granuloma annulare-like papules. J Dermatol 2007 Apr; 34(4):278–279.

Kalogeromitros D, et al: Secondary anetoderma associated with mastocytosis. Int Arch Allergy Immunol 2007; 142(1):86–88.

Kineston DP, et al: Anetoderma: a case report and review of the literature. Cutis 2008 Jun; 81(6):501–506.

Striae distensae

Striae distensae are depressed lines or bands of thin, reddened skin, which later become white, smooth, shiny, and depressed. Elastotic striae have a yellow–gold iridescent appearance. Striae occur in response to changes in weight or muscle mass and skin tension, such as that induced by weight lifting. They are common on the abdomen during and after pregnancy (striae gravidarum) and on the breasts after lactation. They also occur on the buttocks and thighs, the inguinal areas, and over the knees and elbows in children during the growth spurt of puberty. Cushing syndrome, either endogenous or induced by systemic steroid treatment, is a frequent cause of striae, and they may occur after application of potent topical corticosteroid preparations, especially under occlusion or in folds. Striae are common in patients with Marfan syndrome.

The histologic findings are variable and depend on the stage of development. In some early lesions, perivascular and interstitial infiltration of lymphocytes and sometimes eosinophils is noted. In older lesions the primary changes are in the connective tissue. The collagen of the upper dermis is decreased, and thin collagen bundles lie parallel to the overlying epidermis as in a scar. Elastic tissue often appears increased, but this may be due to a loss of collagen in many cases. Dilated upper dermal vessels may be prominent.

Over time striae become less noticeable. Topical tretinoin and vascular lasers may produce some improvement in appearance, although the benefits are more marked in the early erythematous phase. Pulse dye lasers (585 nm) result in a moderate decrease in erythema in striae rubra. Although the total collagen per gram of dry weight increases in striae treated with pulse dye laser, this change may not result in a clinically evidenced change in striae alba. Pulse dye laser has also been used in conjunction with a radiofrequency device. Intense pulsed light has also demonstrated potential for improvement in the appearance of some striae, although darker skin types have greater risk and lower efficacy. Fractional photothermolysis has been used in a variety of skin types.

Kim BJ, et al: Fractional photothermolysis for the treatment of striae distensae in Asian skin. Am J Clin Dermatol 2008; 9(1):33–37.

Suh DH, et al: Radiofrequency and 585-nm pulsed dye laser treatment of striae distensae: a report of 37 Asian patients. Dermatol Surg 2007 Jan; 33(1):29–34.

Taub AF: Fractionated delivery systems for difficult to treat clinical applications: acne scarring, melasma, atrophic scarring, striae distensae, and deep rhytides. J Drugs Dermatol 2007 Nov; 6(11):1120–1128.

Linear focal elastosis (elastotic striae)

This variant presents with asymptomatic, palpable, or atrophic, yellow lines (Fig. 25-9) of the middle and lower back, thighs, arms, and breasts. The condition is more common in males. Histologically, there are increased elastic fibers characterized by thin, wavy, and elongated, as well as fragmented, elastic fiber bundles. Electron microscopy reveals elongated thin, irregularly shaped, swollen elastic fibers with degenerative changes.

Pui JC, et al: Linear focal elastosis: histopathologic diagnosis of an uncommon dermal elastosis. J Drugs Dermatol 2003; 2:79.

Ramlogan D, et al: Linear focal elastosis. Br J Dermatol 2001; 145:188.

Acrodermatitis chronica atrophicans

Patients with acrodermatitis chronica atrophicans present with diffuse thinning of the skin on the extremities, sometimes

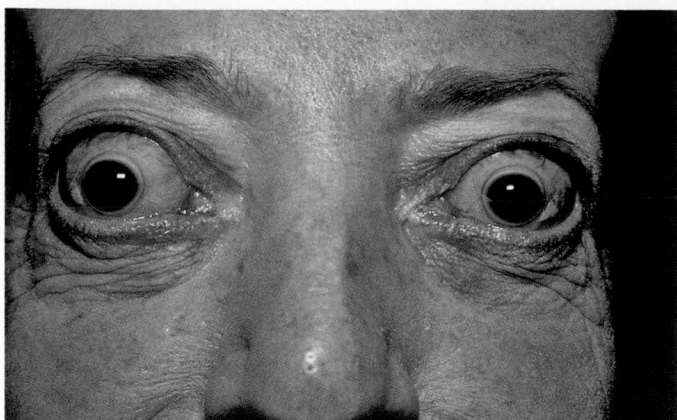

Fig. 25-10 Blue sclera of osteogenesis imperfecta in a patient with Graves' disease. (Courtesy of Lawrence Lieblich, MD)

associated with fibrous bands. It is reviewed in Chapter 14, since it results from infection with *Borrelia*.

Osteogenesis imperfecta

Osteogenesis imperfecta (OI), also known as Lobstein syndrome, affects the bones, joints, eyes, ears, and skin. It is estimated to affect approximately 10 000 persons in the US (4–5 in 100 000). There are seven recognized forms based on differences in clinical presentation and bone architecture. Types I and IV have only an autosomal-dominant inheritance, whereas types II and III have both autosomal-dominant and autosomal-recessive forms. Fifty percent of OI patients have the type I form. The type II form is lethal, and deaths usually occur within the first week of life.

The brittle bones result from a defect in the collagenous matrix. Fractures occur early in life, sometimes in utero. Loose-jointedness may be striking, and dislocation of joints can be a problem. Blue sclerae, when present, are a valuable diagnostic clue (Fig. 25-10). Scoliosis and defective teeth may be present. Deafness develops in many by the second decade of life and is audiologically indistinguishable from otosclerosis. The skin is thin and translucent, and healing wounds result in spreading atrophic scars. Elastosis perforans serpiginosa may occur. Some patients experience unusual bruisability, probably due to a structural defect in either the blood vessel wall or the supporting dermal connective tissue.

The basic defect is abnormal collagen synthesis, resulting in type I collagen of abnormal structure. Most forms of OI result from mutations in the genes for the proα1 or proα2 chains of type I collagen. Types V, VI, and VII are not associated with type I collagen gene defects. In type I (blue scleral dominant) there is diminished type I collagen with a mutation of *COL1A1* gene; in type II (perinatal lethal) there is diminished type I collagen synthesis and decreased integrity of the helical domain of the *α1 (I)* gene; in type III (progressive deforming) there is delayed secretion of type I collagen with altered mannosylation; and in type IV (white sclerae dominant) there is a defective *proα1 (I)* gene. A distinct subset of type IV with clinical improvement over time has been mapped to chromosome 11q.

The major causes of death attributed to OI are respiratory failure secondary to severe kyphoscoliosis and head trauma, mostly observed in type III disease. Aortic dissection has also been described. Patients with type I and type IV disease have a normal lifespan. Brack syndrome is a combination of OI and arthrogryposis multiplex.

Treatment includes surgical intervention, such as intramedullary stabilization. Bisphosphonates and calcitriol are the most effective pharmacologic agents. Specifically, cyclical pamidronate therapy has been shown to suppress bone turnover, reduce bone pain and fracture incidence, and increase bone density and level of ambulation. Gene therapy is promising, but is complicated by the genetic heterogeneity of the disease. Most of the OI mutations result in a mutant allele product that interferes with the function of the normal allele. This sort of abnormality presents greater challenges for gene therapy than simple replacement of a missing enzyme, but gene and stem cell transfer research is ongoing.

Brodsky B, et al: Structural biology: modelling collagen diseases. Nature 2008 Jun 19; 453(7198):998–999.

Brusin JH: Osteogenesis imperfecta. Radiol Technol 2008 Jul–Aug; 79(6):535–548.

Burnei G, et al: Osteogenesis imperfecta: diagnosis and treatment. J Am Acad Orthop Surg 2008 Jun; 16(6):356–366.

Byra P, et al: Osteogenesis imperfecta and aortic dissection. Am J Med Sci 2008 Jul; 336(1):70–72.

Glorieux FH: Treatment of osteogenesis imperfecta: who, why, what? Horm Res 2007; 68(Suppl 5):8–11.

Kamoun-Goldrat A, et al: A new osteogenesis imperfecta with improvement over time maps to 11q. Am J Med Genet A 2008 Jul 15; 146A(14):1807–1814.

Poyrazoglu S, et al: Successful results of pamidronate treatment in children with osteogenesis imperfecta with emphasis on the interpretation of bone mineral density for local standards. J Pediatr Orthop 2008 Jun; 28(4):483–487.

Bonus images for this chapter can be found online at

http://www.expertconsult.com

Fig. 25-1 Cutis laxa.

26 Errors in Metabolism

Amyloidosis

Amyloid is a material deposited in the skin and other organs that is eosinophilic, homogeneous, and hyaline in appearance. It represents beta-pleated sheet forms of various host-synthesized molecules processed into this configuration by host cells.

Amyloidosis can be classified as systemic, localized, and heredofamilial types. The systemic types can deposit amyloid in multiple organs, and are all related to an overproduction of a host protein that cannot be adequately excreted or metabolized by the host. The excess protein is metabolized into amyloid precursors that interact with tissue proteoglycans/glycosaminoglycans, forming soluble amyloid oligomers. These oligomers complex with serum amyloid P (SAP), forming amyloid deposits in the affected organ. In all forms of amyloid, the pattern of deposition is characteristic, although there can be overlap between various forms. The diagnosis of a specific type of amyloid should only be made if the clinical features are characteristic. In atypical cases, the specific amyloid protein being deposited in the tissue should be identified. Primary localized amyloidosis (also called primary cutaneous amyloidosis when the skin is affected) is very common and of importance to the dermatologist. Rare familial syndromes may be complicated by secondary systemic amyloidosis or have genetic defects that lead to amyloid deposition (heredofamilial amyloidosis). Classification of cutaneous amyloidoses is shown below.

I. Systemic amyloidosis
   A. Primary (myeloma-associated) systemic amyloidosis
   B. Secondary systemic amyloidosis
   C. Dialysis-related amyloidosis
II. Cutaneous amyloidosis
   A. Macular amyloidosis
   B. Lichen amyloidosis
   C. Nodular amyloidosis
   D. Secondary (tumor-associated) cutaneous amyloidosis
III. Heredofamilial amyloidosis.

All forms of amyloid have relatively identical histologic and electron microscopic findings. The amyloid in all forms is made up of three distinct components: protein-derived amyloid fibers, amyloid P component (about 15% of amyloid), and ground substance. It is the protein-derived amyloid fibers that differ among the various forms of amyloid.

Amyloid is weakly periodic acid-Schiff (PAS)-positive and diastase-resistant, Congo red-positive, purple with crystal violet, and positive with thioflavin T. Amyloid stained with Congo red exhibits apple-green birefringence under polarized light. Secondary systemic amyloid (AA amyloid) loses its birefringence after treatment with potassium permanganate, whereas primary and localized cutaneous forms do not.

Amyloid stains an intense, bright orange with cotton dyes such as Dylon, Pagoda red, RIT Scarlet No. 5, or RIT Cardinal red No. 9. Ultrastructurally, amyloid has a characteristic fibrillar structure that consists of straight, nonbranching, nonanastomosing, often irregularly arranged filaments 60–100 nm in diameter. In most cases, specific antibodies against the protein component should be used to confirm the type of amyloidosis. Because amyloid substance P is present in all forms of amyloid, immunoperoxidase staining against this component will stain all forms of amyloid. In addition, since SAP is avidly bound to amyloid, radiolabeled, highly purified SAP can be used to localize amyloidosis, determine the extent of organ infiltration, study progression of disease, and see if therapy reduces the amount of amyloid in various organs. Special centers have the capability of doing body scans (radiolabeled SAP scintigraphy) and have the reagents to identify the specific amyloid proteins immunohistochemically. In atypical cases, consulting such centers may be warranted.

Systemic amyloidoses

Primary systemic amyloidosis (AL amyloidosis)

Primary systemic amyloidosis typically involves the kidneys, liver, heart, gastrointestinal tract or peripheral nerve, and skin. Myeloma-associated amyloidosis is included in this category. The amyloid fibril proteins in primary systemic amyloidosis are composed of protein AL, a portion of the immunoglobulin light chain. It is usually of the λ subtype, and certain germline immunoglobulin light chain V chains (6aVλVI and 3rVλIII) are responsible for AL amyloidosis in 40% of patients. Ninety percent of patients will have the immunoglobulin fragment detectable in the serum or urine. Of the 10% that do not have a light chain detected in serum or urine, the serum free light chain assay will detect a clear excess of one of the light chains (κ or λ), confirming the diagnosis. Also, reduction of the urine free light chains by more than 50% correlates with substantial benefit from treatment.

Cutaneous manifestations occur in approximately 40% of cases of primary systemic amyloidosis. The cutaneous eruption usually begins as shiny, smooth, firm, flat-topped, or spherical papules of waxy color, which, because of their tenseness, have the appearance of translucent vesicles. These lesions coalesce to form nodules and plaques of various sizes and, in some cases, bandlike lesions. The regions about the eyes, nose, mouth, and mucocutaneous junctions are commonly involved. Vulvar lesions (Fig. 26-1) may resemble giant condylomata.

Purpuric lesions and ecchymoses occur in about 15% of patients and are the most common cutaneous manifestation of primary systemic amyloidosis. There are several mechanisms by which AL leads to purpura. Amyloid may infiltrate blood vessels, making them fragile. AL may also bind factor X, contributing to the purpura. Lastly, amyloid infiltration of the liver may lead to reduced production of fibrinogen and factor X, adversely affecting clotting. Purpura chiefly involves

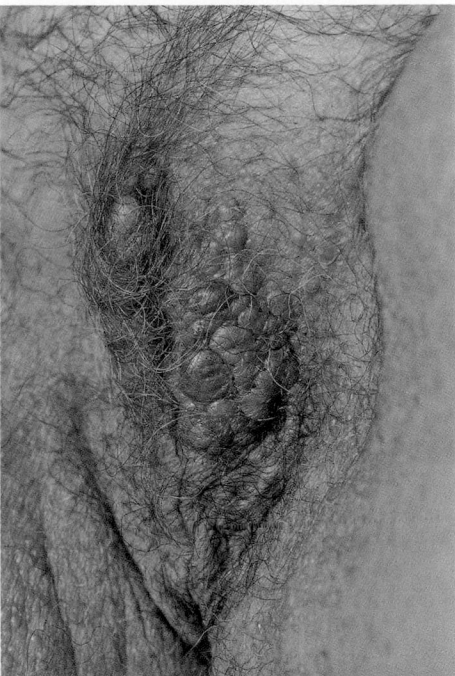

Fig. 26-1 Vulvar amyloid deposits.

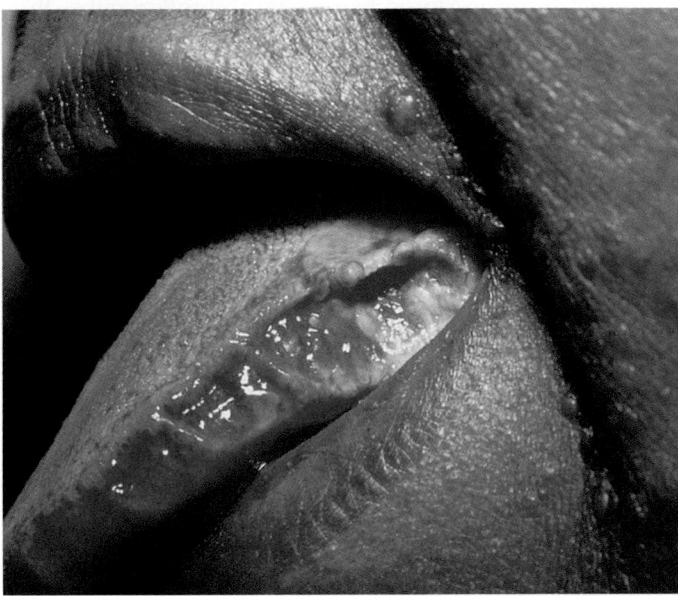

Fig. 26-2 Macroglossia and translucent papules of the tongue. (Courtesy of Lawrence Lieblich, MD)

the eyelids, limbs, and oral cavity. It typically occurs after trauma (pinch purpura). Purpuric lesions also classically appear after actions or procedures that result in increased pressure in the vessels of the face, such as after vomiting, coughing, proctoscopic examination, or pulmonary function testing.

Glossitis, with macroglossia, occurs in at least 20% of cases, may be an early symptom, and can lead to dysphagia. The tongue becomes greatly enlarged, and furrows develop (Fig. 26-2). The lateral aspects show indentations from the teeth. Papules or nodules, sometimes with hemorrhage, occur on the tongue.

Bullous amyloidosis is a rare but important clinical manifestation of amyloidosis. Skin fragility and tense, hemorrhagic or clear, non-inflammatory bullae appear at areas of trauma, usually the hands, forearms, and feet. Lesions heal with scar-

ring and milia. The esophagus and oropharyngeal mucosae may also be involved. Histologically, the lesions are subepidermal and pauci-inflammatory. Epidermolysis bullosa acquisita and porphyria cutanea tarda are the differential diagnoses. Amyloid staining may yield negative results, and direct immunofluorescence (DIF) may be falsely positive (because of AL protein deposition at the dermoepidermal junction). The diagnosis is confirmed by evaluation of the patient's serum and urine for immunoglobulin fragments and by amyloid stains or electron microscopy of the skin biopsies, which will demonstrate the amyloid.

A diffuse or patchy alopecia, cutis verticis gyrata, and a scleroderma-like, scleromyxedema-like, or a cutis laxa-like appearance have also rarely been described. Cutis laxa-like findings may be generalized or localized to the acral parts. The nail matrix may be infiltrated, resulting in atrophy of the nail plate, presenting as longitudinal striae, partial anonychia, splitting, and crumbling of the nail plate. Cordlike thickening along blood vessels can also occur. Bilateral stenosis of the external auditory canals has been reported.

Patients may present with or develop a plethora of systemic findings. Most characteristically, they develop carpal tunnel syndrome, other peripheral neuropathies, a rheumatoid arthritis-like arthropathy of the small joints, orthostatic hypotension, gastrointestinal bleeding, nephrotic syndrome, and cardiac disease. Cardiac troponins are elevated and are powerful prognostic determinants in AL amyloidosis. Elevated troponins are associated with a 6-month survival. AL patients may appear to have prominent deltoid muscles as a result of deposition of amyloid in the muscles (shoulder pad sign). Cardiac arrhythmias and right-sided congestive heart failure are common causes of death.

The prognosis for patients with primary systemic amyloidosis is poor. The median survival averages 43 months. Those presenting with neurologic findings survive longer than patients presenting with cardiac disease. Fifteen percent of patients with AL amyloidosis will have myeloma, and 15% of patients with myeloma will have AL amyloidosis.

Treatment is improving but still relies heavily on systemic chemotherapy (usually melphalan). High-dose melphalan and stem cell reconstitution are the most effective treatments. Most patients with AL amyloidosis cannot undergo this therapy, as the mortality is 12%; patients with cardiomyopathy or at least two organs involved have an even higher mortality. Lower-dose melphalan with dexamethasone, or thalidomide or lenalidomide with or without dexamethasone (at times with cytoxan), can be used in refractory cases.

Secondary systemic amyloidosis (AA amyloidosis)

Secondary systemic amyloidosis is due to a chronic infectious or inflammatory process. In these conditions, the precursor protein, serum amyloid A (SAA), an acute phase reactant, is chronically elevated and cannot be adequately cleared from the body. It is processed to AA amyloid in affected tissues. With adequate control of chronic infections (especially tuberculosis, schistosomiasis, osteomyelitis, bronchiectasis, pyelonephritis, and decubitus ulcer), infection-related AA amyloid is much less common. Most cases are now related to chronic inflammatory conditions, especially rheumatoid arthritis, juvenile idiopathic arthritis, ankylosing spondylitis, adult Still's disease, inflammatory bowel disease, and Behçet's disease. The newer and more aggressive management strategies for these inflammatory conditions have led to reduced numbers or delayed onset of AA amyloidosis in these patients. Maintaining SAA below 4 mg/L is associated with a good outcome in AA amyloidosis. The common organs involved by AA amyloidosis are the kidneys, adrenals, liver, and spleen.

The skin is not involved, but biopsy of skin in patients with AA amyloidosis will detect amyloid deposits in the dermis perivascularly. Certain skin conditions, such as hidradenitis suppurativa, stasis ulcers, psoriatic arthritis, and dystrophic epidermolysis bullosa, may be complicated by AA amyloidosis. Many inherited conditions associated with elevated SAA may be complicated by AA amyloidosis. These include familial Mediterranean fever, cryopyrin-associated periodic syndromes, and tumor necrosis factor (TNF) receptor-associated periodic syndrome (TRAPS).

Dialysis-associated amyloidosis (β_2 microglobulin amyloidosis)

Beta$_2$ microglobulin is excreted primarily by the kidneys. In patients with severe renal failure on dialysis or predialysis, the excess β_2 microglobulin may be processed to amyloid in certain tissues. Nearly 100% of patients on dialysis for 15 years or more will develop this form of amyloidosis. It primarily affects the synovium, causing musculoskeletal symptoms, often carpal tunnel syndrome, and less commonly trigger finger, bone cysts, and spondyloarthropathy. Rarely, the skin may be involved, usually as a subcutaneous tumor, often of the buttocks overlying the sacrum. Pedunculated sacral masses, lichenoid papules, and localized hyperpigmentation can also be seen. The diagnosis is confirmed by biopsy, which demonstrates that the amyloid material is β_2 microglobulin via immunohistochemical stains. The treatment is high-flux dialysis or kidney transplantation.

Cutaneous amyloidosis

Primary localized cutaneous amyloidosis

The primary cutaneous amyloidoses have been divided into three forms—macular, lichen, and nodular amyloid. Nodular and familial cases of cutaneous amyloidosis are rare and have a unique pathogenesis. Non-familial macular and lichen amyloid have the same pathogenic basis (rubbing and friction) and overlap cases (biphasic cutaneous amyloidosis) can be seen, although not commonly. The more common forms have been called primary localized cutaneous amyloidosis (PLCA). Individuals of Asian, Hispanic, or Middle Eastern ancestry seem to be predisposed. In Japan, the use of nylon towels during bathing is often the precipitant. In cases of acquired macular and lichen amyloidosis, the deposited amyloid material contains keratin (primarily keratin 5) as its protein component, strongly suggesting that traumatic damage to basal keratinocytes results in the deposits. Why only certain individuals are affected is unknown. A rare form localized to the conchae has been described. Non-familial macular and lichen amyloidosis may be associated with very pruritic skin conditions such as primary biliary cirrhosis and chronic renal failure.

The histologic picture of acquired macular and lichen amyloidosis is similar, the only difference being the size of the amyloid deposits and the extent of the overlying epidermal changes. The overlying epidermis is frequently hyperkeratotic and focally acanthotic, a result of the chronic rubbing. Focal necrotic keratinocytes may be observed in the basal cell layer. Microscopic and rarely macroscopic bullae (analogous to those seen in lichen planus) may be seen. Dermal papillae are expanded by amorphous deposits of amyloid that abut immediately below the epidermis. Melanin deposits are classically present in the amyloid. In all cases of postinflammatory hyperpigmentation with incontinence of pigment, the texture of the areas of dermal melanosis should be examined carefully to

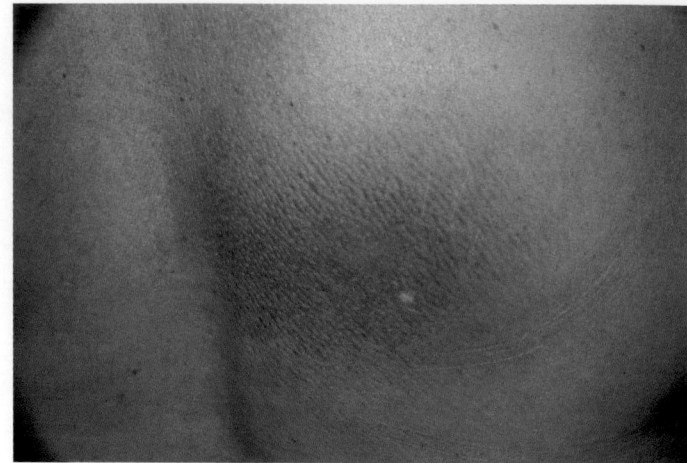

Fig. 26-3 Macular amyloid. (Courtesy of Lawrence Lieblich, MD)

exclude amyloidosis. Systemic amyloidosis is excluded by the absence of amyloid deposits around blood vessels. Special stains may be used to confirm the diagnosis, but this is rarely required if the classic histology is found. In difficult cases, immunoperoxidase stains for keratin will stain the amyloid deposits and confirm the diagnosis of primary cutaneous amyloidosis. DIF may demonstrate immunoglobulin (usually IgM) in a globular pattern in the keratin-derived cutaneous amyloidoses, but this is caused by passive absorption rather than by specific deposition. This phenomenon is seen in all disorders with prominent apoptosis of keratinocytes.

Macular amyloidosis

Typical cases exhibit moderately pruritic, brown, rippled macules characteristically located in the interscapular region of the back (Fig. 26-3). Pigmentation is typically not uniform, giving the lesions a "salt and pepper" or rippled appearance. Notalgia paresthetica is localized to the same sites, and most cases of macular amyloid between the scapulae probably result from rubbing dysesthetic areas of notalgia paresthetica. Occasionally, the thighs, shins, arms, breasts, and buttocks may be involved, and these more diffuse cases are usually associated with diffuse pruritus. Macular amyloidosis is a chronic condition.

Lichen amyloidosis

Lichen amyloidosis is characterized by the appearance of paroxysmally itchy lichenoid papules, typically appearing bilaterally on the shins (Fig. 26-4). Some patients may deny itching. The primary lesions are small, brown, discrete, slightly scaly papules that group to form infiltrated large moniliform plaques. They may, less commonly, occur on the thighs, forearms, face, and even the upper back.

Treatment of the primary localized cutaneous amyloidoses is frequently unsatisfactory. Reducing friction to the skin is critical. Identifying the cause of the rubbing, and whether it is habit, pruritus, or neuropathy (as in notalgia paresthetica), directs treatment. Occlusion plays a major role, because it both enhances topical treatments and provides a physical block to prevent trauma to the skin. Administration of topical high-potency corticosteroid agents can be beneficial, as can intralesional corticosteroid therapy when small areas are involved. Topical tacrolimus 0.1% ointment, psoralen + ultraviolet A (PUVA), re-PUVA, UVB, tar, and calcipotriol benefit individual patients. Oral retinoids, systemic steroids, cyclophosphamide, and dermabrasion have also been reported to be beneficial. The pigmentation of macular amyloidosis has been reported to be improved by laser therapy, especially 532 nm Q-switched Nd:YAG.

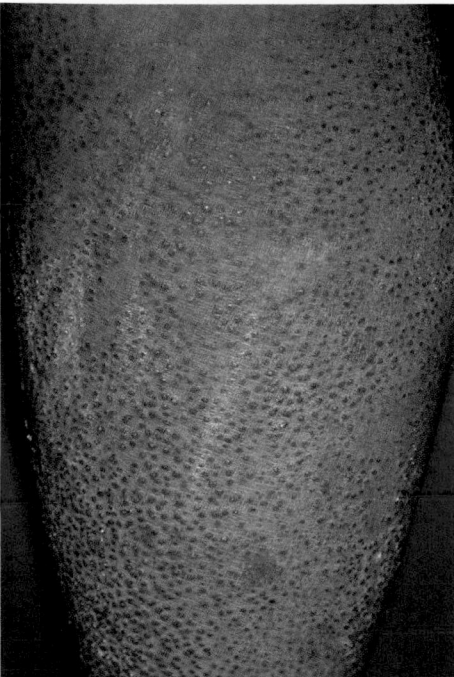

Fig. 26-4 Lichen amyloidosis.

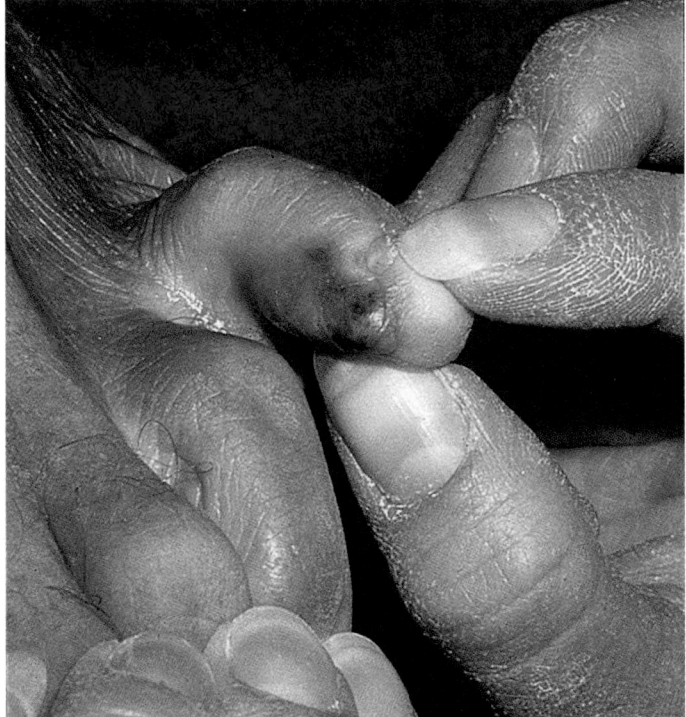

Fig. 26-5 Nodular amyloidosis.

Nodular primary localized cutaneous amyloidosis (NPLCA)

Nodular amyloidosis is a rare form of primary localized cutaneous amyloidosis in which single or, rarely, multiple nodules or tumefactions preferentially involve the acral areas (Fig. 26-5); however, trunk, genital, or facial lesions may be seen. The lesions are asymptomatic. They vary in size from several millimeters to several centimeters, and may grow slowly after their initial appearance. The overlying epidermis may appear atrophic, and lesions may resemble large bullae. Numerous conditions have been reported to be associated with NPLCA, especially Sjögren syndrome, but also systemic sclerosis

(including CREST), and rheumatoid arthritis. Patients with Sjögren syndrome may have elevated serum free light chain concentrations due to their polyclonal B cell hyperactivity. In Sjögren syndrome, the nodular amyloidosis typically appears around age 60, and more commonly in females, and may precede the diagnosis of Sjögren syndrome by many years. The dermis and subcutis may be diffusely infiltrated with amyloid. The lesions may contain numerous plasma cells and are best considered to be isolated plasmacytomas. The amyloid in these patients is immunoglobulin-derived AL, as is seen in primary systemic amyloidosis, and is unrelated to keratinocyte-related amyloid or to AA amyloid. Progression to systemic amyloidosis may occur in around 7% of cases, so they should be regularly evaluated for progression. Treatment is physical removal or destruction of the lesion with shave removal and destruction of the base.

Secondary cutaneous amyloidosis

Following PUVA therapy and in benign and malignant cutaneous neoplasms, deposits of amyloid may be found. Most frequently, the associated neoplasms are nonmelanoma skin cancers or seborrheic keratoses. Discoid lupus and dermatomyositis, as interface dermatoses with apoptosis of keratinocytes, can occasionally demonstrate amyloid in the upper dermis. In all cases, this is keratin-derived amyloid.

Hereditary cutaneous amyloidosis syndromes

Familial primary localized cutaneous amyloidosis (FPLCA) is an autosomal-dominant syndrome associated with chronic itching and cutaneous lesions resembling macular and lichen amyloidosis. It is seen most commonly in Japan, Brazil, and Taiwan. The age of onset is 5–18 years. In some families, sun exposure may be an exacerbating factor. Lesions are often widespread on the limbs, chest, and upper and lower back. The buttocks, conchae, and dorsal feet and hands may also be involved. Some patients may deny pruritus. In some families with FPLCA, a mutation in the *OSMRβ* gene is found. *OSMRβ* is required for IL-31 signalling in keratinocytes. Rare cases of macular amyloidosis in an incontinentia pigmenti-like distribution suggest that mosaicism for FPLCA can be seen, giving this unusual cutaneous distribution.

Amyloidosis cutis dyschromica is a distinct type of FPLCA with onset in childhood, no pruritus, a dotted reticular hyperpigmentation with hypopigmented spots without papulation covering almost all the body, and small foci of amyloid just below the epidermis. The nature of the amyloid is unclear. Most affected families are from Japan, Taiwan, and India. UVB hypersensitivity is reported by these patients. Some FPLCA cases demonstrate extensive poikilodermatous lesions.

Multiple endocrine neoplasia 2A (MEN2A) syndrome and familial medullary thyroid carcinoma (FMTC) are both due to mutations in the *RET* proto-oncogene. Cutaneous amyloidosis, most commonly keratin-derived macular amyloidosis, may be seen in these patients. The macular amyloid may be restricted to the upper back and so unilateral (associated with notalgia paresthetica), or may be bilateral and more extensive. Age of onset is usually before 20. Thirty of 31 patients with MEN2A had cutaneous amyloidosis before the diagnosis of MEN2A was made. In a patient with macular amyloidosis of early onset (before age 20), a careful family history should be taken for endocrine neoplasias, the skin and mucosa should be examined for neuromas, the blood pressure should be taken (looking for pheochromocytoma), and the thyroid should be palpated. A serum calcitonin should be ordered, and if elevated, a thyroid ultrasound should be performed.

Familial syndromes associated with amyloidosis (heredofamilial amyloidosis)

Most forms of familial amyloidosis are due to abnormal host proteins which cannot be adequately processed, resulting in their being deposited in various tissues in the form of amyloid. Only 50% of patients with hereditary amyloidosis will have a positive family history. Liver, kidney, heart, eye, and nervous system may be involved. Several types of hereditary amyloidosis have been identified; two forms are caused by genetic defects in transthyretin. These are autosomal-dominant syndromes, and most affected patients are heterozygotes. Others are caused by a genetic defect in apolipoprotein A-I or A-II, by a defect in gelsolin, fibrinogen A α, cystatin C or lysozyme. These syndromes must often be diagnosed by genetic testing or immunohistochemical identification of the deposited pathogenic protein.

Alvarez-Ruiz SB, et al: Unusual clinical presentation of amyloidosis: bilateral stenosis of the external auditory canal, hoarseness and a rapid course of cutaneous lesions. Int J Dermatol 2007; 46:503.

Arita K, et al: Oncostatin M receptor-beta mutations underlie familial primary localized cutaneous amyloidosis. Am J Hum Genet 2008; 82:73.

Arita K, et al: A novel OSMR mutation in familial primary localized cutaneous amyloidosis in a Japanese family. J Dermatol Sci 2009; 55:64.

Babilas P, et al: Identification of an oncostatin M receptor mutation associated with familial primary cutaneous amyloidosis. Br J Dermatol 2009; 161:944.

Baykal C, et al: Multiple cutaneous neuromas and macular amyloidosis associated with medullary thyroid carcinoma. J Am Acad Dermatol 2007; 56:S33.

Buxbaum JN: The systemic amyloidoses. Curr Opin Rheumatol 2004; 16:67.

Castanedo-Cazares JP: Lichen amyloidosis improved by 0.1% topical tacrolimus. Dermatology 2002; 205:420.

Chang SL, et al: Bullous amyloidosis in a hemodialysis patient is myeloma-associated rather than hemodialysis-associated amyloidosis. Amyloid 2007; 14:153.

Cheung ST, et al: A comparative study of two Congo red stains for the detection of primary cutaneous amyloidosis. J Am Acad Dermatol 2006; 55:363.

Cho TH, et al: A case of lichen amyloidosis accompanied by vesicles and dyschromia. Clin Exp Dermatol 2008; 33:291.

Choi JY, et al: Acitretin for lichen amyloidosis. Australas J Dermatol 2008; 49:109.

Dahdah MJ, et al: Primary localized cutaneous amyloidosis: a sign of immune dysregulation? Int J Dermatol 2009; 48:419.

Dicker TJ, et al: Myeloma-associated systemic amyloidosis presenting with acquired digital cutis laxa-like changes. Australas J Dermatol 2002; 43:144.

Grimmer J, et al: Successful treatment of lichen amyloidosis with combined bath PUVA photochemotherapy and oral acitretin. Clin Exp Dermatol 2007; 32:39.

Gul U, et al: Lichen amyloidosis with face involvement. Int J Dermatol 2008; 47:1201.

Gupta R, et al: Dexamethasone cyclophosphamide pulse therapy in lichen amyloidosis: a case report. J Dermatolog Treat 2007; 18:249.

Huang WH, et al: Amyloidosis cutis dyschromica: four cases from two families. Int J Dermatol 2009; 48:518.

Jhingan A, et al: Lichen amyloidosis in an unusual location. Singapore Med J 2007; 48:e165.

Jin AGT, et al: Comparative study of phototherapy (UVB) vs photochemotherapy (PUVA) vs topical steroids in the treatment of primary cutaneous lichen amyloidosis. Photodermatol Photoimmunol Photomed 2001; 17:42.

Kalajian AH, et al: Nodular primary localized cutaneous amyloidosis after trauma: a case report and discussion of the rate of progression to systemic amyloidosis. J Am Acad Dermatol 2007; 57:S26.

Kaplan B, et al: Biochemical subtyping of amyloid in formalin-fixed tissue samples confirms and supplements immunohistologic data. Am J Clin Pathol 2004; 121:794.

Khoo B-P, et al: Calcipotriol ointment vs betamethasone 17-valerate ointment in the treatment of lichen amyloidosis. Int J Dermatol 1999; 38:539.

Koba S, et al: The occurrence of two types of amyloid in the same patient. Br J Dermatol 2008; 158:860.

Koh M, et al: A rare case of primary cutaneous nodular amyloidosis of the face. J Eur Acad Dermatol Venereol 2008; 22:1011.

Konishi A, et al: Primary localized cutaneous amyloidosis with unusual clinical features in a patient with Sjögren's syndrome. J Dermatol 2007; 34:394.

Love WE, et al: The spectrum of primary cutaneous nodular amyloidosis: two illustrative cases. J Am Acad Dermatol 2008; 58:S33.

Lutz ME, et al: Progressive generalized alopecia due to systemic amyloidosis. J Am Acad Dermatol 2002; 46:434.

Macbeth AE, et al: Calcified subcutaneous nodules: a long-term complication of interferon beta-1a therapy. Br J Dermatol 2007; 157:624.

Matzke TJ, et al: Bullous amyloidosis presenting as naproxen-induced photosensitivity. Int J Dermatol 2007; 46:284.

Meijer JM, et al: Sjögren's syndrome and localized nodular cutaneous amyloidosis: coincidence or a distinct clinical entity? Arthritis Rheum 2008; 58:1992.

Merlini G, et al: The systemic amyloidoses: clearer understanding of the molecular mechanisms offers hope for more effective therapies. J Intern Med 2004; 255:159.

Ostovari N, et al: 532-nm and 1064-nm Q-switched Nd:YAG laser therapy for reduction of pigmentation in macular amyloidosis patches. J Eur Acad Dermatol Venereol 2008; 22:442.

Pardo Arranz L, et al: Familial poikylodermic cutaneous amyloidosis. Eur J Dermatol 2008; 18:289.

Park MY, Kim YC: Macular amyloidosis with an incontinentia pigmenti-like distribution. Eur J Dermatol 2008; 18:477.

Pettersson T, Konttinen YT: Amyloidosis: recent developments. Semin Arthritis Rheum 2008 Nov 18 (Epub ahead of print).

Powell AM, et al: Discoid lupus erythematosus with secondary amyloidosis. Br J Dermatol 2005; 153:746.

Rajkumar SV, et al: Monoclonal gammopathy of undetermined significance, Waldenström macroglobulinemia, AL amyloidosis, and related plasma cell disorders: diagnosis and treatment. Mayo Clin Proc 2006; 81:693.

Rekhtman N, et al: Mucocutaneous bullous amyloidosis with an unusual mixed protein composition of amyloid deposits. Br J Dermatol 2006; 154:751.

Rothberg AE, et al: Familial medullary thyroid carcinoma associated with cutaneous lichen amyloidosis. Thyroid 2009; 19:651.

Sakuma TH, et al: Familial primary localized cutaneous amyloidosis in Brazil. Arch Dermatol 2009; 145:695.

Summers EM, et al: Primary localized cutaneous nodular amyloidosis and CREST syndrome: a case report and review of the literature. Cutis 2008; 82:55.

Sviggum HP, et al: Dermatologic adverse effects of lenalidomide therapy for amyloidosis and multiple myeloma. Arch Dermatol 2006; 142:1298.

Tafarel JR, et al: Cutaneous amyloidosis associated with primary biliary cirrhosis. Eur J Gastroenterol Hepatol 2007; 17:603.

Takayama K, et al: Dialysis-related amyloidosis on the buttocks. Acta Derm Venereol 2008; 88:72.

Tanaka A, et al: New insight into mechanisms of pruritus from molecular studies on familial primary localized cutaneous amyloidosis. Br J Dermatol 2009; May 26 (Epub ahead of print).

Taniguchi Y, et al: Cutaneous amyloidosis associated with amyopathic dermatomyositis. J Rheumatol 2009; 36:1088.

Verga U, et al: Frequent association between MEN 2A and cutaneous lichen amyloidosis. Clin Endocrinol (Oxf) 2003; 59:156.

Vijaikumar M, Thappa DM, et al: Amyloidosis cutis dyschromica in two siblings. Clin Exp Dermatol 2001; 26:674.

Wang XD, et al: Diffuse haemorrhagic bullous amyloidosis with multiple myeloma. Clin Exp Dermatol 2008; 33:94.

Wu JJ, et al: Macular amyloidosis presenting in an incontinentia pigmenti-like pattern with subepidermal blister formation. J Eur Acad Dermatol Venereol 2008; 22:635.

Yasuyuki F, et al: Nail dystrophy and blisters as sole manifestations in myeloma-associated amyloidosis. J Am Acad Dermatol 2006; 54:712.

Yoshida A, et al: Lichen amyloidosis induced on the upper back by long-term friction with a nylon towel. J Dermatol 2009; 36:56.

PORPHYRIAS

Porphyrinogens are the building blocks of all the hemoproteins, including hemoglobin and the cytochrome enzymes. They are produced primarily in the liver and bone marrow. Each form of porphyria has now been associated with a deficiency in an enzyme in the metabolic pathway of heme synthesis. These enzyme deficiencies lead to accumulation of the precursor molecules before the mutation. The precursors are "porphyrins" and the diseases are called "porphyrias."

Understanding the biosynthetic pathway of heme has clarified the biochemical basis of the porphyrias. Delta-aminolevulinic acid (dALA) is synthesized in the mitochondria via dALA synthetase. From it are formed, successively, porphobilinogen, uroporphyrin III, coproporphyrin III, and protoporphyrin IX. This re-enters the mitochondrion, to be acted on by ferrochelatase to produce heme. Each step in this process is catalyzed by a specific enzyme. Heme, by negative feedback, represses the production, or activity, of dALA synthetase. If heme is inadequate, dALA synthetase activity may be increased, leading to the production of more porphyrins. Because this enzyme system is inducible, medications that increase the cytochrome drug-metabolizing system in the liver can lead to exacerbation of the porphyrias by increasing the production of the porphyrin intermediates.

The current grouping of the porphyrias is based on the primary site of increased porphyrin production, either liver or bone marrow—the hepatic or erythropoietic porphyrias, respectively. Some include a hepatoerythropoietic category. Congenital erythropoietic porphyria (CEP), X-linked dominant protoporphyria (XLDPP), and erythropoietic protoporphyria (EPP) are the erythropoietic forms. Acute intermittent porphyria (AIP), ALA dehydratase deficiency (ADP), hereditary coproporphyria (HCP), variegate porphyria (VP), and porphyria cutanea tarda (PCT) are the hepatic forms. Hepatoerythrocytic porphyria (HEP) has been classified as either a hepatic or hepatoerythropoietic type.

Another way to classify the porphyrias is by their symptomatology. This system divides those diseases that have acute episodes, called the acute porphyrias, and those that have skin findings, called the cutaneous porphyrias. Some conditions have both skin disease and acute episodes. The acute porphyrias are ADP, AIP, HCP, and VP. PCT, CEP, XLDPP, and EPP are the cutaneous porphyrias. VP and HCP can have both acute attacks and skin lesions. The acute attacks are induced by conditions that activate the heme biosynthesis pathway. Due to the enzymatic "blocks" as the pathway is activated, large amounts of the heme precursors (specifically dALA and porphobilinogen) are produced by the liver and dumped into the bloodstream. These substances are neurotoxic and affect primarily the autonomic and peripheral nerves. In the cutaneous porphyrias, photosensitivity is observed. The photosensitivity is caused by the absorption of UV radiation in the Soret band (400-410 nm) by increased porphyrins, primarily in the blood vessels of the upper dermis. These activated porphyrins are unstable, and as they return to a ground state, they transfer energy to oxygen, creating reactive oxygen species. These unstable oxygen species interact with biologic systems, primarily plasma and lysosomal membranes, causing tissue damage. Mediators released from mast cells and polymorphonuclear leukocytes, acting through complement, eicosanoids, or factor XII pathways, may augment tissue effects. The primary damage occurs in the blood vessels of the upper dermis and at the dermoepidermal junction.

The porphyrias have classically been diagnosed by identifying characteristic clinical and biochemical abnormalities, typically elevated levels of porphyrins in the urine, serum, red blood cell, or stool. Because there is some clinical overlap, biochemical testing should be performed to confirm any diagnosis of porphyria. In the acute porphyrias, patients are often asymptomatic between attacks. During attacks, porphyrin assays will be abnormal in all forms of porphyria. In between attacks, some patients with AIP may have normal porphyrin assays. The genetic defect and the points of the most common mutations for each gene are now known for most forms of the porphyrias. Genetic testing is now recommended in most forms of the porphyrias, except PCT and EPP. This allows for the diagnosis of AIP between attacks. There is considerable clinical overlap in these rarer porphyrias, dual porphyrias exist (with mutations in two different heme synthesis genes), and low-level mutations causing atypical presentations are now well described. Accurate diagnosis in such cases requires determination of the genetic defect. This also allows for genetic counselling and prenatal diagnosis.

Porphyria cutanea tarda

Porphyria cutanea tarda (PCT) is the most common type of porphyria. Patients present most commonly in midlife, averaging 45 years of age at disease onset. The disease is characterized by photosensitivity resulting in bullae, especially on sun-exposed parts (Fig. 26-6). The dorsal hands and forearms, ears, and face are primarily affected. The bullae are non-inflammatory, and rupture easily to form erosions or shallow ulcers. These heal with scarring, milia, and dyspigmentation. Lesions on the legs, especially the shins and dorsal feet, occur primarily in women. In addition, patients frequently complain of skin fragility in affected areas. There is hyperpigmentation of the skin, especially of the face, neck, and hands. Hypertrichosis of the face, especially over the cheeks and temples, is seen. The face and neck, especially in the periorbital area, may show a pink to violaceous tint. Sclerodermatous thickenings may develop on the back of the neck, in the preauricular areas (Fig. 26-7), or on the thorax, fingers, and scalp. In the latter instance, there is associated alopecia. A direct relationship between the levels of uroporphyrins in the urine and sclerodermatous changes has been reported.

Liver disease is frequently present in patients with PCT. A history of alcoholism is common. Hepatitis C virus (HCV) infection has been found in 17% (Northern Europe), 20% (Australia/New Zealand), 65% (Southern Europe), and 94% (US) of patients with PCT. All PCT patients should be screened for HCV infection. Iron overload in the liver is frequently found in patients with PCT. This may be as a consequence of chemical or viral liver damage, or because 20% of patients with

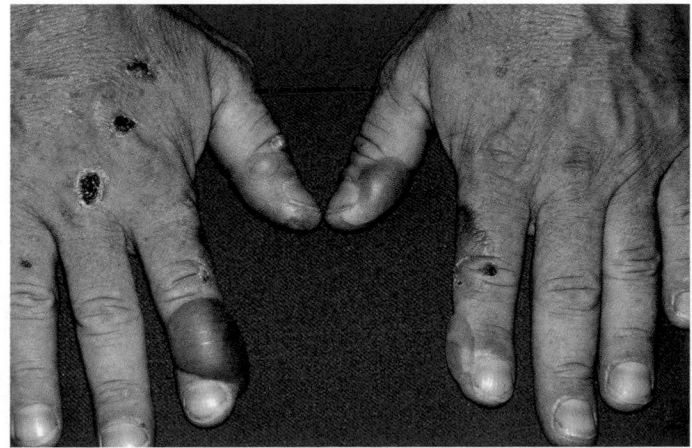

Fig. 26-6 Porphyria cutanea tarda.

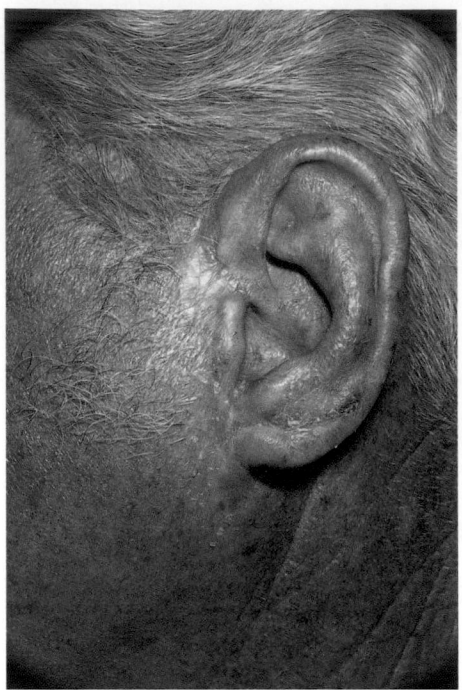

Fig. 26-7 Porphyria cutanea tarda with sclerosis.

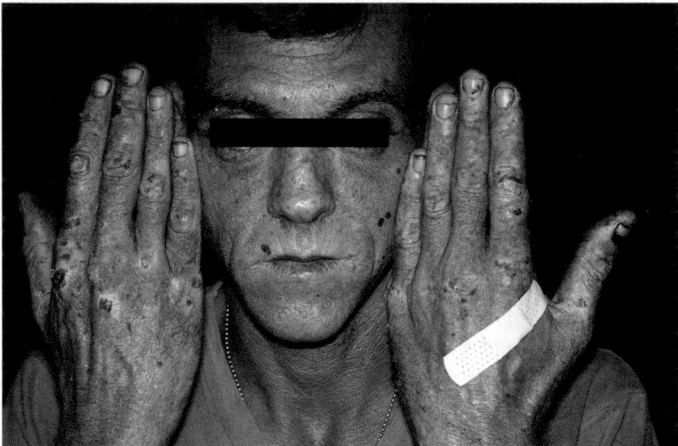

Fig. 26-8 Porphyria cutanea tarda with hemochromatosis. (Courtesy of Curt Samlaska, MD)

PCT are homozygous for the Cys282Tyr mutation (and a few with the His63Asp mutation), causing hemochromatosis (Fig. 26-8). This leads to increases in serum iron and in ferritin, and hepatic iron overload. Hepatocellular carcinoma may rarely produce PCT.

PCT has been frequently associated with other diseases. It is estimated that diabetes mellitus occurs in 15–20% of patients with PCT. Numerous cases of lupus erythematosus concomitant with PCT have been reported. Patients may have systemic and/or purely cutaneous lupus, and either disease may present initially. The pathogenesis of this association is unclear.

PCT occurs not infrequently in patients infected with the human immunodeficiency virus (HIV). This is not solely related to coexistent HCV infection, which is increased in some risk groups of HIV-infected persons. Subtle porphyrin abnormalities are found in HIV disease, but the porphyrin levels are well below those capable of inducing clinical disease. Other risk factors, such as alcoholism, should be evaluated and the existence of PCT should not be attributed to the HIV disease alone. However, effective anti-HIV therapy has led to improvement of PCT in one HIV/HCV-infected patient.

Estrogen treatment is associated with the appearance of PCT by an unknown mechanism. Before oral contraceptives were introduced, PCT cases occurred predominantly among men, but in most recent series, 60% of cases occurred in men and 40% in women. Men treated with estrogens for prostate cancer may develop PCT.

PCT is caused by a deficiency in the enzyme uroporphyrinogen decarboxylase (UROD). Several types have been described. The most common is the sporadic, nonfamilial form, which represents about 80% or more of cases. Enzymatic activity of UROD is abnormal in the liver but normal in other tissues. This is the form associated with the cofactors listed above. The enzyme deficiency is related to loss of enzyme activity due to the liver damage or estrogens triggering the PCT. The enzyme UROD is inhibited by iron, so conditions that lead to iron overload in the liver (cirrhosis, alcoholism, HCV infection, and hemochromatosis) are all associated with PCT. Removal of this iron in the liver can be associated with improvement of PCT as a consequence. With remission, the enzyme activity in the liver may return to normal.

The second or familial type is an autosomal-dominantly inherited deficiency of UROD in the liver and red blood cells of patients, and also of clinically unaffected family members. There is an approximate 50% decrease in both the activity and the concentration of the enzyme. Multiple genetic defects have been reported that produce the same phenotype. Familial PCT tends to present at an earlier age, and development of PCT before age 20 strongly suggests familial PCT.

A third form, acquired toxic PCT, is associated with acute or chronic exposure to hepatotoxins, specifically polyhalogenated hydrocarbons, such as hexachlorobenzene and dioxin. These patients have biochemical and clinical features identical to those of patients with sporadic and familial PCT.

A diagnosis of PCT can be strongly suspected on clinical grounds. A useful confirmatory test that can be performed in the office is the characteristic pink or coral-red fluorescence of a random urine specimen under a Wood's light. A 24-hour collected urine specimen usually contains less than 100 μg of porphyrins in a normal individual; in PCT it may range from 300 to several 1000 μg. The ratio of uroporphyrins to coproporphyrins in PCT is typically 3:1–5:1, distinguishing PCT from variegate porphyria. Plasma porphyrins will also be abnormal. The diagnosis of hereditary PCT is made by demonstrating reduced UROD activity in erythrocytes.

Biopsy of a blister reveals a noninflammatory subepidermal bulla with an undulating, festooned base. PAS-positive thickening of blood vessel walls in the upper and mid-dermis is present. A useful and highly characteristic—but not diagnostic—feature is the presence of the so-called caterpillar bodies. These eosinophilic, elongated, wavy structures are present in the lower and mid-epidermis and lie parallel to the basement membrane zone. They stain positively with PAS and are positive for type IV collagen and laminin, suggesting they represent basement membrane material present in the epidermis. DIF of involved skin shows IgG and C3 at the dermoepidermal junction and in the vessel walls in a granular-linear pattern.

Initial treatment of PCT involves removal of all precipitating environmental agents, such as alcohol and medications. This may lead to sufficient improvement that further therapy is not required. Chemical sunscreens are of little value since they do not typically absorb radiation in the near-visible UVA range. Barrier sunscreens such as titanium dioxide and zinc oxide may be more beneficial, but physical barriers such as hats and gloves may be encouraged while therapy is initiated.

Phlebotomy is the treatment of choice for PCT. UROD is inhibited by iron, and removal of hepatic iron may therefore lead to recovery of enzyme activity. Typically, phlebotomy of

500 mL at 2-week intervals is performed until the hemoglobin reaches 10 g/dL or the serum iron 50–60 µg/dL. Ideally, serum ferritin will become normal also. Urinary porphyrin excretion initially increases, but gradually, 24-hour uroporphyrin levels are markedly reduced, with most patients able to achieve normal levels. This process takes several months, usually requiring a total of 6–10 phlebotomies. As the porphyrins fall, the skin lesions also involute. Initially, blistering improves, then skin fragility decreases, and finally the cutaneous sclerosis and hypertrichosis can eventually reverse. A common error in management is coadministration of oral iron supplementation during the phlebotomies to treat the anemia.

Antimalarials are an alternative to phlebotomy and may be combined with phlebotomy in difficult cases. Full doses of antimalarials may produce a severe hepatotoxic reaction. The initial dose is 125 mg of chloroquine twice a week. Improvement is gradual, but can be more rapid than phlebotomy.

After both phlebotomy and antimalarial therapy, a remission is induced that may last many years. If the patient relapses, these treatments can be repeated. Alternative treatments, which are rarely required, include desferrioxamine (iron chelation) and erythropoietin treatment. Erythropoietin may be combined with phlebotomy. PCT in renal failure may respond to erythropoietin and low-volume phlebotomy, or to renal transplantation. If HCV infection coexists, interferon-α treatment of the HCV infection may lead to improvement of the PCT. The management of PCT associated with hemodialysis is much more difficult. High-flux/high-efficiency hemodialysis should be instituted. Administration of N-acetylcysteine, 400 mg of powder dissolved in orange juice twice a day, can be added to augmented dialysis. Erythropoietin, at times at very high dose, in combination with mini-phlebotomy can be used in anuric patients with PCT not controlled by other methods.

Pseudoporphyria

In certain settings patients develop blistering and skin fragility identical to PCT, with the histologic features of PCT but with normal urine and serum porphyrins. Hypertrichosis, dyspigmentation, and cutaneous sclerosis do not occur. This condition is called pseudoporphyria. Most commonly, this is caused by medications, typically a nonsteroidal anti-inflammatory drug (NSAID), usually naproxen. Other NSAIDs, such as nebumetone and rofecoxib, voriconazole, tetracycline (Fig. 26-9), and multiple other medications can cause a similar picture.

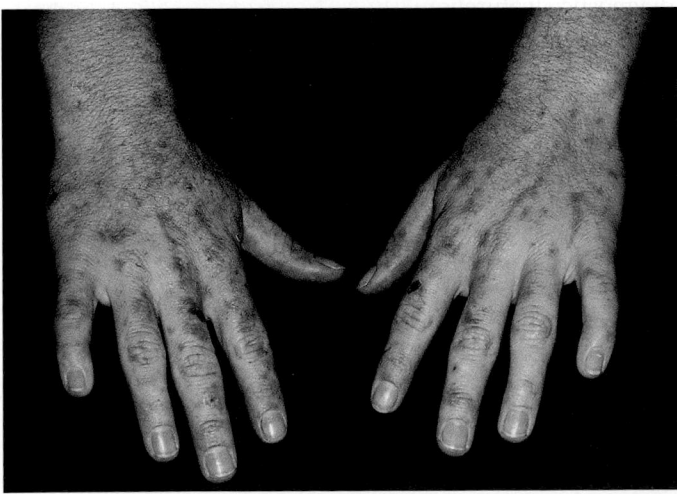

Fig. 26-9 Pseudoporphyria cutanea tarda from tetracycline in a young woman.

Sunbed use can also cause pseudo-PCT. Some patients on hemodialysis develop a similar PCT-like picture. Less commonly, dialysis patients develop true PCT. In the anuric dialysis patient, true PCT and pseudo-PCT are distinguished by analysis of serum porphyrins in a laboratory knowledgeable in the normal porphyrin levels in patients undergoing hemodialysis. The treatment of pseudoporphyria is physical sun protection and discontinuance of any inciting medication. Ibuprofen is a safer alternative NSAID that usually does not cause pseudoporphyria. In medication-induced PCT, blistering resolves over several months once the medication is stopped. Skin fragility may persist for much longer.

Hepatoerythropoietic porphyria

Hepatoerythropoietic porphyria (HEP) is a very rare form of porphyria that is inherited as an autosomal-recessive trait. HEP is the homozygous form of PCT. It is caused by a homozygous or compound heterozygous deficiency of UROD, which is about 10% of normal in both the liver and erythrocytes. The biochemical abnormalities are similar to, but more marked than those in PCT, yet the clinical features are similar to congenital erythropoietic porphyria (CEP). Dark urine is usually present from birth. In infancy vesicles occur in sun-exposed skin, followed by sclerodermoid scarring, hypertrichosis, pigmentation, red fluorescence of the teeth under Wood's light examination, and nail damage. Neurologic disease has been reported in one patient. The diagnosis is confirmed by abnormal urinary uroporphyrins, as seen in PCT, elevated erythrocyte protoporphyrins, and increased coproporphyrins in the feces. In CEP, uroporphyrins are elevated in the erythrocytes, allowing differentiation from HEP. Sun protection is necessary, but often inadequate. Bone marrow transplantation, as in CEP, may be required.

Variegate porphyria

Variegate porphyria (VP) is also known as mixed porphyria, South African genetic porphyria, and mixed hepatic porphyria. VP has an autosomal-dominant inheritance, with a high penetrance. It results from a decrease in activity of protoporphyrinogen oxidase (PPOX). Between 40 and 70% of patients with VP have skin symptoms, 27% have acute attacks, and only 14% have both acute attacks and skin symptoms. Many affected relatives have silent VP, in which there is reduced enzyme activity but no clinical lesions. Such persons should be identified and evaluated.

VP is characterized by the combination of the skin lesions of PCT and the acute gastrointestinal and neurologic disease of acute intermittent porphyria (AIP). In 50% of VP patients skin lesions are the presenting finding. Vesicles and bullae with erosions, especially on sun-exposed areas, are the chief manifestations. In addition, hypertrichosis is seen in the temporal area, especially in women. Hyperpigmentation of sun-exposed areas is also a feature. Facial scarring and thickening of the skin may give the patient a prematurely aged appearance.

The presence of VP should be suspected in a patient when findings indicate both PCT and AIP, especially if he/she is of South African ancestry. Fecal coproporphyrins and protoporphyrins are always elevated, and during attacks urine porphobilinogen and ALA are elevated. Normal excretion of fecal protoporphyrin in adulthood predicts freedom from both skin symptoms and acute attacks. Urinary coproporphyrins are increased over uroporphyrins, distinguishing VP from PCT. Urinary coproporphyrin over 1000 nmol/day predicts increased risk for acute attacks and skin symptoms, and should result in preventive treatment to reduce porphyrins. A finding in the plasma of a unique fluorescence at 626 nm is characteristic of VP and distinguishes it from all other forms of porphyria. Lymphocyte PPOX should be measured. Treatment is symptomatic and as outlined for PCT and AIP. Education of patients and unaffected PPOX-deficient relatives to avoid triggering medications is essential.

Hereditary coproporphyria

Hereditary coproporphyria (HCP) is a rare, autosomal-dominant porphyria resulting from a deficiency of coproporphyrinogen oxidase (CPO). About one-third of patients are photosensitive, with blistering similar to but less severe than in VP. About 35% have acute attacks with gastrointestinal and neurologic symptoms similar to those seen in AIP and VP. Fecal coproporphyrin III is always increased; urinary coproporphyrin, ALA, and porphobilinogen (PBG) are increased only during attacks. Plasma fluorescence at 619 nm is seen. Mutation screening can be used to confirm the diagnosis and identify unaffected but CPO-deficient relatives. Homozygous hereditary coproporphyria, or harderoporphyria is caused by a homozygous defect of CPO, with patients having 10% of normal activity. Children present with photosensitivity, hypertrichosis, and hemolytic anemia. The biochemical findings in plasma, feces, and urine are identical to HCP, but more marked. Harderoporphyrin is the natural intermediate between coproporphyrinogen and protoporphyrinogen.

Erythropoietic protoporphyria

Erythropoietic protoporphyria (EPP) is an autosomal-dominant or autosomal-recessive disorder. The ferrochelatase (FECH) activity is always below 35% and usually 10–25% of normal in affected persons. This low level of enzyme activity, inherited as a dominant trait (which should result in only a 50% reduction in enzyme activity) is due to the fact that all affected persons are in fact compound heterozygotes. In Europe up to 10–15% of the population carries a low-expression (hypomorphic) allele that is only 50% as active as the wild-type enzyme. If the patient also inherits a loss of function mutation, this combination leads to about 25% enzyme activity, below the critical 35% activity required to remain disease-free. Autosomal-recessive EPP results from inheritance of two genes with significant loss of function, but not a common hypomorphic allele.

EPP typically presents early in childhood (3 months to 2 years old), but presentation late in adulthood can occur.

Unique among the more common forms of porphyria is an immediate burning of the skin on sun exposure. Because the elevated protoporphyrin IX absorbs both in the Soret band and at 500–600 nm, visible light through window glass or in the operating room may precipitate symptoms. Infants cry when exposed to sunlight. Erythema, plaque-like edema, and wheals such as those seen in solar urticaria can be seen. These lesions appear solely on sun-exposed areas. In severe cases, purpura is seen in the sun-exposed areas.

With repeated exposure, the skin develops a weather-beaten appearance. Shallow linear or elliptical scars, waxy thickening and pebbling of the skin on the nose and cheeks (Fig. 26-10) and over metacarpophalangeal joints, and atrophy of the rims of the ears have been described. Perioral furrow-like scars are characteristic. The dorsal hands and face of EPP patients look much older than their chronological age.

About 2.5% of patients with EPP have a seasonal palmar keratoderma. It is worse in the summer and resolves in winter or with occlusion of the palm with a plaster cast. The keratoderma is waxy, and may cover the whole palm or be localized

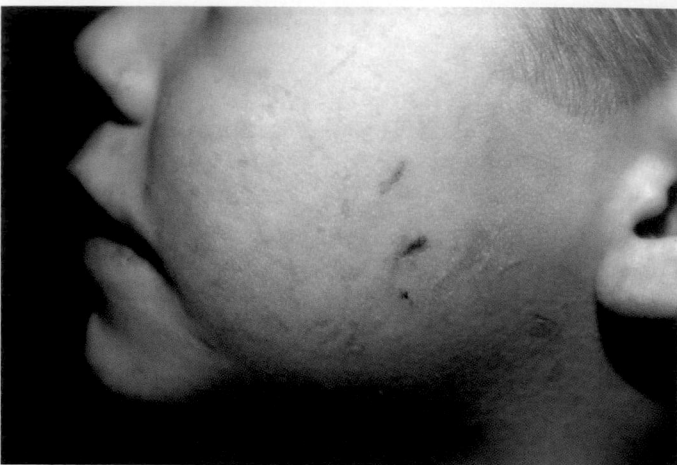

Fig. 26-10 Linear scars and erosions in erythropoietic protoporphyria.

to the first web space. It is sharply demarcated at the wrist and has no red border. The thickening is moderate in severity. The nails are usually unaffected but may show minimal onycholysis. These patients all have autosomal-recessive EPP, with lower levels of erythrocyte protoporphyrin but increased levels of fecal total porphyrin when compared to autosomal-dominant EPP patients. In fact, their erythrocyte protoporphyrin may be near normal. Forty-five percent of patients with autosomal-recessive EPP have this keratoderma. The risk for liver disease appears to be reduced in this form of autosomal-recessive EPP, and may be related to effective hepatobiliary excretion of protoporphyrin. as indicated by the massive elevations in the feces.

Between 20 and 30% of EPP patients have liver complications, due to excessive porphyrin deposits in hepatocytes. This can be anywhere along the spectrum from mild elevation of liver function tests to cirrhosis. Hepatic failure occurs in less than 2% of patients. Autosomal-recessive inheritance of EPP may be a risk factor for the development of liver failure. There is currently no marker for progressive liver disease (not laboratory porphyrins or genetic defect), so all patients must be monitored. Ten percent of patients develop gallstones, often in childhood. A mild microcytic anemia is present in 25% of patients with EPP, but therapy with iron should be used only if iron deficiency is detected, since it may exacerbate symptoms.

The rare syndrome of EPP appearing de novo in adults with an associated myelodysplasia has been reported multiple times. These cases are associated with the deletion of the portion of chromosome 18 containing the ferrochelatase gene, creating a 50% reduction in gene function. If the other gene in that patient is a low-activity common polymorphism, the patient may fall below the 35% activity threshold, resulting in clinical EPP. Bone marrow transplantation is associated with resolution of the EPP.

Histologically, there is prominent ground-glass, PAS-positive material in the upper dermis, mostly perivascularly. This material is type IV collagen. On DIF, IgG and C3 may be found perivascularly.

A diagnosis of EPP can usually be suspected on clinical grounds, especially if both the acute symptoms and chronic skin changes are found. Because protoporphyrin IX is not water-soluble, urine porphyrin levels are normal. Erythrocyte protoporphyrin is elevated, and can be detected by red blood cell (RBC) fluorescence. Erythrocyte, plasma, and fecal protoporphyrin can also be assayed to confirm the diagnosis. Erythrocyte protoporphyrin levels in affected persons may range from several hundred to several thousand μg/100 mL of packed RBCs (normal values, <35 μg/100 mL of packed RBCs). Plasma fluorescence shows a peak at 634 nm.

The differential diagnosis of EPP includes hydroa vacciniforme, xeroderma pigmentosa, and solar urticaria. In infancy, before the appearance of the chronic skin changes, erythrocyte porphyrins may need to be screened to confirm the diagnosis. Once chronic changes are present, a skin biopsy will confirm the diagnosis.

The treatment consists of protection from exposure to sunlight with clothing and barrier sunscreens containing titanium dioxide or zinc oxide. Beta-carotene, 60–180 mg/day in adults and 30–90 mg/day for children, to maintain a serum level of 600 μg/100 mL, provides some protection for most cases. As the child grows, the dose must be increased to maintain adequate tissue levels. Cysteine, at a dose of 500 mg twice a day, can reduce symptoms in some patients. Early spring hardening with narrow-band UVB (NBUVB) or PUVA (wavelengths below the action spectrum of the incriminated porphyrins) is being increasingly used, and is the treatment of choice in some centers. Warfarin treatment may lead to a reduction in symptoms. Transfusions of washed packed RBCs may be used to treat anemia, if the patient is symptomatic. Liver failure requires liver transplantation.

X-linked dominant protoporphyria

X-linked dominant protoporphyria (XLDPP) is due to deletions in the δ-aminolevulinic acid synthetase 2 (ALAS2) gene. These mutations result in gain of function of the ALAS2 gene, with increased production of protoporphyrin. Erythrocyte protoporphyrins are elevated due to this overproduction of protoporphyrin, which exceeds the capacity of the ferrochelatase to incorporate the protoporphyrin into heme, resulting in excess protoporphyrin. Patients present with symptoms identical to EPP. Liver disease may occur in more than 15% of affected patients. Intravenous iron therapy leads to normalization of liver function tests and reduction of skin symptoms.

Congenital erythropoietic porphyria

Congenital erythropoietic porphyria (CEP) is a very rare form of porphyria, also known as erythropoietic porphyria or Gunther's disease. It is inherited as an autosomal-recessive trait and is caused by a homozygous defect of the enzyme uroporphyrinogen III synthase (UROS).

CEP presents soon after birth with the appearance of red urine (noticeable on diapers). Severe photosensitivity occurs, and may result in immediate pain and burning, so that the affected child screams when exposed to the sun. The laser used in pulse oximeters may lead to skin lesions of the nailbed. Redness, swelling, and blistering occur and result in scarring of the face, dorsal hands, and scalp (with subsequent alopecia). Ectropion can occur, with subsequent corneal damage and loss of vision. Erythrodontia (Fig. 26-11) of both deciduous and permanent teeth is also characteristic. This phenomenon is demonstrated by the coral-red fluorescence of the teeth when exposed to a Wood's light. Mutilating scars, especially on the face, and hypertrichosis of the cheeks, with profuse eyebrows and long eyelashes, occur. Other features seen in CEP include growth retardation, hemolytic anemia, thrombocytopenia, porphyrin gallstones, osteopenia, and increased fracturing of bones.

A diagnosis of CEP can be easily suspected when an infant has dark urine and is severely photosensitive. There is a direct correlation of the severity of the disease, the levels of plasma porphyrins, and the residual activity of UROS. Abnormally

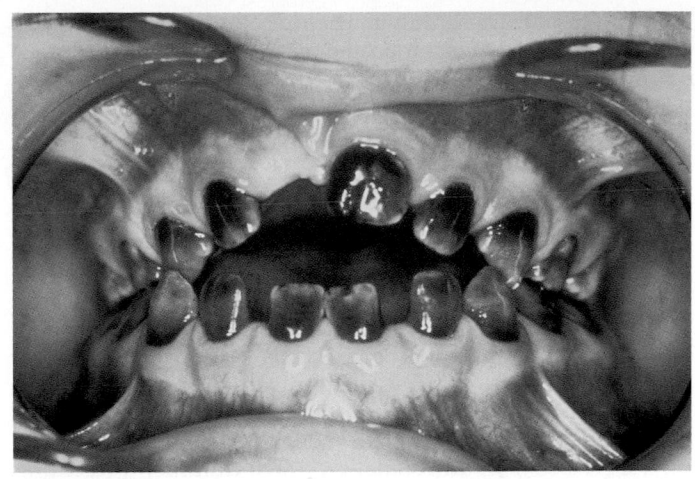

Fig. 26-11 Erythrodontia in congenital erythropoietic porphyria.

high amounts of uroporphyrin I and coproporphyrin I are found in urine, stool, and red cells. There is stable red fluorescence of erythrocytes. On biopsy there is a subepidermal bulla identical to that seen in PCT.

Treatment is strict avoidance of sunlight, and sometimes splenectomy for the hemolytic anemia. Oral activated charcoal is efficacious; presumably it retards the absorption of endogenous porphyrins. Repeated transfusions of packed red cells, enough to maintain the hematocrit level at 33%, turn off the demand for heme and reduce porphyrin production. Bone marrow transplantation should be considered in severely affected children.

Adult-onset CEP is very, very rare. It presents as a mild photosensitive blistering disease resembling PCT. More than half the patients have an associated myelodysplasia.

Acute intermittent porphyria

Acute intermittent porphyria (AIP), the second most common form of porphyria, is characterized by periodic attacks of abdominal pain (up to 95% of patients), gastrointestinal disturbances (up to 90% of patients), pain and paresis (50–70%), seizures (10–20%), and mental symptoms (40–60%) including agitation, hallucinations, and depression. Skin lesions do not occur, since the elevated porphyrin precursors are not photosensitizers. It is inherited as an autosomal-dominant trait and is caused by a deficiency in porphobilinogen deaminase (PBGD), which has 50% activity in affected persons. Only 10% of those with the genetic defect develop disease, but all may be at risk for primary liver cancer. AIP is particularly common in Scandinavia, especially Lapland. AIP usually presents after puberty in young adulthood, and women outnumber men 1.5–2:1.

Severe abdominal colic is most often the initial symptom of AIP. Usually, there is no abdominal wall rigidity, although tenderness and distension are present. Nausea, vomiting, and diarrhea or constipation accompany the abdominal pain. Peripheral neuropathy, mostly motor, is present. Severe pain in the extremities occurs. Optic atrophy, diaphragmatic weakness, respiratory paralysis, flaccid quadriplegia, facial palsy, and dysphagia are but a few of the many neurologic signs.

Attacks of AIP are triggered by certain medications and other conditions. These triggers frequently require increased hepatic heme synthesis (to make the cytochrome P450 enzymes required for metabolism of medications, for example). Progesterone is one trigger, explaining the increased prevalence of AIP in women and the relationship to menses.

Anticonvulsants, griseofulvin, rifampin, and sulfonamides are commonly used drugs implicated in triggering AIP. The implicated medication list is constantly being modified as new drugs enter the market. The website of the European Porphyria Initiative is the best source of an up-to-date list for both patients and healthcare providers (www.porphyria-europe.com). Crash dieting, cigarette smoking, infections and surgery are additional triggers.

A diagnosis of AIP is established by finding elevated levels of urinary PBG and increased dALA in the plasma and urine during attacks. During remissions, the diagnosis can be confirmed in 88% of patients by detecting elevated urinary porphobilinogen. If this test is normal between attacks, it suggests that the likelihood of subsequent attacks is less. Erythrocyte and fecal porphyrin levels are normal. AIP must be distinguished from VP, CP, and ALA dehydratase deficiency porphyria (ALAD), an autosomal-recessive condition presenting in an almost identical manner to AIP. Increased dALA in the urine is found in ALAD and lead poisoning.

No specific treatment is available for AIP. It is important for the patient to avoid such precipitating factors as a wide variety of medications, including sex steroid hormones, and to maintain adequate nutrition. Glucose loading has been used extensively and appears to be beneficial in many cases. Hematin infusions, in the form of heme arginate, result in clinical improvement and a marked decrease in ALA and PBG excretion. Early treatment may ameliorate attacks. The phenothiazines (chlorpromazine) may be helpful for pain; opiates and propoxyphene are also useful for analgesia. Since 10% of patients with AIP die of hepatoma (without the development of cirrhosis), yearly ultrasound and alpha-fetoprotein determination should be undertaken in all AIP patients over the age of 50.

Transient erythroporphyria of infancy (purpuric phototherapy-induced eruption)

Paller et al reported seven infants exposed to 380–700 nm blue lights for the treatment of indirect hyperbilirubinemia who developed marked purpura in skin exposed to UV light. Extensive blistering and erosions occurred in one case. Biopsies of the skin show hemorrhage without epidermal changes in the cases associated with purpura, and a pauci-inflammatory, subepidermal bulla in the case with blistering. The infants had all received transfusions. Elevated plasma coproporphyrins and protoporphyrins were found in the four infants examined. The pathogenesis is unknown.

Anderson KE, et al: Recommendations for the diagnosis and treatment of the acute porphyrias. Ann Intern Med 2005; 142:439.

Cernik C, et al: Adult-onset erythropoietic porphyria in the setting of MDS. Arch Dermatol 2009; 145:948.

Cook NS, McKenna K: A case of haemodialysis-associated pseudoporphyria successfully treated with oral N-acetylcysteine. Clin Exp Dermatol 2007; 32:64.

Crawford RI, et al: Transient erythroporphyria of infancy. J Am Acad Dermatol 1996; 35:833.

Cribier B, et al: Abnormal urinary coproporphyrin levels in patients infected by hepatitis C virus with or without HIV. Arch Dermatol 1996; 132:1448.

DeGiovanni CV, Darley CR: Pseudoporphyria occurring during a course of ciprofloxacin. Clin Exp Dermatol 2008; 33:109.

Gibson GE, et al: Cutaneous abnormalities and metabolic disturbance of porphyrins in patients on maintenance hemodialysis. Clin Exp Dermatol 1997; 22:124.

Gibson GE, et al: Coexistence of lupus erythematosus and porphyria cutanea tarda in 15 patients. J Am Acad Dermatol 1998; 38:569.

Herrero C, et al: Clinical, biochemical, and genetic study of 11 patients with erythropoietic protoporphyria including one with homozygous disease. Arch Dermatol 2007; 143:1125.

Hivnor C, et al: Cyclosporine-induced pseudoporphyria. Arch Dermatol 2003; 139:1373.

Holme SA, et al: Seasonal palmar keratoderma in erythropoietic protoporphyria indicates autosomal recessive inheritance. J Invest Dermatol 2009; 129:599.

Kauppinen R: Porphyrias. Lancet 2005; 365:241.

Lim HW, et al: The cutaneous porphyrias. Semin Cutan Med Surg 1999; 18:285.

Massone C, et al: Successful outcome of haemodialysis-induced pseudoporphyria after short-term oral N-acetylcysteine and switch to high-flux technique dialysis. Acta Derm Venereol 2006; 86:538.

Mathews-Roth MM, et al: A double-blind study of cysteine photoprotection in erythropoietic protoporphyria. Photodermatol Photoimmunol Photomed 1994; 10:244.

Mendez M: A homozygous mutation in the ferrochelatase gene underlies erythropoietic protoporphyria associated with palmar keratoderma. Br J Dermatol 2009; 160:1330.

Oh C, et al: Pseudoporphyria secondary to narrowband UVB phototherapy for psoriasis. Australas J Dermatol 2006; 47:134.

Okano J, et al: Interferon treatment of PCT associated with chronic hepatitis type C. Hepatogastroenterology 1997; 44:525.

Paller AS, et al: Purpuric phototherapy-induced eruption in transfused neonates. Pediatrics 1997; 100:360.

Parsons JL, et al: Neurologic disease in a child with hepatoerythropoietic porphyria. Pediatr Dermatol 1994; 11:216.

Perez-Bustillo A, et al: Torsemide-induced pseudoporphyria. Arch Dermatol 2008; 144:812.

Poblete-Gutierrez P, et al: Dual porphyrias revisited. Exp Dermatol 2006; 15:685.

Sarkany RP: Making sense of the porphyrias. Photodermatol Photoimmunol Photomed 2008; 24:102.

Sarkany RP, et al: Acquired erythropoietic protoporphyria as a result of myelodysplasia causing loss of chromosome 18. Br J Dermatol 2006; 155:464.

Schanbacher CF, et al: Pseudoporphyria. Mayo Clin Proc 2001; 76:488.

Seth AK, et al: Liver transplantation for porphyria: who, when, and how? Liver Transpl 2007; 13:1219.

Sharp MT, Horn TD: Pseudoporphyria induced by voriconazole. J Am Acad Dermatol 2005; 53:341.

Shieh S, et al: Management of porphyria cutanea tarda in the setting of chronic renal failure: a case report and review. J Am Acad Dermatol 2000; 42:645.

Tolland JP, et al: Voriconazole-induced pseudoporphyria. Photodermatol Photoimmunol Photomed 2007; 23:29.

Tremblay J-F, et al: Pseudoporphyria associated with hemodialysis treated with N-acetylcysteine. J Am Acad Dermatol 2003; 49:1189.

Winship I, et al: Antioxidant effect of warfarin therapy: a possible symptomatic treatment for erythropoietic protoporphyria. Arch Dermatol 2009; 145:960.

CALCINOSIS CUTIS

Cutaneous calcification results from deposits of calcium and phosphorus in the skin. Calcinosis cutis is divided into four forms. Dystrophic calcinosis includes conditions in which calcification occurs in damaged tissue (usually collagen or elastic tissue). Serum calcium and phosphorus levels are normal. Dermatomyositis is a classic example. Metastatic calcification refers to deposition of calcium resulting from elevated serum levels of calcium or phosphorus. Hyperparathyroidism is an example of this form of calcification. Iatrogenic and traumatic calcinosis is associated with medical procedures or occupational exposures that may involve both tissue damage and local elevated calcium concentrations. Idiopathic calcinosis cutis refers to those forms of cutaneous calcification of unknown cause with normal serum calcium. In osteoma cutis, true bone is formed in the skin.

Dystrophic calcinosis cutis

This type occurs in a pre-existing lesion or inflammatory process. Systemic calcium metabolism is normal, and lesions

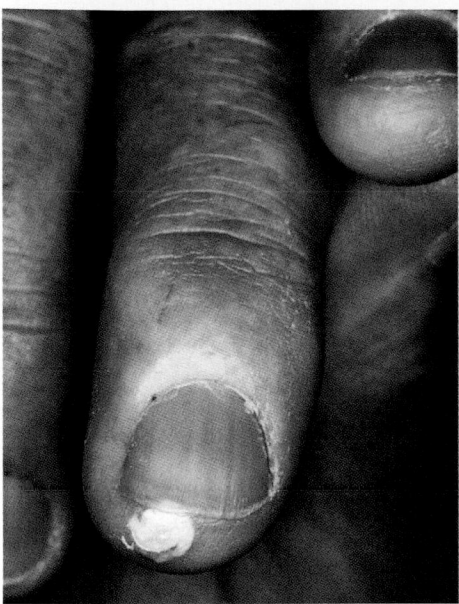

Fig. 26-12 Calcinosis cutis in CREST syndrome.

affect the skin only. Disease may be divided into localized (calcinosis circumscripta) and widespread (calcinosis universalis) types. Localized calcinosis cutis may present as small deposits of chalky granular material around the fingers and on the elbows. They may spontaneously extrude from the skin. This form occurs most commonly in limited scleroderma (the CREST syndrome: calcinosis cutis, Raynaud phenomenon, esophageal disorders, sclerodactyly, and telangiectasia) (Fig. 26-12), but may be seen in progressive systemic sclerosis and systemic lupus erythematosus (SLE). Pancreatic and lupus panniculitis typically demonstrate dystrophic calcification, but the process tends to remain microscopic. Patients with Werner syndrome and PCT may also develop calcifications within the scleroderma-like lesions. As is illustrated by pseudoxanthoma elasticum, dystrophic elastic tissues are often the site of deposition of calcinosis cutis. Even in cases of metastatic calcinosis cutis (see below), the depositions may preferentially or solely affect areas of elastic tissue damage (sun damage, striae, etc.).

Various benign and malignant neoplasms may develop calcification or ossification. Pilomatrixomas, pilar cysts, nevi, mixed tumors, melanomas, and atypical fibroxanthomas are the most commonly reported of these. In the above cases, calcification is in the dermis or subcutaneous tissue; however, in one patient with well-defined infiltrated white plaques of the labia majora and genital mucosa who had chronic irritation from urinary incontinence and a vesicovaginal fistula, calcification occurred in the epithelium.

Calcinosis universalis is seen in 40–70% of children with dermatomyositis. It affects the skin, muscles, and tendons, as well as more occurring diffusely. Dermal and subcutaneous nodules, at times associated with areas of inflammation, are characteristic. This calcification can persist for many years after the dermatomyositis is inactive. Calcinosis cutis in dermatomyositis may occur in adults, particularly those with a delay in diagnosis, or who receive inconsistent treatment, or who have the TNF-α-308A allele. Pseudoxanthoma elasticum and nephrogenic systemic fibrosis, may be complicated by calcinosis universalis, as may Hutchinson–Gilford progeria. Idiopathic cases of calcinosis universalis have been reported. Dystrophic calcification is treated with limited surgical removal as needed to control discomfort. Bisphosphonates, calcium channel-blockers, warfarin, colchicines, probenecid, and a low-calcium, low-phosphate diet combined with alumi-

num hydroxide have been reported to be of benefit in the treatment of calcinosis cutis in individual patients. Treatment of dermatomyositis with IVIG led to improvement of calcinosis cutis in one patient with dermatomyositis. A non-healing leg ulcer with dystrophic calcification in a patient with SLE improved with topical sodium thiosulfate.

Metastatic calcinosis cutis

This rare entity is characterized by calcifications in the skin, elevated serum calcium, and sometimes hyperphosphatemia. Metastatic calcinosis is often associated with bone loss or destruction, the bone providing the source of the elevated serum calcium. Conditions associated with metastatic calcinosis include parathyroid neoplasms, primary hyperparathyroidism, chronic renal failure, hypervitaminosis D, sarcoidosis, and excessive intake of milk and alkali. Destruction of bone by osteomyelitis, leukemia, Paget's disease of the bone, myeloma, and metastatic carcinoma may lead to elevated serum calcium and metastatic calcification. In calcinosis cutis with hyperparathyroidism, the skin manifestations are numerous, small, firm, white papules, about 1–4 mm in diameter, occurring symmetrically in the popliteal fossae, over the iliac crests, and in the posterior axillary lines. At times metastatic calcinosis cutis localizes to areas of damaged elastic tissue (striae, solar elastosis, etc.).

The most common metabolic condition associated with metastatic calcification is renal failure. Usually, there is an elevated phosphorus level and secondary hyperparathyroidism, resulting in high calcium and phosphorus production, and deposition of calcium phosphate in tissues. Less commonly, cutaneous calcification in renal disease can occur with normal serum calcium and phosphorus levels. Three forms of cutaneous calcification in renal disease have been described: tumoral calcinosis, calcifying panniculitis, and calciphylaxis. Tumoral calcinosis is a very rare complication of renal disease. Managing the metabolic abnormalities may lead to resolution of the large deposits of calcium.

Often calcifying panniculitis and calciphylaxis occur in the same patient at the same time, suggesting that they may be of a common pathogenesis. Isolated, firm, indurated nodules, usually on the legs or thighs in the subcutaneous fat, have been called calcifying panniculitis. Usually, they are seen with the most severe complication of the abnormal calcium and phosphorus metabolism of renal disease, calciphylaxis. This life-threatening condition, which leads to livedo reticularis and ischemic tissue necrosis, is discussed in Chapter 35.

Iatrogenic and traumatic calcinosis cutis

Medical procedures that may inadvertently introduce calcium into tissue in association with tissue trauma may lead to cutaneous calcification. This has been reported after extravasation of calcium chloride or calcium gluconate infusion, and after electroencephalography or electromyography. The electrode paste is high in calcium, and the skin is traumatized during the procedure, leading to calcifications at the sites of electrode insertion. The most common setting is on the scalp of children. Lesions spontaneously resolve over months. Performing frequent heel sticks in neonates has led to similar lesions. Injections of low molecular weight calcium-containing heparins in patients suffering from renal failure may result in calcification at the sites of injection. Frequent subcutaneous injection of interferon-β in the abdomen has resulted in localized calcification in the fat.

During liver transplantation, hypocalcemia can occur due to calcium chelation by the citrate in transfused blood products.

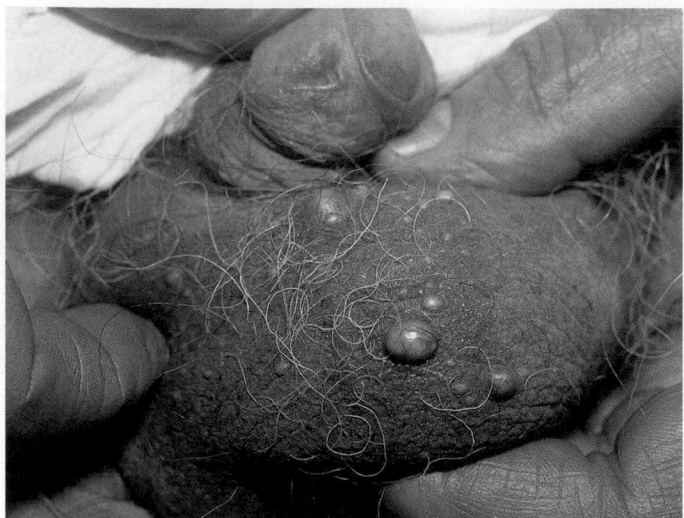

Fig. 26-13 Scrotal calcinosis.

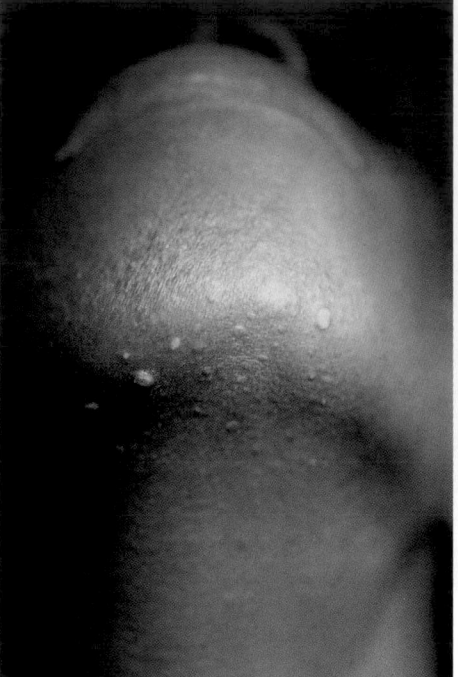

Fig. 26-14 Subepidermal calcified nodules.

Intravenous calcium infusions are regularly given. Calcifications at infusion sites and on the upper extremities, but not at infusion sites, have been reported. They occur 1–3 weeks after transplantation and resolve over 6 months.

Traumatic calcinosis may occur as a result of occupational exposure to calcium-containing materials, as in the cases reported in oil-field workers and coal miners. Exposure of the skin to cloth sacks of calcium chloride, limewater compresses, and refrigerant calcium chloride can all cause calcinosis cutis.

Idiopathic calcinosis cutis

Idiopathic scrotal calcinosis

Idiopathic scrotal calcinosis is the most common form of idiopathic calcinosis cutis. Lesions present in young to middle-aged adult men as multiple, asymptomatic, firm, round, yellow papules from several millimeters up to 1 cm in diameter (Fig. 26-13). The papules resemble infundibular follicular cysts. Similar lesions, usually 1 to several mm in size, may be seen rarely in girls or women on the labia majora. Calcinosis of the areola can have a similar appearance and is very, very rare. Histologically, there are localized deposits of calcium surrounded by a foreign body reaction. At least some are calcified scrotal infundibular cysts. Why they have such a high proclivity to calcification at this anatomic location is unclear. Treatment is not required, but surgical removal cures individual lesions.

Subepidermal calcified nodule

Subepidermal calcified nodule is an uncommon but distinct type of idiopathic calcinosis; it occurs most frequently as one or a few lesions on the scalp or face of children (Fig. 26-14). Males outnumber females by nearly 2:1, and the average age at onset is 7 years. Lesions present as fixed, uninflamed papules that look very much like those of molluscum contagiosum with a central umbilication. The affected children usually do not have an underlying medical condition. A similar condition, milia-like idiopathic calcinosis cutis, has a wider distribution (hands, feet, elbows, and knees are common sites). Two-thirds of patients have Down syndrome. Treatment is not required, but surgical removal will cure any individual lesion.

Tumoral calcinosis

Tumoral calcinosis is a rare disease of unknown cause that can be divided into two forms. The idiopathic, primary, or normophosphatemic form is seen in young adults, primarily in African natives. It is not familial, lesions are usually solitary, and antecedent trauma is frequently present. Hyperphosphatemic familial tumoral calcinosis (HFTC) is characterized by periarticular calcifications. Mutations in two genes have been described as causing this syndrome—fibroblast growth factor 23 (*FGF 23*), *GALNT3* called *KLOTHO*. Most cases present before the second decade of life and occur in black people. Three-quarters of these individuals have affected siblings, but the exact mode of inheritance is unknown. Multiple lesions predominate, and there is no preceding history of trauma. The serum calcium level is normal, but serum phosphorus and calcitriol levels are elevated.

Lesions in both types present as large subcutaneous masses of calcium overlying pressure areas and large joints, usually the hips, elbows, shoulders, or knees. Skin involvement, apart from the tumoral masses, is extremely rare but may occur as localized calcinosis cutis. The internal organs are not involved, and serum calcium levels are generally normal. Surgical excision has been the mainstay of therapy; however, recurrences are frequent after incomplete removal. Various dietary restrictions to lower calcium and phosphorus intake have shown some success. The combination of a phosphate binder, and a carbonic anhydrase inhibitor along with a low-phosphorus diet led to dramatic improvement in one patient, allowing for surgical removal.

Osteoma cutis

Bone formation within the skin may be primary in cases where there was no preceding lesion; metastatic (associated with abnormalities of parathyroid metabolism); or dystrophic, where ossification occurs in a pre-existing lesion or inflammatory process.

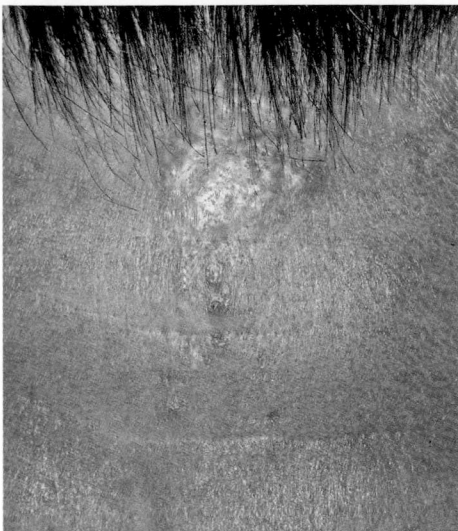

Fig. 26-15 Osteoma cutis. (Courtesy of Curt Samlaska, MD)

Primary osteoma cutis includes four genetic disorders: fibrodysplasia ossificans progressiva, progressive osseous heteroplasia, widespread or single, platelike osteoma cutis, and Albright hereditary osteodystrophy. Additionally, single osteomas may occur as an idiopathic event in later life, or multiple miliary osteomas of the face can be seen, usually in women (Fig. 26-15). Some feel the latter are dystrophic because they occur in patients with acne and are associated with scars. If tetracycline or minocycline is ingested for treatment of the acne, the cutaneous osteomas may be pigmented. Improvement with topical tretinoin, erbium:YAG laser, or with incision, curettage, and primary closure has been reported in these miliary osteomas.

Patients with fibrodysplasia ossificans progressiva develop osteoma cutis as endochondral bone formation associated with deep connective tissue and skeletal muscle involvement. They have dystrophic great toes, baldness, mental retardation, and deafness. The prognosis is poor due to the progressive and deep nature of the lesions, which leads to extreme morbidity and early death because of restricted movement of the chest. The genetic defect is in the *ACVR1* gene.

Progressive osseous heteroplasia is a rare form of cutaneous ossification initially seen between birth and 6 months of age, often in the first month of life. Females are preferentially affected. Lesions begin as small papules that can coalesce to large plaques. Sometimes these plaques will have small, firm, calcified papules overlying them. Lesions are randomly distributed and may be unilateral or involve only one anatomic area. There is no preceding trauma or inflammatory phase. Serum calcium, phosphorus, parathyroid hormone, and calcitriol are normal, but alkaline phosphatase, lactate dehydrogenase (LDH), and creatine phosphokinase (CPK) may be elevated, indicating increased bone formation (alkaline phosphatase) or muscle destruction (CPK and LDH). Histologically, the lesions reveal intramembranous bone formation and can affect the soft tissues as well as skin. Only calcification without ossification may be found in superficial dermal biopsies, so a deep biopsy, including subcutaneous fat, may be required to confirm the diagnosis. The condition is progressive and can lead to serious sequelae, including ulceration, infection, and severe pain. Platelike osteoma cutis also occurs in newborns or young children, is unassociated with dysmorphic features or abnormalities of calcium or phosphorus metabolism, has intramembranous bone formation histologically, but is non-progressive. These disorders are most likely polar ends of a spectrum of disease, as one family has been described with members having either condition. As with Albright hereditary osteodystrophy (see below), the mutation is in the *GNAS1* gene.

Albright hereditary osteodystrophy is described in Chapter 24. It is characterized by childhood development of intramembranous bone formation in the dermis and subcutaneous tissue. The cutaneous ossifications may be noted soon after birth and are usually multiple, small, superficial plaques. They favor the scalp, hands, feet, periarticular regions, abdomen, and chest wall. Small lesions are of little consequence, but large subcutaneous masses may disrupt underlying structures. There may be characteristic dysmorphic features and the presence of pseudo- or pseudopseudo-hypoparathyroidism. It also is associated with mutations of the *GNAS1* gene.

Dystrophic osteoma cutis occurs most frequently in pilomatrixomas; however, other lesions in which bone formation may occur are basal cell epithelioma, intradermal nevi, mixed tumor of the skin, scars, scleroderma, and dermatomyositis.

Abdullah-Lotf M, et al: Regression of cutis calcinosis with diltiazem in adult dermatomyositis. Eur J Dermatol 2005; 15:102.

Altman JF, et al: Treatment of primary miliary osteoma cutis with incision, curettage, and primary closure. J Am Acad Dermatol 2001; 44:96.

Becuwe C, et al: Milia-like idiopathic calcinosis cutis. Pediatr Dermatol 2004; 21:483.

Bernardo BD, et al: Idiopathic calcinosis cutis presenting as labial lesions in children: report of two cases with literature review. J Pediatr Adolesc Gynecol 1999; 12:157.

Chefetz I, et al: GALNT3, a gene associated with hyperphosphatemic familial tumoral calcinosis, is transcriptionally regulated by extracellular phosphate and modulates matrix metalloproteinase activity. Biochim Biophys Acta 2009; 1792:61.

Dominguez-Fernandez I, et al: Calcinosis cutis following extravasation of calcium salts. J Eur Acad Dermatol Venereol 2008; 22:505.

Ehsani AH: Calcinosis cutis complicating liver transplantation. Dermatol Online J 2006; 12:23.

Eich D, et al: Calcinosis of the cutis and subcutis. J Am Acad Dermatol 2004; 50:210.

Federico A, et al: Dystrophic calcinosis cutis in pseudoxanthoma elasticum. J Am Acad Dermatol 2008; 58:707.

Gibney MD, et al: Firm plaque of the forearm in a patient with Hodgkin lymphoma. Arch Dermatol 1999; 134:101.

Goolamali SI, et al: Subcutaneous calcification presenting in a patient with mixed connective tissue disease and cutaneous polyarteritis nodosa. Clin Exp Dermatol 2009; 34:e141.

Kalajian AH, et al: Intravenous immunoglobulin therapy for dystrophic calcinosis cutis: unreliable in our hands. Arch Dermatol 2008; 144:585.

Kupitz S, et al: Chronic ulcers, calcification and calcified fibrous tumours: phenotypic manifestations of a congenital disorder of heterotopic ossification. Int Wound J 2007; 4:273.

Lammoglia JJ, Mericq V: Familial tumoral calcinosis caused by a novel FGF23 mutation: response to induction of tubular renal acidosis with acetazolamide and the non-calcium phosphate binder sevelamer. Horm Res 2009; 71:178.

Larralde M, et al: Calcinosis cutis following liver transplantation in a pediatric patient. Pediatr Dermatol 2003; 20:225.

Lobo IM, et al: Calcinosis cutis: a rare feature of adult dermatomyositis. Dermatol Online J 2008; 14:10.

Macbeth AE, et al: Calcified subcutaneous nodules: a long-term complication of interferon beta-1a therapy. Br J Dermatol 2007; 157:624.

Morris P, et al: Lymphoma arising from a calcinotic lesion in a patient with juvenile dermatomyositis. Pediatr Dermatol 2009; 26:159.

Nagai Y, et al: Nephrogenic systemic fibrosis with multiple calcification and osseous metaplasia. Acta Derm Venereol 2008; 88:597.

Nakamura S, et al: Hutchinson–Gilford progeria syndrome with severe skin calcinosis. Clin Exp Dermatol 2007; 32:525.

Nguyen J, et al: Subepidermal calcified nodule of the eyelid. Ophthal Plast Reconstr Surg 2008; 24:494.

Nico MM, et al: Subepidermal calcified nodule. Pediatr Dermatol 2001; 18:227.

Ochsendorf FR, et al: Erbium:YAG laser ablation of osteoma cutis. Arch Dermatol 1999; 135:1416.

Ogretmen Z, et al: Calcinosis cutis universalis. J Eur Acad Dermatol Venereol 2002; 16:621.

Pecovnik-Balon B, et al: Tumoral calcinosis in patients on hemodialysis. Am J Nephrol 1997; 17:93.

Penate Y, et al: Calcinosis cutis associated with amyopathic dermatomyositis: response to intravenous immunoglobulin. J Am Acad Dermatol 2009; 60:1076.

Rho NK, et al: Calcified nodule on the heel of a child following a single heel stick in the neonatal period. Clin Exp Dermatol 2003; 28:502.

Shah V, Shet T: Scrotal calcinosis results from calcification of cysts derived from hair follicles: a series of 20 cases evaluating the spectrum of changes resulting in scrotal calcinosis. Am J Dermatopathol 2007; 29:172.

Tomazzini E, et al: Vulvar calcinosis in childhood. Int J Gynaecol Obstet 2008; 103:263.

Weinel S, et al: Calcinosis cutis complicating adult-onset dermatomyositis. Arch Dermatol 2004; 140:365.

Wolf EK, et al: Topical sodium thiosulfate therapy for leg ulcers with dystrophic calcification. Arch Dermatol 2008; 144:1560.

Zaka Z, et al: Subcutaneous calcification as a delayed complication of radiotherapy: a case report and review of the literature. Pathol Oncol Res 2008; 14:485.

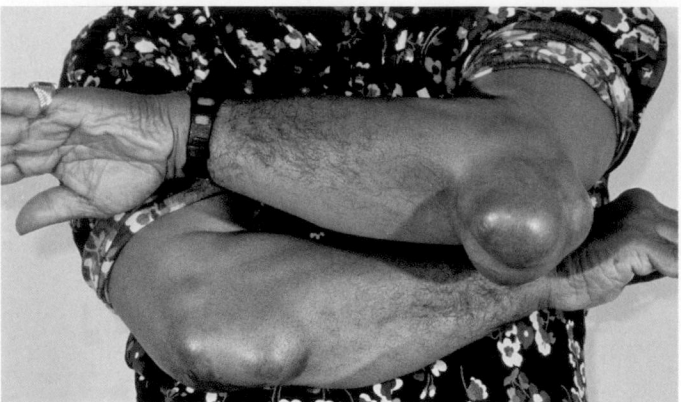

Fig. 26-16 Tuberous xanthomas.

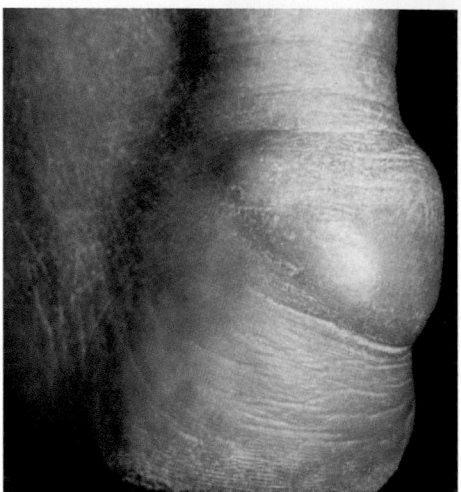

Fig. 26-17 Tendinous xanthomas.

LIPID DISTURBANCES

Xanthomas

Xanthomas are deposits of lipids in tissue. For the dermatologist the important areas to look for lipid deposits are on the skin, tendon, and eyes. Xanthomas appear when there are abnormalities of lipid amount or processing in the body. For this reason, they are important markers of underlying dyslipidemia and potentially increased cardiovascular risk. The histologic features in all varieties of xanthoma are similar, characterized by the presence of numerous large xanthoma or foam cells, which are phagocytes (fat-laden histiocytes). They may be multinucleated. In addition to the foam cells, giant cells of the Touton type occur. Clefts representing cholesterol and fatty acids dissolved by embedding agents may be noted. There is generally a connective tissue reaction about the nests of foam cells, and in old lesions most of the foam cells are replaced with fibrosis. To demonstrate lipids in the histologic sections, frozen sections should be stained with lipid stains (scarlet red). In addition to inherited genetic defects of molecules involved in lipid homeostasis, systemic diseases (such as hypothyroidism and renal failure) and medications (such as systemic retinoids) can also cause hyperlipidemias and result in xanthomas. The names of the various forms of cutaneous xanthomas are based on clinical morphology. Several different genetic diseases may present with similar cutaneous xanthoma patterns. The morphologies are relatively specific for the associated elevated lipid, however, with eruptive xanthomas seen with hypertriglyceridemia and other forms of xanthomas seen with elevations in cholesterol.

Xanthoma tuberosum

Tuberous xanthomas are variously found as flat or elevated and rounded, grouped, yellowish or orange nodules located over the joints, particularly on the elbows and knees (Fig. 26-16). The lesions are indurated and tend to coalesce. They may also occur over the face, knuckles, toe joints, axillary and inguinal folds, and buttocks. Solitary lesions may be found. Early lesions are usually bright yellow or erythematous; older lesions tend to become fibrotic and lose their color. Pedunculated, fissured, and suppurative nodules may also be seen.

Xanthoma tuberosum is associated with elevated low-density lipoprotein (LDL) cholesterol levels, such as in familial hypercholesterolemia. Tuberous xanthomas can also occur in primary biliary cirrhosis, myxedema, phytosterolemia, and normocholesterolemic dysbetalipoproteinemia (HPL3). In the susceptible person, medications may trigger the appearance of tuberous xanthomas.

Xanthoma tendinosum

Papules or nodules 5–25 mm in diameter are found in the tendons, more especially in extensor tendons on the backs of the hands and dorsa of the feet, and in the Achilles tendons (Fig. 26-17). These predominate in conditions with elevated LDL cholesterol, and can be seen in association with tuberous xanthomas and xanthelasma. They also occur in obstructive liver disease, diabetes, myxedema, cerebrotendinous xanthomatosis, and phytosterolemia.

Eruptive xanthoma

Xanthoma eruptivum consists of small, yellowish-orange to reddish-brown papules that appear in crops over the entire body (Fig. 26-18). These occur in association with markedly elevated triglycerides. Certain diseases or drugs raise the triglyceride level by either increased production, decreased

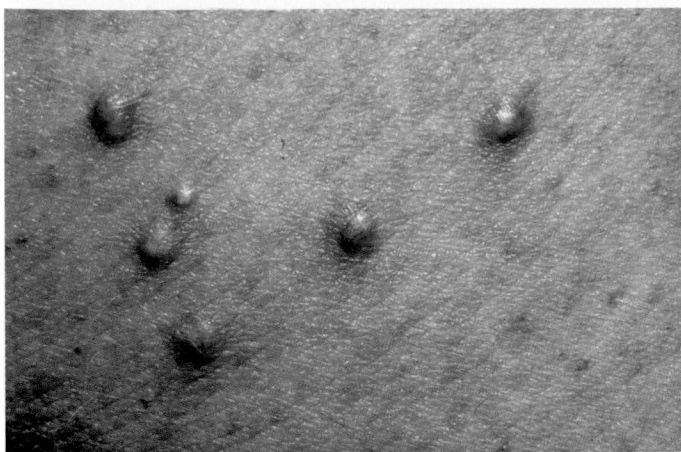

Fig. 26-18 Eruptive xanthomas.

catabolism, or decreased excretion. These include diabetes mellitus, obesity, chronic renal failure, hypothyroidism, and treatment with estrogens, corticosteroids, or systemic retinoids.

The papules may be surrounded by an erythematous halo and may be grouped in various favored locations such as the buttocks, extensor surfaces of the arms and thighs, knees, inguinal and axillary folds, and oral mucosa. Koebnerization may occur. Pruritus is variable.

Xanthoma planum (plane xanthoma)

These xanthomas appear as flat macules or slightly elevated plaques with a yellowish-tan or orange coloration of the skin that is spread diffusely over large areas. They are frequently associated with biliary cirrhosis and myeloma but have been described in patients with high-density lipoprotein (HDL) deficiency monoclonal gammopathy, lymphoma, leukemia, adult T-cell lymphoma/leukemia due to human lymphotropic virus (HTLV)-1, acquired deficiency of C1 esterase inhibitor, disorders with increased activation and consumption of complement, and in xanthomas following erythroderma. In the case of myeloma and monoclonal gammopathy, the paraprotein complexes with LDL and these complexes are phagocytosed by histiocytes in tissue forming the plane xanthomas. Characteristically, plane xanthomas may occur about the eyelids, neck, trunk, shoulders, or axillae (Fig. 26-19). These well-defined macular patches may be situated on the inner surface of the thighs and antecubital and popliteal spaces. A very rare form of normolipemic xanthomatosis can occur in childhood, termed "normolipemic papuloeruptive xanthomatosis." Yellowish papules 2–5 mm in diameter occur on the face. They can coalesce to form large confluent plaques, especially on the face, nape of the neck, and axillae. Spontaneous involution occurs. It is unclear whether this is a rare disease in its own right or a severe variant of benign cephalic histiocytosis or papular xanthoma of childhood.

Palmar xanthomas

These consist of nodules and irregular yellowish plaques involving the palms and flexural surfaces of the fingers (Fig. 26-20). Striated xanthomas appear as yellowish streaks that follow the distribution of creases of the palms and soles. These lesions are seen in familial dysbetalipoproteinemia, multiple myeloma, and biliary cirrhosis.

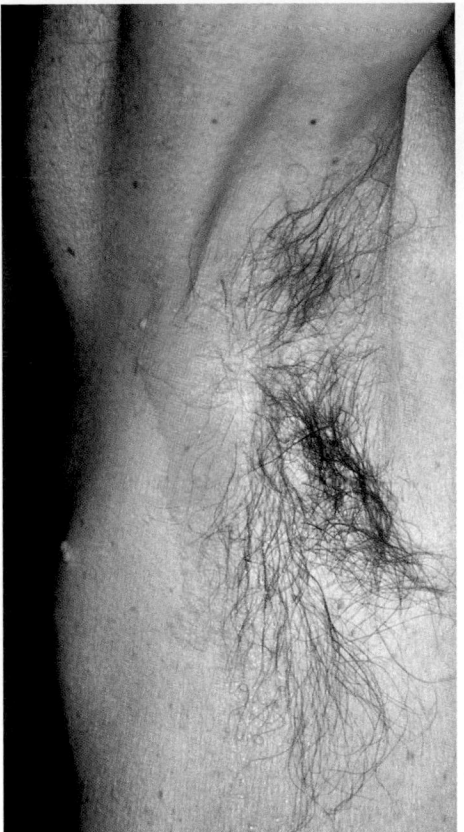

Fig. 26-19 Plane xanthoma.

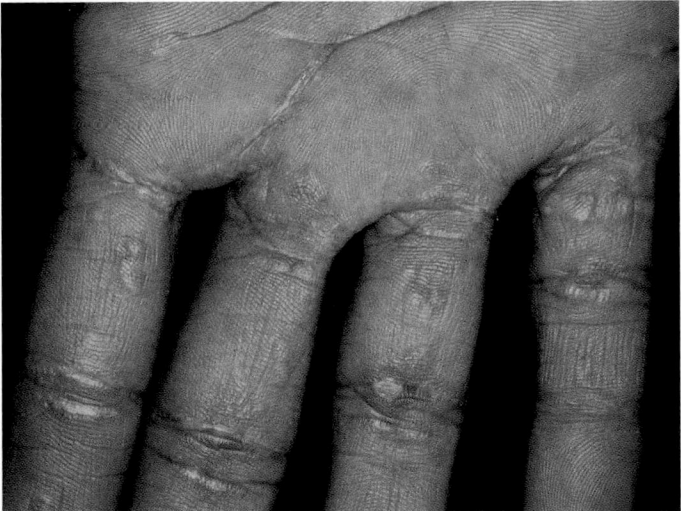

Fig. 26-20 Xanthomas of the palmar striae.

Xanthelasma palpebrarum (xanthelasma)

Xanthelasma is the most common type of xanthoma. It occurs on the eyelids and is characterized by soft, chamois-colored or yellowish-orange oblong plaques, usually near the inner canthi (Fig. 26-21). They tend to appear in middle age. The xanthelasmas vary from 2 to 30 mm in length, and are usually symmetrical. Xanthelasmas are usually seen without other forms of xanthomas, but can be seen in patients with elevated cholesterol, especially familial hypercholesterolemia.

Several studies have found abnormalities in apolipoprotein E phenotypes or other lipoproteins more frequently than in controls. New patients with xanthelasma should be evaluated

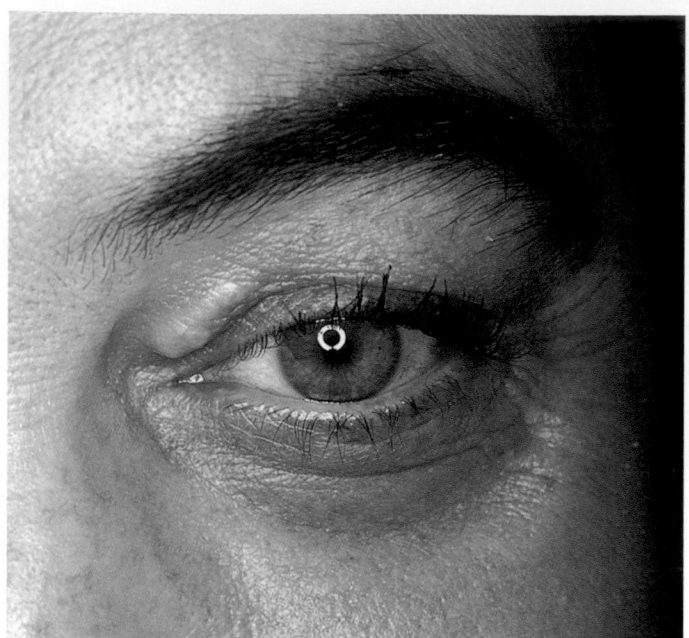

Fig. 26-21 Xanthelasma.

with a full lipoprotein profile, as well as a careful history and physical examination. Patients with a young age at onset and a family history of hyperlipidemias are at higher risk of having lipid abnormalities. The question of whether normolipemic patients with xanthelasma may be at increased risk for atherosclerosis remains controversial.

Treatment of xanthelasma is discussed here because of its uniqueness among the xanthomas, in that surgical therapy is often successful. The best method is surgical excision. The anesthetized lesion is grasped with mouse-tooth forceps and clipped off with scissors, and the skin edges undermined and sutured. Excellent cosmetic results are obtained, even if the wound is not closed. Fulguration, trichloracetic acid cauterization, CO_2 and erbium:YAG and Nd:YAG laser treatments are other methods. Complete removal of the lesions does not preclude the possibility that other new lesions will develop.

Tuberoeruptive xanthomas

These xanthomas are red papules and nodules that appear inflamed and tend to coalesce. They are associated with familial dysbetalipoproteinemia.

Nodular xanthomas

These are multiple, yellowish, dome-shaped lesions, 4–5 mm or larger in diameter; they may be discrete or confluent, and may occur on the earlobes, neck, elbows, and knees. They are usually associated with biliary cirrhosis and atresia of the bile ducts.

Primary hyperlipoproteinemias

Cutaneous xanthomas are usually manifestations of a disorder of lipid metabolism. The blood lipids, with the exception of free fatty acids, are bound to circulating plasma proteins (apoproteins) and are composed of combinations of cholesterol, phospholipid, and triglyceride. The total serum lipids have a range of 400–1000 mg%. Of this, serum cholesterol values vary according to age. The target or ideal cholesterol is now determined by the risk profile of the patient. In a person with no cardiovascular risk factors it is less than 190 mg/dL. Most

patients with hypertriglyceridemia have familial combined hyperlipemia, type II diabetes (even if well controlled), and familial hypoalphalipoproteinemia. These conditions are all associated with increased cardiovascular risk. However, beyond treating massively elevated triglycerides (>1000 mg/dL) to prevent pancreatitis, the value of lowering triglycerides to prevent cardiovascular disease is controversial. In persons with hypertriglyceridemia and cardiovascular risk factors, once LDL cholesterol is normalized in these patients, a triglyceride target level of 200 mg/dL or below is considered ideal. The presence of centrotruncal obesity and diabetes mellitus will exacerbate any inherited metabolic abnormality, leading to higher cholesterol or triglyceride levels.

Lipoprotein fractions may be demonstrated by paper electrophoresis. Four lipoprotein bands may be evident: the α-lipoprotein band (HDL), β-lipoprotein (LDL), preβ-lipoprotein (very low-density lipoprotein, VLDL), and the chylomicron band. When the lipoproteins are subjected to ultracentrifugation, it is found that the HDLs are composed mostly of phospholipid and esterified cholesterol. The LDLs are composed mostly of cholesterols. The VLDL fraction is the main carrier of endogenous triglycerides. The lowest-density chylomicrons are the exogenous triglycerides.

Frederickson classified hyperlipoproteinemias into six types on the basis of electrophoretic patterns, as below. These are now called the WHO ICD hyperlipoprotein (HLP) phenotypes.

- HLP1/Type I: Excess chylomicrons
- HLP2A/Type IIa: Excess β-lipoprotein
- HLP2B/Type IIb: Excess β-lipoprotein with slightly elevated VLDLs
- HLP3/Type III: Increased intermediate-density (remnant) lipoprotein
- HLP4/Type IV: Increased preβ-lipoprotein
- HLP5/Type V: Increased preβ-lipoproteins and chylomicrons

Although this phenotypic classification has been useful for many years, advances in the understanding of lipoprotein metabolism and transport, coupled with new knowledge of molecular defects that result in these phenotypes, has led to the use of a genetic classification of lipoproteinemias. If two or more gene products are required at any point in lipoprotein metabolism, then genetic deficiency of any molecule will lead to a similar phenotype. Multiple genotypes lead to the same phenotype. The discussion below will outline the genotypes and give the corresponding hyperlipoproteinemia type when applicable.

Lipoprotein metabolism may be viewed according to the lipid source: an exogenous and an endogenous category. Exogenous lipids in the diet are absorbed and incorporated into triglyceride-rich chylomicrons. These are hydrolyzed by the action of lipoprotein lipase and certain cofactors, among them apoprotein CII. The resulting remnants are taken up by the liver. Endogenously produced VLDLs are synthesized in the liver and (again through the action of lipoprotein lipase) are connected to cholesterol-rich intermediate-density lipoproteins (IDLs) and eventually into LDLs.

These are then available for uptake by peripheral tissues, as well as by the liver. The uptake of LDL, IDL, and chylomicron remnants is dependent on specific receptors. Abnormalities of lipoprotein lipase, the apolipoproteins, cofactors, receptors, or stimulators or retarders of endogenous production or catabolism, whether on a genetic or sporadic basis, may accelerate or block the pathway in different areas. If blockade occurs early and results in elevation of triglyceride-rich particles, eruptive xanthoma may result. If a defect occurs later in the pathway and cholesterol-rich particles accumulate, xanthelasma,

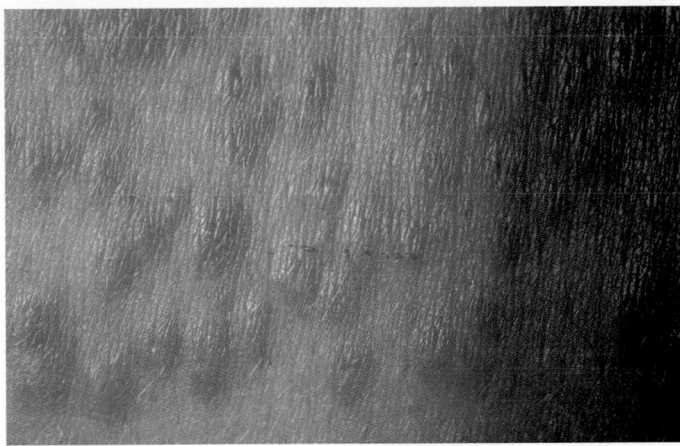

Fig. 26-22 Eruptive xanthomas in lipoprotein lipase deficiency.

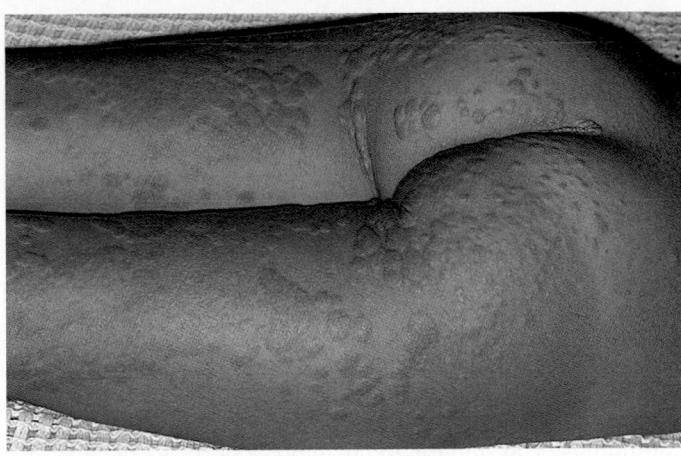

Fig. 26-23 Xanthomas in homozygous familial hypercholesterolemia.

tuberous xanthomas, and tendinous xanthomas are to be expected, along with premature atherosclerotic cardiovascular disease.

Lipoprotein lipase deficiency

Lipoprotein lipase deficiency causes HLP1 disease (chylomicronemia) early in life. It is rare, results from a homozygous defect, and is associated with highly elevated triglycerides. With levels above 1000 mg/dL, a high risk of pancreatitis and eruptive xanthomas (Fig. 26-22) exists. As patients grow older, their VLDLs become elevated.

Familial apoprotein CII deficiency

Patients with the rare familial apoprotein CII deficiency lack lipoprotein lipase activator and have very high triglyceride levels, up to 10 000 mg/dL. They are at risk for pancreatitis and eruptive xanthomas.

Familial hypertriglyceridemia

In familial hypertriglyceridemia, increased hepatic production of VLDLs occurs. Eruptive xanthomas are common. Depending on the cause of this lipid pattern, the risk of atherosclerotic disease may vary. *APOA5* may play a role.

Familial hypercholesterolemia

Familial hypercholesterolemia has an HLP2A (Frederickson type IIa) lipid profile. It is due to mutations in at least four different genes: LDL receptor, apolipoprotein B, proprotein convertase subtilisin-like kexin type 9 (*PCSK9*), and LDL receptor adaptor protein (*LDLRAP1*). Up to one-third of patients with familial hypercholesterolemia do not have defects in any of the known genes described above.

LDL receptor deficiency

In LDL receptor deficiency, the hepatocyte lacks LDL receptors. The frequency of this gene mutation is about 1:500. Between 50 and 75% of patients with monogenic hypercholesterolemia have LDL receptor genetic defects. LDLs are found in high levels in the plasma; there may be a moderate increase in VLDLs and in the triglycerides that they carry. There is overproduction of LDL cholesterol (caused by loss of normal feedback inhibition) and impaired removal of it (because of impaired formation of LDL receptors). There is elevated plasma β-lipoprotein from birth in heterozygotes, and symp-

toms begin in the third to sixth decade, when xanthelasmas, tendinous or, less commonly, tuberous xanthomas, and corneal arcus appear. Atherosclerotic coronary heart disease begins in the thirties and forties in men and a decade later in women.

Homozygotes generally develop coronary atherosclerosis before the age of 20, as their cholesterol levels are in the 800–1000 mg/dL range. Tendinous xanthomas, tuberous xanthomas, and large xanthelasmas (xanthomatous pseudospectacles) appear in childhood. Characteristic xanthomatous plaques occur, which may be generalized (Fig. 26-23), but typically involve intertriginous areas such as the interdigital spaces or the intergluteal cleft. Cultured amniotic fluid cells permit prenatal diagnosis in homozygotes. LDL-apheresis or liver transplantation is the treatment employed for this homozygous type.

Familial defective apolipoprotein B

In this condition, a structural defect in apolipoprotein B-100 means it binds poorly to LDL receptors, allowing for accumulation of LDL. In the more common heterozygous form, hypercholesterolemia occurs, tendinous xanthomas and xanthelasma may be seen, and premature coronary heart disease develops. In the rare homozygous form there are higher levels of cholesterol present but not to the heights seen in homozygous familial hypercholesterolemia. This is because VLDL clearance is unimpaired in these patients.

PCSK9 *deficiency*

This gene codes for a protein that degrades hepatic LDLR in the endosomes. Gain of function mutations result in increased metabolism of LDLR and a consequent deficiency of LDLR. This results in hypercholesterolemia and tendon xanthomas, corneal arcus, and xanthelasma.

LDLRAP1 *deficiency*

This autosomal-recessive hypercholesterolemia (ARH) is due to a defect in the protein that clusters the LDL receptors on the surface of the hepatocytes and is essential for LDL receptor-mediated endocytosis. It is rare, except in Sardinia. The cholesterol levels in these patients can be as high as those with homozygous LDL receptor deficiency, and tuberous xanthomas can occur in childhood.

Familial combined hyperlipidemia

Familial combined hyperlipidemia has an HLP2B (Fredrickson type IIb) lipid profile, with elevated total, LDL and HDL cholesterol, and triglycerides. Multiple etiologies are proposed.

Some cases are due to genetic defects in *APOB*, *LPL*, or *USF1* (upstream factor 1). There is a high risk of atherosclerosis, but xanthomas are not seen.

Dysbetalipoproteinemia (broad beta disease)

In this disorder an HLP3 (Fredrickson type III) hyperlipoproteinemia is seen. LDLs and HDLs are reduced, and triglyceride and cholesterol levels are increased. The cholesterol-rich IDLs form a broad band on electrophoresis, extending from preβ-lipoproteins to β-lipoproteins: hence broad beta disease. The presence of an abnormal form of apolipoprotein E or homozygosity for apolipoprotein E2 (especially in African Americans) is necessary but not sufficient to create this disorder. Drugs can exacerbate the genetic defect, leading to the appearance of xanthomas. The mutant *APOE* binds poorly to hepatic and peripheral cell surface receptors. This results in decreased hepatic uptake of VLDL and chylomicron remnants. These are taken up by macrophages in peripheral tissues, including the skin, where xanthomas can occur. About 40% of affected persons also have a mutation in *APOA5*. Xanthomas (tuberous, palmar, or plantar) are common. Atherosclerosis is premature and increased, especially peripheral vascular disease.

Mixed hyperlipidemia

This polygenic syndrome has an HLP5 (Fredrickson type V) pattern with elevated cholesterol and triglycerides in the form of VLDL and chylomicrons. Mutations in *LPL*, *APOC2*, and *APOA5*, as well as other genes, play a role in creating this phenotype.

Secondary hyperlipoproteinemia

Obstructive liver disease (xanthomatous biliary cirrhosis)

This type of hyperlipoproteinemia shows an increase of the serum phospholipid and cholesterol, giving a type II lipoprotein pattern. This is caused by the presence of lipoprotein X, which is secreted by the liver in cholestasis. It has the ability to carry large quantities of free cholesterol and phospholipids. The triglycerides are not elevated and the plasma is clear, showing no chylomicrons.

The xanthomatous lesions are plane xanthomas, with lesions on the face, flexor surfaces of the extremities, and trunk. Striate palmar and plantar lesions, and xanthelasmas are also seen. Tuberous xanthomas may also occur. Pruritus is extremely severe. Hepatomegaly and jaundice are present. Cholestyramine can be of help in allaying pruritus.

Alagille syndrome is a congenital disorder characterized by intrahepatic bile ductular atresia, patent extrahepatic bile ducts, a characteristic facies (prominent forehead, deeply set eyes, straight nose, and small, pointed chin), cardiac murmur, vertebral and ocular abnormalities, low intelligence, and hypogonadism. It is an autosomal-dominantly inherited condition. There is persistent cholestasis early in life, with pruritus and hyperbilirubinemia. Lipid levels elevate by the age of 2, and planar or papular xanthomas may occur. This is a treatable condition, with cholestyramine and fat-soluble vitamins leading to prolonged improvement.

Hematopoietic diseases (normolipemic xanthomas)

Xanthomas may occur secondarily in myelomas, Waldenström macroglobulinemia, cryoglobulinemia, occasionally lymphoma, and hemochromatosis. These xanthomas are usually generalized plane xanthomas of the eyelids, periorbital areas, sides of the neck, shoulders, and upper back. The lipid levels may be normal in these patients. These xanthomas result from circulating paraproteins that bind to the lipoproteins, preventing their metabolism.

Xanthoma diabeticorum

Eruptive xanthomas may occur secondarily, especially in young persons unresponsive to insulin. Cardiovascular disease and hepatomegaly are common. Insulin is necessary for the normal plasma triglyceride-clearing action of lipoprotein lipase. Therefore, in insulin deficiency, an acquired lipoprotein lipase deficiency exists, which leads to impaired clearance of chylomicrons or VLDLs, or both. This results in a HLP 1, 4, 5 lipoprotein pattern and hypertriglyceridemia. Eruptive xanthomas are seen. Pancreatitis may occur if the triglyceride level is >1000 mg/dL. When the diabetes is brought under control, the triglyceride levels are lowered and prompt involution of the lesions is seen. Weight reduction and carbohydrate intake restriction are also helpful. Identical phenomena may occur in von Gierke's disease, a form of glycogen storage disease in which there is a lack of hepatic glucose-6-phosphatase.

Chronic renal failure

If plasma protein levels are reduced by urinary loss in the nephrotic syndrome (or by plasmapheresis or repeated bleeding), a compensatory increase of lipoproteins may occur, with hyperlipidemia and various kinds of xanthoma. HLP 4 and V profiles are most commonly seen. Renal failure with or without dialysis may cause hypertriglyceridemia.

Myxedema

Lipoprotein lipase needs thyroid hormone to work, and its failure may lead to HLP 1, 4, 5 disease. Thyroid hormone deficiency may lead to hypercholesterolemia because thyroid hormone is needed in the oxidation of hepatic cholesterol to bile salts. Xanthelasma and xanthomas are common in myxedema.

Pancreatitis

Hyperlipidemia in the hyperchylomicronemic syndromes (types I and V) may cause pancreatitis; it may be recurrent, and pancreatic necrosis and death may occur. Alternatively, pancreatitis (perhaps initiated by ethanol) may cause type I or V hyperlipoproteinemia by inducing insulin deficiency and a relative lack of lipoprotein lipase activity. A triglyceride level of 1000 mg/dL is required for pancreatitis to occur in the setting of hypertriglyceridemia. The amylase may be normal, but the lipase will be elevated.

Medication-induced hyperlipoproteinemia

Estrogens, by decreasing lipoprotein lipase activity and increasing VLDL synthesis, may cause HLP 1 or 5 patterns. Eruptive xanthomas may occur. Oral prednisone may induce insulin deficiency and cause HLP 4 or 5 patterns to develop. Oral retinoids, indomethacin, protease inhibitors for HIV, and olanzapine may also cause eruptive xanthomas via hypertriglyceridemia.

Cerebrotendinous xanthomatosis

Cerebrotendinous xanthomatosis is an autosomal-recessive disease caused by an accumulation of cholestanol in plasma lipoproteins and xanthomatous tissue. The underlying abnormality is a mutation in the sterol 27-hydroxylase gene (*CYP27A*) in the mitochondria, leading to incomplete oxidation of cholesterol to bile acids. Cholestanol, an intermediate, accumulates as a result in tendons, brain, heart, lungs, and the lens of the eye. The disorder is characterized by prominent tendinous xanthomas, especially of the Achilles tendons (not present in all cases), macroglossia, and progressive neurologic dysfunction in many forms, as well as cataracts, atherosclerotic coronary disease, and endocrine abnormalities. Plasma cholestanol is elevated and can exceed more than ten times normal levels. The condition is treated with chenodeoxycholic acid, and early treatment can prevent the progressive neurological impairment.

Phytosterolemia (sitosterolemia)

In phytosterolemia, a rare autosomal-recessive disorder, plant sterols (β-sitosterol, stigmasterol, and campesterol) and shellfish sterols (lathosterol and desmosterol) are found in excessive amounts in all tissues except the brain. This disorder is caused by mutations in the genes encoding the ABCG5 and ABCG8 transporters, which are needed to pump sterols out to intestinal cells back into the lumen of the gut, and used to pump plant sterols into the bile. Patients develop tendinous xanthomas, xanthelasma, and tuberous, palmar, and plantar xanthomas. In most patients there is also type IIa hyperlipoproteinemia and accelerated atherosclerosis. Other features are arthritis, splenomegaly, and hematologic disorders. Ezetimibe (an inhibitor of NPC1L1 [Niemann–Pick C1-like 1]), chenodeoxycholic acid, and cholestyramine can be effective in lowering the cholesterol and plant sterols.

Verruciform xanthoma

Verruciform xanthoma (VX) is an uncommon lesion that occurs as a reddish-orange or paler hyperkeratotic plaque or papillomatous growth with a pebbly or verrucous surface. The most common site is the oral mucosa. It has also been reported on other mucosal surfaces, genitalia, lower extremities (Fig. 26-24), and elsewhere. Epidermal nevus-like lesions in CHILD syndrome have characteristics of VX. Recessive dystrophic epidermolysis bullosa, lymphedema, and graft vs host disease have been associated with VX. Additionally, VX has been reported in psoriatic lesions undergoing PUVA therapy and in psoriasiform skin lesions in an HIV-positive patient. Histologically, there is acanthosis without atypia, parakeratosis, and xanthoma cells in the papillary dermis. In a small percentage of VX, a mutation in the *NSDHL* gene (3β-hydroxysteroid dehydrogenase) has been found. This gene is also mutated in CHILD syndrome, explaining why the latter and VX share the same histology.

Familial α-lipoprotein deficiency (hypoalphalipoproteinemia, Tangier disease)

Tangier disease is caused by mutations in the cell-membrane protein ABCA1, which mediates the secretion of excess cholesterol from cells into the HDL metabolic pathway. This results in a profound deficiency of HDL, and accumulation of cholesterol in tissue macrophages. The characteristic clinical finding is yellow, enlarged tonsils from accumulation of lipid in this localized area. Xanthomas do not occur; however, there is diffuse accumulation of cholesterol esters in the skin, as well as the intestines, thymus, bone marrow, lymph nodes, and spleen. Peripheral neuropathy, splenomegaly (with thrombocytopenia) and premature coronary artery disease are other features of Tangier disease. ABC (ATP-binding cassette) transporters generally have transmembrane domains that move substrates across cell membranes. Defects in 14 of the over 50 known ABC transporters cause 13 genetic diseases, including cystic fibrosis, age-related macular degeneration, phytosterolemia, and adrenoleukodystrophy.

Alam M, et al: Tuberous xanthomas in sitosterolemia. Pediatr Dermatol 2000; 17:447.

Bel S, et al: Cerebrotendinous xanthomatosis. J Am Acad Dermatol 2001; 45:292.

Broeshart JH, et al: Normolipemic plane xanthoma associated with adenocarcinoma and severe itch. J Am Acad Dermatol 2003; 49:119.

Brown CA, et al: Tuberous and tendinous xanthomata secondary to ritonavir-associated hyperlipidemia. J Am Acad Dermatol 2005; 52:S86.

Brunzell JD: Clinical practice. Hypertriglyceridemia. N Engl J Med 2007; 357:1009.

Burnside NJ, et al: Type III hyperlipoproteinemia with xanthomas and multiple myeloma. J Am Acad Dermatol 2005; 53:S281.

Chan CC, et al: Xanthelasma is not associated with increased risk of carotid atherosclerosis in normolipidaemia. Int J Clin Pract 2008; 62:221.

Chang HY, et al: Eruptive xanthomas associated with olanzapine use. Arch Dermatol 2003; 139:617.

Chung HG, et al: CD 30 (Ki-1)-positive large-cell cutaneous T-cell lymphoma with secondary xanthomatous changes after radiation therapy. J Am Acad Dermatol 2003; 48:S28.

Connolly SB, et al: Management of cutaneous verruciform xanthoma. J Am Acad Dermatol 2000; 42:343.

Crook M: Xanthelasma and cardiovascular risk. Int J Clin Pract 2008; 62:178.

Dotsch J, et al: Unmasking of childhood hypothyroidism by disseminated xanthomas. Pediatrics 2001; 108:E96.

Garcia MA, et al: Alagille syndrome: cutaneous manifestations in 38 children. Pediatr Dermatol 2005; 22:11.

Garg A, Simha V: Update on dyslipidemia. J Clin Endocrinol Metab 2007; 92:1581.

Geyer AS, et al: Eruptive xanthomas associated with protease inhibitor therapy. Arch Dermatol 2004; 140:617.

Girish MP, Gupta MD: Xanthomatous pseudospectacles in familial hypercholesterolemia. N Engl J Med 2005; 352:2424.

Hegele RA: Plasma lipoproteins: genetic influences and clinical implications. Nat Rev Genet 2009; 10:109.

Horne MK 3rd, et al: In vitro characterization of a monoclonal IgG(kappa) from a patient with planar xanthomatosis. Eur J Haematol 2008; 80:495.

Huang HY, et al: Normolipemic papuloeruptive xanthomatosis in a child. Pediatr Dermatol 2009; 26:360.

Li SG: Images in clinical medicine. Familial hypercholesterolemia. N Engl J Med 2009; 360:1885.

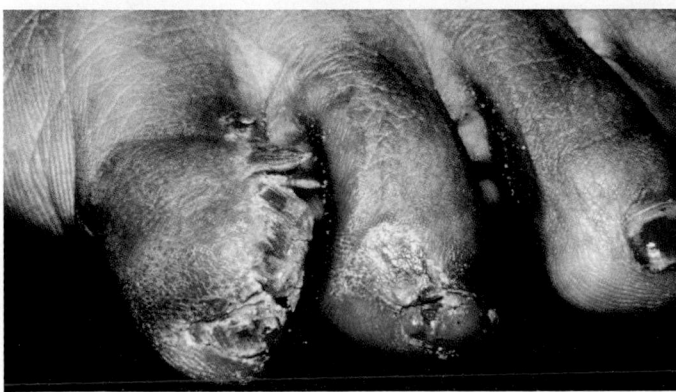

Fig. 26-24 Verruciform xanthoma.

Lorenz S, et al: Treatment of diffuse plane xanthoma of the face with the erbium:YAG laser. Arch Dermatol 2001; 137:1413.

Malbran A, et al: Case report: diffuse plane xanthoma with low C4 and systemic inflammatory symptoms. Dermatol Online J 2009; 15:5.

Mehra S, et al: A novel somatic mutation of the 3beta-hydroxysteroid dehydrogenase gene in sporadic cutaneous verruciform xanthoma. Arch Dermatol 2005; 141:1263.

Mehta BP, Shmerling RH: Teaching neuroimage: cerebrotendinous xanthomatosis. Neurology 2008; 71:e4.

Nayak KR, et al: Eruptive xanthomas associated with hypertriglyceridemia and new-onset diabetes mellitus. N Engl J Med 2004; 350:1235.

Noel B: Premature atherosclerosis in patients with xanthelasma. J Eur Acad Dermatol Venereol 2007; 21:1244.

Ozdöl S, et al: Xanthelasma palpebrarum and its relation to atherosclerotic risk factors and lipoprotein (a). Int J Dermatol 2008; 47:785.

Pilo de la Fuente B, et al: Cerebrotendinous xanthomatosis: neuropathological findings. J Neurol 2008; 255:839.

Rhyne J, et al: Multiple splice defects in ABCA1 cause low HDL-C in a family with hypoalphalipoproteinemia and premature coronary disease. BMC Med Genet 2009; 10:1.

Shirdel A, et al: Diffuse normolipaemic plane xanthomatosis associated with adult T-cell lymphoma/leukaemia. J Eur Acad Dermatol Venereol 2008; 22:1252.

Siddi GM, et al: Multiple tuberous xanthomas as the first manifestation of autosomal recessive hypercholesterolemia. J Eur Acad Dermatol Venereol 2006; 20:1376.

Sinnott BP, Mazzone T: Tuberous xanthomas associated with olanzapine therapy and hypertriglyceridemia in the setting of a rare apolipoprotein E mutation. Endocr Pract 2006; 12:183.

Sopena J, et al: Disseminated verruciform xanthoma. Br J Dermatol 2004; 151:717.

Stalenhoef AF: Phytosterolemia and xanthomatosis. N Engl J Med 2003; 349:51.

Togo M, et al: Identification of a novel mutation for phytosterolemia. Genetic analyses of 2 cases. Clin Chim Acta 2009; 401:165.

Tsuang W: Hypertriglyceridemic pancreatitis: presentation and management. Am J Gastroenterol 2009; 104:984.

Uehara Y, et al: POPC/apoA-I discs as a potent lipoprotein modulator in Tangier disease. Atherosclerosis 2008; 197:283.

von Bergmann K, et al: Cholesterol and plant sterol absorption: recent insights. Am J Cardiol 2005; 96:10D.

Zarubica A, et al: ABCA1, from pathology to membrane function. Pflugers Arch 2007; 453:569.

Niemann–Pick disease

This rare autosomal-recessive condition has three recognized subtypes. The disorder was originally described in Ashkenazi Jews. Type A and type B disease are both caused by mutations in the acid sphingomyelinase gene (*SMPD1*). Type A disease is more severe, presents in infancy with neurovisceral disease, and is often fatal. Type B disease is purely visceral (non-neurologic) and survival into adulthood is characteristic. Skin lesions in type A and B patients include xanthomas (skin-colored to tan papules) and yellow-brown induration of the skin. Histologically, foamy histiocytes are found, which on electron microscopy have characteristic cytoplasmic inclusions. Type C disease (and the former type D disease of Nova Scotia) are due to mutations in the *NPC1* and *NPC2* genes. *NPC1* and 2 are involved in endosomal-lysosomal cholesterol trafficking. Niemann–Pick type C is a neurovisceral disease with a variable age of onset and neurodegenerative course. Patients may present from the perinatal period to adulthood. Cholestatic jaundice is characteristic. Early-onset disease is often associated with severe neurologic disease and death before age 5. Late infantile and juvenile forms have neurologic disease. The adult form may demonstrate visceral involvement and psychiatric and cognitive disorders. Death occurs before age 50. One patient with Niemann–Pick type C developed idiopathic nodular panniculitis.

Bukhari I: Idiopathic nodular panniculitis in Niemann–Pick disease. J Eur Acad Dermatol Venereol 2005; 19:600.

Fancello T, et al: Molecular analysis of NPC1 and NPC2 gene in 34 Niemann–Pick C Italian patients: identification and structural modeling of novel mutations. Neurogenetics 2009; 10:229.

Rodriguez-Pascau L, et al: Identification and characterization of SMPD1 mutations causing Niemann–Pick types A and B in Spanish patients. Hum Mutat 2009; 30:1117.

Sturley SL, et al: Unraveling the sterol-trafficking defect in Niemann–Pick C disease. Proc Natl Acad Sci USA 2009; 106:2093.

Toussaint M, et al: Specific skin lesions in a patient with Niemann–Pick disease. Br J Dermatol 1994; 131:895.

Gaucher's disease

Gaucher's disease is a rare autosomal-recessive disorder caused by insufficient activity of the lysosomal enzyme acid-β glucosidase (glucocerebrosidase, GBA). The disease occurs most frequently among Ashkenazi Jews. Approximately 1 in 20 carry the defective gene. Lysosomal accumulation of glucosylceramide, the substrate of GBA in macrophages, causes the disease manifestations. In rare cases, Gaucher's disease is caused by mutations in the prosaposin gene, which encodes the saposin C activator protein that is necessary for optimal activity of β-glucosidase. Gaucher cells are identified histologically—large macrophages, 20–100 μm in diameter, with one nucleus or a few small nuclei, and pale cytoplasm that stains faintly for fat but is PAS-positive.

The disease occurs at any age but three types are recognized: type 1 (adult type), without neurologic involvement; type 2, the infantile form, with acute early neurologic manifestations; and type 3, the juvenile chronic neuropathic type.

Some type 2 patients have congenital ichthyosis that precedes neurologic manifestations, and some are born with a collodian membrane. Epidermal ultrastructural and biochemical abnormalities occur in all type 2 patients. Hepatosplenomegaly, osteopenia/osteoporosis of the long bones, pingueculae of the sclera, and a distinctive bronze coloration of the skin from melanin characterize the adult type. A deeper pigmentation may extend from the knees to the feet (Fig. 26-25). This is often caused by hemosiderin and may be accompanied by thrombocytopenia and splenomegaly.

The diagnosis is confirmed by DNA testing for the affected gene. Therapy now consists of enzyme replacement therapy with intravenous mannose-terminated glucocerebrosidase, but this is very expensive. Bone marrow transplantation performed before neurologic deficits occur has a high mortality rate (20–50%), but when successful has halted neurologic progression. Enzyme therapy is successful in treating some of the

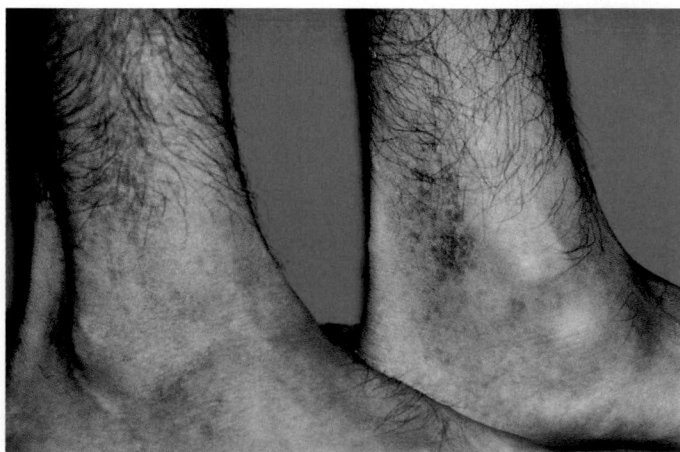

Fig. 26-25 Gaucher pigmentation of the lower leg.

manifestations of the adult form, but it is limited by cost. Substrate reduction therapy using the glycolipid synthesis inhibitor N-butyldeoxynojirimycin (miglustat) is also available.

The intense study of Gaucher's disease has led to two interesting findings. More than 15% of adult patients with Gaucher's disease have monoclonal gammopathy, and in about 20% of these patients there is an associated myelodysplasia (myeloma or lymphoma). More than 7% of adult Gaucher's disease patients will develop myeloma. Heterozygous carriers of GBA mutations are frequently found in patients with Parkinson disease. Parkinson disease is associated with certain "pathogenic" variant GBA mutations.

Grabowski GA: Phenotype, diagnosis, and treatment of Gaucher's disease. Lancet 2008; 372:1263.

Grosbois B, et al: Gaucher disease and monoclonal gammopathy: a report of 17 cases and impact of therapy. Blood Cells Mol Dis 2009; 43:138.

Hughes DA: Enzyme, substrate, and myeloma in Gaucher disease. Am J Hematol 2009; 84:199.

Mitsui J, et al: Mutations for Gaucher disease confer high susceptibility to Parkinson disease. Arch Neurol 2009; 66:571.

Tajima A, et al: Clinical and genetic study of Japanese patients with type 3 Gaucher disease. Mol Genet Metab 2009; 97:272.

Tylki-Szymanska A, et al: Non-neuronopathic Gaucher disease due to saposin C deficiency. Clin Genet 2007; 72:538.

Lipoid proteinosis

Also known as Urbach–Wiethe disease and hyalinosis cutis et mucosae, this rare autosomal-recessive condition usually presents in infancy with a hoarse cry or voice. Mucosal lesions include yellowish-white infiltrative deposits on the inner surfaces of the lips, undersurface of the tongue, fauces, and uvula. Inability to protrude the "woody" tongue fully is characteristic. Xerostomia may occur. In childhood, beaded eyelid papules occur. Uveitis and hyaline deposits on and in the eye may develop. Waxy, yellow papules and nodules with generalized skin thickening occur (Fig. 26-26). Mechanical friction leads to hyperkeratosis of the hands, elbows, knees, buttocks, and axillae, becoming almost verrucous in some patients. Minor trauma leads to bullae that heal with pock-like or acne-like scars, especially on the face (Fig. 26-27). Scalp involvement may lead to mild loss of hair. Neurological sequelae include epilepsy, dystonia, and cognitive impairments.

Distinctive histologic features include extreme dilation of the blood vessels, thickening of their walls, progressive hyalinization of sweat glands, and infiltration of the dermis and subcutaneous tissue with extracellular hyaline deposits. Normal skin and mucous membranes also show changes of endothelial proliferation of the subpapillary vessels and a homogeneous thickening of the walls of the deeper vessels. Type IV collagen and laminin are increased around vessels.

The disease is caused by mutations in the extracellular matrix protein 1. Differentiation from erythropoietic protoporphyria may be difficult, especially histologically. Topical steroids, surgical removal of selected deposits, and occasional reports of improvement with systemic retinoids are treatments of limited benefit. While occasional patients die of respiratory obstruction in infancy, the disease is otherwise compatible with a normal lifespan.

Chan I, et al: The molecular basis of lipoid proteinosis: mutations in extracellular matrix protein 1. Exp Dermatol 2007; 16:881.

Desmet S, et al: Clinical and molecular abnormalities in lipoid proteinosis. Eur J Dermatol 2005; 15:344.

Rao R, et al: Vesiculobullous lesions in lipoid proteinosis: a case report. Dermatol Online J 2008; 14:16.

Toosi S, Ehsani AH: Treatment of lipoid proteinosis with acitretin: a case report. J Eur Acad Dermatol Venereol 2009; 23:482.

Angiokeratoma corporis diffusum (Fabry disease)

Fabry disease is a rare X-linked lysosomal storage disease. It is caused by mutations in the alphagalactosidase A gene (*GLA*), leading to a deficiency in alphagalactosidase A. This results in the inability to catabolize glycosphingolipids, and globotriaosylceramide accumulates in lysosomes in many tissues, including endothelial cells, erector pili muscles, and visceral organs. Although males are affected more severely and earlier, female carriers can have all the stigmata of the full-blown disease.

Skin lesions are common, and in about one-quarter of male patients, a dermatologist makes the diagnosis. The most characteristic skin lesions are widespread punctate telangiectatic

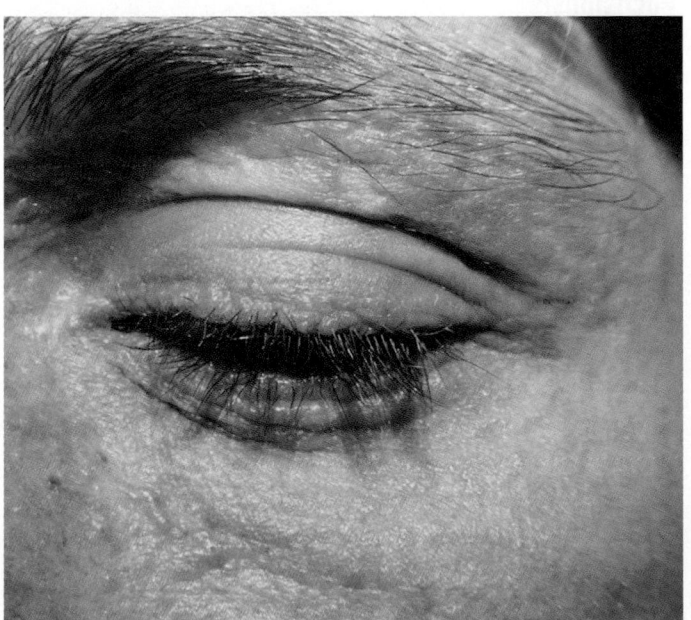

Fig. 26-26 Papules of the eyelid in lipoid proteinosis. (Courtesy of Eric Krause, MD)

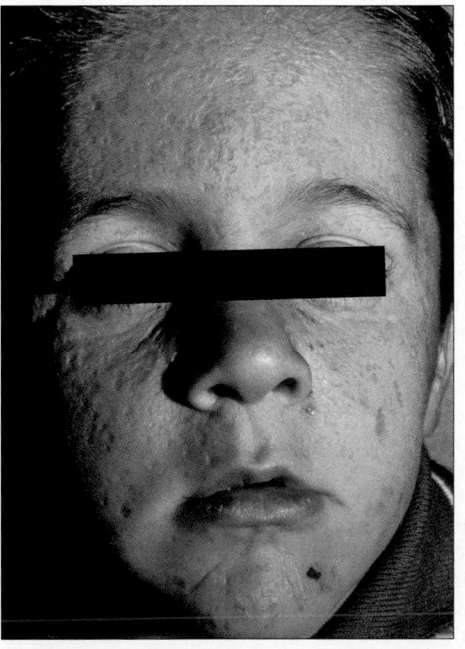

Fig. 26-27 Acneiform scarring in lipoid proteinosis.

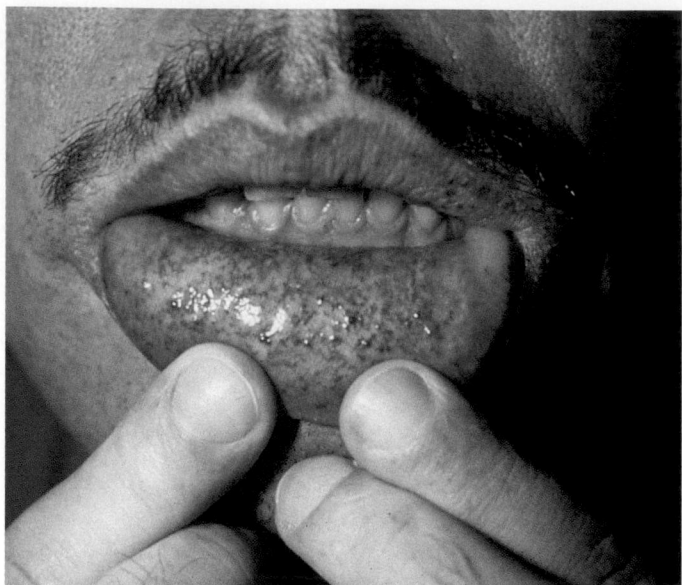

Fig. 26-28 Fabry disease.

vascular papules that on first inspection suggest purpura, but are actually angiokeratomas. Some show hyperkeratotic tops, but these are less prominent than in other forms of angiokeratoma. Angiokeratomas occur in 66% of males and 36% of females with Fabry disease. The average age of onset in males is about age 20; in females it is about 10 years later. Lesions can be present as early as age 1. Lesions tend to occur in the "bathing trunk" area, from the umbilicus to the genitalia (in which areas they may be present in large numbers). Smaller "macular angiomas" are seen, especially on the proximal limbs, palms, and soles, around the nail folds of the digits, and on the vermilion border of the lips (Fig. 26-28). Telangiectasias occur in about 25% of male patients presenting around age 25 and in women around age 40. The vascular lesions can be treated with intense pulse light or various vascular lasers.

Other skin manifestations include lower limb edema and lymphedema. Leg ulceration can occur. Hair growth is scanty. Hypohidrosis is reported by 50% or more of males and more than a quarter of female patients, starting in their twenties. Anhidrosis occurs in 25% of male patients. Heat intolerance can occur. About 13% of females and 6% of males complain of hyperhidrosis.

Visceral disease is common, especially of the kidneys, cardiovascular system, and gastrointestinal tract. Only one organ may be involved. Proteinuria followed by renal failure may begin as early as the second decade and typically presents around age 40. Cardiovascular events (myocardial infarction, arrhythmia, angina, and congestive heart failure) typically appear at around age 40, contributing to premature mortality. About 5% of men and women suffer strokes at around age 40. Abdominal pain, nausea, vomiting and diarrhea can all occur.

Neuropathic pain is the most common initial presentation, affecting around two-thirds of patients. It may begin in childhood, but its nonspecific nature and the lack of physical findings delay the diagnosis, usually by more than a decade, until other stigmata appear. The acroparesthesia or burning pain affects primarily the longest nerves and is most severe on the hands and feet. It may be transient or last for hours. There is a loss of Adelta-fibers. Treatment is as for neuropathy, with tricyclics, gabapentin, capsaicin, and anticonvulsants. Around 25% of Fabry patients develop carpal tunnel syndrome. Cramps and fasciculation may be the presenting neurological symptoms.

Distinctive whorl-like opacities of the cornea occur in 90% of patients, and 50% develop characteristic spokelike cataracts in the posterior capsular location. Telangiectasias may be present on the conjunctiva and in the eye.

The diagnosis may be confirmed by finding diminished levels of α-galactosidase A in leukocytes, serum, fibroblasts, or amniotic fluid cells. Less than 10% enzyme activity is usually detected in affected males. In females the diagnosis requires the identification of a genetic mutation in the *GLA* gene. This can be quite difficult if an affected male relative is not identified, since more than 300 mutations in the *GLA* gene have so far been described that cause Fabry disease.

Histologically, there is dilation of capillaries in the papillary dermis, resulting in endothelium-lined lacunae filled with blood and surrounded by acanthotic and hyperkeratotic epidermis. Electron microscopy reveals characteristic electron-dense bodies in endothelial cells, pericytes, erector pili muscles, and fibroblasts. They are also present in normal skin of affected adults and children.

Enzyme replacement therapy (ERT) is safe and can reverse substrate storage in the lysozyme. ERT leads to a reduction in neuropathic pain, relief of gastrointestinal symptoms, and stabilization of renal function and cardiomyopathy. In patients with a glomerular filtration rate (GFR) below 60 mL/min, renal function may, however, continue to deteriorate. Left ventricular mass decreases, but the vascular coronary disease may not be reversed.

Although widespread angiokeratomas are typical of Fabry disease, patients with other rare autosomal-recessive lysosomal storage diseases, such as galactosialidosis, aspartylglycosaminuria, GM1 gangliosidosis (β-galactosidase deficiency, which may also manifest extensive dermal melanocytosis), and α-N-acetylgalactosaminidase deficiency (Kanzaki disease), have been reported to have Fabry-like angiokeratomas. Finally, several patients without any detectable enzyme deficiency have been reported. Among them was a family with autosomal-dominantly inherited Fabry-like angiokeratomas associated with arteriovenous malformations. It should be emphasized that there are many normal patients who have widespread small petechia-like lesions that erupt in adulthood. This is a variant of cherry angiomas.

Fucosidosis

Angiokeratomas identical to those of Fabry disease occur in types II and III forms of this rare lysosomal storage disease. Fucosidosis can be distinguished clinically by the frequent presence of facial dysmorphism, severe mental retardation, weakness, spasticity, and seizures. The most severely affected die in childhood (type I), without the development of typical angiokeratomas. In type II disease, severe spondyloepiphyseal dysplasia and normal intelligence are found. The adolescent type III type can also have angiokeratomas. The condition is autosomal-recessive and is caused by a deficiency in α-L-fucosidase, usually detected in leukocytes.

Sialidosis

Sialidosis (mucolipidosis type I) is an autosomal-recessive lysosomal storage disease caused by mutations in the sialidase gene, *NEU1*. Two types are described, the most severe of which is the infantile form (type II), in which the children die within the first two years of life. Type I disease is less severe and is characterized by mental retardation, myoclonus, cerebellar ataxia, hypotonia, skeletal abnormalities, and facial dysmorphism. Angiokeratoma can occur.

Beta-mannosidase deficiency

This is a rare autosomal-recessive lysosomal storage disease of glycoprotein metabolism. It is due to a deficiency of β-mannosidase that results in the accumulation of a characteristic disaccharide in the lysosomes, which may also be found in the urine. In addition to the Fabry-like angiokeratomas, mental retardation, hearing loss, aggressive behavior, peripheral neuropathy, recurrent infections, epilepsy, coarse facies, and skeletal abnormalities are often present.

Bodensteiner D, et al: Successful reinstitution of agalsidase beta therapy in Fabry disease patients with previous IgE-antibody or skin-test reactivity to the recombinant enzyme. Genet Med 2008; 10:353.

Calzavara-Pinton PG, et al: Angiokeratoma corporis diffusum and arteriovenous fistulas with dominant transmission in the absence of metabolic disorders. Arch Dermatol 1995; 131:57.

Clarke JT: Narrative review: Fabry disease. Ann Intern Med 2007; 146:425.

Eng CM, et al: Fabry disease: baseline medical characteristics of a cohort of 1765 males and females in the Fabry Registry. J Inherit Metab Dis 2007; 30:184.

Hanson M, et al: Association of dermal melanocytosis with lysosomal storage disease. Arch Dermatol 2003; 139:916.

Heroman JW, et al: Cherry red spot in sialidosis (mucolipidosis type I). Arch Ophthalmol 2008; 126:270.

Kanitakis J, et al: Fucosidosis with angiokeratoma: immuno-histochemical and electron microscopic study of a new case and literature review. J Cutan Pathol 2005; 32:506.

Karen JK, et al: Angiokeratoma corporis diffusum (Fabry disease). Dermatol Online J 2005; 11:8.

Laaksonen SM, et al: Neuropathic symptoms and findings in women with Fabry disease. Clin Neurophysiol 2008; 119:1365.

Molho-Pessach V, et al: Angiokeratoma corporis diffusum in human beta-mannosidosis: report of a new case and a novel mutation. J Am Acad Dermatol 2007; 57:407.

Morais P, et al: Angiokeratomas of Fabry successfully treated with intense pulsed light. J Cosmet Laser Ther 2008; 10:218.

Nakai K, et al: Multiple leg ulcers in a patient with Fabry disease. J Eur Acad Dermatol Venereol 2008; 22:382.

Nance CS, et al: Later-onset Fabry disease: an adult variant presenting with the cramp-fasciculation syndrome. Arch Neurol 2006; 63:453.

Orteu CH, et al: Fabry disease and the skin: data from FOS, the Fabry outcome survey. Br J Dermatol 2007; 157:331.

Pintos-Morell G, Beck M: Fabry disease in children and the effects of enzyme replacement treatment. Eur J Pediatr 2009; 168:1355.

Tsukadaira A, et al: Diagnosis of fucosidosis through a skin rash. Intern Med 2005; 44:907.

SKIN DISORDERS IN DIABETES MELLITUS

Skin lesions are common in diabetic patients, with up to two-thirds having at least one skin finding. Xerosis appears to be particularly common, afflicting 50% of those with type I diabetes. Keratosis pilaris is also common, affecting more than 10% of diabetic patients. Other specific cutaneous findings of diabetes are discussed below.

Necrobiosis lipoidica/necrobiosis lipoidica diabeticorum

Necrobiosis lipoidica (NL) is characterized by well-circumscribed, firm, depressed, waxy, yellow–brown plaques, usually of the anterior shin. Although NL can occur in persons without diabetes mellitus, two-thirds are insulin-dependent diabetics. If it occurs in diabetes, it is called necrobiosis lipoidica diabeticorum (NLD). Women are three times more commonly affected than men; the condition usually appears between the ages of 20 and 40, but may occur in children or the elderly. The average age of onset is 34 years for all diabet-

ics, but 22 years, on average, in insulin-dependent patients, and 49 years in non–insulin-dependent patients. While it is reported to affect only 0.3% of patients with diabetes, the prevalence is much higher (over 2%) in series of patients with type I diabetes. Sixty percent of patients with NL have diabetes mellitus; another 20% will have glucose intolerance or a family history of diabetes. In 15%, NL precedes the onset of frank diabetes by an average of 2 years. Control of the diabetes does not influence the course of the NL.

The earliest changes are sharply bordered, elevated, small red papules; these may be capped by a slight scale and do not disappear under diascopic pressure. Later, the lesions develop into irregularly round or oval lesions with well-defined borders and a smooth, glistening (glazed) surface. The center becomes depressed and sulfur-yellow, so that a firm yellowish lesion forms, surrounded by a broad violet–red or pink border. In the yellow portion, numerous telangiectases and ectatic veins are evident. Ulceration occurs in one-third of NLD cases. In an unusual case, the plaques were studded with exophytic nodules resembling tuberous xanthomas. This patient had marked hyperlipidemia, perhaps contributing to the morphology. Rarely, squamous cell carcinoma may occur in chronic ulcers.

The most common location of the lesions is the shins (Fig. 26-29); about 85% occur on the legs. A much less common site is the forearms, and lesions have been reported on the trunk, face, scalp, palms, and soles. Only rarely are sites other than the legs present.

Histologically, well-developed lesions of NL demonstrate a superficial, deep, and interstitial inflammatory process that involves the whole reticular dermis and often the panniculus. Because the dermis is firm, punch biopsy specimens appear rectangular rather than tapered. The inflammatory cells include lymphocytes, histiocytes, multinucleate giant cells, and plasma cells. At low magnification there are layered palisaded granulomas with pale pink degenerated collagen alternating with ampophilic-staining histiocytes. In contradistinction to granuloma annulare, mucin is not increased in the centers of the granulomas, and there is no normal dermis in NL lesions. Between granulomas in granuloma annulare, the

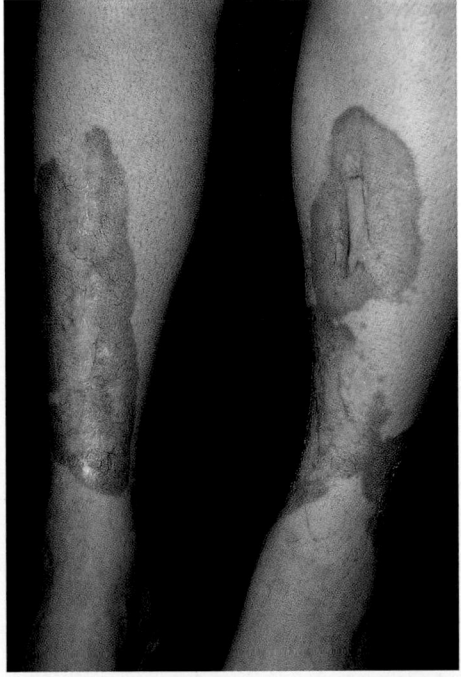

Fig. 26-29 Necrobiosis lipoidica diabeticorum.

collagen pattern is relatively normal, although inflammatory cells may be present. The overlying epidermis tends to be thinned, with loss of the normal rete ridge pattern.

Treatment, after control of the diabetes is achieved, is not completely satisfactory, but NLD has improved in one patient treated with a thiazolidinedione, pioglitazone. Initial therapy is superpotent topical steroids with occlusion. Topical calcineurin inhibitors can also be effective. Intralesional injections of triamcinolone suspension into the inflammatory papules and active advancing edges can be quite effective. Injection into the yellow center is of little benefit and may result in ulceration. It had been proposed that NLD is due to the microangiopathy of diabetes. For this reason, agents designed to improve circulation have been used, at times with success. These include low-dose aspirin, nicotinamide, pentoxifylline, and dipyridamole. The blood flow in lesions of NLD is normal, however, suggesting that this is better considered as an inflammatory dermatosis. Phototherapy, including PUVA and UVA-1, has been effective in selected patients. Oral immunomodulatory therapy should be considered in those patients failing topical treatment. Antimalarial treatment and thalidomide are non-immunosuppressive options that would not alter blood sugar control. Systemic anti-inflammatories reported to be effective in selected cases include systemic steroids, mycophenolate mofetil, and cyclosporine A; TNF inhibitors can be effective in refractory cases. Hyperbaric oxygen may be used for cases with chronic ulceration. In severe cases with persistent ulceration, excision and skin grafting have been effective, although the NLD may recur in or at the edges of the grafts. Despite initial reports of success, photodynamic therapy only improves about one-third of treated patients. Pancreas-kidney transplantation led to resolution in one case, but the patient also received mycophenolate mofetil, prednisone, and tacrolimus orally.

Ahmed I, Goldstein B: Diabetes mellitus. Clin Dermatol 2006; 24:237.

Beattie PE, et al: UVA1 phototherapy for treatment of necrobiosis lipoidica. Clin Exp Dermatol 2006; 31:235.

Berking C, et al: Photodynamic therapy of necrobiosis lipoidica: a multicenter study of 18 patients. Dermatology 2009; 218:136.

Boyd AS: Treatment of necrobiosis lipoidica with pioglitazone. J Am Acad Dermatol 2007; 57:S120.

Clayton TH, et al: Successful treatment of chronic ulcerated necrobiosis lipoidica with 0.1% tacrolimus ointment. Br J Dermatol 2005; 152:581.

Cummins DL, et al: Generalized necrobiosis lipoidica treated with a combination of split-thickness autografting and immunomodulatory therapy. Int J Dermatol 2004; 43:852.

Durupt F, et al: Successful treatment of necrobiosis lipoidica with antimalarial agents. Arch Dermatol 2008; 144:118.

Elmholdt TR, et al: A severe case of ulcerating necrobiosis lipoidica. Acta Derm Venereol 2008; 88:177.

Ferringer T, et al: Cutaneous manifestations of diabetes mellitus. Dermatol Clin 2002; 20:483.

Gullo D, et al: Healing of chronic necrobiosis lipoidica lesions in a type 1 diabetic patient after pancreas-kidney transplantation: a case report. J Endocrinol Invest 2007; 30:259.

Hammami H, et al: Perforating necrobiosis lipoidica in a girl with type 1 diabetes mellitus: a new case reported. Dermatol Online J 2008; 14:11.

Hu SW, et al: Treatment of refractory ulcerative necrobiosis lipoidica diabeticorum with infliximab: report of a case. Arch Dermatol 2009; 145:437.

Kukreja T, Peterson J: Thalidomide for the treatment of refractory necrobiosis lipoidica. Arch Dermatol 2006; 142:20.

Lim C, et al: Squamous cell carcinoma arising in an area of long-standing necrobiosis lipoidica. J Cutan Pathol 2006; 33:581.

Michaels BD, et al: Tuberous necrobiosis lipoidica. Arch Dermatol 2007; 143:546.

Narbutt J, et al: Long-term results of topical PUVA in necrobiosis lipoidica. Clin Exp Dermatol 2006; 31:65.

Ngo B, et al: Skin blood flow in necrobiosis lipoidica diabeticorum. Int J Dermatol 2008; 47:354.

Pavolic MD, et al: The prevalence of cutaneous manifestations in young patients with type 1 diabetes. Diabetes Care 2007; 30:1964.

Peyri J, et al: Necrobiosis lipoidica. Semin Cutan Med Surg 2007; 26:87.

Tan E, et al: Systemic corticosteroids for the outpatient treatment of necrobiosis lipoidica in a diabetic patient. J Dermatolog Treat 2007; 18:246.

Vanhooteghem O, et al: Epidermoid carcinoma and perforating necrobiosis lipoidica: a rare association. J Eur Acad Dermatol Venereol 2005; 19:756.

Wee SA, Possick P: Necrobiosis lipoidica. Dermatol Online J 2004; 10:18.

West EA, et al: A case of recalcitrant necrobiosis lipoidica responding to combined immunosuppression therapy. J Eur Acad Dermatol Venereol 2007; 21:830.

Zeichner JA, et al: Treatment of necrobiosis lipoidica with the tumor necrosis factor antagonist etanercept. J Am Acad Dermatol 2006; 54:S120.

Other diabetic dermadromes

In addition to necrobiosis lipoidica, there are many cutaneous signs in this common endocrinopathy.

Diabetic dermopathy (shin spots)

Dull-red papules that progress to well-circumscribed, small, round, atrophic, hyperpigmented lesions on the shins are a common cutaneous sign of diabetes, occurring in up to 40% of diabetic patients. They are twice as frequent in men. Lesions begin on the lower extremities as crops of four or five dull red macules 0.5–1 cm in diameter. As the lesions resolve, they become shallow, depressed, and hyperpigmented scars. Although they occur individually in people who do not have diabetes, if four or more are present the specificity is high for diabetes.

Diabetic bullae

Noninflammatory, spontaneous, painless blistering, most often in acral locations, is characteristic (Fig. 26-30). Lesions tend to involve the lower legs and be 10 cm or more in

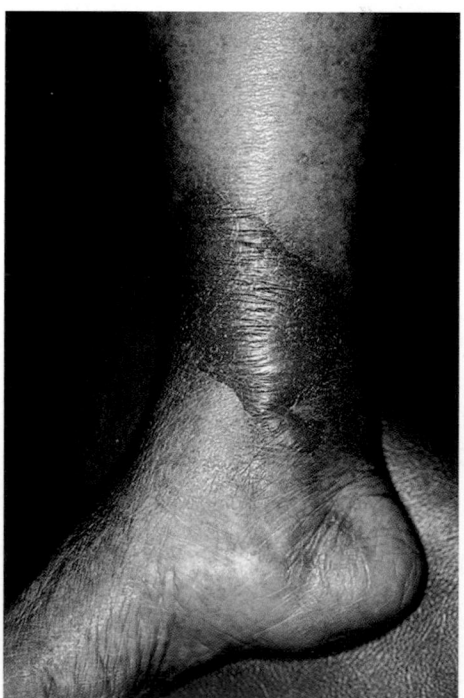

Fig. 26-30 Bullous eruption of diabetes.

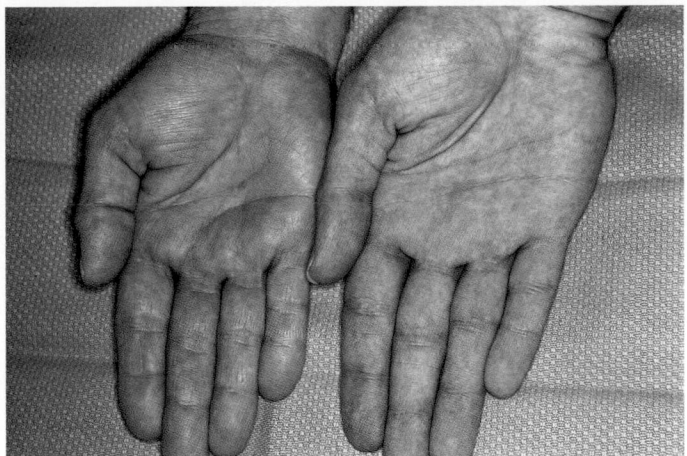

Fig. 26-31 Carotenemia, yellow palm shown next to normal palm.

diameter. The incidence is 0.16% per year. In one series of 5000 persons with diabetes, 25 patients (0.5%) developed diabetic bullae over a 3-year period. In many cases lesions heal spontaneously in 4–5 weeks, usually without scarring. However, lesions may be complicated by chronic ulceration at times. Aggressive and cautious management with dressings and diabetic foot care is required. Minor amputations may be needed. Lesions appear following periods of relative hypoglycemia, perhaps explaining the clinical resemblance of diabetic bullae to pressure bullae.

Both subepidermal and intraepidermal locations have been reported as the site of blister formation, but in the authors' experience lesions are subepidermal. Electron microscopic studies show separation at the lamina lucida level. DIF is negative. There is a reduced threshold to suction-induced blistering in insulin-dependent diabetics.

Carotenosis

Carotenosis is a yellowish discoloration of the skin, especially of the palms and soles (Fig. 26-31), which is sometimes seen in diabetic patients.

Limited joint mobility and waxy skin

Limited joint mobility and waxy skin are important not only because of the 30–50% prevalence of these conditions in diabetic patients with long-standing disease, but also because they are associated with microvascular complications, such as nephropathy and retinopathy. Joint symptoms begin with limitation of joint mobility in the fifth finger at the metacarpophalangeal and proximal joints and progress radially to the other fingers. The condition is bilateral, symmetrical, and painless. Dupuytren's contractures and palmar fibrosis may be associated. Involvement of the feet also occurs and is thought to contribute to the development of chronic ulcerations. Such open sores on the neuropathic, microvascularly compromised, infection-prone diabetic foot pose a constant threat to life and limb.

Other associated conditions in patients with diabetes

Various abnormalities associated with diabetes are erysipelas-like erythema of the legs or feet; sweating disturbances; paresthesias of the legs; mal perforans ulcerations; a predisposition to certain infections such as mucormycosis, group B strepto-

coccal infections, nonclostridial gas gangrene, and malignant external otitis resulting from *Pseudomonas*; disseminated granuloma annulare; eruptive xanthomas; clear cell syringomas; rubeosis of the face; lipoatrophy or lipohypertrophy at sites of insulin injection; acquired perforating disorders; acanthosis nigricans; skin tags; and finger-pebbling.

Anand KP, Kashyap AS: Bullosis diabeticorum. Postgrad Med J 2004; 80:354.

Arkkila PE, et al: Dupuytren's disease in type 1 diabetic patients. Clin Exp Rheumatol 1996; 14:59.

Aye M, et al: Dermatological care of the diabetic foot. Am J Clin Dermatol 2002; 3:463.

Boulton AJM, et al: Neuropathic diabetic foot ulcers. N Engl J Med 2004; 351:48.

Huntley AC: Finger pebbles: a common finding in diabetes mellitus. J Am Acad Dermatol 1986; 14:612.

Jabbour SA: Cutaneous manifestations of endocrine disorders. Am J Clin Dermatol 2003; 4:315.

Kakourou T, et al: Limited joint mobility and lipodystrophy in children and adolescents with insulin-dependent diabetes mellitus. Pediatr Dermatol 1994; 11:310.

Larsen K, et al: Incidence of bullosis diabeticorum: a controversial cause of chronic foot ulceration. Int Wounds J 2008; 5:591.

Lopez PR, et al: Bullosis diabeticorum associated with a prediabetic state. South Med J 2009 May 7 (Epub ahead of print).

OTHER METABOLIC DISORDERS

Citrullinemia

Citrullinemia occurs in two forms. Type I is caused by a deficiency of the enzyme argininosuccinic acid synthetase (*ASS1*) gene. This enzyme converts citrulline and aspartic acid to argininosuccinic acid, as a part of the urea cycle. Low plasma arginine levels result, and the hypothesis is that, since keratin is 16% arginine, dermatitis may occur. Neonates who present with severe deficiencies and hyperammonemic crises may develop erosive, erythematous, scaling patches and plaques prominent in the perioral, lower abdominal, diaper, and buttock regions. This eruption clears with arginine supplementation. Short, sparse hair may also be present. Citrullinemia type II is due to a defect in the *SCL25A13* gene and is seen primarily in East Asia. The deficient enzyme is a liver-type mitochondrial aspartate-glutamate carrier. It presents between adolescence and adulthood.

In carbamyl phosphate synthetase deficiency, low plasma arginine levels may also occur, and similar cutaneous findings have been reported in this second metabolic defect of the urea cycle.

Diets high in arginine will heal the skin lesions.

Engel K, et al: Mutations and polymorphisms in the human argininosuccinate synthetase (ASS1) gene. Hum Mutat 2009; 30:300.

Fiermonte G, et al: An adult with type 2 citrullinemia presenting in Europe. N Engl J Med 2008; 358:1408.

Goldblum OM, et al: Neonatal citrullinemia associated with cutaneous manifestations and arginine deficiency. J Am Acad Dermatol 1986; 14:321.

Takeoka M, et al: Carbamyl phosphate synthetase 1 deficiency. Pediatr Neurol 2001; 24:193.

Hartnup disease

Hartnup disease is an inborn error of tryptophan excretion; it was named after the Hartnup family, in which it was first noted. It is the second most common inherited aminoaciduria after phenylketonuria. The characteristic findings are a pellagra-like dermatitis following exposure to sunlight, intermittent cerebellar ataxia, psychosis, and constant aminoaciduria.

The dermatitis occurs on exposed parts of the skin, chiefly the face, neck, hands, and legs. The erythematous scaly patches flare up into a hot, red, exudative state after exposure to sunlight, followed by hyperpigmentation. Stomatitis and vulvitis also occur. The disease becomes milder with increasing age. Rarely, an acrodermatitis enteropathica-like eruption with normal zinc levels may occur in patients with Hartnup disease.

Hartnup disease is an autosomal-recessive trait. Large amounts of neutral amino acids including tryptophan are present in the urine, establishing the diagnosis. Hartnup disease is caused by mutations in the *SLC6A19* gene. *SLC6A19* transports neutral amino acids across the apical membrane of epithelial cells in the gut and kidneys. The skin lesions respond to niacinamide, but the neurologic disease may not improve.

Azmanov DN, et al: Persistence of the common Hartnup disease D173N allele in populations of European origin. Ann Hum Genet 2007; 71:755.

Azmanov DN, et al: Further evidence for allelic heterogeneity in Hartnup disorder. Hum Mutat 2008; 29:1217.

Sander CS, et al: Severe exfoliative erythema of malnutrition in a child with coexisting coeliac and Hartnup's disease. Clin Exp Dermatol 2009; 34:178.

Seyhan ME, et al: Acrodermatitis enteropathica-like eruptions in a child with Hartnup disease. Pediatr Dermatol 2006; 23:262.

Zheng Y, et al: A novel missense mutation in the SLC6A19 gene in a Chinese family with Hartnup disorder. Int J Dermatol 2009; 48:388.

Prolidase deficiency

Prolidase deficiency is an autosomal-recessive inherited inborn error of metabolism. Prolidase cleaves dipeptides containing C-terminal proline or hydroxyproline. When this enzyme is deficient, the normal recycling of proline residues obtained from collagen degradation is impaired. A build-up of iminodipeptides results, with disturbances in connective tissue metabolism and excretion of large amounts of iminodipeptides in the urine. Also, the absence of prolidase activity causes increased keratinocyte apoptosis, which may be in part responsible for the skin lesions.

Clinically, 85% of patients have some dermatologic manifestations. The most important cutaneous signs, which almost always appear before the affected person is 12 years old, are skin fragility; ulceration and scarring of the lower extremities; photosensitivity and telangiectasia; poliosis; scaly, erythematous, maculopapular, and purpuric lesions; and thickening of the skin with lymphedema of the legs. Systemic signs and symptoms include mental deficiency, splenomegaly, and recurrent infections. An unusual facial appearance is noted at times, with low hairline, frontal bossing, and saddle nose. The nasal septum may be perforated. Some patients with prolidase deficiency meet American Rheumatology Association (ARA) criteria for the diagnosis of SLE, but worsen if immunosuppressive treatment is given. Antinuclear antibodies (ANA) and anti ds-DNA may be positive.

Prolidase measurement may be determined in erythrocytes, leukocytes, or fibroblasts. Many therapeutic options have been described, such as oral supplements of manganese and ascorbic acid, both modulators of prolidase activity; however, results of treatment are highly variable. Topical proline 5% in ointment helped heal chronic leg ulcers in one patient, although it did not prevent the appearance of new ulcerations. Apheresis exchange repeated monthly may improve the leg ulcers. In long-standing ulcerations squamous cell carcinomas may occur.

Bissonnette R, et al: Prolidase deficiency. J Am Acad Dermatol 1993; 29:818.

Di Rocco M, et al: Systemic lupus erythematosus-like disease in a 6-year-old boy with prolidase deficiency. J Inherit Metab Dis 2007; 30:814.

Dunn R, Dolianitis C: Prolidase deficiency: the use of topical proline for treatment of leg ulcers. Australas J Dermatol 2008; 49:237.

Fimiani M, et al: Squamous cell carcinoma of the leg in a patient with prolidase deficiency. Br J Dermatol 1999; 140:362.

Isik D, et al: Nasal reconstruction in a patient with prolidase deficiency syndrome. J Plast Reconstr Aesthet Surg 2008; 61:1256.

Lupi A, et al: Therapeutic apheresis exchange in two patients with prolidase deficiency. Br J Dermatol 2002; 147:1237.

Shrinath M, et al: Prolidase deficiency and systemic lupus erythematosus. Arch Dis Child 1997; 76:441.

Phenylketonuria

Phenylketonuria (PKU) is an autosomal-recessive disorder of phenylalanine metabolism due to a deficiency in the enzyme phenylalanine hydroxylase. Phenylalanine is not metabolized to tyrosine. PKU is the most common form of inherited aminoaciduria, affecting 1 in 15 000 live births in the USA. It is characterized by mental deficiency; epileptic seizures; pigmentary dilution of skin, hair, and eyes; pseudoscleroderma; and dermatitis (Fig. 26-32). It is most common in white persons.

Affected children are blue-eyed, with blond hair and fair skin. They are usually extremely sensitive to light, and about 50% have an eczematous dermatitis. It is clinically similar to atopic dermatitis, with a predilection for the flexures. It is worst in the youngest patients, may improve with dietary treatment, and has been exacerbated by phenylalanine challenge in a carrier of the recessive gene. Skin lesions may be sclerodermatous in nature. Indurations of the thighs and buttocks are present early in infancy and increase with time. After many years the lesions soften and become atrophic.

Blood levels of phenylalanine are high. The presence of phenylpyruvic acid in the urine is demonstrated by a characteristic deep-green color when a few drops of ferric chloride solution are added to it. Green diapers occur in histidinemia, as well as in PKU.

In developed countries universal screening is practiced, so dietary therapy with phenylalanine restriction, combined with supplementation of tyrosine and other amino acids, is instituted. This prevents the manifestations of the disease. If compliance is poor, the manifestations, including eczema, may develop at any age, followed by improvement of the skin with reinstitution of the diet.

Al-Mayouf SM, Al-Owain MA: Progressive sclerodermatous skin changes in a child with phenylketonuria. Pediatr Dermatol 2006; 23:136.

Belloso LM, et al: Cutaneous findings in a 51-year-old man with phenylketonuria. J Am Acad Dermatol 2003; 49:S190.

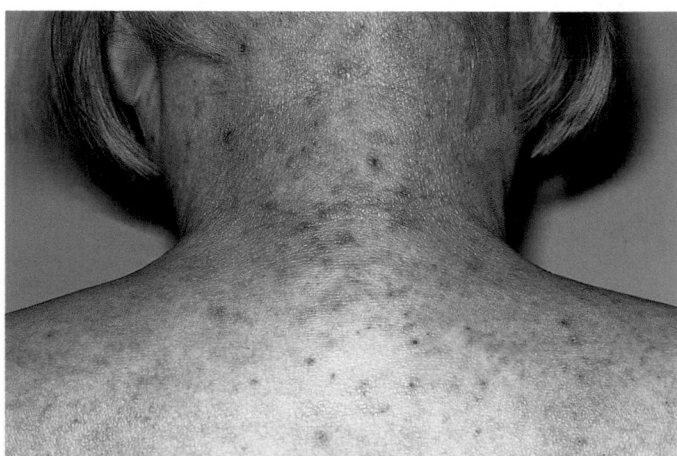

Fig. 26-32 Light-skinned, light-haired phenylketonuria patient with dermatitis. (Courtesy of Jeff Miller, MD)

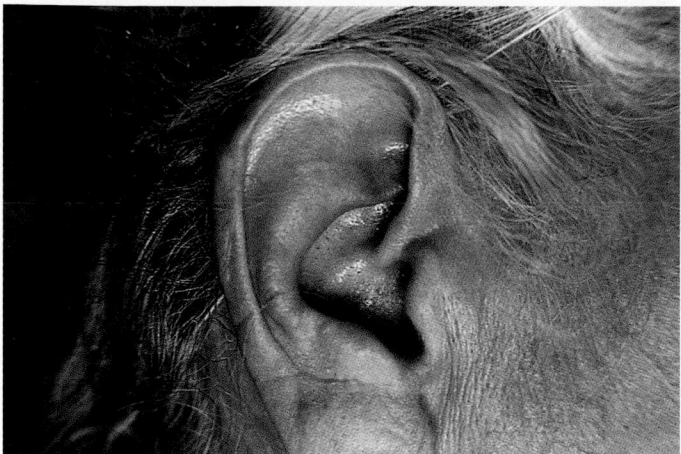

Fig. 26-33 Ochronotic pigmentation of ear cartilage.

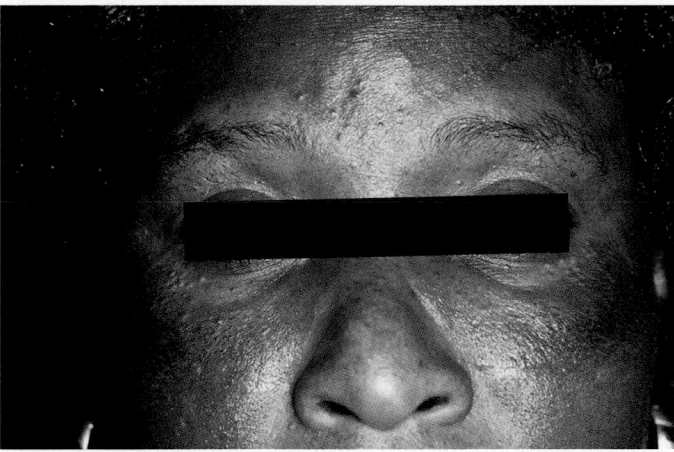

Fig. 26-34 Exogenous ochronosis.

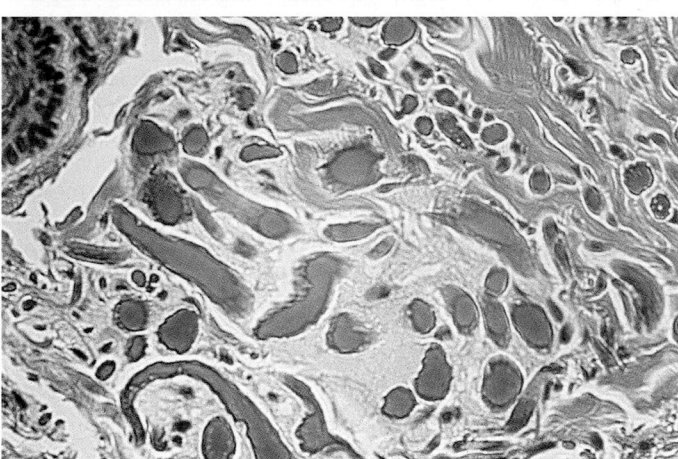

Fig. 26-35 Large ochre bodies in the dermis in exogenous ochronosis.

Alkaptonuria and ochronosis

Alkaptonuria, inherited as an autosomal-recessive trait, is caused by the lack of renal and hepatic homogentisic acid oxidase, the enzyme necessary for the catabolism of homogentisic acid, a product of tyrosine and phenylalanine metabolism. Excess homogentisic acid is excreted in the urine and deposited in connective tissues throughout the body, especially the cartilage. The urine is dark and becomes black on standing.

For many years the dark urine may be the only indication of the presence of alkaptonuria. In the mean time, large amounts of homogentisic acid are accumulated in the body tissues. By the third decade of life the deposition of pigment becomes apparent. The early sign is the pigmentation of the sclera (Osler's sign) and the cartilage of the ears (Fig. 26-33). Later the cartilage of the nose and tendons, especially those on the hands, becomes discolored.

Blue or mottled brown macules appear on the skin. The bluish macules have a predilection for the fingers, ears, nose, genital regions, apices of the axillae, and buccal and vaginal mucosa. Palmoplantar pigmentation may occur. The sweat glands are rich in ochronotic pigment granules, and the intradermal injection of epinephrine into the skin of the axillary vault will yield brown–black sweat droplets in the follicular orifices. The cerumen is often black. Internally, the larynx, great vessels, valves of the heart, kidneys, esophagus, tonsils, and dura mater may be involved.

Histologically, there are large, irregular ochre bodies within the reticular dermis. They represent degenerated elastic fibers with deposition of ochronotic pigment, and stain black with crystal violet or methylene blue.

Ochronotic arthropathy involves the axial spine joints first. Next affected are the knees, shoulders, and hips. Radiographic films show a characteristic appearance of early calcification of the intervertebral disk and later narrowing of the intervertebral spaces with eventual disk collapse.

There is no effective treatment. Dietary restriction of tyrosine and phenylalanine is recommended, but may not prevent progression of disease. Joint and cardiac valve replacement may be necessary.

Exogenous ochronosis

Topically applied phenolic intermediates, such as hydroquinone, carbolic acid (phenol), picric acid, and resorcinol, may produce exogenous ochronosis (Fig. 26-34). Even 2% over-the-counter hydroquinone can produce ochronosis if used regularly for a long period. Hydroquinone specifically inhibits the enzyme homogentisic acid oxidase locally, resulting in accumulation of this substance on the collagen fibers in tissues where it is applied. Most patients affected have high Fitzpatrick phototype (IV–VI). Since most patients use the hydroquinone to treat melasma, findings of melasma may overlay the skin findings of exogenous ochronosis. The typical findings are gray–brown or blue–black macules, usually over the zygomatic regions. Caviar-like hyperchromic pinpoint papules may occur, which on dermoscopy can be seen associated with follicular openings. Confetti-like depigmentation (from the hydroquinone) may be admixed with the hyperpigmentation. Histologically, exogenous ochronosis and alkaptonuria have identical changes on skin biopsy (Fig. 26-35). Treatment is less than satisfactory. Stopping the application of hydroquinone may lead to improvement.

Bellew SG, et al: Treatment of exogenous ochronosis with a Q-switched alexandrite (755 mm) laser. Dermatol Surg 2004; 30:555.

Bongiomo MR, et al: Exogenous ochronosis and striae atrophicae following the use of bleaching creams. Int J Dermatol 2005; 44:112.

Butany JW, et al: Ochronosis and aortic valve stenosis. J Card Surg 2006; 21:182.

Charlin R, et al: Hydroquinone-induced exogenous ochronosis: a report of four cases and usefulness of dermoscopy. Int J Dermatol 2008; 47:19.

Lubics A, et al: Extensive bluish gray skin pigmentation and severe arthropathy. Arch Dermatol 2000; 36:548.

Phornphutkul C, et al: Natural history of alkaptonuria. N Engl J Med 2002; 347:2111.

Tan SK, et al: Hydroquinone-induced exogenous ochronosis in Chinese: two case reports and a review. Int J Dermatol 2008; 47:639.

Wilson's disease (hepatolenticular degeneration)

Wilson's disease is an autosomal-recessive derangement of copper transport. The disease is due to a dysfunction of a copper-transporting enzyme, P-type ATPase (ATP7B), which is required to excrete copper into the bile. This leads to accumulation of copper in the liver, brain, cornea, and kidney. Affected persons develop hepatomegaly, splenomegaly, and neuropsychiatric changes. Slurred speech, a squeaky voice, salivation, dysphagia, tremors, incoordination, and spasticity may all occur. There is progressive, fatal hepatic and central nervous system degeneration.

Azure lunulae (sky-blue moons) of the nails occur in 10% of patients, and the smoky, greenish-brown Kayser–Fleischer rings develop at the edges of the corneas. Hyperpigmentation develops on the lower extremities in most patients. A vague greenish discoloration of the skin on the face, neck, and genitalia may also be present. An idiopathic blistering eruption that ceased with treatment of Wilson's disease has been reported. Skin changes of cirrhosis (vascular spiders and palmar erythema) may occur. Low ceruloplasmin level in the serum leads to suspicion of the diagnosis, along with elevated 24-hour urinary copper excretion and elevated free serum copper. Ten percent of carriers for Wilson's disease have a low ceruloplasmin, so additional tests should be performed to confirm the diagnosis.

The treatment is a low copper diet, often with agents that bind copper and enhance its excretion from the body. D-penicillamine removes copper by chelating it. The dose is 1 or 2 g/day orally. Potential side effects include pemphigus, cutis laxa, and elastosis perforans serpiginosa, which has been reported repeatedly in Wilson patients on penicillamine. Trientine, another copper chelator, enhances copper excretion. It has less toxicity, but is somewhat less effective than D-penicillamine. Zinc supplementation leads to increased metallothionein in the gut and liver. This leads to more copper excretion in the stool and the formation of non-toxic copper complexes in the liver. Zinc cannot be given at the same time as a chelator. Treatment must be continued for life.

Mak CM, Lam CW: Diagnosis of Wilson's disease: a comprehensive review. Crit Rev Clin Lab Sci 2008; 45:263.

Medici V, et al: Wilson disease: a practical approach to diagnosis, treatment and follow-up. Dig Liver Dis 2007; 39:601.

Pfeiffer RF: Wilson's disease. Semin Neurol 2007; 27:123.

Tyrosinemia II (Richner–Hanhart syndrome)

Tyrosinemia is an autosomal-recessive syndrome resulting from a deficiency of hepatic tyrosine aminotransferase, an important enzyme in the degradation of tyrosine and phenylalanine. It is caused by mutations in the *TAT* gene. The diagnosis is confirmed by identifying elevated levels of serum tyrosine. Clinical features are mild to severe keratitis, and hyperkeratotic and erosive lesions of palms and soles, often with mild mental retardation. Photophobia and tearing commonly occur as the keratitis begins, and ultimately neovascularization is seen. Painful palmar and plantar hyperkeratosis may be the only manifestation. The fingertips, and hypothenar and thenar eminences are primarily affected on the palms. Initially, only the soles may be affected, with hyperkeratosis primarily over the tips of the digits and on weight-bearing surfaces. In any child presenting with palmoplantar keratoderma, this diagnosis must be considered. A low-tyrosine, low-phenylalanine diet may improve or prevent the eye and skin lesions, but may or may not benefit established mental retardation.

Meissner T, et al: Richner–Hanhart syndrome detected by expanded newborn screening. Pediatr Dermatol 2008; 25:378.

Pasternack SM, et al: Identification of two new mutations in the TAT gene in a Danish family with tyrosinaemia type II. Br J Dermatol 2009; 160:704.

Tallab TM: Richner–Hanhart syndrome. J Am Acad Dermatol 1996; 35:857.

Hurler syndrome (mucopolysaccharidosis I)

Hurler syndrome, or gargoylism, is an autosomal-recessive lysosomal storage disease of mucopolysaccharide metabolism. A deficiency of α-L-iduronidase is the causative defect. This enzyme is responsible for the breakdown of heparan sulfate and dermatan sulfate. All patients have undetectable enzyme activity by current assays, yet there is significant polymorphism in the severity and age of onset. In general, cases are divided into severe mucopolysaccharidosis (MPS I) (Hurler syndrome) and attenuated MPS I (Hurler–Scheie/Scheie syndrome).

Hurler syndrome is characterized by mental retardation, hepatosplenomegaly, umbilical and inguinal hernia, genital infantilism, corneal opacities, and skin abnormalities. Patients with Hurler syndrome have facial dysmorphism, with a broad saddle nose, thick lips, and a large tongue. The skin is thickened, with ridges and grooves, especially on the upper half of the body. Fine lanugo hair is profusely distributed all over the body. Large, coarse hair is prominent, especially on the extremities. Dermal melanocytosis, characterized by extensive, blue pigmentation with both a dorsal and a ventral distribution, indistinct borders, and a persistent and/or progressive course, occurs in some patients with lysosomal storage disease, including patients with Hurler syndrome, Hunter syndrome, and GM1-gangliosidosis type 1. The skeletal system is deformed, with hydrocephalus, kyphosis, and gibbus (cat-back shape). The hands are broad and have claw-like fingers. The joints are distorted.

The diagnosis of MPS I is made by demonstrating elevated urinary glycosaminoglycan levels, and deficient enzyme activity in fibroblasts, leukocytes, serum, or blood spots. Prenatal diagnosis is possible. Hematopoietic stem cell transplantation (HSCT) is the most effective treatment for Hurler syndrome. It can prevent mental deterioration if performed early enough (before age 2 and before developmental quotients fall below 70). Cardiac and joint complications are not prevented by HSCT. ERT with recombinant human α-L-iduronidase is an option in patients who are not candidates for HSCT.

Hanson M, et al: Association of dermal melanocytosis with lysosomal storage disease. Arch Dermatol 2003; 139:916.

Muenzer J, et al: Mucopolysaccharidosis I: management and treatment guidelines. Pediatrics 2009; 123:19.

Hunter syndrome (mucopolysaccharidosis II)

Hunter syndrome is X-linked recessive lysosomal storage disease. It is due to a deficiency of the enzyme iduronate-2-sulfatase. The pebbly lesions of MPS II in the skin of the upper back, neck, chest, proximal arms, or thighs represent the only diagnostic skin changes of the mucopolysaccharidoses. The lesions are firm, flesh-colored to white papules and nodules, which coalesce into a cobblestone or reticular pattern (Fig. 26-36). They generally occur at about age 10. Histologically, they demonstrate increased dermal mucin and metachromatic granules in the cytoplasm of dermal fibroblasts and at times in eccrine sweat glands and epidermal keratinocytes. Additionally, the dermal melanocytosis described above for Hurler syndrome may occur in Hunter syndrome.

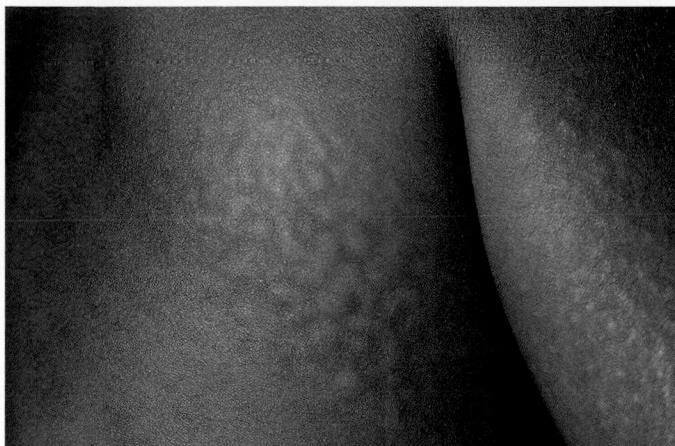

Fig. 26-36 Hunter syndrome papules.

Dermatan sulfate and heparan sulfate are excreted in the urine in large amounts, and the diagnosis can be confirmed by absent iduronate-2-sulphatase in leukocytes. HSCT and ERT can be useful in appropriately evaluated patients.

Guffon N, et al: Bone marrow transplantation in children with Hunter syndrome: outcome after 7 to 17 years. J Pediatr 2009; 154:733.

Ito K, et al: The effect of haematopoietic stem cell transplant on papules with "pebbly" appearance in Hunter's syndrome. Br J Dermatol 2004; 151:207.

Jones SA, et al: Mortality and cause of death in mucopolysaccharidosis type II: a historical review based on data from the Hunter Outcome Survey (HOS). J Inherit Metab Dis 2009; 32:534.

Ochiai T, et al: Significance of extensive Mongolian spots in Hunter's syndrome. Br J Dermatol 2003; 148:1173.

Sakata S, et al: Skin rash with the histological absence of meta-chromatic granules as the presenting feature of Hunter syndrome in a 6-year-old boy. Br J Dermatol 2008; 159:249.

Morquio's disease (mucopolysaccharidosis IV)

This autosomal-recessive disorder is characterized by dwarfism, prognathism, corneal opacities, deafness, progressive kyphoscoliosis, flat feet, and knock-knees. The standing position is a crouch. Sacral dimpling may be present at birth. There is increased excretion of keratan sulfate. The enzyme deficiencies are galactosamine-6-sulfate sulfatase in Morquio A and β-galactosidase in Morquio B.

Ohashi A, et al: Sacral dimple: incidental findings from newborn evaluation. Mucopolysaccharidosis IVa disease. Acta Paediatr 2009; 98:768.

Hyaluronidase deficiency (mucopolysaccharidosis IX)

A deficiency of hyaluronidase, caused by mutations in *HYAL1*, leads to short stature, erosions of the acetabula, and multiple periauricular soft-tissue masses. There is no neurologic or visceral involvement. Hyaluronan is an extracellular matrix component important for cell migration, proliferation, and differentiation, and is a structural component of connective tissue. Turnover of this glycosaminoglycan is dependent upon hyaluronidases, each of which has different tissue expression patterns, likely explaining the mild phenotype of this newly described condition.

Trigs-Raine B, et al: Mutations in HYAL1, a member of a tandemly distributed multigene family encoding disparate hyaluronidase activities, cause a newly described lysosomal disorder, mucopolysaccharidosis IX. Proc Natl Acad Sci USA 1999; 96:6296.

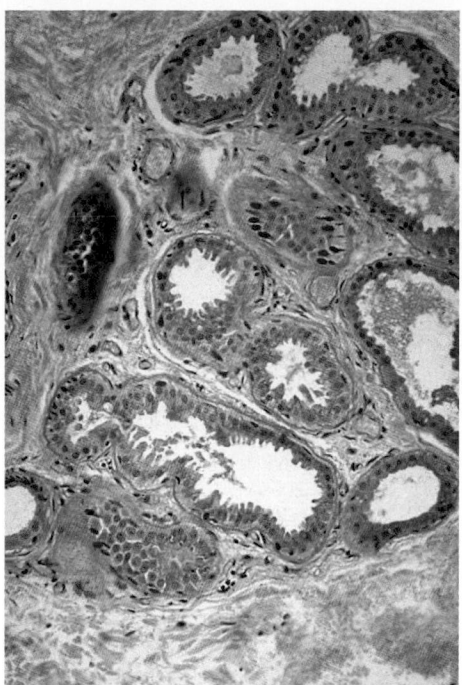

Fig. 26-37 PAS-stained inclusions in Lafora's disease.

Lafora's disease

Lafora's disease is an autosomal-recessive form of progressive myoclonic and tonic-clonic epilepsy beginning at puberty. It is characterized by myoclonic jerks followed by progressive ataxia, dysphagia, dysarthria, dementia, and death in early adulthood. Diagnosis is established in the proper clinical setting by demonstration of characteristic PAS-positive cytoplasmic inclusion bodies in the eccrine ducts, axillary apocrine myoepithelial cells (Fig. 26-37), and peripheral nerves. The best site to biopsy is the axilla. Other conditions in which similar polyglucosan inclusions can be seen include normal aging (amyloid bodies), double athetosis syndrome, amyotrophic lateral sclerosis, and glycogen storage disease type IV.

Cutaneous manifestations are rare. Papulonodular lesions on the ears and indurated, thickened plaques on the arms have been reported. Large amounts of acid mucopolysaccharides were demonstrated histologically in these lesions. The syndrome is caused by mutations of either the *EPM2A* gene (80% of cases) or *NHLRC1*, which encodes ubiquitin ligase. The products of these two genes form a complex critical to the regulation of neuronal function. This explains how mutations in either gene lead to the same phenotype.

Karimipour D, et al: Lafora's disease. J Am Acad Dermatol 1999; 41:790.

Singh S, Ganesh S: Lafora progressive myoclonus epilepsy: a meta-analysis of reported mutations in the first decade following the discovery of the EPM2A and NHLRC1 genes. Hum Mutat 2009; 30:715.

CADASIL syndrome

Cerebral autosomal-dominant arteriopathy with subcortical infarcts and leukoencephalopathy (CADASIL) is a neurovascular disease of young and middle-aged people. It is the most common heritable cause of stroke and vascular dementia in adults. It is caused by mutations in NOTCH3, a transmembrane protein. Children have cognitive impairment, young adults have depression and migraine with aura, and those in their forties and fifties experience apathy, mood disturbances, and motor disability. Executive dysfunction in the late thirties to fifties is followed by dementia in the sixties and seventies. One patient developed generalized hemorrhagic macules and papules. There is deposition of a granular eosinophilic material, NOTCH 3, in the media of arterial walls due to mutations in the NOTCH intercellular signaling pathways. This may be demonstrated on skin biopsy by electron microscopy or by a specific immunostain. However, the recommended diagnostic procedure is genetic testing, screening all 23 exons. Ultrastructural examination of skin biopsy is restricted to patients with negative genetic screening and features highly suggestive of CADASIL.

Chabriat H, et al: CADASIL. Lancet Neurol 2009; 8:643.

Lee YC, et al: The remarkably variable expressivity of CADASIL: report of a minimally symptomatic man at an advanced age. J Neurol 2009; 256:1026.

Ratzinger G, et al: CADASIL: an unusual manifestation with prominent cutaneous involvement. Br J Dermatol 2005; 152:246.

Rumbaugh JA, et al: CADASIL. J Am Acad Dermatol 2000; 43:1128.

Walsh JS, et al: CADASIL. J Am Acad Dermatol 2000; 43:1125.

Farber disease

Also known as fibrocytic dysmucopolysaccharidosis and lipogranulomatosis, Farber disease is characterized by periarticular swellings; a weak, hoarse cry; pulmonary failure; painful joint deformities; and motor and mental retardation. The onset is during the first months of life; death can be expected before the age of 2.

The rubbery subcutaneous nodules have a distinct yellowish hue and are 1–2 cm in diameter. They are usually located over the joints, lumbar spine, scalp, and weight-bearing areas. Histologically, they are granulomas. Diagnosis can be aided by finding Farber bodies (curvilinear bodies) within the cytoplasm or phagosomes of fibroblasts, histiocytes, or endothelial cells, banana-shaped bodies within Schwann cells, and zebra bodies within endothelial cells and neurons. There is an accumulation of ceramide and its degradation products in foam cells due to a specific deficiency of lysosomal ceramidase.

Levade T, et al: Neurodegenerative course in ceramidase deficiency (Farber disease) correlates with the residual lysosomal ceramide turnover in cultured living patient cells. J Neurol Sci 1995; 134:108.

Rauch HJ, et al: Banana bodies in disseminated lipogranulomatosis (Farber disease). Am J Dermatopathol 1983; 5:263.

Adrenoleukodystrophy (Schilder's disease)

Adrenoleukodystrophy (X-ALD) is an X-linked disorder in which cerebral white matter becomes progressively demyelinated and serious adrenocortical insufficiency usually occurs. X-ALD is caused by mutations in the *ALD* gene, which codes for a protein named adrenoleukodystrophy protein (ALDP). The protein defect results in impaired degradation of very long chain fatty acids (>22 carbons). Skin hyperpigmentation often calls attention to the adrenal disease, and mental deterioration indicates the even graver diagnosis of ALD. A mild ichthyotic appearance to the skin of the trunk and legs, and sparse hair with trichorrhexis nodosa-like features may occur. Skin biopsies may show characteristic vacuolization of eccrine secretory coils (duct cells being spared), and biopsies of the skin and conjunctiva may show diagnostic clefts in Schwann cells surrounding myelinated axons. Bone marrow transplantation may benefit a small subset of patients.

Crum BA, et al: 26-year-old man with hyperpigmentation of skin and lower extremity spasticity. Mayo Clin Proc 1997; 72:479.

Unterberger U, et al: Diagnosis of X-linked adrenoleukodystrophy in blood leukocytes. Clin Biochem 2007; 40:1037.

Gout

Classic gout presents as an acute monoarthritis, usually of the great toe or knee, in a middle-aged to elderly man with hyperuricemia. In such patients with chronic disease, usually present for more than 10 years, monosodium urate monohydrate may be deposited in the subcutaneous tissues, forming nodules called tophi. These vary from pinhead- to pea-sized or, rarely, even baseball-sized. They are commonly found on the rims of the ears and over the distal interphalangeal articulations (Fig. 26-38). Tophi are of a yellow or cream color. In the course of time they tend to break down and discharge sodium urate crystals, afterward healing and perhaps breaking down again. The diagnosis is verified histologically by finding the characteristic long, needle-shaped crystals of monosodium urate. Because routine processing dissolves these deposits, fixation in absolute ethanol or freezing is optimal for their demonstration, but is rarely done since most specimens are submitted in formalin. Rather 10 micron unstained sections from formalin fixed specimens can demonstrate characteristic crystals under polarized light. Atypical gout occurs as a polyarticular chronic arthritis, often of the hands. It occurs equally in women and men, and there may be tophi, frequently overlying Heberden nodes, at presentation. Another risk group is organ transplant patients, of whom 10% develop gout. Acute arthritis is treated with NSAIDs, prednisone or colchicines, while long-term management is with uricosuric agents or xanthine oxidase inhibitors.

Lesch–Nyhan syndrome

Also known as juvenile gout, Lesch–Nyhan syndrome is a rare, X-linked, recessively inherited disorder characterized by childhood hyperuricemia, gout, tophi (Fig. 26-39),

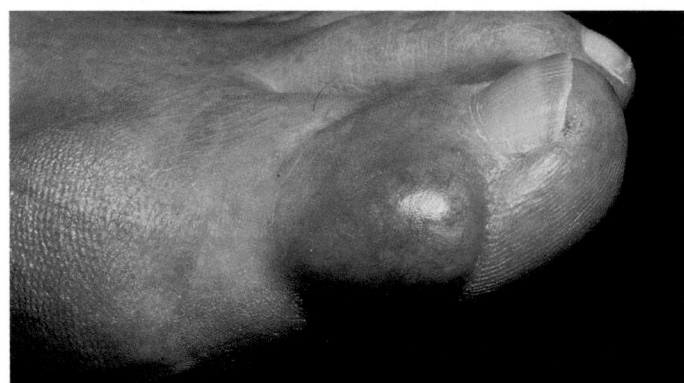

Fig. 26-38 Gouty tophus.

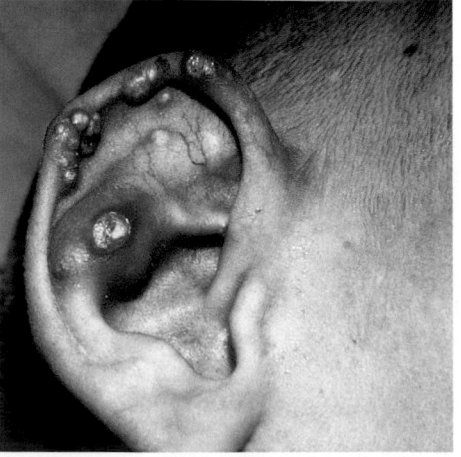

Fig. 26-39 Lesch–Nyhan syndrome.

choreoathetosis, progressive mental retardation, and self-mutilation.

The cutaneous lesions are distinctive. Massive self-mutilation of lips with the teeth occurs. The fingers are also badly chewed. The ears and nose are occasionally mutilated. An early diagnostic clue is orange crystals in the diaper. The blood uric acid is increased and allopurinol, 200–400 mg/day, is given. There is a marked deficiency in an enzyme of purine metabolism, hypoxanthine guanine phosphoribosyl-transferase (HGPRT).

Chopra KF, et al: Finger pad tophi. Cutis 1999; 64:233.
Puig JG, et al: The spectrum of HPRT deficiency. Medicine (Baltimore) 2001; 80:102.
Rott KT, et al: Gout. JAMA 2003; 289:2857.
Terkeltaub RA, et al: Gout. N Engl J Med 2003; 349:1647.
Weaver J, et al: Simple non-staining method to demonstrate urate crystals in formalin-fixed, paraffin-embedded skin biopsies. J Cutan Pathol 2009; 36:560.

 Bonus images for this chapter can be found online at
http://www.expertconsult.com

27 Genodermatoses and Congenital Anomalies

Genetic disorders are often grouped into three categories: chromosomal, single gene, and polygenetic. Chromosomal disorders can be numerical, such as trisomy and monosomy, or structural, resulting from translocations or deletions. Most genodermatoses show single-gene or mendelian inheritance (autosomal-dominant, autosomal-recessive, or X-linked recessive genes). Polygenetic syndromes often involve complex interactions of genes.

Autosomal-dominant conditions require only a single gene to produce a given phenotype. Usually the patient has one affected parent or is affected by a new mutation. The disease is transmitted from generation to generation. Autosomal-recessive traits require a homozygous state to produce the abnormality. The pedigree will often reveal parental consanguinity. Parents will be clinically unaffected but often have affected relatives. X-linked conditions occur when the mutant gene is carried on the X chromosome. If a disease is X-linked recessive, the loss is evident in males (XY), who do not have a second X chromosome to express the normal allele. Therefore, X-linked recessive traits occur almost exclusively in males. They cannot transmit the disease to sons (who inherit their Y chromosome), but all their daughters will be carriers. Carrier females who are heterozygous (having one normal and one abnormal X chromosome) occasionally show some subtle evidence of the disease. This occurs as a result of Lyonization (the physiologic segmental inactivation of one of the X-chromosomes). X-linked dominant disease states are commonly lethal in males. Survival is possible in females who retain a normal allele. As the mutation is lethal in many affected cell lines, females commonly demonstrate loss of normal tissue in the affected segments (loss of digits, microphthalmia, loss of teeth). X-linked dominant traits result in pedigrees in which more than one female is affected but no males express the disease. Rarely, males may survive, especially if they have Klinefelter syndrome (XXY).

Mosaicism is the presence of two or more genetically distinct cell lines in a single individual. It may occur as a result of physiologic inactivation of one X chromosome (Lyonization) or as the result of postzygotic somatic mutation. Mosaicism often presents in a linear and whorled pattern along the lines of Blaschko. In mosaic states, genes that are detrimental to a cell population during fetal development (such as incontinentia pigmenti) typically result in thin segments, as they are overgrown by the adjacent normal tissue. Conversely, genes that confer a growth advantage during fetal development (e.g. a mutated tumor suppressor gene in segmental neurofibromatosis) may result in broad plaque-type lesions that have grown beyond the boundaries of a typical Blaschko segment.

In autosomal-dominant conditions, a normal allele remains, but is not enough to prevent disease. Loss of heterozygosity (LOH) is the segmental loss of this remaining normal allele. LOH may give rise to segments of the body with an exaggerated presentation of the syndrome. The affected area corresponds to a Blaschko segment or plaque. The forehead plaque of tuberous sclerosis is related to a mutation in a tumor suppressor gene. The loss of the tumor suppressor gene imparts a growth advantage and loss of heterozygosity leaves no suppressor gene product in the segment. As a result, the affected segment grows beyond its Blaschko boundaries, forming a broad plaque.

When a patient presents with segmental distribution of a disorder, it is critical to determine if the disorder is a result of mosaicism or LOH. In the latter case, the abnormal allele is present throughout the body, including gonadal tissue. In a patient who presents with segmental neurofibromatosis but has Lisch nodules or axillary freckling, LOH rather than mosaicism is likely to account for the segmental presentation. The risk of passing the gene to a child is roughly 50:50. A geneticist should be involved during discussions of risk of transmission, as the mechanisms may be complex. Patients with mosaicism based on postzygotic somatic gene mutation may have gonadal mosaicism and be capable of passing on the gene. Gonadal mosaicism is more likely when more than one segment is present on different regions of the body. Prior to gastrulation (when a cavity forms in the embryo), every cell is pluripotent and can give rise to an entire organism, or contribute to multiple sites of the body. At the time of gastrulation, cells become dedicated to produce specific segments of the body. Blaschko segments in different regions suggest a mutation that occurred prior to gastrulation when the involved cell lines could contribute to different parts of the body, including the gonads. Polygenetic disorders, such as psoriasis, may also present with limited and linear forms that may relate to segmental LOH.

Happle R: Superimposed segmental manifestation of polygenic skin disorders. J Am Acad Dermatol 2007 Oct; 57(4):690–699.
Irvine AD, et al: The molecular genetics of the genodermatoses: progress to date and future directions. Br J Dermatol 2003; 148:1.
Luu M, et al: Prenatal diagnosis of genodermatoses: current scope and future capabilities. Int J Dermatol 2010 Apr; 49(4):353–361.

X-LINKED, MOSAIC, AND RELATED DISORDERS

Incontinentia pigmenti

Also known as Bloch–Sulzberger disease, incontinentia pigmenti is an X-linked dominant condition characterized by spattered pigmentation on the trunk, preceded by vesicular and verrucous changes. It appears in girls during the first weeks after birth (Fig. 27-1). Most lesions are evident by the time the infant is 4–6 weeks old. A vesicular phase is present in 87% of cases. This first stage begins in most individuals before 6 weeks of age and is replaced by verrucous lesions after several weeks to months in two-thirds of patients. Although these usually resolve by 1 year of age, lesions may persist for many years. In the third, or pigmentary, phase, pigmented macules in streaks, sprays, splatters, and whorls follow the lines of Blaschko. The pigmentary stage may last

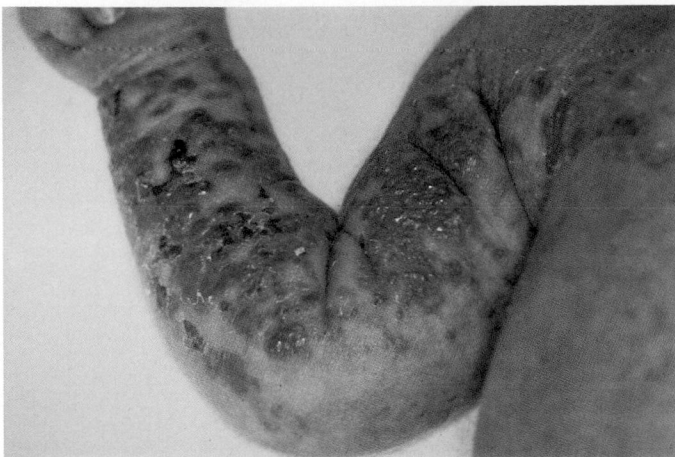

Fig. 27-1 Early incontinentia pigmenti.

for many years and then fade away, leaving no sequelae. A fourth stage may be seen in some adult women, manifesting subtle, faint, hypochromic or atrophic linear lesions, most commonly on the extremities.

Histologically, the vesicular stage is characterized by spongiosis with eosinophils. As the lesions mature, clusters of dyskeratotic cells appear within the epidermis. Dyskeratotic cells predominate in the verrucous stage, and pigmented incontinence (dermal melanophages) predominates in hyperpigmented lesions.

Other cutaneous changes include patchy alopecia at the vertex of the scalp, atrophic changes simulating acrodermatitis chronica atrophicans on the hands, onychodystrophy, subungual tumors with underlying lytic bone lesions, and palmoplantar hyperhidrosis. Extracutaneous manifestations occur in 70–90% of patients. Most commonly involved are the teeth (up to 90%), bones (40%), central nervous system (CNS) (33%), and eyes (35%). Immune dysfunction with defective neutrophil chemotaxis and elevated IgE has been reported. Eosinophilia is common. Incontinentia pigmenti is an important cause of neonatal seizures and encephalopathy.

Dental abnormalities usually manifest by the time the individual is 2 years old. Dental defects include delayed eruption, partial anodontia (43%), microdontia, and cone- or peg-shaped teeth (30%). The most common CNS findings are seizures (13%), mental retardation (12%), spastic paralysis (11%), microcephaly, destructive encephalopathy, and motor retardation. The eye changes include strabismus, cataracts, retinal detachments, optic atrophy, blue sclerae, and exudative chorioretinitis. Skeletal abnormalities include syndactyly, skull deformities, dwarfism, spina bifida, club foot, supernumerary ribs, hemiatrophy, and shortening of the legs and arms.

Incontinentia pigmenti is caused by a mutation in the *NEMO* gene on the X chromosome, localized to Xq28. The gene is generally lethal in male fetuses, although males with Klinefelter syndrome (47,XXY) may survive. Mosaicism may also account for some cases in males. *NEMO* mutations also cause X-linked ectodermal dysplasia with immunodeficiency, characterized by alopecia, hypohidrosis, dental anomalies, and defects in humoral immunity.

Incontinentia pigmenti achromians differs in that it is a negative image, with hypopigmentation (see below). It has autosomal-dominant inheritance, no vesicular or verrucous stages, and a higher incidence of CNS abnormalities. Patients with linear and whorled nevoid hypermelanosis lack the vesicular and verrucous phases.

There is no treatment for incontinentia pigmenti. Use of ruby lasers to treat pigmented lesions in infants and young children is not necessary and may worsen the condition.

Usually, the end stage of streaks of incontinentia pigmenti starts to fade at age 2, and by adulthood there may be little residual pigmentation.

Naegeli–Franceschetti–Jadassohn syndrome

Also known as the chromatophore nevus of Naegeli, Naegeli–Franceschetti–Jadassohn syndrome differs from incontinentia pigmenti in that the pigmentation is reticular and there are no preceding inflammatory changes, vesiculation, or verrucous lesions. Vasomotor changes and hypohidrosis are present. There is reticulate pigmentation involving the neck, flexural skin, and perioral and periorbital areas. Diffuse keratoderma and punctiform accentuation of the palms and soles may occur. Dermatoglyphics are abnormal, producing atrophic or absent ridges on fingerprints. Congenital malalignment of the great toenails may be found. Dental abnormalities are common and many patients are edentulous. Both sexes are equally affected, and the syndrome appears to be transmitted as an autosomal-dominant trait related to mutations in keratin 14, causing increased susceptibility to tumor necrosis factor (TNF)-α-induced apoptosis. The syndrome is allelic to dermatopathia pigmentosa reticularis.

Chang TT, et al: A male infant with anhidrotic ectodermal dysplasia/immunodeficiency accompanied by incontinentia pigmenti and a mutation in the *NEMO* pathway. J Am Acad Dermatol 2008 Feb; 58(2):316–320.

Ehrenreich M, et al: Incontinentia pigmenti (Bloch–Sulzberger syndrome): a systemic disorder. Cutis 2007 May; 79(5):355–362.

Fusco F, et al: Clinical diagnosis of incontinentia pigmenti in a cohort of male patients. J Am Acad Dermatol 2007 Feb; 56(2):264–267.

Lee JH, et al: Serial changes in white matter lesions in a neonate with incontinentia pigmenti. Childs Nerv Syst 2008 Apr; 24(4):525–528.

Loh NR, et al: A genetic cause for neonatal encephalopathy: incontinentia pigmenti with *NEMO* mutation. Acta Paediatr 2008 Mar; 97(3):379–381.

Lugassy J, et al: KRT14 haploinsufficiency results in increased susceptibility of keratinocytes to TNF-alpha-induced apoptosis and causes Naegeli–Franceschetti–Jadassohn syndrome. J Invest Dermatol 2008 Jun; 128(6):1517 1524.

Mancini AJ, et al: X-linked ectodermal dysplasia with immunodeficiency caused by *NEMO* mutation: early recognition and diagnosis. Arch Dermatol 2008 Mar; 144(3):342–346.

Pacheco TR, et al: Incontinentia pigmenti in male patients. J Am Acad Dermatol 2006 Aug; 55(2):251–255.

Incontinentia pigmenti achromians (hypomelanosis of Ito)

Incontinentia pigmenti achromians (IPA) is characterized by various patterns of bilateral or unilateral hypopigmentation following the lines of Blaschko (Fig. 27-2). The lesions suggest the "negative image" of incontinentia pigmenti and usually develop by the first year of life. The female to male ratio is about 2.5:1. Three-quarters of affected individuals have associated anomalies of the CNS, eyes, hair, teeth, skin, nails, musculoskeletal system, or internal organs, including polycystic kidney disease. Patients may manifest psychomotor or mental retardation, autism, microcephaly, coarse facies, and dysmorphic ears. Some patients have had associated Sturge–Weber syndrome-like leptomeningeal angiomatosis.

More than half of these patients have chromosomal abnormalities, with most demonstrating mosaicism for aneuploidy or unbalanced translocations. Several patients have demonstrated trisomy 13 mosaicism. No inflammatory changes or vesiculation are found before the development of the hypopigmentation. There is no treatment, but eventual repigmentation is the rule.

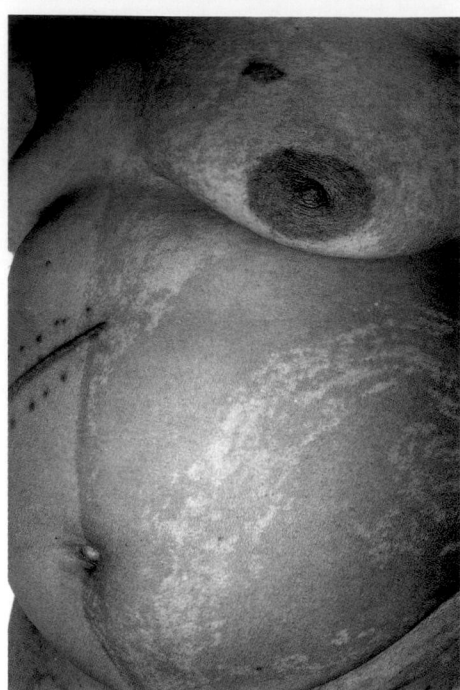

Fig. 27-2 Incontinentia pigmenti achromians.

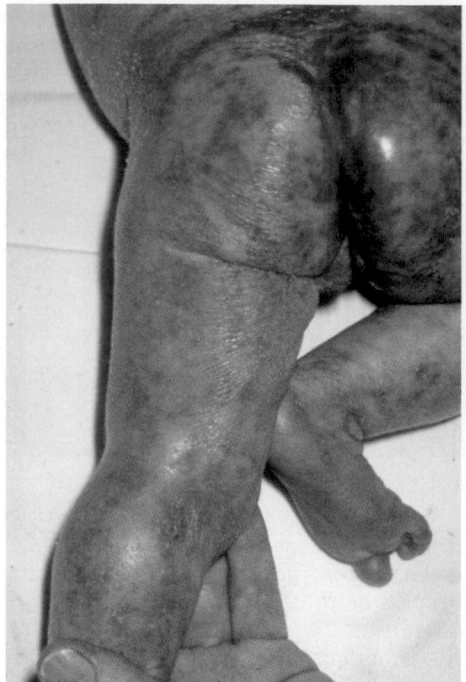

Fig. 27-3 Chondrodysplasia punctata.

Vergine G, et al: Glomerulocystic kidney disease in hypomelanosis of Ito. Pediatr Nephrol 2008 Jul; 23(7):1183–1187.

Linear and whorled nevoid hypermelanosis

This disorder of pigmentation develops within a few weeks of birth and progresses for 1–2 years before stabilizing. There is linear and whorled hyperpigmentation following the lines of Blaschko without preceding bullae or verrucous lesions. Sparing of mucous membranes, eyes, palms, and soles is noted. Congenital anomalies, such as mental retardation, cerebral palsy, atrial septal defects, dextrocardia, auricular atresia, and patent ductus arteriosus may be present. Bilateral giant cerebral aneurysms have been reported. There is no sexual predilection. Biopsy of pigmented areas demonstrates increased pigmentation of the basal layer and prominence of melanocytes without incontinence of pigment.

Most cases appear to be sporadic, although familial cases have been reported. Sporadic forms have been attributed to mosaicism. Because of confusion with other pigmented disorders, such as incontinentia pigmenti, early linear epidermal nevi, hypomelanosis of Ito, and nevus depigmentosus, it is likely that linear and whorled nevoid hypermelanosis may be more common than previously appreciated.

Di Lernia V: Linear and whorled hypermelanosis. Pediatr Dermatol 2007 May–Jun; 24(3):205–210.
Lu Y, et al: Linear and whorled nevoid hypermelanosis complicated with inflammatory linear verrucous epidermal nevus and ichthyosis vulgaris. J Dermatol 2007 Nov; 34(11):765–768.
Yuksek J, et al: Linear and whorled nevoid hypermelanosis. Dermatol Online J 2007 Jul 13; 13(3):23.

Chondrodysplasia punctata

A variant of the original Conradi–Hünermann syndrome or chondrodystrophia calcificans congenita, chondrodysplasia punctata is characterized by ichthyosis of the skin similar to that of the collodion baby, followed by hyperkeratotic "whirl and swirl" patterns on erythematous skin. In addition to reddening, the waxy, shiny skin (Fig. 27-3) has hyperkeratotic scales of a peculiar crushed eggshell configuration. As the child grows, follicular atrophoderma and pseudopelade develop. Usually, the ichthyosis clears within the first year of life but may leave behind hyperpigmentation similar to that seen in incontinentia pigmenti. An additional feature is minor nail defects, such as platonychia and onychoschizia.

There are four forms of chondrodysplasia punctata, which are classified by their inheritance patterns. The Conradi–Hünermann type is associated with autosomal-dominant inheritance, facial dysmorphia with a low nasal bridge, short stature, mild disease, cataracts, and few skin lesions. The rhizomelic form has autosomal-recessive inheritance, marked shortening of the extremities, cataracts, ichthyosis, and nasal hypoplasia; the patient dies in infancy. The X-linked recessive type has been described as part of contiguous gene deletion syndromes, with short stature, telebrachydactyly, and nasal hypoplasia. The X-linked dominant form (Happle syndrome, Conradi–Hünermann–Happle syndrome, or CDPX2) is lethal in males. Happle syndrome (X-linked dominant chondrodysplasia punctata) has ichthyosiform erythroderma along the lines of Blaschko, cataracts, asymmetrical limb shortening, and calcified stippling of the epiphyses of long bones. Follicular atrophoderma replaces the erythroderma after the first year.

The skeletal defects revealed on radiographic evaluation include irregular calcified stippling of the cartilaginous epiphyses in the long bones, costal cartilages, and vertebral diaphysis. The stippling occurs in the fetus and persists until age 3 or 4. The humeri and femurs may be shortened and there may be joint dysplasia. Histologic evaluation of the ichthyotic lesions reveals a thinned, granular cell layer, calcification of keratotic follicular plugs, and focal hyperpigmentation of basal keratinocytes. The keratotic follicular plugs and calcium deposits are characteristic of this disease and very helpful in establishing the diagnosis in newborns. Various types are related to defects in peroxisomal metabolism, plasmalogen, and cholesterol biosynthesis. X-linked recessive chondrodysplasia punctata (CDPX1) is due to a defect in arylsulfatase E, located on Xp22.3. There may be an association between the rhizomelic variety and maternal autoimmunity and connective tissue disease.

Ausavarat S, et al: Two novel EBP mutations in Conradi–Hünermann–Happle syndrome. Eur J Dermatol 2008 Jul–Aug; 18(4):391–393.

Nino M, et al: Clinical and molecular analysis of arylsulfatase E in patients with brachytelephalangic chondrodysplasia punctata. Am J Med Genet A 2008 Apr 15; 146A(8):997–1008.

Pazzaglia UE, et al: The nature of cartilage stippling in chondrodysplasia punctata: histopathological study of Conradi-Hünermann syndrome. Fetal Pediatr Pathol 2008 Aug; 27(2):71–81.

Shanske AL, et al: Chondrodysplasia punctata and maternal autoimmune disease: a new case and review of the literature. Pediatrics 2007 Aug; 120(2):e436–441.

Klinefelter syndrome

Klinefelter syndrome, the most common sex chromosome disorder, consists of hypogonadism, gynecomastia, eunuchoidism, small or absent testicles, and elevated gonadotropins. There may be a low frontal hairline, sparse body hair with only a few hairs in the axillary and pubic areas, scanty or absent facial hair in men, and shortening of the fifth digit of both hands.

Thrombophlebitis and recurrent or chronic leg ulcerations may be a presenting manifestation; these may be more common than previously reported. The cause of the hypercoagulable state is believed to be an increase in plasminogen activator inhibitor-1 levels. Patients are at an increased risk of a variety of cancers, especially male breast cancer, hematologic malignancies, and sarcomas (retinoblastoma and rhabdomyosarcoma).

Many of these patients are tall; some are obese. Dull mentality or misbehavior is frequent, and psychiatric disorders occur in about one-third of these patients. Klinefelter syndrome is most frequently associated with an XXY sex chromosome pattern, although other variations occur as the number of X chromosomes increases. Marked improvement in appearance has been achieved by the injection of testosterone.

XXYY genotype

The XXYY genotype is considered to be a variant of Klinefelter syndrome. In addition to the changes seen in Klinefelter, there are vascular changes, such as cutaneous angiomas, acrocyanosis, and peripheral vascular disease leading to stasis dermatitis. Hypertelorism, clinodactyly, pes planus, and dental abnormalities are common. Systemic manifestations include asthma, cardiac defects, radioulnar synostosis, inguinal hernia, cryptorchidism, CNS defects, attention deficit disorder, autism, and seizures.

Paduch DA, et al: New concepts in Klinefelter syndrome. Curr Opin Urol 2008 Nov; 18(6):621–627.

Tartaglia N, et al: A new look at XXYY syndrome: medical and psychological features. Am J Med Genet A 2008 Jun 15; 146A(12):1509–1522.

Turner syndrome

Turner syndrome, also known as gonadal dysgenesis, is characterized by a webbed neck, low posterior hairline margin, increased carrying angle at the elbow (cubitus valgus), congenital lymphedema, and a triangular mouth. Patients may demonstrate alopecia of the frontal area on the scalp, koilonychia, cutis laxa, cutis hyperelastica, mental retardation, short stature, infantilism, retarded sexual development, primary amenorrhea, numerous melanocytic nevi, and an increased risk of melanoma, pilomatricoma, and thyroid disease. Coarctation of the aorta is frequently found. There may be an increased incidence of alopecia areata and halo nevi in these patients.

Patients with Turner syndrome have only 45 chromosomes rather than the normal 46. An X chromosome is missing, resulting in an XO genotype. Mosaicism, structural abnormalities of the X chromosome, or a partial deficiency of one sex chromosome may account for a number of the variations in gonadal dysgenesis. Several genetic loci have been implicated, including the short stature homeobox gene. Loss of long-arm material (Xq) can result in short stature and ovarian failure, but deletions distal to Xq21 do not appear to affect stature. Loss of the short arm (Xp) produces the full phenotype. Very distal Xp deletions usually have normal ovarian function. No specific treatment is available. Growth hormone (hGH) has been used to treat the short stature. A review of the Cochrane Central Register of Controlled Trials determined that hGH increases short-term growth, but there are few data regarding its effects on final height.

Loscalzo ML: Turner syndrome. Pediatr Rev 2008 Jul; 29(7):219–227.

Wood S, et al: Pilomatricomas in Turner syndrome. Pediatr Dermatol 2008 Jul–Aug; 25(4):449–451.

Noonan syndrome

Noonan syndrome is an autosomal-dominant disease with a webbed neck that mimics Turner syndrome. Males and females are equally affected, and the chromosome number is normal. The major features are a characteristic facies with hypertelorism, prominent ears, webbed neck, short stature, undescended testicles, low posterior neck hairline, cardiovascular abnormalities (pulmonary stenosis and hypertrophic cardiomyopathy), and cubitus valgus. Some 25–40% of patients have dermatologic findings: lymphedema; short, curly hair; dystrophic nails; a tendency toward keloid formation; soft, elastic skin; keratosis pilaris atrophicans (ulerythema of the eyebrows); and abnormal dermatoglyphics. The Noonan syndrome gene, PTPN11, encodes the nonreceptor protein tyrosine phosphatase SHP-2 involved in the RasMAPK (Ras-mitogen-activated protein kinase) pathway. Growth hormone can help patients achieve more normal stature.

Multiple lentigines (LEOPARD) syndrome

The LEOPARD (multiple lentigines, electrocardiographic conduction abnormalities, ocular hypertelorism, pulmonary stenosis, abnormal genitalia, retardation of growth, and sensorineural deafness) syndrome is also known as the multiple lentigines syndrome, Gorlin syndrome II, cardio-cutaneous syndrome, lentiginosis profusa syndrome, or progressive cardiomyopathic lentiginosis. The lentigines are small, dark brown, polygonal, and irregularly shaped macules, usually measuring 2–5 mm in diameter. Individual lesions may be larger, even up to 1–1.5 cm. Melanoma has been described in these patients, so atypical lesions should be biopsied.

LEOPARD syndrome shares many clinical features with Noonan syndrome. They are allelic disorders, as patients with both syndromes demonstrate mutations in the Noonan syndrome gene, PTPN11. Although the "R" in LEOPARD stands for growth retardation, some individuals with the syndrome also exhibit mild mental retardation or speech difficulties. Many cases appear sporadically; however, inheritance as an autosomal-dominant genetic trait has also been reported.

Allanson JE: Noonan syndrome. Am J Med Genet C Semin Med Genet 2007 Aug 15; 145C(3):274–279.

Aoki Y, et al: The RAS/MAPK syndromes: novel roles of the RAS pathway in human genetic disorders. Hum Mutat 2008 Aug; 29(8):992–1006.

Noordam K: Expanding the genetic spectrum of Noonan syndrome. Horm Res 2007; 68(Suppl 5):24–27.

Sarkozy A, et al: LEOPARD syndrome. Orphanet J Rare Dis 2008 May 27; 3:13.

Seishima M, et al: Malignant melanoma in a woman with LEOPARD syndrome: identification of a germline *PTPN11* mutation and a somatic *BRAF* mutation. Br J Dermatol 2007 Dec; 157(6):1297–1299.

Cardio-facio-cutaneous syndrome

Cardio-facio-cutaneous syndrome is a congenital condition manifested by numerous anomalies. Typical features include a characteristic craniofacial appearance, psychomotor and growth retardation, congenital cardiac defects, and skin and hair abnormalities. The most frequent dermatologic findings involve the hair, which may be sparse, curly, fine or thick, woolly or brittle. In more than half of the reported cases, the patient has dry, scaly, or "hyperkeratotic," ichthyotic skin.

Other cutaneous findings include sparse or absent eyebrows and eyelashes, low posterior hairline, patchy alopecia, scant body hair, follicular hyperkeratosis, keratosis pilaris, keratosis pilaris atrophicans faciei, palmoplantar keratoderma, seborrheic dermatitis, eczema, lymphedema, hemangiomas, café-au-lait spots, pigmented nevi, hyperpigmented macules or stripes, cutis marmorata, and sacral dimples. Nail dystrophy, koilonychia, and dysplastic teeth have also been reported. The syndrome is associated with *KRAS*, *BRAF* and *MAP2K1/2* mutations.

The differential diagnosis includes Noonan syndrome, Turner syndrome, Pallister–Killian mosaic aneuploid syndrome (mosaic tetrasomy 12p/trisomy 12p), and Costello syndrome. The difficulty often arises in assessing the facial features, which are similar in all of these syndromes. Exclusion of *PTPN11* mutations in cardio-facio-cutaneous syndrome and Costello syndrome confirms distinct genetic etiologies. Deletion of the long arm of chromosome 12, del(12)(q21.2q22), has been associated with cardio-facio-cutaneous syndrome.

Rodriguez-Viciana P, et al: Biochemical characterization of novel germline *BRAF* and *MEK* mutations in cardio-facio-cutaneous syndrome. Methods Enzymol 2008; 438:277–289.

PHAKOMATOSES

The phakomatoses are the various inherited disorders of the CNS that have congenital retinal tumors and cutaneous involvement. They include tuberous sclerosis, von Recklinghausen's disease (neurofibromatosis), von Hippel–Lindau disease (angiomatosis retinae), ataxia-telangiectasia, nevoid basal cell carcinoma syndrome, nevus sebaceus, and Sturge–Weber syndrome.

Tuberous sclerosis (epiloia, Bourneville disease)

Tuberous sclerosis, described by Desiree-Magloire Bourneville in 1880, is also called epiloia (epi = epilepsy, loi = low intelligence, a = adenoma sebaceum). This classic triad of adenoma sebaceum (Fig. 27-4), mental deficiency, and epilepsy, however, is present in only a minority of patients. Other associated features include periungual fibromas, shagreen plaques (collagenoma), oral papillomatosis (Fig. 27-5), gingival hyperplasia, ash-leaf hypomelanotic macules (Fig. 27-6), skin fibromas, and café-au-lait spots.

Adenoma sebaceum (angiofibromas) are 1–3 mm, yellowish-red, translucent, discrete, waxy papules that are distributed symmetrically, principally over the cheeks, nose, and forehead. They have also been reported in patients with multiple endocrine neoplasia (MEN) 1 and the Birt–Hogg–Dube syndrome. These lesions are present in 90% of patients older than 4 years of age, persist indefinitely, and may increase in number.

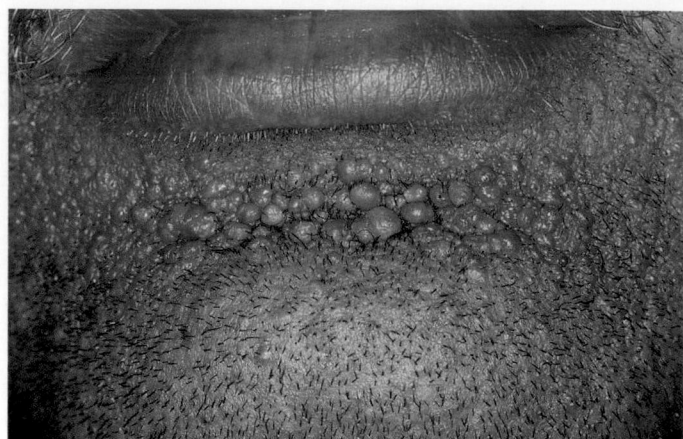

Fig. 27-4 Angiofibromas (adenoma sebaceum).

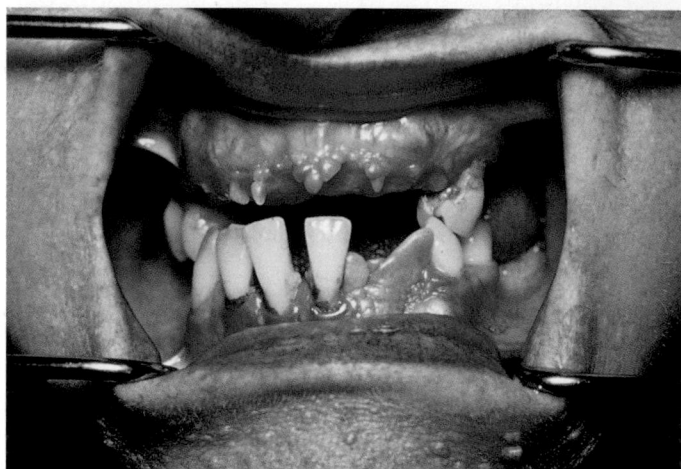

Fig. 27-5 Oral papillomas in tuberous sclerosis.

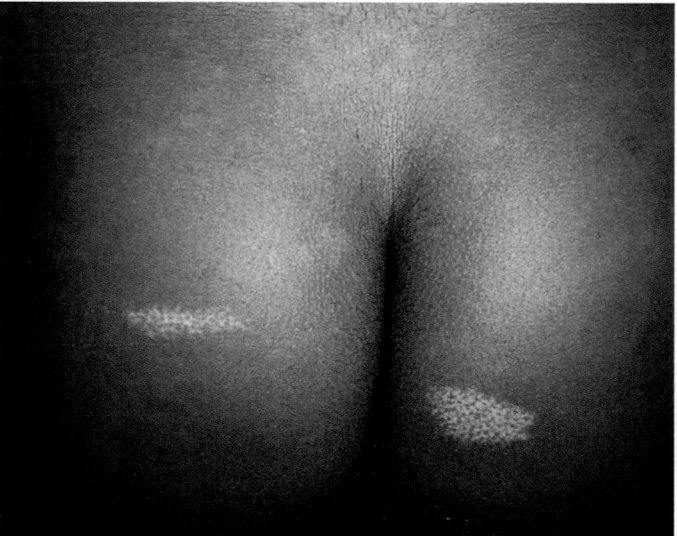

Fig. 27-6 Ash-leaf macules.

Shagreen plaque is named after a type of leather tanned to produce knobs on the surface, resembling shark skin. Patches of this type of "knobby" skin, varying from 1 to 8 cm in diameter, are found on the trunk, most commonly on the lumbosacral area. They are connective tissue nevi composed almost exclusively of collagen, occur in 40% of patients, and develop in the first decade of life.

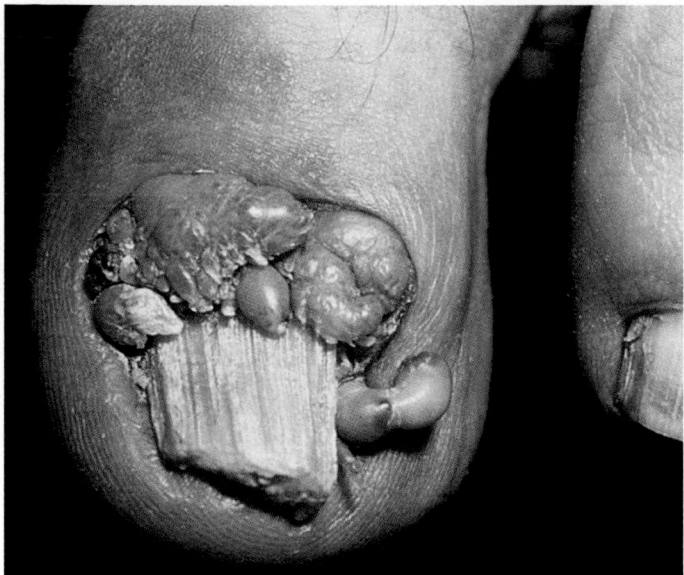

Fig. 27-7 Periungual fibromas.

Koenen tumors (periungual angiofibromas) (Fig. 27-7) occur in 50% of patients. The tumors are small, digitate, protruding, asymptomatic, and periungual and/or subungual. They have their onset at puberty. Similar lesions may occur on the gingiva. Nails may also demonstrate longitudinal groves, long leukonychia and short red streaks.

Congenital white leaf-shaped macules, called hypomelanotic macules, are found in 85% of patients with tuberous sclerosis, their number ranging from 1 to 100. Occasional patients may not develop them until they are 6–8 years of age. They may be shaped like an ash leaf, but linear and confetti-type white macules may also be present. Wood's light examination should be performed when evaluating a patient for tuberous sclerosis. Focal poliosis (localized tufts of white hair) may be present at birth. Solitary ash-leaf macules are not uncommon in the general population and may be confused with other hypopigmented macules, such as nevus depigmentosus.

Mental deficiency, usually appreciated early in life, is present in 40–60% of patients, varying widely in its manifestations. Epilepsy also occurs, is variable in its severity, and usually also presents early in life. Between 80 and 90% of patients have seizures or nonspecific electroencephalographic abnormalities. Hamartomatous proliferations of glial and neuronal tissue produce potato-like nodules in the cortex. X-ray evaluation will reveal these once they are calcified, but computed tomographic (CT) scans, cranial ultrasonography, and magnetic resonance imaging (MRI) may define these lesions as early as 6 weeks of age, and thus are useful in making an early diagnosis. These brain tumors may progress to gliomas. Subependymal nodules (candle drippings) are similar lesions in the ventricular walls. Astrocytomas may also occur. Forehead plaques may be a marker for more serious intracranial involvement.

Retinal tumors (phakomas) occur, which are optic nerve or retinal nerve hamartomas. Various ophthalmologic findings, such as pigmentary changes, nystagmus, and angioid streaks, occur in 50% of patients. Renal hamartomas (angiomyolipomas [45%], cystic disease [18%], fibroadenomas, or mixed tumors) and cardiac tumors (rhabdomyomas [43%]) may also occur. In the familial variety of tuberous sclerosis, 80% of patients have angiomyolipomas, which are often bilateral and frequently cause renal failure. Women of childbearing age may present with pulmonary lymphangioleiomyomatosis with progressive respiratory failure or spontaneous pneumothorax. The condition is characterized by diffuse proliferation of smooth muscle cells and cystic degeneration of the pulmonary parenchyma, and relates to the perivascular epithelioid cells ("PEC" cells) implicated in various PEComas. Nearly half of patients with epiloia have bony abnormalities such as bone cysts and sclerosis, which can be seen on x-ray evaluation. Five or more pits in the enamel of permanent teeth are a marker for this disease.

Tuberous sclerosis is a common inherited autosomal-dominant disease with highly variable penetrance. Prevalence estimates range from 1 in 5800 to 1 in 15000. Up to 50% of cases may occur as a result of spontaneous mutations. There are two genes, the mutations of which produce indistinguishable phenotypes—9q34 (*TSC1*) and 16p13.3 (*TSC2*). *TSC1* and *TSC2* are tumor suppressor genes. *TSC2* encodes for tuberin, a putative GTPase-activating protein for rap1 and rab5. *TSC1* encodes for hamartin, a novel protein with no significant homology to tuberin or any other vertebrate protein. Hamartin and tuberin associate physically in vivo, suggesting that they function in the same complex rather than in separate pathways. This interaction of tuberin and hamartin explains the indistinguishable phenotypes caused by mutations in either gene. Hamartomas frequently demonstrate loss of the remaining normal allele (loss of heterozygosity).

Diagnosis

The ash-leaf macules are usually present at birth and are most easily seen with a Wood's light. If x-ray examination fails to show calcified intracranial nodules, ultrasonography, a CT scan, or MRI should be performed. Fundoscopic examination, hand and foot x-ray evaluation, and renal ultrasonography are often rewarding in a patient with few clinical findings, as up to 31% of asymptomatic parents have been identified using these tests.

Multiple periungual fibromas are highly correlated with the syndrome, but solitary fibromas may occur in unaffected individuals. Molecular analysis for *TSC1* and *TSC2* may be the only way to identify "mildly affected" individuals.

Treatment

Adenoma sebaceum can be treated by shaving, dermabrasion, or laser therapy. Lesions are likely to recur, requiring repeat treatment. Cranial irradiation of astrocytomas should be avoided because this may result in the subsequent development of glioblastomas. Topical and systemic rapamycin shows some promise for prevention of tumor growth, and is effective in models of the disease.

Aldrich SL, et al: Acral lesions in tuberous sclerosis complex: insights into pathogenesis. J Am Acad Dermatol 2010; 63:244–251.

Curatolo P, et al: Tuberous sclerosis. Lancet 2008 Aug 23; 372(9639):657–668.

Datta AN, et al: Clinical presentation and diagnosis of tuberous sclerosis complex in infancy. J Child Neurol 2008 Mar; 23(3): 268–273.

Korol UB, et al: Gingival enlargement as a manifestation of tuberous sclerosis: case report and periodontal management. J Periodontol 2008 Apr; 79(4):759–763.

Rama Rao GR, et al: Forehead plaque: a cutaneous marker of CNS involvement in tuberous sclerosis. Indian J Dermatol Venereol Leprol 2008 Jan–Feb; 74(1):28–31.

Rauktys A, et al: Topical rapamycin inhibits tuberous sclerosis tumor growth in a nude mouse model. BMC Dermatol 2008 Jan 28; 8:1.

Neurofibromatosis (von Recklinghausen's disease)

Neurofibromatosis is an autosomal-dominantly inherited syndrome manifested by developmental changes in the nervous system, bones, and skin. In type 1 neurofibromatosis (NF-1, von Recklinghausen's disease), which includes more than 85% of cases, patients have many neurofibromas (Fig. 27-8), café-au-lait spots, axillary freckles (Fig. 27-9), giant pigmented hairy nevi, sacral hypertrichosis, cutis verticis gyrata, and macroglossia. Neurofibromas of the areolae occur in more than 90% of women with this disease. Lisch nodules are found in the irides of about one-quarter of patients under 6 years of age and in 94% of adult patients. Type 2 neurofibromatosis, central or acoustic neurofibromatosis, is distinguished by bilateral acoustic neuromas, usually in the absence of cutaneous lesions, although neurofibromas and schwannomas may occur. Type 3 (mixed) and 4 (variant) forms resemble type 2 but have cutaneous neurofibromas. Patients with these types are at greater risk for developing optic gliomas, neurilemmomas, and meningiomas. These forms are inherited as autosomal-dominant traits. Segmental neurofibromatosis (Fig. 27-10) may arise from postzygotic somatic mutation or LOH.

Neurofibromas are soft tumors that can be pushed down into the panniculus by light pressure with the finger ("buttonholing") and spring back when released. Histologically, they are well circumscribed, but rarely encapsulated, spindle cell proliferations with a mucinous background and many mast cells. The spindle cells have a wavy appearance. Neurofibromas occur as a result of proliferation of all supporting elements of the nerve fibers. The proliferation is composed of Schwann cells, perineurial cells, endoneurial cells, mast cells, and blood vessels. Axon stains demonstrate individual axons spread randomly throughout the tumor.

Subcutaneous plexiform neurofibromas are virtually pathognomonic of NF-1 and may be a manifestation of LOH. They occur as large nodules containing multiple encapsulated neurofibromas. The overlying skin is usually hyperpigmented (Fig. 27-11). On palpation, they resemble a "bag of worms."

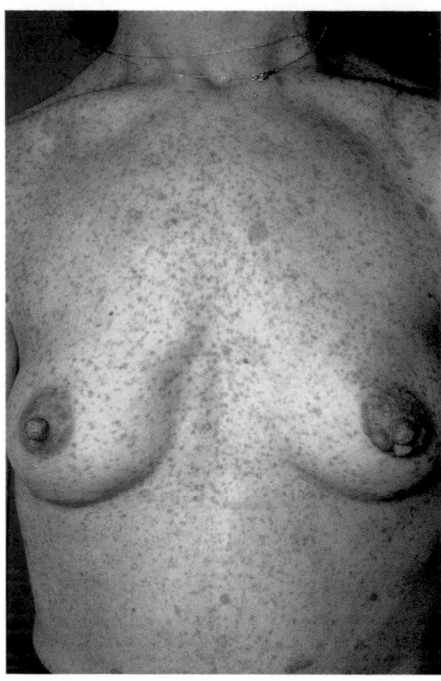

Fig. 27-8 Neurofibromatosis type 1.

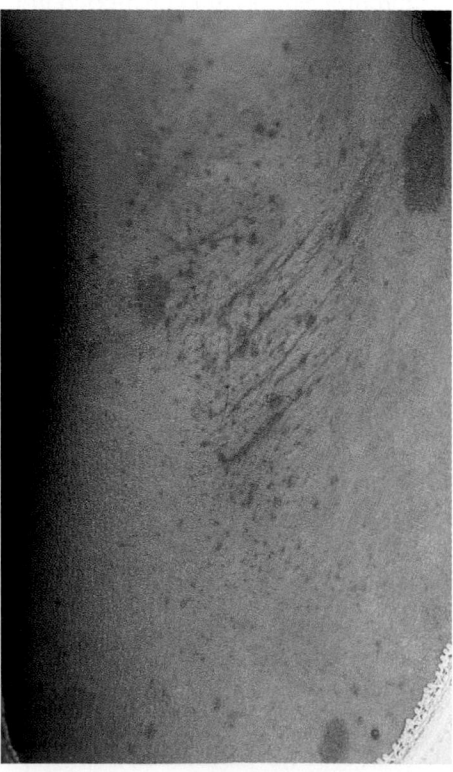

Fig. 27-9 Axillary freckling.

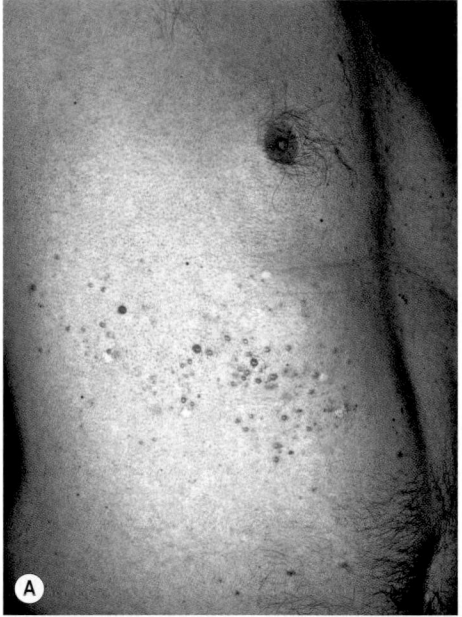

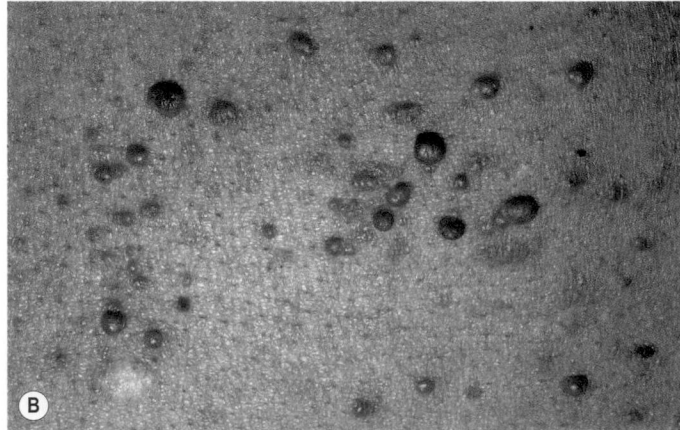

Fig. 27-10 A and B, Segmental neurofibromatosis.

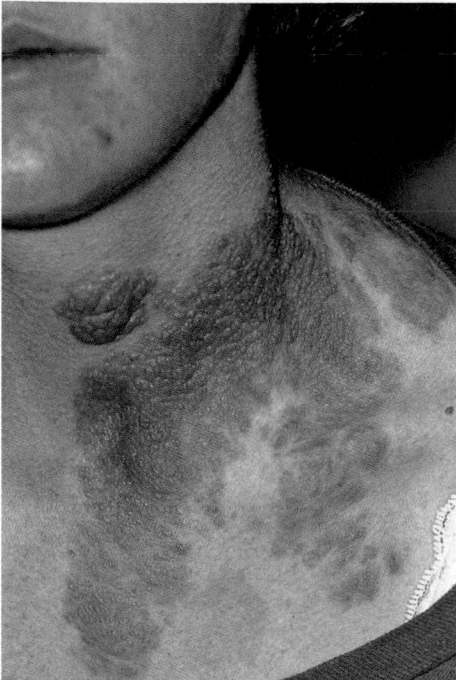

Fig. 27-11 Segmental neurofibromatosis.

Histologically, they demonstrate numerous elongated encapsulated neurofibromas, often embedded in diffuse neurofibroma that involves the dermis and subcutaneous fat.

The café-au-lait macule is a uniformly pigmented, smooth-edged, light brown macule. Most often, these macules are present at birth and almost always present by the time the patient is 1 year of age. The finding of six or more of these lesions measuring at least 1.5 cm in diameter is diagnostic, usually indicating NF-1. In children, the minimum diameter for a significant lesion is 0.5 cm. Histologically, basilar hyperpigmentation is noted and giant melanosomes may be seen. Axillary freckling (Crowe's sign) may occur, extending to the neck and involving the inguinal, genital, and perineal areas.

Many organ systems may be involved. Acromegaly, cretinism, hyperparathyroidism, myxedema, pheochromocytoma (<1%), or precocious puberty may be present. Bone changes (usually erosive) may produce lordosis, kyphosis, and pseudoarthrosis, as well as spina bifida, dislocations, and atraumatic fractures. Neuromas of spinal nerves may cause various paralyses. Patients with NF-1 are four times more likely to develop malignancies than the general population. Cutaneous neurofibromas rarely develop into neurofibrosarcomas (malignant schwannomas), but a growing or hardening lesion is an indication for biopsy. Wilms tumor, rhabdomyosarcomas, gastrointestinal malignancies, and chronic myelogenous leukemia have also been reported. Xanthogranulomas are associated with a higher incidence of chronic myelogenous leukemia. Children with NF-1 are 200–500 times more likely to develop malignant myeloid disorders than age-matched controls.

Mental retardation, dementia, epilepsy, and a variety of intracranial malignancies may occur. Hypertelorism heralds a severe expression of neurofibromatosis with brain involvement. Diffuse interstitial lung disease occurs in 7% of patients.

Approximately 50% of cases of NF-1 represent new mutations. The gene for NF-1 is in the pericentric region of chromosome 17q11.2 and codes for neurofibromin, a protein that negatively regulates signals transduced by Ras proteins. The gene for NF-2 is on the long arm of chromosome 22q11–q13 and encodes for merlin (schwannomin), a protein that links the actin cytoskeleton to cell-surface glycoproteins and functions as a negative growth regulator. Germline loss-of-function mutations in the *SPRED1* gene have been associated with an NF-1-like phenotype with pigmentary changes but no neurofibromas (Legius syndrome).

Diagnosis

The diagnosis of NF-1 requires two or more of the following criteria to be fulfilled:

1. six or more café-au-lait macules with a greatest diameter of more than 5 mm in prepubertal individuals, and a greatest diameter of more than 15 mm in postpubertal individuals
2. two or more neurofibromas of any type or one plexiform neurofibroma
3. freckling in the axillary or inguinal regions
4. optic gliomas
5. two or more Lisch nodules
6. a distinctive osseous lesion, such as a sphenoid dysplasia or thinning of the long bone cortex with or without pseudarthrosis
7. a first-degree relative (parent, sibling, or offspring) with the disease.

A diagnosis of NF-2 requires either of the following:

1. bilateral eighth nerve masses, as demonstrated on CT or MRI
2. a first-degree relative with NF-2 and either unilateral eighth nerve mass or two of the following: a neurofibroma, meningioma, glioma, schwannoma, and juvenile posterior subcapsular lenticular opacity.

Screening and monitoring for complications

In one study of 93 asymptomatic patients with NF-1 who underwent cerebral imaging, 12 optic gliomas were detected, suggesting that screening MRI or CT scans may be of value. However, this is a single study and the results have not been validated by other authors. The National Institutes of Health (NIH) consensus panel concluded that studies should be dictated by findings on clinical evaluation. It concluded that laboratory tests in asymptomatic patients are unlikely to be of value. In the majority of patients with NF-1, imaging studies should only be performed as indicated by signs or symptoms. NF-2 patients, in contrast, often require imaging studies. Screening studies should include an audiogram and brainstem auditory evoked responses. MRI is the best imaging procedure for patients with evidence of hearing impairments or abnormal evoked responses. Tests of vestibular function may be useful, as eighth nerve tumors develop on the vestibular division. A screening MRI should be performed by puberty. Other tests should be performed as dictated by signs and symptoms. Pediatric patients with NF-2 have a worse prognosis, with 75% demonstrating hearing loss, 83% visual impairment, and 25% abnormal ambulation.

Brems H, et al: Germline loss-of-function mutations in *SPRED1* cause a neurofibromatosis 1-like phenotype. Nat Genet 2007 Sep; 39(9): 1120–1126.

Hersh JH, American Academy of Pediatrics Committee on Genetics: Health supervision for children with neurofibromatosis. Pediatrics 2008 Mar; 121(3):633–642.

Proteus syndrome

Although not a phakomatosis, Proteus syndrome may be confused with neurofibromatosis. This rare sporadic disease is named after the Greek god Proteus, who could change shape. The syndrome has protean manifestations that include partial

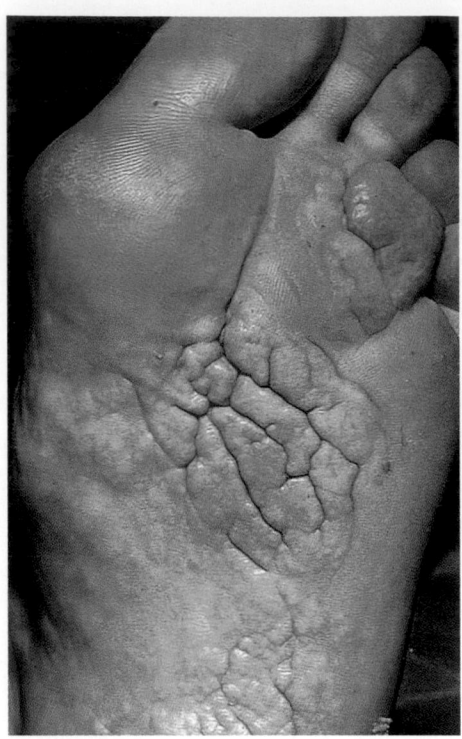

Fig. 27-12 Proteus syndrome. (Courtesy of Michelle Maroon, MD)

gigantism of the hands and feet, cerebriform plantar hyperplasia (Fig. 27-12), hemangiomas, lipomas, lipohypoplasia, linear verrucous epidermal nevi, patchy dermal hypoplasia, macrocephaly, hyperostosis, muscular hypoplasia, and hypertrophy of the long bones. Many investigators believe that Joseph Merrick, who was known as "the Elephant Man," had Proteus syndrome rather than neurofibromatosis. It is believed to be caused by a somatic mutation, lethal in the nonmosaic state. Those patients with a greater number of cutaneous lesions also have the most extracutaneous abnormalities. The findings of both overgrowth (pleioproteus component) and hypoplasia (elattoproteus component) in the same patient may be a manifestation of genetic twin spotting (didymosis), overexpression, and deficiency of a gene product. Linear lesions with PTEN mutations are now classified as segmental Cowden syndrome.

Happle R: The group of epidermal nevus syndromes. J Am Acad Dermatol 2010; 63:1–22.

Satter E: Proteus syndrome: 2 case reports and a review of the literature. Cutis 2007 Oct; 80(4):297–302.

Other Epidermal Nevus Syndromes

Important clues to the diagnosis of specific epidermal nevus syndromes include linear lesions with nevus sebaceus (NS) in Schimmelpenning syndrome, NS and papular nevus spilus in phacomatosis pigmentokeratotica, soft white hair in angora hair nevus syndrome (Schauder syndrome), breast hypoplasia in Becker nevus syndrome, mosaic R248 C mutation in fibroblast growth factor receptor 3 epidermal nevus (EN) syndrome (characterized by soft velvety EN and CNS abnormalities), and acral strawberry papillomatous lesions tips of fingers or toes in CHILD syndrome. Other EN syndromes include nevus trichilemmocysticus (cysts in blaschkoid distribution), didymosis aplasticosebacea (NS with aplasia cutis congenita), SCALP syndrome (NS, CNS malformations, aplasia cutis, limbal dermoid, and pigmented nevus), Gorbello syndrome (systematized linear velvety EN with bone defects, NEVADA syndrome (nevus epidermicus verrucosus with angiodyspla-

sia and aneurysms), and CLOVE syndrome (congenital lipomatous overgrowth, vascular malformations, and EN with non-progressive proportionate overgrowth).

Von Hippel–Lindau syndrome

Von Hippel–Lindau syndrome is an autosomal-dominant disorder consisting of retinal angiomas, cerebellar medullary angioblastic tumors, pancreatic cysts, and renal tumors and cysts. Usually the skin is not involved, although occasionally angiomas may occur in the occipitocervical region. The syndrome is associated with a germline mutation of a tumor suppressor gene on the short arm of chromosome 3.

Ten to 20% of cerebellar hemangioblastomas produce erythropoietin and are accompanied by a secondary polycythemia. Ocular lesions may lead to retinal detachment. Ten percent of hypernephromas and fewer than 8% of renal cysts also produce erythropoietin. Pheochromocytoma has been associated in several kindreds with von Hippel–Lindau disease.

Lonser RR, et al: von Hippel–Lindau disease. Lancet 2003; 361:2059.

Ataxia-telangiectasia

Also known as Louis–Bar syndrome, ataxia-telangiectasia consists of cerebellar ataxia, oculocutaneous telangiectasia, and sinopulmonary infection. It is familial and is usually first noted when the child begins to walk. There is awkwardness and a swaying gait, which results in the child needing to use a wheelchair by about 10 years of age. Choreic and athetoid movements and pseudopalsy of the eyes are other features. Fine telangiectases appear on the exposed surfaces of the conjunctiva at about age 3. Nystagmus is present. Telangiectases also appear later on the butterfly area of the face, inside the helix and over the backs of the ears, in the roof of the mouth, in the necklace area, in the flexures, and over the dorsa of the hands and feet. Other stigmata are café-au-lait patches, hypopigmented macules, seborrheic dermatitis, premature graying and sparsity of the hair, and progeroid features. The skin tends to be dry and coarse, and in time becomes tight and inelastic, as in scleroderma. Atrophic, granulomatous, scarring plaques may occur. Early death from bronchiectasis occurs in more than half of these patients, most of whom suffer from recurrent sinus and lung infections that begin when the patient is between 3 and 8 years of age.

Patients may have a marked IgA deficiency, with decreased lymphocytes and a small to absent thymus. The most common types of malignancy are lymphomas, usually of the B-cell type, and leukemias. It has been shown that homozygous patients also have a higher risk of breast cancer — 100 times higher than age-matched controls. Heterozygous carriers share the defective repair of radiation-induced damage, and there is a three- to five-fold higher risk for development of neoplasms, especially breast cancer, in heterozygotes under the age of 45. The ovaries and testicles do not develop normally. There is deficient thymus development, with absence of Hassall's corpuscles and a lack of T-helper cells. Suppressor T cells are normal. In 80% of cases, IgA is absent or deficient, in 75% absent or deficient IgE is seen, and in 50% IgG is very low.

Ataxia-telangiectasia is transmitted as an autosomal-recessive trait, and heterozygotes, although they lack clinical findings, are cancer-prone. The gene has been designated ATM (ataxia-telangiectasia mutated gene) and is a member of a family of phosphatidylinositol-3-kinase-like enzymes that are involved in cell-cycle control, meiotic recombination, telomere length monitoring, and DNA damage response. Affected cells are hypersensitive to ionizing radiation and are defective at the G1/S checkpoint after radiation damage. They are abnormally resistant to inhibition of DNA synthesis by ionizing radiation. The *ATM* gene is located on chromosome 11q22.3. Translocations are common in these patients, particularly for chromosomes 7 and 14. A high prevalence of *ATM* gene mutations has also been found in a diverse array of sporadic lymphoproliferative disorders.

Early diagnosis can be difficult and the most frequent misdiagnosis is cerebral palsy. Persistently elevated levels of α-fetoprotein and carcinoembryonic antigen occur. These may be useful in early diagnosis. In culture, ataxia-telangiectasia fibroblasts are three times more sensitive to killing by ionizing radiation, but not ultraviolet light. Evaluations for elevated α-fetoprotein and radiosensitivity of fibroblasts used to be the standard for diagnosis of this disorder, but immunoblotting the ATM protein expression is now possible.

Furtado S, et al: A review of the inherited ataxias: recent advances in genetic, clinical and neuropathologic aspects. Parkinsonism Relat Disord 1998 Dec; 4(4):161–169.

Lavin MF: Ataxia-telangiectasia: from a rare disorder to a paradigm for cell signalling and cancer. Nat Rev Mol Cell Biol 2008 Oct; 9(10):759–769.

Epidermolysis bullosa

Epidermolysis bullosa (EB) is a group of rare genetic disorders that have in common the formation of blisters in response to minor physical injury. Treatment consists of prevention of trauma, decompression of large blisters, and treatment of infection. EB acquisita is an autoimmune disease, discussed in Chapter 21. The inherited types of EB are classified as in Box 27-1.

Internal involvement may occur in several of these subtypes of EB. Esophageal and laryngeal complications are seen primarily in recessive dystrophic EB, but may be present in junctional EB (Herlitz). Pyloric atresia is reported to occur in junctional EB. Ocular lesions may be severe in dystrophic EB, and mild lesions have been reported in simplex and junctional disease.

Clinical findings and routine histologic features overlap, and accurate diagnosis depends on genetic mutation mapping, electron microscopic studies, or immunofluorescent mapping. The latter two can identify the level of the epidermal separation, and in addition may define other defects, such as absence of anchoring fibrils or hypoplasia of hemidesmosomes. In recessive dystrophic EB, electron microscopy reveals the cleavage is below the basal lamina and that anchoring fibrils are diminished or absent.

Immunofluorescent mapping may define the level of the split without resorting to electron microscopy. By staining biopsy specimens for normal components of the basement membrane zone, such as bullous pemphigoid antigen, laminin, type IV collagen, or LDA-1 antigen, the level of the split may be determined by whether the antigen localizes at the roof or base of the blister. In simplex types, all of these components will be at the base; in dystrophic types, all will be at the roof; and in junctional types, bullous pemphigoid antigen will be on the roof, while type IV collagen and LDA-1 will be at the base. KF-1 has been found to be absent or diminished in dystrophic EB. The specific keratin abnormalities along with the abnormal genes have been identified for many of these disorders. Many types of EB simplex are caused by defects in genes encoding for keratins 5 and 14. In junctional EB there are defective genes encoding for kallidin/laminin 5. Dystrophic forms result from mutations in type VII collagen gene *COL7A1*.

Intraepidermal forms

Epidermolysis bullosa simplex (Koebner)

The generalized type of EB simplex (EBS), dominantly inherited with complete penetrance, occurs in 1 in 500 000 births. It is characterized by the development of vesicles, bullae, and milia over the joints of the hands, elbows, knees, and feet (Fig. 27-13), and other sites subject to repeated trauma. The child is affected at birth or shortly thereafter, with improvement within the first few months, but with disease recurring when the child begins crawling or later in childhood. The blistering is worse during the summer and improves during the winter. The lesions are sparse and do not lead to severe atrophy. The

---

Box 27-1 Inherited types of epidermolysis bullosa (EB)

Intraepidermal
- EB simplex, generalized (Koebner)
- EB simplex, localized (Weber–Cockayne)
- EB herpetiformis (Dowling–Meara)
- EB simplex (Ogna)
- EB simplex with mottled pigmentation
- EB with muscular dystrophy

Junctional (intralamina lucida)
- Junction EB (JEB) atrophicans generalisata gravis (Herlitz, EB letalis)
- JEB atrophicans generalisata mitis
- JEB atrophicans localisata
- JEB atrophicans inversa
- JEB progressiva
- JEB with pyloric atresia
- Generalized atrophic benign EB (GABEB)
- Cicatricial junctional EB

Dermolytic or dystrophic (sublamina densa)
1. Dominant forms
   - Dystrophic EB, hyperplastic variant (Cockayne–Touraine)
   - Dystrophic EB, albopapuloid variant (Pasini)
   - Bart syndrome
   - Transient bullous dermolysis of the newborn
   - Acrokeratotic poikiloderma (Weary–Kindler)
2. Recessive forms
   - Generalized (gravis or mitis)
   - Localized
   - Inverse

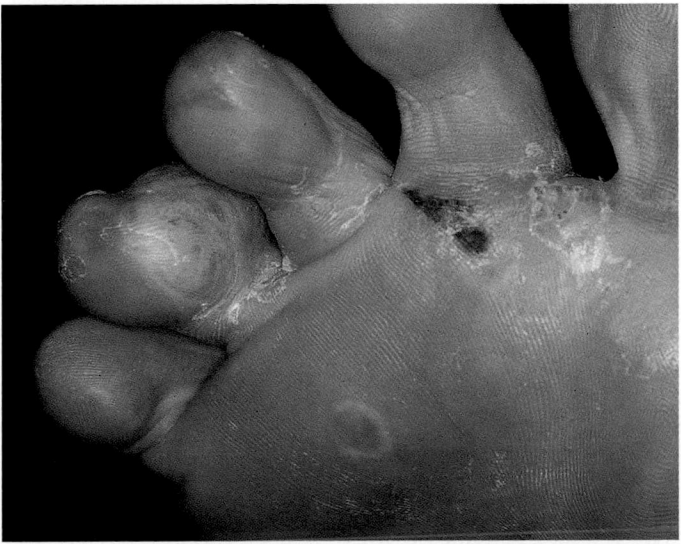

Fig. 27-13 Epidermolysis bullosa simplex.

Nikolsky sign is negative. Usually, the mucous membranes and nails are not involved. EBS is usually milder than other forms of EB.

Inherited as an autosomal-dominant trait, EBS is a disease in which keratin gene mutations cause the production of defective intermediate filaments, which lead to epidermal basal cell fragility and subsequent blistering. Gene mutations produce abnormalities in keratins 5 and 14, keratins expressed in the basal cell layer. Patients heterozygous for abnormal keratin 14 have blistering limited to the hands and feet, but homozygotes have more severe and widespread blistering of the skin and mucous membranes. Separation occurs through the basal cell layer. Rubbing skin with an eraser may lead to a subclinical lesion that demonstrates the split histologically.

Localized epidermolysis bullosa simplex

Recurrent bullous eruption of the hands and feet is autosomal-dominantly determined and appears in a chronic form in infancy or at times later in life. The Weber–Cockayne designation has been dropped in recent classification schemes. The lesions exacerbate during hot weather and when the patient is subjected to prolonged walking or marching, as is experienced in military service. Hyperhidrosis may be an associated finding. In localized EBS, the bullae are intraepidermal and suprabasal, and healing occurs without scarring.

Application of aluminum chloride hexahydrate in anhydrous ethanol (Drysol) on the normal skin of hands and feet twice a day has been shown to reduce blistering in this form of EB. After 2 weeks of daily therapy the patient can be switched to once- or twice-weekly applications.

Epidermolysis bullosa herpetiformis (Dowling–Meara)

In this autosomal-dominant variant of EBS, active blisters with circinate configuration occur in infancy. Milia may develop, but there is no scarring. The oral mucosa is involved. Nails are shed but may regrow, sometimes with dystrophy. Blistering lessens with age. Hyperkeratosis of the palms and soles may occur. Histologically, the split is through the basal layer, and tonofilaments are clumped on electron microscopy. Point mutations have been shown in keratin 5 and 14 genes.

Epidermolysis bullosa simplex (Ogna)

Generalized bruising and hemorrhagic blisters occur. Epidermolysis bullosa simplex is transmitted as an autosomal-dominant trait. At birth there are small, acral, traumatic sanguineous blisters. The basal keratinocytes in this syndrome do not stain with antiplectin antibodies.

Epidermolysis bullosa simplex with mottled pigmentation

One Swedish family has been reported with autosomal-dominant EBS with congenital scattered hyper- and hypopigmented macules that fade slowly after birth. The remaining features are similar to those of generalized EBS. Ultrastructural studies show vacuolization of the basal cell layer.

Epidermolysis bullosa simplex with muscular dystrophy

There is a form of EBS associated with late-onset neuromuscular disease. It is inherited as an autosomal-recessive trait. There is widespread blistering at birth associated with scarring, milia, atrophy, nail dystrophy, dental anomalies, laryngeal webs, and urethral strictures. Progressive muscular dystrophy with weakness and wasting begins in childhood or later. This disease is caused by a mutation in the plectin gene, with affected patients having absent plectin in their skin and muscles.

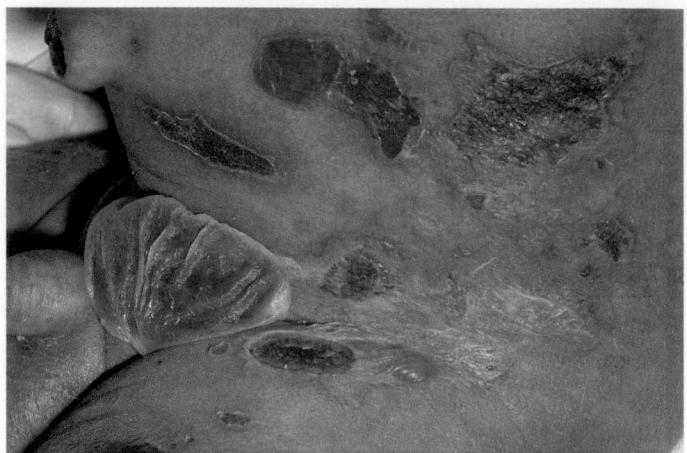

Fig. 27-14 Junctional epidermolysis bullosa.

Junctional forms

Junctional epidermolysis bullosa (epidermolysis bullosa letalis, epidermolysis bullosa Herlitz)

In junctional EB, a rare type that has autosomal-recessive transmission, severe generalized blistering may be present at birth, and extensive denudation may prove fatal within a few months. There is generalized blistering (Fig. 27-14) with relative sparing of the hands, and characteristic perioral and perinasal hypertrophic granulation tissue. Eventually the lesions heal without scarring or milia formation, but erosions may persist for years. Dysplastic teeth are common. Laryngeal and bronchial lesions may cause respiratory distress and even death. Additional systemic complications include gastrointestinal tract, gallbladder, corneal, and vaginal disease. In patients who survive infancy, there is growth retardation, and moderate to severe refractory anemia is frequent. Separation occurs in the lamina lucida, as shown by electron microscopy.

Herlitz junctional EB is caused by mutations in three genes: *LAMA3*, *LAMB3*, or *LAMC2*, which code for polypeptide subunits of laminin 5. In addition to good wound care and control of infection, epidermal autographs of cultured keratinocytes, isolated from clinically uninvolved skin and grown on collagen sponges, may be useful for chronic facial erosions. Complete re-epithelialization can be achieved over 7–10 months.

Junctional epidermolysis bullosa with pyloric atresia

This rare autosomal-recessively inherited form of junctional EB presents at birth with severe mucocutaneous fragility and gastric outlet obstruction. Even if the pyloric atresia is repaired, the neonates may die because of the severity of their skin disease. If they survive the neonatal period, the blistering diminishes. Persistent scarring of the urinary tract may occur, however, with stenosis of the ureteral–vesicular junction, requiring numerous urologic procedures. This syndrome is caused by a genetic mutation in either the α6 or β4 integrin genes (*ITGA6* and *ITGB4*). This α6–β4 integrin complex is uniquely expressed on epithelial surfaces.

Generalized atrophic benign epidermolysis bullosa

Most cases of generalized atrophic benign EB are characterized by onset at birth, generalized blisters and atrophy, mucosal involvement, and thickened, dystrophic, or absent nails. Enamel defects in deciduous and permanent teeth, and atrophic alopecia are prominent features. Multiple cutaneous squamous cell carcinomas have been reported. Cleavage is within the lamina lucida, and hemidesmosomes are reduced or absent. The basal lamina, anchoring fibrils, collagen fibers, and dermal microfibril bundles are unaltered. Inheritance is autosomal-recessive. In contrast to EB Herlitz, patients often survive to adulthood. Studies have shown mutations in the *COL17A1* gene encoding for type XVII collagen (BPAg2), a transmembrane component of hemidesmosomes.

Cicatricial junctional epidermolysis bullosa

In 1985, Haber et al described another type of junctional EB, which they named cicatricial junctional epidermolysis bullosa because the blisters heal with scarring, which may produce syndactyly and contractures; there is also stenosis of the anterior nares. Electron microscopy reveals junctional bullae with rudimentary hemidesmosomes. The bases of the bullae are covered by an intact basal lamina with normal anchoring fibrils.

Dermolytic or dystrophic forms

The cause of dystrophic EB in both autosomal-dominantly and recessively inherited forms is mutations in the *COL7A1* gene encoding for type VII collagen. The anchoring fibrils in these patients are defective or deficient.

Dominant dystrophic epidermolysis bullosa

On the extensor surfaces of the extremities, vesicles and bullae appear; these are most pronounced over the joints, especially over the toes, fingers, knuckles, ankles, and elbows. Spontaneous, flesh-colored, scarlike (albopapuloid) lesions may appear on the trunk, often in adolescence, with no previous trauma. The nails may be thickened. Usually the Nikolsky sign is present, and frequently the accumulated fluid in a bulla can be moved under the skin several centimeters away from the original site. Healing usually occurs with scarring and atrophy. Milia are often present on the rims of the ears, dorsal surfaces of the hands, and extensor surfaces of the arms and legs.

The mucous membranes are frequently involved. Bullae, vesicles, and erosions are encountered on the buccal mucosa, tongue, palate, esophagus, pharynx, and larynx. The latter involvement is manifested by persistent hoarseness in some of these patients. There may be angular contractures at the gingivolabial sulcus and dysphagia from pharyngeal scarring. Scarring on the tip of the tongue is typical. The teeth are normal. Usually the conjunctiva is not involved.

Other changes include nail dystrophy, partial alopecia of the scalp, absence of body hair, dwarfism, and the formation of contractures and clawlike hands, with atrophy of the phalangeal bones and pseudosyndactylism. The albopapuloid type (Pasini) is the more severe expression of dominant dystrophic EB. The Cockayne–Touraine type is more limited in extent and severity, and no albopapuloid lesions are seen.

Histologically, a noninflammatory subepidermal bulla is generally present. On electron microscopy, cleavage occurs beneath the basal lamina, and anchoring fibrils are rudimentary and reduced in number. In blistered areas they are not demonstrable.

Autologous meshed split-thickness skin grafts and allogeneic cultured keratinocytes may be used in treating nonhealing skin defects. In many patients with dominant dystrophic EB, blistering reduces with time and only nail dystrophy may be present in adulthood.

Bart syndrome

Bart described congenital localized defects of the skin (Fig. 27-15), mechanoblisters, and nail deformities with autosomal-dominant inheritance. Although the clinical and histologic

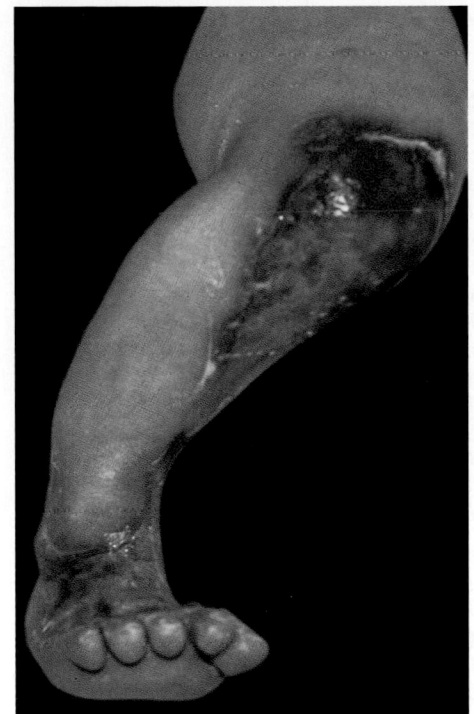

Fig. 27-15 Bart syndrome.

picture of this syndrome is one of a mildly scarring mechanobullous dermatosis with a favorable prognosis, associations with mandibulofacial dysostosis, renal aplasia, and congenital abnormalities of the lower extremities have been reported. Bart syndrome is not a distinct entity, but is a clinical variant of other forms of EB, mostly dominant dystrophic EB, based on identification of a defect in the *COL7A1* gene (chromosome 3p) encoding for type VII collagen.

Transient bullous dermolysis of the newborn

In 1985, Hashimoto et al reported a newborn who developed blisters from every minor trauma. Separation was below the basal lamina, with degeneration of collagen and anchoring fibrils. There was rapid healing by 4 months of age. Nails were not damaged and there was no scarring.

They considered as criteria for this entity:

1. vesiculobullous lesions present at birth or induced by friction
2. spontaneous recovery at a few months of age
3. no dystrophic scars
4. subepidermal blisters beginning in the dermal papillae
5. ultrastructurally observed collagenolysis and damaged anchoring fibrils
6. enormous dilatation of rough endoplasmic reticulum, with stellate bodies of keratinocytes in their vacuoles.

The cause has been shown in one family to be a transversion mutation in the *COL7A1* gene encoding for type VII collagen, and it is therefore allelic with other variants of dominant dystrophic EB. The mechanism for the transient nature of reduced amounts of type VII collagen along the dermoepidermal junction remains to be defined.

Acrokeratotic poikiloderma (Kindler syndrome, Weary–Kindler syndrome)

In 1954, Kindler reported a combination of poikiloderma congenitale and traumatic blistering of the feet from minor trauma. It shares some clinical features with dominant dystrophic EB, but in the largest reported familial cluster, inheritance followed an autosomal-recessive pattern. Characteristic features include skin fragility with blistering, congenital acral bullae, generalized poikiloderma with prominent atrophy, photosensitivity, acral keratoses, severe periodontal disease, and phimosis. Some patients develop intestinal dysfunction or ulcerative colitis. Pseudoainhum and sclerotic bands were reported in one case. The principal histologic change is absence of elastic fibers in the papillary dermis and fragmented ones in the mid-dermis. Ultrastructural studies have shown replication of the lamina densa. The disorder is caused by loss-of-function mutations in fermitin family homologue 1, an actin cytoskeleton-associated protein encoded by the gene *FERMT1* that plays a role in keratinocyte adhesion, migration, and proliferation. The protein is mainly expressed in basal keratinocytes. It binds to fermitin family homologue 2, as well as β1 and β3 integrins.

Ectodermal dysplasia/skin fragility syndrome (McGrath syndrome)

This includes trauma-induced skin fragility and defects of the hair, nails, and sweat glands. Trauma-induced blisters or skin tearing are noted on the pressure points, especially after prolonged standing or walking. Desmosomes in the lower epidermis are small and reduced in number. The disorder is caused by mutations in the plakophilin-1 gene (*PKP1*), gene map locus 1q32.

Recessive dystrophic epidermolysis bullosa (Hallopeau–Siemens)

There are three variants of recessive dystrophic EB—generalized, localized, and inverse. The generalized type has two variants: a mild or mitis form and the severe (Hallopeau–Siemens) variety. All forms result from mutations in the gene encoding type VII collagen, *COL7A1*. Generalized recessive dystrophic EB in its mild (mitis) form has blisters limited primarily to the hands, feet, elbows, and knees, and limited complications. The more severe variety characteristically begins at birth with generalized cutaneous and mucosal blistering. Digital fusion with encasement of the fingers and toes in scar tissues, forming a "mitten-like" deformity (Fig. 27-16), is characteristic of the severe form of recessive dystrophic EB, occurring in up to 90% of patients by age 25. Dental complications may be severe, including rampant dental caries and microstomia. Esophageal stricture may be present. Anemia and growth retardation are frequently seen in the most severe cases, and progressive nutritional deficiency can result in fatal cardiomyopathy. Fatal systemic amyloidosis (AA type) has also been

reported. There is a high risk of developing cutaneous squamous cell carcinomas (SCCs), with up to 50% of patients affected by age 35. These SCCs may be multiple and can metastasize and cause death.

Although gene therapy is promising, treatment remains primarily palliative. Gentle wound care and proper nutrition are critical. Debilitating oral lesions produce pain, scarring, and microstomia. Aggressive dental intervention is recommended. Nutritional support is of critical importance. Autologous meshed split-thickness skin grafts and allogeneic cultured keratinocytes have been shown to be useful in treating non-healing cutaneous defects, or they may be used for closure after removal of large cutaneous malignancies. Family education and referral to DEBRA (Dystrophic Epidermolysis Bullosa Research Association of America, 5 West 36th Street, Room 404, New York, NY 10018, www.debra.org) are strongly recommended.

Bruckner-Tuderman L: European Dermatology Forum: skin diseases in Europe. Skin diseases with a high public health impact: epidermolysis bullosa. Eur J Dermatol 2008 Mar–Apr; 18(2):214–216.

Ferrari S, et al: Towards a gene therapy clinical trial for epidermolysis bullosa. Rev Recent Clin Trials 2006 May; 1(2):155–162.

Fine JD, et al: The classification of inherited epidermolysis bullosa (EB): report of the Third International Consensus Meeting on Diagnosis and Classification of EB. J Am Acad Dermatol 2008 Jun; 58(6):931–950.

Fine JD, et al: The risk of cardiomyopathy in inherited epidermolysis bullosa. Br J Dermatol 2008 Sep; 159(3):677–682.

Fine JD: Inherited epidermolysis bullosa: recent basic and clinical advances. Curr Opin Pediatr 2010 Aug; 22(4):453–458.

Haynes L: Nutritional support for children with epidermolysis bullosa. Br J Nurs 2006 Nov 9–22; 15(20):1097–1101.

Keefe RJ: Inherited epidermolysis bullosa: this dermal disease is beyond skin deep. JAAPA 2008 Jul; 21(7):22–27.

Lai-Cheong JE, et al: Kindler syndrome: a focal adhesion genodermatosis. Br J Dermatol 2009 Feb; 160(2):233–242.

Pillay E: Epidermolysis bullosa. Part 1: Causes, presentation and complications. Br J Nurs 2008 Mar 13–26; 17(5):292–296.

Familial benign chronic pemphigus (Hailey–Hailey disease)

In 1939, Hailey and Hailey described a familial disease characterized by persistently recurrent bullous and vesicular dermatitis of the sides of the neck, axillae, and flexures. The eruption may remain localized or may become widespread. Usually, intact blisters are not evident. Instead, the lesions appear as macerated plaques with a reticulated pattern of fissuring (Fig. 27-17). Lesions may become thickly crusted and

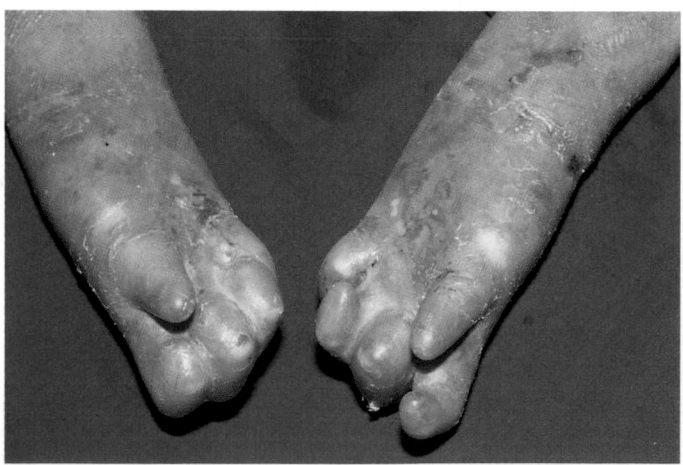

Fig. 27-16 Epidermolysis bullosa, recessive dystrophic type.

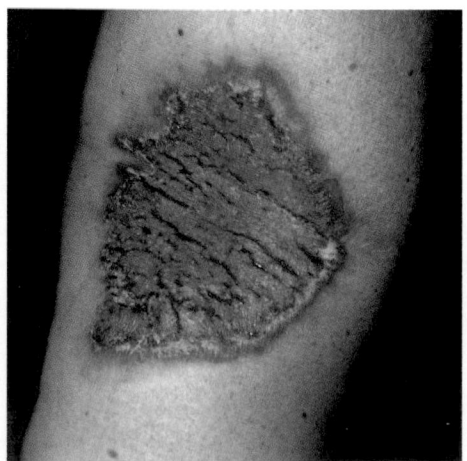

Fig. 27-17 Hailey–Hailey disease.

may resemble impetigo. Sometimes the center becomes dry and crusted and there is an actively inflammatory border that spreads peripherally, producing circinate and figurate patterns. The onset is usually in the late teens or early twenties.

The condition is typically worse during the summer. Lesions tend to recur at sites of prior involvement. A papular variant in the genital area has been described, simulating condylomata. There may be tenderness and enlargement of the regional lymph glands caused by secondary bacterial infection. Longitudinal leukonychia may occur. Involvement of the esophagus, mouth, and labia majora is rare. Hailey–Hailey disease is inherited in an autosomal-dominant manner. Thirty percent of patients express new mutations. The disease is due to a genetic defect in a calcium ATPase (*ATP2C1*) on chromosome 3q21.

In predisposed persons with Hailey–Hailey disease, skin trauma, bacterial or fungal infection, and dermatoses may trigger lesions. Sunburn may also exacerbate the disease. Widespread bullous lesions may occur in response to drug eruptions, and be misdiagnosed as toxic epidermal necrolysis.

The histopathologic picture is unique. There is acanthosis and full-thickness acantholysis resembling a "dilapidated brick wall." The basal cell layer remains attached to the dermis.

The treatment of Hailey–Hailey disease is difficult. Many cases improve with the use of systemic antibiotics effective against *Staphylococcus aureus*, topical clindamycin, antifungal agents, or mupirocin. Corticosteroids, administered topically, systemically, or both, have shown response. Cyclosporine, oral retinoids, topical calcineurin inhibitors, topical calcitriol, botulinum toxin, photodynamic therapy, alefacept, and dapsone have been used in severe cases. Dermabrasion and CO_2 laser vaporization have been shown to be effective, as the epidermis heals from uninvolved adnexal structures. Grafting and electron beam therapy have been helpful in the most severe forms of the disease.

Berger EM, et al: Successful treatment of Hailey–Hailey disease with acitretin. J Drugs Dermatol 2007 Jul; 6(7):734–736.

Guarino MF, et al: Experience with photodynamic therapy in Hailey–Hailey disease. J Dermatolog Treat 2008; 19(5):288–290.

Hurd DS, et al: A case report of Hailey–Hailey disease treated with alefacept (Amevive). Br J Dermatol 2008 Feb; 158(2):399–401.

Koeyers WJ, et al: Botulinum toxin type A as an adjuvant treatment modality for extensive Hailey–Hailey disease. J Dermatolog Treat 2008; 19(4):251–254.

Kumar R, et al: Longitudinal leukonychia in Hailey–Hailey disease: a sign not to be missed. Dermatol Online J 2008 Mar 15; 14(3):17.

Narbutt J, et al: Effective treatment of recalcitrant Hailey–Hailey disease with electron beam radiotherapy. J Eur Acad Dermatol Venereol 2007 Apr; 21(4):567–568.

Nemoto-Hasebe I, et al: Diagnosis of Hailey–Hailey disease facilitated by DNA testing: a novel mutation in *ATP2C1*. Acta Derm Venereol 2008; 88(4):399–400.

Disorders of cornification (ichthyoses and ichthyosiform syndromes)

The term ichthyosis is derived from the Greek word *ichthys*, meaning "fish." Ichthyosis is not one disease but a group of diseases in which the homeostatic mechanism of epidermal cell kinetics or differentiation is altered, resulting in the clinical appearance of scale. Because these disorders manifest as abnormal differentiation of the epidermis, the term disorders of cornification is preferred to ichthyosis.

Treatment

Symptomatic treatment with alphahydroxy acids, such as lactic acid or 12% ammonium lactate lotion, is helpful. Patients with atopic dermatitis and ichthyosis vulgaris may find that these products sting. Other compounds with hydrating and keratolytic properties are also beneficial. Creams containing 10% urea are effective humectants. Response to topical retinoids has been variable. Widespread use of topical salicylic acid in children may lead to salicylism, and salicylic acid products are best reserved for localized thicker areas, when 40% urea has failed. Baths may help by hydrating the horny layer, but the water must be sealed in with an evaporation barrier such as white petrolatum. Topical calcipotriene ointment has proved effective in a variety of ichthyoses and topical maxacalcitol, a vitamin D_3 analogue, has been used successfully in mosaic-type bullous congenital ichthyosiform erythroderma. Application of a 40–60% solution of propylene glycol in water under an occlusive suit removes the scales. Propylene glycol can produce renal failure and cardiac toxicity when given systemically, but few reports of adverse effects have been noted with topical use. Many patients benefit from the use of a sauna suit, even without the use of propylene glycol, so the risk–benefit ratio of adding the propylene glycol to the regimen should be evaluated carefully.

Ichthyosis vulgaris

Ichthyosis vulgaris is autosomal-dominantly inherited and is characterized by onset in early childhood, usually between 3 and 12 months of age, with fine scales that appear "pasted on" over the entire body. Varying degrees of dryness of the skin may be evident. The scales are coarser on the lower extremities than they are on the trunk. The extensor surfaces of the extremities are most prominently involved. The axillary and gluteal folds are usually not affected. Although the antecubital and popliteal fossae are usually spared by ichthyosis vulgaris, atopic changes may be present, as these disorders are frequently associated. Accentuated skin markings and hyperkeratosis of the palms are common features. Keratosis pilaris is frequently associated. The scalp is involved, with only slight scaling. Keratotic lesions may be found on the palmar creases (keratosis punctata). Atopy manifested as hay fever, eczema, asthma, or urticaria is frequently present. The course is favorable, with limited findings by the time the patient is an adult.

Histologically, there is a moderate degree of compact eosinophilic orthokeratosis. The granular layer is reduced or absent, and keratohyalin granules may appear spongy or fragmented on electron microscopy. The spinous layer is of normal thickness. Filaggrin is reduced in involved epidermis, and profilaggrin mRNA is unstable in keratinocytes. This is a retention hyperkeratosis, with a normal rate of epidermal turnover.

The differential diagnosis includes severe xerosis, X-linked ichthyosis, and acquired ichthyosis.

X-linked ichthyosis

X-linked ichthyosis is transmitted only to males by heterozygous mothers as an X-linked recessive trait. This condition results from a deficiency of steroid sulfatase (aryl sulfatase C), and occurs once in every 2000–5000 male births. Onset is usually before 3 months of age. The children are commonly born via cesarian section, with failure of progression of labor owing to a placental sulfatase deficiency. Scales are dark, large, and prominent on the anterior neck, extensor surfaces of the extremities (Fig. 27-18), and the trunk. The sides of the neck are invariably involved, giving the child an unwashed look. The elbow and knee flexures are relatively spared, as are the face and scalp; the palms and soles are nearly always spared.

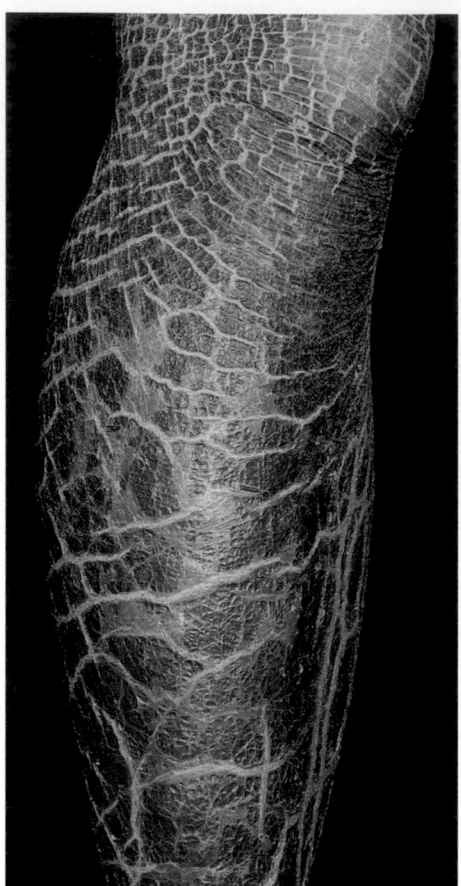

Fig. 27-18 X-linked ichthyosis.

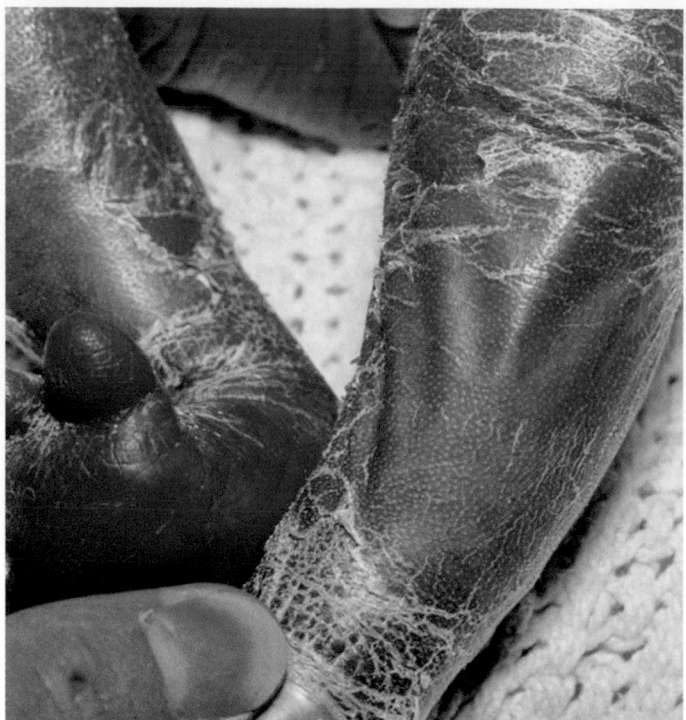

Fig. 27-19 Collodion baby.

The condition may be confused with ichthyosis vulgaris, but typically has darker scales and demonstrates dramatic clearing during the summer months. A diagnosis of X-linked ichthyosis is likely if the abdomen is more involved than the back and if the ichthyosis extends down the entire dorsum of the leg. Keratosis pilaris is not present, and the incidence of atopy is not increased. Corneal opacities (which do not affect vision) are seen by slit-lamp examination on the posterior capsule or Descemet's membrane in about 50% of affected males and female carriers. Another extracutaneous feature is a 12–15% incidence of cryptorchidism and an independently increased risk of testicular cancer. Unlike ichthyosis vulgaris, X-linked ichthyosis does not improve with age, but gradually worsens in both extent and severity.

There is usually a deletion at Xp22.3, and steroid sulfatase is lacking in fibroblasts, leukocytes, and keratinocytes. The diagnosis can be confirmed by lipoprotein electrophoresis, because the increase in cholesterol sulfate makes the low-density lipoproteins (LDLs) migrate much more rapidly, and cholesterol sulfate is elevated in serum, erythrocyte membranes, and keratin. The reduced enzyme activity can be assessed in fibroblasts, keratinocytes, leukocytes, and prenatally in amniocytes.

Multiple sulfatase deficiency

Patients with multiple sulfatase deficiency display an overlap of steroid sulfatase deficiency, mucopolysaccharidosis, and metachromatic leukodystrophy. The scaling is sometimes milder than X-linked recessive ichthyosis. There may be developmental delay, spastic quadriparesis, and coarse facial features. Histologic examination shows hyperkeratosis with a normal granular cell layer. This autosomal-recessive disorder is caused by a lack of or deficiency in all known sulfatases.

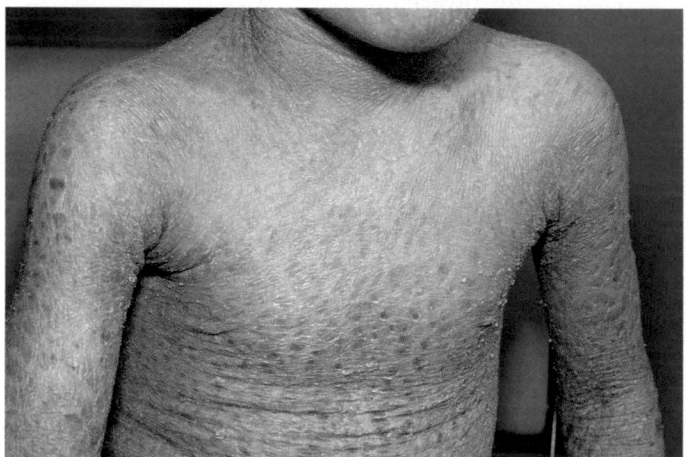

Fig. 27-20 Lamellar ichthyosis.

Autosomal-recessive ichthyosis

Biochemical and genetic studies have helped to define the specific subtypes. Clinical features often overlap, and in the past, the severity of the disease determined the classification. Identification of specific defects, such as transglutaminase 1 and profilaggrin/filaggrin, are important to define each disorder, and are the basis for classification of ichthyotic disorders.

Lamellar ichthyosis

Lamellar ichthyosis is present at birth or becomes apparent soon after, and almost always involves the entire cutaneous surface. Usually, a collodion-like membrane (Fig. 27-19) encases the baby at birth, then desquamates over the first 2–3 weeks of life. The ensuing ichthyosis is characterized by large (5–15 mm), grayish-brown scales (Fig. 27-20), which are strikingly quadrilateral, free at the edges, and adherent in the center. In severe cases, the scales may be so thick that they are

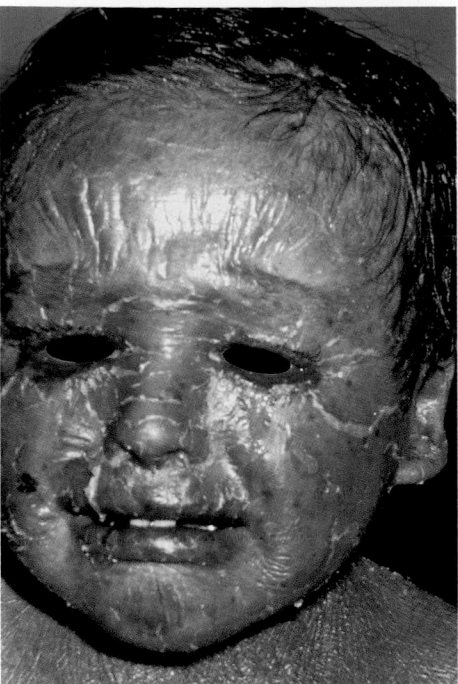

Fig. 27-21 Nonbullous congenital ichthyosiform erythroderma.

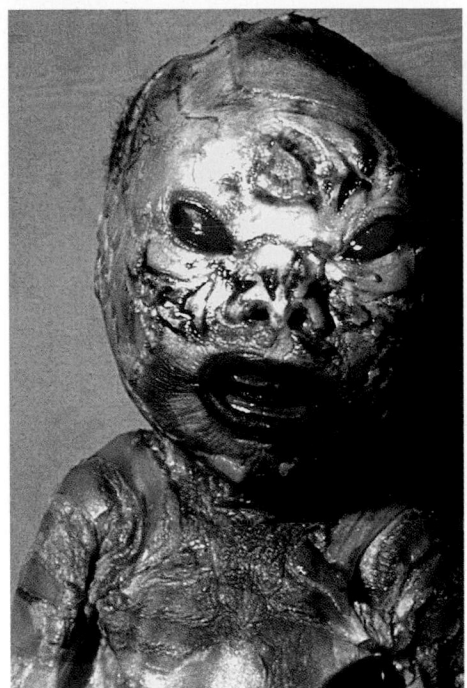

Fig. 27-22 Harlequin fetus.

like armor plate. Moderate hyperkeratosis of the palms and soles is frequently present. The follicles in most instances have a crateriform appearance. Ectropion is almost always present and is a helpful diagnostic sign.

Lamellar ichthyosis is inherited as an autosomal-recessive trait. About half the patients have decreased or absent transglutaminase 1 (TGM1) activity. *ALOXE3* and *ALOX12B* mutations can produce a similar appearance. Lamellar ichthyosis type 2 has been associated with mutations in the *ABCA12* gene.

In addition to the topical agents recommended for the treatment of other ichthyoses, tazarotene (Tazorac) and orally administered retinoids can improve symptoms. The adverse effects of prolonged oral retinoid therapy make their use for long-term maintenance therapy difficult.

Nonbullous congenital ichthyosiform erythroderma

Most infants with nonbullous congenital ichthyosiform erythroderma are born enclosed in a constricting parchment- or collodion-like membrane. They also have ectropion of the eyelids, which has led to confusion with lamellar ichthyosis, and at one time the term lamellar ichthyosis was used for almost all patients with nonbullous autosomal-recessive ichthyoses. As mutations in *TGM1*, *ALOXE3*, or *ALOX12B* can lead to either congenital ichthyosiform erythroderma or lamellar ichthyoses, the separation of the entities is largely on the basis of the clinical phenotype.

Within 24 h of birth, fissuring and peeling begin, and large keratinous lamellae are cast off in 10–14 days, coincident with rapid improvement. As the membrane is shed, underlying redness and scaling are apparent (Fig. 27-21). Generalized involvement is the rule, including the face, palms, soles, and flexures. Cicatricial alopecia, nail dystrophy, and some ectropion are common. Scales may be large and platelike on the legs but are likely to be fine on the trunk, face, and scalp. The condition has been found in association with neutral lipid storage disease.

Histologically, parakeratosis and inflammation are seen more frequently in congenital ichthyosiform erythroderma than in lamellar ichthyoses. The stratum corneum is usually thicker in lamellar ichthyoses, and is usually not parakeratotic.

Harlequin fetus

Harlequin fetus is a severe disorder that affects the skin in utero, causing thick, horny, armor-like plates covering the entire surface (Fig. 27-22). The ears are rudimentary or absent, and eclabium and ectropion are severe. The child is often stillborn or dies soon after delivery; however, with aggressive management, there have been long-term survivors. These survivors develop features of congenital ichthyosiform erythroderma or lamellar ichthyosis. Absent or abnormal lamellar granules, a lack of extracellular lipid lamellae, and lipid droplets in the stratum corneum have been reported. Abnormalities of profilaggrin and of K6 and K16 expression have been reported. Recessive inheritance has been favored, and is supported by reports of consanguinity. Some reports suggest a dominant mutation with parental mosaicism.

Bullous ichthyosiform erythroderma

An autosomal-dominantly inherited disorder, bullous congenital ichthyosiform erythroderma (epidermolytic hyperkeratosis, EHK) is usually manifested by blisters at or shortly after birth. Later, thickened, horny, warty, or spine-like, ridged scales predominate (Fig. 27-23). They are particularly prominent at the flexures. There is remarkable heterogeneity, particularly in regard to the degree of hyperkeratosis, the extent of body surface involvement, presence or absence of erythroderma, and palm and sole involvement. An association with hypocalcemic vitamin D-resistant rickets has been reported. Epidermal nevi of the epidermolytic type are mosaic expressions of epidermolytic hyperkeratosis.

Epidermolytic hyperkeratosis is caused by mutations in the genes for keratins K1 and K10. Keratin distribution patterns in keratinocytes are abnormal, suggesting that there is an altered assembly process of cornified cell envelopes in epidermolytic hyperkeratosis.

Histologically, the lesional skin demonstrates compact hyperkeratosis. The granular layer is markedly thickened and

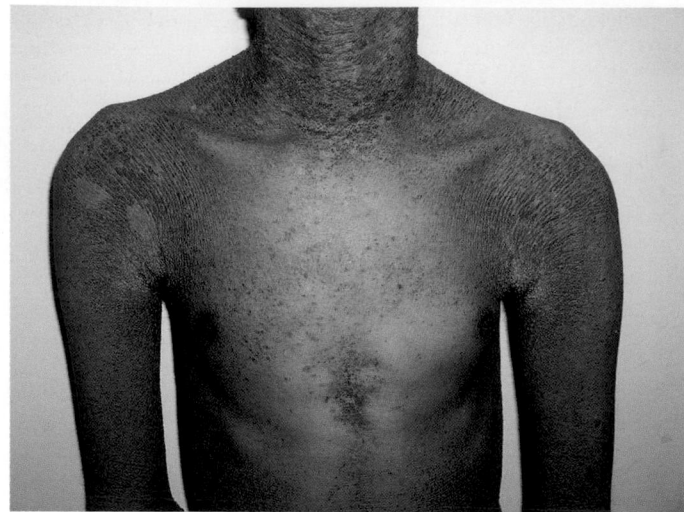

Fig. 27-23 Epidermolytic hyperkeratosis. (Courtesy of Shyam Verma, MD)

contains coarse keratohyaline granules. Epidermal cells detach in the granular cell layer and may appear disrupted. Electron microscopy reveals the formation of perinuclear haloes. These findings allow prenatal diagnosis by fetal skin biopsy. Epidermolytic hyperkeratosis has been described as an incidental finding in normal skin, skin adjacent to benign and malignant epidermal tumors, and normal oral mucosa. It may be more commonly seen in association with dysplastic nevi than with banal nevi.

Short, intensive therapy with high-dose vitamin A, 750 000 U of Aquasol A daily for 2 weeks, produces modest clinical improvement. Others have tried administering systemic retinoids, with similar results; however, the patient's blistering may worsen, despite clinical improvement of the scales. Decisions regarding systemic retinoid therapy must therefore be made on a case-by-case basis. Application of 0.1% retinoic acid (Retin-A cream) has been used successfully. Pyogenic infection is a common problem, and appropriate antibiotics should be administered. A water solution of 10% glycerin and 3% lactic acid applied to wet skin can result in clinical improvement. The disease tends to become less severe with age.

Ichthyosis bullosa of Siemens

Once classified as a subtype of epidermolytic hyperkeratosis, this condition is characterized by a lack of erythema, relatively mild hyperkeratosis usually limited to the flexures, and superficial molting or peeling of the skin (the "mauserung" phenomenon). Ichthyosis bullosa of Siemens is caused by mutations in the gene for keratin 2e.

Akiyama M, et al: An update on molecular aspects of the non-syndromic ichthyoses. Exp Dermatol 2008 May; 17(5):373–382.

DiGiovanna JJ, et al: Ichthyosis: etiology, diagnosis, and management. Am J Clin Dermatol 2003; 4:81.

Elias PM, et al: Pathogenesis of permeability barrier abnormalities in the ichthyoses: inherited disorders of lipid metabolism. J Lipid Res 2008 Apr; 49(4):697–714.

el-Khateeb EA: Bullous congenital ichthyosiform erythroderma associated with hypocalcemic vitamin D-resistant rickets. Pediatr Dermatol 2008 Mar–Apr; 25(2):279–282.

Ross R, et al: Histopathologic characterization of epidermolytic hyperkeratosis: a systematic review of histology from the National Registry for Ichthyosis and Related Skin Disorders. J Am Acad Dermatol 2008 Jul; 59(1):86–90.

Schmuth M, et al: Ichthyosis update: towards a function-driven model of pathogenesis of the disorders of cornification and the role of corneocyte proteins in these disorders. Adv Dermatol 2007; 23:231–256.

Umekoji A, et al: A case of mosaic-type bullous congenital ichthyosiform erythroderma successfully treated with topical maxacalcitol, a vitamin D3 analogue. Clin Exp Dermatol 2008 Jul; 33(4):501–502.

Vahlquist A, et al: Congenital ichthyosis: an overview of current and emerging therapies. Acta Derm Venereol 2008; 88(1):4–14.

Restrictive dermopathy

Restrictive dermopathy is a rare, lethal, autosomal-recessively inherited laminopathy characterized by abnormal facies, tight skin, sparse or absent eyelashes, and secondary joint changes. Virtually all cases are associated with polyhydramnios, reduced fetal movements, and premature delivery. Infants exhibit a fixed facial expression, with blurring of groove between nose and cheek, sometimes described as an "Asiatic porcelain doll" appearance. Patients also exhibit micrognathia, mouth in the "O" position, rigid and tense skin with erosions and denudations, and multiple joint contractures. Some patients have wide cranial sutures, small pinched nose, low-set ears, microstomia, rocker-bottom feet, scaly skin, and respiratory insufficiency. Pulmonary hypoplasia, microcolon, vessel transposition, natal teeth, ectropion, submucous cleft palate, hypospadias, urethral duplication, dysplasia of clavicles, adrenal hypoplasia, and an enlarged placenta with short umbilical cord may be noted.

Histopathologic features include hyperkeratosis, parakeratosis, abnormal keratohyaline granules, and effacement of the rete ridge pattern. The dermis is attenuated with collagen fibers parallel to the epidermis, resembling a scar or tendon. Elastic fibers are absent. The subcutis demonstrates hypoplastic eccrine and sebaceous glands. The disease is usually caused by mutations in *ZMPSTE24*, causing loss of function of the encoded zinc metalloproteinase STE24 and resulting in accumulation of prelamin A at the nuclear periphery. Dominant forms may be related to *LMNA* mutations.

Khanna P, et al: Restrictive dermopathy: report and review. Fetal Pediatr Pathol 2008 Aug; 27(2):105–118.

Sander CS, et al: A newly identified splice site mutation in *ZMPSTE24* causes restrictive dermopathy in the Middle East. Br J Dermatol 2008 Sep; 159(4):961–967.

Thill M: Restrictive dermopathy: a rare laminopathy. Arch Gynecol Obstet 2008 Sep; 278(3):201–208.

Ichthyosis linearis circumflexa

Ichthyosis linearis circumflexa is an inherited autosomal-recessive disorder of cornification in which migratory annular and polycyclic patches occur (Fig. 27-24). It may first appear as severe congenital generalized exfoliative erythroderma. Later, lesions predominate on the trunk and extremities, and appear as a polycyclic serpiginous eruption characterized by constantly changing patterns. In about a week the lesions attain their maximum diameter and involute, leaving no atrophy, scarring, or pigmentation. The lesions may clear almost completely during the summer. Most patients are found to have bamboo hair (trichorrhexis invaginata). The association of ichthyosiform dermatitis, hair abnormality, and atopic diathesis is called Netherton syndrome. Because of coexistent atopic dermatitis, the scalp, face, and eyebrow regions are erythematous and scaly. Hairs may fracture below the surface of the scalp, so that the patient appears bald. Mutations in *SPINK5*, which encodes the serine protease inhibitor Kazal-type 5 protein, have been identified in Netherton syndrome.

Histologic examination shows hyperkeratosis, parakeratosis, and acanthosis. The granular layer is typically absent.

Acitretin has been effective in some patients, but should be avoided in erythrodermic neonates; long-term use is limited

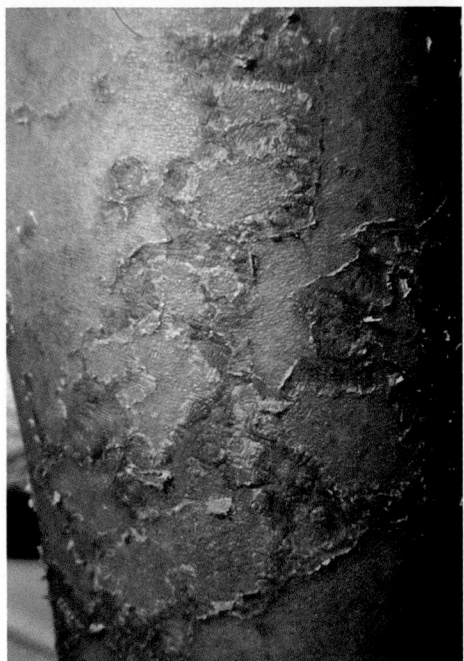

Fig. 27-24 Ichthyosis linearis circumflexa.

by toxicity. Topical tacrolimus has also been reported as effective, but in one report, three patients treated twice with 0.1% tacrolimus ointment were found to have significant tacrolimus blood levels. Although none of these patients developed signs or symptoms of toxic effects, monitoring of blood levels is advised if tacrolimus is used in this setting.

Allen A, et al: Significant absorption of topical tacrolimus in 3 patients with Netherton syndrome. Arch Dermatol 2001; 137:747.

Saif GB, et al: Netherton syndrome: successful use of topical tacrolimus and pimecrolimus in four siblings. Int J Dermatol 2007 Mar; 46(3):290–294.

Neutral lipid storage disease

Dorfman–Chanarin syndrome is a rare autosomal-recessive disorder characterized by an ichthyosiform eruption, myopathy, and vacuolated leukocytes. Lipid vacuoles are present in all circulating granulocytes and monocytes, as well as dermal fibroblasts, Schwann cells, smooth muscle cells, and sweat gland cells. Other organ systems, such as the CNS, liver, muscles, ears, and eyes, may also have deposits. Associated cutaneous disorders include poikiloderma atrophicans vasculare and bullous congenital ichthyosiform erythroderma. The disorder is caused by a regulatory defect that alters the rates of synthesis and degradation of the major cellular phospholipids, particularly triacylglycerol-derived diacylglycerol. Electron microscopic findings show electron-lucent globular inclusions in lamellar structures. Dietary intervention, with modulation of dietary fats, has been shown to aid in controlling the disease.

Pena-Penabad C, et al: Dorfman–Chanarin syndrome (neutral lipid storage disease): new clinical features. Br J Dermatol 2001; 144:430.

Ichthyosis follicularis

Ichthyosis follicularis is characterized by noncicatricial universal alopecia, severe photophobia, and generalized cutaneous follicular projections that are flesh-colored and spiny. There is xerosis of nonspiny skin, and absence of sebaceous glands has been noted histologically. Hepatosplenomegaly, undescended testicles, nail dystrophy, inguinal hernia, short stature, seizures, psychomotor developmental delay, digital anomalies, and ptosis have been reported. It has also been called ichthyosis follicularis, alopecia, and photophobia (IFAP) syndrome. Males outnumber females 5:1. The main considerations in differential diagnosis are the keratitis-ichthyosis-deafness (KID) syndrome and keratosis follicularis spinulosa decalvans (KFSD). The disorder may be transmitted by an X-linked recessive gene, although an autosomal-dominant form has also been reported.

Rai VM, et al: Ichthyosis follicularis with alopecia and photophobia (IFAP) syndrome. Indian J Dermatol Venereol Leprol 2006 Mar–Apr; 72(2):136–138.

Sjögren–Larsson syndrome

Sjögren–Larsson syndrome is characterized by ichthyosis, spastic paralysis, oligophrenia, mental retardation, and a degenerative retinitis. The ichthyosis is usually generalized, with little or no involvement of the scalp, hair, or nails. There is a flexural and lower abdominal accentuation. The central face is spared, ectropion is unusual, and palms and soles are involved. Mongolian spots may be present. Beginning by the age of 2 or 3, there is spastic paralysis consisting of a stiff, awkward movement of the extremities. Gluten sensitivity has been reported. Electron microscopy reveals prominent Golgi apparatus and increased numbers of mitochondria in keratinocytes. Usually, a severe mental deficiency is present. The epilepsy is of the grand mal type. This syndrome is of autosomal-recessive inheritance, localized to chromosome 17p11.2. These patients have a fibroblast and leukocyte deficiency in fatty aldehyde dehydrogenase.

Lidén M, et al: Gluten sensitivity in patients with primary Sjögren's syndrome. Scand J Gastroenterol 2007 Aug; 42(8):962–967.

Lloyd MD, et al: Characterisation of recombinant human fatty aldehyde dehydrogenase: implications for Sjögren–Larsson syndrome. J Enzyme Inhib Med Chem 2007 Oct; 22(5):584–590.

Willemsen MA, et al: Mongolian spots in Sjögren–Larsson syndrome. Pediatr Dermatol 2008 Mar–Apr; 25(2):285.

Refsum syndrome

Refsum syndrome (heredopathia atactica polyneuritiformis) is an autosomal-recessively inherited ichthyosis with atypical retinitis pigmentosa, hypertrophic peripheral neuropathy, cerebellar ataxia, nerve deafness, and various electrocardiographic changes. The ichthyosis resembles ichthyosis vulgaris. It may be generalized or localized to the palms and soles. It is of delayed onset and shows lipid vacuoles in the basal layer. The epidermal cell turnover rate is increased. Biochemically, the disease is a peroxisomal disorder characterized by excessive accumulation of phytanic acid, pristanic acid, and picolinic acid in fatty tissues, myelin sheaths, heart, kidneys, and retinal tissues. The disease is caused by a deficiency of phytanolyl/pristanoyl-CoA-hydroxilase. In most patients, mutations in the *PHYH* gene have been identified, and a second locus has been found on chromosome 6q22–24 with mutations in *PEX7* (a gene also associated with rhizomelic chondrodysplasia punctata type 1) and *PAHX*. Dietary restriction of phytanic acid-containing vegetables can lead to an improvement of neurologic symptoms, but does not affect retinal changes. Unfortunately, in many patients, dietary restriction is not sufficient to prevent acute attacks or stabilize the progressive course. The acids are localized within very low-density lipoprotein (VLDL), LDL, and high-density lipoprotein (HDL) particles, and may be removed by extracorporeal LDL-apheresis.

Finsterer J, et al: Non-manifesting Refsum heterozygotes carrying the c.135-2A>G *PAHX* gene transition. Neurol Sci 2008 Jun; 29(3):173–175.

Straube R, et al: Membrane differential filtration is safe and effective for the long-term treatment of Refsum syndrome—an update of treatment modalities and pathophysiological cognition. Transfus Apheresis Sci 2003; 29:85.

Rud syndrome

Rud syndrome is characterized by ichthyosis, hypogonadism, small stature, mental retardation, acanthosis nigricans, epilepsy, macrocytic anemia, and, rarely, retinitis pigmentosa. Most kindreds have shown autosomal-recessive inheritance and may be atypical variants of well-described disorders, such as Sjögren–Larsson syndrome or Refsum syndrome, rather than representing a distinct inherited disorder. Some patients have X-linked steroid sulfatase deficiency.

Rajagopalan B: Non-bullous ichthyosiform erythroderma associated with retinitis pigmentosa. Am J Med Genet 2001; 99:181.

Stoll C, et al: A syndrome of congenital ichthyosis, hypogonadism, small stature, facial dysmorphism, scoliosis and myogenic dystrophy. Ann Genet 1999; 42:45.

Keratitis-ichthyosis-deafness syndrome

The keratitis-ichthyosis-deafness (KID or Senter) syndrome is characterized by vascularization of the cornea, an extensive congenital ichthyosiform eruption, neurosensory deafness, reticulated hyperkeratosis of the palms and soles, hypotrichosis, partial anhidrosis, nail dystrophy, and tight heel cords. Distinctive leathery, verrucoid plaques involve the central portion of the face and ears. These changes, with absent eyebrows and eyelashes (Fig. 27-25), and furrows about the mouth and chin, give the children a unique facies. Occasionally, hairs may demonstrate bright and dark bands with polarized microscopy, as seen in trichothiodystrophy. Some kindreds lack deafness. The disorder is related to missense mutations in the *GJB2* gene that encodes connexin-26 (Cx26). Most cases are sporadic.

Isotretinoin treatment may exacerbate and promote corneal vascularization. Treatment with acitretin has been reported to clear the hyperkeratotic ichthyotic lesions with little effect on the cornea or hearing. Cyclosporine A eye drops have been used to treat corneal neovascularization.

De Raeve L, et al: Trichothiodystrophy-like hair abnormalities in a child with keratitis ichthyosis deafness syndrome. Pediatr Dermatol 2008 Jul–Aug; 25(4):466–469.

Mazereeuw-Hautier J, et al: Keratitis-ichthyosis-deafness syndrome: disease expression and spectrum of connexin 26 (*GJB2*) mutations in 14 patients. Br J Dermatol 2007 May; 156(5):1015–1019.

Nemoto-Hasebe I, et al: Keratitis-ichthyosis-deafness syndrome lacking subjective hearing impairment. Acta Derm Venereol 2008; 88(4):406–408.

Congenital hemidysplasia with ichthyosiform erythroderma and limb defects syndrome

Present at birth, congenital hemidysplasia with ichthyosiform erythroderma and limb defects (CHILD) syndrome is characterized by unilateral inflammatory epidermal nevi and ipsilateral limb hypoplasia or limb defects (Fig. 27-26). Features may vary widely, from complete absence of an extremity to defects of internal organs involving the musculoskeletal, cardiovascular, or central nervous systems. Biopsy may demonstrate abnormal lamellar granules in the upper stratum spinosum. The condition is believed to be X-linked dominant and lethal in hemizygous males. Survival in males has been reported as a result of mosaicism. In females, Lyonization may produce cutaneous patterns following the lines of Blaschko, similar to incontinentia pigmenti or X-linked dominant chondrodysplasia. The pathogenesis is related to mutations in the *NSDHL* gene that is localized at Xq28 and involved in cholesterol metabolism. When unilateral epidermal nevi show features of verruciform xanthoma, CHILD syndrome should be suspected. The CHILD nevus is distinguished by ptychotropism (flexural involvement), waxy yellowish scaling, lateralization showing both diffuse and linear involvement, and the presence of foamy macrophages in the dermal papillae.

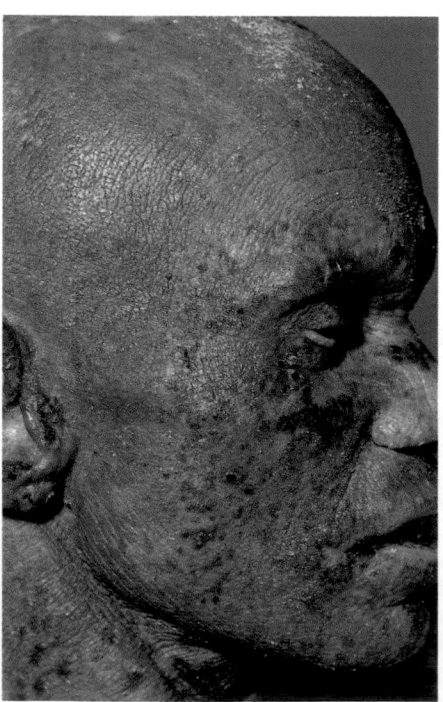

Fig. 27-25 KID syndrome.

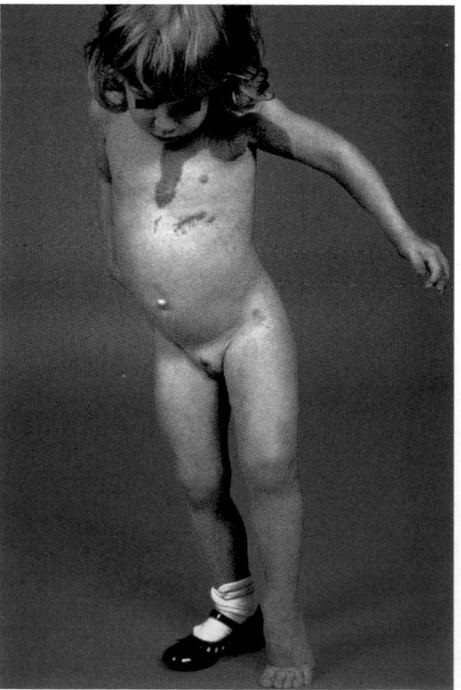

Fig. 27-26 CHILD syndrome, left hand has a bony defect.

Ishibashi M, et al: Abnormal lamellar granules in a case of CHILD syndrome. J Cutan Pathol 2006 Jun; 33(6):447–453.

Kim CA, et al: CHILD syndrome caused by a deletion of exons 6–8 of the *NSDHL* gene. Dermatology 2005; 211(2):155–158.

Erythrokeratodermia variabilis

Erythrokeratodermia variabilis, also called erythrokeratodermia figurata variabilis, and Mendes da Costa-type erythrokeratodermia, is a rare autosomal-dominant disorder characterized by erythematous patches and hyperkeratotic plaques of sparse but generalized distribution. The erythematous patches may assume bizarre geographic configurations that are sharply demarcated (Fig. 27-27). Over time, they change their shape or size, or involute completely. The keratotic plaques are reddish-brown, often polycyclic, and fixed in location. The extensor surfaces of the limbs, buttocks, axillae, groins, and face are most often involved. Approximately 50% of patients display a palmoplantar keratoderma associated with peeling. Hair, nails, and mucous membranes are spared.

The onset of the condition is shortly after birth or, rarely, at birth, or in early adult life. There may be some improvement with age, particularly after menopause. Exacerbations have been seen during pregnancy. The figurate erythematous component may be accentuated by exposure to heat, cold, or wind. Emotional upsets may also be a factor.

The gene has been mapped to 1p34–p35, the gene *GJB3* coding for a gap junction protein α-4 (connexin 31). Histologically, there is hyperkeratosis and parakeratosis, and a diminished granular layer. Acanthosis may occur. Ultrastructurally, epidermal keratinosomes are diminished.

Systemic retinoids such as acitretin or isotretinoin can restore the deficient keratinosomes and partially clear the hyperkeratotic plaques. The disease often relapses when therapy is discontinued. Urea, salicylic acid, and lactic acid have proved useful for the hyperkeratotic plaques.

Schnichels M, et al: The connexin31 F137L mutant mouse as a model for the human skin disease erythrokeratodermia variabilis (EKV). Hum Mol Genet 2007 May 15; 16(10):1216–1224.

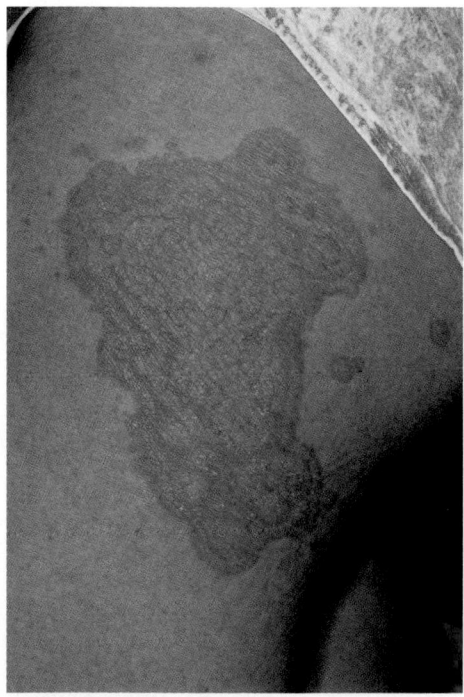

Fig. 27-27 Erythrokeratoderma variabilis.

Stănescu L, et al: Erythrokeratodermia variabilis variant with circumscribed variable erythema and periorificial fixed Bazex Dupré erythema. Rom J Morphol Embryol 2007; 48(4):443–447.

Progressive symmetric erythrokeratodermia

Progressive symmetric erythrokeratodermia (erythrokeratodermia progressiva symmetrica) is a rare, autosomal-dominantly inherited disorder that manifests soon after birth with erythematous, hyperkeratotic plaques that are symmetrically distributed on the extremities, buttocks, and face, sparing the trunk. Palmoplantar keratoderma may be present. The lesions may regress at puberty. Occipital alopecia, oligodontia, and severe caries have been reported. The cause in one kindred was related to an insertion mutation in the loricrin gene. A novel locus has been identified—21q11.2–21q21.2 Topical treatments, including keratolytics, corticosteroids, and retinoids, have had variable success.

Bongiorno MR, et al: Progressive symmetric erythrokeratodermia associated with oligodontia, severe caries, disturbed hair growth and ectopic nail: a new syndrome? Dermatology 2008 Sep 18; 217(4):347–350.

Cui Y, et al: Identification of a novel locus for progressive symmetric erythrokeratodermia to a 19.02-cM interval at 21q11.2–21q21.2. J Invest Dermatol 2006 Sep; 126(9):2136–2139 (Epub 2006).

Acquired ichthyosis

Ichthyosis clinically similar to ichthyosis vulgaris may develop in patients with several systemic diseases. Acquired ichthyosis has been reported with Hodgkin disease, and may be a presenting symptom. It has also occurred in non-Hodgkin lymphoma, mycosis fungoides, multiple myeloma, and carcinomatosis. In hypothyroidism, patients may develop fine scaling of the trunk and extremities, as well as carotenemia and diffuse alopecia. Characteristic ichthyosiform lesions may develop in patients with sarcoidosis, particularly over the lower extremities. Biopsy of the lesion will often show granulomas. Ichthyosiform changes have also been reported in patients with Hansen's disease, nutritional deficiency, acquired immune deficiency syndrome (AIDS), human T-cell lymphotropic virus infection, lupus erythematosus, and dermatomyositis. Drug-induced ichthyosis may occur with nicotinic acid, statins, triparanol, and butyrophenones.

Sparsa A, et al: Acquired ichthyosis with pravastatin. J Eur Acad Dermatol Venereol 2007 Apr; 21(4):549–550.

Pityriasis rotunda

Pityriasis rotunda (pityriasis circinata) manifests as perfectly circular scaly patches on the torso and proximal portions of the extremities (Fig. 27-28). The scale is adherent and resembles that of icthyosis vulgaris. There is a strong ethnic predisposition, with a preponderance of reports in black persons, Japanese, Koreans, and Italians. Some cases are associated with systemic illnesses, especially in darker-skinned patients. Associated illnesses include tuberculosis, other pulmonary disorders, liver disease, malnutrition, leukemia, lymphoma, and carcinoma of the esophagus or stomach. Familial cases with autosomal-dominant transmission have also been described.

Two forms of the disease occur. Type I is found in black or Asian persons, usually has fewer than 30 hyperpigmented lesions, is nonfamilial, and may be associated with systemic disease. Type II disease occurs in white persons, has larger numbers of hypopigmented lesions, is often familial, and usually is not associated with internal disease.

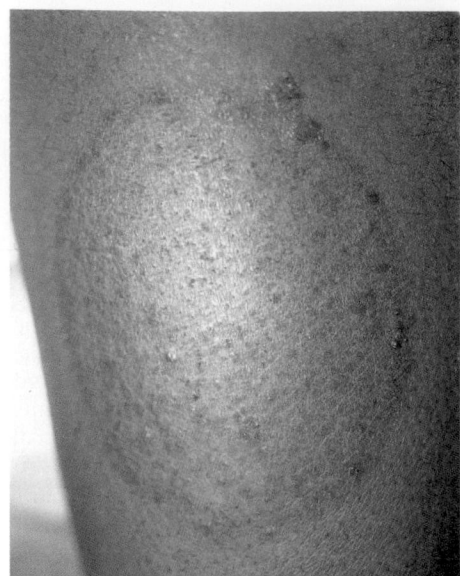

Fig. 27-28 Pityriasis rotunda.

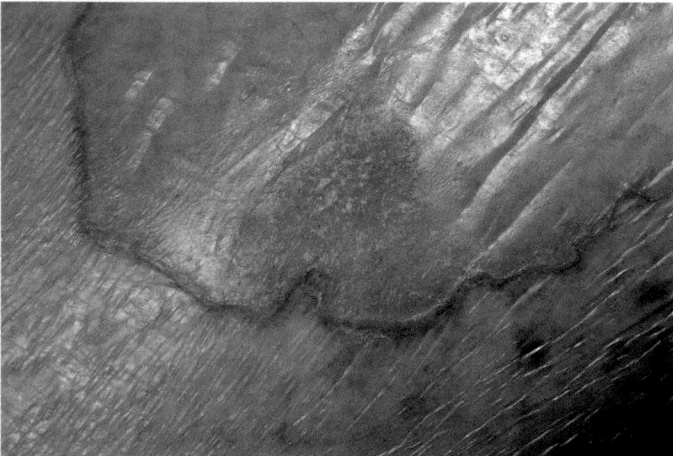

Fig. 27-29 Porokeratosis with keratotic ridge. (Courtesy of Curt Samlaska, MD)

The differential diagnosis includes tinea versicolor, tinea corporis, erythrasma, Hansen's disease, fixed drug eruptions, and pityriasis alba. Some patients note a seasonal improvement during the summer, and some respond to emollients during the winter months. Low levels of steroid sulfatase have been identified in some patients and familial cases have been observed. Topical and systemic retinoids have been used successfully, but often the condition is unresponsive unless there is an underlying systemic illness that can be treated.

Friedmann AC, et al: Familial pityriasis rotunda in black-skinned patients; a first report. Br J Dermatol 2007 Jun; 156(6):1365–1367.

Yoshida Y, et al: Pityriasis rotunda with low levels of steroid sulfatase. Eur J Dermatol 2007 May–Jun; 17(3):248.

Porokeratosis

Porokeratosis comprises a heterogeneous group of disorders that are inherited in an autosomal-dominant fashion. Except for the punctate type, they are characterized by distinct clinical findings of a keratotic ridge with a central groove that corresponds to the cornoid lamella on histology (Fig. 27-29). The groove may be accentuated by the application of gentian violet followed by removal with alcohol. The dye remains in the groove. Povidone iodine has been used in a similar fashion.

Immunosuppression, ultraviolet exposure, and radiation therapy may exacerbate porokeratosis and promote the development of skin cancers within the lesions. The linear type has the greatest risk of malignant transformation. Segmental forms have been reported in a blaschkoid distribution and following radiation therapy.

Topical 5-fluorouracil (5-FU) is generally effective in destroying individual lesions. It may have to be applied under occlusion but may result in scarring. In disseminated superficial actinic porokeratosis (DSAP), where the risk of malignant transformation is very low, the risks of treatment with 5-FU must be weighed against the generally indolent course of the lesions. Sun protection, emollients, and observation for signs of malignant degeneration may be the most suitable course of action for many patients with DSAP. Other agents that have been shown to be effective for some patients with DSAP include topical vitamin D_3 analogs, diclofenac gel, and topical retinoids, including tazarotene. Salicylic acid and α-hydroxyl acids may make the lesions less noticeable. Topical imiquimod has been used for porokeratosis, including porokeratosis of Mibelli. Oral retinoids have shown efficacy, but the lesions commonly recur after treatment, and long-term treatment with these agents is impractical. Combinations of oral retinoids and topical 5-FU have been effective for refractory DSAP and porokeratosis plantaris, palmaris, et disseminata, but the side effects of treatment may be considerable. Destructive modalities must extend into the dermis and produce scarring. More superficial treatment is commonly followed by recurrence. Other effective modalities include photodynamic therapy, cryotherapy, electrodesiccation and curettage, CO_2 laser ablation, Q-switched ruby laser, fractional photothermolysis, flashlamp-pumped pulsed dye laser, frequency-doubled Nd:YAG laser, dermabrasion, and Grenz ray.

Plaque-type porokeratosis (Mibelli)

Plaque-type porokeratosis is a chronic, progressive disease characterized by the formation of slightly atrophic patches surrounded by an elevated, warty border. The lesion begins as a small keratotic papule, which spreads peripherally and becomes depressed centrally. Eventually, it becomes a circinate or serpiginous, well-defined plaque surrounded by a keratotic wall or collar. This wall is grayish or brownish, and frequently is surmounted by a tiny groove or linear ridge running along its summit. The enclosed central portion of the plaque consists of dry, smooth, atrophic skin, the lanugo hairs generally being absent when the patches occur in hairy areas. Linear or zosteriform distribution of the lesions may also occur. If the nail matrix is involved, nail dystrophy may develop. Lesions may appear during chemotherapy for malignancy, after renal transplantation, while on PUVA treatment, and in areas of chronic sun damage or chemical exposure, such as benzylhydrochlorothiazide.

Sites of predilection are the surfaces of the hands and fingers, and the feet and ankles. The disease also occurs on the face and scalp (where it produces bald patches), on the buccal mucosa (where the ridge becomes macerated by moisture and appears as a milky white, raised cord), and on the glans penis (where it causes erosive balanitis).

Histologically, the principal diagnostic changes are in the area of the cornoid lamella. This area demonstrates a column of parakeratotic keratin extending at about a 45° angle from a focus of dyskeratotic cells in the malpighian layer. The column trails behind the focus of dyskeratosis as the focus expands peripherally. The granular cell layer is absent beneath the parakeratotic column. The central portion of the lesion may demonstrate atrophy with loss of the rete ridge pattern, lichenoid dermatitis, or psoriasiform hyperplasia.

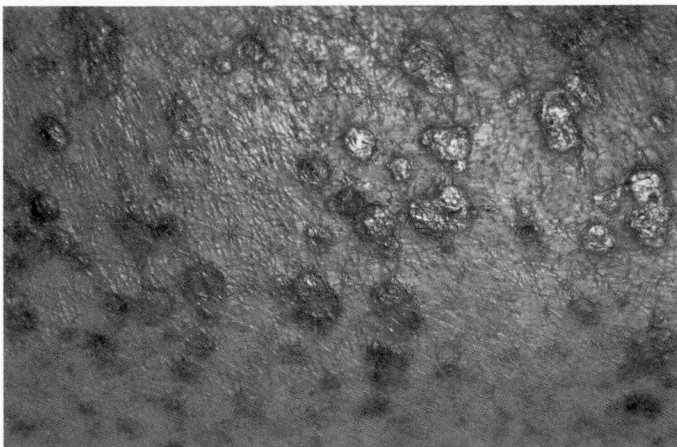

Fig. 27-30 Disseminated superficial actinic porokeratosis.

Disseminated superficial actinic porokeratosis

Disseminated superficial actinic porokeratosis (DSAP) is characterized by numerous superficial, circinate, keratotic, brownish-red macules found on sun-exposed skin (Fig. 27-30). It is more common in women. The keratotic ridge is thin and thread-like, but may be accentuated by application of gentian violet followed by removal with alcohol. A surgical skin-marking pen or cotton-tipped applicator works equally well for dye application.

The distribution of the lesions on the sun-exposed areas indicates that actinic radiation is an important factor in the pathogenesis, and new lesions have been induced by exposure at commercial tanning salons. Exacerbations occur in up to two-thirds of patients during summer. Immunosuppression is also well documented as exacerbating the disease. It has been seen in patients with AIDS, cirrhosis, and Crohn's disease. Organ transplant patients may develop DSAP. Improvement of the immunosuppression may lead to resolution of the lesions. Gene loci for DSAP have been localized to chromosomes 12q23.2–24.1 and 15q25.1–26.1, suggesting that DSAP is a genetically heterogeneous disorder.

Linear porokeratosis

Linear porokeratosis may be segmental or generalized. It may be identified during the newborn period, and when found in the segmental pattern, may follow the lines of Blaschko. Ulcerations and erosions involving the face or extremities may delay the correct diagnosis, and linear porokeratosis should be included in the differential diagnosis of ulcerative lesions in the neonatal period. This form of porokeratosis has the highest risk of developing cutaneous malignancies, including squamous cell carcinoma (Fig. 27-31), Bowen's disease, and basal cell carcinoma.

Porokeratosis palmaris, plantaris, et disseminata

In this distinctive form of porokeratosis, lesions first appear on the palms or soles, or more often both. Onset is frequently noted when patients are in their twenties. Slowly, the lesions may extend over the entire body. In porokeratotic eccrine ostial and dermal duct nevus, the presentation clinically appears like a nevus comedonicus of the palm or sole (Fig. 27-32), but histologic analysis reveals multiple coronoid, lamella-like, parakeratotic columns. In porokeratosis punctata, palmaris, et plantaris or punctate porokeratosis, lesions are limited to the hands and feet.

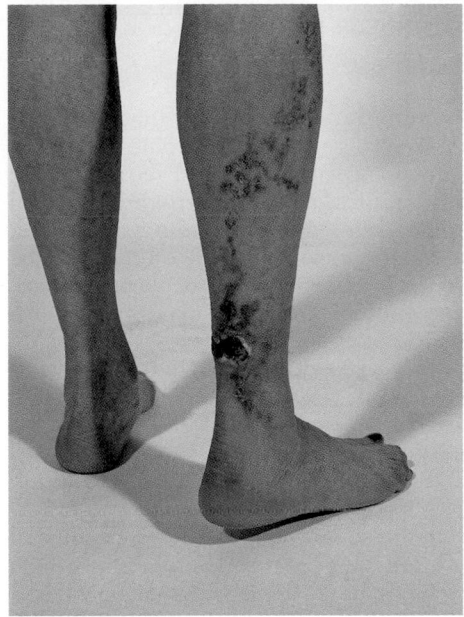

Fig. 27-31 Linear porokeratosis with squamous cell carcinoma.

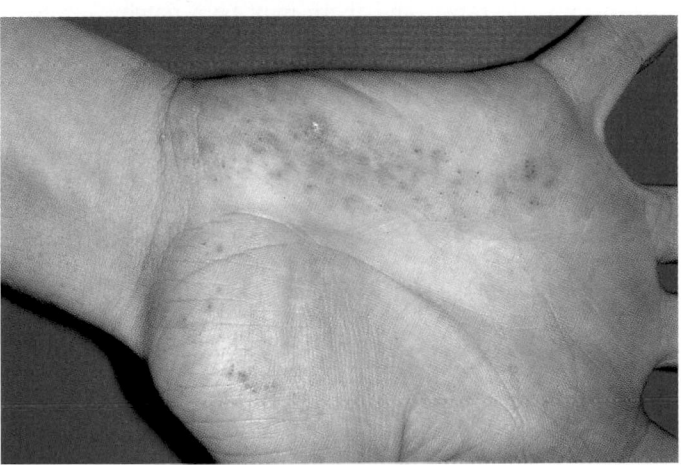

Fig. 27-32 Porokeratotic eccrine ostial and dermal duct nevus.

Porokeratotic eccrine ostial and dermal duct nevus

This is a related condition that affects the eccrine ostia and typically presents with volar keratoses.

Ahn SJ, et al: Case of linear porokeratosis: successful treatment with topical 5% imiquimod cream. J Dermatol 2007 Feb; 34(2):146–147.

Chrastil B, et al: Fractional photothermolysis: a novel treatment for disseminated superficial actinic porokeratosis. Arch Dermatol 2007 Nov; 143(11):1450–1452.

Itoh M, et al: Successful treatment of disseminated superficial actinic porokeratosis with Q-switched ruby laser. J Dermatol 2007 Dec; 34(12):816–820.

James AJ, et al: Segmental porokeratosis after radiation therapy for follicular lymphoma. J Am Acad Dermatol 2008 Feb; 58(2 Suppl): S49–50.

Kluger N, et al: Genital porokeratosis: treatment with diclofenac topical gel. J Dermatolog Treat 2007; 18(3):188–190.

Lorenz GE, et al: Linear porokeratosis: a case report and review of the literature. Cutis 2008 Jun; 81(6):479–483.

Montes de Oca-Sánchez G, et al: Porokeratosis of Mibelli of the axillae: treatment with topical imiquimod. J Dermatolog Treat 2006; 17(5):319–320.

Suárez-Amor O, et al: Coexistence of linear porokeratosis and disseminated superficial actinic porokeratosis: a type 2 segmental manifestation. Acta Derm Venereol 2007; 87(4):363–364.

Darier's disease (keratosis follicularis, Darier–White disease)

Darier's disease is an autosomal-dominantly inherited skin disorder characterized by brown keratotic papules that tend to coalesce into patches in a seborrheic distribution. Early lesions are small, firm papules, almost the color of normal skin. Each papule becomes covered with a greasy, gray–brown crust that fits into a small concavity in the summit of the papule. As the lesions grow older, their color darkens. Over the course of years, the papules grow and may fuse to form malodorous, papillomatous, vegetating growths.

The neck, shoulders, face, extremities, front of the chest, and midline of the back are sites of predilection for the disease. A frequent site for the earliest lesions is behind the ears. As the eruption spreads, the entire trunk, buttocks, genitals, and other parts of the skin may be involved. Usually, the eruption is symmetrical and widespread, but striking unilateral or segmental involvement may also occur. Cases with segmental distribution probably represent postzygotic mutations.

Vegetations appear chiefly in the axillae, gluteal crease, and groin, and behind the ears. The scalp is generally covered with greasy crusts. Lesions on the face are often prominent about the nose. The lips may be crusted, fissured, swollen, and superficially ulcerated, and there may be a patchy keratosis with superficial erosions on the dorsum of the tongue. Small white papules or pebbling may be present on the gingiva and palate. Involvement of the oropharynx, esophagus, hypopharynx, larynx, and anorectal mucosa has been reported. Punctate keratoses are frequently noted on the palms and soles. A general horny thickening of the palms and soles may be present because of innumerable, closely set, small papules. On the dorsa of the hands and on the shins the flat verrucous papules may resemble verrucae planae. The nails show subungual hyperkeratosis, fragility, and splintering, with longitudinal alternating white and red streaks, and triangular nicking of the free edges (Fig. 27-33). Esophageal involvement has been described.

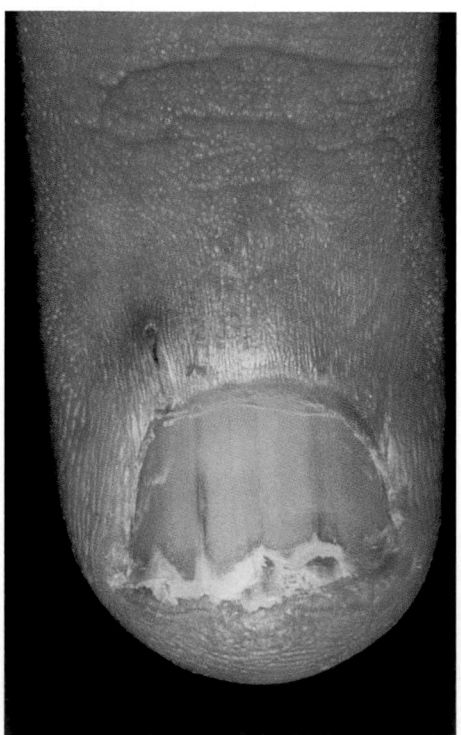

Fig. 27-33 Darier nail.

Darier's disease is usually worse in the summer. It may begin after severe sunburn, and in some patients the lesions may be reproduced with suberythema doses of UVB. Lithium carbonate has been shown to induce Darier's disease in some individuals. Disseminated cutaneous herpes simplex may be a complication of the disease.

Abnormal dissolution of desmosomal plaque proteins is seen, specifically desmoplakin I and II, plakoglobin, and desmoglein. Acantholysis occurs as a result of deficiency in the tonofilament/desmosome attachment. Ca^{2+}-dependent cell–cell adhesion molecules (epithelial cadherins) are markedly reduced on the acantholytic cells of patients with Darier's disease. The Darier gene (*ATP2A2*) has been localized to 12q23–24.1 and codes for the second isoform of a calcium ATPase of the sarco-/endoplasmic reticulum (SERCA2) pump, which transports Ca^{2+} from the cytosol into the endoplasmic reticulum. Inhibition of SERCA impairs trafficking of desmoplakin to the cell surface, contributing to acantholysis.

Histology

Darier's disease is characterized by acantholytic dyskeratosis with overlying hyperkeratosis. Abnormally keratinizing cells appear as round eosinophilic or basophilic cells (corps ronds), which often demonstrate a pale halo surrounding the nucleus. Grains are flat, deeply basophilic, dyskeratotic cells, seen most frequently in the stratum granulosum and stratum corneum. Both grains and corps ronds are separated from the surrounding cells as a result of acantholysis. Formation of a suprabasal cleft (lacuna) is noted, and may involve hair follicles as well as the surface epidermis. Dermal papillae covered by a single layer of basal cells project as villi into the acantholytic space.

Treatment

During flares, topical antibacterial agents, oral antibiotics, and short-term application of a corticosteroid may be of benefit. For localized disease, topical retinoids may be effective, but papules often occur at the periphery of the treated region. Oral retinoids are the drugs of choice for most severe cases. Cyclosporine may control severe flares, and topical sunscreens and ascorbic acid can prevent disease flares in some patients. For hypertrophic lesions, dermabrasion, laser vaporization, or excision and grafting can be considered. Photodynamic therapy using topical 5-aminolaevulinic acid produces an initial inflammatory response that lasts 2–3 weeks. In some patients, this is followed by sustained improvement. Because of the initial inflammatory response, it is only appropriate for patients who have failed most other options.

Pani B, et al: Darier's disease: a calcium-signaling perspective. Cell Mol Life Sci 2008 Jan; 65(2):205–211.

Sanderson EA, et al: Localized Darier's disease in a Blaschkoid distribution: two cases of phenotypic mosaicism and a review of mosaic Darier's disease. J Dermatol 2007 Nov; 34(11):761–764.

Stewart LC, et al: Vulval Darier's disease treated successfully with ciclosporin. J Obstet Gynaecol 2008 Jan; 28(1):108–109.

Vieites B, et al: Darier's disease with esophageal involvement. Scand J Gastroenterol 2008 Apr; 2:1–2.

Acrokeratosis verruciformis

This rare autosomal-dominant genodermatosis is characterized by numerous flat verrucous papules occurring on the backs of the hands, insteps, knees, and elbows. The papules are closely grouped and resemble warts, except that they are flatter and more localized. The verrucous lesions are identical to those in Darier's disease, and some, but not all, cases of acrokeratosis verruciformis of Hopf are caused by mutations in the *ATP2A2* gene.

Histologically, hyperkeratosis, thickening of the granular layer, acanthosis, and church spire papillomatosis characterize the disease. Available treatments are liquid nitrogen therapy, shave excision, and CO_2 laser ablation. Recurrence is common. Acitretin has been used successfully.

Serarslan G, et al: Acitretin treatment in acrokeratosis verruciformis of Hopf. J Dermatolog Treat 2007; 18(2):123–125.

Wang PG, et al: Genetic heterogeneity in acrokeratosis verruciformis of Hopf. Clin Exp Dermatol 2006 Jul; 31(4):558–563.

Pachyonychia congenita

In 1906, Jadassohn and Lewandowsky described a rare, often familial, anomaly of the nails, to which they gave the name pachyonychia congenita. It is characterized by thickened nailbeds of all fingers and toes, palmar and plantar hyperkeratosis, blistering under the callosities, palmar and plantar hyperhidrosis, spiny follicular keratoses, and benign leukokeratosis of the mucous membranes. The nail plates are extremely hard and are firmly attached to the nailbeds. The nailbed is filled with yellow, horny, keratotic debris, which may cause the nail to project upward at the free edge (Fig. 27-34). Paronychial inflammation is frequently present. Delayed onset of pachyonychia in young adulthood has been described, as has acro-osteolysis.

On the extensor surfaces of the extremities, buttocks, and lumbar regions spine-like follicular keratotic papules are found. Removal of these central cores leaves a slightly bleeding cavity. The eruption on the outer aspects of the upper and lower extremities is also follicular, resembling keratosis pilaris. This latter condition is not constant and disappears at times.

Painful friction blisters may develop on the plantar aspects of the toes or heels, or along the edges of the feet, and cases have been misdiagnosed as epidermolysis bullosa. Leukokeratosis of the tongue and oral mucosa, as well as occasional laryngeal involvement with hoarseness, may occur. This oral leukokeratosis resembles an oral white sponge nevus histologically and is not predisposed to the development of malignancy.

Pachyonychia congenita is divided into four types. Type I (Jadassohn–Lewandowsky syndrome) is the most common and is described above. Type II (Jackson–Sertoli syndrome)

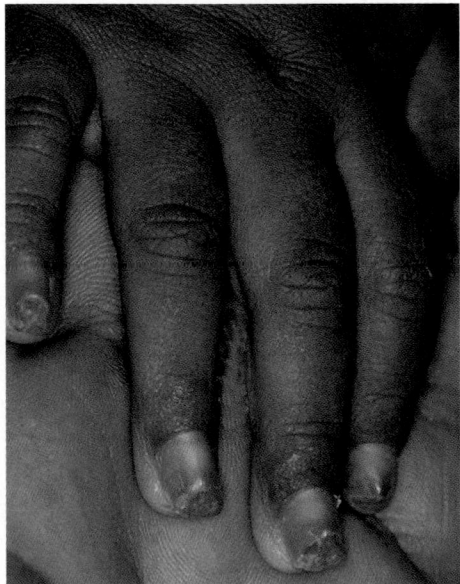

Fig. 27-34 Pachyonychia congenita.

has the same features as type I, with the additional features of natal teeth and steatocystoma multiplex. Patients with type II syndrome typically have less severe palmoplantar keratoderma, and oral lesions may be absent. Type III (Schafter–Branauer syndrome) is like type I, with the addition of leukokeratosis of the corneas. Pachyonychia congenita tarda was suggested as the name for late-onset disease (type IV). Type IV disease has been described with hyperpigmentation around the neck, waist, axillae, thighs, flexures of the knees, buttocks, and abdomen. Pigmentary incontinence and amyloid deposition are seen in biopsy specimens.

Pachyonychia congenita is usually inherited as an autosomal-dominant trait, although recessive forms have been reported. There is a genetic mutation of keratin 6a or 16 in type I disease, and of keratin 6b or 17 in type II disease. Mutant-specific small inhibitory RNAs (siRNAs) and hedgehog signaling may be important in disease expression.

Avulsion of the nails brings about only temporary relief. Vigorous curettage of the matrix and nailbed is the simplest and most effective therapy. Destruction of the nail matrix with phenol may be partially effective, but recurrence of nailbed hyperkeratosis is common. The keratoderma is difficult to treat, but topical lactic acid, ammonium lactate, salicylic acid, or urea may be of some benefit. Isotretinoin has been reported to clear the keratotic papules and the oral leukokeratosis, but not the palms or soles. Acitretin has been shown to be effective in treating the late-onset form.

Gu LH, et al: Hedgehog signaling, keratin 6 induction, and sebaceous gland morphogenesis: implications for pachyonychia congenita and related conditions. Am J Pathol 2008 Sep; 173(3):752–761.

Leachman SA, et al: Therapeutic siRNAs for dominant genetic skin disorders including pachyonychia congenita. J Dermatol Sci 2008 Sep; 51(3):151–157.

Murugesh SB, et al: Acro-osteolysis: a complication of Jadassohn–Lewandowsky syndrome. Int J Dermatol 2007 Feb; 46(2):202–205.

Zamiri M, et al: Pachyonychia congenita type 2: abnormal dentition extending into adulthood. Br J Dermatol 2008 Aug; 159(2):500–501.

Dyskeratosis congenita (Zinsser–Cole–Engman syndrome)

Dyskeratosis congenita is a rare congenital syndrome characterized by cutaneous poikiloderma, nail dystrophy, and premalignant leukoplakia. Atrophy and telangiectasia are accompanied by tan–gray, mottled, hyper- and hypopigmented macules or reticulated patches (Fig. 27-35). These lesions are located typically on the upper torso, neck, and face, although the extremities may also be involved.

The nails may be thin and dystrophic, although only ridging and longitudinal fissuring may be seen in mild cases. This is the first component of the syndrome to appear, becoming apparent between the ages of 5 and 15. The other cutaneous lesions generally follow within 3–5 years. Leukoplakia occurs mostly on the buccal mucosa, where extensive involvement with verrucous thickening may be present. The anus, vagina, conjunctiva, and urethral meatus can be involved. Malignant neoplasms of the skin, mouth, nasopharynx, esophagus, rectum, and cervix may occur in sites of leukoplakia. Other manifestations of dyskeratosis congenita include hyperhidrosis of the palms and soles, bullous conjunctivitis, gingival disorders, dental caries, hypodontia, thin tooth enamel, periodontitis, dysphagia resulting from esophageal strictures and diverticula, skeletal abnormalities, aplastic anemia, mental deficiency, and hypersplenism. In many cases, a Fanconi type of anemia develops, beginning with leukopenia and thrombocytopenia, and progressing to severe pancytopenia. Pulmonary complications include interstitial fibrosis and *Pneumocystis jirovecii* (formerly *carinii*) pneumonia.

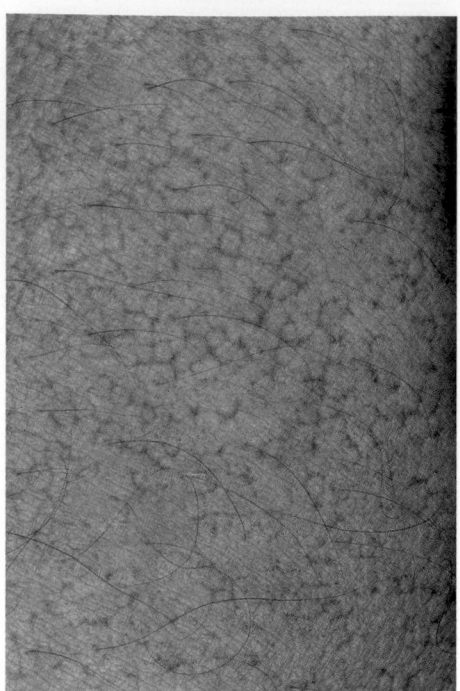

Fig. 27-35 Dyskeratosis congenita. (Courtesy of Lawrence Lieblich, MD)

Patients with the disorder have short telomeres, related to mutations in genes that encode components of the telomerase complex. These include dyskerin, *TERC*, *TERT*, *NHP2*, and *NOP10*. The genetic defect for the X-linked form is located on Xq28 and associated with the *DKC1* gene for dyskerin, a protein implicated in both telomerase function and ribosomal RNA processing. Autosomal-dominant inheritance is often associated with mutations in hTR (*hTERC*), involved in the RNA component of telomerase. Some autosomal-dominant cases have anemia and reticulated pigmentation following the lines of Blaschko. Of interest, some patients with idiopathic aplastic anemia or myelodysplastic syndrome without skin findings demonstrate *hTERC* mutations. Autosomal-recessive inheritance of dyskeratosis congenita has also been reported.

Granulocyte colony-stimulating factor and erythropoietin may provide short-term benefits in treating bone marrow failure. Bone marrow transplantation or hematopoietic stem-cell transplantation with nonmyeloablative conditioning affords the best outcomes.

Hoyeraal–Hreidarsson syndrome is characterized by intrauterine growth retardation, cerebellar hypoplasia, mental retardation, microcephaly, progressive combined immune deficiency, and aplastic anemia. The syndrome is genetically heterogeneous. Some patients demonstrate *DKC1* gene mutations and are therefore allelic to dyskeratosis congenita.

Atkinson JC, et al: Oral and dental phenotype of dyskeratosis congenita. Oral Dis 2008 Jul; 14(5):419–427.

Röth A, et al: Dyskeratosis congenita. Br J Haematol 2008 May; 141(4):412.

Vulliamy T, et al: Mutations in the telomerase component NHP2 cause the premature ageing syndrome dyskeratosis congenita. Proc Natl Acad Sci U S A 2008 Jun 10; 105(23):8073–8078.

Fanconi syndrome

Also known as familial pancytopenia or familial panmyelophthisis, Fanconi syndrome may be associated with diffuse pigmentation of the skin (hypopigmentation, hyperpigmentation, and café-au-lait macules), absence of the thumbs, aplasia of the radius, severe hypoplastic anemia, thrombocytopenia, retinal hemorrhage, strabismus, generalized hyperreflexia, and testicular hypoplasia. The syndrome is associated with increased risk of myelomonocytic leukemia, squamous cell carcinoma, and hepatic tumors. No hypersensitivity to UV light, x-rays, or chemical agents is present. Human papilloma-virus DNA is often found in the squamous cell carcinomas. Both cutaneous and pulmonary manifestations of associated Sweet's syndrome have been reported. Some patients manifest short stature, failure to thrive, absent thumbs, short palpebral fissures, and typical skin abnormalities, but no hematologic abnormalities.

The syndrome is inherited in an autosomal-recessive fashion. Complementation analysis has shown five complementation groups (FA-A, FA-B, FA-C, FA-D, and FA-E) and therefore five associated genes. The genes play an important role in hematopoiesis, and abnormal gene expression has been shown to increase apoptosis. FA-A has been localized to 16q24.3, and FA-D to 3p22.26. Chromosome patterns are frequently abnormal.

Chatham-Stephens K, et al: Metachronous manifestations of Sweet's syndrome in a neutropenic patient with Fanconi anemia. Pediatr Blood Cancer 2008 Jul; 51(1):128–130.

Dokal I, et al: Inherited aplastic anaemias/bone marrow failure syndromes. Blood Rev 2008 May; 22(3):141–153.

Ectodermal dysplasia

The ectodermal dysplasias are a clinically and genetically heterogenous group of genodermatoses in which the cardinal features are the abnormal, absent, incomplete, or delayed development during embryogenesis of one or more of the epidermal or mucosal appendages (hair, sebaceous glands, nails, teeth, or mucosal glands). Some patients with ectodermal dysplasia also have features of mucous membrane pemphigoid with mucosal anti-basement membrane zone BP-180 autoantibodies and severe bilateral cicatrizing conjunctivitis with blindness. Craniofacial reconstruction and dental implants can improve quality of life for patients with ectodermal dysplasia, but the failure rate of dental implants is high in this population.

Hypohidrotic ectodermal dysplasia (anhidrotic ectodermal dysplasia, Christ–Siemens–Touraine syndrome)

The classic triad of this disorder consists of hypotrichosis, anodontia, and hypohidrosis or anhidrosis. Febrile seizures may occur in childhood. Biopsy confirms that eccrine glands are absent or rudimentary. Prenatal skin biopsy may be diagnostic.

Patients with the disorder have facies suggestive of congenital syphilis. The cheekbones are high and wide, whereas the lower half of the face is narrow. The supraorbital ridges are prominent and the nasal bridge is depressed, forming a saddle nose. The tip of the nose is small and upturned, and the nostrils are large and conspicuous. The eyebrows are scanty and the eyes slant upward. The lips are thickened, with the upper lip particularly protrusive. At the buccal commissures there may be radiating furrows (pseudorhagades), and on the cheeks there may be telangiectases. Sebaceous gland hyperplasia may be noted on the cheeks and forehead. Absence of mammary glands and nipples has been reported.

Generalized hypotrichosis is present with thin, sparse hair on the scalp. The skin is soft, thin, dry, and smooth. There is

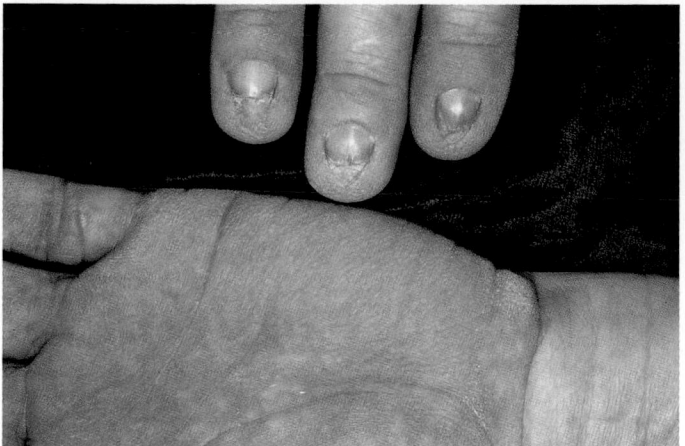

Fig. 27-36 Hidrotic ectodermal dysplasia.

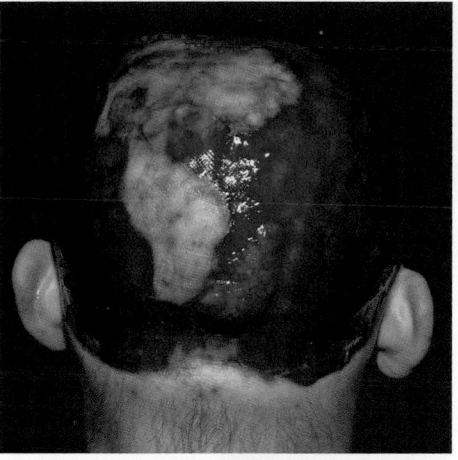

Fig. 27-37 AEC syndrome with scalp dermatitis.

partial or total anodontia, and nails may be thinned, brittle, and ridged. The teeth may be conical in shape. Mental retardation has been reported but may be a consequence of hyperthermic episodes in childhood.

The inheritance pattern is almost always X-linked recessive. Three genes, ectodysplasin (*EDA1*), EDA-receptor (*EDAR*), and EDAR-associated death domain (*EDARADD*), have been described. They are all involved in nuclear factor (NF)-κB activation. Female carriers may have segmental expression that can be demonstrated with a starch iodide test for sweating. Both autosomal-recessive and dominant modes of inheritance have been described. The gene for autosomal-dominant hypohidrotic ectodermal dysplasia has been mapped to 2q11–q13.

X-linked anhidrotic ectodermal dysplasia with immunodeficiency is caused by mutations in the gene encoding NF-κB modulator, *NEMO*, or inhibitor of κB kinase (*IKK-γ*). Stop codon mutations are associated with a severe phenotype with associated osteopetrosis and lymphedema.

Hidrotic ectodermal dysplasia

The hidrotic type of congenital ectodermal dysplasia is often referred to as Clouston syndrome. Inheritance is autosomal-dominant. Eccrine sweat glands function normally and facial features are normal. Alopecia, nail dystrophy, palmoplantar hyperkeratosis (Fig. 27-36), and eye changes, such as cataracts and strabismus, are seen. Some patients have features resembling pachyonychia congenita. Widespread poromas and palmoplantar syringofibroadenomas have been described. The defective gene has been identified as *GJB6*, encoding the gap junction protein connexin 30 on the pericentromeric region of chromosome 13q (13q11–q12.1).

AEC syndrome (Hay–Wells syndrome)

Ankyloblepharon (fusion or partial fusion of the lids), ectodermal defects, and cleft lip and/or palate constitute the AEC syndrome. It has an autosomal-dominant pattern of inheritance. Ankyloblepharon may be present at birth. Sparse hair, dental defects, cleft palate and lip, dystrophic nails, hypospadias, syndactyly, absent lacrimal puncta, stenotic auditory canals, and short stature may be present. An erosive scalp dermatitis is more likely to be observed in AEC than in other ectodermal disorders and occurs at an early age. The scalp dermatitis is often extensive (Fig. 27-37) and difficult to treat, and persists or recurs. Low-frequency ultrasound has been successful in treating scalp wounds unresponsive to other

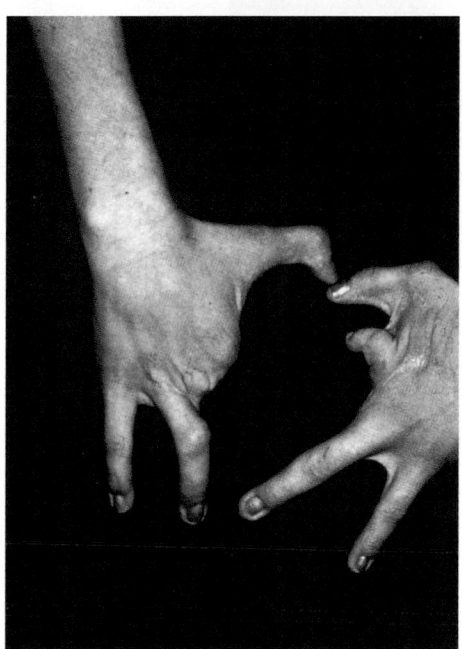

Fig. 27-38 Ectrodactyly in EEC syndrome.

measures. The syndrome is associated with mutations in the *p63* gene.

EEC syndrome

Ectodermal dysplasia, ectrodactyly, and cleft lip/palate are defining features of EEC syndrome. EEC lacks scalp dermatitis, has mild hypohidrosis, and ectrodactyly (congenital absence of all or part of a digit) (Fig. 27-38) is a prominent feature. Folliculitis with scarring may be noted during puberty. Like the AEC syndrome, EEC syndrome is associated with mutations in the *p63* gene.

Rapp–Hodgkin ectodermal dysplasia syndrome

Characteristic features of Rapp–Hodgkin ectodermal dysplasia syndrome include anomalies of hair (pili torti, pili canaliculi, alopecia, erosive folliculitis, thinning of eyebrows/lashes), cleft lip/palate, onychodysplasia, dental caries, hypodontia, craniofacial abnormality (Fig. 27-39), hypohidrosis, otitis media (hearing deficits), and hypospadias. It is usually inherited in an autosomal-dominant manner. The syndrome is

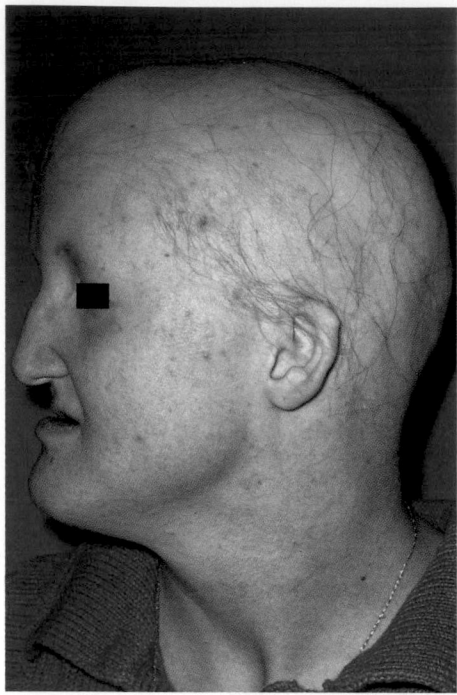

Fig. 27-39 Rapp–Hodgkin syndrome.

allelic to AEC and EEC, and mutations in the *p63* gene have been demonstrated in all three.

Ectodermal dysplasia with corkscrew hairs

Abramovits–Ackerman et al described this disorder in 27 patients from seven families who live on Margarita Island, northeast of Venezuela. Salient features include corkscrew hairs (exaggerated pili torti), scalp keloids, follicular plugging, keratosis pilaris, xerosis, eczema, palmoplantar keratodermia, syndactyly, onychodysplasia, and conjunctival neovascularization. Typical facies, anteverted pinnae, malar hypoplasia, cleft lip and palate, and dental abnormalities may also be found. Inheritance is autosomal-recessive. Anhidrosis and hypohidrosis are not features.

Odonto-tricho-ungual-digital-palmar syndrome

First described by Mendoza et al, the salient clinical features are natal teeth, trichodystrophy, prominent interdigital folds, simian-like hands with transverse palmar creases, and ungual digital dystrophy, inherited as an autosomal-dominant trait. Hypoplasia of the first metacarpal and metatarsal bones and distal phalanges of the toes may also occur.

Costello syndrome

Costello syndrome is characterized by growth retardation, failure to thrive in infancy, coarse facies, redundant skin on the neck, palms, soles, and fingers, acanthosis nigricans, and nasal papillomata. Ventricular dilation is observed in more than 40% of cases. Hydrocephalus, brain atrophy, Chiari malformation, and syringomyelia may occur. Mild to moderate mental deficiency is frequently discovered, and most patients exhibit a characteristic sociable and friendly personality.

Lenz–Majewski syndrome

Lenz–Majewski syndrome is characterized by hyperostosis, craniodiaphyseal dysplasia, dwarfism, cutis laxa, proximal symphalangism, syndactyly, brachydactyly, mental retardation, enamel hypoplasia, and hypertelorism.

CHIME syndrome

The CHIME syndrome, a rare neuroectodermal disorder, comprises colobomas of the eye, heart defects, ichthyosiform dermatosis, mental retardation, and ear defects. Other features may include facial anomalies, epidermal nevi, developmental delay, infantile macrostomia, recurrent infections, acute lymphoblastic leukemia, and duplicated renal collecting system. The inheritance is believed to be autosomal-recessive.

Lelis syndrome

The Lelis syndrome is a form of ectodermal dysplasia with acanthosis nigricans, palmoplantar hyperkeratosis, hypotrichosis, hypohidrosis, nail dystrophy, early loss of adult teeth, and mental retardation.

Acarturk TO, et al: Correction of saddle nose deformity in ectodermal dysplasia. J Craniofac Surg 2007 Sep; 18(5):1179–1182.
Baujat G, et al: Ellis–van Creveld syndrome. Orphanet J Rare Dis 2007 Jun 4; 2:27.
Bergendal B, et al: Implant failure in young children with ectodermal dysplasia: a retrospective evaluation of use and outcome of dental implant treatment in children in Sweden. Int J Oral Maxillofac Implants 2008 May–Jun; 23(3):520–524.
Birgfeld CB, et al: Midface growth in patients with ectrodactyly-ectodermal dysplasia-clefting syndrome. Plast Reconstr Surg 2007 Jul; 120(1):144–150.
Cabiling DS, et al: Cleft lip and palate repair in Hay–Wells/ankyloblepharon-ectodermal dysplasia-clefting syndrome. Cleft Palate Craniofac J 2007 May; 44(3):335–339.
Caswell D, et al: Low-frequency, therapeutic ultrasound treatment for congenital ectodermal dysplasia in toddlers. Ostomy Wound Manage 2008 Oct; 54(10):58–61.
Saw VP, et al: Cicatrising conjunctivitis with anti-basement membrane autoantibodies in ectodermal dysplasia. Br J Ophthalmol 2008 Oct; 92(10):1403–1410.
Stanford CM, et al: Perceptions of outcomes of implant therapy in patients with ectodermal dysplasia syndromes. Int J Prosthodont 2008 May–Jun; 21(3):195–200.

Pachydermoperiostosis (idiopathic hypertrophic osteoarthropathy, Touraine–Solente–Gole syndrome)

Pachydermoperiostosis is characterized by thickening of the skin in folds and accentuation of creases on the face and scalp, clubbing of the fingers, and periostosis of the long bones. The changes are especially prominent on the forehead, where the horizontal lines are deepened and the skin becomes shiny (Fig. 27-40). The eyelids, particularly the upper ones, are thickened. Likewise, there is thickening of the ears and lips, and the tongue is enlarged. The scalp may be thickened and show cutis verticis gyrata (pachydermie vorticelle). The extremities, especially the elbows, knees, and hands, are enlarged and spade-shaped. The fingers become club-shaped. The palms are rough, and the thenar and hypothenar eminences are enlarged. Hyperhidrosis is common. Hyperkeratotic linear lesions of the palms and soles may be present. These lines are rippled, resembling sand of the "wind-blown desert." Movements of the muscles may be painful. An association with gynecomastia and osteoporosis has been described.

There are inherited and acquired forms. The acquired form may occur with chronic pulmonary, mediastinal, and cardiac diseases that are associated with chronic hypoxia in peripheral tissues. Some cases have been associated with bronchogenic

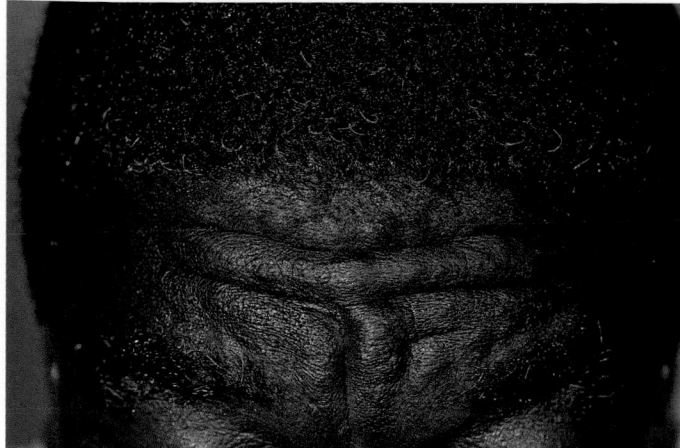

Fig. 27-40 Pachydermoperiostosis.

carcinoma. When such an association occurs, enlargement of the forehead, hands, and fingers may antedate the recognition of the tumor or may develop after the tumor is known to be present. Bronchogenic carcinoma-associated pachydermoperiostosis occurs almost exclusively in men over the age of 40, whereas inherited Touraine–Solente–Gole syndrome usually occurs as an autosomal-dominant disorder with onset in late adolescence. It is not associated with malignant disease. More prominent signs are seen in males. Autosomal-recessive inheritance with cleft palate and congenital heart defects has been described. Frontal rhytidectomy has been used to treat associated leonine facies, and bone manifestations have shown some response to oral bisphosphonate therapy and arthroscopic synovectomy.

Cutis verticis gyrata

Cutis verticis gyrata is characterized by folds and furrows on the scalp, usually in an anteroposterior direction. Most frequently the vertex is involved, but other areas may have the distinctive furrowing. There may be 2–20 folds. The hair itself is normal.

Cutis verticis gyrata has been reported primarily in males, with a male to female ratio of 6:1. Onset is usually at puberty, with more than 90% of patients developing it before age 30. The condition may be familial when it occurs as a component of pachydermoperiostosis. It has been reported to be the result of developmental anomalies, inflammation, trauma, tumors, nevi, amyloidosis, syphilis, myxedema, Ehlers–Danlos syndrome, Turner syndrome, Klinefelter syndrome, fragile X syndrome, and the insulin resistance syndrome. Biopsy findings can be normal or show thick collagen bundles and hypertrophy of adnexal structures.

Cutis verticis gyrata is frequently found in patients with mental retardation, seizures, and schizophrenia. Rarely, a cerebriform intradermal nevus may be mistaken for this disorder. In severely involved cases, excision with grafting or scalp reduction may be indicated. Surgical excision has been used successfully to improve facial involvement.

Beier JP, et al: Surgical treatment of facial cutis verticis gyrata with direct excision. J Cutan Med Surg 2007 Jan–Feb; 11(1):4–8.

George L, et al: Frontal rhytidectomy as surgical treatment for pachydermoperiostosis: a case report. J Dermatolog Treat 2008; 19(1):61–63.

Jojima H, et al: A case of pachydermoperiostosis treated by oral administration of a bisphosphonate and arthroscopic synovectomy. Mod Rheumatol 2007; 17(4):330–332.

Ukinc K, et al: Pachydermoperiostosis with gynecomastia and osteoporosis: a rare case with a rare presentation. Int J Clin Pract 2007 Nov; 61(11):1939–1940.

Aplasia cutis congenita

Aplasia cutis congenita has a predilection for the midline of the vertex of the scalp. It presents with localized absence of skin and is rarely associated with full-thickness defects of the cranium. An association with thyroid disease and thyroid medications has been noted. Rarely, multiple symmetrical defects may occur in the skin of the lower extremities. Distal radial epiphyseal dysplasia has been associated with localized aplasia cutis congenita.

The "hair collar sign" refers to a ring of long, dark hair encircling the lesion. It is commonly seen with membranous aplasia cutis, which may represent a forme fruste of a neural tube defect. Bullous aplasia cutis congenita demonstrates a fibrovascular or edematous stroma similar to that seen in encephaloceles and meningoceles, suggesting it may also be related to a neural tube defect. Focal preauricular dermal dysplasia is a form of aplasia cutis congenita not typically associated with any extracutaneous anomalies. The SCALP syndrome is a nevus sebaceus syndrome with CNS malformations, aplasia cutis congenita, limbal dermoid, and a giant congenital pigmented melanocytic nevus with neurocutaneous melanosis.

Krathen MS, et al: Focal preauricular dermal dysplasia: report of two cases and a review of literature. Pediatr Dermatol 2008 May–Jun; 25(3):344–348.

Lam J, et al: SCALP syndrome: sebaceous nevus syndrome, CNS malformations, aplasia cutis congenita, limbal dermoid, and pigmented nevus (giant congenital melanocytic nevus) with neurocutaneous melanosis: a distinct syndromic entity. J Am Acad Dermatol 2008 May; 58(5):884–888.

Adams–Oliver syndrome

Features of Adams–Oliver syndrome include severe aplasia cutis congenita of the scalp, which may involve both skin and skull ossification defects, limb defects (brachydactyly, syndactyly of toes two and three, and hypoplastic toenails), extensive cutis marmorata telangiectatica congenita, cryptorchidism, and cardiac abnormalities. Other associations include hemangiomas, retro- and micrognathia, strabismus, and atrial septal defect. It is a rare autosomal-dominantly inherited neuroectodermal syndrome.

Narang T, et al: Adams–Oliver syndrome: a sporadic occurrence with minimal disease expression. Pediatr Dermatol 2008 Jan–Feb; 25(1):115–116.

Focal dermal hypoplasia (Goltz syndrome)

Goltz syndrome is characterized by multiple abnormalities of mesodermal and ectodermal tissues. Reddish-tan, atrophic, often linear or cribriform patches are commonly present on the buttocks, axillae, and thighs (Fig. 27-41). Later, lipocytes accumulate in the lesions in a nevoid fashion, resulting in yellowish-brown nodules. The lesions are strikingly linear and often serpiginous, following lines of Blaschko. They are often narrower than typical Blaschko segments, suggesting that the genetic defect is lethal in many of the affected cells during development. Telangiectases are commonly present. Papillomas may occur around the orifices of the mouth, anus, and vulva. They may be misdiagnosed as condyloma acuminata. An early inflammatory vesicular stage has been described along with cleft lip and palate. Eighty percent of patients have skeletal defects. Bone changes most commonly involve the extremities, where there may be syndactyly, oligodactyly, and adactyly (Fig. 27-42). Scoliosis, spina bifida, and hypoplasia of the clavicle have also been reported. Forty to 50% of patients

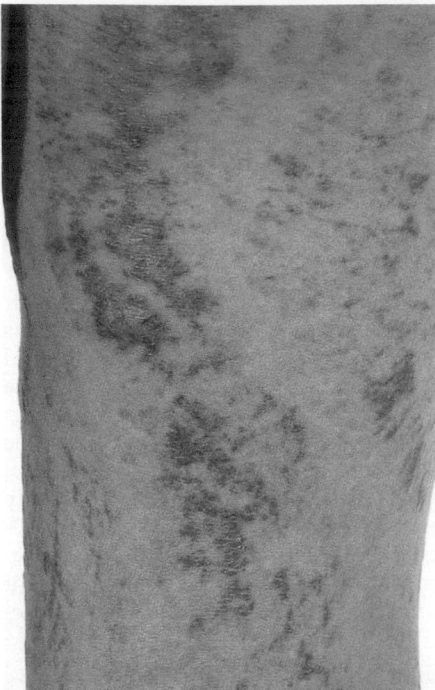

Fig. 27-41 Goltz syndrome.

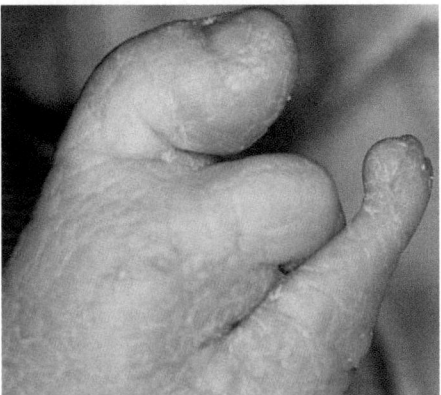

Fig. 27-42 Goltz syndrome.

have ocular or dental abnormalities, with coloboma being the most common ocular defect. Van Allen–Myhre syndrome appears to represent a severe form of Goltz syndrome with split foot and split hand anomalies. MIDAS syndrome (microphthalmia, dermal aplasia, and sclerocornea) is also an X-linked phenotype, but distinct from Goltz syndrome. It has been mapped to Xp22.3. Patients have bilateral microphthalmia with blepharophimosis and linear dermal aplasia often involving the face.

Goltz syndrome is related to defects in *PORCN*, a regulator of Wnt signaling. The large majority of patients with Goltz syndrome have been female. X-linked dominant inheritance, with lethality in males, is likely. Females are protected by X-chromosome mosaicism, identical to the situation in incontinentia pigmenti. Treatment of atrophic erythematous patches has been successful using a flashlamp-pumped pulsed dye laser.

Grzeschik KH, et al: Deficiency of *PORCN*, a regulator of Wnt signaling, is associated with focal dermal hypoplasia. Nat Genet 2007 Jul; 39(7):833–835.

Maymí MA, et al: Focal dermal hypoplasia with unusual cutaneous features. Pediatr Dermatol 2007 Jul–Aug; 24(4):387–390.

Paller AS: Wnt signaling in focal dermal hypoplasia. Nat Genet 2007 Jul; 39(7):820–821.

Petrides G, et al: Caudal appendage in focal dermal hypoplasia (Goltz syndrome). Clin Dysmorphol 2008 Apr; 17(2):129–131.

Werner syndrome (adult progeria)

Werner syndrome is a premature aging syndrome characterized by many metabolic and structural abnormalities involving the skin, hair, eyes, muscles, fatty tissues, bones, blood vessels, and carbohydrate metabolism. Cells demonstrate genomic instability. Because most of these signs are not fully manifested before the age of 30, the diagnosis is usually made in middle age. These patients usually die before the age of 50 from malignant disease or vascular accidents.

The most characteristic findings are premature aging and arrest of growth at puberty, senile cataracts developing in the late twenties and thirties, premature balding and graying, and scleroderma-like lesions of the skin. A characteristic change is the loss of subcutaneous tissue and wasting of muscles, especially the extremities, so that the legs become spindly and the trunk becomes stocky. Osteoporosis and aseptic necrosis are frequent in the small bones of the hands. The skin changes include poikiloderma, scleroderma, atrophy, hyperkeratoses, and leg ulcers. The skin has a dark gray or blackish diffuse pigmentation. A high-pitched voice and hypogonadism in both sexes are distinctive in this syndrome.

Painful callosities with ulcerations may occur around the malleoli, Achilles tendons, heels, and toes. The hair thins on the eyebrows, axillae, and pubis. The skin over the cheekbones becomes taut, producing proptosis and beaking of the nose. Cataracts develop early, and the vocal cords become thickened so that a weak, high-pitched voice ensues. Premature arteriosclerosis and sexual impotence are frequently observed. Diabetes is frequent, and areas of calcinosis circumscripta occur. Gene expression mimics normal aging.

A high rate of malignancy is associated with Werner syndrome. Uterine sarcoma, hepatoma, carcinoma of the breast, fibrosarcoma, and thyroid adenocarcinoma have occurred. Histologic changes in the skin may include atrophy of the epidermis and fibrosis of the dermis.

Consanguinity and familial incidence are encountered, suggesting a mendelian recessive mode of transmission. Werner syndrome is molecularly heterogeneous. The Werner protein confers adhesive properties to macromolecular proteins and is required for genomic stability. It belongs to the RecQ family of DNA helicases and appears to play a role in telomere maintenance, homologous recombination, and DNA repair. Mutant LMNA encoding nuclear lamin A/C is associated with atypical Werner syndrome with a more severe phenotype. Mutations in LMNA also cause Hutchinson–Gilford progeria, Emery–Dreifuss muscular dystrophy, and dilated cardiomyopathy.

Progeria (Hutchinson–Gilford syndrome)

Progeria, or Hutchinson–Gilford syndrome, is characterized by accelerated aging, dwarfism, alopecia, generalized atrophy of the skin and muscles, enlarged head with prominent scalp veins, and a high incidence of generalized atherosclerosis, usually fatal by the second decade. The large bald head and lack of eyebrows and eyelashes are distinctive (Fig. 27-43). The skin is wrinkled, pigmented, and atrophic. The nails are thin and atrophic. Most patients lack subcutaneous fat, which produces the appearance of premature senility. There are usually sclerodermatous plaques on the extremities. The intelligence remains intact. Arteriosclerosis, anginal attacks, and hemiplegia may occur, followed by death from coronary heart disease at an early age. Mutations in LMNA and mosaicism have been identified. Treatment is symptomatic: chiefly, control of diabetes mellitus and treatment of leg ulcerations.

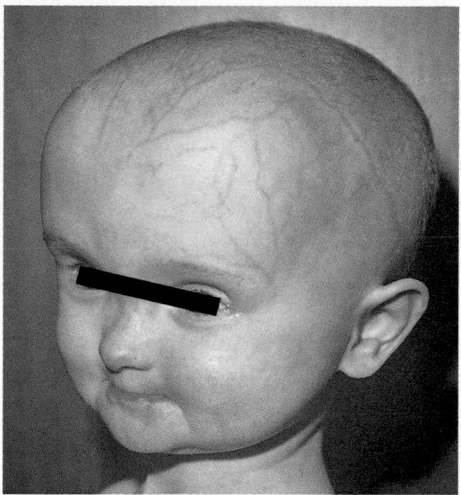

Fig. 27-43 Progeria.

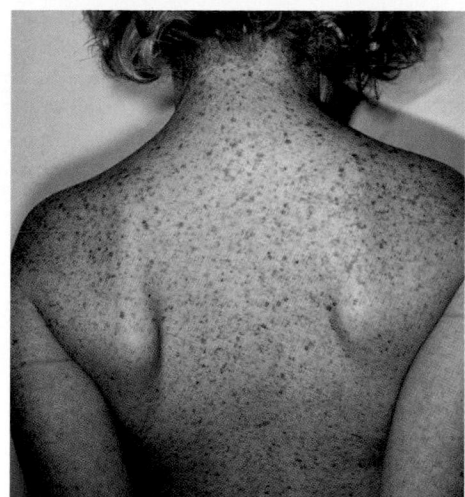

Fig. 27-44 Xeroderma pigmentosum. (Courtesy of Ken Kraemer, MD)

Davis T, et al: The role of cellular senescence in Werner syndrome: toward therapeutic intervention in human premature aging. Ann N Y Acad Sci 2007 Apr; 1100:455–469.

Kudlow BA, et al: Werner and Hutchinson–Gilford progeria syndromes: mechanistic basis of human progeroid diseases. Nat Rev Mol Cell Biol 2007 May; 8(5):394–404.

Makrantonaki E, et al: Molecular mechanisms of skin aging: state of the art. Ann N Y Acad Sci 2007 Nov; 1119:40–50.

Opresko PL: Telomere ResQue and preservation—roles for the Werner syndrome protein and other RecQ helicases. Mech Ageing Dev 2008 Jan–Feb; 129(1-2):79–90.

Sidorova JM: Roles of the Werner syndrome RecQ helicase in DNA replication. DNA Repair 2008 Nov 1; 7(11):1776–1786.

Xeroderma pigmentosum

Xeroderma pigmentosum is an autosomal-recessive disorder characterized by defective DNA thymidine dimer excision repair, extreme sun sensitivity, freckling, and skin cancer. Sun sensitivity and lentigines (Fig. 27-44) are early skin findings, with the median onset before the age of 2. Skin cancers often appear before 10 years of age, and an increase in internal cancer has been noted as well. In a study of 830 patients, 45% had basal cell carcinoma or squamous cell carcinoma, and melanoma was noted in 5%. Most of the tumors occur on the head and neck. Ocular abnormalities were found in 40% and included ectropion, corneal opacity, and neoplasms. Progressive neurologic degeneration is seen in about 20% of patients. Xeroderma pigmentosum patients in complementation group C remain free of neurologic problems. Complementation groups are defined by correction of excision repair when fibroblasts from patients in different groups are fused. A variant type with normal excision repair has also been described. Retinoids can prevent the appearance of new cancers, but side effects are significant, and a rebound in the number of cancers occurs when the drug is stopped, suggesting that the tumors are merely suppressed. Photoprotection remains essential for management. Individual tumors may be excised or destroyed with cryotherapy. Some may be treated with topical imiquimod or 5-FU. Topical application of recombinant liposomal encapsulated T4 endonuclease V repairs UV-induced cyclobutane–pyrimidine dimers and is a promising form of therapy. Gene therapy is also being pursued. Guidelines for evaluation and management from the XP Society can be found at www.xps.org. A publication from the National Institutes of Health (NIH) can be found at www.cc.nih.gov/ccc/patient_education/pepubs/xeroderma.pdf.

Xeroderma pigmentosum, Cockayne syndrome, and trichothiodystrophy are all associated with defects in nucleotide excision repair (NER). Global genome NER repairs DNA lesions throughout the genome, preventing the accumulation of mutations. Transcription-coupled NER prevents cell death caused by stalled transcription by rapidly identifying and repairing defects in the transcribed strand of DNA. Skin tumors in xeroderma pigmentosum patients have sunlight-induced mutations in *ras*, *p53*, and *ptch* genes. Mutations in the *XPG* gene give rise to the complementation group G form of xeroderma pigmentosum, as well as early-onset Cockayne syndrome. Prenatal diagnosis is possible via cultured chorionic villus cells or amniocytes.

The De Sanctis–Cacchione syndrome consists of xeroderma pigmentosum with mental deficiency, dwarfism, and gonadal hypoplasia. It occurs most often in patients in complementation group D. Mutations in the *ERCC6* gene, which also cause Cockayne syndrome type B, have been demonstrated as well.

Cockayne syndrome

Cockayne syndrome is an autosomal-recessive syndrome with sun sensitivity and neurologic degeneration. It differs from xeroderma pigmentosum in the lack of freckling and skin cancer, and in the presence of dwarfism, beaked nose, loss of subcutaneous tissue, deafness, basal ganglia calcification, failure of brain growth, and retinopathy.

Cockayne described the syndrome as dwarfism with retinal atrophy and deafness. Dermatologic features include photodermatitis with telangiectasia, atrophy, and scarring. The hands and feet are large and cyanotic. Microcephaly, sunken eyes, severe flexion contractures, dorsal kyphosis, cryptorchidism, cataracts, growth retardation, mental retardation, hypothalamic and cerebellar dysfunction, and retinitis pigmentosa with optic atrophy may be seen. There is progressive neurologic disturbance with a shortened lifespan. Dermal fibroblasts and lymphoblastoid cell lines, as well as cultured amniotic fluid cells from an affected fetus, demonstrate impaired colony-forming ability, and decreased DNA and RNA synthesis after UV light exposure (254 nm).

DNA helicases unwind DNA and are important in DNA replication, DNA repair, and RNA transcription. Mutations in XPB or XPD DNA helicase can result in xeroderma pigmentosum, Cockayne syndrome, or trichothiodystrophy. The

Cockayne syndrome complementation group A (CSA) and CSB genes responsible for Cockayne syndrome are associated with RNA polymerase. CSB protein plays a role in transcription as well as global nucleotide excision repair. Cockayne syndrome has also been associated with mutations in *XPG*.

Xeroderma pigmentosum/Cockayne syndrome complex

Some patients have skin features of xeroderma pigmentosum and neurologic features of Cockayne syndrome. Patients in complementation groups B, D, and G have presented with the complex. Mutations in the associated genes may give rise to clinical manifestations of xeroderma pigmentosum, Cockayne syndrome, or the xeroderma pigmentosum/Cockayne syndrome complex.

Trichothiodystrophy

Trichothiodystrophy is an autosomal-recessive disorder characterized by photosensitivity, ichthyosis, brittle hair, intellectual impairment, decreased fertility, and short stature (PIBIDS). A review of 112 patients noted a wide spectrum of clinical features that varied from patients with only hair involvement to those with profound developmental defects. Common features included intellectual impairment (86%), short stature (73%), ichthyosis (65%), ocular abnormalities (51%), infections (46%), and photosensitivity (42%). More than half of the patients had abnormal characteristics at birth and 19 patients died before the age of 10.

Tay syndrome is similar but lacks photosensitivity. Abnormalities in nucleotide excision repair of UV-damaged DNA are present in about 50% of those with the disorder. The UV sensitivity and defective excision repair are similar to those of xeroderma pigmentosum patients, but these patients do not experience an increased incidence of skin cancer. Two of the three described complementation groups match xeroderma pigmentosum groups B and D, with the *XPD* gene accounting for most photosensitive trichothiodystrophy. A combined xeroderma pigmentosum/trichothiodystrophy complex has been described. Patients with trichothiodystrophy without xeroderma pigmentosum do not have an increase in skin cancer formation.

The hair, with sulfur reduced to 50% of the normal value, has distinctive features under polarizing, light, and scanning electron microscopy. With polarizing microscopy, the hair shows alternating bright and dark regions that give a striking striped, or tiger tail, appearance, but the pattern may not be evident at birth. A similar pattern of bright and dark bands has been described in the keratitis ichthyosis deafness syndrome. With light microscopy, hairs from patients with trichothiodystrophy demonstrate trichoschisis (clean fractures). Trichorrhexis nodosa-like fractures may also be seen. In addition, the hair is markedly flattened and folds over itself like a thick ribbon. The hair shaft outline is irregular and slightly undulating, and the melanin granules are distributed in a wavy pattern. With scanning electron microscopy, the surface shows marked ridging and fluting, and the cuticle scales may be absent or greatly reduced.

Bath-Hextall F, et al: Interventions for preventing non-melanoma skin cancers in high-risk groups. Cochrane Database Syst Rev 2007 Oct 17; (4):CD005414.

Charles CA, et al: A rare presentation of squamous cell carcinoma in a patient with PIBIDS-type trichothiodystrophy. Pediatr Dermatol 2008 Mar–Apr; 25(2):264–267.

Cleaver JE, et al: Clinical implications of the basic defects in Cockayne syndrome and xeroderma pigmentosum and the DNA lesions responsible for cancer, neurodegeneration and aging. Mech Ageing Dev 2008 Jul–Aug; 129(7–8):492–497.

De Raeve L, et al: Trichothiodystrophy-like hair abnormalities in a child with keratitis ichthyosis deafness syndrome. Pediatr Dermatol 2008 Jul–Aug; 25(4):466–469.

Faghri S, et al: Trichothiodystrophy: a systematic review of 112 published cases characterises a wide spectrum of clinical manifestations. J Med Genet 2008 Oct; 45(10):609–621.

Horkay I, et al: Photosensitivity skin disorders in childhood. Photodermatol Photoimmunol Photomed 2008 Apr; 24(2):56–60.

Kleijer WJ, et al: Prenatal diagnosis of xeroderma pigmentosum and trichothiodystrophy in 76 pregnancies at risk. Prenat Diagn 2007 Dec; 27(12):1133–1137.

Kraemer KH, et al: Xeroderma pigmentosum, trichothiodystrophy and Cockayne syndrome: a complex genotype-phenotype relationship. Neuroscience 2007 Apr 14; 145(4):1388–1396.

Malhotra AK, et al: Multiple basal cell carcinomas in xeroderma pigmentosum treated with imiquimod 5% cream. Pediatr Dermatol 2008 Jul–Aug; 25(4):488–491.

Niedernhofer LJ: Tissue-specific accelerated aging in nucleotide excision repair deficiency. Mech Ageing Dev 2008 Jul–Aug; 129(7–8):408–415.

Rapin I, et al: Cockayne syndrome in adults: review with clinical and pathologic study of a new case. J Child Neurol 2006 Nov; 21(11):991–1006.

Stevnsner T, et al: The role of Cockayne syndrome group B (CSB) protein in base excision repair and aging. Mech Ageing Dev 2008 Jul–Aug; 129(7–8):441–448.

Wang F, et al: DNA repair gene XPD polymorphisms and cancer risk: a meta-analysis based on 56 case-control studies. Cancer Epidemiol Biomarkers Prev 2008 Mar; 17(3):507–517.

Webb S: Xeroderma pigmentosum. BMJ 2008 Feb 23; 336(7641):444–446.

Bloom syndrome (Bloom–Torre–Machacek syndrome)

Bloom syndrome is transmitted as an autosomal-recessive trait, chiefly among Jewish persons of Eastern European origin. It is characterized by photosensitive telangiectatic erythema in the butterfly area of the face and dwarfism. Telangiectatic erythematous patches resembling lupus erythematosus develop in the first 2 years of life (Fig. 27-45). Bullous, crusted lesions may be present on the lips. Exacerbation of skin lesions occurs during the summer. Other changes that may be noted are café-au-lait spots, ichthyosis, acanthosis nigricans, syndactyly, irregular dentition, lens opacities, prominent ears, hypospadias, and cryptorchidism. The stunted growth is

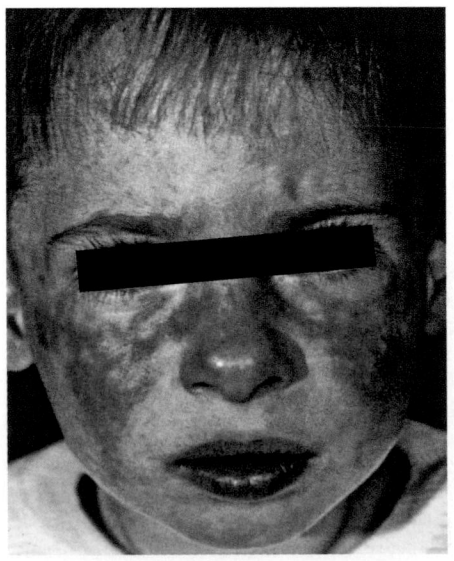

Fig. 27-45 Bloom syndrome.

characterized by normal body proportions, no endocrine abnormalities (except diabetes mellitus), and low birth weight at full term. Dolichocephaly and narrow, delicate facies are present. Immune functions are abnormal, and gastrointestinal and respiratory infections occur frequently. Cancer of all cell types and sites is increased in frequency. Leukemia, lymphoma, adenocarcinoma of the sigmoid colon, and oral and esophageal squamous cell carcinoma, as well as other malignancies, have been associated with Bloom syndrome. About one-quarter of patients under the age of 20 develop a neoplasm. Regular use of a broad-spectrum sunscreen, as well as photoprotection, is recommended.

The gene mutated in Bloom syndrome, *BLM*, codes for a RecQ DNA-helicase. BLM is localized to the nuclear bodies and the nucleolus and is critical for genomic stability. BLM interacts with WRN, the DNA helicase mutated in Werner syndrome, and is part of a large BRCA-1-containing complex containing DNA repair factors. BLM expression is highest during the S and G2 phases of the cell cycle. BLM associates with telomeres and ribosomal DNA. BLM interacts directly with ATM (the protein product of the gene mutated in ataxia-telangiectasia) and together they recognize abnormal DNA structures.

Cefle K, et al: Lens opacities in Bloom syndrome: case report and review of the literature. Ophthalmic Genet 2007 Sep; 28(3):175–178.
Holman JD, et al: Genodermatoses with malignant potential. Curr Opin Pediatr 2007 Aug; 19(4):446–454.
Thomas ER, et al: Surveillance and treatment of malignancy in Bloom syndrome. Clin Oncol (R Coll Radiol) 2008 Jun; 20(5):375–379.

Rothmund–Thomson syndrome (poikiloderma congenitale)

Rothmund–Thomson syndrome is a rare autosomal-recessive disorder. Poikiloderma begins at 3–6 months of age, with tense, pink, edematous patches on the cheeks, hands, feet, and buttocks, sparing the chest, back, and abdomen (acute phase). Sensitivity to sunlight may be manifested by the development of bullae or intense erythema after brief sun exposure. There follows fine reticulated or punctate atrophy associated with telangiectasia and reticulated pigmentation (chronic phase) (Fig. 27-46). Characteristically, the arms and legs are affected, with sparing of the antecubital and popliteal fossae. The skin lesions are characteristic. Otherwise, patients with Rothmund–Thomson syndrome may have a broad range of noncutaneous

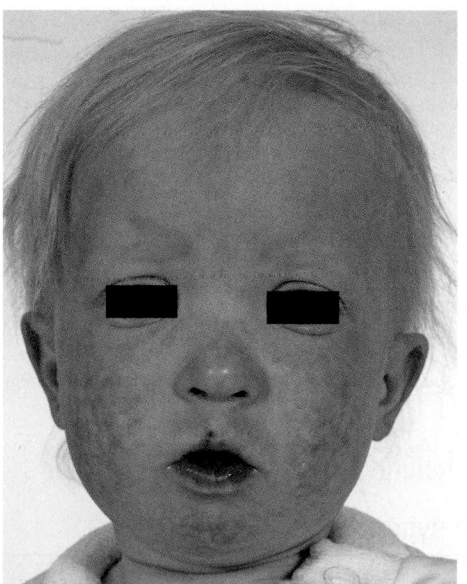

Fig. 27-46 Rothmund–Thomson syndrome.

lesions. Short stature (two-thirds of patients), small hands with radial ray defects, saddle nose, absence or sparseness of eyebrows and eyelashes (73%), alopecia of the scalp (50%), and numerous bone defects (75%) are frequently observed. Hypogonadism, dystrophic nails, and defective dentition are seen in a significant proportion of patients (25–60%). Cataracts occur in a small percentage of patients in childhood or young adult life. Associated cutaneous neoplasms include squamous cell carcinoma, Bowen's disease, basal cell carcinoma, and melanoma, but it is the risk for osteosarcoma of bone that is particularly high (>30%). Several patients with compound heterozygous mutations in *RECQL4*, a human helicase gene, have been reported. Thus, at least a subset of patients with Rothmund–Thomson syndrome has abnormal DNA helicase activity, as do patients with Werner and Bloom syndromes.

Cabral RE, et al: Identification of new *RECQL4* mutations in Caucasian Rothmund–Thomson patients and analysis of sensitivity to a wide range of genotoxic agents. Mutat Res 2008 Aug 25; 643(1–2):41–47.
Howell SM, et al: Amelanotic melanoma in a patient with Rothmund–Thomson syndrome. Arch Dermatol 2008 Mar; 144(3):416–417.
Stinco G, et al: Multiple cutaneous neoplasms in a patient with Rothmund–Thomson syndrome: case report and published work review. J Dermatol 2008 Mar; 35(3):154–161.

Hereditary sclerosing poikiloderma and mandibuloacral dysplasia

Hereditary sclerosing poikiloderma is an autosomal-dominant condition. The skin changes consist of generalized poikiloderma appearing in childhood (but not at birth), with hyperkeratotic and sclerotic cutaneous bands extending across the antecubital spaces, axillary vaults, and popliteal fossae. In addition, the palms and soles may show sclerosis resembling shiny scotch-grain leather. Aortic stenosis, clubbing of the fingers, and localized calcinosis of the skin have also been noted. There is no treatment. The cases described by Weary were subsequently reported later in life as mandibuloacral dysplasia, a rare autosomal-recessive syndrome characterized by mandibular hypoplasia, delayed cranial suture closure, dysplastic clavicles, abbreviated, club-shaped terminal phalanges, myopathy, lipodystrophy, acro-osteolysis, atrophy of the skin of the hands and feet, and typical facial changes. Mandibuloacral dysplasia must be distinguished from progeria and Werner syndrome.

A distinct subtype has been described in two generations of a South African family. The characteristics included poikiloderma, tendon contracture, and pulmonary fibrosis, with apparent autosomal-dominant inheritance. Sparse fine hairs are present on the scalp, face, and body.

Khumalo NP, et al: Poikiloderma, tendon contracture and pulmonary fibrosis: a new autosomal dominant syndrome? Br J Dermatol 2006 Nov; 155(5):1057–1061.
Lombardi F, et al: Compound heterozygosity for mutations in *LMNA* in a patient with a myopathic and lipodystrophic mandibuloacral dysplasia type A phenotype. J Clin Endocrinol Metab 2007 Nov; 92(11):4467–4471.

Scleroatrophic syndrome of Huriez

Huriez syndrome, a very rare autosomal-dominant disorder, is characterized by:

1. scleroatrophy of the hands, with sclerodactyly
2. ridging, clubbing, or hypoplasia of the nails
3. lamellar keratoderma of the hands and, to a lesser extent, the soles.

Patients with Huriez syndrome may also have multiple telangiectasias of the lips and face, and flexion contractures of the little finger. Aggressive squamous cell carcinomas occur in the scleroatrophic skin, including that of the palms and soles (13% lifetime risk, 5% mortality in affected persons). Affected patients have reduced Langerhans cells in affected skin, but normal dermal dendritic cells.

Franceschetti–Klein syndrome (mandibulofacial dysostosis)

This syndrome includes palpebral antimongoloid fissures, hypoplasia of the facial bones, macrostomia, vaulted palate, malformations of both the external and internal ear, buccal–auricular fistula, abnormal development of the neck with stretching of the cheeks, accessory facial fissures, and skeletal deformities. Patients who have the complete syndrome usually die in infancy, but patients with the abortive type may live to an old age. The syndrome is allelic to the Treacher Collins syndrome and caused by the Treacher Collins–Franceschetti (*TCOF1*) gene.

Treacher Collins syndrome

This syndrome includes midface hypoplasia with micrognathia, microtia, conductive hearing loss, and cleft palate. It is inherited as an autosomal-dominant trait and caused by mutations in the *TCOF1* gene, which encodes a protein called treacle.

Oculoauriculofrontonasal syndrome

This syndrome is sporadic in nature, although autosomal-recessive inheritance has been suggested by some authors. Features include hemifacial microsomia, microtia, ocular hypertelorism, upper palpebral colobomata, preauricular tags, lateral face clefting, and nasal clefting.

Popliteal pterygium syndrome

Pterygia or skinfolds may extend from the thigh down to the heel and thus prevent extension or rotation of the legs. Crural pterygia, cryptorchidism, bifid scrotum, agenesis of the labia majora, cleft lip and palate, adhesions between the eyelids, syndactyly, and talipes equinovarus may be present. Autosomal-dominant inheritance has been described, and the syndrome is allelic to the van der Woude syndrome.

Van der Woude syndrome

The syndrome is an autosomal-dominant craniofacial disorder characterized by hypodontia, pits of the lower lip, and cleft palate. It is associated with mutations in the *IRF6* gene. Other reported associations include natal teeth, ankyloglossia, syndactyly, equinovarus foot deformity, and congenital heart disease. Lower lip pits may be found in other congenital disorders, such as popliteal pterygium syndrome, and occasionally in orofaciodigital syndrome type I (oral frenula and clefts, hypoplasia of alae nasi, and digital asymmetry). Surgical correction is the treatment of choice.

Apert syndrome (acrocephalosyndactyly)

Apert syndrome is autosomal-dominantly inherited and is characterized by craniosynostosis and fusion of the digits (syndactyly). Patients present with synostosis of the feet, hands, carpi, tarsi, cervical vertebrae, and skull. The facial features are distorted and the second, third, and fourth fingers are fused into a bony mass with a single nail. Neurologic defects may be due in part to brain compression by the abnormal skull.

Oculocutaneous albinism and severe acne vulgaris have been reported with Apert syndrome, although some of the acneiform lesions actually represent follicular hamartomas. Mutations in the fibroblast growth factor receptor (*FGFR2*) gene are responsible for Apert syndrome, Crouzon syndrome, and Pfeiffer syndrome.

Pfeiffer syndrome

The syndrome is autosomal-dominantly inherited and consists of osteochondrodysplasia and craniosynostosis. Type 1 has normal intelligence and generally good outcome. Types 2 and 3 have severe neurologic compromise, a poor prognosis, and sporadic occurrence. Respiratory compromise may occur as a result of tracheal stenosis and fibrous cartilaginous rings.

Crouzon syndrome

The syndrome includes craniosynostosis and acanthosis nigricans. It is associated with mutations in the *FGFR2* gene. The crouzonodermoskeletal syndrome with choanal atresia and hydrocephalus is caused by mutations in *FGFR3*, a gene associated with achondroplastic dwarfism.

Carpenter syndrome

Carpenter syndrome is an acrocephalopolysyndactyly syndrome with an autosomal-recessive pattern of inheritance. Patients present with craniosynostosis and acral deformities that include syndactyly.

Whistling face syndrome

In this rare disorder, also known as craniocarpotarsal syndrome, Freeman–Sheldon syndrome, Windmill–Vane–Hand syndrome, and distal arthrogryposis type 2, the child appears to be whistling all the time. This configuration is the result of microstomia, deep-set eyes, flattened midface, coloboma, contracted joint muscles of the fingers and hands, and alterations of the nostrils. Ulnar deviation of the fingers, kyphoscoliosis, and talipes equinovarus may be present. Brain anomalies have also been reported. Autosomal-dominant, autosomal-recessive, and sporadic variants have been reported. Prenatal diagnosis can be made on ultrasound. Surgical intervention may be required for some patients.

Chen CP, et al: Craniosynostosis and congenital tracheal anomalies in an infant with Pfeiffer syndrome carrying the W290C *FGFR2* mutation. Genet Couns 2008; 19(2):165–172.

Gabbett MT, et al: Characterizing the oculoauriculofrontonasal syndrome. Clin Dysmorphol 2008 Apr; 17(2):79–85.

Horbelt CV: Physical and oral characteristics of Crouzon syndrome, Apert syndrome, and Pierre Robin sequence. Gen Dent 2008 Mar–Apr; 56(2):132–134.

Perlyn CA, et al: Craniofacial dysmorphology of Carpenter syndrome: lessons from three affected siblings. Plast Reconstr Surg 2008 Mar; 121(3):971–981.

Rice DP: Clinical features of syndromic craniosynostosis. Front Oral Biol 2008; 12:91–106.

Saadeh PB, et al: Microsurgical correction of facial contour deformities in patients with craniofacial malformations: a 15-year experience. Plast Reconstr Surg 2008 Jun; 121(6):368e–378e.

Syndromes that include abnormalities of the hair

Hallerman–Streiff syndrome

This syndrome includes characteristic "bird facies," congenital cataracts, microphthalmia, mandibular hypoplasia, hypotrichosis, and dental abnormalities. The nose is thin, sharp, and hooked, and the chin is absent. The hair is diffusely sparse and brittle. Baldness may occur frontally or at the scalp margins, but sutural alopecia—hair loss following the lines of the cranial sutures—is characteristic of this syndrome. The small face is in sharp contrast with a disproportionately large-appearing head. The lips are thin; some of the teeth may be absent while others are dystrophic, resulting in malocclusion. Nystagmus, strabismus, and other ocular abnormalities are present. Cleft palate and syndactyly may be present, representing overlap with oculodentodigital dysplasia associated with *GJA1* gene mutation.

Polyostotic fibrous dysplasia (Albright's disease)

This may present as slowly progressive lifelong unilateral hair loss: scalp, pubic, axillary, and palpebral. Sickle-cell disease is often characterized by scantiness of body and facial hair.

Cronkhite–Canada syndrome

The Cronkhite–Canada syndrome is characterized by alopecia, skin pigmentation, onychodystrophy, malabsorption, and generalized gastrointestinal polyposis.

Marinesco–Sjögren syndrome

This syndrome consists of cerebellar ataxia, mental retardation, congenital cataracts, inability to chew food, thin brittle fingernails, and sparse hair. The dystrophic hairs do not have the normal layers (cortex, cuticle, and medulla), and 30% of the hair shafts show narrow bands of abnormal incomplete keratinization. There is an autosomal-recessive type of inheritance in this syndrome and the gene has been mapped to chromosome 5q31.

Trichothiodystrophy

This is discussed above with xeroderma pigmentosum.

Generalized trichoepitheliomas

Generalized trichoepitheliomas, alopecia, and myasthenia gravis may be a variant of the generalized hair follicle hamartoma syndrome. There is a report of a localized variant of this syndrome. Histologically, there is replacement of the hair follicles by trichoepithelioma-like epithelial proliferations associated with hyperplastic sebaceous glands.

Crow–Fukase (POEMS) syndrome

This acquired syndrome is characterized by polyneuropathy, organomegaly, endocrinopathy, M-protein, and skin changes such as diffuse hyperpigmentation, dependent edema, skin thickening, hyperhidrosis, and hypertrichosis.

Cartilage–hair hypoplasia (McKusick-type metaphyseal chondrodysplasia)

This encompasses short-limbed dwarfism and abnormally fine and sparse hair in children. These children are especially susceptible to viral infections and recurrent respiratory infections. A high incidence of non-Hodgkin lymphoma, leukemia, squamous cell carcinoma, and basal cell carcinoma has been reported. A functional defect of small lymphocytes, with impaired cell-mediated immunity, may occur (Fig. 27-47).

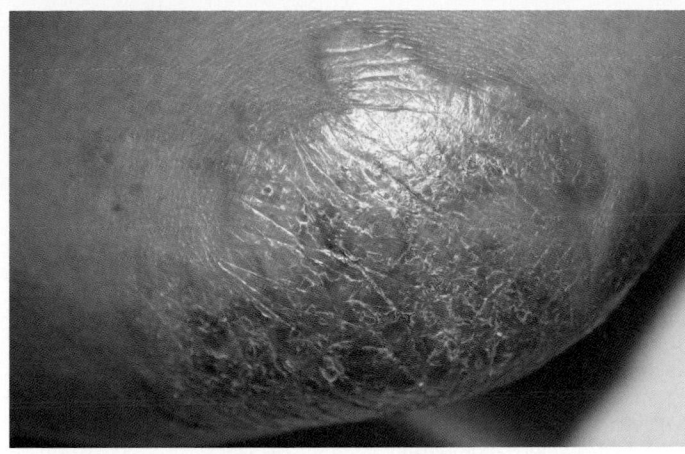

Fig. 27-47 Non-infectious granuloma in cartilage–hair hypoplasia. (Courtesy of J. Treat, MD and A Yan, MD)

Most patients are anergic to skin-test panels and have increased numbers of natural killer (NK) cells. The major mutation involves the *RMRP* gene, which encodes a component of mitochondrial RNA-processing endoribonuclease.

Trichorhinophalangeal syndrome

This is a genetic disorder consisting of fine and sparse scalp hair, thin nails, pear-shaped broad nose, and cone-shaped epiphyses of the middle phalanges of some fingers and toes. Supernumerary teeth have been reported. There is an autosomal-dominant and also a recessive inheritance type. The syndrome can result from either single base-pair mutations or deletion of the *TRPS1* gene, which encodes a GATA zinc-finger transcription factor located on chromosomal band 8q24.1.

Papillon–Lefèvre syndrome

This is characterized by hyperkeratosis palmaris et plantaris, periodontosis, and sparsity of the hair. Hyperhidrosis and other signs and symptoms begin early in life. Inheritance of this disease is of an autosomal-recessive type.

Klippel–Feil syndrome

This syndrome consists of a low posterior scalp hairline extending on to the shoulders, with a short neck, limiting movement of the neck and suggestive of webbing. The cervical vertebrae are fused. This syndrome is caused by faulty segmentation of the mesodermal somites between the third and seventh weeks in utero. Strabismus, nystagmus, cleft palate, bifid uvula, and high palate are other features. Ear abnormalities include microtia, external ear canal stenosis, and chronic ear inflammation. This syndrome occurs mostly in girls.

McKusick syndrome

Features of this syndrome include short-limbed dwarfism and fine, sparse, hypoplastic, and dysmorphic hair.

Atrichia with papules

This is a rare disorder characterized by loss of hair beginning shortly after birth and the development of cutaneous cystic papules. Mutations in the hairless gene have been identified in both humans and mice, but a similar phenotype has also been reported with a normal hairless gene but with vitamin D-resistant rickets type IIA and mutations in the vitamin D receptor gene. The cyst epithelium demonstrates keratin-15 and 17, suggesting derivation from the follicular bulge and the presence of stem cells. Both the hairless gene and the vitamin D receptor gene produce zinc-finger proteins and may have overlapping functions.

Kantaputra P, et al: Tricho-rhino-phalangeal syndrome with supernumerary teeth. J Dent Res 2008 Nov; 87(11):1027–1031.

Matesic D, et al: Cartilage-hair hypoplasia. Mayo Clin Proc 2007 Jun; 82(6):655.

Taskinen M, et al: Extended follow-up of the Finnish cartilage-hair hypoplasia cohort confirms high incidence of non-Hodgkin lymphoma and basal cell carcinoma. Am J Med Genet A 2008 Sep 15; 146A(18):2370–2375.

Yildirim N, et al: Klippel–Feil syndrome and associated ear anomalies. Am J Otolaryngol 2008 Sep–Oct; 29(5):319–325.

Keratosis pilaris

Keratosis pilaris may be limited in mild cases to the posterior upper arms, and manifests as a horny plug in each hair follicle. The thighs are the next most common site, but lesions may occur on the face, forearms, buttocks, trunk, and legs. Facial involvement may be mistaken for acne vulgaris and may leave small, pitted scars, even when the condition does not scar elsewhere. Variants of keratosis pilaris with more prominent scarring are included under the heading of keratosis pilaris atrophicans.

The individual lesions are small, acuminate, follicular papules. They may or may not be erythematous. Sometimes the keratotic plugs are the most prominent feature of the eruption, whereas at other times most of the lesions are punctate erythematous papules. Occasionally, inflammatory acneiform pustules and papules may appear.

Forcible removal of one of the plugs leaves a minute cup-shaped depression at the apex of the papule, which is soon filled by new keratotic material. The lesions tend to be arranged in poorly defined groups, dotting the otherwise normal skin in a fairly regular pattern. They are prone to appear in xerotic or atopic subjects. Autosomal-dominant inheritance has been described.

Other conditions associated with keratosis pilaris are ichthyosis follicularis, atrichia with papular lesions, mucoepidermal dysplasia, cardiofacio-cutaneous syndrome (keratosis pilaris, curly hair, sparse hair with pulmonary valve stenosis, hypertrophic cardiomyopathy, or atrial septal defect), ectodermal dysplasia with corkscrew hairs, and KID syndrome. Keratosis pilaris rubra has prominent erythema and widespread areas of skin involvement, but no atrophy or hyperpigmentation.

Treatment is difficult, but some patients respond to topical retinoids. Twelve percent ammonium lactate can produce some smoothing of the lesions but seldom results in improvement of the erythema. Topical calcipotriene is effective in some patients.

Erythromelanosis follicularis faciei et colli

Patients with the condition present with well-demarcated erythema, follicular papules, and hyperpigmentation. Itching and photosensitivity may be prominent.

Follicular atrophoderma

Follicular atrophoderma consists of follicular indentations without hairs, notably occurring on extensor surfaces of the hands, legs, and arms. Scrotal (fissured) tongue may also be found. It has been described repeatedly in association with other genetically determined abnormalities, including X-linked dominant chondrodysplasia punctata, Bazex syndrome (follicular atrophoderma type), and keratosis palmoplantaris disseminata. Bazex (Bazex–Dupré–Christol) syndrome is characterized by congenital hypotrichosis, follicular atrophoderma, multiple milia, hypohidrosis, and basal cell carcinomas. Both trichorrhexis nodosa and pili bifurcati have been described in patients with the syndrome.

Keratosis pilaris atrophicans

Keratosis pilaris atrophicans is seen in three syndromes: keratosis pilaris atrophicans faciei, atrophodermia vermiculata, and keratosis pilaris follicularis spinulosa decalvans. Keratosis pilaris atrophicans has been reported as being associated with woolly hair and Noonan syndrome. Overlap between the three entities may occur.

Response to therapy is often limited, but some success has been noted with keratolytics and retinoids. Pulsed dye laser has led to improvement in erythema, but not skin roughness.

Keratosis pilaris atrophicans faciei and ulerythema ophryogenes

Keratosis pilaris atrophicans faciei is characterized by persistent erythema and small, horny, follicular papules with onset during childhood. On involution these leave pitted scars and atrophy, with resulting alopecia. The disorder involves the eyebrows, from which it may rarely spread to the neighboring skin and even to the scalp. The term ulerythema ophryogenes is used to describe cases with involvement limited to the lateral third of the eyebrows.

Lesions may also begin on the cheeks or temples, rather than the eyebrows. The follicles become reddened (Fig. 27-48), then develop papules, and finally, follicular atrophy. In keratosis pilaris atrophicans faciei the follicular involvement extends to the cheeks and forehead.

Histologically, follicular hyperkeratosis of the upper third of the hair follicle is seen. A small depressed scar forms when the lesion heals. It may occur with atopy or woolly hair, and may be seen in Noonan syndrome and the cardio-facio-cutaneous syndrome. Transmission is autosomal-dominant.

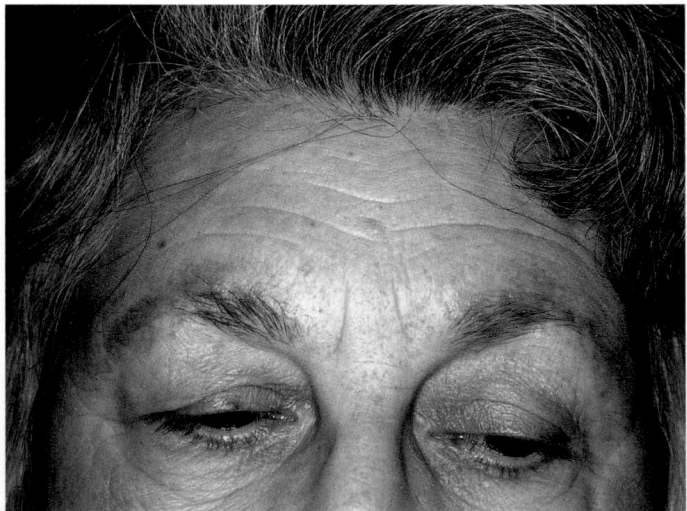

Fig. 27-48 Ulerythema ophryogenes.

Atrophodermia vermiculata

Atrophodermia vermiculata is also known as atrophoderma vermiculata, atrophodermia ulerythematosa, folliculitis ulerythematosa reticulata, and honeycomb atrophy. It is characterized by symmetrical involvement of the face by numerous, closely crowded, small areas of atrophy separated by narrow ridges, producing a cribriform or honeycomb surface. This worm-eaten (vermiculate) appearance results from atrophy of the follicles and surrounding skin. Each atrophic area is an abrupt, pitlike depression 1–3 mm in diameter. Among the ridges a few milia may be seen.

The skin covering the ridges is even with the normal skin but is contrasted with it by being somewhat waxy, firmer, and apparently stretched. The cause of the disease is undetermined but familial occurrence has been noted, and it may be associated with other diseases, such as congenital heart block, other cardiac anomalies, neurofibromatosis, oligophrenia, or Down syndrome.

Histologically, the epidermis is slightly atrophic, with diminution in size of the interpapillary projections. In the dermis the capillaries are dilated and the vessels have a moderate lymphocytic perivascular infiltration. Follicles may be enlarged, tortuous, dilated, and hyperkeratotic.

Rombo syndrome

Rombo syndrome is a rare disorder characterized by atrophodermia vermiculata, cyanosis of the hands and feet, milia, telangiectases, hypotrichosis, multiple basal cell carcinomas, and trichoepitheliomas. The associated vermicular atrophoderma produces a coarse, grainy skin texture. The syndrome is inherited in an autosomal-dominant fashion. It must be distinguished from Bazex syndrome, Rasmussen syndrome (milia, trichoepithelioma, and cylindroma), and multiple trichoepitheliomas.

Keratosis follicularis spinulosa decalvans (Siemens-1 syndrome)

In keratosis follicularis spinulosa decalvans, keratosis pilaris begins on the face and progresses to involve the scalp, limbs, and trunk. There is hyperkeratosis of the palms and soles. Cicatricial alopecia of the scalp and eyebrows is characteristic. Atopy, photophobia, and corneal abnormalities are commonly associated. Deafness, physical and mental retardation, recurrent infections, nail abnormalities, acne keloidalis nuchae, tufted hair folliculitis and aminoaciduria have also been purported associations. The disorder is genetically heterogeneous. Although inheritance in large kindreds has been X-linked recessive, X-linked dominant and autosomal-dominant inheritance have also been suggested. In one X-linked form, the defective genetic site is on Xp22.13–p22.2 in the region of the gene for spermidine/spermine N(1)-acetyltransferase.

Armour CM, et al: Further delineation of cardio-facio-cutaneous syndrome: clinical features of 38 individuals with proven mutations. J Med Genet 2008 Apr; 45(4):249–254.

Barcelos AC, et al: Bazex-Dupré-Christol syndrome in a 1-year-old boy and his mother. Pediatr Dermatol 2008 Jan–Feb; 25(1):112–113.

Bellet JS, et al: Keratosis follicularis spinulosa decalvans in a family. J Am Acad Dermatol 2008 Mar; 58(3):499–502.

Chien AJ, et al: Hereditary woolly hair and keratosis pilaris. J Am Acad Dermatol 2006 Feb; 54(2 Suppl):S35–39.

Di Lernia V, et al: Folliculitis spinulosa decalvans: an uncommon entity within the keratosis pilaris atrophicans spectrum. Pediatr Dermatol 2006 May–Jun; 23(3):255–258.

Hwang S, et al: Keratosis pilaris: a common follicular hyperkeratosis. Cutis 2008 Sep; 82(3):177–180.

Janjua SA, et al: Keratosis follicularis spinulosa decalvans associated with acne keloidalis nuchae and tufted hair folliculitis. Am J Clin Dermatol 2008; 9(2):137–140.

Marqueling AL, et al: Keratosis pilaris rubra: a common but underrecognized condition. Arch Dermatol 2006 Dec; 142(12):1611–1616.

Sardana K, et al: An observational analysis of erythromelanosis follicularis faciei et colli. Clin Exp Dermatol 2008 May; 33(3):333–336.

H syndrome

The "H syndrome" is an inherited syndrome characterized by hyperpigmentation, hypertrichosis, and indurated patches of skin involving the lower two-thirds of the body, with hearing loss, hypogonadism, hepatosplenomegaly, short stature, cardiac anomalies, and scrotal masses. The patients exhibit growth hormone deficiency and hypergonadotropic hypogonadism with azoospermia. Biopsies of involved skin demonstrate acanthosis with dermal and subcutaneous infiltration by histiocytes, plasma cells, and mast cells.

Molho-Pessach V, et al: The H syndrome: a genodermatosis characterized by indurated, hyperpigmented, and hypertrichotic skin with systemic manifestations. J Am Acad Dermatol 2008 Jul; 59(1):79–85.

Bonus images for this chapter can be found online at **http://www.expertconsult.com**

28 Dermal and Subcutaneous Tumors

The dermis and subcutaneous tissue contain many cellular elements, all capable of both reactive and neoplastic proliferation. In this chapter, proliferations derived from vascular endothelial cells, fibroblasts, myofibroblasts, smooth muscle cells, Schwann cells, and lipocytes are reviewed. Also discussed are several neoplasms of cells invading or aberrantly present in the dermis, such as metastatic cancer, endometriosis, and meningioma.

Cutaneous vascular anomalies

Clear differentiation between infantile hemangiomas and vascular malformations is helpful when planning therapy, as infantile hemangiomas involute spontaneously while vascular malformations are persistent. The biology of vascular lesions remains a fertile area for research. Blie et al reported six kindreds in which infantile hemangiomas and/or vascular malformations occurred in various family members in an autosomal-dominant fashion. This unexpected finding clinically links malformations and hemangiomas. The nature of underlying angiogenic etiologic factors awaits elucidation. PHACE syndrome is another instance where hemangiomas and vascular malformations segregate together. Pediatric patients with vascular abnormalities benefit from multidisciplinary evaluation by experts, as the diagnosis and management may be difficult.

Garzon MC, et al: Vascular malformations. Part I. J Am Acad Dermatol 2007 Mar; 56(3):353–370.
Garzon MC, et al: Vascular malformations. Part II: associated syndromes. J Am Acad Dermatol 2007 Apr; 56(4):541–564.
Goh SG, et al: Cutaneous vascular tumours: an update. Histopathology 2008 May; 52(6):661–673.

Hamartomas

Hamartomas are characterized by an abnormal arrangement of tissues normally present in a given site. This is in contrast to a nevus, which has an increase in tissue normally present at a given site, but in an orderly "normal" arrangement.

Phakomatosis pigmentovascularis

Patients with a combination of vascular malformations and melanocytic or epidermal nevi are grouped into this disorder, and are manifestations of genetic twin spotting. In the traditional classification, types I–IV have nevus flammeus. Those with a coexisting epidermal nevus have type I; if aberrant Mongolian spots are present, it is classified as type II; if a nevus spilus is seen, it is classified as type III; and when both ectopic Mongolian spots and nevus spilus are present, it is classified as type IV. The last three categories may have associated nevus anemicus. The association of extensive cutis marmorata telangiectatica congenita and aberrant Mongolian spots has been classified as type V. If only cutaneous disease is present, the patient's condition is designated subtype a; if there is associated systemic disease, subtype b is appended. A revised classification includes only three types: phakomatosis cesioflammea (blue spots and nevus flammeus), phakomatosis spilorosa (nevus spilus and a pale pink spot), and phakomatosis cesiomarmorata (blue spots and cutis marmorata telangiectatica congenita). Associated systemic findings may include intracranial and visceral vascular anomalies, ocular abnormalities, choroidal melanoma, and hemihypertrophy of the limbs. Type II is the most common (85%). Half of patients with this type have serious manifestations, such as Klippel–Trenaunay–Parkes–Weber syndrome or Sturge–Weber syndrome. Bilateral deafness and malignant hypertension have also been described. Some authors have suggested that particularly extensive and aberrant Mongolian spots may be a marker for more severe systemic involvement. Type III has been associated with multiple granular cell tumors. Most patients are Asian. Phacomatosis pigmentokeratotica may be associated with linear connective tissue nevus and pinhead-sized angioma-like lesions superimposed on a speckled lentiginous nevus.

Boente Mdel C, et al: Phacomatosis pigmentokeratotica: a follow-up report documenting additional cutaneous and extracutaneous anomalies. Pediatr Dermatol 2008 Jan–Feb; 25(1):76–80.
Fernández-Guarino M, et al: Phakomatosis pigmentovascularis: clinical findings in 15 patients and review of the literature. J Am Acad Dermatol 2008 Jan; 58(1):88–93.
Hall BD, et al: Phakomatosis pigmentovascularis: implications for severity with special reference to Mongolian spots associated with Sturge–Weber and Klippel–Trenaunay syndromes. Am J Med Genet A 2007 Dec 15; 143A(24):3047–3053.

Eccrine angiomatous hamartoma

Eccrine angiomatous hamartoma usually appears as a solitary nodular lesion on the acral areas of the extremities, particularly the palms and soles, but identical lesions also occur on areas of the body that normally have few eccrine glands. This lesion appears at birth or in early childhood, and is often associated with pain and hyperhidrosis. The lesion is a dome-shaped, tender, bluish nodule. Hypertrichosis may be present. When it is stroked or pinched, drops or beaded rings of perspiration may be seen.

Histologically, there is a combination of lobules of mature eccrine glands and ducts with thin-walled blood vessels. Excessive mucin, fat, smooth muscle, and terminal hairs may be present. The lesion has been associated with spindle cell hemangioma, arteriovenous malformation, and verrucous hemangioma. Excision may be necessary because of pain.

Galan A, et al: Eccrine angiomatous hamartoma with features resembling verrucous hemangioma. J Cutan Pathol 2007 Dec; 34 Suppl 1:68–70.
Toll A, et al: Multifocal segmental hyperthermic and hyperhidrotic naevus flammeus: a peculiar variant of eccrine angiomatous hamartoma? Clin Exp Dermatol 2007 Nov; 32(6):696–698.

Malformations

These are abnormal structures that result from an aberration in embryonic development or trauma. The abnormality may stem from an anatomic malformation or from functional alteration (as in nevus anemicus). The former are subdivided according to the type of vessel involved: capillary, venous, arterial, lymphatic, or combined. The term "capillary malformation" is sometimes used as a synonym for nevus flammeus, but is best used as a term encompassing a variety of other entities, such as nevus anemicus and cutis marmorata telangiectatica congenita.

Happle R: What is a capillary malformation? J Am Acad Dermatol 2008 Dec; 59(6):1077–1079.

Nevus anemicus

Nevus anemicus is a congenital disorder characterized by macules of varying size and shape that are paler than the surrounding skin and cannot be made red by trauma, cold, or heat. The nevus resembles vitiligo, but there is a normal amount of melanin. Wood's light does not accentuate it, and diascopy causes it to merge into the surrounding blanched skin. The patches are usually well defined with irregular edges. Rarely, it may occur in neurofibromatosis, tuberous sclerosis, or as one component of phakomatosis pigmentovascularis. In nevus anemicus the triple response of Lewis lacks a flare, but outside the nevus a flare does develop after rubbing the skin. The underlying defect is an increased sensitivity of the blood vessels to catecholamines.

Nevus oligemicus

Nevus oligemicus presents as a patch of livid skin that is cooler than the normal skin, as a result of decreased blood flow. Vasoconstriction of deep vessels is thought to be the underlying defect.

Davies MG, et al: Nevus oligemicus. Arch Dermatol 1981; 117:111.
Plantin P, et al: Nevus oligemicus. J Am Acad Dermatol 1992; 26:268.

Cutis marmorata telangiectatica congenita (congenital phlebectasia, van Lohuizen syndrome)

Cutis marmorata telangiectatica congenita is characterized by the presence of a purplish, reticulated, vascular network with a segmental distribution, usually involving the extremities. The mottling is pronounced and is made more distinct by crying, vigorous activity, and cold; at birth, it may resemble a port wine stain. Lesions usually improve by 2 years of age but may remain stable. The condition occurs sporadically and there is a female preponderance. The segmental distribution suggests mosaicism, and occasional familial occurrence could be explained by paradominant inheritance, where heterozygous individuals are phenotypically normal and the mutation is transmitted unperceived, only becoming manifest when a postzygotic mutation gives rise to loss of heterozygosity.

Associated anomalies occur in more than half of patients. Common anomalies include varicosities, nevus flammeus, ulceration, macrocephaly, and hypoplasia and hypertrophy of soft tissue and bone. Unusual associations include generalized congenital fibromatosis, premature ovarian failure, Chiari I malformation, and rectal and genital anomalies. These lesions are associated with Mongolian spots as type 5 phakomatosis pigmentovascularis. They have also been reported in association with features of the Adams–Oliver syndrome (limb abnormalities, scalp defects, skull ossification defects). High copper levels and increased elastolysis have been described.

The differential diagnosis includes residual vascular lesions from neonatal lupus and Bockenheimer syndrome.

Bockenheimer syndrome appears in childhood and shows progressive development of large venous ectasias involving one limb. No treatment is required. Many will become less noticeable with time.

Hinek A, et al: High copper levels and increased elastolysis in a patient with cutis marmorata telangiectasia congenita. Am J Med Genet A 2008 Oct 1; 146A(19):2520–2527.
Imafuku S, et al: Cutis marmorata telangiectatica congenita manifesting as port wine stain at birth. J Dermatol 2008 Jul; 35(7):471–472.
Katugampola R, et al: Macrocephaly-cutis marmorata telangiectatica congenita: a case report and review of salient features. J Am Acad Dermatol 2008 Apr; 58(4):697–702.

Nevus flammeus (port wine stain)

Nevus flammeus nuchae (stork bite) is a congenital capillary malformation present in 25% of newborns. It may persist in at least 5% of the population. It usually is a pink–red macule situated on the posterior midline between the occipital protuberance and the tip of the spine of the fifth cervical vertebra. The long axis is usually up and down. A similar-appearing midline nevus flammeus (salmon patch or angel's kiss) on the glabellar region or on one upper eyelid is present in approximately 15% of newborns. It tends to fade during childhood.

Other port wine stains occur in an estimated 3 in 1000 children. They are present at birth, and vary in color from pink to dark or bluish red. The lesions are usually unilateral and located on the face and neck, although they may be widespread and involve as much as half the body. The most common site is a unilateral distribution on the face. The mucous membrane of the mouth may be involved (Fig. 28-1). Although the surface of a nevus flammeus is usually smooth, small vascular nodular outgrowths or warty excrescences may develop over time. These lesions often become more bluish or purple with age. Several reports document multiple basal cell carcinomas occurring in adult life over sites of long-standing nevus flammeus. Rarely, nevus flammeus may appear as an acquired condition, usually with onset after trauma.

Nevus flammeus in the area supplied by the ophthalmic division of the trigeminal cranial nerve is a component of the Sturge–Weber syndrome (encephalotrigeminal angiomatosis), but the leptomeningeal component is present in only 10% of patients with all or most of the V1 branch of the trigeminal nerve involved. Leptomeningeal angiomatosis may clinically manifest as epilepsy, mental retardation, hemiplegia, hemisensory defects, and homonymous hemianopsia. Characteristic

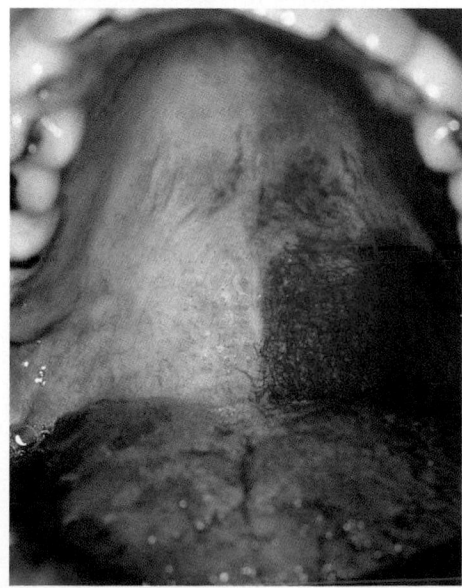

Fig. 28-1 Port wine stain.

calcifications are present in the outer layers of the cerebral cortex; these consist of double-contoured "tram tracks" that follow the brain convolutions. Ocular abnormalities, such as glaucoma, buphthalmos (infantile glaucoma, related to abnormal development of the angle formed by cornea and iris), retinal detachment, and blindness, affect approximately 50% of patients. These may be present without leptomeningeal involvement. The syndrome results from the persistence of the primitive embryonal vascular plexus that develops during the sixth fetal week around the cephalic neural tube and in the region destined to become facial skin. Normally, the plexus regresses during the ninth week, but in the Sturge–Weber syndrome it persists. Fibronectin gene expression is increased in lesional fibroblasts.

Overgrowth of soft tissue and underlying bone may occur in an affected extremity, giving rise to the Klippel–Trenaunay–Parkes–Weber syndrome. The Klippel–Trenaunay syndrome is characterized by port wine malformations, and the Parkes–Weber syndrome by deep arteriovenous malformations.

Port wine stains are components of many rare congenital disorders. Occasionally, nevus flammeus may be associated with nevus anemicus, nevus spilus, atypical Mongolian spots, or epidermal nevi. Such patients have a condition called phakomatosis pigmentovascularis. The Beckwith–Wiedemann syndrome may comprise facial port wine stain, macroglossia, omphalocele, visceral hyperplasia, occasionally hemihypertrophy, and hypoglycemia. Cobb syndrome (cutaneous meningospinal angiomatosis) is a nonfamilial disorder characterized by a port wine hemangioma or other vascular malformation in a dermatome supplied by a segment of the spinal cord containing a venous or arteriovenous malformation. Kyphoscoliosis is common, and multiple neurologic, gastrointestinal, urologic, and skeletal abnormalities may also be present. Proteus syndrome is characterized by vascular malformations including nevus flammeus, hemihypertrophy, macrodactyly, verrucous epidermal nevus, soft-tissue subcutaneous masses, and cerebriform overgrowth of the plantar surface. Roberts syndrome consists of a facial port wine stain and hypomelia, hypotrichosis, growth retardation, and cleft lip. The Wyburn–Mason syndrome consists of unilateral retinal arteriovenous malformation associated with ipsilateral port wine stain near the affected eye. This may be present in association with Sturge–Weber syndrome. The TAR syndrome is defined by congenital thrombocytopenia, bilateral absence or hypoplasia of the radius, and port wine stain. Coats' disease manifests with retinal telangiectasia and ipsilateral facial port wine stain.

Lesional skin demonstrates overexpression of vascular endothelial growth factor (VEGF) and its receptor (VEGF-R2). Occasional familial segregation of port wine stains has been noted, and a large associated gene locus, CMC1, has been identified on chromosome 5q. RASA1, a gene encoding p120–RasGAP, is found within this region and heterozygous inactivating RASA1 mutations have been found in affected families.

Histologically, port wine stains demonstrate dilatation of capillaries in the subpapillary network. Laser therapy has been used with satisfactory results, but a number of treatments are required and recurrence is common. The flashlamp pulsed dye laser has the best record of safety and efficacy. Commonly, a pulse duration of 0.45 ms is used. A study of cryogen spray-cooled laser treatment at wavelengths of 585 versus 595 nm, both with 7 mm spot size in a range of 7–10 J/cm^2, demonstrated better blanching at 585 nm. In another study, purple lesions responded best to 585 nm at 0.5 ms, while red and pink lesions showed similar results with either 585 nm at 0.5 ms or 595 nm for 20 ms. In this study, 595 nm at 0.5 ms was less effective than the other settings. Optical–thermal models predict that for vessel diameters of 40, 80, and 120 μm,

effective pulse durations should be approximately 1.5, 6, and 20 ms, respectively. Cryospray cooling and fluence can be varied to produce optimal results. For darker-skinned patients, multiple pulse stacking with multiple cryogen spurts provides better epidermal protection. Intense pulsed light has been effective in some patients resistant to multiple pulsed dye laser treatments. Long-pulse pulsed alexandrite lasers work best for hypertrophic, purple lesions, while pulsed dye lasers work best for flat, pink lesions. The variable pulse pulsed dye laser may be effective in lesions refractory to standard pulse dye laser treatment. Other modalities that have been studied include 810 nm diode and 1064 nm neodymium:yttrium-aluminum-garnet (Nd:YAG), as well as intense pulse light systems. Photodynamic therapy shows some promise.

Goldberg DJ: Treatment of port wine stains. J Cosmet Laser Ther 2010 Feb; 12(1):1.

Jasim ZF, et al: Treatment of pulsed dye laser-resistant port wine stain birthmarks. J Am Acad Dermatol 2007 Oct; 57(4):677–682.

Kelly K: Current treatment options for port wine stain birthmarks. Photodiagn Photodyn Ther 2007 Sep; 4(3):147–148.

Li L, et al: Comparison study of a long-pulse pulsed dye laser and a long-pulse pulsed alexandrite laser in the treatment of port wine stains. J Cosmet Laser Ther 2008 Mar; 10(1):12–15.

MacFie CC, et al: Diagnosis of vascular skin lesions in children: an audit and review. Pediatr Dermatol 2008 Jan–Feb; 25(1):7–12.

Stier MF, et al: Laser treatment of pediatric vascular lesions: port wine stains and hemangiomas. J Am Acad Dermatol 2008 Feb; 58(2):261–285.

Vural E, et al: The expression of vascular endothelial growth factor and its receptors in port wine stains. Otolaryngol Head Neck Surg 2008 Oct; 139(4):560–564.

Angiokeratoma circumscriptum naeviforme

This is a malformation of dermal and subcutaneous capillaries and veins, and is variably classified as a capillary or venous malformation. The vascular malformation is congenital. Over time, a verrucous component appears. The lesions are bluish-red and well defined, and occur on the lower extremities mostly, but also on the chest or forearm. Linear segmental lesions have been described. Associated spinal lesions (Cobb syndrome) have been reported. Klippel–Trenaunay syndrome has also been reported in association with verrucous vascular malformation. Superficial ablative therapy is typically followed by recurrence, regardless of whether ablation is performed by excision, laser, cryotherapy, or electrocautery. Full-thickness excision is generally effective, and may be used in combination with laser therapy.

Deep venous malformations including cavernous venous malformation

Cavernous venous malformations present as rounded, bright red or deep purple, spongy nodules. They occur chiefly on the head and neck and may involve both the skin and the mucous membranes. There is usually a deep component with a connection to the venous circulation. Calcified phleboliths and localized hyperhidrosis may occasionally be present, but the lesions are generally asymptomatic. The deep components are not amenable to laser therapy. Results of surgical resection are generally poor. Compression may be helpful. Customized, snug-fitting garments are preferable to elastic bandages.

Several syndromes are associated with venous malformations. The Bannayan–Riley–Ruvalcaba syndrome is described later in this chapter. Maffucci syndrome, also known as dyschondroplasia with hemangiomata, is characterized by multiple vascular malformations with dyschondroplasia (Fig. 28-2). The dyschondroplasia is manifested by uneven bone growth as a result of the defects of ossification, with enchondromatosis that results in multiple and frequent fractures in the period of bone growth. During the prepubertal

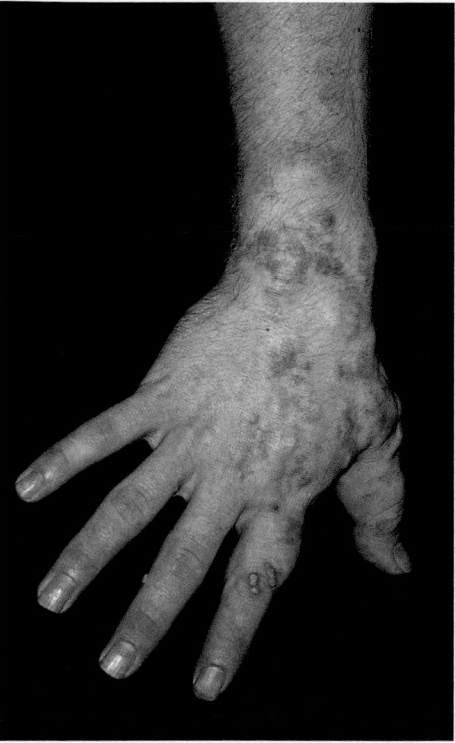

Fig. 28-2 Maffucci syndrome.

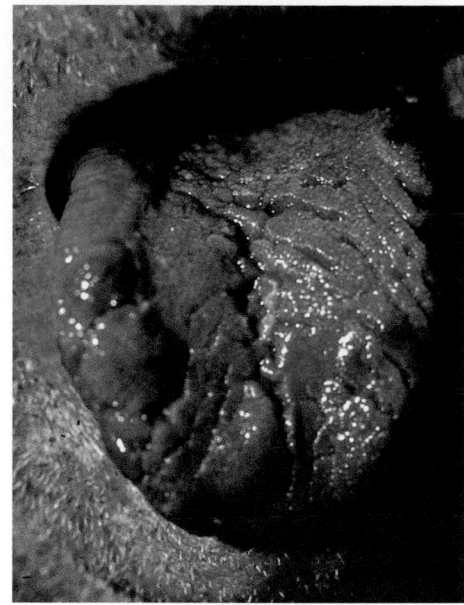

Fig. 28-3 Blue rubber bleb nevus syndrome.

years, 1–2 cm nodules appear on the small bones of the hand or foot. Later, larger nodules, the enchondromas, appear on the long bones. Much later, similar lesions appear on the trunk. Sarcomatous degeneration occurs in 50% of patients. The distribution of the lesions is mostly unilateral. Multiple venous malformations of the skin and mucous membranes are present in this nonhereditary mesodermal dysplasia disorder. Lymphangiomas may also occur. Pigmentary changes, such as vitiligo and café-au-lait macules, have been noted. In Ollier disease, the enchondromatosis is present without the cutaneous abnormalities. Human enchondromatosis has been associated with abnormalities in parathyroid hormone-related protein (PTHrP), its receptor, and the Indian hedgehog (IHH) gene. PTHrP delays differentiation of proliferating chondrocytes, whereas IHH promotes proliferation.

The blue rubber bleb nevus syndrome is characterized by cutaneous and gastrointestinal venous malformations. The skin lesions have a cyanotic, bluish appearance with a soft, elevated, nipple-like center, but deeper lesions may also occur. They can be emptied by firm pressure, leaving them flaccid. They are located predominantly on the trunk and arms. Nocturnal pain may occur and is a characteristic symptom. Gastrointestinal hemangiomas are found throughout the gastrointestinal tract (Fig. 28-3), but are numerous in the small intestines. Rupture of a lesion may produce melena. Occasionally, other organs may express venous malformations and symptomatic central nervous system (CNS) lesions have been described. This syndrome generally occurs as a sporadic condition. It may be present as an autosomal-dominant familial trait. Treatment of bleeding or painful lesions is destruction or excision. Minimally invasive surgical techniques are well suited to the treatment of numerous lesions. For patients who continue to have bleeding episodes that require blood transfusions, octreotide, a somatostatin analog known to decrease splanchnic blood flow, may be effective. ε-Aminocaproic acid has also been used.

Gorham's disease (Gorham's sign) is characterized by cutaneous and osseous venous and lymphatic malformations associated with massive osteolysis or "disappearing bones." Although multiple areas of the skeletal system may be involved, usually only a single bone is destroyed. There is complete or partial replacement of the bone with fibrous tissue. The cutaneous malformation may be the initial sign of the disease, which appears commonly in young children, usually in areas adjacent to involved bones.

Sinusoidal hemangioma is a vascular malformation that usually presents in adults as a bluish-purple nodule, less than 4 cm in diameter, on the trunk or breasts. Multiple lesions may occur and a facial location has also been reported. Histologically, it appears as a lobular, circumscribed mass with dilated interconnected vascular channels filled with blood.

A familial condition of multiple cutaneous and mucosal venous malformations that show abnormal venous channels with decreased or absent smooth muscle has been shown to be the result of an activating mutation in the receptor tyrosine kinase TIE-2 endothelial gene. It is located on chromosome 9p and is the result of a single amino acid substitution in the kinase domain of the TIE-2 receptor.

Cerebral cavernomas are vascular malformations that may be inherited in an autosomal-dominant fashion. The gene, CCM1, has been mapped to chromosome 7. Cutaneous malformations are sometimes present, including hyperkeratotic cutaneous capillary venous malformations.

Venous malformations (VM) should be distinguished from glomuvenous malformations (GM, glomangioma). VMs are usually sporadic, while GMs are frequently inherited. VM is linked to chromosome 9p21, while GM is linked to 1p21 and loss-of-function mutations in glomulin. GM can be pink at initial presentation, but evolves to blue–black with a cobblestone appearance and minimal hyperkeratosis. Involvement of an extremity is typical and the lesions are often painful if compressed. VM is an isolated mucosal or subcutaneous blue lesion that may involve muscle. The lesion often shrinks with external pressure and is typically painful in the morning due to congestion. Increased pain may be noted at puberty, during menstruation, with pregnancy, or with oral contraceptives. VM may be associated with intravascular coagulopathy. Sclerotherapy is more effective in VM than in GM. Ethanolamine oleate has been reported as a novel sclerotherapy agent. Both soft tissue injury and neuropathy have been reported after various forms of embolization or sclerotherapy. Absence of deeper tissue involvement noted with magnetic resonance imaging (MRI) is associated with a higher rate of skin necrosis and alcohol embolization.

Fayad LM, et al: Venous malformations: MR imaging features that predict skin burns after percutaneous alcohol embolization procedures. Skeletal Radiol 2008 Oct; 37(10):895–901.

Lee KB, et al: Incidence of soft tissue injury and neuropathy after embolo/sclerotherapy for congenital vascular malformation. J Vasc Surg 2008 Nov; 48(5):1286–1291.

Klippel–Trenaunay syndrome (hemangiectatic hypertrophy, angio-osteohypertrophy syndrome)

Klippel–Trenaunay syndrome (KTS) is characterized as a triad of nevus flammeus, venous and lymphatic malformations, and soft tissue hypertrophy of the affected extremity (Fig. 28-4). The lower limb is affected in approximately 95% of patients. When there is an associated arteriovenous fistula, Parkes–Weber is appended to the diagnosis.

The earliest and most common presenting sign is a nevus flammeus that is confined to the skin of an extremity. The port wine stain often stops abruptly at the midline with a sharp, linear border, but it may be patchy and extend over the buttocks and trunk, and may occasionally be seen with a bilateral or generalized distribution. Varicose veins may be present. The deeper venous malformation in this sporadic syndrome may be confined to the skin; however, it is common for the malformation to extend to muscle and bone. Venous thromboembolism has been reported with an incidence as high as 22%. In other patients, the deep venous system is hypoplastic.

The involved limb is usually larger and longer than normal. Other less frequent features include intermittent claudication, venous ulcers, increased skin temperature, diffuse hair loss, hypertrichosis, lymphedema, altered sweating, lacrimation, or salivation. Gait abnormalities are common. Hemihypertrophy of the face; cutaneous lymphangioma; varicose pulmonary, bladder, and colonic veins; and recurrent pulmonary emboli have been reported. Intradural spinal cord arteriovenous malformations, epidural hemangioma, and epidural angiomyolipoma have been reported to occur at the same segmental level as cutaneous lesions of KTS. Clinical evaluation consists of color duplex ultrasonography to evaluate the patency of the deep venous system, MRI for visualization of hypertrophic muscle and bone, arteriography when an arteriovenous fistula

is suspected, and conventional radiography of both extremities. Early venography may be performed, if the deep venous system is not hypoplastic, to determine whether there are defects that might be amenable to surgical correction. Thick-slice dynamic magnetic resonance projection angiography (MRPA) and intra-arterial digital subtraction angiography can be used to detect arteriovenous shunting in Parkes–Weber syndrome. Mutations associated with the angiogenic factor, VG5Q, have been described in KTS. A balanced translocation involving chromosomes 8q22.3 and 14q13 has also been reported.

Flashlamp-pumped pulsed dye laser treatments may be used for the nevus flammeus component. The varicosities and malformations may respond to microfoam sclerosis, endovenous thermal ablation, or surgical stripping. Edema is managed through elevation, graded compression pumps, fitted garments, and diuretics. Surgery may be performed to correct the inequality in limb length, to relieve deep venous obstruction, or to correct an associated arteriovenous fistula. Skin ulcers have responded to sunitinib. The Klippel–Trenaunay Support Group website can be found at www.k-t.org.

Gloviczki P, et al: Klippel–Trenaunay syndrome: current management. Phlebology 2007; 22(6):291–298.

Nguyen S, et al: Skin ulcers in Klippel–Trenaunay syndrome respond to sunitinib. Transl Res 2008 Apr; 151(4):194–196.

Redondo P, et al: Microfoam treatment of Klippel–Trenaunay syndrome and vascular malformations. J Am Acad Dermatol 2008 Aug; 59(2):355–356.

Arteriovenous fistulas

An arteriovenous (AV) fistula is a route from artery to vein, bypassing the capillary bed. AV fistulas may be congenital or acquired. Congenital AV fistulas occur mostly on the extremities and may be recognized, or at least suspected, in the presence of varicose veins, ulcerations, hemangiomas, and nevus flammeus. They may occur internally as a component of Osler–Weber–Rendu disease (hereditary hemorrhagic telangiectasia). Acquired fistulas are usually the result of trauma (Fig. 28-5), but may be created intentionally for hemodialysis access.

The skin over these fistulas is warmer, hair may grow faster, and the affected limb may be larger than the other; thrills and bruits may be discerned in some cases. There may be changes resulting from stasis, a vascular steal syndrome, edema, a vascular mass, increased sweating, or paresthesias. At times, reddish-purple nodules or a plaque may be present with a clinical resemblance to Kaposi sarcoma; this has been called pseudo-Kaposi sarcoma (Stewart–Bluefarb syndrome). It may

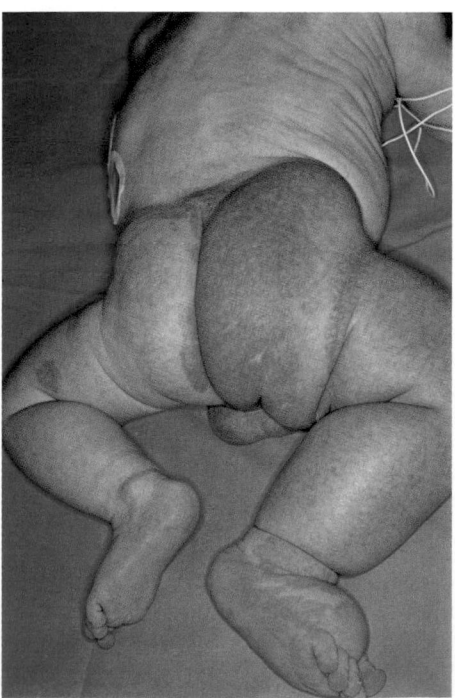

Fig. 28-4 Klippel–Trenaunay syndrome.

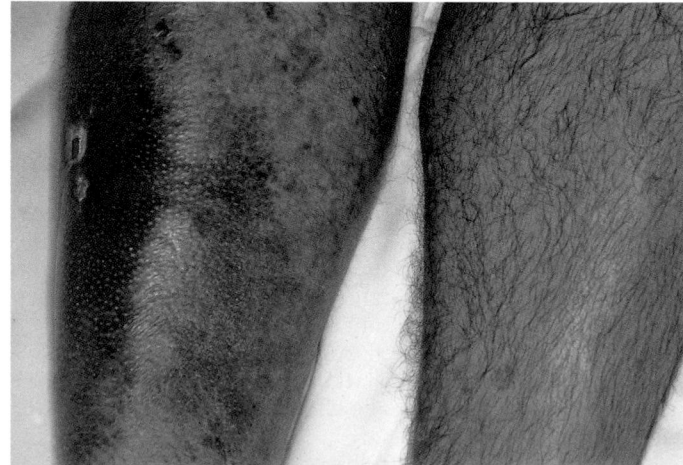

Fig. 28-5 Stasis-like changes below an acquired arteriovenous fistula.

occur because of congenital malformations, in which case a unilateral purplish discoloration of the skin over or distal to the AV anomaly begins to appear in the second or third decade of life. This type accounts for 80% of cases; the remainder are secondary to fistulas caused by trauma. Iatrogenic AV fistulas, such as those produced to facilitate hemodialysis, may also bring about skin changes, including reactive angioendothelio-matosis. Histologically, there is an increase in thick-walled vessels lined by plump endothelial cells, extravasated erythrocytes, and deposits of hemosiderin. Proliferating endothelial cells may occlude the lumen.

Cirsoid aneurysms (angioma arteriale racemosum) are uncommon congenital AV fistulas of the scalp or face. They may appear on the skin as a pulsating mass that may extend over the neck and scalp and may penetrate into the cranium, or they may simply manifest as a solitary blue or red papule in the mid-adult period.

Diagnosis of an AV fistula is established by plethysmography, thermography, determination of oxygen saturation of venous blood, or arteriography.

Treatment of traumatically induced AV fistulas by excision is curative. Because the congenital malformation variety consists of multiple small distal lesions, surgical intervention is not feasible in most cases. Color echo-Doppler ultrasonography-guided sclerotherapy with polidocanol microfoam has been used successfully in this setting. Pressure and elevation as supportive measures may limit ulceration, infection, and other secondary complications. Cirsoid aneurysms of the scalp have been treated by embolization and injection of sodium tetra-decyl sulfate.

Benito-Ruiz J, et al: Steal syndrome of the hand complicating an arteriovenous fistula. Plast Reconstr Surg 2006 Apr; 117(4):1361–1363.
Lee S, et al: Stasis dermatitis associated with arteriovenous fistula. Kidney Int 2007 Nov; 72(9):1171–1172.

Prominent inferior labial artery

The arteries supplying the lips are normally tortuous to accommodate the movements of the mouth. Howell and Freeman reported a potentially troublesome arterial anomaly of the lower lip characterized by the appearance of a pulsating papule in the lower vermilion, a centimeter or two from the oral commissure, formed by an especially tortuous segment of the inferior labial artery. A similar anomaly may involve the upper lip. Caliber-persistent labial artery may be misdiagnosed as squamous cell carcinoma, and the biopsy may produce significant bleeding. On the lip, it is best to "palpate for pulsation prior to puncture."

Acral arteriolar ectasia

Paslin and Heaton reported a man with purple serpiginous ectatic arterioles on the backs of his fingers, which appeared in the fifth decade of life.

Howell JB, Freeman RG: The potential peril from caliber-persistent arteries of the lips. J Am Acad Dermatol 2002; 46:256.
Paslin DA, Heaton CL: Acral arteriolar ectasia. Arch Dermatol 1972; 106:906.

Superficial lymphatic malformation (lymphangioma circumscriptum)

The old term for superficial lymphatic malformation was lymphangioma circumscriptum; however, this is not a tumor but rather a congenital malformation of the superficial lymphatics. A superficial lymphatic malformation presents as groups of deep-seated, vesicle-like papules (Fig. 28-6), resembling frog spawn, at birth or shortly thereafter. The lesions are usually yellowish but may be pink, red, or dark. When the papules are punctured, they exude clear, colorless lymph. The

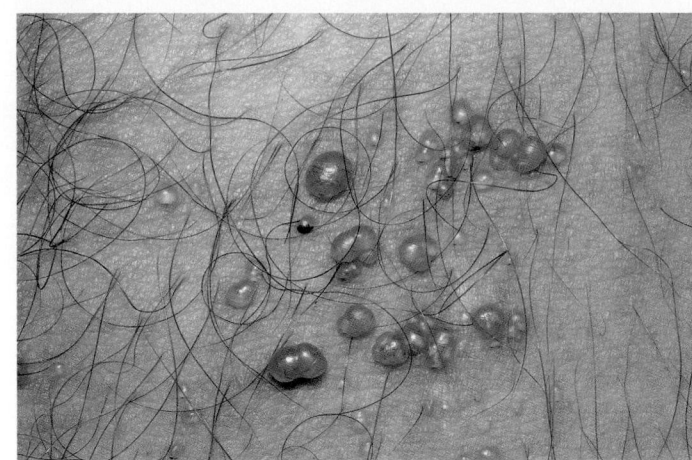

Fig. 28-6 Superficial lymphatic malformation.

papules are arranged irregularly in groups that may be interconnected by sparsely scattered lymph cysts. The entire process, however, is as a rule localized to one region. The sites of predilection are the abdomen, axillae, genitalia, and mouth, particularly the tongue. The scrotum is subject to multifocal lymphatic malformations presenting as clear, thick-walled, vesicle-like lesions. At times the surface is verrucous, in which instance the color may be brownish, and the lesions may be mistaken for warts. Lesions resembling molluscum contagiosum have also been described.

Frequently, the lesions consist of a combination of blood and lymph element, so that purple areas are sometimes seen scattered within the vesicle-like papules. The lesions are also frequently associated with a deep component that occupies the subcutaneous tissues and muscles. In the course of time, these lymphatic malformations show only slight changes.

Excision and grafting, fulguration, or coagulation is frequently unsatisfactory because of recurrences resulting from vascular connections between the surface lesions and deep-seated lymphatic cisterns. The deeper component should be evaluated by MRI or other suitable radiologic imaging procedure to delineate the extent of deep involvement before planned procedures. Vaporization with the CO_2 laser may be successful if deeper components are not present. Pulsed dye laser and intense pulse light systems have also been reported as effective. Keloid formation has been described after laser vaporization of genital lymphangiomas. Sclerotherapy has been reported as successful, and radiotherapy has been employed successfully in selected refractory cases.

Bikowski JB, et al: Lymphangioma circumscriptum: treatment with hypertonic saline sclerotherapy. J Am Acad Dermatol 2005; 53:442.
Bond J, et al: Lymphangioma circumscriptum: pitfalls and problems in definitive management. Dermatol Surg 2008 Feb; 34(2):271–275.
Heller M, et al: Lymphangioma circumscriptum. Dermatol Online J 2008 May 15; 14(5):27.
Thissen CA, et al: Treatment of lymphangioma circumscriptum with the intense pulsed light system. Int J Dermatol 2007 Nov; 46 Suppl 3:16–18.
Yildiz F, et al: Radiotherapy in congenital vulvar lymphangioma circumscriptum. Int J Gynecol Cancer 2008 May–Jun; 18(3):556–559.

Cystic lymphatic malformation

Cystic lymphatic malformations are deep-seated, typically multilocular, ill-defined, soft tissue masses that are painless and covered by normal skin. They are most common in the oral cavity and on the extremities, and have been described in Maffucci syndrome. Cystic hygromas are clinically better circumscribed, occurring usually in the neck (Fig. 28-7), axilla, or groin. The posterior neck lesions may be associated with

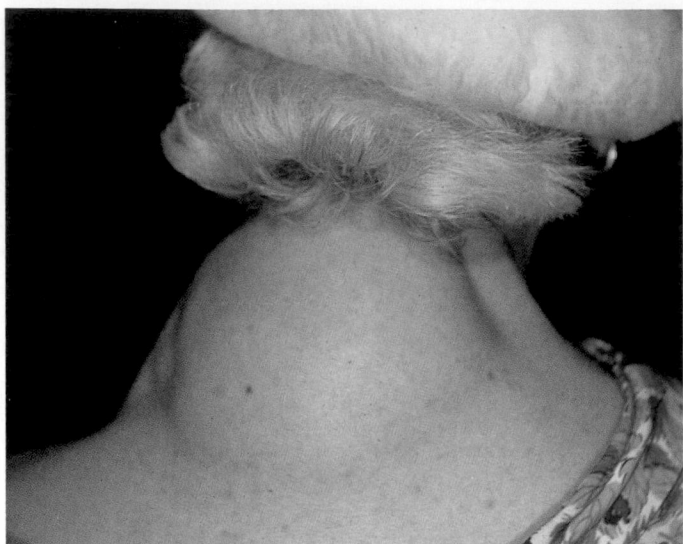

Fig. 28-7 Cystic hygroma.

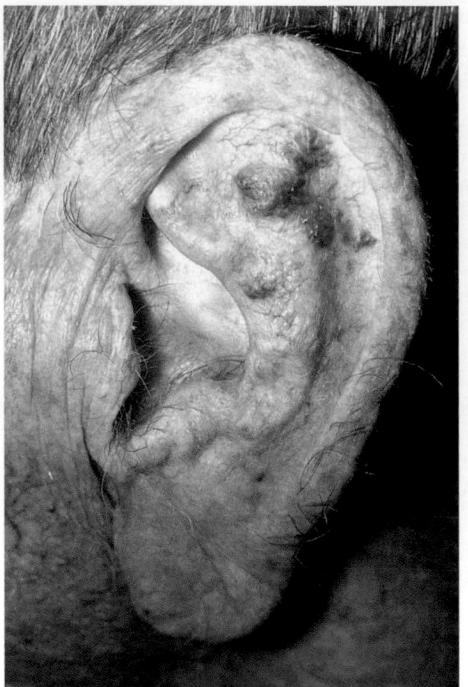

Fig. 28-8 Venous lake.

Turner syndrome, other chromosomal aneuploidy conditions, hydrops fetalis, or other congenital abnormalities. Cytogenic analysis of children born with cystic hygromas is indicated, as aneuploidy may recur in subsequent pregnancies. Transabdominal or transvaginal sonography can visualize these lesions in utero. Usually these lesions will recur after surgical treatments because of their depth, but injection sclerotherapy with agents such as OK-432 (picibanil) may result in regression.

Fujino A, et al: A role of cytokines in OK-432 injection therapy for cystic lymphangioma: an approach to the mechanism. J Pediatr Surg 2003; 38:1806.
Lille ST, et al: The surgical management of giant cervicofacial lymphatic malformations. J Pediatr Surg 1996; 31:1648.
Mosca RC, et al: Cystic hygroma: characterization by computerized tomography. Oral Surg Oral Med Oral Pathol Oral Radiol Endod 2008 May; 105(5):e65–e69.
Woolley SL, et al: Adult cystic hygroma: successful use of OK-432 (Picibanil). J Laryngol Otol 2008 Nov; 122(11):1260–1264.

Lymphangiomatosis

Diffuse or multifocal dilated lymphatic channels involving the skin, soft tissues, bone, and parenchymal organs are a rare congenital condition. If an extremity is affected, the prognosis is good; however, when vital internal organs are involved, the prognosis is poor. Skin lesions are presenting signs in 7% of patients with thoracic lymphangiomatosis. These patients have a high incidence of complications, including chylothorax (49%), pulmonary infiltrates (45%), bone lesions (39%), splenic lesions (19%), cervical involvement (15%), and disseminated intravascular coagulation (9%).

Gorham–Stout syndrome

Gorham–Stout syndrome is characterized by lymphangiomatosis and chylous effusions, with osteolytic changes resulting in "vanishing bones." Response to pegylated interferon (IFN)-α2b was noted in a 9-year-old boy with systemic disease, Response to bisphosphonates has also been noted.

Meltzer E, et al: Diffuse lymphangiomatosis—a fatal case with atypical skeletal features. Am J Med Sci 2008 Nov; 336(5):445–448.
Ozeki M, et al: Clinical improvement of diffuse lymphangiomatosis with pegylated interferon alpha-2b therapy: case report and review of the literature. Pediatr Hematol Oncol 2007 Oct–Nov; 24(7):513–524.
Wong CS, et al: Clinical and radiological features of generalised lymphangiomatosis. Hong Kong Med J 2008 Oct; 14(5):402–404.

Dilation of pre-existing vessels

Spider angioma (vascular spider, spider nevus, nevus araneus)

The lesion of spider angioma is suggestive of a red spider; hence its name. The ascending central arteriole represents the "body" of the spider, and the radiating fine vessels are suggestive of the multiple legs. These small telangiectases occur singly or severally, most frequently on the face and neck, with decreasing frequency on the upper trunk and upper extremities. In young children, the sites of predilection are the backs of the hands and forearms, and the face.

Young children and pregnant women show these lesions most frequently. In pregnant women, palmar erythema is usually present with the vascular spiders. The presence of vascular spiders in otherwise healthy children is common.

The vascular spiders of childhood usually involute without treatment; however, several years may elapse before that happens. In pregnant women, most lesions will involute soon after delivery.

Vascular spiders also occur in patients with cirrhosis, hepatitis C, malignant disease of the liver, and other hepatic dysfunctions. The common denominator has been shown to be an elevated blood estrogen level. Elevations in VEGF and basic fibroblastic growth factor are also significant predictors for spider angiomas in cirrhotic patients. When vascular spiders occur with palmar erythema and pallid nails with distal hyperemic bands, cirrhosis of the liver should be considered. AV hemangioma has also been reported to be associated with chronic liver disease.

If active therapy is to be performed, either obliteration by electrodesiccation of the central punctum or laser treatment produces excellent results. Laser treatment has produced good results in some patients.

Venous lakes

Venous lakes (phlebectases) are small, dark blue, slightly elevated blebs (Fig. 28-8). They are easily compressed, and are located on the face, ears, lips, neck, forearms, and backs of the hands. These manifestations of chronic sun damage are markedly dilated, blood-filled spaces that are lined with thin, elongated endothelial cells, and are usually surrounded by prominent solar elastosis.

Venous lakes may be treated by light electrocautery, laser ablation, fulguration, infrared coagulation, intralesional injection of 1% polidocanol, and cryotherapy. Sometimes they must be treated because of traumatic bleeding.

Capillary aneurysms

These flesh-colored solitary lesions, resembling an intradermal nevus, may suddenly grow larger and darker and become blue–black or black as a result of thrombosis. They are surrounded by a zone of erythema. The lesions may be clinically indistinguishable from malignant melanoma. Histologically, these are thrombotic, dilated capillaries lying just below the epidermis. Shave excision in stages will expose the clot and eliminate the uncertainty.

Telangiectasia

A telangiectasis is a dilated cutaneous blood vessel—venule, capillary, or arteriole. Telangiectases are fine, linear vessels coursing on the surface of the skin; the name given to them collectively is telangiectasia. Telangiectasia may occur in normal skin at any age, in both sexes, and anywhere on the skin and mucous membranes. Fine telangiectases may be seen on the alae nasi of most adults. They are prominent in areas of chronic actinic damage seen in fair-skinned persons. Persons long exposed to wind, cold, or heat are also subject to telangiectasia.

Telangiectases can be found in such conditions as radiodermatitis, xeroderma pigmentosum, lupus erythematosus, dermatomyositis, scleroderma and the CREST syndrome, rosacea, cirrhosis of the liver, acquired immunodeficiency syndrome (AIDS), poikiloderma, basal cell carcinoma, necrobiosis lipoidica diabeticorum, sarcoid, lupus vulgaris, adenoma sebaceum, keloid, angioma serpiginosum, angiokeratoma corporis diffusum, ataxia-telangiectasia, pregnancy, Osler–Weber–Rendu disease, and Bloom syndrome. These entities are discussed in other sections with the disease states in which they occur.

Altered capillary patterns on the fingernail folds (cuticular telangiectases) are indicative of collagen vascular disease, such as lupus erythematosus, scleroderma, or dermatomyositis. Tortuous glomeruloid loops are characteristic of lupus erythematosus, whereas dilated loops and avascular areas are typical of scleroderma and dermatomyositis. Reticular telangiectatic erythema may occur overlying implantable cardioverter defibrillators.

Electrodessication and laser ablation can be effective. Pulsed dye laser and other vascular lasers, such as the 532 nm Nd:YAG laser, are usually well tolerated and associated with a low risk of scarring. Larger vessels require a longer pulse duration. Contact or cryospray cooling can reduce the incidence of complications. Pulse stacking (multiple pulses of low fluences) has been used to reduce the incidence of side effects, such as purpura, hyperpigmentation, hypopigmentation, and scar formation.

Generalized essential telangiectasia

Generalized essential telangiectasia (GET) is characterized by the dilation of veins and capillaries over a large segment of the body without preceding or coexisting skin lesions. The telangiectases may be distributed over the entire body or be localized to some large area such as the legs, arms, and trunk. They may be discrete or confluent. Distribution along the course of the cutaneous nerves may occur. This type of telangiectasia is not associated with systemic disease, although patients with a similar appearance may have autoimmune

disease. One report documented gastrointestinal bleeding from a watermelon stomach in a woman with GET.

GET develops most frequently in women in their forties and fifties. The initial onset is on the lower legs and then spreads to the upper legs, abdomen, and arms. The dilations persist indefinitely. Generally, this is a sporadic condition, although it has been described in families as an autosomal-dominant condition. In the latter case, it has been termed hereditary benign telangiectasia.

It has been reported that GET may be differentiated from telangiectasia associated with systemic disease by the presence of alkaline phosphatase activity. Telangiectatic vessels in GET do not have alkaline phosphatase activity in the endothelium of the terminal arteriole and the arterial portion of the capillary loops.

Individual areas may be treated with laser ablation. High-energy, high-frequency, long-pulse Nd:YAG laser and the 585 nm flashlamp-pumped pulsed dye laser have been reported to produce good results. Tetracycline, ketoconazole, and the treatment of a chronic sinus infection have led to involution in individual reports.

Universal angiomatosis

Universal angiomatosis, called generalized telangiectasia by Bean, is a bleeding disease that affects the blood vessels of the skin and mucous membranes, as well as other parts of the body. Bean and Rather reported a 13-year-old boy who had frequent nose bleeds, and ear and upper respiratory infections. He had mottled skin, with redness that blanched on pressure. Finely dilated blood vessels were universal, suggesting the term "pink man." Some irregular white patches were also present. Continual bleeding into the skin was evident despite normal coagulation of the blood. This type of angiomatosis differs from generalized telangiectasia because of its hemorrhagic tendency, especially epistaxis.

Unilateral nevoid telangiectasia

In unilateral nevoid telangiectasia, fine, threadlike telangiectases develop in a unilateral, sometimes dermatomal, distribution. The areas most often involved are the trigeminal and C3 and C4 or adjacent areas, with the right side involved slightly more often than the left. In some cases the condition is congenital, but more often it is acquired. Increased estrogen appears to play a role in the onset of acquired cases, e.g. pregnancy, puberty in women, adrenarche in men, and hepatitis/alcohol-related cases have all been reported. Lesions have responded to pulse dye laser treatment.

Angiokeratomas

Angiokeratomas are essentially telangiectases that have an overlying hyperkeratotic surface (Fig. 28-9). These are dilations of pre-existing papillary dermal vessels. Angiokeratoma circumscriptum is discussed in the malformations section above. Angiokeratoma corporis diffusum is discussed in Chapter 26.

Angiokeratoma of Mibelli

The lesions of angiokeratoma of Mibelli consist of 1–5 mm red vascular papules, the surfaces of which become hyperkeratotic in the course of time. The papules are dull red or purplish-black, verrucous, and rounded, and are usually situated on the dorsum of the fingers and toes, the elbows, and the knees. Frequently, these are called telangiectatic warts. The patient often has cold, cyanotic hands and feet.

This is a rare genodermatosis with an autosomal-dominant trait for vascular lesions located over bony prominences and a family history of chilblains. The condition is most frequently discovered in prepubertal children.

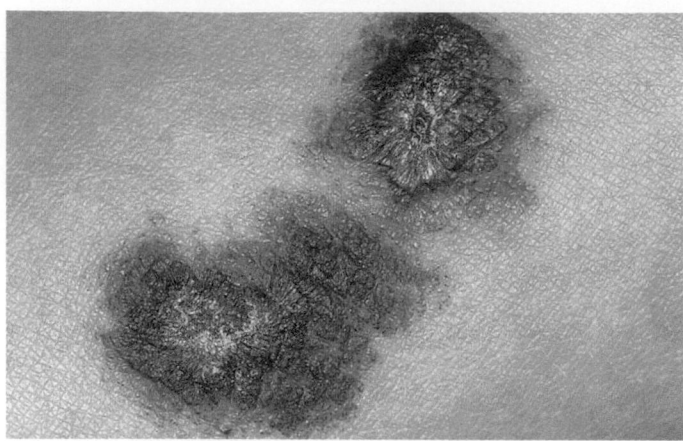

Fig. 28-9 Angiokeratoma.

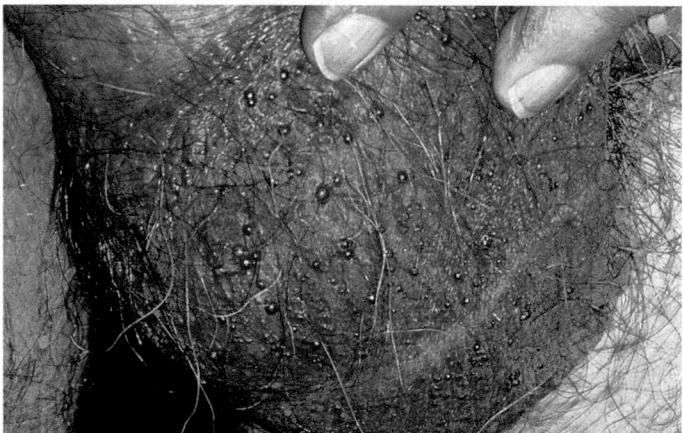

Fig. 28-10 Fordyce angiokeratomas.

Histologically, hyperkeratosis, increased thickness of the granular layer, and dilation of the subpapillary vessels to form lacunae are the chief features.

In the differential diagnosis of angiokeratomas of the dorsal hands in children is acral pseudolymphomatous angiokeratoma in children (APACHE). However, APACHE is unilateral and sporadic in nature, without associated cold sensitivity; on histologic examination there is a dense, nodular, lymphohistiocytic infiltrate with occasional plasma cells, eosinophils, and multinucleated giant cells. It is a variant of pseudolymphoma and not primarily a vascular lesion. Similar lesions may occur in adolescents and adults, and the term acral angiokeratoma-like pseudolymphoma has been proposed for these lesions in all age groups.

Angiokeratoma may be treated with electrocautery, fulguration, CO_2 laser ablation, long-pulse vascular laser therapy, or cryotherapy, with fairly good results.

Angiokeratoma of the scrotum (Fordyce)

The angiomas are multiple small vascular papules that stud the scrotum (Fig. 28-10) and sometimes the vulva in middle-aged and elderly individuals. There is often a diffuse redness of the involved area that may be a source of concern to the patient. Urethral or clitoral lesions may also be seen. Infrequently, the keratotic part may be involuntarily scratched off to produce considerable bleeding. Rarely, they may bleed spontaneously. Histologically, the many communicating lacunae in the subpapillary layer are lined with endothelium and connected underneath by dilated veins. Treatment is best accomplished by shave excision, cautery, laser ablation, or fulguration of troublesome lesions. The primary therapy is reassurance.

Solitary angiokeratoma

Described by Imperial and Helwig in 1967, solitary angiokeratoma is a single small, bluish-black, warty papule that occurs predominantly on the lower extremities. It is not a hereditary lesion and probably follows trauma, with subsequent telangiectasia before the formation of the angiokeratoma. The mode of acquiring this lesion, and its small size, solitary nature, and location, distinguish it from other forms of angiokeratoma. Solitary angiokeratoma is to be considered in the differential diagnosis of seborrheic keratosis, melanoma, pigmented basal cell carcinoma, and ordinary hemangioma. Treatment is by electrosurgery, laser ablation, or excision.

Karabudak O, et al: Acquired unilateral nevoid telangiectasia syndrome. J Dermatol 2006 Nov; 33(11):825–826.

Karen JK, et al: Generalized essential telangiectasia. Dermatol Online J 2008 May 15; 14(5):9.

Sharma VK, et al: Unilateral nevoid telangiectasia—response to pulsed dye laser. Int J Dermatol 2006 Aug; 45(8):960–964.

Wenzel SM, et al: Progressive disseminated essential telangiectasia and erythrosis interfollicularis colli as examples for successful treatment with a high-intensity flashlamp. Dermatology 2008; 217(3):286–290.

Lymphangiectasis (lymphangioma)

Lymphangiectases are acquired dilations of lymph vessels. Some forms are discussed under malformations (above). Solitary lymphangiomas have an appearance resembling frog's eggs. Like angiokeratomas, they may be seen adjacent to café-au-lait macules. This may represent a twin spotting phenomenon. Acquired lesions occur on women's arms, axillae, chest, and back after lymph node dissection and irradiation for breast cancer, and on the scrotum, penis, thighs, and pubic region of men treated aggressively for prostate cancer. Other cancers treated similarly, such as cervical carcinoma, may result in similar lesions. If cancers obstruct outflow from an extremity, lymphangiectases may occur and may be the presenting sign of disease. At times, benign disease, such as scrofuloderma or recurrent erysipelas, which leads to progressive scarring of the lymphatic vessels, may induce lymphangiectasia. Rarely, degenerative changes to the supporting connective tissue may allow lymphangiectasia to develop. A peculiar penicillamine-induced dermopathy may result from damage to the underlying supporting structures of the dermis and allow dilation of lymph vessels within areas of trauma, such as the dorsal hands and knees. Central facial involvement may be seen in variegate porphyria, and sites of chronic high-potency steroid application may develop lymphangiectasia.

The lesions are thick-walled, translucent, 2–5 mm white vesicles. They are multiple, and when present on the penis, may mimic condylomata. Spontaneous drainage of a straw-colored to milky-white fluid may occur. Such chylous discharge may induce surface irritation and erythema of the site. At times, recurrent erysipelas may complicate the moist, superficially eroded flexural skin. In penicillamine-induced dermopathy there is a hemorrhagic macular stain that is often surmounted by milia.

The method of treatment depends on the cause. If lymphangiectasis results from cancer infiltration and pressure, treatment of the primary process may reopen the lymphatic drainage and lead to resolution. If the condition results from penicillamine or topical steroid application, decreasing the dose or discontinuance may result in improvement. If the underlying process is fibrosis and scarring, and the involved part is amenable to pressure dressings or a pump, the chylous discharge may be improved. If erysipelas is a recurrent complication, long-term oral antibiotic prophylaxis may prevent this.

Pena JM, et al: Cutaneous lymphangiectases associated with severe photoaging and topical corticosteroid application. J Cutan Pathol 1996; 23:175.

Stone MS: Central-facial papular lymphangiectases. J Am Acad Dermatol 1997; 36:493.

Hyperplasias

Angiolymphoid hyperplasia with eosinophilia

Patients with angiolymphoid hyperplasia with eosinophilia (ALHE) usually present with pink to red–brown, dome-shaped, dermal papules or nodules of the head or neck, especially about the ears and on the scalp. ALHE may also occur in the mouth, and on the trunk, extremities, penis, and vulva. Grouped lesions merge to form plaques or grapelike clusters. There is a female preponderance, and the average age of onset is 32 years. Symptoms can be pain or pruritus; these may occur after trauma. An underlying AV shunt is present as a result of damage to and repair of an artery or vein. Histologically, central thick-walled vessels with hobnail endothelium are noted. Surrounding hyperplasia of smaller vessels and nodular lymphoid aggregates with eosinophils are present.

Lesions do not spontaneously regress. Treatment with surgical excision is successful in 65% of cases. The lesions may recur if the underlying AV shunt is not excised. Intralesional corticosteroids, pulsed dye laser therapy with conventional or ultra-long pulsed systems, Nd:YAG laser, cryotherapy, pentoxifylline, indomethacin, imiquimod, and electrodesiccation have been successful in some cases. Difficult cases have been controlled with IFN-α2b, isotretinoin, or vinblastine, and partial responses to intralesional bleomycin have been reported.

Much confusion in the literature has centered on distinguishing ALHE from Kimura's disease (Fig. 28-11). The latter is an inflammatory disorder that presents as massive subcutaneous swelling in the periauricular and submandibular region in young Asian men. Histologically, prominent germinal centers with eosinophils are present in the subcutaneous tissue. Although blood vessels are abundant, changes are less prominent than in ALHE. Additionally, Kimura's disease is associated with allergic conditions such as asthma, rhinitis, and eczema, and is frequently accompanied by lymphadenopathy, peripheral blood eosinophilia, and an elevated IgE level. Overlap of the two syndromes may occur. Although clonal T-cell gene rearrangement has been reported in both ALHE and Kimura's disease, heteroduplex polymerase chain reaction (PCR) has disproved clonality in some cases positive by conventional PCR. Coexistence of ALHE and peripheral T-cell lymphoma has been reported.

Akdeniz N, et al: Intralesional bleomycin for angiolymphoid hyperplasia. Arch Dermatol 2007 Jul; 143(7):841–844.

Carlesimo M, et al: Angiolymphoid hyperplasia with eosinophilia treated with isotretinoin. Eur J Dermatol 2007 Nov–Dec; 17(6):554–555.

Choi JE, et al: Successful treatment of Kimura's disease with a 595-nm ultra-long pulsed dye laser. Acta Derm Venereol 2008; 88(3):315–316.

Cunha Filho RR, et al: Angiolymphoid hyperplasia with eosinophilia: excellent response to intralesional triamcinolone. Braz J Otorhinolaryngol 2008 Jan–Feb; 74(1):160.

Esmaili DD, et al: Simultaneous presentation of Kimura disease and angiolymphoid hyperplasia with eosinophilia. Ophthal Plast Reconstr Surg 2008 Jul–Aug; 24(4):310–311.

Gencoglan G, et al: Angiolymphoid hyperplasia with eosinophilia successfully treated with imiquimod. A case report. Dermatology 2007; 215(3):233–235.

Gonzalez-Cuyar LF, et al: Angiolymphoid hyperplasia with eosinophilia developing in a patient with history of peripheral T-cell lymphoma: evidence for multicentric T-cell lymphoproliferative process. Diagn Pathol 2008 May 29; 3:22.

Kadurina MI, et al: Angiolymphoid hyperplasia with eosinophilia: successful treatment with the Nd:YAG laser. J Cosmet Laser Ther 2007 Jun; 9(2):107–111.

Oguz O, et al: Angiolymphoid hyperplasia with eosinophilia responding to interferon-alpha2B. J Eur Acad Dermatol Venereol 2007 Oct; 21(9):1277–1278.

Pyogenic granuloma

A pyogenic granuloma is a small, eruptive, usually solitary, sessile or pedunculated, friable papule (Fig. 28-12). The lesion is common in children, but may occur at any age. It occurs most often on an exposed surface: on the hands, forearms, or face, or at sites of trauma. The lesion also occurs in the mouth, especially on the gingiva, most often in pregnant women (granuloma gravidarum). On the sole of the foot or nailbed, it may be mistaken for a melanoma. Pyogenic granulomas bleed easily on the slightest trauma and, if cut off superficially, promptly recur. Recurring lesions may have one or many satellite lesions.

Pyogenic granulomas may be seen in patients treated with isotretinoin, capecitabine, or indinavir. Isotretinoin treatment of acne vulgaris can be complicated by numerous exuberant pyogenic granuloma-like lesions of the trunk

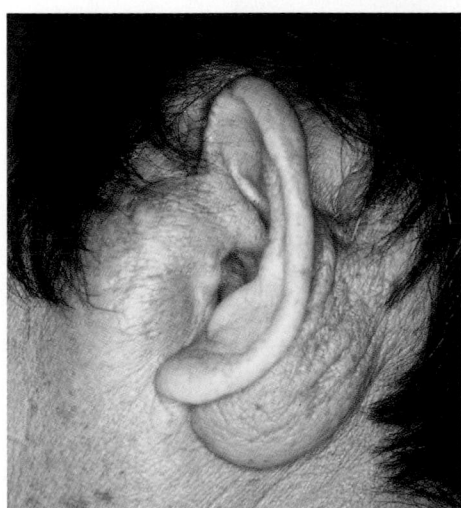

Fig. 28-11 Kimura's disease. (Courtesy of Department of Dermatology, Keio University School of Medicine)

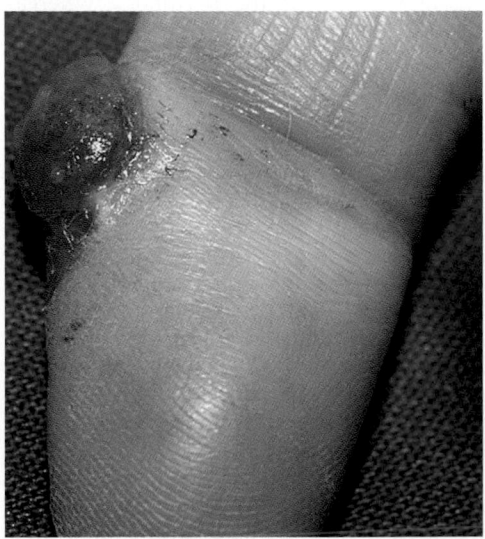

Fig. 28-12 Pyogenic granuloma.

or periungual lesions. Some data suggest that patients with pyogenic granuloma have a statistically higher prevalence of *Bartonella* seropositivity compared with controls, but a definite etiologic role has not been established.

Histologically, pyogenic granuloma is a lobular capillary hemangioma, with lobules separated by connective tissue septae. With time, the epidermis becomes thinned, then eroded. Heavy secondary staphylococcal colonization is common. Intravascular pyogenic granuloma appears as a lobular capillary proliferation within a vein.

Treatment is by curettage or shave excision, followed by destruction of the base by fulguration or silver nitrate. Silver nitrate alone may be sufficient to treat smaller lesions. Imiquimod under occlusion has been successful, and sclerotherapy with monoethanolamine oleate has also been used successfully. At times, a recalcitrant lesion may require excision or laser ablation. The drug-induced variety will regress after lowering of the dose or discontinuation of the medication. Systemic steroids have been used to treat recurrent giant pyogenic granulomas.

Georgiou S, et al: Pyogenic granuloma: complete remission under occlusive imiquimod 5% cream. Clin Exp Dermatol 2008 Jul; 33(4):454–456.

Piqué-Duran E, et al: Pyogenic granuloma-like lesions caused by capecitabine therapy. Clin Exp Dermatol 2008 Aug; 33(5):652–653.

Intravascular papillary endothelial hyperplasia

Masson described this intravascular papillary proliferation that may mimic angiosarcoma. The lesions appear as red or purplish 5 mm to 5 cm papules or deep nodules on the head, neck, or upper extremities. The condition represents recanalization of a thrombosed vessel. Histologic examination reveals intravascular papillary projections lined by endothelial cells. Thrombi may still be present, and the papillary projections may have a fibrinous or hyaline core. High-resolution ultrasound imaging may be useful in establishing the diagnosis, although the diagnosis is usually made by biopsy. Excision is curative.

Schwartz SA, et al: Intravascular papillary endothelial hyperplasia: sonographic appearance with histopathologic correlation. J Ultrasound Med 2008 Nov; 27(11):1651–1653.

Angioma serpiginosum

Angioma serpiginosum, first described by Hutchinson in 1889, is characterized by minute, copper-colored to bright red angiomatous puncta that have a tendency to become papular. These puncta occur in groups, which enlarge through the constant formulation of new points at the periphery, whereas those at the center fade. In this manner, linear arrays, small rings, or serpiginous patterns are formed. No purpura is present, but a netlike or diffuse erythema forms the background. In the areas undergoing involution, a delicate tracery of rings and lines, a fine desquamation, and, at times, a semblance of atrophy are seen. Slight lichenification and scaling may be evident in the papular lesions. The eruption predominates on the lower extremities. Although it affects both sexes at all ages, 90% of cases occur in girls under 16. It is usually slowly progressive and chronic, and although involution may occur, it is probably never complete. Treatment with a pulsed dye laser will improve or eliminate such lesions. Angioma serpiginosum following Blaschko's lines, with associated esophageal papillomatosis, has been reported as an X-linked dominant condition with mild features of Goltz–Gorlin syndrome, including hair and nail dystrophy. The condition maps to Xp11.3–Xq12.

Angioma serpiginosum must be differentiated from the progressive pigmentary disease of Schamberg. In the latter, pin-point areas of purpura, the so-called cayenne pepper spots, form macules that tend to coalesce and form diffusely pigmented patches. The pigment is hemosiderin. Purpura annularis telangiectodes (Majocchi) is often bilateral and is characterized by acute outbreaks of telangiectatic points that spread peripherally and form small rings. In lichenoid purpuric and pigmentary dermatosis of Gougerot and Blum, the primary lesion is a minute, lichenoid, reddish-brown papule that is sometimes hemorrhagic. It has a tendency toward central involution and residual pigmentation.

In angioma serpiginosum, the most important histologic finding is dilated and tortuous capillaries in the dermal papillae and the upper dermis. No inflammatory infiltrate or extravasation of red cells is observed. The dilated capillaries show no alkaline phosphatase activity, in contrast to normal capillaries.

Blinkenberg EO, et al: Angioma serpiginosum with oesophageal papillomatosis is an X-linked dominant condition that maps to Xp11.3–Xq12. Eur J Hum Genet 2007 May; 15(5):543–547.

Kalisiak MS, et al: Angioma serpiginosum with linear distribution: case report and review of the literature. J Cutan Med Surg 2008 Jul–Aug; 12(4):180–183.

Benign neoplasms

Infantile hemangioma (strawberry hemangioma)

Strawberry (capillary) hemangiomas, the most common benign tumors of childhood, are present at birth in one-third of cases. The remainder appear shortly thereafter. Sixty percent are on the head and neck, but they may occur anywhere. The dome-shaped lesion is dull to bright red, and when involution begins, streaks or islands of white appear in the lesion as it flattens. The lesions have sharp borders; they are soft and easily compressed (Fig. 28-13). Generally, they tend to grow over the first year or so, remain stable for a period of months, and then slowly involute spontaneously. The period of greatest growth is the first 5 months. Ulceration occurs in nearly 16% of lesions, usually by 4 months of age. Approximately 30% resolve by the third year, 50% by age 5, and 70% by the

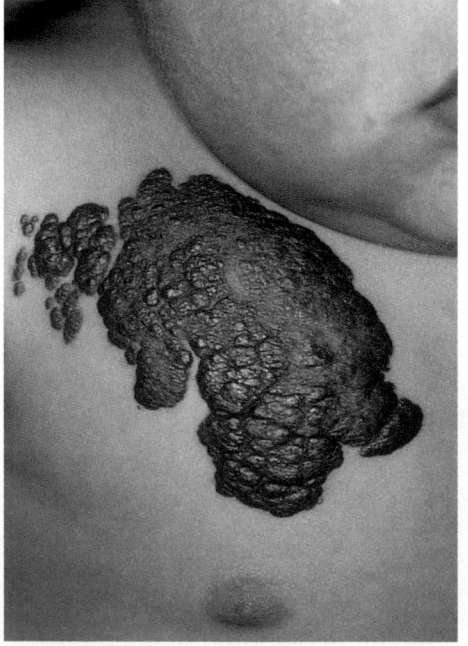

Fig. 28-13 Infantile hemangioma.

time the patient is 7 years of age. The skin may appear normal after involution, but more commonly, atrophy, telangiectasia, or anetoderma-type redundancy is present.

The majority of these lesions occur sporadically, but kindreds with autosomal-dominant inheritance of infantile hemangiomas and/or vascular malformations have been described. Approximately 7% of hemangiomas may occur in association with structural malformations. One grouping of associated abnormalities is the PHACE syndrome. This acronym, proposed by Frieden et al in 1996, denotes the association of posterior fossa brain malformations (primarily the Dandy–Walker malformation), hemangiomas, arterial anomalies, coarctation of the aorta and cardiac defects, and eye abnormalities. When sternal clefting and abdominal raphae are present, the designation PHACES is used. The hemangiomas tend to be large, plaquelike, and facial in location, frequently involving more than one dermatome. Frieden et al recommended that brain imaging studies be performed in all infants with such hemangiomas. Solitary segmental hemangiomas of the skin are also associated with visceral hemangiomatosis involving the liver, gastrointestinal tract, lung, brain, and mediastinum; 40% have PHACE(S) syndrome.

Multiple hemangiomas, usually 1–10 mm in size, may appear in the first few weeks to months of life and can be large in number. If they are purely cutaneous, they generally involute without sequelae, and the term benign neonatal hemangiomatosis is applied. However, visceral lesions may be present in the CNS, lungs, liver, or other organs. When internal lesions are present, complications may occur, such as gastrointestinal or CNS bleeding, high-output cardiac failure, obstructive jaundice, or respiratory failure; this results in a high mortality rate among untreated patients. This more ominous variant is called diffuse neonatal hemangiomatosis. Flat lumbar hemangiomas are often associated with occult spinal dysraphism.

Rapidly involuting congenital hemangioma (RICH) and noninvoluting congenital hemangioma (NICH) are rare vascular tumors that present fully grown at birth and either involute rapidly or fail to involute. Whereas smooth muscle actin (SMA)-positive cells are common in the walls of infantile hemangiomas, they are rare in RICH. Children with RICH or NICH coexisting with infantile hemangioma have been described, as have children with RICH showing rapid but incomplete regression. In these cases, the residuum was NICH.

The pathogenesis of infantile hemangiomas is complex. CD133+ stem cells within the hemangioma differentiate into mature blood vessels that express GLUT-1 (a glucose transporter normally restricted to endothelial cells with blood–tissue barrier function, such as in brain and placenta). The vessels proliferate, then involute. Some have suggested that the stem cells could originate from placental trophoblast. Some data suggest that local hypoxia may lead to upregulation of hypoxia-inducible factor-1α responsive chemokines, including stromal cell-derived factor-1α (SDF-1α) and VEGF. These cytokines promote recruitment and proliferation of endothelial progenitor cells. Reduced activity of a pathway involving β1 integrin, the integrin-like receptor tumor endothelial marker-8 (TEM8), VEGF receptor-2 (VEGF-R2), and NFAT has been shown to reduce VEGF receptor-1 (VEGF-R1) expression. This produces a VEGF-dependent activation of VEGF-R2.

Histologically, strawberry marks are composed of primitive endothelial cells similar to those found before the embryonic development of true venous channels. Ultrastructurally, they lack typical Weibel–Palade bodies but do have crystalloid inclusions typical of embryonic endothelium and stain for GLUT-1. They also stain for Fc-γ-RII, Lewis Y antigen (LeY),

and merosin. Some subgroups, such as rapidly involuting hemangiomas and noninvoluting hemangiomas, lack GLUT-1 staining. Young hemangiomas show evidence of endothelial progenitor cells that stain with CD133 and CD34. In late stages, the endothelium flattens and the lumina are more apparent because of increased blood flow. In time, fibrosis becomes pronounced as involution progresses.

In most cases, intervention produces a cosmetic result no better or worse than that achieved with simple observation. Proponents of early treatment point out that many of these hemangiomas remain significant body image factors to children when they enter school. Cryotherapy or laser ablation of early lesions has generally not been successful. The pulsed dye laser can improve the appearance of residual involuted lesions with prominent telangiectasia; however, the depth of the hemangiomas does not allow the lasers to be effective in growing or stable childhood hemangiomas. Vascular lasers have been used to treat ulcerated hemangiomas, but have also caused ulceration.

The so-called Cyrano defect, a hemangioma that causes the end of the nose to become bulbous, may be successfully approached surgically in many cases before the patient begins school. Additionally, surgical intervention in small pedunculated hemangiomas and eyelid tumors may also be an excellent option. Finally, compressive wraps may improve extremity hemangiomas.

Specific circumstances necessitate treatment. Indications for intervention include severe hemorrhage, thrombocytopenia, threatened cardiovascular compromise from high-output cardiac failure, nasal or auditory canal obstruction, hepatic hemangiomatosis, skin ulceration, or threatened interference with vital functions, such as feeding, respiration, passage of urine or stool, limb function, tissue destruction, or vision. There is a risk of occlusion amblyopia, astigmatism, and myopia from periorbital hemangiomas. Additionally, strong consideration should be given to treatment of those hemangiomas that may lead to permanent disfigurement or long-term psychological consequences, such as large hemangiomas of the ear, nose, glabellar area, or lips.

Oral prednisone and beta blockers are used most commonly. Beta blockers can produce rapid involution of hemangiomas, but treatment can be complicated by bradycardia or hypoglycemia. Some very thin hemangiomas may respond to topical beta blockers. Intralesional corticosteroid treatment has been used, but carries some risk of embolization and occlusion of ocular vessels. Injection regularly produces pressures exceeding the systemic arterial pressure, leading to the possibility of embolization.

Oral treatment with prednisone requires a dose of 2–4 mg/kg/day. In the 30% of patients who respond well to treatment, the enlarging hemangioma stops growing in 3–21 days. Ulcerations will heal within 2 weeks. The lesion will usually shrink if treatment is continued for 30–90 days. Laryngeal involvement and stridor, if present, are usually dramatically relieved by treatment. Repeated courses of treatment may be undertaken if rebound of growth occurs on discontinuation of the steroidal agent. Some experts recommend prolonged low-dose oral steroids over a 12-month period to prevent this rebound phenomenon. In another 40%, the clinical situation will stabilize with this treatment; however, the remaining 30% do not respond to treatment with prednisone. Treatment with recombinant IFN-α2a or 2b may result in a good response in 80% of patients, but is rarely used because of the risk of spastic diplegia. Topical imiquimod, low-frequency ultrasound, and selective arterial embolization have also been used. Both Nd:YAG and Potassium Titanyl Phosphate (KTP) lasers have been used to deliver intralesional laser therapy.

Balakrishnan K, et al: Management of airway hemangiomas. Expert Rev Respir Med 2010 Aug; 4(4):455–462.

Barry RB, et al: Involution of infantile haemangiomas after imiquimod 5% cream. Clin Exp Dermatol 2008 Jul; 33(4):446–449.

Chamlin SL, et al: Multicenter prospective study of ulcerated hemangiomas. J Pediatr 2007 Dec; 151(6):684–689, 689.e1.

Chang LC, et al: Growth characteristics of infantile hemangiomas: implications for management. Pediatrics 2008 Aug; 122(2):360–367.

Holland KE, et al: Hypoglycemia in children taking propranolol for the treatment of infantile hemangioma. Arch Dermatol 2010 Jul; 146(7):775–778.

Pandey A, et al: Evaluation and management of infantile hemangioma: an overview. Ostomy Wound Manage 2008 May; 54(5):16–18, 20, 22–26, 28–29.

Pope E, et al: Oral versus high-dose pulse corticosteroids for problematic infantile hemangiomas: a randomized, controlled trial. Pediatrics 2007 Jun; 119(6):e1239–e1247.

Serena T: Wound closure and gradual involution of an infantile hemangioma using a noncontact, low-frequency ultrasound therapy. Ostomy Wound Manage 2008 Feb; 54(2):68–71.

Sun ZY, et al: Infantile hemangioma is originated from placental trophoblast, fact or fiction? Med Hypotheses 2008 Sep; 71(3):444–448.

Cherry angiomas (senile angiomas, de Morgan spots)

These round, slightly elevated, 0.5–6 mm diameter, ruby-red papules are the most common vascular anomalies. It is a rare 30-year-old person who does not have a few, and the number increases with age. Probably every 70-year-old person has some. Most are on the trunk; they are rarely seen on the hands, feet, or face. Early lesions may mimic petechiae. When lesions are surrounded by a purpuric halo, amyloidosis should be suspected. Eruptive lesions have been described after nitrogen mustard therapy.

Light electrodesiccation or laser ablation with intense pulsed light (IPL) and long-pulse Nd:YAG systems can be effective. Shave excision can also be performed, but most patients accept reassurance and do not request their removal.

Fodor L, et al: A side-by-side prospective study of intense pulsed light and Nd:YAG laser treatment for vascular lesions. Ann Plast Surg 2006 Feb; 56(2):164–170.

Ma HJ, et al: Eruptive cherry angiomas associated with vitiligo: provoked by topical nitrogen mustard? J Dermatol 2006 Dec; 33(12):877–879.

Targetoid hemosiderotic hemangioma

In 1988, Santa Cruz and Aronberg described a lesion characterized by a central brown or violaceous papule that is surrounded by an ecchymotic halo (Fig. 28-14). The term hobnail hemangioma has been proposed, as many lesions are not targetoid. These acquired hemangiomas occur in the young to middle-aged and are present on the trunk or extremities. They likely represent trauma to a pre-existing hemangioma, with thrombosis and subsequent recanalization. Histologically, a biphasic growth pattern is seen, with central superficial dilated vascular structures lined by prominent hobnail endothelial cells, and collagen-dissecting, narrow vessels in deeper parts of the lesion. The endothelial cells commonly stain for CD31, but not CD34. D2-40 staining suggests lymphangiomatous proliferation. Carlson et al studied 33 cases and concluded that targetoid hemosiderotic hemangiomas are variants of solitary angiokeratomas. They found episodic changes of swelling, darkening, and/or involution in three patients.

Franke FE, et al: Hobnail hemangiomas (targetoid hemosiderotic hemangiomas) are true lymphangiomas. J Cutan Pathol 2004 May; 31(5):362–367.

Morales-Callaghan AM, et al: Targetoid hemosiderotic hemangioma: clinical and dermoscopical findings. J Eur Acad Dermatol Venereol 2007 Feb; 21(2):267–269.

Glomeruloid hemangioma

This distinctive benign vascular neoplasm was described in 1990 and has been reported in patients with POEMS (polyneuropathy, organomegaly, endocrinopathy, monoclonal gammopathy, and skin changes) syndrome (Crow–Fukase syndrome) and Castleman's disease. Some have also been associated with idiopathic thrombocytopenic purpura and Sjögren syndrome. Similar lesions have been reported in patients who are otherwise healthy.

POEMS syndrome consists of polyneuropathy (severe sensorimotor), organomegaly (heart, spleen, kidneys), endocrinopathy, M protein, and skin changes (hyperpigmentation, hypertrichosis, thickening, sweating, clubbed nails, leukonychia, and angiomas). Small, firm, red to violaceous papules appear on the trunk and proximal extremities in approximately one-third of patients. Histologically, the lesions may be microvenular hemangiomas, cherry angiomas, multinucleated cell angiohistiocytomas, or glomeruloid hemangiomas. The latter consist of ectatic vascular structures containing aggregates of capillary loops within a dilated lumen, simulating the appearance of a renal glomerulus. Sequestered degenerating red blood cells are a characteristic finding. Two types of endothelial cell have been noted within the lesions: a capillary-type endothelium with large vesicular nuclei, open chromatin pattern, and a large amount of cytoplasm; and sinusoidal endothelium with small basal nuclei, dense chromatin, and scant cytoplasm. Lesions associated with POEMS syndrome demonstrate increased expression of VEGF and its receptor, Flt-1.

Forman SB, et al: Glomeruloid hemangiomas without POEMS syndrome: series of three cases. J Cutan Pathol 2007 Dec; 34(12):956–957.

Yamamoto T, et al: Increased expression of vascular endothelial growth factor and its receptor, Flt-1, in glomeruloid haemangioma associated with Crow–Fukase syndrome. J Eur Acad Dermatol Venereol 2007 Mar; 21(3):417–419.

Yuri T, et al: Glomeruloid hemangioma. Pathol Int 2008 Jun; 58(6):390–395.

Microvenular hemangioma

This recently described, acquired, benign, vascular neoplasm presents as an asymptomatic, slowly growing, 0.5–2.0 cm reddish lesion on the forearms or other sites of young to middle-aged adults. Dermoscopic examination reveals multiple, well-demarcated, red globules. Monomorphous, elongated blood vessels with small lumina involve the entire reticular dermis. In many areas, the podoplanin (D2-40)-negative endothelial cells are surrounded by

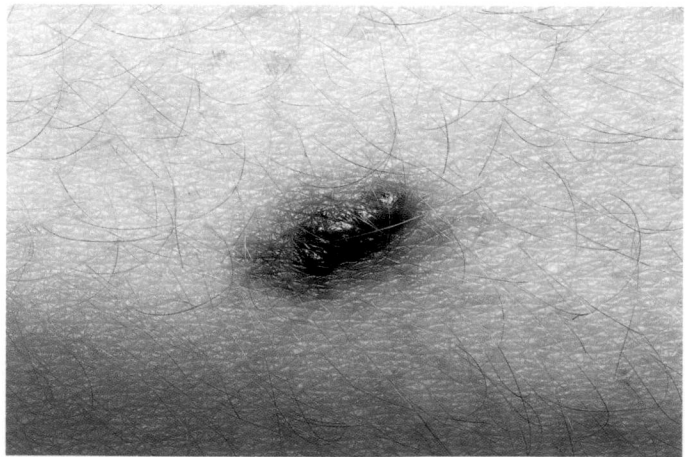

Fig. 28-14 Targetoid hemosiderotic hemangioma.

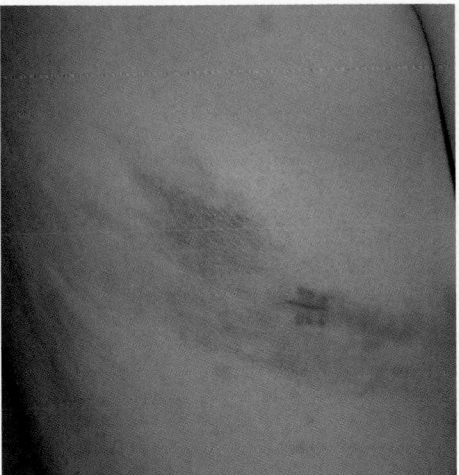

Fig. 28-15 Tufted angioma.

pericytes. The main differential diagnosis is that of Kaposi sarcoma. Along with glomeruloid hemangioma, they may sometimes be present in POEMS syndrome.

Fernandez-Flores A: Lack of expression of podoplanin by microvenular hemangioma. Pathol Res Pract 2008; 204(11):817–821.

Scalvenzi M, et al: Dermoscopy of microvenular hemangioma: report of a case. Dermatology 2007; 215(1):69–71.

Tufted angioma (angioblastoma)

This lesion usually develops in infancy or early childhood on the neck and upper trunk. Adult onset has also been described. The lesions present as ill-defined, dull red macules with a mottled appearance; they vary from 2 to 5 cm in diameter. Some show clusters of smaller angiomatous papules superimposed on the main macular area (Fig. 28-15), and associated hypertrichosis has been noted. The lesions are usually sporadic, although familial cases have been reported. Histologic examination reveals small, circumscribed angiomatous tufts and lobules scattered in the dermis in a so-called cannon-ball pattern. Tumors with features of both tufted angioma and kaposiform hemangioendothelioma (KHE) have been described, and transformation between the tumors has also been noted. Immunostaining can be helpful in distinguishing these tumors. Tufted angioma is characterized by a proliferation of CD34+ endothelial cells with few actin-positive cells. KHE shows CD34 staining only in the luminal endothelial cells. In infantile hemangiomas, actin-positive cells outnumber CD34+ cells.

Most lesions slowly extend with time, being progressive but benign in nature. Occasional spontaneous regression is documented; however, treatment with pulsed dye laser, intense pulsed light, excision, high-dose steroids, and IFN-α has been successful in individual cases. Lesions associated with Kasabach–Merritt syndrome have also been treated with embolization and vincristine.

The term angioblastoma has also been used for a rare pediatric tumor often associated with destruction of regional structures, including bone. Basic fibroblast growth factor has been reported to be elevated, and some patients have responded to treatment with IFN-α2b.

Chiu CS, et al: Treatment of a tufted angioma with intense pulsed light. J Dermatolog Treat 2007; 18(2):109–111.

Lee B, et al: Adult-onset tufted angioma: a case report and review of the literature. Cutis 2006 Nov; 78(5):341–345.

Yesudian PD, et al: Tufted angioma-associated Kasabach–Merritt syndrome treated with embolization and vincristine. Plast Reconstr Surg 2008 Feb; 121(2):692–693.

Kaposiform hemangioendothelioma

Kaposiform hemangioendothelioma (KHE) is an uncommon vascular tumor that affects infants and young children. Rare cases have been reported in adults. It was first designated KHE in 1993. Although it frequently occurs in the retroperitoneum, it may present as multinodular soft tissue masses, purpuric macules, plaques, and multiple telangiectatic papules. The lesions extend locally and usually involve the skin, soft tissues, and even bone. The cutaneous variant may be associated with lymphangiomatosis. KHE is locally aggressive and may be complicated by platelet trapping and consumptive coagulopathy (Kasabach–Merritt syndrome), but distant metastases have not yet been reported. It has also been reported in association with Milroy–Nonne disease (primary hereditary lymphedema).

Histologically, there are combined features of cellular infantile hemangioma and Kaposi sarcoma. Additionally, in some tumors, lymphangiomatosis is seen sharply separated from the vascular lesion. There is a multilobular appearance that closely resembles that of tufted angioma, but in KHE lesions are larger, less circumscribed, and involve the deep soft tissue and even bone. Transition between these tumors has been described. The transcription factor Prox-1 has been shown to induce proliferation and deep extension in a mouse model of the disease.

The prognosis depends on the depth and location of the lesion. Significant morbidity and mortality may occur as a result of the compression and invasion of surrounding structures. If localized to the skin, lesions may be successfully excised. However, because of their tendency for deep and infiltrative growth this is usually not possible. Prednisone may shrink the tumor or limit tumor expansion. Successful treatment has also been reported with IFN-α, vincristine, and radiation. If Kasabach–Merritt phenomenon occurs, prognosis is linked to this complication.

Dadras SS, et al: Prox-1 promotes invasion of kaposiform hemangioendotheliomas. J Invest Dermatol 2008 Dec; 128(12):2798–2806.

Harper L, et al: Successful management of a retroperitoneal kaposiform hemangioendothelioma with Kasabach–Merritt phenomenon using alpha-interferon. Eur J Pediatr Surg 2006 Oct; 16(5):369–372.

Vetter-Kauczok CS, et al: Kaposiform hemangioendothelioma with distant lymphangiomatosis without an association to Kasabach–Merritt syndrome in a female adult! Vasc Health Risk Manag 2008; 4(1):263–266.

Multifocal lymphangioendotheliomatosis

Patients with multifocal lymphangioendotheliomatosis present at birth with hundreds of red–brown plaques as large as several centimeters. Similar lesions may occur in the gastrointestinal tract and are associated with severe bleeding. Severe thrombocytopenic coagulopathy (Kasabach–Merritt syndrome) occurs in affected children. Treatment with corticosteroids and/or IFN-α results in little to no improvement. The histology is distinctive, with delicate thin-walled vessels lined by hobnailed endothelium with papillary tufting. The endothelial cells demonstrate a high proliferative fraction with Ki-67 staining, and are reactive with LYVE-1, suggesting lymphatic differentiation.

Piggott KD, et al: Multifocal lymphangioendotheliomatosis with thrombocytopenia: a rare cause of gastrointestinal bleeding in the newborn period. Pediatrics 2006 Apr; 117(4):e810–e813.

Yeung J, et al: Multifocal lymphangioendotheliomatosis with thrombocytopenia. J Am Acad Dermatol 2006 May; 54(5 Suppl): S214–S217.

Kasabach–Merritt syndrome (hemangioma with thrombocytopenia)

Kasabach-Merritt syndrome (KMS) is seen in infants at an average age of 7 weeks. Before the onset of the acute event, the infant will often have a reddish or bluish plaque or tumor on the limb or trunk, or in rare instances, no visible lesion at all. The lesions usually have an associated lymphatic component and most are KHEs. KMS also occurs in tufted angiomas and multifocal lymphangioendotheliomatosis, lesions that both demonstrate lymphatic differentiation. It is rarely reported in association with capillary hemangiomas or angiosarcoma. Some patients with venous malformations will have a chronic low-grade consumptive coagulopathy that occurs throughout life, and this is not to be confused with KMS.

Infants with KMS suddenly develop a painful violaceous mass in association with purpura and thrombocytopenia. The most striking sign is the bleeding tendency, especially in the hemangioma itself or into the chest or abdominal cavities. The spleen may be enlarged. Hemoglobin, platelets, fibrinogen, and factors II, V, and VIII are all reduced. Prothrombin time and partial thromboplastin time are prolonged, and fibrin split products may be elevated. Cases of microangiopathic hemolytic anemia have also been described. Repeated episodes of bleeding may occur, and although these may be spontaneous, it is not uncommon for bleeding to be precipitated by surgery, directed either at the hemangioma or elsewhere. The mortality may be as high as 30%, most deaths being secondary to bleeding complications.

As KMS may be a self-limited disorder, expectant observation may be the best approach initially. Systemic steroids, IFN-α2a, vincristine, vinblastine, cyclophosphamide, actinomycin D, embolization, ε-aminocaproic acid, antiplatelet agents, irradiation, excision, and compression therapy have been utilized alone or in combination, but treatment is often difficult and some patients respond poorly to all attempted modalities.

Abass K, et al: Successful treatment of Kasabach–Merritt syndrome with vincristine and surgery: a case report and review of literature. Cases J 2008 May 23; 1(1):9.

Berkley EM, et al: Consumptive coagulopathy associated with Gorham syndrome and subsequent Kasabach–Merritt syndrome during pregnancy: a case report. J Reprod Med 2007 Dec; 52(12):1103–1106.

Imafuku S, et al: Kasabach–Merritt syndrome associated with angiosarcoma of the scalp successfully treated with chemoradiotherapy. Acta Derm Venereol 2008; 88(2):193–194.

Wang Z, et al: Kasabach–Merritt syndrome caused by giant hemangiomas of the spleen in patients with Proteus syndrome. Blood Coagul Fibrinolysis 2007 Jul; 18(5):505–508.

Acquired progressive lymphangioma (benign lymphangioendothelioma)

The term acquired progressive lymphangioma was introduced by Wilson-Jones in 1976 to designate a group of lymphangiomas that occur anywhere in young individuals, grow slowly, and present as bruise-like lesions or erythematous macules. Rarely, the lesion is yellow or alopecic. The histologic appearance is that of delicate endothelium-lined spaces dissecting between collagen bundles. A similarity to the plaque stage of Kaposi sarcoma may be striking. Simple excision is curative. Prednisone has caused some extensive lesions to regress.

Kim HS, et al: Acquired progressive lymphangioma. J Eur Acad Dermatol Venereol 2007 Mar; 21(3):416–417.

Paik AS, et al: Acquired progressive lymphangioma in an HIV-positive patient. J Cutan Pathol 2007 Nov; 34(11):882–885.

Glomus tumor (glomangioma)

The solitary glomus or neuromyoarterial tumor is most frequently a skin-colored or slightly dusky blue, firm nodule 1–20 mm in diameter. Subungual tumors show a bluish tinge through the translucent nail plate. The tumor is usually extremely tender and paroxysmal pain occurs frequently. Sensitivity is likely to be present constantly, and when touched,

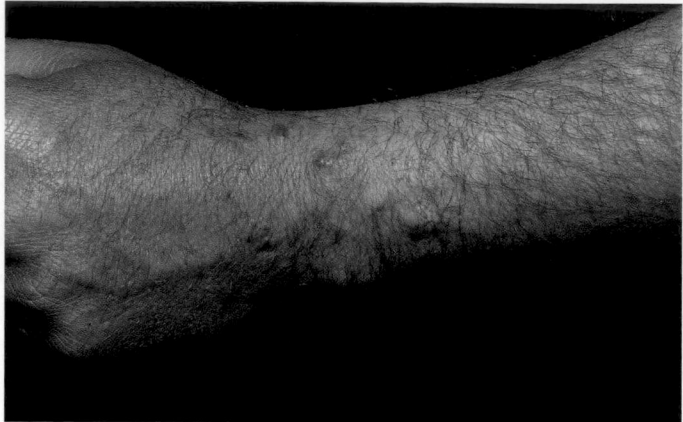

Fig. 28-16 Multiple glomangiomas.

the tumor responds with severe radiating pain. However, nontender glomus tumors are encountered. The characteristic location is subungual, but tumor may occur on the fingers and arms, or elsewhere. Digital lesions are more common in women, and there is a male predominance of nondigital lesions. High-resolution MRI, high-resolution ultrasonography (5–9 MHz), and color duplex sonography may be used to define the limits of the tumor before surgery is undertaken. Progressive growth may lead to ulceration.

Multiple glomangiomas are usually nontender and are generally widely distributed over the body. These may be inherited as an autosomal-dominant trait and can be congenital. Clinically, they may resemble lesions of blue rubber bleb nevus (Fig. 28-16). When grouped in one area, they may appear as a confluent mass. Hereditary multiple glomus tumors may represent an autosomal-dominant mosaic trait and may be congenital. The glomus coccygeum is a normal structure that may be seen in pilonidal sinus excision specimens.

Histologically, glomus tumors contain numerous vascular lumina lined by a single layer of flattened endothelial cells. Peripheral to the endothelial cells are layers of glomus cells. Generally, these are round and arranged in distinct rows resembling strings of black pearls. Rarely, the cells have a somewhat spindled morphology. Multiple glomangiomas tend to have only one or two layers of glomus cells. Glomangiomyomas have a prominent muscularis media in addition to one or two layers of glomus cells. Both solitary and multiple glomus tumors are related to the arterial segment of the cutaneous glomus, the Sucquet–Hoyer canal. The glomus cells are modified vascular smooth muscle cells and stain with vimentin rather than desmin. Smooth muscle actin is often positive.

Treatment of solitary glomus tumors is best carried out by complete excision, which immediately produces relief from pain. The subungual tumors are most difficult to locate and eradicate since they are usually small, seldom more than a few millimeters in diameter.

Rare reports of glomangiosarcomas describe large, deeply located extremity lesions that consist of sarcomatous areas intermingled with areas of benign glomus tumor.

Anakwenze OA, et al: Clinical features of multiple glomus tumors. Dermatol Surg 2008 Jul; 34(7):884–890.

Fong ST, et al: A modified periungual approach for treatment of subungual glomus tumour. Hand Surg 2007; 12(3):217–221.

Gombos Z, et al: Glomus tumor. Arch Pathol Lab Med 2008 Sep; 132(9):1448–1452.

Hemangiopericytoma

True hemangiopericytomas are rare. The term is now reserved for lesions that demonstrate differentiation towards pericytes and cannot be otherwise classified. Many lesions formerly classified as hemangiopericytomas are now classified as examples of solitary fibrous tumor or giant cell angiofibroma. Remaining lesions can often be classified as glomangiopericytoma/myopericytoma or infantile myofibromatosis.

Clinically, the typical lesion is a nontender, bluish red tumor that occurs on the skin or in the subcutaneous tissues on any part of the body. The firm, usually solitary nodule may be up to 10 cm in diameter. Histologically, the tumor is composed of endothelium-lined vessels that are filled with blood and surrounded by cells with oval or spindle-shaped nuclei (pericytes). The pericytes often form a concentric perivascular pattern. Staghorn-like ectatic spaces are often encountered. Wide local excision is the treatment of choice, but radiation therapy may produce excellent palliation.

It is difficult to distinguish between benign and malignant forms of hemangiopericytoma, although large lesions and those with numerous mitoses are more likely to metastasize. Nearly half of the malignant hemangiopericytomas of deep soft tissues metastasize. The rate of metastasis from lesions of the skin is closer to 20%. The most common cause of death is pulmonary metastasis. Infantile tumors are almost always cutaneous or subcutaneous, and do not metastasize.

Lesions formerly classified as hemangiopericytomas

Various soft tissue tumors can present with a hemangiopericytoma-like staghorn vascular pattern, the most common being solitary fibrous tumor and giant cell angiofibroma. Myofibromas demonstrate nodular, pale blue, hypocellular zones with surrounding hypercellular zones that contain staghorn vessels. Some examples lack the hypocellular zones and present only with a hemangiopericytoma-like pattern. Myopericytoma is a rare mesenchymal neoplasm that typically involves the extremities. The tumor demonstrates concentric perivascular spindle cells with myoid differentiation. Glomangiopericytoma is a closely related lesion composed of perivascular spindle cells with myoid differentiation. The tumor combines features of glomus tumors and a hemangiopericytoma-like vascular pattern.

Gengler C, et al: Solitary fibrous tumour and haemangiopericytoma: evolution of a concept. Histopathology 2006 Jan; 48(1):63–74.

Proliferating angioendotheliomatosis

Diseases designated angioendotheliomatosis have historically been divided into two groups: a reactive, involuting type and a malignant, rapidly fatal type. "Malignant angioendotheliomatosis" has been shown to be intravascular (angiotropic) lymphoma, rather than a true vascular lesion.

The reactive type of angioendotheliomatosis is uncommon. It occurs in patients who have subacute bacterial endocarditis, Chagas' disease, pulmonary tuberculosis, cryoproteinemia, severe atherosclerotic disease, periodontal disease, and antiphospholipid antibodies, as well as in patients with no identifiable underlying process. Patients present with red–purple patches, plaques, nodules, petechiae, and ecchymoses, usually of the lower extremities. Some may present with a livedoid pattern or lesions resembling atrophie blanche. Diffuse dermal angiomatosis is a variant associated with atherosclerosis. The lesion occurs most often on the thigh in areas of vascular insufficiency (Fig. 28-17) and clears with revascularization. It has also been described in association with an AV fistula and with anticardiolipin antibodies.

Histologically, the vessels in benign reactive angioendotheliomatosis are dilated and are filled with proliferating endothelial cells, usually without atypia. Some cases demonstrate a proliferation of capillaries in the dermis, with diffuse, lobular,

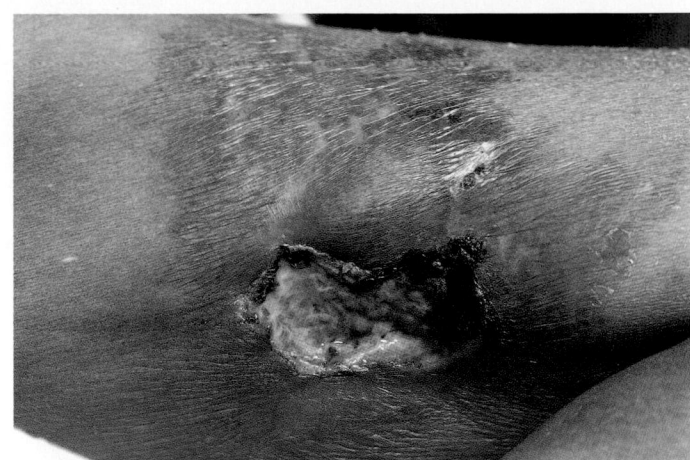

Fig. 28-17 Diffuse dermal angiomatosis.

or mixed patterns. Fibrin microthrombi are common, and some cases show amyloid deposits or positive immunohistochemical staining for human herpesvirus (HHV)-8 in lesional endothelial cell nuclei. The course in this type is characterized by involution over 1–2 years. Therapy for the underlying condition has been considered as hastening involution.

The malignant type of "angioendotheliomatosis" is actually a large-cell, intravascular lymphoma. This is a rapidly progressive disease; usually death ensues within 10 months of diagnosis. The mean age at onset is 55 years. Reddish-purple plaques, nodules, or patches develop in the skin. Multisystem disease is characteristic, with the CNS often involved. There may be progressive dementia or focal signs that reflect ischemic infarcts. Kidney, heart, lung, and gastrointestinal lesions may occur. Biopsy will show a proliferation of atypical cells that fill the lumen of cutaneous vessels. Immunochemical stains for leukocyte/common antigen have confirmed the lymphomatous nature of these cells. Angioendotheliomatosis is usually B-cell in phenotype, but cases of T-cell lineage have been reported. Some organs may show diffuse large-cell lymphoma.

Doxorubicin alone, as well as in combination with vincristine, prednisone, and cyclophosphamide, has been effective in isolated cases. Rituximab has also been useful in CD20+ B-cell intravascular lymphoma.

Kawaoka J, et al: Coexistence of diffuse reactive angioendotheliomatosis and neutrophilic dermatosis heralding primary antiphospholipid syndrome. Acta Derm Venereol 2008; 88(4):402–403.
Kirke S, et al: Localized reactive angioendotheliomatosis. Clin Exp Dermatol 2007 Jan; 32(1):45–47.
Misago N, et al: Simultaneous occurrence of reactive angioendotheliomatosis and leukocytoclastic vasculitis in a patient with periodontitis. Eur J Dermatol 2008 Mar–Apr; 18(2):193–194.

Hemangioendotheliomas

Hemangioendotheliomas (HEs) are a group of tumors that spans the spectrum from benign to low-grade malignancy. Composite lesions occur and kaposiform hemangioendotheliomas are associated with tufted angiomas and Kasabach–Merritt syndrome and discussed along with those entities.

Spindle cell hemangioma (spindle cell hemangioendothelioma) is a vascular tumor that was first described in 1986. The condition commonly presents in a child or young adult who develops blue nodules of firm consistency on a distal extremity (Fig. 28-18). Usually, multifocal lesions occur within an anatomic region. Histologically, a well-circumscribed dermal nodule will contain dilated vascular spaces with fascicles of spindle cells between them. Areas of the tumor will have an open alveolar pattern resembling hemorrhagic lung tissue. Phleboliths are common. A thrombosed large adjacent vessel

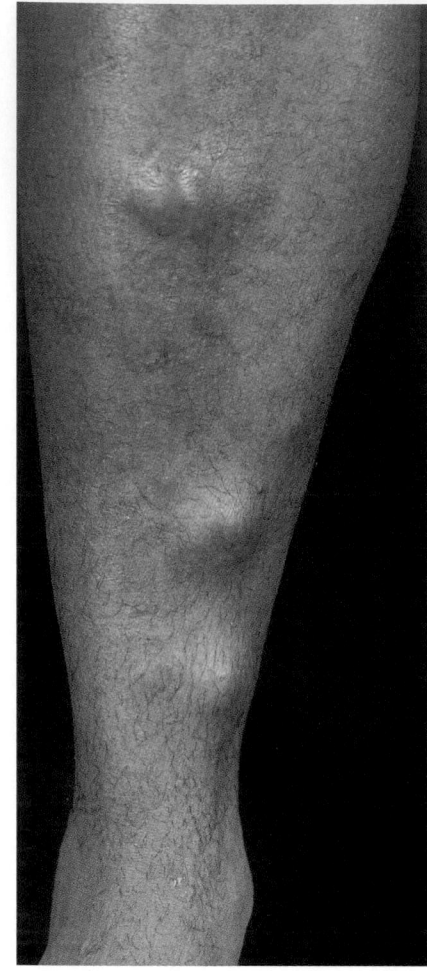

Fig. 28-18 Spindle-cell hemangioendotheliomas. (Courtesy of Timothy Gardner, MD)

with recanalization may be identified. The lesions appear to represent benign vascular proliferations in response to trauma to a larger vessel. They may repeatedly recur focally after excision. Epithelioid HEs are solid tumors composed of epithelioid cells with intracellular lumens. Retiform HEs resemble rete testis at scan. Both tumors behave as low grade malignancies. Composite hemangioendotheliomas may have epithelioid or retiform features and behave as borderline malignant tumors. Immunoreactivity for Prox-1 suggests lymphatic differentiation.

Requena L, et al: Cutaneous composite hemangioendothelioma with satellitosis and lymph node metastases. J Cutan Pathol 2008 Feb; 35(2):225–230.

Tejera-Vaquerizo A, et al: Composite cutaneous hemangioendothelioma on the back. Am J Dermatopathol 2008 Jun; 30(3):262–264.

Malignant neoplasms

Kaposi sarcoma

Moritz Kaposi described this vascular neoplasm in 1872 and called it multiple benign pigmented idiopathic hemorrhagic sarcoma. Since his description, the disease has been reported in five separate clinical settings, with different presentations, epidemiology, and prognoses. The five subtypes are:

1. classic Kaposi sarcoma (KS), an indolent disease seen chiefly in middle-aged men of Southern and Eastern European origin
2. African cutaneous KS, a locally aggressive process affecting middle-aged Africans in tropical Africa

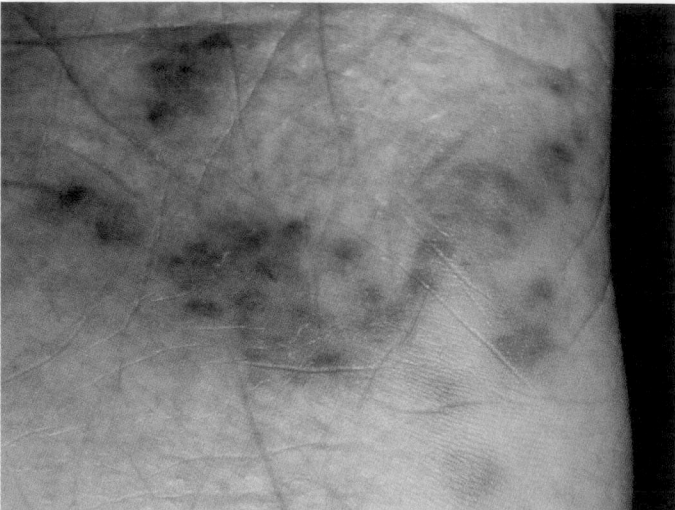

Fig. 28-19 Kaposi sarcoma.

3. African lymphadenopathic KS, an aggressive disease of young patients, chiefly children under age 10
4. KS in patients immunosuppressed by AIDS
5. lymphoma or immunosuppressive therapy.

Clinical features

Classic Kaposi sarcoma The early lesions appear most commonly on the toes or soles as reddish, violaceous, or bluish-black macules and patches that spread and coalesce to form nodules or plaques (Fig. 28-19). These have a rubbery consistency. There may be brawny edema of the affected leg. Macules or nodules may appear, usually much later, on the arms and hands, and rarely may extend to the face, ears, trunk, genitalia, or buccal cavity, especially the soft palate. The course is slowly progressive and may lead to great enlargement of the lower extremities as a result of lymphedema. However, there may be periods of remission, particularly in the early stages of the disease, when nodules may undergo spontaneous involution. After involution there may be an atrophic and hyperpigmented scar.

African cutaneous Kaposi sarcoma Nodular, infiltrating, vascular masses occur on the extremities, mostly of men between the ages of 20 and 50. This form of KS is endemic in tropical Africa, and has a locally aggressive but systemically indolent course.

African lymphadenopathic Kaposi sarcoma Lymph node involvement, with or without skin lesions, may occur in children under 10 years of age. The course is aggressive, often terminating fatally within 2 years of onset.

AIDS-associated Kaposi sarcoma Cutaneous lesions begin as one or several red to purple–red macules, rapidly progressing to papules, nodules, and plaques. There is a predilection for the head, neck, trunk, and mucous membranes. A fulminant, progressive course with nodal and systemic involvement is expected. This may be the presenting manifestation of human immunodeficiency virus (HIV) infection.

Immunosuppression-associated Kaposi sarcoma The lesion's morphology resembles that of classic KS; however, the site of presentation is more variable.

Internal involvement

The gastrointestinal tract is the most frequent site of internal involvement in classic KS. The small intestine is probably the most commonly involved viscus. In addition, the lungs, heart, liver, conjunctiva, adrenal glands, and lymph nodes of the abdomen may be affected. Skeletal changes are characteristic and diagnostic. Bone involvement is always an indication of widespread disease. Changes noted are rarefaction, cysts, and cortical erosion.

African cutaneous KS is frequently accompanied by massive edema of the legs and frequent bone involvement.

African lymphadenopathic KS has been reported among Bantu children, who develop massive involvement of the lymph nodes, especially the cervical nodes, preceding the appearance of skin lesions. The children also develop lesions on the eyelids and conjunctiva, from which masses of hemorrhagic tissue hang down. Eye involvement is often associated with swelling of the lacrimal, parotid, and submandibular glands, with a picture similar to Mikulicz syndrome.

In AIDS-associated KS, 25% of patients have cutaneous involvement alone, whereas 29% have visceral lesions only. The most frequent sites of visceral involvement are the lungs (37%), gastrointestinal tract (50%), and lymph nodes (50%). Visceral involvement ultimately occurs in more than 70% of patients with AIDS-associated KS. Other immunosuppressed patients with KS may have visceral involvement in a variable percentage of cases.

Epidemiology

KS is worldwide in distribution. In Europe there are foci of classic KS in Galicia, near the Polish–Russian border, and extending southward to Austria and Italy. In New York City, KS has occurred mostly in elderly male Galician Jewish and southern Italian persons. In Africa, KS occurs largely south of the Sahara. Northeast Congo and Rwanda–Burundi areas have the highest prevalence, and to a lesser extent, West and South Africa.

The prevalence of AIDS-related KS has decreased since the 1980s. Most cases are in men who have sex with men. Very few reports have documented the exceptional occurrence of KS in patients with AIDS who acquired their infection from intravenous drug use, or in Haitians, children, or people with hemophilia. Patients at risk for developing KS associated with other causes of immunosuppression include those with iatrogenic suppression from oral prednisone or other chronic immunosuppressive therapies, as may be given to transplant patients. Endemic disease in southern Europe is strongly associated with oral corticosteroid use and diabetes, and inversely associated with cigarette smoking.

KS is associated with an increased risk of developing second malignancies, such as malignant lymphomas (Hodgkin disease, T-cell lymphoma, non-Hodgkin lymphoma), leukemia, and myeloma. The risk of lymphoreticular malignancy is about 20 times greater in KS patients than in the normal population.

Etiopathogenesis

KS is formed by proliferation of abnormal vascular endothelial cells. HHV-8 was first found in tissue of a patient with KS and was reported in 1994. Now it has been found in KS lesional tissue irrespective of clinical type. Detection of HHV-8 in HIV-infected individuals who do not have KS is predictive of the development of KS, usually within 2–4 years. It is considered at this time that sexual or fecal–oral transmission is the most likely means of acquiring this infection. The HHV-8 genome has many open reading frames that encode products that lead to growth dysregulation or evasion of immune surveillance. How these orchestrate the formation and proliferation of spindle cells is under active investigation. Primary effusion lymphoma, solid lymphoma, and Castleman's disease are other confirmed associations with HHV-8 infection.

Histology

There is considerable variation in the histopathology according to the stage of the disease. Early lesions demonstrate irregularly shaped ectatic vessels with scattered lymphocytes and plasma cells. The endothelial cells of the capillaries are large and protrude into the lumen, like buds. Later lesions show proliferation of vessels around pre-existing vessels and adnexal structures. The pre-existing structure may jut into the vascular space, forming a promontory sign. Dull pink globules, extravasated erythrocytes, and hemosiderin are present. Nodular lesions are composed of spindle cells with erythrocytes that appear to line up between spindle cells with no apparent vascular space.

Treatment

All types of KS are radiosensitive. Radiation therapy has been used with considerable success, either in small fractionated doses, in larger single doses to limited or extended fields, or by electron beam radiation. Local excision, cryotherapy, alitretinoin gel (Panretin), locally injected chemotherapy or IFN, and laser ablation have been used for troublesome, localized lesions.

Vincristine solution, 0.1 mg/mL injected intralesionally, not more than 3 mL at one time and at intervals of 2 weeks, produces involution of tumors, some for as long as 8 months. These studies indicate that adequate control of the lesions may be achieved, at least for periods of 6–12 months. The development of resistance to medication seems to be inevitable.

Many other agents have been found to be effective; among the best are IFN, vinblastine, and actinomycin D. The response rate initially is high, but recurrent lesions, which are common, are generally less responsive. Systemic therapy is usually needed if more than ten new KS lesions develop in 1 month, or if there is symptomatic lymphedema, symptomatic pulmonary disease, or symptomatic visceral involvement.

In the setting of HIV, protease inhibitors have been shown to have anti-angiogenic effects; however, the results of non-nucleoside reverse transcriptase inhibitor-based regimens are not inferior to protease inhibitor-based therapy in the prevention of KS. This suggests that regression of KS is mediated by an overall improvement in immune function and not by the effects of specific antiretrovirals. Liposomal anthracyclines and paclitaxel have been approved by the US Food and Drug Administration (FDA) as first- and second-line monotherapy, respectively, for advanced KS.

Rapamycin (sirolimus), an inhibitor of the mammalian target of rapamycin (mTOR), is an effective immunosuppressant for the prevention of transplant rejection, with benefits as a treatment for Kaposi's sarcoma. Dual inhibition of PI3Kα and mTOR by PI-103 looks promising.

Course

Classic KS progresses slowly, with rare lymph node or visceral involvement. Death usually occurs years later from unrelated causes. African cutaneous KS is aggressive, with early nodal involvement, and death from KS is expected within 1–2 years. AIDS-related KS, although widespread, is almost never fatal; nearly all patients die of intercurrent infection. The course of the disease is variable in patients who develop immunosuppression-related KS from causes other than AIDS. Removal of the immunosuppression may result in resolution of the KS without therapy.

Anderson LA, et al: Risk factors for classical Kaposi sarcoma in a population-based case-control study in Sicily. Cancer Epidemiol Biomarkers Prev 2008 Dec; 17(12):3435–3443.

Bower M, et al: Immune reconstitution inflammatory syndrome associated with Kaposi's sarcoma. J Clin Oncol 2005; 23:5224.

Chaisuparat R, et al: Dual inhibition of PI3Kalpha and mTOR as an alternative treatment for Kaposi's sarcoma. Cancer Res 2008 Oct 15; 68(20):8361–8368.

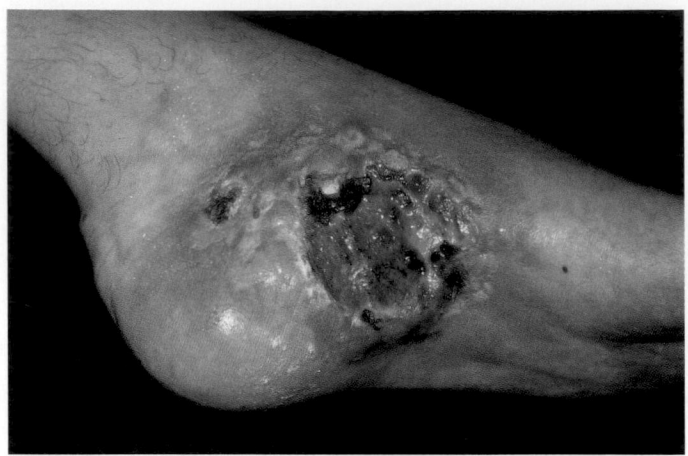

Fig. 28-20 Large ulcerated epithelioid hemangioendothelioma.

O'Mahony D, et al: Imaging techniques for Kaposi's sarcoma. J HIV Ther 2008 Sep; 13(3):65–71.

Epithelioid hemangioendothelioma

In 1982, Weiss et al described this rare tumor, which, both clinically and histologically, is intermediate between angiosarcoma and hemangioma (Fig. 28-20). It is usually a solitary, slowly growing papule or nodule on a distal area of an extremity. There is a male preponderance, and onset is frequently before the individual is 25 years of age. Histologically, there are two components: dilated vascular channels and solid epithelioid and spindle-cell elements with intracytoplasmic lumens. Some may have cellular pleomorphism and mitotic activity. Wide excision is recommended with evaluation of regional lymph nodes. This is the usual site of metastases, and if they occur here, further surgery may be curative. In the minority of cases in which distant metastatic lesions develop, chemotherapy, radiation, or both may be employed. Of the 31 patients from the original series who had follow-up at an average of 18 months, 20 were alive and well.

Epithelioid sarcoma-like hemangioendothelioma demonstrates round to slightly spindled cells in sheets and nests. The cells demonstrate immunohistochemical evidence of endothelial differentiation. Local recurrence and regional soft tissue metastases may occur.

Retiform hemangioendothelioma

Retiform hemangioendothelioma is a low-grade angiosarcoma, first described in 1994. It presents as a slow-growing exophytic mass, dermal plaque, or subcutaneous nodule. It most commonly occurs on the upper or lower extremities of young adults. Histologically, there are arborizing blood vessels reminiscent of normal rete testis architecture. HHV-8 DNA sequences have been reported in this tumor. Wide excision is recommended, although local recurrences are common. To date, no widespread metastases have occurred, although regional lymph nodes may develop tumor infiltrates.

Composite hemangioendothelioma

This low-grade angiosarcoma typically occurs in adults, although it has been described in infancy. The tumor exhibits a mix of retiform hemangioendothelioma-like, spindle cell hemangioma-like, cavernous hemangioma-like, epithelioid hemangioendothelioma-like, and angiosarcoma-like patterns. Labeling for Prox-1 suggests a lymphatic line of differentiation. The lesions may be associated with Kasabach–Merritt or Maffucci syndrome. Local recurrences and regional lymph

node metastasis have been noted. Excision is the usual treatment, but response to IFN has been reported.

Fukunaga M, et al: Composite hemangioendothelioma: report of 5 cases including one with associated Maffucci syndrome. Am J Surg Pathol 2007 Oct; 31(10):1567–1572.
Goh SG, et al: Cutaneous vascular tumours: an update. Histopathology 2008 May; 52(6):661–673.
Parsons A, et al: Retiform hemangioendotheliomas usually do not express D2-40 and VEGFR-3. Am J Dermatopathol 2008 Feb; 30(1):31–33.
Requena L, et al: Cutaneous composite hemangioendothelioma with satellitosis and lymph node metastases. J Cutan Pathol 2008 Feb; 35(2):225–230.
Tan D, et al: Retiform hemangioendothelioma: a case report and review of the literature. J Cutan Pathol 2005 Oct; 32(9):634–637.
Uta S, et al: Composite cutaneous haemangioendothelioma treated with interferon. J Eur Acad Dermatol Venereol 2008 Apr; 22(4):503–505.

Endovascular papillary angioendothelioma (Dabska tumor)

Endovascular papillary angioendothelioma, a rare low-grade angiosarcoma, presents as a slow-growing tumor on the head, neck, or extremity of infants or young children. It shows multiple vascular channels with papillary plugs of endothelial cells surrounding central hyalinized cores that project into the lumina, sometimes forming a glomeruloid pattern. The entity is controversial, as similar histologic features have been observed in other vascular tumors, such as angiosarcoma, retiform hemangioendothelioma, and glomeruloid hemangioma. The tumor may be a distinct entity, or demonstrate a histologic pattern seen in other vascular tumors. One patient with this histologic pattern developed KMS, and others have developed regional metastasis. Wide excision and excision of the regional lymph nodes, in cases where they are involved, are usually curative.

Schwartz RA, et al: The Dabska tumor: a thirty-year retrospect. Dermatology 2000; 201:1.

Angiosarcoma

Angiosarcomas of the skin occur in four clinical settings. First and most common are those that occur in the head and neck of elderly people. The male to female ratio is 2:1. The lesion often begins as an ill-defined bluish macule that may be mistaken for a bruise. Distinguishing features are the frequent occurrence of a peripheral erythematous ring, satellite nodules, the presence of intratumoral hemorrhage, and the tendency for the lesion to bleed spontaneously, or after minimal trauma. The tumor progressively enlarges asymmetrically, often becomes multicentric, and develops indurated bluish nodules and plaques. The sudden development of thrombocytopenia may herald metastatic disease or an enlarging primary tumor.

Solid sheets of atypical epithelioid cells may be present, but more commonly, the pattern is that of subtle infiltration in the dermis, producing the appearance of cracks between collagen bundles. The spaces are lined by hyperchromatic nuclei. Immunoperoxidase staining for endothelial markers such as CD31, CD34, and *Ulex europeus* lectin aids in the diagnosis. Virtually all malignant vascular tumors are positive for podoplanin.

Early diagnosis and complete surgical excision, followed by moderate-dose, very wide-field radiotherapy, offer the best prognosis for limited disease. Chemotherapy and radiation therapy for extensive disease are often only palliative, especially when dealing with scalp lesions and high-grade lesions. Doxorubicin–ifosfamide chemotherapy produces a modest response rate. Paclitaxel and IFN have shown some response for scalp and facial angiosarcomas. Because of the multicentricity of lesions, the frequent occurrence on the face or scalp, and the rapid growth with early metastasis, death occurs in most patients within 2 years. Spieth et al reported a dramatic response in a 77-year-old man with recurrent angiosarcoma of the face and scalp after combination treatment with IFN-α2a and 13-cis-retinoic acid.

The second classic clinical situation in which angiosarcoma develops is in chronic lymphedematous areas, such as that which occurs in the upper arm after mastectomy, the so-called Stewart–Treves syndrome (Fig. 28-21). This tumor appears approximately 11–12 years after surgery in an estimated 0.45% of patients. The prognosis is poor for these patients, with a mean survival of 19–31 months, and a 5-year survival rate of 6–14%. Metastases to the lungs are the most frequent cause of death. Early amputation offers the best hope.

A third setting includes tumors that develop in previously irradiated sites. If the condition for which radiation therapy was given was a benign one, the average interval between radiation and development of angiosarcoma is 23 years. If the preceding illness was a malignant condition, the interval is shortened to 12 years. Again, the prognosis is poor, with survival time generally between 6 months and 2 years after diagnosis. Many patients with the Stewart–Treves syndrome received radiation, and radiation may play a pathogenic role.

Angiosarcomas develop in settings other than those previously described, and this small miscellaneous subset comprises the fourth category. An angiosarcoma producing granulocyte colony-stimulating factor was associated with prominent peripheral leukocytosis.

Buschmann A, et al: Surgical treatment of angiosarcoma of the scalp: less is more. Ann Plast Surg 2008 Oct; 61(4):399–403.

Gkalpakiotis S, et al: Successful radiotherapy of facial angiosarcoma. Int J Dermatol 2008 Nov; 47(11):1190–1192.

Kikuchi A, et al: Primary cutaneous epithelioid angiosarcoma. Acta Derm Venereol 2008; 88(4):422–423.

Köhler HF, et al: Cutaneous angiosarcoma of the head and neck: report of 23 cases from a single institution. Otolaryngol Head Neck Surg 2008 Oct; 139(4):519–524.

Fibrous tissue abnormalities

Keloid

A keloid is a firm, irregularly shaped, fibrous, hyperpigmented, pink or red excrescence. The growth usually arises as the result of a cut, laceration, or burn—or, less often, an acne pustule on the chest or upper back—and spreads beyond the limits of the original injury, often sending out clawlike (cheloid) prolongations. The overlying epidermis is smooth, glossy, and thinned from pressure. The early, growing lesion is red and tender, and has the consistency of rubber. It is often surrounded by an erythematous halo, and the keloid may be telangiectatic. Lesions may be tender, painful, and pruritic, and may rarely ulcerate or develop draining sinus tracts.

Keloids are often multiple. They may be as tiny as pinheads or as large as an orange. Those that follow burns and scalds are large. Lesions are often linear, frequently having bulbous expansions at each end. The surface may be larger than the base, so that the edges are overhanging. The most common location is the sternal region, but keloids also occur frequently on the neck, ears, extremities, or trunk, and rarely on the face, palms, or soles. The earlobes are frequently involved as a result of ear piercing, but involvement of the central face is rare. They are much more common, and grow to larger dimensions, in black persons than in other races.

Why certain individuals develop keloids still remains unsolved. Trauma is usually the immediate causative factor, but this induces keloids only in those with a predisposition for their development. There is also a regional predisposition.

Histologically, a keloid is a dense and sharply defined nodular growth of myofibroblasts and collagen with a whorl-like arrangement resembling hypertrophic scar. Centrally, thick hyalinized bundles of collagen are present, and distinguish keloids from hypertrophic scars. There is a paucity of elastic tissue, just as in a scar. By pressure, the tumor causes thinning of the normal papillary dermis and atrophy of adjacent appendages, which it pushes aside. Mucopolysaccharides are increased, and often there are numerous mast cells.

Keloids are usually distinctive. They may be distinguished from hypertrophic scars by their clawlike projections (Fig. 28-22), which are absent in the hypertrophic scar, the extension of the lesion beyond the confines of the original injury, and the

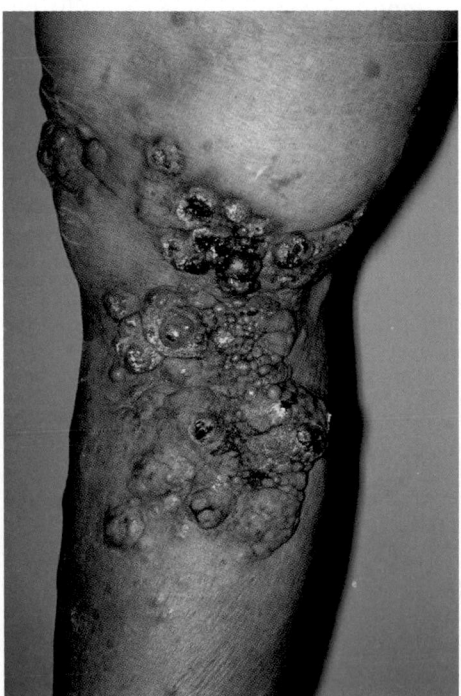

Fig. 28-21 Stewart–Treves syndrome.

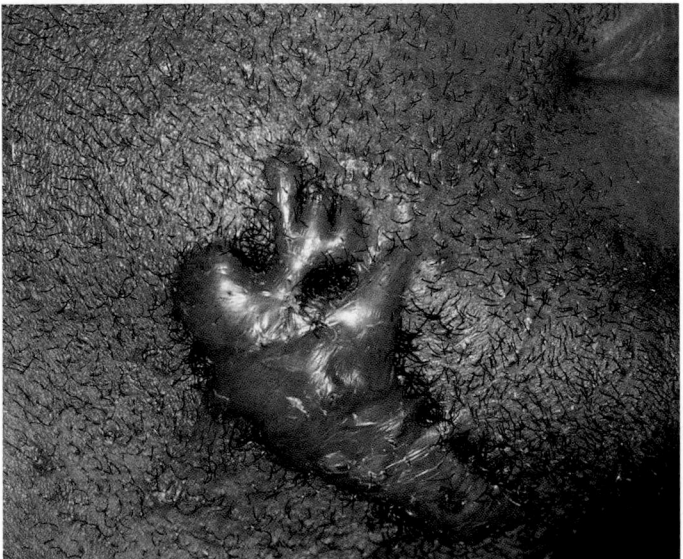

Fig. 28-22 Keloid.

presence of thick hyalinized collagen bundles histologically. Frequently there is a spontaneous improvement of the hypertrophic scar over a period of months, whereas in the keloid this does not occur. Atypical lesions should be biopsied, as carcinoma en cuirasse may mimic keloid.

Initial treatment is usually by means of intralesional injection of triamcinolone suspension alone or in combination with 5-fluorouracil (5-FU). Using a 30-gauge needle on a 1 mL tuberculin Luer syringe, triamcinolone suspension is injected into various parts of the lesion; 40 mg/mL is generally used for initial treatment, although, as the lesion softens, 10–20 mg/mL may be sufficient to produce involution with less risk of surrounding hypopigmentation and atrophy related to lymphatic spread of the corticosteroid. Injections are repeated at intervals of 6–8 weeks, as required. Flattening and cessation of itching are reliably achieved by this approach, and may sometimes even be achieved with topical corticosteroids. The lesions are never made narrower, however, and hyperpigmentation generally persists. Transforming growth factor (TGF)-β is known to be involved in keloid formation, and triamcinolone acetonide-induced decreases in cellular proliferation and collagen production are associated with a statistically significant decrease in the level of TGF-β1 in both normal and keloid fibroblast cell lines. Anti-TGF-β1 therapy looks promising, as does NF-κB inhibition and green tea polyphenol epigallocatechin-3-gallate.

Other approaches to treatment include flashlamp pulsed dye laser treatment, which is also associated with reduced expression of TGF-β1. Cryosurgery (including contact, intralesional needle cryoprobe, and spray cryosurgery), intralesional 5-FU, intralesional etanercept, and calcium channel-blockers have some demonstrated efficacy in the treatment of keloids. Fibroblasts derived from the central part of keloids grow faster than peripheral keloid and nonkeloid fibroblasts. Verapamil has been shown to decrease interleukin (IL)-6 and VEGF in these cultured cells, and to inhibit cell growth.

If surgical removal by excision is feasible, and if narrowing of the keloid is a vitally important goal, the keloid may be excised. After the excision, intralesional injection of triamcinolone or IFN-α2b may be combined with postoperative x-ray irradiation or topical application of imiquimod. Silicone sheeting and pressure are other adjunctive methods used to limit recurrences. Results with these modalities have been mixed. Silicone gel-sheet treatment has been shown to reduce lesional mast cell numbers and decrease itching. Banding at the base of the keloid with a suture ligature for a 5-week period has been used successfully to treat pedunculated lesions.

Pierced-ear keloids occur with considerable frequency. When the keloid is young, intralesional injection of triamcinolone is frequently sufficient to control the problem. In old keloids, excision of the lesion using lidocaine with triamcinolone, followed by injections at 2-week intervals, produces good results. CO$_2$ laser excision has also been successful in old mature keloids in this site.

Berman B, et al: Prevention and management of hypertrophic scars and keloids after burns in children. J Craniofac Surg 2008 Jul; 19(4):989–1006.

Berman B, et al: Evaluating the tolerability and efficacy of etanercept compared to triamcinolone acetonide for the intralesional treatment of keloids. J Drugs Dermatol 2008 Aug; 7(8):757–761.

Butler PD, et al: Current progress in keloid research and treatment. J Am Coll Surg 2008 Apr; 206(4):731–741 (Epub 2008 Feb 1).

Chike-Obi CJ, et al: Keloids: pathogenesis, clinical features, and management. Semin Plast Surg 2009 Aug; 23(3):178–184.

Hochman B, et al: Intralesional triamcinolone acetonide for keloid treatment: a systematic review. Aesthetic Plast Surg 2008 Jul; 32(4):705–709.

Makino S, et al: DHMEQ, a novel NF-kappaB inhibitor, suppresses growth and type I collagen accumulation in keloid fibroblasts. J Dermatol Sci 2008 Sep; 51(3):171–180.

Park G, et al: Green tea polyphenol epigallocatechin-3-gallate suppresses collagen production and proliferation in keloid fibroblasts via inhibition of the STAT3-signaling pathway. J Invest Dermatol 2008 Oct; 128(10):2429–2441.

Robles DT, et al: Keloids: pathophysiology and management. Dermatol Online J 2007 Jul 13; 13(3):9.

Tan KT, et al: The influence of surgical excision margins on keloid prognosis. Ann Plast Surg 2010 Jan; 64(1):55–58.

Dupuytren contracture

Dupuytren contracture is a fibromatosis of the palmar aponeurosis. The lesion arises most commonly in men between the ages of 30 and 50 as multiple firm nodules in the palm. Usually, 3–5 nodules about 1 cm in diameter develop, proximal to the fourth finger. Later, the fibromatosis produces contractures, which may be disabling. The condition occurs at times with alcoholic cirrhosis, diabetes mellitus, and chronic epilepsy. It is also associated with Peyronie's disease, plantar fibromatosis, and knuckle pads. In some cases there is a familial predisposition. The fibrous nodules are composed of myofibroblasts that express androgen receptors. 5-α-Dihydrotestosterone induces an increase in Dupuytren fibroblast proliferation. In contrast to deep fibromatoses, which behave more aggressively, superficial fibromatoses lack β-catenin and adenomatous polyposis coli (APC) gene mutations.

Early intralesional triamcinolone may help, but surgical excision of the involved palmar fascia may be the only way to liberate severely contracted fingers. Androgen blockade represents a potential avenue of pharmacologic therapy. As with keloids, matrix metalloproteinase and TGF-β2 inhibition appear promising.

Plantar fibromatosis

The plantar analog of Dupuytren contracture, plantar fibromatosis (Ledderhose's disease) occurs as slowly enlarging nodules on the soles that ultimately cause difficulty in walking or even weight-bearing. The diagnosis is usually made clinically, but both biopsy and MRI can be used to confirm the diagnosis. The usual treatment, as for Dupuytren contracture, is wide excision of the plantar fascia. Subtotal excision is associated with a high rate of recurrence. Although adjuvant radiotherapy is effective in decreasing the recurrence rate, it has a significant complication rate with functional impairment. Improvement by the intralesional injection of triamcinolone acetonide, 30 mg/mL monthly for 5 months, has been reported. The triamcinolone can be diluted with lidocaine solution.

Hindocha S, et al: Revised Tubiana's staging system for assessment of disease severity in Dupuytren's disease—preliminary clinical findings. Hand (N Y) 2008 Jun; 3(2):80–86.

Ostlere S, et al: Masses of the foot closely related to the plantar fascia. Foot Ankle Int 2007 Jan; 28(1):145.

Townley WA, et al: Matrix metalloproteinase inhibition reduces contraction by Dupuytren fibroblasts. J Hand Surg [Am] 2008 Nov; 33(9):1608–1616.

Zhang AY, et al: Gene expression analysis of Dupuytren's disease: the role of TGF-β2. J Hand Surg Eur Vol 2008 Dec; 33(6):783–790.

Peyronie's disease

Plastic induration of the penis is a fibrous infiltration of the intercavernous septum of the penis. This fibrosis results in the formation of nodules or plaques. As a result of these plaques, a fibrous chordee is produced, and curvature of the penis occurs on erection, sometimes so severe as to make intromission difficult or impossible. Sometimes pain may be severe. The association of this disease with Dupuytren contracture has been recognized.

Injection of IFN-α2b, verapamil, or collagenase has been employed, with the strongest evidence supporting IFN use. Intralesional triamcinolone suspension injected or iontophoresed into the plaques and nodules has shown mixed results. Oral therapies include tocopherol (vitamin E), para-aminobenzoate, colchicine, tamoxifen, and acetyl-L-carnitine, but data supporting oral therapy are weak. Surgical correction tailored to the degree of deformity is often successful. Extracorporeal shock wave therapy may reduce penile pain and improve sexual function, although objective changes in plaque size and curvature have not been demonstrated.

Smith JF, et al: Peyronie's disease: a critical appraisal of current diagnosis and treatment. Int J Impot Res 2008 Sep–Oct; 20(5):445–459.

Tran VQ, et al: Review of the surgical approaches for Peyronie's disease: corporeal plication and plaque incision with grafting. Adv Urol 2008:263450.

Knuckle pads

Knuckle pads (heloderma) are well-defined, round, plaque-like, fibrous thickenings that develop on the extensor aspects of the proximal interphalangeal joints (Fig. 28-23) of the toes and fingers, including the thumbs. They develop at any age and grow to be some 10–15 mm in diameter in the course of a few weeks or months, then persist permanently. They are flesh-colored or somewhat brown, with normal or slightly hyperkeratotic epidermis overlying and adherent to them. They are a part of the skin and are freely movable over underlying structures.

Knuckle pads are sometimes associated with Dupuytren contracture, clubbing, or camptodactylia (irreducible flexion contracture of one or more fingers). Some cases are familial and some are related to trauma or frequent knuckle cracking. An autosomal-dominant association of knuckle pads, mixed hearing loss (sensorineural and conductive), and total leukonychia has been reported. Knuckle pads have also been

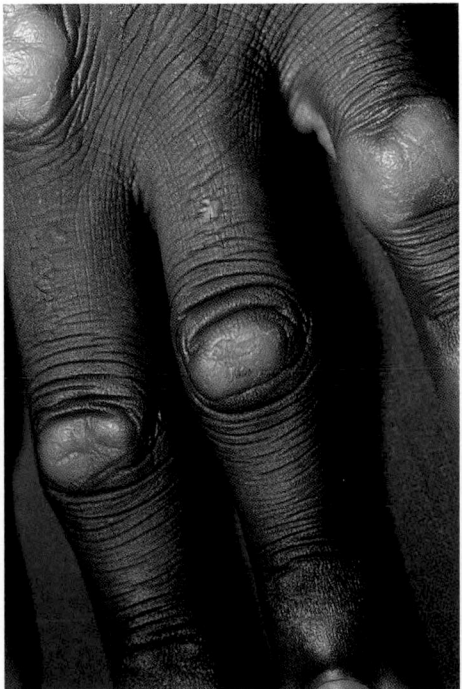

Fig. 28-23 Knuckle pads.

associated with autosomal-dominant epidermolytic palmoplantar keratoderma with a mutation in keratin 9.

Histologically, the lesions are fibromas. They are to be differentiated clinically from the nodular type of neurodermatitis and from the small hemispherical pitted papules that may develop over the knuckles after frostbite or in acrocyanosis, and from rheumatic nodules. Treatment with intralesional injection of corticosteroids may be beneficial. As with keloids, intralesional 5-FU may be beneficial.

Akiyama M, et al: A novel GJB2 mutation p.Asn54His in a patient with palmoplantar keratoderma, sensorineural hearing loss and knuckle pads. J Invest Dermatol 2007 Jun; 127(6):1540–1543.

Koba S, et al: Knuckle pads associated with clubbed fingers. J Dermatol 2007 Dec; 34(12):838–840.

Weiss E, et al: A novel treatment for knuckle pads with intralesional fluorouracil. Arch Dermatol 2007 Nov; 143(11):1458–1460.

Pachydermodactyly

Pachydermodactyly represents a benign fibromatosis of the fingers. There is a fullness of the medial and lateral digit just proximal to the proximal interphalangeal joint. This asymptomatic process is most often first noted in adolescence and usually involves multiple fingers. Five types have been described: classic pachydermodactyly, localized pachydermodactyly, transgrediens pachydermodactyly in which the abnormality extends to the metacarpophalangeal areas, familial pachydermodactyly, and pachydermodactyly associated with tuberous sclerosis. Some instances may result from repetitive tic-like obsessive-compulsive behaviors. Increased collagen or mucin accounts for the swelling. Cases associated with repetitive tics respond to treatment for the obsessive-compulsive disorder.

Al Hammadi A, et al: Pachydermodactyly: case report and review of the literature. J Cutan Med Surg 2007 Sep–Oct; 11(5):185–187.

Desmoid tumor

Desmoid tumors occur as large, deep-seated, well-circumscribed masses arising from the muscular aponeurosis. They most commonly occur on the abdominal wall, especially in women during or soon after pregnancy. Desmoid tumors have been divided into five types: abdominal wall, extra-abdominal, intra-abdominal, multiple, and those occurring in Gardner syndrome/familial adenomatous polyposis. They recur locally and can kill if they invade, surround, or compress vital structures. The most dangerous, then, are those at the root of the neck and the intra-abdominal type. MRI will aid in the evaluation of soft tissue extension and recurrence following treatment. Mutations in the β-catenin gene correlate with local recurrence.

Treatment may be with wide local excision, radiotherapy, or hormonal manipulation. High-dose tamoxifen in combination with sulindac has been effective. Mesenteric desmoid tumors have been treated with anti-angiogenic therapy with toremifene and IFN-α2b. Imatinib mesylate looks promising.

Lazar AJ, et al: Specific mutations in the beta-catenin gene (CTNNB1) correlate with local recurrence in sporadic desmoid tumors. Am J Pathol 2008 Nov; 173(5):1518–1527.

Collagenous fibroma (desmoplastic fibroblastoma)

This slow-growing, deep-set, benign fibrous tumor is usually located in the deep subcutis, fascia, aponeurosis, or skeletal muscle of the extremities, limb girdles, or head and neck regions. It is characterized by hypocellularity and dense bands of hyalinized collagen that may infiltrate into skeletal muscle.

Despite this, no tumors have been reported to metastasize or recur after excision. Chromosomal translocation (2; 11)(q31; q12) has been reported. Tumor cells stain for vimentin, and may stain for actin, but have been negative for CD34, S-100 protein, keratin, CD68, desmin, and β-catenin.

Sakamoto A, et al: Desmoplastic fibroblastoma (collagenous fibroma) with a specific breakpoint of 11q12. Histopathology 2007 Dec; 51(6):859–860.

Watanabe H, et al: Desmoplastic fibroblastoma (collagenous fibroma). J Dermatol 2008 Feb; 35(2):93–97.

Aponeurotic fibroma

Aponeurotic fibroma has also been called juvenile aponeurotic fibroma (calcifying fibroma). It is a tumor-like proliferation characterized by the appearance of slow-growing, cystlike masses that occur on the limbs, especially the hands and feet.

Histologically, the distinctive lesions are sharply demarcated and composed of collagenous stroma showing acid mucopolysaccharides infiltrated by plump mesenchymal cells with oval nuclei. Hyalinized areas are also present, suggesting chondroid or osteoid metaplasia. An aid to the diagnosis is stippled calcification, readily seen on roentgenograms. Surgical excision is the treatment of choice and can be guided by MRI.

Morii T, et al: Clinical significance of magnetic resonance imaging in the preoperative differential diagnosis of calcifying aponeurotic fibroma. J Orthop Sci 2008 May; 13(3):180–186.

Infantile myofibromatosis

Infantile myofibromatosis is the most common fibrous tumor of infancy. Eighty percent of patients have solitary lesions, with half of these occurring on the head and neck. About 60% are present at or soon after birth.

Congenital generalized fibromatosis is an uncommon condition that presents at birth or soon after. It is characterized by multiple, firm, dermal and subcutaneous nodules. Skeletal lesions, primarily of the metaphyseal regions of the long bones, occur in 50% of patients. If only the skin and bones develop fibromas, the prognosis is excellent, with spontaneous resolution of the lesions without complications expected within the first 1–2 years of life. Some refer to this limited disease as congenital multiple fibromatosis. Females more commonly contract the generalized disease.

The fibromas may involve the viscera, including the gastrointestinal tract, breast, lungs, liver, pancreas, tongue, serosal surfaces, lymph nodes, or kidney. Autosomal-dominant inheritance has been reported. Histologically, fascicles of spindle cells occur in a whorled pattern. These nodules are composed of myofibroblasts.

Mortality in this more widespread subset is high. Eighty percent of affected individuals die from obstruction or compression of vital organs. Those who survive past 4 months have spontaneous regression of their disease. Some life-threatening cases have responded to low-dose chemotherapy.

Diffuse infantile fibromatosis

This process occurs within the first 3 years of life and is usually confined to the muscles of the arms, neck, and shoulder area. There is a multicentric infiltration of muscle fibers with fibroblasts resembling those seen in aponeurotic fibromas. Calcification does not occur. Recurrence after excision occurs in about one-third of cases.

Aggressive infantile fibromatosis

The clinical presentation of this locally recurring, nonmetastasizing lesion involves single or multiple fast-growing masses that are present at birth or occur within the first year of life. Infantile fibromatosis may be seen in any location, although the arms, legs, and trunk are the usual sites. Histologically, it is hypercellular and mimics malignancy.

Alaggio R, et al: Morphologic overlap between infantile myofibromatosis and infantile fibrosarcoma: a pitfall in diagnosis. Pediatr Dev Pathol 2008 Sep–Oct; 11(5):355–362.

Azzam R, et al: First-line therapy of generalized infantile myofibromatosis with low-dose vinblastine and methotrexate. Pediatr Blood Cancer 2008 Oct 20; 52(2):308.

Martín JM, et al: Self-healing generalized infantile myofibromatosis. J Eur Acad Dermatol Venereol 2008 Feb; 22(2):236–238.

Juvenile hyaline fibromatosis and infantile systemic hyalinosis

Juvenile hyaline fibromatosis and infantile systemic hyalinosis are allelic autosomal-recessive conditions characterized by multiple subcutaneous skin nodules, hyaline deposition, gingival hypertrophy, osteolytic bone lesions, and joint contractures. Nodular tumors of the scalp, face, and extremities usually appear in early childhood. Pink confluent papules may occur on the paranasal folds, and periauricular (Fig. 28-24) and perianal regions. The gene has been mapped to chromosome 4q21 with at least 15 different mutations in the gene encoding capillary morphogenesis protein 2, a transmembrane protein that is induced during capillary morphogenesis and that binds laminin and collagen IV.

Histologically, there are fibroblasts with fine intracytoplasmic eosinophilic granules, embedded in a homogeneous eosinophilic dermal ground substance. Ultrastructurally, the fibroblasts demonstrate defective synthesis of collagen, deposited as fibrillogranular material.

Antaya RJ, et al: Juvenile hyaline fibromatosis and infantile systemic hyalinosis overlap associated with a novel mutation in capillary morphogenesis protein-2 gene. Am J Dermatopathol 2007; 29:99.

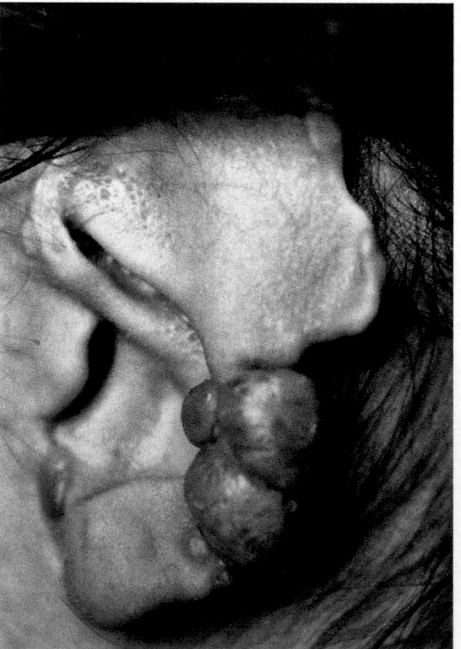

Fig. 28-24 Juvenile hyaline fibromatosis.

Dhingra M, et al: Juvenile hyaline fibromatosis and infantile systemic hyalinosis: divergent expressions of the same genetic defect? Indian J Dermatol Vencreol Leprol 2008 Jul–Aug; 74(4):371–374.

Infantile digital fibromatosis (infantile digital myofibroblastoma, inclusion body fibroma)

Infantile digital fibromatosis is a rare neoplasm of infancy and childhood that usually occurs on the dorsal or lateral aspects of the distal phalanges of the toes and fingers. The thumb and great toe are usually spared. These asymptomatic, firm, red, smooth nodules occur during the first year of life, 47% in the first month. Rare congenital lesions have been noted. The lesions do not metastasize, but may infiltrate deeply.

Histologically, the epidermis is normal, but the dermis is infiltrated with proliferating myofibroblasts and collagen bundles. Eosinophilic cytoplasmic inclusions in many of the fibroblasts are characteristic. Treatment by surgical excision has a high risk of recurrence, and conservative, nonsurgical management is often appropriate. Spontaneous regression is generally noted, but the lesion may cause functional impairment and may infiltrate deeply before regression occurs. Mohs micrographic surgery has been performed successfully using both trichrome staining and smooth muscle actin staining to demonstrate the inclusion bodies within tumor cells.

Campbell LB, et al: Mohs micrographic surgery for a problematic infantile digital fibroma. Dermatol Surg 2007 Mar; 33(3):385–387.
Grenier N, et al: A range of histologic findings in infantile digital fibromatosis. Pediatr Dermatol 2008 Jan–Feb; 25(1):72–75.
Taylor HO, et al: Infantile digital fibromatosis. Ann Plast Surg 2008 Oct; 61(4):472–476.

Fibrous hamartoma of infancy

Fibrous hamartoma of infancy is a single dermal or subcutaneous firm nodule of the upper trunk that is present at birth or shortly thereafter. Overlying skin changes are uncommon, but may include increased hair, alteration in pigmentation, and eccrine gland hyperplasia. Most cases are solitary, but multiple tumors have been reported. Ninety-one percent are noted within the first year of life and 23% are congenital. The male to female ratio is 2.4:1. Most lesions occur in the axillary region, upper arm, upper trunk, inguinal region, and external genital area. An association with Williams syndrome has been reported. Biopsy shows an organoid pattern with different types of tissue organized in whorls or bands. In early lesions, lobules of mature fat are interspersed between myxoid and fibrous areas. Myxoid zones have primitive mesenchymal cells with stellate nuclei. Fibrosing areas demonstrate delicate collagen bundles and many elongated fibroblast nuclei. A complex chromosomal translocation (6; 12; 8)(q25; q24.3; q13) has been reported. Over time, both the myxoid and fibrosing areas develop into cell-poor fibrous areas with thick collagen bundles. There is no recurrence after excision.

Gupta R, et al: Cytologic diagnosis of fibrous hamartoma of infancy: a case report of a rare soft tissue lesion. Acta Cytol 2008 Mar–Apr; 52(2):201–203.
Togo T, et al: Fibrous hamartoma of infancy in a patient with Williams syndrome. Br J Dermatol 2007 May; 156(5):1052–1055.

Fibromatosis colli

In fibromatosis colli there is a fibrous tissue proliferation infiltrating the lower third of the sternocleidomastoid muscle at birth. Fine needle aspiration is useful to confirm the diagnosis. Spontaneous remission occurs within a few months. Occasionally, some patients are left with a wryneck deformity; however, this complication is amenable to surgery.

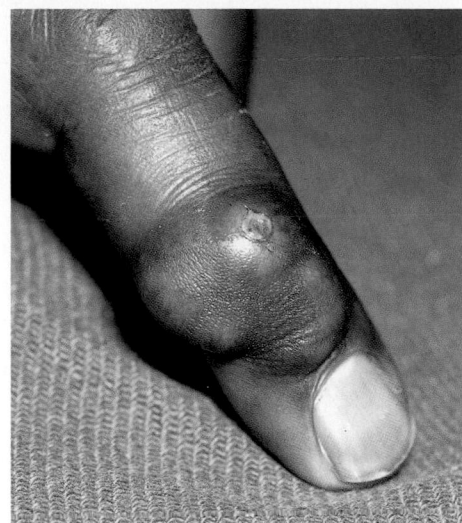

Fig. 28-25 Giant cell tumor of the tendon sheath.

Nayak SP, et al: Cytodiagnosis of fibromatosis colli. Cytopathology 2007 Aug; 18(4):266–268.

Giant cell tumor of the tendon sheath

This tumor, which is most commonly attached to the tendons of the fingers (Fig. 28-25), hands, and wrists, has a predilection for the flexor surfaces. It is firm, measures from 1 to 3 cm in diameter, and does not spontaneously involute. It recurs after excision in approximately 25% of cases. Another tumor of the tendon sheath, fibroma of the tendon sheath, may represent a variant of the giant cell tumor. It also affects the flexural tendons of the fingers and hands, and morphologically, it and the giant cell tumor are identical. The condition tends to occur in younger men (the average age at onset is 30) than does the giant cell variety. When a proliferation similar to giant cell tumor of the tendon sheath occurs in deeper tissues, it is referred to as pigmented villo-nodular tenosynovitis. The pigment is hemosiderin.

Histologically, the giant cell tumor consists of lobules of densely hyalinized collagen. The characteristic osteoclast-like giant cells have deeply eosinophilic cytoplasm that moulds to adjacent cells. A variable number of randomly distributed nuclei are present. Lipophages and siderophages may be numerous, and hemosiderin deposition may impart a brown color to the lesions on gross examination. The fibroma of the tendon sheath generally lacks lipophages, siderophages, and giant cells, with the lobules being composed of dense fibrocollagenous tissue.

The rate of recurrence depends on the presence or absence of a pseudocapsule, lobulation of the tumor, extra-articular location, and the presence of satellite lesions. Local recurrence has been treated with more extensive surgery, and imaging studies can define the extent of the tumor. Radiation therapy has been reported anecdotally.

Gholve PA, et al: Giant cell tumor of tendon sheath: largest single series in children. J Pediatr Orthop 2007 Jan–Feb; 27(1):67–74.
Wang Y, et al: The value of sonography in diagnosing giant cell tumors of the tendon sheath. J Ultrasound Med 2007 Oct; 26(10): 1333–1340.

Ainhum

Ainhum is also known as dactylolysis spontanea, bankokerend, and sukhapakla. It is a disease affecting the toes, especially the fifth toe, characterized by a linear constriction around the affected digit, which leads ultimately to the spontaneous amputation of the distal part. It occurs chiefly among black men in Africa. Usually it is unilateral, but it may be bilateral.

The disease begins with a transverse groove in the skin on the flexor surface of the toe, usually beneath the first interphalangeal articulation. The furrow is produced by a ringlike fibrosis and an induration of the dermis. It deepens and extends laterally around the toe until the two ends meet, so that the digit becomes constricted, as if in a ligature. The constricted part becomes swollen, soft, and after a time, greatly distended. Ulceration may result in a malodorous discharge, with pain and gangrene. The course of the disease is slow, but in 5–10 years spontaneous amputation occurs, generally at a joint.

The cause is unknown. The condition may result from chronic trauma and exposure to the elements by walking barefoot in the tropics. Fissuring followed by chronic inflammation and fibrosis may then result.

Treatment in early cases by cutting the constricting band is unsuccessful; in advanced cases amputation of the affected member is advisable. Surgical correction by Z-plasty has produced good results. Intralesional injection of betamethasone (total, 15 injections) has also been successful.

Pseudo-ainhum

Pseudo-ainhum has been a term used in connection with certain hereditary and nonhereditary diseases in which annular constriction of digits occurs. Hereditary disorders include hereditary palmoplantar keratodermas, especially Vohwinkel syndrome and mal de Meleda, pachyonychia congenita, Ehlers–Danlos syndrome, erythropoietic protoporphyria, and congenital ectodermal defect. Nonhereditary disorders associated with constriction of digits are ainhum, Hansen's disease, cholera, ancylostomiasis, scleroderma, Raynaud syndrome, pityriasis rubra pilaris, psoriasis, Olmsted syndrome, Reynold syndrome (scleroderma and primary biliary cirrhosis with antimitochondrial antibodies), syringomyelia, ergot poisoning, and tumors of the spinal cord. Factitial pseudo-ainhum may be produced by self-application of a rubber band, string, or other ligature. Congenital cases have been reported that may affect digits or limbs. It may occur as a familial condition or may be secondary to amniotic bands.

Treatment may be with surgery or intralesional injection of corticosteroids, as in ainhum. Retinoids may be used in diseases responsive to them.

Almond SL, et al: Pseudoainhum in chronic psoriasis. Br J Dermatol 2003; 149:1064.

Rashid RM, et al: Destructive deformation of the digits with auto-amputation: a review of pseudo-ainhum. J Eur Acad Dermatol Venereol 2007 Jul; 21(6):732–737.

Connective tissue nevi

These uncommon lesions may present as acquired isolated plaques, as multiple lesions—either acquired or congenital, or as one finding in a more generalized disease. Biopsy findings in many cases do not appear very different from normal skin, although in some cases altered amounts of collagen or elastin may be identified.

These lesions characteristically occur on the trunk, most often in the lumbosacral area (Fig. 28-26). They may be solitary, but are often multiple, in which case they may show a linear or zosteriform arrangement. Individual lesions are slightly elevated plaques 1–15 cm in diameter, varying in color

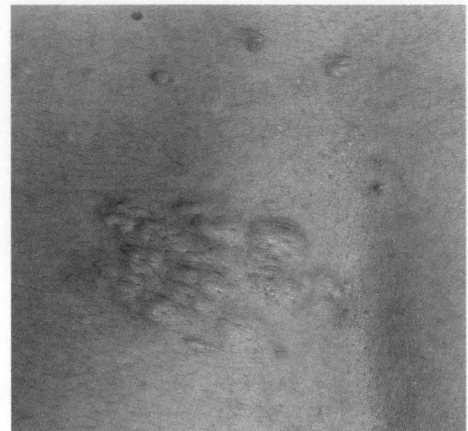

Fig. 28-26 Connective tissue nevus.

from light yellow to orange, with a surface texture resembling shagreen leather. In Proteus syndrome, the connective tissue nevi are present as plantar, or occasionally, palmar masses with a cerebriform surface.

Connective tissue nevi of the acquired type have been classified as eruptive collagenomas, isolated collagenomas, or isolated elastomas, depending on the number of lesions and the predominant dermal fibers present. They cannot be differentiated clinically.

Hereditary types of connective tissue nevi include dermatofibrosis lenticularis disseminata in the Buschke–Ollendorff syndrome, familial cutaneous collagenoma, and the shagreen patches seen in tuberous sclerosis.

Buschke–Ollendorff syndrome is an autosomal-dominantly inherited disorder in which widespread dermal papules and plaques develop asymmetrically over the trunk and limbs. Elastic fiber thickening, highly variable fiber diameter, and desmosine increases 3–7-fold above normal have been described in these patients. The associated feature of osteopoikilosis is asymptomatic, but it is diagnostic in x-ray evaluation. Focal sclerotic densities are seen, primarily in the long bones, pelvis, and hands. The syndrome is highly variable, and familial inheritance of elastic tissue nevi without evidence of osteopoikilosis has been reported.

Papular elastorrhexis is characterized by multiple white, evenly scattered papules, usually occurring on the trunk. There is a decrease of elastic fibers, which may appear thin and fragmented. Most reported cases are sporadic but familial occurrence has been described.

Patients with familial cutaneous collagenomas may present with numerous symmetric asymptomatic dermal nodules on the back. The age of onset is usually in the mid- to late teens. In patients with the inherited disease, multiple endocrine neoplasia type I multiple collagenomas were reported in 23 of 32 patients. These were less than 3 mm in diameter and were on the upper torso, neck, and shoulders. They occurred in association with numerous other cutaneous findings, such as angiofibromas, café-au-lait macules, and lipomas. Atrioseptal defect has also been reported in association with familial collagenomas.

The collagenomas of tuberous sclerosis are associated with adenoma sebaceum, periungual fibromas, and ash-leaf macules. Because at least half the cases of tuberous sclerosis result from new mutations, all patients with connective tissue nevi should be carefully studied for evidence of tuberous sclerosis, even in the absence of a family history of the disease. Isolated plantar collagenoma may exhibit a cerebriform appearance and resemble plantar fibromas of Proteus syndrome.

Eruptive collagenomas may be widespread or localized. They have rarely been associated with infectious diseases such as syphilis.

Mucinous nevus is a form of connective tissue nevus characterized by increased ground substance without increases in collagen or elastin. Histologically, collagen bundles are widely separated by mucin and may be attenuated. Overlying follicular induction similar to that seen in dermatofibromas may be present.

Asano Y, et al: Linear connective tissue nevus. Pediatr Dermatol 2007 Jul–Aug; 24(4):439–441.

Brazzelli V, et al: Zosteriform connective tissue nevus in a pediatric patient. Pediatr Dermatol 2007 Sep–Oct; 24(5):557–558.

Gurel MS, et al: Familial cutaneous collagenoma: new affected family with prepubertal onset. J Dermatol 2007 Jul; 34(7):477–481.

Elastofibroma dorsi

Elastofibroma dorsi is a benign tumor usually located in the deep soft tissues in the subscapular region, but sometimes at other sites. The tumor is firm and unencapsulated, and measures up to several centimeters in diameter. It is believed to represent an unusual response to repeated trauma. Histologically, the tumor consists of abundant compact sclerotic collagen mixed with large, swollen, irregular elastic fibers, often appearing as globules of elastic tissue. It commonly appears on nuclear medicine scans, suggesting it is not as uncommon as once believed. Computed tomography (CT) and MRI can define the extent of the lesion, and excision is curative.

Mortman KD, et al: Elastofibroma dorsi: clinicopathologic review of 6 cases. Ann Thorac Surg 2007 May; 83(5):1894–1897.

Angiofibromas

These skin-colored to reddish papules, which show fibroplasia and varying degrees of vascular proliferation in the upper dermis, may occur as a solitary nonhereditary form, the fibrous papule of the nose, as multiple nonhereditary lesions, pearly penile papules, or as multiple hereditary forms as in tuberous sclerosis, Birt–Hogg–Dube syndrome (in combination with the specific lesion, the fibrofolliculoma), and multiple endocrine neoplasia type I. There have been reports of agminated or segmental angiofibromas that may represent a segmental form of tuberous sclerosis. The multiple hereditary types are discussed in other chapters.

Cellular angiofibroma typically occurs in the genital region of older women. It is composed of small spindle cells arranged in short fascicles and relatively abundant small rounded vessels. They may express estrogen and progesterone receptors, and also CD34.

Hall MR, et al: Unilateral facial angiofibromas without other evidence of tuberous sclerosis: case report and review of the literature. Cutis 2007 Oct; 80(4):284–288.

Val-Bernal JF, et al: Extragenital subcutaneous cellular angiofibroma. Case report. APMIS 2007 Mar; 115(3):254–258.

Fibrous papule of the nose (fibrous papule of the face, benign solitary fibrous papule)

These lesions occur in adults as dome-shaped, sessile, skin-colored, white or reddish papules, 3–6 mm in diameter, on or near the nose (Fig. 28-27). Fibrous papule is usually solitary, but it is not uncommon for a few lesions to occur. It may be confused with a nevocytic nevus, neurofibroma, granuloma pyogenicum, or a basal cell carcinoma. Like other angiofibromas, fibrous papules demonstrate concentric fibrosis surrounding vessels and adnexal structures. Stellate dermal

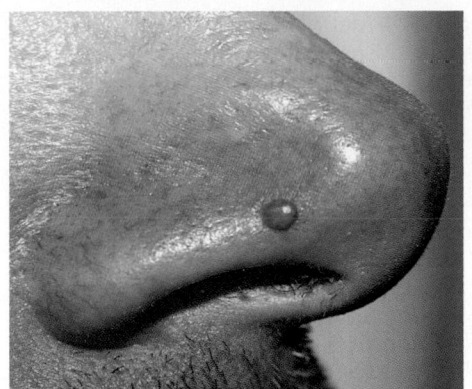

Fig. 28-27 Fibrous papule.

dendrocytes are often prominent. Clear cell, granular, and epithelioid variants have been described. They stain for factor XIIIa. Large pyramidal junctional melanocytes are often noted overlying the lesion, and a superficial shave biopsy may be mistaken for a melanocytic lesion. Conservative excision is curative; recurrence is rare. Multiple lesions should prompt a search for other stigmata of tuberous sclerosis.

Jacyk WK, et al: Fibrous papule of the face with granular cells. Dermatology 2008; 216(1):56–59.

Kucher C, et al: Epithelioid fibrous papule—a new variant. J Cutan Pathol 2007 Jul; 34(7):571–575.

Pearly penile papules

This is the term given to pearly-white, dome-shaped papules occurring circumferentially on the coronal margin and sulcus of the glans penis. The lesions may be firm or soft and filiform. Occasionally, lesions are also present on the penile shaft. Pearly penile papules are not uncommon. Patients usually present around the age of 20–30 years, concerned that these are condylomata, or are referred as having treatment-resistant venereal warts. These lesions should be distinguished from papillomas, hypertrophic sebaceous glands, and condyloma acuminatum. No treatment is necessary, only reassurance. If treatment is desired, laser ablation or shave excision is effective.

Acral fibrokeratoma

Acral fibrokeratoma, often called acquired digital fibrokeratoma, is characterized by a pinkish, hyperkeratotic, horn-like projection occurring on a finger, toe, or palm. The projection usually emerges from a collarette of elevated skin. The average age of the patient is 40. The lesion resembles a rudimentary supernumerary digit, cutaneous horn, or a neuroma. Onset during immunosuppressive therapy has been reported.

Histologic sections show a central core of thick collagen bundles interwoven closely in a vertical position. This is surrounded by capillaries and a fine network of reticulum fibers. Stellate dermal dendrocytes may be present, as in fibrous papule. Simple surgical excision or laser ablation at the level of the skin surface is effective.

Qiao J, et al: Acquired digital fibrokeratoma associated with ciclosporin treatment. Clin Exp Dermatol 2009 Mar; 34(2):257–259.

Familial myxovascular fibromas

Multiple verrucous papules on the palms and fingers, which on biopsy show focal neovascularization and mucin-like changes in the papillary dermis, have been described. Clinically, these lesions closely resemble warts. They have been reported in several family members, with a probable autosomal-dominant inheritance.

Superficial acral fibromyxoma

Superficial acral fibromyxoma typically appears in the superficial soft tissues of the acral extremity of an adult. Most are painless. Histologically, they are characterized by a moderately cellular proliferation of bland spindled and stellate fibroblasts with a loose storiform or fascicular growth pattern. Mucin and small blood vessels are prominent. Spindle cells commonly express CD34, CD99, and epithelial membrane antigen. CD10 and nestin expression have also been reported.

Al-Daraji WI, et al: Superficial acral fibromyxoma: a clinicopathological analysis of 32 tumors including 4 in the heel. J Cutan Pathol 2008 Nov; 35(11):1020–1026.

Tardío JC, et al: Superficial acral fibromyxoma: report of 4 cases with CD10 expression and lipomatous component, two previously underrecognized features. Am J Dermatopathol 2008 Oct; 30(5):431–435.

Subungual exostosis

Subungual exostosis is closely related to solitary osteochondroma and both are found beneath the distal edge of the nail, most commonly of the great toe. Rarely, the terminal phalanges of other toes, particularly the little toe or even the fingers, may be involved. The exostosis is seen chiefly in women between the ages of 12 and 30. The first appearance is a small pinkish growth projecting slightly beyond the inner free edge of the nail. The overlying nail becomes brittle and either breaks or is removed, after which the tumor, being released, mushrooms upward and distally above the level of the nail. It grows slowly to a maximum diameter of about 8 mm. Pressure of the shoe on the lesion causes great pain.

Subungual exostosis must be differentiated from pyogenic granuloma, verruca vulgaris, pterygium inverum unguis, ingrowing nail, and glomus tumor. If subungual exostosis is suspected, the diagnosis can be confirmed by radiographic examination. Complete excision or curettage is the proper method of treatment.

Campanelli A, et al: Images in clinical medicine. Subungual exostosis. N Engl J Med 2008 Dec 18; 359(25):e31.

Lee SK, et al: Two distinctive subungual pathologies: subungual exostosis and subungual osteochondroma. Foot Ankle Int 2007 May; 28(5):595–601.

Chondrodermatitis nodularis chronica helicis

This is a small, nodular, tender, chronic inflammatory lesion occurring on the helix of the ear. Most patients are men. The lesions are not uncommon, and sometimes as many as 12 nodules may arrange themselves along the edge of the upper helix. The lesions are 2–4 mm in diameter, well defined, slightly reddish, and extremely tender. At times, the surface is covered by an adherent scale or a shallow ulcer. After the masses have reached a certain size, growth ceases, but the lesions persist unchanged for years. There is no tendency to malignant change. Similar lesions may occur on the anthelix, predominantly in women.

The lesion is produced by ischemic necrosis of the dermis, and generally occurs on the side the patient favors during sleep. There may be a history of frostbite, chronic trauma, or chronic actinic exposure with concomitant actinically induced lesions of the face and dorsal hands.

Histologically, a zone of eosinophilic necrosis of collagen is flanked by granulation tissue. Overlying acanthosis and hyperkeratosis and central ulceration may be present. The histologic changes resemble those of a decubitus ulcer, but on a smaller scale. Occasionally, bizarre reactive fibroblasts are noted, as in atypical decubital fibroplasia.

The lesions may be excised. The underlying cartilage may be excised or fenestrated to reduce pressure on the overlying skin during sleep. The patient may be encouraged to change sleeping positions, but many find this difficult. Pillows with an ear slot are also available.

Affleck AG: Surgical treatment of chondrodermatitis nodularis chronica helicis: conservation of normal tissue is important for optimal esthetic outcome. J Oral Maxillofac Surg 2008 Oct; 66(10):2194.

Rajan N, et al: The punch and graft technique: a novel method of surgical treatment for chondrodermatitis nodularis helicis. Br J Dermatol 2007 Oct; 157(4):744–747.

Oral submucous fibrosis

A distinctive fibrosis of the oral mucosa occurs in the western Pacific basin and south Asia among persons whose diet is heavily seasoned with chili or who chew betel, a compound of the nut of the areca palm, the leaf of the betel pepper, and lime. The irritation produced first causes a thickening of the palate, tonsillar pillars, and fauces secondary to dermal and muscular fibrosis (Fig. 28-28). As the disease progresses, opening of the mouth and protrusion of the tongue develop, such that eating, swallowing, and speech are impaired. Later, ulceration and leukoplakic areas occur, and finally, in approximately 7% of patients, malignant transformation to squamous cell carcinoma develops. Treatment consists of the intralesional injection of dexamethasone and hyaluronidase, and in advanced cases surgical excision and grafting or laser ablation have been used. Discontinuance of the offending substance and physical therapy are also needed.

Aziz SR: Oral submucous fibrosis: case report and review of diagnosis and treatment. J Oral Maxillofac Surg 2008 Nov; 66(11):2386–2389.

Isaac U, et al: Histopathologic features of oral submucous fibrosis: a study of 35 biopsy specimens. Oral Surg Oral Med Oral Pathol Oral Radiol Endod 2008 Oct; 106(4):556–560.

Nayak DR, et al: Role of KTP-532 laser in management of oral submucous fibrosis. J Laryngol Otol 2008 Oct 10:1–4.

Fascial hernia

Evanescent herniations in the form of nodules appear in the skin where the deep and superficial veins meet as they go

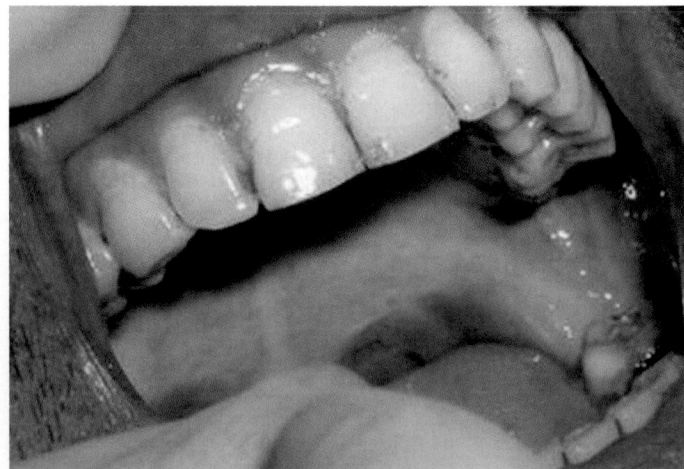

Fig. 28-28 Oral submucous fibrosis. (Courtesy of Shyam Verma, MD)

through the fascia. These herniated nodules, seen most frequently on the lower extremities, become prominent when the underlying muscles contract, and pain may occur with prolonged exertion. Treatment is not indicated unless the area is chronically painful. Light compression may be effective.

Harrington AC, et al: Hernias of the anterior tibialis muscle. J Am Acad Dermatol 1990; 22:123.

Perineal skin tag (infantile perianal pyramidal protrusion)

Perineal skin tags may be congenital or acquired. They are generally asymptomatic, but may require surgical intervention if inflamed or traumatized. A similar appearance may occur as a manifestation of lichen sclerosus.

Cutaneous pseudosarcomatous polyp and umbilical polyp

Cutaneous pseudosarcomatous polyps and umbilical pseudosarcomatous polyps are benign proliferations with a tag-like configuration, but dramatic cytologic atypia and pleomorphism. The cells stain positive for vimentin and variably for CD34 and factor XIIIa. Their clinical behavior is benign.

Bord A, et al: Prenatal sonographic diagnosis of congenital perineal skin tag: case report and review of the literature. Prenat Diagn 2006 Nov; 26(11):1065–1067.

Cathro HP, et al: Cutaneous pseudosarcomatous polyp: a recently described lesion. Ann Diagn Pathol 2008 Dec; 12(6):440–444.

Acrochordon (cutaneous tag, papilloma colli, fibroma pendulum, cutaneous papilloma, fibroma molluscum, Templeton skin tags, skin tags)

Small, flesh-colored to dark brown, pinhead-sized and larger, sessile and pedunculated papillomas commonly occur on the neck, often in association with small seborrheic keratoses. These tags are also seen frequently in the axillae and on the eyelids, and less often on the trunk and groins, where the soft, pedunculated growths often hang on thin stalks. These flesh-colored, teardrop-shaped tags feel like small bags. Occasionally, as a result of twisting of the pedicle, one will become inflamed, tender, and even gangrenous. Both sexes have the same incidence, with nearly 60% of individuals acquiring them by the age of 69. They often increase in number when the patient is gaining weight or during pregnancy, and may be related to the growth hormone-like activity of insulin. They may be associated with diabetes mellitus. In patients preselected for gastrointestinal complaints, skin tags appear to be more prevalent in those with colonic polyps. This association has not been proved for the general population.

Histologically, acrochordons are characterized by epidermis enclosing a dermal fibrovascular stalk. The baglike papillomas generally show a flattened epidermis. Smaller lesions often demonstrate seborrheic keratosis-like acanthosis and horn cysts.

Small lesions can be clipped off at the base with little or no anesthesia. Aluminum chloride may be applied for hemostasis if needed. Light electrodesiccation can also be effective. For larger lesions, anesthesia and snip excision are preferred.

An entity that is frequently reported as perianal acrochordons or skinfolds has now been named infantile perianal pyramidal protrusions. This occurs in young children, usually girls, in the midline anterior to the anus. It reduces with time and no treatment is necessary. Child abuse, genital warts, hemorrhoids, granulomatous lesions of inflammatory bowel disease, or rectal prolapse must be considered in the differential diagnosis of these lesions.

Tag-like basal cell carcinomas in childhood should suggest a diagnosis of nevoid basal cell carcinoma syndrome (NBCCS). Biopsy should be performed on acrochordons in children because the lesions are uncommon in this age group, and they may be the presenting sign of NBCCS.

Dermatofibroma (fibrous histiocytoma)

This common skin lesion's appearance is usually sufficiently characteristic to permit clinical diagnosis. It is generally a single round or ovoid papule or nodule, about 0.5–1 cm in diameter, which is reddish-brown, sometimes with a yellowish hue. The sharply circumscribed nodule is more evident on palpation than expected from inspection. The larger lesions may present an abrupt elevation at the border to form an exteriorized tumor resting on a sessile base.

Dermatofibroma may be elevated or slightly depressed. The hard lesion is adherent to the overlying epidermis, which may be thinner from pressure or even indented, so that there is a dell-like depression over the nodule (Fig. 28-29). In such cases only the depression is seen, but on palpation the true nature of the lesion is found. Fitzpatrick proposed the term dimple sign for the depression created over a dermatofibroma when it is grasped gently between thumb and forefinger.

Dermatofibromas seldom occur in children; they are encountered mostly in middle-aged adults. Their size generally varies from 4 to 20 mm, although giant lesions greater than 5 cm occur. After they reach this size, growth ceases and the harmless lump remains stationary. The principal locations are on the lower extremities, above the elbows, or on the sides of the trunk. Systemic lupus erythematosus, treatment with prednisone or immunosuppressive drugs, chronic myelogenous leukemia, and HIV infection have been associated with the development of multiple dermatofibromas. It is suspected that many dermatofibromas are initiated by injuries to the skin, such as insect bites or blunt trauma.

On histologic examination there is a dermal mass composed of close whorls of fibrous tissue in which there are numerous spindle or histiocytic cells. The cells have features of fibroblasts and myofibroblasts, but are probably of primitive mesenchymal origin. Immunohistochemical studies show that most cells are positive for factor XIIIa and CD10, and negative for MAC387, S-100, and CD34. The tumor is not well circumscribed and may extend into adjacent structures and surround individual collagen bundles at the periphery

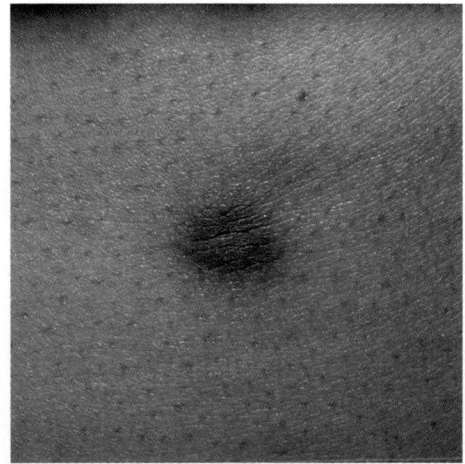

Fig. 28-29 Dermatofibroma. (Courtesy of Lawrence Lieblich, MD)

(collagen trapping). Overlying acanthosis is typical, and induction of primitive epithelial germs or mature follicular structures may be noted. Basal cell carcinoma-like changes commonly overlie dermatofibromas, but true basal cell carcinoma is quite rare.

At times, large histiocytic cells within the lesion are strikingly atypical (monster cells). Occasionally, granular cytoplasm may predominate. Hemosiderin may be present, and foam cells and lipid deposits may be seen. The presence of Touton giant cells containing hemosiderin is pathognomonic of dermatofibroma. There is a great variation in the vascular components. Rarely, the vascularization is pronounced and suggests a kind of hemangioma (sclerosing hemangioma). Deep penetrating dermatofibromas may grow into the subcutaneous tissue via the fibrous septa or with a pushing front of tumor. They lack the extensive lacy and lamellar infiltrative growth pattern of dermatofibrosarcoma protuberans. Deep fascial fibrous histiocytomas may involve the fat or muscle at times. Signet ring and plaque-type variants have been described. A pigmented variant has been described showing histologic overlap with Bednar tumor (pigmented dermatofibrosarcoma protuberans). The lesion stained positive for CD34, a marker usually absent in dermatofibromas.

The clinical appearance of the lesion and its location, chiefly on the lower extremities, are distinctive. Clinically, granular cell tumor, dermatofibrosis lenticularis disseminata, clear-cell acanthoma, and melanoma are some of the lesions to be considered. At times only a biopsy can differentiate these. Progressive enlargement beyond 2 or 3 cm in diameter suggests a malignant fibrous histiocytoma or dermatofibrosarcoma protuberans, and excisional biopsy is indicated.

These lesions usually are asymptomatic and do not require treatment. Involution may occur after many years if the lesion is left alone. Simple reassurance is suggested.

Epithelioid cell histiocytoma

Usually solitary, but occasionally multiple, these lesions appear as dome-shaped papules composed of bland epithelioid cells. They typically stain for factor XIIIa and are considered by many to be closely related to dermatofibromas.

Cangelosi JJ, et al: Unusual presentation of multiple epithelioid cell histiocytomas. Am J Dermatopathol 2008 Aug; 30(4):373–376.

de Feraudy S, et al: Evaluation of CD10 and procollagen 1 expression in atypical fibroxanthoma and dermatofibroma. Am J Surg Pathol 2008 Aug; 32(8):1111–1122.

Garrido-Ruiz MC, et al: Signet-ring cell dermatofibroma. Am J Dermatopathol 2009 Feb; 31(1):84–87.

Leow LJ, et al: Plaque-like dermatofibroma: a distinct and rare benign neoplasm? Australas J Dermatol 2008 May; 49(2):106–108.

McAllister JC, et al: CD34+ pigmented fibrous proliferations: the morphologic overlap between pigmented dermatofibromas and Bednar tumors. Am J Dermatopathol 2008 Oct; 30(5):484–487.

Dermal dendrocyte hamartoma

This presents as a rounded, medallion-like lesion on the upper trunk; it is composed of fusiform CD34, factor XIIIa-positive cells in the mid- and reticular dermis. The lesions are asymptomatic, brown or erythematous in color, and may have a slightly atrophic, wrinkled surface (Fig. 28-30). The major differential diagnosis is congenital atrophic dermatofibrosarcoma protuberans (DFSP), but to date there has been no evidence of chromosomal abnormalities such as the t(17; 22)(q22; q13) translocation with the DFSP fusion gene *COL1A1-PDGFB*.

Marque M, et al: Medallion-like dermal dendrocyte hamartoma: the main diagnostic pitfall is congenital atrophic dermatofibrosarcoma. Br J Dermatol 2009 Jan; 160(1):190–193.

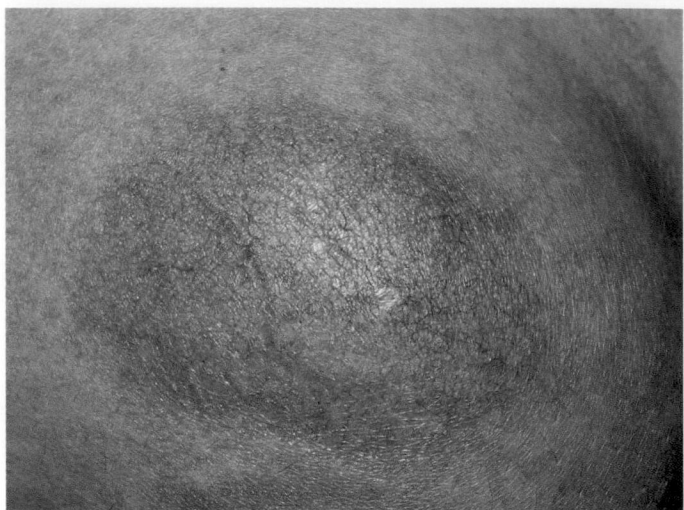

Fig. 28-30 Dermal dendrocyte hamartoma.

Shah KN, et al: Medallion-like dermal dendrocyte hamartoma. Pediatr Dermatol 2007 Nov–Dec; 24(6):632–636.

Nodular fasciitis (nodular pseudosarcomatous fasciitis)

Also known as subcutaneous pseudosarcomatous fibromatosis, this benign mesenchymal neoplasm occurs most often on the arms. Clinically, a firm, solitary, sometimes tender nodule develops in the deep fascia, and often extends into the subcutaneous tissue. It usually measures 1–4 cm in diameter. The lesion appears suddenly over a period of a few weeks, without apparent cause, in normal, healthy persons. Sex distribution is equal and the average age at onset is 40.

Microscopic findings consist of well-defined, loose nodules of stellate and spindled cells that may have a myxoid "tissue culture" appearance. Capillary proliferation is typical, and erythrocyte extravasation between spindle cells is common. Nodular lymphoid infiltrates are often noted within the lesion. On electron microscopic examination, the component cells in the neoplasm have proved to be myofibroblasts.

Dermal, intravascular, and proliferating variants (proliferative fasciitis) have been described. These are designated when the nodular masses arise in the dermis, in intimate association with blood vessels, or show ganglion-like giant cells and infiltration of collagen. The proper treatment is complete excision. Recurrence is rare and the prognosis is excellent. A rapid response to intralesional corticosteroids has been reported in one case.

Cranial fasciitis of childhood is an uncommon variant of nodular fasciitis, manifesting as a rapidly enlarging mass in the subcutaneous tissue of the scalp, which may invade the cranium. It occurs in infants and children, resembles nodular fasciitis histologically, and usually does not recur after surgical excision. Some lesions have demonstrated dysregulation of the Wnt/β-catenin pathway.

Proliferative fasciitis and proliferative myositis are closely related entities. Proliferative fasciitis demonstrates irregular extension into the fibrous septae with collagen trapping and ganglion-like nuclei. Proliferative myositis has a similar appearance, but extends into adjacent muscle.

Pseudosarcomatous ischemic fasciitis (atypical decubital fibroplasia) is a manifestation of pressure-induced necrosis. The histologic appearance is similar to that of chondrodermatitis nodularis of the ear, only on a much larger scale. A wide zone of fibrinoid necrosis is bordered by granulation tissue and large atypical fibroblast nuclei that resemble radiation fibroblasts.

Hussein MR: Cranial fasciitis of childhood: a case report and review of literature. J Cutan Pathol 2008 Feb; 35(2):212–214.
Johnson KK, et al: Diagnosing cranial fasciitis based on distinguishing radiological features. J Neurosurg Pediatrics 2008 Nov; 2(5):370–374.
Numajiri T, et al: Nodular fasciitis of the upper eyelid. Eur J Dermatol 2009 Jan–Feb; 19(1):85–86.
Rakheja D, et al: A subset of cranial fasciitis is associated with dysregulation of the Wnt/beta-catenin pathway. Mod Pathol 2008 Nov; 21(11):1330–1336.
Reitzen SD, et al: Nodular fasciitis: a case series. J Laryngol Otol 2008 Jun 13:1–4.

Solitary fibrous tumor

Solitary fibrous tumors occur in the mediastinum, but may also be found in many other parts of the body. They have a diffuse "patternless" growth pattern and stain strongly positive for CD34. Some express progesterone receptor. Their behavior is unpredictable and complete excision is recommended. Spindle cell lipomas with few or no lipocytes ("low-fat" and "non-fat" spindle cell lipomas) may be misinterpreted as solitary fibrous tumors because they are also CD34-positive.

Billings SD, et al: Diagnostically challenging spindle cell lipomas: a report of 34 "low-fat" and "fat-free" variants. Am J Dermatopathol 2007 Oct; 29(5):437–442.
Insabato L, et al: Extrapleural solitary fibrous tumor: a clinicopathologic study of 19 cases. Int J Surg Pathol 2009 Jun; 17(3):250–254.

Plexiform fibrohistiocytic tumor

This rare tumor arises primarily on the upper extremities of children and young adults. There is a strong female predisposition. It presents as a slowly growing, painless growth in the subcutaneous tissue. There is usually extension into the dermis or the underlying skeletal muscle. Histologically, it is a distinctly biphasic tumor, with a fibroblastic component mixed with aggregates of mononuclear histiocyte-like cells and multinucleated osteoclast-like cells. The multinucleated cells label for vimentin and CD68, while the spindle cells express smooth muscle actin but not factor XIIIa. While most patients are cured with excisional surgery, some tumors will recur locally, and uncommonly, regional and systemic metastases can occur.

Moosavi C, et al: An update on plexiform fibrohistiocytic tumor and addition of 66 new cases from the Armed Forces Institute of Pathology, in honor of Franz M. Enzinger, MD. Ann Diagn Pathol 2007 Oct; 11(5):313–319.

Dermatofibrosarcoma protuberans

Dermatofibrosarcoma protuberans (DFSP) is characterized by bulky, protuberant, neoplastic masses. Between 50 and 60% occur on the trunk, with less common involvement of the proximal extremities and the head and neck. The disease begins with one or multiple elevated, erythematous, firm nodules or plaques, often associated with a purulent exudate or with ulceration. Patients, usually middle-aged, complain of a firm, painless lump in the skin that has been slowly increasing in size for several years. The course is slowly progressive, with pain becoming prominent as the lesion grows, and frequent recurrence after initial conservative surgical intervention (Fig. 28-31). In untreated patients, severe pain and contractures may result. There is little tendency to metastasize, although wide dissemination has been reported.

Histologically, the tumor shows a subepidermal fibrotic plaque with uniform spindle cells and variable vascular

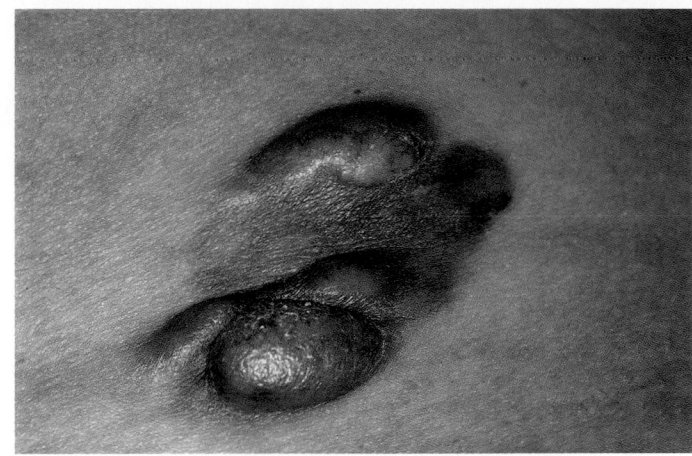

Fig. 28-31 Recurrent dermatofibrosarcoma protuberans.

spaces. In many instances, there is a pronounced matlike woven pattern of spindle cells. Cytogenetic studies commonly demonstrate a t(17; 22)(22; q13) fusion involving the *COL1A1* gene on chromosome 17 and the *PDGFB* gene on chromosome 22. Giant cells may be present in small numbers. Pigmented DFSPs, in which the cells contain melanin, predominantly affect persons of color and are called Bednar tumors. CD34, nestin, and stromelysin 3 positivity are characteristic and serve as markers to distinguish DFSP from dermatofibroma. S-100 is negative and may be used to separate spindle cell melanoma from a Bednar tumor. Recurrent DFSP can be myxoid and resembles the diffuse type of neurofibroma histologically. A juvenile variant, called giant cell fibroblastoma, is characterized by a loose arrangement of spindle cells, and by multinucleated giant cells adjacent to dilated spaces that resemble dilated lymphatic vessels.

The differential diagnosis, especially in the early stage, is that of keloid and a large dermatofibroma. CD34-positive myxoid dermatofibrohistiocytoma of the skin occurs as an indolent post-traumatic tumor. It resembles myxoid DFSP.

Mohs surgical excision technique is the treatment of choice for DFSP. In a series of 50 patients the recurrence rate was 2%; with wide local excision, recurrence is 11–50%. A preoperative MRI may assist in planning successful clearance. Imatinib mesylate has been effective in some unresectable tumors.

Al-Quran SZ, et al: CD34-positive myxoid dermatofibrohistiocytoma of the skin: an indolent post-traumatic tumor that can be mistaken for dermatofibrosarcoma protuberans. J Cutan Pathol 2009 Jan; 36(1):84–86.
Dimitropoulos VA: Dermatofibrosarcoma protuberans. Dermatol Ther 2008 Nov–Dec; 21(6):428–432.
Kimmel Z, et al: Peripheral excision margins for dermatofibrosarcoma protuberans. Ann Surg Oncol 2008 Sep; 15(9):2617.
Lemm D, et al: Remission with imatinib mesylate treatment in a patient with initially unresectable dermatofibrosarcoma protuberans—a case report. Oral Maxillofac Surg 2008 Dec; 12(4):209–213.
Mori T, et al: Expression of nestin in dermatofibrosarcoma protuberans in comparison to dermatofibroma. J Dermatol 2008 Jul; 35(7):419–425.
Nelson RA, et al: Mohs micrographic surgery and dermatofibrosarcoma protuberans: a multidisciplinary approach in 44 patients. Ann Plast Surg 2008 Jun; 60(6):667–672.
Thomison J, et al: Hyalinized collagen in a dermatofibrosarcoma protuberans after treatment with imatinib mesylate. J Cutan Pathol 2008 Nov; 35(11):1003–1006.

Atypical fibroxanthoma

Atypical fibroxanthoma (AFX) of the skin is a low-grade malignancy that occurs chiefly on the sun-exposed parts of the head or neck in white persons over age 50. Most cases appear

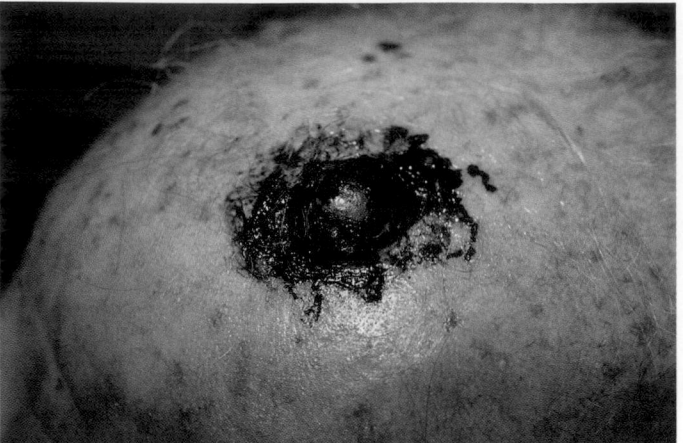

Fig. 28-32 Atypical fibroxanthoma. (Courtesy of Daniel Loo, MD)

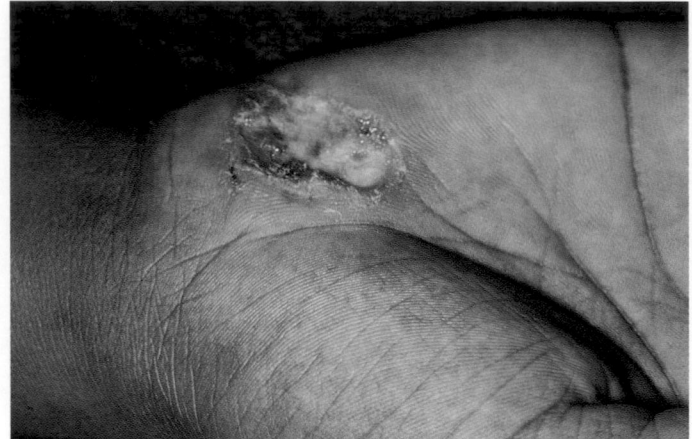

Fig. 28-33 Epithelial sarcoma.

to be related to undifferentiated pleomorphic sarcoma (malignant fibrous histiocytoma), which it resembles histologically. Its smaller size and more superficial location account largely for its more favorable prognosis. Some cases probably represent spindled or anaplastic squamous cell carcinoma that has lost the ability to express keratin. Clinically, the tumor begins as a small, firm nodule, often with an eroded or crusted surface without characteristic morphologic features (Fig. 28-32). A distinct clinical variant has a different presentation as a slowly enlarging tumor on a covered area, in patients with an average age of 39. This variant accounts for 25% of cases.

The lesion develops in the dermis and is separated from the epidermis by a thin band of collagen. The tumor consists of bizarre spindle cells mingled with atypical histiocytic cells. The cytoplasm may be vacuolated and resembles the xanthoma cell. Mitotic figures, prominent eosinophilic nucleoli, and the presence of a biphasic tumor cell population are characteristic findings, but purely spindle cell variants also occur. S-100 staining is sparse when compared with melanoma, and prekeratin staining is negative; this helps to distinguish AFX from squamous cell carcinoma. Variants with clear cells, granular cells, and osteoclast-type cells have been described. Tumor cells stain for CD10, S100A6, and procollagen I, but none of these markers is specific for the tumor.

The treatment of choice is complete surgical excision. Mohs microsurgery results in fewer recurrences and smaller defects than conventional excision. Although the prognosis is excellent, local recurrence after inadequate excision is usual, and cases of metastasizing AFX have been reported.

de Feraudy S, et al: Evaluation of CD10 and procollagen 1 expression in atypical fibroxanthoma and dermatofibroma. Am J Surg Pathol 2008 Aug; 32(8):1111–1122.
Marcet S: Atypical fibroxanthoma/malignant fibrous histiocytoma. Dermatol Ther 2008 Nov–Dec; 21(6):424–427.

Undifferentiated pleomorphic sarcoma (malignant fibrous histiocytoma)

This is the most common soft tissue sarcoma of middle and late adulthood. It arises deeply and is more likely to appear in deep fascial planes than in subcutaneous tissue. One-third occur on the thigh or buttock. Peak incidence is in the seventh decade. They sometimes arise in an area of radiodermatitis or in a chronic ulceration.

Several histologic variants have been described, including myxoid, inflammatory, and giant cell types. Gene expression profiling is now being used to define subtypes of pleomorphic sarcoma. Cell staining is positive for vimentin and factor XIIIa.

Pleomorphic cellular elements and bizarre mitotic figures are characteristic. AFXs are smaller and more superficial tumors of the dermis, compared with the deeper location of malignant fibrous histiocytoma (MFH). Epithelioid sarcoma lacks the large, bizarre, multinucleated cells often seen in MFH.

The prognosis in MFH is related to the site; deeper and more proximally located tumors have a poorer prognosis. The myxoid variant is less likely to metastasize. An especially poor prognosis attends tumors arising in sites of radiodermatitis. Local recurrence after excision occurs in 25%, 35% metastasize, and the overall survival rate is 50%. Mohs surgical removal may result in fewer recurrences.

The angiomatoid type may have a different presentation on the extremities of children as a slowly growing dermal or subcutaneous mass. It has been separated, as it has a relatively good prognosis.

Cutaneous myxofibrosarcoma

The diagnosis of cutaneous myxofibrosarcoma is often delayed because the tumor may appear indolent clinically and may mimic an interstitial granuloma histologically. Areas of atypical spindle cells within a prominent myxoid stroma and pleomorphic multinucleated cells suggest the diagnosis.

Kwong RA, et al: Histopathological evolution of a cutaneous myxofibrosarcoma. Australas J Dermatol 2008 Aug; 49(3):169–172.
Park SW, et al: Malignant fibrous histiocytoma of the head and neck: CT and MR imaging findings. Am J Neuroradiol 2009 Jan; 30(1):71–76.

Epithelioid sarcoma

Epithelioid sarcoma occurs chiefly in young adults, with onset usually being from 20 to 40 years of age. Two-thirds of cases are in men. Nearly all lesions are on the extremities, half of them on the hands or wrists (Fig. 28-33). They have, however, been reported from a wide variety of locations, including the genital region ("proximal type").

The tumor grows slowly among fascial structures and tendons, often with central necrosis of the tumor nodules and ulceration of the overlying skin. Initial clinical diagnoses may include granuloma annulare, rheumatoid nodule, or ganglion cyst. Histologically, irregular nodular masses of large, deeply acidophilic polygonal cells merge with spindle cells in a biphasic pattern. Central necrosis within masses of epithelioid cells may give the impression of a palisaded granuloma. Absence of staining for CD68 (KP-1) and co-expression of keratins and vimentin confirm the diagnosis. Absence of INI1 expression is also helpful diagnostically, but has no prognostic implications.

Wide local excision of small, early lesions may achieve a cure. Recurrence after attempted excision occurs in three of four cases, and late metastasis in 45% of patients. There is a propensity for lymph node and lung metastases, and in one series of eight patients, 5- and 10-year survival rates of 25% were reported. Women have a more favorable prognosis; the proximal lesions have a worse prognosis.

Chbani L, et al: Epithelioid sarcoma: a clinicopathologic and immunohistochemical analysis of 106 cases from the French sarcoma group. Am J Clin Pathol 2009 Feb; 131(2):222–227.

Myxomas

Cutaneous myxomas may be solitary, and appear as flesh-colored nodules on the face, trunk, or extremities. They may also occur as part of Carney complex. This has also been reported under the acronyms NAME (nevi, atrial myxoma, myxoid neurofibromas, and ephelides) and LAMB (lentigines, atrial myxoma, mucocutaneous myxomas, blue nevi), and simply as cutaneous lentiginosis with atrial myxoma.

The Carney complex consists of patients who have two or more of the following:

1. cardiac myxomas (79%)
2. cutaneous myxomas (not myxoid neurofibromas) (45%)
3. mammary myxoid fibromas (30%)
4. spotty mucocutaneous pigmentation, including lentiginoses (not ephelides) and blue nevi, often of a distinctive epithelioid variety (65%)
5. primary pigmented nodular adrenocortical disease (45%), which results in Cushing syndrome
6. testicular tumors (56% of male patients)
7. pituitary growth hormone-secreting tumors (10%).

A peculiar type of schwannoma featuring melanin and psammoma bodies may also be present.

The cutaneous myxomas occur as small (<1 cm), multiple, skin-colored papules having a predilection for development by a mean age of 18 years, and a tendency to occur on the ears, eyelids, and nipples. The lentigines are prominent on the face, lips, conjunctival mucosa (Fig. 28-34), rectal mucosa, and genital mucosa. Cardiac myxomas may occur in any of the four chambers of the heart and are recurrent in 20%. They may embolize to the skin, producing acral necrotic lesions.

Recognition of this syndrome, with diagnosis and removal of the atrial myxomas, can be lifesaving. The first-degree family members should be examined, as this is an autosomal-dominantly inherited condition. The disease has been mapped to two loci and a third is likely. Mutations in the gene coding for the protein kinase A type I-a regulatory subunit (*PPKAR1A*) on chromosome 17 have been documented in about half of the families.

A malignant counterpart, the myxosarcoma, is a tumor that arises in the subcutaneous fat and underlying soft tissues. There is a tendency for local recurrence after wide and deep excision. Metastases are rare.

Mateus C, et al: Heterogeneity of skin manifestations in patients with Carney complex. J Am Acad Dermatol 2008 Nov; 59(5):801–810.
Misago N, et al: Digital superficial angiomyxoma. Clin Exp Dermatol 2007 Sep; 32(5):536–538.

Aggressive angiomyxoma

Aggressive angiomyxoma is an uncommon soft tissue neoplasm that usually involves the vulvoperineal and pelvic regions of young women. Any angiomyxoid tumor in this area is suspect for aggressive behavior. The tumor is mucinous and deeply infiltrative, but does not demonstrate nuclear atypia or mitosis. The rate of local recurrence is high despite wide surgical resection.

Sereda D, et al: Aggressive angiomyxoma of the vulva: a case report and review of the literature. J Low Genit Tract Dis 2009 Jan; 13(1):46–50.

Mastocytosis

Mastocytosis is a general term applied to local and systemic accumulations of mast cells. Mast cells are bone marrow-derived CD34+ cells. These cells carry preformed mediators, such as histamine, heparin, and various cytokines, which, when released, may cause symptoms such as flushing, urticaria, diarrhea, abdominal pain, headache, dyspnea, syncope, and palpitations.

Mastocytosis is divided into childhood- and adult-onset disease. The condition varies in these two age groups, in terms of clinical presentation, prognosis, and pathogenic factors. Studies have revealed mutations in the *c-KIT* proto-oncogene in many adult-onset cases. Its protein product is the transmembrane tyrosine kinase KIT receptor (CD117), whose ligand is stem cell factor (also known as mast cell growth factor). Both clonality studies and mutational analysis indicate that many adult cases of mastocytosis result from a neoplastic proliferation of mast cells, with a mutation at codon 816 in the *c-KIT* gene. This mutation is activating, resulting in the proliferation of mast cells. A second mutation, a chromosomal deletion on 4q12, results in the juxtaposition of platelet-derived growth factor receptor-α and FIP1L1. This fusion gene activates hematopoietic cells and is pathogenic in a subset of patients with systemic mastocytosis and eosinophilia. This subset of patients has also been considered as having a type of "hypereosinophilic syndrome." Thus, the vast majority of adults with mastocytosis have systemic disease that may be viewed as a fundamentally myelodysplastic disorder.

Children often do not express any *c-KIT* mutation; nor do the uncommon familial cases. The latter is usually transmitted by autosomal-dominant inheritance with reduced expressivity, although other patterns may occur. The mutations leading to familial disease have not been defined. It appears that spontaneous childhood disease may occur from either cytokine-derived hyperplasias, from mutations other than the activating 816 type, or from mutations yet to be described. Some pediatric cases, however, are known to have inactivating mutations of *c-KIT* and a few have the adult-type activating mutations.

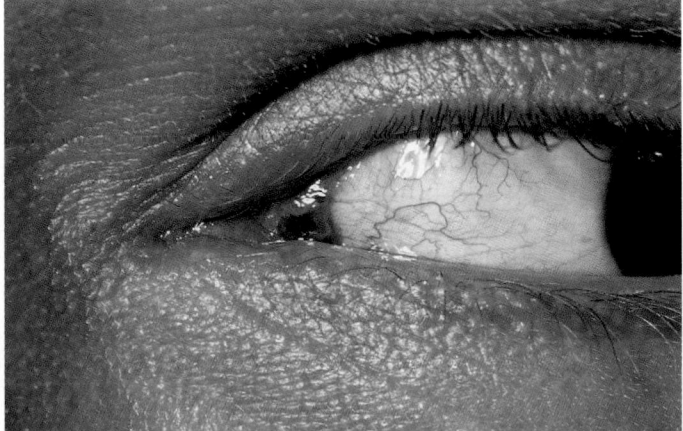

Fig. 28-34 Characteristic pigmentation on the medial conjunctiva in Carney syndrome.

Childhood disease is defined as occurring before age 15. The majority of children develop their disease before the age of 2, and in most of them the condition spontaneously involutes.

Clinical classification

Mast cell disease is divided into two broad categories—cutaneous and systemic. Cutaneous mastocytosis describes those cases with involvement of the skin only, and includes most cases of childhood mastocytosis and infrequent adult cases. Childhood cases usually fall into one of three categories of cutaneous mastocytosis. The most common (60–80% of patients) is urticaria pigmentosa or so-called "maculopapular" cutaneous mastocytosis; fewer (10–35%) patients present with solitary mastocytosis; the remainder have the rare forms of diffuse cutaneous mastocytosis or the telangiectatic type. A classification has been proposed by Akin and Metcalfe, which incorporates the World Health Organization (WHO) criteria (Box 28-1).

The vast majority of adult patients with mastocytosis are classified as having systemic mastocytosis, since they typically have clonal proliferation of the bone marrow-derived mast cells. Of adult patients with systemic mastocytosis not associated with hematopoietic disease, 60% have indolent mastocytosis and 40% have aggressive mastocytosis. Patients with aggressive systemic mastocytosis usually lack skin lesions. Mast cell leukemia and sarcoma are very rare. Many patients who present to the dermatologist with only skin lesions will have the indolent variety. Symptoms and signs of systemic disease are classified as those related to organ infiltration by mast cells, and those due to mediator release from mast cells. Direct organ involvement is most frequently bone pain from lytic bone lesions, hepatosplenomegaly, lymphadenopathy, or cytopenia from bone marrow involvement. For the dermatologists, the most important symptoms are those related to mediator release, usually acting on the gastrointestinal tract, respiratory tree, or blood vessels. These include pruritus, flushing, urticaria, angioedema, headache, nausea, vomiting, abdominal cramps, diarrhea, gastric and/or duodenal ulcer, malabsorption, asthma-like symptoms, presyncope, syncope, and anaphylaxis. These may occur spontaneously or be the result of massive histamine release after ingestion of known mast cell degranulators, such as alcohol, morphine, codeine, or extended rubbing of the skin. *Hymenoptera* stings may induce anaphylaxis. Mast cells also produce heparin, which may result in hematemesis, epistaxis, melena, and ecchymoses. Osteoporosis may also occur from chronic heparin release, resulting in fractures.

Cutaneous mastocytosis

Cutaneous mastocytosis is relatively common, representing about 1 in 500 initial consultations to pediatric dermatologists.

Solitary mastocytoma

About 10–40% of childhood mastocytosis presents in this way. The solitary lesion may be present at birth or may develop during the first weeks of life. It originates as a brown macule that urticates on stroking. It may develop into a papule, a raised round or oval plaque, or a tumor. The size is usually less than 1 cm, but occasionally may reach two or three times this diameter. The surface is usually smooth, but may have a peau d'orange appearance. Although the mastocytoma may occur anywhere on the body, its favorite location is on the dorsum of the hand near the wrist. Edema, urtication, vesiculation, and even bulla formation may be observed in the lesion. Even a solitary lesion may produce systemic symptoms, usually flushing.

Although the generalized form may begin with a single lesion, dissemination usually occurs within 3 months of its appearance. Most solitary mastocytomas involute spontaneously by the age of 10 or earlier. They also respond favorably to excision, or the application of a hydrocolloid dressing to prevent the rubbing that triggers mediator release and symptomatology. Progression to malignant disease does not occur.

Generalized eruption, childhood type (urticaria pigmentosa)

This form of cutaneous mastocytosis represents 60–90% of childhood cases. In this type, the eruption usually begins during the first weeks of life, presenting with rose-colored, pruritic, urticarial, slightly pigmented macules, papules, or nodules. The lesions are oval or round, and vary in diameter between 5 and 15 mm and may coalesce. The color varies from yellowish-brown to yellowish-red. Occasionally, the lesions are a pale yellow color and this has been called xanthelasmoidea. Vesicle and bulla formation is a frequent prominent feature early in the disease (Fig. 28-35). Indeed, vesicles and bullae may be the initial presenting signs, but they usually persist no longer than 3 years. In the older age groups vesiculation rarely occurs.

At their onset, lesions are similar to urticaria, except that they are not evanescent. The lesions persist and gradually become chamois- or slate-colored (Fig. 28-36). When they are firmly stroked or vigorously rubbed, urticaria with a surrounding erythematous flare (Darier's sign) usually develops. Dermatographism of clinically uninvolved skin is present in

---

Box 28-1 Classification of mastocytosis

Cutaneous and systemic mastocytosis

1. Indolent systemic mastocytosis (ISM)
   • Isolated bone marrow mastocytosis
   • Smouldering systemic mastocytosis (SSM)
2. Systemic mastocytosis with associated hematopoietic disease (SM-AHD, AHNMD [*associated* hematological non mast cell disorder]): systemic mastocytosis with leukaemia, myelodysplastic syndrome/disease, or non-Hodgkin lymphoma
3. Aggressive systemic mastocytosis (ASM)
4. Mast cell leukemia
5. Mast cell sarcoma
6. Extracutaneous mastocytoma

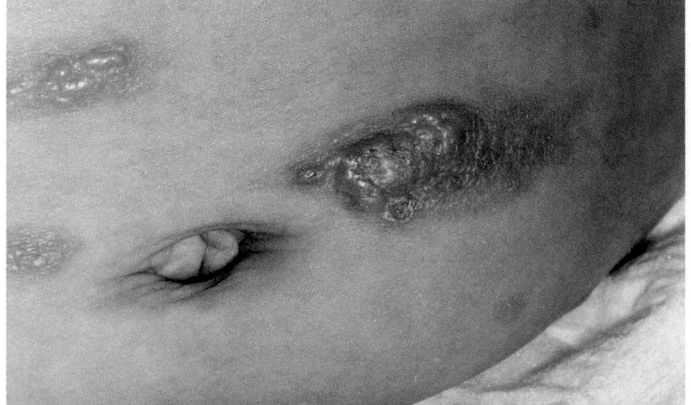

Fig. 28-35 Bullous mastocytosis.

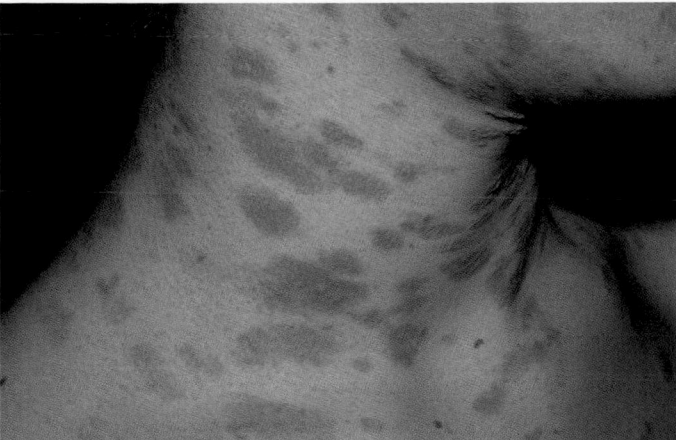

Fig. 28-36 Urticaria pigmentosa.

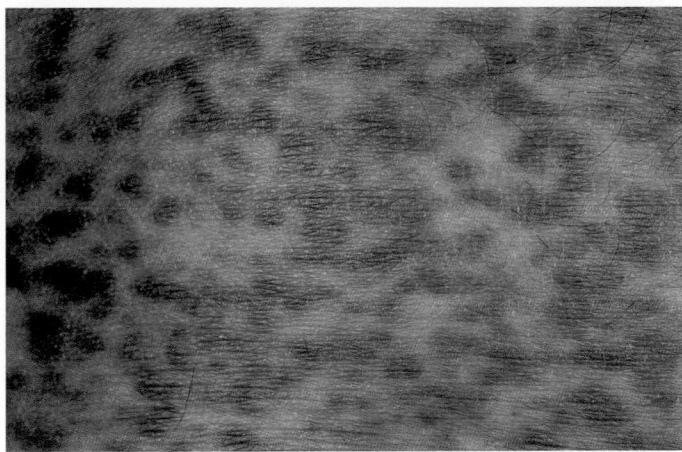

Fig. 28-37 Adult generalized mastocytosis.

one-third to one-half of patients. For many years, the brown, waxy skin lesions may persist before they begin to involute. Pigmentation and all evidence of the disease commonly disappear within a few years, generally before puberty. The eruption, however, may uncommonly persist into adult life. Although systemic involvement is possible, malignant systemic disease is extremely rare.

Diffuse cutaneous mastocytosis

In this rare form, with diffuse involvement, the entire integument may be thickened and infiltrated with mast cells to produce a peculiar orange color, giving rise to the term homme orange. There is an infiltrated doughy or boggy consistency to the skin, and lichenification may be present. In the neonatal period, diffuse cutaneous blistering may occur, leading to the diagnosis of epidermolysis bullosa or some other primary bullous disorder. This is termed "bullous mastocytosis."

Systemic mastocytosis

Systemic mastocytosis is diagnosed by fulfilling the one major criterion and one minor criterion, or three minor criteria. The major criterion is the finding of dense infiltrates of mast cells (aggregates of 15 or more) in bone marrow or other extracutaneous tissues. The four minor criteria are:

1. atypical mast cell morphology
2. aberrant mast cell surface phenotype (CD25 or CD2)
3. serum/plasma tryptase greater than 20 ng/mL
4. a codon 816 *c-KIT* mutation in peripheral blood, bone marrow, or lesional tissue.

Patients with a history of *Hymenoptera*-induced anaphylaxis and an elevated tryptase should be evaluated for systemic mastocytosis.

The most common type of systemic mastocytosis in adults is indolent systemic mastocytosis. These patients lack evidence of an associated non-mast cell hematologic disorder; lack end-organ dysfunction such as ascites, malabsorption, cytopenias, and pathologic fractures; and lack mast cell leukemia. The disorder is then diagnosed through physical and histopathologic examination of skin lesions. Several different patterns of cutaneous involvement have been described.

Generalized eruption, adult type

This is the most common pattern of mastocytosis presenting to the dermatologist. The most common lesions are macules, papules, or nodules disseminated over most of the body, but especially on the upper arms, legs, and trunk. The upper arms and upper inner thighs may be the only areas involved on presentation. These may be reddish-purple (Fig. 28-37), rust-colored, or brown. In the latter case, they may closely resemble common nevi. They may urticate upon rubbing, as is seen in children with urticaria pigmentosa.

Erythrodermic mastocytosis

There is generalized erythroderma and the skin has a leather-grain appearance. Urtication can be produced over the entire surface.

Telangiectasia macularis eruptiva perstans

This is a persistent, pigmented, asymptomatic eruption of macules usually less than 0.5 cm in diameter, with a slightly reddish-brown tinge. Despite the name, little or no telangiectasia may evident. Darier's sign may not be demonstrable, as the number of mast cells in the skin may not be greatly increased.

Classification and prognosis in adult systemic mastocytosis

Patients with systemic mastocytosis with an associated hematologic non-mast cell lineage disorder (SM-AHNMD) are typically older adults with signs and symptoms of systemic disease. A variety of associated non-mast cell hematologic conditions, including polycythemia vera, hypereosinophilic syndrome, chronic myelogenous or monocytic leukemia, lymphocytic leukemia, primary myelofibrosis, and Hodgkin disease, may be seen. Typically, this type does not have skin lesions. The prognosis in these patients is that of their underlying hematologic condition. Smoldering systemic mastocytosis is characterized by a slow progression and lack of end-organ dysfunction due to mast cell infiltration. It describes patients with 30% or more infiltration of the bone marrow cavity by mast cells, a serum tryptase of greater than 200 ng/mL, and hepatosplenomegaly. Adult systemic mastocytosis has a more fulminant course and describes the condition of those patients with end-organ dysfunction due to mast cell infiltration (bone marrow failure, liver dysfunction, splenomegaly with hypersplenism, pathologic fractures, and gastrointestinal involvement with malabsorption and weight loss). This group of patients has a poor prognosis. Mast cell leukemia occurs when the atypical mast cells (multilobular or multiple nuclei) represent 10% of circulating cells or 20% of bone marrow cells. The prognosis is poor.

Mast cell sarcoma and extracutaneous mastocytoma

These are rare findings of isolated tumors of either atypical mast cells in mast cell sarcoma, or benign-appearing mast cells in extracutaneous mastocytoma. They occur in sites other than the skin or bone marrow. Mast cell sarcomas are aggressive, locally destructive lesions, as opposed to the benign mastocytomas, which carry a good prognosis.

Biochemical studies

Mast cells produce tryptase. It has become the preferred laboratory test to demonstrate evidence of increased mast cell burden, replacing urinary histamine and urinary histamine metabolites. It is of prognostic significance in some cases. Tryptase is measured as a total serum tryptase level. This should be obtained when the patient is in his/her normal state of health, as anaphylaxis will increase it transiently. Mastocytosis patients may have a persistently and significantly elevated level. Results above 20 ng/mL are a minor criterion for the diagnosis of systemic mastocytosis.

Histopathology

The typical skin lesion shows a dense dermal aggregate of mononuclear cells with abundant amphophilic cytoplasm. When these large mononuclear cells are stained with Giemsa or toluidine blue, the metachromatic granules are observed. A Leder stain will stain the cells diffusely red. When blisters are present, the roof of the vesicle or bulla is subepidermal. The mast cells collect in a band below the vesicle. Infiltration of local anesthetic adjacent to the lesion rather than directly into it and the use of anesthetic without epinephrine may help to avoid mast cell degranulation. Monoclonal antibodies against tryptase and CD117 (KIT) are available and are very sensitive.

Diagnosis

The typical case of cutaneous mastocytosis is easily diagnosed by the presence of solitary or multiple pigmented macules, papules, or nodules that urticate when irritated by stroking or scratching. The diagnosis is confirmed by biopsy of the lesion with the demonstration of increased numbers of mast cells. The bullous and vesicular lesions may be more difficult to diagnose clinically; however, scrapings from the base of the bulla when stained with Giemsa or Wright stain will show mast cells in profusion.

Once the diagnosis of skin lesions of mastocytosis is made, the decision to assess for bone marrow involvement is key. While therapy to reduce the disease burden of proliferating clonal mast cells is not effective, bone marrow examination will provide information about the extent of the disease and the presence or absence of a non-mast cell hematologic disorder, and will assist in the counseling concerning prognosis. All adult patients and children with the unexplained presence of an abnormal complete blood count (CBC), hepatomegaly, splenomegaly, lymphadenopathy, or a serum baseline tryptase of greater than 20 ng/mL should be offered a bone marrow examination. In asymptomatic adults whose only sign or symptom of mastocytosis is skin lesions, and who do not desire a bone marrow examination, serum tryptase and CBC should be repeated at least yearly during a complete history and physical examination. Elevation of the tryptase level, a drop in the platelet count or hemoglobin, a rise in the monocytes, or the onset of organomegaly should trigger a bone marrow examination. In children with early-onset disease, the prognosis is good; usually tryptase evaluations or mutational analysis is reserved for those with the above findings, or with persistent localized bone pain, severe gastrointestinal symptoms, or biochemical evidence of hepatic insufficiency.

Differential diagnosis

Clinically, a small solitary mastocytoma most frequently resembles a pigmented nevus or juvenile xanthogranuloma. Urtication establishes the diagnosis. The disseminated lesions are also distinctive enough to give little or no difficulty in the diagnosis. The nodular form may resemble xanthomas; however, the presence of urtication is distinctive. The vesicular and bullous lesions are to be distinguished from various hereditary and nonhereditary bullous diseases. The main histologic similarity is to Langerhans cell histiocytosis.

Prognosis

Most cases of early-onset, skin-limited disease in children clear completely. The solitary mastocytoma involutes spontaneously, usually within 3 years of onset. In those children and adults with indolent systemic mastocytosis, the prognosis is also good. This is the most common category of patients presenting for diagnosis in the dermatology clinic. Patients with AHNMD have the prognosis of the associated disease. In the newly described patients with smoldering systemic mastocytosis, the prognosis is intermediate and not yet well defined. Aggressive systemic mastocytosis, mast cell leukemia, and mast cell sarcoma patients have a poor prognosis.

Treatment

Symptomatic relief of histamine-mediated symptoms may be achieved in many cases by the use of antihistamines. Both H_1 and H_2 blockers and antiserotonin drugs, such as cyproheptadine, may alleviate urtication, pruritus, and flushing. Nifedipine, 10 mg three times a day, may also be effective in isolated cases. Psoralen with ultraviolet A (PUVA) or medium-dose UVA1 alone produces excellent clearing of the skin in most cases. Most patients will have sustained benefit for at least 6 months following treatment. Approximately 25% will have a remission lasting longer than 5 years, and in others the frequency of phototherapy may be tapered to once or twice a month and patients still remain clear. Intralesional triamcinolone or potent topical steroids under occlusion may also clear cutaneous lesions; however, the lesions do recur after discontinuance. Also, concern about local atrophy, striae, and systemic absorption limit the utility of this treatment.

It cannot be overemphasized that avoidance of physical stimuli, such as extremes of temperature, pressure/friction, and chemical degranulators of mast cells, is important. The application of a hydrocolloid dressing over an isolated mastocytoma in an infant may reduce the flushing it produces. The chemicals patients with mastocytosis must avoid include opiates, aspirin, alcohol, quinine, scopolamine, gallamine, decamethonium, reserpine, amphotericin B, polymyxin B, and d-tubocurarine. *Hymenoptera* stings may induce anaphylaxis; the patient (and parents, if the affected individual is a child) should be taught to recognize the signs of anaphylactic shock, given a premeasured dose of epinephrine (Epipen) for emergency use, and taught about its use. After such an event it is prudent to treat for several days with 20–40 mg of prednisone to avoid recurrent attacks.

Control of diarrhea in systemic mastocytosis may be achieved by orally administered disodium cromoglycate. Gastrointestinal ulcers may be treated with proton pump inhibitors and H_2 antagonists. The treatment of systemic mast cell disease is of limited efficacy. For patients with indolent systemic mastocytosis and severe osteoporosis, IFN-α may be considered. In patients with smoldering systemic mastocytosis, watchful waiting is recommended, although IFN-α, with or without glucocorticoids, may be considered for progressive

"B" findings. In aggressive systemic mastocytosis, IFN-α may also be used, with or without glucocorticoids. 2-Chlorodeoxyadenosine (as used in Langerhans cell histiocytosis) can also be effective in aggressive systemic mastocytosis. A gain-of-function D816V point mutation in the transmembrane receptor KIT kinase domain is found in the majority of patients with systemic mastocytosis. Patients with the mutation do not generally respond to imatinib mesylate. Patients with systemic mastocytosis who have the *FIP1L1–PDGFRA* translocation, lack the *c-KIT* mutation, or have novel mutations may respond to imatinib. Bone marrow transplantation for the most severely affected patients with systemic mastocytosis is being investigated.

Aichberger KJ, et al: Treatment responses to cladribine and dasatinib in rapidly progressing aggressive mastocytosis. Eur J Clin Invest 2008 Nov; 38(11):869–873.

Brockow K, et al: Mastocytosis. Chem Immunol Allergy 2010; 95:110–124.

Heide R, et al: Mastocytosis in children: a protocol for management. Pediatr Dermatol 2008 Jul–Aug; 25(4):493–500.

Hoffmann KM, et al: Successful treatment of progressive cutaneous mastocytosis with imatinib in a 2-year-old boy carrying a somatic KIT mutation. Blood 2008 Sep 1; 112(5):1655–1657.

Metcalfe DD: Mast cells and mastocytosis. Blood 2008 Aug 15; 112(4):946–956.

Pardanani A, et al: Systemic mastocytosis in adults: a review on prognosis and treatment based on 342 Mayo Clinic patients and current literature. Curr Opin Hematol 2010 Mar; 17(2):125–132.

Abnormalities of neural tissue

Solitary neurofibroma

The ordinary solitary cutaneous neurofibroma may be 2–20 mm in diameter. It is soft, flaccid, and pinkish-white. Frequently, the soft small tumor can be invaginated, as if through a ring in the skin, by pressure with the finger (this is called "button-holing").

Neurofibroma is either solitary or multiple. When only one or two lesions are present, they are typically spontaneous tumors without any internal manifestations. When three or more are present, a diagnosis of neurofibromatosis should be considered. Uncommonly, large pendulous masses occur, in which numerous, tortuous, thickened nerves can be felt; this has been likened to a "bag of worms." These plexiform neurofibromas, which often have overlying pigmentation, usually occur in neurofibromatosis. Neurofibromatosis is discussed in Chapter 27.

Histologically, the lesion demonstrates wavy spindled nuclei and fine collagen fibers. The stroma is often myxoid and contains many mast cells. Cholinesterase activity is markedly positive in the neurofibromas. Immunochemical staining shows positivity for S-100, vimentin, and myelin basic protein, markers for schwannian tissue.

Treatment of those lesions that are particularly objectionable is by surgical excision.

Granular cell tumor

About one-third of reported cases occur on the tongue (Fig. 28-38), one-third involve the skin, and one-third occur in the internal organs. The tumor is usually a well-circumscribed, solitary, firm nodule ranging from 5 to 30 mm, with a brownish-red or flesh tint, depending on nearness to the surface. Its surface may be smooth, rough, or verrucous. Rarely, the lesions may ulcerate. They are multiple in 10–15% of cases.

The solitary lesion may be located anywhere on the body, but nearly half of all tumors appear on the head or neck.

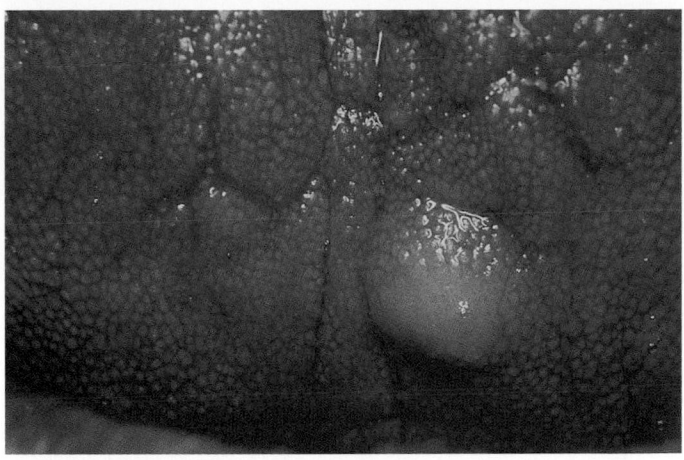

Fig. 28-38 Granular cell tumor of the tongue.

Usually, the patients are in their third to fifth decade. About two-thirds of patients are black and two-thirds are women. In most cases the tumor grows very slowly, and when completely removed, does not usually recur. However, local or multicentric recurrence may at times cause confusion in determining if a granular cell tumor is malignant.

The histologic picture is distinctive. The cells are large, pale, and irregularly polygonal, with a poorly defined cellular membrane, and contain coarsely granular cytoplasm with scattered giant lysosomal granules. Some of the cells are multinucleated or contain vacuoles or small pyknotic or eosinophilic inclusions. At times, the arrangement is in cords or sheets, in irregular alveolar masses, or even organoid. Pseudo-epitheliomatous hyperplasia is a regular feature. The cells stain positively with vimentin, neuron-specific enolase, S-100, myelin protein, p75 nerve growth factor, calretinin, NKI/C3, and PGP9.5. Hybrid forms that overlap with perineurioma have been described.

Malignant granular cell tumor is uncommon. Most are much larger than the benign granular cell tumors, with an average diameter of 9 cm; benign lesions average less than 2 cm. Most malignant granular cell tumors demonstrate cytologic atypia, but some are quite bland cytologically. Other factors that correlate with malignant behavior are an infiltrative growth pattern, history of local recurrence, older patient age, presence of necrosis, increased mitotic activity, spindling of tumor cells, and nuclear staining with the proliferation marker Ki67 (MIB 1) in more than 10% of tumor nuclei. Mutant p53 protein has been identified in more than half of malignant granular cell tumors studied. About one-third are aneuploid, one-third hyperdiploid, and one-third diploid. In contrast, almost all benign tumors are diploid.

Because of the difficulties in distinguishing benign from some malignant granular cell tumors, complete excision is advisable whenever possible. Malignant granular cell tumors often have an infiltrative growth pattern and perineural extension. Mohs micrographic surgery may be helpful in ensuring complete excision.

Vered M, et al: Granular cell tumor of the oral cavity: updated immunohistochemical profile. J Oral Pathol Med 2009 Jan; 38(1):150–159.

Zarineh A, et al: Multiple hybrid granular cell tumor-perineuriomas. Am J Surg Pathol 2008 Oct; 32(10):1572–1577.

Perineurioma

The normal perineurium is composed of flattened cells that surround the nerve. Perineuriomas are derived from these cells. They appear as nondescript papules clinically. Sclerosing perineuriomas demonstrate concentric lamellar fibrosis and are EMA-positive. Reticular, granular, and lipomatous variants have been described.

Al-Daraji WI: Granular perineurioma: the first report of a rare distinctive subtype of perineurioma. Am J Dermatopathol 2008 Apr; 30(2):163–168.
Piña-Oviedo S, et al: The normal and neoplastic perineurium: a review. Adv Anat Pathol 2008 May; 15(3):147–164.

Neuroma cutis

Cutaneous neuromas are uncommon. Three true neuromas exist in the skin and mucous membranes: traumatic neuromas, multiple mucosal neuromas, and solitary palisaded encapsulated neuromas.

Traumatic neuromas result from the overgrowth of nerve fibers in the severed ends of peripheral nerves. The lesion may be tender or painful, and when scarring has occurred or the distal stump has been removed, a phantom limb syndrome may result. These often occur on the fingers, at sites of amputation of supernumerary digits, or on the sole, usually at the third metatarsal space.

Multiple mucosal neuromas (Fig. 28-39) occur as part of the autosomal-dominantly inherited multiple mucosal neuroma syndrome (multiple endocrine neoplasia type 2b). These patients have a marfanoid habitus, thickened protruding lips, and multiple neuromas of the oral mucosa (lips, tongue, and gingiva), conjunctiva, and sometimes sclera. A few have multiple cutaneous neuromas, usually limited to the face. There is a strong association with medullary carcinoma of the thyroid, bilateral pheochromocytomas, and diffuse gastrointestinal tract ganglioneuromatosis. Disease is caused by a mutation in the *RET* proto-oncogene. Infants at risk should be screened for this mutation, and total thyroidectomy performed if positive.

The palisaded, encapsulated neuroma of the skin is a solitary, large, encapsulated tumor, usually of the face. It is a slow-growing, flesh-colored, dome-shaped, firm lesion, usually appearing around the mouth or nose. It closely resembles a basal cell carcinoma or an intradermal nevus.

Newman MD, et al: Palisaded encapsulated neuroma (PEN): an often misdiagnosed neural tumor. Dermatol Online J 2008 Jul 15; 14(7):12.
Rishpon A, et al: Neuroma formation and toe amputation resulting from stonefish envenomation. Arch Dermatol 2008 Aug; 144(8):1076–1077.

Neurothekeoma (nerve sheath myxoma)

Neurothekeoma, meaning a tumor of the nerve sheath, is composed of cords and nests of large cells packed among collagen bundles in close proximity to small nerves. Mitotic figures and nuclear atypia are sometimes seen, but the tumor is benign. These benign intradermal or subcutaneous tumors are divided histologically into two distinct subtypes: the classic or myxoid variant and the cellular type. An intermediate or mixed variety is also recognized. The myxoid variant (nerve sheath myxoma) is characterized by large islands of stellate and spindled cells in a mucinous matrix. The cells stain strongly for S-100 protein. Myxoid neurothekeoma occurs in middle-aged adults, primarily on the head, neck, and upper extremities. It is twice as common in women. The cellular type occurs in childhood, with a high female preponderance, and has a predilection for the head, neck, or shoulders. The cellular type does not stain for S-100 protein, but does stain for S-100A6, PGP9.5, MITF, and NK1C3. It is unclear if these tumors really demonstrate nerve sheath differentiation, but for now they are grouped with the myxoid neurothekeomas. Examples of cellular neurothekeoma with high mitotic rate and atypia mimic malignant spindle cell tumors. They have a significant rate of recurrence but at this point are not known to have a clear metastatic potential.

Campanati A, et al: Atypical neurothekeoma: a new case and review of the literature. J Cutan Pathol 2007 May; 34(5):435–437.
Fetsch JF, et al: Neurothekeoma: an analysis of 178 tumors with detailed immunohistochemical data and long-term patient follow-up information. Am J Surg Pathol 2007 Jul; 31(7):1103–1114.
Hornick JL, et al: Cellular neurothekeoma: detailed characterization in a series of 133 cases. Am J Surg Pathol 2007 Mar; 31(3):329–340.
Wu RC, et al: Cellular neurothekeoma with melanocytosis. J Cutan Pathol 2008 Feb; 35(2):241–245.

Schwannoma (neurilemmoma)

Peripheral schwannomas are usually solitary nerve sheath tumors, most often seen in women. They occur almost exclusively in deep tissues, along the main nerve trunks of the extremities, especially the flexor surface of the arms, wrists, and knees. They are also seen on the scalp, sides of the neck, and tongue. The solitary tumor is a nodule of 3–30 mm in diameter (Fig. 28-40). It is soft or firm, and pale pink or yellowish; it may or may not be painful. Schwannomas involve many other organs, and brain tumors such as meningiomas, gliomas, and astrocytomas may occur.

Sometimes the tumors are multiple. When this is so, they may be seen with neurofibromatosis type 1 (NF-1) or, more commonly, type 2, or as an entity independent of neurofibromatosis. The independent type may be congenital or have a delayed onset. It may be sporadic or familial. Three clinical patterns are described: elevated, dome-shaped nodules; pale

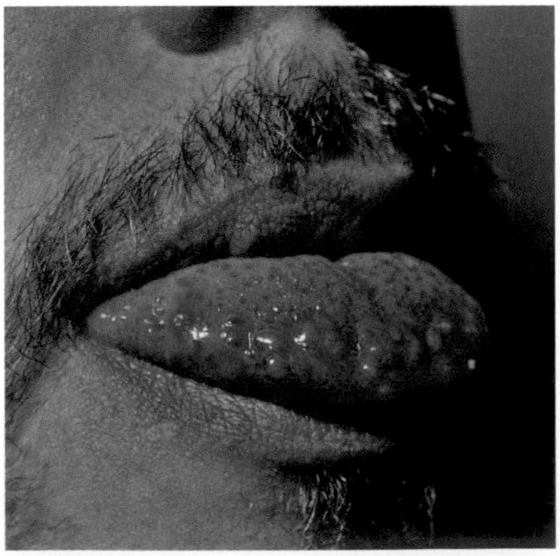

Fig. 28-39 Multiple mucosal neuromas.

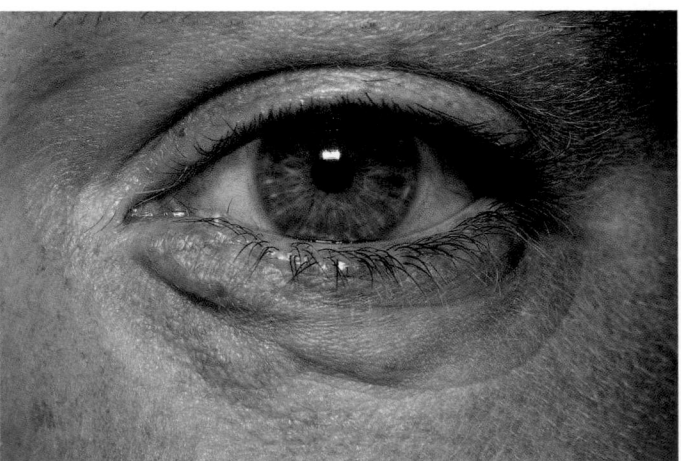

Fig. 28-40 Schwannoma. (Courtesy of Curt Samlaska, MD)

brown, indurated macules; and multiple papules coalescing into plaques from 2 to 100 mm in diameter, with a predilection for the trunk. Cases have occurred that appeared to be unassociated with NF-2, but on further investigation of the individual or family revealed other signs of NF-2 and the gene abnormality on chromosome 22.

Plexiform schwannomas may occur as single or multiple lesions, localized to a single anatomic site or more generalized, and arise in the dermis or subcutaneous tissue. They may occur as a solitary lesion, or be associated with NF-1, NF-2, or multiple schwannomas. Another subtype of schwannoma is the melanotic psammomatous type that is seen in association with Carney syndrome featuring spotty pigmentation, myxomas, and endocrine overactivity.

Histologically, the classic forms are well encapsulated and composed of two types of tissue, referred to as Antoni types A and B. Hard schwannomas are firm on gross examination, and are composed of Antoni A tissue — palisades of basophilic Schwann cell nuclei separated by brightly eosinophilic zones (Verocay bodies). Soft schwannomas are edematous. They are composed mostly or entirely of Antoni B tissue, a degenerative change characterized by loose, edematous connective tissue and ectatic blood vessels. S-100, vimentin, and myelin basic protein stains are positive in hard schwannomas. Staining is variable in soft schwannomas. A Bodian or neurofilament stain reveals very few or no nerve fibers within the bulk of the tumor, although a compressed nerve may be present at one edge of the mass in a subcapsular location. Ancient schwannomas may demonstrate remarkable nuclear atypia, which represents a benign degenerative change. Mitoses are absent. Ancient schwannomas should not be confused with malignant schwannoma (neurofibrosarcoma), a tumor that generally arises in long-standing neurofibromas in the setting of NF-1. Excision is almost invariably curative, except in the malignant variety, for which combined wide resection and radiotherapy is needed.

Fong KL, et al: Ancient schwannoma of the vulva. Obstet Gynecol 2009 Feb; 113(2 Pt 2):510–512.

Infantile neuroblastoma

Neuroblastoma is the most common malignant tumor of early childhood. Cutaneous nodules are most often seen in younger patients, being present in 32% of infants with the disease. These occur as multiple 2–20 mm, firm blue nodules that, when rubbed, blanch and form a halo of erythema. The blanching persists for 1–2 h and is followed by a refractory period of several hours. Biopsy shows clusters of basophilic cells with a high nuclear to cytoplasmic ratio, surrounded by eosinophilic fine fibrillar material. Two other findings that may be present are periorbital ecchymoses (the so-called raccoon eyes) and heterochromia of the irises.

For infants with skin involvement the prognosis is good, with either spontaneous remission or spontaneous transformation into benign ganglioneuromas expected. Prognostic factors other than age, based upon molecular genetic characteristics such as the status of the oncogene *MYCN* and chromosome 1p deletion, are helping to stratify prognosis and therapeutic recommendations.

Monclair T, et al: The International Neuroblastoma Risk Group (INRG) staging system: an INRG Task Force report. J Clin Oncol 2009 Jan 10; 27(2):298–303.

Ganglioneuroma

Ganglioneuroma has only rarely been described in the skin as an isolated entity. These tumors are composed of mature ganglion cells comingled with fascicles of spindle cells. They arise most often in von Recklinghausen neurofibromatosis or with neuroblastomas, and usually occur in childhood. The tissue stains positively for both argyrophilic and argentaffin granules.

Furmanczyk PS, et al: Cutaneous ganglioneuroma associated with overlying hyperkeratotic epidermal changes: a report of 2 cases. Am J Dermatopathol 2008 Dec; 30(6):600–603.

Murphy M, et al: Cutaneous ganglioneuroma. Int J Dermatol 2007 Aug; 46(8):861–863.

Nasal glioma (cephalic brainlike heterotopias)

Nasal gliomas are rare, benign, congenital tumors. When they occur extranasally, they are easily confused with hemangiomas. The tumor is usually a firm, incompressible (unlike a hemangioma and encephalocele), reddish-blue to purple lesion occurring on the nasal bridge or midline near the root. It does not transilluminate or enlarge with crying, unlike some encephaloceles. It may also occur intranasally.

Nasal gliomas differ from encephaloceles in that the latter are connected to the subarachnoid space by a sinus tract, while the former usually lose this connection before birth. Clinically, these cannot be absolutely differentiated, so a biopsy should not be performed. Skull radiographs, MRI, ultrasound, and Doppler flow studies may be performed; these will help define the lesion and detect possible skull involvement. Neurosurgical consultation is advisable.

Histologically, the nodule consists of glial tissue associated with glial giant cells, fibrous tissue, and numerous blood vessels. It is unencapsulated. The lesion does not involute spontaneously.

Niedzielska G, et al: Nasal ganglioglioma—difficulties in radiological imaging. Int J Pediatr Otorhinolaryngol 2008 Feb; 72(2):285–287.

Cutaneous meningioma

Primary cutaneous meningioma, also known as rudimentary meningocele, is a developmental defect. It results from the presence of meningocytes outside the calvarium. If actual brain remnants are present, the lesion is called a rudimentary cephalocele. Small, hard, fibrous, calcified nodules occur along the spine, in the scalp, on the forehead, or rarely in the external ear canal. Most occur over the scalp, some have an underlying connection to the CNS or an underlying bony abnormality, and usually come to medical attention in the first year of life. On the scalp they may present with a dark tuft of hair or an alopecic area surrounded by a dark collar of hair (hair collar sign).

Cutaneous meningiomas may develop in the scalp secondary to an intracranial meningioma, either by means of erosion of the skull, or by extension through an operative defect of the skull. Finally, they may also arise from cranial or spinal nerves. Clinically, these lesions have no distinctive appearance. They are firm subcutaneous nodules adherent to the skin.

Diagnosis is made by histologic examination. The tumors consist of strands of cells with large oval vesicular nuclei and granular cytoplasm. Lamellar, calcified psammoma bodies are commonly present. Psammoma bodies are not specific for meningiomas, and may also be found in intradermal nevi, juvenile xanthogranuloma, the pituitary of the fetus and newborn, schwannomas associated with Carney syndrome, meninges, choroid plexus, pineal gland, papillary carcinoma of the thyroid, ovarian neoplasms, and mammary intraductal papilloma.

Hussein MR, et al: Primary cutaneous meningioma of the scalp: a case report and review of literature. J Cutan Pathol 2007 Dec; 34 Suppl 1: 26–28.

Zeikus P, et al: Primary cutaneous meningioma in association with a sinus pericranii. J Am Acad Dermatol 2006 Feb; 54(2 Suppl):S49–S50.

Encephalocele and meningocele

Primary defects in the neural tube may lead to encephaloceles, meningoceles, or meningomyeloceles. They present in infancy along the midline of the face, scalp, neck, or back as soft, compressible masses that may transilluminate or enlarge with crying. Tufts of long, dark hair, or alopecia with a surrounding collar of dark hair may overlie them.

Many cutaneous lesions of the midline of the back, most commonly at the base of the spine, suggest that malformations of the spinal cord and associated structures are present. Cutaneous manifestations of spinal dysraphism include depressed or polypoid lesions; dyschromic or hairy lesions; dermal or subcutaneous lesions; vascular malformations; or neoplasms of many types. Midline masses require intensive radiologic and neurosurgical evaluation before biopsy because of the possible connection to the CNS. MRI is the imaging modality of choice. Approximately 10% of patients will have evidence of occult spinal dysraphism if one abnormality is present, whereas the majority will have dysraphism if two or more abnormalities are present.

Chordomas

These slow-growing, locally invasive neoplasms present as firm, smooth nodules in the sacrococcygeal region or at the base of the skull in middle-aged patients. They arise from notochord remnants. The pathologic appearance is that of incompletely encapsulated sheets, nests, and cords of large epithelioid cells with fibrous trabeculae present. They may metastasize late in their course to various sites, including the skin. Wide excision with postoperative radiation therapy is the treatment of choice.

Persichetti G, et al: Chordoma cutis. Dermatol Surg 2007 Dec; 33(12):1520–1524.
Vergara G, et al: Metastatic disease from chordoma. Clin Transl Oncol 2008 Aug; 10(8):517–521.

Abnormalities of fat tissue

Lipomas

Lipomas, subcutaneous tumors composed of fat tissue, may occur as a solitary sporadic lesion or as multiple lesions with or without a familial component. There are multiple histologic subtypes, and these frequently have an associated clinical correlation. Most have specific chromosomal alterations that help in their identification in difficult cases. Protease inhibitors given for HIV disease may induce lipomas, angiolipomas, or benign symmetric lipomatosis, as well as lipodystrophy.

Lipomas are most commonly found on the trunk. They also occur frequently on the neck, forearms, and axillae. They are soft, single or multiple, small or large, lobulated, compressible growths, over which the skin on traction often becomes dimpled, although otherwise unchanged. They usually stop growing after attaining a certain size, then remain stationary indefinitely. Frontalis-associated lipomas of the forehead are relatively large lesions arising either within or deep to the frontalis muscle.

A lipoma located in the midline of the sacral region may be a marker for spinal dysraphism or other embryologic malformation. Other midline lesions, such as tufts of hair ("fawn's tail"), hemangiomas (Cobb syndrome), skin tags, sinuses, or pigmented lesions, should also raise suspicion for occult embryologic malformations. MRI is the most sensitive imaging

modality. If spinal dysraphism is diagnosed, early treatment may be possible before irreversible damage has occurred. Do not attempt to biopsy a sacrococcygeal lipoma; call a neurosurgeon into consultation. It may be a lipomeningocele with communicating sinuses to the dura.

Histologically, the lipoma is an encapsulated, lobulated tumor containing normal fat cells held together by strands of connective tissue. Occasionally, eccrine sweat glands may be associated and then they are called adenolipomas. Alterations in chromosomes 12q13–15 and chromosomes 13q12–22 may be detected in benign lipomas.

In the differential diagnosis, the epidermoid cyst should always be considered. At times it is difficult to distinguish the two. Many soft, deep, single, nongrowing lesions of the skin do not require biopsy. The appearance of multiple lesions or progressive growth indicates the need for biopsy. Large solitary lesions should be investigated for malignancy, especially when they occur on the upper thigh.

Lipomas may be left untreated, unless they are large enough to be objectionable. They may be excised, removed with liposuction, extruded through a 3 mm incision after being freed with a cutting curette, or segmentally extracted through a stab incision. More advanced surgical technique is necessary to remove the deep lesions on the forehead, which may lie below the fascial plane. Injection with phosphatidylcholine has also been reported as successful.

Multiple lipomas may occur in groups of two to hundreds of confluent painless tumors of various sizes over any part of the body (Fig. 28-41). These lesions are sometimes painful when growing rapidly. When present in certain patterns, special designations are applied. Madelung's disease (benign symmetric lipomatosis or multiple symmetric lipomatosis) occurs most commonly in middle-aged men, who may develop multiple, large, painless, coalescent lipomas around the neck, shoulders, and upper arms. Familial multiple lipomatosis is a dominantly-inherited syndrome in which multiple asymptomatic lipomas of the forearms and thighs appear in the third decade of life. The shoulders and neck are spared, and the lipomas are encapsulated and movable. Diffuse lipomatosis is characterized by an early age of onset, usually before the age of 2; diffuse infiltration of muscle by an unencapsulated mass of histologically mature lipocytes; and progressive enlargement and extension of the tumor mass. It usually involves a large portion of the trunk or an extremity. Some cases are associated with distant lipomas or hemangiomas, or with hypertrophy of underlying bone.

Dercum's disease (adiposis dolorosa) is seen most often in obese or corpulent menopausal women who develop

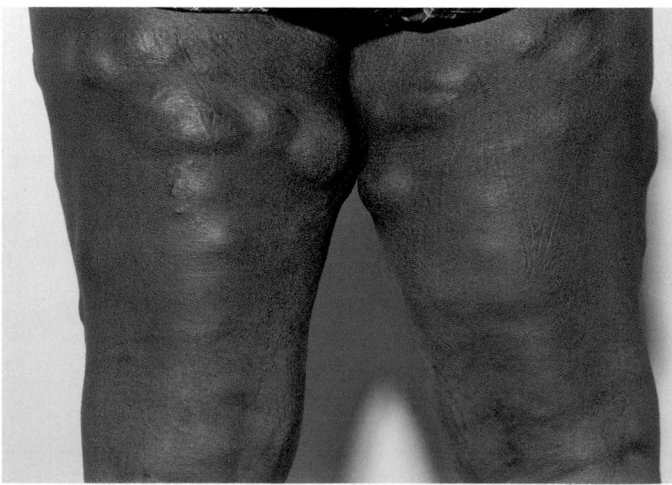

Fig. 28-41 Multiple lipomas.

symmetrical, tender, circumscribed fatty lesions. They are often accompanied by weakness and psychiatric disturbances. Relief of pain lasting for weeks after intravenous infusions of lidocaine, 1.3 g/day for 4 days, has been reported.

Several other conditions are characterized by multiple abnormalities including lipomas. Encephalocraniocutaneous lipomatosis is a rare neurocutaneous syndrome characterized by unilateral porencephalic cysts with cortical atrophy, ipsilateral facial and scalp lesions, ocular abnormalities, cranial asymmetry, and neurologic complications. The skin changes consist of unilateral lipomatous scalp tumors with overlying alopecia and connective tissue nevi. Ipsilateral lipodermoids, choristomas, and calcifications are the eye findings. CNS abnormalities are unilateral cerebral atrophy, dilated ventricles, porencephaly, cerebral calcifications, and lipomas of the leptomeninges. Seizures and mental retardation may occur. Some cases may have overlapping features of Proteus syndrome—multiple lipomas, epidermal nevi, cerebriform lesions of the plantar surfaces, vascular malformations, macrodactyly, hemihypertrophy, exostoses, and scoliosis.

Bannayan–Riley–Ruvalcaba syndrome is characterized by multiple subcutaneous lipomas and vascular malformations, lentigines of the penis and vulva, verrucae, and acanthosis nigricans. There is overlap in some of these cases with Cowden syndrome. Both have been found to have allelic mutations of the *PTEN* gene.

Multiple endocrine neoplasia type 1 has been found to have skin lesions consisting of multiple facial angiofibromas, collagenomas, café-au-lait spots, lipomas, confetti-like hypopigmented macules, and multiple gingival papules, in addition to the tumors of the parathyroid glands, endocrine pancreas, and anterior pituitary.

Fröhlich syndrome consists of multiple lipomas, obesity, and sexual infantilism.

Gardner syndrome consists of multiple osteomas, fibromas, desmoid tumors, lipomas, fibrosarcomas, epidermal inclusion cysts, and leiomyomas, associated with intestinal polyposis exclusively in the colon and rectum. The coexistence of cutaneous cysts, leiomyomas, and osteomas (mostly on the skull) with intestinal polyposis is frequently not recognized until malignant degeneration of one of the polyps occurs and operative removal brings the syndrome to notice. Half of such patients develop carcinoma of the colon before the age of 30, and practically all these patients die before the age of 50, unless they have surgical treatment. In general, total colectomy is advised. Bony exostoses occur in 50% of patients and usually involve the membranous bones of the face and head. Cysts occur in 63% of patients, and again most commonly involve the face and scalp. These are epidermal inclusion cysts; two-thirds have within them foci of pilomatrical differentiation. Pigmented lesions of the ocular fundus occurred in 90% of 41 patients with Gardner syndrome and 46% of 43 first-degree relatives. They are usually multiple and bilateral, and, having been seen in a 3-month-old infant, are probably congenital. Gardner syndrome is transmitted as an autosomal-dominant disease. The defect is a mutation in the *APC* gene located at chromosome 5q21. In some families polyposis and carcinoma may occur without the skin and bone tumors. Lipomas have also been noted in the Carney complex, along with myxomas and pigmented lesions.

Subtypes

Angiolipomas present as painful subcutaneous nodules, having all the other features of a typical lipoma. Multiple subcutaneous angiolipomas are common, and have no invasive or metastatic potential. They may be associated with capillary malformations and may be induced by protease inhibitor therapy of HIV disease.

The angiolipoleiomyoma (angiomyolipoma of the skin) affects the acral skin of middle-aged men. No signs of tuberous sclerosis or renal angiomyolipoma are present. Mature adipocytes, thick-walled blood vessels, and smooth muscle cells in fascicles around blood vessels are present.

Neural fibrolipoma is an overgrowth of fibro-fatty tissue along a nerve trunk that often leads to nerve compression. Patients are usually aged 30 or younger and note a slowly enlarging subcutaneous mass with associated tenderness, decreased sensation, or paresthesia. The median nerve is most commonly involved. At times, macrodactyly appears, with elongation and splaying of the phalanges. MRI will provide the diagnosis, but unfortunately there is no effective treatment.

Chondroid lipomas are deep-seated, firm, yellow tumors that characteristically occur on the legs of women. Histologically, there is a thin capsule around mature lipocytes that have a single large vacuole and multivacuolated S-100, vimentin-positive cells within a chondromyxoid matrix.

The spindle cell lipoma is an asymptomatic, slow-growing subcutaneous tumor that has a predilection for the posterior back, neck, and shoulders of older men. It is usually solitary, although multiple lesions may occur. Some patients have a familial background of similar lesions. The neoplasm consists of lobulated masses of mature adipose tissue with areas of spindle cell proliferation. The spindle cells stain positively for CD34. Abnormalities of chromosome 16 and 13 have been reported. The spindled component of young spindle cell lipomas may be myxoid or cellular. The nuclei may be wavy and accompanied by mast cells, as in a neurofibroma. Examples with little fat may be misdiagnosed as solitary fibrous tumors. In old spindle cell lipomas (fibrolipomas), the spindle cell component has matured into dense collagen bundles.

Pleomorphic lipomas, like spindle cell lipomas, occur for the most part on the backs or necks of elderly men. There are floret giant cells with overlapping nuclei. Occasional lipoblast-like cells and atypical nuclei may be present and require differentiation from a liposarcoma. There is loss of chromosome 16q material. Despite this alarming appearance, the lesions behave in a perfectly benign manner. Pleomorphic lipomas lack the size, depth, infiltrative growth, and arborizing vascular pattern of liposarcoma. The term atypical lipomatous tumor is used to describe well-differentiated, low-grade liposarcoma. Extensive or deeply infiltrating tumors should be reviewed by an expert in soft tissue pathology.

The intradermal spindle cell/pleomorphic lipoma is distinct in that it most commonly affects women and has a wide distribution, occurring with relatively equal frequency on the head and neck, trunk, and the upper and lower extremities. Histologically, these lesions are unencapsulated and have infiltrative margins. Again, the spindle cells stain positively with CD34.

Hibernoma (lipoma of brown fat) is a form of lipoma composed of finely vacuolated fat cells of embryonic type. Hibernomas have a distinctive brownish color and a firm consistency, and usually occur singly. These tumors are benign. They occur chiefly in the mediastinum and the interscapular region of the back, but they also occur on the scalp, sternal region, and legs. They are usually about 3–12 cm in breadth and the onset is most often in adult life. Abnormalities of chromosomes 10 and 11 have been reported in the lesions. Epidural lipomatosis, collections of fat in the epidural space, may cause acute chord compression in the course of systemic corticosteroid treatment. A case of this distinctive, uncommon side effect proved to be the result of deposits of brown fat.

Bechara FG, et al: Fat tissue after lipolysis of lipomas: a histopathological and immunohistochemical study. J Cutan Pathol 2007 Jul; 34(7):552–557.

Blanes M, et al: Angiolipomas, a rare manifestation of HIV-associated lipodystrophy. AIDS 2008 Feb 19; 22(4):552–554.

Dalal KM, et al: Diagnosis and management of lipomatous tumors. J Surg Oncol 2008 Mar 15; 97(4):298–313.

Kacerovska D, et al: Carney complex: a clinicopathologic and molecular biological study of a sporadic case, including extracutaneous and cutaneous lesions and a novel mutation of the PRKAR1A gene. J Am Acad Dermatol 2009 Jul; 61(1):80–87.

Lapidoth M, et al: Capillary malformation associated with angiolipoma: analysis of 127 consecutive clinic patients. Am J Clin Dermatol 2008; 9(6):389–392.

Nevus lipomatosus superficialis

Soft, yellowish papules or cerebriform plaques, usually of the buttock or thigh, less often of the ear or scalp, with a wrinkled rather than warty surface, characterize this tumor. The distribution may be either zonal (as in the multiple lesions reported by Hoffmann and Zurhelle) or solitary. Solitary lesions appear as plaque, or linear array, but some resemble broad, fatty acrochordons. Onset before the age of 20 is the rule. Most do not require treatment, but diagnostic biopsy is sometimes performed and intralesional phosphatidylcholine has been reported as successful.

de Paula Mesquita T, et al: Histologic resolution of naevus lipomatosus superficialis with intralesional phosphatidylcholine. J Eur Acad Dermatol Venereol 2009 Jun; 23(6):714–715.

Folded skin with scarring (Michelin tire baby syndrome)

In this rare syndrome, there are numerous deep, conspicuous, symmetrical, ringed creases around the extremities (Fig. 28-42). The underlying skin may manifest a smooth muscle hamartoma, a nevus lipomatosis, or elastic tissue abnormalities. It may occur as an autosomal-dominant trait, a sporadic condition, an isolated finding, or in association with congenital facial and limb abnormalities, or with severe neurologic defects.

Kharfi M, et al: Michelin tire syndrome: a report of two siblings. Pediatr Dermatol 2005; 22:245.

Benign lipoblastoma

This tumor, frequently confused with a liposarcoma, affects infants and young children exclusively, with approximately 90% of cases occurring before 3 years of age. It most commonly involves the soft tissues of the upper and lower extremities. A circumscribed and a diffuse form can be distinguished. The circumscribed form is superficially located and clinically comparable to a lipoma. The diffuse form is more deeply situated

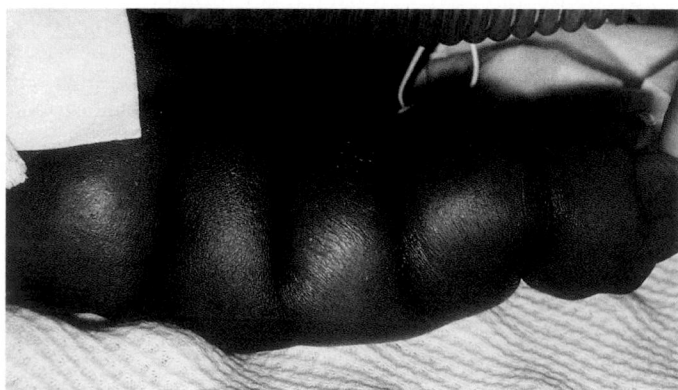

Fig. 28-42 Michelin tire baby.

and is analogous to diffuse lipomatosis. Microscopically, both forms consist of lobulated immature adipose tissue composed of lipoblasts, a plexiform capillary pattern, and a richly myxoid stroma. Cytogenetic studies for rearrangements of chromosome 8q11–q13 or fluorescence in situ hybridization (FISH) analysis for the *PLAG1–HAS2* fusion gene help to distinguish this tumor from liposarcoma, a distinction that can be difficult histologically. Complete local excision is the treatment of choice; however, recurrences may occur in as many as one-quarter of patients.

Ende L, et al: Lipoblastoma: appreciation of an expanded spectrum of disease through cytogenetic analysis. Arch Pathol Lab Med 2008 Sep; 132(9):1442–1444.

Morerio C, et al: Differential diagnosis of lipoma-like lipoblastoma. Pediatr Blood Cancer 2009 Jan; 52(1):132–134.

Liposarcoma

Liposarcomas are the most common soft tissue sarcoma. They usually arise from the intermuscular fascia, and only rarely from the subcutaneous fat. They do not arise from pre-existing lipomas. The usual course is an inconspicuous swelling of the soft tissue that undergoes an imperceptibly gradual enlargement. When a fatty tumor becomes larger than 10 cm in diameter, liposarcoma should be seriously considered. The upper thigh is the most common site. Other frequent sites are the buttocks, groin, and upper extremities. Adult males are affected mostly.

Liposarcomas may be well differentiated; subtypes include the adipocytic, sclerosing, inflammatory, spindle cell, and dedifferentiate variants. In this category there are aberrations of chromosome 12. Myxoid and round-cell variant liposarcoma often shows poorly differentiated histology. In most cases there is a reciprocal translocation t(12; 16)(q13; q11). The third major class is pleomorphic liposarcoma.

Treatment is adequate radical excision of the lesion. In well-differentiated superficial lesions the prognosis is good; for deeper, high-grade lesions, the extension between fascial planes and presence of small satellite nodules require carefully planned surgery, which may be assisted by MRI guidance. For metastatic liposarcomas, radiation therapy may be effective.

Shoji T, et al: Giant primary liposarcoma of the chest. Gen Thorac Cardiovasc Surg 2009 Mar; 57(3):159–161.

Abnormalities of smooth muscle

Leiomyoma

Cutaneous leiomyomas are smooth muscle tumors characterized by painful nodules that occur singly or multiply. They may be separated conveniently into solitary and multiple cutaneous leiomyomas arising from arrectores pilorum muscles (piloleiomyomas); solitary genital leiomyomas arising from the dartoic, vulvar, or mammillary muscle; and solitary angioleiomyomas arising from the muscles of veins.

Solitary cutaneous leiomyoma

The typical lesion is a deeply circumscribed, rounded nodule ranging from 2 to 15 mm in diameter. It is freely movable. The overlying skin may have a reddish or violaceous tint. Although the lesion is insensitive at first, painful paroxysms may occur. Once pain commences, the tendency is for it to intensify.

Multiple cutaneous leiomyomas

These brownish, grouped, papular lesions vary from 2 to 23 mm in diameter and are the most common variety of

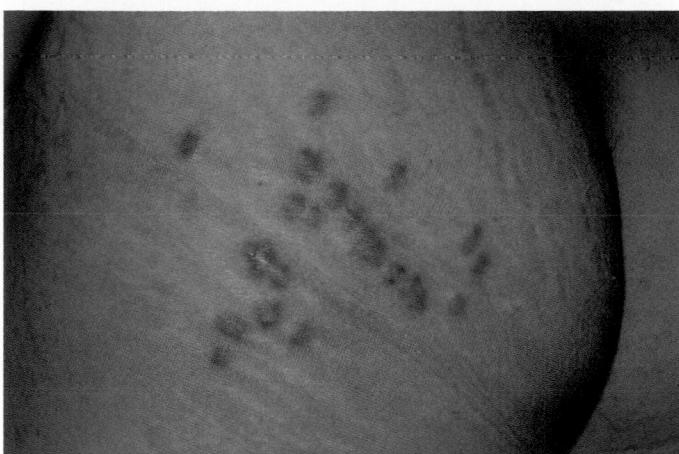
Fig. 28-43 Multiple leiomyomas.

leiomyoma (Fig. 28-43). Two or more sites of the skin surface may be involved. The firm, smooth, superficial, sometimes translucent, and freely movable nodules are located most frequently on the trunk and extremities. They often form linear or dermatomal patterns, either alone or with scattered isolated nonsegmental lesions elsewhere. These leiomyomas may occur on the tongue or, less often, elsewhere in the mouth as well. The usual age at onset is the teens to the fourth decade. Eruptive lesions have been described in chronic lymphocytic leukemia.

Multiple leiomyomas are inherited in an autosomal-dominant fashion. Women with this inherited type often have uterine leiomyomas as well. This is part of an inherited syndrome in which some patients also have a predisposition to type II papillary renal carcinomas or renal collecting duct cancer. Mutations in the fumarate hydratase gene are present in 75% of patients with this syndrome. Fumarate hydratase gene mutations may also be inherited in an autosomal-recessive manner. Fully affected children have severe neurologic impairment. The adult carriers may develop leiomyomas. Sporadic leiomyoma, leiomyosarcomas, renal cancers, and uterine leiomyomas have a very low frequency of fumarate hydratase mutations.

Genital leiomyomas

These lesions are located on the scrotum, on the labia majora, or rarely, on the nipples. They may be intra- or subcutaneous in location. Most genital leiomyomas are painless and solitary. Alport syndrome is an X-linked dominant syndrome consisting of hematuric nephropathy, deafness, and maculopathy due to mutations in type IV collagen. Some of these patients will have diffuse leiomyomatosis, which may affect the esophagus, tracheobronchial tree, perirectal area, and genital tract and vulva.

Angioleiomyoma (vascular leiomyoma)

This variety of leiomyoma arises from the muscle of veins. Pain, either spontaneous or provoked by pressure or cold, occurs in roughly half the cases. It is found mostly on the lower leg in middle-aged women. Solid tumors occur three times more frequently in women, and cavernous tumors occur four times more frequently in men. Solid lesions on the extremities are commonly painful; tumors of the head are rarely painful. In AIDS, multiple skin and visceral angioleiomyomas may occur. These tumors cells possess the Epstein–Barr virus genome.

Histologically, the leiomyoma is made up of bundles and masses of smooth muscle fibers. Varying amounts of collagen are intermingled. The smooth muscle cells are finely fibrillated

and contain a glycogen vacuole adjacent to the nucleus. The nuclei are typically long, thin, and cigar-shaped.

Angiolipoleiomyoma

Fitzpatrick et al reported eight patients with acquired, solitary, asymptomatic acral nodules. Seven were men and all were adults. Histologically, they had well-circumscribed subcutaneous tumors composed of smooth muscle cells, blood vessels, connective tissue, and fat.

Treatment

Leiomyomas are benign. Solitary painful lesions may be excised. When they are multiple and familial, monitoring for renal cell or collecting duct carcinoma is important. When multiple lesions are present and painful, as they may be especially in the winter, relief of pain may be achieved by giving doxazosin, an oral α-1 adrenoceptor antagonist. This is better tolerated than phenoxybenzamine, an α-adrenergic blocker, which also has been reported to provide pain relief. Nifedipine, 10 mg three times a day, gabapentin, oral nitroglycerin, and α-blockers have also had variable success. An ice cube applied over the lesions often induces pain, and the effectiveness of therapy may be assessed by the length of time it takes for the ice cube to cause pain. Botox injection has also been reported as effective.

Akay BN, et al: Congenital pilar leiomyoma. Am Acad Dermatol 2008 Nov; 59(5 Suppl):S102–S104.
Onder M, et al: A new indication of botulinum toxin: leiomyoma-related pain. J Am Acad Dermatol 2009 Feb; 60(2):325–328.
Stewart L, et al: Association of germline mutations in the fumarate hydratase gene and uterine fibroids in women with hereditary leiomyomatosis and renal cell cancer. Arch Dermatol 2008 Dec; 144(12):1584–1592.

Congenital smooth muscle hamartoma

Congenital smooth muscle hamartoma is typically a skin-colored or lightly pigmented patch or plaque with hypertrichosis (Fig. 28-44). It is often present at birth, usually on the trunk, with the lumbosacral area involved in two-thirds of patients. Older patients may have perifollicular papules. They vary in size from 2 × 3 to 10 × 10 cm. The Michelin tire baby syndrome may result from a diffuse smooth muscle hamartoma. One patient presented with a linear reddish-purple plaque. The incidence is approximately 1 in 2600 newborns. Transient elevation on rubbing may be seen (pseudo-Darier's sign) in 80%. An association with multiple adult myofibromas has been reported, as has association with congenital melanocytic nevus.

Histologically, numerous thick, long, well-defined bundles of smooth muscle are seen in the dermis at various angles of orientation. There may be an increase in hair follicles.

In some cases there is clinical and histologic overlap with Becker nevus. Classically, Becker nevus is a unilateral (rarely bilateral) acquired hyperpigmentation, usually beginning as a tan macule on the shoulder or pectoral area of a teenage male. Over time, hypertrichosis develops within it. Biopsy of such lesions shows acanthosis, papillomatosis, and increased basal cell pigmentation. Occasional congenital lesions manifesting hyperpigmentation and hypertrichosis have shown biopsy findings consistent with those of a Becker nevus (no smooth muscle proliferation), and lesions with a typical late-onset history compatible with Becker nevus have occasionally shown smooth muscle hamartoma-like changes in the dermis. Other cases of late-onset smooth muscle hamartomas are occasionally reported that are not hyperpigmented or hypertrichotic. No treatment is necessary.

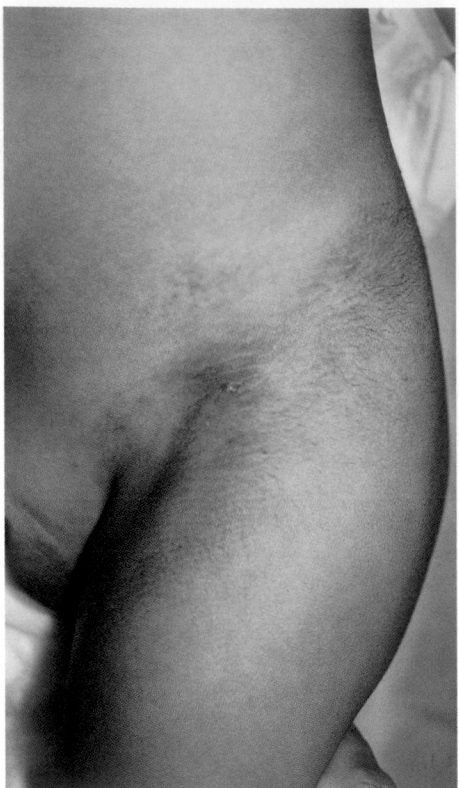

Fig. 28-44 Smooth muscle hamartomas.

Holland KE, et al: Generalized congenital smooth muscle hamartoma presenting with hypertrichosis, excess skin folds, and follicular dimpling. Pediatr Dermatol 2008 Mar–Apr; 25(2):236–239.

Kim DS, et al: Multiple adult myofibromas with congenital smooth muscle hamartoma. Clin Exp Dermatol 2009 Mar; 34(2):254–256.

Zarineh A, et al: Smooth muscle hamartoma associated with a congenital pattern melanocytic nevus, a case report and review of the literature. J Cutan Pathol 2008 Oct; 35 Suppl 1:83–86.

Leiomyosarcoma

Superficial leiomyosarcomas (those originating in the dermis or subcutaneous tissue) comprise approximately 2% of all soft tissue sarcomas. Occasionally, a lesion may present in the skin that is a metastasis from an internal source. The cutaneous leiomyosarcoma appears in the dermis as a solitary nodule. It may originate from the arrector pili or genital dartoic muscle. This has a good prognosis. Recurrence rates with Mohs surgery are approximately 15%, with metastases a rare event. Subcutaneous leiomyosarcomas, on the contrary, have a guarded prognosis, since hematogenous metastases occur in approximately 35% of patients. These prove fatal in about one-third of cases. Lung metastases are frequent, so chest imaging is an important part of monitoring these patients.

The clinical appearance of these lesions is not distinctive, so that the diagnosis is established by the histopathologic findings. These differ from the leiomyoma by dense cellularity, nuclear pleomorphism, numerous mitotic figures, and disarray of the smooth muscle bundles. Collagen is found only in the septa. Desmin, smooth muscle actin, and h-caldesmon are helpful in differentiating leiomyosarcoma from other spindle cell or pleomorphic tumors.

The preferred method of treatment is wide local excision. The Mohs surgical approach is useful in limiting recurrences and sparing tissue. Radiation therapy and chemotherapy are generally not effective.

Rouhani P, et al: Cutaneous soft tissue sarcoma incidence patterns in the U.S.: an analysis of 12,114 cases. Cancer 2008 Aug 1; 113(3):616–627.

Miscellaneous tumors and tumor-associated conditions

Cutaneous endometriosis

Endometriosis of the skin is characterized by the appearance of brownish papules at the umbilicus or in lower abdominal scars after gynecologic surgery in middle-aged women. The usually solitary tumor ranges from a few to 60 mm (average, 5 mm) in diameter. The tender or painful lesion is bluish-black from the bleeding that occurs cyclically in many patients.

Histopathologic findings are glandular structures with a decidualized stroma typically containing extravasated red blood cells and hemosiderin. Treatment of choice is surgical excision. Preoperative treatment with danazol or leuprolide may reduce its size.

Lee A, et al: Cutaneous umbilical endometriosis. Dermatol Online J 2008 Oct 15; 14(10):23.

Teratoma

Teratomas may develop in the skin but are most common in the ovaries or testes. Occurrence with a myelomeningocele has been reported. They have no characteristic clinical features, but on microscopic examination many types of tissue, representative of all three germ layers, are present. Hair, teeth, and functioning thyroid tissue are examples of fully differentiated tissues that may develop. Occasionally, malignancy may occur.

Habibi Z, et al: Teratoma inside a myelomeningocele. J Neurosurg 2007 Jun; 106(6 Suppl):467–471.

Kim MK, et al: A suprapubic dermoid cyst confused with cutaneous endometriosis: a case report. Fertil Steril 2008 Mar; 89(3):724.e5–724.e7.

Metastatic carcinoma

Malignant tumors are able to grow at sites distant from the primary site of origin; thus, dissemination to the skin may occur with any malignant neoplasm. These infiltrates may result from direct invasion of the skin from underlying tumors, may extend by lymphatic or hematogenous spread, or may be introduced by therapeutic procedures.

Five to 10% of patients with cancer develop skin metastases. The reported incidence figures vary widely according to the type of study undertaken and the site of primary tumor studied. The frequency of involvement of the skin is low when other sites are considered, such as the lung, liver, lymph nodes, and brain.

Usually, metastases occur as numerous firm, hard, or rubbery masses, with a predilection for the chest, abdomen, or scalp, in an adult over the age of 40 who has had a previously diagnosed carcinoma. Many variations in morphology, number of lesions, site of growth, age at onset, and timing of metastases exist, however. They are most commonly intradermal papules, nodules, or tumors that are firm, skin-colored to reddish, purplish, black or brown; may be fixed to underlying tissues; and rarely ulcerate.

Several unusual morphologic patterns occur. Carcinoma en cuirasse is a diffuse infiltration of the skin that imparts an indurated and hidebound leathery quality to it. This sclerodermoid change, also referred to as scirrhous carcinoma,

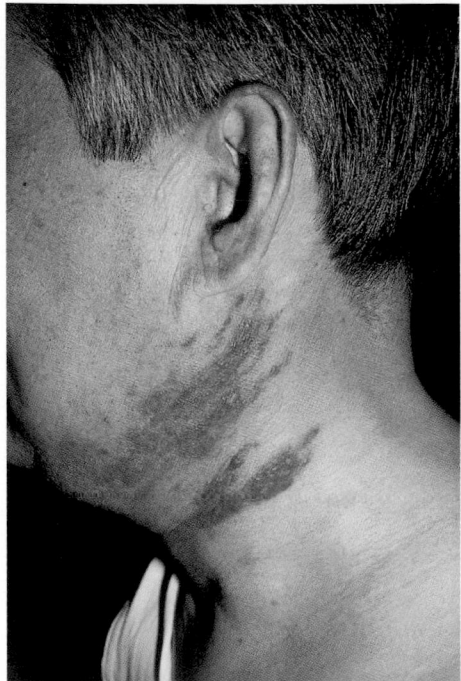

Fig. 28-45 Metastatic rectal cancer presenting as inflammatory carcinoma.

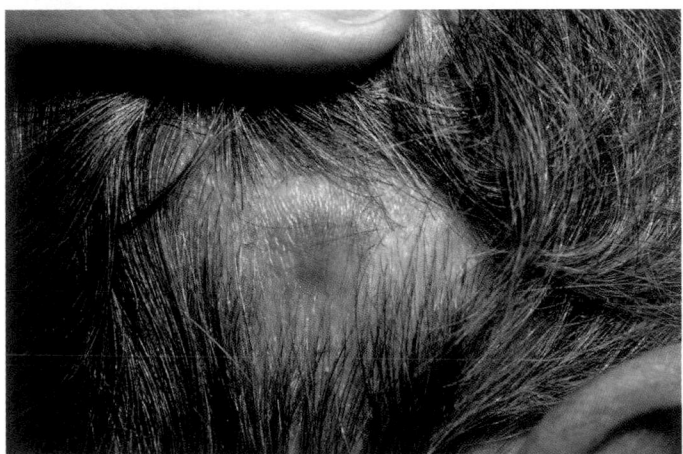

Fig. 28-46 Alopecia neoplastica secondary to breast carcinoma.

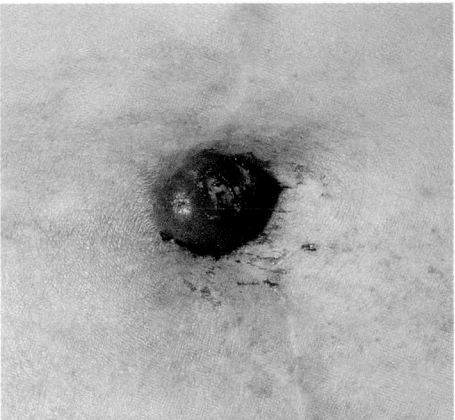

Fig. 28-47 Sister Mary Joseph nodule.

is produced by fibrosis and single rows of tumor cells. This type primarily occurs with breast carcinoma. Carcinoma telangiectaticum is another unusual type of cutaneous metastasis from breast carcinoma that presents as small pink to purplish papules, pseudovesicles, and telangiectases.

Inflammatory carcinoma (carcinoma erysipelatoides) is characterized by erythema, edema, warmth, and a well-defined leading edge, similar to erysipelas in appearance (Fig. 28-45). This is usually caused by breast carcinoma, but has been reported with many other primary tumors. Histologically, there is little to no inflammation, but rather neoplastic cells within dilated superficial dermal vessels.

Alopecia neoplastica (Fig. 28-46) may present as a cicatricial localized area of hair loss, which, on biopsy, is usually seen to be caused by breast metastases in women, and lung or kidney carcinoma in men. Metastatic breast cancer may be darkly pigmented, as may Paget's disease of the breast.

The so-called Sister Mary Joseph nodule is formed by localization of metastatic tumors to the umbilicus (Fig. 28-47). The most common primary sites are the stomach, large bowel, ovary, and pancreas. Zosteriform, linear, or chancroidal ulcerations of the genitalia, and verrucous nodules of the legs, are other rarely reported clinical presentations.

The primary tumor is usually diagnosed before the appearance of metastases, and dissemination to the skin is often a late finding. Metastases to other more commonly involved organs, such as the lung and liver, have usually occurred. A poor prognosis is thus the rule. Skin infiltrates may, however, be the first harbinger of a malignant visceral neoplasm and are often the first clinically apparent metastatic site.

The principal anatomic sites to which metastases localize are the chest, abdomen, and scalp, with the back and extremities being relatively uncommon areas. Involvement of the skin is likely to be near the area of the primary tumor. Thus, chest lesions are usually caused by breast carcinoma in women and lung carcinoma in men, abdominal or perineal lesions by colonic carcinoma, and the face by squamous cell carcinoma of the oral cavity. Extremity lesions, when they occur, are most commonly caused by melanoma.

Because of its overall high prevalence, breast cancer is the type most commonly metastatic to the skin in women, and melanoma, followed by lung cancer, is the type seen most commonly in men. Colon carcinoma is also common because of its high incidence in both sexes. Renal cell carcinoma, while less common, has a predilection for scalp metastases. Metastatic lesions are uncommon in children, but when they do occur, neuroblastoma and leukemia are the most frequent causes.

Lymphangiosarcoma (Stewart–Treves syndrome) develops in a site of chronic lymphedema, such as in breast cancer patients who have had lymph node resection. Antikeratin antibodies are useful in identifying metastatic breast carcinoma, while CD34, CD31, and *Ulex europeus* lectin are positive in Stewart–Treves angiosarcoma.

Benmously R, et al: Cutaneous metastases from internal cancers. Acta Dermatovenerol Alp Panonica Adriat 2008 Dec; 17(4):167–170.

Paraneoplastic syndromes

Some cancers produce findings in the skin that indicate that an underlying internal malignancy may be present. These may range from a specific eruption characteristic of a particular type of cancer, such as necrolytic migratory erythema, to a nonspecific cutaneous reaction pattern, among the causes of which may be an internal malignancy. Although many of these syndromes are discussed in other sections of the book, a few are mentioned here as illustrative examples of this phenomenon.

Bazex syndrome, or acrokeratosis paraneoplastica, is characterized by violaceous erythema and scaling of the fingers, toes, nose, and aural helices. Nail dystrophy and palmoplantar

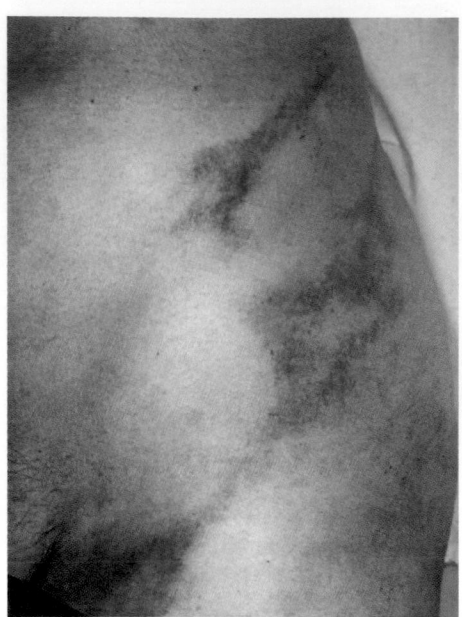

Fig. 28-48 Superficial migratory thrombophlebitis secondary to breast cancer.

keratoderma may be seen. These cases are secondary to primary malignant neoplasms of the upper aerodigestive tract or metastatic cancer to lymph nodes, often in the cervical region.

The glucagonoma syndrome is characterized by weight loss, glucose intolerance, anemia, glossitis, and necrolytic migratory erythema. Erythematous patches with bullae and light brown papules with scales involving the face, groin, and abdomen characterize the skin eruption. This is seen with glucagon-secreting tumors of the pancreas.

Erythema gyratum repens is a gyrate serpiginous erythema with characteristic wood grain-pattern scales; it is nearly always associated with an underlying malignancy. Hypertrichosis lanuginosa acquisita, or malignant down, is the sudden growth of profuse, soft, nonmedullated, nonpigmented, downy hair in an adult. The most common sites of associated carcinoma were the lung and colon.

The sign of Leser–Trélat is the sudden appearance of multiple pruritic seborrheic keratoses, associated with an internal malignancy. Trousseau's sign, or migratory thrombophlebitis (Fig. 28-48), is usually associated with pancreatic carcinoma. A form of pemphigus, paraneoplastic pemphigus, is most commonly associated with lymphoma, chronic lymphocytic leukemia, and Castleman's disease.

Several cutaneous diseases that are not associated with internal malignancy with the frequency of the above conditions, but that may be a sign of internal malignancy in some cases, are exfoliative erythroderma (lymphoproliferative disease), acanthosis nigricans (adenocarcinoma), multicentric reticulohistiocytosis, Sweet syndrome (acute myelogenous leukemia), nodular fat necrosis (pancreatic carcinoma), Paget's disease (underlying adnexal or breast carcinoma, or adenocarcinoma of the genitourinary tract or colon), dermatomyositis in patients over the age of 40, palmar fasciitis and polyarthritis syndrome, and acquired ichthyosis (lymphoproliferative).

A variant of acquired ichthyosis, pityriasis rotunda, manifests circular, brown, scaly patches from 1 to 28 cm in diameter and varying in number from 1 to 20. They may occur on the trunk or extremities. These symptomless patches may be a clue to the diagnosis of hepatocellular carcinoma in South African black patients. Tripe palms, considered by some to be acanthosis nigricans of the palms, are associated with carcinoma in more than 90% of cases. Filiform hyperkeratosis of the palms may present in patients who develop cancer.

El Tal AK, et al: Cutaneous vascular disorders associated with internal malignancy. Dermatol Clin 2008 Jan; 26(1):45–57.
Hospach T, et al: Acute febrile neutrophilic dermatosis (Sweet's syndrome) in childhood and adolescence: two new patients and review of the literature on associated diseases. Eur J Pediatr 2009 Jan; 168(1):1–9.
Moore RL, et al: Epidermal manifestations of internal malignancy. Dermatol Clin 2008 Jan; 26(1):17–29.
Pipkin CA, et al: Cutaneous manifestations of internal malignancies: an overview. Dermatol Clin 2008 Jan; 26(1):1–15.
Weenig RH, et al: Dermal and pannicular manifestations of internal malignancy. Dermatol Clin 2008 Jan; 26(1):31–43.
Yoo KH, et al: Cutaneous paraneoplastic syndrome in a patient with adenocarcinoma of unknown primary site syndrome. J Clin Oncol 2009 Jan 10; 27(2):309–311.

Carcinoid

Carcinoid involves the lungs, heart, and gastrointestinal tract, as well as the skin. The outstanding feature of the skin is flushing, usually lasting 5–10 min. It most prominently involves the head and neck, but also produces a diffuse, scarlet color, with mottled red patches on the thorax and abdomen. Striking color changes may occur, with salmon red, bluish white, and other colors appearing simultaneously on various portions of the skin. Cyanosis may also be present. As the episodic flushing continues over months to years, telangiectases and plethora appear, as though the patient has polycythemia vera. Gyrate and serpiginous patches of erythema and cyanosis flare up and subside, not only on the face but also on all parts of the body and extremities.

Pellagroid changes may appear as a result of shunting of dietary tryptophan away from the kynurenine–niacin pathway and into the 5-hydroxyindole pathway. Periorbital swelling, edema of the face, neck, and feet, and sclerodermatous changes may occur. Disseminated deep dermal and subcutaneous metastatic nodules from a primary bronchial carcinoid tumor have been documented.

The clinical features of the carcinoid syndrome become evident only after hepatic metastases have occurred, or when the primary tumor is a bronchial carcinoid, or if the carcinoid arises in an ovarian teratoma, where the venous drainage bypasses the hepatic circulation.

The release of excessive amounts of serotonin and bradykinin into the circulation produces attacks of flushing of the skin, weakness, abdominal pain, nausea, vomiting, sweating, bronchoconstriction, palpitation, diarrhea, and collapse. These attacks may last a few hours. Right-sided cardiac valvular fibrosis occurs in 60% of chronically affected patients. Symptoms may be induced in these patients by the injection of epinephrine, at which time kinin peptide is released. Alcohol, hot beverages, exercise, and certain foods, among others, may induce flushing. The patient will provide the relevant triggers by history.

Etiologic factors

Carcinoid, also called argentaffinoma, is a tumor that arises from the argentaffin Kulchitsky chromaffin cells in the appendix or terminal ileum, and also in other parts of the gastrointestinal tract, from the lungs as bronchial adenomas, and rarely from ovarian or testicular teratomas. Some of these produce large amounts of serotonin (5-hydroxytryptamine), a derivative of tryptophan, and others do not. The primary lesion is more active in the production of serotonin than are the metastases. The tumor frequently metastasizes to the draining lymph glands or to neighboring organs, especially the liver, and rarely to more distal sites.

Laboratory findings

The diagnosis may be established by finding a high level of 5-hydroxyindolacetic acid (5-HIAA) in the urine. The normal urinary excretion of 5-HIAA is 3–8 mg/day, but in the presence of carcinoid it may reach 300 mg. Urinary values greater than 25 mg/day are diagnostic of carcinoid. Any value above the normal output is considered suspicious. The ingestion of bananas may cause significant elevations of 5-HIAA in the urine within a few hours, because banana pulp contains serotonin (4 mg/banana) and catecholamines. Tomatoes, red plums, pineapples, avocados, and eggplants also contain serotonin, but in much smaller amounts.

A screening test for 5-HIAA is the addition of nitrosonaphthol to the urine. A purple color is produced when 40 mg/day of 5-HIAA is excreted. Other serotonin metabolites besides 5-HIAA are found in the urine. The blood also contains serotonin in amounts of 0.2–0.4 mg%. In the presence of carcinoid the amount may be 10 times normal.

Metastatic carcinoid may appear in the skin. A high index of suspicion is needed, as metastatic carcinoid has been reported to mimic apocrine poroma on shave biopsy.

Treatment

In the rare cases where there is only a primary tumor without metastases, this should be removed. Excision of metastatic lesions in the liver may also be considered. If this is impossible, long-acting somatostatin analogs provide good long-term symptomatic control of the flushing and diarrhea. Injections are given monthly. Vitamin supplementation with niacin and avoidance of known trigger factors to flushing are recommended. Restriction of tryptophan-containing foods for short periods may limit serotonin production.

Puri PK, et al: Metastatic cutaneous carcinoid tumor mimicking an adnexal poroid neoplasm. J Cutan Pathol 2008 Jan; 35(1):54–57.
Santi R, et al: Skin metastasis from typical carcinoid tumor of the lung. J Cutan Pathol 2008 Apr; 35(4):418–422.

29 Epidermal Nevi, Neoplasms, and Cysts

Epidermal nevi

The term "epidermal nevus" can be used to include several entities, including keratinocytic epidermal nevi, nevus sebaceus, and nevus comedonicus. Although it is usually possible to classify epidermal nevi into one type, it is not uncommon to find local elements of various types within the same epidermal nevus. The epidermal nevus should be classified by its predominant histological and clinical feature (keratinocytic, comedonal, or sebaceous). Some syndromes have also been included in this classification, such as Proteus, CHILD, and phakomatosis pigmentokeratotica, since localized lesions and widespread systematized presentations are due to the same genetic mutations. This suggests that all "epidermal nevi" should be classified according to their histological phenotype. Epidermal nevi of all types are considered an expression of mosaicism with genetic mutation in the affected skin, but sparing the unaffected skin in widespread lesions; much less commonly, the mutation is found not only in the skin but also in other tissues. Lesions follow the lines of Blaschko, suggesting that they represent postzygotic mutations. In general, larger lesions, more widespread lesions, and lesions of the head and neck are more likely to have associated internal complications. The combination of an epidermal nevus and an associated internal problem is called "epidermal nevus syndrome." For each histological type, the frequency and nature of associated systemic problems may be characteristic. Overall, about 1:1000 children have an epidermal nevus of some type.

Keratinocytic epidermal nevi

Keratinizing epidermal nevi are described by a great variety of terms, such as linear epidermal nevus, hard nevus of Unna, soft epidermal nevus, and nevus verrucosus (verrucous nevus). If the lesion is widespread on half the body, the term nevus unius lateris has been used. The term ichthyosis hystrix is used if the lesions are bilateral and widespread.

The most common pattern of keratinocytic epidermal nevus is linear epidermal nevus. The individual lesions are verrucous, skin-colored, dirty-gray or brown papules, which coalesce to form a serpiginous plaque (Fig. 29-1). Interspersed in the localized patch may be horny excrescences and, rarely, comedones. The age of onset of epidermal nevi is generally at birth, but they may also develop within the first 10 years of life. They follow the lines of Blaschko.

The histologic changes in the epidermis are hyperplastic and affect chiefly the stratum corneum and stratum malpighii. There is variable hyperkeratosis, acanthosis, and papillomatosis. Up to 62% of biopsies of epidermal nevi have this pattern, so called non-epidermolytic epidermal nevi (NONEEN). About 16% show epidermolytic hyperkeratosis. At times, other histologic patterns may be found, including a psoriatic type, an acrokeratosis verruciformis-like type, and a Darier's disease-like type. It is assumed that each of these types would be associated with a specific mutation in the affected skin that,

if widespread, would give rise to the cutaneous disorder with the same histology. For example, epidermal nevi that show epidermolytic hyperkeratosis would have the same gene mutation as the disorder of cornification, bullous congenital ichthyosiform erythroderma, i.e. keratins K1 and K10. In a significant portion of the classic and common keratinocytic epidermal nevi that simply shows hyperkeratosis, papillomatosis, and acanthosis histologically, there is an activating gene mutation in fibroblast growth factor receptor 3 (FGFR3) and/or PI3K, a downstream effector of FGFR signaling. FOXN1 is highly expressed in these lesions. These same gene mutations are found in sporadic seborrheic keratoses, which, not surprisingly, have the same histology.

Keratinocytic epidermal nevi, as a part of an "epidermal nevus syndrome," may be associated with internal manifestations, including primarily skeletal abnormalities and less commonly central nervous system (CNS) manifestations. Various abnormalities of the bones, vessels, and brain are associated with these clinical findings. CNS manifestations appear to be more common when the lesions are large and located on the head and neck. Large keratinocytic epidermal nevi of the trunk and extremities are more frequently associated with skeletal abnormalities. Since, in the original and large reports of epidermal nevus syndrome, both nevus sebaceus and keratinocytic epidermal nevi were included, the precise characterization of the "keraticocytic epidermal nevus syndrome" waits to be defined.

Both Proteus syndrome and CLOVE syndrome (congenital lipomatous overgrowth, vascular malformations, and epidermal nevi) can have skin lesions of epidermal nevus. CLOVE is distinguished from Proteus syndrome by congenital overgrowth of a ballooning nature, which grows proportionately with the patient and typically affects the feet.

CHILD syndrome and verruciform xanthoma are both characterized by the presence histologically of elongated and widened dermal papillae filled with xanthoma-like cells. Epidermal hyperplasia, with acanthosis, papillomatosis, parakeratosis, and hyperkeratosis, is also present (the features of a keratinocytic epidermal nevus). In rare cases, instead of half the body being affected, large quadrants of the body, favoring folds, are the sites of the epidermal growths (ptychotropism). CHILD and verruciform xanthoma (in some cases) contain mutations in the NSDHL gene, located on the X chromosome and required for cholesterol biosynthesis.

Rarely, keratinocytic and adnexal malignancies occur in keratinocytic epidermal nevi. Any newly appearing lesion within a stable epidermal nevus should be biopsied to exclude this possibility. Management of keratinocytic epidermal nevi is difficult, since, unless the treatment also affects the dermis (and hence may cause scarring), the lesion recurs. The use of a combination of 5% 5-fluorouracil (5-FU) plus 0.1% tretinoin creams once a day may be beneficial and the response may be enhanced by occlusion. CO_2 and Er:YAG laser treatment may also be effective. If the lesion is small, simple excision can be considered.

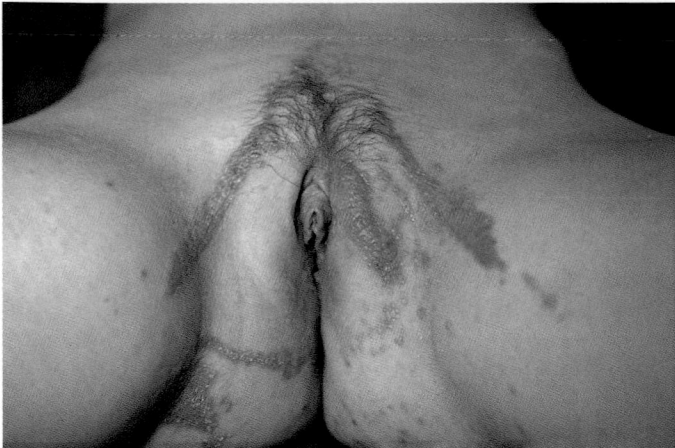

Fig. 29-1 Linear epidermal nevus.

Alam M, Arndt KA: A method for pulsed carbon dioxide laser treatment of epidermal nevi. J Am Acad Dermatol 2002; 46:554.

Avgerinou GP, et al: CHILD syndrome: the *NSDHL* gene and its role in CHILD syndrome, a rare hereditary syndrome. J Eur Acad Dermatol Venereol 2009 Nov 2 (Epub ahead of print).

Bittar M, Happle R: CHILD syndrome avant la lettre. J Am Acad Dermatol 2004; 50:S34.

Garcia-Vargas A, et al: An epidermal nevus syndrome with cerebral involvement caused by a mosaic *FGFR3* mutation. Am J Med Genet A 2008; 146A:2275.

Gucev ZS, et al: Congenital lipomatous overgrowth, vascular malformations, and epidermal nevi (CLOVE) syndrome: CNS malformations and seizures may be a component of this disorder. Am J Med Genet A 2008; 146A:2688.

Hafner C, et al: Oncogenic *PIK3CA* mutations occur in epidermal nevi and seborrheic keratoses with a characteristic mutation pattern. Proc Natl Acad Sci U S A 2007; 104:13450.

Hafner C, et al: Mosaicism of activating *FGFR3* mutations in human skin causes epidermal nevi. J Clin Invest 2006; 116:2201.

Hamanaka S, et al: Multiple malignant eccrine poroma and a linear epidermal nevus. J Dermatol 1996; 23:469.

Ichikawa T, et al: Squamous cell carcinoma arising in a verrucous epidermal nevus. Dermatology (Switzerland) 1996; 193:135.

Kim JJ, et al: Topical tretinoin and 5-fluorouracil in the treatment of linear verrucous epidermal nevus. J Am Acad Dermatol 2000; 43:129.

Ko JY, et al: A verruciform xanthoma-like phenomenon in a linear epidermal naevus in the absence of a syndromic association. Br J Dermatol 2008; 159:493.

Mehra S, et al: A novel somatic mutation of the 3beta-hydroxysteroid dehydrogenase gene in sporadic cutaneous verruciform xanthoma. Arch Dermatol 2005; 141:1263.

Park JH, et al: Er:YAG laser treatment of verrucous epidermal nevi. Dermatol Surg 2004; 30:378.

Nevus comedonicus

Nevus comedonicus is characterized by closely arranged, grouped, often linear, slightly elevated papules that have at their center keratinous plugs resembling comedones. Cysts, abscesses, fistulas, and scars develop in about half the cases, which have been described as "inflammatory" nevus comedonicus. As with other epidermal nevi, lesions may be localized to a small area or have an extensive distribution. They are most commonly unilateral; however, bilateral cases are also seen. Lesions occur mostly on the trunk and follow the lines of Blaschko. The lesions may develop any time from birth to age 15, but are usually present by the age of 10. Follicular tumors, including trichofolliculoma and pilar sheath acanthoma, can appear with the lesion. An "epidermal nevus syndrome" or "nevus comedonicus syndrome" has been reported with electroencephalogram (EEG) abnormalities, ipsilateral cataract, corneal changes, and skeletal anomalies (hemivertebrae, scoliosis, and absence of the fifth ray of a hand).

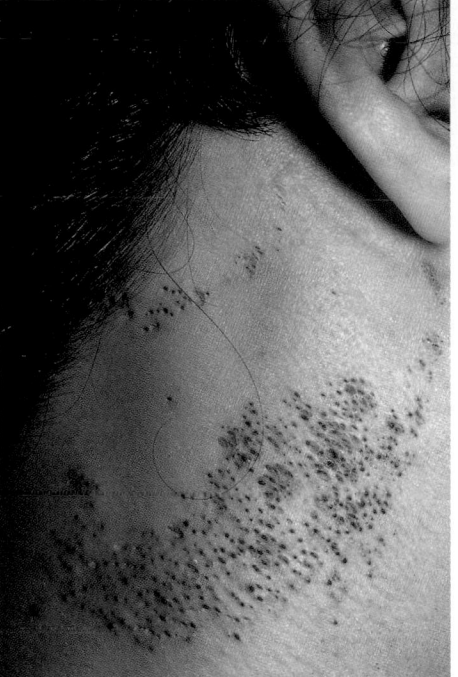

Fig. 29-2 Nevus comedonicus.

The pilosebaceous follicles are dilated and filled with keratinous plugs (Fig. 29-2). On the palms, pseudocomedones are present. Histologic examination reveals large dilated follicles filled with orthokeratotic horny material and lined by atrophic squamous epithelium. The interfollicular epidermis is papillomatous, as is seen in typical epidermal nevi. Hair follicle differentiation, well-formed follicular structures, and normal sebaceous glands are not common in well-formed lesions.

Apert's syndrome is characterized by skeletal anomalies and acne. It is due to a mutation in *FGFR2*. A mutation has also been found in *FGFR2* in at least one case of nevus comedonicus, suggesting that nevus comedonicus may be a mosaic form of Apert's.

Treatment of lesions not complicated by inflammatory cysts and nodules is primarily cosmetic. Pore-removing cosmetic strips and comedone expression may improve the cosmetic appearance. Topical tretinoin may be beneficial. Patients with inflammatory lesions are much more difficult to manage. If the area affected is limited, surgical excision may be considered. Oral isotretinoin, chronically at the minimum effective dose (0.5 mg/kg/day or less if possible), may partially suppress the formation of cysts and inflammatory nodules; however, many cases of nevus comedonicus fail to respond. The comedonal lesions are not improved by the oral isotretinoin.

Ioue Y, et al: Two cases of nevus comedonicus: successful treatment of keratin plugs with a pore strip. J Am Acad Dermatol 2000; 43:927.

Kirtak N, et al: Extensive inflammatory nevus comedonicus involving half of the body. Int J Dermatol 2004; 43:434.

Melnik B, Schmitz G: FGFR2 signaling and the pathogenesis of acne. J Dtsch Dermatol Ges 2008; 6:721.

Milburn S, et al: The treatment of naevus comedonicus. Br J Plast Surg 2004; 57:805.

Munro CS, Wilkie A: Epidermal mosaicism producing localised acne: somatic mutation in FGFR2. Lancet 1998; 352:704.

Wakahara M, et al: Bilateral nevus comedonicus: efficacy of topical tacalcitol ointment. Acta Dermatol Venereol 2003; 83:51.

Epidermal nevus syndrome

Epidermal nevus syndrome does not represent a single entity, but rather multiple syndromes characterized by keratinocytic or organiod nevi at times associated with internal organ involvement. Each variant has characteristic cutaneous findings, and at times relatively specific internal findings. There are at least 5 variants of organoid epidermal nevus syndrome:

1. Schimmelpenning syndrome: Nevus sebaceus with cerebral, ocular and skeletal defects. Lesions of the head and neck may lack prominent sebaceous hyperplasia. Coloboma and lipodermoid of the conjunctiva can occur. Vitamin D–resistant hypophosphatemic rickets may be present.
2. Phacomatosis pigmentokeratotica: Nevus sebaceus and papular nevus spilus coexist. The nevus sebaceus may have a flat erythematous central area with an elevated margin showing features of a nonorganoid epidermal nevus. Multiple angiomas may be found in the nevus spilus component. True basal cell carcinomas develop in the nevus sebaceus of this syndrome. CNS complications can occur, along with hyperhidrosis, weakness, and sensory or motor neuropathy. Vitamin D-resistant rickets may also be present.
3. Nevus comedonicus syndrome: Nevus comedonicus with ipsilateral ocular, skeletal, or neurologic defects defines this syndrome.
4. Angora hair nevus syndrome: A linear epidermal nevus covered with long white hair growing out from dilated follicular pores. CNS, eyes, and skeletal abnormalities may be found.
5. Becker nevus syndrome: Becker nevus associated with ipsilateral hypoplasia of the breast.

Keratinocytic nevi are seen in at least 4 epidermal nevus syndromes:

1. Proteus syndrome.
2. Type 2 segmental Cowden disease. A linear soft, thick, papillomatous keratinocytic nevus in the absence of cerebriform hyperplasia of the palms and soles, but with segmental glomerulosclerosis. It is caused by loss of heterozygosity in an embryo carrying a PTEN germline mutation. Associated anomalies include lipomas, connective tissue nevi, vascular nevi, hemihypertrophy, seizures, hydrocephalus, and GI polyps.
3. CHILD syndrome: X-linked dominant, male lethal trait. It is caused by a mutation in NSDHL. Chondrodysplasia

punctata is characteristic. There is a marked affinity of the nevus for the body folds (ptychotropism). There is a tendency to spontaneous involution.

4. Fibroblast growth factor receptor 3 epidermal nevus syndrome (Garcia-Hafner-Happle syndrome). A velvety type nonepidermolytic epidermal nevus and cerebral defects identify this syndrome.

Less well defined syndromes include:

1. Nevus trichilemmocysticus: Multiple trichilemmal cysts along Blaschko's lines associated with osteomalacia and fractures.
2. Didymosis aplasticosebacea: Sebaceous nevus coexisting with aplasia cutis, usually in close proximity to each other.
3. SCALP syndrome: Sebaceous nevus, CNS malformations, aplasia cutis congenital, limbal dermoid and pigmented nevus. It is a combination of didymosis aplasticosebacea and a large melanocytic nevus.
4. Gobellos syndrome: Systematized, linear, velvety, orthokeratotic nevus with hypertrichosis and follicular hyperkeratosis. Multiple bony defects are present.
5. Bafverstedt syndrome: Horny excrescences in a linear pattern with mental retardation and seizures. Diffuse icthyosis-like hyperkeratosis covers the entire body including the palms and soles.
6. NEVADA syndrome: Keratinocytic, verrucous nevus with angiodysplasia.
7. CLOVE syndrome: Congenital lipomatous overgrowth, vascular malformation and epidermal nevus. Extensive truncal vascular malformations and overgrown feet are characteristic.

Happle R: The group of epidermal nevus syndromes. J Am Acad Dermatol 2010; 63:1.

Happle R: The group of epidermal nevus syndromes. J Am Acad Dermatol 2010; 63:25.

Inflammatory linear verrucous epidermal nevus

The term inflammatory linear verrucous epidermal nevus (ILVEN) may encompass as many as four separate conditions. The most common form is the classic ILVEN or "dermatitic" epidermal nevus. At least three-quarters of these cases appear before age 5 years, most before age 6 months. Later onset in adulthood has been reported. ILVEN is characteristically pruritic and pursues a chronic course. Lesions follow the lines of Blaschko. The individual lesions comprising the affected region are erythematous papules and plaques with fine scale (Fig. 29-4). The lesions are morphologically nondescript and, if the distribution is not recognized, could be easily overlooked as an area of dermatitis. Multiple widely separated areas may be affected, usually on only one side of the body; this may be bilateral, analogous to other epidermal nevi. Familial cases have been reported. Rarely, systemic involvement, with musculoskeletal and neurologic sequelae (developmental delay, epilepsy), has been reported.

Histologically, classic ILVEN demonstrates abruptly alternating areas of hypergranulosis with orthokeratosis, and parakeratosis with agranulosis. An inflammatory infiltrate of lymphocytes is present in the upper dermis. At times, the histology may simply be that of a subacute dermatitis. While the histologic diagnosis of psoriasis can be considered, the correct diagnosis can be established if the dermatopathologist is made aware of ILVEN as a consideration. If there is a question, the presence of involucrin expression in the parakeratotic areas can distinguish ILVEN from psoriasis.

Three other types of inflammatory nevus have been included in this group. Some cases of "linear" lichen planus have been considered as "epidermal nevi," as they commonly follow lines of Blaschko. CHILD syndrome, also considered a type of

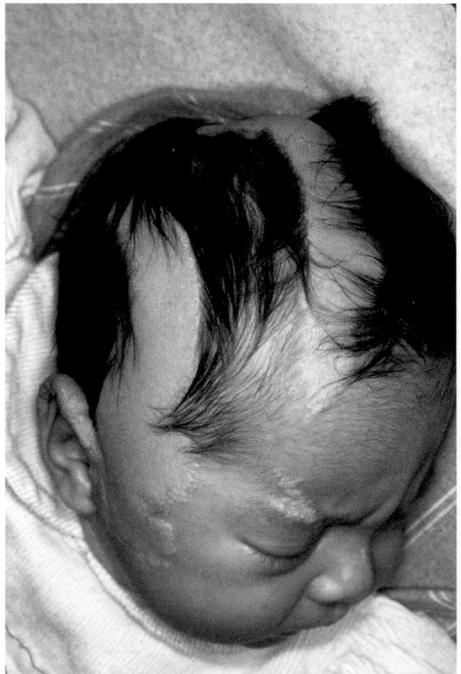

Fig. 29-3 Schimmelpenning syndrome.

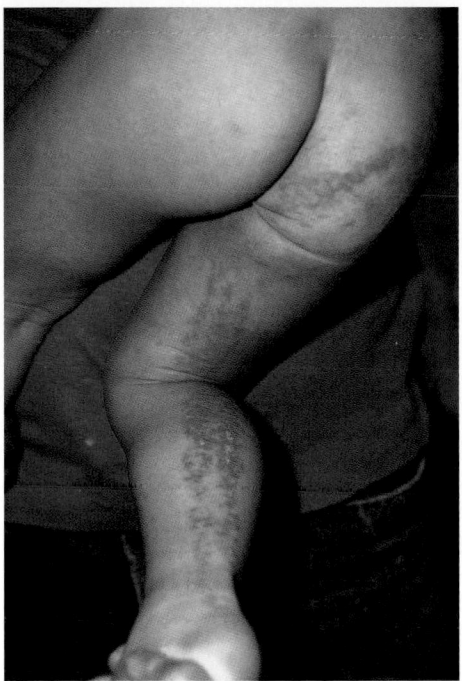

Fig. 29-4 Inflammatory linear verrucous epidermal nevus.

"inflammatory" epidermal nevus, is usually clinically distinct, demonstrating its characteristic hemidysplasia. The most confusing entity has been the so-called "nevoid" or "linear" psoriasis. These cases are of two types. The first type is a child with a family history of psoriasis who has a nevoid lesion at or near birth. The child later develops psoriasis which "koebnerizes" into the ILVEN lesion, suggesting it is a "locus minoris resistensiae" for psoriasis. Treatment of the psoriasis clears the psoriasis overlying the ILVEN, but not the ILVEN. Arthritis developed in one such case. The second type is one in which psoriasis initially presents in one band or area. Histologically, it resembles psoriasis. Most of these cases later develop typical psoriasis later in life, suggesting a mosaicism that allowed expression of the psoriasis earlier in the initially affected area.

ILVEN is differentiated from other epidermal nevi by the presence of erythema and pruritus clinically and by histologic features. Lichen striatus can be distinguished by its histology and natural history. Topical steroids and topical retinoids appear to have limited benefit in ILVEN. Topical vitamin D (calcipotriol and calcitriol) and topical anthralin have been beneficial, however. Surgical modalities include excision, cryotherapy, and pulsed dye laser. In cases of "nevoid," "linear," or "blaschkolinear" psoriasis, acitretin, narrow-band ultraviolet (UV)B and calcipotriene have been beneficial, but etanercept has failed.

Al-Enezi S, et al: Inflammatory linear verrucous epidermal nevus and arthritis: a new association. J Pediatr 2001; 138:602.
Chien P Jr, et al: Linear psoriasis. Dermatol Online J 2009; 15.4.
Ginarte M, et al: Unilateral psoriasis: a case individualized by means of involucrin. Cutis 2000; 65:167.
Hofer T: Does inflammatory linear verrucous epidermal nevus represent a segmental type 1/type 2 mosaic of psoriasis? Dermatology 2006; 212:103.
Khachemoune A, et al: Inflammatory linear verrucous epidermal nevus: a case report and short review of the literature. Cutis 2006; 78:261.
Le K, et al: Vulval and perianal inflammatory linear verrucous epidermal naevus. Australas J Dermatol 2009; 50:115.
Lee SH, Rogers M: Inflammatory linear verrucous epidermal naevi: a review of 23 cases. Australas J Dermatol 2001; 42:252.
Lopez N, et al: Unilateral blaschkolinear psoriasis. Eur J Dermatol 2008; 18:457.
Mazereeuw-Hautier J, et al: Familial inflammatory linear verrucous epidermal naevus in a father and daughter. Australas J Dermatol 2009; 50:115.

Ozdemir M, et al: Acitretin narrow-band TL-01 phototherapy but not etanercept treatment improves a localized inflammatory linear verrucous epidermal naevus with concomitant psoriasis. J Eur Acad Dermatol Venereol 2009 Mar 10 (Epub ahead of print).
Renner R, et al: Acitretin treatment of a systematized inflammatory linear verrucous epidermal naevus. Acta Derm Venereol 2005; 85:348.
Sidwell RU, et al: Pulsed dye laser treatment for inflammatory linear verrucous epidermal naevus. Br J Dermatol 2001; 144:1262.
Sotiriadis D, et al: Is inflammatory linear verrucous epidermal naevus a form of linear naevoid psoriasis? J Eur Acad Dermatol Venereol 2006; 20:483.
Ulkur E, et al: Carbon dioxide laser therapy for an inflammatory linear verrucous epidermal nevus: a case report. Aesthetic Plast Surg 2004; 28:428.

Hyperkeratosis of the nipple and areola

Hyperkeratosis of the nipple and areola (HNA) is an uncommon benign, asymptomatic, acquired condition of unknown pathogenesis. Women represent 80% of cases and it presents in their second or third decade. In men, the time of presentation is variable. Most cases are bilateral, although unilateral cases can occur. In about half the cases, both the areola and nipple are involved. Breastfeeding is usually not affected. Clinically, there is verrucous thickening and brownish discoloration of the nipple and/or areola. Histologically, there is orthokeratotic hyperkeratosis with occasional keratinous cysts in the filiform acanthotic epidermis. The course is chronic. Treatment with cryotherapy, electrosurgical superficial removal of hyperkeratosis, low-dose acitretin, and calcipotriol have benefitted some patients. A similar clinical manifestation has been seen in graft versus host disease (GVHD), malignant acanthosis nigricans, and candidiasis of the nipple associated with mucocutaneous candidiasis. Painful areolar hyperkeratosis may be seen as a complication of sorafenib therapy. It must be distinguished from acanthosis nigricans, nipple eczema with lichenification, and Darier's disease. Isolated papules or small plaques in this location probably represent seborrheic keratoses affecting the nipple or areola. The relationship of HNA and areolar melanosis is unclear; these conditions have significant clinical similarity, except for the absence of hyperkeratosis in those lesions described as areolar melanosis.

Baykal C, et al: Nevoid hyperkeratosis of the nipple and areola: a distinct entity. J Am Acad Dermatol 2002; 46:414.
Bayramgürler D, et al: Nevoid hyperkeratosis of the nipple and areola: treatment of two patients with topical calcipotriol. J Am Acad Dermatol 2002; 46:131.
Frigerio M, et al: Hyperkeratosis of nipple skin during sorafenib treatment. Dig Liver Dis 2009; 41:611.
Kartal Durmazlar SP, et al: Hyperkeratosis of the nipple and areola: 2 years of remission with low-dose acitretin and topical calcipotriol therapy. J Dermatolog Treat 2008; 19:337.
Kavak K, et al: Hyperkeratosis of the nipple and areola in a patient with chronic mucocutaneous candidiasis. J Dermatol 2006; 33:510.
Lee HW et al: Hyperkeratosis of the nipple and areola as a sign of malignant acanthosis nigricans. Clin Exp Dermatol 2005; 30:721.
Lee HW, et al: Hyperkeratosis of the nipple associated with acanthosis nigricans: treatment with topical calcipotriol. J Am Acad Dermatol 2005; 52:529.
Lee HW, et al: Unilateral nevoid hyperkeratosis of the nipple and areola: excellent response to cryotherapy. Dermatol Surg 2005; 31:611.
Mikhail M, et al: Four views of areolar melanosis: clinical appearance, dermoscopy, confocal microscopy, and histopathology. Dermatol Surg 2008; 34:1101.
Ozyazgan I, et al: Treatment of nevoid hyperkeratosis of the nipple and areola using a radiofrequency surgical unit. Dermatol Surg 2005; 31:703.
Sanli H, et al: Hyperkeratosis of the nipple associated with chronic graft versus host disease after allogeneic haematopoietic cell transplantation. Acta Derm Venereol 2003; 83:385.
Sceppa JA, et al: Melanosis of the areola and nipple. J Am Acad Dermatol 2008; 59:S33.

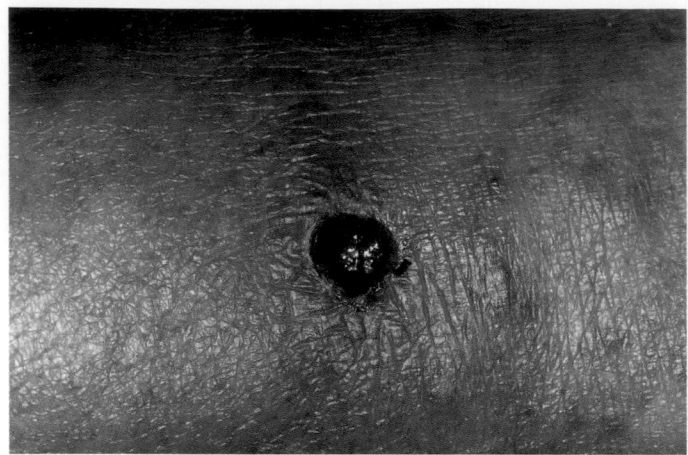

Fig. 29-5 Clear cell acanthoma.

Sengul N, et al: Nevoid hyperkeratosis of the nipple and areola: a diagnosis of exclusion. Breast J 2006; 12:383.

Clear cell acanthoma (pale cell acanthoma)

Clear cell acanthoma is also known as Degos acanthoma. The typical lesion is a circumscribed, reddish, moist nodule with some crusting and peripheral scales (Fig. 29-5); it is usually about 1–2 cm in diameter. A collarette is commonly observed and there may be pigmented variants. Exophytic nodules have been reported. The favorite site is on the shin, calf, or occasionally the thigh, although other sites have been reported, such as the abdomen and scrotum. The lesion is asymptomatic and slow-growing, and can occur in either sex, usually after the age of 40. Solitary lesions are most common, but multiple ones have been described. Rarely, an eruptive form of the disease occurs, producing up to 400 lesions. Squamous cell carcinoma (SCC) arising from clear cell acanthoma has also been reported. Lesions occurring in plaques of psoriasis on the buttocks have been described.

The acanthotic epidermis consists of pale, edematous cells and is sharply demarcated. The basal cell layer is normal. Neutrophils are scattered within the acanthoma and in groups below and within the stratum corneum, a finding similar to the micropustules of psoriasis. The dermal blood vessels are dilated and tortuous, as seen in psoriasis. The clear keratinocytes abound in glycogen, staining positive with periodic acid-Schiff (PAS). Several centers have reported identification of human papillomavirus (HPV) in clear cell acanthomas, making distinction of these lesions from warts difficult.

Clear cell acanthoma must be differentiated from eccrine poroma, which appears most frequently on the hair-free part of the foot, and from clear cell hidradenoma, which occurs most frequently on the head, especially on the face and eyelids. Treatment is surgical, either with cryotherapy or excision.

Finch TM, Tan CY: Clear cell acanthoma developing on a psoriatic plaque: further evidence of an inflammatory aetiology? Br J Dermatol 2000; 142:842.

Garrido-Rios AA, et al: Human papillomavirus detection in multiple large-cell acanthomas. J Eur Acad Dermatol Venereol 2009; 23:454.

Kavanagh GM, et al: Multiple clear cell acanthomas treated by cryotherapy. Australas J Dermatol 1995; 36:33.

Langer K, et al: Pigmented clear cell acanthoma. Am J Dermatol 1994; 16:134.

Murphy R, et al: Giant clear cell acanthoma. Br J Dermatol 2000; 143:1114.

Parsons ME, et al: Squamous cell carcinoma in situ arising within clear cell acanthoma. Dermatol Surg 1997; 23:487.

Tanaka T, et al: Pedunculated clear cell acanthoma. Report of a case with dermoscopic observation. Eur J Dermatol 2009 Nov 4 (Epub ahead of print).

Waxy keratoses of childhood (kerinokeratosis papulosa)

Waxy keratoses of childhood is a genodermatosis that is either sporadic or familial. It may be generalized or segmental. Clinically, the lesions are keratotic, flesh-colored papules, which affect the trunk and extremities. They appear before the age of 3 years. Histologically, there is papillomatosis with focal "church-spire" tenting of the epidermis and marked hyperkeratosis. The natural history of this rare disorder is unknown. Clinically and histologically, the lesions must be distinguished from warts.

Happle R, et al: Kerinokeratosis papulosa with a type 2 segmental manifestation. J Am Acad Dermatol 2004; 50:S84.

Mehrabi D, et al: Waxy keratoses of childhood in a segmental distribution. Pediatr Dermatol 2001; 18:415.

Multiple minute digitate hyperkeratosis

Multiple minute digitate hyperkeratosis (MMDH) is a rare disorder. About half of cases are familial, inherited in an autosomal-dominant fashion, and the other half are sporadic. This condition has also been called digitate keratoses, disseminated spiked hyperkeratosis, minute aggregate keratosis, and familial disseminated piliform hyperkeratosis. Clinically, hundreds of asymptomatic tiny digitate keratotic papules appear on the trunk and proximal extremities. They are not associated with follicular structures. Histologically, each lesion represents a spiked, digitate, or tented area of acanthotic epidermis with overlying orthohyperkeratosis. Similar lesions can be seen after inflammation and radiation therapy. The relationship of the familial/sporadic cases and the postinflammatory condition is unclear. In some adult cases, an underlying malignancy is found.

Pimentel CL, et al: Multiple minute digitate hyperkeratosis. J Eur Acad Dermatol Venerol 2002; 16:422.

Rubegni P, et al: Two sporadic cases of idiopathic multiple minute digitate hyperkeratosis. Clin Exp Dermatol 2001; 26:53.

Takagawa S, et al: Multiple minute digitate hyperkeratoses. Br J Dermatol 2000; 142:1044.

Acantholytic acanthoma, epidermolytic acanthoma, acantholytic dyskeratotic acanthoma

These three conditions represent benign, usually solitary, but at times multiple papules that are nondescript and may be mistaken for basal cell carcinoma (BCC), SCC, or HPV infection. Histological examination shows epidermal hyperplasia with acantholysis resembling pemphigus vulgaris, pemphigus foliaceus, or Hailey–Hailey disease. The condition multiple epidermolytic acanthoma usually occurs in the genital area and histologically resembles Hailey–Hailey disease. This probably represents a localized variant of that condition.

Cho S, et al: Acantholytic acanthoma clinically resembling a molluscum contagiosum. J Eur Acad Dermatol Venereol 2007; 21:119.

Jang BS, et al: Multiple scrotal epidermolytic acanthomas successfully treated with topical imiquimod. J Dermatol 2007 Apr; 34:267.

Ko CJ, et al: Acantholytic dyskeratotic acanthoma: a variant of a benign keratosis. J Cutan Pathol 2008; 35:298.

Kukreja T, Krunic A: Multiple epidermolytic acanthomas must not be confused with genital human papillomavirus infection. Acta Derm Venereol 2009; 89:169.

Omulecki A, et al: Plaque form of warty dyskeratoma—acantholytic dyskeratotic acanthoma. J Cutan Pathol 2007 Jun; 34:494.

Sass U, et al: Acantholytic tumor of the nail: acantholytic dyskeratotic acanthoma. J Cutan Pathol 2009; 36:1308.

Warty dyskeratoma

Warty dyskeratomas are most commonly solitary and found on the head and neck (70%), trunk (20%), or extremities. Rare oral lesions occur. The lesion is a brownish-red papule or nodule with a soft, yellowish, central keratotic plug. Histologically, a cuplike depression filled with a keratotic plug is most common. The epithelium lining the invagination shows the features of Darier's disease, with intraepidermal clefts, acantholytic cells, and pseudovilli. Keratin pearls, corps ronds, and grains may be seen. Cystic lesions with prominent keratinous cysts can occur. Cutaneous lesions appear to originate from a hair follicle. Warty dyskeratoma must be distinguished histologically from keratoacanthoma and acantholytic SCC. Acantholytic acanthoma has a similar histology but dyskeratosis is absent, distinguishing it from warty dyskeratoma. Treatment is surgical.

Kaddu S, et al: Warty dyskeratoma—"follicular dyskeratoma": analysis of clinicopathologic features of a distinctive follicular adnexal neoplasm. J Am Acad Dermatol 2002; 47:423.

Seborrheic keratosis

Seborrheic keratoses are incredibly common and usually multiple. They present as oval, slightly raised, tan/light brown to black, sharply demarcated papules or plaques, rarely more than 3 cm in diameter. They appear "stuck on" the skin, as if they could be removed with the flick of a fingernail (Fig. 29-6). They are located mostly on the chest and back, but also commonly involve the scalp, face, neck, and extremities. An inframammary accumulation is common. Occasionally, genital lesions are seen. The palms and soles are spared; "seborrheic keratoses" in these areas are usually eccrine poromas. The surface of the warty lesions often becomes crumbly, like a crust that is loosely attached. When this is removed, a raw, moist base is revealed. Seborrheic keratoses may be associated with itching. Some patients have hundreds of these lesions on the trunk. While it had been thought that the age of onset is generally in the fourth to fifth decade, in Australia the prevalence of seborrheic keratoses was 20% in males and 25% in females aged 15–25 years. Typical lesions of the trunk are much more common in white persons; however, the "dermatosis papulosa nigra" variant of the central face is common in African Americans and Asians.

The pathogenesis of seborrheic keratoses is unknown. Clinically, they usually originate de novo or appear initially as a lentigo. A sudden eruption of many seborrheic keratoses

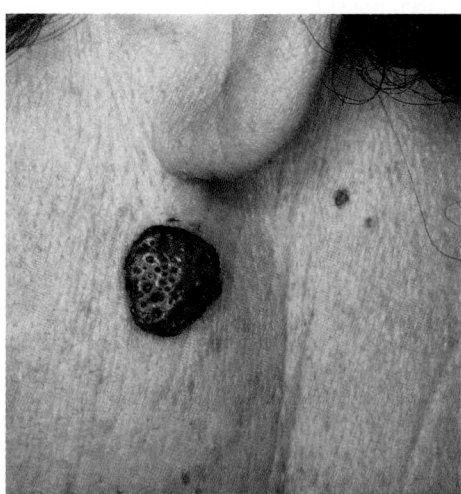

Fig. 29-6 Seborrheic keratosis.

may follow an exfoliative erythroderma, erythrodermic psoriasis, or an erythrodermic drug eruption. These lesions may be transient. Seborrheic keratoses are more common in areas of sun exposure, including favoring the driver's side in truck drivers. In about one-third or more of cases, solar lentigines and seborrheic keratoses both have gain-of-function mutations in *FGFR3* and *PI3K*, the genes mutated in keratinocytic epidermal nevi. This supports the concept that some seborrheic keratoses begin as flat lesions that cannot be distinguished from solar lentigines.

Histologically, most seborrheic keratoses demonstrate acanthosis, varying degrees of papillomatosis, hyperkeratosis, and at times keratin accumulations within the acanthotic epidermis (pseudo-horn cysts). The epidermal cells lack cytologic atypia, except at times in the irritated variant where typical normal mitoses may occur. Six histologic types—hyperkeratotic, acanthotic, adenoid or reticulated, clonal, irritated, and melanoacanthoma—are distinguished. There is a poor correlation between the clinical appearance and the observed histology, unlike for inverted follicular keratosis, dermatosis papulosa nigra, and stucco keratosis, where the histologic features are characteristic and match the clinical lesion. Melanoacanthoma differs from regular seborrheic keratosis by the presence of numerous dendritic melanocytes within the acanthotic epidermis. Oral melanoacanthoma, which has also been called melanoacanthosis, is clinically a reactive pigmented lesion seen primarily in young black patients (see Chapter 34). Many cases of inverted follicular keratosis represent irritated seborrheic keratoses. Granular parakeratotic acanthoma is considered by some to be a variant of irritated seborrheic keratosis, and a separate entity by others.

The differential diagnosis usually poses no problems in most cases, but clinically atypical lesions can be a challenge. The most difficult, especially for the nondermatologist, is to differentiate the solitary black seborrheic keratosis from melanoma. The regularly shaped verrucous lesion is often different from the smooth-surfaced and slightly infiltrating pattern of melanoma. Dermoscopy can at times be of great value; however, at times seborrheic keratoses may demonstrate dermatoscopic features typical of melanocytic lesions, and the presence of horn cysts does not exclude a melanocytic lesion. Actinic keratoses are usually erythematous, more sharply rough, and slightly scaly. The edges are not sharply demarcated, and they occur most often on the face, bald scalp, and backs of the hands. Nevi may be closely simulated. Clonal seborrheic keratoses demonstrate intraepidermal nests suggestive of intraepidermal epithelioma of Jadassohn. Rarely, Bowen's disease, SCC, BCC, trichilemmal carcinoma, or melanoma arises within typical-appearing seborrheic keratosis. Some of these may represent collision lesions, not cancers arising from seborrheic keratoses. It is prudent to biopsy any lesion that appears atypical, since even the most seasoned dermatologist has been humbled by the occasional diagnosis of melanoma in low-suspect lesions.

Seborrheic keratoses are easily removed with liquid nitrogen, curettage, or the combination of the two to avoid the need for local anesthesia to perform the curettage. The spray freezes the lesion to make it brittle enough for easy removal with the curette. Scarring is not produced by this method. Light freezing with liquid nitrogen alone is also effective, as is simple curettage with local anesthesia. Light fulguration and shave removal are other acceptable methods.

Sign of Leser–Trélat

The sudden appearance of numerous seborrheic keratoses in an adult may be the cutaneous finding of internal malignancy. Sixty percent of the neoplasms have been adenocarcinomas, primarily of the gastrointestinal tract. Other common malignancies are lymphoma, breast cancer, and SCC of the lung, but many other types have been reported. To be considered a case of Leser–Trélat, the keratoses should begin at approximately the same time as the development of the cancer, have a rapid onset, and run a parallel course in regard to growth and remission. The lesions are often pruritic, and acanthosis nigricans and tripe palms may accompany the appearance of the seborrheic keratoses of Leser–Trélat.

Barron LA, et al: The sign of Leser–Trélat in a young woman with osteogenic sarcoma. J Am Acad Dermatol 1992; 26:344.

Braun RP, et al: Dermoscopy of pigmented seborrheic keratosis: a morphological study. Arch Dermatol 2002; 138:1556.

Ceylan C, et al: Leser–Trélat. Int J Dermatol 2002; 41:687.

da Costa Franca AF: Acanthosis nigricans, tripe palms and the sign of Leser–Trélat in a patient with a benign hepatic neoplasia. J Eur Acad Dermatol Venereol 2007; 21:846.

da Rosa AC, et al: Three simultaneous paraneoplastic manifestations (ichthyosis acquisita, Bazex syndrome, and Leser–Trélat sign) with prostate adenocarcinoma. J Am Acad Dermatol 2009; 61:538.

Dasanu CA, Alexandrescu DT: Bilateral Leser–Trélat sign mirroring lung adenocarcinoma with early metastases to the contralateral lung. South Med J 2009; 102:216.

Dunwell P, Rose A: Study of the skin disease spectrum occurring in an Afro-Caribbean population. Int J Dermatol 2003; 42:287.

Flugman SL, et al: Transient eruptive seborrheic keratoses associated with erythrodermic psoriasis and erythrodermic drug eruption: report of two cases. J Am Acad Dermatol 2001; 45:S212.

Gill D, et al: The prevalence of seborrheic keratoses in people aged 15 to 30 years. Arch Dermatol 2000; 136:759.

Hafner C, et al: *FGFR3* and *PIK3CA* mutations are involved in the molecular pathogenesis of solar lentigo. Br J Dermatol 2009; 160:546.

Hirata SH, et al: "Globulelike" dermoscopic structures in pigmented seborrheic keratosis. Arch Dermatol 2004; 140:128.

Hsu C, et al: Sign of Leser–Trélat in a heart transplant recipient. Br J Dermatol 2005; 153:861.

Kavak A, et al: Preliminary study among truck drivers in Turkey: effects of ultraviolet light on some skin entities. J Dermatol 2008; 35:146.

Kilickap S, Yalcin B: Images in clinical medicine. The sign of Leser–Trélat. N Engl J Med 2007; 356:2184.

Kluger N, Guillot B: Sign of Leser–Trélat with an adenocarcinoma of the prostate: a case report. Cases J 2009; 2:8868.

Kocyigit P, et al: Post-renal transplantation Leser–Trélat sign associated with carcinoma of the gallbladder: a rare association. Scand J Gastroenterol 2007; 42:779.

Kwon OS, et al: Seborrheic keratosis in the Korean males: causative role of sunlight. Photodermatol Photoimmunol Photomed 2003; 19:73.

Li M, et al: The Leser–Trélat sign is associated with nasopharyngeal carcinoma: case report and review of cases reported in China. Clin Exp Dermatol 2009; 34:52.

Moore RL, Devere TS: Epidermal manifestations of internal malignancy. Dermatol Clin 2008; 26:17.

Nanda A, et al: Sign of Leser–Trélat in newly diagnosed advanced gastric adenocarcinoma. J Clin Oncol 2008; 26:4992.

Oyama N, Kaneko F: Trichilemmal carcinoma arising in seborrheic keratosis: a case report and published work review. J Dermatol 2008; 35:782.

Pentenero M, et al: Oral acanthosis nigricans, tripe palms and sign of Leser–Trélat in a patient with gastric adenocarcinoma. Int J Dermatol 2004; 43:530.

Resnik KS: Granular parakeratotic acanthoma is not adenoid seborrheic keratosis. Am J Dermatopathol 2005; 27:393.

Rubegni P, et al: False Leser–Trélat sign. Int J Dermatol 2009; 48:912.

Scully C, et al: Oral acanthosis nigricans, the sign of Leser–Trélat and cholangiocarcinoma. Br J Dermatol 2001; 145:506.

Shamsadini S, et al: Surrounding ipsilateral eruptive seborrheic keratosis as a warning sign of intraductal breast carcinoma and Paget's disease (Leser–Trélat sign). Dermatol Online 2006; 12:27.

Tomich CE, et al: Melanoacanthosis (melanoacanthoma) of the oral mucosa. J Dermatol Surg Oncol 1990; 16:231.

Wieland CN, Kumar N: Sign of Leser–Trélat. Int J Dermatol 2008; 47:643.

Zabel RJ, et al: Malignant melanoma arising in a seborrheic keratosis. J Am Acad Dermatol 2000; 42:831.

Dermatosis papulosa nigra

Dermatosis papulosa nigra occurs in about 35% of black persons and is also relatively common in Asians. It usually begins in adolescence, appearing first as minute, round, skin-colored or hyperpigmented macules or papules that develop singly or in sparse numbers on the malar regions or on the cheeks below the eyes. It has been described in patients as young as age 3. The lesions increase in number and size over time, so that over the course of years the patient may have hundreds of lesions. They are distributed over the periorbital regions initially, but may occur on the rest of the face, neck, and upper chest. Lesions do not spontaneously resolve. They closely simulate seborrheic keratoses. They are asymptomatic and do not develop scaling, crusting, or ulceration.

Microscopically, the chief alterations are in the epidermis. Irregular acanthosis, papillomatosis, and deposits of uncommonly large amounts of pigment throughout the rete, and particularly in the basal layer, are characteristic. Many believe this to be a form of seborrheic keratosis. This concept is supported by the finding of *FGFR3* mutations in the lesions of dermatosis papulosis nigra, similar to those found in seborrheic keratoses.

Treatment is made difficult by the tendency for the development of dyspigmentation. Light curettage with or without anesthesia; light, superficial liquid nitrogen application; and light electrodesiccation are effective, but may result in hyper- or hypopigmentation. KTP and Nd:YAG laser have been reported as effective, but not superior to simple electrodesiccation. Aggressive treatment should be avoided to minimize dyspigmentation and scarring.

Stucco keratosis

Stucco keratoses have been described as "stuck on" lesions occurring on the lower legs, especially in the vicinity of the Achilles tendon. They are also seen on the dorsa of the feet (Fig. 29-7), forearms, and dorsal hands. The palms, soles, trunk, and head are never affected. Varying in diameter from 1 to 5 mm, the lesions are loosely attached, so that they can easily be scratched off. They vary in number from a few to more than 50. Stucco keratoses are common in the US and Australia. They occur mostly in men over 40 years old. Histologically, the picture is that of a hyperkeratotic type of seborrheic keratosis, with no hypergranulosis and no wart particles seen by electron microscopy. The presence of *PIK3CA* mutations in stucco keratoses suggests they are a variant of seborrheic keratosis. The treatment, if any is required, consists of emollients, which soften the skin and cause the scaly lesions

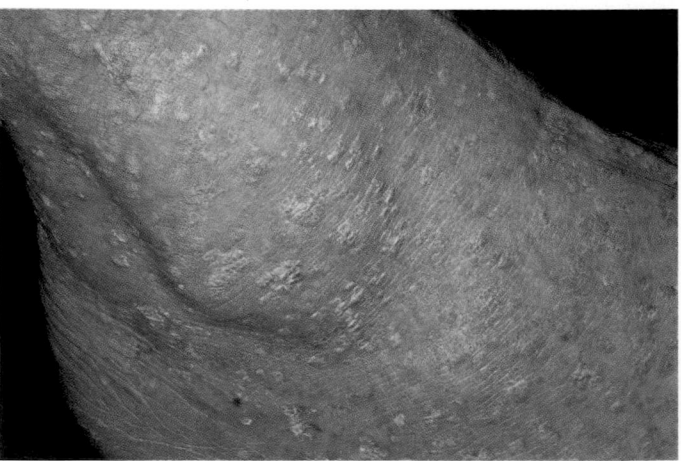

Fig. 29-7 Stucco keratosis.

to fall off. Ammonium lactate lotion, 12%, may be effective in improving the appearance of the lesions. Stucco keratoses must be distinguished from Flegel's disease.

Babapour R, et al: Dermatosis papulosa nigra in a young child. Pediatr Dermatol 1993; 10:356.

Hafner C, et al: *FGFR3* and *PIK3CA* mutations in stucco keratosis and dermatosis papulosa nigra. Br J Dermatol 2009 Sep 1 (Epub ahead of print).

Katz TM, et al: Dermatosis papulosa nigra treatment with fractional photothermolysis. Dermatol Surg 2009; 35:1840.

Kundu RV, et al: Comparison of electrodesiccation and potassium-titanyl-phosphate laser for treatment of dermatosis papulosa nigra. Dermatol Surg 2009; 35:1079.

Niang SO, et al: Dermatosis papulosa nigra in Dakar, Senegal. Int J Dermatol 2007; 46:45.

Schwartzberg JB, et al: Eruptive dermatosis papulosa nigra as a possible sign of internal malignancy. Int J Dermatol 2007; 46:186.

Schweiger ES, et al: Treatment of dermatosis papulosa nigra with a 1064 nm ND:YAG laser; report of two cases. J Cosmet Laser Ther 2008; 10:120.

Hyperkeratosis lenticularis perstans (Flegel's disease)

Rough, yellow–brown keratotic, flat-topped papules, 2–5 mm in diameter and found primarily on the dorsal feet and lower legs, are characteristic. The palms, soles, and oral mucosa may rarely be involved. Familial cases have been reported.

The histologic findings are distinctive, with hyperkeratosis and parakeratosis overlying a thinned epidermis, and irregular acanthosis at the periphery. A bandlike inflammatory infiltrate occurs in the papillary dermis. Topical emollients, topical keratolytics, topical steroids, zinc bandages, topical 5-FU, and PUVA have been reported as useful. Oral retinoids may cause improvement, but are hard to justify in this chronic asymptomatic condition. Both benefit and failure with topical vitamin D analogs have been reported. The lesions do not recur after shallow shave excision.

Ando K, et al: Histopathological differences between early and old lesions of hyperkeratosis lenticularis perstans (Flegel's disease). Am J Dermatopathol 2006; 28:122.

Bayramgurler D, et al: Flegel's disease: treatment with topical calcipotriol. Clin Exp Dermatol 2002; 27:161.

Blaheta HJ, et al: Hyperkeratosis lenticularis perstans (Flegel's disease)—lack of response to treatment with tacalcitol and calcipotriol. Dermatology 2001; 202:255.

Cooper SM, George S: Flegel's disease treated with psoralen ultraviolet A. Br J Dermatol 2000; 142:340.

Jang KA, et al: Hyperkeratosis lenticularis perstans (Flegel's disease): histologic, immunohistochemical, and ultrastructural features in a case. Am J Dermatopathol 1999; 21:395.

Lindsay E: Zinc paste bandages and the treatment of Flegel's disease. Br J Community Nurs 2005; 10:S14.

Miranda-Romero A, et al: Unilateral hyperkeratosis lenticularis perstans (Flegel's disease). J Am Acad Dermatol 1998; 39:655.

Sterneberg-Vos H, et al: Hyperkeratosis lenticularis perstans (Flegel's disease)—successful treatment with topical corticosteroids. Int J Dermatol 2008; 47:38.

Benign lichenoid keratoses (lichen planus-like keratosis)

Benign lichenoid keratoses are usually solitary, dusky-red to violaceous, papular lesions up to 1 cm in diameter, but are at times larger (Fig. 29-8). They occur most often on the distal forearms, hands, or chest of middle-aged white women. The lesions are commonly biopsied, since the clinical features are identical to those of a superficial BCC. A slight violaceous hue or the presence of an adjacent solar lentigo can raise the suspicion of lichen planus-like keratosis. Multiple lesions may simulate a photodermatitis, such as lupus erythematosus.

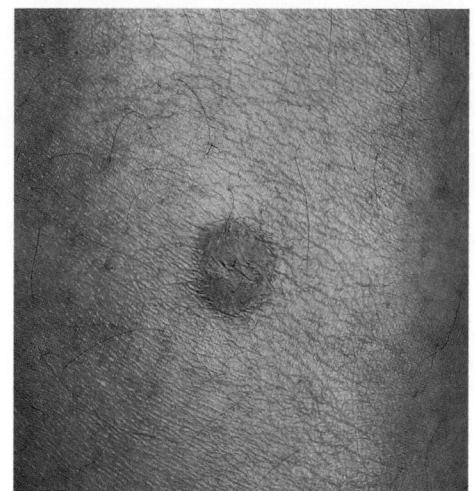

Fig. 29-8 Lichen planus-like keratosis.

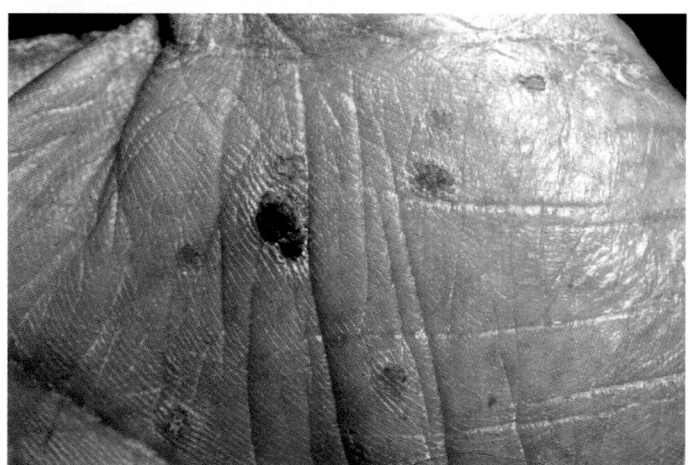

Fig. 29-9 Arsenical keratosis of the palm.

Evolution from pre-existing solar lentigines is often noted histologically or by history.

Histologically, the lesion may be indistinguishable from idiopathic lichen planus. While idiopathic lichen planus rarely demonstrates parakeratosis, plasma cells, or eosinophils, these may be present in lichen planus-like keratosis. The remnants of a solar lentigo may be seen at the periphery. These features, plus the clinical information that this represents a solitary lesion, suggest the correct diagnosis. Clinical correlation is essential, as similar histologic findings may be seen in lichenoid drug eruptions, acral lupus erythematosus, and lichenoid regression of melanoma. Direct immunofluorescence is positive, with clumped deposits of IgM in a lichen planus-like pattern at the dermoepidermal junction. This differs from the continuous granular immunoglobulin deposition of acral lupus erythematosus. Cryotherapy with liquid nitrogen is effective.

Jang K, et al: Lichenoid keratosis: a clinicopathologic study of 17 patients. J Am Acad Dermatol 2000; 43:511.

Ramesh V, et al: Benign lichenoid keratosis due to constant pressure. Australas J Dermatol 1998; 39:177.

Arsenical keratoses

Arsenical keratoses are keratotic, pointed, 2–4 mm wartlike lesions on the palms, soles, and sometimes ears of persons who have a history of drinking contaminated well water or taking medications containing arsenic trioxide, usually for asthma (Fowler's solution, Bell's Asthma Mixture), atopic dermatitis, or psoriasis, often years previously (Fig. 29-9). These lesions resemble palmar pits, but may have a central hyperkeratosis. When the keratosis is picked off with the fingernails, a small dell-like depression is seen.

Bowen's disease and invasive arsenical SCC may be present, with the latent period being 10 and 20 years, respectively. The profound increase in Bowen's disease and SCC appears to be characteristic of patients with arsenic exposure from well water. In patients exposed to arsenic via elixirs, BCCs are more characteristically seen. The latency period for development of BCC is also 20 years. Lesions are most common on the scalp and trunk.

Boonchai W, et al: Basal cell carcinoma in chronic arsenicism occurring in Queensland, Australia, after ingestion of an asthma medication. J Am Acad Dermatol 2000; 43:664.

Boonchai W, et al: Expression of p53 in arsenic-related and sporadic basal cell carcinoma. Arch Dermatol 2000; 136:195.

Col M, et al: Arsenic-related Bowen's disease, palmar keratosis, and skin cancer. Environ Health Perspect 1999; 107:687.

Elmariah SB, et al: Invasive squamous-cell carcinoma and arsenical keratoses. Dermatol Online J 2008; 14:24.

Khandpur S, et al: Chronic arsenic toxicity from Ayurvedic medicines. Int J Dermatol 2008; 47:618.

Lien H, et al: Merkel cell carcinoma and chronic arsenicism. J Am Acad Dermatol 1999; 41:641.

Son SB, et al: Successful treatment of palmoplantar arsenical keratosis with a combination of keratolytics and low-dose acitretin. Clin Exp Dermatol 2008; 33:202.

Wong SS, et al: Cutaneous manifestations of chronic arsenicism: review of seventeen cases. J Am Acad Dermatol 1998; 38:179.

Nonmelanoma skin cancers and their precursors

Nonmelanoma skin cancers (NMSCs) are the most common form of cancer diagnosed in the US, with more than 1.3 million cases diagnosed annually. One in 2 men and 1 in 3 women in the US will develop NMSC in their lifetime, usually after the age of 55. While these result in only about 2000–2500 deaths annually, due to their sheer numbers NMSCs represent about 5% of all Medicare cancer expenditures. Those at risk for skin cancer are fair-skinned individuals who tan poorly and who have had significant chronic or intermittent sun exposure. Red hair phenotype with loss-of-function mutations in the melanocortin-1 receptor may be a risk factor as well. Additional risk factors include a prior history of skin cancer, prior radiation therapy, PUVA treatment, arsenic exposure, and systemic immunosuppression (Fig. 29-10). Once an individual has developed an NMSC, his/her risk for a second is increased 10-fold. Over the 3-year period following the initial NMSC diagnosis, more than 40% of BCC and SCC patients develop a BCC, and 18% of SCC patients develop another SCC. By 5 years, as many as 50% of women and 70% of men will develop a second NMSC. The rate of developing NMSCs is no different 3 years or 10 years after the initial NMSC diagnosis. Patients with a history of NMSC should be examined for NMSCs on a regular basis.

Ultraviolet radiation (UVR) is the major cause of nongenital NMSCs and actinic keratoses. The effect of UVR appears to be mediated through mutation of the *p53* gene, which is found mutated in a substantial percentage of NMSCs and actinic keratoses. Most skin cancers are highly immunogenic, but the immune response is suppressed by continued actinic exposure. Both chronic sun exposure and intermittent intense exposure are risk factors for the development of NMSCs. It is believed that avoiding sun exposure reduces the risk for NMSC. The use of sunscreens in the prevention of NMSCs has been controversial, as they may inadvertently lead to prolonged intentional sun exposure, negating their possible beneficial effect. None the less, dermatologists and their societies recommend a program of sunscreen use together with sun

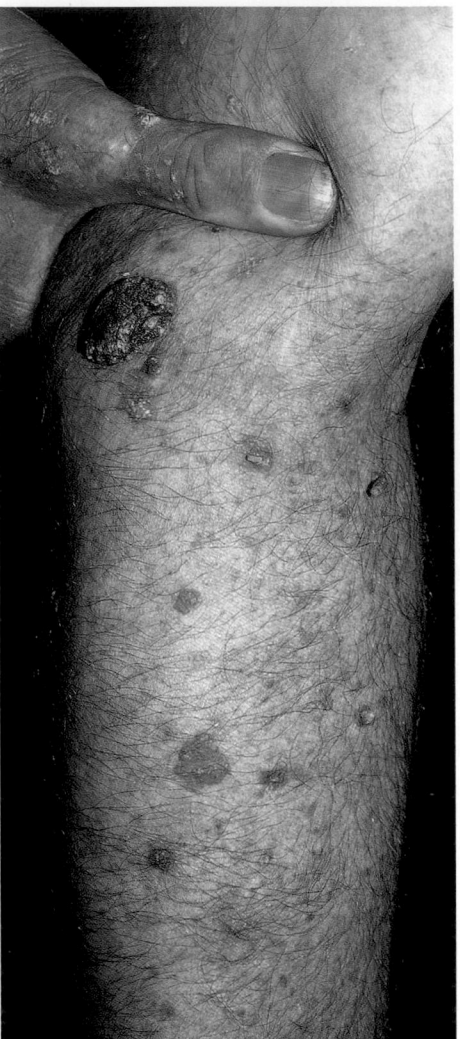

Fig. 29-10 Actinic keratosis/Bowen's disease in a transplant recipient.

avoidance to patients at risk for skin cancer. This includes avoiding midday sun, seeking shade, wearing protective clothing, and regularly applying a sunblock of sun protection factor (SPF) 15–30 with both UVB and UVA coverage. This program, which was pioneered in Australia, has led to improvements in some skin cancer rates in that country.

Chuang T, Brashear R: Risk factors of non-melanoma skin cancer in United States veteran patients: a pilot study and review of literature. J Eur Acad Dermatol Venereol 1999; 12:126.

Czarnecki C, Czarnecki D: Patients who have multiple skin cancers develop new skin cancers at a constant rate. Arch Dermatol 2002; 138:125.

Diepgen TL, Mahler V: The epidemiology of skin cancer. Br J Dermatol 2002; 146:1.

Higashi MK, et al: Health economic evaluation of non-melanoma skin cancer and actinic keratosis. Pharmacoeconomics 2004; 22:83.

Housman TS, et al: Skin cancer is among the most costly of all cancers to treat for the Medicare population. J Am Acad Dermatol 2003; 48:425.

Leffell D: The scientific basis of skin cancer. J Am Acad Dermatol 2000; 42:S18.

Lewis KG, Weinstock MA: Nonmelanoma skin cancer mortality (1988–2000). Arch Dermatol 2004; 140:837.

Lichter MD, et al: Therapeutic ionizing radiation and the incidence of basal cell carcinoma and squamous cell carcinoma. Arch Dermatol 2000; 136:1007.

Marcil I, Stern RS: Risk of developing a subsequent nonmelanoma skin cancer in patients with a history of nonmelanoma skin cancer. Arch Dermatol 2000; 136:1524.

MMWR: Preventing skin cancer: findings of the task force on community preventive services on reducing exposure to ultraviolet light. Arch Dermatol 2004; 140:251.

Schaffer JV, Bolognia JL: The melanocortin-1 receptor: red hair and beyond. Arch Dermatol 2001; 137:1477.

Veien K, Veien NK: Risk of developing subsequent nonmelanoma skin cancers. Arch Dermatol 2001; 137:1251.

Actinic keratosis (solar keratosis)

Actinic keratoses represent in situ dysplasias resulting from sun exposure. They are found chiefly on the chronically sun-exposed surfaces of the face (Fig. 29-11), ears, balding scalp, dorsal hands, and forearms. They are usually multiple, discrete, flat or elevated, verrucous or keratotic, red, pigmented, or skin-colored. Usually, the surface is covered by an adherent scale, but sometimes it is smooth and shiny. On palpation the surface is rough, like sandpaper, and at times lesions are more easily felt than seen. The patient may complain of tenderness when the lesion is rubbed or shaved over with a razor. The lesions are usually relatively small, measuring 3 mm to 1 cm in diameter, most being less than 6 mm. Rarely, lesions may reach 2 cm in size, but a lesion larger than 6 mm should only be considered an actinic keratosis if this is confirmed by biopsy or if it completely resolves with therapy. The hypertrophic type, which may lead to cutaneous horn formation, is most frequently present on the dorsal forearms and hands.

Actinic keratoses are the most common epithelial precancerous lesions. While lesions typically appear in persons over 50 years of age, actinic keratoses may occur in the twenties or thirties in patients who live in areas of high solar irradiation and are fair-skinned. Patients with actinic keratoses have a propensity for the development of nonmelanoma cutaneous malignancies. Actinic keratoses can be prevented by the regular application of sunscreen and by a diet low in fats. Beta-carotene is of no benefit in preventing actinic keratoses.

Six types of actinic keratosis can be recognized histologically: hypertrophic, atrophic, bowenoid, acantholytic, pigmented, and lichenoid. The epidermis may be acanthotic or atrophic. Keratinocyte maturation may be disordered, with overlying parakeratosis sometimes present. The basal cells are most frequently dysplastic, although in more advanced lesions dysplasia may be seen throughout the epidermis, simulating Bowen's disease (bowenoid actinic keratosis).

The clinical diagnosis of actinic keratosis is usually straightforward. Early lesions of chronic cutaneous lupus erythematosus, erosive and pustular dermatosis of the scalp, and pemphigus foliaceus are sometimes confused with actinic keratoses. Seborrheic keratoses, even when they lack pigmentation, are usually more "stuck on" in appearance and more sharply marginated than actinic keratoses. Dermoscopy may aid in this distinction. It is difficult to distinguish hypertrophic actinic keratoses from early SCC, and a low threshold for biopsy is recommended. Similarly, actinic keratoses, which present as red patches, cannot easily be distinguished from Bowen's disease or superficial BCC. If there is a palpable dermal component, or if on stretching the lesion there is a pearly quality, a biopsy should be considered. Any lesion larger than 6 mm, and any lesion that has failed to resolve with appropriate therapy for actinic keratosis should also be carefully evaluated for biopsy.

Since some percentage of actinic keratoses will progress to NMSC, their treatment is indicated. There are many effective therapeutic modalities. Cryotherapy with liquid nitrogen is most effective and practical when there are a limited number of lesions. A bulky cotton applicator dipped into liquid nitrogen or a handheld nitrogen spray device can be used. If the cotton-tip applicator method is used, the liquid nitrogen into which the applicator is dipped should be used for only one patient, as there is theoretical risk of cross-contamination from one patient to another. Infectious agents are not killed by freezing. For this reason, many dermatologists now use the spray devices. We recommend using a small opening tip with continuous bursts of nitrogen spray in a circular motion, depending on the size of the lesion, attempting an even frosting. Only the lesion should be frosted and the duration of cryotherapy must be carefully controlled. A long freeze that results in significant epidermal–dermal injury produces white scars, which are easily seen on the fair skin of those at risk for actinic keratoses. When correctly performed, healing usually occurs within a week on the face, but may require up to 4 weeks on the arms and legs. Caution should be exercised when treating below the knee, since wound healing in these regions is particularly poor and a chronic ulcer can result. Also, use caution in persons at risk for having a cryoprotein (hepatitis C virus-infected patients, and patients with connective tissue disease or lymphoid neoplasia). They may have an excessive reaction to cryotherapy. It is better on the first visit to "under-treat" until the tolerance of a patient's skin to cryotherapy is known. Application of 0.5% 5-FU for 1 week prior to cryotherapy improves the response to cryotherapy.

For extensive, broad, or numerous lesions, topical chemotherapy is recommended. Any lesion that potentially might represent an NMSC should be biopsied prior to beginning topical chemotherapy for actinic keratoses. Self-treatment with 5-FU without a doctor's supervision should be discouraged. The diagnosis of NMSC may be delayed by ineffective topical chemotherapy. The two agents most commonly used are 5-FU cream, 0.5–5%, or imiquimod 5% cream. Topical tretinoin and adapalene do not have the efficacy of these two agents, but can be used for prolonged periods and represent an option for patients with a few early lesions. Three percent diclofenac in 2.5% hyaluronan gel can also be effective when used for 60 days for actinic keratoses. Topical resiquimod and ingenol mebutate are less frequently used topical therapeutic options.

The frequency and duration of treatment are determined by the individual's reaction and the anatomic site of application. 5-FU is applied once a day in most cases. For the face, 0.5% 5-FU tends to give a predictable response, which is a bit less severe than that produced by the 1–5% concentrations. Some patients prefer the stronger concentration for a briefer period, while others favor a slower onset of the reaction and a more prolonged course. For the 5% cream, treatment duration rarely needs to exceed 2–3 weeks. For the 0.5% cream, the treatment course is usually 3–6 weeks. Usually, the central face will respond more briskly than the temples and forehead, which

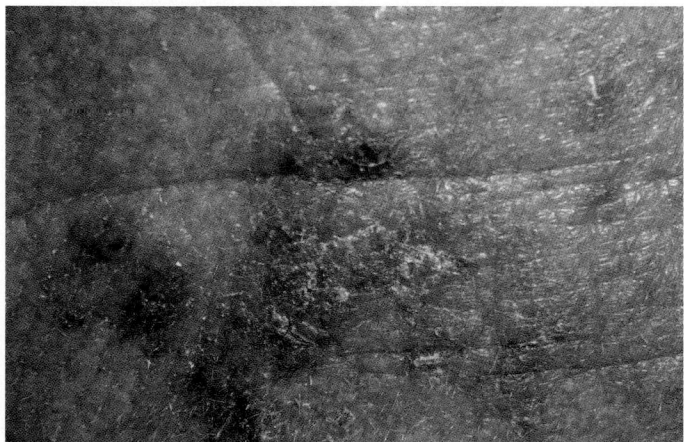

Fig. 29-11 Actinic keratosis.

may require a longer duration of treatment. If the reaction is brisk, the treatment can be stopped and restarted at a lower concentration. Depending on the individual's sensitivity, an erythematous burning reaction will occur within several days. Treatment is stopped when a peak response occurs, characterized by a change in color from bright to dusky-red, by re-epithelialization, and by crust formation. Healing usually occurs within another 2 weeks of stopping treatment, depending on the treatment site. Certain areas of the face are prone to intense irritant dermatitis when exposed to 5-FU and tolerance can be improved if the patient avoids application to the glabella, melolabial folds, and chin. For the scalp, the 0.5% concentration may be adequate, but often prolonged or multiple treatment courses are required if this low concentration is used. The 5% cream produces a more predictable, albeit brisk, reaction. A thick cutaneous horn can prevent penetration of 5-FU, and hypertrophic actinic keratoses on the scalp, dorsal hand, and forearm may respond poorly unless the area is pretreated with an agent to remove excessive keratin overlying the lesions. Pretreatment with tretinoin for 2–3 weeks can improve efficacy and shorten the duration of subsequent 5-FU treatment. It has been observed that 5-FU "seeks out" lesions that may not be clinically apparent. The use of topical 5-FU to the face can also reverse photoaging. Clinically inapparent BCCs may be detected during or on completion of the treatment. Rarely, patients who have had multiple courses of 5-FU topical chemotherapy will develop a true allergic contact dermatitis to the 5-FU. This is manifested by the redness, edema, or vesiculation extending beyond the area of application and by the patient developing pruritus rather than tenderness on the treated areas. Patch testing can be confirmatory.

Imiquimod is an interferon (IFN) inducer and apparently eradicates actinic keratoses by producing a local immunologic reaction against the lesion. The ideal protocol for application of imiquimod may not yet be determined. About 80% of patients respond to imiquimod and 20% may not respond at all, perhaps due to the fact that they lack some genetic component required to induce an inflammatory cascade when imiquimod is applied. If it is applied three times a week, patients develop an inflammatory reaction similar to that seen with daily application of 5-FU. The severity of the reaction is somewhat unpredictable, with a small subset of patients (especially fair-skinned women) developing a severe burning and crusting reaction after only one or a few applications. In others, no reaction at all occurs. With twice a week application, the treatment course is prolonged, up to 16 weeks. Severe erythema occurs in 17.7% and scabbing/crusting in 8.4% of patients so treated. The median percentage reduction in actinic keratoses is 83.3% with this treatment protocol. However, only 7% of patients treating actinic keratoses on the arms and hands with imiquimod three times per week achieved complete clearance. Applying it more frequently led to increased toxicity. Overall, while the reaction is less predictable with imiquimod, it is also typically less severe than with high concentrations of 5-FU. The adverse event rates are similar to those with low-concentration (0.5%) 5-FU. Another regimen is to apply imiquimod for long periods at a reduced frequency (once or twice a week). Applications can be in alternating 1-month cycles or continuous for many months. This may allow management of some patients who require treatment but cannot tolerate any significant changes in appearance. In the end, the choice between topical 5-FU and imiquimod will be based on patient preference, prior physician and patient experience with the modalities, and the cost of the medication. Imiquimod is significantly more expensive per gram than any form of 5-FU. A paired comparative trial would be of great value in determining the optimal and most cost-effective strategy for the treatment of extensive actinic keratoses. Surgical management of actinic keratoses with chemical peels, laser resurfacing, and photodynamic therapy is discussed in Chapters 37 and 38.

Anderson L, et al: Randomized, double-blind, double-dummy, vehicle-controlled study of ingenol mebutate gel 0.025% and 0.05% for actinic keratosis. J Am Acad Dermatol 2009; 60:934.

Askew DA, et al: Effectiveness of 5-fluorouracil treatment for actinic keratosis—a systematic review of randomized controlled trials. Int J Dermatol 2009; 48:453.

Bagatin E, et al: 5-fluorouracil superficial peel for multiple actinic keratoses. Int J Dermatol 2009; 48:902.

Fernandez-Vozmediano J, et al: Infiltrative squamous cell carcinoma of the scalp after treatment with 5% imiquimod cream. J Am Acad Dermatol 2005; 152:716.

Gebauer K, et al: Effect of dosing frequency on the safety and efficacy of imiquimod 5% cream for treatment of actinic keratosis on the forearms and hands: a phase II, randomized placebo-controlled trial. Br J Dermatol 2009; 161:897.

Hughes MC, et al: Food intake, dietary patterns, and actinic keratoses of the skin: a longitudinal study. Am J Clin Nutr 2009; 89:1246.

Jorizzo J, et al: Effect of a 1-week treatment with 0.5% topical fluorouracil on occurrence of actinic keratosis after cryosurgery. Arch Dermatol 2004; 140:813.

Kaminaka C, et al: Phenol peels as a novel therapeutic approach for actinic keratosis and Bowen disease: prospective pilot trial with assessment of clinical, histologic, and immunohistochemical correlations. J Am Acad Dermatol 2009; 60:615.

Korman N, et al: Dosing with 5% imiquimod cream 3 times per week for the treatment of actinic keratosis. Arch Dermatol 2005; 141:467.

Kose O, et al: Comparison of the efficacy and tolerability of 3% diclofenac sodium gel and 5% imiquimod cream in the treatment of actinic keratosis. J Dermatolog Treat 2008; 19:159.

Lebwohl M, et al: Imiquimod 5% cream for the treatment of actinic keratosis: results from two phase III, randomized, double-blind, parallel group, vehicle-controlled trials. J Am Acad Dermatol 2004; 50:714.

Mastrolonardo M: Topical diclofenac 3% gel plus cryotherapy for treatment of multiple and recurrent actinic keratoses. Clin Exp Dermatol 2009; 34:33.

Park MY, et al: Photorejuvenation induced by 5-aminolevulinic acid photodynamic therapy in patients with actinic keratosis: a histologic analysis. J Am Acad Dermatol 2010; 62:85.

Sachs DL, et al: Topical fluorouracil for actinic keratoses and photoaging: a clinical and molecular analysis. Arch Dermatol 2009; 145:659.

Salasche SJ, et al: Cycle therapy of actinic keratoses of the face and scalp with 5% topical imiquimod cream: an open-label trial. J Am Acad Dermatol 2002; 47:571.

Siller G, et al: PEP005 (ingenol mebutate) gel, a novel agent for the treatment of actinic keratosis: results of a randomized, double-blind, vehicle-controlled, multicentre, phase IIa study. Australas J Dermatol 2009; 50:16.

Sotiriou E, et al: Intraindividual, right-left comparison of topical 5-aminolevulinic acid photodynamic therapy vs. 5% imiquimod cream for actinic keratoses on the upper extremities. J Eur Acad Dermatol Venereol 2009; 23:1061.

Stockfleth E, et al: Development of a treatment algorithm for actinic keratoses: a European consensus. Eur J Dermatol 2008; 18:651.

Szeimies RM, et al: A phase II dose-ranging study of topical resiquimod to treat actinic keratosis. Br J Dermatol 2008; 159:205.

Szeimies RM, et al: Long-term follow-up of photodynamic therapy with a self-adhesive 5-aminolaevulinic acid patch: 12 months data. Br J Dermatol 2009 June 30 (Epub ahead of print).

Unis ME: Short-term intensive 5-fluorouracil treatment of actinic keratoses. Dermatol Surg 1995; 21:121.

Vaccaro M, et al: Erosive pustular dermatosis of the scalp following treatment with topical imiquimod for actinic keratosis. Arch Dermatol 2009; 145:1340.

Weinstock MA, et al: Quality of life in the actinic neoplasia syndrome: the VA Topical Tretinoin Chemoprevention (VATTC) Trial. J Am Acad Dermatol 2009; 61:207.

Yentzer B, et al: Adherence to a topical regimen of 5-fluorouracil, 0.5% cream for the treatment of actinic keratoses. Arch Dermatol 2009; 145:203.

Zeichner JA, et al: Placebo-controlled, double-blind, randomized pilot study of imiquimod 5% cream applied once per week for 6 months for the treatment of actinic keratoses. J Am Acad Dermatol 2009; 60:59.

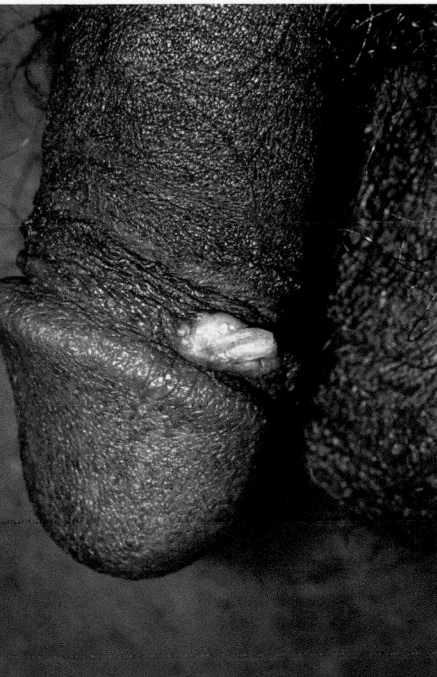

Fig. 29-12 Cutaneous horn of the palm overlying a human papillomavirus-positive squamous cell carcinoma.

Cutaneous horn (cornu cutaneum)

Cutaneous horns are encountered most frequently on the dorsal hands and scalp. Lesions may also occur on the hands, penis (Fig. 29-12), and eyelids. They are skin-colored, horny excrescences, 2–60 mm long, sometimes divided into several antler-like projections.

These lesions are most often benign, with the hyperkeratosis being superimposed on an underlying seborrheic keratosis, verruca vulgaris, angiokeratoma, molluscum contagiosum, or trichilemmoma about 60% of the time. However, 20–30% may overlie premalignant keratoses and 20% may overlie SCCs or BCCs. The risk for a cutaneous horn overlying a malignancy is much higher in elderly fair-complexioned persons. Hyperkeratotic actinic plaques less than 1 cm in diameter on the dorsum of the hand, wrist, or forearms in white patients have been shown to have a malignancy rate of 50%. One-third of penile horns are associated with underlying malignancies. Excisional biopsy with histologic examination of the base is necessary to determine the best therapy, which would be dictated by the diagnosis of the underlying lesion and by the apparent adequacy of removal.

Copcu E, et al: Cutaneous horns: are these lesions as innocent as they seem to be? World J Surg Oncol 2004; 2:18.
Solivan GA, et al: Cutaneous horn of the penis: its association with squamous cell carcinoma and HPV-16 infection. J Am Acad Dermatol 1990; 23:269.
Yu RC, et al: A histopathological study of 643 cutaneous horns. Br J Dermatol 1991; 124:449.

Keratoacanthoma

Clinical features

There are four types of keratoacanthoma: solitary, multiple, eruptive, and keratoacanthoma centrifugum marginatum. The exact biologic behavior of keratoacanthoma remains controversial. In the past it had been considered a reactive condition or pseudomalignancy, which could be treated expectantly. Now the favored view is that keratoacanthomas are low-grade

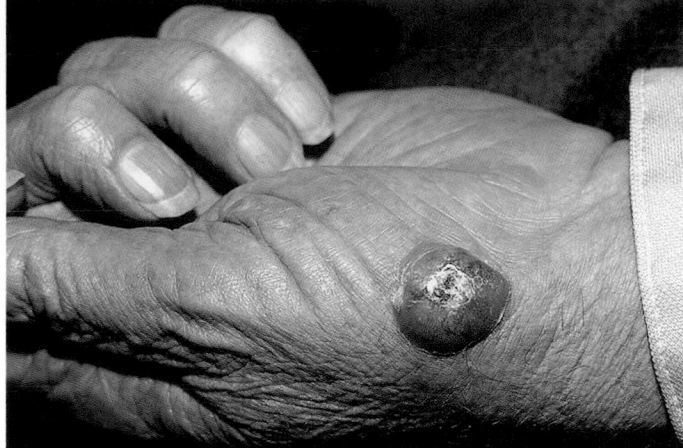

Fig. 29-13 Keratoacanthoma.

squamous cell carcinomas, which in many cases will regress. The regression may be partially mediated by immunity, but takes the form of terminal differentiation. The course of these tumors is unpredictable. Even those that ultimately involute can cause considerable destruction before they regress. Any lesions with the histologic features of keratoacanthoma and which appear in an immunosuppressed host should be managed as an SCC, with complete eradication.

Sunlight appears to play an important role in the etiology, especially in the solitary types, with light-skinned persons being predominately affected. Instances of keratoacanthomas following trauma, hypertrophic lichen planus, discoid lupus erythematosus, tattoos, fractional thermolysis, and imiquimod erosions, and along the distal ends of surgical excisions suggest that an isomorphic phenomenon is common. The keratoacanthomas appear about 1 month after the traumatic injury. All these associated conditions result in damage to the dermis, especially along the dermoepidermal junction, and necessitate wound healing. The biologic behavior of these lesions is unknown, but they have added to the controversy of keratoacanthoma as a reactive versus a malignant process. In Muir–Torre syndrome, sebaceous tumors and keratoacanthomas occur in association with multiple internal malignancies. A second, less common cancer scenario is the keratoacanthoma visceral carcinoma syndrome (KAVCS). Only a handful of cases have been reported. Patients have multiple or large keratoacanthomas that appear at the same time as an internal malignancy, always of the genitourinary tract. The relationship of Muir–Torre syndrome to KAVCS awaits identification of the genetic basis of both syndromes.

Solitary keratoacanthoma

This type of keratoacanthoma is a rapidly growing papule that enlarges from a 1 mm macule or papule to as large as 25 mm in 3–8 weeks. When fully developed, it is a hemispheric, dome-shaped, skin-colored nodule in which there is a smooth crater, filled with a central keratin plug (Fig. 29-13). The smooth shiny lesion is sharply demarcated from its surroundings. Telangiectases may run through the lesion. Subungual keratoacanthomas are tender subungual tumors, which usually cause significant nail dystrophy. Subungual lesions often do not regress spontaneously and induce early underlying bony destruction, characterized on radiograph as a crescent-shaped lytic defect without accompanying sclerosis or periosteal reaction.

The solitary keratoacanthoma occurs mostly on sun-exposed skin, with the central portion of the face, backs of the hands, and arms being the most commonly involved sites. Less frequently, other sites are involved, such as the buttocks, thighs, penis, ears, and scalp. Elderly fair-skinned individuals most commonly develop keratoacanthomas. Lesions of the dorsal hands are more common in men, and keratoacanthomas of the lower legs are more common in women. The most interesting feature of this disease is the rapid growth for some 2–6 weeks, followed by a stationary period for another 2–6 weeks, and finally a spontaneous involution over another 2–6 weeks to leave a slightly depressed scar. The stationary period and involuting phase are variable; some lesions may take 6 months to a year to resolve completely. It has been estimated that some 5% of treated lesions recur. Invasion along nerve trunks has been documented and may result in recurrence after a seemingly adequate excision.

Histopathology

The histologic findings of keratoacanthoma and a low-grade SCC are so similar that it is frequently difficult to make a definite diagnosis on the histologic findings alone. When a properly sectioned specimen is examined under low magnification, the center of the lesion shows a crater filled with eosinophilic keratin. Over the sides of the crater, which seems to have been formed by invagination of the epidermis, a "lip" or "marginal buttress" of epithelium extends over the keratin-filled crater. At the base and sides of the crater, the epithelium is acanthotic and composed of keratinocytes, which are highly keratinized and have an eosinophilic, glassy cytoplasm. Surrounding the keratinocyte proliferation, a dense inflammatory infiltrate is frequently seen. Neutrophilic microabscesses are common within the tumor, and trapping of elastic fibers is commonly identified at the periphery of the tumor. These features favor a diagnosis of keratoacanthoma. The most definitive histologic feature is evidence of terminal differentiation, where the scalloped outer border of the tumor has lost its infiltrative character and is reduced to a thin rim of keratinizing cells lining a large keratin-filled crater. The presence of acantholysis within the tumor is incompatible with a diagnosis of keratoacanthoma. It is also important to distinguish keratoacanthoma from marked pseudoepitheliomatous hyperplasia, as seen in prurigo nodularis. Unfortunately, histology does not completely correlate with biological behavior. The diagnosis of benign-behaving keratoacanthoma versus a potentially aggressive SCC may not always be possible. Even if the classic histological features of keratoacanthoma are seen, the diagnosis of SCC should be contemplated if the lesion does not behave as expected.

Treatment

Although keratoacanthomas spontaneously involute, it is impossible to predict how long this will take. The patient may be faced with destructive growth of a tumor for as long as a year. More importantly, SCC cannot always be excluded clinically. Therefore, excisional biopsy of the typical keratoacanthoma of less than 2 cm in diameter should be considered in most cases. If the history is characteristic or multiple lesions have appeared simultaneously, less aggressive interventions may be considered. Nonsurgical therapy may also be considered in certain sites to preserve function or improve cosmetic outcome.

Intralesional injections of 5-FU solution, 50 mg/mL (undiluted from the ampoule) at weekly intervals; bleomycin, 0.5 mg/mL; or methotrexate, 25 mg/mL, can be effective. For a typical lesion, four injections along the base at each pole are recommended. Low-dose systemic methotrexate can be considered if multiple lesions are present and there is no contraindication. For clinically typical lesions, these modalities may be tried before resorting to surgical removal, especially if the latter presents any problem. Excision is recommended if there is not at least 50% involution of the lesion after 3 weeks. Radiation therapy may also be used on giant keratoacanthomas when surgical excision or electrosurgical methods are not feasible.

Multiple keratoacanthomas (Ferguson Smith type)

This type of keratoacanthoma is frequently referred to as the Ferguson Smith type of multiple self-healing keratoacanthoma. These lesions are identical clinically and histologically to the solitary type. There is frequently a family history of similar lesions. The condition has been traced to two large Scottish kindreds. Affected families from other countries have also been reported. Beginning on average at about the age of 25, but possibly as early as the second decade, patients develop crops of keratoacanthomas that begin as small red macules and rapidly become papules that evolve to typical keratoacanthomas. Lesions may number from a few to hundreds, but generally only 3–10 lesions are noted at any one time. Sun-exposed sites are favored, especially the ears and nose, and in most cases scalp lesions occur. In addition, these patients typically develop keratoacanthomas at sites of trauma, often at the ends of surgical excisions. Lesions grow over 2–4 weeks, reaching a size of 2–3 cm, then remain stable for 1–2 months before slowly involuting. They leave a prominent crateriform scar. If the early lesions are aggressively treated with cryotherapy, shave removal, or curettage, the scar may be less marked than that induced by spontaneous involution. Treatment with an oral retinoid can be effective in stopping the appearance of new lesions and causing involution of existing ones.

Generalized eruptive keratoacanthomas (Grzybowski variant)

This type of keratoacanthoma is very rare and sporadic, with most patients having no affected family members. The usual age of onset is between 40 and 60. The patients are usually in good health and are not immunosuppressed. The cause of this condition is unknown. Human papillomavirus has not been detected in most cases in which it was sought. The clinical features are characteristic and unique. The Grzybowski type of multiple keratoacanthoma is characterized by a generalized eruption of numerous dome-shaped, skin-colored papules from 2 to 7 mm in diameter. Multiple larger typical keratoacanthomas may also appear. Thousands of lesions may develop. The eruption is usually generalized, but spares the palms and soles. The oral mucous membranes and larynx can be involved. Severe pruritus may be a feature. Clinically, pityriasis rubra pilaris or widespread lichen planopilaris are often considered. Bilateral ectropion, narrowing of the oral aperture, and severe facial disfigurement can result. Linear arrangement of some lesions, especially over the shoulders and arms, has also been noted. Despite the multiplicity of lesions, no case of "metastasis" from a skin lesion or increased risk of internal malignancy has been reported in the Grzybowski variant of keratoacanthoma. Dr Grzybowski's original patient died of a myocardial infarction 16 years after diagnosis. Treatment with oral retinoids, oral methotrexate, and oral cyclophosphamide can prove effective.

Keratoacanthoma centrifugum marginatum

This uncommon variant of keratoacanthoma is most commonly solitary, but multiple lesions can occur. Keratoacanthoma centrifugum marginatum is characterized by progressive peripheral expansion and concomitant central healing, leaving

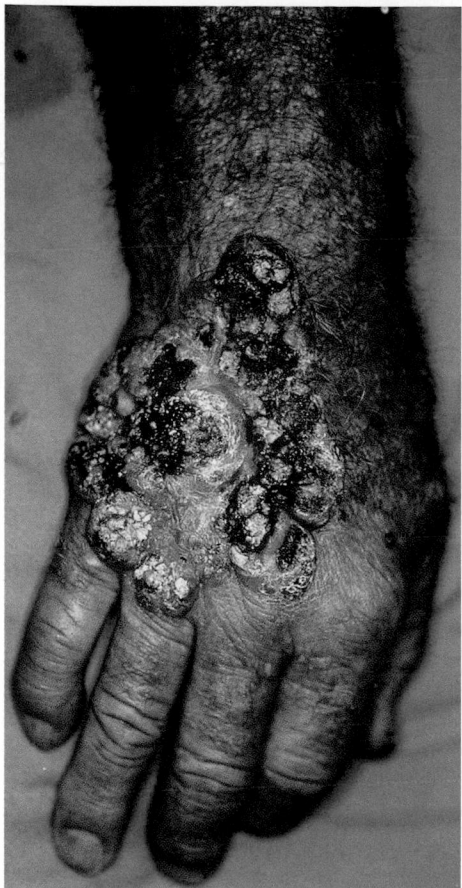

Fig. 29-14 Keratoacanthoma centrifugum marginatum.

atrophy. Spontaneous involution, as may be seen in other variants of keratoacanthoma, does not occur. Lesions range from 5 to 30 cm in diameter (Fig. 29-14). The dorsum of the hands and pretibial regions are favored sites. Treatment with oral etretinate and oral methotrexate with prednisone have been effective in isolated cases.

Andreassi A, et al: Guess what! Keratoacanthoma treated with intralesional bleomycin. Eur J Dermatol 1999; 9:403.

Chorny JA, et al: Eruptive keratoacanthomas in a new tattoo. Arch Dermatol 2007; 143:1457.

Consigli JE, et al: Generalized eruptive keratoacanthoma (Grzybowski variant). Br J Dermatol 2000; 142:800.

Cuesta-Romero C, et al: Intralesional methotrexate in solitary keratoacanthoma. Arch Dermatol 1998; 134:513.

de la Torre C, et al: Keratoacanthoma centrifugum marginatum: treatment with intralesional bleomycin. J Am Acad Dermatol 1997; 37:1010.

Esser AC, et al: Acute development of multiple keratoacanthomas and squamous cell carcinomas after treatment with infliximab. J Am Acad Dermatol 2004; 50:S75.

Gewirtzman A, et al: Eruptive keratoacanthomas following carbon dioxide laser resurfacing. Dermatol Surg 1999; 25:666.

Goldberg LH, et al: Keratoacanthoma as a postoperative complication of skin cancer excision. J Am Acad Dermatol 2004; 50:753.

Goldenberg G, et al: Eruptive squamous cell carcinomas, keratoacanthoma type, arising in a multicolor tattoo. J Cutan Pathol 2008; 35:62.

Haas N, et al: Nine-year follow-up of a case of Grzybowski type multiple keratoacanthomas and failure to demonstrate human papillomavirus. Br J Dermatol 2002; 147:793.

Kato N, et al: Ferguson Smith type multiple keratoacanthomas and a keratoacanthoma centrifugum marginatum in a woman from Japan. J Am Acad Dermatol 2003; 49:741.

Keeney GL, et al: Subungual keratoacanthoma. Arch Dermatol 1988; 124:1074.

LeBoit PE: Can we understand keratoacanthoma? Am J Dermatopathol 2002; 24:166.

Mamelak AJ, et al: Eruptive keratoacanthomas on the legs after fractional photothermolysis: report of two cases. Dermatol Surg 2009; 35:513.

Mangas C, et al: A case of multiple keratoacanthoma centrifugum marginatum. Dermatol Surg 2004; 30:803.

Ming ME: Multiple hyperkeratotic nodules on the arms—diagnosis: keratoacanthoma visceral carcinoma syndrome (KAVCS). Arch Dermatol 2003; 139:1363.

Oakley A, Ng S: Grzybowski's generalized eruptive keratoacanthoma: remission with cyclophosphamide. Australas J Dermatol 2005; 46:118.

Ogasawara Y, et al: A case of multiple keratoacanthoma centrifugum marginatum: response to oral etretinate. J Am Acad Dermatol 2003; 48:282.

Pattee SF, Silvis NG: Keratoacanthoma developing in sites of previous trauma: a report of two cases and review of the literature. J Am Acad Dermatol 2003; 48:S35.

Pini AM, et al: Eruptive keratoacanthoma following topical imiquimod for in situ squamous cell carcinoma of the skin in a renal transplant recipient. J Am Acad Dermatol 2008; 59:S116.

Sanders S, et al: Intralesional corticosteroid treatment of multiple eruptive keratoacanthomas: case report and review of a controversial therapy. Dermatol Surg 2002; 28:954.

Schwartz RA, et al: Generalized eruptive keratoacanthoma of Grzybowski: follow-up of the original description and 50-year retrospect. Dermatology 2002; 205:348.

Singal A, et al: Unusual multiple keratoacanthoma in a child successfully treated with 5-fluorouracil. J Dermatol 1997; 24:546.

Tamir G, et al: Synchronous appearance of keratoacanthomas in burn scar and skin graft donor site shortly after injury. J Am Acad Dermatol 1999; 40:870.

Vandergriff T, et al: Generalized eruptive keratoacanthomas of Grzybowski treated with isotretinoin. J Drugs Dermatol 2008; 7:1069.

Basal cell carcinoma

Basal cell carcinoma (BCC) is the most common cancer in the US, Australia, New Zealand, and many other countries with a largely white, fair-skinned population with the opportunity to expose their skin to sunlight. In Hawaii, the incidence of BCC is 14-fold higher in persons of European ancestry (especially Celtic) than in Japanese, and 34-fold higher than in Filipinos. Still, persons of color can develop BCCs, especially fair-skinned Asians and Hispanics who have accumulated significant lifetime sun exposure from occupational sources, usually farm work. White Hispanics have less skin cancer awareness, use sun protection less frequently, and are more likely to use tanning beds than darker-skinned Hispanics. They represent a prevalent at-risk population for skin cancer over the next decades. Intermittent intense sun exposure, as identified by prior sunburns; radiation therapy; a positive family history of BCC; immunosuppression; a fair complexion, especially red hair; easy sunburning (skin types I or II); and blistering sunburns in childhood are risk factors for the development of BCC. Of interest, actinic elastosis and wrinkling are not risk factors for the development of BCC. In fact, BCCs are relatively rare on the dorsal hand, where sun exposure is high, while actinic keratoses and SCCs abound. SCC is three times more common than BCC on the dorsum of the hand. These findings suggest that the mechanism by which UVR induces BCC is not related solely to the total amount of UVR received. The regular use of sunscreens cannot be proven to reduce the risk for BCC, as opposed to actinic keratoses and SCCs, which are clearly related to the amount of lifetime sun exposure. The ratio of BCC:SCC decreases as one moves from the northern US (about 10) to the southern US (about 2). Once a person has had a BCC, their risk for a subsequent BCC is high: 44% in the next 3 years.

Many clinical morphologies of BCC exist. Clinical diagnosis is dependent on the clinician being aware of the many forms BCC may take. Since these clinical types may also have different biologic behavior, histologic classification of the type of BCC may also influence the form of therapy chosen.

Nodular basal cell carcinoma (classic basal cell carcinoma)

The classic or nodular BCC comprises 50–80% of all BCCs. Nodular BCC is composed of one or a few small, waxy, semi-translucent nodules, forming around a central depression that may or may not be ulcerated, crusted, and bleeding. The edge of larger lesions has a characteristic rolled border. Telangiectases course through the lesion. Bleeding on slight injury is a common sign.

As growth progresses, crusting appears over a central erosion or ulcer, and when the crust is knocked or picked off, bleeding occurs and the ulcer becomes apparent. This ulcer is characterized by chronicity and gradual enlargement over time. The lesions are asymptomatic and bleeding is the only difficulty encountered. The lesions are most frequently found on the face (85–90% on the head and neck) and especially on the nose (25–30%). The forehead, ears (Fig. 29-15), periocular areas, and cheeks are also favored sites. Any part of the body may be involved, however.

Cystic basal cell carcinoma

These dome-shaped, blue–gray cystic nodules are clinically similar to eccrine and apocrine hidrocystomas (Fig. 29-16).

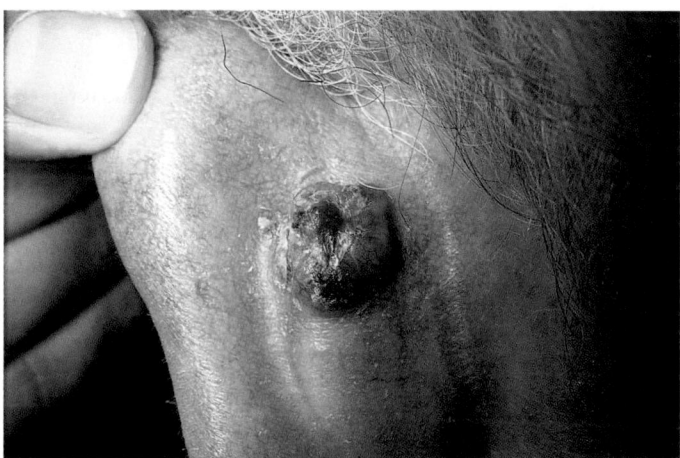

Fig. 29-15 Basal cell carcinoma, nodular type.

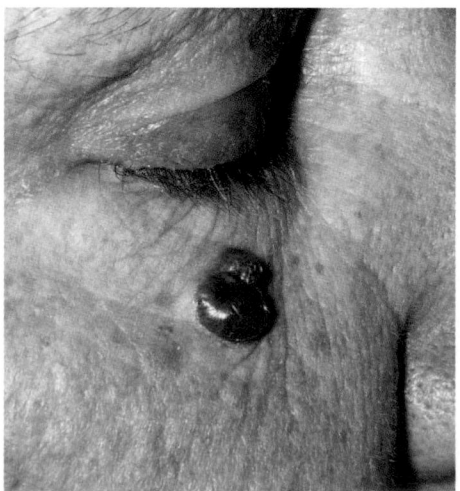

Fig. 29-16 Basal cell carcinoma, cystic.

Morpheic, morpheaform, or cicatricial basal cell carcinoma

This type of BCC presents as a white sclerotic plaque. Ninety-five percent of these BCCs occur on the head and neck. Ulceration, a pearly rolled border, and crusting are usually absent. Telangiectasia is variably present. For this reason, the lesion is often missed or misdiagnosed for some time. The differential diagnosis includes desmoplastic trichoepithelioma, a scar, microcystic adnexal carcinoma, and desmoplastic melanoma. The unique histologic feature is the strands of basal cells interspersed amid densely packed, hypocellular connective tissue. Morpheic BCCs constitute 2–6% of all BCCs.

Infiltrative basal cell carcinoma

Infiltrative BCC is an aggressive subtype characterized by deep infiltration of spiky islands of basaloid epithelium in a fibroblast-rich stroma. Clinically, it lacks the scarlike appearance of morpheic BCC. Histologically, the stroma is hypercellular, the islands are jagged in outline, and squamous differentiation is common.

Micronodular basal cell carcinoma

These tumors are not clinically distinctive, but the micronodular growth pattern makes them less amenable to curettage.

Superficial basal cell carcinoma

Superficial BCC is also termed superficial multicentric BCC. This is a very common form of BCC, comprising at least 15% of the total. It favors the trunk (45%) or distal extremities (14%). Only 40% occur on the head and neck. The multicentricity is merely a histologic illusion created by the passing of the plane of section through the branches of a single, multiply branching lesion.

This type of BCC most frequently presents as a dry, psoriasiform, scaly lesion. It is usually a superficial flat growth, which in many cases exhibits little tendency to invade or ulcerate. The lesions enlarge very slowly and may be misdiagnosed as patches of eczema or psoriasis. They may grow to be 10–15 cm in diameter. Close examination of the edges of the lesion will show a thread-like raised border. These erythematous plaques with telangiectasia may show atrophy or scarring occasionally. Some lesions may develop an infiltrative component in their deeper aspect and grow into the deeper dermis. When this occurs, they may induce dermal fibrosis and multifocal ulceration, forming a "field of fire" type of large BCC. Sometimes the lesion will heal at one place with a white atrophic scar and then spread actively to the neighboring skin. It is not uncommon for a patient to have several of these lesions simultaneously or with time. This form of BCC is the most common pattern seen in patients with human immuno-deficiency virus (HIV) infection and BCC.

Pigmented basal cell carcinoma

This variety has all the features of nodular BCC, but in addition, brown or black pigmentation is present (Fig. 29-17). When dark-complexioned persons, such as Latin Americans, Hispanics, or Asians, develop BCC, this is the type they tend to develop. Pigmented BCCs comprise 6% of all BCCs. In the management of these lesions it should be known that, if ionizing radiation therapy is chosen as the therapeutic modality, the pigmentation remains at the site of the lesion.

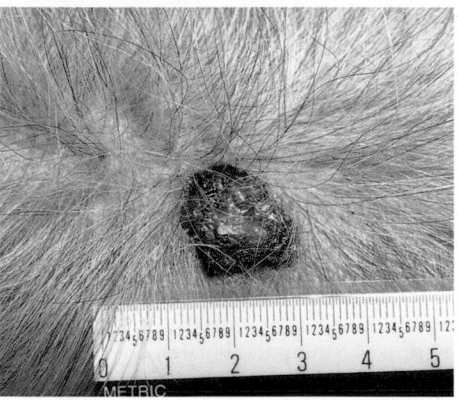

Fig. 29-17 Basal cell carcinoma, pigmented.

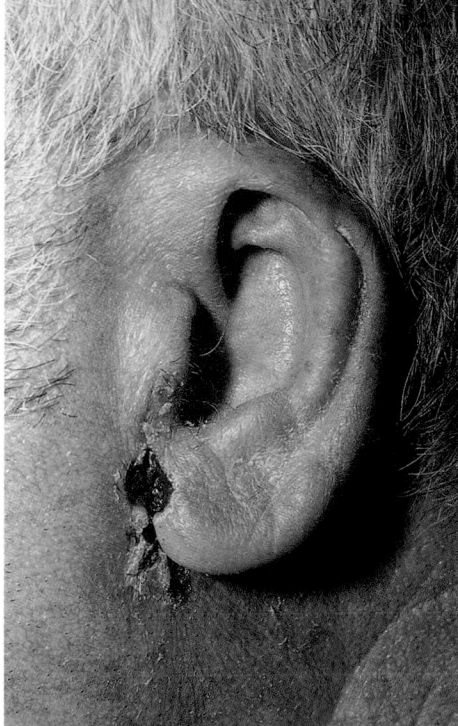

Fig. 29-18 Basal cell carcinoma, rodent ulcer.

Rodent ulcer

Also known as Jacobi ulcer, rodent ulcer is a neglected BCC that has formed an ulceration (Fig. 29-18). The pearly border of the lesion may not be recognized. If it occurs on the lower extremity, it may be misdiagnosed as a vascular ulceration.

Fibroepithelioma of Pinkus

First described by Pinkus as premalignant fibroepithelial tumor, this is usually an elevated, skin-colored, sessile lesion on the lower trunk, lumbosacral area, groin, or thigh, and may be as large as 7 cm. The lesion is superficial and resembles a fibroma or papilloma.

Histologically, there are interlacing basocellular sheets that extend downward from the surface to form an epithelial meshwork enclosing a hyperplastic mesodermal stroma. Like infundibulocystic BCC, fibroepithelioma is composed of pink epithelial strands with blue basaloid buds. Fibroepithelioma has a more prominent fibromucinous stroma and lacks the horn cysts characteristic of infundibulocystic BCC.

Fibroepithelioma often demonstrates sweat ducts within the pink epithelial strands. A slight inflammatory infiltrate may also be present. Simple removal by excision or electrosurgery is the treatment of choice.

Polypoid basal cell carcinoma

These tumors present as exophytic nodules of the head and neck.

Pore-like basal cell carcinoma

Patients with thick sebaceous skin of the central face may develop a BCC that resembles an enlarged pore or stellate pit. The lesions virtually always occur on the nose, melolabial fold, or lower forehead. Affected patients are generally men and the majority are smokers. Many years pass from the appearance of the lesion until a diagnostic biopsy is taken because the lesion is considered inconsequential.

Aberrant basal cell carcinoma

Even in the absence of any apparent carcinogenic factor, such as arsenic, radiation, or chronic ulceration, BCC may occur in odd sites, such as the scrotum, vulva, perineum, nipple, and axilla.

Solitary basal cell carcinoma in young persons

These curious lesions are typically located in the region of embryonal clefts in the face and are often deeply invasive. Complete surgical excision is much safer than curettage for their removal. Cases in children and teenagers, unassociated with the basal cell nevus syndrome or nevus sebaceus, are well documented.

Natural history

BCCs run a chronic course as the lesion slowly enlarges and tends to become more ulcerative. As a rule, there is a tendency for the lesions to bleed without pain or other symptoms. Some of the lesions tend to heal spontaneously and to form scar tissue as they extend. Peripheral spreading may produce configurate, somewhat serpiginous patches. The ulceration may burrow deep into the subcutaneous tissues or even into cartilage and bone, causing extensive destruction and mutilation. At least half of the deaths that occur from BCC result from direct extension into a vital structure rather than metastases.

Metastasis

Metastasis is extremely rare, occurring in 0.0028–0.55% of BCCs. This low rate is believed to be due to the fact that the tumor cells require supporting stroma to survive. The following criteria are now widely accepted for the diagnosis of metastatic BCC:

1. The primary tumor must arise in the skin.
2. Metastases must be demonstrated at a site distant from the primary tumor and must not be related to simple extension.
3. Histologic similarity between the primary tumor and the metastases must exist.
4. The metastases must not be mixed with SCC.

Metastatic BCC is twice as common in men as in women. Immunosuppression does not appear to increase the risk of metastasis of BCC. Most BCCs that metastasize arise on the head and neck, and tend to be large tumors that have recurred despite multiple surgical procedures or radiation therapy. The histologic finding of perineural or intravascular BCC increases the risk for metastasis. The regional lymph nodes are the most frequent site of metastasis, followed by the lung, bone, skin, liver, and pleura. Spread is equally distributed between hematogenous and lymphatic. An average of 9 years elapses between the diagnosis of the primary tumor and metastatic disease, but the interval for metastasis ranges from under 1 year to 45 years. Although the primary tumor may be present for many years before it metastasizes, once metastases occur the course is rapidly downhill. Fewer than 20% of patients survive 1 year and fewer than 10% will live for more than 5 years after metastasis.

Association with internal malignancies

Frisch et al reported a series of 37 674 patients with BCCs, followed over 14 years. Comparison of cancer rates for the general population was remarkable, with 3663 new cancers as opposed to 3245 in the control population. Malignant melanoma and lip cancers were the most frequently found; however, internal malignancies were also noted to be excessive, involving the salivary glands, larynx, lung, breast, kidney, and lymphatics (non-Hodgkin lymphoma). The rate of non-Hodgkin lymphoma was particularly high. Patients receiving the diagnosis of BCC before the age of 60 were found to have a higher rate of breast cancer, testicular cancer, and non-Hodgkin lymphoma.

Immunosuppression

Immunosuppression for organ transplantation increases the risk for the development of BCC by about 10-fold. Some increased risk for BCC is considered also to occur in HIV infection and in persons on immunosuppressive medications for other reasons. Patients with chronic lymphocytic leukemia are also at increased risk for BCC. In the immunosuppressed population, a history of blistering sunburns in childhood is a strong risk factor for the development of BCC following immunosuppression.

Etiology and pathogenesis

It appears that BCCs arise from immature pluripotential cells associated with the hair follicle. Mutations that activate the hedgehog signaling pathway, which controls cell growth, are found in most BCCs. The affected genes are *sonic hedgehog*, *Patched 1*, and *Smothened (SMO)* genes. Inactivation of the *Patched 1* gene is most common, while *SMO* mutations are associated with 10–20% of sporadic BCCs.

Histopathology

There is a general belief that there is a correlation between histologic subtype of BCC and biologic behavior. BCCs are considered as being of low or high risk, depending on their probability of causing problems in the future: subclinical extension, incomplete removal, aggressive local invasive behavior, and local recurrence. Therefore, the dermatopathology report of a BCC should include a subtype descriptor when possible. Unfortunately, many shave biopsy specimens do not allow for accurate typing and the presence of an indolent growth pattern superficially does not exclude the possibility of a more aggressive deeper growth pattern. The common histologic patterns are nodular, superficial, infiltrative, morpheic, micronodular, and mixed. The nodular type is a low-risk type. High-risk types include the infiltrative, morpheic, and micronodular types, due to aggressive local invasive

behavior and a tendency to recurrence. Superficial BCC is prone to increased recurrence due to inadequate removal. When evaluating the histologic margin of superficial BCC, tumor stroma involving the margin should be considered a positive margin.

The early lesion shows small, dark-staining, polyhedral cells resembling those of the basal cell layer of the epidermis, with large nuclei and small nucleoli. These occur within the epidermis as thickenings or immediately beneath the epidermis as downgrowths connected with it. After the growth has progressed, regular compact columns of these cells fill the tissue spaces of the dermis, and a connection with the epidermis may be difficult to demonstrate. At the periphery of the masses of cells, the columnar cells may be characteristically arranged like fence posts (palisading). This may be absent when the tumor cells are in cord arrangement or in small nests. Cysts may form. The interlacing strands of tumor cells may present a lattice-like pattern. The dermal stroma is an integral and important part of the BCC. The stroma is loose and fibromyxoid, with a sparse lymphoid infiltrate commonly present. The stroma can be highlighted by metachromatic toluidine blue staining, which can be useful during Mohs surgery.

Differential diagnosis

Distinguishing between small BCCs and small SCCs is largely an intellectual exercise. Both are caused chiefly by sunlight; neither is likely to metastasize; and both will have to be removed, usually by simple surgical excision or curettage. A biopsy is always indicated, but may be performed at the time of the definitive procedure when the likelihood of the diagnosis of NMSC is high and the patient is fully informed and gives consent.

A waxy, nodular, rolled edge is fairly characteristic of BCC (Fig. 29-19). The SCC is a dome-shaped, elevated, hard, and infiltrated lesion. The early BCC may easily be confused with sebaceous hyperplasia, which has a depressed center with yellowish small nodules surrounding the lesion. These lesions never bleed and do not become crusted.

Bowen's disease, Paget's disease, amelanotic melanoma, and actinic and seborrheic keratoses may also simulate BCC. Ulcerated BCC on the shins is frequently misdiagnosed as a stasis ulcer, and a biopsy may be the only way to differentiate the two. Pigmented basal cell epithelioma is frequently misdiagnosed as melanoma or as a pigmented nevus. The superficial BCC is easily mistaken for psoriasis or eczema. The careful search for the rolled edge of the peripheral nodules is important in differentiating BCC from all other lesions.

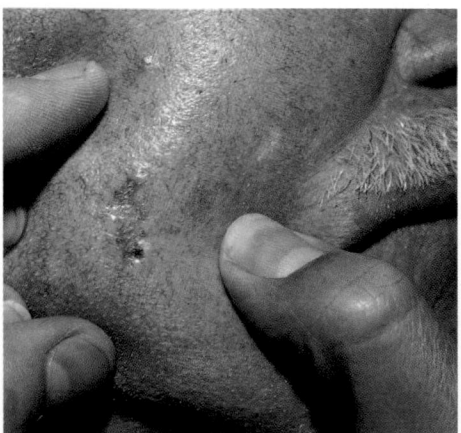

Fig. 29-19 Basal cell carcinoma, accentuation of the pearly border when the skin is stretched.

Treatment

Each lesion of BCC must be thoroughly evaluated individually. Age and sex of the patient, as well as the size, site, and type of lesion, are important factors to be considered when choosing the proper method of treatment. No single treatment method is ideal for all lesions or all patients. The choice of treatment will also be influenced by the experience and ability of the treating physician in the various treatment modalities. A biopsy should be performed in all cases of suspected BCC, to determine the histologic subtype and to confirm the diagnosis.

The aim of treatment is for a permanent cure with the best cosmetic results. This is important because the most common location of BCC is the face. Recurrences result from inadequate treatment and are usually seen during the first 4–12 months after treatment. A minimum 5-year follow-up is indicated, however, to continue a search for new lesions, since the development of a second BCC is common.

Treatment of BCC is usually surgical (see Chapter 37), but some forms of BCC are amenable to medical treatment.

Topical therapy

Topical treatment appears to be most effective in the treatment of superficial BCC. For nodular BCCs the cure rates are only 65%, which is unacceptable given the other options available. On the other hand, superficial BCCs may be cured 80% of the time with topical treatment. Topical 5-FU is not extraordinarily effective and recurrence rates are high. Imiquimod applied three times a week with occlusion, or five times a week without occlusion, is the favored form of topical, patient-applied treatment for superficial BCC. Duration of treatment is 6 weeks, but may be extended if the lesion does not appear to have been eradicated. Cosmetic results are excellent, especially for lesions of the anterior chest and upper back, where significant scarring usually results from surgical procedures. Photodynamic therapy has also emerged as a treatment option for BCC.

Annemans L, et al: Real-life practice study of the clinical outcome and cost-effectiveness of photodynamic therapy using methyl aminolevulinate (MAL-PDT) in the management of actinic keratosis and basal cell carcinoma. Eur J Dermatol 2008; 18:539.

Benedetto AV, et al: Basal cell carcinoma presenting as a large pore. J Am Acad Dermatol 2002; 47:727.

Betti R, et al: Basal cell carcinoma of covered and unusual sites of the body. Int J Dermatol 1997; 36:503.

Boyd AS, et al: Basal cell carcinoma in young women: an evaluation of the association of tanning bed use and smoking. J Am Acad Dermatol 2002; 46:706.

Brooke RCC, et al: Discordance between facial wrinkling and the presence of basal cell carcinoma. Arch Dermatol 2001; 137:751.

Byrd-Miles K, et al: Skin cancer in individuals of African, Asian, Latin-American, and American-Indian descent: differences in incidence, clinical presentation, and survival compared to Caucasians. J Drugs Dermatol 2007; 6:10.

Corona R, et al: Risk factors for basal cell carcinoma in a Mediterranean population: role of recreational sun exposure early in life. Arch Dermatol 2001; 137:1162.

Donovan J: Review of the hair follicle origin hypothesis for basal cell carcinoma. Dermatol Surg 2009; 35:1311.

Epstein EH: Basal cell carcinomas: attack of the hedgehog. Nat Rev Cancer 2008; 8:743.

Esquivias Gomez JI, et al: Basal cell carcinoma of the scrotum. Australas J Dermatol 1999; 40:141.

Frisch M, et al: Risk for subsequent cancer after diagnosis of basal-cell carcinoma. Ann Intern Med 1996; 125:815.

Geisse J, et al: Imiquimod 5% cream for the treatment of superficial basal cell carcinoma: results from two phase III, randomized, vehicle-controlled studies. J Am Acad Dermatol 2004; 50:722.

Gloster HM Jr, Neal K: Skin cancer in skin of color. J Am Acad Dermatol 2006; 55:741.

Goldberg LH: Basal-cell carcinoma as a predictor of other cancers. Lancet 1997; 349:664.

Gottlöber P, et al: Basal cell carcinomas occurring after accidental exposure to ionizing radiation. Br J Dermatol 1999; 141:383.

Heckmann M, et al: Frequency of facial basal cell carcinoma does not correlate with site-specific UV exposure. Arch Dermatol 2002; 138:1494.

Kahn HS, et al: Increased cancer mortality following a history of nonmelanoma skin cancer. JAMA 1998; 280:910.

Lin LK, et al: Pigmented basal cell carcinoma of the eyelid in Hispanics. Clin Ophthalmol 2008; 2:641.

Ma F, et al: Skin cancer awareness and sun protection behaviors in white Hispanic and white non-Hispanic high school students in Miami, Florida. Arch Dermatol 2007; 143:983.

McCormack CJ, et al: Differences in age and body site distribution of the histological subtypes of basal cell carcinoma: a possible indicator of differing causes. Arch Dermatol 1997; 133:593.

Megahed M: Polypoid basal cell carcinoma: a new clinicopathological variant. Br J Dermatol 1999; 140:701.

Naldi L, et al: Host-related and environmental risk factors for cutaneous basal cell carcinoma: evidence from an Italian case-control study. J Am Acad Dermatol 2000; 42:446.

Requena L, et al: Keloidal basal cell carcinoma: a new clinicopathological variant of basal cell carcinoma. Br J Dermatol 1996; 134:953.

Robinson JK, Dahiya M: Basal cell carcinoma with pulmonary and lymph node metastasis causing death. Arch Dermatol 2003; 139:643.

Rosso S, et al: The multicentre south European study "Helios." II: Different sun exposure patterns in the aetiology of basal cell and squamous cell carcinomas of the skin. Br J Cancer (Scot) 1996; 73:1447.

Saldanha G, et al: Basal cell carcinoma: a dermatopathological and molecular biological update. Br J Dermatol 2003; 148:195.

Scrivener Y, et al: Variations of basal cell carcinomas according to gender, age, location and histopathological subtype. Br J Dermatol 2002; 147:41.

Tilli CMLJ, et al: Molecular aetiology and pathogenesis of basal cell carcinoma. Br J Dermatol 2005; 152:1108.

Walther U, et al: Risk and protective factors for sporadic basal cell carcinoma: results of a two-centre case-control study in southern Germany. Clinical actinic elastosis may be a protective factor. Br J Dermatol 2004; 151:170.

Nevoid basal cell carcinoma syndrome (Gorlin syndrome)

Clinical features

The nevoid BCC syndrome (NBCCS) or basal cell nevus syndrome is an autosomal-dominantly inherited disorder. The major diagnostic criteria include:

1. development of multiple BCCs (>5) or a BCC before age 30 (Fig. 29-20)
2. odontogenic keratocysts of the jaws
3. pitted depressions on the hands and feet (palmar plantar pits) (two or more)
4. lamellar calcification of the falx under age 20
5. first-degree relative with NBCCS.

Minor criteria include:

1. childhood medulloblastoma
2. lympho-mesenteric or pleural cysts
3. macrocephaly (97th percentile)
4. cleft lip/palate
5. vertebral/rib abnormalities
6. preaxial or postaxial polydactyly
7. ovarian/cardiac fibromas
8. ocular abnormalities.

The diagnosis is made if the affected individual has two major criteria and one minor criterion, or one major criterion and three minor criteria. Genetic testing has revealed that some

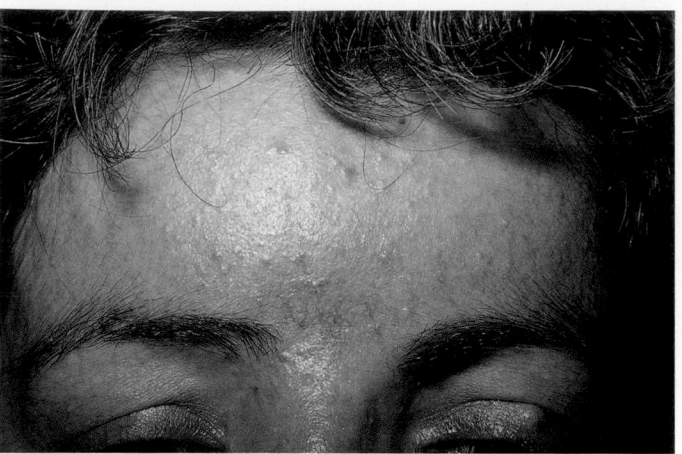

Fig. 29-20 Multiple basal cell carcinomas in nevoid basal cell carcinoma syndrome.

persons carrying the genetic mutation do not meet the diagnostic criteria.

Essentially, all cases of NBCCS are due to mutations in the *PTCH* (or *PTCH1*) gene. One family with a mutation in the *SUFU* gene has been reported. *SUFU* mutations have been reported with meduloblastoma susceptibility. Mutations occur throughout the *PTCH* gene and there does not appear to be a correlation between the site of the mutation and the clinical phenotype. Most mutations result in premature termination and production of shortened gene product. Loss of the *PTCH* gene can also occur by deletions of part of the long arm of chromosome 9, where the *PTCH* gene is located (region q22). This represents about 6% of NBCCS patients

The clinical findings seen with this syndrome are dependent on two characteristics: the race of the patient and the form of mutation (nucleotide point mutation or chromosome deletion). Of 105 patients reported in one series, 80% were white. The first tumor developed by the mean age of 23 years for white patients. Palmar pits were seen in 87%. Jaw cysts were found in 74%, with 80% manifested by the age of 20. The total number of cysts ranged from 1 to 28. Medulloblastomas developed in four patients and three had cleft lip or palate. Physical findings in this series included "coarse face" (54%), macrocephaly (50%), hypertelorism (42%), frontal bossing (27%), pectus deformity (13%), and Sprengel deformity (11%). In Japanese and African American patients with NBCCS, palmar and plantar pits, odontogenic keratocysts, and skeletal abnormalities are most common, with BCCs not appearing until much later in life. Those patients with NBCCS due to deletions of chromosome 9q22 have all the stigmata of typical NBCCS patients, and in addition often have severe mental retardation, hyperactivity, overfriendliness with strangers, short stature, and less commonly, neonatal hypotonia, epicanthic folds, short neck, pectus, scoliosis, and epilepsy.

Skin tumors

The BCCs occur at an early age or any time thereafter as multiple lesions, usually numerous. The usual age of appearance is between 17 and 35 years. Although any area of the body may be affected, there is a marked tendency toward involvement of the central facial area, especially the eyelids, periorbital area, nose, upper lip, and cheeks. Persons with fair skin (type 1) and prior excessive UV exposure are particularly prone to develop many BCCs. Lesions typically appear as 1–10 mm, hyperpigmented or skin-colored, dome-shaped papules. They have a striking resemblance to typical compound or intradermal nevi. Polypoid BCC or acrochordon-like BCC is a more unusual variant that tends to occur in NBCCS

patients in childhood. Among the many BCCs an NBCCS patient may have, some sit indolently and others may grow more aggressively.

Jaw cysts

Jaw cysts occur in approximately 90% of patients. They occur as early as age 5 years and rarely after age 30. Both the mandible and the maxilla may show cystic defects on x-ray, with mandibular involvement occurring twice as often. Jaw cysts most commonly present as painless swelling. They usually have a keratinized lining (keratocysts) but uncommonly a cyst may be an ameloblastoma.

Pits of palms and soles

An unusual pitting of palms and soles is a distinguishing feature of the disease. This usually becomes apparent in the second decade of life. Up to 87% of patients with NBCCS will have pits. Histologically, they show basaloid proliferation, but the lesions do not progress or behave like a BCC.

Skeletal defects/birth defects

Most NBCCS patients have skeletal anomalies that are easily detected by x-ray. Macrocephaly is the first feature observed, and explains the high rate of cesarian section delivery of NBCCS-affected fetuses. Other skeletal defects include bifid, fused, missing, or splayed ribs; scoliosis; and kyphosis. Radiographic evidence of multiple lesions is highly suggestive of this syndrome; and since most are present congenitally, radiology may be useful in diagnosing this syndrome in patients too young to manifest other abnormalities. Cleft lip/ palate is seen in 5% of patients, lamellar calcification of the falx will be evident in 90% of patients by age 20, and polydactyly also occurs. Numerous ocular findings have been reported, and if NBCCS is suspected or confirmed, an ophthalmologic evaluation should be performed. Spina bifida is, fortunately, uncommon.

Histopathology

The histology of BCCs arising in syndrome patients is identical to that arising in nonsyndromic patients, with the solid and superficial types being most common.

Differential diagnosis

Several other unique types of BCC presentation should not be confused with NBCCS. One is the linear unilateral BCC syndrome, in which a linear arrangement of close-set papules, sometimes interspersed with comedones, is present at birth. Biopsy reveals basal cell epitheliomas; however, they do not increase in size with the age of the patient. The second type, referred to as Bazex syndrome, is an X-linked dominantly inherited disease comprising follicular atrophoderma of the extremities, localized or generalized hypohidrosis, hypotrichosis, and multiple BCCs of the face, which often arise at an early age. The third type consists of multiple hereditary infundibulocystic BCCs; this is an autosomal-dominant syndrome. It is distinguished from NBCCs by the absence of palmar pits and jaw cysts in most cases. Clinically, patients appear to have multiple trichoepitheliomas. Numerous skincolored pearly papules affect the central face, accentuated in the nasolabial folds. The generalized basaloid follicular hamartoma syndrome differs from NBCCS by having basaloid follicular hamartomas instead of BCCs. It is reported from a large kindred in the southeastern US (see below). Tiny palmar pits are present. Histologically, infundibulocystic BCC and basaloid follicular hamartoma may be indistinguishable, so the two familial syndromes may be difficult to separate. Rombo syndrome, reported in one large Swedish family, has multiple BCCs, vermiculate atrophoderma, and hypotrichosis. A patient with multiple BCCs and myotonic dystrophy has been reported, suggesting yet another genodermatosis associated with multiple BCCs.

Treatment

Genetic counseling is essential. Strict sun avoidance and maximum sun protection, as recommended for xeroderma pigmentosum patients, is advised. Treatment involves very regular monitoring and biopsy of suspicious lesions. Topical therapy with tazarotene and imiquimod may be of some use in preventing and treating the superficial tumors. Oral retinoid therapy may reduce the frequency of new BCCs appearing, and the existing small BCCs stop growing. However, once the oral retinoids are stopped, the lesions again begin to grow. Surgical treatments are used for most lesions, either curettage and desiccation or excisions. At times, megasessions, with removal of multiple tumors under general anesthesia in the operating room, are needed to keep up with the large number of BCCs that these patients develop. Photodynamic therapy appears to be particularly beneficial when used to treat areas that have had multiple BCCs in the past.

Abe S, et al: Coincident two mutations and one single nucleotide polymorphism of the *PTCH1* gene in a family with naevoid basal cell carcinoma syndrome. Acta Derm Venereol 2008; 88:635.

Bañuls J, et al: Tissue and tumor mosaicism of the myotonin protein kinase gene trinucleotide repeat in a patient with multiple basal cell carcinomas associated with myotonic dystrophy. J Am Acad Dermatol 2004; 50:S1.

Dalati T, Zhou H: Gorlin syndrome with ameloblastoma: a case report and review of the literature. Cancer Invest 2008; 26:975.

de Ravel TJ, et al: Early detection of chromosome 9q22.32q31.1 microdeletion and the nevoid basal cell carcinoma syndrome. Eur J Med Genet 2009; 52:145.

El Sobky RA, et al: Successful treatment of an intractable case of hereditary basal cell carcinoma syndrome with paclitaxel. Arch Dermatol 2001; 137:827.

Evans DG, Farndon PA, et al: Nevoid basal cell carcinoma syndrome (updated January 25, 2008). In: GeneReviews at GeneTests: Medical Genetics Information Resource (database online). Copyright, University of Washington, Seattle. 1997–2010. Available at http://www.genetests.org.

Feito-Rodriguez M, et al: Dermatoscopic characteristics of acrochordon-like basal cell carcinomas in Gorlin–Goltz syndrome. J Am Acad Dermatol 2009; 60:857.

Gilchrest BA, et al: Photodynamic therapy for patients with basal cell nevus syndrome. Dermatol Surg 2009; 35:1576.

Glaessl A, et al: Sporadic Bazex–Dupré–Christol-like syndrome: early onset basal cell carcinoma, hypohidrosis, hypotrichosis, prominent milia. Dermatol Surg 2000; 26:152.

Kimonis VE, et al: Clinical manifestations in 105 persons with nevoid basal cell carcinoma syndrome. Am J Med Genet 1997; 69:299.

Kulkarni P, et al: Nevoid basal cell carcinoma syndrome in a person with dark skin. J Am Acad Dermatol 2003; 49:332.

Lo Muzio L: Nevoid basal cell carcinoma syndrome (Gorlin syndrome). Orphanet J Rare Dis 2008; 3:32.

Micali G, et al: The use of imiquimod 5% cream for the treatment of basal cell carcinoma as observed in Gorlin's syndrome. Clin Exp Dermatol 2003; 28:19.

Nakamura M, Tokura Y: A novel missense mutation in the *PTCH1* gene in a premature case of nevoid basal cell carcinoma syndrome. Eur J Dermatol 2009; 19:262.

Pastorino L, et al: Identification of a *SUFU* germline mutation in a family with Gorlin syndrome. Am J Med Genet A 2009; 149A:1539.

Requena L, et al: Multiple hereditary infundibulocystic basal cell carcinomas. Arch Dermatol 1999; 135:1227.

Takahashi C, et al: Germline *PTCH1* mutations in Japanese basal cell nevus syndrome patients. J Hum Genet 2009; 54:403.

van der Geer S, et al: Treatment of basal cell carcinomas in patients with nevoid basal cell carcinoma syndrome. J Eur Acad Dermatol Venereol 2009; 23:308.

van der Geer S, et al: Treatment of the patient with nevoid basal cell carcinoma syndrome in a megasession. Dermatol Surg 2009; 35:709.

Vered M, et al: The immunoprofile of odontogenic keratocyst (keratocystic odontogenic tumor) that includes expression of *PTCH*, *SMO*, *GLI-1* and *bcl-2* is similar to ameloblastoma but different from odontogenic cysts. J Oral Pathol Med 2009; 38:597.

Wheeler CE, et al: Autosomal dominantly inherited generalized basaloid follicular hamartoma syndrome: report of a new disease in a North Carolina family. J Am Acad Dermatol 2000; 43:189.

Yamamoto K, et al: Further delineation of 9q22 deletion syndrome associated with basal cell nevus (Gorlin) syndrome: report of two cases and review of the literature. Congenit Anom (Kyoto) 2009; 49:8.

Squamous cell carcinoma

Squamous cell carcinoma (SCC) is the second most common form of skin cancer. Most cases of SCC of the skin are induced by UVR. Chronic, long-term sun exposure is the major risk factor, and areas that have had such exposure (the face, scalp, neck, and dorsal hands) are favored locations. SCC becomes relatively more common as the annual amount of UVR increases, so SCC is more common in Texas than in Minnesota, for example. Immunosuppression greatly enhances the risk for the development of SCC, with azathioprine exposure especially associated with greater risk for development of cutaneous SCC. Sorafenib and possibly the tumor necrosis factor (TNF) inhibitors may be associated with increased risk of cutaneous SCC. High-risk genital human papillomaviruses (HPV-16, 18, 31, and 35, primarily) play a role in SCCs that develop on the genitalia and periungually. A chronic ulcer, hidradenitis suppurativa, prior x-radiation exposure, PUVA treatment, recessive dystrophic epidermolysis bullosa, lesions of discoid lupus, and erosive lichen planus are skin conditions or treatments that appear to enhance the risk for the development of SCC. Metastasis, with a mortality rate of 18%, is very uncommon for SCCs arising in sites of chronic sun damage, whereas it is relatively high (20–30%) in SCCs occurring in the various scarring processes. Patients with epidermodysplasia verruciformis (EDV) also develop SCCs on sun-exposed sites, associated with unique HPV types. These unique EDV HPV types (HPV-5, 8, and others) may also play a role in SCCs that develop in immunosuppressed persons. SCC of the oral mucosa is discussed in Chapter 34. Because the vast majority of cutaneous SCCs are induced by UVR, sun protection, with avoidance of the midday sun, protective clothing, and the regular application of a sunblock of SPF 30, is recommended. Some researchers have suggested that smoking is also a risk factor for cutaneous SCC, but this is controversial.

Clinical features

Frequently, SCC begins at the site of actinic keratosis on sun-exposed areas such as the face and backs of the hands. BCCs far outnumber SCCs on the facial skin, but SCCs on the hand occur three times more commonly than BCCs. The lesion may be superficial, discrete, and hard, and arises from an indurated, rounded, elevated base (Fig. 29-21). It is dull-red and contains telangiectases. In the course of a few months the lesion becomes larger, deeply nodular, and ulcerated. The ulcer is at first superficial and is hidden by a crust. When this is removed, a well-defined, papillary base is seen, and on palpation a discrete hard disk is felt. In the early phases this tumor is localized, elevated, and freely movable on the underlying structures; later it gradually becomes diffuse, more or less depressed, and fixed. The growth eventually invades the underlying tissues. The tumor above the level of the skin may

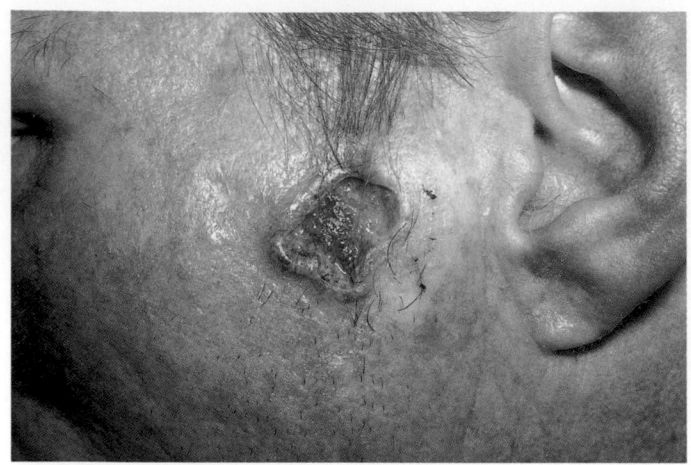

Fig. 29-21 Squamous cell carcinoma, preauricular ulceration in a patient with AIDS.

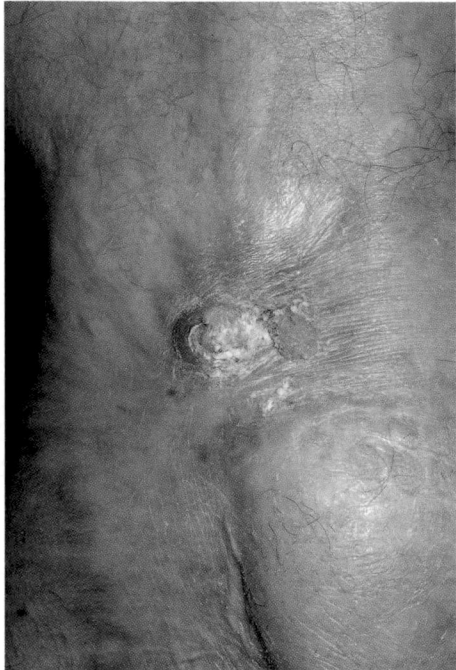

Fig. 29-22 SCC in a burn scar. (Courtesy of Curt Samlaska, MD)

be dome-shaped, with a core-like center that later ulcerates. The surface in advanced lesions may be cauliflower-like, composed of densely packed, filamentous projections, between which are clefts filled with a viscid, purulent, malodorous exudate.

In black patients SCCs are 20% more common than BCCs. The most favored sites are the face and lower extremities, with involvement of non-sun-exposed areas more common. Elderly women (mean age 77) are primarily affected in cases involving the lower legs. Prior direct heat exposure from open fireplaces may be the predisposing factor. In contrast, the most frequently found predisposing conditions in white patients are scarring processes, such as burns (Fig. 29-22), leg ulcers, and hidradenitis suppurativa.

On the lower lip, SCC often develops on actinic cheilitis. From repeated sunburn the vermilion surface becomes dry, scaly, and fissured. At the beginning only a local thickening is noticeable. This then becomes a firm nodule. It may grow outward as a sizable tumor or inward with destructive ulceration. A history of smoking is also frequent and a significant predisposing factor. Lower lip lesions far outnumber upper lip lesions, men far outnumber women (12:1), and the median age

is the late sixties. SCCs occurring on the lower lip metastasize approximately 10–15% of the time. SCC of the lip may also occur in areas of discoid lupus erythematosus (DLE) in black patients. Neoplastic transformation into SCC may develop in 0.3–3% of patients with DLE of the lip.

Periungual SCC frequently presents with signs of erythema and scaling, which can superficially appear as a wart. The patient may even have periungual warts on other digits. Early on, pain and ulceration are uncommon. Fifty percent of those x-rayed show changes in the terminal phalanx. There is a low rate of metastases (3%), but local excision with Mohs microsurgery is recommended, as it reduces the risk of recurrence. Periungual SCC is strongly associated with genital HPV types, primarily 16, 18, 31, and 35.

Given the numerous presentations of SCC on the skin, there should be a low threshold for biopsy of any suspicious keratotic, ulcerated or nodular lesions, especially on the background of chronic sun exposure.

Histopathology

SCC is characterized by irregular nests, cords, or sheets of neoplastic keratinocytes invading the dermis to various depths. Thickness is an important risk factor for metastasis, with thickness >2 mm associated with 4% metastases and >6 mm with a 16% metastatic rate. Less than 5% of patients with metastatic SCC had a primary cutaneous SCC <2 mm in thickness. Immunosuppression, ear location, and increased horizontal size all increase risk of metastasis by 2–4-fold. Desmoplasia and tumor thickness also increase local recurrence risk, 16 and 6 times respectively. Although histological differentiation should be reported, it seems less important than these other tumor features in predicting prognosis. In tumors that are poorly differentiated or of primary clear cell morphology, there are other types of neoplasm that must be excluded, including melanoma. Immunoperoxidase staining for keratins is very useful in this setting. Desmoplastic SCCs by light microscopy have prominent trabecular growth patterns, narrow columns of atypical epithelial cells, and marked desmoplastic stromal reaction. These tumors tend to recur. Acantholytic SCC is a recognized histologic subtype, but of no prognostic importance. The finding of perineural and vascular invasion, and recurrence are bad prognostic features.

Differential diagnosis

The differentiation of SCC from keratoacanthoma is of academic interest in most cases, as simple surgical excision is performed on most of these lesions. However, if nonsurgical modalities are contemplated, a biopsy confirming the diagnosis of keratoacanthoma is recommended. In the setting of immunosuppression, keratoacanthoma-like lesions should be managed as SCCs. The rapid growth and presence of a rolled border with a keratotic central plug suggest the diagnosis of keratoacanthoma, as does explosive growth. An early SCC may be confused with a hypertrophic actinic keratosis and indeed the two may be indistinguishable clinically. Biopsy to include the base of the lesion is necessary to make the diagnosis.

Pseudoepitheliomatous hyperplasia (PEH) must be distinguished histologically from true SCC. Marked PEH may be seen in granular cell tumor, bromoderma, blastomycosis, granuloma inguinale, and chronic pyodermas. It is frequently mistaken for SCC in chronic stasis ulcers, ulcerations occurring in thermal burns, lupus vulgaris, leishmaniasis, and even sporotrichosis. PEH arises from adnexal structures, as well as the surface epidermis. Hyperkeratosis and hypergranulosis of adjacent hair follicles are often present. Strands of epidermal cells may extend into the reticular dermis and commonly trap elastic fibers, a finding also seen in keratoacanthoma, but rarely in conventional SCCs. A potential diagnostic pitfall is the presence of benign PEH adjacent to and overlying invasive SCC. This is particularly common in lesions that have been picked or scratched.

Metastases

The rate of SCC metastasis from all skin sites ranges from 0.5% to 5.2%. Careful attention should be paid to regional lymph nodes draining the site of the SCC. These should be examined at the time of the initial evaluation when the suspicious lesion is identified, and at the regular visits that follow the treatment of the SCC.

Patients with SCC are at increased risk of developing other malignancies, such as cancers of the respiratory organs, buccal cavity, pharynx, small intestines (in men), non-Hodgkin lymphoma, and leukemia.

Prevention/treatment

The primary treatment of SCC of the skin is surgical (see Chapter 37). Oral retinoids may be useful as a preventive strategy in patients with immunosuppression who develop frequent cancers. Photodynamic therapy might be beneficial to reduce the number of SCCs occurring in areas of prior UV damage where SCCs have already been sited. Organ transplant recipients should be educated about sun protection and skin cancer risk, ideally *before* their transplantation, and should have regular skin examinations by a trained dermatologist. The use of sirolimus instead of other immunosuppressives appears to reduce the prevalence of SCCs in organ transplant recipients.

Alam M, et al: Human papillomavirus-associated digital squamous cell carcinoma: literature review and report of 21 new cases. J Am Acad Dermatol 2003; 48:305.

Breuninger H, et al: Desmoplastic squamous cell carcinoma of skin and vermilion surface: a highly malignant subtype of skin cancer. Cancer 1997; 79:915.

Campistol JM: Minimizing the risk of posttransplant malignancy. Transplantation 2009; 87:S19.

Chen SJ, et al: Activation of the mammalian target of rapamycin signalling pathway in epidermal tumours and its correlation with cyclin-dependent kinase 2. Br J Dermatol 2009; 160:442.

Clowers-Webb HE, et al: Educational outcomes regarding skin cancer in organ transplant recipients. Arch Dermatol 2006; 142:712.

Cooper JZ, Brown MD: Special concern about squamous cell carcinoma of the scalp in organ transplant recipients. Arch Dermatol 2006; 142:755.

Dinehart SM, et al: Metastatic cutaneous squamous cell carcinoma derived from actinic keratosis. Cancer 1997; 79:920.

Donovan JC, Shaw JC: Compliance with sun protection following organ transplantation. Arch Dermatol 2006; 142:1232.

Dubauskas Z, et al: Cutaneous squamous cell carcinoma and inflammation of actinic keratoses associated with sorafenib. Clin Genitourin Cancer 2009; 7:20.

English DR, et al: Case-control study of sun exposure and squamous cell carcinoma of the skin. Int J Cancer 1998; 77:347.

Fernandez A, et al: Sirolimus: a potential chemopreventive agent. J Invest Dermatol 2008; 128:2352.

Fritsch C, et al: New primary cancers after squamous cell skin cancer. Am J Epidemiol 1995; 141:916.

Gonzalez-Perez R, et al: Metastatic squamous cell carcinoma arising in Bowen's disease of the palm. J Am Acad Dermatol 1997; 36:635.

Harwood CA, et al: Low dose retinoids in the prevention of cutaneous squamous cell carcinomas in organ transplant recipients. Arch Dermatol 2005; 141:456.

Hemminki K: Smoking overlooked as an important risk factor for squamous cell carcinoma. Arch Dermatol 2004; 140:362.

Hofbauer GL, et al: Swiss clinical practice guidelines for skin cancer in organ transplant recipients. Swiss Med Wkly 2009; 139:407.

Iaria G, et al: Conversion to rapamycin immunosuppression for malignancy after kidney transplantation: case reports. Transplant Proc 2007; 39:2036.

Ingvar A, et al: Immunosuppressive treatment after solid organ transplantation and risk of post-transplant cutaneous squamous cell carcinoma. Nephrol Dial Transplant 2009 Sep 3 (Epub ahead of print).

Kerbleski JF, Gottlieb AB: Dermatological complications and safety of anti-TNF treatments. Gut 2009; 58:1033.

Khanna M, et al: Histopathologic evaluation of cutaneous squamous cell carcinoma: results of a survey among dermatopathologists. J Am Acad Dermatol 2003; 48:721.

Koch A, et al: Polydactylous Bowen's disease. J Eur Acad Dermatol Venereol 2003; 17:213.

Lindelöf B, et al: Cutaneous squamous cell carcinoma in organ transplant recipients. Arch Dermatol 2005; 141:447.

McCall CO, Chen SC: Squamous cell carcinoma of the legs in African Americans. J Am Acad Dermatol 2002; 47:524.

McQuillan RF, et al: The effect of switching from calcineurin inhibitor to sirolimus on the incidence of skin cancers in kidney transplant recipients. J Eur Acad Dermatol Venereol 2009; 23:330.

Mendonca H, et al: Squamous cell carcinoma arising in hidradenitis suppurativa. J Dermatol Surg Oncol 1991; 17:830.

Motley R, Lawrence C: Multiprofessional guidelines for the management of the patient with primary cutaneous squamous cell carcinoma. Br J Dermatol 2002; 146:18.

Nijsten TEC, Stern RS: Oral retinoid use reduces cutaneous squamous cell carcinoma risk in patients with psoriasis treated with psoralen-UVA: a nested cohort study. J Am Acad Dermatol 2003; 49:644.

Paghdal KV, Schwartz RA: Sirolimus (rapamycin): from the soil of Easter Island to a bright future. J Am Acad Dermatol 2007; 57:1046.

Rival-Tringali AL, et al: Conversion from calcineurin inhibitors to sirolimus reduces vascularization and thickness of post-transplant cutaneous squamous cell carcinomas. Anticancer Res 2009; 29:1927.

Schulz TF: Cancer and viral infections in immunocompromised individuals. Int J Cancer 2009; 125:1755.

Sheppard J, et al: Skin cancer in psoriatic arthritis treated with anti-TNF therapy. Rheumatology (Oxford) 2007; 46:1622.

Takeda H, et al: Multiple squamous cell carcinomas in situ in vitiligo lesions after long-term PUVA therapy. J Am Acad Dermatol 1998; 38:268.

van Leeuwen MT, et al: Immunosuppression and other risk factors for lip cancer after kidney transplantation. Cancer Epidemiol Biomarkers Prev 2009; 18:561.

Wennberg AM, et al: Photodynamic therapy with methyl aminolevulinate for prevention of new skin lesions in transplant recipients: a randomized study. Transplantation 2008; 86:423.

Wisgerhof HC, et al: Trends of skin diseases in organ-transplant recipients transplanted between 1966 and 2006: a cohort study with follow-up between 1994 and 2006. Br J Dermatol 2009 Oct 3 (Epub ahead of print).

Verrucous carcinoma (carcinoma cuniculatum)

Verrucous carcinoma is a distinct, well-differentiated, low-grade SCC. It affects mostly elderly men. The primary characteristic of these lesions is their close resemblance, clinically and histologically, to a wart. The lesions present as a bulbous mass with a soft consistency and often multiple sinuses opening to the surface, resembling "rabbit burrows." Lesions of this type are most common on the sole, but also occur in the genital area (Fig. 29-23) (giant condyloma of Buschke and Lowenstein), and in the oral mucosa. In some cases, as in the Buschke–Lowenstein tumor, verrucous carcinomas are induced by HPV. These HPV may be of the "low-risk" types, such as HPV-6 or 11, or the high-risk types, such as HPV-16. In other cases no HPV can be found, and pressure or other factors (but not UV light) are felt to play a role. The natural history is of a slow-growing mass that over years may invade the bones beneath the tumor.

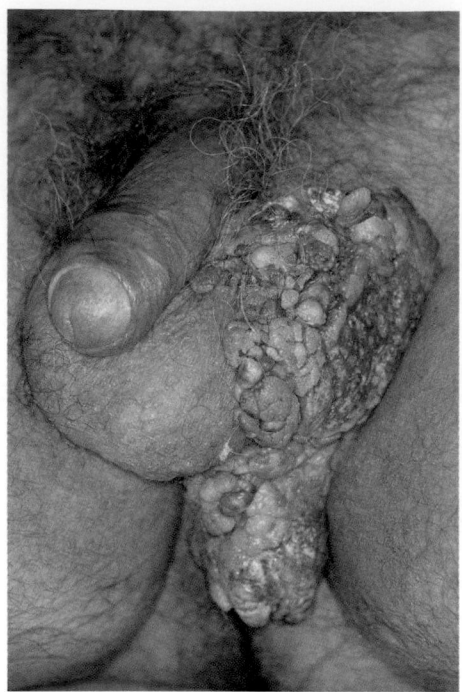

Fig. 29-23 Giant condyloma of Buschke and Lowenstein.

Histologically, the lesion shows a characteristic picture of bulbous rete ridges that are topped by an undulating keratinized mass. The squamous epithelium is well differentiated and cytologic atypia is minimal. The cytoplasm is often apple-pink and may have a glassy appearance. The tumor border is smooth and bulldozing, rather than spiky and infiltrative.

Excision is the best treatment and Mohs microsurgery may be a helpful technique. Radiotherapy may induce anaplastic transformation and is best avoided if other treatment options exist. Lymph node metastasis is rare and the prognosis is favorable when complete excision is accomplished.

Assaf C, et al: Verrucous carcinoma of the axilla: case report and review. J Cutan Pathol 2004; 31:199.

Bhushan M, et al: Carcinoma cuniculatum of the foot assessed by magnetic resonance scanning. Clin Exp Dermatol 2001; 26:419.

Cassarino DS, et al: Cutaneous squamous cell carcinoma: a comprehensive clinicopathologic classification. Part one. J Cutan Pathol 2006; 33:191.

Castano E, et al: Verrucous carcinoma in association with hypertrophic lichen planus. Clin Exp Dermatol 1997; 22:23.

D'Aniello C, et al: Verrucous "cuniculatum" carcinoma of the sacral region. Br J Dermatol 2000; 143:459.

Ho J, et al: An ulcerating verrucous plaque on the foot. Arch Dermatol 2000; 136:547.

Kanik AB, et al: Penile verrucous carcinoma in a 37-year-old circumcised man. J Am Acad Dermatol 1997; 37:329.

Koch H, et al: Verrucous carcinoma of the skin: long-term follow-up results following surgical therapy. Dermatol Surg 2004; 30:1124.

Lee KY, et al: Verrucous carcinoma of the foot from chronic pressure ulcer. Spinal Cord 2004; 42:431.

Bowen's disease (squamous cell carcinoma in situ)

Bowen's disease (BD) is intraepidermal SCC. There are multiple possible agents that can induce BD: HPV of certain types, arsenic exposure, and sun exposure. An association with the Merkel cell polyomavirus has been reported in immunosuppressed patients. The origin of the cells developing into BD is unknown, but might be a pluripotential epidermal cell. BD may ultimately become invasive. When it does, it may have an aggressive biological behavior.

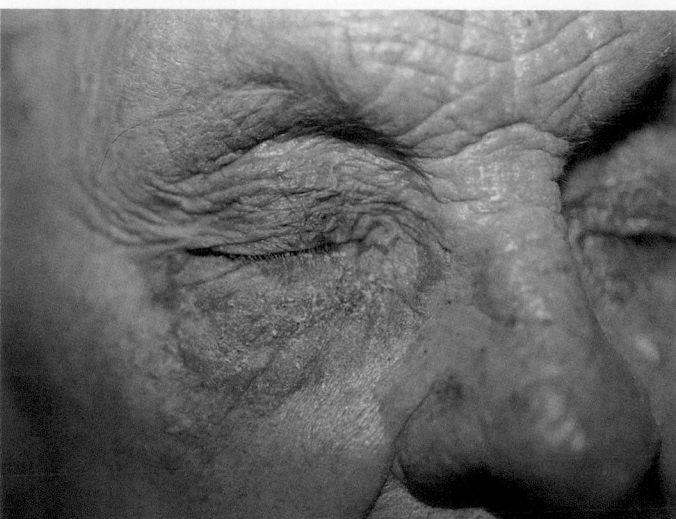

Fig. 29-24 Bowen's disease.

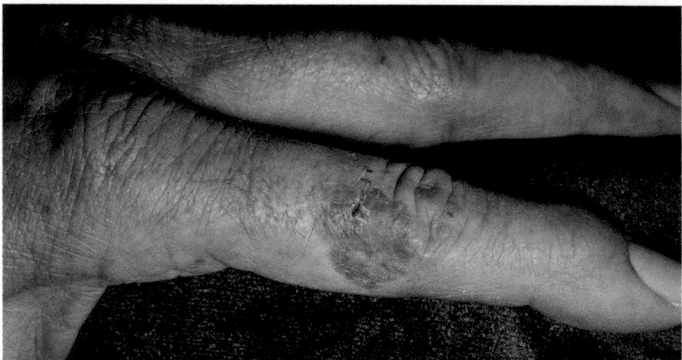

Fig. 29-25 Bowen's disease.

Clinical features

BD may be found on any part of the body as an erythematous, slightly scaly and crusted, noninfiltrated patch from a few millimeters to many centimeters in diameter (Figs 29-24 and 29-25). The lesion is sharply defined. The scale may be pronounced enough for the lesions to be mistaken for psoriasis, or the plaque may have a stuck on appearance and may be mistaken for a broad sessile seborrheic keratosis. Papillated keratotic lesions can occur. Invasion is often indicated by the development of an exophytic, endophytic, or ulcerative component. A rare but particularly difficult clinical scenario is the elderly female patient with multicentric BD of the shins.

As the lesion slowly enlarges, spontaneous cicatrization may develop in portions of the lesion. When the intraepithelial growth becomes invasive, the lesion may appear ulcerated and fungating. The squamous carcinoma that evolves from BD tends to be more aggressive than SCC arising in actinic keratosis. When SCC in situ occurs as a velvety plaque on the glans penis, it is referred to as erythroplasia of Queyrat (see below).

BD around or beneath the nail can be difficult to diagnose. It can present as a red (erythronychia) or black/brown (melanonychia) longitudinal band of several millimeters in width. HPV may be associated with these lesions, which should be biopsied.

Histopathology

The atypical keratinocytes may invade the adjacent epidermis in a buckshot or clonal nested pattern. With time, they may replace the entire epidermis, often with deep, full-thickness involvement of adnexal structures, especially the hair follicles. The epidermis shows hyperkeratosis, parakeratosis, and broad acanthosis or anastomosis of adjacent rete ridges. Epidermal maturation is absent, so the epidermis appears disorganized, and individually keratinizing cells and atypical cells are seen at all levels of the epidermis. There is, however, a sharp delineation between dermis and epidermis, and the basement membrane is intact. The upper dermis usually shows a chronic inflammatory infiltrate. Although the cells tend to be anaplastic with a high nuclear to cytoplasmic ratio, variants with smaller nuclei and abundant cytoplasm exist and transitional areas between the patterns may be seen. Invasive lesions of BD tend to have a squamoid to basaloid appearance, with central necrosis. Adnexal differentiation may be present.

Differential diagnosis

BD is frequently misdiagnosed as psoriasis, superficial multicentric BCC, tinea corporis, nummular eczema, seborrheic keratosis, and actinic keratosis. Paget's disease, especially the extramammary type, may mimic Bowen's disease, not only clinically but also histologically. There is no dyskeratosis in Paget's disease and the intervening nonvacuolated epidermal cells are not atypical in Paget's disease. Stains for mucin and carcinoembryonic antigen are positive in Paget's disease and negative in pagetoid BD. BD may be heavily pigmented, especially when occurring in the anogenital region. Lesions of bowenoid papulosis show a histologic spectrum from genital warts with buckshot atypia to full-thickness atypia indistinguishable from BD. If the lesions are multicentric and behave like genital warts, the term bowenoid papulosis may be applied. Treatment is guided completely by the clinical pattern. Since genital SCC is induced by high-risk HPV, bowenoid papulosis represents the initial clinical lesion in the progression from HPV infection to carcinoma. There is no clear boundary where bowenoid papulosis stops and SCC in situ begins.

Treatment

Topical treatment of SCC in situ with cryotherapy and topical 5-FU has been disappointing due to a high rate of recurrence. Imiquimod 5% cream, applied once a day for up to 16 weeks, seems to be effective enough to be recommended as a therapeutic option. Response rates have been as high as 90%. It may allow treatment of large lesions that might be difficult to approach surgically. Combination treatment with imiquimod 5% cream, three times a week, and 5% 5-FU, twice a day (except at the times of the imiquimod application), has also been reported as effective. Tazarotene could be added to this treatment for hyperkeratotic lesions or to enhance penetration. Photodynamic therapy can be considered.

Simple excision of small lesions is a reasonable treatment option. Large, ill-defined lesions, or lesions in which preservation of normal tissue is critical, are indications for Mohs microsurgery. Other surgical techniques to treat SCC in situ are described in Chapter 37. Curettage and desiccation may also be performed, but recurrence may occur if the extension down the follicles is not eradicated. Lesions of the lower legs are particularly problematic, as they are often multiple, and in the elderly are often found in conjunction with significant venous insufficiency. Any form of therapy may result in chronic leg ulceration in this setting. Consideration should be given to using a compression bandage after surgery identical to one applied to a chronic leg ulcer. This may prevent ulceration.

Ball SB, et al: Treatment of cutaneous Bowen's disease with particular emphasis on the problem of lower leg lesions. Australas J Dermatol 1998; 39:63.

Calzavara-Pinton PG, et al: Methylaminolaevulinate-based photodynamic therapy of Bowen's disease and squamous cell carcinoma. Br J Dermatol 2008; 159:137.

Cassarino DS, et al: Cutaneous squamous cell carcinoma: a comprehensive clinicopathologic classification. Part one. J Cutan Pathol 2006; 33:191.

Cassarino DS, et al: Cutaneous squamous cell carcinoma: a comprehensive clinicopathologic classification. Part two. J Cutan Pathol 2006; 33:261.

Chen K, Shumack S: Treatment of Bowen's disease using a cycle regimen of imiquimod 5% cream. Clin Exp Dermatol 2003; 28:10.

Chen S, et al: Immunohistochemical analysis of the mammalian target of rapamycin signalling pathway in extramammary Paget's disease. Br J Dermatol 2009; 161:357.

Christensen E, et al: Guidelines for practical use of MAL-PDT in non-melanoma skin cancer. J Eur Acad Dermatol Venereol 2009 Oct 6 (Epub ahead of print).

Cox NH, et al: Guidelines for management of Bowen's disease. Br J Dermatol 1999; 141:633.

de Berker DA, et al: Localized longitudinal erythronychia: diagnostic significance and physical explanation. Arch Dermatol 2004; 140:1253.

Gonzalez-Perez R, et al: Metastatic squamous cell carcinoma arising in Bowen's disease of the palm. J Am Acad Dermatol 1997; 36:635.

Kassem A, et al: Merkel cell polyomavirus sequences are frequently detected in nonmelanoma skin cancer of immunosuppressed patients. Int J Cancer 2009; 125:356.

Mackenzie-Wood A, et al: Imiquimod 5% cream in the treatment of Bowen's disease. J Am Acad Dermatol 2001; 44:462.

Modi G, et al: Combination therapy with imiquimod, 5fluorouracil, and tazarotene in the treatment of extensive radiation-induced Bowen's disease of the hands. Dermatol Surg 2009 Sep 1 (Epub ahead of print).

Muzio G, et al: Occlusive medication with imiquimod in Bowen's disease. Acta Derm Venereol 2004; 84:168.

Prinz BM, et al: Treatment of Bowen's disease with imiquimod 5% cream in transplant recipients. Transplantation 2004; 15:790.

Shimizu A, et al: Detection of human papillomavirus type 56 in Bowen's disease involving the nail matrix. Br J Dermatol 2008; 158:1273.

Sun JD, Barr RJ: Papillated Bowen disease, a distinct variant. Am J Dermatopathol 2006; 28:395.

Takahagi S, et al: Metastatic extramammary Paget's disease treated with paclitaxel and trastuzumab combination chemotherapy. J Dermatol 2009; 36:457.

Erythroplasia of Queyrat

Erythroplasia of Queyrat is SCC in situ of the glans penis or prepuce. SCC in situ on the penile shaft also occurs. Both conditions are caused by high-risk HPV types (16, 18, 31, 35). Clinically, erythroplasia of Queyrat is characterized by single or multiple, fixed, well-circumscribed, erythematous, moist, velvety or smooth, red-surfaced plaques on the glans penis (Fig. 29-26). Uncircumcised men, usually over age 40, are most commonly affected, and when SCC in situ affects the penile shaft it is usually distally under the foreskin. The differential diagnosis includes Zoon's balanitis, candidiasis, penile psoriasis, irritant balanitis, and extramammary Paget's disease. A biopsy is usually indicated to confirm the diagnosis. The intensity of the inflammatory infiltrate under lesions of erythroplasia of Queyrat can be great and plasma cells can be numerous. This may lead to the histological misdiagnosis of both erythroplasia and Zoon's balanitis occurring simultaneously or sequentially.

Since red lesions on the glans of elderly uncircumcised men are common, the following factors suggest that a biopsy is indicated:

1. The lesion is fixed (does not move or resolve).
2. The patient lacks other stigmata of psoriasis or another skin disease that could affect the glans penis.

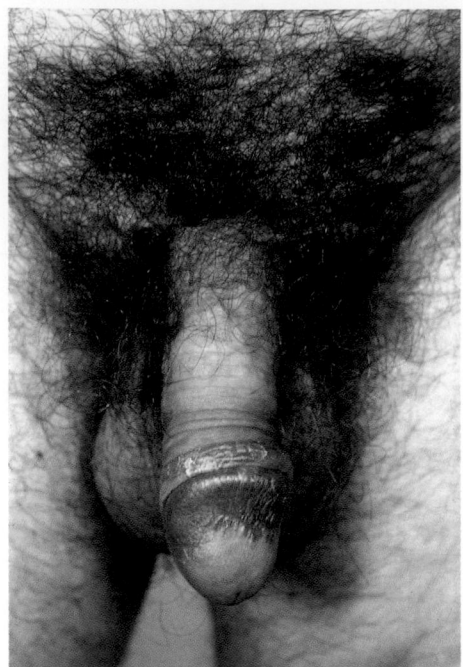

Fig. 29-26 Erythroplasia of Queyrat.

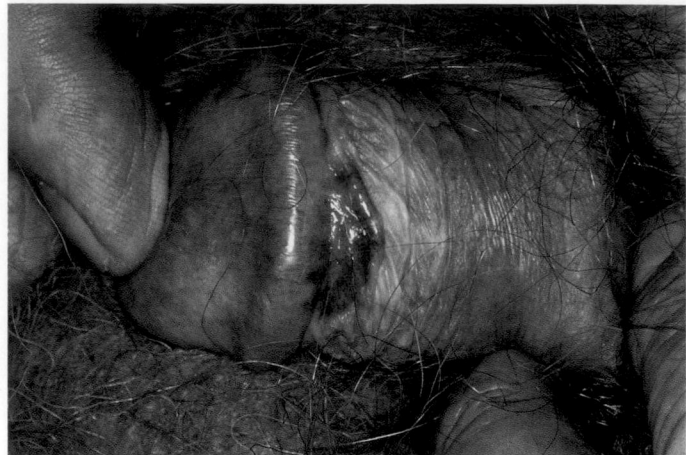

Fig. 29-27 Zoon's balanitis.

3. The patient's sexual partner has cervical dysplasia.
4. The lesion does not resolve with effective topical therapy for irritant balanitis, candidiasis, and psoriasis.

Once the diagnosis of SCC in situ of the penis is made, the patient's sex partner(s) should be referred for evaluation. Sexual partners of men with SCC of the penis are more likely to develop preinvasive and invasive cancer of the cervix or anus.

Progression to invasive SCC is more common in erythroplasia of Queyrat than in Bowen's disease of the nongenital skin, and the resulting SCCs are more aggressive and tend to metastasize earlier than those that develop in Bowen's disease of the nongenital skin. There is no evidence of an increase in internal malignancy in patients with erythroplasia.

Topical therapy can be effective in the treatment of erythroplasia of Queyrat and has the advantage that it can identify and treat areas not visible clinically. Topical 5% 5-FU cream applied once a day under occlusion (with the foreskin or a condom) can be effective. It will induce a brisk reaction and superficial erosion, which can be uncomfortable. Treatment is continued for 3–12 weeks, depending on the response. Imiquimod cream 5%, applied between once a day and three times a week, will similarly induce a significant reaction, but after 3–12 weeks may clear the lesion. Careful follow-up is required, especially for the first few years. Surgical modalities such as excision, laser treatments, and photodynamic therapy are reserved for cases failing topical treatments. Radiation therapy can also be effective.

Arlette JP: Treatment of Bowen's disease and erythroplasia of Queyrat. Br J Dermatol 2003; 149:43.

Danielsen AG, et al: Treatment of Bowen's disease of the penis with imiquimod 5% cream. Clin Exp Dermatol 2003; 28:7.

Divakaruni AK, et al: Erythroplasia of Queyrat with Zoon's balanitis: a diagnostic dilemma. Int J STD AIDS 2008; 19:861.

Orengo I, et al: Treatment of squamous cell carcinoma in situ of the penis with 5% imiquimod cream: a case report. J Am Acad Dermatol 2002; 47:S225.

Schroeder TL, Sengelmann RD: Squamous cell carcinoma in situ of the penis successfully treated with imiquimod 5% cream. J Am Acad Dermatol 2002; 46:545.

Balanitis plasmacellularis (Zoon's balanitis)

Balanitis plasmacellularis is also known as balanoposthitis chronica circumscripta plasmacellularis or Zoon's balanitis. Zoon's balanitis represents about 7% of persistent genital lesions biopsied for diagnosis. It is a benign inflammatory lesion of the glans penis, which histologically demonstrates a plasma cell-rich infiltrate. The plasma cell infiltrate, while characteristic, may not be present in all lesions of this type, and in fact, some researchers feel there is a spectrum of histology in idiopathic, benign, nonscarring balanitis, from lesions containing few plasma cells to lesions containing many plasma cells. Clinically, Zoon's balanitis is characterized by a red patch, which is usually sharply demarcated and usually on the inner surface of the prepuce or on the glans penis (Fig. 29-27). The lesion is erythematous, moist, and shiny. It occurs as a single lesion, but may consist of several confluent macules. It is asymptomatic and does not produce inguinal adenopathy. Uncircumcised men from ages 24 to 85 are most often affected.

Vulvitis chronica plasmacellularis is the counterpart of balanitis in women. The vulva shows a striking lacquer-like luster. Erosions, punctate hemorrhage, synechiae, and a slate to ochre pigmentation may supervene.

Plasmacytosis circumorificialis is the same disease on the oral mucosa, lips, cheeks, and tongue. The differential diagnosis of Zoon's balanitis is penile psoriasis, lichen planus, lichen sclerosus, and SCC in situ. Histologically, the epidermis is atrophic, with flattened diamond-shaped keratinocytes and mild spongiosis. In the papillary dermis a band of infiltrate consisting almost exclusively of plasma cells is present. Dilated vessels are also seen. This picture is strikingly different from that of the main clinical differential diagnosis, erythroplasia of Queyrat, in which the epidermis is principally involved, with atypia of keratinocytes throughout the entire epithelium. HPV has not been detected. Topical steroids, alone or in combination with anticandidal treatment, are helpful. Potent topical steroids, pimecrolimus cream 1%, tacrolimus ointment 0.1%, and imiquimod cream 5% have all been reported as effective in selected cases. Circumcision may be curative. Laser ablation can also be effective.

Albertini JG, et al: Zoon's balanitis treated with erbium:YAG laser ablation. Lasers Surg Med 2002; 30:123.

Alessi E, et al: Review of 120 biopsies performed on the balanopreputial sac. From Zoon's balanitis to the concept of a wider spectrum of inflammatory non-cicatricial balanoposthitis. Dermatology 2004; 208:120.

Bardazzi F, et al: Two cases of Zoon's balanitis treated with pimecrolimus 1% cream. Int J Dermatol 2008; 47:198.

Ferrandiz C, et al: Zoon's balanitis treated with circumcision. J Dermatol Surg Oncol 1984; 10:622.

Hague J, Ilchyshyn A: Successful treatment of Zoon's balanitis with topical tacrolimus. Int J Dermatol 2006; 45:1251.

Marconi B, et al: Zoon's balanitis treated with imiquimod 5% cream. Eur J Dermatol 2010; 20:134.

Palamaras I, et al: The usefulness of a diagnostic biopsy clinic in a genitourinary medicine setting: recent experience and a review of the literature. J Eur Acad Dermatol Venereol 2006; 20:905.

Retamar RA, et al: Zoon's balanitis: presentation of 15 patients, five treated with a carbon dioxide laser. Int J Dermatol 2003; 42:305.

Tang A, et al: Plasma cell balanitis of Zoon: response to Trimovate cream. Int J STD AIDS 2001; 12:75.

Virgili A, et al: Tacrolimus 0.1% ointment: is it really effective in plasma cell vulvitis? Report of four cases. Dermatology 2008; 216:243.

Pseudoepitheliomatous keratotic and micaceous balanitis

Pseudoepitheliomatous keratotic and micaceous balanitis was described by Lortat-Jacob and Civatte in 1966. The lesions occurring on the glans penis are verrucous excrescences with scaling. Ulcerations, cracking, and fissuring on the surface of the glans are frequently present. The keratotic scale is usually micaceous and resembles psoriasis. Most patients are over the age of 50 and frequently have been circumcised for phimosis in adult life.

Histologically, there is marked hyperkeratosis and para-keratosis, as well as pseudoepitheliomatous hyperplasia. Acanthotic masses give rise to a crater-like configuration. HPV has not been detected. This is probably best considered as a form of verrucous carcinoma. The treatment is usually surgical and might include Mohs microsurgery. Topical 5-FU has been effective, but the hyperkeratotic scale may make penetration suboptimal. If topical chemotherapy is utilized, post-treatment biopsies are recommended.

Child FJ, et al: Verrucous carcinoma arising in pseudoepitheliomatous keratotic and micaceous balanitis, without evidence of human papillomavirus. Br J Dermatol 2000; 143:183.

Ganem JP, et al: Pseudo-epitheliomatous keratotic and micaceous balanitis. J Urol 1999; 161:217.

Perry D, et al: Pseudoepitheliomatous, keratotic, and micaceous balanitis: case report and review of the literature. Dermatol Nurs 2008; 20:117.

Zawar V, et al: "Watering-can penis" in pseudoepitheliomatous, keratotic and micaceous balanitis. Acta Derm Venereol 2004; 84:329.

Paget's disease of the breast

Clinical features

Paget's disease (PD) of the nipple affects largely women (there are very rare male cases). It is how between 1% and 4% of breast carcinomas present. PD is characterized by a unilateral, sharply marginated, erythematous, and at times crusted patch or plaque affecting the nipple and occasionally the areola (Fig. 29-28). At times it may be hyperpigmented. As the lesion grows, it may spread to the areola, and even beyond, making the areolae appear asymmetric. Over the course of months or years it may become eroded. The nipple may or may not be retracted. In advanced cases, a subjacent mass and ipsilateral axillary adenopathy may be palpable. About 5% of patients have PD without confirmed evidence of underlying carcinoma, and the remaining 95% have either an invasive or an intraductal carcinoma in proportions between 35% and 65%, depending on the reporting center. In rare cases, even when no underlying carcinoma is found on surgical removal, the sentinel node may be positive.

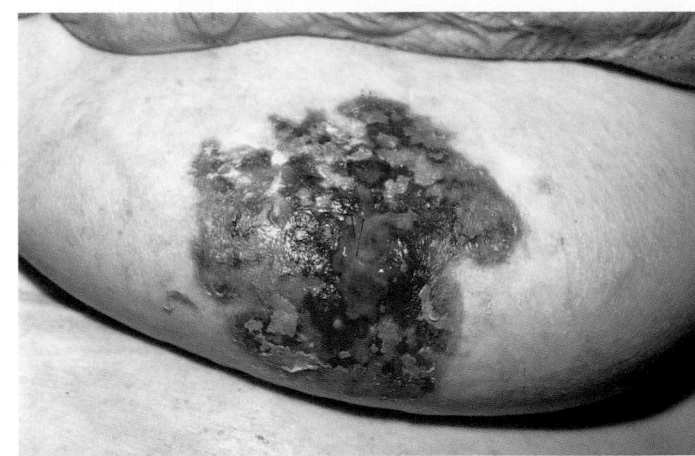

Fig. 29-28 Paget's disease of the breast.

Histopathology

PD is characterized by the presence of Paget cells: large, round, pale-staining cells with large nuclei. Intercellular bridges are absent. The cells appear singly or in small nests between the squamous cells. Usually, acanthosis is present, the granular layer is preserved, and there is no parakeratosis, but atypical cells may be "spat out" into the stratum corneum. Frequently, a layer of basal cells separates the Paget cells from the basement membrane and is seen crushed beneath the nests of Paget cells. This histologic feature helps to distinguish PD from pagetoid melanoma and Bowen's disease. In the dermis an inflammatory reaction is often present. Unusual variants include PD with marker intraepidermal melanin and an acantholytic anaplastic form.

The Paget cell is PAS-positive, diastase-resistant, almost always HER-2/neu-positive, and EMA-positive; it stains with CAM 5.2 and CK 7. This staining profile and negativity for S-100 and cytokeratins 5/6 allow clear distinction from pagetoid melanoma and pagetoid Bowen's disease. Carcinoembryonic antigen (CEA) positivity is variable in PD of the breast, being positive in only 0–50% of PD cases, but virtually 100% of extramammary PD cases (see below). The Toker cell, a normal clear cell of the breast, stains similarly, but is Her-2/neu-negative. It has been proposed as the precursor cell of PD, and may be so for some cases of PD with no underlying breast cancer.

Diagnosis

The presence of unilateral eczema of the nipple recalcitrant to simple treatment should lead to suspicion of PD and the lesion should be biopsied. The presence of bilateral lesions suggests a benign process, usually atopic dermatitis. Papillary adenoma of the nipple clinically resembles PD, but on biopsy shows a papillary and adenomatous growth in the dermis with connection to the surface. There is a lining of apocrine-type secretory epithelium. Hyperkeratosis of the nipple and areola may occasionally be unilateral, but histologically reveals only hyperkeratosis, acanthosis, and papillomatosis.

Treatment

Patients with PD of the breast should be referred to a center with expertise in the management of breast cancer.

Bernardi M, et al: Paget disease in a man. Arch Dermatol 2008; 144:1660.

Brummer O, et al: HER-2/neu expression in Paget's disease of the vulva and the female breast. Gynecol Oncol 2004; 95:336.

Caliskan M, et al: Paget's disease of the breast: the experience of the European Institute of Oncology and review of the literature. Breast Cancer Res Treat 2008; 112:513.

Faten Z, et al: Pigmented mammary Paget's disease mimicking melanoma: a further case in a man. Breast J 2009; 15:420.

Garijo MF, et al: An overview of the pale and clear cells of the nipple epidermis. Histol Histopathol 2009; 24:367.

Hanna W, et al: The role of HER-2/neu oncogene and vimentin filaments in the production of the Paget's phenotype. Breast J 2003; 9:485.

Lau J, Kohler S: Keratin profile of intraepidermal cells in Paget's disease, extramammary Paget's disease, and pagetoid squamous cell carcinoma in situ. J Cutan Pathol 2003; 30:449.

Lester T, et al: Different panels of markers should be used to predict mammary Paget's disease associated with in situ or invasive ductal carcinoma of the breast. Ann Clin Lab Sci 2009; 39:17.

Liu W, et al: Mammary Paget's disease and extra-mammary Paget's disease: two morphologically similar but biologically different diseases. J Cutan Pathol 2009 Aug 27 (Epub ahead of print).

Miller L, et al: Erosive adenomatosis of the nipple: a benign imitator of malignant breast disease. Cutis 1997; 59:91.

Mobini N: Acantholytic anaplastic Paget's disease. J Cutan Pathol 2009; 36:374.

Montemarano AD, et al: Superficial papillary adenomatosis of the nipple: a case report and review of the literature. J Am Acad Dermatol 1997; 36:871.

Nofech-Mozes S, Hanna W: Toker cells revisited. Breast J 2009; 15:394.

Oiso N, et al: Pigmented spots as a sign of mammary Paget's disease. Clin Exp Dermatol 2009; 34:36.

Petersson F, et al: Pigmented Paget disease—a diagnostic pitfall mimicking melanoma. Am J Dermatopathol 2009; 31:223.

Tanaka VD, et al: Mammary and extramammary Paget's disease: a study of 14 cases and the associated therapeutic difficulties. Clinics (Sao Paulo) 2009; 64:599.

Wang CC, et al: Pigmented mammary Paget's disease presenting as an enlarged areola. Breast J 2009; 15:421.

Extramammary Paget's disease

Extramammary Paget's disease (EMPD) is much less common than PD. It affects adults, usually between 65 and 70 years of age. The vulva is the most common location, except perhaps in China, where penoscrotal EMPD is reported in large numbers. Penoscrotal EMPD is uncommon in black persons. EMPD presents most commonly as a unifocal process, but multifocal lesions may occur (including cases involving as many as four anatomic locations simultaneously). Axillary lesions typically appear with or after genital lesions and are more frequent in men. Lesions typically affect apocrine sites, including the groin (vulva, scrotum, perianal area, penis, and inguinal folds) (Fig. 29-29) and axilla, but rare cases can affect other anatomic locations. The lesions of EMPD are typically erythematous, well-demarcated plaques measuring several centimeters in diameter. They may involve any region of the genitalia, including the penis, scrotum, vulva, or perianal skin. The condition often goes undiagnosed for months to years, as the misdiagnoses of pruritus ani, a fungal infection, contact dermatitis, lichen sclerosus, or intertrigo are made. A nonhealing banal eczematous patch persisting in the anogenital or axillary region should raise concern about EMPD, and trigger a biopsy. Intense pruritus is common. Bleeding, nodularity, and induration are late signs. Underpants erythema, or redness in the whole genital area, may be indicative of widespread lymphatic involvement in the pelvic basin and is a poor prognostic sign. Lesions may be hyperpigmented or hypopigmented.

EMPD can be divided into four forms:

1. primary EMPD (arising intraepidermally), with or without invasion

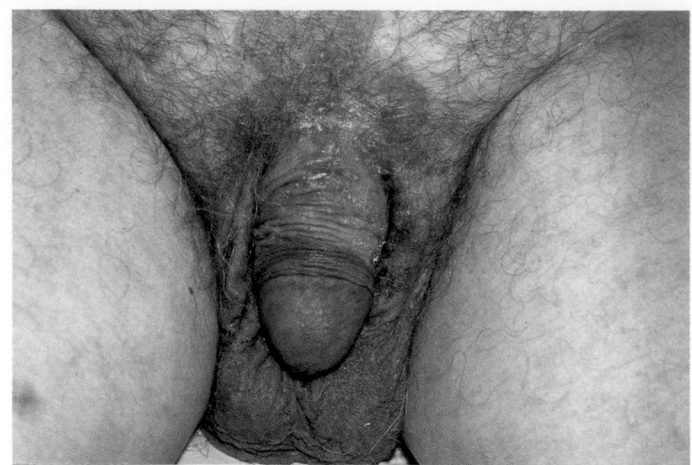

Fig. 29-29 Extramammary Paget's disease.

2. EMPD associated with an underlying apocrine carcinoma
3. EMPD associated with an underlying adjacent malignancy
4. EMPD associated with an underlying distant carcinoma.

The majority of patients with EMPD do not have underlying carcinoma, and the process apparently begins as an intraepidermal neoplasm, which can then invade (invasive EMPD). The clinical appearance of all types of EMPD is identical. The location of the EMPD determines the percentage of patients who have other associated malignancies. In vulvar EMPD 4–17% have an associated adnexal neoplasm, and 11–20% have a distant carcinoma of the breast, cervix, vagina, bladder, colon, rectum, ovary, liver, gallbladder, or skin. In perianal EMPD an underlying adnexal carcinoma occurs in 7–10% of cases, and a distant carcinoma of the rectum, stomach, breast, or ureter in 15–45%. Penoscrotal EMPD has an associated carcinoma of the prostate, bladder, testicles, ureter, or kidney in 11% of cases. In a large series from the Netherlands, underlying malignancy was found in 35% of patients with EMPD. In all patients with EMPD, an extensive and targeted cancer workup should be undertaken, depending on the histological staining pattern (see below) and the location.

Histologically, the findings are similar to those found in mammary PD: acanthosis hyperkeratosis, parakeratosis, or both, and pale, vacuolated Paget cells in suprabasilar levels of the epithelium. Signet ring Paget's cells are present in a small minority of cases. Paget cells can form nests that compress basal keratinocytes. Conventional histopathologic findings are similar in both primary cutaneous EMPD and most cases in which EMPD is due to an underlying malignancy. Mucin, stainable by alcian blue or colloidal iron, is present in the majority of cases. The finding of cytoplasmic mucin makes a urothelial origin unlikely. Significant effort has been put into developing a series of stains that would clearly distinguish PD from EMPD and identify those cases that have underlying carcinomas, either local apocrine cancers or distant neoplasms. This involves looking at the expression of various cytokeratins, mucins, and other products specific to certain organ systems. RCAS1 may be very sensitive for EMPD cells, and measurement of serum levels of this marker can be used to monitor patients with invasive disease (analogous to following the prostate-specific antigen in patients with treated prostate cancer). In vulvar and perianal EMPD, two distinct staining patterns have been defined. CK7+/CK20+/GCDFP15-negative is called the type I or endodermal pattern. It is associated with EMPD and distant cancers. Ectodermal or cutaneous pattern (type II) stains the atypical cells CD7+/CK20-/GCDFP15-positive. This is associated with a cutaneous origin for the EMPD. In addition, tissue-specific markers may at times identify the distant tumor responsible for the EMPD. Immunohistochemical studies can provide some guidance in distinguishing between these possibilities, largely through identifying antigens that are not found on the cells of primary cutaneous EMPD. The specificity of these studies is limited, but a positive finding of an immunoprofile that differs from that of typical primary EMPD should lead to a thorough investigation. Primary cutaneous EMPD has an immunophenotype similar to that of apocrine epithelium: cytokeratin 7-positive, cytokeratin 20-negative, and CEA-positive. Cases due to spread from an underlying bladder carcinoma are typically uroplakin- and p63-positive. Those due to rectal carcinoma are usually CK7-negative, CDX2-positive, and CK20-positive. Prostatic adenocarcinoma can also result in extramammary PD, and can be identified by staining for PSA or the marker, P504S. Unfortunately, PSA positivity can be seen in female patients with EMPD, and not all males with PSA positivity of the EMPD cells have underlying prostate cancer. p63 staining in vulvar EMPD suggests an underlying urothelial carcinoma. Staining with AKT, CDK2, mTOR, and other proteins in the mTOR pathway suggests that this pathway may be important in the pathogenesis of EMPD.

EMPD can remain within the epithelium or "invade" the dermis. "Invasive" EMPD has a high rate of metastasis and a very poor prognosis. Sentinel node examination of patients with "invasive" EMPD should be considered, as it predicts the risk for metastases.

Surgical removal is the treatment of choice, with Mohs microsurgery having a better outcome than fixed surgical margins. Despite what appears to be adequate margins, recurrence rates are high because of the discontinuous and microscopic wide extension of EMPD. The recurrence rate following micrographic surgery is around 25%, and over 30% for standard 2 cm margins. Imiquimod has been used with success in multiple reports, but follow-up is limited. Radiation therapy, photodynamic therapy, and laser treatments have also been used. Intralesional IFN-α2b was beneficial in one case. Some cases of genital EMPD are HER-2/neu-positive and have responded to trastuzumab, a monoclonal antibody directed against HER2.

Abe S, et al: Quadruple extra-mammary Paget's disease. Acta Derm Venereol 2007; 87:80.

Anolik R, et al: Extramammary Paget disease. Dermatol Online J 2008; 14:15.

Bagby CM, MacLennan GT: Extramammary Paget's disease of the penis and scrotum. J Urol 2009; 182:2908.

Berman B, et al: Successful treatment of extramammary Paget's disease of the scrotum with imiquimod 5% cream. Clin Exp Dermatol 2003; 28:36.

Brummer O, et al: HER-2/neu expression in Paget's disease of the vulva and the female breast. Gynecol Oncol 2004; 95:336.

Challenor R, et al: Multidisciplinary treatment of vulval extramammary Paget's disease to maintain sexual function: an imiquimod success story. J Obstet Gynaecol 2009; 29:252.

Chen S, et al: Immunohistochemical analysis of the mammalian target of rapamycin signalling pathway in extramammary Paget's disease. Br J Dermatol 2009; 161:357.

Chen YH, et al: Depigmented genital extramammary Paget's disease: a possible histogenetic link to Toker's clear cells and clear cell papulosis. J Cutan Pathol 2001; 28:105.

Fujisawa Y, et al: Penile preservation surgery in a case of extramammary Paget's disease involving the glans penis and distal urethra. Dermatol Surg 2008; 34:823.

Fukui T, et al: Photodynamic therapy following carbon dioxide laser enhances efficacy in the treatment of extramammary Paget's disease. Acta Derm Venereol 2009:89:150.

Hammer A, et al: Prostate-specific antigen-positive extramammary Paget's disease—association with prostate cancer. APMIS 2008; 116:81.

Hatta N, et al: Sentinel lymph node biopsy in patients with extramammary Paget's disease. Dermatol Surg 2004; 30:1329.

Hatta N, et al: Extramammary Paget's disease: treatment, prognostic factors and outcome in 76 patients. Br J Dermatol 2008; 158:313.

Hendi A, et al: Unifocality of extramammary Paget disease. J Am Acad Dermatol 2008; 59:811.

Hilliard NJ, et al: Pigmented extramammary Paget's disease of the axilla mimicking melanoma: case report and review of the literature. J Cutan Pathol 2009; 36:995.

Im M, et al: Extramammary Paget's disease of the scrotum with adenocarcinoma of the stomach. J Am Acad Dermatol 2007; 57:S43.

Kanitakis J: Mammary and extramammary Paget's disease. J Eur Acad Dermatol Venereol 2007; 21:581.

Karam A, et al: HER-2/neu targeting for recurrent vulvar Paget's disease. A case report and literature review. Gynecol Oncol 2008; 111:568.

Kim TH, et al: Extramammary Paget's disease of scrotum treated with radiotherapy. Urology 2009; 74:474.e1.

Kondo Y, et al: The ectopic expression of gastric mucin in oxtramammary and mammary Paget's disease. Am J Surg Pathol 2002; 26:617.

Kuan SF, et al: Differential expression of mucin genes in mammary and extramammary Paget's disease. Am J Surg Pathol 2001; 25:1469.

Lee KY, et al: Comparison of Mohs micrographic surgery and wide excision for extramammary Paget's disease: Korean experience. Dermatol Surg 2009; 35:34.

Liegl B, et al: Mammary and extramammary Paget's disease: an immunohistochemical study of 83 cases. Histopathology 2007; 50:439.

Minicozzi A, et al: Perianal Paget's disease: presentation of six cases and literature review. Int J Colorectal Dis 2010; 25:1.

Miyamoto T, et al: Axillary apocrine carcinoma with Paget's disease and apocrine naevus. Clin Exp Dermatol 2009; 34:e110.

Murata Y, et al: Underpants-pattern erythema. J Am Acad Dermatol 1999; 40:949.

Murata Y, Kumano K: Multicentricity of extramammary Paget's disease. Eur J Dermatol 2007; 17:164.

Pascual JC, et al: Extramammary Paget's disease of the groin with underlying carcinoma and fatal outcome. Clin Exp Dermatol 2008; 33:595.

Panasiti V, et al: Intralesional interferon alfa-2b as neoadjuvant treatment for perianal extramammary Paget's disease. J Eur Acad Dermatol Venereol 2008; 22:522.

Plaza JA, et al: HER-2/neu expression in extramammary Paget disease: a clinicopathologic and immunohistochemistry study of 47 cases with and without underlying malignancy. J Cutan Pathol 2009; 36:729.

Salamanca J, et al: Paget's disease of the glans penis secondary to transitional cell carcinoma of the bladder: a report of two cases and review of the literature. J Cutan Pathol 2004; 31:341.

Sendagorta E, et al: Successful treatment of three cases of primary extramammary Paget's disease of the vulva with imiquimod—proposal of a therapeutic schedule. J Eur Acad Dermatol Venereol 2009 Oct 15 (Epub ahead of print).

Shan SJ, et al: Expression of survivin and human telomerase reverse transcriptase in extramammary Paget's disease. J Cutan Pathol 2009 Sep 24 (Epub ahead of print).

Shi C, Argani P: Synchronous primary perianal Paget's disease and rectal adenocarcinoma: report of a hitherto undescribed phenomenon. Int J Surg Pathol 2009; 17:42.

Siesling S, et al: Epidemiology and treatment of extramammary Paget disease in the Netherlands. Eur J Surg Oncol 2007; 33:951.

Spiliopoulos D, et al: Vulvar and breast Paget's disease with synchronous underlying cancer: a unique association. Arch Gynecol Obstet 2009; 280:313.

St Peter SD, et al: Wide local excision and split-thickness skin graft for circumferential Paget's disease of the anus. Am J Surg 2004; 187:413.

Tsujino Y, et al: Fluorescence navigation with indocyanine green for detecting sentinel nodes in extramammary Paget's disease and squamous cell carcinoma. J Dermatol 2009; 36:90.

Virich G, et al: Extramammary Paget's disease—occupational exposure to used engine oil and a new skin grafting technique. J Plast Reconstr Aesthet Surg 2008; 61:1528.

Wang Z, et al: Penile and scrotal Paget's disease: 130 Chinese patients with long-term follow-up. BJU Int 2008; 102:485.

Wright JL, et al: Primary scrotal cancer: disease characteristics and increasing incidence. Urology 2008; 72:1139.

Yanai H, et al: Immunohistochemistry of p63 in primary and secondary vulvar Paget's disease. Pathol Int 2008; 58:648.

Yeh MH, Hu SL: Treatment of double ectopic extramammary Paget's disease of bilateral chest with imiquimod 5% cream. J Eur Acad Dermatol Venereol 2007; 21:997.

Yoon SN, et al: Extramammary Paget's disease in Korea: its association with gastrointestinal neoplasms. Int J Colorectal Dis 2008; 23:1125.

Yoshida Y, et al: Potential utility of the tumour marker RCAS1 for monitoring patients with invasive extramammary Paget's disease. Acta Derm Venereol 2008; 88:296.

Yoshii N, et al: Expression of mucin core proteins in extramammary Paget's disease. Pathol Int 2002; 52:390.

Zawislak AA, et al: Successful photodynamic therapy of vulval Paget's disease using a novel patch-based delivery system containing 5-aminolevulinic acid. Br J Obstet Gynaecol 2004; 111:1143.

Zhu Y, et al: Clinicopathological characteristics, management and outcome of metastatic penoscrotal extramammary Paget's disease. Br J Dermatol 2009; 161:577.

Clear cell papulosis

Clear cell papulosis is an uncommon disorder that presents with multiple, minimally elevated, hypopigmented papules. Most cases have been reported in Asian or Hispanic children. Onset is usually before age 6 and may be as soon as 4 months of age. The eruption favors the pubic region, lower abdomen and along the milk lines. Histology demonstrates mild acanthosis, decreased epidermal pigmentation, and the presence of single or small clusters of large clear cells in the basal and occasionally suprabasal layers of the epidermis. The cells are EMA-, CEA-, and CD7-positive, identical to Toker cells.

Farley-Loftus R, et al: Clear cell papulosis. Dermatol Online J 2008; 14:19.

Gianotti R, et al: Clear cell papulosis (pagetoid papulosis) in a non-Asian patient. Dermatology 2001; 203:260.

Kim YC, et al: Clear cell papulosis: an immunohistochemical study to determine histogenesis. J Cutan Pathol 2002; 29:11.

Mohanty SK, et al: Clear cell papulosis of the skin. Ann Diag Pathol 2002; 6:385.

Yu Y, et al: Clear cell papulosis: a connection of clear cells to Toker cells or Paget disease. Arch Dermatol 2009; 145:1066.

Merkel cell carcinoma (trabecular carcinoma)

Merkel cell carcinoma (MCC) was first described by Toker in 1972. The cell of origin is the Merkel cell, a slow-acting mechanoreceptor in the basal layer of the epidermis. MCC, while still a rare tumor occurring at an incidence of about 0.44/100 000 population, has increased three-fold over the last 15 years, i.e. has an increased incidence of 8% per year. Melanoma, by comparison, increased at a rate of only 3% per year over the same period. More than 1500 MCCs occur yearly in the US. This is a tumor of the elderly, with 90% of cases found in persons over the age of 50 years, 76% in persons over the age of 65 years, and 72% in persons over the age of 70. The mean age is 76 years in women and 74 years in men. Sixty percent of MCC patients are men. Ninety-five percent of MCCs occur in white people. There is strong evidence that MCC is induced by sun exposure. Ninety percent of cases occur on sun-exposed sites, with 27% of cases on the face, 9% on the scalp and neck (or 36% on the head and neck), 22% on the upper extremity, 15% on the lower extremity (37% on the extremities), and only 11% on the trunk. About 3% occur on the ear, eyelid, or lip. PUVA therapy is associated with an increased risk for MCC. Immunosuppression by organ transplantation, chronic lymphatic leukemia, and HIV infection all substantially increase the risk for developing MCC, so that in some series, 8–15% of patients with MCC have some form of immune impairment.

Clinically, this tumor presents as a rapidly growing, nontender, red to violaceous nodule with a shiny surface (Fig.

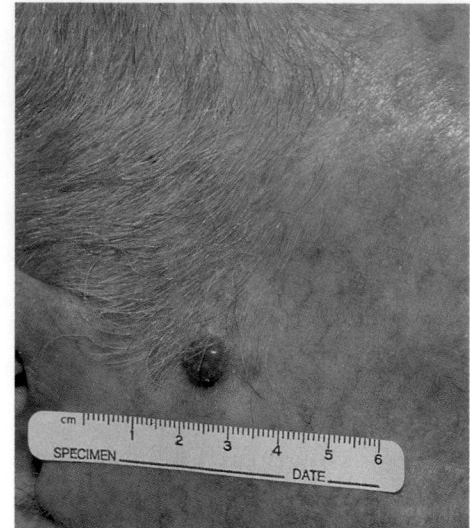

Fig. 29-30 Merkel cell carcinoma.

29-30) and overlying telangiectasia. Most cases are *not* considered by the dermatologist as being malignant at the time of biopsy The acronym AEIOU has been suggested: (asymptomatic/lack of tenderness, expanding rapidly, immune suppression, older than 50 years, and ultraviolet-exposed site on a person with fair skin). MCC is an aggressive tumor with a propensity for local recurrence and nodal and distant metastases. At presentation, about one-third of cases have regional node involvement, and hematogenous spread will eventuate in at least one-third of patients. Spontaneous remissions have been reported, primarily in women with head and neck tumors; this is most often associated with reducing iatrogenic immunosuppression. The regression is rapid, but the MCC can recur after "spontaneous resolution." MCC can present as a metastatic disease without an evident primary tumor.

Approximately 80% of MCCs in North America and 25% of MCCs in Australia are associated with a virus, the Merkel cell polyomavirus (MCPyV). The virus is found integrated into the genome of the MCC when present, and all progenitor cells have the same viral genome, suggesting that the viral infection began at the time the neoplasia was developing, or before. MCC patients are more likely to be seropositive for the MCPyV. Infection with this virus is widespread, with seroprevalence increasing from 30% in children less than 5 years of age to almost 80% in persons older than 50. Lymphoid tissue, especially the tonsils, seems to be the reservoir. The virus may behave like HPV, with increasing seroprevalence with exposure over time, and spontaneous clearance in most adults. The virus can be recovered from about 4% of immunocompetent persons, but 36% of immunosuppressed patients. This may explain the high risk for MCC with immunosuppression, analogous to the high risk of HPV-related neoplasia in the immunosuppressed. MCPyV has also been reported in non-melanoma skin cancers in both immunocompetent and immunosuppressed patients. Bowen's disease, BCC, and SCC have been associated with viral infection in up to 40% of cases in some laboratories, but these results have not been reproduced and may represent laboratory over-identification. At the University of California, San Francisco (UCSF), the figure is <1%. Normal skin infection has also been reported, and the viral copies in these NMSCs are much fewer than in MCC. The pathogenic role of MCPyV in NMSCs other than MCC is speculative. Visceral tumors, and other small-cell neuroendocrine tumors of other organ systems do *not* contain MCPyV, substantiating its role in the development of MCC.

Patients should be staged for therapy and prognosis. As expected, staging predicts prognosis and guides therapy. Sentinel lymph node biopsy (SLNB) should be performed, prior to the definitive excision of the primary tumor. One-third of patients with no palpable adenopathy have a positive SLNB. The SLNB sample must be examined with CK20 (if the primary tumor is positive) to detect micrometastases. Computed tomography (CT) will detect metastatic disease in only 20% of MCC patients. SLNB-positive patients have a 0% survival rate if not given additional therapy for the lymphatic involvement. Whether tumors less than 1 cm in diameter require SLNB is controversial, but even in small tumors, lymph node metastases can be found. Imaging with CT, MRI, or positron emission tomography (PET) may be used to search for metastatic disease. Palpable lymph nodes must be sampled to exclude the presence of metastatic disease. MCC patients who harbor the MCPyV have a better prognosis (45% vs 15%, 5-year survival), and the MCC is more likely to present on an extremity. MCC should be treated expeditiously, as patients have developed metastatic disease in the weeks awaiting definitive surgery.

The treatment of MCC should be directed by persons with expertise in managing this rare tumor. Therapy may need to be individualized, depending on various risk factors present. Many of these patients are elderly and may not be able to tolerate some of the recommended treatments. The goal of treatment for patients with only local disease or regional nodal metastases is cure and local control. This involves the combined use of surgery and radiation therapy in most cases. Radiation therapy alone can be efficacious and is recommended for patients unable to tolerate surgery. Radiation therapy is directed at both the primary site and the draining and or regional lymph node basins in most cases. Untreated lymph nodes experience recurrence 46–76% of the time. Even after Mohs surgery, radiation therapy reduces the recurrence rate from 16% to near 0%. Prophylactic lymph node dissection enhances local control but does not improve survival. It is gradually being replaced with radiation therapy of the affected nodal basin. Adjuvant chemotherapy has been disappointing, as it does not prevent later development of metastatic, regional, or local disease; it is therefore not recommended. MCC may be initially responsive to chemotherapy but disease progression occurs. In the setting of metastatic MCC, chemotherapy would be considered palliative. There has been a partial response with the use of a multikinase inhibitor, pazopanib.

Histologically, MCC is a dermal tumor that may extend into the subcutaneous tissue. The cells are about 15 μm in diameter and have very scanty cytoplasm and hyperchromatic nuclei with a distinctive smudged chromatin pattern. Mitoses and apoptotic cells are numerous. The cells are arranged in sheets and cords. Depth of invasion, lymphovascular involvement, and mitotic index may be poor prognostic histological features. MCC must be distinguished from small-cell lung cancer, lymphoma, neuroblastoma, small-cell endocrine carcinoma, Ewing sarcoma, melanoma, and even BCC. Immunoperoxidase confirmation of the diagnosis and exclusion of other small-cell tumors are required to establish the diagnosis. The tumor should be CK20-positive and thyroid transcription factor-1 (TTF-1)-negative. CK20 staining is of the "perinuclear dot pattern." CK7 tends to stain small-cell lung cancer and not MCC, and can also be used. Other markers are used to exclude other small-cell cancers. MCC is negative for S-100 and leukocyte common antigen (LCA).

Albores-Saavedra J, et al: Merkel cell carcinoma demographics, morphology, and survival based on 3870 cases: a population based study. J Cutan Pathol 2009 Jul 21 (Epub ahead of print).

Andres C, et al: Prevalence of MCPyV in Merkel cell carcinoma and non-MCC tumors. J Cutan Pathol 2009 Jul 14 (Epub ahead of print).

Assouline A, et al: Clinical and therapeutic aspects in elderly patients with Merkel cell carcinoma: special focus on radiotherapy. J Am Geriatr Soc 2009; 57:1946.

Boyer JD, et al: Local control of primary Merkel cell carcinoma: review of 45 cases treated with Mohs micrographic surgery with and without adjuvant radiation. J Am Acad Dermatol 2002; 47:885.

Busam KJ: Merkel cell polyomavirus expression in Merkel cell carcinomas and its absence in combined tumors and pulmonary neuroendocrine carcinomas. Am J Surg Pathol 2009; 33:1378.

Carter JJ, et al: Association of Merkel cell polyomavirus-specific antibodies with Merkel cell carcinoma. J Natl Cancer Inst 2009; 101:1510.

Connelly T: Regarding complete spontaneous regression of Merkel cell carcinoma. Dermatol Surg 2009; 35:721.

Davids M, et al: Response to a novel multitargeted tyrosine kinase inhibitor pazopanib in metastatic Merkel cell carcinoma. J Clin Oncol 2009; 27:e97.

DeCaprio JA: Does detection of Merkel cell polyomavirus in Merkel cell carcinoma provide prognostic information? J Natl Cancer Inst 2009; 101:905.

Dworkin AM, et al: Merkel cell polyomavirus in cutaneous squamous cell carcinoma of immunocompetent individuals. J Invest Dermatol 2009; 129:2868.

Feng H, et al: Clonal integration of a polyomavirus in human Merkel cell carcinoma. Science 2008; 319:1096.

Foulongne V, et al: Merkel cell polyomavirus DNA detection in lesional and nonlesional skin from patients with Merkel cell carcinoma or other skin diseases. Br J Dermatol 2009 Jul 6 (Epub ahead of print).

Garneski KM, et al: Merkel cell polyomavirus is more frequently present in North American than Australian Merkel cell carcinoma tumors. J Invest Dermatol 2009; 129:246.

Gass JK, et al: Multiple primary malignancies in patients with Merkel cell carcinoma. J Eur Acad Dermatol Venereol 2009 Nov 9 (Epub ahead of print).

Heath M, et al: Clinical characteristics of Merkel cell carcinoma at diagnosis in 195 patients: the AEIOU features. J Am Acad Dermatol 2008; 58:375.

Herrmann G, et al: Complete remission of Merkel cell carcinoma of the scalp with local and regional metastases after topical treatment with dinitrochlorbenzene. J Am Acad Dermatol 2004; 50:965.

Kantola K, et al: Merkel cell polyomavirus DNA in tumor-free tonsillar tissues and upper respiratory tract samples: implications for respiratory transmission and latency. J Clin Virol 2009; 45:292.

Karkos PD, et al: Spontaneous regression of Merkel cell carcinoma of the nose. Head Neck 2009 Apr 16 (Epub ahead of print).

Kassem A, et al: Merkel cell polyomavirus sequences are frequently detected in nonmelanoma skin cancer of immunosuppressed patients. Int J Cancer 2009; 125:356.

Koh CS, Veness MJ: Role of definitive radiotherapy in treating patients with inoperable Merkel cell carcinoma: the Westmead Hospital experience and a review of the literature. Australas J Dermatol 2009; 50:249.

Koljonen V, et al: Chronic lymphocytic leukaemia patients have a high risk of Merkel-cell polyomavirus DNA-positive Merkel-cell carcinoma. Br J Cancer 2009; 101:1444.

Longo MI, Nghiem P: Merkel cell carcinoma treatment with radiation: a good case despite no prospective studies. Arch Dermatol 2003; 139:1641.

Miller SJ, et al: Merkel cell carcinoma. J Natl Compr Canc Netw 2009; 7:322.

Mortier L, et al: Radiotherapy alone for primary Merkel cell carcinoma. Arch Dermatol 2003; 139:1587.

Ohnishi Y, et al: Merkel cell carcinoma and multiple Bowen's disease: incidental association or possible relationship to inorganic arsenic exposure? J Dermatol 1997; 24:310.

Peloschek P, et al: Diagnostic imaging in Merkel cell carcinoma; lessons to learn from 16 cases with correlation of sonography, CT, MRI and PET. Eur J Radiol 2008 Dec 22 (Epub ahead of print).

Poulsen M: Merkel-cell carcinoma of the skin. Lancet Oncol 2004; 5:593.

Poulsen M, et al: Factors influencing relapse-free survival in Merkel cell carcinoma of the lower limb—a review of 60 cases. Int J Radiat Oncol Biol Phys 2009 Jun 8 (Epub ahead of print).

Ridd K, et al: The presence of polyomavirus in non-melanoma skin cancer in organ transplant recipients is rare. J Invest Dermatol 2009; 129:250.

Sarnaik AA, et al: Routine omission of sentinel lymph node biopsy for Merkel cell carcinoma ≤1 cm is not justified. J Clin Oncol 2010; 28:e7.

Shuda M, et al: Human Merkel cell polyomavirus infection I. MCV T antigen expression in Merkel cell carcinoma, lymphoid tissues and lymphoid tumors. Int J Cancer 2009; 125:1243.

Sihto H, et al: Clinical factors associated with Merkel cell polyomavirus infection in Merkel cell carcinoma. J Natl Cancer Inst 2009; 101:938.

Stokes JB, et al: Patients with Merkel cell carcinoma tumors ≤1.0 cm in diameter are unlikely to harbor regional lymph node metastasis. J Clin Oncol 2009; 27:3772.

Tolstov YL, et al: Human Merkel cell polyomavirus infection II. MCV is a common human infection that can be detected by conformational capsid epitope immunoassays. Int J Cancer 2009; 125:1250.

Turk T, et al: Spontaneous regression of Merkel cell carcinoma in a patient with chronic lymphocytic leukemia: a case report. J Med Case Reports 2009; 3:7270.

Urbatsch A, et al: Merkel cell carcinoma occurring in renal transplant patients. J Am Acad Dermatol 1999; 41:289.

Veness M, et al: The role of radiotherapy alone in patients with Merkel cell carcinoma: reporting the Australian experience of 43 patients. Int J Radiat Oncol Biol Phys 2009 Nov 23 (Epub ahead of print).

Warnick M, et al: Merkel cell carcinoma presenting as lymphadenopathy without a primary cutaneous lesion: a report of 2 cases. Arch Dermatol 2008; 144:1397.

Wetzels CT, et al: Ultrastructural proof of polyomavirus in Merkel cell carcinoma tumour cells and its absence in small cell carcinoma of the lung. PLoS One 2009; 4:e4958.

Wieland U, et al: Merkel cell polyomavirus DNA in persons without Merkel cell carcinoma. Emerg Infect Dis 2009; 15:1496.

Zhan FQ, et al: Merkel cell carcinoma: a review of current advances. J Natl Compr Canc Netw 2009; 7:333.

Sebaceous nevi and tumors

Nevus sebaceus (organoid nevus)

Nevus sebaceus of Jadassohn presents as a sharply circumscribed, yellow–orange hamartoma, varying from a few millimeters to several centimeters in size. These lesions are usually solitary, congenital, and linear in configuration. The scalp is the most common location (50%), but other areas of the head and neck (45%) are also common. The trunk is involved in 5% or less of cases. The lesions persist throughout life and are usually alopecic. In childhood, they are only very slightly papillated or velvety (Fig. 29-31), but in adulthood, with hyper-

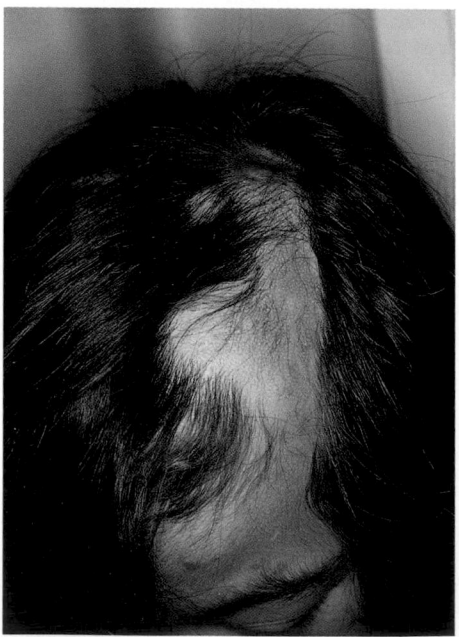

Fig. 29-31 Nevus sebaceus in a prepubescent child.

plasia of the sebaceous elements, the lesions become more elevated and cerebriform. Large, pedunculated lesions presenting as exophytic tumors at birth are an unusual phenotype. Numerous neoplasms, most of them adnexal, have been described arising in nevus sebaceus. The most common tumors are trichoblastoma and syringocystadenoma papilliferum, each occurring in about 5% of nevus sebaceus. Both of these tumors present as new, often pigmented papules or nodules arising in the nevus sebaceus. BCC is uncommon, occurring in less than 1% of lesions. Many cases previously diagnosed as BCC are actually trichoblastomas. Many of the tumors are difficult to classify precisely as a well-described entity. Development of benign tumors occurs in less than 5% of nevus sebaceus before the age of 16, and malignant tumors are rare in childhood or adolescence. The risk for tumor development increases with age. Rarely, aggressive malignant adnexal neoplasms may arise, usually in older adults. Familial cases have been described.

Nevus sebaceus may be associated with multiple internal abnormalities, making it one of the cutaneous abnormalities to be included within the epidermal nevus syndrome (see above). Schimmelpenning syndrome is a synonym for sebaceous nevus syndrome (SNS). In cases of SNS, the nevus sebaceus is usually on the scalp, and is linear and of larger size (10 cm or larger). The sebaceous nevi usually occupy more than one dermatome. Ocular colobomas and choristomas are characteristic. Neurologic findings are present in 7% of all patients with nevus sebaceus and up to two-thirds of patients with SNS. Epilepsy is seen about two-thirds of cases, usually beginning in the first year of life. Mental retardation is unfortunately not uncommon. While numerous anatomic abnormalities of the brain have been described in SNS, the CT and MRI are frequently normal in children with seizures and mental retardation. Urological and cardiovascular defects have also been reported. A very rare variant of SNS is the SCALP syndrome: sebaceus nevus syndrome, CNS malformations, aplasia cutis congenita, limbal dermoid, and pigmented nevus (giant congenital melanocytic nevus). The aplasia cutis and sebaceus nevus are adjacent and on the scalp. This syndrome is also called didymosis aplasticosebacea.

A rare but frequently reported association is that of nevus sebaceus and hypophosphatemic rickets. Most patients have large sebaceous nevi and evidence of "SNS." If the rickets goes unrecognized, permanent bone loss and orthopedic injury result. Serum phosphate is low and there is excess phosphate in the urine. Serum calcium is normal. It is now clear that the nevus sebaceus itself secretes some factor responsible for the phosphorus wasting. Fibroblast growth factor-23 (FGF-23) and matrix extracellular phosphoglycoprotein (MEPE) are both elevated in the blood of patients with this syndrome, and the levels of these substances parallel the hypophosphatemia. Surgical removal of the nevus sebaceus is the treatment of this syndrome. When the nevus sebaceus is removed, the metabolic abnormalities normalize, and FGF-23 and MEPE levels return to normal. Partial removal can ameliorate the condition. Octreotide can also be used in these cases if the surgical removal is not possible.

Histologically, in prepubertal lesions, the epithelium is acanthotic and papillomatous. Pilosebaceous structures are immature and resemble the fetal pilar germ. After puberty, the epidermis is more hyperplastic and at times papillomatous. It may resemble a seborrheic keratosis or acanthosis nigricans, or have features of an epidermal nevus. Sebaceous glands are usually abundant, placed high in the dermis, and connect directly to the epidermal surface. Follicular structures, if present, are usually vellous or partially formed. Apocrine glands are present in about half of the lesions. The dermis is thickened, with increased vascularity and fibrous connective tissue. Mature lesions have been described as broad, bald, bumpy (papillomatous), and bubbly (sebaceous). The finding of epidermodysplasia verruciformis (EDV)-associated and genital-mucosal HPV DNA in nevus sebaceus is of unclear significance.

Although the risk of development of malignancy exists, it is small, and virtually always occurs after adolescence. For this reason, surgical removal can be delayed until adulthood, when the patient can make an informed decision regarding removal. If the lesion leads to disfigurement, stigmatization, or symptomatology, it may be removed at any age.

Carlson JA, et al: Epidermodysplasia verruciformis-associated and genital-mucosal high-risk human papillomavirus DNA are prevalent in nevus sebaceus of Jadassohn. J Am Acad Dermatol 2008; 59:279.

Correale D, et al: Large, papillomatous, pedunculated nevus sebaceus: a new phenotype. Pediatr Dermatol 2008; 25:355.

Cribier B, et al: Tumors arising in nevus sebaceus: a study of 596 cases. J Am Acad Dermatol 2000; 42:263.

Dalle S, et al: Apocrine carcinoma developed in nevus sebaceus of Jadassohn. Eur J Dermatol 2003; 13:487.

De Giorgi V, et al: Sebaceous carcinoma arising from nevus sebaceus: a case report. Dermatol Surg 2003; 29:105.

Demerdjieva Z, et al: Epidermal nevus syndrome and didymosis aplasticosebacea. Pediatr Dermatol 2007; 24:514.

Diwan AH, et al: Mucoepidermoid carcinoma arising within nevus sebaceus of Jadassohn. J Cutan Pathol 2003; 30:652.

Duncan A, et al: Squamous cell carcinoma developing in a naevus sebaceus of Jadassohn. Am J Dermatopathol 2008; 30:269.

Goldblum JR, Headington JT: Hypophosphatemic vitamin D-resistant rickets and multiple spindle and epithelioid nevi associated with linear nevus sebaceus syndrome. J Am Acad Dermatol 1993; 29:109.

Guhan B, Duncan RD: Linear sebaceous naevus syndrome and resistant rickets. J Bone Joint Surg Br 2004; 86:151.

Happle R, König A: Familial naevus sebaceus may be explained by paradominant transmission. Br J Dermatol 1999; 141:377.

Hoffman WH, et al: Elevated fibroblast growth factor-23 in hypophosphatemic linear nevus sebaceus syndrome. Am J Med Genet A 2005; 134:233.

Hoffman WH, et al: Matrix extracellular phosphoglycoprotein (MEPE) correlates with serum phosphorus prior to and during octreotide treatment and following excisional surgery in hypophosphatemic linear sebaceous nevus syndrome. Am J Med Genet A 2008; 146A:2164.

Hosalkar HS, et al: Linear sebaceous naevus syndrome and resistant rickets. J Bone Joint Surg Br 2003; 85:578.

Lam J, et al: SCALP syndrome: sebaceous nevus syndrome, CNS malformations, aplasia cutis congenita, limbal dermoid, and pigmented nevus (giant congenital melanocytic nevus) with neurocutaneous melanosis: a distinct syndromic entity. J Am Acad Dermatol 2008; 58:884.

Manonukul J, et al: Mucoepidermoid (adenosquamous) carcinoma, trichoblastoma, trichilemmoma, sebaceous adenoma, tumor of follicular infundibulum and syringocystadenoma papilliferum arising within 2 persistent lesions of nevus sebaceus: report of a case. Am J Dermatopathol 2009; 31:658.

Santibanez-Gallerani A, et al: Should nevus sebaceus of Jadassohn in children be excised? A study of 757 cases, and literature review. J Craniofac Surg 2003; 14:658.

Wiedemeyer K, et al: Trichoblastomas with Merkel cell proliferation in nevi sebacei in Schimmelpenning–Feuerstein–Mims syndrome— histological differentiation between trichoblastomas and basal cell carcinomas. J Dtsch Dermatol Ges 2009; 7:612.

Zutt M, et al: Schimmelpenning–Feuerstein–Mims syndrome with hypophosphatemic rickets. Dermatology 2003:207:72.

Sebaceous hyperplasia

The age of onset is usually past 40, and the prevalence increases with age. The areas of predilection are the forehead, infraorbital regions, and temples. The lesions are small, creamcolored or yellowish, umbilicated papules, 2–6 mm in diameter. Dermoscopy can be helpful in confirming the diagnosis and identifies the central crater, the yellow lobules, and the associated telangiectasia. Unusual sites may be affected, such as the areolas, nipples, penis, neck, and chest, where disease occurs as solitary lesions, clustered papules, or beaded lines. Prominent sebaceous hyperplasia occurs in 15% of patients taking cyclosporine and may involve ectopic sites such as the oral mucosa. It often appears many years after the cyclosporine is begun. Histologically, sebaceous hyperplasia demonstrates hyperplasia of one sebaceous gland, with the surrounding glands being of normal size. The glands are multilobulated, each dividing into smaller lobules to produce a cluster resembling a bunch of grapes. Clinically, they may mimic an early BCC.

Premature sebaceous hyperplasia, also known as familial presenile sebaceous hyperplasia, presents with extensive sebaceous hyperplasia with onset at puberty and worsening with age. Familial patterns have been reported, inherited in an autosomal-dominant fashion. It involves the face, neck, and upper thorax but spares the periorificial regions.

Treatment is solely for cosmetic purposes and employs electrosurgery, laser treatment, photodynamic therapy, or even shallow shave biopsy. Isotretinoin will reduce lesions, but they immediately recur when it is stopped, so it is probably not indicated for this condition.

Belinchon I, et al: Areolar sebaceous hyperplasia. Cutis 1996; 58:63.

Boonchai W, et al: Familial presenile sebaceous gland hyperplasia. J Am Acad Dermatol 1997; 36:120.

Boschnakow A, et al: Ciclosporin A-induced sebaceous gland hyperplasia. Br J Dermatol 2003; 149:193.

de Berker DA, et al: Sebaceous hyperplasia in organ transplant recipients: shared aspects of hyperplastic and dysplastic processes? J Am Acad Dermatol 1996; 35:696.

Grimalt R, et al: Premature familial sebaceous hyperplasia: successful response to oral isotretinoin in three patients. J Am Acad Dermatol 1997; 37:996.

Kumar A, et al: Band-like sebaceous hyperplasia over the penis. Australas J Dermatol 1999; 40:47.

Pang SM, Chau YP: Cyclosporin-induced sebaceous hyperplasia in renal transplant patients. Ann Acad Med Singapore 2005; 34:391.

Perrett CM, et al: Topical photodynamic therapy with methyl aminolevulinate to treat sebaceous hyperplasia in an organ transplant recipient. Arch Dermatol 2006; 142:781.

Sebaceous adenoma

This slow-growing tumor usually presents as a pink, flesh-colored, or yellow papule or nodule. It occurs primarily on the head and neck (70%) in the elderly (mean age 60 years). Histologically, the tumor is composed of multiple, sharply marginated, sebaceous lobules. Each lobule has a basal layer of darker germinative cells, but the maturation is not as well developed as in a normal sebaceous gland. The basaloid cells occupy more than the typical 1–2 cell layers seen in the normal sebaceous gland or in sebaceous hyperplasia. Multiple openings directly to the overlying epidermis may be found. Sebaceous adenoma may be a cutaneous marker of the Muir–Torre syndrome.

Sebaceoma (sebaceous epithelioma)

Clinically, sebaceomas have the same morphologic characteristics as BCCs. They appear as yellow or orange papules, nodules, or plaques (Fig. 29-32), usually on the scalp, face, and neck. They may be associated with Muir–Torre syndrome. Histologically, the tumor consists of oval nests of irregularly shaped basaloid cells with differentiation toward sebaceous cells. The basaloid cells should outnumber the differentiated

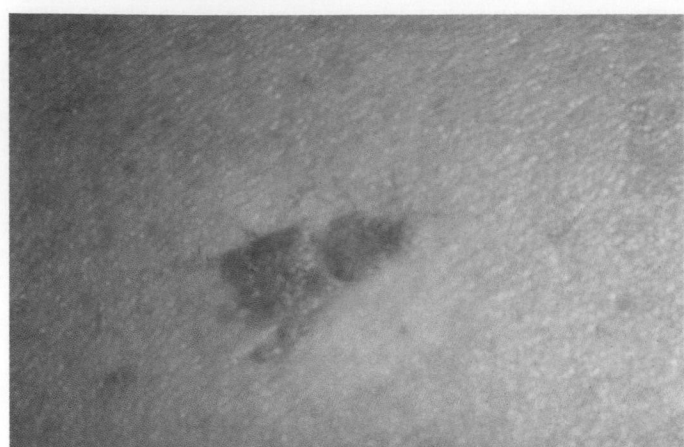

Fig. 29-32 Sebaceoma.

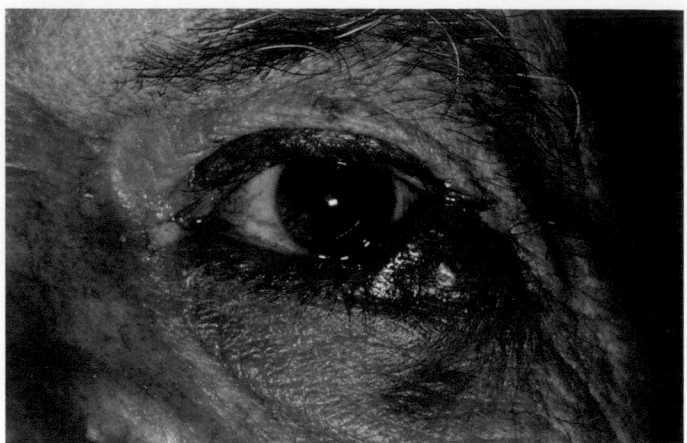

Fig. 29-33 Sebaceous carcinoma in a patient with Muir–Torre syndrome.

sebocytes in a sebaceoma. Also, there may be cystic spaces containing vacuolated amorphous material.

Reticulated acanthoma with sebaceous differentiation

This rare tumor presents as an enlarging, erythematous to brown plaque, often on the back. Histologically, the tumor has a reticulated seborrheic keratosis-like pattern, being broad and well circumscribed. There are clusters of sebocytes at the bases of the rete ridges. Sebaceous ducts may also be seen. These ductal elements are EMA-positive and CEA-negative. This tumor can also be associated with Muir–Torre syndrome.

Sebaceous carcinoma

Sebaceous carcinoma is a rare neoplasm, and 75% of cases occur on the eyelid or around the eye. It most frequently arises on the eyelids from the meibomian or Zeis glands. It usually appears in the tarsal region of the upper eyelids (75%) and represents 1% or more of eyelid malignancies. It is frequently misdiagnosed as a chalazion, delaying appropriate treatment. The scalp, other areas of the face, and the trunk are the next most common areas involved. Lesions present as a painless subcutaneous nodule or, less commonly, a pedunculated growth. Rarely, sebaceous carcinoma has been reported as involving the feet, external genitalia, and the oral mucosa. Fatal metastatic disease occurs in 9–50% of cases (30% of eyelid cases), and the 5-year survival for this tumor is 80%. Sebaceous carcinomas arising in nonocular locations can also metastasize, usually to regional lymph nodes. Sebaceous carcinoma may be seen in Muir–Torre syndrome (Fig. 29-33).

Histologically, the tumor is composed of lobules or sheets of cells that extend deeply into the dermis, subcutaneous fat, or muscle. The tumor cells are pleomorphic and show various degrees of sebaceous differentiation, manifested by a vacuolated rather than clear cytoplasm. Undifferentiated cells with mitotic figures can be found. The cells vary greatly in size and shape. A characteristic feature in ocular tumors is pagetoid or bowenoid spread of the tumor on to the overlying conjunctiva or skin. Sebaceous differentiation may be minimal in this in situ component, leading to the misdiagnosis of SCC in situ. Treatment is surgical, with Mohs microsurgery having had good results; there is an 11% recurrence rate after Mohs and 30% after standard excision. Given the extent of these tumors, oculoplastic reconstruction is usually required. In extraocular cases, complete excision, as for an adnexal carcinoma, and careful follow-up are recommended.

Muir–Torre syndrome

Sebaceous tumors of the skin were first reported by Muir in 1967 and Torre in 1968 as being associated with the development of internal malignancy, a combination that has been called the Muir–Torre syndrome (MTS). The cutaneous lesions may be sebaceous adenomas, sebaceomas, or sebaceous carcinomas. Keratoacanthomas (KAs) are also frequent and multiple. The KAs may show sebaceous differentiation. The combination of a sebaceous tumor and a KA should be highly suggestive of MTS. The recognition of the association of sebaceous neoplasms and MTS is highlighted by one report, in which 42% of persons with a sebaceous neoplasm had MTS. Between 22% and 32% of patients with MTS present with the sebaceous neoplasm before the development of the internal malignancy. About 60% have already had an internal malignancy by the time the sebaceous neoplasm occurs. Since the mean age of presentation of the sebaceous neoplasm is 63 years, the confirmation of MTS becomes important for genetic counseling of the patient's children.

MTS is now recognized to be a subset of the Lynch syndrome or hereditary nonpolyposis coli cancer syndrome (HNCCS). HNCCS and MTS are caused by mutations in mismatch repair (MMR) genes (*MLH1*, *MSH2*, and *MSH6* for MTS and Lynch syndrome, and *PMS2* only in Lynch syndrome). *MSH2* mutations are responsible for 60% of MTS families. The most common malignancy is colonic adenocarcinoma (47%), usually proximal to the splenic flexor. Multiple polyps are not present. Genitourinary tumors (21%), breast cancer (12%), and hematological disorders (9%) are also common.

The absence of an MMR enzyme results in microsatellite instability (MSI). MSI can be detected in routinely processed pathology specimens. MSI is found in about 60% of sebaceous neoplasms, and more than half of those patients will have MTS. This allows for the suspicion of MTS to be raised during the pathological evaluation of a sebaceous neoplasm. Any pathology report regarding a sebaceous tumor should include this information, as it is essential for directing the patient's further evaluation and care. The visceral tumors also contain the MSI. The finding of MSI on the biopsy should lead to germline testing of the patient, and subsequently of his/her family if he/she has the mutation. Hypermethylations of *MLH1* promoter and *BRAF-600E* mutations can lead to immunohistochemical results suggesting MLH1 deficiency and should be screened for before undertaking genetic testing of the patient who shows MLH1 deficiency on his/her biopsy. Once the diagnosis is confirmed, the patient and his/her genetically related family members should be appropriately screened for underlying malignancies of the gastrointestinal and genitourinary systems. This screening should begin at a much younger age than is standard: 20–25 years for colonoscopy and 30–35 years for transvaginal ultrasound. Other organs are screened if the affected family has such cancers: for example, using endoscopy, urine cytology, or abdominal ultrasound. The value of screening for non-colonic carcinomas has not been demonstrated. Genetic counseling should be provided.

Abbas O, Mahalingam M: Cutaneous sebaceous neoplasms as markers of Muir–Torre syndrome: a diagnostic algorithm. J Cutan Pathol 2009; 36:613.

Abbott JJ, et al: Cystic sebaceous neoplasms in Muir–Torre syndrome. Arch Pathol Lab Med 2003; 127:614.

Bassetto F, et al: Biological behavior of the sebaceous carcinoma of the head. Dermatol Surg 2004; 30:472.

Eisen DB, Michael DJ: Sebaceous lesions and their associated syndromes: part I. J Am Acad Dermatol 2009; 61:549.

Eisen DB, Michael DJ: Sebaceous lesions and their associated syndromes: part II. J Am Acad Dermatol 2009; 61:563.

Fiorentino DF, et al: Muir–Torre syndrome: confirmation of diagnosis by immunohistochemical analysis of cutaneous lesions. J Am Acad Dermatol 2004; 50:476.

Fukai K, et al: Reticulated acanthoma with sebaceous differentiation. Am J Dermatopathol 2006; 28:158.

Haake DL, et al: Reticulated acanthoma with sebaceous differentiation. Lack of association with Muir–Torre syndrome. Am J Dermatopathol 2009; 31:391.

Harrington CR, et al: Extraocular sebaceous carcinoma in a patient with Muir–Torre syndrome. Dermatol Surg 2004; 30:817.

Jones B, et al: Muir–Torre syndrome: diagnostic and screening guidelines. Australas J Dermatol 2006; 47:266.

Kruse R, et al: Frequency of microsatellite instability in unselected sebaceous gland neoplasias and hyperplasias. J Invest Dermatol 2003; 120:858.

Lai TF, et al: Eyelid sebaceous carcinoma masquerading as in situ squamous cell carcinoma. Dermatol Surg 2004; 30:222.

Mangold E, et al: A genotype-phenotype correlation in HNPCC: strong predominance of MSH2 mutations in 41 patients with Muir–Torre syndrome. J Med Genet 2004; 41:567.

Ponti G, et al: Different phenotypes in Muir–Torre syndrome: clinical and biomolecular characterization in two Italian families. Br J Dermatol 2005; 152:1335.

Ponti G, Ponz de Leon M: Muir–Torre syndrome. Lancet Oncol 2005; 6:980.

Tanyi M, et al: A new mutation in Muir–Torre syndrome associated with familiar transmission of different gastrointestinal adenocarcinomas. Eur J Surg Oncol 2009; 35:1128.

Sweat gland tumors

Syringoma

Syringomas are very common neoplasms demonstrating sweat duct differentiation. They present as small papules 1–3 mm in diameter. They may be yellow, brown, or pink. They are virtually always multiple and most frequently occur on the eyelids and upper cheeks (Fig. 29-34). They are disproportionately common in these sites in Japanese women. Other sites of involvement include the axillae, abdomen, forehead, penis, and vulva. Genital syringomas may cause genital pruritus and be mistaken for genital warts. Rarely, they may be unilateral or linear. Symmetrical distal extremity involvement has also been reported. Eruptive syringomas are histologically identical to syringomas of the eyelid, but appear suddenly as numerous lesions on the neck, chest, axillae, upper arms, and periumbilically, usually in young persons (Fig. 29-35). Some have suggested that eruptive syringomas represent a proliferative process of inflamed normal eccrine glands, analogous to traumatic neuroma being a proliferation of normal peripheral nerve. The fact that numerous lesions appear after

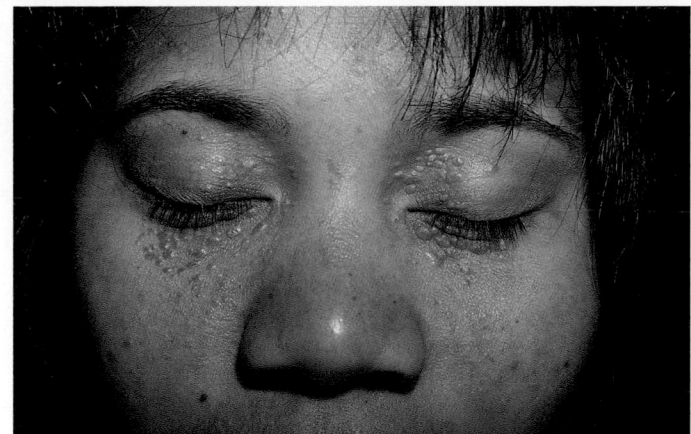

Fig. 29-34 Syringomas.

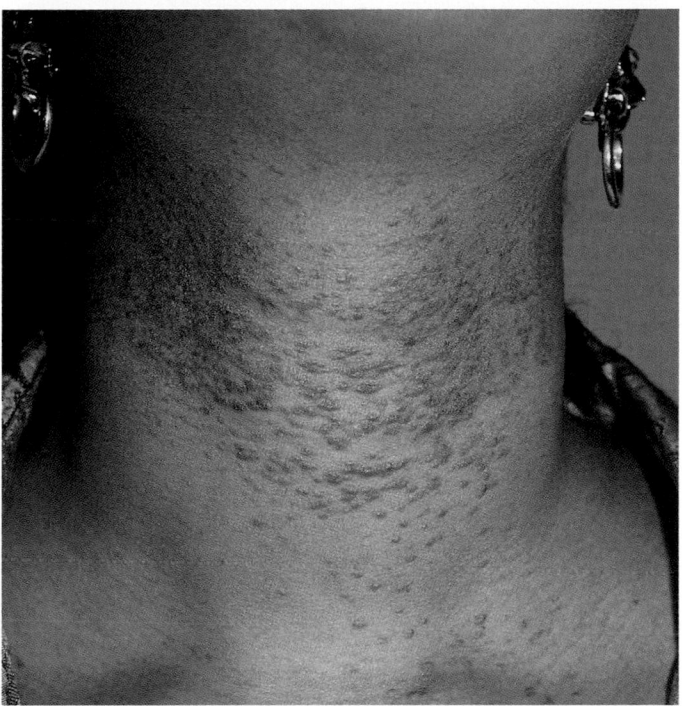

Fig. 29-35 Syringomas.

"waxing" in the pubic areas supports this hypothesis. Many individual case reports document unusual clinical variants of syringomas. These include types limited to the scalp, associated with alopecia; a unilateral linear or nevoid distribution; those limited to the vulva or penis; those limited to the distal extremities; and the lichen planus- and milia-like types. Syringomas may calcify and be mistaken for subepidermal calcified nodules. The rare "plaque-type" syringoma may be mistaken for a microcystic adnexal carcinoma.

Familial cases of syringomas occur. In general, except in eruptive cases, syringomas develop slowly and persist indefinitely without symptoms. Acral lesions are often present. Syringomas occur in 18% of adults with Down syndrome, particularly females. This is approximately 30 times the frequency seen in patients with other syndromes.

Histologically, syringomas are characterized by dilated cystic spaces lined by two layers of cuboidal cells and epithelial strands of similar cells. Some of the cysts have small comma-like tails, which produce a distinctive picture, resembling tadpoles or the pattern of a paisley tie. There is a dense fibrous stroma. At times, the cells of the syringoma have abundant clear cytoplasm, which represents accumulated glycogen. This has been called "clear cell syringoma." Syringomas stain positive for keratins 5, 6, 14, 6, 16, 19, and 77 on the inner cell layer, and K5 and K14 on the outer cell layer, in a pattern identical to the intraglandular eccrine duct. The microscopic differential diagnosis of "paisley tie" epithelial islands embedded in a sclerotic stroma includes microcystic adnexal carcinoma (sclerosing sweat duct carcinoma), desmoplastic trichoepithelioma, and morpheiform BCC.

Treatment is difficult, but many lesions respond to very light electrodessication or shave removal. For larger lesions, surgical removal may be considered. Carbon dioxide laser treatment by the pinhole method or fractional thermolysis has been reported as effective.

Akita H, et al: Syringoma of the face treated with fractional photothermolysis. J Cosmet Laser Ther 2009; 11:216.

Ceulen RP, et al: Multiple unilateral skin tumors suggest type 1 segmental manifestation of familial syringoma. Eur J Dermatol 2008; 18:285.

Draznin M: Hereditary syringomas: a case report. Dermatol Online J 2004; 10:19.

Garrido-Ruiz MC, et al: Eruptive syringoma developed over a waxing skin area. Am J Dermatopathol 2008; 30:377.

Huang YH, et al: Vulvar syringoma: a clinicopathologic and immunohistologic study of 18 patients and results of treatment. J Am Acad Dermatol 2003; 48:735.

Karam P, et al: Intralesional electrodesiccation of syringomas. Dermatol Surg 1998; 24:692.

Kavala M, et al: Vulvar pruritus caused by syringoma of the vulva. Int J Dermatol 2008; 47:831.

Langbein L, et al: New concepts on the histogenesis of eccrine neoplasia from keratin expression in the normal eccrine gland, syringoma and poroma. Br J Dermatol 2008; 159:633.

Martyn-Simmons CL, Ostlere LS: Papular eruption on a patient with Down syndrome. Arch Dermatol 2004; 140:1161.

Marzano AV, et al: Familial syringoma: report of two cases with a published work review and the unique association with steatocystoma multiplex. J Dermatol 2009; 36:154.

Missall TA, et al: Immunohistochemical differentiation of four benign eccrine tumors. J Cutan Pathol 2009; 36:190.

Nguyen DB, et al: Syringoma of the moustache area. J Am Acad Dermatol 2003; 49:337.

Nosrati N, et al: Axillary syringomas. Dermatol Online J 2008; 14:13.

Olson JM, et al; Multiple penile syringomas. J Am Acad Dermatol 2008; 59:S46.

Park HJ, et al: The treatment of syringomas by CO(2) laser using a multiple-drilling method. Dermatol Surg 2007; 33:310.

Petersson F, et al: Eruptive syringoma of the penis. A report of 2 cases and a review of the literature. Am J Dermatopathol 2009; 31:436.

Sacoor MF, Medley P: Eruptive syringoma in four black South African children. Clin Exp Dermatol 2004; 29:686.

Schepis C, et al: Eruptive syringomas with calcium deposits in a young woman with Down's syndrome. Dermatology 2001; 203:345.

Seo SH, et al: A case of milium-like syringoma with focal calcification in Down syndrome. Br J Dermatol 2007; 157:612.

Soler-Carrillo J, et al: Eruptive syringoma: 27 new cases and review of the literature. J Eur Acad Dermatol Venereol 2001; 15:242.

Suwattee P, et al: Plaque-type syringoma: two cases misdiagnosed as microcystic adnexal carcinoma. J Cutan Pathol 2008; 35:570.

Wang KH, et al: Milium-like syringoma: a case study on histogenesis. J Cutan Pathol 2004; 31:336.

Wu CY: Multifocal penile syringoma masquerading as genital warts. Clin Exp Dermatol 2009; 34:e290.

Hidrocystomas

Hidrocystomas are 1–3 mm translucent papules that occasionally have a bluish tint. They usually are solitary, occur on the face or scalp, and are more common in women. In some patients, multiple lesions may be present (Fig. 29-36) and they may be pigmented. They may become more prominent during hot weather. They most typically occur periocularly. Multiple

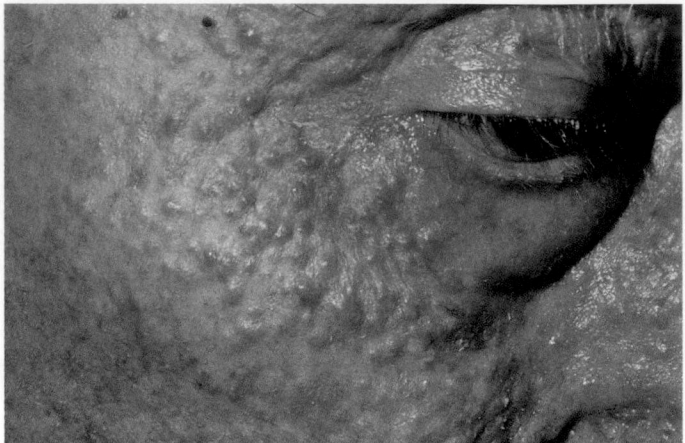

Fig. 29-36 Hidrocystomas.

hidrocystomas with apocrine secretion on the eyelids are the hallmark of Schopf–Schulz–Passarge syndrome (SSPS), an adult-onset syndrome resembling focal dermal hypoplasia. Other features include hypodontia, hypotrichosis, nail dystrophy, and palmoplantar keratoderma. Multiple palmoplantar syringofibroadenomas are present in most cases of SSPS, and can present as a palmoplantar keratoderma. Up to 44% of patients have other adnexal tumors. Skin and visceral malignancy are not increased in SSPS.

Microscopically, a single cystic cavity lined by two layers of small cuboidal epithelial cells is present. Apocrine differentiation in the form of decapitation secretion is common. Lesions with papillary proliferations of the lining are classified as cystadenomas. Treatment, if desired, is by excision for solitary lesions. Laser treatment may be effective, both with CO_2 and pulsed dye laser. Topical atropine ointment 1% or scopolamine cream 0.01% (1.2 mL of 0.25% scopolamine eyedrops in 30 g of Eucerin), once daily, has been used with variable success in patients with multiple lesions. Pupil size may increase with these agents. Oral glycopyrrolate, 1 mg twice daily, may be useful in suppressing exercise- and hot weather-induced enlargement. Botulinum toxin may also be effective.

Castori M, et al: Schopf–Schulz–Passarge syndrome: further delineation of the phenotype and genetic considerations. Acta Derm Venereol 2008; 88:607.

Choi JE, et al: Lack of effect of the pulsed-dye laser in the treatment of multiple eccrine hidrocystomas: a report of two cases. Dermatol Surg 2007; 33:1513.

Correia O, et al: Multiple eccrine hidrocystomas—from diagnosis to treatment: the role of dermatoscopy and botulinum toxin. Dermatology 2009; 219:77.

Hampton PJ, et al: A case of Schopf Schulz–Passarge syndrome. Clin Exp Dermatol 2005; 30:528.

Lee HW, et al: Multiple eccrine hidrocystomas: successful treatment with the 595 nm long-pulsed dye laser. Dermatol Surg 2006; 32:296.

Madan V, et al: Multiple eccrine hidrocystomas—response to treatment with carbon dioxide and pulsed dye lasers. Dermatol Surg 2009; 35:1015.

Ozkan Z: Multiple eccrine hidrocystomas of the vulva. Int J Gynaecol Obstet 2009; 105:65.

Sanz-Sanchez T, et al: Efficacy and safety of topical atropine in treatment of multiple eccrine hidrocystomas. Arch Dermatol 2001; 137:670.

Sheth HG, Raina J: Giant eccrine hidrocystoma presenting with unilateral ptosis and epiphora. Int Ophthalmol 2008; 28:429.

Shimokawa M, et al: Successful treatment of multiple eccrine hidrocystoma with topical atropine sulfate ointment. J Dermatol 2009; 36:114.

Smith DR, et al: Multiple eccrine hidrocystomas treated with glycopyrrolate. J Am Acad Dermatol 2008; 59:S122.

Woolery-Lloyd H, et al: Treatment for multiple periorbital eccrine hidrocystomas: botulinum toxin A. J Drugs Dermatol 2009; 8:71.

Acrospiromas (poroma, hidroacanthoma simplex, dermal duct tumor, nodular hidradenoma, clear cell hidradenoma)

Acrospiromas are benign tumors with acrosyringial differentiation. A poroma presents as a slow-growing, 2–12 mm, slightly protruding, sessile, soft, reddish tumor that occurs most often on the sole (Fig. 29-37) or side of the foot. Palmar lesions may also occur, and more rarely lesions appear wherever sweat glands are found. The lesion will bleed on slight trauma. A distinctive finding is the cup-shaped shallow depression from which the tumor grows and protrudes. Poromas tend to occur singly, but multiple lesions may also occur. A rare variant is called eccrine poromatosis, in which more than 100 lesions may involve the palms and soles and may be associated with hidrotic ectodermal dysplasia. These may represent acrosyringeal nevi. Dermal duct tumors present deep nodules that may involve any part of the body. Nodular and clear cell hidradenomas are larger nodules that often involve the head or neck, but may occur anywhere. Hybrid combinations of different patterns of acrospiroma are very common.

Histologically, poromas demonstrate solid masses of uniform, cuboidal epithelial cells with ample cytoplasm and focal duct differentiation. The cells are smaller than those in the contiguous epidermis and tend to arrange themselves in cords and broad columns extending downward from the normal epidermis. Areas of clear cell and cystic degeneration may be present, and an underlying dermal duct tumor or hidradenoma may be present. Melanocytes may be dispersed throughout the tumor and be clinically hyperpigmented. The surrounding stroma is highly vascular, with telangiectatic vessels. Hidroacanthoma simplex represents an intraepidermal eccrine poroma. These lesions resemble clonal seborrheic keratoses, except for the presence of focal duct differentiation. Dermal duct tumors are composed of the same small acrosyringeal cells as other acrospiromas. The cells form small dermal islands with ductal differentiation. When the cells form a large nodule, the tumor is referred to as a nodular hidradenoma. When clear cells and cystic degeneration are prominent, the tumor is referred to as a clear cell hidradenoma. A distinctive feature of the latter two tumors is the presence of areas of eosinophilic hyalized stroma. All the cells in a poroma, except entrapped ducts, stain with K5/14. Focally, they are K1/10-positive and uniformly K77-negative. This is the staining pattern of the sweat duct ridge and acrosyringium (the intraepidermal portions of the sweat duct). The clinical differential diagnosis includes porocarcinoma, granuloma pyogenicum, melanoma (amelanotic and melanotic), Kaposi sarcoma, BCC, and seborrheic keratosis. The lesions are benign, but often recur following inadequate excision. Malignant degeneration may occur, and atypia is sometimes minimal within tumors that have metastasized. For these reasons, simple complete excision is recommended when feasible.

Malignant acrospiroma (malignant poroma, porocarcinoma)

This represents the most common form of sweat duct carcinoma. Most malignant acrospiromas appear clinically similar to poromas, but may also manifest as a blue or black nodule, plaque, or ulcerated tumor. Porocarcinoma affects men and women equally at an average age of 70 years. The most frequent sites of involvement are the legs (30%), feet (20%), face (12%), thighs (8%), and arms (7%). Of interest is the rare involvement of the palms and soles, despite these having the greatest concentration of sweat glands. The average age from onset to treatment is 8 years. These tumors are of intermediate aggressiveness, with metastases usually occurring to regional lymph nodes and, less commonly, hematogenously.

Histologically, the tumor may be seen adjoining benign acrospiroma. Atypia may be marked or minimal, with pleomorphic or monomorphous nuclei, and abundant or scant eosinophilic cytoplasm. Most commonly, the cells are smaller and more basophilic than those in benign acrospiromas with a high mitotic rate. Focal squamous or sarcomatous differentiation may be present. Pagetoid spread within the adjacent epidermis may be seen, just as in benign acrospiromas clear cell and cystic degeneration may be present. The degree of ductal differentiation is variable. The tumors can be deeply infiltrative. Perineural and lymphovascular involvement by the tumor can be present and should be noted on the dermatopathology report. The epidermis may be invaded by metastatic porocarcinoma. Mohs surgery can be a valuable technique, particularly on the face. As with other cutaneous neoplasms, margins should be free of tumor islands and tumor stroma to be considered negative. Local recurrence approaches 20%, and lymph node metastases occur in about 20% of patients. Sentinel lymph node biopsy could be considered. Distant metastases occur in 10% of cases, often at a distant skin site.

Altamura D, et al: Eccrine poroma in an unusual site: a clinical and dermoscopic simulator of amelanotic melanoma. J Am Acad Dermatol 2005; 53:539.

Barzi AS, et al: Malignant metastatic eccrine poroma: proposal for a new therapeutic protocol. Dermatol Surg 1997; 23:267.

Brown CW Jr, Dy LC: Eccrine porocarcinoma. Dermatol Ther 2008; 21:433.

Burra UK, et al: Eccrine porocarcinoma (malignant eccrine poroma): a case report. Dermatol Online J 2005; 11:17.

Chiu HH, et al: Origin of poroid hidradenoma and pigmentation mechanism of eccrine poroma: critical analysis of a unique presentation. J Eur Acad Dermatol Venereol 2009; 23:597.

Feldman AH, et al: Clear cell hidradenoma of the second digit: a review of the literature with case presentation. J Foot Ankle Surg 1997; 36:21.

Ferrari A, et al: Eccrine poroma: a clinical-dermoscopic study of seven cases. Acta Derm Venereol 2009; 89:160.

Gerber PA, et al: Eccrine porocarcinoma of the head: an important differential diagnosis in the elderly patient. Dermatology 2008; 216:229.

Goh SG, et al: Sarcomatoid eccrine porocarcinoma: report of two cases and a review of the literature. J Cutan Pathol 2007; 34:55.

Hu SC, et al: Pigmented eccrine poromas: expression of melanocyte-stimulating cytokines by tumour cells does not always result in melanocyte colonization. J Eur Acad Dermatol Venereol 2008; 22:303.

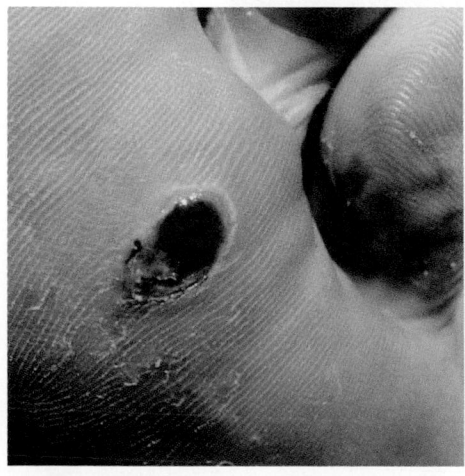

Fig. 29-37 Poroma.

Jagdeo J, et al: Unusual clinical presentation of benign eccrine poroma. J Am Acad Dermatol 2006; 54:733.

Jo JH, et al: A case of eccrine poroma treated with 5% imiquimod cream. J Dermatol 2005; 32:691.

Kurt M, et al: Malignant eccrine poroma presenting with pulmonary and liver metastases. Int J Dermatol 2006; 45:1263.

Langbein L, et al: New concepts on the histogenesis of eccrine neoplasia from keratin expression in the normal eccrine gland, syringoma and poroma. Br J Dermatol 2008; 159:633.

Ohta M, et al: Nodular hidradenocarcinoma on the scalp of a young woman: case report and review of the literature. Dermatol Surg 2004; 30:1265.

Orlandi C, et al: Eccrine poroma in a child. Pediatr Dermatol 2005; 22:279.

Sidro-Sarto M, et al: Eccrine poroma arising in chronic radiation dermatitis. J Eur Acad Dermatol Venereol 2008; 22:1517.

Urso C, et al: Carcinomas of sweat glands: report of 60 cases. Arch Pathol Lab Med 2001; 125:498.

Wakamatsu J, et al: The occurrence of eccrine poroma on a burn site. J Eur Acad Dermatol Venereol 2007; 21:1128.

Spiradenoma

Spiradenoma presents clinically as a solitary, 1 cm, deep-seated nodule, occurring most frequently on the ventral surface of the body, especially over the upper half. Normal-appearing skin covers the nodule, which may be skin-colored, blue, or pink. Occasionally, multiple lesions may be present and may occur in a linear or segmental pattern. Giant lesions that are very vascular are rarely seen. Lesions may be painful, but not universally. Spiradenoma has a generally benign clinical course and occurs most frequently between the ages of 15 and 35, although it has also been reported in infancy and childhood. Familial cases have been described. Rarely, malignant transformation occurs, and the subsequent tumor may also have features of a cylindroma (spiradenocylindrocarcinoma).

Microscopically, it demonstrates either a single nodule or multiple basophilic nodules within the dermis. Tumor cells have little to no visible cytoplasm. They are often arranged in characteristic small rosettes. Three cell types are present: cells with large, pale gray nuclei; those with smaller, darker gray nuclei; and jet-black lymphocytes peppered throughout the nodule. Duct-like structures are often present, as are large pink hyaline globules that resemble the bright red hyaline basement membrane material that outlines the islands of cylindromas. In fact, spiradenomas and cylindromas commonly occur together in the same patient, and hybrid collision tumors are quite common.

When painful, eccrine spiradenoma may be mistaken for leiomyoma, glomus tumor, neuroma, and angiolipoma. Treatment is simple excision. Spiradenocylindrocarcinoma presents as a solitary nodule that may have experienced an abrupt change in size. Histologically, these lesions have focal areas of atypia, mitoses, and invasion. They may metastasize to regional lymph nodes, or hematogenously. Local recurrence occurs with inadequate, primarily local control.

Altinyazar HC, et al: Multiple eccrine spiradenoma in zosteriform distribution. Plast Reconstr Surg 2003; 112:927.

Ben Brahim E, et al: Malignant eccrine spiradenoma: a new case report. J Cutan Pathol 2009 Jul 10 (Epub ahead of print).

Bumgardner AC, et al: Trichoepitheliomas and eccrine spiradenomas with spiradenoma/cylindroma overlap. Int J Dermatol 2005; 44:415.

Carlsten JR: Spiradenocylindrocarcinoma: a malignant hybrid tumor. J Cutan Pathol 2005; 32:166.

Ekmekci TR, et al: Congenital blaschkoid eccrine spiradenoma on the face. Eur J Dermatol 2005; 15:73.

Fernandez-Acenero MJ, et al: Malignant spiradenoma: report of two cases and literature review. J Am Acad Dermatol 2001; 44:395.

Jukic DM, et al: Carcinoma ex spiradenoma/cylindroma confirmed by immunohistochemical and molecular loss-of-heterozygosity profiling. Am J Dermatopathol 2009; 31:702.

Kazakov DV, et al: Low-grade adnexal carcinoma of the skin with multidirectional (glandular, trichoblastomatous, spiradenocylindromatous) differentiation. Am J Dermatopathol 2006; 28:341.

Kazakov DV, et al: Morphologic diversity of malignant neoplasms arising in preexisting spiradenoma, cylindroma, and spiradenocylindroma based on the study of 24 cases, sporadic or occurring in the setting of Brooke–Spiegler syndrome. Am J Surg Pathol 2009; 33:705.

Kurokawa I, et al: Eccrine spiradenoma: co-expression of cytokeratin and smooth muscle actin suggesting differentiation toward myoepithelial cells. J Eur Acad Dermatol Venereol 2007; 21:121.

Leach BC, Graham BS: Papular lesion of the proximal nail fold. Eccrine spiradenoma. Arch Dermatol 2004; 140:1003.

Lobo I, et al: Multiple nodules of the head—clinicopathologic challenge. Int J Dermatol 2009; 48:237.

Petersson F, et al: Adenoid cystic carcinoma-like pattern in spiradenoma and spiradenocylindroma: a rare feature in sporadic neoplasms and those associated with Brooke–Spiegler syndrome. Am J Dermatopathol 2009; 31:642.

Poorten T, et al: Familial eccrine spiradenoma: a case report and review of the literature. Dermatol Surg 2003; 29:411.

Rodriguez-Martin M, et al: An unusual case of congenital linear eccrine spiradenoma. Pediatr Dermatol 2009; 26:180.

Tanese K, et al: Malignant eccrine spiradenoma: case report and review of the literature, including 15 Japanese cases. Clin Exp Dermatol 2010; 35:51.

Turhan-Haktanir N, et al: A case of eccrine spiradenoma arising in nevus sebaceus in an adolescent girl. Am J Dermatopathol 2008; 30:196.

Yamakoshi T, et al: A case of giant vascular eccrine spiradenoma with unusual clinical features. Clin Exp Dermatol 2009; 34:e250.

Yoshida A, et al: Two cases of multiple eccrine spiradenoma with linear or localized formation. J Dermatol 2004; 31:564.

Cylindroma

Cutaneous cylindroma, also known as dermal eccrine cylindroma, occurs predominantly on the scalp and face as a solitary lesion. The tumor is firm, but rubber-like and pinkish to blue; it ranges in size from a few millimeters to several centimeters (Fig. 29-38). The solitary cylindroma is considered to be nonhereditary and may at times be found in areas other than the head and neck. Women are affected more than men.

The dominantly inherited form, Brooke–Spiegler syndrome (BSS), appears soon after puberty as numerous rounded masses of various sizes on the scalp. The lesions resemble bunches of grapes or small tomatoes. Lesions appear in the second or third decade. Sometimes they cover the entire scalp like a turban. BSS is characterized by the presence of multiple adnexal neoplasms, including cylindroma, trichoepitheliomas, spiradenomas, trichoblastomas, follicular cysts, and milia.

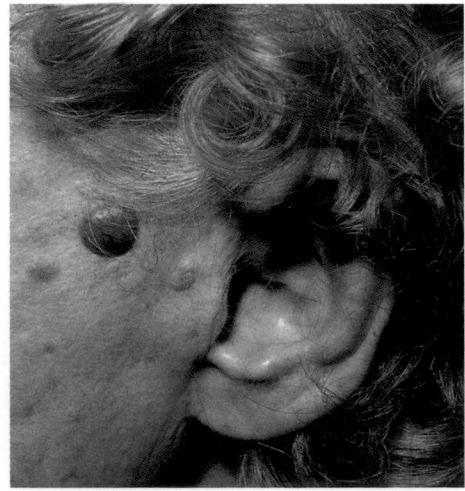

Fig. 29-38 Cylindroma.

Familial cylindroma is now considered a variant of BSS since it harbors the same mutation. There is no genotypic/phenotypic correlation in these two syndromes. BSS is due to a mutation in the *CYLD* tumor suppressor gene.

Histologically, these are cylindrical masses of epithelial cells surrounded and segmented by thick bands of a hyaline material. Cylindroma may be mistaken for pilar cyst, but the distinctive appearance and consistency make diagnosis easy, especially in the multiple type. Treatment is surgical.

Bowen S, et al: Mutations in the *CYLD* gene in Brooke–Spiegler syndrome, familial cylindromatosis, and multiple familial trichoepithelioma: lack of genotype-phenotype correlation. J Invest Dermatol 2005; 124:919.

Chaer RA, Lipnick S: Images in clinical medicine: cylindroma. N Engl J Med 2004; 351:2530.

Kakagia D, et al: Brooke–Spiegler syndrome with parotid gland involvement. Eur J Dermatol 2004; 14:139.

Kim C, et al: Brooke–Spiegler syndrome. Dermatol Online J 2007; 13:10.

Ly H, et al: Case of the Brooke–Spiegler syndrome. Australas J Dermatol 2004; 45:220.

Tarstedt M, Molin L: Nd:YAG laser for effective treatment of multiple cylindroma of the scalp. J Cosmet Laser Ther 2004; 6:41.

Mixed tumor (chondroid syringoma)

Cutaneous mixed tumor is an uncommon skin tumor, representing about 1 in 1000 skin lesions removed electively. It favors men between the ages of 25 and 65. Mixed tumor presents clinically as a firm intradermal or subcutaneous nodule, virtually always located on the head and neck. These tumors are usually asymptomatic and measure 5–30 mm in diameter, but may be much larger.

Histologically, nests of cuboidal or polygonal epithelial cells in the dermis give rise to tubuloalveolar and ductal structures, and occasionally, keratinous cysts. These structures are embedded in a matrix varying from a faint, bluish, chondroid substance to an acidophilic hyaline material. Myoepithelial and lipomatous elements may also be found in the tumor, in addition to the chondroid stroma. Ossification may occur. The treatment is surgical. Mixed tumors may also occur in other organs, especially salivary glands. In salivary and rarely in cutaneous chondroid syringoma, tyrosine crystals may be seen in the tumor. Tumors with only focal glandular elements, or with no epithelial elements, have been called "cutaneous myoepitheliomas." They are tumors of the myoepithelial cells. Myoepithelial cells surround the sweat glands and, by their contraction, help deliver the product of the glands to the surface.

Malignant mixed tumor (malignant chondroid syringoma)

This rare tumor favors the trunk and extremities (whereas benign mixed tumor of the skin favors the head and neck). At presentation, the masses range from 1 to 10 cm, with a median size of 4 cm, and often grow rapidly. The chance of metastasis is more than 50%, with a predilection for visceral spread. Metastases usually take the form of an adenocarcinoma, and the chondroid stroma found in primary lesions is often not found. Histologic features that distinguish malignant mixed tumor from chondroid syringoma include cytologic atypia, pleomorphism, increased mitotic activity, and focal necrosis. Treatment is surgical.

Agrawal A, et al: Chondroid syringoma. Singapore Med J 2008; 49:e33–e34.

Awasthi R, et al: Benign mixed tumour of the skin with extensive ossification and marrow formation: a case report. J Clin Pathol 2004; 57:1329.

Constantinescu MB, et al: Chondroid syringoma with tyrosine crystals: case report and review of the literature. Am J Dermatopathol 2009 Oct 21 (Epub ahead of print).

Hafezi-Bakhtiari S, et al: Benign mixed tumor of the skin, hypercellular variant: a case report. J Cutan Patol 2009 Jul 10 (Epub ahead of print).

Kakitsubata Y, et al: Giant chondroid syringoma presenting as a growing subcutaneous mass in the upper arm: MRI findings with pathologic correlation. Joint Bone Spine 2009:76:711.

Laxmisha C, et al: Chondroid syringoma of the ear lobe. J Cutan Pathol 2009 Jul 10 (Epub ahead of print).

Mentzel T, et al: Cutaneous myoepithelial neoplasms: clinicopathologic and immunohistochemical study of 20 cases suggesting a continuous spectrum ranging from benign mixed tumor of the skin to cutaneous myoepithelioma and myoepithelial carcinoma. J Cutan Pathol 2003; 30:294.

Miracco C, et al: Lipomatous mixed tumour of the skin: a histological, immunohistochemical and ultrastructural study. Br J Dermatol 2002; 146:899.

Radhi JM: Chondroid syringoma with small tubular lumina. J Cutan Med Surg 2004; 8:23.

Sivamani R, et al: Chondroid syringoma: case report and review of the literature. Dermatol Online J 2006; 12:8.

Ceruminoma

Ceruminous glands, modified apocrine glands of the external ear, may give rise to both benign and malignant tumors. Distinguishing these may be very difficult; hence both the malignant and benign tumors have been termed ceruminomas. The tumors present as a firm papule or nodule in the external auditory canal. Ulceration and crusting may occur, and continued growth may obstruct the meatus.

Histologically, glands and cysts are present, lined by a tuboglandular proliferation with two layers—an inner layer of ceruminous cells (containing cerumen and with decapitation secretion) and a basal spindled or cuboidal myoepithelial layer. Treatment is excision, which is curative if margins are clear.

Schenk P, et al: Ultrastructural morphology of a middle ear ceruminoma. J Otorhinolaryngol Relat Spec 2002; 64:358.

Thompson LD, et al: Ceruminous adenomas: a clinicopathologic study of 41 cases with a review of the literature. Am J Surg Pathol 2004; 28:308.

Hidradenoma papilliferum

Hidradenoma papilliferum is a benign apocrine adenoma that is located almost exclusively in the vulvar and perianal areas. The tumor is covered by normal skin. On palpation it is a firm papule less than 1 cm in diameter. Malignant transformation is rare and can resemble a focus of ductal carcinoma in situ.

Microscopically, hidradenoma papilliferum is encapsulated and lies in the dermis, having no connection with the epidermis. There is a cyst-like cavity lined with villi. The walls of the cavity and the villi are lined, occasionally with a single, but usually with a double layer of cells—luminal secretory cells and myoepithelial cells. This is a benign lesion and the diagnosis and treatment are accomplished by excisional biopsy.

Daniel F, et al: An uncommon perianal nodule: hidradenoma papilliferum. Gastroenterol Clin Biol 2007; 31:166.

Fernandez-Acenero MJ, et al: Ectopic hidradenoma papilliferum: a case report and literature review. Am J Dermatopathol 2003; 25:176.

Handa Y, et al: Large ulcerated perianal hidradenoma papilliferum in a young female. Dermatol Surg 2003; 29:790.

Moon JW, et al: Giant ectopic hidradenoma papilliferum on the scalp. J Dermatol 2009; 36:545.

Nishie W, et al: Hidradenoma papilliferum with mixed histopathologic features of syringocystadenoma papilliferum and anogenital mammary-like glands. J Cutan Pathol 2004; 31:561.

Smith FB, et al: Hidradenoma papilliferum of nasal skin. Arch Pathol Lab Med 2003; 127:E86.

Vazmitel M, et al: Hidradenoma papilliferum with a ductal carcinoma in situ component: case report and review of the literature. Am J Dermatopathol 2008; 30:392.

Veeranna S, Vijaya: Solitary nodule over the labia majora. Hidradenoma papilliferum. Indian J Dermatol Venereol Leprol 2009; 75:327.

Syringadenoma papilliferum (syringocystadenoma papilliferum)

This lesion develops in a nevus sebaceus of Jadassohn on the scalp (Fig. 29-39) or face in about one-third of cases. Around half are present at birth, while approximately 25% arise on the trunk and genital and inguinal regions during adolescence. The lesions are rose-red papules of firm consistency; they vary from 1 to 3 mm and may occur in groups. Vesicle-like inclusions are seen, pinpoint to pinhead in size, filled with clear fluid. Some of the papules may be umbilicated and simulate molluscum contagiosum. Extensive verrucous or papillary plaques may also be present.

Histologically, the tumor shows ductlike structures that extend from the surface epithelium. Numerous papillary projections may extend into the lumina, which may be cystic. The papillary projections are lined by glandular epithelium, often consisting of two rows of cells. The tumor cells stain positively for carcinoembryonic antigen. The dermal stroma contains numerous plasma cells. Rarely, malignant transformation may occur. Excision is recommended.

Arai Y, et al: A case of syringocystadenocarcinoma papilliferum in situ occurring partially in syringocystadenoma papilliferum. J Dermatol 2003; 30:146.

Askar S, et al: Syringocystadenoma papilliferum mimicking basal cell carcinoma on the lower eyelid: a case report. Acta Chir Plast 2002; 44:117.

Chi CC, et al: Syringocystadenocarcinoma papilliferum: successfully treated with Mohs micrographic surgery. Dermatol Surg 2004; 30:468.

Dawn G, Gupta G: Linear warty papules on the neck of a young woman: syringocystadenoma papilliferum (SP) in a sebaceous nevus (SN). Arch Dermatol 2002; 138:1091.

Gonul M, et al: Linear syringocystadenoma papilliferum of the arm: a rare localization of an uncommon tumour. Acta Derm Venereol 2008; 88:528.

Goshima J, et al: Syringocystadenoma papilliferum arising on the scrotum. Eur J Dermatol 2003; 13:271.

Hoekzema R, et al: Syringocystadenocarcinoma papilliferum in a linear nevus verrucosus. J Cutan Pathol 2009 (Epub ahead of print).

Karg E, et al: Congenital syringocystadenoma papilliferum. Pediatr Dermatol 2008; 25:132.

Laximisha C, et al: Linear syringocystadenoma papilliferum of the scalp. J Eur Acad Dermatol Venereol 2007; 21:275.

Li A, et al: Syringocystadenoma papilliferum contiguous to a verrucous cyst. J Cutan Pathol 2003; 30:32.

Malhotra P, et al: Syringocystadenoma papilliferum on the thigh: an unusual location. Indian J Dermatol Venereol Leprol 2009; 75:170.

Monticciolo NL, et al: Verrucous carcinoma arising within syringocystadenoma papilliferum. Ann Clin Lab Sci 2002; 32:434.

Nakai K, et al: Sebaceoma, trichoblastoma and syringocystadenoma papilliferum arising within a nevus sebaceus. J Dermatol 2008; 35:365.

Narang T, et al: Linear papules and nodules on the neck. Syringocystadenoma papilliferum (SP). Arch Dermatol 2008; 144:1509.

Philipone E, Chen S: Unique case: syringocystadenoma papilliferum associated with an eccrine nevus. Am J Dermatopathol 2009; 31:806.

Rosen H, et al: Management of nevus sebaceus and the risk of basal cell carcinoma: an 18-year review. Pediatr Dermatol 2009 Jul 20 (Epub ahead of print).

Saricaoglu H, et al: A case of syringocystadenoma papilliferum: an unusual localization on postoperative scar. J Eur Acad Dermatol Venereol 2002; 16:534.

Schaffer JV, et al: Syringocystadenoma papilliferum in a patient with focal dermal hypoplasia due to a novel *PORCN* mutation. Arch Dermatol 2009; 145:218.

Stewart CJ: Syringocystadenoma papilliferum-like lesion of the vulva. Pathology 2008; 40:638.

Townsend TC, et al: Syringocystadenoma papilliferum: an unusual cutaneous lesion in a pediatric patient. J Pediatr 2004; 145:131.

Yaghoobi R, et al: Giant linear syringocystadenoma papilliferum on scalp. Indian J Dermatol Venereol Leprol 2009; 75:318.

Papillary eccrine adenoma (tubular apocrine adenoma)

This uncommon benign sweat gland neoplasm presents clinically as dermal nodules located primarily on the extremities of black patients, especially on the dorsal hand or foot. Histologic findings consist of a well-circumscribed, dermal, unencapsulated growth composed of dilated ductlike structures lined by two or more layers of cells. Intraluminal papillations may project into the cystic spaces. Because of this lesion's tendency to recur locally, complete surgical excision with clear margins is recommended. Hybrid or overlapping lesions with a superficial component resembling syringocystadenoma papilliferum and a deep component resembling tubular adenoma can occur.

Ahn BK, et al: A case of tubular apocrine adenoma with syringocystadenoma papilliferum arising in nevus sebaceous. J Dermatol 2004; 31:508.

Jackson EM, Cook J: Mohs micrographic surgery of a papillary eccrine adenoma. Dermatol Surg 2002; 28:1168.

Kazakov DV, et al: Tubular adenoma and syringocystadenoma papilliferum: a reappraisal of their relationship. An interobserver study of a series, by a panel of dermatopathologists. Am J Dermatopathol 2007; 29:256.

Syringofibroadenoma (acrosyringeal nevus of Weedon and Lewis)

First described by Mascaro in 1963, four variants of eccrine syringofibroadenoma (ESFA) are now recognized:

1. solitary
2. multiple, in Schopf syndrome
3. multiple, without other skin manifestations
4. nonfamilial unilateral linear.

The solitary type presents frequently as a hyperkeratotic nodule or plaque involving the extremities. The linear type may be linear, blaschkoid, or zosteriform in appearance and some cases may represent an acrosyringeal nevus. Multiple lesions have been termed eccrine syringofibroadenomatosis (ESFA) and occur in both variants of hidrotic ectodermal

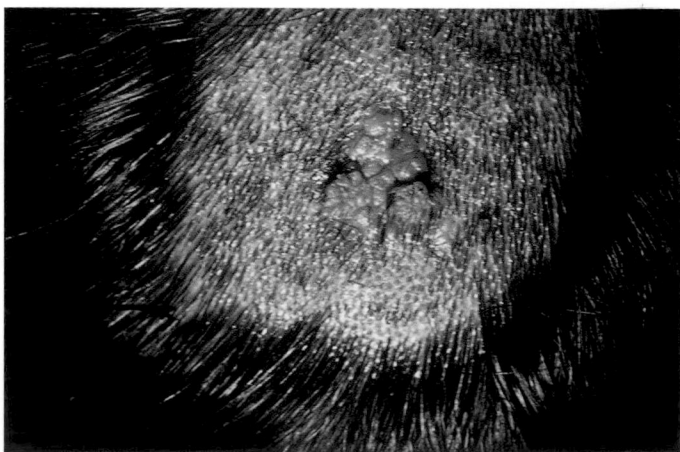

Fig. 29-39 Syringocystadenoma papilliferum.

dysplasia, Schopf syndrome, and Clouston syndrome. The multiple ESFAs may appear in a mosaic pattern. In Clouston syndrome (due to mutation in the *GJB6* gene), HPV-10 has been detected in the tumors. Multiple lesions have also been reported without any other associated cutaneous findings. Many cases represent a reactive epithelial proliferation, whereas others represent a true neoplasm of acrosyringeal cells. Histologically, the strands resemble those of the fibroepithelial tumor of Pinkus, but with broader anastomosing cords without the basaloid buds. "Reactive eccrine syringofibroadenoma" most commonly occurs on the lower leg and may show adjacent changes of an associated dermatosis. Carcinomatous transformation of ESFA has been reported.

Kawaguchi M, et al: Eccrine syringofibroadenoma with diffuse plantar hyperkeratosis. Br J Dermatol 2003; 149:885.

Poonawalla T, et al: Clouston syndrome and eccrine syringofibroadenomas. Am J Dermatopathol 2009; 31:157.

Schadt CR, Boyd AS: Eccrine syringofibroadenoma with co-existent squamous cell carcinoma. J Cutan Pathol 2007; 34:71.

Starink TM: Eccrine syringofibroadenoma: multiple lesions representing a new cutaneous marker of the Schopf syndrome, and solitary nonhereditary tumors. J Am Acad Dermatol 1997; 36:569.

Utani A, et al: Reactive eccrine syringofibroadenoma: an association with chronic foot ulcer in a patient with diabetes mellitus. J Am Acad Dermatol 1999; 41:650.

Microcystic adnexal carcinoma (sclerosing sweat duct carcinoma)

The tumor generally presents as a very slow-growing plaque or nodule. It occurs most commonly on the head and neck (87%), face (73%), and scalp (10%). Lesions favor the central face and periorbital area. The upper lip (Fig. 29-40) is involved nine times more often than the lower lip. Microcystic adnexal carcinomas have occurred at sites of prior therapeutic radiation. They are very locally aggressive, with local recurrences in 50% of cases. Metastasis rarely occurs. Microcystic adnexal carcinoma is reported in Japanese and African Americans; in the latter, it may be found in atypical locations. Histologically, the superficial part of the tumor is composed of ducts, keratinous cysts, and small cords of cells, superficially resembling a syringoma. The deeper component consists of nests and strands in a dense stroma. Perineural invasion is common and may be extensive. This explains the frequent recurrence after initial excision. Specific immunohistochemical markers have been proposed to distinguish microcystic adnexal carcinoma from infiltrative BCC , desmoplastic trichoepithelioma, and SCC. BCC stains almost universally with Ber-EP4, while microcystic adnexal carcinoma stains in 0–31% of cases. Mohs microsurgery is the treatment of choice. Radiation treatment of the tumor is ineffective and may lead to recurrence, with more aggressive behavior.

Gabillot-Carre M, et al: Microcystic adnexal carcinoma: report of seven cases including one with lung metastasis. Dermatology 2006; 212:221.

Hansen T, et al: Extrafacial microcystic adnexal carcinoma: case report and review of the literature. Dermatol Surg 2009; 35:1835.

Hoang MP, et al: Microcystic adnexal carcinoma: an immunohistochemical reappraisal. Mod Pathol 2008; 21:178.

Krahl D, Selheyer K: Monoclonal antibody Ber-EP4 reliably discriminates between microcystic adnexal carcinoma and basal cell carcinoma. J Cutan Pathol 2007; 34:782.

Leibovitch I, et al: Microcystic adnexal carcinoma: treatment with Mohs micrographic surgery. J Am Dermatol 2005; 52:295.

Leibovitch I, et al: Periocular microcystic adnexal carcinoma: management and outcome with Mohs' micrographic surgery. Ophthalmologica 2006; 220:109.

Matsushita S, et al: Giant microcystic adnexal carcinoma of the scalp. J Dermatol 2008; 35:726.

Nadiminti H, et al: Microcystic adnexal carcinoma in African-Americans. Dermatol Surg 2007; 33:1384.

Ohtsuka H, Nagamatsu S: Microcystic adnexal carcinoma: review of 51 Japanese patients. Dermatology 2002; 204:190.

Redd MA, et al: Asymptomatic cutaneous lip plaque. Diagnosis: microcystic adnexal carcinoma (MAC). Arch Dermatol 2007; 143:791.

Stein JM, et al: The effect of radiation therapy on microcystic adnexal carcinoma: a case report. Head Neck 2003; 25:251.

Wang SQ, et al: The merits of adding toluidine blue-stained slides in Mohs surgery in the treatment of a microcystic adnexal carcinoma. J Am Acad Dermatol 2007; 56:1067.

Wetter R, Goldstein GD: Microcystic adnexal carcinoma: a diagnostic and therapeutic challenge. Dermatol Ther 2008; 21:452.

Yu JB, et al: Surveillance, epidemiology, and end results (SEER) database analysis of microcystic adnexal carcinoma (sclerosing sweat duct carcinoma) of the skin. Am J Clin Oncol 2009 Aug 11 (Epub ahead of print).

Eccrine carcinoma (syringoid carcinoma)

Eccrine carcinoma is rare and presents as a plaque or nodule on the scalp (Fig. 29-41), trunk, or extremities. Local recurrence is common, but metastases are rare. It is composed of ducts and tubules with atypical basaloid cells. A more cellular tumor with numerous tubules and ducts has been termed polymorphous sweat gland carcinoma. Overlap features with microcystic adnexal carcinoma occur, but in general eccrine carcinoma has a less desmoplastic stroma.

Mucinous carcinoma

This tumor is commonly a round, elevated, reddish, and sometimes ulcerated mass, usually located on the head and neck

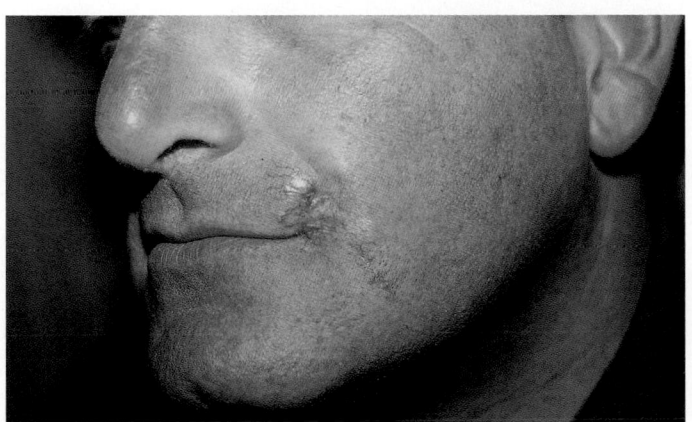

Fig. 29-40 Microcystic adnexal carcinoma.

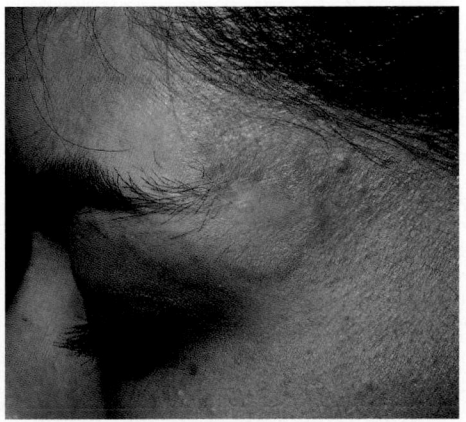

Fig. 29-41 Eccrine carcinoma.

(75%). Forty percent occur on the eyelid. It grows slowly and is usually asymptomatic. Local recurrence is seen in 36%, but the rate of metastasis and widespread dissemination is low (15%). Rare tumors on the eyelid (derived from the glands of Moll) may express estrogen and progesterone receptors, analogous to mucinous carcinoma of the breast. Mucinous gut carcinomas may also metastasize to skin and must be excluded before diagnosing a primary cutaneous mucinous carcinoma.

Histologically, tumors are characterized by the presence of large areas of mucin, in which small islands of basophilic epithelial cells are embedded (blue islands floating in a sea of mucus). Basaloid cells in a cribriform pattern, with duct-like structures, are typical. The recommended treatment is local surgical excision.

Cecchi R, Rapicano V: Primary cutaneous mucinous carcinoma: report of two cases treated with Mohs' micrographic surgery. Australas J Dermatol 2006; 47:192.

Ivan D, et al: Use of *p63* expression in distinguishing primary and metastatic cutaneous adnexal neoplasms from metastatic adenocarcinoma to skin. J Cutan Pathol 2007; 34:474.

Kwatra KS, et al: Oestrogen and progesterone receptors in primary mucinous carcinoma of skin. Australas J Dermatol 2005; 46:246.

Lennerz JK, et al: *CRTC1* rearrangements in the absence of t(11; 19) in primary cutaneous mucoepidermoid carcinoma. Br J Dermatol 2009; 161:925.

Marra DE, et al: Mohs micrographic surgery of primary cutaneous mucinous carcinoma using immunohistochemistry for margin control. Dermatol Surg 2004; 30:799.

Terada T, et al: Primary cutaneous mucinous carcinoma initially diagnosed as metastatic adenocarcinoma. Tohoku J Exp Med 2004; 203:345.

Wako M, et al: Mucinous carcinoma of the skin with apocrine-type differentiation: immunohistochemical studies. Am J Dermatopathol 2003; 25:66.

Aggressive digital papillary adenocarcinoma (digital papillary adenocarcinoma)

This aggressive malignancy involves the digit between the nailbed and the distal interphalangeal joint spaces in most cases, or occurs just proximal to this region. It presents as a solitary cystic nodule. Ulceration and bleeding can occur and rarely the malignancy may be fixed to underlying tissues. Most patients are men in their fifties. The tumor is locally aggressive, with a 50% local recurrence rate. Metastases occur in about 15% of cases, particularly pulmonary. The tumor is poorly circumscribed and is composed of tubuloalveolar and ductal structures with areas of papillary projections. The tumor is positive for S-100, and the cystic contents are positive for CEA and EMA. Complete excision is the treatment of choice. Cases previously called aggressive digital papillary "adenoma" are best regarded as adenocarcinoma.

Keramidas EG, et al: Aggressive digital papillary adenoma-adenocarcinoma. Scand J Plast Reconstr Surg Hand Surg 2006; 40:189.

Mori O, et al: Aggressive digital papillary adenocarcinoma arising on the right great toe. Eur J Dermatol 2002; 12:491.

Primary cutaneous adenoid cystic carcinoma

This rare cutaneous tumor usually presents on the chest, scalp, or vulva of middle-aged to older persons. It is similar histologically to adenoid cystic carcinoma of the salivary gland, with a proliferation of small duct-like islands and larger islands with a "Swiss cheese" or cribriform pattern. It may recur locally or rarely metastasizes. Surgical excision, perhaps with Mohs micrographic surgery, is the treatment of choice.

Doganay L, et al: Primary cutaneous adenoid cystic carcinoma with lung and lymph node metastases. J Eur Acad Dermatol Venereol 2004; 18:383.

Krunic AL, et al: Recurrent adenoid cystic carcinoma of the scalp treated with Mohs micrographic surgery. Dermatol Surg 2003; 29:647.

Marback EF, et al: Eyelid skin adenoid cystic carcinoma: a clinicopathological study of one case simulating sebaceous gland carcinoma. Br J Ophthalmol 2003; 87:118.

Apocrine gland carcinoma

Apocrine gland carcinoma, unrelated to Paget's disease, is rare. The axilla or anogenital region is the most common site, but occasionally other areas with apocrine glands may be involved. Lesions present as a mass. Widespread metastases occur in at least 40% of cases.

Bratthauer GL, et al: Androgen and estrogen receptor mRNA status in apocrine carcinomas. Diagn Mol Pathol 2002; 11:113.

Chintamani, et al: Metastatic sweat gland adenocarcinoma: a clinico-pathological dilemma. World J Surg Oncol 2003; 1:13.

Kiyohara T, et al: Apocrine carcinoma of the vulva in a band-like arrangement with inflammatory and telangiectatic metastasis via local lymphatic channels. Int J Dermatol 2003; 42:71.

Shintaku M, et al: Apocrine adenocarcinoma of the eyelid with aggressive biological behavior: report of a case. Pathol Int 2002; 52:169.

Sugita K, et al: Primary apocrine adenocarcinoma with neuroendocrine differentiation occurring on the pubic skin. Br J Dermatol 2004; 150:371.

Hair follicle nevi and tumors

Pilomatricoma (calcifying epithelioma of Malherbe)

Also known as Malherbe calcifying epithelioma and pilomatrixoma, this benign tumor is derived from hair matrix cells. It usually occurs as a single lesion, which is most commonly found on the face, neck, or proximal upper extremity. Lesions may also be located on the scalp, trunk, and lower extremities. Pilomatricoma is an asymptomatic, deeply seated, 0.5–7 cm, firm nodule, covered by normal or pink skin, which on stretching may show the "tent sign," with multiple facets and angles (Fig. 29-42). Overlying epidermal atrophy is common, leading to an appearance that may resemble anetoderma or striae. In a review of 209 patients, the youngest was 18 months and the oldest 86 years. There is a bimodal age

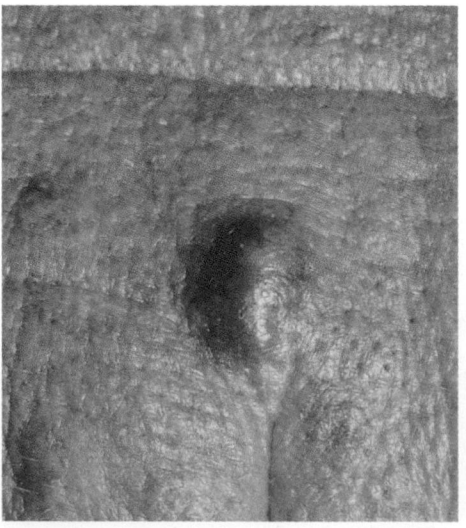

Fig. 29-42 Pilomatricoma.

distribution, in the first and sixth decades. Females are more commonly affected than males.

Multiple pilomatricomas are uncommon. They are usually seen in association with myotonic dystrophy—Steinert syndrome. They may also occur in Rubinstein–Taybi syndrome, trisomy 9, and Turner syndrome. Patients with Gardner syndrome have epidermoid cysts with focal areas of pilomatricoma-like changes. Rarely, multiple pilomatricomas will be inherited in an autosomal-dominant pattern with no other association.

The histopathology shows an encapsulated mass. Basophilic cells with little cytoplasm resemble those of the hair matrix. They evolve into eosinophilic "shadow" cells. Calcification occurs commonly. Ossification, melanin deposits, and foreign body reaction with giant cells may all be present. Activating mutations in β-catenin are present in the majority of pilomatricomas. It is expressed in the basophilic but not the shadow cells. "Melanocytic matricoma" is a rare lesion presenting as a small papule, which histologically is composed of metrical cells, some shadow cells, and numerous dendritic melanocytes containing melanin.

Clinical differential diagnosis is usually impossible in the adult, but in children, since epidermoid cysts are rare, this diagnosis should be considered for any firm cystic mass of the face and upper body. When palpated, pilomatricomas are firmer and more faceted than epidermoid and pilar cysts. Fine needle aspiration has led to misdiagnosis, with the basophilic cells being interpreted as carcinoma. Treatment is surgical excision.

Malignant pilomatricoma (pilomatrix carcinoma, pilomatrical carcinoma)

Malignant pilomatricomas are rare tumors. Described as being locally aggressive, but with limited metastatic potential, many cases labeled "malignant" may actually have been "proliferating" pilomatricomas. Metastases to regional lymph nodes are most frequent. Mohs micrographic surgery may be considered to obtain clear margins.

Ahern NJ, et al: Pilomatrix carcinoma presenting as an extra axial mass: clinicopathological features. Diagn Pathol 2008; 3:47.

Barberio E, et al: Guess what! Multiple pilomatricomas and Steinert disease. Eur J Dermatol 2002; 12:293.

Bassarova A, et al: Pilomatrix carcinoma with lymph node metastases. J Cutan Pathol 2004; 31:330.

Berberian BJ, et al: Multiple pilomatricomas in association with myotonic dystrophy and a family history of melanoma. J Am Acad Dermatol 1997; 37:268.

Blaya B, et al: Multiple pilomatricomas in association with trisomy 9. Pediatr Dermatol 2009; 26:482.

Chan EF, et al: A common skin tumor is caused by activating mutations in beta-catenin. Nat Genet 1999; 21:410.

de Giorgi V, et al: Bullous pilomatricoma: a particular and rare dermal bullous disorder. Acta Derm Venereol 2009; 89:189.

Demircan M, et al: Pilomatricoma in children: a prospective study. Pediatr Dermatol 1997; 14:430.

Fender AB, et al: Anetodermic pilomatricoma with perforation. J Am Acad Dermatol 2008; 58:535.

Fernandez BF, et al: Anetodermic variant of a periorbital pilomatricoma. Ophthal Plast Reconstr Surg 2008; 24:419.

Fujioka M, et al: Secondary anetoderma overlying pilomatrixomas. Dermatology 2003; 207:316.

Hassanein AM, Glanz SM: Beta-catenin expression in benign and malignant pilomatrix neoplasms. Br J Dermatol 2004; 150:511.

Hubbard VG, Whittaker SJ: Multiple familial pilomatricomas: an unusual case. J Cutan Pathol 2004; 31:281.

Julian CG, et al: A clinical review of 209 pilomatricomas. J Am Acad Dermatol 1998; 39:191.

Krishna SM, et al: Anetodermic pilomatricoma in a patient with tuberous sclerosis. Clin Exp Dermatol 2009; 34:e307.

Lemos LB, Brauchle RW: Pilomatrixoma: a diagnostic pitfall in fine-needle aspiration biopsies. A review from a small county hospital. Ann Diagn Pathol 2004; 8:130.

Nakai K, et al: Giant pilomatricoma and psoriasis vulgaris with myotonic dystrophy. Eur J Dermatol 2009; 19:507.

Niiyama S, et al: Proliferating pilomatricoma. Eur J Dermatol 2009; 19:188.

Piel S, et al: Giant pilomatricoma: a benign tumor in an uncommon presentation. J Pediatr 2009; 154:623.

Sable D, Snow SN: Pilomatrix carcinoma of the back treated by Mohs micrographic surgery. Dermatol Surg 2004; 30:1174.

Sherrod QJ, et al: Multiple pilomatricomas: cutaneous marker for myotonic dystrophy. Dermatol Online J 2008; 14:22.

Yiqun J, Jianfang S: Pilomatricoma with a bullous appearance. J Cutan Pathol 2004; 31:558.

Trichofolliculoma

Trichofolliculoma is a benign, highly structured tumor of the pilosebaceous unit, characterized by a small, dome-shaped nodule some 5 mm in diameter on the face or scalp. From the center of the flesh-colored nodule a small wisp of fine, vellus hairs protrudes through a central pore (Fig. 29-43). It may occur at any age but mostly affects adults.

Histologically, the tumor consists of one or more large follicles with smaller radiating secondary follicular structures (sometimes referred to as the mother follicle with her babies). The secondary follicles range from an immature rudimentary matrix to well-formed follicles with papillae, matrix, trichohyaline, and fine hairs ("fingers of fully formed follicles forming fiber"). The tumor may have little stroma or may be embedded in a fibrous orb. Sebaceous glands may be prominent, a variant termed "sebaceous trichofolliculoma." The follicular structures in trichofolliculomas transition through phases of the hair cycle. In telogen, they may resemble fibrofolliculomas. The presence of hair shafts helps distinguish the two. Folliculosebaceous cystic hamartoma may closely resemble a sebaceous trichofolliculoma. Treatment is surgical removal.

Kurokawa I, et al: Trichofolliculoma: case report with immunohistochemical study of cytokeratins. Br J Dermatol 2003; 148:593.

Misago N, et al: A revaluation of trichofolliculoma: the histopathological and immunohistochemical features. Am J Dermatopathol 2009 Sep 1 (Epub ahead of print).

Misago N, et al: A revaluation of folliculosebaceous cystic hamartoma: the histopathological and immunohistochemical features. Am J Dermatopathol 2009 Sept 7 (Epub ahead of print).

Tanimura S, et al: Two cases of folliculosebaceous cystic hamartoma. Clin Exp Dermatol 2006; 31:68.

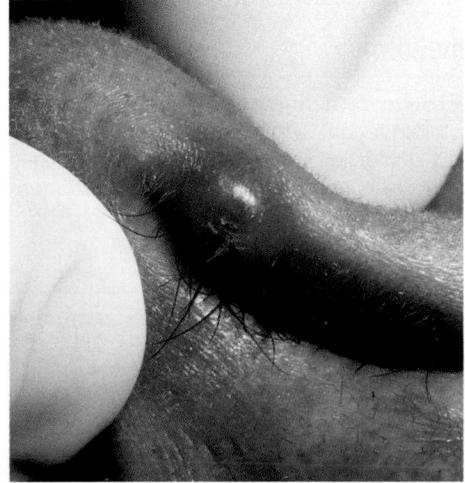

Fig. 29-43 Trichofolliculoma.

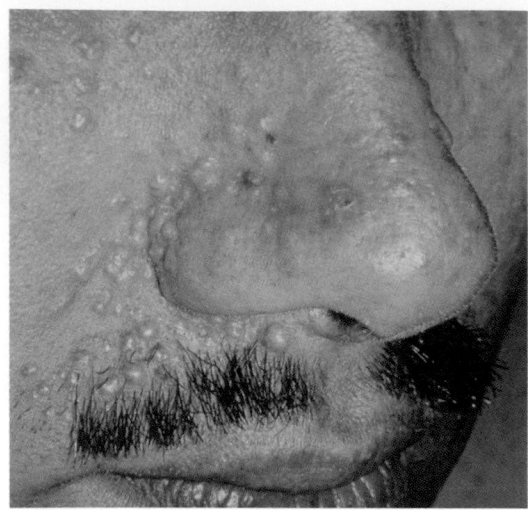

Fig. 29-44 Trichoepitheliomas.

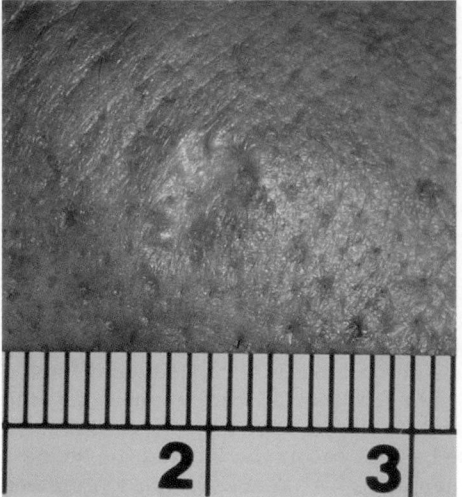

Fig. 29-45 Trichoepithelioma, desmoplastic type.

Multiple familial trichoepithelioma (epithelioma adenoides cysticum, Brooke–Spiegler syndrome)

This autosomal-dominant condition usually presents in childhood or around puberty. Familial cylindroma, multiple familial trichoepithelioma, and Brooke–Spiegler syndrome are all variants of the same condition. The favored term is Brooke–Spiegler syndrome (BSS). There is a variable phenotypic expression among and within families and patients. The multiple trichoepitheliomas present as multiple cystic and solid papules on the face, favoring the upper lip, nasolabial folds, and eyelids. The individual lesions are small, round, smooth, shiny, slightly translucent, firm, circumscribed papules or nodules. The individual lesions average 2–4 mm in diameter. The center may be slightly depressed. Most frequently, the lesions are grouped but discrete. On the face they are often symmetrical (Fig. 29-44). Other sites may be the scalp, neck, and trunk. Multiple linear and dermatomal trichoepitheliomas may rarely be seen. Multiple cylindromas and spiradenomas, epidermoid cysts, and milia may occur in association with multiple trichoepitheliomas. BSS is due to mutations in the *CYLD* gene. *CYLD* functions as a tumor suppressor gene. It has a critical role in deubiquinating proteins, which is important in controlling their biological function. Some individuals in these families have primarily trichoepitheliomas, others have primarily cylindromas, and others have a panoply of adnexal tumors, including cylindromas, trichoepitheliomas, and spiradenomas. BSS patients seem to be at particular risk for degeneration of their cylindromas and spiradenomas to carcinomas.

Solitary trichoepithelioma

The singly occurring trichoepithelioma is nonhereditary and mostly favors the face; however, it may also be found on the scalp, neck, trunk, and proximal extremities. It presents as a firm dermal papule or nodule and must be distinguished from BCC.

Giant solitary trichoepithelioma

The lesions may be several centimeters in diameter, occurring most commonly on the thigh or perianal regions. They are found in older adults.

Desmoplastic trichoepithelioma

This lesion, which is difficult to differentiate from morpheiform BCC histologically, occurs as solitary or multiple lesions on the face. Desmoplastic trichoepitheliomas are firm and slightly indented (central dell sign), with a raised, annular border (Fig. 29-45). Young women are most commonly affected, and familial solitary and multiple desmoplastic trichoepitheliomas have been described.

Histology

Trichoepitheliomas are dermal tumors with multiple nests of basaloid cells, some of which show abortive follicular differentiation. Keratinous cysts, calcification, and amyloid may all be seen. The stroma in most trichoepitheliomas resembles the fibrous sheath of a normal hair follicle. It contains many fine collagen fibers and fibroblasts that surround the tumor islands in a concentric array. Clusters of plump nuclei resembling the cells of the follicular papilla (papillary mesenchymal bodies) are common. In the desmoplastic variety, the tumor is composed of small cords of epithelium embedded in a dense eosinophilic stroma with fewer fibroblasts. The islands often present a "paisley tie" appearance, and the microscopic differential diagnosis includes morpheiform BCC, syringoma, and microcystic adnexal carcinoma. The clinical features may distinguish these entities. Focal calcification, horn cysts, and a central dell favor trichoepithelioma. In desmoplastic trichoepithelioma, clefts form between collagen fibers in the stroma, while in BCC, clefts form between the tumor islands and stroma. Trichoepitheliomas are best classified as benign tumors of the hair germ. As such, they may be considered variants of trichoblastoma. Histologically, trichoepithelioma must be differentiated from keratotic BCC, with which it is frequently confused.

Treatment

Solitary lesions can be treated by surgical excision. Multiple lesions can be smoothed down by resurfacing the skin with laser surgery, dermabrasion, or electrosurgery. This procedure must be repeated at regular intervals, as the lesions gradually recur.

Trichoblastoma

These benign neoplasms of follicular germinative cells usually present as asymptomatic nodules 0.5–1 cm in size in the deep dermis or subcutaneous tissue. The scalp is the most common location, especially if associated with nevus sebaceus of Jadassohn. Trichoblastomas usually occur in male and female adults, but children can also develop them. The lesions may be pigmented. Trichoblastomas arise in organoid nevi and represent the majority of basaloid neoplasms described as "basal cell carcinomas" in nevus sebaceus. The rare Curry–Jones syndrome, with cutaneous streaky hypopigmentation, hyperpigmented linear atrophic lines on the soles, and many other musculoskeletal, ocular, and gastrointestinal defects, can feature multiple trichoblastomas. Histologically, trichoblastoma is a dermal or subcutaneous tumor composed of basaloid cells with areas of follicular differentiation of the tumor. The islands may connect with the overlying epidermis, especially in the setting of an organoid nevus. The stroma is identical to that seen in trichoepithelioma and typically contains papillary mesenchymal bodies. Merkel cells may be prominent within the tumor and amyloid can be found. Cutaneous lymphadenoma is a variant of trichoblastoma with extensive infiltration of the tumor islands by lymphocytes and histiocytes. The stroma resembles that of other trichoblastomas. A single or double row of basaloid tumor cells is seen at the periphery of each island, while the center is composed of histiocytes and lymphocytes. Surgical excision is curative.

Blake PW, Toro JR: Update of cylindromatosis gene (CYLD) mutations in Brooke–Spiegler syndrome: novel insights into the role of deubiquitination in cell signaling. Hum Mutat 2009; 30:1025.

De Giorgi V, et al: Multiple pigmented trichoblastomas and syringocystadenoma papilliferum in naevus sebaceus mimicking a malignant melanoma: a clinical dermoscopic-pathological case study. Br J Dermatol 2003; 149:1067.

Grange DK, et al: Two new patients with Curry–Jones syndrome with trichoblastoma and medulloblastoma suggest an etiologic role of the sonic hedgehog-patched-GLI pathway. Am J Med Genet A 2008; 146A:2589.

Hu G, et al: A novel missense mutation in CYLD in a family with Brooke–Spiegler syndrome. J Invest Dermatol 2003; 121:732.

Johnson H, et al: Trichoepithelioma. Dermatol Online J 2008; 14:5.

Kanda A, et al: A case of multiple trichoepithelioma with an unusual appearance. Br J Dermatol 2003; 149:655.

Kang TW, et al: Trichoblastoma in a child. Pediatr Dermatol 2009; 26:476.

Koay JL, et al: Asymptomatic annular plaque of the chin: desmoplastic trichoepithelioma. Arch Dermatol 2002; 138:1091.

Layegh P, et al: Brooke–Spiegler syndrome. Indian J Dermatol Venereol Leprol 2008; 74:632.

Ly H, et al: Case of the Brooke–Spiegler syndrome. Australas J Dermatol 2004; 45:220.

Parren LJ, et al: Brooke–Spiegler syndrome complicated by unilateral hearing loss. Int J Dermatol 2008; 47:56.

Salhi A, et al: Multiple familial trichoepithelioma caused by mutations in cylindromatosis tumor suppressor gene. Cancer Res 2004; 64:5113.

Szepietowski J, et al: Brooke–Spiegler syndrome. J Eur Acad Dermatol Venereol 2001; 15:346.

Takai T, et al: Two cases of subcutaneous trichoblastoma. J Dermatol 2004; 31:232.

Vollmer RT: Panel vs. single marker for discriminating desmoplastic trichoepithelioma from morpheaform/infiltrative basal cell carcinoma. J Cutan Pathol 2009; 36:283.

Trichilemmoma and Cowden syndrome (Cowden's disease, multiple hamartoma syndrome)

Trichilemmoma is a benign neoplasm that differentiates toward cells of the outer root sheath. It usually occurs as a small solitary papule on the face, particularly the nose and cheeks. Most lesions are clinically misdiagnosed as BCC or benign keratosis.

Trichilemmomas may also occur as multiple facial lesions. When they do, this is a specific cutaneous marker for Cowden syndrome (CS), an autosomal-dominantly inherited condition. The prevalence of CS is 1/200 000 to 1/250 000. The penetrance is nearly complete, with 90% of affected patients having stigmata by age 20. Diagnostic criteria for CS have been established and certain of the mucocutaneous manifestations are considered pathognomonic, including mucocutaneous lesions, trichilemmomas of the face, acral keratoses, papillomatous papules (Figs 29-46 and 29-47), and mucosal lesions. The trichilemmomas, or "facial papules," are present in 86% of CS patients and appear on average at 22 years, but can appear anytime from childhood to advanced age (75 years). Trichilemmomas are generally limited to the head and neck, especially the central face, around the orifices; however, other sites may be involved—ears, for example. Since not all facial papules have characteristic histology, the presence of "papillomatous" lesions is a diagnostic criterion. The other pathognomonic mucocutaneous benign features are acral keratoses, which present as either verrucous hyperkeratosis on the extensor extremities, or palmoplantar translucent keratoses in 28% and 20% of CS patients respectively. Acral neuromatosis may present as translucent papules on the backs and sides of the fingers. The mucous membranes are involved in more than 80% of patients and usually in multiple anatomic locations, favoring the buccal and gingival mucosa. They can coalesce and form the characteristic cobblestone pattern seen in 40% of CS patients. Involvement of the respiratory mucosa can occur, with an acanthosis nigricans-like appearance. The mucosal lesions develop after the cutaneous lesions and have a persistent but benign course. Other cutaneous lesions include lipomas, hemangiomas, xanthomas, acanthosis nigricans, and various hyperpigmented macules. Macrocephaly with head circumference of >97% is a major criterion for the diagnosis.

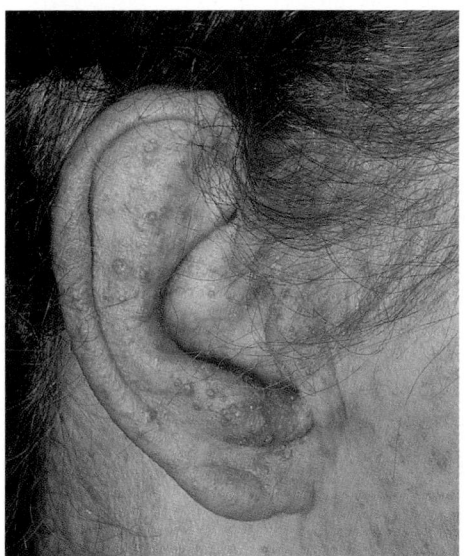

Fig. 29-46 Cowden syndrome.

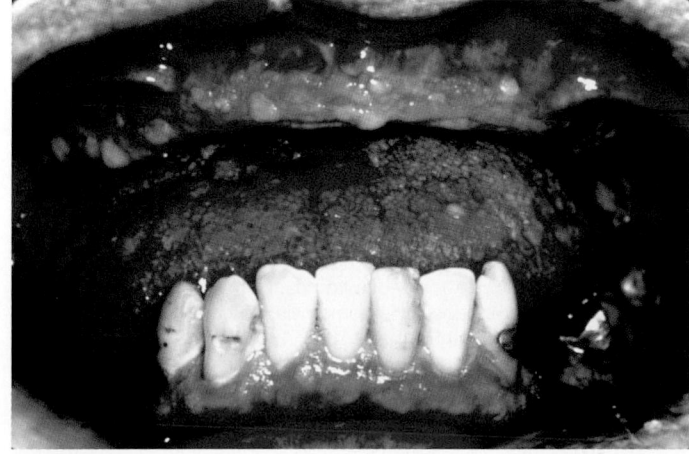

Fig. 29-47 Oral papillomas in Cowden syndrome.

Malignancies develop in up to 40% of patients with CS. They are major criteria for the diagnosis and include breast, endometrial, and thyroid carcinoma. Breast cancer occurs in 25–50% of female patients and has been reported in male patients with CS. For breast cancer the average age at diagnosis is 36 years. Around 75% of affected females have fibrocystic disease of the breast. Endometrial cancer occurs in 6% of women with CS and has appeared as early as adolescence. Although not criteria for the diagnosis, multiple gastrointestinal polyps (in 70–85%) and gastrointestinal malignancies also occur. Minor criteria include thyroid lesions (including adenomas or goiter, and thyroiditis, in two-thirds of patients), mental retardation, lipomas, fibromas (multiple sclerotic fibromas or storiform collagenomas), and genitourinary tumors. Multiple lipomatosis of the testicles is a common manifestation. The adult form of Lhermitte–Duclos disease, or dysplastic gangliocytoma of the cerebellum, represents the neurologic manifestation of CS. Lhermitte–Duclos disease is another pathognomonic criterion for the diagnosis of CS. A number of mucocutaneous malignancies have been found in patients with CS, including melanoma, BCC, SCC, Merkel cell carcinoma, and trichilemmal carcinoma.

Mutations in the tumor suppressor gene *PTEN* are responsible for CS. Patients who do not have a mutation in *PTEN* have mutations in the promoter region for *PTEN*. In 10% of cases, the mutation is not in *PTEN* or the promoter, and may be in the succinate dehydrogenase genes. Another disorder caused in 65% of cases by mutations in *PTEN* is Bannayan–Riley–Ruvalcaba syndrome (BRRS) (autosomal-dominantly inherited, macrocephaly, genital lentigines, motor and speech delay, mental retardation, hamartomatous polyps, myopathies, lipomas, and hemangiomas). BRRS is now considered a variant of CS that presents earlier in life, and patients having overlap syndromes with features of both CS and BRRS have been described. Some patients with a Proteus-like syndrome also have mutations in *PTEN*. These diseases have been called the "*PTEN* hamartoma tumor syndrome."

Microscopically, trichilemmomas show variable hyperkeratosis and parakeratosis. Tumor lobules extend downward from the epidermis and demonstrate glycogen-rich clear cells, peripheral palisading, and a thick hyalinized basement membrane.

Facial papillomas can be removed with surgical procedures, but new lesions continue to appear throughout life. Some patients achieve satisfactory cosmetic results from dermabrasion or CO_2 laser. Regular cancer screening and genetic counseling are paramount in CS. Rapamycin prevents the development of mucocutaneous lesions and premature death in the animal model for CS, suggesting that the mTOR pathway is involved in the development of the cutaneous lesions and the later complications of CS.

Al-Daraji WI, et al: Storiform collagenoma as a clue for Cowden disease or *PTEN* hamartoma tumour syndrome. J Clin Pathol 2007; 60:840.

Blumenthal GM, Dennis PA: *PTEN* hamartoma tumor syndromes. Eur J Hum Genet 2008; 16:1289.

Caux F, et al: Segmental overgrowth, lipomatosis, arteriovenous malformation and epidermal nevus (SOLAMEN) syndrome is related to mosaic *PTEN* nullizygosity. Eur J Hum Genet 2007; 15:767.

Devi M, et al: Testicular mixed germ cell tumor in an adolescent with Cowden disease. Oncology 2007; 72:194.

Eng C: *PTEN*: one gene, many syndromes. Hum Mutat 2003; 22:183.

Ferran M, et al: Acral papular neuromatosis: an early manifestation of Cowden syndrome. Br J Dermatol 2008; 158:174.

Ferran M, et al: Bilateral and symmetrical palmoplantar punctate keratoses in childhood: a possible clinical clue for an early diagnosis of *PTEN* hamartoma-tumour syndrome. Clin Exp Dermatol 2009; 34:e28.

Jarrett R, et al: Dermoscopy of Cowden syndrome. Arch Dermatol 2009; 145:508.

Jornayvaz FR, Philippe J: Mucocutaneous papillomatous papules in Cowden's syndrome. Clin Exp Dermatol 2008; 33:151.

Lachlan KL, et al: Cowden syndrome and Bannayan–Riley–Ruvalcaba syndrome represent one condition with variable expression and age-related penetrance: results of a clinical study of *PTEN* mutation carriers. J Med Genet 2007; 4:579.

McGarrity TJ, et al: GI polyposis and glycogenic acanthosis of the esophagus associated with *PTEN* mutation positive Cowden syndrome in the absence of cutaneous manifestations. Am J Gastroenterol 2003; 98:1429.

Merks JHM, et al: *PTEN* hamartoma tumour syndrome: variability of an entity. J Med Genet 2003; 40:e111.

Ni Y, et al: Germline mutations and variants in the succinate dehydrogenase genes in Cowden and Cowden-like syndromes. Am J Hum Genet 2008; 83:261.

Nishizawa A, et al: Cowden syndrome: a novel mutation and overlooked glycogenic acanthosis in gingiva. Br J Dermatol 2009; 160:1116.

Orloff MS, Eng C: Genetic and phenotypic heterogeneity in the *PTEN* hamartoma tumour syndrome. Oncogene 2008; 27:5387.

Pérez-Núñez A, et al: Lhermitte–Duclos disease and Cowden disease: clinical and genetic study in five patients with Lhermitte–Duclos disease and literature review. Acta Neurochir (Wien) 2004; 146:679.

Pilarski R: Cowden syndrome: a critical review of the clinical literature. J Genet Couns 2009; 18:13.

Pinzone JJ, et al: A novel *PTEN* mutation in Cowden syndrome is associated with a mixed degenerative-erosive arthritic process: potential molecular pathogenic mechanisms. Am J Med Genet A 2007; 143A:1522.

Schmeler KM, et al: Endometrial cancer in an adolescent: a possible manifestation of Cowden syndrome. Obstet Gynecol 2009; 114:477.

Shukuya T, et al: Squamous papillomas in the trachea and main bronchi found in a Cowden's disease patient. Intern Med 2006; 45:987.

Soysal Y, et al: Analysis of *PTEN* gene mutations in a Turkish patient with Cowden syndrome. Genet Test Mol Biomarkers 2009; 13:547.

Squarize CH, et al: Chemoprevention and treatment of experimental Cowden's disease by mTOR inhibition with rapamycin. Cancer Res 2008; 68:7066.

Umemura K, et al: Gastrointestinal polyposis with esophageal polyposis is useful for early diagnosis of Cowden's disease. World J Gastroenterol 2008; 14:5755.

Uppal S, et al: Cowden disease: a review. Int J Clin Pract 2007; 61:645.

Vasovcak P, et al: A novel mutation of *PTEN* gene in a patient with Cowden syndrome with excessive papillomatosis of the lips, discrete cutaneous lesions, and gastrointestinal polyposis. Eur J Gastroenterol Hepatol 2007; 19:513.

Woodhouse J, Ferguson MM: Multiple hyperechoic testicular lesions are a common finding on ultrasound in Cowden disease and represent lipomatosis of the testis. Br J Radiol 2006; 79:801.

Trichilemmal carcinoma

Trichilemmal carcinomas are reported to arise on sun-exposed areas, most commonly the face and ears. They present as a slow-growing papule, indurated plaque, or nodule with a tendency to ulcerate. They may arise in the association of immunosuppression. It may be difficult to distinguish trichilemmal carcinoma from invasive Bowen's disease (which often shows adnexal differentiation) or a clear cell SCC. Surgical removal is recommended; Mohs micrographic surgery has been used successfully.

Allee JE, et al: Multiply recurrent trichilemmal carcinoma with perineural invasion and cytokeratin 17 positivity. Dermatol Surg 2003; 29:886.

Cecchi R, et al: Malignant proliferating trichilemmal tumour of the scalp managed with micrographic surgery and sentinel lymph node biopsy. J Eur Acad Dermatol Venereol 2008; 22:1258.

Garrett AB, et al: Trichilemmal carcinoma: a rare cutaneous malignancy: a report of two cases. Dermatol Surg 2004; 30:113.

Kanitakis J, et al: Trichilemmal carcinoma of the skin mimicking a keloid in a heart transplant recipient. J Heart Lung Transplant 2007; 26:649.

Masui Y, et al: Proliferating tricholemmal cystic carcinoma: a case containing differentiated and dedifferentiated parts. J Cutan Pathol 2008; 35:55.

Satyaprakash AK, et al: Proliferating trichilemmal tumors: a review of the literature. Dermatol Surg 2007; 33:1102.

Trichodiscoma, fibrofolliculoma, perifollicular fibromas, mantleomas and Birt–Hogg–Dubé syndrome

These benign tumors form a spectrum of neoplasms combining a follicular element and the specialized periadventitial dermis of the upper portion of the hair follicle. They may represent variations of the same tumor cut in different planes of section. All these lesions clinically appear as 2–4 mm, asymptomatic, skin-colored, dermal papules, affecting the face and upper trunk. They may be single, but are frequently multiple. When multiple, they are often numerous and are a marker for Birt–Hogg–Dubé syndrome (BHD) (Fig. 29-48). The histomorphology of these hair follicle tumors is identical in patients with BHD and in cases unassociated with BHD. Fibrofolliculoma demonstrates cords and strands of 2–4-cell epithelium emanating from a follicular structure. The epithelial elements may anastomose and sebaceous elements may be present. This follicular structure is surrounded by a collagenous or fibromucinous orb. Trichodiscomas represent a sectioning artifact that demonstrates only the tumor stroma.

BHD syndrome is caused by a mutation in the gene folliculin (FLCN), which is located on chromosome 17p. Many of the mutations occur in a hypermutable region of the gene. This gene is conserved in many species and expressed in many tissues, but its exact function is unknown. Homozygous loss of function of the folliculin gene is embryonically lethal, suggesting that it has important functions.

Cutaneous lesions are common in patients with BHD, affecting more than 80% of persons 30 years or older. The fibrofolliculomas appear in adulthood and usually precede other stigmata, but can be quite subtle. In the vast majority of cases they are multiple and often very numerous. They can be widespread, but always affect the nose, paranasal area, the back of the pinna, and behind the ear. Comedo-like papules with keratinous plugs may be seen. Lesions can coalesce into plaques and be grouped. Multiple epidermoid cysts can occur. Hyperseborrhea may be seen, with numerous facial fibrofolliculomas. Skin tags are present in 100% of patients, most commonly in the axilla. Small, discrete, soft, mucosa-colored or white papules of the lips, gingiva, tongue, and/or buccal mucosa are present in about 40% of patients and families with BHD. Biopsies of the oral lesions reveal an acanthotic epithelium overlying a fibrotic process.

In addition to the cutaneous lesions noted above, patients are at risk for the development of renal tumors and spontaneous pneumothorax. The renal tumor risk is seven times that of the general population and especially affects men (at twice the risk) and those over 40. At least 30% of patients with BHD develop renal tumors, and these can appear after age 20 years. Renal tumors may be multiple and bilateral, a clinical scenario that should suggest the diagnosis of BHD. BHD patients develop renal oncocytomas and chromophobe renal carcinomas, or a mixed type that is characteristic of BHD. These are otherwise rare histological variants of renal cell carcinoma. Multiple renal cysts may also occur.

Persons with BHD have greater than 30 times the risk of developing a spontaneous pneumothorax compared to unaffected persons—a lifetime risk of 24%. Pneumothorax can occur at a young age in BHD—17% of BHD patients under 40 will have a spontaneous pneumothorax. Median age of pneumothorax is 38 years. Spontaneous pneumothorax results from multiple pulmonary cysts, which affect 83% of BHD patients. The cysts are at the lung base and subpleural. Recurrent pneumothorax is common, and should raise the possibility of BHD. BHD patients do not seem to have progressive pulmonary failure, and severe chronic obstructive pulmonary disease (COPD) is not associated with FLCN mutations. Colonic polyps and neoplasms, which were initially reported to be associated with BHD syndrome, do not appear to be increased in BHD syndrome. Thyroid nodules are seen in 90% of affected families and 65% of patients with BHD.

The treatment of the fibrofolliculomas is surgical debulking. In most patients, the lesions are small and can be cosmetically removed by shave removal, curettage, or resurfacing if the lesions are numerous. Smoking is proscribed, as it may worsen lung complications. Renal imaging should be periodically performed, but the best method is unclear. CT is more accurate than ultrasound, especially for smaller lesions, but repeat scans lead to unacceptable radiation exposure. MRI is expensive, but diagnostically most accurate. Although there is no genotype/phenotype correlation known at this time for FLCN mutations, certain families seem to be predisposed to certain complications of BHD. In those families, more aggressive screening for the particularly prevalent complication seems warranted. Since the FLCN gene seems to interact with the mTOR pathway, it has been suggested that the use of rapamycin has potential benefit in BHD.

Baba M, et al: Folliculin encoded by the BHD gene interacts with a binding protein, FNIP1, and AMPK, and is involved in AMPK and mTOR signaling. Proc Natl Acad Sci U S A 2006; 103:15552.

Cho MH, et al: Folliculin mutations are not associated with severe COPD. BMC Med Genet 2008; 9:120.

Collins GL, et al: Histomorphologic and immunophenotypic analysis of fibrofolliculomas and trichodiscomas in Birt–Hogg–Dubé syndrome and sporadic disease. J Cutan Pathol 2002; 29:529.

Diamond JM, Kotloff RM: Recurrent spontaneous pneumothorax as the presenting sign of the Birt–Hogg–Dubé syndrome. Ann Intern Med 2009; 150:289.

Farrant PB, Emerson R: Hyfrecation and curettage as a treatment for fibrofolliculomas in Birt–Hogg–Dubé syndrome. Dermatol Surg 2007; 33:1287.

Imada K, et al: Birt–Hogg–Dubé syndrome with clear-cell and oncocytic renal tumour and trichoblastoma associated with a novel FLCN mutation. Br J Dermatol 2009; 160:1350.

Jacob CI, Dover JS: Birt–Hogg–Dubé syndrome: treatment of cutaneous manifestations with laser skin resurfacing. Arch Dermatol 2001; 137:98.

Jarrett R, et al: Dermoscopic features of Birt–Hogg–Dubé syndrome. Arch Dermatol 2009; 145:1208.

Kluger N, et al: Birt–Hogg–Dubé syndrome: clinical and genetic studies of 10 French families. Br J Dermatol 2009 Sep 26 (Epub ahead of print).

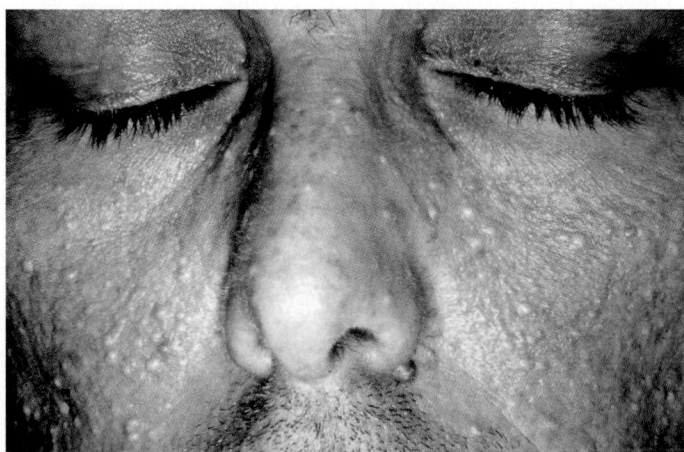

Fig. 29-48 Birt–Hogg–Dubé syndrome.

Kluijt I, et al: Early onset of renal cancer in a family with Birt–Hogg–Dubé syndrome. Clin Genet 2009; 75:537.

Menko FH, et al: Birt–Hogg–Dubé syndrome: diagnosis and management. Lancet Oncol 2009; 10:1199.

Misago N, et al: Fibrofolliculoma/trichodiscoma and fibrous papule (perifollicular fibroma/angiofibroma): a revaluation of the histopathological and immunohistochemical features. J Cutan Pathol 2009; 36:943.

Okimoto K, et al: A germ-line insertion in the Birt–Hogg–Dubé (BHD) gene gives rise to the Nihon rat model of inherited renal cancer. Proc Natl Acad Sci U S A 2004; 101:2023.

Painter JN, et al: A 4-bp deletion in the Birt–Hogg–Dubé gene (*FLCN*) causes dominantly inherited spontaneous pneumothorax. Am J Hum Genet 2005; 76:522.

Tobino K, et al: Characteristics of pulmonary cysts in Birt–Hogg–Dubé syndrome: thin-section CT findings of the chest in 12 patients. Eur J Radiol 2009 Sep 24 (Epub ahead of print).

Toro JR, et al: Lung cysts, spontaneous pneumothorax, and genetic associations in 89 families with Birt–Hogg–Dubé syndrome. Am J Respir Crit Care Med 2007; 175:1044.

Toro JR, et al: BHD mutations, clinical and molecular genetic investigations of Birt–Hogg–Dubé syndrome: a new series of 50 families and a review of published reports. J Med Genet 2008; 45:321.

Vincent A, et al: Birt–Hogg–Dubé syndrome: a review of the literature and the differential diagnosis of firm facial papules. J Am Acad Dermatol 2003; 49:698.

Vinson-Spencer DJ, Christiansen LR: A 40-year-old woman with facial papules and flank pain. Birt–Hogg–Dubé syndrome. Arch Pathol Lab Med 2006; 130:e66.

Other hair follicle tumors

Dilated pore (Winer)

This lesion typically presents as a solitary, prominent, open comedo on the face or upper trunk of an elderly individual. Histologically, it is composed of a markedly dilated follicular pore lined by outer root sheath epithelium. Multiple short, bulbous, acanthotic projections extend from the central infundibulum-like pore.

Pilar sheath acanthoma

Pilar sheath acanthoma is most often found on the face, particularly above the upper lip in adults. Patients present with a solitary 5–10 mm skin-colored nodule with a central keratinous plug. Histologically, pilar sheath acanthoma differs from a dilated pore by having larger tumor lobules radiating from the central infundibulum-like pore.

Trichoadenoma

Presenting as a solitary growth ranging from 3 to 15 mm in diameter, this lesion may be clinically mistaken for a seborrheic keratosis, having a vegetative or verrucous appearance. Although most frequently found on the face, it may occur at other sites, especially the buttock, which is the second most common location. Trichoadenomas also differentiate towards the follicular infundibulum. Histologically, they are quite distinctive, being composed of a collection of ringlike eosinophilic structures that often occur in pairs (resembling spectacles). No hair shafts are present.

Basaloid follicular hamartoma

Basaloid follicular hamartoma (BFH) is a distinctive benign adnexal tumor that has four described variants: solitary papule, localized plaque of alopecia, linear or blaschkoid unilateral plaque, and generalized papules. This latter form has also been termed "generalized hair follicle hamartoma." Most often affecting the skin of the face and scalp, BFHs are solitary or multiple skin-colored, 2–3 mm papules (Fig. 29-49) or infiltrating plaques associated with progressive hair loss in the affected areas. Congenital and adult appearance has been

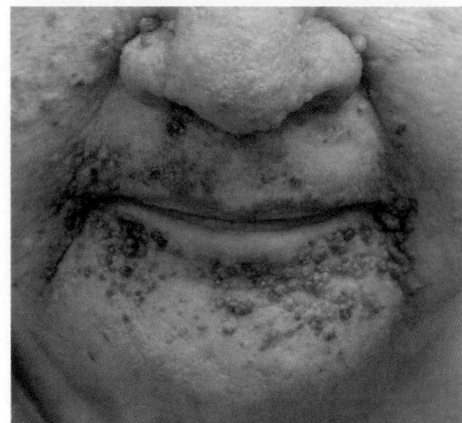

Fig. 29-49 Basaloid follicular hamartoma. (Courtesy of J. English, MD)

described. In some generalized cases, there is an association with alopecia, myasthenia gravis, and/or circulating autoantibodies (antinuclear and antiacetylcholine receptor antibodies). Cystic fibrosis and generalized follicular hamartomas have been reported in three siblings, suggesting a possible genetic linkage. A familial, autosomal-dominant form has been described, with numerous milia; comedo-like lesions; hyperpigmented papules of the face, scalp, ears, neck, and trunk; hypotrichosis; hypohidrosis; and pinpoint palmar pits. It presents in early childhood. Happle–Tinschert syndrome is segmentally arranged BFH, linear atrophoderms with hypo- and hyperpigmentation, enamel defects, ipsilateral hypertrichosis, and skeletal and cerebral anomalies.

Histologically, BFH may be indistinguishable from infundibulocystic BCC. Lesions are characterized by thin, branching eosinophilic strands and thick cords with associated basaloid buds and keratin cysts. Unlike most other pilar tumors, the stroma is loose, fibrillar, or mucinous. In nevoid and generalized forms, apparently normal skin may also demonstrate small islands of basaloid cells. Trichoblastomas may occur within nevoid lesions. *PTCH* gene signaling is upregulated in the cells contacting the dermis in BFH. Generalized BFH syndrome must be distinguished from Bazex–Dupré–Christol syndrome, Brown–Crounse syndrome, Rombo syndrome, basal cell nevus syndrome, and Brooke–Spiegler syndrome. Its differentiation from multiple hereditary infundibulocystic basal cell carcinoma syndrome may be difficult.

Folliculosebaceous cystic hamartoma

Folliculosebaceous cystic hamartoma is a benign hamartoma of epithelial and mesenchymal elements. It presents as a solitary 0.5–1.5 cm papule or nodule virtually always on the head, with two-thirds occurring on or adjacent to the nose. Rare giant lesions up to 15 cm in diameter have been reported. Age of onset ranges from infancy to the sixth decade. Histologically, the lesion is composed of three elements: an intradermal cystic structure lined by squamous epithelium identical to that of the infundibulum; numerous sebaceous lobules radiating from the cystic structure; and a surrounding stroma with fibrous, adipose, vascular, and neural tissues. Stromal spindle cells are positive for CD34. The tumor may represent a sebaceous trichofolliculoma biopsied during telogen phase.

Tumors of the follicular infundibulum

These flat, keratotic papules of the head and neck are usually solitary but may be multiple. They appear in adulthood. The term eruptive infundibulomas and infundibulomatosis has been used to describe the cases with multiple lesions. In the rare generalized cases, there is a strong clinical resemblance to Darier's disease, with accentuation on the neck, central chest, groin, and axillae. Histologically, the solitary and multiple cases are identical. There is a platelike proliferation of epidermal cells growing parallel to the epidermis and connecting to it at multiple sites. Clear gylogenated cells like those of a trichilemmoma, sebaceous differentiation, cystic and ductal structures, and papillary mesenchymal bodies may be seen.

Cheng AC, et al: Multiple tumors of the follicular infundibulum. Dermatol Surg 2004; 30:1246.

Choi YS, et al: Pilar sheath acanthoma—report of a case with review of the literature. Yonsei Med J 1989; 30:392.

El-Darouti MA, et al: Basaloid follicular hamartoma. Int J Dermatol 2005; 44:361.

Happle R, Tinschert S: Segmentally arranged basaloid follicular hamartomas with osseous, dental and cerebral anomalies: a distinct syndrome. Acta Derm Venereol 2008; 88:382.

Itin PH: Happle–Tinschert syndrome. Segmentally arranged basaloid follicular hamartomas, linear atrophoderma with hypo- and hyperpigmentation, enamel defects, ipsilateral hypertrichosis, and skeletal and cerebral anomalies. Dermatology 2009; 218:221.

Jakobiec FA, et al: Winer's dilated pore of the eyelid. Ophthal Plast Reconstr Surg 2009; 25:411.

Katayama I, et al: Basaloid follicular hamartoma with eruptive milia and hypohidrosis: is there a pathogenic relationship? Eur J Dermatol 2003; 13:505.

Kurokawa I, et al: Trichoadenoma: cytokeratin expression suggesting differentiation towards the follicular infundibulum and follicular bulge regions. Br J Dermatol 2005; 153:1084.

Lee JH, et al: Unusual presentation of trichoadenoma in an infant. Acta Derm Venereol 2008; 88:291.

Lee MW, et al: Linear basaloid follicular hamartoma on the Blaschko's line of the face. Clin Exp Dermatol 2005; 30:30.

Lee WS, et al: Congenital trichoadenoma with an unusual clinical manifestation. J Am Acad Dermatol 2007; 57:905.

Mahalingam M, et al: Tumor of the follicular infundibulum with sebaceous differentiation. J Cutan Pathol 2001; 28:314.

Mascaro JM, et al: Congenital generalized follicular hamartoma associated with alopecia and cystic fibrosis in three siblings. Arch Dermatol 1995; 131:454.

Miller CJ, et al: Sebaceous carcinoma, basal cell carcinoma, trichoadenoma, trichoblastoma, and syringocystadenoma papilliferum arising within a nevus sebaceus. Dermatol Surg 2004; 30:1546.

Naeyaert HM, et al: CD-34 and Ki-67 staining patterns of basaloid follicular hamartoma are different from those in fibroepithelioma of Pinkus and other variants of basal cell carcinoma. J Cutan Pathol 2001; 28:538.

Patel AB, et al: Familial basaloid follicular hamartoma: a report of one family. Dermatol Online J 2008; 14:14.

Ramos-Deballos FI, et al: Bcl-2, CD34 and CD10 expression in basaloid follicular hamartoma, vellus hair hamartoma and neurofollicular hamartoma demonstrate full follicular differentiation. J Cutan Pathol 2008; 35:477.

Ricks M, et al: Multiple basaloid follicular hamartomas associated with acrochordons, seborrhoeic keratoses and chondrosarcoma. Br J Dermatol 2002; 146:1068.

Saxena A, et al: Basaloid follicular hamartoma: a cautionary tale and review of the literature. Dermatol Surg 2007; 33:1130.

Steffen C: Winer's dilated pore: the infundibuloma. Am J Dermatopathol 2001; 23:246.

Sturtz DE, et al: Giant folliculosebaceous cystic hamartoma of the upper extremity. J Cutan Pathol 2004; 31:287.

Swaroop K, et al: Trichoadenoma of Nikolowski. Indian J Pathol Microbiol 2008; 51:277.

Yebenes M, et al: Linear unilateral hamartomatous basal cell naevus with glandular and follicular differentiation. Clin Exp Dermatol 2008; 33:429.

Epithelial cysts and sinuses

Epidermal cyst (epidermal inclusion cyst, infundibular cyst)

Epidermal inclusion cyst is one of the most common benign skin tumors. It presents as a compressible, but not fluctuant,

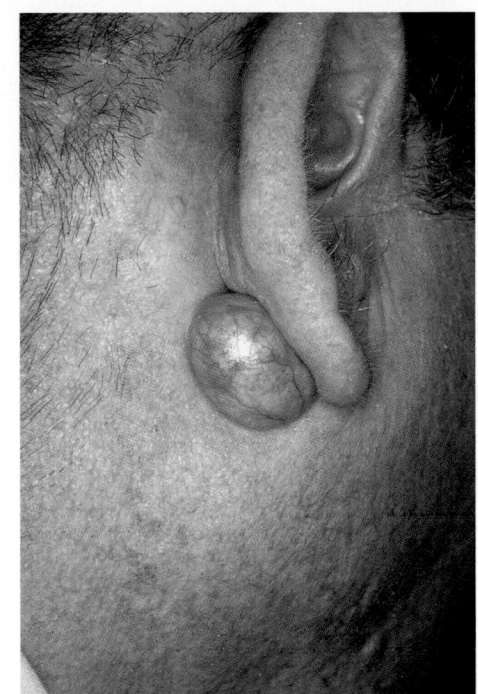

Fig. 29-50 Epidermal inclusion cyst.

cystic mass from 0.5 to several centimeters in diameter (Fig. 29-50). The surface of the overlying skin is usually smooth and shiny from the upward pressure. These nodules are freely movable over underlying tissue and are attached to the normal skin above them by a comedo-like central infundibular structure or punctum. The pasty contents of the cysts are formed mostly of macerated keratin, which has a cheesy consistency and pungent odor. Epidermal inclusion cysts occur most commonly on the face, neck, and trunk, but may be found almost anywhere. They frequently result from plugging of the follicular orifice, often in association with acne vulgaris. They may also occur by epidermal implantation. Deep penetrating injuries, such as with a sewing machine needle or stapler, may result in epidermoid cysts growing within bone. In pigmented races, the lining of the epidermoid cyst and its contents may be pigmented. Epidermoid cysts rarely appear before puberty and earlier onset should suggest an alternative diagnosis (e.g. pilomatricoma, dermoid cyst, or Gardner syndrome). Lesions of the scalp are usually trichilemmal cysts. Rare cysts of the soles are due to infection by HPV-60.

Epidermoid cysts may rupture and induce a vigorous foreign body inflammatory response, after which they are firmly adherent to surrounding structures and are more difficult to remove. Rupture is associated with the sudden onset of redness, pain, swelling, and local heat, simulating an abscess. Incision and drainage will confirm the diagnosis of inflamed cyst, when the smelly, cheesy material is evacuated. This will also lead to rapid resolution of symptoms. These episodes are often misdiagnosed as "infection" of the cyst, but cultures are usually negative and antibiotic treatment is not required. Intralesional triamcinolone may hasten resolution of the symptoms.

The epidermoid cyst is a keratinizing cyst, the wall of which is stratified squamous epithelium containing keratohyalin granules. It is differentiated from the pilar cyst by the different pattern of keratinization, although hybrid cysts with infundibular, trichilemmal, and even pilomatrical differentiation can be seen. Idiopathic scrotal calcinosis is the end stage of calcification of epidermoid cysts of the scrotum. Pilomatrical differentiation within an epidermoid cyst should raise the suspicion of Gardner syndrome.

Surgical excision is curative, but the complete cyst and any associated "daughter" cysts must be removed. Enucleation of the cyst through a small incision or a hole made with a 4 mm or even a 2 mm biopsy punch may be attempted. A curette may be used to scrape out and snag all the fragments of the cyst wall. Alternatively, the lining of the cyst can be eradicated by cauterizing it with 20% trichloroacetic acid. Inflamed cysts may also be treated in this way, but the inflammation makes complete removal of the cyst more difficult. If any fragment of the cyst wall is left behind, the cyst may recur.

Proliferating epidermoid cyst

These tumors, derived from epidermoid cysts, occur more commonly in men (64%), and the most frequent sites are the pelvic/anogenital areas (36%), scalp (21%), upper extremities (18%), and trunk (15%). In rare cases, carcinomatous changes on histology, with anaplasia, high mitotic rate, and deep invasion, occur. They are locally aggressive, but distant metastasis is rare. Malignant onycholemmal cyst may describe a rare slow-growing tumor arising from a subungual keratinous cyst.

Akasaka T, et al: Pigmented epidermal cyst. J Dermatol (Japan) 1997; 24:475.

Diven DG, et al: Bacteriology of inflamed and uninflamed epidermal inclusion cysts. Arch Dermatol 1998; 134:49.

Fujiwara M, et al: Multilocular giant epidermal cyst. Br J Dermatol 2004; 151:927.

May SA, et al: Follicular hybrid cysts with infundibular, isthmic-catagen, and pilomatrical differentiation: a report of 2 patients. Ann Diagn Pathol 2006; 10:110.

Okeke LI: Epidermal inclusion cyst as a rare complication of neonatal male circumcision: a case report. J Med Case Reports 2009; 3:7321.

Poonawalla T, et al: Survey of antibiotic prescription use for inflamed epidermal inclusion cysts. J Cutan Med Surg 2006; 10:79.

Ramagosa R, et al: Human papillomavirus infection and ultraviolet light exposure as epidermoid inclusion cyst risk factors in a patient with epidermodysplasia verruciformis? J Am Acad Dermatol 2008; 58:S68. e1.

Ramakrishna Y, et al: Post-traumatic epidermoid inclusion cyst in the chin region. J Clin Pediatr Dent 2009; 33:251.

Sau P, et al: Proliferating epithelial cysts: clinicopathological analysis of 96 cases. J Cutan Pathol 1995; 22:394.

Smoot EC: Removal of large inclusion cysts with minimal incisional scars. Plast Reconstr Surg 2007; 119:1395.

Sukal SA, Myskowski PL: Safer and less unpleasant incision and drainage of epidermal inclusion cysts. Dermatol Surg 2006; 32:1214.

Yang HJ, Yang KC: A new method for facial epidermoid cyst removal with minimal incision. J Eur Acad Dermatol Venereol 2009; 23:887.

Pilar cyst (trichilemmal cyst, isthmus-catagen cyst)

The trichilemmal cyst, also known as a wen, is similar clinically to the epidermoid cyst, except for the fact that about 90% of pilar cysts occur on the scalp (Fig. 29-51). Women over the age of 60 are predominantly affected. The cyst may be found rarely on the face, trunk, and extremities. An overlying punctum is not present and lesions tend to be more mobile and firmer than epidermoid cysts. Hereditary trichilemmal cysts link to the short arm of chromosome 3, but not to β-catenin or MLH1.

The trichilemmal cyst is lined by stratified squamous epithelium, which is derived from the outer root sheath. The lining cells demonstrate trichilemmal keratinization, increasing in size as they approach the cyst cavity and abruptly keratinizing without forming a granular cell layer. The cyst contents are homogenous and commonly calcify. Hybrid cysts with features of both an epidermoid cyst and a pilar cyst can be seen.

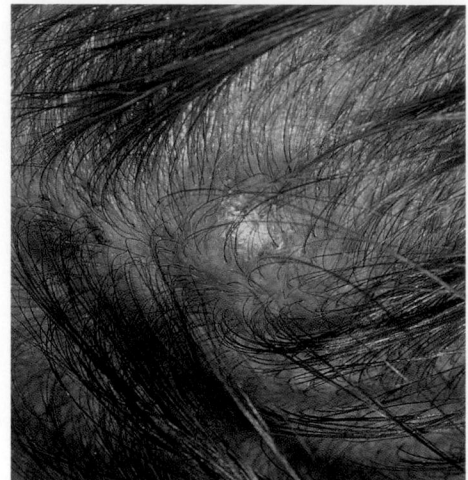

Fig. 29-51 Pilar cyst.

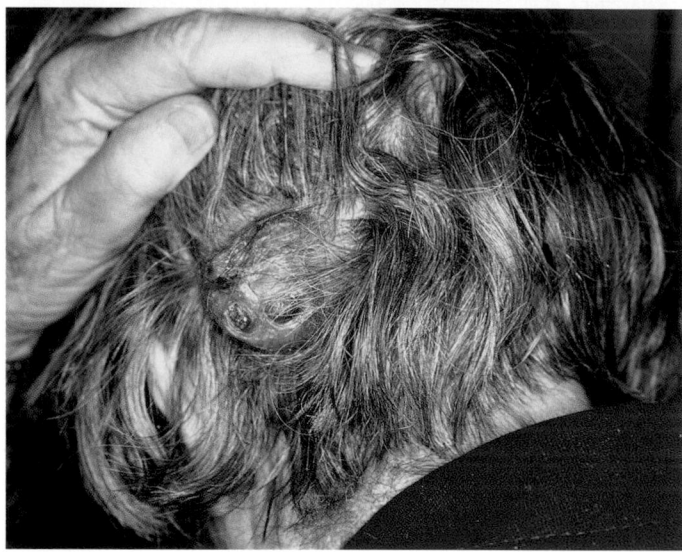

Fig. 29-52 Pilar cyst, proliferating type.

Treatment is the same as that for the epidermoid cyst. They are much more easily enucleated, so more limited incision is required to remove the lesion.

Proliferating trichilemmal cyst/malignant trichilemmal cyst

There is a spectrum of lesions ranging from typical pilar cysts with focal areas of epithelial proliferation to solid proliferating growths with atypia that are best considered SCCs. The typical proliferating pilar cyst or proliferating pilar tumor is a large (up to 25 cm), exophytic neoplasm confined almost exclusively to the scalp and back of the neck. These lesions are approximately five times more common in women, and the mean age of patients is 65 years. They gradually enlarge and may undergo ulceration (Fig. 29-52). The vast majority of lesions are cured by local excision. Some lesions may recur and, less commonly, they may be locally aggressive. Focal areas of atypia and mitoses may be seen in benign-behaving, proliferating pilar tumors. In uncommon cases, there are focal areas that show frank SCC. These lesions should be called malignant proliferating pilar tumor. Areas of SCC are characterized by increased cellularity, atypia, frequent mitoses, and most importantly, invasion of the surrounding stroma. These tumors may behave aggressively. The clinical features that should raise the suspicion of potential aggressive behavior are non-scalp location, recent rapid growth, size greater than 5 cm, and an infiltrative growth pattern clinically and histologically. In KID (keratosis, ichthyosis, deafness) syndrome the development of malignant proliferating pilar tumor may occur in young adulthood and be fatal.

Proliferating trichilemmal cysts are composed of proliferations of squamous cells with trichilemmal differentiation, forming scroll-like structures or small cysts. Lesions are usually well circumscribed. Focal cellular atypia, mitoses, and necrosis may be present and do not necessarily predict aggressive behavior. Cases with aggressive growth and metastases usually have cytologic atypia, as well as an invasive growth pattern. The presence of a clearly benign component and a second anaplastic component growing outward suggests the development of a carcinoma. Proliferating pilar cysts and their malignant counterparts express hair cytokeratins (cytokeratin 7), and malignant trichilemmal tumors express CD34, suggesting fetal hair root phenotype and trichilemmal differentiation.

Chang SJ, et al: Proliferating trichilemmal cysts of the scalp on CT. Am J Neuradiol 2006; 27:712.

Eiberg H, et al: Mapping of hereditary trichilemmal cyst (*TRICY1*) to chromosome 3p24–p21.2 and exclusion of β-catenin and MLH1. Am J Med Genet 2005; 133A:44.

Folpe AL, et al: Proliferating trichilemmal tumors: clinicopathologic evaluation is a guide to biologic behavior. J Cutan Pathol 2003; 30:492.

Hayashi I, et al: Malignant proliferating trichilemmal tumour and CAV (cisplatin, adriamycin, vindesine) treatment. Br J Dermatol 2004; 150:155.

Karaman E, et al: Giant trichilemmal cyst at the neck region. J Craniofac Surg 2009; 20:961.

Nyquist GG, et al: Malignant proliferating pilar tumors arising in KID syndrome: a report of two patients. Am J Med Genet A 2007; 143:734.

Satyaprakash AK, et al: Proliferating trichilemmal tumors: a review of the literature. Dermatol Surg 2007; 33:1102.

Dermoid cyst

Cutaneous dermoid cysts, also called congenital inclusion dermoid cysts, result from local anomalies in embryonic development and occur along embryonic closure zones. On the face they occur above the lateral end of the eyebrow (external angular dermoid) (Fig. 29-53), at the nasal root, along the midline of the forehead, over the mastoid process on the floor of the mouth, and anywhere along the midline of the scalp

from the frontal to the occipital region. They may also be found on the chest, back, abdomen, and perianally. Nasal and external angular dermoids may be seen in multiple members of a family, suggesting a genetic component. Lesions usually present within the first year of life, although only 70% of lesions have been identified by age 5 years. The typical lesion is a few millimeters to several centimeters in diameter and located in the subcutaneous fat. A tethering to the underlying tissues and an underlying bony defect may be noted. They are nonpulsatile, firm, and cystic, and do not transilluminate. A punctum or opening to the skin surface may sometimes be present, but they are commonly not attached to the overlying skin. A tuft of hair may project from a pit, signifying the presence of an underlying sinus or cyst. Inflammation of the cyst due to rupture (with extrusion of hair and a foreign body reaction) or infection may first bring the patient to the physician. Since the dermoid may connect to underlying structures, including the pleura and CNS, infection may spread to the CNS or lungs, causing potentially serious infections. Patients with spina bifida frequently develop dermoid cysts of the repaired portion of their spinal column. Dermoids overlying the lower spine may be associated with tethered cord and late development of ambulating difficulties. A times dermoids may be on the lateral buttocks. Dermal sinuses/dermoids may be associated with other findings of occult spinal dysraphism, including hyperpigmented patches, "skin tags," hemangiomas, and hairy nevi.

Histologically, the cyst wall is lined with keratinizing stratified squamous epithelium containing skin appendages, including lanugo hair. Portions of the cyst lining may demonstrate a wavy eosinophilic (shark tooth) pattern like that of a steatocystoma.

In a child, attempts at surgical removal or biopsy of a cyst over cleavage planes (including along the midline of the back) should not be attempted without proper assessment to rule out an intraspinal or intracranial communication. CT or MRI is required for this. Any underlying bony changes detected by CT scan should be followed up with an MRI scan, since the cranial penetration by the cyst may at times be difficult to identify by CT. If an intracranial connection is detected, the patient should be referred to a neurosurgeon.

Ackerman LL, et al: Cervical and thoracic dermal sinus tracts. A case series and review of the literature. Pediatr Neurosurg 2002; 37:137.

Akhaddar A, et al: Cerebellar abscesses secondary to occipital dermoid cyst with dermal sinus. Surg Neurol 2002; 58:266.

Bodkin PA, et al: Beware of the midline scalp lump. J R Soc Med 2004; 97:239.

Cambiaghi S, et al: Nasal dermoid sinus cyst. Pediatr Dermatol 2007; 24:646.

Ikwueke I, et al: Congenital dermal sinus tract in the lateral buttock: unusual presentation of a typically midline lesion. J Pediatr Surg 2008; 43:1200.

Mazzola CA, et al: Dermoid inclusion cysts and early spinal cord tethering after fetal surgery for myelomeningocele. N Engl J Med 2002; 347:256.

McIntyre JD, et al: Familial external angular dermoid: evidence for a genetic link? J Craniofac Surg 2002; 13:311.

Misago N, et al: Intradermal dermoid cyst associated with occult spinal dysraphism. J Dermatol 1996; 23:275.

Muto J, et al: Congenital dermoid fistula of the anterior chest region. Clin Exp Dermatol 2004; 29:91.

Pilonidal sinus

Pilonidal cyst or sinus occurs in the midline sacral region at the upper end of the cleft of the buttocks. A pit may be all that is visible before puberty. Pilonidal cysts/sinuses usually become symptomatic during adolescence. The lesion becomes inflamed due to rupture or, less commonly, infection. Pilonidal

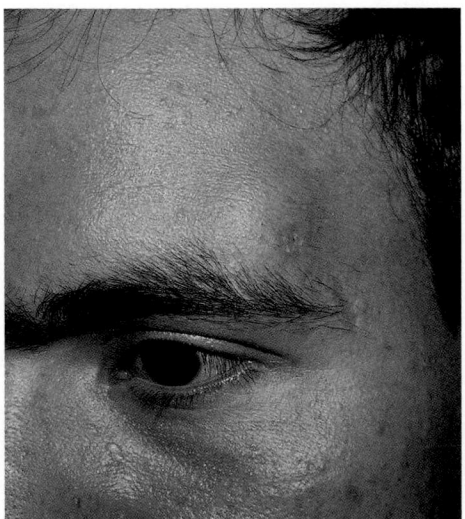

Fig. 29-53 Dermoid, cystic nodule of the lateral eyebrow.

sinus/cyst often occurs with nodulocystic acne, dissecting cellulitis, and hidradenitis suppurativa (the acne tetrad). Histologically, the cyst/sinus is lined by stratified squamous epithelium of the type seen in normal epidermis or follicular infundibulum. Some pilonidal cysts/sinuses are composed of epithelium, which keratinizes without formation of a granular cell layer, analogous to outer root sheath. Referral to a general surgeon is recommended, as recurrences may follow simple cystectomy and marsupialization. SCCs have been reported to arise from chronic inflammatory pilonidal disease.

Gur E, et al: Squamous cell carcinoma in perineal inflammatory disease. Ann Plast Surg 1997; 38:653.
Kurokawa I, et al: Cytokeratin expression in pilonidal sinus. Br J Dermatol 2002; 146:409.

Steatocystoma simplex

Solitary steatocystoma (simple sebaceous duct cyst, steatocystoma simplex) occurs with equal frequency in adult women and men, and can be sited on the face, trunk, or extremities. The oral mucosa may also be involved. It is not familial, and solitary lesions are much less common than multiple ones. The cysts are usually 0.5–1.5 cm in size, although rarely solitary steatocystomas over 8 cm have been reported. The cyst contains an oily, yellow fluid and may contain vellus hairs. Histologically, the cyst is lined by stratified squamous epithelium. Small, mature, sebaceous lobules are present along the cyst wall and empty into the cyst. The luminal surface of the cyst is eosinophilic, wavy (shark tooth pattern), and ribbon-like, analogous to the sebaceous duct. "Hydrid" cysts may have portions of their lining of the steatocystoma type, with the other portions resembling pilar cyst, epidermoid cyst, or even pilomatricoma. Simple excision is curative.

Cunningham SC, et al: Steatocystoma simplex. Surgery 2004; 136:95.
Dailey T: Pathology of intraoral sebaceous glands. J Oral Pathol Med (Denmark) 1993; 22:241.
Monshizadeh R, et al: Perforating follicular hybrid cyst of the tarsus. J Am Acad Dermatol 2003; 48:S33.

Steatocystoma multiplex

Steatocystoma multiplex (SM) consists of multiple, uniform, yellowish, cystic papules usually 2–6 mm in diameter (Fig. 29-54), located principally on the upper anterior portion of the trunk, upper arms, axillae, and thighs. The lesions lack a punctum. The majority of cases present with dermal lesions, but multiple subcutaneous masses resembling multiple lipomas can occur. Lesions usually appear in adolescence or early adulthood, when sebaceous activity is at its peak. Development of SM can first occur in late adulthood. In severe cases, the lesions may be generalized, with sparing only of the palms and soles. At times, the lesions may be limited to the face or scalp, a distinct form termed the facial papular variant. Lesions limited to the genital area have also been reported. Congenital and adolescent-onset linear lesions are rare. Steatocystoma may be larger (up to 2 cm), and prone to rupture and suppuration (steatocystoma multiplex suppurativum). If these lesions are widespread, the condition can be very disfiguring. Steatocystomas contain a syrup-like, yellowish, odorless, oily material. In the suppurative type, colonization with bacteria can occur, leading to foul odor and social isolation.

Histologically, the lining of the cyst is stratified squamous epithelium, with the cyst lining containing mature sebaceous glands. The epithelial lining is identical to the sebaceous duct. The luminal surface is wavy and eosinophilic, and may stain with calretinin (perhaps only in the late-onset facial type). The

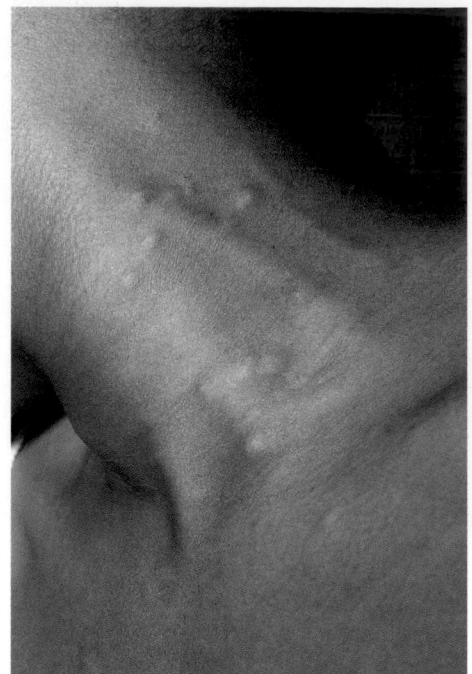

Fig. 29-54 Steatocystoma multiplex.

granular layer is absent, but large basophilic granules may be seen focally in the epithelial cells in the upper layers of the cyst lining. In some instances, hair follicles occur in the cyst wall and vellus hairs may be present in the cavity. A relationship with eruptive vellus hair cysts has been suggested because of a similar clinical appearance, time of onset, and overlapping histologic features. It has been proposed that these clinical entities are a spectrum of the same disease process and should be classified as multiple pilosebaceous cysts.

SM is often familial, demonstrating an autosomal-dominant mode of inheritance. Sporadic cases are not uncommon, however. Keratin 17 missense mutations occur in familial (but not sporadic) SM, usually in a hypermutable site of exon 1 of the gene (the helix initiation motif). Keratin 17 is specialization keratin expressed in the nailbed, hair follicles, and sebaceous glands. This same genetic mutation also causes pachyonychia congenita type 2 (PC-2). This form of pachyonychia congenita has milder keratoderma, but also natal teeth, pili torti, angular cheilosis, and hoarseness. These patients have multiple cysts, some of which are steatocystomas and some eruptive vellus hair cysts. Milia, flexural abscesses identical to hidradenitis, and scrotal and vulvar cysts can also be seen in these kindreds. Hybrid cysts may occur. It is unclear why patients with hereditary SM and keratin 17 mutations identical to those seen in PC-2 have no other stigmata of PC-2. Oligodontia and partial persistent primary dentition can be seen in some kindreds with SM and keratin 17 mutations.

The definitive treatment of individual lesions is removal. This may be accomplished with small incisions and gentle extraction. However, the sheer number of the cysts usually precludes this type of treatment, and the location on the chest makes healing with cosmetically acceptable scars an issue. Laser incision of the cysts may also be effective. They may remain clinically improved for many months; however, eventual recurrence is the rule. Isotretinoin orally, at a dose of 0.75–1 mg/kg, has been reported to benefit the suppurative variant of steatocystoma. Long-term follow-up has not been reported.

Ahn SK, et al: Steatocystoma multiplex localized only in the face. Int J Dermatol 1997; 36:372.

Apaydin R, et al: Steatocystoma multiplex suppurativum: oral isotretinoin treatment combined with cryotherapy. Australas J Dermatol 2000; 41:98.

Chu DH: Steatocystoma multiplex. Dermatol Online J 2003; 9:18.

de Almeida HL Jr, Basso P: Linear unilateral steatocystoma multiplex. J Eur Acad Dermatol Venereol 2009; 23:213.

Gass JK, et al: Steatocystoma multiplex, oligodontia and partial persistent primary dentition associated with a novel keratin 17 mutation. Br J Dermatol 2009; 161:1396.

Hollmig T, Menter A: Familial coincidence of hidradenitis suppurativa and steatocystoma multiplex. Clin Exp Dermatol 2009 Nov 3 (Epub ahead of print).

Jeong SY, et al: Giant steatocystoma multiplex limited to the scalp. Clin Exp Dermatol 2009; 34:e318.

Kanda M, et al: Morphological and genetic analysis of steatocystoma multiplex in an Asian family with pachyonychia congenita type 2 harbouring a KRT17 missense mutation. Br J Dermatol 2009; 160:465.

Laquer VT, et al: Pruritic bluish-black subcutaneous papules on the chest. Dermatol Online J 2008; 14:14.

Lee SJ, et al: The vein hook successfully used for eradication of steatocystoma multiplex. Dermatol Surg 2007; 33:82.

Park YM, et al: Congenital linear steatocystoma multiplex of the nose. Pediatr Dermatol 2000; 17:136.

Riedel C, et al: Late onset of a facial variant of steatocystoma multiplex—calretinin as a specific marker of the follicular companion cell layer. J Dtsch Dermatol Ges 2008; 6:480.

Rossi R, et al: CO_2 laser therapy in a case of steatocystoma multiplex with prominent nodules on the face and neck. Int J Dermatol 2003; 42:302.

Wang JF, et al: Novel missense mutation of keratin in Chinese family with steatocystoma multiplex. J Eur Acad Dermatol Venereol 2009; 23:723.

Yamada A, et al: Acquired multiple pilosebaceous cysts on the face having the histopathological features of steatocystoma multiplex and eruptive vellus hair cysts. Int J Dermatol 2005; 44:861.

Yanagi T, Matsumura T: Steatocystoma multiplex presenting as acral subcutaneous nodules. Acta Derm Venereol 2006; 86.374.

Eruptive vellus hair cysts

Eruptive vellus hair cysts (EVHCs) appear as multiple (up to hundreds), 1–4 mm, skin-colored or hyperpigmented, dome-shaped papules of the mid-chest and proximal upper extremities. They may be congenital but usually have their onset between ages 4 and 18 (in the first and second decades). Disseminated lesions have been reported. Lesions are localized to the face only, and a unilateral distribution can occur. Facial lesions can be distinctly hyperpigmented and simulate a primary melanocytic disorder, such as nevus of Ota. The pinna of the ear may rarely be affected. Hidrotic and anhidrotic ectodermal dysplasia and Lowe syndrome have been associated with EVHC. Onset in later adulthood with chronic renal failure has been reported multiple times. Clinically, EVHCs tend to be smaller than steatocystomas and may have an area of central hyperkeratosis or umbilication, a feature lacking in steatocystoma. Acne is distinguished by the lack of inflammatory lesions. Histologically, the cystic epithelium is of the stratified squamous type; the cyst contents are composed of laminated keratin and multiple vellus hairs, and follicle-like invaginations may be present in the cyst wall. Steatocystoma may at times have vellus hairs, and EVHCs may have sebaceous glands in their lining. About 25% of EVHC lesions spontaneously resolve by transepidermal elimination. Topical tazarotene has been effective, but with no long-term follow-up. Similarly, lactic acid 12% and topical tretinoin can lead to improvement. Most treatments are surgical, including extraction, and CO_2 laser. Erbium:YAG laser is inferior to tazarotene and associated with recurrence.

Chan KH, et al: Eruptive vellus hair cysts presenting as bluish-grey facial discoloration masquerading as naevus of Ota. Br J Dermatol 2007; 157:188.

Coras B, et al: Early recurrence of eruptive vellus hair cysts after Er:YAG laser therapy: case report and review of the literature. Dermatol Surg 2005; 31:1741.

Fernandez-Torres R, et al: Treatment of multiple eruptive vellus hair cysts with carbon dioxide laser vaporization and manual lateral pressure. Clin Exp Dermatol 2009; 34:e716.

Hong SD, Frieden IJ: Diagnosing eruptive vellus hair cysts. Pediatr Dermatol 2001; 18:258.

Karen JK, et al: Eruptive vellus hair cysts. Dermatol Online J 2007; 13:14.

Kaya TI, et al: Eruptive vellus hair cysts: an effective extraction technique for treatment and diagnosis. J Eur Acad Dermatol Venereol 2006; 20:264.

Köse O, et al: Anhidrotic ectodermal dysplasia with eruptive vellus hair cysts. Int J Dermatol 2001; 40:401.

Lew BL, et al: Unilateral eruptive vellus hair cysts occurring on the face. J Eur Acad Dermatol Venereol 2006; 20:1314.

Mieno H, et al: Eruptive vellus hair cyst in patients with chronic renal failure. Dermatology 2004; 208:67.

Nandedkar MA, et al: Eruptive vellus hair cysts in a patient with Lowe syndrome. Pediatr Dermatol 2004; 21:54.

Reep MD, Robson KJ: Eruptive vellus hair cysts presenting as multiple periorbital papules in a 13-year-old boy. Pediatr Dermatol 2002; 19:26.

Saks K, Levitt JO: Tazarotene 0.1 percent cream fares better than erbium:YAG laser or incision and drainage in a patient with eruptive vellus hair cysts. Dermatol Online J 2006; 12:7.

Yamada A, et al: Acquired multiple pilosebaceous cysts on the face having the histopathological features of steatocystoma multiplex and eruptive vellus hair cysts. Int J Dermatol 2005; 44:861.

Yanik ME, et al: Eruptive vellus hair cysts occurring on the ears. J Dermatol 2009; 36:360.

Milia

Milia are white keratinous cysts, 1–4 mm in diameter. They are white and easily seen as cystic through the overlying attenuated skin. Milia are common and multiple clinical patterns of milia have been described. Milia can be considered primary, appearing spontaneously, or secondary, appearing secondary to trauma, a skin disease, or medication.

Primary milia occur congenitally (or a little after birth in preterm neonates) in up to 50% of newborns. They favor the face, especially the nose, scalp, upper trunk, and proximal extremities of all races and both genders. They resolve over weeks. Rare kindreds with an autosomal-dominant inheritance have profuse, essentially confluent, congenital milia on the face. These also spontaneously resolve. Adults and children commonly develop milia, especially on the cheeks, eyelids, forehead, and genitalia. In infants, milia localized to the areola may be seen. These milia tend to persist. Multiple eruptive milia is a term applied to lesions that occur spontaneously in too large a number to be considered benign primary milia of children and adults. Cases favor the head and erupt over weeks to months. This can be idiopathic or familial. Nasal crease milia describe a row of milia in the nasal crease in nonatopics. Some cases are congenital. Pseudoacne of the nasal crease may be related. Milia cn plaque describes a rare disorder characterized by an erythematous plaque containing numerous milia. They are usually on the head and neck, especially the periauricular or periorbital regions. It is most common in middle-aged females. One 3-year-old had widespread depigmented macules and patches with numerous milia in the depigmented areas (termed generalized milia with nevus depigmentosus).

Secondary milia can develop as a consequence of blistering skin diseases, such as epidermolysis bullosa, pemphigus, bullous pemphigoid, porphyria cutanea tarda, herpes zoster, polymorphous light eruption, lupus erythematosus, Stevens–Johnson syndrome, contact dermatitis, and many other conditions. They also tend to occur after trauma, such as dermabrasion, chemical peel, ablative laser therapy, skin grafts, and radiotherapy. Long-term topical corticosteroid therapy and the use of occlusive moisturizers may result in the appearance of milia. Cyclosporine and 5-FU have been associated with the development of milia.

Multiple milia have been reported in a number of genodermatoses, such as congenital ectodermal defect; reticular pigmented genodermatosis with milia (Naegeli–Franceschetti–Jadassohn syndrome); congenital absence of dermal ridges, syndactyly, and facial milia; generalized basaloid follicular hamartoma syndrome; basal cell nevus syndrome; atrichia with papular lesions; pachyonychia congenita type 2; Rombo syndrome; Brooke–Spiegler syndrome; and Bazex syndrome.

Primary milia are small epidermoid cysts, derived from the infundibulum of the vellus hair (Fig. 29-55). Like epidermoid cysts, they are fixed and persistent. Secondary milia may be derived from eccrine ducts or hair follicles as they attempt to re-epithelialize eroded epidermis. They are often transient and spontaneously disappear. Milia must be distinguished from milia-like idiopathic calcinosis cutis, military osteomas, syringomas with milia-like structures, trichoepitheliomas, comedonal acne, flat warts, and xanthelasma. Lesions of cutaneous T-cell lymphoma with prominent follicular mucinosis may have many milia. Treatment is incision and expression of the contents with a beveled cutting tipped hypodermic needle, 11 blade, or comedo extractor. No anesthesia is needed for most patients. Topical tretinoin (Retin-A) has been reported as effective in treating milia en plaque and more generalized forms of milia involving the face. Minocycline has been used to treat milia en plaque.

Belhadjali H, et al: Milia en plaque and discoid lupus erythematosus. Clin Exp Dermatol 2009; 34:e356.

Berk DR, Bayliss SJ: Milia: a review and classification. J Am Acad Dermatol 2008; 59:1050.

Berk DR, Bayliss SJ: Milium of the areola: a novel regional variant of primary milia. Pediatr Dermatol 2009; 26:485.

Bryden AM, et al: Milia complicating photocontact allergy to absorbent sunscreen chemicals. Clin Exp Dermatol 2003; 28:666.

Bulai Livideanu C, et al: Milia complicating bullous polymorphic light eruption. Photodermatol Photoimmunol Photomed 2009; 25:51.

Connelly T: Eruptive milia and rapid response to topical tretinoin. Arch Dermatol 2008; 144:816.

Diba VC, et al: Multiple eruptive milia in a 9-year-old boy. Pediatr Dermatol 2008; 25:474.

Fujita H, et al: Milia en plaque on the forehead. J Dermatol 2008; 35:39.

Kalayciyan A, et al: Milia in regressing plaques of mycosis fungoides: provoked by topical nitrogen mustard or not? Int J Dermatol 2004; 43:953.

Kautz O, et al: Milia en plaque in a linear pattern. J Eur Acad Dermatol Venereol 2009; 23:1335.

Kouba DJ, et al: Milia en plaque: a novel manifestation of chronic cutaneous lupus erythematosus. Br J Dermatol 2003; 149:419.

Risma KA, Lucky AW: Pseudoacne of the nasal crease? a new entity? Pediatr Dermatol 2004; 21:427.

Rose RF, et al: Retroauricular milia en plaque: a rare presentation of lupus erythematosus. Clin Exp Dermatol 2008; 33:715.

Rutter KJ, Judge MR: Profuse congenital milia in a family. Pediatr Dermatol 2009; 26:62.

Stefanidou MP, et al: Milia en plaque: a case report and review of the literature. Dermatol Surg 2002; 28:291.

Thami GP, et al: Surgical pearl: enucleation of milia with a disposable hypodermic needle. J Am Acad Dermatol 2002; 47:601.

Tzermias C, et al: Reticular pigmented genodermatosis with milia: special form of Naegeli–Franceschetti–Jadassohn syndrome or a new entity? Clin Exp Dermatol 1995; 20:331.

Verrucous cysts (cystic papillomas)

Verrucous cysts resemble epidermoid cysts, except that the lining demonstrates papillomatosis and coarse hypergranulosis. Koilocytes may be present. On the sole, red granules resembling those in myrmecia are commonly seen. They have been shown to contain HPV and probably form as a result of HPV infection of a follicular unit or sweat duct (see Chapter 19).

Pseudocyst of the auricle (auricular endochondral pseudocyst)

Pseudocyst of the auricle presents clinically as a fluctuant, tense, noninflammatory swelling on the upper half of the ear (Fig. 29-56). Most affected persons are between the ages of 20 and 45, and up to 90% are male. Pruritic disorders such as atopic dermatitis and systemic lymphoma, hard pillows in

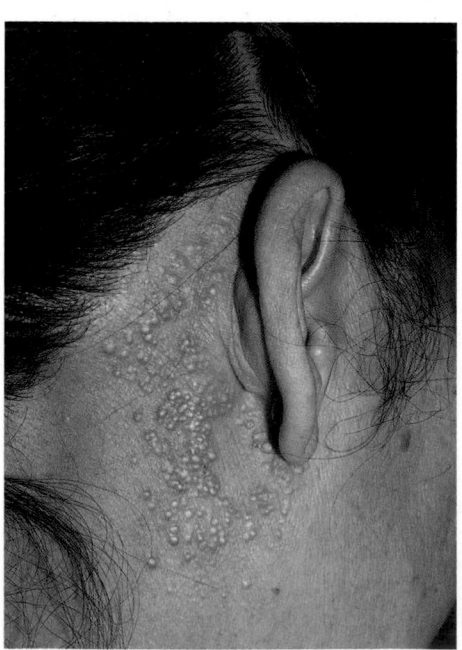

Fig. 29-55 Milia en plaque.

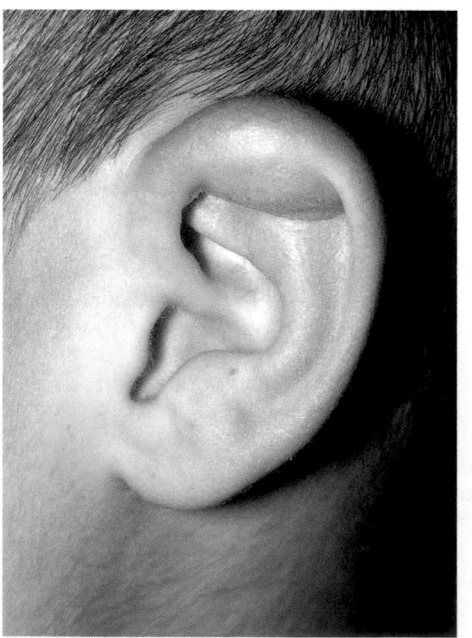

Fig. 29-56 Pseudocyst of the auricle.

China, carrying heavy objects on the shoulder, helmet and earphone wearing, and a slap to the side of the head have all been associated with auricular pseudocysts. This strongly suggests that trauma plays a role, although patients will frequently deny trauma. The fluid collection is between the two layers of the bilaminate cartilage of the pinna. There is no cyst lining, with the affected cartilage showing focal degeneration and granulation tissue. Needle aspiration yields serous or bloody fluid. Simple aspiration is ineffective. Aspiration or drainage, followed by the application of a bolster or pressure dressing for several weeks, is usually effective. Since application of pressure for several weeks is required, a sutured-on bolster with buttons or gauze is easier for the patient than an externally applied dressing. Intracystic injections of corticosteroids, fibrin glue, or minocycline have been used in recurrent cases. Surgical intervention involves removal of the inner anterior portion of the cyst.

Kanotra SP, Lateef M: Pseudocyst of pinna: a recurrence-free approach. Am J Otolaryngol 2009; 30:73.

Kim TY, et al: Treatment of a recurrent auricular pseudocyst with intralesional steroid injection and clip compression dressing. Dermatol Surg 2009; 35:245.

Miyamoto H, et al: Lactate dehydrogenase isozymes in and intralesional steroid injection therapy for pseudocyst of the auricle. Int J Dermatol 2001; 40:380.

Ng W, et al: Pseudocysts of the auricle in a young adult with facial and ear atopic dermatitis. J Am Acad Dermatol 2007; 56:858.

Oyama N, et al: Treatment of recurrent auricle pseudocyst with intralesional injection of minocycline: a report of two cases. J Am Acad Dermatol 2001; 45:554.

Paul AY, et al: Pseudocyst of the auricle: diagnosis and management with a punch biopsy. J Am Acad Dermatol 2001; 45:S230.

Pereira FC, et al: Bilateral pseudocyst of the auricle in a man with pruritus secondary to lymphoma. Int J Dermatol 2003; 42:818.

Salgado CJ, et al: Treatment of auricular pseudocyst with aspiration and local pressure. J Plast Reconstr Aesthet Surg 2006; 59:1450.

Tan BYB, Hsu PP: Auricular pseudocyst in the tropics: a multi-racial Singapore experience. J Laryngol Otol 2004; 118:185.

Tuncer S, et al: Recurrent auricular pseudocyst: a new treatment recommendation with curettage and fibrin glue. Dermatol Surg 2003; 29:1080.

Vano-Galvan S: Dermacase. Auricular pseudocyst. Can Fam Physician 2009; 55:271.

Cutaneous columnar cysts

Five types of cyst that occur in the skin are lined by columnar epithelium.

Bronchogenic cysts

These are small, solitary cysts or sinuses, most typically located in the region of the suprasternal notch or over the manubrium sterni. They can also occur on the chin, neck, and abdominal wall. A scapular location is rarely described. Boys are four times more commonly affected than girls. Lesions are typically subcutaneous and rarely connect to deeper structures. Histologically, the cyst is composed of a wall lined by respiratory epithelium, and may contain seromucinous glands and underlying fibromuscular connective tissue or cartilage. Gastric mucosa may also be seen.

Branchial cleft cysts

These present as cysts, sinuses, or skin tags along the anterior border of the sternocleidomastoid muscle or near the angle of the mandible (Fig. 29-57). Branchial cysts are lined primarily with stratified squamous epithelium. Lymphoid follicles are often present and smooth muscle is absent, distinguishing them from bronchogenic cysts, although some evidence suggests that these cysts are related.

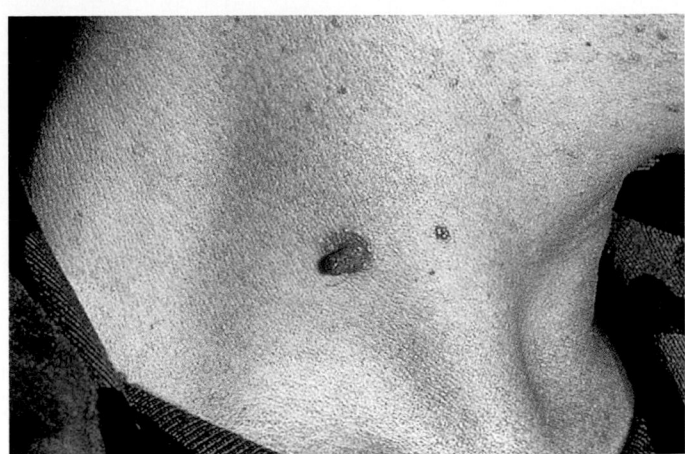

Fig. 29-57 Branchial cleft cyst.

Thyroglossal duct cysts

These virtually always occur on the anterior portion of the neck, near the hyoid bone. They present as a sinus, cyst, or recurrent abscess of the neck. They are the most common cause of congenital neck anomalies in childhood. Presentation in adult life can occur. Malignancies (papillary adenocarcinoma, follicular adenocarcinoma, mixed papillary/follicular adenocarcinoma, adenocarcinoma, and SCCs) arising from cysts have been reported in 1% of cases. Clinically, thyroglossal duct cysts are deep to subcutaneous tissue and usually are not managed by dermatologists.

Cutaneous ciliated cysts

These are usually solitary and located on the legs of females. Men account for only 10% of cases. These cysts have also been described in the perineum and vulva (vulvar ciliated cysts). The epithelium lining the cysts is cuboidal to columnar, with pseudostratified areas. Cilia are seen and the lining cells stain strongly for dynein. This histology is similar to the normal fallopian tube, suggesting that the cysts are of müllerian origin. Ciliated metaplasia of eccrine duct has been proposed for those lesions occurring on the upper half of the body and in men. Like the median raphe cyst, the cavity is often filled with debris.

Median raphe cysts

Median raphe cysts of the penis are developmental defects lying in the ventral midline of the perineum from the anus to the urethra, but most commonly on the distal shaft near the glans. They most commonly present as dermal lesions of less than 1 cm in young men, and may appear suddenly after sexual intercourse-associated trauma. These cysts may appear as a cord or a series of beads (termed canal-like). They are lined by pseudostratified columnar epithelium with focal areas of mucin-secreting epithelium present. Ciliated cells may be present and, like ciliated cysts in females, the cavity is typically filled with debris. Melanocytes may occasionally be present in the cyst wall, giving the cysts a pigmented appearance. Median raphe cysts do not stain with human milk fat globulin 1, distinguishing them from apocrine cystadenomas. Median raphe cysts do not connect with the urethra and can be treated with surgical excision.

Congenital preauricular fistula

This anomaly occurs as a pit in the preauricular region, often in several members and generations of a family. On each side, just anterior to the external ear, there is a small dimple, pore, or fistulous opening that may extend as far as the middle ear. Most of these fistulas are benign and do not require surgery. Complications of surgery are frequent, and complete excision of both the pit and sinus tract should be the goal if surgery is attempted.

Aceñero MJF, García-González J: Median raphe cyst with ciliated cells: report of a case. Am J Dermatopathol 2003; 25:175.

Brousseau VJ, et al: Thyroglossal duct cysts: presentation and management in children versus adults. Int J Pediatr Otorhinolaryngol 2003; 67:1285.

Carden C, et al: An unusual midline swelling—case report of a cutaneous bronchogenic cyst. Eur J Pediatr Surg 2008; 18:345.

Cardoso R, et al: Median raphe cyst of the penis. Dermatol Online J 2005; 11:37.

Dehner LP, et al: Median raphe cyst in the scrotum after orchiopexy. Int J Urol 2007; 14:573; author reply 574.

Dini M, et al: Median raphe cyst of the penis: a report of two cases with immunohistochemical investigation. Am J Dermatopathol 2001; 23:320.

Giannakopoulos S, et al: Two unusual cases of median raphe penile cysts. Eur J Dermatol 2007; 17:342.

Hara N, et al: Median raphe cyst in the scrotum, mimicking a serous borderline tumor, associated with cryptorchidism after orchiopexy. Int J Urol 2004; 11:1150.

Kang IK, et al: Ciliated cyst of the vulva. J Am Acad Dermatol 1995; 32:514.

Kim NR, et al: Cutaneous bronchogenic cyst of the abdominal wall. Pathol Int 2001; 51:970.

Koga K, et al: Median raphe cyst with ciliated cells of the penis. Acta Derm Venereol 2007; 87:542.

Krauel L, et al: Median raphe cysts of the perineum in children. Urology 2008; 71:830.

Motamed M, McGlashan JA: Thyroglossal duct carcinoma. Curr Opin Otolaryngol Head Neck Surg 2004; 12:106.

Ohba N, et al: Cutaneous ciliated cyst on the cheek in a male. Int J Dermatol 2002; 41:48.

Ohnishi T, Watanabe S: Immunohistochemical analysis of human milk fat globulin 1 and cytokeratin expression in median raphe cyst of the penis. Clin Exp Dermatol 2001; 26:88.

Ozel SK, et al: Scapular bronchogenic cysts in children: case report and review of the literature. Pediatr Surg Int 2005; 21:843.

Park CO, et al: Median raphe cyst on the scrotum and perineum. J Am Acad Dermatol 2006; 55:S114.

Persaud R, et al: Thyroglossal duct cyst masquerading as a haematoma. J Laryngol Otol 2004; 118:240.

Pradeep KE: Cutaneous bronchogenic cyst: an under-recognised clinicopathological entity. J Clin Pathol 2009; 62:384.

Turkyilmaz Z, et al: Management of thyroglossal duct cysts in children. Pediatr Int 2004; 46:77.

Urahashi J, et al: Pigmented median raphe cysts of the penis. Acta Derm Venereol 2000; 80:297.

Vadmal M, Makarewicz K: Cutaneous ciliated cyst of the abdominal wall. Am J Dermatopathol 2002; 24:452.

Verma SB: Canal-like median raphe cysts: an unusual presentation of an unusual condition. Clin Exp Dermatol 2009; 34:e857.

Vlodavsky E, et al: Gastric mucosa in a bronchogenic cutaneous cyst in a child: case report and review of literature. Am J Dermatopathol 2005; 27:145.

Yokozaki H, et al: Cutaneous ciliated cyst of the right lower leg. Pathol Int 1999; 4:354.

Bonus images for this chapter can be found online at **http://www.expertconsult.com**

Melanocytic Nevi and Neoplasms

30

Melanocytes originate in the embryonal neural crest and migrate to the epidermis, dermis, leptomeninges, retina, mucous membrane epithelium, and inner ear, cochlea, and vestibular system. Nevus cells are a form of melanocyte with a tendency to aggregate into clusters of cells. They lack dendritic processes, but are otherwise similar to other melanocytes.

Epidermal melanocytic lesions

The melanocytes occurring at the dermoepidermal junction are dendritic cells that supply melanin to the skin. These cells contain pigment granules (melanosomes). They stain with the dopa reaction and silver stains because they contain melanin. Immunohistochemical stains, such as S100, HMB-45 and Mart-1, do not depend on the presence of melanin. These stains have largely replaced silver stains for the identification of melanocytes in biopsy specimens. Melanocytes of the epidermis transfer melanosomes through their thin dendritic processes, where they are actively taken up by keratinocytes. Melanocyte numbers vary by anatomic site and are increased in sun-damaged skin, but vary little among racial groups. The type, number, size, dispersion, and degree of melanization of the melanosomes determine the pigmentation of the skin and hair.

Treatment of epidermal pigmented lesions can be directed at pigmented keratinocytes, melanocytes, or melanosomes. Q-switched lasers target the melanosome. Lasers with a longer pulse duration lasting milliseconds result in melanocyte destruction. Laser treatment produces consistent lightening of ephelides, but the response is variable for café-au-lait macules, Becker nevus, and nevus spilus.

Ephelis

The common freckle occurs in light-skinned individuals in response to sun exposure. Histologically, freckles demonstrate pigmented basilar keratinocytes, and a mild increase in the number of melanocytes.

Nevus spilus

Nevus spilus (speckled lentiginous nevus) presents as a light brown or tan macule, speckled with smaller, darker macules or papules (Fig. 30-1). It frequently occurs on the trunk and lower extremities, tends to follow Blaschko lines, and is noted in approximately 2% of the population. The nevus spilus may be small, measuring less than 1 cm in diameter, or may be quite large and follow a segmental distribution, referred to as a zosteriform lentigo. Multiple sites may be involved in the same individual, and may be widely separated by normal skin. Happle has suggested dividing the entity into two forms, a macular type and a papular type. The dark speckles in the former are more evenly distributed and represent junctional lentiginous nevi. Malignant melanoma has been reported more commonly in this type and it is consistently found in phakomatosis spilorosea, whereas nevus spilus papulosus demonstrates compound or intradermal nevi and is seen in phakomatosis pigmentokeratotica.

Nevus spilus in combination with a nevus flammeus is called phakomatosis pigmentovascularis (see Chapter 28). Phakomatosis pigmentokeratotica includes a speckled lentiginous nevus, organoid nevus, hemiatrophy, and neurologic findings such as muscular weakness. Generalized nevus spilus has been associated with nevus anemicus and primary lymphedema. Nevus spilus has also been reported in association with nevus depigmentosus and with bilateral nevus of Ito.

Histologically, the flat, tan background may show only basilar hyperpigmentation, such as is present in a café-au-lait spot, or lentiginous proliferation of the epidermis with bulbous rete ridges. The darker speckles usually contain nevus cells and may occasionally demonstrate blue nevi or Spitz nevi.

Because nevus cells are often present in the dark speckles, melanoma may rarely arise in them. A changing lesion should be biopsied. Removal by Q-switched (QS) ruby laser or QS alexandrite laser rarely has been reported as effective, but may require many sessions for acceptable results.

Hanayama H, et al: Congenital melanocytic nevi and nevus spilus have a tendency to follow the lines of Blaschko: an examination of 200 cases. J Dermatol 2007 Mar; 34(3):159–163.

Happle R: Nevus spilus maculosus vs. partial unilateral lentiginosis. J Eur Acad Dermatol Venereol 2007 May; 21(5):713.

Happle R: Speckled lentiginous naevus: which of the two disorders do you mean? Clin Exp Dermatol 2009 Mar; 34(2):133–135.

Meguerditchian AN, et al: Nevus spilus with synchronous melanomas: case report and literature review. J Cutan Med Surg 2009; 13(2):96–101.

Ramolia P, et al: Speckled lentiginous nevus syndrome associated with musculoskeletal abnormalities. Pediatr Dermatol 2009; 26(3):298–301.

Trindade F, et al: Bilateral nevus of Ito and nevus spilus in the same patient. J Am Acad Dermatol 2008 Aug; 59(2 Suppl 1):S51–S52.

Lentigo

Lentigo simplex

These lesions occur as sharply defined, round to oval, brown or black macules. They usually arise in childhood but may appear at any age. There is no predilection for areas of sun exposure. Multiple lentigines may appear after clearing of plaques of psoriasis, including during biologic therapy.

Histologically, lentigo simplex shows hyperpigmentation of basilar keratinocytes and an increase in the number of melanocytes in the basal layer. Melanophages are commonly present in the upper dermis.

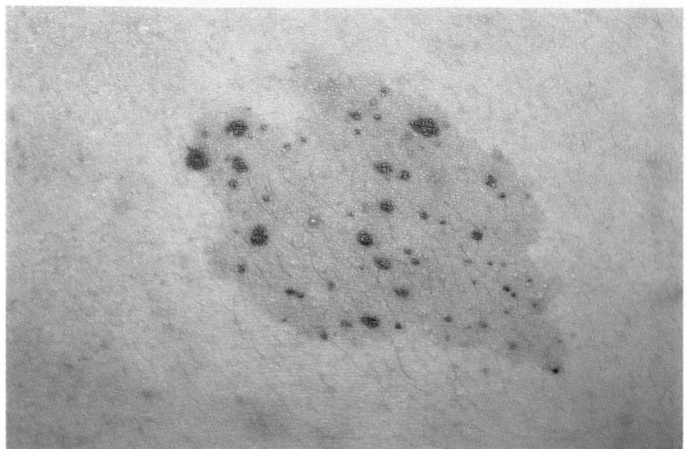

Fig. 30-1 Nevus spilus. (Courtesy of Rui Tavares-Bello, MD)

Solar lentigo (lentigo senilis)

Solar lentigines are commonly known as liver spots. They are persistent, benign, discrete, hyperpigmented, round to oval macules occurring on sun-damaged skin. The backs of the hands, cheeks, and forehead are favorite sites in the typical older patient. Red-haired, light-skinned individuals, especially those with high solar exposure, may develop many of these on the shoulders and central upper chest, even at an early age. Solar lentigines may be accompanied by depigmented macules, actinic purpura, and other chronic actinic degenerative changes in the skin. They may evolve into benign lichenoid keratoses and reticulated seborrheic keratoses.

Histologically, the rete ridges appear club-shaped or show narrow, budlike extensions. There is a marked increase in pigmentation in the basal cell layer, especially at the tips of the bulbous rete. The number of melanocytes is slightly increased, and the upper dermis often contains melanophages.

Application of liquid nitrogen with a cotton-tip applicator or cryospray unit is often effective. Argon, Q-switched Nd:YAG, frequency-doubled Nd:YAG, Q-switched and long-pulse alexandrite, Q-switched ruby, and Er:YAG lasers have been reported as effective. Intense-pulsed light has also been used. Post-inflammatory pigment alteration is the major complication seen with destructive modalities. Sun protection will reduce the number of new lesions. Bleaching creams containing 4% or 5% hydroquinone, used over a period of several months, will induce temporary lightening. Hydroquinone-cyclodextrin (2%), 4-hydroxyanisole (4-HA), chemical peels, local dermabrasion, topical tretinoin, and adapalene are other treatment options. The combination of 2% 4-HA and 0.01% tretinoin is superior to either active component alone, and a commercial preparation containing these two ingredients plus 2% mequinol has been shown to lighten lesions.

Early lesions of lentigo maligna (melanoma in situ) may be light to medium brown and mimic solar lentigines. When in doubt, a biopsy is appropriate. Lentigo maligna, benign solar lentigo, and pigmented actinic keratosis all occur on sun-damaged skin, and collision lesions are common. If a lesion is not homogeneous clinically, representative biopsies should be taken from each area.

PUVA lentigines

Individuals receiving oral methoxsalen photochemotherapy (PUVA) may develop persistent pigmented macules in which there may be melanocytic atypia. These lesions may occur on sites that are normally protected from sunlight. High-dose single exposures to radiation may result in similar radiation lentigines in exposed skin.

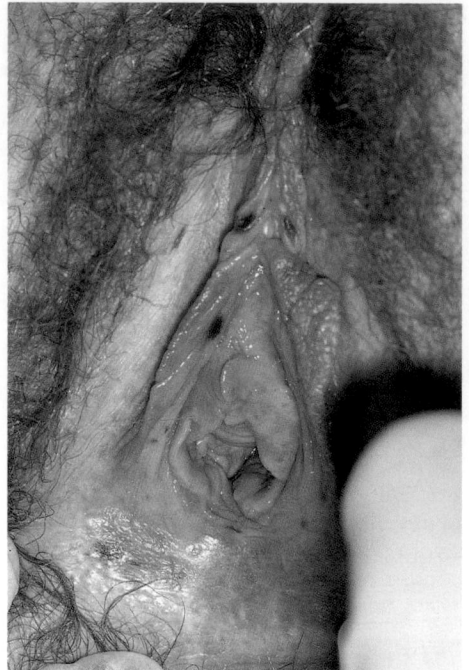

Fig. 30-2 Vulvar melanosis.

Ink spot lentigo (sunburn lentigo)

These lesions commonly occur on the shoulders as small markedly irregular, reticulated, dark gray–black macules resembling spots of ink on the skin. Histologically, there is a mild increase in the number of melanocytes and increased melanin in both the basilar keratinocytes and the stratum corneum.

Labial, penile, and vulvar melanosis (melanotic macules, mucosal lentigines)

Melanotic macules are usually light brown on the oral labial mucosa, but may be strikingly irregular and darkly pigmented in the genitalia. In females, the labia minora are most often affected (Fig. 30-2), while in males, the glans and prepuce are most frequently involved. Histologically, these lesions demonstrate broad "box car" rete ridges with prominent basilar hyperpigmentation, and a normal to slightly increased number of melanocytes. The melanocytes are usually morphologically normal.

Multiple lentigines syndrome

The lesions appear shortly after birth and develop a distinctive speckled appearance that has given rise to the designation LEOPARD syndrome. LEOPARD is Gorlin's mnemonic acronym for lentigines, electrocardiographic abnormalities, ocular hypertelorism, pulmonary stenosis, abnormalities of genitalia, retardation of growth, and deafness. Inheritance is autosomal-dominant. Multiple lentigines occur mainly on the trunk, but other areas may also be involved, such as the palms and soles, buccal mucosa, genitalia, and scalp. *PTPN11* gene mutations are seen in both LEOPARD syndrome and Noonan syndrome. Café noir spots noted in these patients are larger and darker than café au lait spots. Histologically, some are melanocytic nevi while others demonstrate histologic features of lentigo simplex.

Moynahan syndrome

Moynahan syndrome consists of multiple lentigines, congenital mitral stenosis, dwarfism, genital hypoplasia, and mental deficiency.

Generalized lentiginosis

An occasional patient will have generalized lentiginosis without associated abnormalities.

Centrofacial lentiginosis

Centrofacial lentiginosis is characterized by lentigines on the nose and adjacent cheeks, variously associated with status dysraphicus, multiple skeletal anomalies, and central nervous system (CNS) disorders. Mucous membranes are spared. Onset is in the first years of life. Lentigines of the central face are also typical of Carney complex.

Carney complex

Carney complex is also known as NAME syndrome and LAMB syndrome. This designation comprises cardiocutaneous myxomas, lentigines, blue nevi, and endocrine abnormalities. It is discussed in more detail with myxomas in Chapter 28.

Inherited patterned lentiginosis in black persons

O'Neill and James reported 10 light-complexioned black patients with autosomal-dominant lentigines beginning in infancy or early childhood, but no internal abnormalities (Fig. 30-3). The lentigines were distributed over the central face and lips, with variable involvement of the dorsal hands and feet, elbows, and buttocks. The mucous membranes were spared.

Partial unilateral lentiginosis

Partial unilateral lentiginosis is a rare disorder of cutaneous pigmentation characterized by the presence of multiple simple lentigines, wholly or partially involving half of the body. Conjunctival involvement has been reported. Agminated lentiginosis appears to be a similar if not identical entity.

Peutz–Jeghers syndrome

Peutz–Jeghers syndrome is an autosomal-dominant syndrome consisting of pigmented macules on the lips, oral mucosa, and perioral and acral areas. Gastrointestinal polyps, especially prominent in the jejunum, are frequently associated. It is discussed further under disorders of pigmentation in Chapter 36.

Bujaldón AR: LEOPARD syndrome: what are café noir spots? Pediatr Dermatol 2008 Jul–Aug; 25(4):444–448.

Costa LA, et al: Multiple lentigines arising in resolving psoriatic plaques after treatment with etanercept. Dermatol Online J 2008 Jan 15; 14(1):11.

Piérard-Franchimont C, et al: Analytic quantification of the bleaching effect of a 4-hydroxyanisole-tretinoin combination on actinic lentigines. J Drugs Dermatol 2008 Sep; 7(9):873–878.

Raziee M, et al: Efficacy and safety of cryotherapy vs. trichloroacetic acid in the treatment of solar lentigo. J Eur Acad Dermatol Venereol 2008 Mar; 22(3):316–319.

Sadighha A, et al: Efficacy and adverse effects of Q-switched ruby laser on solar lentigines: a prospective study of 91 patients with Fitzpatrick skin type II, III, and IV. Dermatol Surg 2008 Nov; 34(11):1465–1468.

Trafeli JP, et al: Use of a long-pulse alexandrite laser in the treatment of superficial pigmented lesions. Dermatol Surg 2007 Dec; 33(12):1477–1482.

Becker nevus

Becker nevus presents as a hyperpigmented, hypertrichotic patch on the upper trunk (Fig. 30-4) or proximal upper extremity. The lesion usually begins before puberty, and almost all patients are males. The lesion may be associated with a smooth muscle hamartoma on histology. Usually the lesion is asymptomatic and of little consequence, but some lesions have also been associated with connective tissue nevus, inflammatory linear verrucous epidermal nevus, basal cell carcinoma, and phakomatosis pigmentovascularis. The pathogenesis may be related to increased expression of androgen receptors within lesional skin.

Kim YJ, et al: Androgen receptor overexpression in Becker nevus: histopathologic and immunohistochemical analysis. J Cutan Pathol 2008 Dec; 35(12):1121–1126.

Patrizi A, et al: Becker naevus associated with basal cell carcinoma, melanocytic naevus and smooth-muscle hamartoma. J Eur Acad Dermatol Venereol 2007 Jan; 21(1):130–132.

Melanoacanthoma

Cutaneous melanoacanthoma is an uncommon lesion first described by Bloch. Clinically, it resembles a pigmented seborrheic keratosis or pigmented basal cell carcinoma, and tends to occur in older white males. Histologically, it is a benign epidermal neoplasm composed of keratinocytes and dendritic melanocytes. It is best considered a form of seborrheic keratosis. The starburst dermatoscopic appearance can be confused with that of Spitz nevus.

Oral melanoacanthoma is also a proliferation of two cell types, melanocytes and epithelial cells, but appears to be a reactive lesion. It occurs as a macular or slightly raised

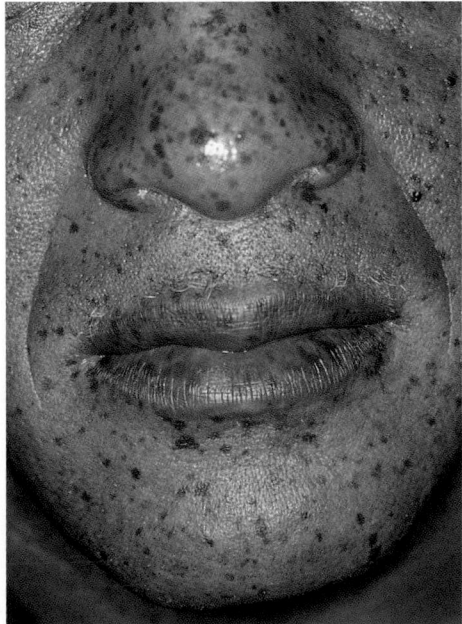

Fig. 30-3 Inherited patterned lentiginosis of black persons.

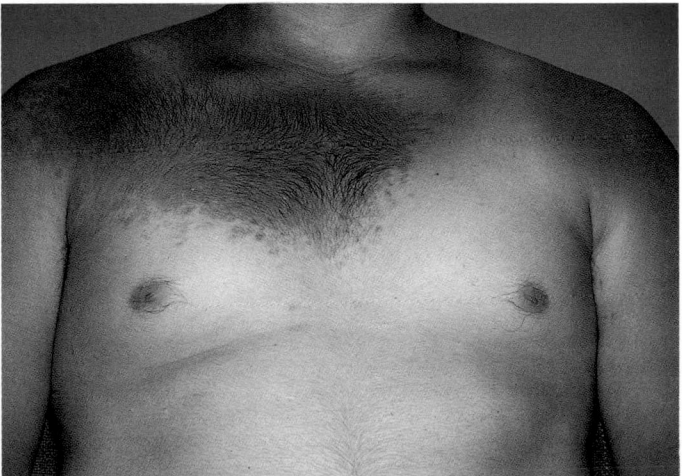

Fig. 30-4 Becker nevus.

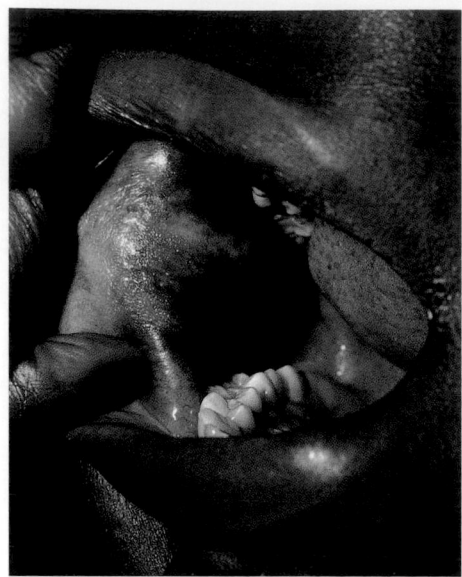

Fig. 30-5 Melanoacanthoma.

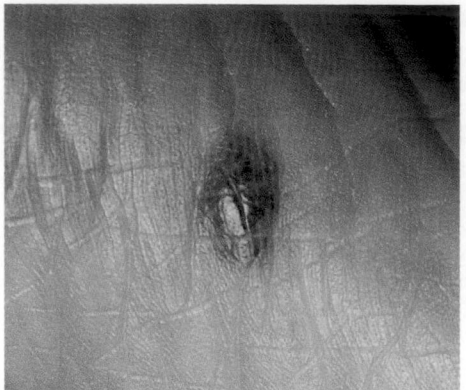

Fig. 30-6 Acral nevus.

pigmented area on the buccal mucosa, predominantly in young adult black women (Fig. 30-5). Rapid onset and spontaneous resolution are typical.

Carlos-Bregni R, et al: Oral melanoacanthoma and oral melanotic macule: a report of 8 cases, review of the literature, and immunohistochemical analysis. Med Oral Patol Oral Cir Bucal 2007 Sep 1; 12(5):E374–E379.

Rossiello L, et al: Melanoacanthoma simulating pigmented Spitz nevus: an unusual dermoscopy pitfall. Dermatol Surg 2006 May; 32(5):735–737.

Benign melanocytic nevi

Common moles, also known as nevocytic nevi or banal nevi, tend to increase in number during the first three decades of life. They are less common in doubly covered areas, such as the buttocks. They typically begin as sharply defined macular lesions, become papular, then gradually become soft and lose their pigment.

Sun exposure increases the number of moles in the exposed skin. Australians have more moles than Europeans. White persons have more than black persons, and individuals with a light complexion have more nevi than those with a dark complexion. Women have more total nevi and more nevi on the legs. Men have more on the trunk. Black persons have more nevi on the palms, soles, conjunctivae, and nailbeds. A study of young British women showed an association of holidays overseas with an increased nevus count. The association was greatest in anatomical sites intermittently exposed to sunlight.

Eruptive nevi may occur in association with bullous diseases, severe sunburn, immunosuppression, or sulfur mustard gas exposure. The cheetah phenotype refers to patients with more than 100 uniform dark-brown to black pigmented macules 4 mm or smaller. The evaluation of these patients can be challenging, as similar-appearing lesions range from junctional nevi to melanoma histologically.

Melanocytic lesions with a junctional component are more commonly removed during the summer months, while excision of intradermal nevi is relatively constant during the year. This suggests that some change in these lesions draws more attention during the summer months. Nevi may darken during pregnancy, but other changes should prompt consideration of a biopsy.

Clinical and histologic features

Features of benign nevi include a diameter of 6 mm or less, perfectly uniform pigmentation, flaccid epidermis, smooth, uniform border, and an unchanging size and color. Benign nevi tend to be round to oval, and undergo a predictable course of maturation.

Junctional nevi are smooth brown macules, varying in diameter from 1 to 6 mm. They usually appear between 3 and 18 years of age. During adolescence and adulthood, some become compound or intradermal. Small, well-nested junctional melanocytic proliferations are almost invariably benign. Benign junctional nevi associated with bulbous hyperplasia of the rete ridges are referred to as junctional lentiginous nevi. Lentigo maligna can appear well nested with an appearance similar to that of junctional lentiginous nevi. Any broad junctional melanocytic lesion on sun-damaged skin should be viewed with suspicion.

Compound nevi demonstrate both junctional and intradermal melanocytes. Benign compound nevi are well nested at the junction, with dispersion of individual melanocytes at the base of the lesion. They demonstrate bilateral symmetry, but are not symmetrical from top to bottom. Instead, with descent into the dermis, the melanocytes become smaller and spindled in appearance. Nests at the junction tend to be round to oval and are roughly equidistant from one another. Dermal nests are generally smaller than the junctional nests, and become progressively smaller deeper in the dermis. Individual cells rather than nests are present at the base. Pigment is most prominent at the junction, and becomes progressively less prominent deeper in the dermis. Intradermal nevi look similar to compound nevi without the junctional nests.

In most benign nevi, there are no melanocytes above the dermoepidermal junction. Individual melanocytes in a "buckshot" scatter throughout the epidermis are typical of superficial spreading melanoma. Sunburned benign nevi may demonstrate buckshot intraepidermal scatter of melanocytes. Buckshot scatter may also be seen in the central portion of acral nevi and Spitz nevi. Genital nevi often demonstrate large, poorly cohesive nests. They may also resemble dysplastic nevi histologically. A histologic resemblance to dysplastic nevi is also common in nevi from the scalp, ears, dorsal foot, and breast, even in patients with no other evidence of the dysplastic nevus syndrome.

On the palms and soles, the rete pattern follows the dermatoglyphs (Fig. 30-6). Nests in these locations tend to run along the rete ridges. If a benign palmar nevus is bisected across the dermatoglyphs, the nests will appear round to oval. If the same lesion is sectioned parallel to the dermatoglyphs, the nests will appear elongated and may mimic those of melanoma as an artifact of sectioning. Careful communication with the pathologist is essential when submitting an acral melanocytic lesion to the laboratory.

Malignant degeneration

Almost half of melanomas occur in pre-existing nevi, and an increased number of nevi represents a risk factor for melanoma. The signs of malignant transformation in pigmented nevi are recent enlargement, an irregular or scalloped border, asymmetry, changes or variegation in color (especially red, white, or blue), surface changes (scaling, erosion, oozing, crusting, ulceration, or bleeding), development of a palpable thickening, signs of inflammation, or the appearance of satellite pigmentation. Symptoms may include development of pain, itch, or tenderness. The "ugly duckling" sign refers to the fact that nevi in an individual generally tend to share a similar appearance. Any mole that does not share the same characteristics should be considered for biopsy. Moles with small dark dots that do not lie entirely within the lesion, but produce a small extension beyond the border, may represent melanoma arising in association with a pre-existing nevus. The clinician should alert the pathologist to the presence of these dots and the pathologist should section through the appropriate area. Perifollicular hypopigmentation is a common finding in benign nevi. When it occurs at the edge of the nevus it may give the lesion a notched appearance. Dermatoscopic examination may be of value in this setting. Lesions with changing clinical or dermatoscopic features should be biopsied.

Nevi commonly darken with pregnancy or with oral contraceptive use. Nevi from normal persons have no estrogen or progesterone receptors, but there may be positive estrogen receptor binding in nevi from pregnant women, as is also found in malignant melanoma. The development of what appears to be a new pigmented nevus in a patient over 35 years of age should alert the physician to possible melanoma, as patients without the dysplastic nevus syndrome usually do not develop new nevi at this age.

Treatment

Acquired nevi should be removed if they show signs of malignant transformation. Nevi of the neckline, beltline, or other areas that are irritated may be removed to relieve the patient of the irritation. Nevi may also be removed if they are in a location where it is impractical to observe them. If a solitary darkly pigmented lesion is present on the oral or genital mucous membrane, a biopsy should be performed, because nevi are uncommon in these locations. Nail matrix nevi and lentigines produce a pigmented nail band. The proximal matrix gives rise to the dorsal nail plate, and the distal matrix gives rise to the ventral nail plate. When the nail is observed end-on, the level of the pigment may be evident, and indicates the location of the pigmented lesion in the matrix. A widening band indicates a matrix lesion increasing in diameter. Biopsy of a solitary expanding acquired longitudinal pigmented band in an adult is typically necessary to ascertain the cause. Hutchinson's sign (pigmentation of the nailfold) is an indicator of melanoma. Nail matrix melanoma in children is exceptional.

Conjunctival nevi occur, and most can be followed serially if the lesion has been present since childhood or has shown no evidence of growth. Changing pigmented lesions and those acquired after childhood are best evaluated by an ophthalmologist or other physician skilled in the evaluation of ocular pigmented lesions. Most conjunctival nevi occur on the bulbar conjunctiva and commonly abut the nasal or temporal corneoscleral limbus. Suspicion of melanoma should arise if a pigmented lesion occurs in the palpebral or forniceal conjunctiva, if lesions are not hinged at the limbus and are immovable, if they extend into the cornea, if there is canalicular obstruction that leads to tearing, or if adjacent dilated vessels are noted.

Combined melanocytic nevi are common. They consist of a banal nevus together with a blue nevus, Spitz nevus, or deep penetrating nevus. Two or more distinct populations of melanocytes are evident.

Melanocytic nevi may occur in lymph nodes and are present in about 10% of sentinel node biopsies. Nodal nevi typically occur in the capsule, in contrast to melanoma metastases, which are typically subcapsular. Nodal nevi are commonly associated with cutaneous nevi in the draining basin, especially nevi with congenital features.

Arevalo A, et al: The significance of eccentric and central hyperpigmentation, multifocal hyper/hypopigmentation, and the multicomponent pattern in melanocytic lesions lacking specific dermoscopic features of melanoma. Arch Dermatol 2008 Nov; 144(11):1440–1444.

Barnhill RL, et al: State of the art, nomenclature, and points of consensus and controversy concerning benign melanocytic lesions: outcome of an international workshop. Adv Anat Pathol 2010; 17(2):73–90.

Driscoll MS, et al: Nevi and melanoma in the pregnant woman. Clin Dermatol 2009 Jan–Feb; 27(1):116–121.

Fabrizi G, et al: Atypical nevi of the scalp in adolescents. J Cutan Pathol 2007 May; 34(5):365–369.

Hosler GA, et al: Nevi with site-related atypia: a review of melanocytic nevi with atypical histologic features based on anatomic site. J Cutan Pathol 2008 Oct; 35(10):889–898.

Pellacani G, et al: In vivo confocal microscopic and histopathologic correlations of dermoscopic features in 202 melanocytic lesions. Arch Dermatol 2008 Dec; 144(12):1597–1608.

Ribé A: Melanocytic lesions of the genital area with attention given to atypical genital nevi. J Cutan Pathol 2008 Nov; 35 Suppl 2:24–27.

Silva Idos S, et al: Overseas sun exposure, nevus counts, and premature skin aging in young English women: a population-based survey. J Invest Dermatol 2009 Jan; 129(1):50–59.

Tran KT, et al: Biopsy of the pigmented lesion: when and how. J Am Acad Dermatol 2008 Nov; 59(5):852–871.

Zalaudek I, et al: The epidermal and dermal origin of melanocytic tumors: theoretical considerations based on epidemiologic, clinical, and histopathologic findings. Am J Dermatopathol 2008 Aug; 30(4):403–406.

Zalaudek I, et al: The morphologic universe of melanocytic nevi. Semin Cutan Med Surg 2009; 28(3):149–156.

Zalaudek I, et al: Using dermoscopic criteria and patient-related factors for the management of pigmented melanocytic nevi. Arch Dermatol 2009; 145(7):816–826.

Pseudomelanoma (recurrent nevus)

Melanotic lesions clinically resembling a superficial spreading melanoma may occur at the site of a recent shave removal of a melanocytic nevus. Melanocytic nevi occurring in areas of lichen sclerosus or bullous disease often have similar features. On dermatoscopic examination, a regular network and the presence of streaks suggest reactive pigmentation. Any truly suspicious lesion should be removed. Histologically, the junctional component often demonstrates a predominance of non-nested melanocytes, confluence of nests, and nests that vary in size and shape. The presence of a superficial dermal scar with remnants of the original nevus beneath this zone of fibrosis is an important clue to the correct diagnosis. Although atypical in appearance, the junctional proliferation remains entirely confined to the area overlying the scar.

Recurrent Spitz nevus is a particular problem because many of the histologic features of benign Spitz nevi overlap with those of melanoma. In benign recurrent Spitz nevi, the dermal component typically retains cytologic maturation, dispersion at the base of the lesion, and an immunostaining pattern typical for benign nevi. Recurrent blue nevi also present special difficulties. High cellularity, cellular pleomorphism, mitotic figures, and a lymphoid host response may be present. In the absence of marked cytologic atypia, frequent mitotic figures or necrosis en mass, the lesions are likely to be benign. Because of the special problems posed by recurrent Spitz and blue nevi, the initial biopsy of these lesions should be a complete excisional biopsy whenever possible. Congenital nevi have a higher rate of recurrence when surgery is done at a younger age.

Botella-Estrada R, et al: Clinical, dermoscopy and histological correlation study of melanotic pigmentations in excision scars of melanocytic tumours. Br J Dermatol 2006 Mar; 154(3):478–484.

Mérigou D, et al: Management of congenital nevi at a dermatologic surgical paediatric outpatient clinic: consequences of an audit survey 1990–1997. Dermatology 2009; 218(2):126–133.

Balloon cell nevus

Clinically, balloon cell nevi are indistinguishable from ordinary nevi. Histologically, they are composed of large, pale, polyhedral balloon cells. Generally, foci of ordinary nevus cells are also evident. Rarely, the lesions are composed entirely of balloon cells. Balloon cell change has been reported in cellular blue nevus as well. Balloon cell melanoma does exist, but the nuclei are large and pleomorphic, and the architecture of the lesion is that of melanoma. Balloon cell nodal nevi may be seen in sentinel node specimens.

Cagnano E, et al: Compound nevus with congenital features and balloon cell changes: an immunohistochemical study. Ann Diagn Pathol 2008 Oct; 12(5):362–364.

Urso C: Nodal melanocytic nevus with balloon-cell change (nodal balloon-cell nevus). J Cutan Pathol 2008 Jul; 35(7):672–676.

Halo nevus

Halo nevus is also known as Sutton nevus, perinevoid vitiligo, and leukoderma acquisitum centrifugum. The lesions are characterized by a pigmented nevus with a surrounding depigmented zone (Fig. 30-7). Halo nevi tend to be multiple and occur most frequently on the trunk, mostly in teenagers. The central nevus gradually loses its pigmentation, turns pink, and then disappears, leaving a round to oval area of depigmentation. Over time, the area repigments. Darkening of the central

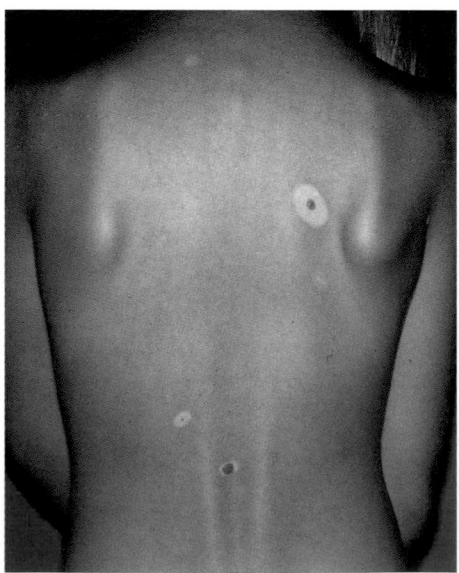

Fig. 30-7 Halo nevus.

nevus rather than lightening has also been reported in association with the halo phenomenon. Halo nevi have been reported during infliximab therapy. Target-like pigmented nevi present with the appearance of an inverse halo-nevus phenomenon.

The infiltrate contains many cytotoxic T cells, and may represent immunologically induced rejection. The peripheral blood has been shown to contain activated adhesive lymphocytes that disappear when the lesion is excised. Patients also demonstrate antibodies to melanocytes and cell-mediated immunity to melanoma cells. There may be associated vitiligo.

Regressing melanoma may also have associated leukoderma, but the pattern is usually haphazard and confined to the pigmented lesion. Other lesions that may also have a surrounding zone of leukoderma include blue nevi and neurofibromas.

Histologically, halo nevi demonstrate a band of lymphocytes that extends throughout the lesion, intimately mingling with the melanocytes. In contrast, the lymphoid infiltrate associated with melanoma tends to aggregate at the periphery of the lesion. In early halo nevi, amelanotic melanocytes may be found in the leukodermic halo. Later, melanocytes are absent until repigmentation occurs. A granulomatous infiltrate may rarely be present. The term Myerson's nevus has been applied to eczematous change associated with a nevus. Hypopigmentation may be present.

A full mucocutaneous examination at the time of diagnosis is indicated to exclude a concurrent melanoma, but this is rarely found. The decision to remove the nevus at the center of the halo is based on its morphologic features, just as with any other nevus.

Denianke KS, et al: Granulomatous inflammation in nevi undergoing regression (halo phenomenon): a report of 6 cases. Am J Dermatopathol 2008 Jun; 30(3):233–235.

Fabre C, et al: Worsening alopecia areata and de novo occurrence of multiple halo nevi in a patient receiving infliximab. Dermatology 2008; 216(2):185–186.

Loh J: Meyerson phenomenon. J Cutan Med Surg 2010; 14(1):30–32.

Nashan D, et al: Multiple target-like pigmented nevi: an inverse halo-nevus phenomenon. J Eur Acad Dermatol Venereol 2010; 24(1):104–105.

Congenital melanocytic nevus

Giant pigmented nevus (giant hairy nevus, bathing trunk nevus)

Giant pigmented nevi appear as large, darkly pigmented hairy patches in which smaller, darker patches may be interspersed or present as small satellite lesions. The skin may be thickened and verrucous. The trunk is a favored site, especially the upper or lower parts of the back (Fig. 30-8). Giant hairy nevi are present at birth and grow proportionally with the body. Widespread congenital dermal nevus with large nodules may affect the entire body, including the palms, soles, and oral mucous membrane. Some congenital melanocytic nevi have associated placental infiltration by benign melanocytes.

The incidence of melanomas developing in giant congenital pigmented nevi is between 2% and 15%. Approximately 60% of these melanomas appear within the first decade of life, and the majority arise in the dermis or subjacent tissue, rather than at the dermoepidermal junction. About 40% of the malignant melanomas seen in children occur in large congenital nevi. The risk is greatest for axial lesions. Large axial lesions may be associated with neurocutaneous melanocytosis. The risk is greatest for large axial lesions with many satellite lesions, and almost half of patients with symptomatic neurocutaneous melanosis develop leptomeningeal melanoma. Neurocutaneous

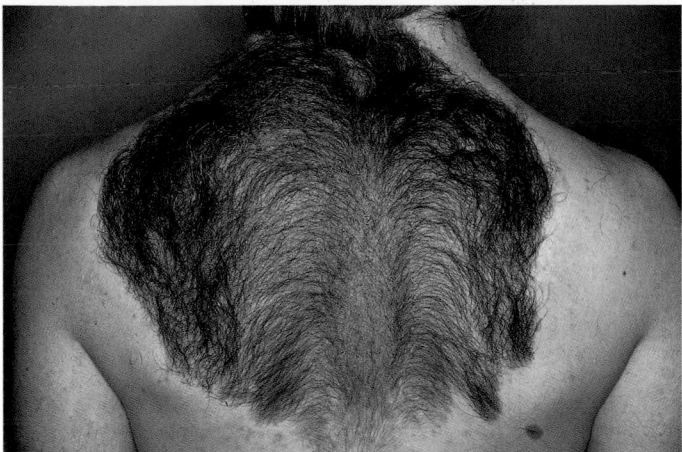

Fig. 30-8 Giant hairy nevus.

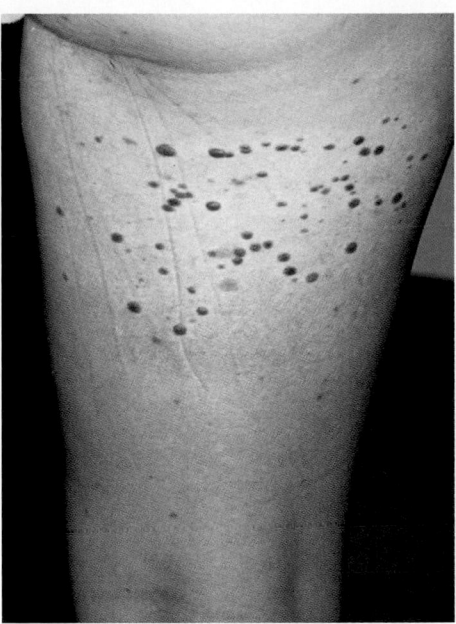

Fig. 30-9 Agminated Spitz nevi. (Courtesy of Brooke Army Medical Center Teaching File)

melanosis can be detected by magnetic resonance imaging (MRI).

Histologically, giant congenital nevi extend into the deep dermis, and may involve the subcutis, fascia, muscle, and other underlying structures. Nevus cells are found in a patchy perivascular distribution and often extend in a patchy single-file fashion between collagen bundles. Nests are commonly seen in association with adnexal structures or nerves. Extensive desmoplasia has been described. Estrogen and progesterone binding has been noted in congenital nevi. These receptors are generally absent from common acquired nevi.

Benign "proliferative" nodules within giant congenital nevi may be confused histologically with malignant change. Features useful in distinguishing the two include lack of high-grade atypia, lack of necrosis, rarity of mitoses, a lack of Ki-67 expression, evidence of transition between the cells of the nodule and those of the adjacent nevus, and lack of compressive expansile growth. Comparative genomic hybridization has demonstrated chromosomal aberrations in atypical nodular proliferations in congenital nevi, but many of these are numerical aberrations of whole chromosomes, suggesting a mitotic spindle defect. These differ from the chromosomal aberrations seen in melanoma.

Treatment decisions must be individualized. Half of all melanomas in giant congenital nevi occur in deep structures. Extensive surgery to remove the upper portions of the lesion reduces, but does not eliminate, the risk of melanoma. In patients with leptomeningeal melanosis, the risk of melanoma remains high. Satellite lesions and extremity lesions have a lower incidence of neoplastic conversion than large axial lesions, and the risk to benefit ratio of extensive surgery on these lesions differs accordingly. Some lesions are not amenable to excision, as they involve functionally critical areas.

Serial excision is the method of choice whenever possible. Tissue expansion, cultured autologous cultured skin substitutes, and flap closure are especially useful in the head and neck region. Alternative approaches to treatment, such as dermabrasion, curettage, CO_2 laser ablation or treatment with Q-switched Nd:YAG, ruby, and alexandrite lasers can lead to improvement in appearance. They may also eliminate some nevus cells, with theoretic lowering of the melanoma risk. It is important to note that most melanomas in giant congenital nevi occur in the dermal component, rather than at the dermo-epidermal junction. Any treatment that alters the surface may alter detection of deep melanoma. Malignant transformation has been reported 20 years after dermabrasion. Regardless of the method of choice, lifelong periodic cutaneous examinations and general medical evaluations are indicated.

Small and medium-sized congenital nevocytic nevus

Small congenital nevocytic nevi are generally defined as less than 2 cm in greatest diameter, and medium-sized lesions measure more than 2 cm but less than 20 cm. They are found in about 1% of newborns. About half eventually become hairy.

Histologically, they share many features with giant congenital nevi, but usually do not extend into the subcutaneous tissue. Many of the histologic features associated with congenital nevi also occur in acquired nevi.

The risk of melanoma in small to medium-sized congenital nevi is extremely low. It may be no greater or only slightly greater than the risk of melanoma arising in ordinary acquired nevi. One important difference is that malignant degeneration may occur in the deep dermal component of small congenital nevi, rather than at the dermoepidermal junction. Most of the melanomas that do occur do so after puberty. Excision is recommended for changing lesions, and may be considered for those of cosmetic concern, and those in areas that are difficult to observe.

Kovalyshyn I, et al: Congenital melanocytic naevi. Australas J Dermatol 2009 Nov; 50(4):231–240.

Marghoob AA, et al: Congenital melanocytic nevi: treatment modalities and management options. Semin Cutan Med Surg 2007 Dec; 26(4):231–240.

Margulis A, et al: Congenital melanocytic nevi of the eyelids and periorbital region. Plast Reconstr Surg 2009; 124(4):1273–1283.

Warner PM, et al: An 18-year experience in the management of congenital nevomelanocytic nevi. Ann Plast Surg 2008 Mar; 60(3):283–287.

Zhang W, et al: Neurocutaneous melanosis in an adult patient with diffuse leptomeningeal melanosis and a rapidly deteriorating course: case report and review of the literature. Clin Neurol Neurosurg 2008 Jun; 110(6):609–613.

Spindle and epithelioid cell nevus (benign juvenile melanoma, Spitz nevus)

Spitz nevi commonly appear as pink, smooth-surfaced, raised, round, firm papules. Most frequently, Spitz nevi occur during the first two decades of life, although they occur in adulthood in about one-third of cases. Infrequently, multiple lesions present as agminate (clustered) (Fig. 30-9) or disseminated

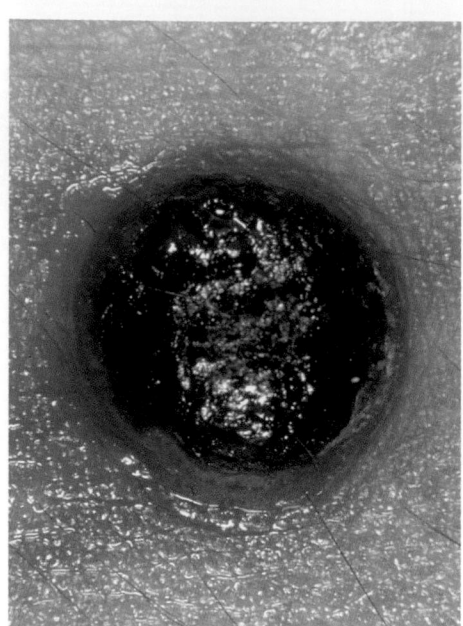

Fig. 30-10 Spitz nevus. (Courtesy of Brooke Army Medical Center Teaching File)

lesions in children and adults. Although they usually contain no visible pigment, some lesions are pigmented. Occasionally, Spitz nevi can be blue–black in color (Fig. 30-10). A starburst pattern is characteristic on dermatoscopic examination. Although dermoscopy and confocal microscopy are being used in this setting, both false-positive and false-negative studies occur and histologic examination remains the gold standard for evaluation of suspicious lesions.

Like other nevi, Spitz nevi may be junctional, compound, or intradermal. Compound nevi are most common, and are characterized by compact hyperkeratosis, hypergranulosis, and pseudoepitheliomatous hyperplasia. The cells are large, with round to spindled nuclei. Epithelioid cells have large vesicular nuclei with prominent nucleoli and ample pink cytoplasm. Adjacent to the nucleus, the cytoplasm typically has a more amphophilic hue, giving it a characteristic two-tone appearance, similar to the cytoplasm of the cells in reticulohistiocytic granuloma. The nests tend to be oval, and oriented in a vertical direction, as are the nuclei within the nests, so that they appear to be "raining down" the adjacent rete ridges. Clefts are typically present adjacent to some of the nests, and superficial vascular ectasia is characteristic. Dull pink globules (Kamino bodies) are seen within the epidermis. These represent trapped basement membrane zone material, and stain like collagen with a trichrome stain as well as with immunostains for type IV collagen. Buckshot scatter of melanocytes may be noted within the epidermis overlying the center of the lesion, but the lesion is sharply circumscribed, and cells disperse as individual units between collagen bundles at the base of the lesion. Rosette-like structures may occur. In a review of 349 Spitz nevi, the presence of epithelioid and/or spindled cells was the only feature present in 100% of cases. Other findings, in descending order, included maturation (72%), inflammatory infiltrate (70%), epidermal hyperplasia (66%), melanin (50%), telangiectasias (40%), Kamino bodies (34%), desmoplastic stroma (26%), mitosis (23%), pagetoid extension (13%), and hyalinization of the stroma (8%).

Melanomas may have many of the above features, but generally lack Kamino bodies, and often demonstrate broad lateral extension, deep mitoses, and large nests at the base of the lesion. In questionable cases, adjunctive studies may be of value. S100A6 shows strong and diffuse expression in Spitz nevi. Other melanocytic nevi often express S100A6 weakly or not at all. Melanomas may express S100A6, but the expression tends to be weak and patchy in the dermal component and is often negative in the junctional component. HMB-45 typically stains Spitz nevi in a top-heavy fashion, while melanomas stain uniformly top to bottom. MIB-1 (Ki-67), a proliferation marker, may also be helpful as an adjunct to the histopathologic diagnosis of Spitz nevi. MIB-1+ nuclei are rare in the deep portion of a Spitz nevus, while they are often numerous in melanoma. Comparative genomic hybridization demonstrates chromosomal aberrations in the majority of melanomas, but most Spitz nevi show no aberrations. A minority of Spitz nevi show an isolated gain of chromosome 11p, but this aberration is not observed in melanoma. Specific gains or losses can be demonstrated with fluorescent in situ hybridization probes. Studies of the mitogen-activated protein kinase (MAPK) pathway and genomic gains and losses may also prove helpful in this setting.

Junctional Spitz nevi commonly show some degree of buckshot scatter of melanocytes, and share many histologic features with melanoma. Lesions that lack sharp lateral circumscription are more likely to represent melanoma. Intradermal Spitz nevi lack overlying hyperkeratosis, hypergranulosis, and pseudoepitheliomatous hyperplasia, but the cells disperse as individual units at the deep margin. Dermal spitzoid lesions that remain nested at the deep margin are likely to represent melanoma. Desmoplastic Spitz nevi may be compound or intradermal, and are characterized by a dense hypocellular collagenous stroma.

Pigmented spindle cell nevus is regarded by many as a variant of Spitz nevus. The lesions tend to be pigmented macules on the legs of young women. The cells are smaller and uniformly spindled, but other histologic features are similar to those of Spitz nevi. In contrast to Spitz nevi, they stain poorly with S100A6. Desmoplastic Spitz nevi are moderately to strongly positive for p16, while most desmoplastic melanomas are negative. Both Spitz naevi and spitzoid melanoma have a lower incidence of *BRAF* and *NRAS* mutations than common acquired nevi and conventional melanomas. *HRAS* mutations are typical of Spitz nevi, but are rare to absent in spitzoid melanoma.

Although new molecular techniques may allow better differentiation, because of the histologic overlap with melanoma, the biopsy technique for suspected Spitz nevi should be complete excision whenever possible. Critical differentiating histologic features include sharp lateral circumscription and dispersion at the base of the lesion. An incomplete excision will fail to demonstrate either the lateral or deep aspect of the tumor, and these diagnostic features will not be evident. When a lesion is incompletely excised, most authorities recommend re-excision of the site to ensure complete removal. However, there are times when the dogma that all Spitz nevi should be completely excised must be tempered in the best interest of the patient. An otherwise typical Spitz nevus that extends to the deep margin on a young child's nose may be difficult to excise without disfigurement. The risks of anesthesia must also be weighed against the likelihood that the lesion is anything but a benign Spitz nevus. Data suggest that children and teenagers with atypical spitzoid neoplasms and positive sentinel nodes have a less aggressive clinical course than those with unambiguous melanoma, but this may merely reflect mixed outcomes of benign and malignant lesions that were classified together.

Busam KJ, et al: Atypical spitzoid melanocytic tumors with positive sentinel lymph nodes in children and teenagers, and comparison with histologically unambiguous and lethal melanomas. Am J Surg Pathol 2009; 33(9):1386–1395.

Da Forno PD, et al: Understanding spitzoid tumours: new insights from molecular pathology. Br J Dermatol 2008 Jan; 158(1):4–14.

Da Forno PD, et al: BRAF, NRAS and HRAS mutations in spitzoid tumours and their possible pathogenetic significance. Br J Dermatol 2009; 161(2):364–372.

Haenssle HA, et al: Large speckled lentiginous naevus superimposed with Spitz naevi: sequential digital dermoscopy may lead to unnecessary excisions triggered by dynamic changes. Clin Exp Dermatol 2009 Mar; 34(2):212–215.

Hilliard NJ, et al: p16 expression differentiates between desmoplastic Spitz nevus and desmoplastic melanoma. J Cutan Pathol 2009; 36(7):753–759.

Kamino H: Spitzoid melanoma. Clin Dermatol 2009; 27(6):545–555.

Kantrow S, et al: Spitz nevus with rosette-like structures: a new histologic variant. J Cutan Pathol 2008 May; 35(5):510–512.

Lyon VB: The Spitz nevus: review and update. Clin Plast Surg 2010; 37(1):21–33.

Nino M, et al: Spitz nevus: follow-up study of 8 cases of childhood starburst type and proposal for management. Dermatology 2009; 218(1):48–51.

Pellacani G, et al: Spitz nevi: in vivo confocal microscopic features, dermatoscopic aspects, histopathologic correlates, and diagnostic significance. J Am Acad Dermatol 2009 Feb; 60(2):236–247.

Requena C, et al: Spitz nevus: a clinicopathological study of 349 cases. Am J Dermatopathol 2009; 31(2):107–116.

Dysplastic nevus

In 1978, Clark et al described families with unusual nevi and multiple inherited melanomas, a condition they referred to as the B-K mole syndrome (after Family B and Family K). About the same time, Lynch et al recognized similar findings in other families, and they designated this the familial atypical multiple mole-melanoma syndrome. The most widely accepted term for the marker lesions is dysplastic nevus, with the patient's condition called the dysplastic nevus syndrome (DNS). The lesions may also be referred to as atypical nevi, Clark's nevi, or nevi with architectural disorder. Patients with dysplastic nevi who have at least two blood relatives with dysplastic nevi and melanoma have the worst prognosis for development of melanoma. In these individuals, there may be a 100% lifetime risk of melanoma. An associated increased risk of developing pancreatic carcinoma is present in some families. Some studies have indicated that ocular melanomas may occur in these patients.

The genetic basis for familial melanoma is being elucidated. A quarter to a third of patients have germline mutations on chromosome 9p in the *CDKN2A* tumor-suppressor gene (also known as *p16*, *MTS1*, and *p16INK4A*). It encodes for an inhibitor of a cyclin-dependent kinase 4 (CDK4), which functions to suppress proliferation. In patients with mutations that impair the function of the p16 suppressor protein, referred to as the p16M alleles, there is a concomitant predisposition to pancreatic cancer. In other families where this is not present and who have 16W alleles, the predisposition to melanoma does not correlate with an elevated risk of pancreatic cancer. Mutations in the *CDK4* gene have also been found to be responsible for a lesser number of cases of familial melanomas. The products of this gene interact with the same cell growth cycle process as *p16*.

Dysplastic nevi also occur commonly in patients without a personal or family history of melanoma, with 5–20% of patients having at least one clinically dysplastic nevus, depending on the criteria used. During the growth phase, many nevi demonstrate junctional extension beyond the dermal component. This "shouldering" phenomenon is also one of the criteria for dysplastic nevi, and many growing nevi will have some histologic features of dysplastic nevi. The same is true for many congenital nevi, genital nevi, and those on the breast, dorsal foot, and scalp.

When a biopsy specimen is read as a dysplastic nevus, clinical correlation is needed to determine if the patient has the dysplastic nevus syndrome. Examination of the patient, personal and family history of moles and melanoma, and inspection of other family members may be important in establishing the diagnosis. The presence of many moles and atypical moles is a risk factor for melanoma. Other risk factors include skin type, freckle density, eye color, and history of blistering sunburns.

Dysplastic nevi differ from common acquired nevi in several respects. Clinically, dysplastic nevi are characterized by a variegated tan, brown, and pink coloration, with the pink hues seen mainly in the macular portion of the nevus. A macular component is always present and may comprise the entire lesion, but frequently surrounds a papular center. The nevi are larger than common nevi, usually 5–12 mm in diameter (common nevi usually measure 6 mm or less). The shape of dysplastic nevi is often irregular, with indistinct borders. Atypical nevi are most commonly seen on the back (Fig. 30-11), and exposure to sun promotes the development of these lesions in individuals with DNS. In patients with the familial variety, it is not uncommon to see 75 to more than 100 pigmented lesions on the trunk. Although dysplastic nevi may not be evident until puberty in affected children, these nevi continue to develop over a lifetime, whereas common nevocytic nevi usually develop only in childhood or the early adult years. Atypical moles are associated with an increased risk of melanoma, which may be as much as 150-fold greater than that of the general population. Familial atypical moles with inherited melanoma confer a 500-fold greater risk.

The lesions appear to be precursors for melanoma, as well as serving as a marker for an increased risk of de novo melanoma. Most of the melanomas that occur in these patients will arise in normal-appearing skin. Nuclear minichromosome maintenance protein expression is low in banal nevi (roughly 1%), higher in dysplastic nevi (roughly 6%), and highest in cutaneous melanomas (roughly 50% of cells). Survivin is present in 85.2% of dysplastic nevi. These are only two of a battery of tests that have been proposed to help distinguish these lesions. To date, none has replaced H&E sections.

Criteria for histologic diagnosis of dysplastic nevi vary. The National Institutes for Health (NIH) consensus conference published the following as characteristic histologic features: basilar melanocytic hyperplasia with bulbous elongation of the rete ridges; spindle-shaped or epithelioid melanocytes arranged horizontally and aggregating in nests that fuse with adjacent rete ridges; lamellar and concentric superficial dermal fibrosis; and cytologic atypia (usually present but not essential for diagnosis). In compound dysplastic nevi, the junctional component generally extends at least three rete ridges beyond the dermal component. Grading of atypia is variable from one observer to another. Much of the atypia is focal, and localized to the periphery (shoulder region) of the lesion. Atypia that extends throughout the lesion is more significant, and lesions with high-grade atypia may be difficult to distinguish from melanoma arising in conjunction with a dysplastic nevus. Lesions with the architecture of a dysplastic (Clark) nevus but cytologic features of a Spitz nevus have been referred to as "Spark" nevus (Spitz/Clark), "spastic" nevus (Spitz/dysplastic), or "ditz" (dysplastic/Spitz).

When a patient with clinically dysplastic nevi is seen, initial examination should include a total body inspection, including the scalp. A family history should be obtained with special attention paid to items such as moles, skin cancer, and melanoma. In general, excision of individual atypical nevi should be limited to those suspicious for melanoma. In some patients, many lesions may be suspicious for melanoma, and very irregular lesions may be difficult to follow clinically. It is

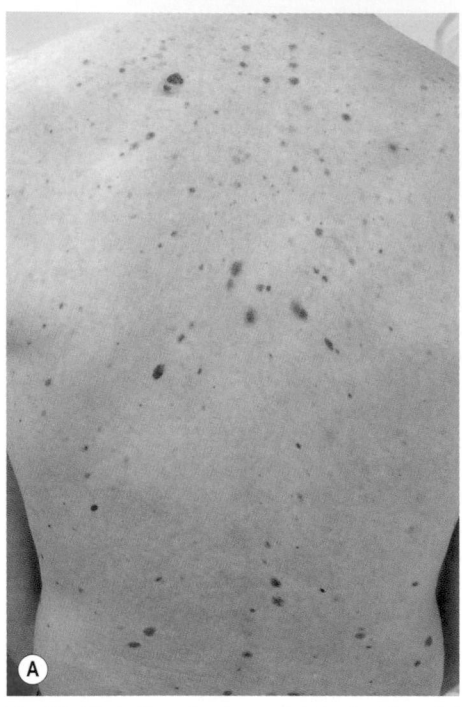 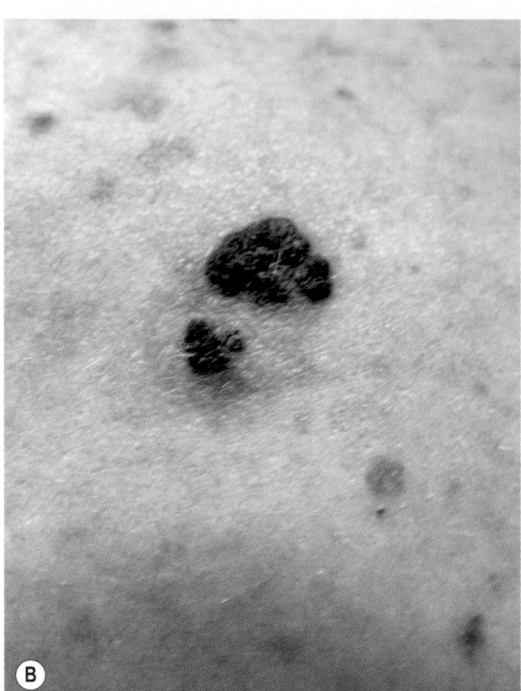

Fig. 30-11 A, Dysplastic nevi ugly duckling, left shoulder. B, Close up of left shoulder lesion, superficial spreading melanoma.

not unreasonable to excise the worst-looking lesions in such cases, but this does not eliminate the need for surveillance for changing moles and de novo melanoma. There should be prudent sun avoidance and sunscreen use. Patients should be educated in self-examination and encouraged to examine themselves monthly. Physician examination every year is also prudent. Baseline dermatologic photography may aid surveillance examinations. This is particularly helpful for detecting new lesions. Digital epiluminescence microscopic surveillance of atypical nevi may also be of value. Indications for removal of a lesion include an increase in diameter, focal enlargement, radial streaming, peripheral black dots, and clumping within the pigment network. Individual patients often demonstrate a consistent nevus phenotype clinically and on dermatoscopic examination. Lesions that differ from this "signature pattern" should generally be removed for histologic examination.

In patients with dysplastic nevi and a positive family or personal history of melanoma, physician examination every 3–6 months is recommended, with excision of those nevi that change in clinical appearance and of new lesions suspicious for melanoma. The use of photographs or digital images is particularly helpful in patients with the familial syndrome.

Narrow excisional biopsies of dysplastic nevi often fail to remove the subclinical junctional component of the lesion. The pathologist is left to comment on a specimen with melanocytic atypia at a positive margin. When the lesions recur, they often appear atypical both clinically and histologically. Recurrent lesions may easily be misinterpreted as melanoma by someone unfamiliar with the preceding lesion. In general, the most appropriate biopsy technique for a dysplastic nevus is a broad saucerization that extends 2 mm beyond the clinically evident border of the lesion. After wound contraction, the 2 mm margin results in little difference in the appearance of the final scar, and the risk of a recurrent lesion is far lower. Especially on the upper shoulders and limb girdle area, saucerized biopsies often result in scars with a better appearance than those produced by suture closure. When faced with a positive lateral margin, it is best to re-excise lesions with significant atypia. The re-excision may take the form of a wider saucerization. When a lesion with low-grade atypia extends to a lateral margin, it is reasonable to observe the lesion for signs of recurrence. Because recurrent lesions can be confused with melanoma, it is best to advise the patient to return to a physician who is familiar with the original lesion. It is also best to send the specimen from the recurrence to a pathologist who is familiar with the original specimen. Clearly indicate on the laboratory request form that the lesion is a recurrence of a dysplastic nevus with low-grade atypia.

Adamkov M, et al: Expression pattern of anti-apoptotic protein survivin in dysplastic nevi. Neoplasma 2009; 56(2):130–135.

Boyd AS, et al: Minichromosome maintenance protein expression in benign nevi, dysplastic nevi, melanoma, and cutaneous melanoma metastases. J Am Acad Dermatol 2008 May; 58(5):750–754.

Ferrara G, et al: Desmoplastic nevus: clinicopathologic keynotes. Am J Dermatopathol 2009 Oct; 31(7):718–722.

Fleming MG: Pigmented lesion pathology: what you should expect from your pathologist, and what your pathologist should expect from you. Clin Plast Surg 2010; 37(1):1–20.

Friedman RJ, et al: The "dysplastic" nevus. Clin Dermatol 2009 Jan–Feb; 27(1):103–115.

Kmetz EC, et al: The role of observation in the management of atypical nevi. South Med J 2009 Jan; 102(1):45–48.

Ko CJ: Melanocytic nevi with features of Spitz nevi and Clark's/dysplastic nevi ("Spark's" nevi). J Cutan Pathol 2009; 36(10):1063–1068.

Mesters I, et al: Skin self-examination of persons from families with familial atypical multiple mole melanoma (FAMMM). Patient Educ Couns 2009; 75(2):251–255.

Scope A, et al: The "ugly duckling" sign: agreement between observers. Arch Dermatol 2008 Jan; 144(1):58–64.

Epidermolysis bullosa-associated nevus

Patients with epidermolysis bullosa (EB) may develop large acquired melanocytic nevi with a clinical and dermoscopic appearance that resembles melanoma. Long-term follow-up suggests benign behavior. Biopsy findings can be similar to those of a persistent/recurrent nevus.

Cash SH, et al: Epidermolysis bullosa nevus: an exception to the clinical and dermoscopic criteria for melanoma. Arch Dermatol 2007 Sep; 143(9):1164–1167.

Gallardo F, et al: Large atypical melanocytic nevi in recessive dystrophic epidermolysis bullosa: clinicopathological, ultrastructural, and dermoscopic study. Pediatr Dermatol 2005 Jul–Aug; 22(4):338–343.

Melanoma (malignant melanoma)

Except in the setting of giant congenital nevi, melanomas typically originate from melanocytes at the dermoepidermal junction. Almost half will develop in pre-existing nevi, but the rest will develop on previously normal-appearing skin. Usually, there is a prolonged, noninvasive, radially oriented growth phase in which the lesion enlarges asymmetrically. Eventually, a tumor nodule develops, reflecting a vertical growth phase. Although the presence of a vertical growth phase may represent an independent risk factor for metastasis, the single greatest risk factor is the depth of invasion.

The ABCD criteria for melanoma are imperfect, but are simple for lay individuals to understand and have proved helpful for the detection of melanoma. The letters stand for asymmetry, border irregularity, color variegation, and a large diameter (greater than 6 mm). Epiluminescence microscopy is a noninvasive technique for examining pigmented lesions that makes subsurface structures visible. In the hands of experienced users, it can be a helpful technique.

The incidence of melanoma has increased dramatically, probably because of patterns of sun exposure. It occurs most often in light-skinned people, often at the most productive time of their lives. Melanoma is not commonly encountered in the darker races, and acral lesions account for a greater share of melanomas in dark-skinned individuals. The lowest incidence is found among Asians. The incidence of melanoma is low until after puberty. Children rarely manifest congenital or acquired melanoma. The former may occur because of transplacental transmission from an affected mother, as a primary intrauterine lesion, as a melanoma that occurs on a congenital nevus in utero, or as prenatal metastatic lesions from neurocutaneous melanosis. All of these have a poor prognosis. In children, melanomas occur at least half of the time from pre-existing normal skin, where the clues to diagnosis are the same as in adults, but there is often delayed recognition because of the overall low incidence in this population. Melanomas may also develop in pre-existing nevi, most importantly deep within giant congenital nevi.

During pregnancy, pigmented nevi often become uniformly darker, and may enlarge symmetrically. Estrogen and progesterone receptors develop on the melanocytes and these changes are likely to be hormonally induced. If, however, changes occur that would normally incite worry about melanoma, such as irregular pigmentation or asymmetrical growth, a biopsy should be performed. Women who develop melanoma during pregnancy have a shorter disease-free interval following excision; however, there is no adverse survival effect.

Etiologic factors

A light complexion, light eyes, blond or red hair, the occurrence of blistering sunburns in childhood, heavy freckling, and a tendency to tan poorly and sunburn easily indicate increased risk for melanoma. Large numbers of common nevi, the presence of large nevi, and the presence of clinically dysplastic lesions all increase the risk of melanoma. Axial giant congenital nevi or mutations in the *p16-cyclin-dependent kinase 4 (CDK4)* gene are potent risk factors. The risk of developing multiple primary melanomas is elevated if there is a family history of melanoma, if there are clinically or histologically atypical nevi, if there are more than 50 benign nevi, and if the patient is a nonuser of sunscreen. Sunscreens should be applied daily to sun-exposed areas, but must be used in conjunction with sun avoidance. Mutations of the *BRAF* gene are frequent in melanomas on non-chronically sun-exposed skin in Caucasians. Acral and mucosal lentiginous melanomas are associated with mutations of the *KIT* gene and amplifications of *cyclin D1* or *CDK4* gene. Amplifications of the *cyclin D1* gene are also detected in normal-looking melanocytes adjacent to these melanomas, suggesting field cancerization, as has been postulated for head and neck carcinomas where early mutations impart a selective growth advantage, leading to expansion of the population of cells and creating a field of cells ripe for secondary mutations.

Other implicated factors include psoralen + UVA (PUVA), tanning lamps, xeroderma pigmentosum, burn scars, and immunodeficiency. An association between administration of levodopa therapy for Parkinson's disease and the onset of melanoma remains unproved.

Melanoma types

Clinicopathologic types of melanoma include lentigo maligna, superficial spreading melanoma, acral-lentiginous melanoma, nodular melanoma, desmoplastic melanoma, mucosal melanoma, ocular melanoma, primary CNS melanoma, and primary soft tissue malignant melanoma. Clinically, melanomas may be pedunculated, polypoid, amelanotic, or hyperkeratotic. Some authors recognize animal-type melanoma as a distinct subtype. It resembles dendritic melanoma seen in horses and demonstrates low nuclear expression of glutathione S-transferase.

Lentigo maligna (lentiginous melanoma on sun-damaged skin)

Lentigo maligna begins as a tan macule that extends peripherally, with gradual uneven darkening over the course of years. It is more common in older patients with heavily sun-damaged skin, and is more common in sunny climates. It appears to be increasing in frequency and some data suggest it is now the most common form of melanoma. The spread and darkening are usually so slow that the patient pays little attention to this insidious lesion. After a radial growth period of 5–20 years, a vertical growth phase of invasive melanoma can develop (Fig. 30-12). The lesion is then referred to as lentigo maligna melanoma. A palpable nodule within the original macular lesion is the best evidence that this has occurred, though there may be darkening or bleeding as well. Lentiginous types of melanoma also give rise to desmoplastic melanoma, which may appear as a papule, firm plaque, or inconspicuous area of induration.

The lentiginous melanomas (lentigo maligna and acral lentiginous melanoma) proliferate principally at the dermoepidermal junction, with little buckshot scatter into the overlying epidermis. Because the junctional involvement is often only

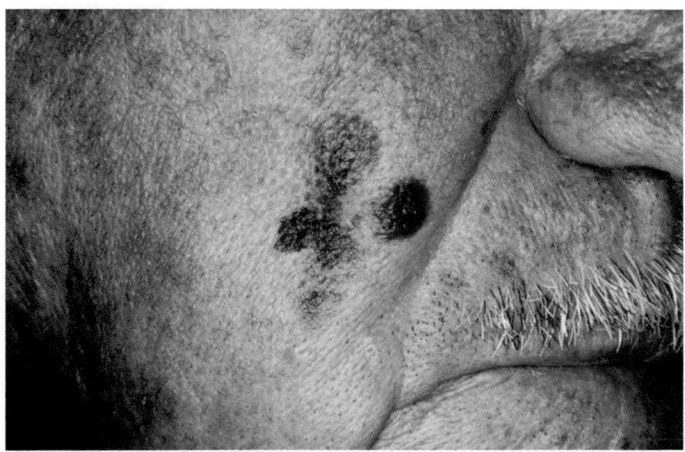

Fig. 30-12 Lentigo maligna melanoma.

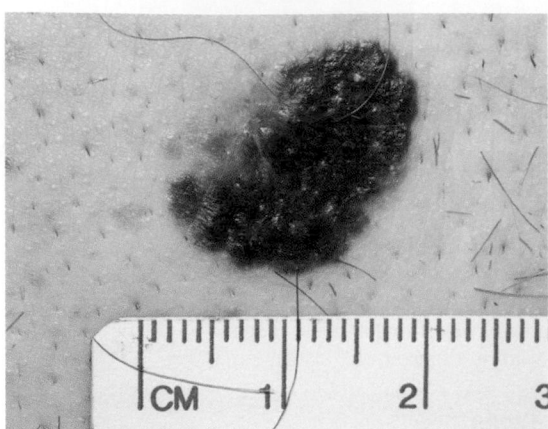

Fig. 30-13 Superficial spreading malignant melanoma.

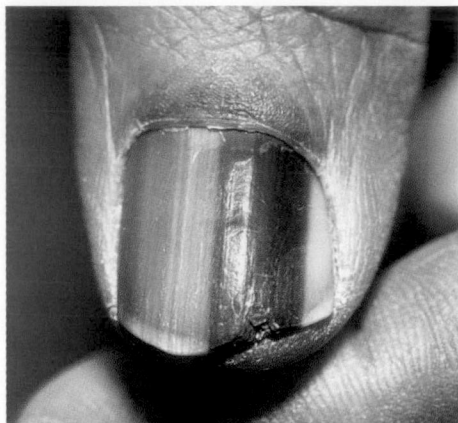

Fig. 30-14 Malignant melanoma.

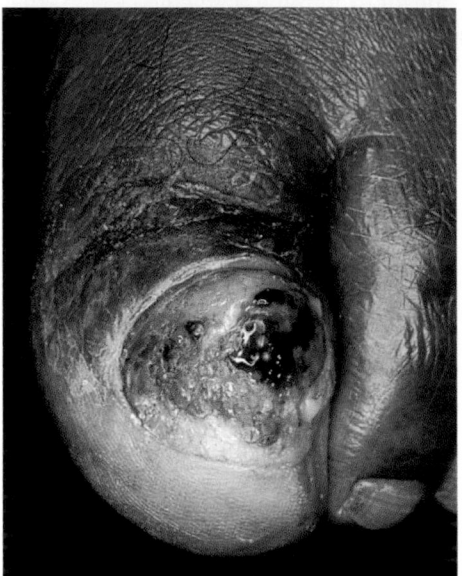

Fig. 30-15 Malignant melanoma.

one cell thick, they often extend laterally far beyond the clinically apparent margin. The lateral subclinical extension frequently exceeds the "standard" 5 mm margin for in situ melanoma, and asymmetrical growth is common.

Superficial spreading melanoma

Superficially spreading melanoma used to be the most common form of melanoma and affects adults of all ages, with the median age in the fifth decade. Unlike lentigo maligna, it has no preference for sun-damaged skin. The upper back in both sexes and the legs in women are the most common sites. There is a tendency to multicoloration, not just with different shades of tan, but variegated black, red, brown, blue, and white (Fig. 30-13). Lesions may arise de novo or in association with a pre-existing nevus. Areas of color change within a nevus, especially dark areas that extend beyond the border of the remainder of the lesion, are suspicious for melanoma arising in a nevus. As a vertical growth phase develops, a papule or nodule usually appears. Skin markings disappear as the lesion expands. Regression may appear as variation in pigmentation or a scalloped margin. The radial growth phase is characterized by buckshot scatter of melanocytes throughout the epidermis. Because of this, the borders tend to be more sharply defined than those of lentiginous types of melanoma.

Acral-lentiginous melanoma

Acral-lentiginous melanoma is the most common type of melanoma in dark-skinned and Asian populations. This is because the frequency of the other types is low in these patients, not because the incidence of acral-lentiginous melanoma is any higher than in white persons. The median age of patients is 50 years, with equal sex distribution. The most common site of melanoma in black persons is the foot, with 60% of patients having subungual or plantar lesions. All lentiginous melanomas demonstrate a junctional growth pattern and tend to have indistinct margins. Over time, a vertical growth phase develops. Periungual hyperpigmentation, Hutchinson's sign, a black discoloration of the proximal nailfold at the end of a pigmented streak (melanonychia striata), is an ominous sign suggesting melanoma in the matrix of the nail (Fig. 30-14).

The early changes of acral-lentiginous melanoma may be light brown and uniformly pigmented. The thumb and hallux are more frequently involved than the other digits. In time, the lesion becomes darker and nodular, and may ulcerate. Metastases to the epitrochlear and axillary nodes are common, because there is often a delay in diagnosis. Subungual melanoma (Fig. 30-15) may be misdiagnosed as onychomycosis, verruca vulgaris, chronic paronychia, subungual hyper-

keratosis, pyogenic granuloma, Kaposi sarcoma, glomus tumor, or subungual hematoma. Nests in acral nevi tend to follow dermatoglyphs. If ink is applied to an acral melanocytic lesion and then wiped off (leaving ink in the furrows), the presence of pigment between the inked furrows suggests the possibility of melanoma. A biopsy demonstrating large dendritic melanocytes in an acral location is highly suggestive of acral-lentiginous melanoma, even in the absence of irregular junctional nests or confluent melanocytic growth.

Mucosal melanoma

Primary melanoma of the mucous membranes is rare, and typically demonstrates a lentiginous (junctional) growth pattern. In the mouth, especially the palate, the lesion is usually pigmented and may be ulcerated. It may occur in the nasal mucosa as a polypoid tumor. On the lip it is apt to be an indolent ulcer. Melanoma of the vulva is manifested by a tumor, and is often ulcerated, with bleeding and pruritus. It is most often detected after metastasis to the groin has occurred.

Nodular melanoma

These lesions arise without a clinically apparent radial growth phase, but usually large atypical melanocytes can be found in the epidermis beyond the region of vertical growth. Primary dermal melanomas in congenital nevi are also nodular, and lack a radial growth phase. Nodular melanoma constitutes

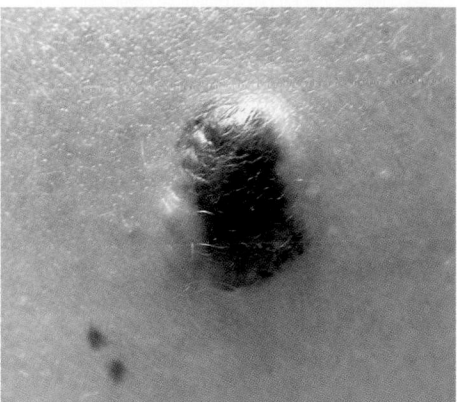

Fig. 30-16 Desmoplastic melanoma.

about 15% of all melanomas. It occurs twice as often in men as in women, primarily on sun-exposed areas of the head, neck, and trunk. The tumors may be smooth and dome-shaped, fungating, friable, or ulcerated. Bleeding is usually a late sign.

Polypoid melanoma

This is a variant of nodular melanoma, presenting as a pedunculated tumor. At its base the polypoid melanoma does not appear to descend for any appreciable distance into the dermis. Nevertheless, the 5-year survival rate is only 42%, compared with 57% for other nodular melanomas. The prognosis relates to the thickness (a measure of the volume of the tumor), and the presence of a vertical growth phase.

Desmoplastic melanoma

This deeply infiltrating type of melanoma usually has a spindle-cell pattern histologically in which collagen fibers extend between the tumor cells. It most often occurs on the head or neck of older men (Fig. 30-16), many times within a subtle lentigo maligna. The lesions may also occur on the digits, in association with a subtle acral lentiginous melanoma. One-third of cases present with only a palpable dermal irregularity and are amelanotic. The biopsy demonstrates a spindle cell proliferation with a dense fibrous stroma. Atypia is variable. The lesions are commonly neurotropic, and demonstrate extensive growth along the perineurium beyond the bulk of the tumor. Nodular lymphoid aggregates are frequently present and are an important clue to the diagnosis. S-100 protein is the most reliable immunostain. HMB-45 and Mart-1 are commonly negative. Pure desmoplastic melanomas have a low risk of metastasis while hybrid tumors have a much greater risk.

Amelanotic melanoma

Nonpigmented melanoma differs from other melanomas only in its lack of pigment. The lesion is pink (Fig. 30-17), erythematous, or flesh-colored, and commonly mimics basal cell carcinoma or granuloma pyogenicum. Amelanotic melanoma is the typical variant seen in albinos. Dermatoscopic features may still be of diagnostic value, even in amelanotic melanomas.

Soft-tissue melanoma and clear cell sarcoma

Primary soft-tissue melanoma is rare and distinguished from clear cell sarcoma by the presence of BRAF mutations and the absence of the characteristic t(12;22)(q12;q12) translocation that is seen in clear cell sarcoma. Like melanoma, clear cell sarcoma contains melanosomes and stains positively for S-100 and HMB-45. It occurs most frequently on the lower extremities of young people. The average age at onset is 27. The history is of an enlarging, often painful mass on an extremity,

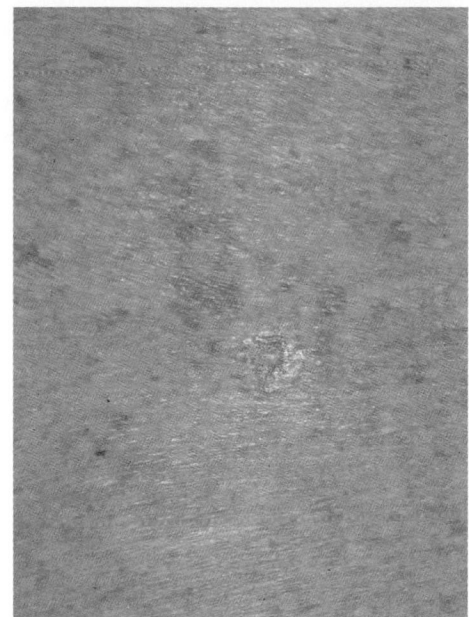

Fig. 30-17 Amelanotic malignant melanoma.

with the foot or ankle involved 43% of the time. The tumors arise in and are bound to the aponeuroses, tendons, or fascia, and only uncommonly invade the overlying skin. Histologically, there are compact nests and fascicles of polygonal or fusiform cells with a clear cytoplasm present between dense fibrous tissue septa that connect with tendinous or aponeurotic tissue. Multinucleated cells are common. Frequently, there are translocations of chromosomes 12 and 22. Metastases are often present at first diagnosis and the prognosis is poor. Local recurrence or distant metastases after the initial excision are frequent and result in death in more than 50% of reported cases. Treatment is with wide excision and lymph node dissection. Radiotherapy and chemotherapy are used as an adjunct in some cases. The lesion appears to arise from neural crest cells.

Differential diagnosis

Melanoma may clinically simulate a wide variety of lesions, including pigmented basal cell carcinoma, darkly pigmented seborrheic keratosis, pyogenic granuloma, and Kaposi sarcoma. Melanomas may appear pearly, contain horn cysts, and exhibit a collarette, and none of these is sufficient to forego a biopsy. Other melanoma-simulating lesions include subungual traumatic hematoma, cherry angioma, pigmented Bowen's disease, and pigmented Paget's disease. Histologic differentiation from Spitz nevi, epithelioid blue nevi, and deep penetrating nevi may be difficult and some dermatopathologists use the term MELTUMP (melanocytic tumor of uncertain malignant potential) for this group of disorders. Genomic and immunohistochemical analysis can aid in the differential diagnosis, and the presence of deep mitoses and a host inflammatory response correlate with malignant behavior in such tumors. When the lesions are grouped, outcomes are better than expected for conventional melanoma. Controversy persists as to whether this group represents a uniform group of low-grade malignancies or whether the intermediate outcomes merely reflect a mix of malignant and benign tumors.

Biopsy

Complete excision with a 1–3 mm margin of skin is the preferred method of biopsy for a lesion suspected to be melanoma.

Although the National Comprehensive Cancer Network (NCCN) recommends avoiding wider margins to permit accurate lymphatic mapping for sentinel node biopsy, some evidence suggests that accurate mapping is usually still possible even after wide excision.

In lesions too large for simple excision, an incisional or punch biopsy, deep enough to permit measurement of thickness, has no effect on prognosis. When melanoma is suspected in a giant pigmented nevus, an incisional biopsy should be performed. Biopsy of lentigo maligna is problematic, as the lesions tend to be quite large and arise in cosmetically sensitive areas. Skip areas are common in these lesions and may lead to misdiagnosis. Areas of the tumor may undergo lichenoid regression and resemble benign lichenoid keratosis. Collision with other pigmented lesions, such as benign solar lentigo, pigmented large-cell acanthoma, and pigmented actinic keratosis, is common. Because of the potential for sampling error, small biopsies frequently result in misdiagnosis. The best biopsy technique in the setting of suspected lentigo maligna is generally a broad superficial shave biopsy. This results in minimal scarring and provides the pathologist with a broad area of dermoepidermal junction for examination. If the lesion is heterogeneous, multiple areas may need to be sampled with smaller shave biopsies. If lentigo maligna melanoma or desmoplastic melanoma is suspected, an incisional biopsy should be performed. Punch biopsies are more prone to sampling error.

Histopathology

Biopsies should be read by a dermatopathologist or other pathologist experienced in pigmented lesions. The report should include thickness and an assessment of the deep and peripheral margins. The presence of ulceration should be noted. Several studies demonstrate that concordance for assessment of Clark's level is poor, but as Clark's level may add prognostic information, it was still noted in many cases. More recently, reporting of Clark's level has been replaced by mitotic rate. The presence of satellitosis is a powerful adverse prognostic indicator, and it should be noted in the report. Other factors that may be important to note include regression, tumor-infiltrating lymphocytes, vertical growth phase, angiolymphatic invasion, neurotropism, and histologic subtype.

Whereas benign nevi are well nested at the junction, melanomas usually demonstrate junctional areas where non-nested melanocytes predominate. Benign nevi demonstrate dispersion of individual melanocytes at the base of the lesion, while melanomas remain nested at the base. Melanomas may be asymmetrical, but metastatic and nodular melanoma may present as perfectly symmetrical spheres. Benign nevi demonstrate bilateral symmetry and show maturation (smaller, more neuroid cells) with descent into the dermis. Most melanomas lack bilateral symmetry and show little maturation with descent into the dermis. In nevi, nests at the junction tend to be round to oval and are roughly equidistant from one another. In melanoma, junctional nests are often elongated or have irregular shapes. They are randomly distributed, and often involve the arches over the dermal papillae, as well as the tips and sites of the rete ridges. Confluent runs of melanocytes are frequently seen at the dermoepidermal junction, and often continue down the adnexal structures. In nevi, dermal nests are generally smaller than the junctional nests, and become progressively smaller deeper in the dermis. In melanoma, dermal nests generally fail to become smaller in the deeper dermis. In nevi, pigment is most prominent at the junction, and becomes progressively less prominent deeper in the dermis. Melanomas often retain pigment deep in the lesion. In superficial spreading melanoma, individual melanocytes are present in a "buckshot" scatter throughout the epidermis.

Lentiginous types of melanoma tend to proliferate at the dermoepidermal junction with little associated buckshot scatter. Invasive melanoma is commonly associated with a lymphoid infiltrate that forms a band at the periphery of the lesion. Plasma cells may be numerous. A vertical growth phase is identified by the presence of a dermal nest larger than the largest junctional nest, or invasion of the reticular dermis or solar elastotic band. Melanoma depth is measured from the granular layer or base of the ulcer. If invasion has taken place from follicular extension of the tumor, the lesion is measured from the inner root sheath. Rare variants of melanoma include balloon cell melanoma and dendritic "equine-type" melanoma.

Some types of benign nevus mimic individual features of melanoma. Sunburned nevi, acral nevi, and Spitz nevi may demonstrate buckshot intraepidermal scatter of melanocytes. Blue nevi typically are pigmented to the base of the lesion, and extend into the dermis as a bulbous projection with little maturation and no dispersion of cells at the base. The silhouette, sclerotic stroma, and bland cytology are key to the diagnosis.

Comparative genomic hybridization has shown that chromosomal aberrations are common in melanoma. They occur earlier in the progression of acral melanoma than in melanomas on the trunk. In general, melanomas tend to have abnormalities involving chromosomes 9, 10, 7, and 6. Acral melanomas are more likely to have aberrations involving chromosomes 5p, 11q, 12q, and 15, and many amplifications are found at the *cyclin D1* locus. Lentigo maligna melanomas are more likely to show losses of chromosomes 17p and 13q. Chromosomal aberrations are rare in benign banal nevi. A minority of Spitz nevi may show an isolated gain involving the entire short arm of chromosome 11.

Metastasis

Early metastases typically occur via the lymphatics, and regional lymphadenopathy may be the first sign. Satellite metastases appear as pigmented nodules around the site of the excision (Fig. 30-18). Later, metastases occur via the bloodstream and may become widespread. The chief site for metastatic melanoma is the skin, but all other organs are at risk.

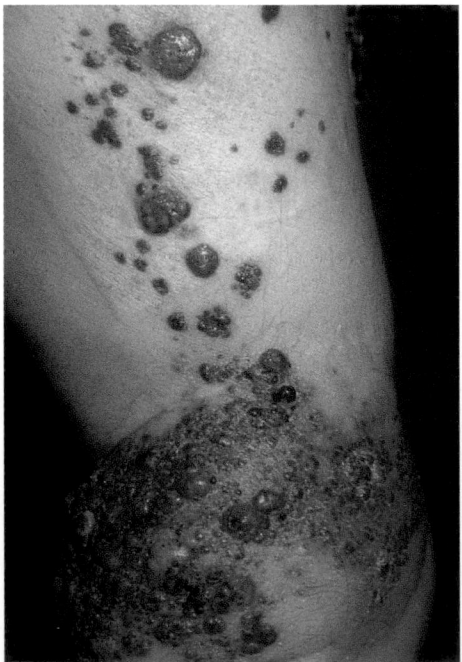

Fig. 30-18 Metastatic malignant melanoma. (Courtesy of Brooke Army Medical Center Teaching File)

CNS metastasis is the most common cause of death. Although most metastatic spread occurs in the first 5 years after diagnosis, late-onset metastases occur, especially in premenopausal women. Melanemia, melanuria, and cachexia are likely to occur in terminal disease. In extreme cases, the entire integument may become deeply pigmented (generalized melanosis), with melanin in melanophages, endothelial cells, and tissue histiocytes. Occasionally, patients present with metastatic melanoma from an unknown source. Full-body skin examination may reveal a depigmented or irregularly pigmented atrophic patch consistent with a regressed primary lesion. Such patients are estimated to have a 40% chance of 5-year survival. Estrogen receptors may play a role in melanoma progression and metastasis, with lower levels of expression of receptors in thicker lesions.

Staging

The American Joint Committee on Cancer (AJCC) developed a staging system for cutaneous melanoma. The system's categories depend on definitions for primary tumors, lymph node involvement, and distant metastases (Box 30-1; www.cancerstaging.net). The NCCN consensus statement regarding staging and management of melanoma can be found at www.nccn.org/physician_gls/f_guidelines.html.

Prognosis

The prognosis for a patient with stage I melanoma is primarily related to tumor thickness. Cure rates by stage are:

> **Box 30-1** Summary of American Joint Committee on Cancer melanoma staging
>
> - T0: No evidence of primary tumor
> - Tis: Melanoma in situ
> - T1: Up to 1.0 mm in thickness
>   - T1a: Level II or III
>   - T1b: Level IV or V or with ulceration
> - T2: 1.01–2.0 mm in thickness
>   - T2a: No ulceration
>   - T2b: Ulceration
> - T3: 2.01–4.0 mm in thickness
>   - T3a: No ulceration
>   - T3b: Ulceration
> - T4: >4.0 mm in thickness
>   - T4a: No ulceration
>   - T4b: Ulceration
>
> - N0: No regional lymph node metastasis
> - N1: Metastasis in one lymph node
>   - N1a: Clinically occult
>   - N1b: Clinically apparent
> - N2: Two to three regional nodes or in-transit metastasis
>   - N2a: Clinically occult
>   - N2b: Clinically apparent
>   - N2c: Satellite or in-transit metastases
> - N3: Four or more nodes, matted nodes or in-transit metastasis with positive nodes
>
> - M0: No distant metastases
> - M1: Distant metastases
>   - M1a: Skin or nodes
>   - M1b: Lung
>   - M1c: All other viscera or any distant metastases with elevated lactic acid dehydrogenase (LDH)

- Stage I (T1 or T2a, N0, M0): >80%
- Stage II (T2b-4, N0, M0): 60–80%
- Stage III (N1–3, M0): 10–60%
- Stage IV (M1): <10%

Many variables have been reported to influence survival, including:
- the presence of tumor-infiltrating lymphocytes (brisk response is best)
- mitotic rate (0 is best and $>6/mm^2$ is worst)
- ulceration (adverse effect)
- location (hair-bearing limbs yield a better prognosis than when lesions are present on the trunk, head, neck, palm, or sole)
- sex (women have a better prognosis than men)
- age (younger patients have a better prognosis)
- the presence of leukoderma at distal sites (improves the prognosis)
- regression (associated with a poorer prognosis).

Multivariant analysis shows that some are not independently predictive and others are of variable significance in different series. Pregnancy does not have an adverse effect on survival in patients with clinically localized melanoma. Tumor thickness, ulceration, and lymph node involvement have the greatest predictive value and are used to determine therapy.

The presence or absence of melanoma in regional lymph nodes is the single most important prognostic factor for melanoma. Sentinel lymph node dissection using lymphoscintigraphy with ^{99m}Tc-labeled colloids is widely used for the staging of clinically node-negative melanomas. The success rate in localizing the sentinel lymph node approaches 98% at centers experienced in the technique. When combined with the vital blue dye technique the success rate can approach 99%. About 20% of patients with melanoma between 1.5 and 4 mm in depth will have metastasis in their sentinel node(s). For desmoplastic and neurotropic melanoma (mean Breslow depth, 4.0 mm; median, 2.8 mm), published data suggest that up to 12% have at least one positive sentinel lymph node, although recent data suggests those with metastases are likely to be hybrid tumors rather than pure desmoplastic melanomas. Tumor thickness and ulceration are the major independent predictors of sentinel lymph node metastases. Age and axial tumor location are also significant. Patients with larger metastases to the sentinel node (metastatic deposits greater than 2 mm in diameter) have significantly decreased survival.

Local recurrence related to a positive margin should not be equated with local recurrence representing dermal in-transit lymphatic metastasis. The latter is associated with a poor prognosis, while the former may be cured in many cases by re-excision.

Work-up and follow-up

There is no definite proof that any routine laboratory work or imaging studies affect longevity. Some advocate only ordering studies as prompted by signs or symptoms. Other guidelines recommend limited studies varying by stage. For all stages, studies should be ordered if signs or symptoms occur. Lactic acid dehydrogenase (LDH) is not a sensitive screening tool, but has prognostic value. The yield of computed tomography (CT), MRI, and positron emission tomography (PET) is low. There is broad consensus that no x-rays or blood work are routinely indicated for those with stage 0 or Ia melanoma. For stages Ib and II, a baseline chest x-ray and LDH level are optional in the NCCN guidelines. For stage IIIa disease, a chest x-ray and LDH are recommended by NCCN guidelines. For stage IIIb or IIIc disease, fine needle aspiration should be attempted to confirm nodal involvement. A chest x-ray and LDH are recommended by NCCN guidelines. A pelvic CT scan is recommended in those with inguinofemoral lymphadenopathy. For stage IV disease, the work-up should be similar to that for stage IIIb disease, along with consideration of abdominal and pelvic CT scan, head MRI, or PET. The highest yield for CT scans is in the area adjacent to nodal disease. As glucose metabolism is increased in malignant tumors, PET using the glucose analog fluorine-18-fluorodeoxyglucose (F18-FDG) can be used to detect metastases. Periodic skin examinations are important to detect second primary tumors, as well as metastatic disease. Skin and lymph node examination should be performed at least yearly. Tumor recurrence occurs sooner in patients with thick melanomas than those with thin melanomas. Some authors have suggested follow-up schedules based on AJCC staging, to include annual examinations for patients with stage I disease, 6-monthly examinations for 2 years and then annually for those with stage IIa disease, and 4-monthly examinations for 2 years, 6-monthly in the third year and annually thereafter, for those with stage IIb–IIc disease. Those with other risk factors may need more frequent examinations.

Treatment

Early excision remains the most important determinant of outcome. Most published guidelines are based on data that relate largely to superficial spreading melanoma, and may not be applicable to all melanomas. A margin of 0.5 cm is recommended for excision of a melanoma in situ, a 1.0 cm margin for melanomas less than or equal to 1.0 mm thick, a 1–2 cm margin for those less than or equal to 2 mm, and a 2 cm margin for those thicker than 2.0 mm. In the case of lentigo maligna and acral lentiginous melanoma, subclinical extension of the in situ tumor commonly exceeds 0.5 cm, and asymmetrical growth is common. In such cases, a symmetrical "standard" margin may do a disservice to the patient. It may result in a positive lateral margin, and difficult closure because excessive uninvolved skin was sacrificed. Mohs micrographic surgery may be useful in this setting. Although H&E-stained frozen sections have been used, immunostains such as MelanA or MITF are easier to interpret. "Slow Mohs" staged excision with permanent sections is another option. In patients who are poor surgical candidates, nonsurgical treatments such as topical imiquimod and radiotherapy may be utilized. Nail apparatus melanoma may necessitate amputation of a digit or skin grafting. This is another setting where Mohs micrographic surgery may be considered as a tissue-sparing technique.

Sentinel node biopsy (SNB) should be discussed with patients whose melanomas are 1 mm or greater in thickness. SNB should be considered for thinner lesions in patients who have ulceration, Clark level IV or V invasion, regression, a vertical growth phase, or a positive deep margin on initial biopsy. Dual-basin drainage from the trunk is not independently associated with an increased risk of nodal metastases, but each basin must be identified and sampled. Those with a positive SNB or nodal metastasis confirmed by fine needle aspiration should receive counseling regarding dissection of the remainder of the nodal basin. An analysis of SNB results in 422 Swedish patients with a mean thickness of 3.2 mm suggests that SN-negative patients have better disease-free survival (p < 0.0001), but the false-negative rate may be as high as 14%.

Ipilimumab blocks the CTLA-4 protein, reducing tumor tolerance. It has shown impressive results in some patients with melanoma and trials of this agent with other immunomodulat-

ing drugs and vaccines are ongoing. Oncogenic mutations in KIT occur in mucosal and acral melanomas, as well as those on chronically sun-damaged skin. Imatinib may have a role in treating tumors in these sites. For in-transit metastases, surgical excision, interferon (IFN), hyperthermic isolated limb perfusion with melphalan, CO_2 laser ablation, and intralesional bacille Calmette–Guérin (BCG) are used. Dinitrochlorobenzene in the setting of in-transit melanoma metastases has been reported to induce local remission but did not prevent metastatic lymph node and liver involvement. For stage IV disease, treatment options include resection, radiation, dacarbazine, temozolomide, interleukin-2, paclitaxel, and combination chemotherapy. Before surgical intervention, a period of observation to rule out more widespread metastasis may be reasonable.

Adjuvant therapy should be discussed with patients who have positive nodes or node-negative melanoma that is 4 mm thick, or ulcerated or Clark's level IV or V. IFN-α 2b is Food and Drug Administration (FDA)-approved as adjuvant therapy and is used most commonly. Although meta-analysis suggests that IFN therapy may increase relapse-free survival, an advantage for overall survival is uncertain. Systemic symptoms may require discontinuation of therapy in some patients, and lipodystrophy has been reported with IFN therapy. The results of trials have been mixed. Reports of long-term survival after resection of distant melanoma metastases suggest that cytoreductive surgery may play a role in selected patients.

Clinical vaccine trials are ongoing and some have shown promising results. However, despite numerous trials, only a few patients have been shown to exhibit strong antigen-specific cellular responses.

Barnhill RL, et al: Unusual variants of malignant melanoma. Clin Dermatol 2009; 27(6):564–587.

Braun RP, et al: The furrow ink test: a clue for the dermoscopic diagnosis of acral melanoma vs nevus. Arch Dermatol 2008 Dec; 144(12):1618–1620.

Busam KJ, et al: Distinction of conjunctival melanocytic nevi from melanomas by fluorescence in situ hybridization. J Cutan Pathol 2010 Feb; 37(2):196–203.

Cadili A, et al: Predictors of sentinel lymph node metastasis in melanoma. Can J Surg 2010; 53(1):32–36.

Carlson JA, et al: New techniques in dermatopathology that help to diagnose and prognosticate melanoma. Clin Dermatol 2009 Jan–Feb; 27(1):75–102.

Curtin JA, et al: Somatic activation of KIT in distinct subtypes of melanoma. J Clin Oncol 2006; 24:4340–4346.

de Giorgi V, et al: Estrogen receptor expression in cutaneous melanoma: a real-time reverse transcriptase-polymerase chain reaction and immunohistochemical study. Arch Dermatol 2009 Jan; 145(1):30–36.

Driscoll MS, et al: Hormones, nevi, and melanoma: an approach to the patient. J Am Acad Dermatol 2007 Dec; 57(6):919–931.

Driscoll MS, et al: Nevi and melanoma in the pregnant woman. Clin Dermatol 2009; 27(1):116–121.

Erickson C, et al: Treatment options in melanoma in situ: topical and radiation therapy, excision and Mohs surgery. Int J Dermatol 2010 May; 49(5):482–491.

Forman SB, et al: Is superficial spreading melanoma still the most common form of malignant melanoma? J Am Acad Dermatol 2008 Jun; 58(6):1013–1020.

Francken AB, et al: Follow-up schedules after treatment for malignant melanoma. Br J Surg 2008 Nov; 95(11):1401–1407.

Gambichler T, et al: Minichromosome maintenance proteins are useful adjuncts to differentiate between benign and malignant melanocytic skin lesions. J Am Acad Dermatol 2009; 60(5):808–813.

Ghosh P, et al: Genetics and genomics of melanoma. Expert Rev Dermatol 2009; 4(2):131–143.

Hansson J: Familial cutaneous melanoma. Adv Exp Med Biol 2010; 685:134–145.

Hodi FS, et al: Improved survival with ipilimumab in patients with metastatic melanoma. N Engl J Med 2010; 363:711–723.

Jen M, et al: Childhood melanoma. Clin Dermatol 2009; 27(6):529–536.

Mattsson J, et al: Sentinel node biopsy in malignant melanoma: Swedish experiences 1997–2005. Acta Oncol 2008; 47(8):1519–1525.

Menzies SW, et al: Dermoscopic evaluation of amelanotic and hypomelanotic melanoma. Arch Dermatol 2008 Sep; 144(9): 1120–1127.

Orlandi A, et al: Relation between animal-type melanoma and reduced nuclear expression of glutathione S-transferase pi. Arch Dermatol 2009 Jan; 145(1):55–62.

Rivers JK, et al: The case for early detection of melanoma. J Cutan Med Surg 2010; 14(1):24–29.

Shokrollahi K, et al: Malignant melanoma: perspectives, diagnostics and treatment. Ann Plast Surg 2010 Feb; 64(2):132–133.

Spatz A, et al: The biology of melanoma prognostic factors. Discov Med 2010 Jul; 10(50):87–93.

Takata M, et al: Molecular pathogenesis of malignant melanoma: a different perspective from the studies of melanocytic nevus and acral melanoma. Pigment Cell Melanoma Res 2010; 23(1):64–71.

Tucker MA: Melanoma epidemiology. Hematol Oncol Clin North Am 2009; 23(3):383–395.

Weedon D: Lentiginous melanoma. J Cutan Pathol 2009; 36(11):1232.

Dermal melanocytic lesions

Mongolian spot

The Mongolian spot is a bluish-gray macule that varies in diameter from 2 to 8 cm. It occurs typically in the sacral region of the newborn (Fig. 30-19), in 80–90% of Asian, southern European, American black, and Native American persons. The Mayan Indians uniquely take great pride in it as an indicator of pure Mayan inheritance. The Mongolian spot may be situated in other locations. Multiple spots may occur in a widespread distribution, and overlapping spots have been described. These have been called generalized dermal melanocytosis or dermal melanocytic hamartomas. They may occur in phakomatosis pigmentovascularis types II, IV, and V, and have been described in the setting of Sjögren–Larsson syndrome. Extensive Mongolian spots have been associated with Hunter syndrome and with trisomy 20 mosaicism.

Histologically, the Mongolian spot shows elongated dendritic dermal melanocytes, widely scattered among normal collagen bundles. It usually disappears during childhood, although rarely, it may persist into adulthood.

Q-switched ruby laser and Q-switched neodymium-doped yttrium aluminium garnet (Nd:YAG) lasers have been used to treat Mongolian spots. Application of bleaching creams should be considered prior to treatment to reduce overlying pigmentation. The outcome of laser treatment tends to be better for lesions treated before the age of 20.

Kagami S, et al: Laser treatment of 26 Japanese patients with Mongolian spots. Dermatol Surg 2008 Dec; 34(12):1689–1694.

Leung AK, et al: Superimposed Mongolian spots. Pediatr Dermatol 2008 Mar–Apr; 25(2):233–235.

Nevus of Ota (oculodermal melanocytosis)

This nevus is also known as nevus fuscoceruleus ophthalmo-maxillaris. It is usually present at birth in the two-thirds of patients who have ocular involvement. Other lesions may not appear until the teen years. The conjunctiva and skin about the eye supplied by the first and second branch of the trigeminal nerve, as well as the sclera, ocular muscles, retrobulbar fat, periosteum, and buccal mucosa, may be involved. On the skin, brown, slate gray, or blue–black macules grow slowly larger and deeper in color (Fig. 30-20). It persists throughout life. Eighty percent occur in females; 5% are bilateral. Glaucoma or ipsilateral sensorineural hypoacusia may also occasionally complicate nevus of Ota. Malignant melanoma rarely occurs in nevus of Ota. Malignant degeneration is more frequent in white patients. The most common site of malignancy is the choroid. Histologically, elongated dendritic dermal melanocytes are seen scattered in the upper portion of the dermis. Acquired unilateral nevus of Ota-like macules are known as Sun nevus. Some express hormone receptors. Q-switched lasers have been used successfully to treat nevus of Ota. Nd:YAG laser at 1064 nm is suitable for use in a wide range of skin types. Acquired dermal melanocytosis (acquired bilateral nevus of Ota-like macules or Hori nevus) is recalcitrant to laser therapy compared with nevus of Ota. Good results have been reported after treatment with Q-switched ruby laser. Initial topical bleaching with 0.1% tretinoin and a 5% hydroquinone ointment containing 7% lactic acid can be used to reduce epidermal melanin prior to laser treatment. Epidermal cooling has been advocated in the past, but some data suggest an increased incidence of hyperpigmentation with epidermal

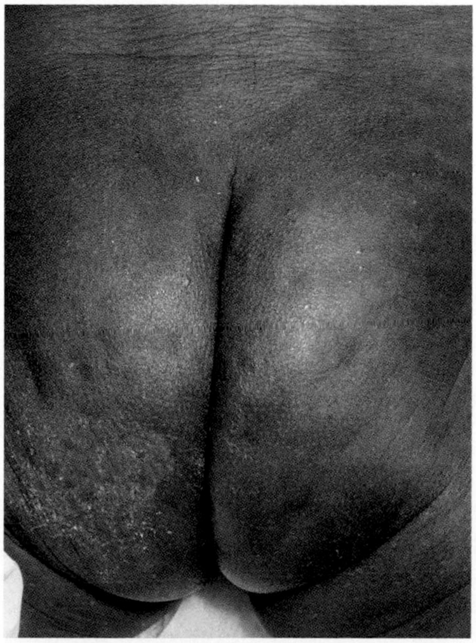

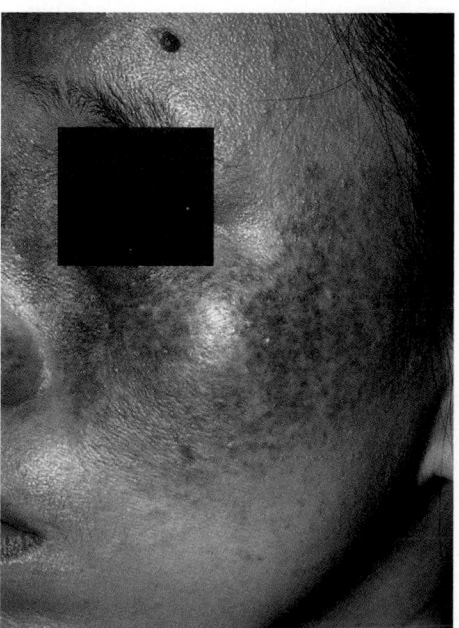

Fig. 30-19 Mongolian spot.

Fig. 30-20 Nevus of Ota.

cooling. Q-switched ruby laser has also been used after epidermal ablation using a scanned CO_2 laser. Lesions of phakomatosis pigmentovascularis have been treated successfully with Q-switched ruby laser and Q-switched alexandrite laser, with flashlamp pumped pulsed dye laser for the vascular component. Intense pulse light systems have been combined with the Q-switched ruby laser for complex dyspigmentation among Asian patients. Fractional photothermolysis using a fractionated 1440 nm Nd:YAG laser has also been reported as successful.

Nevus of Ito

Also known as nevus fuscoceruleus acromiodeltoideus, the nevus of Ito has the same features as nevus of Ota except that it occurs in the distribution of the posterior supraclavicular and lateral cutaneous brachial nerves, to involve the shoulder, side of the neck, and supraclavicular areas.

Ee HL, et al: Characteristics of Hori naevus: a prospective analysis. Br J Dermatol 2006 Jan; 154(1):50–53.

Harrison-Balestra C, et al: Clinically distinct form of acquired dermal melanocytosis with review of published work. J Dermatol 2007 Mar; 34(3):178–182.

Kouba DJ, et al: Nevus of Ota successfully treated by fractional photothermolysis using a fractionated 1440-nm Nd:YAG laser. Arch Dermatol 2008 Feb; 144(2):156–158.

Long TF, et al: Androgen, estrogen and progesterone receptors in acquired bilateral nevus of Ota-like macules. Pigment Cell Melanoma Res 2010 Feb; 23(1):144–146.

Manuskiatti W, et al: Effect of cold air cooling on the incidence of postinflammatory hyperpigmentation after Q-switched Nd:YAG laser treatment of acquired bilateral nevus of Ota-like macules. Arch Dermatol 2007 Sep; 143(9):1139–1143.

Park JM, et al: Combined use of intense pulsed light and Q-switched ruby laser for complex dyspigmentation among Asian patients. Lasers Surg Med 2008 Feb; 40(2):128–133.

Blue nevus

Blue nevi appear as well-defined blue papules or nodules (Fig. 30-21). Histologically, they share the silhouette of a bulbous finger-like or wedge-shaped protrusion into the dermis. All variants show little maturation, and no dispersion of melanocytes in the deep portion of the lesion. All except epithelioid blue nevi and some cellular blue nevi are associated with a dense sclerotic stroma. They commonly occur as combined nevi (combinations of various types of blue nevus, blue nevus combined with banal nevus, or blue nevus combined with Spitz nevus).

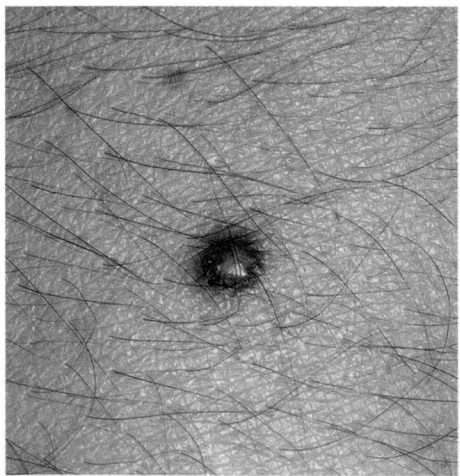

Fig. 30-21 Blue nevus.

Blue nevus of Jadassohn–Tiche (common blue nevus, nevus ceruleus)

The typical lesion is a steel-blue papule or nodule that begins in early life. Some may be large and congenital. The slowly growing lesion is rarely more than 2–10 mm in diameter, and occurs most frequently on the dorsal hands, feet, and face. Histologically, the lesion is composed of dendritic dermal melanocytes and melanophages. The sclerotic stroma is particularly prominent in this variant.

Cellular blue nevus

Usually, a cellular blue nevus is a large, firm, blue or blue–black nodule. It is most frequently seen on the buttock and sacrococcygeal region, and occasionally is present at birth. Women have cellular blue nevus 2.5 times as frequently as men, and the average age of the patient seen with this lesion is 40 years. Uncommonly, these may invade underlying structures such as the skull in scalp lesions. Occasionally, cellular blue nevi may occur on the eyelids. Histologically, in addition to deeply pigmented melanophages, islands of cells are observed with large fusiform vesicular nuclei, prominent nucleoli, and abundant pale cytoplasm. The cellular islands contain little or no pigment. Important diagnostic criteria for benign blue nevi include a low mitotic rate, absence of necrosis, a low Ki-67-+ proliferative fraction, and uniform HMB45 labeling. Cytologic atypia may be present in benign blue nevi, but mitotic figures should not been seen. Such "ancient" blue nevi frequently demonstrate edematous stromal areas and hyaline changes in vessels, suggesting a degenerative phenomenon.

Epithelioid blue nevus

Epithelioid blue nevi are mostly seen in patients with the Carney complex (myxomas, spotty skin pigmentation, endocrine overactivity, and schwannomas). They occur on the extremities and trunk, and less frequently on the head and neck. They may also be noted in the absence of Carney complex, and may occur on the genital mucosa. The lesions are composed of large polygonal and epithelioid melanocytes often laden with melanin. These cells are admixed with heavily pigmented dendritic melanocytes, spindled melanocytes, and melanophages. Some melanocytes are situated among the dermal collagen bundles singly, in short rows, and small groups. The nuclei are vesicular with very pale chromatin and a single prominent nucleolus. They may demonstrate moderate pleomorphism and rare mitotic figures. In contrast with other blue nevi, they lack the usual sclerotic stroma. Some have grouped these lesions with dendritic and epithelioid melanomas under the designation pigmented epithelioid melanocytoma, which they regard as a borderline malignancy or low-grade melanoma. One problem with this designation is the lack of data suggesting that the lesions in patients with the Carney complex behave in a malignant fashion.

Deep penetrating nevus

This unique type of nevus is commonly seen in combination with other forms of blue nevus. The fascicles of cells have small hyperchromatic nuclei with a smudged chromatin pattern and inconspicuous nucleoli. Adjacent melanophages are noted.

Amelanotic blue nevus (hypomelanotic blue nevus)

In the amelanotic or hypomelanotic variant of cellular blue nevus, mild cytologic atypia and pleomorphism may be present. Mitotic activity (up to three mitoses/mm) may also be observed. It is important to recognize the entity so as not to confuse it with a malignant lesion.

"Malignant blue nevus"

The term "malignant blue nevus" has been used to refer to melanomas arising in a blue nevus (usually a cellular blue nevus). It has also been used for de novo melanoma resembling a cellular blue nevus. When melanoma occurs in a blue nevus, an abrupt transition can be seen between the nevus and the melanoma. The melanoma demonstrates a sheet-like growth pattern, mitoses, necrosis, and nuclear atypia.

Treatment

Excision is the mainstay of treatment for blue nevi. Successful results have been reported with the Q-switched ruby laser. Treatment of the malignant variety is the same as for a malignant melanoma. Intratumoral therapy with IFN-β has also been used.

Berman EL, et al: Multifocal blue nevus of the conjunctiva. Surv Ophthalmol 2008 Jan–Feb; 53(1):41–49.

Cerroni L, et al: "Ancient" blue nevi (cellular blue nevi with degenerative stromal changes). Am J Dermatopathol 2008 Feb; 30(1):1–5.

Fleming MG: Pigmented lesion pathology: what you should expect from your pathologist, and what your pathologist should expect from you. Clin Plast Surg 2010; 37(1):1–20.

Murali R, et al: Blue nevi and related lesions: a review highlighting atypical and newly described variants, distinguishing features and diagnostic pitfalls. Adv Anat Pathol 2009; 16(6):365–382.

von Moos R, et al: Intratumoral therapy with interferon-alpha in a locoregional advanced malignant blue nevus: a brief communication. J Immunother 2010; 33(1):92–95.

Wang Q, et al: Cellular blue nevi of the eyelid: a possible diagnostic pitfall. J Am Acad Dermatol 2008 Feb; 58(2):257–260.

Bonus images for this chapter can be found online at
http://www.expertconsult.com

Fig. 30-1 Solar lentigines.

Fig. 30-2 Benign nevi.

Fig. 30-3 Medium-sized congenital nevus.

Fig. 30-4 Spitz nevus.

Fig. 30-5 Multiple spindle cell nevi.

Fig. 30-6 Fried egg appearance of a dysplastic nevus.

Fig. 30-7 Melanoma.

Fig. 30-8 Palatal melanoma.

Fig. 30-9 Congenital common blue nevus.

Fig. 30-10 Nevus spilus.

Fig. 30-11 Becker nevus.

Fig. 30-12 Halo nevus.

Fig. 30-13 Spitz nevus.

Fig. 30-14 Amelanotic malignant melanoma.

31 Macrophage/Monocyte Disorders

Palisaded granulomatous dermatoses

Granuloma annulare

Granuloma annulare (GA) is a relatively common idiopathic disorder of the dermis and subcutaneous tissue. It occurs in all races and at all ages, but much more frequently affects women (2:1). GA may exhibit the isomorphic response of Koebner, affect healed areas of herpes zoster, and may be restricted to sun-exposed areas. While most cases spontaneously resolve, leaving entirely normal skin, loss of elastic tissue may occur, leaving atrophic lesions resembling mid-dermal elastolysis or anetoderma. GA lesions will sometimes spontaneously resolve when biopsied. Long-term follow-up of at least 20 years in patients with GA reveals that lesions usually heal, and that the patients remain healthy and do not develop unusual diseases. Case reports of associations as described below demonstrate that GA can be a reactive condition associated with a variety of underlying disorders and medications. In most patients, however, it is a benign, self-limited (although not soon enough for the dermatologist or patient) condition affecting only the skin.

Many clinical morphologies of GA exist. Usually, patients exhibit primarily one clinical type during the course of their illness, except in the subcutaneous form, in which typical papular or localized GA may also occur.

Localized granuloma annulare

This form of GA tends to affect children and young to middle-aged adults. Usually only one or a few lesions are present at any one time. Localized GA usually appears on the lateral or dorsal surfaces of the fingers or hands, elbows, dorsal feet, and ankles (Figs 31-1 to 31-3). Rarely, the eyelid or even a Becker

nevus may be affected. Lesions are erythematous, fawn-colored or violaceous, thinly bordered plaques or papules, which slowly spread peripherally, at the same time undergoing central involution, so that roughly annular lesions are formed. The overlying skin usually remains completely normal. Lesions may coalesce and sometimes form scalloped patterns or firm plaques. The lesions never ulcerate and on resolving virtually always leave no residua. They develop slowly and often involute spontaneously. Although more than

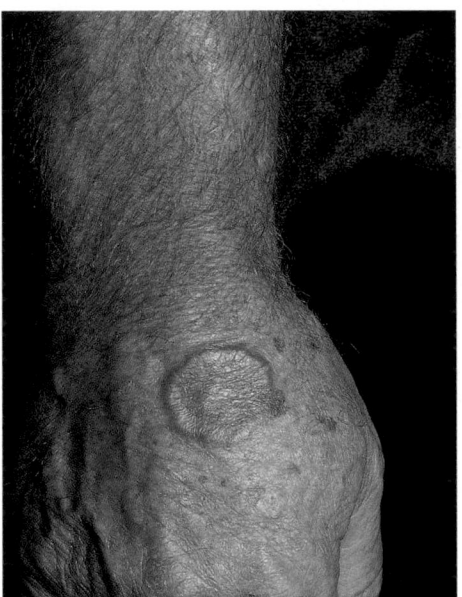

Fig. 31-2 Granuloma annulare, annular, localized type.

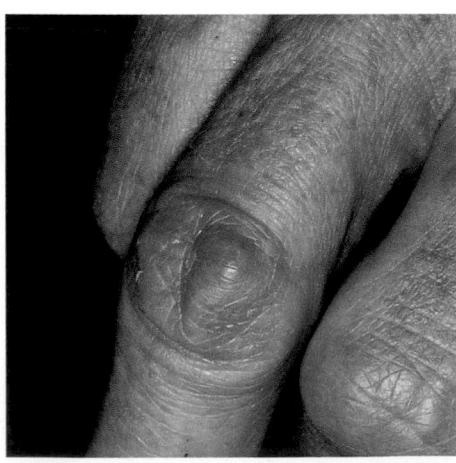

Fig. 31-1 Granuloma annulare, dermal papule on the knuckle.

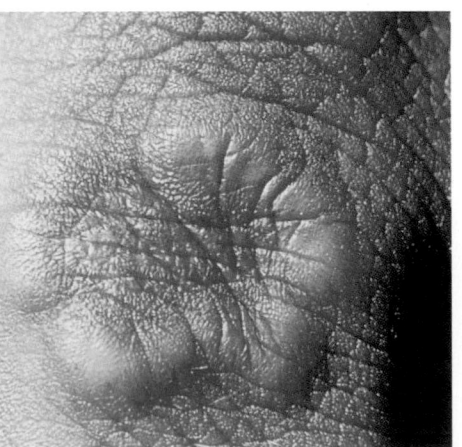

Fig. 31-3 Granuloma annulare, annular plaque composed of coalescing papules.

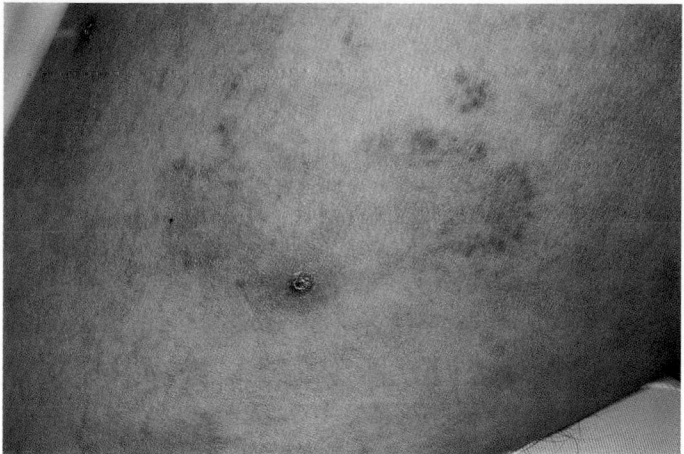

Fig. 31-4 Granuloma annulare, macular lesion of the medial thigh.

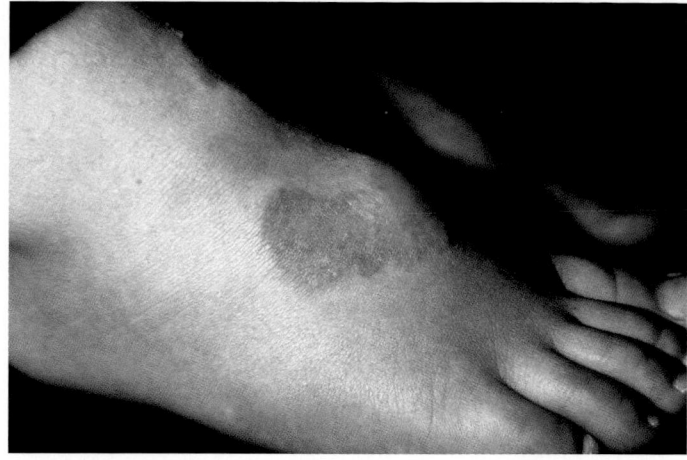

Fig. 31-5 Granuloma annulare, subcutaneous and dermal lesion.

50% of patients clear within 2 years, lesions will recur in 40%. Autoimmune thyroiditis may be present in women with localized GA.

Generalized granuloma annulare

This form of GA affects mostly women in the fifth and sixth decades, adolescents and children. The association of generalized GA with diabetes mellitus has been questioned. The eruption presents as a diffuse but symmetrical, papular or annular eruption of more than 10 lesions, and often hundreds. Lesions favor the nape of the neck, upper trunk, and proximal upper extremities, and rarely exceed 5 cm in diameter. The palms, soles, and eyelids may be affected. The face and genital area are usually spared. In some cases sun exposure seems to be a trigger (see section on actinic granuloma below). Some patients are completely asymptomatic, whereas others complain of severe pruritus. Spontaneous clearing usually occurs but at variable times. The average duration is 3–4 years but may be as short as 4 months or longer than a decade.

Patch-type or macular granuloma annulare

This form of GA is significantly more common in women, usually between 30 and 70 years of age. Flat or only slightly palpable erythematous or red–brown lesions occur (Fig. 31-4), especially on the upper medial thighs and in bathing-trunk distribution. Lesions may closely simulate cutaneous T-cell lymphoma or morphea. Individual lesions average at least several centimeters in diameter but may be much larger. On careful palpation, small papules can be felt in some cases and on stretching the skin the papules or small annular lesions can be seen. Such papules are the most fruitful sites for biopsies. Both well-formed necrobiotic granulomas and the interstitial pattern of GA may be seen on biopsy.

Subcutaneous granuloma annulare (deep granuloma annulare, pseudorheumatoid nodule)

Subcutaneous GA is most common in children, with boys affected twice as frequently as girls. Childhood cases appear at any age from 1 year to adolescence, with one congenital case reported. Lesions tend to occur on the lower legs, especially the dorsal foot, but may also occur on the distal upper extremity or scalp. Multiple lesions are usually present. There is often a history of trauma to the affected area preceding the appearance of a lesion. Typically, lesions are skin-colored, deep dermal or subcutaneous nodules, up to several centimeters in diameter (Fig. 31-5). Superficial papular lesions are present in about one-quarter of patients with subcutaneous GA. Lesions in general are asymptomatic and resolve over a few years. The major clinical problem occurs when the initial pathologic interpretation is rheumatoid nodule and an unnecessary extensive rheumatologic work-up is performed. An unusual variant is one that remains localized to the penis or scrotum, an atypical location for GA in general. Adult women without rheumatoid arthritis may develop similar lesions around the joints.

Perforating granuloma annulare

Perforating GA usually appears on the dorsal hands and presents as papules with a central keratotic core. This core represents transepidermal elimination of the degenerated material in the center of GA lesions and clinically can resemble a pustule.

Acute-onset painful acral granuloma annulare

This recently described clinical variant of GA does not resemble other forms of the disease. Female patients present with the sudden onset of painful lesions on the hands and feet, and a scattering of lesions at other sites. The lateral, dorsal, and marginal hands and, to less extent, the feet are affected. Palm and sole lesions are characteristic. Lesions are tender to palpation and, when present on the palms, are dusky and may vaguely resemble erythema multiforme. Patients may have associated arthralgias and diarrhea, and feel feverish, features of a "cytokine storm." The erythrocyte sedimentation rate (ESR) may be elevated, even above 50 mm/hr. Lesions resolve over months, at times after having been treated with systemic corticosteroids or hydroxychloroquine. The authors have seen one such case associated with Hodgkin disease.

Granuloma annulare in human immunodeficiency (HIV) disease

GA may occur in persons with HIV infection at all stages of disease. Lesions are typically papular and generalized GA is more common (60%) than localized GA (40%). Photodistributed and perforating lesions may also occur. The histology is identical to GA in the normal host. The natural history of GA in HIV is unknown.

Granuloma annulare and malignant neoplasms

The occurrence of GA and a cancer in the same patient is rare, but has been reported many times. Most of these patients are between 35 and 75, older than the typical GA patient. Half the cases occur in lymphoma/leukemia patients and half in solid tumor patients. The diagnosis of the neoplasm usually predates the diagnosis of GA, but may precede it. In some cases, lesions are described as "atypical" in that they may be painful (see above).

Other conditions associated with granuloma annulare

Since these reports are anecdotal, causality cannot be ascribed in every case. However, these cases do show trends that parallel our concept of the pathogenesis of GA. Numerous medications have been reported to cause GA. Many of these medications are immunomodulatory—interferon (IFN)-α, IFN-β, and tumor necrosis factor (TNF) inhibitors. GA may follow a bee sting, waxing in a patient with pseudofolliculitis, and injections at a medispa for mesotherapy. Two groups of infectious diseases have been described as having GA-like lesions either histologically or clinically: borreliosis and tuberculosis. Both Lyme disease in the USA and *Borrelia* infections in Europe have been described rarely as demonstrating interstitial granulomatous inflammation; clinically, however, at least in Europe, the lesions resemble morphea rather than GA. Despite laboratory evidence of infection, treatment of the patient with appropriate antibiotics may not lead to resolution of the skin lesions. A tuberculid can closely resemble disseminated GA, although histologically caseous necrosis may be seen in the center of the granulomas. Treatment for tuberculosis leads to resolution of the skin lesions. In the appropriate patient evaluation for tuberculosis and anti-tuberculous treatment may be indicated.

Granuloma annulare and eye disease

Anterior and chronic intermediate uveitis has been described in patients with localized GA. The uveitis can be unilateral or bilateral, may be mild and respond to topical therapy, or may be aggressive, resulting in visual impairment. The frequency of uveitis in patients with GA seems to be too low to recommend that all patients with GA be screened by an ophthalmologist. However, GA patients should be questioned about visual symptoms, including reduced visual acuity. If these are present, ophthalmologic evaluation would be appropriate.

Histology

Because there are many clinical patterns of GA, skin biopsies are often performed to confirm the diagnosis. In general, there are two histopathologic patterns that often coexist in the same patient. The classic pattern of GA is a palisading granuloma characterized by histiocytes and epithelioid cells surrounding a central zone of altered collagen. In well-developed lesions, there is mucin deposition within the foci of altered collagen. Fibrin and nuclear dust may also be present in the degenerated foci. Lesions are most typically located in the upper and mid-reticular dermis, but may involve the deep dermis or subcutaneous tissue. At the periphery of lesions a leukocytoclastic vasculitis may rarely be found. IgM and C3 in the blood vessels of the skin lesions are found in about half of patients.

The second pattern of GA is the interstitial pattern. Lesions may be entirely interstitial, or an interstitial pattern may be seen adjacent to well-formed palisaded lesions. A patchy dermal infiltrate of histiocytes and other mononuclear cells with occasional neutrophils is interspersed between collagen bundles. The patchy distribution within the dermis is best appreciated at scanning magnification. Interstitial mucin is often present in the affected areas, and is best demonstrated with a colloidal iron stain. Although these features are sufficient to confirm the diagnosis of GA, further sectioning may reveal typical palisaded granulomas. If the number of histiocytes in the infiltrate is small and lymphocytes predominate, the diagnosis of interstitial cutaneous T-cell lymphoma should be considered.

Treatment

Patients regularly report that a biopsy of the lesion will cause its involution. Because the lesions are often asymptomatic and spontaneous involution occurs, no treatment is required in many mild cases. Numerous modalities have been reported to improve GA, suggesting that no one treatment is uniformly efficacious and the "treatment of choice." It is best to develop a therapeutic ladder for both localized and generalized cases of GA. For localized cases, the intralesional injection of triamcinolone suspension is effective and is a reasonable initial treatment. Most cases relapse within 3–7 months. Superpotent topical steroids or topical calcineurin inhibitors, or imiquimod, may be effective in some patients, especially those with more macular lesions. Localized phototherapy in the form of pulsed dye laser, high-intensity UV therapy with a laser designed to treat psoriasis, PUVA, photodynamic therapy, or even fractional photothermolysis could be considered.

Generalized cases represent a major therapeutic challenge. Although systemic steroids may be very effective, the high doses required and the usual immediate relapse as the steroids are tapered make this approach untenable in most situations. In addition, because diabetes may be present, systemic steroids may complicate the management of the diabetes. Many systemic agents have been reported as effective, but few have been tested in large numbers of cases or in blinded or controlled fashion. For any treatment, 3–6 months of therapy appear to be necessary for efficacy or failure to be demonstrated. With all treatments, the GA may clear, only to recur when the treatment is stopped. Antibiotics such as doxycycline; the combination of rifampin, ofloxacin, and minocycline, once monthly; pentoxiphylline, 400 mg three times daily; or high-dose nicotinamide, potassium iodide, or dapsone, 100 mg per day, can be effective. Fumaric acid esters over 1–18 months have also shown efficacy. Oral retinoids, especially isotretinoin, can be considered at a dose of 0.5 mg/kg or slightly more. Hydroxychloroquine in very high doses (9 mg/kg initially) reportedly cleared all nine patients so treated. Phototherapy in the form of NB-UVB, PUVA, or UVA-1 can be effective in selected patients. With UVA-1 about half of treated patients have a "satisfactory response"; however, stopping treatment led to relapse. Photodynamic therapy will clear or "almost clear" some lesions and can be used for multiple lesions in a localized area. For patients with severe or disabling disease, TNF inhibitors can be considered. Etanercept, infliximab, and adalimumab have all been reported to be effective. It is of interest that these medications can also cause GA. Systemic agents, such as cyclosporine, IFN-γ, and hydroxyurea, have been reported to be effective in small series of patients. The potential toxicity of these medications limits their use to patients with significant GA.

Adams BB, Mutasim DF: Colocalization of granuloma annulare and mid-dermal elastolysis. J Am Acad Dermatol 2003; 48:S25.

Adams DC, Hogan DJ: Improvement of chronic generalized granuloma annulare with isotretinoin. Arch Dermatol 2002; 138:1518.

Asano Y, et al: Generalized granuloma annulare treated with short-term administration of etretinate. J Am Acad Dermatol 2006; 54:S245.

Badavanis G, et al: Successful treatment of granuloma annulare with imiquimod cream 5%: a report of four cases. Acta Derm Venereol 2005; 85:547.

Barzilai A, et al: Pseudorheumatoid nodules in adults: a juxta-articular form of nodular granuloma annulare. Am J Dermatopathol 2005; 27:1.

Baskan EB, et al: A case of granuloma annulare in a child following tetanus and diphtheria toxoid vaccination. J Eur Acad Dermatol Venereol 2005; 19:639.

Baskan EB, et al: A case of generalized granuloma annulare with myelodysplastic syndrome: successful treatment with systemic isotretinoin and topical pimecrolimus 1% cream. J Eur Acad Dermatol Venereol 2007; 21:693.

Batchelor R, Clark S: Clearance of generalized papular umbilicated granuloma annulare in a child with bath PUVA therapy. Pediatr Dermatol 2006; 23:72.

Brey NV, et al: Acute-onset, painful acral granuloma annulare: a report of 4 cases and a discussion of the clinical and histologic spectrum of the disease. Arch Dermatol 2006; 142:49.

Brey NV, et al: Association of inflammatory eye disease with granuloma annulare? Arch Dermatol 2008; 144:803.

Cannistraci C, et al: Treatment of generalized granuloma annulare with hydroxychloroquine. Dermatology 2005; 211:167.

Chiu ML, Tang MB: Generalized granuloma annulare associated with gastrointestinal stromal tumour: case report and review of clinical features and management. Clin Exp Dermatol 2008; 33:469.

Cohen PR: Granuloma annulare, relapsing polychondritis, sarcoidosis, and systemic lupus erythematosus: conditions whose dermatologic manifestations may occur as hematologic malignancy-associated mucocutaneous paraneoplastic syndromes. Int J Dermatol 2006; 45:70.

Czarnecki DB, et al: The response of generalized granuloma annulare to dapsone. Acta Dermatol Venereol (Stockh) 1986; 66:82.

Dadban A, et al: Widespread granuloma annulare and Hodgkin's disease. Clin Exp Dermatol 2008; 33:465.

Dahl MV: Granuloma annulare: long-term follow-up. Arch Dermatol 2007; 143:946.

De Aloe G, et al: Congenital subcutaneous granuloma annulare. Pediatr Dermatol 2005; 22:234.

Duarte AF, et al: Generalized granuloma annulare—response to doxycycline. J Eur Acad Dermatol Venereol 2009; 23:84.

Forman SB, et al: Penile granuloma annulare of an adolescent male—case report and review of the literature. Pediatr Dermatol 2008; 25:260.

Frigerio E, et al: Multiple localized granuloma annulare: ultraviolet A1 phototherapy. Clin Exp Dermatol 2007; 32:762.

Grundmann-Kollmann M, et al: Cream psoralen plus ultraviolet A therapy for granuloma annulare. Br J Dermatol 2001; 144:996.

Gualco F, et al: Interstitial granuloma annulare and borreliosis: a new case. J Eur Acad Dermatol Venereol 2007; 21:1117.

Hacihamdioglu B, et al: Subcutaneous granuloma annulare in a child: a case report. Clin Pediatr 2008; 47:306.

Hall CS, et al: Treatment of recalcitrant disseminated granuloma annulare with hydroxyurea. J Am Acad Dermatol 2008; 58:525.

Herron MD, Florell SR: Disseminated granuloma annulare accompanying mycobacterium tuberculosis lymphadenitis. Int J Dermatol 2004; 43:961.

Hertl MS, et al: Rapid improvement of recalcitrant disseminated granuloma annulare upon treatment with the tumour necrosis factor-α inhibitor, infliximab. Br J Dermatol 2005; 152:552.

Hinckley MR, et al: Generalized granuloma annulare as an initial manifestation of chronic myelomonocytic leukemia: a report of 2 cases. Am J Dermatopathol 2008; 30:274.

Hsu S, et al: Granuloma annulare localized to the palms. J Am Acad Dermatol 1999; 41:287.

Inui S, et al: Disseminated granuloma annulare responsive to narrowband ultraviolet B therapy. J Am Acad Dermatol 2005; 53:533.

Karsai S, et al: Fractional photothermolysis for the treatment of granuloma annulare: a case report. Lasers Surg Med 2008; 40:319.

Kawakami T, et al: Granuloma annulare-like skin lesions as an initial manifestation in a Japanese patient with adult T-cell leukemia/lymphoma. J Am Acad Dermatol 2009; 60:848.

Kiremitci U, et al: Generalized granuloma annulare resolving to anetoderma. Dermatol Online J 2006; 12:16.

Kluger N, et al: Generalized interstitial granuloma annulare induced by pegylated interferon-alpha. Dermatology 2006; 213:248.

Knoell KA: Efficacy of adalimumab in the treatment of generalized granuloma annulare in monozygotic twins carrying the 8.1 ancestral haplotype. Arch Dermatol 2009; 145:610.

Levin NA, et al: Resolution of patch-type granuloma annulare lesions after biopsy. J Am Acad Dermatol 2002; 46:426.

Li A, et al: Granuloma annulare and malignant neoplasms. Am J Dermatopathol 2003; 25:113.

Lopez-Navarro N, et al: Successful treatment of perforating granuloma annulare with 0.1% tacrolimus ointment. J Dermatolog Treat 2008; 19:376.

Ma A, et al: Response of generalized granuloma annulare to high-dose niacinamide. Arch Dermatol 1983; 119:836.

Madan V, et al: Multiple asymptomatic scrotal nodules. Clin Exp Dermatol 2009; 34:433.

Marcus DV, et al: Granuloma annulare treated with rifampin, ofloxacin, and minocycline combination therapy. Arch Dermatol 2009; 145:787.

Marie I, et al: Rosai–Dorfman disease and granuloma annulare. Acta Derm Venereol 2007; 87:375.

Mehta LR, Rose JW: Recurrent granuloma annulare during treatment with daclizumab. Mult Scler 2009; 15:527.

Moreno C, et al: Interstitial granulomatous dermatitis with histiocytic pseudorosettes: a new histopathologic pattern in cutaneous borreliosis. Detection of Borrelia burgdorferi DNA sequences by a highly sensitive PCR-ELISA. J Am Acad Dermatol 2003; 48:376.

Nebesio CL, et al: Lack of an association between granuloma annulare and type 2 diabetes mellitus. Br J Dermatol 2002; 146:122.

Neto Pimentel DR, et al: Multiple deep granuloma annulare limited to the cephalic segment in childhood. Pediatr Dermatol 2008; 25:407.

Özkan S, et al: Anetoderma secondary to generalized granuloma annulare. J Am Acad Dermatol 2000; 42:335.

Pasmatzi E, et al: Temporary remission of disseminated granuloma annulare under oral isotretinoin therapy. Int J Dermatol 2005; 44:169.

Piaserico S, et al: Generalized granuloma annulare treated with methylaminolevulinate photodynamic therapy. Dermatology 2009; 218:282.

Reddy HS, et al: Granuloma annulare anterior uveitis. Ocul Immunol Inflamm 2008; 16:55.

Requena L, Fernandez-Figueras MT: Subcutaneous granuloma annulare. Semin Cutan Med Surg 2007; 25:96.

Sandwich JT, Davis LS: Granuloma annulare of the eyelid: a case report and review of the literature. Pediatr Dermatol 1999; 16:373.

Schnopp C, et al: UVA1 phototherapy for disseminated granuloma annulare. Photodermatol Photoimmunol Photomed 2005; 21:68.

Setoyama M, et al: Granuloma annulare associated with Hodgkin's disease. Int J Dermatol 1997; 36:445.

Shimizu S, et al: Atypical generalized granuloma annulare associated with two visceral cancers. J Am Acad Dermatol 2006; 54:S236.

Shupack J, Siu K: Resolving granuloma annulare with etanercept. Arch Dermatol 2006; 142:394.

Sidwell RU, et al: Subcutaneous granuloma annulare of the penis in 2 adolescents. J Pediatr Surg 2005; 40:1329.

Simon M, et al: Antimalarials for control of disseminated granuloma annulare in children. J Am Acad Dermatol 1994; 31:1064.

Sliger BN, et al: Treatment of granuloma annulare with the 595 nm pulsed dye laser in a pediatric patient. Pediatr Dermatol 2008; 25:196.

Smith JB, et al: Potassium iodide in the treatment of disseminated granuloma annulare. J Am Acad Dermatol 1994; 30:791.

Sniezek PJ, et al: Treatment of granuloma annulare with the 585 nm pulsed dye laser. Dermatol Surg 2005; 31:1370.

Spadino S, et al: Disseminated granuloma annulare: efficacy of cyclosporine therapy. Int J Immunopathol Pharmacol 2006; 19:433.

Strahan JE, et al: Granuloma annulare as a complication of mesotherapy: a case report. Dermatol Surg 2008; 34:836.

Takayama K, et al: Papular granuloma annulare with subcutaneous granulomatous reaction induced by a bee sting. Acta Derm Venereol 2008; 88:519.

Toro JR, et al: Granuloma annulare and human immunodeficiency virus infection. Arch Dermatol 1999; 135:1341.

Tsai J, et al: Cutaneous tuberculid clinically resembling generalized granuloma annulare. Clin Exp Dermatol 2007; 32:450.

Uenotsuchi T, et al: Seasonally recurrent granuloma annulare on sun-exposed areas. Br J Dermatol 1999; 141:367.

Vázquez-López F, et al: Localized granuloma annulare and autoimmune thyroiditis in adult women: a case-control study. J Am Acad Dermatol 2003; 48:517.

Villegas RG, et al: Pustular generalized perforating granuloma annulare. Br J Dermatol 2003; 149:866.

Voulgari PV, et al: Granuloma annulare induced by anti-tumour necrosis factor therapy. Ann Rheum Dis 2008; 67:567.

Webber HO, et al: Treatment of disseminated granuloma annulare with low-dose fumaric acid. Acta Derm Venereol 2009; 89:295.

Weinberg JM, et al: Granuloma annulare restricted to Becker's nevus. Br J Dermatol 2004; 151:245.

Weisenseel P, et al: Photodynamic therapy for granuloma annulare: more than a shot in the dark. Dermatology 2008; 217:329.

Weiss JM, et al: Treatment of granuloma annulare by local injections with low-dose recombinant human interferon gamma. J Am Acad Dermatol 1998; 39:117.

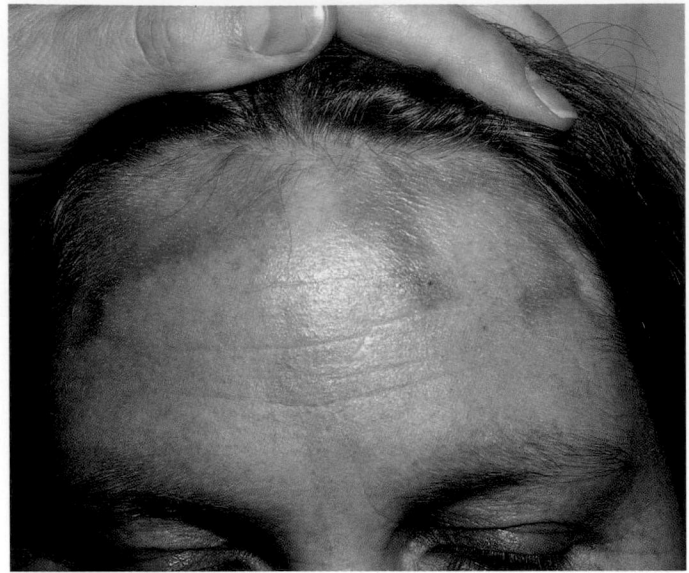

Fig. 31-6 Granuloma annulare, annular elastolytic giant cell granuloma (Meischer), atrophic annular plaque.

Whelan JP, Zembowicz A: Case records of the Massachusetts General Hospital. Case 19-2000: a 22-month-old boy with the rapid growth of subcutaneous nodules. N Engl J Med 2006; 254:2697.

Wu H, et al: Granuloma annulare with a mycosis fungoides-like distribution and palisaded granulomas of CD68-positive histiocytes. J Am Acad Dermatol 2004; 51:39.

Young HS, Coulson IH: Granuloma annulare following waxing induced pseudofolliculitis—resolution with isotretinoin. Clin Exp Dermatol 2000; 25:274.

Ziemer M, et al: Granuloma annulare—a manifestation of infection with *Borrelia*? J Cutan Pathol 2008; 35:1050.

Annular elastolytic giant cell granuloma (Meischer's) and actinic granuloma (O'Brien)

Annular elastolytic giant cell granuloma (AEGCG) and actinic granuloma are unified by their histopathologic appearance. Non-diabetes-associated necrobiosis lipoidica of the face has been included in this category. It is currently unclear whether they simply represent variants of GA occurring on sun-damaged skin or are distinct diseases.

AEGCG have been reported in two patterns. One is a single, asymptomatic, atrophic-appearing, yellow, thin plaque on the forehead (Meischer's Granuloma) (Fig. 31-6). Fine wrinkling and loss of elasticity characterize the skin within the ring. Clinically, this pattern resembles facial necrobiosis lipoidica more than GA. The second variant is of multiple extensor upper extremity and sometimes trunk lesions, and occurs more frequently in women and largely in sun-exposed areas. In these cases the lesions have an active erythematous border with central clearing. A papular variant has been described. While the vast majority of cases occur in adults, children and even an infant have been affected. Except for temporal arteritis as described below, most patients are otherwise well. However, AEGCG has been described in association with acute myelogenous leukemia (which resolved with remission and recurred with relapse of the leukemia) and pleomorphic cutaneous T-cell lymphoma, At times, as in GA, the lesions may heal with loss of elastic tissue and clinical features of skin laxity and anetoderma. The condition is chronic.

Actinic granuloma, as described by O'Brien, may represent the same disorder as AEGCG. It presents as papules and plaques on sun-exposed skin (Fig. 31-7). Lesions are frequently numerous and may coalesce to cover much of the exposed

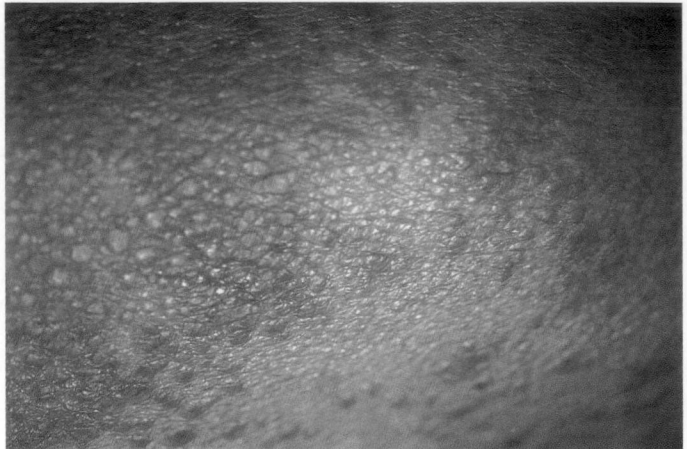

Fig. 31-7 Granuloma annulare, generalized papular lesions localized to sun-exposed sites.

skin. A history of onset after significant sun exposure and the distribution on physical examination should lead to suspicion of the diagnosis. A few lesions may occur on sun-protected sites or spill over from affected areas to more photoprotected sites. Rarely, open comedones, scarring, and milia formation may be present clinically. This may be associated with transepidermal elimination of damaged connective tissue or loss of elastic tissue surrounding the follicular ostia, leading to a Favre–Racouchot-like appearance. This condition affects older adults (usually over age 50) and can be intensely pruritic. It is not associated with diabetes mellitus, but there are numerous reports of it occurring in patients with temporal arteritis. It is speculated that the vasculitis is also due to actinic injury to the connective tissue surrounding the temporal artery.

Histologically, all these conditions show a characteristic histology. The dermal infiltrate of macrophages is largely interstitial and well-formed palisaded granulomas are uncommon. Multinucleated giant cells, often quite large, are numerous. Mucin is scant or lacking. The macrophages characteristically contain fragments of actinically damaged elastic tissue (elastophagocytosis). When this typical histology is seen in concert with the classic clinical features noted above, it may be reasonable to make these specific diagnoses. These conditions cannot, however, be diagnosed on clinical or histologic grounds alone. Some cases with the clinical features of AEGCG or actinic granuloma will show a histology more characteristic of typical GA, suggesting that there is a spectrum of both clinical and histologic features in these patients.

Treatment of these conditions has been difficult. Cases with an active erythematous border tend to respond to systemic steroids, but relapse immediately when the steroids are tapered or discontinued. Tranilast, 300 mg/day, and chloroquine, 250 mg/day, have been reported as effective. Insulin improved diabetic control and the actinic granuloma in one case. Other anecdotal treatments include oral retinoids, fumaric acid, PUVA, pentoxiphylline, cyclosporine, and methotrexate.

Boussault P, et al: Primary cutaneous CD4+ small/medium-sized pleomorphic T-cell lymphoma associated with an annular elastolytic giant cell granuloma. Br J Dermatol 2009; 160:1126.

Davies MG, et al: Actinic granuloma in a young woman following prolonged sunbed usage. Br J Dermatol 1997; 136:797.

Garg A, et al: Annular elastolytic giant cell granuloma heralding onset and recurrence of acute myelogenous leukemia. Arch Dermatol 2006; 142:532.

Gass JK, et al: Generalized granuloma annulare in a photosensitive distribution resolving with scarring and milia formation. Clin Exp Dermatol 2009; 34:e53.

Klemke CD, et al: Generalized annular elastolytic giant cell granuloma. Dermatology 2003; 207:420.

Lau H, et al: Actinic granuloma in association with giant cell arteritis. Pathology 1997; 29:260.

Lee HW, et al: Annular elastolytic giant cell granuloma in an infant: improvement after treatment with oral tranilast and topical pimecrolimus. J Am Acad Dermatol 2005; 53:S244.

Morita K, et al: Papular elastolytic giant cell granuloma: a clinical variant of annular elastolytic giant cell granuloma or generalized granuloma annulare? Eur J Dermatol 1999; 9:647.

Muller FB, Groth W: Annular elastolytic giant cell granuloma: a prodromal stage of mid-dermal elastolysis? Br J Dermatol 2007; 156:1377.

Özkaya-Bayazit E, et al: Annular elastolytic giant cell granuloma: sparing of a burn scar and successful treatment with chloroquine. Br J Dermatol 1999; 140:525.

Sniezek PJ, et al: Annular atrophic plaques on the arms of a 57-year-old woman. Arch Dermatol 2006; 142:775.

Stein JA, et al: Actinic granuloma. Dermatol Online J 2007; 13:19.

Sudy E, et al: Open comedones overlying granuloma annulare in a photoexposed area. Photodermatol Photoimmunol Photomed 2006; 22:273.

Interstitial granulomatous drug reaction

Interstitial granulomatous drug reaction (IGDR) is an uncommon, and increasingly recognized, pattern of adverse reactions to medication. While it may occur within a few days of starting the medication, most patients with IGDR have been on the offending medication for months to years. A wide variety of medications have been implicated, including calcium channel-blockers (most common cause reported), lipid-lowering agents, angiotensin-converting enzyme (ACE) inhibitors, diuretics, nonsteroidal anti-inflammatory drugs (NSAIDs), antihistamines, anticonvulsants, antidepressants, allopurinol, thalidomide, lenalidomide, darifenacin, anakinra, ganciclovir, strontium ranelate, sennoside (a common over-the-counter laxative), Chinese herbs, and even soy. The TNF inhibitors have been implicated as causal in IGDR in many cases, mostly in patients being treated for rheumatoid arthritis. Since rheumatoid arthritis patients may develop similar lesions independent of medication exposure, it suggests that rheumatoid arthritis patients may be predisposed to developing this reaction pattern. In cases of IGDR from TNF inhibitors, stopping the medication led to resolution of the eruption over several months, strongly supporting the association.

Clinically, the lesions are erythematous annular plaques with an indurated border and sometimes a tendency to central clearing. Lesions favor the creases (groin, axillae, popliteal fossae), but may also affect the trunk, proximal extremities, palms, and soles. Lesions may be photodistributed, affecting the face and dorsal extensor forearm and hands. Pruritus is minimal or absent. Mucous membranes are spared. Histologically, there is a diffuse deep dermal infiltrate that is perivascular but has a prominent interstitial component. The inflammatory infiltrate is centered in the lower two-thirds of the dermis; it contains neutrophils, eosinophils, histiocytes, and multinucleated giant cells. Degenerated collagen bundles may be surrounded by histiocytes, neutrophils, and eosinophils, forming "Churg–Strauss" granulomas, and mucin is usually scant or absent. Necrobiotic granulomas are usually incomplete, but have at times been reported to resemble those seen in GA. Unique features that should suggest IGDR over GA include an interface component and "atypical" lymphocytes in the infiltrate. The histologic differential diagnosis includes interstitial granulomatous dermatitis associated with arthritis, palisaded neutrophilic granulomatous dermatitis, papular eruption of methotrexate, and interstitial GA. Lesions resolve over months once the offending ingestant is stopped.

Chen YC, et al: Interstitial granulomatous drug reaction presenting as erythroderma: remission after discontinuation of enalapril maleate. Br J Dermatol 2008; 158:1143.

Deng A, et al: Interstitial granulomatous dermatitis associated with the use of tumor necrosis factor alpha inhibitors. Arch Dermatol 2006; 142:198.

Dyson SW, et al: Interstitial granulomatous dermatitis secondary to soy. J Am Acad Dermatol 2004; 51:S105.

Fujita Y, et al: A case of interstitial granulomatous drug reaction due to sennoside. Br J Dermatol 2004; 150:1028.

Groves C, et al: Interstitial granulomatous reaction to strontium ranelate. Arch Dermatol 2008; 144:268.

Lee HW, et al: Interstitial granulomatous drug reaction caused by Chinese herbal medication. J Am Acad Dermatol 2005; 52:712.

Lim AC, et al: A granuloma annulare-like eruption associated with the use of amlodipine. Australas J Dermatol 2002; 45:24.

Marcollo Pini A, et al: Interstitial granulomatous drug reaction following intravenous ganciclovir. Br J Dermatol 2008; 158:1391.

Mason HR, et al: Interstitial granulomatous dermatitis associated with darifenacin. J Drugs Dermatol 2008; 7:895.

Regula CG, et al: Interstitial granulomatous drug reaction to anakinra. J Am Acad Dermatol 2008; 59:S25.

Yazganoglu KD, et al: Interstitial granulomatous drug reaction due to thalidomide. J Eur Acad Dermatol Venereol 2009; 23:490.

Granuloma multiforme (Leiker)

Granuloma multiforme is seen most commonly in central Africa, where it is a common disorder, and rarely elsewhere. It affects adults aged over 40 and is more common in females. Lesions are most frequently found on the upper trunk and arms, and in sun-exposed areas. It begins as small papules that evolve within a year into round or oval plaques up to 15 cm in diameter. The active edge of lesions may be elevated to as much as 4 mm in height and the center may be slightly depressed and hypopigmented. Pruritus can occur and coalescing lesions may form unusual polycyclic shapes. The course is chronic. It is, most importantly, separated from tuberculoid leprosy. Histologically, it resembles GA, but multinucleated giant cells are prominent. Giant cells typically contain phagocytosed connective tissue and elastic tissue is decreased in the areas affected by the granulomas. GM shares many features with AEGCG and actinic granuloma/GA of sun-exposed skin, and in fact may be considered identical to those disorders.

Kumari R, et al: Granuloma multiforme: a report from India. Indian J Dermatol Venereol Leprol 2009; 75:296.

Necrobiotic xanthogranuloma

Necrobiotic xanthogranuloma is an uncommon multisystem disease with prominent skin findings. The cause is unknown. Disease is gradually progressive, affecting men and women equally, and beginning on average at around age 50 (range 25–80 years or more). The most common site affected is the periorbital area (65–80% of cases). Multicentric involvement is typical. The characteristic skin lesions are yellow (xanthomatous) plaques and nodules. Periorbitally, they may be mistaken for xanthelasma, but they are deep, firm, and indurated, and may extend into the orbit. The trunk and proximal extremities may have orange–red plaques that have an active red border and an atrophic center with superficial telangiectasias (Fig. 31-8). These plaques may grow to 25 cm in diameter. The skin lesions ulcerate in 50% of cases, leading to atrophic scarring. Acral nodules may also occur, some localized solely to the subcutaneous tissue. Extracutaneous involvement most commonly affects the eyes. Patients may complain of burning, itching, or pain around or in the eyes. Diplopia and inflammation in various compartments of the eye can occur, including

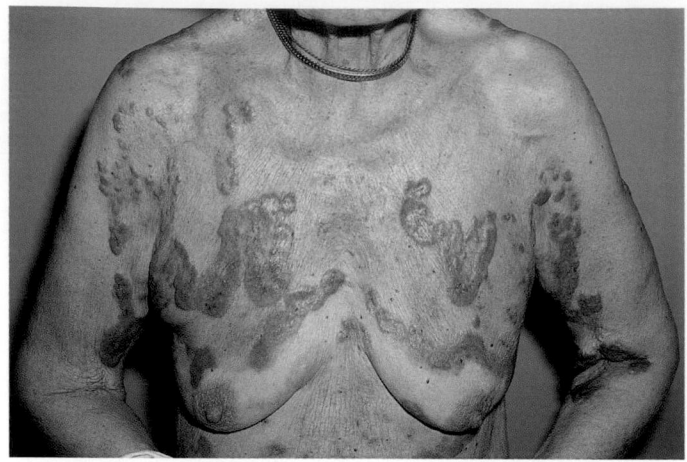

Fig. 31-8 Necrobiotic xanthogranuloma.

Newman B, et al: Aggressive histiocytic disorders that can involve the skin. J Am Acad Dermatol 2007; 56:302

Spicknall, KE, Mehregan DA: Necrobiotic xanthogranuloma. Int J Dermatol 2009; 48:1.

Venencie PY, et al: Recombinant interferon alfa-2b treatment of necrobiotic xanthogranuloma with paraproteinemia. J Am Acad Dermatol 1995; 32:666.

Wood AJ, et al: Necrobiotic xanthogranuloma: a review of 17 cases with emphasis on clinical and pathologic correlation. Arch Dermatol 2009; 145:279.

Yasukawa K, et al: Necrobiotic xanthogranuloma: isolated skeletal muscle involvement and unusual changes. J Am Acad Dermatol 2005; 52:729.

conjunctivitis, keratitis, scleritis, uveitis, iritis, ectropion, or proptosis. Ulceration and scarring of the plaques and distortion of the eye may lead to visual occlusion. Blindness may result. Lymphadenopathy, hepatosplenomegaly, and mucosal, myocardial, and pulmonary lesions may occur. There is a monoclonal IgG (usually κ) paraproteinemia in 80% of cases, and rarely an IgA paraproteinemia (one patient had both). Thrombocytopenia, neutrophilia, neutropenia, and eosinophilia may be present. The bone marrow may show leukopenia, plasmacytosis (25–50% of patients), or frank myeloma (10–20% of patients). In some cases a myelodysplastic syndrome may be present or develop (chronic lymphocytic lymphoma, Hodgkin or non-Hodgkin lymphoma). The necrobiotic xanthogranuloma predates the development of the myeloma or myelodysplastic syndrome by an average of 2.5 years.

Histologically, there are extensive zones of degenerated collagen surrounded by palisaded macrophages. These macrophages are of various forms—foamy, Touton cells, epithelioid, and giant cells, sometimes with more than 50 nuclei. Atypical multinucleated giant cells with multiple nuclei clustered at one end of the cell (polarized nuclei) are seen in 80% or more of cases. The process extends into the fat, obliterating fat lobules. Cholesterol clefts and extracellular lipid deposits are prominent. Within this process is a perivascular and interstitial infiltrate of lymphocytes and plasma cells. Lymphoid follicles are present. In the skin, the lymphoid aggregates are polytypic. The histologic differential diagnosis includes necrobiosis lipoidica and other histiocytoses. Necrobiotic xanthogranuloma has more atypical and Touton giant cells, lymphoid nodules, and cholesterol clefts.

The treatment is usually directed at the paraprotein or underlying malignancy and consists of systemic corticosteroids, alkylating agents (including chlorambucil, cyclophosphamide, and melphalan), plasmapheresis, or local radiation therapy (for eye lesions). Anecdotally, high dose intravenous immunoglobin (0.5 g/kg/d for 4 consecutive days 2 g/kg total) at 4 week intervals, IFN-α 2b, 3–6 MU three times a week, in combination with systemic corticosteroids, and pulse cytoxan with dexamethasone both led to improvement. Simple excision is an option, but lesions may recur.

Chave TA, et al: Recalcitrant necrobiotic xanthogranuloma responding to pulsed high-dose oral dexamethasone plus maintenance therapy with oral prednisolone. Br J Dermatol 2001; 144:158.

Flann S, et al: Necrobiotic xanthogranuloma with paraproteinaemia. Clin Exp Dermatol 2006; 31:248.

Hallerman C, et al: Successful treatment of necrobiotic xanthogranuloma with intravenous immunoglobin. Arch Dermatol 2010; 146:957.

Meyer S, et al: Cyclophosphamide-dexamethasone pulsed therapy for treatment of recalcitrant necrobiotic xanthogranuloma with paraproteinemia and ocular involvement. Br J Dermatol 2005; 153:443.

Sarcoidosis

Sarcoidosis is a systemic granulomatous disease that involves the skin and many of the internal organs with an acute or persistent course. In addition to the skin, which is involved in approximately 25% of cases, other sites of involvement are the lungs, mediastinal and peripheral lymph nodes, eyes, phalangeal bones, myocardium, central nervous system (CNS), kidneys, spleen, liver, and parotid glands.

Sarcoidosis occurs worldwide. In Europe it is most prevalent in Scandinavia, especially in Sweden, with a prevalence of 64 in 100 000. In the UK, the rate is 20 in 100 000, and in France and Germany about 10 in 100 000, with lower rates in Spain and Japan of 1.4 in 100 000. In the US the southeastern states and certain urban centers (New York City, Detroit, and Washington DC) show the highest prevalence. In the US there is a marked racial variation with a rate of 10–14 in 100 000 for white persons and 35–64 in 100 000 for African Americans. The highest annual incidence is in African American women between the ages of 30 and 39, who have an annual incidence of 107 in 100 000. The lifetime risk for the development of sarcoidosis is 0.85% for white US residents, and 2.4% for African Americans. The disease begins most frequently between the ages of 20 and 40, and is slightly more common in women. Children may also develop sarcoidosis. There are two distinct forms of pediatric sarcoidosis. Early-onset disease, usually before the age of 4, is unique and characterized by the triad of skin lesions, uveitis, and arthritis. It is due to a defined genetic deficiency. It may be confused with juvenile rheumatoid arthritis. Older children, aged 8–14, present similarly to adults, with lymphadenopathy and pulmonary disease.

Several genetic associations have been made with sarcoidosis, but the underlying cause still remains a mystery. *HLA-DQB1*0201* and *HLA-DRB1*0301* are strongly associated with acute disease and a good prognosis. The butyrophilin-like 2 (*BTNL2*) gene is associated with sarcoidosis, but the mechanism of this association is unknown. Mutations in the promoter region of TNF are associated with erythema nodosum in sarcoidosis in white Caucasians, and a variant in intron 1 of the lymphotoxin alpha (*LTA*) gene is associated with erythema nodosum in Caucasian female sarcoidosis patients.

Cutaneous involvement in sarcoidosis may be classified as specific, which reveals granulomas on biopsy, or nonspecific, which is mainly reactive, such as erythema nodosum. In about 20% of cases the skin lesions appear before the systemic disease, in 50% there is simultaneous appearance of the skin and systemic lesions, and in 30% the skin lesions appear up to 10 years after the systemic disease has occurred. This is often coincidental with the tapering of systemic steroids for pulmonary sarcoidosis. The cutaneous manifestations of sarcoidosis are quite varied and numerous morphologic lesion types have been described. The morphology of the lesions in sarcoidosis might include papules, nodules, plaques, subcutaneous nodules, scar sarcoidosis, erythroderma, and ulcerations. The lesions may be verrucous, ichthyosiform, hypomelanotic, psoriasiform, or alopecic. They are usually multiple, firm, and

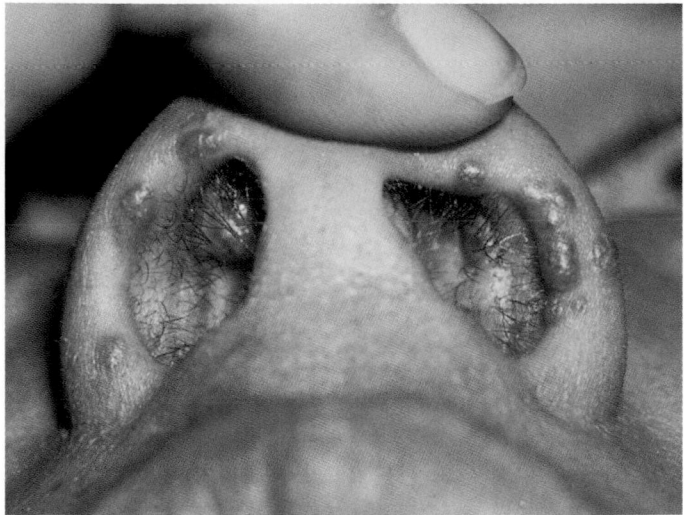

Fig. 31-9 Sarcoidosis, characteristic papules on the nares.

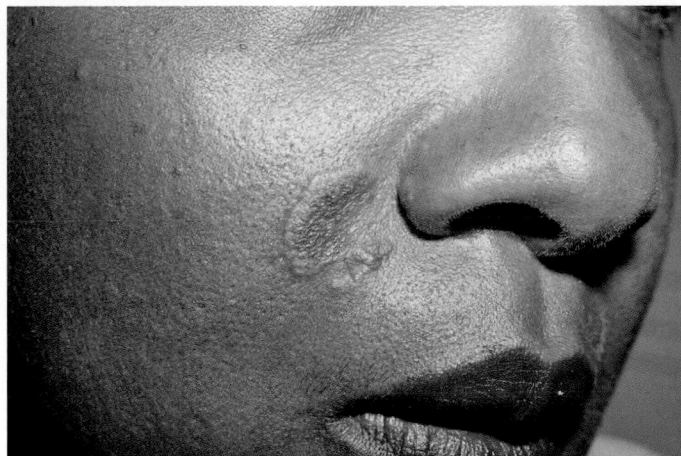

Fig. 31-10 Sarcoidosis, annular plaque.

elastic when palpated. They extend to involve the entire thickness of the dermis. The overlying epidermis may be slightly thinned, discolored, telangiectatic, or scaly. The color is faint, showing dull tints of red, purple, brown, or yellow according to the stage of development. Usually the lesions are asymptomatic, but approximately 10–15% of patients itch. There is a racial difference in the frequency of cutaneous lesions in sarcoidosis. Among white patients erythema nodosum is as frequent as the specific cutaneous manifestations and both types of cutaneous involvement occur in about 10% of white patients with sarcoidosis. In black patients, erythema nodosum is much less common; however, specific cutaneous manifestations occur in 50% or more of patients. The skin lesions in general do not correlate with the extent or nature of systemic involvement or with prognosis. The exceptions are erythema nodosum, which is associated with a good prognosis, and subcutaneous sarcoidosis and lupus pernio. The morphologic types of sarcoidosis are discussed below, and when possible, the relationship to systemic sarcoidosis is discussed.

Erythema nodosum in sarcoidosis

Erythema nodosum is the most common nonspecific cutaneous finding in sarcoidosis. Sarcoidosis may first appear with fever, polyarthralgias, uveitis, bilateral hilar adenopathy, fatigue, and erythema nodosum. This combination, known as Lofgren syndrome, occurs frequently in Scandinavian white persons and is uncommon in American blacks. The typical red, warm, and tender subcutaneous nodules of the anterior shins are distinctive and are most frequently seen in young women. The face, upper back, and extensor surfaces of the upper extremities may less commonly be involved. There is a strikingly elevated ESR, frequently above 50 mm/hr. Erythema nodosum is associated with a good prognosis, with the sarcoidosis involuting within 2 years of onset in 80% of cases. Conversely, the absence of erythema nodosum is a risk factor for persistent disease activity. Sweet's syndrome may also rarely be seen in association with sarcoidosis as a non-specific finding.

Papular sarcoid

Papules are the most common morphology of cutaneous sarcoidosis and are usually less than 1 cm in diameter. Lesions may be localized or generalized, in which case small papules predominate (Fig. 31-9). This is also known as miliary sarcoid.

The papules are especially numerous over the face, eyelids, neck, and shoulders. Plaques may occur by the expansion or coalescence of papules. In time the lesions involute to faint macules. Hyperkeratosis may rarely be prominent, giving the lesions a verrucous appearance. "Papular sarcoidosis of the knee" is distinctive, in that disease is often limited to this site. In this region the sarcoidal granulomas often contain foreign bodies. In Caucasians it often occurs in the context of Lofgren syndrome (see above) and has a good prognosis. Papular lesions along the alar rim in African Americans, in contrast, may be the first evidence of lupus pernio (see below) and portend a bad prognosis.

Annular sarcoidosis

Papular lesions may coalesce or be arranged in annular patterns, usually with a red–brown hue (Fig. 31-10). On palpation the lesions are indurated. Central clearing with hypopigmentation, atrophy, and scarring may occur. Lesions favor the head and neck, and are usually associated with chronic sarcoidosis. Alopecia may result in the center of the lesion. Annular plaques of sarcoidosis can preferentially develop in sun-exposed areas.

Hypopigmented sarcoidosis

Hypopigmentation may be the earliest sign of sarcoidosis and is usually diagnosed in darkly pigmented races. Lesions vary from a few millimeters to more than a centimeter in diameter and favor the extremities. Although they appear macular by visual inspection, on palpation a dermal or subcutaneous component is often palpable in the center of the lesion.

Lupus pernio

Lesions typically are brown to violaceous, smooth, shiny plaques on the head and neck, especially the nose (Fig. 31-11), cheeks, lips, forehead, and ears. They can be very disfiguring. Involvement of the nasal mucosa and underlying bone may occur and lead to nasal perforation and collapse of the nasal bridge. Upper aerodigestive tract involvement is also common. Ear, nose, and throat (ENT) evaluation is recommended. In three-quarters of cases of lupus pernio, chronic fibrotic respiratory tract involvement is found. In 43% of cases, lupus pernio is associated with granulomas in the bones (punched-out cysts), most commonly of the fingers. Chronic ocular lesions occur in 37% of cases. Sarcoid involving the sinus is

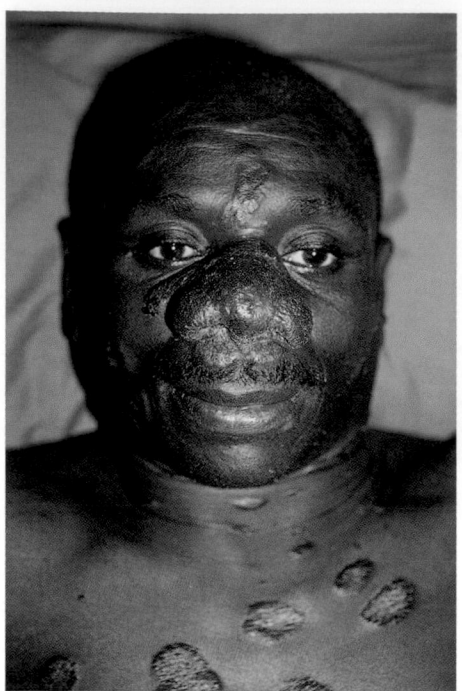

Fig. 31-11 Sarcoidosis, lupus pernio with rhinophymatous nasal changes.

associated with lupus pernio 50% of the time. Lupus pernio is typically seen in women in their fourth or fifth decade of life. The skin lesions rarely involve spontaneously. At times, lupus pernio may resemble rhinophyma. It is important to make the correct diagnosis, as ulceration of sarcoidal lesions may occur with laser treatment, even with pulsed dye laser.

Ulcerative sarcoidosis

Ulcerative sarcoidosis is very rare, affecting about 0.5% of patients with sarcoidosis. It affects primarily blacks, but it is also well recognized in Japanese. It is 2–3 times more common in women than men. In one-third of cases it is the presenting finding of sarcoidosis, except in Japan where it is commonly a late finding in patients with known sarcoidosis. The ulcerations may occur de novo or in sarcoidal plaques. Lesions favor the lower extremities, but most patients have lesions in more than one anatomic region. Trauma may be the inciting event. The clinical appearance may not be specific, but skin biopsies are diagnostic. Lupus pernio may also be present. Many patients have multisystem sarcoidosis, although uncommonly no other evidence of sarcoidosis is found. Biopsies may show necrosis in the center of sarcoidal granulomas. Methotrexate, which can be therapeutic in sarcoidosis, may also lead to ulceration in sarcoidosis patients.

Subcutaneous sarcoidosis

About 10% of patients with cutaneous sarcoidosis will have subcutaneous lesions. They may also have other types of specific lesion, along with subcutaneous lesions. Subcutaneous sarcoidosis is also known as Darier–Roussy sarcoid and consists of a few to numerous 0.5–3 cm, deep-seated nodules on the trunk and extremities; only rarely do they appear on the face. The overlying epidermis may be normal (30%), erythematous (50%), or slightly violaceous (10%). The lesions are usually asymptomatic. Ninety percent of patients will have multiple lesions, and the upper extremity is most frequently affected (virtually 100% of patients). Lesions on the upper extremity have a tendency to form indurated linear bands from the elbow to the hand on the cubital side of the forearm. The amount of subcutaneous involvement in the upper extremity may be so extensive as to simulate chronic cellulitis. A biopsy is usually required to confirm the diagnosis. About 90% of patients will have systemic involvement, usually bilateral hilar adenopathy, but the overall prognosis is good.

Plaques

These distinctive lesions are flat-surfaced, slightly elevated plaques that appear with greatest frequency on the cheeks, limbs, and trunk symmetrically. Superficial nodules may be superimposed and coalescence of plaques may lead to serpiginous lesions. Involvement of the scalp may lead to permanent alopecia. The finding of alopecia in an annular plaque with a raised border should raise the diagnostic consideration of sarcoidosis.

Erythrodermic sarcoidosis

Erythrodermic sarcoidosis is an extremely rare form of sarcoidosis. A diffuse infiltrative erythroderma of the skin usually begins as erythematous, scaling patches that merge to involve large portions of the body. A biopsy is confirmatory, but the diagnosis can be clinically suspected if small apple jelly papules are seen on diascopy throughout the erythroderma.

Ichthyosiform sarcoidosis

Ichthyosiform sarcoidosis resembles ichthyosis vulgaris or acquired ichthyosis, with fine scaling usually on the distal extremities (Fig. 31-12). It is virtually always seen in non-white persons, especially African Americans. Nearly all patients have or will develop systemic disease. In 75% of patients, the skin lesions follow or occur at the same time as the diagnosis of systemic sarcoidosis. Although the lesions have no palpable component, a biopsy will reveal dermal noncaseating granulomas.

Alopecia

Alopecia on the scalp due to sarcoidosis can have multiple morphologies. Plaques may extend into and involve the scalp, leading to scarring hair loss (Fig. 31-13). More rarely, macular lesions from one to several centimeters in diameter appear on the scalp and closely resemble alopecia areata. This form may be permanent or reversible. Diffuse alopecia, scaly plaques resembling seborrheic dermatitis, and cicatricial lesions resembling discoid lupus erythematosus or pseudopelade may also occur. A biopsy of all forms of alopecic sarcoid will reveal dermal granulomas and sometimes loss of follicular structures. Scalp sarcoidosis is virtually always seen in African or African American women. In cases where sarcoidosis affects the scalp, causing alopecia, the patient virtually always has other cutaneous lesions and the vast majority of cases will demonstrate systemic involvement.

Morpheaform sarcoidosis

Very rarely, specific cutaneous lesions of sarcoidosis may be accompanied by substantial fibrosis and simulate morphea. Less than 10 cases have been described to date. Most typically, the lesions are localized and resemble linear morphea. Skin biopsy will demonstrate noncaseating granulomas. African American women are most commonly affected. This form of sarcoidosis responds favorably to antimalarial therapy.

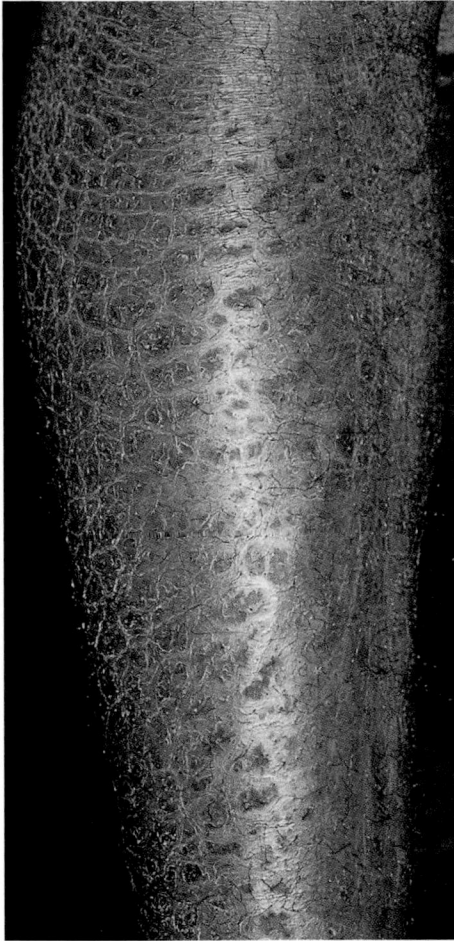

Fig. 31-12 Sarcoidosis, ichthyosiform type; biopsy showed noncaseating granuloma, although there was no palpable dermal component to the lesions.

Sarcoidosis in scars (scar sarcoid)

Infiltration and elevation of tattoos and old flat scars are two variants of scar sarcoid. Previously flat scars become raised and may become erythematous or violaceous. These lesions may be confused with hypertrophic scars. Infiltration of tattoos may be the first manifestation of sarcoidosis and can be confused with a granulomatous hypersensitivity reaction to the tattoo pigment (Fig. 31-14). Cosmetic tattooing, as may be performed in a dermatology office, may result in sarcoidal granulomas in patients with pulmonary sarcoidosis. Hyaluronic acid injections can also be complicated by the development of sarcoidal lesions in patients with sarcoidosis. As noted below, patients with hepatitis C virus (HCV) infection receiving IFN therapy are at high risk for developing sarcoidosis and can develop disfiguring sarcoidal reactions following cosmetic filler injections. Similar granulomatous reactions may occur in the earlobe following ear piercing, and represent granulomatous dermatitis to metals introduced by the procedure or the earring. Titanium, nickel, cobalt, zinc, gold, and palladium can all be the allergen.

From 22 to 77% of biopsies from patients with cutaneous sarcoidosis will contain polarizable foreign material, suggesting that scar sarcoidosis is very common. The foreign material seems to be a nidus that favors the development of sarcoidal granulomas when sarcoidosis develops. Scar sarcoid may sometimes occur in patients with acute disease and erythema nodosum, especially if the lesions are small papules on the knees. It may also occur in patients with chronic sarcoidosis. The presence of polarizable material in a granulomatous

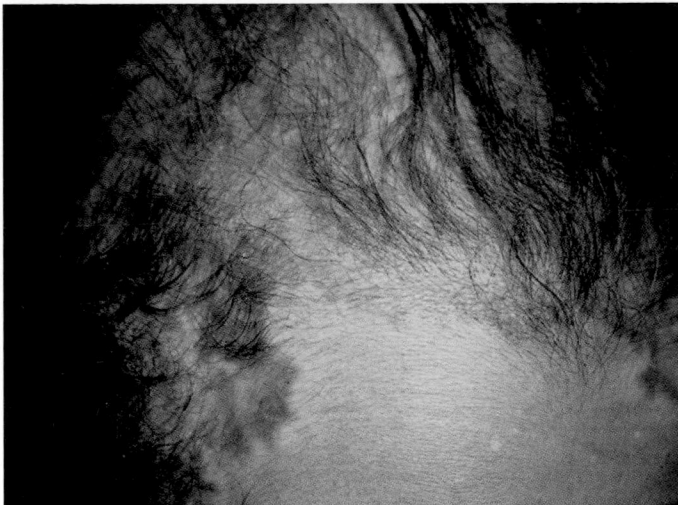

Fig. 31-13 Sarcoidosis, scarring alopecia of the scalp.

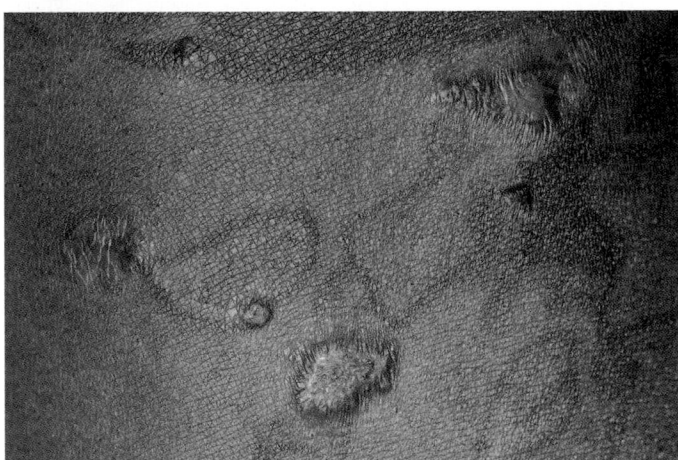

Fig. 31-14 Sarcoidosis, papules and plaques arising in a tattoo.

process does not confirm the diagnosis of "foreign body granuloma," but rather should result in evaluation of the patient for evidence of systemic sarcoidosis. When foreign material is found, infection must be carefully excluded if no other features of sarcoidosis are found.

Mucosal sarcoidosis

The lesions in the mouth are characterized by pinhead-size papules that may be grouped and fused together to form a flat plaque. The hard palate, tongue, buccal mucosa, or posterior pharynx may be involved. They may simulate Fordyce spots. In lupus pernio the nasal mucosa is frequently involved. Rarely, in ulcerative sarcoidosis, the oral mucosa may be involved. Sarcoidosis may also infiltrate the gingiva, causing "strawberry gums" that simulate Wegener's granulomatosis.

Systemic sarcoidosis

Sarcoidosis may involve virtually every internal organ and its presentations are protean. Many instances of sarcoidosis are asymptomatic and it is only when routine radiographs of the chest reveal some abnormality that sarcoidosis is suspected. Fever may be the only symptom of the disease or be accompanied by weight loss, fatigue, and malaise.

Intrathoracic lesions, including parenchymal lung lesions and hilar adenopathy, are the most common manifestation of the disease, occurring in 90% of cases of sarcoidosis. Pulmonary changes are staged as follows:

Stage 0: normal

Stage I: bilateral hilar and/or paratracheal adenopathy

Stage II: adenopathy with pulmonary infiltrates

Stage III: pulmonary infiltrates only

Stage IV: pulmonary fibrosis.

Transbronchial lung biopsy and needle aspiration have a high yield in confirming the diagnosis of sarcoidosis, even in patients with only stage I changes on chest x-ray. Gallium-67 scanning is useful in the diagnosis of sarcoidosis since typical patterns of uptake are seen. The panda sign correlates with gallium uptake in the nasopharynx and lacrimal and parotid glands; the lambda sign correlates with uptake in the paratracheal lymph nodes. These characteristic findings, plus a skin biopsy demonstrating typical sarcoidal granulomas, can be used as presumptive evidence for sarcoidosis.

Lymphadenopathy, especially of the mediastinal and hilar nodes, and generalized adenopathy, or adenopathy confined to the cervical or axillary areas, may be an initial sign of sarcoidosis or may occur during the course of the disease.

Polyarthralgias may be seen with acute sarcoidosis or as a component of chronic disease. Chronic arthritis may occur (Fig. 31-15). Osseous involvement is often present in chronic disease. The most characteristic changes are found radiographically in the bones of the hands and feet, particularly in the phalanges. They consist of round, punched-out, lytic, cystic lesions. These are seen frequently in patients with lupus pernio. The bone lesions represent epithelioid granulomas.

Ocular involvement is present in 30–50% of patients, with granulomatous uveitis the most characteristic lesion. The lacrimal gland may be involved unilaterally or bilaterally by painless nodular swellings. Lesions of the iris are nodular and painless. There may also be lesions of the retina, choroid, sclera, and optic nerve. Ophthalmic disease is highly correlated with systemic involvement. All patients, even those who have no ocular symptoms, should be seen by an ophthalmologist. Sarcoidal involvement of the eye can progress to blindness. Conjunctival biopsy is positive in about 50% of patients with sarcoidosis, making it an easy site to sample and confirm the diagnosis.

Parotid gland and lacrimal gland enlargement with uveitis and fever may occur in sarcoidosis; this is known as uveoparotid fever or Heerfordt syndrome, and usually lasts 2–6 months if not treated. Facial nerve palsy and CNS disease are frequently seen in this syndrome. Mikulicz syndrome is bilateral sarcoidosis of the parotid, submandibular, sublingual, and lacrimal glands.

Clinically apparent hepatic involvement occurs in about 20% of patients; however, a blind liver biopsy will reveal granulomas in 60% of cases. Hepatomegaly with elevation of serum alkaline phosphatase, biliary cirrhosis with hypercholesterolemia, and portal hypertension with esophageal varices are some of the manifestations. Liver biopsy showing hepatic granulomas is an excellent means of confirming the diagnosis of sarcoidosis.

Renal disease may be due to direct involvement with granulomas or secondary to hypercalcemia. Hypercalcemia is due to the macrophage in the granulomas having large amounts of 25-hydroxyvitamin D-1α-hydroxylase, which converts 25-hydroxyvitamin D to the more active 1,25 dihydroxyvitamin D. Nephrolithiasis may result. Cardiac involvement occurs in 5% of cases, but in a higher percentage of autopsy cases.

Neurosarcoidosis occurs in 5–10% of patients. It can present in numerous ways, from focal cranial nerve involvement (most commonly facial nerve palsy) to aseptic meningitis, seizures, psychiatric changes, stroke, and space-occupying lesions. Neurosarcoidosis tends to be chronic and relapsing, with a higher mortality rate. Vision loss in sarcoidosis after heat exposure is called the Uhthoff phenomenon. Magnetic resonance imaging (MRI) with gadolinium is useful for detecting CNS lesions of sarcoidosis and following therapy. Treatment is recommended with corticosteroids and an immunosuppressive agent until all MRI-visible lesions are eradicated.

Measuring ACE levels in sarcoidosis patients has little utility. ACE levels may be elevated in all granulomatous diseases, including infectious granulomatous disorders. An elevated ACE level is suggestive of, but not diagnostic for granulomatous inflammation. A normal ACE level cannot be used to rule out sarcoidosis and an elevated level does not necessarily indicate the presence of multisystem involvement. The use of 18FDG positron emission tomography (PET) is more accurate in identifying extent of involvement and monitoring response to treatment.

Pediatric sarcoidosis

Childhood sarcoidosis is rare. The clinical features are very age-dependent. In children under 4 years, the triad of skin, joint, and eye involvement is characteristic, and often confused with juvenile rheumatoid arthritis. In older children, lung, lymph node, and eye involvement is typical. Calcium abnormalities are present in 30% of children with sarcoidosis. Older children develop specific sarcoidal skin lesions at the same rate as adults, about 30% of the time. One presentation resembles granulomatous peri-orificial dermatitis.

Blau syndrome is due to mutations in the *NOD2* gene and is associated with early-onset sarcoidosis (age <4 years). It is more common in white patients. Skin lesions are typically small papules and are the first clinical feature in more than half of patients, starting at a median age of 1 year. The skin lesions are often generalized and may be flat-topped, giving them a lichenoid appearance. They are red–brown to tan and can occur in clusters or linear arrays. The face may have confluent lesions. Infliximab can be beneficial in early-onset sarcoidosis/Blau syndrome.

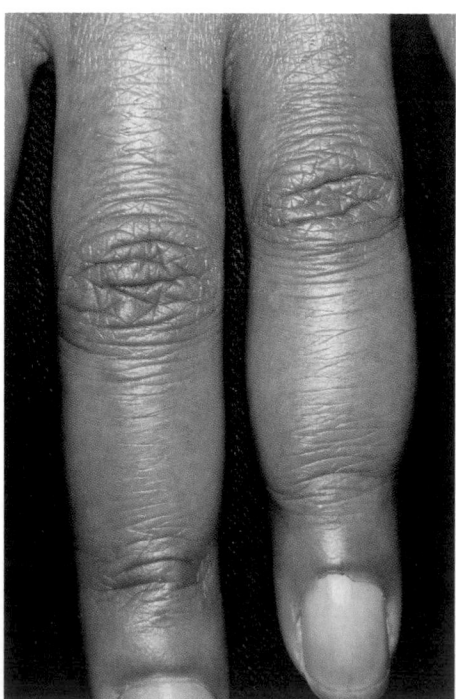

Fig. 31-15 Sarcoidosis, fusiform swelling of the digits.

Histopathology

The histology of sarcoidosis in all affected tissues is identical. The characteristic finding is that of the "naked tubercle," composed of collections of large, pale-staining, epithelioid histiocytes. There may be small foci of necrosis in the center of the granulomas, and multinucleate giant cells, sometimes with inclusions (asteroid bodies and Schaumann bodies), may be present. Although classically there are few lymphocytes around the granulomas, they may be numerous. The granulomas may be nodular, diffuse, or tubular along neurovascular structures. Perifollicular and other periadnexal involvement can be seen in sarcoidosis.

The histologic differential diagnosis is broad and the diagnosis of sarcoidosis cannot be definitely made histologically. Allergic granulomas caused by metals are histologically identical to sarcoidosis. Other foreign body granulomas (especially as a result of silica), granulomatous rosacea, granulomatous secondary syphilis, tuberculoid leprosy, atypical mycobacterial infections, and leishmaniasis may closely simulate sarcoidosis.

The diagnosis of sarcoidosis is established by the demonstration of involvement consistent with sarcoidosis in two different organ systems. This is usually done histologically, or by characteristic findings with radiological techniques (including gallium scans, PET scans, and MRI). If cutaneous sarcoidal granulomas are identified in a patient with no prior history of sarcoidosis, the first diagnostic test to be performed should be a chest radiograph. If this is abnormal, further pulmonary evaluation is indicated. Ophthalmologic evaluation and conjunctival biopsy may be useful. Since many patients with sarcoidosis may develop ocular involvement that may be asymptomatic, every patient should see an ophthalmologist. Blind biopsy of the minor salivary glands may demonstrate sarcoidal granulomas in about 50% of patients with systemic sarcoidosis. Otherwise, histologic evaluation of any involved tissue may be considered. The site for biopsy may be guided by PET scans, which, if characteristic, can be used to support the diagnosis.

Sarcoidosis in the setting of immunologic abnormalities

Numerous reports document sarcoidosis occurring in patients with various forms of spontaneous or iatrogenic immunological aberrations. Sarcoidosis may be associated with lymphoma, especially Hodgkin disease ("sarcoidosis–lymphoma syndrome"). B-cell lymphoma, chronic myeloid and lymphoid leukemia, and MALT lymphoma have all been described in patients with sarcoidosis. Sarcoidosis patients are about 40–60% more likely to develop malignancy, including solid tumors such as non-melanoma skin cancers (three-fold risk), renal cancer, and nonthyroid endocrine tumors. In addition, adenopathy in patients with lymphoma or solid tumors may demonstrate sarcoidal granulomas without tumor. This is important to know when a patient with a cancer develops an enlarged node, and makes sampling of the node important to avoid unnecessary therapy. Sézary syndrome with extensive cutaneous granulomas has been described.

Alteration of the immune system with medications can lead to the development of systemic sarcoidosis. These typically cause a constellation of pulmonary and cutaneous disease. Etanercept, adalimumab, and infliximab (the TNF inhibitors) have all been reported to trigger sarcoidosis. This is ironic, since they are also often therapeutic in sarcoidosis (analogous to the situation with TNF inhibitors and psoriasis). There are numerous reports documenting the appearance of sarcoidosis in association with IFN-α therapy, usually for the treatment of HCV infection. HCV alone may also trigger sarcoidosis. Cutaneous lesions (60% of patients), pulmonary findings (75% of patients), or both, as well as other features of sarcoidosis, occur in 5% of patients treated with IFN-α for HCV. The addition of ribavirin may increase the risk. In more than 80% of cases the sarcoidosis resolves after the treatment is discontinued. Treatment of HIV infection with highly active antiretroviral therapy (HAART) has led to the appearance of sarcoidosis or tattoo granulomas, apparently by enhancing the number and function of helper T cells. Sarcoidosis is now well recognized as a feature of immune reconstitution syndrome (IRIS). Hematopoietic stem cell transplantation, both allogenic or autologous, has been associated with the appearance of pulmonary sarcoidosis. If the transplantation is performed for malignant disease, the presence of hilar adenopathy may be interpreted as recurrent or metastatic disease, and inappropriate treatment may be given. Other medications causing sarcoidosis include alemtuzumab (anti-CD52 monoclonal antibody for CTCL) and ipilimumab (anti CTLA4 monoclonal antibody for malignant melanoma).

Differential diagnosis

Granulomatous secondary syphilis may closely simulate sarcoidosis both clinically and histologically. Blau syndrome, an autosomal-dominant granulomatous disease, is similar to childhood sarcoidosis. It can be distinguished from sarcoidosis by the lack of pulmonary involvement. Granulomatous cutaneous T-cell lymphoma can usually be distinguished histologically and by the presence of pulmonary involvement in sarcoidosis.

Treatment

Numerous therapies have been reported as beneficial in cutaneous sarcoidosis, usually after anecdotal observation. There is virtually no information regarding what types of therapy are best for which of the various cutaneous manifestations. The cutaneous disease may spontaneously remit without treatment. Because most skin lesions are asymptomatic, the major indication for treatment is cosmetic.

Systemic corticosteroids are virtually always beneficial in cutaneous sarcoidosis. Unfortunately, the doses required to control cutaneous disease may be too high (usually in excess of 15 mg/day) to be ideal for long-term use. For limited skin disease, intralesional injection of 2.5–5.0 mg/mL of triamcinolone acetonide suspension is very effective. For thinner lesions, superpotent topical steroids, topical tacrolimus, and UVA1 phototherapy may be effective. A trial of minocycline or doxycycline, up to 100 mg twice a day, may be considered in patients with skin lesions in whom systemic disease does not require treatment. Maximum response is reported to occur at 3 months of therapy.

Local surgical procedures can be beneficial for some forms of sarcoidosis. Pulsed dye laser, used repeatedly, photodynamic therapy, and even CO_2 laser remodeling may be effective in the appropriate cases. In severe lupus pernio, nasal skin excision followed by flap reconstruction can lead to dramatic improvement.

Systemic corticosteroid therapy is indicated when there is acute systemic involvement with fever and weight loss, in active eye disease, in sarcoidal involvement of the myocardium, in active pulmonary disease with functional disability, in hypersplenism, in hypercalcemia, and in symptomatic CNS involvement.

Antimalarials, both chloroquine and hydroxychloroquine, have been used to treat extensive cutaneous sarcoidosis, in doses of 250 mg/day or 200–400 mg/day, respectively. About three-quarters of patients appear to respond partially or completely. In some cases the associated CNS disease or hypercalcemia also improves. These agents may also be used to reduce the dose of systemic steroids required.

Methotrexate, in doses of 15–25 mg/week, is also efficacious and seems to help patients with severe lupus pernio or ulcerative sarcoidosis who are otherwise very difficult to treat. Methotrexate-induced hepatitis occurs in 15% of patients with sarcoidosis treated with methotrexate. Leflunomide may be given in analogous fashion to methotrexate and may be used in patients with gastrointestinal intolerance for methotrexate. Response rates are about 75%. The retinoids, principally isotretinoin, have been reported as beneficial in some patients, usually at doses of 0.5–1.0 mg/kg. Response is only seen after 6 weeks or more. Thalidomide, 50–200 mg/day, has led to improvement of the skin lesions after several months. It should not be used to treat pregnant patients, however, because of possible teratogenic effects on the fetus. Venous thrombosis may complicate thalidomide therapy, especially if doses above 100 mg/day are used. While azathioprine and cyclophosphamide had been used for refractory disease, mycophenolate mofetil has shown efficacy in mucocutaneous disease and may be considered as an effective form of rescue and steroid-sparing therapy. The combination of thalidomide, an immunosuppressive agent, with an antimalarial may be effective when these agents fail individually. Such combination therapy in addition to anti-TNF agents may be necessary in severe sarcoidosis. TNF is an important cytokine in the formation of granulomas. Not surprisingly, TNF inhibitors, including infliximab, etanercept, and adalimumab, can be effective in refractory cutaneous and systemic sarcoidosis. Infliximab appears to be particularly beneficial in controlling severe lupus pernio.

Ahmed I, Harshad SR: Subcutaneous sarcoidosis: is it a specific subset of cutaneous sarcoidosis frequently associated with systemic disease? J Am Acad Dermatol 2006; 54:55.

Antonovich DD, Callen JP: Development of sarcoidosis in cosmetic tattoos. Arch Dermatol 2005; 141:869.

Arostequi JI, et al: NOD2 gene-associated pediatric granulomatous arthritis: clinical diversity, novel and recurrent mutations, and evidence of clinical improvement with interleukin-1 blockade in a Spanish cohort. Arthritis Rheum 2007; 56:3805

Bachelez H, et al: The use of tetracyclines for the treatment of sarcoidosis. Arch Dermatol 2001; 137:69.

Badgwell C, Rosen T: Cutaneous sarcoidosis therapy updated. J Am Acad Dermatol 2007; 56:69.

Baughman RP, et al: Infliximab therapy in patients with chronic sarcoidosis and pulmonary involvement. Am J Respir Crit Care Med 2006; 174:795.

Bhagat R, et al: Pulmonary sarcoidosis following stem cell transplantation: is it more than a chance occurrence? Chest 2004; 126:642.

Caras WE, et al: Coexistence of sarcoidosis and malignancy. South Med J 2003; 96:918.

Cardoso JC, et al: Cutaneous sarcoidosis: a histopathological study. J Eur Acad Dermatol Venereol 2009; 23:678.

Choi HJ, et al: Papular sarcoidosis limited to the knees: a clue for systemic sarcoidosis. Int J Dermatol 2006; 45:169.

Coto-Segura P, et al: A sporadic case of early-onset sarcoidosis resembling Blau syndrome due to the recurrent R334W missense mutation on the NOD2 gene. Br J Dermatol 2007; 157:1257.

Dadban A, et al: Association of Sweet's syndrome and acute sarcoidosis: report of a case and review of the literature. Clin Exp Dermatol 2009; 34:189.

Daien CI, et al: Sarcoid-like granulomatosis in patients treated with tumor necrosis factor blockers: 10 cases. Rheumatology (Oxford) 2009; 48:883.

Dal Sacco D, et al: Scar sarcoidosis after hyaluronic acid injection. Int J Dermatol 2005; 44:411.

Dash SS, et al: Discoid lupus erythematosus-like sarcoidosis. Clin Exp Dermatol 2007; 32:442.

Descamps V, et al: Facial cosmetic filler injections as possible target for systemic sarcoidosis in patients treated with interferon for chronic hepatitis C: two cases. Dermatology 2008; 217:81.

Eckert A, et al: Anti-CTLA4 monoclonal antibody induced sarcoidosis in a metastatic melanoma patient. Dermatology 2009; 218:69.

Garrido-Ruiz MC, et al: Lichenoid sarcoidosis: a case with clinical and histopathological lichenoid features. Am J Dermatopathol 2008; 30:271.

Ginarte M, et al: Morpheaform sarcoidosis. Acta Derm Venereol 2006; 86:264.

Goossens A, et al: Allergic contact granuloma due to palladium following ear piercing. Contact Dermatitis 2006; 55:338.

Green JJ, Lawrence N: Generalized ulcerative sarcoidosis induced by therapy with the flashlamp-pumped pulsed dye laser. Arch Dermatol 2000; 137:507.

Gregg PJ, et al: Sarcoidal tissue reaction in Sézary syndrome. J Am Acad Dermatol 2000; 43:372.

Haley H, et al: Infliximab therapy for sarcoidosis (lupus pernio). Br J Dermatol 2004; 150:146.

Heffernan MP, Anadkat MJ: Recalcitrant cutaneous sarcoidosis responding to infliximab. Arch Dermatol 2005; 141:910.

Heffernan MP, Smith DI: Adalimumab for treatment of cutaneous sarcoidosis. Arch Dermatol 2006; 142:17.

High WA, et al: Granulomatous reaction to titanium alloy: an unusual reaction to ear piercing. J Am Acad Dermatol 2006; 55:716.

Hurst EA, Mauro T: Sarcoidosis associated with pegylated interferon alfa and ribavirin treatment for chronic hepatitis C: a case report and review of the literature. Arch Dermatol 2005; 141:865.

Iannuzzi MC, et al: Sarcoidosis. N Engl J Med 2007; 357:2153.

Ichiki Y, Kitajima Y: Ulcerative sarcoidosis: a case report and review of the Japanese literature. Acta Derm Venereol 2008; 88:526.

Ji J, et al: Cancer risk in hospitalized sarcoidosis patients: a follow-up study in Sweden. Ann Oncol 2009; 20:1121.

Ji R, et al: Cutaneous sarcoidosis. Ann Acad Med Singapore 2007; 36:1044.

Kalajian AH, et al: Sarcoidal anemia and leucopenia treated with methotrexate and mycophenolate mofetil. Arch Dermatol 2009; 145:905.

Kapoor S: Cutaneous and systemic malignancies in patients with sarcoidosis: a close association. Ann Acad Med Singapore 2009; 38:179.

Katoh N, et al: Cutaneous sarcoidosis successfully treated with topical tacrolimus. Br J Dermatol 2002; 147:154.

Katta R, et al: Sarcoidosis of the scalp: a case series and review of the literature. J Am Acad Dermatol 2000; 42:690.

Khanna D, et al: Etanercept ameliorates sarcoidosis arthritis and skin disease. J Rheumatol 2003; 30:1864.

Kim C, Long WT: Sarcoidosis. Dermatol Online J 2004; 10:24.

Kouba DJ, et al: Mycophenolate mofetil may serve as a steroid-sparing agent for sarcoidosis. Br J Dermatol 2003; 148:147.

Kowalczyk JP, et al: "Strawberry gums" in sarcoidosis. J Am Acad Dermatol 2008; 59:S118.

Kwon EJ, et al: Interstitial granulomatous lesions as part of the spectrum of presenting cutaneous signs in pediatric sarcoidosis. Pediatr Dermatol 2007; 24:517.

Liu DTL, et al: Ophthalmology for diagnosis of sarcoidosis. Lancet 2004; 3:578.

Lodha S, et al: Sarcoidosis of the skin: a review for the pulmonologist. Chest 2009; 136:583.

Mahnke N, et al: Cutaneous sarcoidosis treated with medium-dose UVA1. J Am Acad Dermatol 2004; 50:978.

Mangas C, et al: Clinical spectrum and histological analysis of 32 cases of specific cutaneous sarcoidosis. J Cutan Pathol 2006; 33:772.

Marcoval J, et al: Subcutaneous sarcoidosis—clinicopathological study of 10 cases. Br J Dermatol 2005; 153:790.

McDougal KE, et al: Variation in the lymphotoxin-alpha/tumor necrosis factor locus modifies risk of erythema nodosum in sarcoidosis. J Invest Dermatol 2009; 129:1921.

Milman N, et al: Favourable effect of TNF-alpha inhibitor (infliximab) on Blau syndrome in monozygotic twins with a de novo CARD15 mutation. APMIS 2006; 114:912.

Morales-Callaghan AM Jr, et al: Sarcoid granuloma on black tattoo. J Am Acad Dermatol 2006; 55:S71.

Mortimer NJ, et al: Childhood sarcoidosis presenting with extensive cutaneous lesion, bilateral hilar lymphadenopathy and severe hypercalcaemia. Australas J Dermatol 2007; 48:233.

Moss J, et al: Mycobacterial infection masquerading as cutaneous sarcoidosis. Clin Exp Dermatol 2009; 34:e199.

Mutlu GM, Rubinstein I: Clinical manifestations of sarcoidosis among inner-city African-American dwellers. J Natl Med Assoc 2006; 98:1140.

Nguyen YT, et al: Treatment of cutaneous sarcoidosis with thalidomide. J Am Acad Dermatol 2004; 50:235.

O'Donoghue NB, Barlow RJ: Laser remodeling of nodular nasal lupus pernio. Clin Exp Dermatol 2006; 31:27.

Osawa R, et al: Chain saw blade granuloma: reaction to a deeply embedded metal fragment. Arch Dermatol 2006; 142:1079.

Papadavid E, et al: Subcutaneous sarcoidosis masquerading as cellulitis. Dermatology 2008; 217:212.

Pascual JC, et al: Sarcoidosis after highly active antiretroviral therapy in a patient with AIDS. Clin Exp Dermatol 2004; 29:156.

Perez-Gala S, et al: Cutaneous sarcoidosis limited to scars following pegylated interferon alfa and ribavirin therapy in a patient with chronic hepatitis C. J Eur Acad Dermatol Venereol 2007; 21:393.

Philips MA, et al: Ulcerative cutaneous sarcoidosis responding to adalimumab. J Am Acad Dermatol 2005; 53:917.

Ramos-Casals M, et al: Sarcoidosis in patients with chronic hepatitis C virus infection: analysis of 68 cases. Medicine (Baltimore) 2005; 84:69.

Reich JM: Concurrent sarcoidosis and lung cancer. Chest 2009; 136:943.

Roos S, et al: Successful treatment of cutaneous sarcoidosis lesions with the flashlamp pumped pulsed dye laser: a case report. Dermatol Surg 2009; 35:1139.

Rosen T, Doherty C: Successful long-term management of refractory cutaneous and upper airway sarcoidosis with periodic infliximab infusion. Dermatol Online J 2007; 13:14.

Rosenberg B: Ichthyosiform sarcoidosis. Dermatol Online J 2005; 11:15.

Schaffter JV, et al: Widespread granulomatous dermatitis of infancy: an early sign of Blau syndrome. Arch Dermatol 2007; 143:386.

Shetty AK, et al: Pediatric sarcoidosis. J Am Acad Dermatol 2003; 48:150.

Shigemitsu H, et al: Is sarcoidosis frequent in patients with cancer? Curr Opin Pulm Med 2008; 14:478.

Shinya C, et al: Cutaneous sarcoidosis presenting with pinhead-sized papules. Eur J Dermatol 2008; 18:191.

Smith R, et al: Improving cosmesis of lupus pernio by excision and forehead flap reconstruction. Clin Exp Dermatol 2009; 34:e25.

Stagaki E, et al: The treatment of lupus pernio: results of 116 treatment courses in 54 patients. Chest 2009; 135:468.

Thachil J, et al: The development of sarcoidosis with the use of alemtuzumab—clues to T-cell immune reconstitution. Br J Haematol 2007; 138:559.

Trevenzoli M, et al: Sarcoidosis and HIV infection: a case report and a review of the literature. Postgrad Med J 2003; 79:535.

Trokhan EQ, et al: Destructive lupus pernio masquerading as rhinophyma in a patient with eruptive syringoma. J Am Acad Dermatol 2004; 50:P40.

Wilsmann-Theis D, et al: Photodynamic therapy as an alternative treatment for cutaneous sarcoidosis. Dermatology 2008; 217:343.

Histiocytoses

These disorders are characterized by infiltrates which contain either Langerhans cells (the X-type histiocytoses) or infiltrates of non-Langerhans cell histiocytes (the non-X histiocytoses).

Non-X histiocytoses

Zelger and Burgdorf proposed classifying this group of disorders as the "xanthogranuloma family." Their classification scheme relies on the morphology of the monocyte/macrophage composing the lesion. Weitzman and Jaffe refined this concept and outlined the immunohistochemical features of the cells involved. These classification schemas are useful for this uncommon group of disorders. However, since the histiocytes within any disorder can change their appearance, no one specific morphological cell type absolutely characterizes these disorders. There are three large families of histiocytoses based on these classification schema—X-type histiocytosis or Langerhans cell histiocytosis (LCH); non-LCH histiocytoses of the juvenile xanthogranuloma (JXG) family (which have the phenotype of dermal dendritic cells, being positive for factor XIIIa, fascin, MS-1, and CD68); and multicentric reticulohistiocytosis and sinus histiocytosis with massive lymphadenopathy (SHML; Rosai–Dorfman disease), which are felt to not be in the JXG family of non-X histiocytoses. In the end, the final diagnosis is established by typical clinical features, a compatible histology, and an evolution typical for that disorder (Fig. 31.16).

The non-X histiocytoses are divided clinically into three groups: those involving primarily or only the skin (JXG); those that affect the skin but have a major systemic component (Erdheim–Chester disease); and those that are primarily a systemic disease with occasional skin lesions as a part of the disease (SHML). At any level of differentiation or appearance of the histiocyte there may be a disease in any category. Conceptually, this allows one to think of the JXG group of non-X histiocytoses as lying along a spectrum: benign cephalic histiocytosis, JXG, Erdheim–Chester disease, generalized eruptive histiocytosis, xanthoma disseminatum, and progressive nodular histiocytosis. Most diseases at the beginning of the spectrum are localized benign disorders; as one progresses through the diseases they tend to become more generalized but are still benign; at the end of the spectrum lie diseases that are less likely to involute and may have visceral involvement. This parallels the histological appearance of the infiltrating histiocyte, which progresses from scalloped to vacuolated to xanthomatized and finally spindled. In any disease, however, many morphologies of the histiocyte may be seen.

Weitzman S, Jaffe R: Review: uncommon histiocytic disorders. The non-Langerhans cell histiocytoses. Pediatr Blood Cancer 2005; 45:256.

Zelger B, Burgdorf WHC: The cutaneous "histiocytoses." In: Advances in Dermatology, vol. 17, ch 4. St Louis: Mosby, 2001.

Juvenile xanthogranuloma

Juvenile xanthogranuloma (JXG) is the most common non-LCH. Between 20 and 35% of lesions are congenital. The vast majority of lesions (70%) are diagnosed within the first year of life. The mean age of onset is 22 months, and the median 5 months (demonstrating the proclivity for early onset). Eighty percent of cases are solitary (Fig. 31-17). Boys are slightly more commonly affected than girls (1.5:1). In adults, lesions tend to occur in the late twenties to early thirties, and the gender distribution is equal. JXG is 10 times more common in white than black persons, but occurs in all races. Multiple cutaneous lesions affect male children much more commonly (12:1).

JXGs begin as well-demarcated, firm, rubbery, round to oval dermal papules or nodules from 5 to 10 mm in diameter. Early lesions are pink to red with a yellow tinge and become tan-brown over time. By dermoscopy, the lesions have an orange-yellow background, a subtle erythematous border with branched and linear vessels running from the edge to the center of the lesion, and "clouds" of paler yellow areas representing areas of xanthomatized histiocytes. Most lesions are asymptomatic. The head and neck are the most common locations, followed by the upper trunk and upper extremities. Lesions have been divided into three forms: small nodular (2–5 mm; Fig. 31-18); large nodular (5–20 mm; Fig. 31-19); and giant xanthogranuloma (>20 mm) types. The small-type lesions are more numerous than the large type. However, often one patient will have both types of lesion, and the proposed increased risk for ocular involvement in the

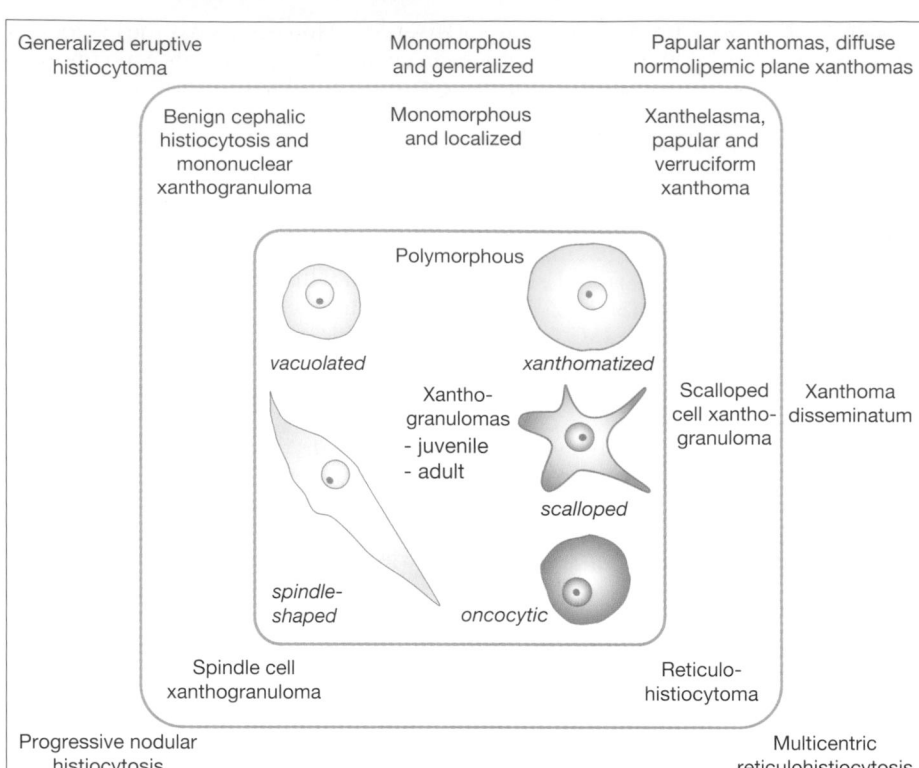

Fig. 31-16 Schematic drawing of unifying concept of non-X histiocytoses.

Generalized eruptive histiocytoma

Monomorphous and generalized

Papular xanthomas, diffuse normolipemic plane xanthomas

Benign cephalic histiocytosis and mononuclear xanthogranuloma

Monomorphous and localized

Xanthelasma, papular and verruciform xanthoma

Polymorphous

vacuolated

xanthomatized

Xantho-granulomas
- juvenile
- adult

Scalloped cell xantho-granuloma

Xanthoma disseminatum

scalloped

spindle-shaped

oncocytic

Spindle cell xanthogranuloma

Reticulo-histiocytoma

Progressive nodular histiocytosis

Multicentric reticulohistiocytosis

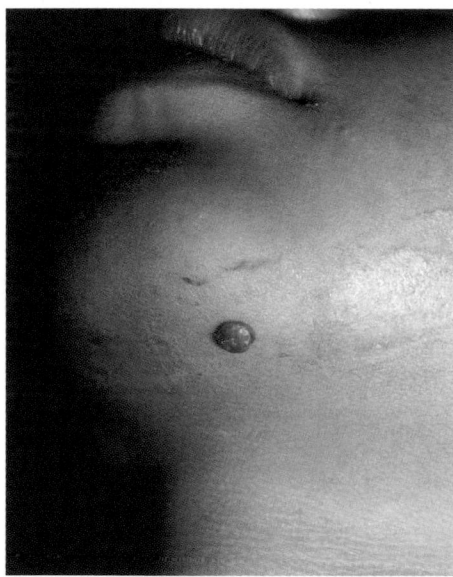

Fig. 31-17 Juvenile xanthogranuloma, solitary.

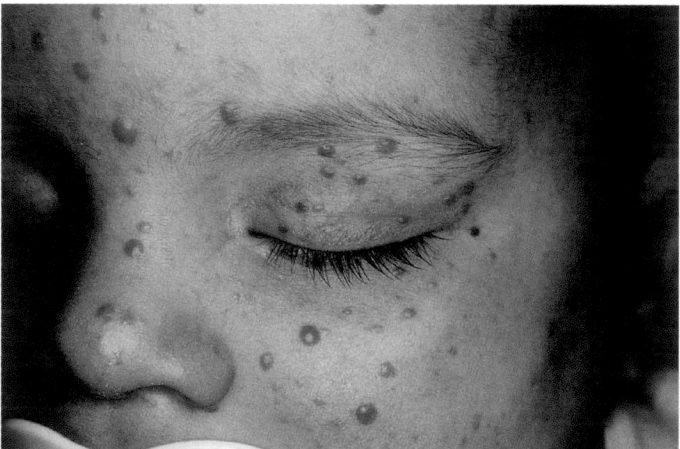

Fig. 31-18 Juvenile xanthogranuloma, multiple small papules.

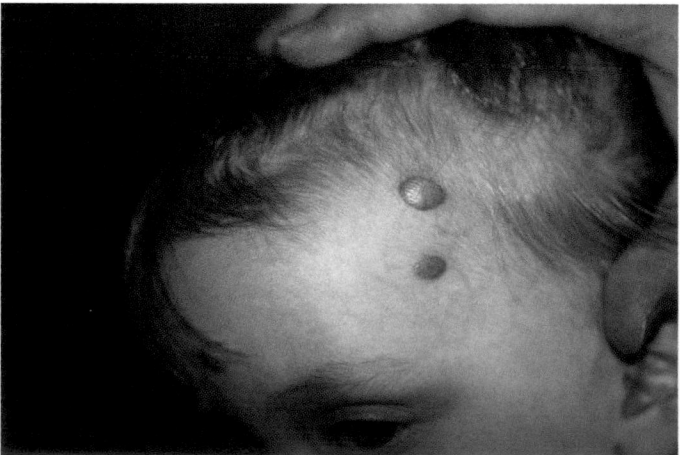

Fig. 31-19 Juvenile xanthogranuloma, multiple nodules.

micronodular type and other internal involvement in the macronodular type has been refuted. Skin lesions regress spontaneously within 3–6 years in children. In adults, lesions are usually persistent. Hyperpigmentation, atrophy, or aneto-derma may remain after lesions resolve.

Multiple atypical presentations have been described. These include hyperkeratotic nodules; macronodular tumors from 2 to 10 cm in diameter; clustered (agminated) forms; linear lesions; flat, plaque-like lesions; and pedunculated or cylindri-cal exophytic lesions. Atypical sites of involvement include the genitalia, lips, palms, soles, earlobes, and fingers. The most common location for JXGs after the dermis is the subcutaneous tissue, again most commonly on the head and neck. About 15% of JXGs present in this manner, usually as a solitary mobile mass up to 3 cm in diameter. Subcutaneous JXG most commonly appears before age 1 and often before age 3 months. Oral JXG may develop in infancy or childhood, and is most frequently a solitary lesion of the tongue, lip, or palate.

Extracutaneous JXG is uncommon and occurs as visceral involvement, in association with either multiple cutaneous lesions or a solitary extracutaneous lesion. Visceral disease of both types accounts for only 4% of childhood JXGs, and for 5–10% of all JXG cases. Ocular involvement occurs in about 0.3–0.4% of children with multiple JXGs, and 41% of children with ocular JXGs have skin lesions. Skin lesions appear after eye lesions in 45% of cases. In 92% of cases, eye lesions occur during the first 2 years of life. The most common location is the iris, where JXG can present as a tumor, unilateral glaucoma, unilateral uveitis with spontaneous hyphema, or as heterochromia iridis. The eyelid or posterior eye may also be involved. Ocular screening is recommended for all children with multiple cutaneous lesions before the age of 2 years.

Mass lesions of the nasal, orbital, and paranasal sinus region can occur and can cause erosion of the orbit and extend to the skull. Other extracutaneous sites and their presentations, in order of frequency, include the lung (respiratory distress and nodular opacities on chest radiograph), liver (hepatomegaly and, rarely, fatal giant cell hepatitis), testis (mass), and rarely, the CNS, kidney, spleen, and retroperitoneum. Other evaluations for extracutaneous JXGs are not indicated unless there are symptoms or findings suggesting their presence. Extracutaneous lesions also spontaneously regress. If surgical intervention is required, extracutaneous lesions tend not to recur, even if they are incompletely excised. Rarely, the burden of visceral JXGs may be so great that the patient's life is threatened. These cases have been called "disseminated JXG," "systemic JXG," or "systemic xanthogranuloma." In 25% of these cases, no skin lesions are found. Progressive CNS, liver, or bone marrow involvement usually mandates aggressive therapy. These cases may simulate hemophagocytic lymphohistiocytosis syndrome. Locally aggressive tumors may be radiated. Systemic steroids, chemotherapy, and even liver or bone marrow transplantation may be required. Even more rarely, a visceral lesion may behave malignantly, spreading to previously unaffected organs and killing the patient.

JXGs have been reported in association with neurofibromatosis (NF-1) and juvenile myelomonocytic leukemia (JMML). Patients with NF-1 and JXG are 20–32 times more likely to develop JMML. JMML and NF-1 are known to be linked, but since JMML occurs in infancy or early childhood, often café-au-lait macules are the only findings of NF-1 at the time. Sometimes all three conditions affect the same patient, with males having a 3:1 predominance and commonly a maternal history of NF-1. Children with JXG should be examined for stigmata of NF-1. If these stigmata are found, especially in a boy with a maternal history of NF-1, the pediatrician should be alert to the possible, although uncommon, occurrence of JMML. Rarely, JXG in childhood may be associated with mastocytosis or childhood acute lymphoblastic leukemia. Multiple xanthogranulomas are rare in adults and it is quite unusual for them to occur in an eruptive manner. At least six cases have been associated with hematologic malignancy (chronic lymphocytic leukemia, essential thrombocytosis, large B-cell lymphoma, adult T-cell lymphoma/leukemia, and monoclonal gammopathy).

Lesions appear histologically as nonencapsulated but circumscribed proliferations in the upper and mid-reticular dermis, and may extend more deeply into the subcutaneous tissue or abut directly on the epidermis with no Grenz zone. Epidermotropism does not occur. Classically, it has been proposed that the histopathology varies in accordance with the age of the lesion. Very early lesions are composed of mono-

nuclear cells with abundant amphophilic cytoplasm that is poorly lipidized or vacuolated. Later, the cells become more vacuolated and multinucleated forms appear. In mature lesions, foam cells, multinucleated foam cells (Touton giant cells), and foreign-body giant cells are present. Touton giant cells are characteristic of JXG but not specific for it. The inflammatory infiltrate consists of lymphocytes, eosinophils, and neutrophils, and lacks plasma cells. Fibrosis occurs in the older lesions. The histology described above is characteristic of cutaneous JXGs. Soft-tissue and visceral JXGs present with more monomorphous cytology, may have very few of the characteristic Touton giant cells, and can have a prominent spindle cell appearance. Immunohistochemistry is especially valuable in confirming the diagnosis of extracutaneous JXG. The cells of JXG of all anatomic locations stain with factor XIIIa, vimentin, fascin, MS-1, and CD68, not with CD1, S-100, or other specific markers for Langerhans cells.

The treatment for most cases of JXG is observation. By age 6 most lesions have resolved, often leaving normal or only slightly hyperpigmented skin. In adults spontaneous involution is slower, and local removal with surgery or CO_2 laser could be considered.

It is noteworthy that the patterns of involvement by JXG and LCH are similar, with childhood onset and primary cutaneous involvement; when visceral disease occurs, the liver, bone, and lungs are commonly involved. Without histologic confirmation, isolated JXG of the bone would be most likely diagnosed as isolated LCH, a much more common condition. These clinical similarities between JXG and LCH may be explained by the fact that both diseases are caused by antigen-presenting dendritic cells. JXG is a proliferation of dermal dendrocytes and LCH is a proliferation of Langerhans cells. The clinical features favoring JXG include lack of crusting or scale and the distribution and uniformity of size of lesions. Histologic evaluation is definitive in difficult cases, since JXGs are negative for the Langerhans cell marker CD1. Unlike LCH, JXGs are usually negative for S-100, although a few S-100-positive JXGs have been reported. Benign cephalic histiocytosis (BCH) may be difficult to distinguish both clinically and histologically, but in BCH lesions tend to be flatter and are mainly on the head and neck. Papular xanthoma can be distinguished histologically. Clinically, mastocytosis will urticate when scratched (Darier's sign) and can be distinguished histologically. Solitary JXG appearing in a child must be distinguished from a Spitz nevus, usually requiring a biopsy.

Aparicio G, et al: Eruptive juvenile xanthogranuloma associated with relapsing acute lymphoblastic leukemia. Pediatr Dermatol 2008; 25:487.

Bowling JC, et al: Solitary anogenital xanthogranuloma. Clin Exp Dermatol 2005; 30:716.

Bradford RK, Choudhary AK: Imaging findings of juvenile xanthogranuloma of the penis. Pediatr Radiol 2009; 39:176.

Chantorn R, et al: Severe congenital systemic juvenile xanthogranuloma in monozygotic twins. Pediatr Dermatol 2008; 25:470.

Chantranuwat C: Systemic form of juvenile xanthogranuloma: a report of a case with liver and bone involvement. Pediatr Dev Pathol 2004; 7:646.

Clayton TH, et al: Congenital plaque on the chest. Diagnosis: solitary giant congenital juvenile xanthogranuloma. Clin Exp Dermatol 2007; 32:613.

Dehner LP: Juvenile xanthogranulomas in the first two decades of life: a clinicopathologic study of 174 cases with cutaneous and extracutaneous manifestations. Am J Surg Pathol 2003; 27:579.

Dincaslan HU, et al: An infant with giant juvenile xanthogranuloma presenting as an axillary mass. Pediatr Blood Cancer 2008; 51:713.

Dolken R, et al: Treatment of severe disseminated juvenile systemic xanthogranuloma with multiple lesions in the central nervous system. J Pediatr Hematol Oncol 2006; 28:95.

Gamo R, et al: Anetoderma developing in juvenile xanthogranuloma. Int J Dermatol 2005; 44:503.

Gunson TH, Birchall NM: Symmetrical giant facial plaque-type juvenile xanthogranuloma. J Am Acad Dermatol 2008; 59:S56.

Hara T, et al: Prolonged severe pancytopenia preceding the cutaneous lesions of juvenile xanthogranuloma. Pediatr Blood Cancer 2006; 47:103.

Haughton AM, et al: Disseminated juvenile xanthogranulomatosis in a newborn resulting in liver transplantation. J Am Acad Dermatol 2008; 58:S12.

Hirata M, et al: A case of adult limbal xanthogranuloma. Jpn J Ophthalmol 2007; 51:302.

Hsiao PF, et al: An infant with juvenile xanthogranuloma, multiple café-au-lait macules, acute myeloid leukaemia: an incomplete, rare form of triple association? J Eur Acad Dermatol Venereol 2008; 22:1378.

Hu JY, et al: An infant with extensive cutaneous nodular juvenile xanthogranuloma and hyperlipidemia. J Am Acad Dermatol 2007; 56:S54.

Hughes DB, et al: Juvenile xanthogranuloma of the finger. Pediatr Dermatol 2006; 23:53.

Imiela A, et al: Juvenile xanthogranuloma: a congenital giant form leading to a wide atrophic sequela. Pediatr Dermatol 2004; 21:121.

Janssen D, Harms D: Juvenile xanthogranuloma in childhood and adolescence: a clinicopathologic study of 129 patients from the Kiel pediatric tumor registry. Am J Surg Pathol 2005; 29:21.

Kaur MR, et al: Disseminated clustered juvenile xanthogranuloma: an unusual morphological variant of a common condition. Clin Exp Dermatol 2008; 33:575.

Kim EJ, et al: Juvenile xanthogranuloma of the finger: an unusual localization. J Dermatol 2007; 34:590.

Kiopelidou D, et al: Linear-agminated juvenile xanthogranulomas. Int J Dermatol 2008; 47:387.

Kirke S, et al: Juvenile xanthogranuloma associated with contralateral lymphadenopathy. Pediatr Dermatol 2005; 22:424.

Klemke CD, et al: Multiple juvenile xanthogranulomas successfully treated with CO laser. J Dtsch Dermatol Ges 2007; 5:30.

Kolivras A, et al: Congenital disseminated juvenile xanthogranuloma with unusual skin presentation and renal involvement. J Cutan Pathol 2009; 36:684.

Liang S, et al: Juvenile xanthogranuloma with ocular involvement. Pediatr Dermatol 2009; 26:232.

Matcham NJ, et al: Systemic juvenile xanthogranulomatosis imitating a malignant abdominal wall tumor with lung metastases. J Pediatr Hematol Oncol 2007; 29:72.

Mocan MC, et al: Juvenile xanthogranuloma of the corneal limbus: report of two cases and review of the literature. Cornea 2008; 27:739.

Motegi S, et al: An unusual presentation of juvenile xanthogranuloma. Pediatr Dermatol 2007; 24:576.

Mowbray M, Schofield OM: Juvenile xanthogranuloma en plaque. Pediatr Dermatol 2007; 24:670.

Nishi T, et al: A case of juvenile limbal xanthogranuloma. Jpn J Ophthalmol 2007; 51:301.

Orsey A, et al: Central nervous system juvenile xanthogranuloma with malignant transformation. Pediatr Blood Cancer 2008; 50:927.

Rajendra B, et al: Successful treatment of central nervous system juvenile xanthogranulomatosis with cladribine. Pediatr Blood Cancer 2009; 52:413.

Redbord KP, Sheth AP: Multiple juvenile xanthogranulomas in a 13-year-old. Pediatr Dermatol 2007; 24:238.

Rubegni P, et al: Juvenile xanthogranuloma: dermoscopic pattern. Dermatology 2009; 218:380.

Savasan S, et al: Successful bone marrow transplantation for life-threatening xanthogranuloma disseminatum in neurofibromatosis type-1. Pediatr Transplant 2005; 9:534.

Shoo BA, et al: Xanthogranulomas associated with hematologic malignancy in adulthood. J Am Acad Dermatol 2008; 59:488.

Sidwell RU, et al: Is disseminated juvenile xanthogranulomatosis benign cephalic histiocytosis? Pediatr Dermatol 2005; 22:40.

Stover DG, et al: Treatment of juvenile xanthogranuloma. Pediatr Blood Cancer 2008; 51:130.

Torrelo A, et al: Multiple lichenoid juvenile xanthogranuloma. Pediatr Dermatol 2009; 26:238.

Tsutsui K, et al: Urticaria pigmentosa occurring with juvenile xanthogranuloma. Br J Dermatol 1999; 140:990.

Unuvar E, et al: Successful therapy of systemic xanthogranuloma in a child. J Pediatr Hematol Oncol 2007; 29:425.

Vendal Z, et al: Glaucoma in juvenile xanthogranuloma. Semin Ophthalmol 2006; 21:191.

Benign cephalic histiocytosis

BCH is a rare condition affecting boys and girls of all races equally. The onset is between 2 and 34 months of age (rarely up to 5 years), with 50% of cases beginning between ages 5 and 12 months. The disease begins initially on the head in virtually all cases, often the cheeks, eyelids, forehead, and ears. Lesions may later appear on the neck and upper trunk, and less commonly more caudad. There are always multiple lesions, but often few in number (5–20), although they can number more than 100. Individual lesions are slightly raised, reddish-yellow papules, 2–4 mm in diameter. Lesions may coalesce to give a reticulate appearance. The lesions cause no symptoms. The mucosa and viscera are not involved. Lesions spontaneously involute over 2–8 years, leaving behind hyper-pigmented macules. Some cases of BCH have evolved to become JXGs, and one patient later developed generalized eruptive histiocytoma many years after the involution of BCH. This supports the concept outlined above that these conditions lie along a spectrum and all derive from the same cell type, a dermal dendritic cell. Histologically, there is a diffuse dermal infiltration of monomorphous macrophages, which stain posi-tively for CD68 and factor XIIIa and negatively with S-100 and CD1a.

Dadzie O, et al: Benign cephalic histiocytosis in a British-African child. Pediatr Dermatol 2005; 22:444.

Hasegawa S, et al: Japanese case of benign cephalic histiocytosis. J Dermatol 2009; 36:69.

Jih DM, et al: Benign cephalic histiocytosis: a case report and review. J Am Acad Dermatol 2002; 47:908.

Generalized eruptive histiocytoma (generalized eruptive histiocytosis)

Generalized eruptive histiocytosis (GEH) is a rare disease, usually presenting in young adulthood. The diagnostic criteria are:

1. widespread, erythematous, essentially symmetrical papules, particularly involving the trunk and proximal extremities, sparing the flexors, and rarely involving the mucous membranes (there is no visceral involvement)
2. progressive development of new lesions, often in crops, over several years with eventual spontaneous involution to hyperpigmented macules
3. a benign histologic picture of monomorphous, vacuolated macrophages.

Lesions appear in crops, and may be grouped or clustered. (Since Winkelmann's initial report of this entity, several cases with grouped lesions have been reported, so finding grouped lesions does not exclude the diagnosis of GEH.) They are skin-colored, brown, or violaceous. GEH is rare in childhood. It may be difficult to distinguish from widespread BCH in child-hood, if indeed it is a separate condition. In adults and chil-dren, GEH may suddenly appear several weeks following a bacterial or viral illness; in adults it may be associated with underlying malignancy, usually leukemia or lymphoma. GEH is distinguished from xanthoma disseminatum by the lack of visceral disease, the benign course, and by the scalloped appearance of the macrophages in xanthoma disseminatum. Histologically, there is a dermal infiltrate of monomorphous vacuolated macrophages and mononuclear histiocytes. The GEH cells stain positively for vimentin, CD68, and usually factor XIIIa, and negatively for S-100, and CD1a. The natural history of GEH is unpredictable, with complete resolution in some cases and persistence in others. Some cases have progressed to widespread xanthogranulomas, xanthoma disseminatum, or progressive nodular histiocytosis, again supporting the concept that these diseases all fall along a spectrum and derive from the same cell type. In childhood, no treatment may be required. In adulthood, treatment with PUVA or isotretinoin could be considered.

Deng YJ, et al: Generalized eruptive histiocytosis: a possible therapeutic cure? Br J Dermatol 2004; 150:155.

Fernandez-Jorge B, et al: A case of generalized eruptive histiocytosis. Acta Derm Venereol 2007; 87:533.

Klemke C, et al: Atypical generalized eruptive histiocytosis associated with acute monocytic leukemia. J Am Acad Dermatol 2003; 49:233.

Lan Ma H, et al: Successful treatment of generalized eruptive histiocytoma with PUVA. J Dtsch Dermatol Ges 2007; 5:131.

Misery L, et al: Generalized eruptive histiocytoma in an infant with healing in summer: long-term follow-up. Br J Dermatol 2001; 144:435.

Seward JL, et al: Generalized eruptive histiocytosis. J Am Acad Dermatol 2004; 50:116.

Tamiya H, et al: Generalized eruptive histiocytoma with rapid progression and resolution following exanthema subitum. Clin Exp Dermatol 2005; 30:300.

Xanthoma disseminatum (Montgomery syndrome)

Xanthoma disseminatum (XD) is a very rare, potentially progressive non-LCH that preferentially affects males in childhood or young adulthood. It is characterized by the insidious onset of small, yellowish-red to brown papules and nodules that are discrete and disseminated. They characteristically involve the eyelids and flexural areas of the axillary and inguinal folds, and the antecubital and popliteal fossae. Over years the lesions increase in number, forming coalescent xanthomatous plaques and nodules. About 30–50% of cases have mucous membrane involvement, most commonly of the oropharynx (causing dysphagia), larynx (causing dysphonia and airway obstruction), and conjunctiva and cornea (causing blindness). Diabetes insipidus, usually transient, occurs in 40%. CNS involvement, with epilepsy, hydrocephalus, and ataxia, can occur. Synovitis and osteolytic bone lesions have been described. In some cases, the disease may spontaneously involute.

The serum lipids are abnormal in 20% of cases, which may lead to confusion with hyperlipidemic xanthomatosis. Histologic examination of early lesions shows surprisingly nonfoamy, scalloped macrophages. Later lesions show xanthoma cells, Touton giant cells, and frequently, a mild inflammatory cell infiltrate of lymphocytes, plasma cells, and neutrophils. The macrophages stain with CD68 and factor XIIIa.

Disseminated xanthosiderohistiocytosis is a variant of XD in which there is a keloidal consistency to the lesions; they have annular borders, a cephalad distribution, and extensive iron and lipid deposition in the macrophages and connective tissue.

Progressive XD can produce considerable morbidity and can even be fatal. Therefore, aggressive therapy may be indicated. Systemic steroids have led to improvement in one case. In a patient with XD and dyslipidemia, the combination of rosiglitazone, simvastatin, and acipimox led to partial remission and stabilization of mucosal and osseous disease. Cyclophosphamide has led to dramatic improvement in two of three patients so treated.

Eisendle K, et al: Inflammation and lipid accumulation in xanthoma disseminatum: therapeutic considerations. J Am Acad Dermatol 2008; 58:S47.

Goodenberger ME, et al: Xanthoma disseminatum and Waldenstrom's macroglobulinemia. J Am Acad Dermatol 1990; 23:1015.

Heald P, et al: Xanthoma disseminatum. N Engl J Med 1998; 338:1138.

Seaton ED, et al: Treatment of xanthoma disseminatum with cyclophosphamide. Br J Dermatol 2004; 150:346.

Yusuf SM, et al: Xanthoma disseminatum in a black African woman. Int J Dermatol 2008; 47:1145.

Progressive nodular histiocytosis

Progressive nodular histiocytosis (PNH) is a very rare disorder that affects men and women equally and usually begins between the ages of 40 and 60 years. The characteristic clinical feature is the development of two types of lesion: superficial papules and deeper, larger, subcutaneous nodules. The superficial lesions are small xanthomatous papules up to 5 mm in diameter. They are diffusely distributed on the body, but spare the flexors. The larger deep lesions can be up to 5 cm in diameter and are associated with pain, ulceration, and disfigurement. On the face, lesions may coalesce, giving the patient a leonine facies and creating ectropion. New lesions progressively appear and spontaneous resolution does not occur. Most patients have no mucosal or visceral lesions, although one patient had a hypothalamic lesion leading to precocious puberty and growth hormone deficiency. Histologically, the superficial lesions show foamy macrophages and the deeper lesions a densely cellular proliferation of spindle-shaped histiocytes with multinucleated giant cells. It is the development of these deep lesions composed of primarily spindled histiocytes that is the diagnostic feature of PNH. Local excision may be used for symptomatic lesions.

Beswick SJ, et al: Progressive nodular histiocytosis in a child with a hypothalamic tumour. Br J Dermatol 2002; 146:138.

Gonzalez A, et al: Progressive nodular histiocytosis accompanied by systemic disorders. Br J Dermatol 2000; 143:628.

Lufti M, et al: Progressive nodular histiocytosis—rare variant of cutaneous non-Langerhans cell histiocytosis. J Dtsch Dermatol Ges 2006; 4:236.

Nogueras SV, et al: An indolent and progressive papulonodular eruption. Int J Dermatol 2009; 48:751.

Watanabe T, et al: Progressive nodular histiocytosis—a five-year follow up. Eur J Dermatol 2008; 18:200.

Papular xanthoma

Papular xanthoma (PX) is a rare form of non-LCH that is poorly defined. The disease can occur at any age, but usually appears in early childhood or after adolescence. PX usually presents as a solitary lesion favoring men 4:1 over women. The primary lesion is a small, yellow papule from 1 to 10 mm in diameter. If there are multiple lesions they are generalized, not grouped, and do not favor the flexors. There is no visceral involvement and no abnormalities are found on lipid profile examination. Histologically, there are aggregates of xanthomatized foamy macrophages in the dermis, with Touton giant cells. Inflammatory cells are scant or absent. Cells stain positively for markers of monocytes/macrophages such as CD68, but are negative for factor XIIIa. The differential diagnosis includes normolipemic plane xanthomas and normolipemic papuloeruptive xanthomatosis. In infants the natural history is for spontaneous involution. In one adult patient, treatment with doxycycline was effective.

Bastida J, et al: Adult disseminated primary papular xanthoma treated with doxycycline. Arch Dermatol 2007; 143:667.

Breier F, et al: Papular xanthoma: a clinicopathological study of 10 cases. J Cutan Pathol 2002; 29:200.

Chen CG, et al: Primary papular xanthoma of children. Am J Dermatopathol 1997; 19:596.

Kim SH, et al: Congenital papular xanthoma. Br J Dermatol 2000; 142:569.

Singla A: Normolipemic papular xanthoma with xanthelasma. Dermatol Online J 2006; 12:19.

Erdheim–Chester disease

This rare non-LCH is primarily a visceral disorder with cutaneous manifestations. It can begin at any age from childhood to the ninth decade. The characteristic feature is bilateral and symmetrical sclerosis of the metaphyseal and diaphyseal regions of the long bones. These radiologic findings are considered pathognomonic. Diabetes insipidus from involvement of the pituitary and retroperitoneal fibrosis affecting the kidneys may occur. Despite a normal gross appearance, many internal organs are affected. The course is progressive with infiltration of many visceral organs, followed by fibrosis. This is often fatal, usually from pulmonary fibrosis and cardiac failure. In one series, 60% of patients had died, 36% within 6 months of diagnosis, with a mean survival of less than 3 years. Skin lesions occur in 25% of patients, typically presenting as red–brown or xanthomatous 2–15 mm papules or nodules. Lesions favor the eyelids, axilla, groin, neck, trunk (inframammary areas), and face. As opposed to plane xanthomas and xanthelasmas, the lesions can be elevated or tubelike, resembling sausages or keloids.

Dickson BC, et al: Systemic Erdheim–Chester disease. Virchows Arch 2008; 452:221.

Taguchi T, et al: Erdheim–Chester disease: report of a case with PCR-based analysis of the expression of osteopontin and surviving in xanthogranulomas following glucocorticoid treatment. Endocr J 2008; 55:217.

Vanichaniramol N, et al: Erdheim–Chester disease. Intern Med 2008; 47:1633.

Progressive mucinous histiocytosis in women

Progressive mucinous histiocytosis is an autosomal-dominant or X-linked hereditary disorder described only in women. The skin lesions consist of a few to numerous skin-colored to red–brown papules, ranging from pinhead- to pea-sized, which tend to appear on the face, arms, forearms, hands, and legs. Onset is in the second decade of life, with slow progression and no tendency to spontaneous involution. Visceral and mucosal lesions have not been reported. Histologically, in the mid-dermis there is a proliferation of spindle-shaped and epithelioid monocytes. Superficial telangiectatic vessels and increased mast cells are found. Abundant mucin is demonstrated by alcian blue staining, indicating the presence of acid mucopolysaccharides. This condition can be distinguished from the other non-LCHs by its familial pattern, lack of lipidized and multinucleated cells, and presence of mucin. Immunoperoxidase studies have been conflicting, but most consistently show positivity for factor XIIIa and CD68, and negativity for CD1a, S-100, and CD34.

Sass U, et al: A sporadic case of progressive mucinous histiocytosis. Br J Dermatol 2000; 142:133.

Young A, et al: Two sporadic cases of adult-onset progressive mucinous histiocytosis. J Cutan Pathol 2006; 33:166.

Reticulohistiocytosis

Two distinct forms of reticulohistiocytosis occur: reticulohistiocytoma and multicentric reticulohistiocytosis. The two forms have identical histology but distinct clinical manifestations.

Reticulohistiocytoma

Reticulohistiocytoma usually occurs as a solitary, firm dermal lesion of less than 1 cm in diameter. Lesions favor the trunk and extremities. Multiple lesions may rarely occur and can be quite extensive and diffuse. Solitary lesions and multiple lesions without systemic involvement, in contrast to multicentric reticulohistiocytosis, have been described, mainly in adult men and rarely in children.

Multicentric reticulohistiocytosis

Multicentric reticulohistiocytosis (MRH) is a multisystem disease beginning usually around age 50 (range 6–86). It is twice as common in women as in men and affects all races. The primary manifestations are skin lesions and a potentially

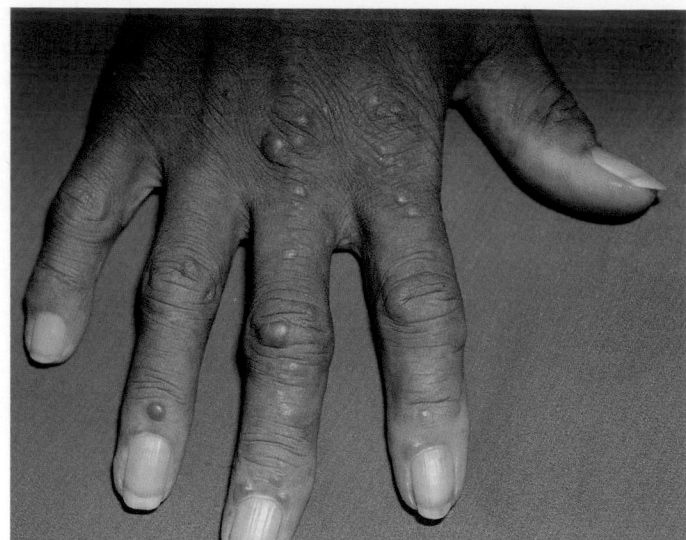

Fig. 31-20 Multicentric reticulohistiocytosis.

destructive arthritis. In 40% of cases the joint disease occurs first, in 30% the skin lesions precede the joint symptoms, and in 40% the joint and skin disease appear simultaneously.

Clinically, there may be a few to a few hundred firm, skin-colored to red–brown papules and nodules, mostly 2–10 mm in diameter, but some reaching several centimeters in size (Fig. 31-20). These occur most frequently on the fingers and hands, with a tendency to cause paronychial lesions. In about half the cases, lesions will be arranged about nailfolds, giving a so-called "coral bead" appearance, which may be associated with nail dystrophy. The upper half of the body, including the arms, scalp, face, ears, and neck, are also common sites. Ninety percent of patients have lesions on the face and hands. Nodular and papular involvement of the pinnae and a symmetrical distribution of the lesions, especially over joints, are characteristic. The nodules on the arms, elbows, and knees may resemble rheumatoid nodules. Diffuse erythematous lesions can occur, at times simulating erythroderma. Lesions may ulcerate. Xanthelasma occurs in 30% of patients. Atypical patchy areas of hypopigmentation over the face and upper limbs have been noted. About 10% of MRH patients may complain of pruritus. The itching is not localized to the lesions and may precede the appearance of the skin lesions.

Mucous membrane involvement is seen in one-third of cases and is most common on the lips and tongue; other sites are the gingiva, palate, buccal mucosa, nasopharynx, larynx, and sclera. Lesions of the esophagus can lead to dysphagia. One-third of cases have hypercholesterolemia and xanthelasma. Rheumatoid factor is usually negative.

Osteoarticular changes are the most important aspect of MRH. There is no association between the extent, size, or severity of the skin eruption and the course of the joint disease. The associated arthropathy is an inflammatory, symmetrical, polyarticular arthritis that can affect many joints, including the hands, knees, shoulders, wrists, hips, ankles, elbows, feet, and spine. The arthritis can be rapidly destructive and mutilating, with absorption and telescopic shortening of the phalanges and digits—doigts en lorgnette (opera-glass fingers). In older reports at least 50% of cases developed arthritis mutilans, but this has been reduced to about 11%. The infiltrating cells in the skin and joints are identical on microscopic examination and immunophenotypic evaluation. The clinical course varies. In many instances there is complete involution after about 8 years. The joint destruction is permanent, however, and is a cause of severe disability. The joint involvement may resemble rheumatoid arthritis and psoriatic arthritis. Weight loss and fever occur in one-third of patients.

About 15% of patients with MRH have associated autoimmune disorders. Thyroiditis, Sjögren's, ulcerative colitis, and vitiligo have all been reported. At least six patients have been described with myopathy closely simulating dermatomyositis.

About 25% of reported cases have had an associated malignancy. Given this high rate of malignancy, every patient with MRH should have a complete age-appropriate cancer screening, repeated at regular intervals (similar to the protocol followed for patients with dermatomyositis). No specific tumor type has been associated. There are reports involving breast, colon, cervix, stomach, melanoma, and ovary, as well as leukemia and lymphoma. The skin lesions usually appear before the diagnosis of the malignancy, but synchronous behavior of the skin lesions and the underlying malignancy is only occasionally reported. In one case, tuberculosis was identified, and treatment of the tuberculosis led to resolution of the MRH.

Other organs and tissues may be involved, such as bone, muscle, lymph nodes, liver, myocardium, pericardium, lungs, pleura, and stomach. Myocardial involvement may be fatal. Gallium is a method to screen for extent of disease.

Histologically, the skin lesions are usually centered in the mid-dermis and tend to occupy much or all of the dermis. The infiltrating cells are mononuclear and multinucleate monocyte/macrophages. The giant cells are most characteristic, with an abundant smooth or slightly granular, eosinophilic or amphophilic, "ground-glass" cytoplasm. Their cytoplasm is darker in the center than at the periphery. These cells stain positive for periodic-acid Schiff (PAS) after diastase digestion. The overlying epidermis may be thinned but is usually separated from the dermal process by a narrow zone of collagen (Grenz zone). Characteristically, there is a polymorphous infiltrate of lymphocytes, neutrophils, eosinophils, and plasma cells within the lesions. By immunohistochemistry the monocyte/macrophage cells stain positively for CD68, vimentin, and CD163. In MRH the cells in the skin and joints stain positively for acid phosphatase that is tartrate-resistant (TRAP) and cathepsin K, markers for osteoclasts. This may explain the response of MRH to bisphosphonates, which cause apoptosis of osteoclasts and are taken up by cells in the reticuloendothelial system.

Given the aggressive nature of the arthritis, early and adequate treatment should be considered. However, associated malignancy is frequent and can be worsened by immunosuppressive therapy. The same would be true if there were underlying asymptomatic tuberculosis. Initially, the patient should be screened for these two conditions and they should be adequately treated if found. In patients free of neoplasia and tuberculosis, the treatment is individualized. Spontaneous remissions are common, making efficacy of treatment hard to determine. The major goal of treatment is to prevent the destruction of the joints that are the cause of disability. If systemic therapy is considered, two approaches can be taken. One is the use of the combination of systemic steroids, methotrexate, and a TNF inhibitor. In the case of TNF inhibitors, infliximab has proven more effective than etanercept and should probably be the initial agent used. The other approach is to use a combination of immunosuppressives and a bisphosphonate. Since the infiltrating cells in MRH seem phenotypically to be osteoclastic in behavior, this therapy is logical and appears to be joint-sparing. In refractory cases, the use of a bisphosphonate and TNF inhibitor with methotrexate and systemic steroids could be considered. For patients with skin lesions only, therapy is not required. PUVA, antimalarials, topical nitrogen mustard, and low-dose methotrexate, a bisphosphonate, or a TNF inhibitor could be considered if symptoms are severe.

Baghestani S, et al: Multicentric reticulohistiocytosis presenting with papulonodular skin eruption and polyarthritis. Eur J Dermatol 2005; 15:196.

Bogle MA, et al: Multicentric reticulohistiocytosis with pulmonary involvement. J Am Acad Dermatol 2003; 49:1125.

Chen CH, et al: Multicentric reticulohistiocytosis presenting with destructive polyarthritis, laryngopharyngeal dysfunction, and a huge reticulohistiocytoma. J Clin Rheumatol 2006; 12:252.

Codriansky KA, et al: Multicentric reticulohistiocytosis: a systemic osteoclastic disease? Arthritis Rheum 2008; 59:444.

Gajic-Veljic M, et al: Multicentric reticulohistiocytosis—a case with minimal articular changes. J Eur Acad Dermatol Venereol 2006; 20:108.

Goto H, et al: Successful treatment of multicentric reticulohistiocytosis with alendronate. Arthritis Rheum 2003; 48:3538.

Ho SG, Yu RC: A case of multicentric reticulohistiocytosis with multiple lytic skull lesions. Clin Exp Dermatol 2005; 30:515.

Hsiung SH, et al: Multicentric reticulohistiocytosis presenting with clinical features of dermatomyositis. J Am Acad Dermatol 2003; 48:S11.

Hsu S, et al: Multicentric reticulohistiocytosis with neurofibroma-like nodules. J Am Acad Dermatol 2001; 44:373.

Kalajian AH, Callen JP: Multicentric reticulohistiocytosis successfully treated with infliximab: an illustrative case and evaluation of cytokine expression supporting anti-tumor necrosis factor therapy. Arch Dermatol 2008; 144:1350.

Kishikawa T, et al: Multicentric reticulohistiocytosis associated with ovarian cancer. Mod Rheumatol 2007; 17:422.

Liu YU, Fang K: Multicentric reticulohistiocytosis with generalized systemic involvement. Clin Exp Dermatol 2004; 29:373.

Lovelace K, et al: Etanercept and the treatment of multicentric reticulohistiocytosis. Arch Dermatol 2005; 141:1167.

Luz FB, et al: Multicentric reticulohistiocytosis: a proliferation of macrophages with tropism for skin and joints, part I. Skinmed 2007; 6:172.

Mavragani CP, et al: Alleviation of polyarticular syndrome in multicentric reticulohistiocytosis with intravenous zoledronate. Ann Rheum Dis 2005; 64:1521.

McIlwain KL, et al: Multicentric reticulohistiocytosis with prominent cutaneous lesions and proximal muscle weakness masquerading as dermatomyositis. J Rheumatol 2005; 32:193.

Miettinen M, Fetsch JF: Reticulohistiocytoma (solitary epithelioid histiocytoma): a clinicopathologic and immunohistochemical study of 44 cases. Am J Surg Pathol 2006; 30:521.

Millar A, et al: Multicentric reticulohistiocytosis: a lesson in screening for malignancy. Rheumatology (Oxford) 2008; 47:1102.

Morris-Jones R, et al: Multicentric reticulohistiocytosis associated with Sjögren's syndrome. Br J Dermatol 2000; 143:649.

Outland JD, et al: Multicentric reticulohistiocytosis in a 14-year-old girl. Pediatr Dermatol 2002; 19:527.

Poochareon VN, et al: Multiple pink papules in the setting of arthritis and fever. Multicentric reticulohistiocytosis (MRH). Arch Dermatol 2008; 144:1383.

Rentsch JL, et al: Prolonged response of multicentric reticulohistiocytosis to low dose methotrexate. J Rheumatol 1998; 25:1012.

Satoh M, et al: Treatment trial of multicentric reticulohistiocytosis with a combination of prednisolone, methotrexate and alendronate. J Dermatol 2008; 35:168.

Shannon SE, et al: Multicentric reticulohistiocytosis responding to tumor necrosis factor-alpha inhibition in a renal transplant patient. J Rheumatol 2005; 32:565.

Simpson EM, et al: Multicentric reticulohistiocytosis: diagnosis at the nailbeds. J Rheumatol 2008; 35:2272.

Webb-Detiege T, et al: Infiltration of histiocytes and multinucleated giant cells in the myocardium of a patient with multicentric reticulohistiocytosis. J Clin Rheumatol 2009; 15:25.

Yang HJ, et al: Multicentric reticulohistiocytosis with lungs and liver involved. Clin Exp Dermatol 2009; 34:183.

Indeterminate cell histiocytosis

Indeterminate cells are felt to represent dermal precursors of Langerhans cells. They are positive for S-100 and CD1a but do not contain Birbeck granules. Indeterminate cell histiocytosis (ICH) is the term used to describe disorders that are composed of cells that immunophenotypically stain as Langerhans cells but lack Birbeck granules. Since electron microscopy is rarely employed, it is difficult to use this criterion to establish the diagnosis of a disorder. Langerin immunostaining might be substituted.

ICH cases are quite rare, and there is little homogeneity among the reports to reassure one that all these cases actually describe a single disease. In addition, S-100 staining is variable in the various non-Langerhans cell histiocytoses (NLCH), making S-100 positivity a soft criterion to use. In addition, reactive conditions are associated with tissue infiltration by S-100-positive cells. Indeterminate cells may be found as a minor component of the dermal infiltrate in nodular scabies and rarely following pityriasis rosea. Some authors favor classifying ICH as a generalized eruptive histiocytosis. This being said, it appears that both children and adults are affected by ICH, with males outnumbering females. Solitary and multiple lesions may occur, and the color of lesions varies from yellow to red–brown. Lesions may be papules, plaques, or nodules from 3 mm to 10 cm in size. These clinical features are not specific, and resemble the papular lesions seen in many forms of NLCH. Conjunctival involvement has been reported. Solitary malignant tumors with similar immunohistochemistry have been described, clinically resembling atypical fibroxanthoma. Histologically, while the cells in these cases do stain with S-100 and at times with CD1a, the staining is never as intense as in Langerhans cells. ICH seems to have a benign course in the vast majority of cases, and no therapy is required. Broad-band UVB, PUVA, and total skin electron beam have each been effective in limited number(s) of cases with severe skin involvement. Many cases have been treated with numerous chemotherapeutic agents similar to those used for LCH, including cyclophosphamide, etoposide, vinblastine, systemic corticosteroids, and 2-chlorodeoxyadenosine, but therapeutic response has been equivocal. Acute myelogenous leukemia has followed some of these courses of chemotherapy. Solitary lesions with malignant histology should be managed with surgical excision ensuring adequate margins. The utility of adjunctive therapy and sentinel lymph node sampling is not known.

Amo Y, et al: A case of solitary indeterminate cell histiocytosis. J Dermatol 2003; 30:751.

Calatayud M, et al: Ocular involvement in a case of systemic indeterminate cell histiocytosis: a case report. Cornea 2001; 20:769.

Caputo R, et al: Chemotherapeutic experience in indeterminate cell histiocytosis. Br J Dermatol 2005; 153:206.

Ferran M, et al: Acquired mucosal indeterminate cell histiocytoma. Pediatr Dermatol 2007; 24:253.

Frater JL, et al: Histiocytic sarcoma with secondary involvement of the skin and expression of CD1a: evidence of indeterminate cell differentiation? J Cutan Pathol 2006; 33:437.

Hashimoto K, et al: Post-scabietic nodules: a lymphohistiocytic reaction rich in indeterminate cells. J Dermatol 2000; 27:181.

Ishibashi M, et al: Indeterminate cell histiocytosis successfully treated with ultraviolet B phototherapy. Clin Exp Dermatol 2008; 33; 301.

Malhomme de la Roche H, et al: Indeterminate cell histiocytosis responding to total skin electron beam therapy. Br J Dermatol 2008; 158:838.

Ratzinger G, et al: Indeterminate cell histiocytosis: fact or fiction? J Cutan Pathol 2005; 32:552.

Rezk SA, et al: Indeterminate cell tumors: a rare dendritic neoplasm. Am J Surg Pathol 2008; 32:1868.

Rodriguez-Jurado R, et al: Indeterminate cell histiocytosis: clinical and pathologic study in a pediatric patient. Arch Pathol Lab Med 2003; 127:748.

Rosenberg AS, Morgan MB: Cutaneous indeterminate cell histiocytosis: a new spindle cell variant resembling dendritic cell sarcoma. J Cutan Pathol 2001; 28:531.

Vener C, et al: Indeterminate cell histiocytosis in association with later occurrence of acute myeloblastic leukaemia. Br J Dermatol 2007; 156:1357.

Wollenberg A, et al: Long-lasting "Christmas tree rash" in an adolescent: isotopic response of indeterminate cell histiocytosis in pityriasis rosea? Acta Derm Venereol 2002; 82:288.

Sea-blue histiocytosis

Sea-blue histiocytosis may occur as a familial inherited syndrome or as an acquired secondary or systemic infiltrative process. The characteristic and diagnostic cell is a histiocytic cell containing cytoplasmic granules that stain blue–green with Giemsa stain and blue with May–Gruenwald stain. The disorder is characterized by infiltration of these cells into the marrow, spleen, liver, lymph nodes, and lungs, as well as the skin in some cases. Skin lesions include papules or nodules, facial waxy plaques, eyelid swelling, and patchy gray pigmentation of the face and upper trunk. Similar histologic findings have occurred in patients with myelogenous leukemia, light chain deposition disease, adult Niemann–Pick disease (type B), sphingomyelinase deficiency, or mutations in the apolipoprotein E gene, and following the prolonged use of intravenous fat supplementation. The unifying feature in all these conditions is an abnormal lipid metabolism by the infiltrating histiocytes. This condition has been seen in the infiltrate of a case of cutaneous T-cell lymphoma.

Bigorgne C, et al: Sea-blue histiocyte syndrome in the bone marrow secondary to total parenteral nutrition. Leukemia Lymphoma 1998; 28:523.

Candoni A, et al: Sea-blue histiocytosis secondary to Niemann–Pick disease type B: a case report. Ann Hematol 2001; 80:620.

Caputo R, et al: Unusual variants of non-Langerhans cell histiocytosis. J Am Acad Dermatol 2007; 57:1031.

Naghashpour M, Cualing H: Splenomegaly with sea-blue histiocytosis, dyslipidemia, and nephropathy in a patient with lecithin-cholesterol acyltransferase deficiency: a clinicopathologic correlation. Metabolism 2009; 58:1459.

Newman B, et al: Aggressive histiocytic disorders that can involve the skin. J Am Acad Dermatol 2007; 56:302.

Suzuki O, Abe M: Secondary sea-blue histiocytosis derived from Niemann–Pick disease. J Clin Exp Hematop 2007; 47:19.

X-type histiocytoses (Langerhans cell histiocytosis—LCH)

This group of disorders is caused by infiltration of the skin, and in some cases other organs, by Langerhans cells. The spectrum of disease is broad, with solitary, usually benign and autoinvoluting lesions at one end, and multicentric, multiorgan visceral and skin disease at the other. While not completely worked out, it appears that most cases of LCH demonstrate clonality. In addition, the Langerhans cells in LCH demonstrate telomere shortening. Clonality and telomere shortening are features of preneoplastic conditions and cancer.

Histologically, in all cases of LCH in the skin, there is a dense dermal infiltrate of Langerhans cells. This can be superficial and immediately below the epidermis (usually corresponding to small papules or scaly patches clinically), folliculocentric, or deep and diffuse (in papular and nodular lesions). The Langerhans cells are recognized by their abundant, amphophilic cytoplasm and eccentric round or kidney bean-shaped nucleus. There is frequently exocytosis of the abnormal cells into the overlying epidermis. If this is extensive, macroscopic vesicles can be seen, and erosion can occur secondarily. The dermal infiltrate is accompanied by many other inflammatory cells, including neutrophils, eosinophils, lymphocytes, and plasma cells. Dermal edema and hemorrhage are characteristically present. In larger and older lesions the infiltrating histiocytic cells become foamy and fibrosis may be present.

The histologic features of the Langerhans cells, such as nuclear atypia and mitotic indices, do not predict prognosis and are not reproducible. Histology is not predictive of biological behavior. Immunohistochemistry is useful in confirming the diagnosis. The infiltrating cells in LCH are positive for S-100 and CD1a. Langerin is a protein expressed in the Birbeck granule and stained with CD207. Electron microscopy is rarely required to diagnose LCH due to this panel of Langerhans cell "characteristic" markers.

Congenital self-healing reticulohistiocytosis (Hashimoto–Pritzker disease)

Congenital self-healing reticulohistiocytosis (CSHR) is an autoinvoluting, self-limited form of LCH. It can be considered as one end of the spectrum of LCH, and although cases continue to be described, it is best approached as a variant of LCH, not a separate entity. CSHR is usually present at birth or appears very soon thereafter, although a case in an 8-year-old has been reported. It has been described in two forms: a solitary and a multinodular variant. Solitary or generalized lesions can affect any part of the cutaneous surface. Lesions range from 0.2 to 2.5 cm in diameter (Fig. 31-21). Lesions may grow postnatally. Exceptionally large tumors up to 8 cm in diameter can occur. At presentation the lesions can be papules or nodules, with or without erosion or ulceration. Individual lesions are red, brown, pink, or dusky. Lesions may rarely appear as hemorrhagic bullae. Lesions greater than 1 cm characteristically ulcerate as they resolve. Lesions are asymptomatic and spontaneously involute over 8–24 weeks, leaving atrophic scarring from the ulcerated nodules. Internal involvement is not found. Histologically, the skin lesions are composed of Langerhans cells and no histological features identify this variant of LCH. Because LCH with systemic involvement may present in identical fashion, systemic evaluation is recommended, including a physical examination, complete blood count, liver function tests, and radiological evaluation of the bones. The affected child must be followed regularly because, as in other forms of LCH, late recurrences can occur.

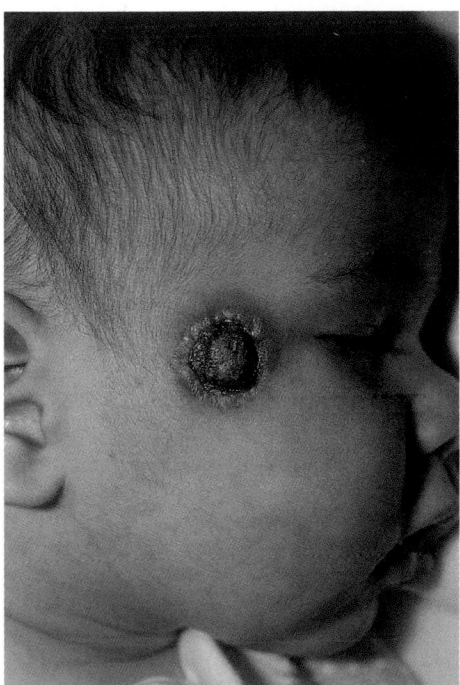

Fig. 31-21 Congenital self-healing reticulohistiocytosis, solitary lesion.

Belhadjali H, et al: Self-healing Langerhans cell histiocytosis (Hashimoto–Pritzker disease): two Tunisian cases. Acta Dermatovenerol Alp Panonica Adriat 2008; 17:188.

Inuzuka M, et al: Congenital self-healing reticulohistiocytosis presenting with hemorrhagic bullae. J Am Acad Dermatol 2003; 48:S75.

Kapur P, et al: Congenital self-healing reticulohistiocytosis (Hashimoto–Pritzker disease): ten-year experience at Dallas Children's Medical Center. J Am Acad Dermatol 2007; 56:290.

Nakahigashi K, et al: Late-onset self-healing reticulohistiocytosis: pediatric case of Hashimoto–Pritzker type Langerhans cell histiocytosis. J Dermatol 2007; 34:205.

Riva B, et al: Two cases of a solitary congenital ulcerated nodule. Pediatr Dermatol 2009; 26:473.

Thong HY, et al: An unusual presentation of congenital self-healing reticulohistiocytosis. Br J Dermatol 2003; 149:191.

Weidner KR, et al: JAAD Grand Rounds quiz. Necrotic, ulcerated papules on a newborn male. J Am Acad Dermatol 2009; 61:544.

Zwerding T, et al: Congenital, single system, single site, Langerhans cell histiocytosis: a new case, observations from the literature, and management considerations. Pediatr Dermatol 2009; 26:121.

Langerhans cell histiocytosis (LCH)

LCH is a rare disease characterized by proliferation of Langerhans cells in many organs. The rarity of the disease and a lack of understanding of how to manage patients appropriately have inspired the formation of the "Histiocyte Society." Many patients throughout the world are entered in large standardized treatment protocols (LCH-I to IV). This has led not only to standardized approaches to management, but also to standardized terminology and classification of patients. It is clear that age of onset is an important determinant of the nature of the disease, and childhood and adult forms of LCH are considered separately. It is also quite clear that patients may begin with any pattern of disease and evolve or relapse to another pattern. This is especially true of younger children. Up to 50% of children under the age of 1 year diagnosed with skin-limited LCH progress to have multisystem disease. Repeated evaluation and close follow-up are required.

Childhood LCH

In childhood LCH, boys are slightly more commonly affected than girls. The incidence in children is about 2.6 cases per million, with a greater rate in children under 1 year of age (9 cases per million), 5 cases per million in 1–4-year-olds, and about 1 per million in 5–14-year-olds. Neonatal disease occurs in 6% of cases but at times is unrecognized, especially if it were to involve an internal organ asymptomatically but not affect its function. Thus many of the neonatal cases have predominantly cutaneous lesions. Overall, in childhood LCH bone lesions represent about two-thirds of cases and skin disease about one-third. Only 10% of cases have neither skin nor bone involvement. In children under 1 year of age, the skin is involved in three-quarters of cases, with ear and bone being involved in about one-third of cases. Two-thirds of children under 1 year of age have multisystem disease, with half having involvement of liver, lungs, or bone marrow. In children aged 1–4, bone disease is most common, but two-thirds or more have multisystem disease. In children aged 5–14, bone disease is almost always seen, and multisystem disease is seen in less than 20%.

Skin lesions About 10% of children have single-organ disease involving only the skin and 50% of children with multisystem LCH have skin involvement, making skin the second most commonly involved organ in childhood LCH. Almost 90% of children less than 1 year old with multisystem LCH have skin lesions. The pattern of skin disease does not predict the presence or extent of systemic disease. The most common form of skin disease in children is that described in Abt–Letterer–Siwe disease. The skin lesions are tiny red,

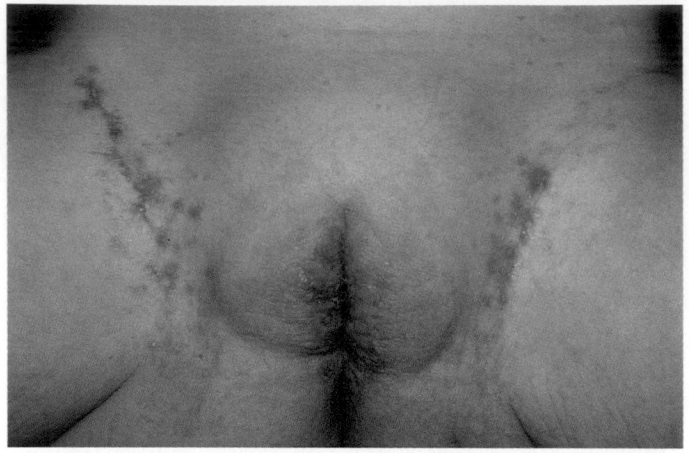

Fig. 31-22 Langerhans cell histiocytosis, erythematous eruption accentuated in the groin folds.

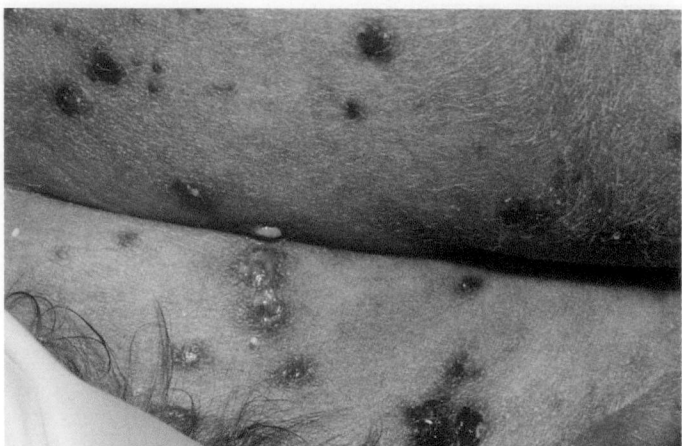

Fig. 31-24 Langerhans cell histiocytosis, bullous lesions.

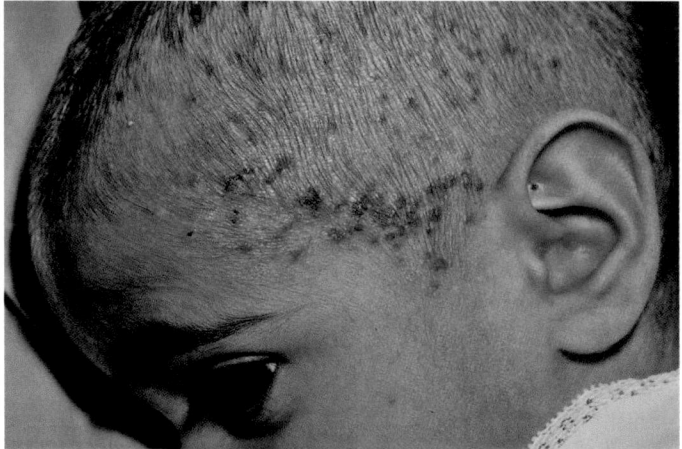

Fig. 31-23 Langerhans cell histiocytosis, seborrheic dermatitis-like eruption with hemorrhage.

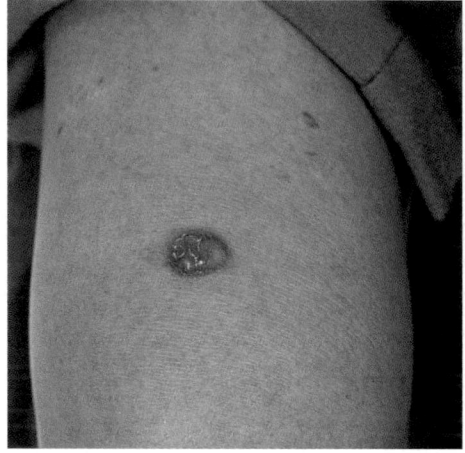

Fig. 31-25 Langerhans cell histiocytosis, xanthomatous nodule in a patient with diabetes insipidus.

red–brown, or yellow papules that are widespread but favor the intertriginous areas, behind the ears, and the scalp (Figs 31-22 and 31-23). There is a superficial resemblance to seborrheic dermatitis, but on careful inspection the lesions are individual papules and there is focal hemorrhage in the lesions. The papules are often folliculocentric. Lesions may erode or weep. In children this pattern is frequently associated with multisystem disease. A rare variant of this pattern of LCH is one in which vesicles appear (Fig. 31-24), usually in infants. The vesicles rupture easily, resulting in widespread erosions. This presentation may be confused with other bullous diseases, especially congenital candidiasis, herpes virus infections, bullous impetigo, bullous mastocytosis, primary immunobullous diseases, and epidermolysis bullosa. The vesicles are due to large intraepidermal collections of Langerhans cells, and a Tzanck smear may lead to suspicion of the diagnosis. A less common presentation is with slightly larger papules up to 1 cm in diameter. These lesions tend to be yellow–red and resemble xanthomas or xanthogranulomas (Fig. 31-25). They can be numerous and widespread. A rare variant resembling lichen planopilaris has been reported. Congenital lesions with hemorrhage have been reported as resembling "blueberry muffin" babies, but the biopsies show typical LCH.

Nail changes can occur, but are uncommon and can include longitudinal grooving, purpuric striae, hyperkeratosis, sub-ungual thinning, deformities, loss of nail plate, and paronychia. Both fingernails and toenails may be affected. Most patients with nail involvement have multisystem disease.

LCH restricted to the genitalia is rare, but vulvar, inguinal, and perianal disease may be the initial manifestation of LCH. It tends to be painful and ulcerative, and may simulate hidradenitis suppurativa, since axillary and scalp involvement may also be present.

Oral mucosa lesions The oral mucosa may be involved. Lesions may be mucosal ulcerations that are painful and inflamed. They affect primarily the buccal mucosa. Most oral disease is due to alveolar bone lesions. These osteolytic lesions can lead to significant periodontitis. Gingival ulceration can result (Fig. 31-26). Teeth detach from the underlying bone and on x-ray appear to be "floating." Palpable masses and gingival lesions should be looked for and a dental evaluation completed in all patients. Cervical adenopathy is common. Bilateral parotid swelling may occur.

Visceral involvement The most commonly involved organ is the bone (Fig. 31-27). The lesions may be asymptomatic or cause pain. The skull is most commonly involved, followed by the long bones, then the flat bones. Bony lesions tend to occur in older children and young adults. Lesions are treated with curettage, intralesional corticosteroids, or radiation. Endocrine dysfunction occurs, usually in the form of diabetes insipidus, which is more common in patients with bone disease of the

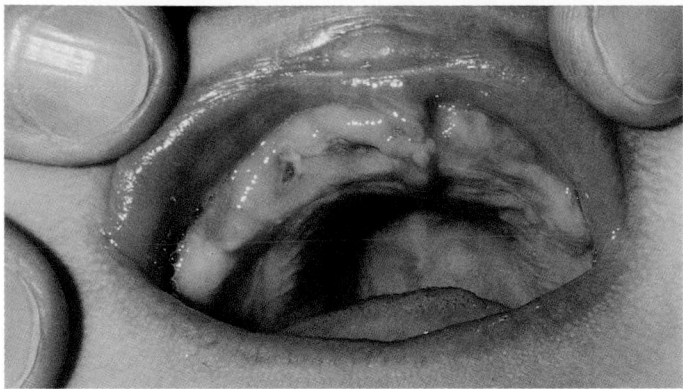

Fig. 31-26 Langerhans cell histiocytosis, gingival lesions.

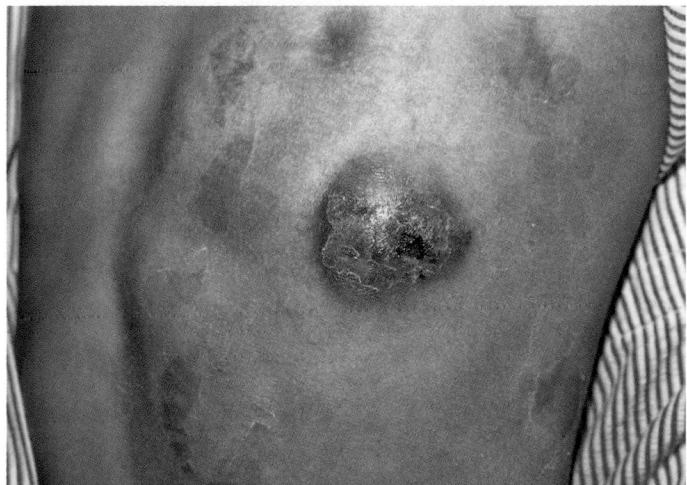

Fig. 31-27 Langerhans cell histiocytosis, eosinophilic granuloma of rib that eroded through to the skin.

skull and in patients with extensive disease. Diabetes insipidus is one of the common long-term sequelae of children recovering from LCH.

Lymph nodes are characteristically involved, especially the cervical nodes. The bone marrow may be affected, resulting in cytopenias. This may present as purpura in the skin. The liver may be involved directly by infiltration with Langerhans cells, or may be affected indirectly by enlarged nodes in the porta hepatis, leading to obstructive disease. Either pattern can lead to biliary cirrhosis. Pulmonary disease with diffuse micronodular infiltrates and cysts occurs less commonly in childhood LCH than in adults with LCH.

Adult LCH

In adults the peak age of presentation is between 20 and 35 years, with multisystem disease in between one-third and two-thirds of adults with LCH. Bones are the most common organ involved in adults with LCH, and 12% of adult LCH patients have disease limited to one or several bones. Skin and mucosal involvement is the second most common manifestation in adults. In the skin, lesions can be papular or diffuse, sometimes with both forms of lesion present at different sites. Acneiform lesions of the chest and back, identical clinically to acne vulgaris, can occur. Xanthomatous lesions may be found. A pattern that has been repeatedly reported in the skin of adults with LCH is a red, erosive, intertriginous eruption, with a close resemblance to deficiency dermatitis. It favors the groin and inframammary areas, especially in elderly women.

Box 31-1 Classification system for Langerhans cell histiocytosis (LCH)

1. Monosystem disease
   a. Focal disease of bone, skin, or lymph node
   b. Multifocal disease of skeleton or lymph nodes
2. Multisystem disease
   a. Low risk—age over 2, without involvement of lungs, liver, spleen, or hematopoietic system
   b. High risk—age under 2 and involvement of multiple organs, or age over 2 years and involvement of lungs, liver, spleen, or hematopoietic system

Pulmonary LCH occurs on average at age 33 years. A diffuse micronodular pattern on chest radiograph may progress to cyst formation (honeycomb lung), large bullae, and pneumothorax. More than 90% of adults with pulmonary LCH are tobacco or marijuana smokers. Pneumothorax occurs in 25% of cases. High-resolution CT is useful for diagnosis. Five-year survival is 88%. Lung transplantation may be required. It is unclear if isolated pulmonary LCH is a reactive process or a variant of LCH.

Treatment/prognosis

In childhood LCH, outcome is determined by the extent of involvement and, more importantly, the function of affected organs. Children younger than 1 year with multisystem disease have the worst prognosis, with mortality approaching 50%, children aged 1–4 have a 30% or lower mortality, and mortality is only 6% in children 5 years or older. Not only is the organ system involved important, but also the extent of involvement. Liver function tests greater than five times normal are associated with a 5-year survival of only 25%, with most deaths occurring within 1 year. Without liver involvement, the 5-year survival is more than 75%. Involvement of the ear and lung is also a poor prognostic finding in patients with multisystem disease. Early initial response to multidrug chemotherapy in childhood multisystem LCH is an important predictor of survival, with survival of 92% of responders and 11% of nonresponders after 6 weeks of treatment. Baseline and repeated evaluation is important. Lesions in one organ system may resolve while disease progresses in another organ. Skin lesions may spontaneously resolve, only for the disease to recur, even years later, so patients must be followed regularly.

For treatment children with LCH are classified into four groups (Box 31.1). Monosystem disease 1a and 1b involves local therapies to the skin, and surgery alone for bone lesions. These patients may be observed, as spontaneous resolution may occur. Treatment is not required. Low-risk patients are treated with a combination of vinblastine and prednisone over months. High-risk patients receive prednisone and vinblastine as initial treatment, followed by maintenance therapy with methotrexate and 6-mercaptopurine. Multisystem LCH in adults has a 5-year survival of more than 90%. Pulmonary LCH in adults can be progressive and fatal, especially in smokers. Adults with multisystem disease who require treatment are given a combination of vinblastine and prednisone induction, followed by maintenance treatment with 6-mercaptopurine and methotrexate. Relapses or progression may be treated with 2-chlorodeoxyadenosine. Imatinib mesylate, thalidomide, cyclosporine, and anti-TNF agents can be considered experimental approaches. Rarely, hematopoietic stem cell transplantation and solid organ (liver, lung) transplantation have been performed as life-saving measures in refractory or progressing patients.

Various skin-directed treatments have been reported for children and adults with skin-predominant disease, who do not require systemic therapy. These include topical nitrogen mustard, topical steroids, imiquimod, systemic steroids, PUVA, narrow-band UVB, excimer laser, isotretinoin, thalidomide, low-dose methotrexate, and IFN-α. Associated lymphomas, solid tumors, and myelodysplasias have occurred in patients with LCH, with acute lymphoblastic leukemia and myelodysplastic syndrome preceding the appearance of LCH, and acute myelogenous leukemia and acute lymphoblastic leukemia following it. The role of the preceding lymphoma or myelodysplasia in the appearance of LCH in adults is unknown. The appearance of acute leukemia and possibly solid tumors following the diagnosis of LCH is felt to be a complication of the chemotherapeutic regimens and is seen predominantly in LCH patients so treated. In some cases of cutaneous and systemic lymphomas, aggregates of polyclonal Langerhans cells are seen in the tissue affected by the lymphoma. Whether this represents the coexistence of LCH and lymphoma (unlikely) or a reactive proliferation of Langerhans cells within the tissue affected by the lymphoma (more likely) is unknown. Reactive proliferations of histiocytes resembling sarcoidosis can also be seen in lymphoma, suggesting this is a reactive phenomenon.

Differential diagnosis

The diffuse small papular form is frequently misdiagnosed as seborrheic dermatitis. The yellow color of the lesions and the presence of hemorrhage in the small papules, if present, should suggest the diagnosis of LCH. Nodular lesions of scabies can closely simulate LCH. This includes the finding of Langerhans or indeterminate cells in the dermal infiltrate by electron microscopy and S-100 and CD1a staining. The larger papules resemble juvenile xanthogranulomas and xanthomas. Erosive genital disease may simulate deficiency dermatitis.

Alston RD, et al: Incidence and survival of childhood Langerhans cell histiocytosis in Northwest England from 1954 to 1998. Pediatr Blood Cancer 2007; 48:555.

Aviner S, et al: Langerhans cell histiocytosis in a premature baby presenting with skin-isolated disease: case report and literature review. Acta Paediatr 2008; 97:1751.

Avram MM, et al: Case records of the Massachusetts General Hospital. Case 20-2007: a newborn girl with skin lesions. N Engl J Med 2007; 357:1327.

Aydogan K, et al: Adult-onset Langerhans cell histiocytosis confined to the skin. J Eur Acad Dermatol Venereol 2006; 20:890.

Bechan GI, et al: Telomere length shortening in Langerhans cell histiocytosis. Br J Haematol 2008; 140:420.

Billings SD, et al: Langerhans cell histiocytosis associated with myelodysplastic syndrome in adults. J Cutan Pathol 2006; 33:171.

Broekaert SM, et al: Multisystem Langerhans cell histiocytosis: successful treatment with thalidomide. Am J Clin Dermatol 2007; 8:311.

Campanati A, et al: Purely cutaneous Langerhans' cell histiocytosis in an adult woman. Acta Derm Venereol 2009; 89:299.

Campos MK, et al: Langerhans cell histiocytosis: a 16-year experience. J Pedatri (Rio J) 2007; 83:79.

Chander R, et al: Pulmonary disease with striking nail involvement in a child. Pediatr Dermatol 2008; 25:633.

Chi DH, et al: Eruptive xanthoma-like cutaneous Langerhans cell histiocytosis in an adult. J Am Acad Dermatol 1996; 34:688.

Chiles LR, et al: Langerhans cell histiocytosis in a child while in remission for acute lymphocytic leukemia. J Am Acad Dermatol 2001; 45:S233.

Christie LJ, et al: Lesions resembling Langerhans cell histiocytosis in association with other lymphoproliferative disorders: a reactive or neoplastic phenomenon? Hum Pathol 2006; 37:32.

Escardó-Paton JA, et al: Late recurrence of Langerhans cell histiocytosis in the orbit. Br J Ophthalmol 2004; 88:838.

Fernandez Flores A, Mallo S: Langerhans cell histiocytosis of vulva. Dermatol Online J 2006; 12:15.

Hagiuda J, et al: Langerhans cell histiocytosis on the penis: a case report. BMC Urol 2006; 6:28.

Hancox JG, et al: Adult onset folliculocentric Langerhans cell histiocytosis confined to the scalp. Am J Dermatopathol 2004; 26:123.

Hatakeyama N, et al: An infant with self-healing cutaneous Langerhans cell histiocytosis followed by isolated thymic relapse. Pediatr Blood Cancer 2009; 53:229.

Honda R, et al: Langerhans' cell histiocytosis after living donor liver transplantation: report of a case. Liver Transpl 2005; 11:1435.

Imafuku S, et al: Cutaneous Langerhans cell histiocytosis in an elderly man successfully treated with narrowband ultraviolet B. Br J Dermatol 2007; 157:1277.

Iqbal Y, et al: Langerhans cell histiocytosis presenting as a painless bilateral swelling of the parotid glands. J Pediatr Hematol Oncol 2004; 26:276.

Kartono F, et al: Crusted Norwegian scabies in an adult with Langerhans cell histiocytosis: mishaps leading to systemic chemotherapy. Arch Dermatol 2007; 143:626.

Kwong YL, et al: Widespread skin-limited Langerhans cell histiocytosis: complete remission with interferon alfa. J Am Acad Dermatol 1997; 36:628.

Lau L, et al: Cutaneous Langerhans cell histiocytosis in children under one year. Pediatr Blood Cancer 2006; 46:66.

Madrigal-Martinez-Pereda C, et al: Langerhans cell histiocytosis: literature review and descriptive analysis of oral manifestations. Med Oral Patol Oral Cir Bucal 2009; 14:E222.

Mataix J, et al: Nail changes in Langerhans cell histiocytosis: a possible marker of multisystem disease. Pediatr Dermatol 2008; 25:247.

McElligott J, et al: Spontaneous regression of Langerhans cell histiocytosis in a neonate with multiple bony lesions. J Pediatr Hematol Oncol 2008; 30:85.

Moravvej H, et al: An unusual case of adult disseminate cutaneous Langerhans cell histiocytosis. Dermatol Online J 2006; 12:13.

Mosterd K, et al: Neonatal Langerhans' cell histiocytosis: a rare and potentially life-threatening disease. Int J Dermatol 2008; 47:10.

Mottl H, et al: Treatment results of Langerhans cell histiocytosis according to the LCH II protocol. Cas Lek Cesk 2005; 144:753.

Nagarajan R, et al: Successful treatment of refractory Langerhans cell histiocytosis with unrelated cord blood transplantation. J Pediatr Hematol Oncol 2001; 23:629.

Pollono D, et al: Reactivation and risk of sequelae in Langerhans cell histiocytosis. Pediatr Blood Cancer 2007; 48:696.

Querings K, et al: Clinical spectrum of cutaneous Langerhans' cell histiocytosis mimicking various diseases. Acta Derm Venereol 2006; 86:39.

Sankilampi U, et al: Congenital Langerhans cell histiocytosis mimicking a "blueberry muffin baby". J Pediatr Hematol Oncol 2008; 30:245.

Satter EK, et al: Langerhans cell histiocytosis: a case report and summary of the current recommendations of the Histiocyte Society. Dermatol Online J 2008; 14:3.

Satter EK, et al: Diffuse xanthogranulomatous dermatitis and systemic Langerhans cell histiocytosis: a novel case that demonstrates bridging between non-Langerhans cell histiocytosis and Langerhans cell histiocytosis. J Am Acad Dermatol 2009; 60:841.

Saven A, et al: 2-chlorodeoxyadenosine-induced complete remission in Langerhans-cell histiocytosis. Ann Intern Med 1994; 121:430.

Shaffer MP, et al: Langerhans cell histiocytosis presenting as blueberry muffin baby. J Am Acad Dermatol 2005; 53; S143.

Steen AE, et al: Successful treatment of cutaneous Langerhans cell histiocytosis with low-dose methotrexate. Br J Dermatol 2001; 145:137.

Stefanos CM, et al: Langerhans cell histiocytosis in the elderly. J Am Acad Dermatol 1998; 39:375.

Tantiwongkosi B, et al: Congenital solid neck mass: a unique presentation of Langerhans cell histiocytosis. Pediatr Radiol 2008; 38:575.

Tatevossian R, et al: Adults with LCH—orphans with an orphan disease. Clin Med 2006; 6:404.

Teng CL, et al: Rapidly fatal Langerhans' cell histiocytosis in an adult. J Formos Med Assoc 2005; 104:955.

Vogel CA, et al: Excimer laser as adjuvant therapy for adult cutaneous Langerhans cell histiocytosis. Arch Dermatol 2008; 144:1287.

Von Stebut E, et al: Successful treatment of adult multisystemic Langerhans cell histiocytosis with psoralen-UV-A, prednisone, mercaptopurine, and vinblastine. Arch Dermatol 2008; 144:649.

Wagner C, et al: Langerhans cell histiocytosis: treatment failure with imatinib. Arch Dermatol 2009; 145:949.

Yazc N, et al: Langerhans cell histiocytosis with involvement of nails and lungs in an adolescent. J Pediatr Hematol Oncol 2008; 30:77.

Bonus images for this chapter can be found online at

http://www.expertconsult.com

Fig. 31-1 Granuloma annulare, generalized small papules and annular plaques.

Fig. 31-2 Sarcoidosis, hypopigmented papules.

Fig. 31-3 Sarcoidosis, hypopigmented and annular plaques.

Histiocytoses

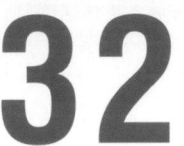
32

Cutaneous Lymphoid Hyperplasia, Cutaneous T-cell Lymphoma, Other Malignant Lymphomas, and Allied Diseases

Cutaneous lymphoid hyperplasia (lymphocytoma cutis, lymphadenosis benigna cutis, pseudolymphoma)

The term cutaneous lymphoid hyperplasia refers to a group of benign disorders characterized by collections of lymphocytes, macrophages, and dendritic cells in the skin. These processes can be caused by known stimuli (such as medications, injected foreign substances, infections, or the bites of arthropods) or they may be idiopathic. They may have a purely benign histologic appearance or resemble cutaneous lymphoma. If there is a histologic resemblance to lymphoma, the term pseudolymphoma is sometimes used. Most cases contain a mixed population of T and B cells, but they may contain mostly T cells. By standard techniques, most cases of cutaneous lymphoid hyperplasia will be found to lack clonality. Cases of monoclonal B- and T-cell cutaneous lymphoid hyperplasia do occur. Thus, a finding of monoclonality does not equate to the diagnosis of malignancy or lymphoma, nor does it predict biologic behavior. A subset of polyclonal or monoclonal (T- or B-cell) cutaneous lymphoid hyperplasias does progress to cutaneous B-cell and, less commonly, T-cell lymphoma. Even when the initial evaluation detects a T-cell rich infiltrate (>90%), which may be monoclonal, the lymphoma that eventuates from this form of cutaneous lymphoid hyperplasia may be B-cell. Thus, as in many cancer syndromes, cutaneous lymphoid hyperplasia represents the benign end of a spectrum of cutaneous lymphoid proliferation, with cutaneous lymphoma at the other end, and cases falling everywhere along that spectrum of progression. Unfortunately, current techniques cannot always predict which cases will progress.

Two clinical patterns of cutaneous lymphoid hyperplasia exist. The nodular form consists of nodular and diffuse dermal aggregates of lymphocytes, macrophages, and dendritic cells. The clinical and histologic differential diagnosis is cutaneous B-cell lymphoma. The diffuse type is usually associated with drug exposure or photosensitivity (actinic reticuloid). Histologically, it is to be distinguished from cutaneous T-cell lymphoma.

Cutaneous lymphoid hyperplasias—nodular B-cell pattern

The nodular pattern of cutaneous lymphoid hyperplasia is the most common pattern. It usually presents in adults and is 2–3 times more common in women. It favors the face (cheek, nose, or earlobe), and the majority of cases present as a solitary or localized cluster of asymptomatic, erythematous to violaceous papules or nodules (Fig. 32-1). Less commonly, lesions may affect the trunk (36%) or extremities (25%). At times, the lesions may coalesce into a plaque or be widespread in one region, in which case they present as miliary papules. Systemic symptoms are absent and, except for rare cases with regional lymphadenopathy, there are no other physical or laboratory abnormalities. It is usually idiopathic, but can be caused by tattoos, *Borrelia* infections, herpes zoster scars, antigen injections, acupuncture, and, in rare cases, drug reactions, tumor necrosis factor (TNF)-α inhibitors, and persistent insect bite reactions. Lesions that result from a known stimulus tend to be localized to the site of the original process—tattoo, injection, or insect bite.

Borrelia-induced cutaneous lymphoid hyperplasia is an uncommon manifestation of this infection, occurring in 0.6–1.3% of cases reported from Europe. The lack of borrelial pseudolymphoma in the US compared with Europe may relate to the fact that there are different borrelial species in Europe, specifically *Borrelia afzelii*, that cause borreliosis. Lesions occur at the site of the tick bite or close to the edge of a lesion of erythema migrans. They may appear up to 10 months after infection. Lesions may be multiple and favor the earlobes, nipple and areola, nose, and scrotal area, and vary from 1 to 5 cm in diameter. Usually, there are no symptoms, but associated regional lymphadenopathy may be present. Late manifestations of *Borrelia* infection are uncommon. The diagnosis is suspected from a history of a tick bite or erythema migrans, the location (earlobe or nipple), and the histologic picture. The diagnosis is confirmed by an elevated anti-*Borrelia* antibody (present in 50% of cases) and the finding of borrelial DNA in the affected tissue. The treatment is penicillin. Some cases progress to true lymphoma.

Histologic examination of nodular cutaneous lymphoid hyperplasia reveals a dense, nodular infiltrate that occupies primarily the dermis and lessens in the deeper dermis and subcutaneous fat, i.e. it is "top-heavy." The process is usually separated from the epidermis by a clear Grenz zone. The infiltrate is composed chiefly of mature small and large lymphocytes, histiocytes, plasma cells, dendritic cells, and eosinophils. In the deeper portions, well-defined germinal centers are usually seen, with central large lymphoid cells with abundant cytoplasm and tingible body macrophages, and a peripheral cuff of small lymphocytes. A plasma cell-predominant variant has been described. Reactive hyperplasia of adnexal epithelium is common and characteristic, but may also occasionally be seen in true lymphomas. Germinal centers are symmetrical and surrounded by a mix of B and T cells. BCL-6 and CD10 expression is limited to the germinal centers, which also have an intact CD21+ network of dendritic cells. Typically, more than 90% of the cells in the germinal center express the proliferative marker Ki-67 (MIB-1). There is no evidence of light chain restriction by in situ hybridization. CD30+ cells may occasionally be prominent, raising concern about the development of a CD30+ lymphoproliferative disorder.

As most lesions are asymptomatic, treatment is often not required. If the process has been induced by a medication, use of the medication should be discontinued. Infection should be

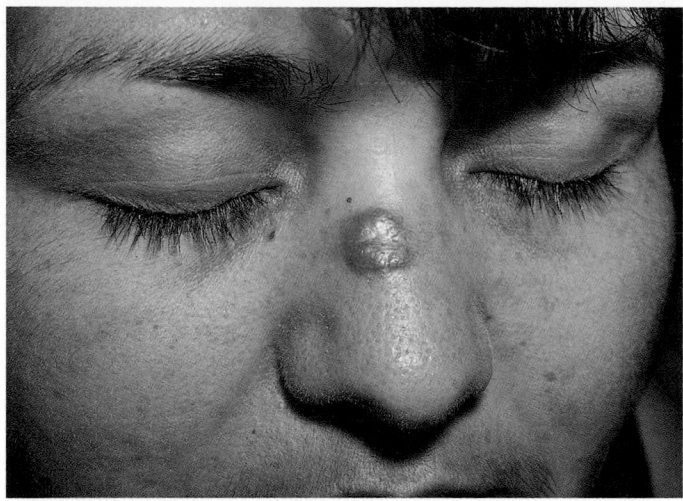

Fig. 32-1 Reactive lymphoid hyperplasia.

treated and localized foci of infection removed. Intralesional steroidal agents are sometimes beneficial, but lesions may recur in a few months. Potent topical steroids may also be tried for superficial lesions. Intralesional corticosteroids, cryosurgery, thalidomide, 100 mg/day for a few months, interferon (IFN)-α, IFN-α 2b, laser ablation, and surgical excision can all produce good results. Low-dose radiation therapy is usually very effective and may be used on refractory facial lesions that cannot be satisfactorily removed surgically. If monoclonality is detected in a localized lesion, complete removal and local radiation have been recommended, but there is no evidence that this improves outcome, and lesions that are not initially monoclonal may also progress to lymphoma.

Cutaneous lymphoid hyperplasias—bandlike T-cell pattern

Cutaneous lymphoid hyperplasias may histologically show a bandlike and perivascular dermal infiltrate, at times with epidermotropism. They may be idiopathic, or caused by photosensitivity (formerly called actinic reticuloid; now called chronic actinic dermatitis), medications (usually anticonvulsants, but also many others), or contact dermatitis (so-called lymphomatoid contact dermatitis).

Clinically, these patients have lesions that clinically resemble mycosis fungoides: widespread erythema with scaling. Thicker plaques may occur as well and these cases are frequently caused by medications. The treatment is to stop any implicated medication. If stopping the medication is ineffective, topical and intralesional steroids, PUVA, and, for persistent localized lesions, radiotherapy may be considered.

Histologically, a T cell-rich band of lymphocytes is present. Epidermotropism, atypia, and even clonality may suggest mycosis fungoides, but the lesions resolve when the drug or other inciting agent is withdrawn.

Jessner lymphocytic infiltrate of the skin

The existence of this entity has recently been challenged. Even the coauthors of the original paper feel their cases would now best be classified as a variant of lupus erythematosus. Clinically, Jessner infiltrate is a persistent papular and plaque-like eruption that is photosensitive and occurs primarily on the face. Histologically, there is a superficial and deep perivascular and periadnexal lymphocytic infiltrate. Interface dermatitis is absent. The infiltrating lymphocytes are suppressor T cells (CD8+). Features that suggest this may be distinct from

other forms of cutaneous lupus erythematosus include the absence of an interface dermatitis, lack of mucin, and negative direct immunofluorescence. Tumid lupus erythematosus also lacks interface dermatitis but has ample mucin. Polymorphous light eruption (PMLE) is distinguished from Jessner infiltrate by having edematous papules and plaques that are more transient, and by the presence of dermal edema. In PMLE the infiltrating cells are CD8+. There may still exist true cases of lymphocytic infiltration of the skin. To distinguish them clearly from lupus erythematosus and PMLE, the lesions must contain predominantly CD8+ suppressor T cells, lack dermal mucin and dermal edema, and be fixed (not transient like PMLE); patients must have negative direct immunofluorescence and serologic testing for lupus erythematosus. Both Jessner and chronic cutaneous lupus erythematosus can respond to antimalarials.

Belousova IE, et al: Atypical histopathological features in cutaneous lymphoid hyperplasia of the scrotum. Am J Dermatopathol 2008 Aug; 30(4):407–408.

Böer A, et al: Pseudoclonality in cutaneous pseudolymphomas: a pitfall in interpretation of rearrangement studies. Br J Dermatol 2008 Aug; 159(2):394–402.

Cerroni L, et al: Cutaneous B-cell pseudolymphoma at the site of vaccination. Am J Dermatopathol 2007 Dec; 29(6):538–542.

Guis S, et al: Cutaneous pseudolymphoma associated with a TNF-alpha inhibitor treatment: etanercept. Eur J Dermatol 2008 Jul–Aug; 18(4):474–476.

Kazakov DV, et al: Hyperplasia of hair follicles and other adnexal structures in cutaneous lymphoproliferative disorders: a study of 53 cases, including so-called pseudolymphomatous folliculitis and overt lymphomas. Am J Surg Pathol 2008 Oct; 32(10):1468–1478.

Nervi SJ, et al: Plasma cell predominant B cell pseudolymphoma. Dermatol Online J 2008 Oct 15; 14(10):12.

Shin JB, et al: Cutaneous T cell pseudolymphoma at the site of a semipermanent lip-liner tattoo. Dermatology 2009; 218(1):75–78.

Tomar S, et al: Treatment of cutaneous pseudolymphoma with interferon alfa-2b. J Am Acad Dermatol 2009 Jan; 60(1):172–174.

Cutaneous lymphomas

Because cutaneous Hodgkin disease is very rare, the term non-Hodgkin lymphoma has little meaning when speaking of a lymphoma in the skin, because virtually all cutaneous lymphomas are "non-Hodgkin lymphomas." Cutaneous lymphoma can be considered to be either primary or secondary. Primary cutaneous lymphomas are those that occur in the skin and where no evidence of extracutaneous involvement is found for some period after the appearance of the cutaneous disease. Secondary cutaneous lymphoma includes cases that have simultaneous or preceding evidence of extracutaneous involvement. These cases are best classified and managed as lymph node-based lymphomas with skin involvement. This conceptual separation is not ideal, but it has been important in developing classification schemes and determining prognosis in cutaneous lymphomas.

For many years classification of lymphomas has been based on their histologic appearance, and lesions from all organ systems were classified histomorphologically in an identical manner to lymphomas arising in lymph nodes. It had been recognized that these classification schemes have major shortcomings when applied to extranodal lymphomas. Specifically, they did not uniformly predict clinical behavior. The new World Health Organization (WHO) classification scheme recognizes distinct forms of primary cutaneous lymphoma.

Cutaneous lymphomas are classified based on their cell type. There are B-cell lymphomas and T-cell lymphomas, but B-cell lymphomas can be T cell-rich. In such cases, atypia is restricted to the B-cell population and immunoglobulin gene rearrangements are detected. Histologic features used in the classification system include cell size (large versus small), nuclear morphology (cleaved or non-cleaved), and immunophenotype. Because appropriate classification may be prognostically important, experienced dermatopathology consultation should be sought in cases of cutaneous lymphoma.

Primary cutaneous T-cell lymphomas

A major insight into cutaneous lymphoma was the finding that the majority of lymphomas in the skin were of T-cell origin. This is logical, since T cells normally traffic through the skin and are important in "skin-associated lymphoid tissue." Unfortunately, dermatologists frequently use the term cutaneous T-cell lymphoma synonymously with mycosis fungoides. Although mycosis fungoides represents the large majority of primary cutaneous T-cell lymphomas, up to 30% of primary cutaneous T-cell lymphomas are not mycosis fungoides. The following discussion is divided into mycosis fungoides and related conditions, Sézary syndrome, lymphomatoid papulosis, and non-mycosis fungoides primary cutaneous T-cell lymphomas.

Mycosis fungoides

Mycosis fungoides is a malignant neoplasm of T-lymphocyte origin, almost always a memory T-helper cell. The incidence has been cited as 1 in 300 000 per year, but has been increasing. Mycosis fungoides affects all races. In the US black persons are relatively more commonly affected than white persons. The condition is twice as common in males as in females.

Natural history

In most cases, mycosis fungoides is a chronic, slowly progressive disorder. It usually begins as flat patches (patch stage), which may or may not be histologically diagnostic of mycosis fungoides. This inability to diagnose early cases has more to do with the limits of diagnostic capabilities, rather than a transformation from some non-neoplastic (premycotic) condition to mycosis fungoides, and these cases are best considered mycosis fungoides from the onset. Pruritus, sometimes severe, is usually present at this stage. Over time, sometimes years, the lesions become more infiltrated, and the diagnosis is usually confirmed with repeated histologic evaluation. Infiltrated plaques occur eventually (plaque stage). In some cases, tumors may eventually appear (tumor stage). Some patients may present with or progress to erythroderma. Most rarely, patients may present with tumors de novo, the so-called d'emblée form. With immunophenotyping, many of these cases are now recognized as non-mycosis fungoides T-cell lymphomas. Eventually, in some patients, noncutaneous involvement is detected. This is most commonly first identified in lymph nodes. Peripheral blood involvement and visceral organ involvement may also occur.

In general, mycosis fungoides affects elderly patients and has a long evolution. However, once tumors develop or lymph node involvement occurs, the prognosis is guarded and mycosis fungoides can be fatal. In most fatal cases the patient dies of septicemia. Early, aggressive chemotherapy in an attempt to "cure" mycosis fungoides is associated with excessive morbidity and mortality, and is not indicated.

Evaluation and staging

The North American Mycosis Fungoides Cooperative Group has developed a staging system. Because mycosis fungoides is a systemic disease from the onset (as lymphocytes naturally traffic throughout the body), concepts used for solid tumors, such as tumor burden and metastasis, cannot be readily applied. The TNMB system scores involvement in the skin (T), lymph node (N), viscera (M), and peripheral blood (B), and is

in evolution. Skin involvement is divided into less than 10% (T1), more than 10% (T2), tumors (T3), and erythroderma (T4). Node involvement is normal clinically and pathologically (N0), palpable but pathologically not mycosis fungoides (N1), not palpable but pathologically mycosis fungoides (N2), or clinically and pathologically involved (N3). Viscera and blood are either not involved (M0 and B0) or involved (M1 and B1).

- Stage IA is T1,N0,M0.
- Stage IB is T2,N0,M0.
- Stage IIA is T1–2,N1,M0.
- Stage IIB is T3,N0–1,M0.
- Stage IIIA is T4,N0,M0.
- Stage IIIB is T4,N1,M0.
- Stage IVA is T1–4, N2–3,M0.
- Stage IVB is T1–4,N0–3,M1.

The "B" or blood status does not alter staging of the disease.

A staging work-up would include a complete history and physical examination, with careful palpation of lymph nodes and mapping of skin lesions; a complete blood cell count with assays for circulating atypical cells (Sézary cells); serum chemistries, including renal and liver function tests with lactic dehydrogenase; a chest radiograph evaluation; and a skin biopsy. If lymph nodes are palpable, they should be examined histologically. Fine-needle aspiration is not an ideal mode of evaluation, since early lymph node involvement may be localized to certain areas of the affected nodes, and architectural evaluation is often required to detect early lymph node involvement. If any abnormalities are detected through the above evaluations, they should be pursued. Computed tomography (CT) can be performed to assess chest, abdominal, and pelvic lymph nodes, and visceral organs. These are useful in patients with stage II–IV disease, but are not indicated in patients with stage IA disease. Whether patients with stage IB disease should undergo these tests is unknown.

The value of this staging system is confirmed in large series. Stage IA patients have a life expectancy identical to that of a control population; only 8–9% progress to have more advanced disease; and only 2% die of their disease. By contrast, patients with T2 disease have a shorter survival time than control subjects (median survival of 11.7–15.6 years). Twenty-four percent of T2 patients progress to more advanced disease. T3 patients have a median survival of 3.2–8.4 years, and T4 patients 1.8–3.7 years. Palpable adenopathy is associated with a median survival of only 7.7 years, whereas patients without adenopathy have a survival of 21.8 years. Lymphadenopathy, tumors, and cutaneous ulceration are cardinal prognostic factors; no patient dies without having developed one of them and patients with all three (in any order) survive a median of 1 year.

Clinical features

In the early patch/plaque stage, the lesions are macular or slightly infiltrated patches or plaques varying in size from 1 to 5 cm or more. Folliculotropic disease can resemble lichen nitidus. Except for the folliculotropic variant, lesions >5 cm in size are virtually always present in true cases of mycosis fungoides. In contrast, most histologic simulators present with smaller skin lesions. The eruption may be generalized or begin localized to one area and then spread. The lower abdomen, buttocks, upper thighs, and breasts of women are preferentially affected. The lesions may have an atrophic surface, or present as true poikiloderma with atrophy, mottled dyspigmentation, and telangiectasia. Poikiloderma vasculare atrophicans most commonly represents a clinical form of patch-stage mycosis fungoides. Likewise, large-plaque parapsoriasis and cases of small-plaque parapsoriasis with poikilodermatous change are early patch-stage lesions of mycosis fungoides. In contrast, typical digitate dermatosis probably never evolves into mycosis fungoides. "Invisible" mycosis fungoides is generalized skin involvement that is not visible to the naked eye but can be documented histologically. With current diagnostic methods, this can usually be confirmed. In general, the patch-stage lesions resemble an eczema, being round or ovoid, but annular, polycyclic, or arciform configurations can occur. Less common forms are the verrucous or hyperkeratotic form, the hypopigmented form (Fig. 32-2), lesions resembling a pigmented purpura, and the vesicular, bullous, or pustular form. The hypopigmented form seems to be more common in persons of color and is a common presentation for adolescents and children with mycosis fungoides. Subtle lesions of mycosis fungoides may manifest clinically during anti-TNF therapy.

In the plaque stage, lesions are more infiltrated and may resemble psoriasis (Fig. 32-3), a subacute dermatitis, or a granulomatous dermal process such as granuloma annulare. The palms and soles may be involved, with hyperkeratotic, psoriasiform, and fissuring plaques. The infiltration of the plaques, at first recognized by light palpation, may be present in only a few of the lesions. It is a manifestation of diagnostic importance. Different degrees of infiltration may exist even in the same patch and sometimes it is more pronounced peripherally, the central part of the plaque being depressed to the level of the surrounding skin. The infiltration becomes more marked and leads to discoid patches or extensive plaques, which may be as wide as 30 cm.

Eventually, through coalescence of the various plaques, the involvement becomes widespread, but there are usually patches of apparently normal skin interspersed. When the involvement is advanced, painful superficial ulcerations may occur. During this phase, enlarged lymph nodes usually develop. They are nontender, firm, and freely movable.

The tumor stage is characterized by large, various-sized and shaped nodules on infiltrated plaques and on apparently normal skin. These nodules have a tendency to break down early and to form deep oval ulcers, whose bases are covered with a necrotic grayish substance and which have rolled edges (Fig. 32-4). The lesions generally have a predilection for the trunk, although they may be seen anywhere on the skin or may involve the mouth and upper respiratory tract. Uncommonly, tumors may be the first sign of mycosis fungoides.

The erythrodermic variety of mycosis fungoides is a generalized exfoliative process, with universal redness. The hair is scanty, nails are dystrophic, palms and soles are hyperkeratotic, and at times there may be generalized hyperpigmentation (Fig. 32-5). Erythroderma may be the presenting feature.

Alopecia mucinosa The infiltrating cells of mycosis fungoides can demonstrate a predilection for involving the hair follicle (Fig. 32-6). This may be observed simply by

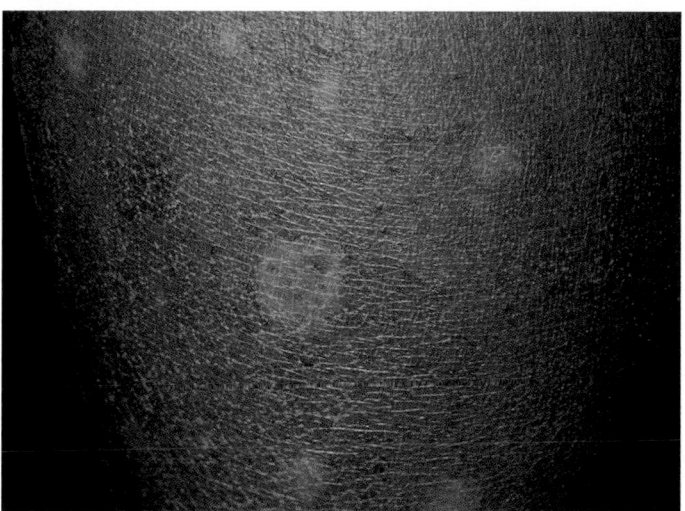

Fig. 32-2 Mycosis fungoides, hypopigmented patches.

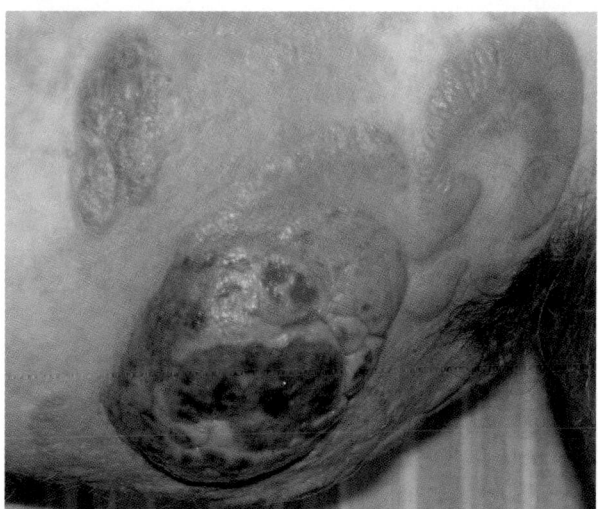

Fig. 32-4 Tumor-stage mycosis fungoides. (Courtesy of Ellen Kim, MD)

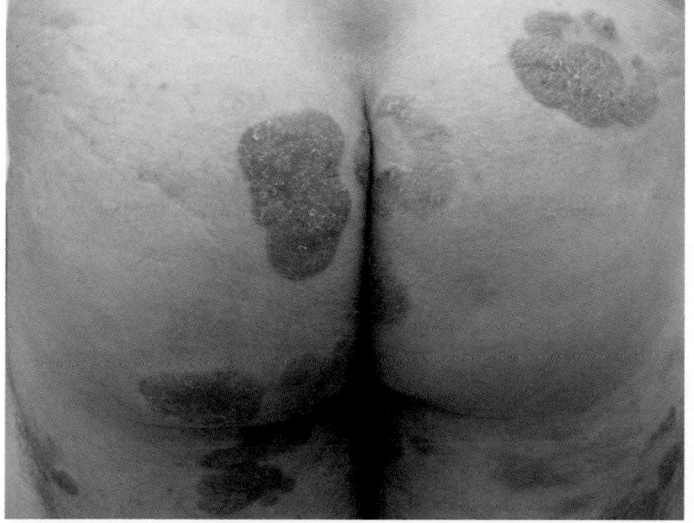

Fig. 32-3 Plaque stage mycosis fungoides. (Courtesy of Ellen Kim, MD)

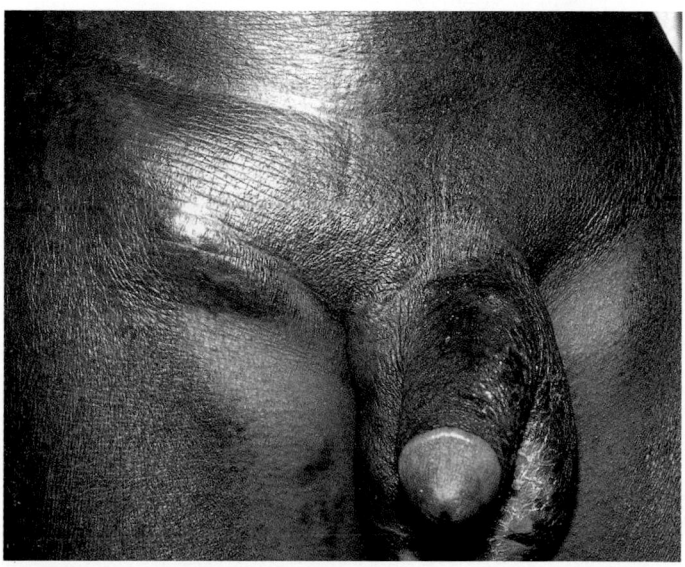

Fig. 32-5 Erythrodermic mycosis fungoides.

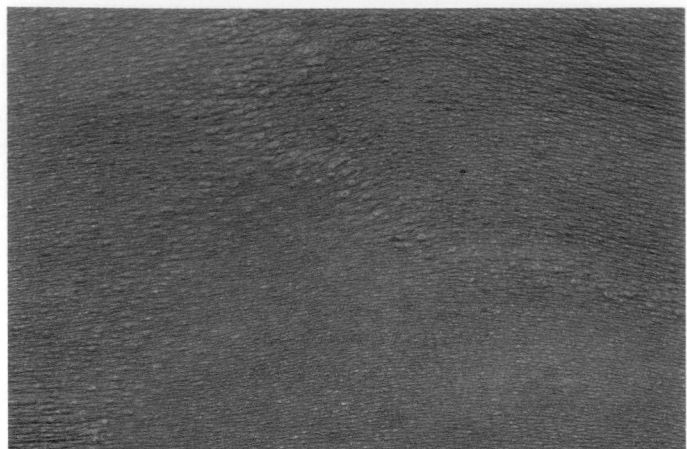

Fig. 32-6 Follicular mycosis fungoides.

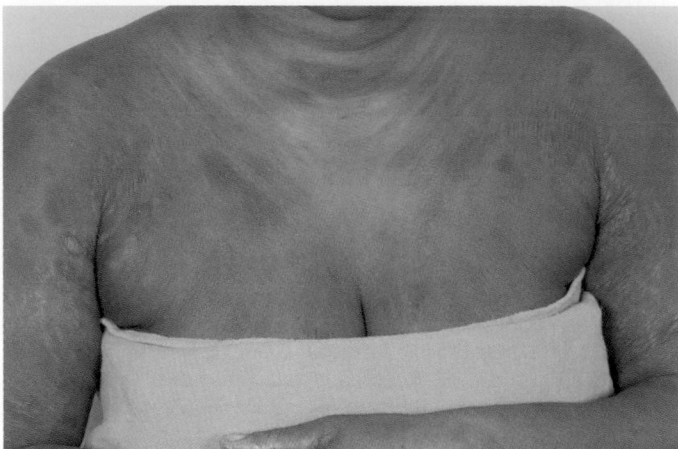

Fig. 32-8 Syringotropic mycosis fungoides.

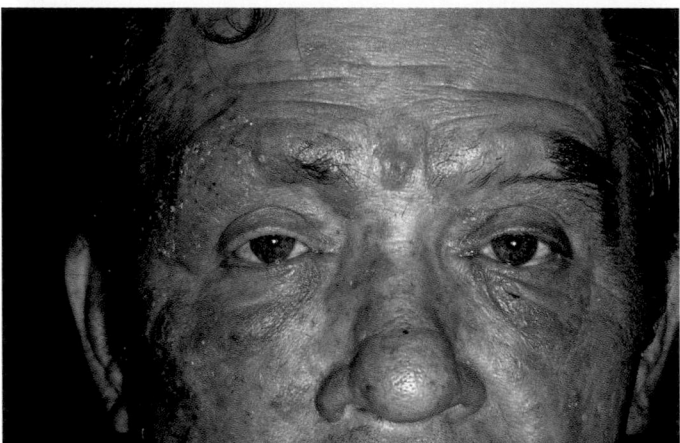

Fig. 32-7 Alopecia mucinosa.

folliculotropism of the cells (pilotropic or follicular mycosis fungoides) or by the appearance of follicular mucinosis (Fig. 32-7). In all cases of follicular mucinosis, the histologic specimen should be carefully examined and the diagnosis of mycosis fungoides considered. Among patients older than 40 years of age who have follicular mucinosis, a large percentage will have mycosis fungoides or go on to develop it. However, the finding of a T-cell clone in lesions of follicular mucinosis without mycosis fungoides is not predictive of the development of cutaneous T-cell lymphoma.

Selective tropism of the cutaneous T-cell lymphoma cells to the sweat glands and ducts is termed syringotropic cutaneous T-cell lymphoma (Fig. 32-8). This is often seen in conjunction with follicular involvement. Syringolymphoid hyperplasia may be seen in these cases histologically and may mimic eccrine carcinoma. Cases previously termed "syringolymphoid hyperplasia with alopecia" are now considered to be cutaneous T-cell lymphoma. Clinically, the lesions present as discrete follicular and nonfollicular erythema, along with alopecia, milia, and follicular cysts. The initial clinical diagnosis in such cases is often discoid lupus erythematosus. The prognosis in mycosis fungoides with adnexal involvement is as predicted by the staging system for other forms of mycosis fungoides.

Systemic manifestations

Mycosis fungoides as a form of malignant lymphoma may progress to include visceral involvement. Lymph node involvement is most common; it predicts progression of the disease in at least one-quarter of patients and reduces survival to about 7 years. Any other evidence of visceral involvement is a grave prognostic sign. An abnormal result on liver–spleen scan, chest radiograph or CT evaluation, abdominal or pelvic CT scans, or bone marrow biopsy is associated with a survival of about 1 year. The prognosis is worse in non-Caucasian patients with early-onset mycosis fungoides, especially African American women.

Pathogenesis

Mycosis fungoides is a neoplasm of memory helper T cells in most cases. Rare cases of suppressor cell (CD8+) mycosis fungoides have been reported. These CD8+ cases may behave indolently, like mycosis fungoides, or aggressively. The latter aggressive subset tends to present with plaques rather than patches. The events leading to the development of the malignant T cells are unknown. It has been speculated that it is caused by chronic exposure to an antigen, but this has yet to be confirmed. Patients with atopic dermatitis appear to be at increased risk for the development of mycosis fungoides, suggesting that persistent stimulation of T cells may lead to development of a malignant clone.

The inflammatory nature of the skin lesions has led to investigation of the interactions of the malignant T cells and both keratinocytes and antigen-presenting cells (including Langerhans cells) in mycosis fungoides. Mycosis fungoides skin lesions have many features of skin that is immunologically "activated." Mycosis fungoides cells express cutaneous lymphocyte antigen (CLA), the ligand for E selectin, which is expressed on the endothelial cells of inflamed skin. This allows the malignant cells to traffic into the skin from the peripheral blood. CCR4, another homing molecule, is expressed on mycosis fungoides cells, and the ligand for this receptor is on basal keratinocytes. Antigen-presenting cells are increased in mycosis fungoides lesions and have increased functional capacity to activate T cells. There is increased expression of major histocompatibility complex (MHC) class II antigens on the surface of the antigen-presenting cells. Through cytokines, infiltration of neoplastic and reactive T cells is increased. The pattern in early mycosis fungoides is more T-helper 1 (Th1)-like and the non-neoplastic infiltrating cells (tumor infiltrating lymphocytes [TILs]) may play a role in downregulating and controlling the neoplastic cells. There are more CD8+ cells in these early lesions and these TILs may control the malignant clone. In fact, mycosis fungoides patients with more than 20% CD8+ cells in their skin survive longer than those with less than 15%. In summary, early mycosis fungoides is a condition in which host immunity is intact and the host immune system effectively limits proliferation of the malignant T-cell clone. In more advanced mycosis fungoides and in Sézary syndrome, perhaps through interleukin (IL)-4 and 10, a Th2 environment exists. This downregulates suppressor cell function and allows the malignant clone to proliferate. In addition, the Th2-dominant environment reduces effective helper T-cell function, explaining the increased risk of infection and secondary cancer in patients with advanced cutaneous T-cell lymphoma. Correcting the aberrant immune response in advanced cutaneous T-cell lymphoma is the basis of some treatment approaches.

Common chromosomal alterations in mycosis fungoides include gain of 7q36 and 7q21–7q22, and loss of 5q13 and 9p21. This characteristic pattern differs from that seen in Sézary syndrome, suggesting that the two disorders are distinct. Low levels of human herpesvirus (HHV) 8 have been detected in large-plaque parapsoriasis as well as mycosis fungoides, but an etiologic link has not been established.

As mycosis fungoides advances, the number of circulating malignant T cells increases. Standard cytologic evaluation (the Sézary preparation) is expensive and not very accurate, even when enhanced by specific labeling techniques. Use of standard laboratory tests, such as the CD4/CD8 ratio test, which increases as mycosis fungoides progresses, and assessment of the number of CD4+,CD7– or CD4+,CD26– circulating cells, which relatively specifically identify mycosis fungoides cells, yield indicators of tumor burden with advanced disease but are of limited value in early disease.

Histopathology

Perhaps more than in any other situation in dermatopathology, the ability to diagnose mycosis fungoides histologically correlates closely with the skill, training, and experience of the reviewing pathologist. When the clinician is considering a diagnosis of mycosis fungoides, consultation with a skilled dermatopathologist should be strongly considered if original histologic reports are nonconfirmatory or nonspecific.

In patch-stage lesions there is subtle epidermotropism of lymphocytes that resembles a vacuolar interface dermatitis with a lymphocyte in every vacuole. As lesions progress, there is a distinct bandlike distribution of lymphocytes with epidermotropism. At this stage, there is a large dark lymphocyte in every vacuole. The lymphocytes within the epidermis may be numerous or few in number, but are typically larger, darker, and more angulated than those in the dermis. Papillary dermal fibrosis is typically present. The superficial perivascular lymphoid infiltrate that surrounds the postcapillary venule is typically more prominent above the vessel than below the vessel (bare under-belly sign).

Plaques of mycosis fungoides show a more prominent superficial bandlike lymphoid infiltrate and a deeper perivascular dermal component than patch-stage lesions. Papillary dermal fibrosis is more prominent and the subpapillary plexus is shifted downward. Epidermotropism is much more marked and is typically associated with very little spongiosis. This helps distinguish patch-stage mycosis fungoides from spongiotic dermatitis. Vesicular variants are an exception to this rule. In vesicular variants, spongiosis is prominent and results in intraepidermal and subcorneal vesiculation. Eosinophils are common in folliculotropic mycosis fungoides (with or without follicular mucinosis), but are uncommon in other forms of mycosis fungoides.

In thick plaques and tumors, epidermotropism may be substantially diminished. The diagnosis is confirmed by the presence of dense sheets of infiltrating lymphocytes in the dermis and subcutaneous fat. These cells may have cerebriform nuclei.

Cardinal features that should suggest a diagnosis of mycosis fungoides include the following:

- solitary or small groups of lymphocytes in the basal cell layer

- epidermotropism of lymphocytes, with disproportionately scant spongiosis
- more lymphocytes within the epidermis than would normally be seen in an inflammatory dermatosis, with little accompanying acanthosis or spongiosis
- lymphocytes in the epidermis larger than those in the dermis
- papillary dermal fibrosis with bundles of collagen arranged haphazardly
- prominent folliculotropism or syringotropism of the lymphocytes, especially with intrafollicular mucin deposition (follicular mucinosis).

Features that should suggest a diagnosis of inflammatory dermatosis over mycosis fungoides include the following:
- prominent upper dermal and papillary edema
- marked epidermal spongiosis
- accumulation of the intraepidermal inflammatory cells in flask-shaped collections, with the top open to the stratum corneum.

Immunohistochemistry is of some value in assessing mycosis fungoides. Mycosis fungoides cells characteristically are CD4+, but lose the CD7 and CD26 antigens, i.e. they are CD4+,CD7–,CD26–. This phenotype is very unusual for nonmalignant T cells and thus is useful in evaluating biopsy specimens and peripheral blood lymphocytes. Loss of CD7 expression within the large dark lymphocytes in the epidermis, with normal expression in the benign recruited lymphocytes in the infiltrate below, suggests a diagnosis of mycosis fungoides. DNA hybridization or a Southern blot test is frequently performed in equivocal cases to detect clonal rearrangement of the T-cell receptor (TCR). However, these data must be interpreted with caution; clonality does not confirm a diagnosis of malignancy. Benign processes may contain clonal TCR rearrangements. In early lesions of mycosis fungoides, the number of infiltrating cells may be insufficient for a clone to be detected, so a negative test does not exclude the diagnosis of mycosis fungoides. Testing with fresh tissue is somewhat more sensitive than with fixed tissue using current methods. Similar techniques can be used to evaluate lymph nodes in mycosis fungoides patients. Lymph node involvement can be detected by these molecular methods, while the routine histologic evaluation yields normal results. Patients with more advanced disease are more likely to have clones in their lymph nodes, and the presence of clonality is predictive of shorter survival.

Differential diagnosis

In the early patch stage, mycosis fungoides may be difficult to diagnose. The skin lesions usually resemble a nondescript form of eczema with some scale. Interestingly, despite the itching, scratch marks and lichenification are usually absent. Mycosis fungoides presenting as papuloerythroderma of Ofuji is an obvious exception. The multiple morphologies of mycosis fungoides make the differential diagnosis vast. Plaque-like lesions may resemble subacute dermatitis or psoriasis. Tumors must be differentiated from other forms of lymphoreticular malignancy and metastases.

Treatment

Effective therapy that reliably prolongs survival has not yet been documented. Many forms of therapy induce remissions of variable length. The choice between them depends on extent of disease, the patient's overall health and physical status, the physician's experience and preference, and the availability of various options. Topical steroids, topical nitrogen mustard or 1,3-bis (2-chloroethyl)-l-nitrosourea (carmustine) (BCNU), bexarotene gel 1%, and PUVA (or narrow-band UVB) are generally good choices for stages IA, IB, and IIA disease. Patch-stage mycosis fungoides has responded to alefacept. Total skin electron beam (TSEB) therapy can be used for refractory stage IIA and IIB cases. Single-agent chemotherapy or photophoresis can be employed as initial management for stage III patients. Low-dose methotrexate may control the skin lesions of mycosis fungoides, but has been associated with the development of a secondary aggressive lymphoma in a few patients. Pegylated liposomal doxorubicin and combinations of IFN-α, retinoids (bexarotene or isotretinoin), photophoresis, IFN-γ, skin-directed PUVA, sargramostim (granulocyte macrophage colony-stimulating factor), alemtuzumab, and perhaps IL-2, IL-12, and IFN-α may be effective in stage IV disease, and for patients who have failed the above therapies for stages IIB and III mycosis fungoides. Multiagent systemic chemotherapy is used much less commonly with the advent of immunomodulatory treatments for mycosis fungoides. It should only be considered when all other treatment options have failed. Treatment of early-stage disease is in general restricted to skin-directed treatments. More advanced disease is treated with different modalities at different institutions. Combinations of agents are often used, and those combinations and their order of use vary from one institution to the next. In general, therapies that also enhance the patient's immune system are favored in persons with more advanced disease. Complete remission has been noted following a severe reaction to combined therapy with bexarotene, vorinostat, and high-dose fenofibrate. The reaction included fever, extensive skin necrosis, and granuloma formation.

Topical corticosteroids The availability of superpotent class I topical corticosteroids has led to a reassessment of their possible role in the management of early (patch-stage, T1 and T2) mycosis fungoides. Zackheim reported a 63% complete remission for patients with T1 disease and a total response rate of 94% in T1 patients. In T2 patients, complete responses were only 25% but total responses were 82%. The predominant side effect was a temporary and reversible suppression of the hypothalamic–pituitary axis in about 13% of patients. The responses were short-lived if therapy was stopped, but given the limited toxicity, this is not necessary in many patients. The adjunctive value of topical corticosteroids in T1 mycosis fungoides requires reappraisal because the response rates are similar to other modalities used for early mycosis fungoides and the toxicity is very low.

Topical nitrogen mustard The contents of a 10 mg vial of mechlorethamine hydrochloride (Mustargen-MSD) are dissolved in 60 mL of tap water and applied to the entire skin surface, except the face, axillae, and genitalia, with a 2 inch paint brush or gauze pad. The last milliliter may be diluted to half-strength or greater dilution for application to the face, axillae, and genitalia. Daily applications are made until complete clearing occurs, which usually takes several months or longer, and may be continued indefinitely. Such treatment leads to complete responses in 80% of patients with stage IA disease, 68% in patients with stage IB, 61% in stage IIA, 49% in stage IIB, and 60% in stage III patients. About 10% of patients obtain a durable and long-lasting remission of over 8 years. The major side effects of topical nitrogen mustard (NH2) therapy are cutaneous intolerance, which occurs in almost 50% of patients, and allergic contact dermatitis, which occurs in 15%. Short (1 h) contact does not reduce this rate of sensitization. This can be reduced by the use of an ointment formulation, but response rates have been reported to be inferior with the ointment form. At least half of patients will relapse when therapy is stopped, but frequently will respond again to NH2.

The duration of maintenance therapy after achieving remission varies in different centers. Some treat for an additional 6 months and others taper treatment over a year

or more, or continue treatment indefinitely. In many centers, topical nitrogen mustard has been a proven mainstay of therapy for patch- or plaque-stage mycosis fungoides without lymphadenopathy.

Topical BCNU (carmustine) BCNU, 2 mg/mL in 150 mL aliquots, dissolved in ethanol, is dispensed to the patient. From this stock solution the patient takes 5 mL and adds it to 60 mL of water at room temperature. This is applied once a day to the whole body, sparing the folds, genitals, hands, and feet (if they do not have lesions). If the extent of disease is limited, only the affected areas are treated. The average treatment course is 8–12 weeks. If, after 3–6 months, the patient's condition is not responding, the concentration may be doubled and the treatment repeated for 12 weeks. For small or persistent lesions, the straight stock solution may be applied daily. Patients tolerate BCNU better than nitrogen mustard, contact sensitization is uncommon, and responses are more rapid. Complete blood counts should be monitored monthly during treatment, but marrow suppression occurs in less than 10% of patients treated with the low concentrations. Telangiectasia, which may be persistent and severe, can occur after prolonged BCNU therapy or following an adverse cutaneous reaction to the medication.

Ultraviolet therapy Both UVB (narrow- or broad-band) and PUVA (systemic or bath) have been effective in the management of mycosis fungoides. About 75% of patients with patch-stage disease will have a complete clinical remission with UVB therapy. Home therapy is successful. PUVA has been used more extensively and, because of its deeper penetration, is perhaps better suited to the treatment of a disorder with a dermal component. Complete clearing is seen in 88% of patients with limited patch/plaque disease and in 52% of patients with extensive disease. Tumor-stage patients do not clear. Erythrodermic patients have poor tolerance for PUVA. Up to 50% of patients with a complete response to PUVA may have a remission of up to 10 years. Retinoids and IFN-α may be added to PUVA. Retinoids may reduce the total number of PUVA treatments required. Low-dose IFN-α plus PUVA may be used in patch-stage patients in whom topical therapy and PUVA alone are ineffective. The excimer laser may be used once or twice a week to deliver the phototherapy if the patient has a limited number of lesions. On average, 5–6 weeks of treatment are required, and remissions of up to 2 years or more can be achieved.

Extracorporeal photochemotherapy (photophoresis, ECP) is a therapeutic modality in which the circulating cells are extracted and treated with UVA outside the body; the patient ingests psoralen before the treatment. Complete responses are seen in a small percentage of mycosis fungoides patients, about 20%, and a partial response occurs in a similar percentage of patients. In the original reports, the overall response rate for erythrodermic patients was 80%, but many of these patients failed to have at least the 50% clearing required to be considered a partial response. In one comparative trial, standard PUVA was significantly more effective than photophoresis alone, and photophoresis was judged ineffective in plaque-stage (T2) mycosis fungoides. ECP is now used in combination with other agents, especially IFN-α, and appears to have better efficacy. Insulin-dependent diabetics respond poorly.

Radiation TSEB therapy in doses in excess of 3000 Gy is very effective in the management of mycosis fungoides. Stage T1 patients have a 98% complete response; stage T2, 71%; stage T3, 36%; and stage T4, 64%. Long-term remissions occur in about 50% of T1 patients and 20% of T2 patients. Erythrodermic patients tolerate TSEB therapy poorly; other modalities should be attempted initially. Adjuvant therapy with a topical agent or PUVA can be considered if the patient relapses, which is a frequent occurrence. The most common side effects of TSEB therapy are erythema, edema, worsening of lesions, alopecia, and nail loss. Persistent hyperpigmentation and chronically dry skin are also problems after TSEB therapy. Orthovoltage radiation may be used to control tumors or resistant thick plaques in patients whose conditions have been otherwise controlled with another modality.

Biologic response modifiers (multimodality immunomodulatory therapy) The appearance of circulating malignant T cells in mycosis fungoides may indicate failure of the host immune system to control the disease. Immunomodulatory agents are used in an attempt to enhance host immune function and gain control of the disease. It is often combined with treatments that increase malignant cell apoptosis, so that the "tumor antigens" released will be recognized and immunologically "attacked" by the host immune system. These immunomodulatory agents both activate antigen-presenting cells and enhance Th1 immune function directed against the malignant T-cell clone. IFN-α and IFN-γ have been shown to have efficacy against mycosis fungoides. IFN-α is associated with a positive response in about 60% of patients and a complete response in 19%. If it is used as a single agent, toxicity is high and includes fever, chills, myalgias, neutropenia, and depression. Low-dose IFN-α and IFN-γ treatments and granulocyte macrophage colony-stimulating factor are now used in an adjunctive fashion in combination with retinoid therapy, phototherapy, and other modalities. This is termed multimodality immunomodulatory therapy. IL-2 and 12 may be used in a similar fashion in the future.

Retinoids Both isotretinoin and etretinate have efficacy in the treatment of mycosis fungoides. A clinical response is noted in about 44% of patients. Dosage of isotretinoin is about 1 mg/kg/day to start, and may be increased up to 3 mg/kg/day as tolerated. Retinoids may be effective in stage IB (T2) and stage III patients, and as a palliative treatment in those with stage IVA disease. Bexarotene (Targretin), a synthetic retinoid that is bound preferentially by the retinoid X receptor (RXR), is felt to work by inducing apoptosis in the malignant T cells. It is available as a 1% topical gel and as an oral tablet. Topical therapy is used in patients with stage IA–IIA cutaneous T-cell lymphoma. Patients improve about 50% with this treatment. Oral bexarotene at a dose of 300 mg/m^2 also has a response rate of about 50% in early-stage cutaneous T-cell lymphoma. This dose is complicated by hypercholesterolemia, marked hypertriglyceridemia (at times complicated by pancreatitis), central hypothyroidism, and leukopenia. It may be combined with PUVA and other forms of treatment at a lower dose.

Systemic chemotherapy For most forms of cancer, combinations of chemotherapeutic agents are given. In mycosis fungoides, however, multidrug chemotherapy often exacerbates the ongoing immune imbalance and may prevent the patient's immune system from attacking the malignant T cells. For this reason, and due to the enhanced efficacy of combination immunomodulatory treatment regimens, systemic chemotherapy is now very uncommonly used for mycosis fungoides. Methotrexate, in doses from 5 to 125 mg/week, is effective for the management of T3 patients. In these patients, Zackheim et al demonstrated that 41% had a complete response, and an additional 17% a partial response, giving a total response of 58%. The median overall survival was 8.4 years and 69% of patients were alive at 5 years. For advanced mycosis fungoides, higher doses of methotrexate with citrovorum-factor rescue were successful in obtaining a response, which was then maintained with lower doses of methotrexate, not requiring rescue. Similarly, pentostatin, etoposide, fludarabine, and 2-chlorodeoxyadenosine have been used. Systemic chemotherapy beyond methotrexate, especially multiagent chemotherapy, is best managed by an oncologist. Systemic chemotherapy is only indicated in stage III and IVA patients who have failed all the available immunoenhancing treatment

protocols noted above. A number of new agents are being evaluated for the treatment of mycosis fungoides. Histone deacetylase inhibitors including vorinostat demonstrate responses in a subgroup of patients. Forodesine is a novel inhibitor of purine nucleoside phosphorylase and pralatrexate is a novel targeted antifolate agent.

Fusion toxin DAB389IL-2 is the fusion of a portion of the diphtheria toxin to recombinant IL-2. This selectively binds to cells expressing the IL-2 receptor and leads to their death. A series of mycosis fungoides cases that expressed the IL-2 receptor demonstrated a response rate of 37%, including a complete response in 14% of cases. These patients had failed conventional therapies. Patients in stages I–III achieved response, but no patient with stage IV disease did so. Fever, chills, hypotension, nausea, and vomiting were common and at high doses a vascular leak syndrome occurred. This agent is reserved for advanced-stage patients who have failed other modalities.

Arulogun SO, et al: Long-term outcomes of patients with advanced-stage cutaneous T-cell lymphoma and large cell transformation. Blood 2008 Oct 15; 112(8):3082–3087.

Carter J, et al: Phototherapy for cutaneous T-cell lymphoma: online survey and literature review. J Am Acad Dermatol 2009 Jan; 60(1):39–50.

Enke CA: New options in diagnosis and management of mycosis fungoides and Sézary syndrome. Oncology (Williston Park) 2010 May; 24(6):507–508.

Galper SL, et al: Diagnosis and management of mycosis fungoides. Oncology (Williston Park) 2010 May; 24(6):491–501.

Gerami P, et al: Folliculotropic mycosis fungoides: an aggressive variant of cutaneous T-cell lymphoma. Arch Dermatol 2008 Jun; 144(6):738–746.

Green WH, et al: Patch-stage mycosis fungoides in remission after therapy with alefacept. J Am Acad Dermatol 2008 May; 58(5 Suppl 1): S110–S112.

Kempf W, et al: Granulomatous mycosis fungoides and granulomatous slack skin: a multicenter study of the Cutaneous Lymphoma Histopathology Task Force Group of the European Organization for Research and Treatment of Cancer (EORTC). Arch Dermatol 2008 Dec; 144(12):1609–1617.

Lansigan F, et al: Current and emerging treatment strategies for cutaneous T cell lymphoma. Drugs 2010 Feb 12; 70(3):273–286.

Lafaille P, et al: Exacerbation of undiagnosed mycosis fungoides during treatment with etanercept. Arch Dermatol 2009 Jan; 145(1):94–95.

McGirt LY, et al: Predictors of response to extracorporeal photopheresis in advanced mycosis fungoides and Sézary syndrome. Photodermatol Photoimmunol Photomed 2010 Aug; 26(4):182–191.

Novelli M, et al: Flow cytometry immunophenotyping in mycosis fungoides. J Am Acad Dermatol 2008 Sep; 59(3):533–534.

Olsen E, et al: Revisions to the staging and classification of mycosis fungoides and Sézary syndrome: a proposal of the International Society for Cutaneous Lymphomas (ISCL) and the cutaneous lymphoma task force of the European Organization for Research and Treatment of Cancer (EORTC). Blood 2007 Sep 15; 110(6):1713–1722.

Quereux G, et al: Prospective multicenter study of pegylated liposomal doxorubicin treatment in patients with advanced or refractory mycosis fungoides or Sézary syndrome. Arch Dermatol 2008 Jun; 144(6): 727–733.

Steinhoff M, et al: Complete clinical remission of tumor-stage mycosis fungoides after acute extensive skin necroses, granulomatous reaction, and fever under treatment with bexarotene, vorinostat, and high-dose fenofibrate. J Am Acad Dermatol 2008 May; 58(5 Suppl 1):S88–91.

Sun G, et al: Poor prognosis in non-Caucasian patients with early-onset mycosis fungoides. J Am Acad Dermatol 2009 Feb; 60(2):231–235.

Pagetoid reticulosis

Localized epidermotropic reticulosis, Pagetoid reticulosis, or Woringer–Kolopp disease is an uncommon lymphoproliferative disorder considered be a form of mycosis fungoides. Other terms suggested for these cases have been acral mycosis fungoides or mycosis fungoides palmaris et plantaris. In large mycosis fungoides clinics, such cases represent about 0.6% of all mycosis fungoides cases. Pagetoid reticulosis is divided into classic Woringer–Kolopp, which usually describes solitary lesions, and cases with multiple lesions (Ketron–Goodman variant). The unique features of Woringer–Kolopp disease are clinical. The disease presents as a solitary lesion that is often located on an extremity and frequently has a keratotic rim. If there is more than a single lesion, there is often a propensity for lesions to involve both the palms and soles. Frequently, over months to years, the lesion gradually enlarges, reaching a size of over 10 cm. In some cases, the lesions spontaneously come and go over many years. Twenty percent of cases occur in patients who are younger than 15 years of age. The long duration without progression has been a clinical hallmark of Woringer–Kolopp disease. Histologically, there is prominent epidermotropism of lymphocytes, with many lining up in the basal cell layer. This histologic pattern correlates with strong αE–β7 and α4–β7 integrin expression by the infiltrating cells. This integrin expression is also seen in the epidermotropic cells of classic mycosis fungoides and contact dermatitis. In mycosis fungoides, most cases are CD4+, but in the acral mycosis fungoides cases they may be CD4+, CD8+, or negative for both. TCR gene rearrangements can be detected in many cases of Woringer–Kolopp disease. Therapeutically, local excision and radiation therapy have been "curative" in many cases. Topical and systemic PUVA has also proved effective. Local recurrence is possible.

Sézary syndrome

Sézary syndrome is the leukemic phase of mycosis fungoides. The characteristic features are generalized erythroderma, superficial lymphadenopathy, and atypical cells in the circulating blood. Although patients with classic mycosis fungoides may progress to Sézary syndrome, usually patients with Sézary syndrome are erythrodermic from the onset. The skin shows a generalized or limited erythroderma of a typical fiery red color. Associated features can include leonine facies, eyelid edema, ectropion, diffuse alopecia, hyperkeratosis of the palms and soles, and dystrophic nails. Some patients develop lesions identical to vitiligo, especially on the lower legs. The symptoms are those of severe pruritus and burning, with episodes of chills. Prognosis is poor, with an average survival of about 5 years.

Superficial lymphadenopathy is usually found in the cervical, axillary, and inguinal areas. Leukocytosis up to 30 000/mm³ is usually present. In the peripheral blood, skin infiltrate, and lymph nodes, helper T cells with deeply convoluted nuclei are found—the so-called Sézary cells. Chromosomal aberrations are common, but differ from the typical pattern seen in mycosis fungoides. Resistance to Fas-ligand and TNF-related apoptosis has been demonstrated.

Histologically, and by immunohistochemistry, there are no reproducible differences between cases of mycosis fungoides and Sézary syndrome. In a fair number of cases of the latter, the cutaneous histology may be nonspecific, showing a spongiotic dermatitis. Additional hematologic evaluation may be necessary to confirm the diagnosis in the erythrodermic patient. T-cell gene rearrangement studies are frequently used to confirm the diagnosis of Sézary syndrome. In addition, an increased CD4/CD8 ratio in the blood, with an increase in the number of CD3+/CD4+/CD7–/CD26– circulating cells, is suggestive of leukemic mycosis fungoides.

The erythroderma of Sézary syndrome must be distinguished from chronic lymphocytic leukemia (CLL), psoriasis, atopic dermatitis, photodermatitis, seborrheic dermatitis, contact dermatitis, drug reaction, and pityriasis rubra pilaris. This is done primarily by histopathologic and immunopathologic examination. In Sézary syndrome, the infiltrating T cells in the skin have a Th2 phenotype, and Th2 cytokines are produced by these cells. This explains the reduced delayed-type hypersensitivity, elevated IgE, and eosinophilia seen in these patients.

Sézary syndrome is difficult to treat. Low-dose methotrexate has a reasonable response rate of about 50% and an overall survival of 101 months, suggesting a survival benefit with its use. Photophoresis, used in combination with other agents, is effective in some patients, but the median survival time is only between 39 and 60 months (see above). TSEB radiation has produced some complete cutaneous responses, as well as improvement in the blood burden of malignant cells. Zanolimumab has also been used in this setting.

Arulogun S, et al: Extracorporeal photopheresis for the treatment of Sézary syndrome using a novel treatment protocol. J Am Acad Dermatol 2008 Oct; 59(4):589–595.

Contassot E, et al: Resistance to FasL and tumor necrosis factor-related apoptosis-inducing ligand-mediated apoptosis in Sézary syndrome T-cells associated with impaired death receptor and FLICE-inhibitory protein expression. Blood 2008 May 1; 111(9):4780–4787.

Dores GM, et al: Assessment of delayed reporting of mycosis fungoides and Sézary syndrome in the United States. Arch Dermatol 2008 Mar; 144(3):413–414.

Introcaso CE, et al: Total skin electron beam therapy may be associated with improvement of peripheral blood disease in Sézary syndrome. J Am Acad Dermatol 2008 Apr; 58(4):592–595.

Granulomatous slack skin

Granulomatous slack skin is a rare variant lymphoma that typically presents in middle-aged adults and gradually progresses over years. It occurs more often in men. Lesions are erythematous, atrophic, bulky, infiltrated, pendulous, and redundant plaques in the axillae and groin (Fig. 32-9). Unusual presentations may resemble Hansen's disease or acquired ichthyosis. Histologically, there is a lymphohistiocytic infiltrate extending through the dermis into the subcutaneous fat. Focal collections of huge, multinucleated cells with 20–30 nuclei arranged in a wreath-like pattern are characteristic. Elastophagocytosis is prominent and elastic tissue is absent in areas of inflammation. Lymphocytes are also found within the multinucleate giant cells and are arranged around them. Epidermotropic lymphocytes are also seen. Immunohistologically, the cells are CD4+. T-cell gene rearrangements can be detected. In most patients, the condition evolves into mycosis fungoides, but about one-third of patients with granulomatous slack skin develop Hodgkin disease after years to decades.

Hsiao PF, et al: Granulomatous slack skin presenting as acquired ichthyosis and muscle masses. Am J Clin Dermatol 2009; 10(1):29–32.

Pratchyapruit W, et al: Granulomatous slack skin clinically and histologically masquerading as borderline leprosy in its early stages. Eur J Dermatol 2009 Jan–Feb; 19(1):88–89.

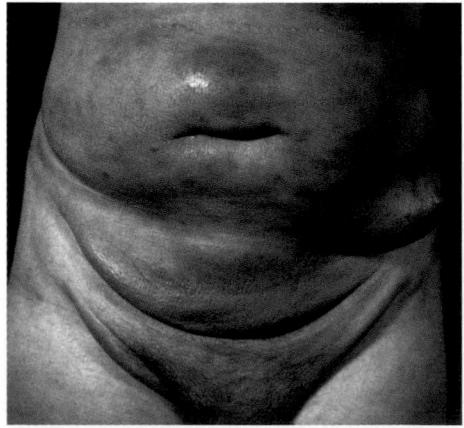

Fig. 32-9 Granulomatous slack skin.

Lymphomatoid papulosis

Lymphomatoid papulosis (LyP) is an uncommon, but not rare disorder. It occurs at any age, including childhood, but is most common in adults with a mean age of 44. In most typical cases, the lesions and course are very similar to that of Mucha–Habermann disease (pityriasis lichenoides et varioliformis acuta), except that the lesions tend to be slightly larger and fewer in number, and have a greater propensity to necrosis. Symptoms are usually minimal. The primary lesion is a red papule up to about 1 cm in diameter (Fig. 32-10). The lesions evolve to papulovesicular, papulopustular, or hemorrhagic, then necrotic papules over days to weeks. They typically heal spontaneously within 8 weeks, somewhat longer in larger lesions. Lesions are usually generalized, although cases limited to one anatomic region have been reported.

There may be crops of lesions or a constant appearance of a few lesions. In most patients, however, the condition tends to be chronic, and lesions are present most of the time if no treatment is given. The average number of lesions present at any one time is usually 10–20, but cases with more than 100 lesions occur. Lesions heal with varioliform, hyperpigmented, or hypopigmented scars. Cases previously reported as solitary, large nodules of lymphomatoid papulosis would now be classified as CD30+ large-cell lymphomas or as overlaps between LyP and lymphoma, termed borderline cases. Localized agminated LyP may be seen in areas typical for mycosis fungoides.

The diagnosis of LyP is confirmed histologically. There is a dermal infiltrate that is wedge-shaped, patchy, and perivascular. In larger lesions, the infiltrate may occupy the whole dermis. It may also be bandlike. The infiltrate may involve the epidermis, with epidermotropism of inflammatory cells. As lesions evolve, epidermal necrosis and ulceration may occur. The dermal vessels may demonstrate fibrin deposition and, more rarely, a lymphocytic "vasculitis." The dermal infiltrate is composed of lymphoid cells, eosinophils, neutrophils, and larger mononuclear cells. Atypical large or small lymphoid cells are present and may represent up to 50% of the infiltrate. Histologically, lesions have been classified into type A, type B, and type C lesions.

Type A lesions contain atypical large cells with abundant cytoplasm and prominent nuclei, with prominent eosinophilic nucleoli. If these cells contain two nuclei, they closely resemble Reed–Sternberg cells. In type B lesions, the atypical cells are smaller, with a smaller cerebriform, hyperchromatic nucleus. These resemble the atypical cells of mycosis fungoides. In both types of lesion, atypical mitotic figures may be observed.

Immunophenotypically, the large atypical cells mark as T cells, usually of the helper type. The atypical cells, especially those of the type A lesions, stain for the activation marker Ki-1 or CD30. Bcl-2 expression occurs in about 50% of cases. When clonal rearrangement studies are performed, clonal rearrangements may be found in up to 40% of LyP lesions, but this finding is not predictive of the behavior of that lesion or the case in general. Type C lesions overlap with primary cutaneous large-cell lymphoma with no clear distinction between the two. CD8+ LyP is a rare variant in which the Tc2 subset of CD8+ T cells proliferates and attracts eosinophils.

Lymphomatoid papulosis types A and B are associated with lymphoma. In the general literature this number is about 5–10%, but some reports have documented rates as high as 20%, and at the University of California at San Francisco (UCSF) up to 40% of cases of LyP have an associated lymphoma. The lymphoma may occur before, concurrently with, or after the appearance of the LyP. In most cases, the LyP precedes the development of lymphoma, sometimes by a long period—up to 20 years. The associated lymphoma is most commonly mycosis fungoides (40%), a CD30+ T-cell lymphoma (30%), or Hodgkin disease (25%). The lymphoma and LyP may behave quite independently. If the lymphoma is successfully treated and cleared, the LyP typically continues. Despite this independent behavior, the lymphoma and the LyP may contain the same clonal TCR gene rearrangement. Patients with pure type B lesions are much less likely to develop lymphoma than patients with type A lesions. Lesions of LyP may occur on a background of mycosis fungoides and must be distinguished from CD30-positive large-cell transformation of mycosis fungoides. Papular lesions of LyP tend to occur in crops. Even though the LyP lesions may demonstrate the same clonal rearrangements as the mycosis fungoides, they often continue to appear in crops, even when the mycosis fungoides lesions respond to therapy.

Therapy may not be necessary; there is no evidence that treatment of LyP prevents the development of secondary lymphoma. When any therapy is stopped, the LyP invariably returns. Therefore, patients only need to be treated if they are moderately symptomatic and the treatment has fewer potential complications than the benefits gained. Superpotent topical corticosteroids have been beneficial in some childhood cases. Topical bexarotene may abort early lesions, and oral bexarotene may suppress lesion formation. PUVA systemically or topically may be effective, although maintenance treatment is usually required. Both narrow- and broad-band UVB may be successful. Of all the systemic agents, methotrexate gives the most dependable response, with up to 90% of LyP patients improving significantly. It is given in weekly doses similar to those used for rheumatoid arthritis—usually 7.5–15 mg/week. Higher doses may be required in some patients. Response is rapid. Some patients treated with methotrexate may have remissions of the LyP. In most, however, maintenance therapy is required.

Heald P, et al: Persistent agmination of lymphomatoid papulosis: an equivalent of limited plaque mycosis fungoides type of cutaneous T-cell lymphoma. J Am Acad Dermatol 2007 Dec; 57(6):1005–1011.

Kamstrup MR, et al: Potential involvement of Notch1 signalling in the pathogenesis of primary cutaneous CD30-positive lymphoproliferative disorders. Br J Dermatol 2008 Apr; 158(4):747–753.

Slone SP, et al: IL-4 production by CD8+ lymphomatoid papulosis, type C, attracts background eosinophils. J Cutan Pathol 2008 Oct; 35(Suppl 1):38–45.

Pityriasis lichenoides

Both the acute and chronic forms of pityriasis lichenoides are lymphocytic vasculitides. The lymphoid infiltrate may contain

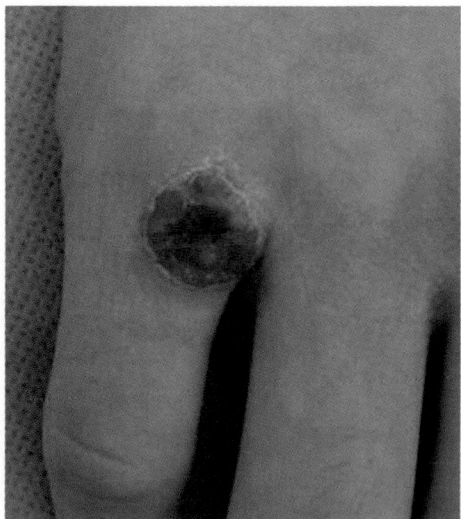

Fig. 32-10 Lymphomatoid papulosis. (Courtesy of M. Rosenbach, MD)

a clonal proliferation. However, progression to cutaneous lymphoma is rare.

Pityriasis lichenoides et varioliformis acuta (Mucha–Habermann disease)

Pityriasis lichenoides et varioliformis acuta (PLEVA) is a disorder that usually appears suddenly in children or young adults. Individual lesions are erythematous macules, papules, or papulovesicles. Lesions tend to be brownish-red and evolve through stages of crusting, necrosis, and varioliform scarring. Lesions tend to appear in crops, and may number from a few to more than 100 (Fig. 32-11). In general, PLEVA patients have more and smaller lesions than patients with LyP. The trunk is favored, but even the palms and soles may infrequently be involved. The patient feels otherwise well. The natural history is benign, with spontaneous involution occurring over 1–3 years. In children, diffuse cases resolved more quickly than cases that were purely central; cases with primarily peripheral lesions took almost twice as long to resolve.

Histologically, PLEVA is characterized by epidermal necrosis, together with prominent hemorrhage and a dense perivascular infiltrate in the upper and mid-dermis in a wedge-shaped pattern. Lymphocytic vasculitis may be seen. T-cell gene rearrangements may be detected, but the significance of that finding is unclear at this time. Treatment of PLEVA may include oral erythromycin or tetracyclines and phototherapy (broad- or narrow-band UVB, PUVA, or photodynamic therapy). Topical tacrolimus may be effective. Low-dose methotrexate, 5.0–15 mg/week, may be required in severe cases. A rapid response to azithromycin has been reported. Etanercept has been reported as effective, but infliximab has been reported to cause pityriasis lichenoides.

An unusually severe form of PLEVA (febrile ulceronecrotic Mucha–Habermann disease) is characterized by the acute onset of diffuse, coalescent, large, ulceronecrotic skin lesions associated with high fever and constitutional symptoms. The condition may begin as typical PLEVA, but the ulceronecrotic lesions usually begin to appear within a few weeks. Skin necrosis may be extensive, especially in the intertriginous regions. Associated symptoms include gastrointestinal and central nervous system (CNS) symptoms, pneumonitis, myocarditis, and even death (in adult cases). The condition favors boys who are 18 years of age or younger. This severe form of PLEVA usually lasts several months with successive outbreaks, then resolves or converts to more classic PLEVA. Reported triggers include viral infections and radiocontrast injection. Treatment is systemic steroids, and if response is limited, methotrexate. Dapsone may also be useful, for maintenance and as a steroid-sparing agent.

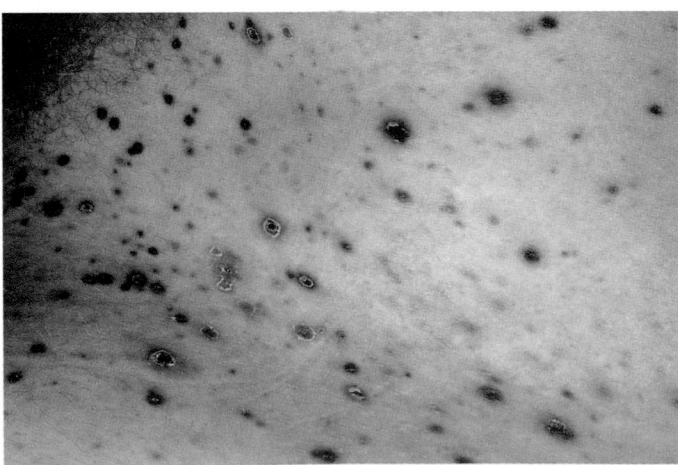

Fig. 32-11 Mucha–Habermann disease.

Pityriasis lichenoides chronica

Pityriasis lichenoides chronica (PLC) is a chronic form of pityriasis lichenoides, related to PLEVA by its common histology. Lesions are erythematous, scaly macules and flat papules with very slow evolution. Lesions each last several months. The eventual resolution of lesions of PLC distinguishes it from guttate parapsoriasis, which it may resemble clinically. Lesions of small-plaque parapsoriasis do not spontaneously resolve. Lesions of PLC favor the lateral trunk and proximal extremities. Patients may have from 10 to hundreds of lesions, but usually fewer than 50. Resolution may leave persistent areas of hypopigmentation, which last for months to years. In many patients, the hypopigmented macules are the most prominent clinical finding. Unlike PLEVA, PLC tends to last for many years. Lesions may occur at any age. The condition commonly affects children, and onset at birth has been described.

Histologically, the changes are similar to PLEVA but much more subtle. A mild interface or perivascular lymphocytic infiltrate with overlying parakeratosis may be present. T-cell gene rearrangement studies may demonstrate monoclonality; however, the meaning of this finding is unclear at this time. Treatment with phototherapy (natural sunlight, UVB, UVA1, or PUVA) is most effective. Topical steroids or tacrolimus may be tried. No treatment is required.

PLC is generally a benign disease. There are rare patients who have progressed to develop cutaneous T-cell lymphoma. The authors recommend that patients with PLC be followed regularly and changes in lesion morphology, including induration, erosion, atrophy, persistent erythema, or poikiloderma, should trigger repeat pathologic evaluation.

Aydogan K, et al: Narrowband UVB (311 nm, TL01) phototherapy for pityriasis lichenoides. Photodermatol Photoimmunol Photomed 2008 Jun; 24(3):128–133.

Ersoy-Evans S, et al: Narrowband ultraviolet-B phototherapy in pityriasis lichenoides chronica. J Dermatolog Treat 2008 Nov; 14:1–5.

Fernandes NF, et al: Pityriasis lichenoides et varioliformis acuta: a disease spectrum. Int J Dermatol 2010 Mar; 49(3):257–261.

Fernández-Guarino M, et al: Pityriasis lichenoides chronica: good response to photodynamic therapy. Br J Dermatol 2008 Jan; 158(1):198–200.

López-Ferrer A, et al: Pityriasis lichenoides chronica induced by infliximab, with response to methotrexate. Eur J Dermatol 2010 Jul–Aug; 20(4):511–512.

Nikkels AF, et al: Etanercept in therapy multiresistant overlapping pityriasis lichenoides. J Drugs Dermatol 2008 Oct; 7(10):990–992.

Skinner RB, et al: Rapid resolution of pityriasis lichenoides et varioliformis acuta with azithromycin. J Am Acad Dermatol 2008 Mar; 58(3):524–525.

Smith JJ, et al: Febrile ulceronecrotic Mucha–Habermann disease associated with herpes simplex virus type 2. J Am Acad Dermatol 2009 Jan; 60(1):149–152.

Sotiriou E, et al: Febrile ulceronecrotic Mucha–Habermann disease: a case report and review of the literature. Acta Derm Venereol 2008; 88(4):350–355.

Primary cutaneous T-cell lymphomas other than mycosis fungoides

Once a cutaneous lymphoma has been identified as being of T-cell origin and the diagnosis of mycosis fungoides and its variants has been excluded, the most important evaluation is to determine the CD30-staining pattern. CD30 is a marker found on some activated, but not resting T and B cells. It also marks the Reed–Sternberg cells of Hodgkin disease. Monoclonal antibodies Ki-1 and Ber H2 are used to identify CD30 positivity. A cutaneous lymphoma is considered to be CD30+ if there are large clusters of CD30+ cells or more than 75% of the anaplastic T cells are CD30+. Systemic CD30+ lymphoma with cutaneous involvement has a poor prognosis. Those cases that express anaplastic lymphoma kinase (ALK-1) associated with a 2:5 translocation have a somewhat better prognosis. Primary cutaneous large T-cell lymphomas that are CD30+ are typically ALK-1-negative, have a very good prognosis, and tend to run a relapsing course similar to that of lymphomatoid papulosis. Individual lesions respond to irradiation and the relapsing course may remit with low-dose methotrexate. Large-cell lymphomas of the skin have similar histologic and clinical features, so immunophenotyping is essential for prognosis. Clonal TCR gene rearrangements are present in large-cell T-cell lymphoma. The group of T-cell lymphomas that are not large-cell and CD30+ are classified in the WHO system as peripheral T-cell lymphomas.

CD56 is rapidly becoming the second most important immunophenotypic marker for cutaneous lymphomas. Four important variants of CD56+ cutaneous lymphomas have been identified: a subset of subcutaneous panniculitis-like T-cell lymphoma; natural killer (NK)/T-cell lymphoma; blastic NK cell lymphoma; and CD8+ aggressive epidermotrophic cytotoxic T-cell lymphoma.

Peripheral T-cell lymphoma is a heterogeneous grouping that includes primary cutaneous CD30+ nonanaplastic large-cell lymphoma, primary cutaneous CD30− anaplastic and nonanaplastic large-cell lymphoma, and primary cutaneous CD30− pleomorphic small-/medium-cell lymphoma.

CD30+ cutaneous T-cell lymphoma (primary cutaneous anaplastic large-cell lymphoma)

Clinically, these lymphomas present as solitary or localized skin lesions that have a tendency to ulcerate (50%), spontaneously regress (25%), and relapse. They are rare in children and occur with slightly greater frequency in males. Lesions are usually firm, red to violaceous tumors up to 10 cm in diameter (Fig. 32-12). Tumors may grow in a matter of weeks. There is no favored anatomic site. Onset has been reported during glatiramer acetate treatment of multiple sclerosis.

Relapses in the skin are common, but the development of extracutaneous, bone marrow, or lymph node involvement is uncommon. Clonal populations may occasionally be demonstrated in peripheral blood, but differ from those in the skin. Lymph node involvement is associated with a poorer prognosis. The "pyogenic lymphoma" of the skin is a neutrophil-rich CD30+ lymphoma with skin lesions that clinically resemble Sweet syndrome, pyoderma gangrenosum, halogenoderma, leishmaniasis, or deep fungal infection. IL-8 overexpression by the anaplastic CD30+ cells causes the neutrophilic infiltration. The number of neutrophils present may make histologic interpretation difficult. Cases with features of both lymphomatoid

papulosis and CD30+ anaplastic T-cell lymphoma have been described, sometimes under the designation type C lymphomatoid papulosis. Histologically, there is a dense dermal non-epidermotropic infiltrate with atypical tumor cells whose large nuclei have one or several prominent nucleoli and abundant cytoplasm. The malignant cells can be further characterized as anaplastic, pleomorphic, and immunoblastic, but this distinction may be difficult and has yet to be determined to be of prognostic or therapeutic value. This form of primary cutaneous T-cell lymphoma has an excellent prognosis, with a 5-year survival of 90%. Lesions are highly responsive to radiotherapy. Early individual lesions can even be surgically excised. Topical imiquimod has been therapeutically successful. Chemotherapy causes regression of lesions, but a rapid relapse usually occurs. Other than low-dose methotrexate, chemotherapy generally has little role in the treatment of this disease. Local hyperthermia has been used successfully, as has inhibition of the mammalian target of rapamycin.

Secondary cutaneous CD30+ large-cell lymphoma

CD30+ large-cell lymphomas may arise in cases of mycosis fungoides, in patients with lymphomatoid papulosis, and in patients who have documented extracutaneous disease (secondary cutaneous anaplastic large-cell lymphoma). Skin lesions of pyogenic lymphoma may be seen secondary to a pyogenic lymphoma of other organs. The prognosis is poor in patients who have extracutaneous disease preceding or near the time of cutaneous involvement. Among those with systemic disease, the expression of Alk-1 associated with a t(2; 5) translocation is a favorable prognostic feature. Kempf et al reported that MUM1 expression is common in secondary anaplastic large-cell lymphoma and in LyP, but uncommon in primary cutaneous anaplastic large-cell lymphoma. Other authors have disputed that MUM1 is a useful marker. Patients with lymphomatoid papulosis, who develop cutaneous CD30+ lymphoma and who do not have systemic lymphoma or mycosis fungoides, typically have an excellent prognosis. The prognosis for patients with mycosis fungoides who develop CD30+ anaplastic large-cell lymphoma is poor.

Non-mycosis fungoides CD30− cutaneous large T-cell lymphoma

Non-mycosis fungoides CD30− cutaneous large T-cell lymphomas usually present as solitary or generalized plaques, nodules, or tumors of short duration. There is no preceding patch stage that distinguishes it from mycosis fungoides. The prognosis is poor, with a 5-year survival rate of 15%. The malignant cells are pleomorphic large or medium cell types or are immunoblastic. The cells may be cerebriform and epidermotropism may be present. Some cases previously called d'emblée mycosis fungoides are better classified in this group. Multiagent chemotherapy is recommended.

Pleomorphic T-cell lymphoma (non-mycosis fungoides CD30− pleomorphic small/medium-sized cutaneous T-cell lymphoma)

This group comprises about 3% of all primary cutaneous lymphomas. Pleomorphic small/medium-sized cutaneous T-cell lymphoma is distinguished from the large-cell type by having less than 30% large pleomorphic cells. It is distinguished from mycosis fungoides by clinical features (lack of patch or plaque lesions). These primary cutaneous lymphomas usually present with one or several red–purple papules, nodules, or tumors (5 mm to 15 cm in size). Immunophenotypically, they are usually of helper T-cell origin and clonal rearrangements of the TCR gene are usually present. A CD4 phenotype, as opposed to a CD8 phenotype, is associated with a more

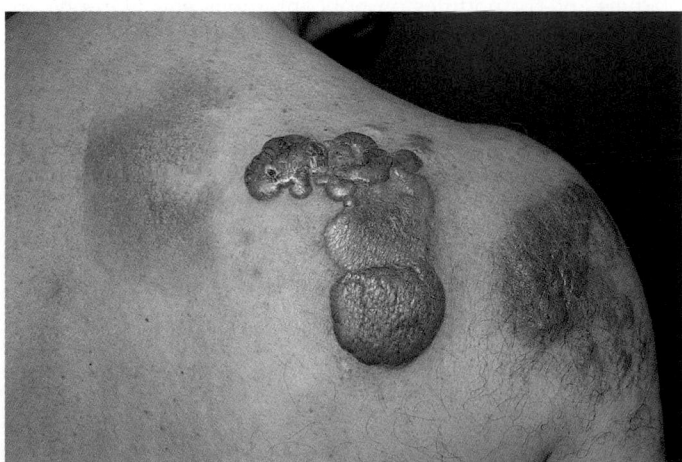

Fig. 32-12 Large-cell anaplastic lymphoma.

favorable prognosis, but a CD4/CD56 phenotype has a poorer prognosis. The presence of a mixed population of suppressor cells, B cells, and histiocytes usually favors the diagnosis of reactive lymphoid hyperplasia. The overall prognosis is intermediate, with a 5-year survival rate of 62%. The optimal therapy for this form of lymphoma has not been determined. Therapeutically, localized lesions have been treated with radiation therapy or surgical excision. Chemotherapy, retinoids, interferons, and monoclonal antibodies have been used in widespread or progressive disease.

Lennert lymphoma (lymphoepithelioid lymphoma)

Lennert lymphoma is a rare CD4+ systemic T-cell lymphoma. Cutaneous lesions occur in less than 10% of cases and present as papules, plaques, or nodules. The skin lesions may not represent lymphoma cutis because palisaded granulomatous and nonspecific dermal infiltrates may occur. The clinical and histologic appearance may resemble granuloma annulare very closely. The course is low-grade until the lymphoma transforms to a high-grade, large-cell lymphoma.

Subcutaneous (panniculitis-like) T-cell lymphoma

Clinically, patients are usually young adults who present with subcutaneous nodules (Fig. 32-13), usually on the lower extremities, and are frequently diagnosed as having erythema nodosum or some other form of panniculitis. Weight loss, fever, and fatigue are common and may herald the onset of a rapidly progressive hemophagocytic syndrome, which is often fatal. Extracutaneous involvement is rare, even in fatal cases. An indolent chronic course can also be seen, but even in these cases the prognosis is poor. This variant of lymphoma may also rarely be seen in childhood.

Histologically, there is a lace-like infiltration of the lobules of adipocytes, mimicking panniculitis, especially lupus profundus. A characteristic feature is rimming of neoplastic cells around individual adipocytes. The infiltrate contains primarily small cells with hyperchromatic, irregular nuclei and large anaplastic cells in varying proportions. The small cells are atypical, karyorrhexis is prominent, and mitotic figures are

frequent. Benign histiocytes are present in large or small numbers and demonstrate erythrophagocytosis (bean-bag cells). Immunophenotypically, the neoplastic cells mark as T cells (CD2+, CD3+). Most cases are derived from α/β T cells and are CD56–. They have a less aggressive course. A subset of subcutaneous T-cell lymphomas are derived from γ/δ T cells and are CD56+. These cases have been misdiagnosed as lupus profundus or alopecia areata; histologically prominent dermal and even epidermal (interface) involvement may be seen. They have a more aggressive course and are now classified separately. SPTCL may evolve from the benign variant of cytophagic histiocytic panniculitis, which may also have a hemophagocytic syndrome. Multiagent chemotherapy is recommended, at times with stem-cell support. Denileukin diftitox (Ontak) was reported to produce a favorable response.

Nasal/nasal-type NK/T-cell lymphoma (angiocentric lymphoma)

NK/T-cell lymphoma most frequently presents in extranodal tissue and is characterized by a high incidence of nasal involvement. It is more common in Asia, where it affects primarily women with a mean age of 40. In Korea it is reported to be the most common form of cutaneous lymphoma after mycosis fungoides. It is uncommon in the US. It presents clinically as dermal or subcutaneous papules or nodules that may ulcerate. Lesions are usually widespread and involve the lower extremities. A hydroa vacciniforme-type has been described in children in Mexico and in adults and children in Japan and Korea. Skin lesions are facial and extremity papulo-vesicles ulcerate and heal with scarring. Skin lesions are exacerbated by sun exposure and are reproduced with UVA irradiation.

Histologically, the dermis and subcutaneous fat are infiltrated with intermediate-sized, atypical lymphocytes, within and around the walls of small and medium-sized vessels. Epidermotropism may be noted. The lymphoma cells express a spectrum of T- and NK-cell immunophenotypic markers, variably expressing CD2, CD3, CD4, CD8, and the NK-cell marker CD56. CD56 is not cell lineage-specific, and a subset of CD56 cutaneous lymphoma cases is classified under the SPTCL category. Epstein–Barr virus is present in the NK variants and variably present in the T-cell variants. T-cell clonality is detected if the T-cell immunophenotype is present. The prognosis is poor.

Blastic plasmacytoid dendritic cell neoplasm (blastic NK-cell lymphoma, CD4, CD56+ hematodermic neoplasm)

The majority of patients are males, with a mean age of about 60 years. All patients present with multiple, rapidly expanding plaques and/or nodules on noncontiguous sites. Lesions are characteristically purple in color. The course is aggressive in most patients, with rapid cutaneous relapse after chemotherapy with systemic involvement. Histologically, the cells infiltrate the dermis or subcutaneous fat, with a tendency for the neoplastic cells to "Indian file" in dermal collagen. There is usually a Grenz zone below the epidermis. The lymphoma cells are small/medium to large blastic lymphocytes. Angiocentricity may be noted, but is not prominent. Immunophenotyping is usually CD4+,CD56+. MIB-1 shows a proliferation activity of over 50%. T-cell gene rearrangements are negative. A response to pralatrexate has been reported, but in general the results with radiation therapy and chemotherapy have been poor. Bone marrow transplantation (BMT) may play an important role in therapy.

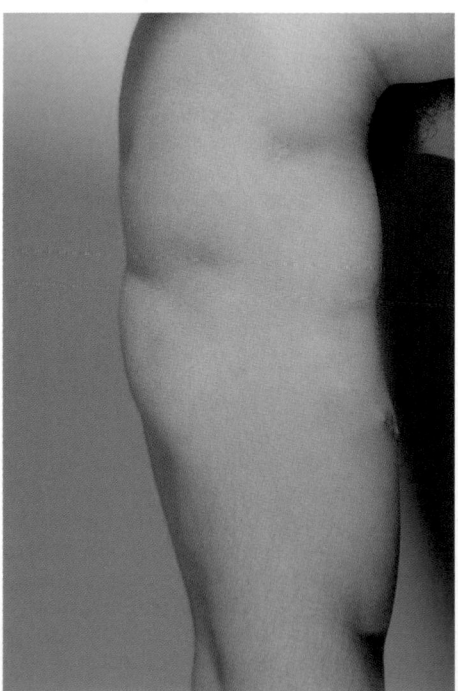

Fig. 32-13 Subcutaneous T-cell lymphoma.

Benner MF, et al: Bone marrow examination has limited value in the staging of patients with an anaplastic large cell lymphoma first presenting in the skin. Retrospective analysis of 107 patients. Br J Dermatol 2008 Nov; 159(5):1148–1151.

Chumsri S, et al: Inhibition of the mammalian target of rapamycin (mTOR) in a case of refractory primary cutaneous anaplastic large cell lymphoma. Leuk Lymphoma 2008 Feb; 49(2):359–361.

Ehst BD, et al: Primary cutaneous CD30+ anaplastic large cell lymphoma responds to imiquimod cream. Eur J Dermatol 2008 Jul–Aug; 18(4):467–468.

Fernández-Torres R, et al: Extranodal NK/T-cell lymphoma, nasal type presenting as a pyogenic granuloma-like on a fingertip. Eur J Dermatol 2009 Jan–Feb; 19(1):79–80.

Fujita H, et al: Primary cutaneous anaplastic large cell lymphoma successfully treated with low-dose oral methotrexate. Eur J Dermatol 2008 May–Jun; 18(3):360–361.

Herling M, et al: CD4+/CD56+ hematodermic tumor: the features of an evolving entity and its relationship to dendritic cells. Am J Clin Pathol 2007 May; 127(5):687–700.

Honma M, et al: Primary cutaneous anaplastic large cell lymphoma successfully treated with local thermotherapy using pocket hand warmers. J Dermatol 2008 Nov; 35(11):748–750.

Humme D, et al: Dominance of nonmalignant T-cell clones and distortion of the TCR repertoire in the peripheral blood of patients with cutaneous CD30+ lymphoproliferative disorders. J Invest Dermatol 2009 Jan; 129(1):89–98.

Kempf W, et al: MUM1 expression in cutaneous CD30+ lymphoproliferative disorders: a valuable tool for the distinction between lymphomatoid papulosis and primary cutaneous anaplastic large-cell lymphoma. Br J Dermatol 2008 Jun; 158(6):1280–1287.

Leitenberger JJ, et al: CD4+ CD56+ hematodermic/plasmacytoid dendritic cell tumor with response to pralatrexate. J Am Acad Dermatol 2008 Mar; 58(3):480–484.

Madray MM, et al: Glatiramer acetate-associated, CD30+, primary, cutaneous, anaplastic large-cell lymphoma. Arch Neurol 2008 Oct; 65(10):1378–1379.

Massone C, et al: The morphologic spectrum of primary cutaneous anaplastic large T-cell lymphoma: a histopathologic study on 66 biopsy specimens from 47 patients with report of rare variants. J Cutan Pathol 2008 Jan; 35(1):46–53.

Parveen Z, et al: Subcutaneous panniculitis-like T-cell lymphoma: redefinition of diagnostic criteria in the recent World Health Organization-European Organization for Research and Treatment of Cancer classification for cutaneous lymphomas. Arch Pathol Lab Med 2009 Feb; 133(2):303–308.

Querfeld C, Khan I, Mahon B, Nelson BP, Rosen ST, Evens AM: Primary cutaneous and systemic anaplastic large cell lymphoma: clinicopathologic aspects and therapeutic options. Oncology (Williston Park) 2010 Jun; 24(7):574–587.

Savage KJ: Prognosis and primary therapy in peripheral T-cell lymphomas. Hematology Am Soc Hematol Educ Program 2008; 2008:280–288.

Savage KJ, et al: ALK– anaplastic large-cell lymphoma is clinically and immunophenotypically different from both ALK+ ALCL and peripheral T-cell lymphoma, not otherwise specified: report from the International Peripheral T-Cell Lymphoma Project. Blood 2008 Jun 15; 111(12):5496–5504.

Adult T-cell leukemia/lymphoma

Infection with human lymphotropic virus type 1 (HTLV-1) may lead to acute T-cell leukemia/lymphoma (ATL) in 0.01–0.02% of infected persons. This virus is endemic in Japan, Southeast Asia, the Caribbean, Latin America, and equatorial Africa. ATL usually has an acute onset, with leukocytosis, lymphadenopathy, and HOTS (hypercalcemia, osteolytic bone lesions, T-cell leukemia, and skin lesions). Lesions resemble mycosis fungoides, except that patches are uncommon and plaques and nodules predominate. Histologically, the skin lesions contain lichenoid infiltrates of medium-sized lymphocytes with convoluted nuclei. Epidermotropism and involvement around and within adnexa occur. Granuloma formation may occur in the dermis. ATL cells are usually CD4+/CD7– and show T-cell gene rearrangements.

Cutaneous B-cell lymphoma

Primary cutaneous B-cell lymphomas (Fig. 32-14) occur less commonly than cutaneous T-cell lymphomas (25% of cases of primary cutaneous non-Hodgkin lymphomas are B-cell in origin). Although the morphologic appearance of the malignant lymphocytes composing these primary cutaneous lymphomas is identical to lymphomas based in lymph nodes, they have a distinctly different clinical behavior and immunophenotypic profiles. This renders the classification systems based on lymph node histology of limited benefit in the diagnosis of primary cutaneous B-cell lymphomas. More simplified schemes have thus been proposed that apply to primary cutaneous lymphomas only. While most entities classified by the European Organization for Research and Treatment of Cancer (EORTC) have now been accepted in the WHO classification, some remain provisional entities.

The great majority of primary cutaneous B-cell lymphomas are composed of cells with the morphologic characteristics of the B cells normally found in the marginal zone or germinal centers of lymph nodes. Classification schemes used primarily for lymph node-based lymphomas divide these lymphomas into multiple types based on histomorphology. Secondary cutaneous involvement can occur with all forms of B-cell lymphoma based primarily in lymph node or other sites. The clinical features are similar to those of primary cutaneous lymphoma, with violaceous papules or nodules (Fig. 32-15). Typically, the histologic structure of secondary lesions in the skin is similar to that of the lymphoma at the site of origin, usually the lymph nodes. The pattern in the skin may not, however, be sufficient to classify the lymphoma, making lymph node biopsy necessary in most cases. In secondary cutaneous B-cell lymphomas the prognosis is generally poor. It is therefore critical to evaluate any patient suspected of having primary cutaneous B-cell lymphoma to exclude involvement at another site. Radiation is most commonly used for indolent forms of cutaneous B-cell lymphoma, but excision, rituximab, intralesional corticosteroids, and systemic chemotherapy have also been used in selected cases. Higher-grade lymphomas, including leg-type lymphoma, primary cutaneous follicle center lymphoma occurring on the leg, and precursor B-cell lymphoblastic lymphoma, are typically treated with systemic chemotherapy regimens including combinations of anthracycline-containing chemotherapies and rituximab.

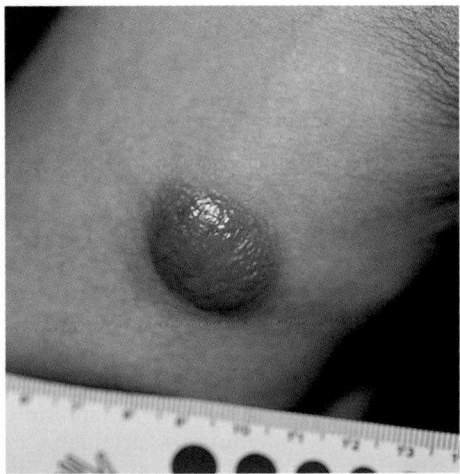

Fig. 32-14 Lymphoma, B-cell.

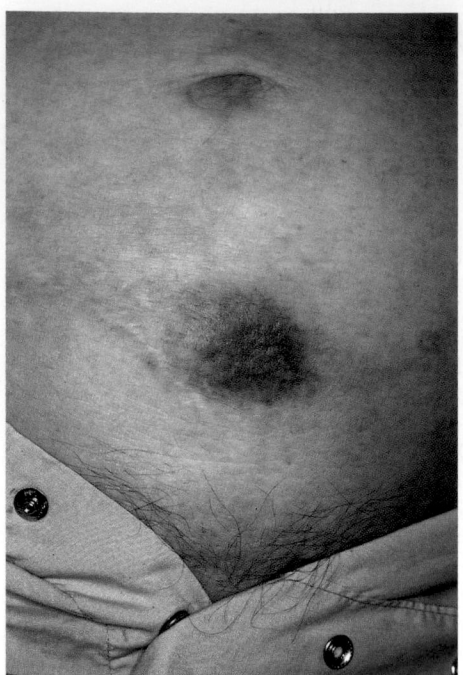

Fig. 32-15 Secondary cutaneous B-cell lymphoma.

Primary cutaneous marginal zone lymphoma (PCMZL, MALT-type lymphoma, including primary cutaneous immunocytoma)

These lymphomas present as solitary or multiple dermal or subcutaneous nodules or tumors primarily on the upper part of the body, trunk, or extremities. Widespread lesions suggest secondary skin involvement by systemic lymphoma. Women are affected more than men. Immunocytomas are associated with European *Borrelia* and occur as tense, shiny, pink to red nodules on the legs of older patients.

Histologically, the infiltrate may be nodular or diffuse. The neoplastic cells are medium-sized gray cells with predominantly cleaved nuclei that proliferate within the space surrounding and between benign germinal centers. Plasma cells are typically present and may be numerous. Light chain restriction is easiest to identify in the plasma cell population by means of in situ hybridization. The lymphoma cells may contain "Dutcher bodies," intranuclear collections of immunoglobulin. Initially, the malignant cells may represent a very small proportion of the infiltrate and an incorrect diagnosis of pseudolymphoma may be made. Over time, the "marginal zone" cells predominate and the germinal centers are diminished. Immunophenotypically, the cells are CD20+, CD79+, and BCL-2+. Clonal immunoglobulin gene rearrangements can usually be demonstrated. The prognosis is excellent, with 5-year survival close to 100%. Local radiation therapy, or excision if lesions are few, is recommended. In some *Borrelia*-endemic areas in Europe, immunocytomas are common. They present with sheets of plasmacytoid B cells with Dutcher bodies. Treatment is similar to other forms of PCMZL.

Primary cutaneous follicle center cell lymphoma (PCFCCL, diffuse and follicular types)

Clinically, most patients present with single or multiple papules, plaques, or nodules, with surrounding erythema, in one anatomic region. About two-thirds of cases present on the trunk, about one-fifth on the head and neck (the vast majority of these on the scalp), and about 15% on the leg. These lym-

phomas are more common in men than women. Males outnumber females 4:1 in trunk lesions, whereas women disproportionately have head and leg lesions. Untreated, the lesions gradually increase in size and number, but extracutaneous involvement is uncommon. The prognosis is excellent, 5-year survival with treatment approaching 100%. Secondary cutaneous involvement of systemic follicular lymphoma has a poor prognosis.

Histologically, the neoplasm is composed of centroblasts (uncleaved nuclei with a peripheral nucleolus) and centrocytes (cleaved nuclei with a peripheral nucleolus). The diffuse form is more common than the follicular form. In the diffuse form, the neoplastic cells retain the normal BCL-6+ phenotype of a follicle center cell, but typically lose expression of CD10. The follicular growth pattern is composed of irregularly shaped asymmetrical follicles that crowd together like pieces of a jigsaw puzzle. The cells typically stain for both BCL-6 and CD10, and these stains demonstrate neoplastic cells that have "wandered" beyond the confines of the follicle center. Elongated "carrot-shaped" nuclei are often present within the follicular centers, and CD21 staining shows defects in the net of dendritic cells in the follicle center.

In early lesions, the neoplastic cells are of smaller size and there is a substantial portion of normal T cells surrounding and mixed with the neoplastic B cells. Over time, the neoplastic B cells become a more predominant portion of the infiltrate, the neoplastic cells are larger in size, and tumor-infiltrating T cells diminish. Immunophenotypically, the neoplastic cells stain with B-cell markers (CD20) and may be monotypic for immunoglobulin production, i.e. they stain for either κ or λ light chains, but not both. Immunoglobulin staining is commonly negative in tumorous lesions, but clonal rearrangement of the immunoglobulin gene can be demonstrated by polymerase chain reaction (PCR). The absence of expression of BCL-2, lack of adenopathy, and lack of involvement of the bone marrow help to exclude nodal follicular center lymphoma. Nodal follicular lymphoma usually expresses BCL-2 and there is a t(14:18) translocation in more than 80% of cases. BCL-2 expression is usually lacking in primary cutaneous follicular lymphoma.

Radiation therapy totaling 30–40 Gy and including all erythematous skin and a 2 cm margin of normal skin is very effective for lesions of the head and trunk. A combination of intralesional IFN-α, 5 MU every 4 weeks, and topical bexarotene gel, 1% twice, has also been used. Anthracycline-based chemotherapy or rituximab may be used for relapses, as well as for more aggressive lesions of the leg. In Europe, a few cases of PCFCL are associated with *Borrelia* infection and may arise in lesions of acrodermatitis chronica atrophicans.

Diffuse large B-cell lymphoma (primary cutaneous large B-cell lymphoma)

Clinically, lesions present as solitary or localized red or purple papules, nodules, or plaques. In general, solitary or localized lesions are typical of primary disease, and widespread lesions suggest secondary cutaneous involvement of primary nodal lymphoma. Lesions on the head and neck have an excellent prognosis. Lesions on the leg have a poorer prognosis, with a 5-year survival of about 50%, and are considered in some classifications as a separate entity (Fig. 32-16).

This group of lymphomas is composed of large lymphocytes. Tumors made up of sheets of centroblasts and immunoblasts (non-cleaved nuclei with peripheral or central nucleoli, respectively) should be stained for MUM1, a marker for leg-type lymphoma. If the tumor cells express MUM1, the prognosis is worse. Immunophenotypically, cells usually express CD20 and

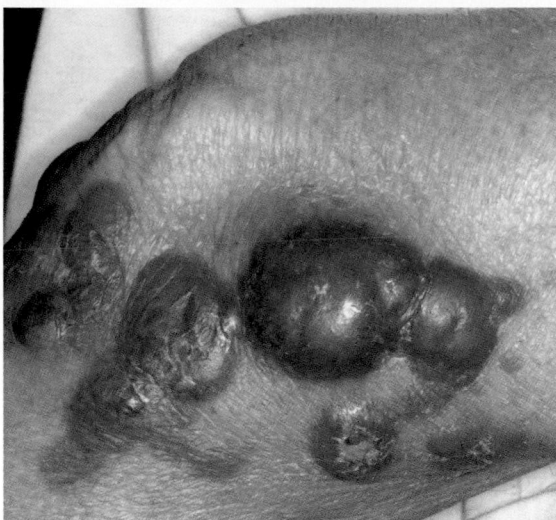

Fig. 32-16 B-cell lymphoma of the leg.

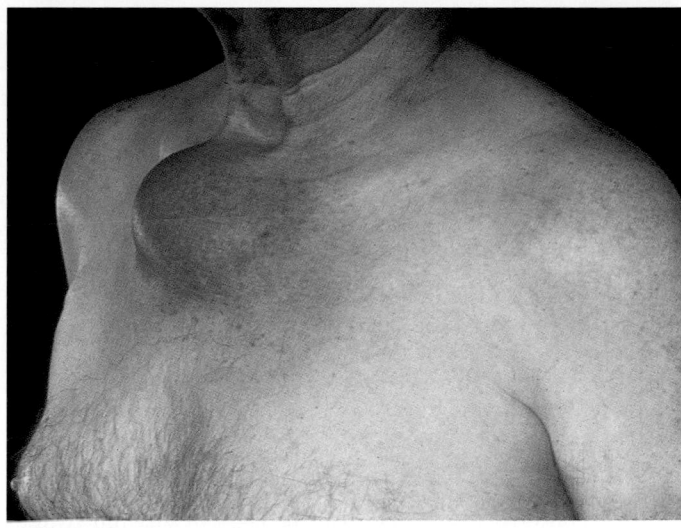

Fig. 32-17 Plasmacytoma extending from the sternum.

monotypic immunoglobulin, and leg-type lymphoma expresses BCL-2. Secondary cutaneous involvement with nodal large B-cell lymphoma is also associated with a poor prognosis.

Richter transformation of chronic lymphocytic leukemia into a high-grade lymphoma occurs in 3–10% of patients with chronic lymphocytic leukemia. Its onset is often heralded by fever, night sweats, and weight loss. The lymphoma commonly arises in the lymph nodes or bone marrow, but can also present in the skin or internal organs.

Intravascular large B-cell lymphoma (malignant "angioendotheliomatosis," angiotropic large-cell lymphoma)

Clinically, these patients present with variable cutaneous morphologies, often very subtle and nonspecific. Some cases resemble classic lymphoma with violaceous papules or nodules. Others more closely resemble intravascular thrombotic disorders, with livedo reticularis-like lesions or telangiectatic patches. Sclerotic plaques may also occur. Even normal skin can show the characteristic changes on biopsy. Patients often present with fever of unknown origin. CNS symptoms are prominent, with progressive dementia or multiple cerebrovascular ischemic events that may precede skin findings by many months.

Histologically, the features are characteristic and diagnostic. Dermal and subcutaneous vessels are dilated and filled with large neoplastic cells. Focal extravascular accumulations may be seen. The neoplastic cells are CD20+ and CD79a+, and monotypic for immunoglobulin. Clonal immunoglobulin gene rearrangements may be detected. Despite the large number of intravascular cells in the skin and other affected organs, the peripheral blood smears and bone marrow may be normal histologically. The prognosis is very poor. Multiagent chemotherapy is recommended. Rare cases of intravascular lymphoma may be of T-cell origin.

Adam DN, et al: Review of intravascular lymphoma with a report of treatment with allogenic peripheral blood stem cell transplant. Cutis 2008 Oct; 82(4):267–272.

Gerami P, et al: Applying the new TNM classification system for primary cutaneous lymphomas other than mycosis fungoides and Sézary syndrome in primary cutaneous marginal zone lymphoma. J Am Acad Dermatol 2008 Aug; 59(2):245–254.

Grange F, et al: Primary cutaneous diffuse large B-cell lymphoma, leg type: clinicopathologic features and prognostic analysis in 60 cases. Arch Dermatol 2007 Sep; 143(9):1144–1150.

Hallermann C, et al: New prognostic relevant factors in primary cutaneous diffuse large B-cell lymphomas. J Am Acad Dermatol 2007 Apr; 56(4):588–597.

Morales AV, et al: Indolent primary cutaneous B-cell lymphoma: experience using systemic rituximab. J Am Acad Dermatol 2008 Dec; 59(6):953–957.

Senff NJ, et al: Results of radiotherapy in 153 primary cutaneous B-cell lymphomas classified according to the WHO-EORTC classification. Arch Dermatol 2007 Dec; 143(12):1520–1526.

Senff NJ, et al: European Organization for Research and Treatment of Cancer and International Society for Cutaneous Lymphoma consensus recommendations for the management of cutaneous B-cell lymphomas. Blood 2008 Sep 1; 112(5):1600–1609.

Shafer D, et al: Cutaneous precursor B-cell lymphoblastic lymphoma in 2 adult patients: clinicopathologic and molecular cytogenetic studies with a review of the literature. Arch Dermatol 2008 Sep; 144(9):1155–1162.

van Tuyll van Serooskerken AM, et al: Coincidence of cutaneous follicle center lymphoma and diffuse large B-cell lymphoma. Int J Dermatol 2008 Nov; 47(Suppl 1):21–24.

Yamazaki ML, et al: Primary cutaneous Richter syndrome: prognostic implications and review of the literature. J Am Acad Dermatol 2009 Jan; 60(1):157–161.

Plasmacytoma (multiple myeloma)

True cutaneous plasmacytomas are seen most commonly in the setting of myeloma. They are, however, rare, occurring in only 2% of myeloma cases. These cases are called secondary cutaneous plasmacytoma. They may also occur by direct extension from an underlying bone lesion (Fig. 32-17). They may appear at sites of trauma, such as biopsies or intravenous catheters (inflammatory oncotaxis). Most commonly, secondary cutaneous plasmacytomas occur in the setting of advanced myeloma and the prognosis is poor. Less commonly, the skin lesions may be the initial clinical finding, leading to the diagnosis of myeloma. Many cutaneous lesions formerly classified as primary cutaneous plasmacytomas are now classified as plasma cell-rich primary cutaneous marginal zone lymphoma.

Anetoderma may show plasmacytoma on biopsy. A rare manifestation of a solitary plasmacytoma of bone is an overlying erythematous skin patch that may be 10 cm or more in diameter. The chest is the most common location. Lymphadenopathy is present and some of the patients have or develop POEMS syndrome (polyneuropathy, organomegaly, endocrinopathy, monoclonal protein, and skin changes). This syndrome has been called adenopathy and extensive skin patch overlying a plasmacytoma, or AESOP.

Histologically, there are nodular and diffuse collections of plasma cells with varying degrees of pleomorphism and atypia. The degree of atypia may predict prognosis. The cells are monotypic for immunoglobulin production and produce the same light chain as the myeloma. The immunoglobulin produced is most commonly IgG or IgA, and rarely IgD or IgE. CD79 is positive, but CD19 and CD20 are negative.

In addition to plasmacytomas, patients with myeloma may develop a vast array of cutaneous complications. These include normolipemic plane xanthomas, amyloidosis, vasculitis, and calcinosis cutis. An unusual but characteristic skin finding in myeloma is multiple follicular spicules of the nose, forehead, cheeks, and chin. They are yellowish and firm to palpation, and can be removed without bleeding. Numerous small ulcerations may occur on the trunk. Both the spicules and ulcers contain an eosinophilic material composed of the abnormal monoclonal protein produced by the malignant cells. The spicules are not made of keratin. Clinically similar cutaneous spicules composed of keratin can be seen in vitamin A deficiency, chronic renal failure, acquired immunodeficiency syndrome (AIDS), Crohn's disease, and other malignant diseases.

The appropriate treatment of plasmacytomas is determined by the presence or absence of associated systemic disease. Solitary or paucilesional primary cutaneous plasmacytomas have been treated successfully with local surgery and radiation therapy. Systemic chemotherapy may be required if these modalities fail. The treatment for secondary plasmacytomas and for patients with numerous primary cutaneous plasmacytomas is chemotherapy.

Cutaneous and systemic plasmacytosis

Cutaneous plasmacytosis and systemic plasmacytosis occur largely in Asians, slightly favoring males. They typically occur between the ages of 20 and 55. These conditions are characterized by polyclonal proliferations of plasma cells and hyperglobulinemia, and were originally considered variants of Castleman's disease. Cutaneous plasmacytosis affects only the skin but patients may have lymphadenopathy and systemic symptoms of fever and malaise. Systemic plasmacytosis has involvement in two or more organ systems, usually, in addition to skin, the lung, bone marrow, and liver. Dyspnea may occur due to interstitial pneumonia. Uncommonly, cases of systemic plasmacytosis may progress to lymphoma. The course is chronic and benign, and response to various cytostatic and immunosuppressive treatments has been poor. PUVA and topical tacrolimus have been reported to be effective for skin lesions. The skin lesions in cutaneous and systemic plasmacytosis are identical. They consist of multiple brown–red plaques, mostly of the central upper trunk, but also of the face. Lesions range from 1 to 3 cm in diameter. They are often considered simply postinflammatory hyperpigmentation until they are palpated. Histologically, they show a dense perivascular infiltrate of mature plasma cells, which stain for both κ and λ light chains (polyclonality). Elevated IL-6 has been reported in some patients.

Hodgkin disease

The vast majority of reports of cutaneous Hodgkin disease actually represent type A lymphomatoid papulosis (LyP). These two diseases have a considerable number of overlapping features. The type A cells of LyP have similar morphology and share immunophenotypic markers with Reed–Sternberg cells. LyP can be seen in patients with Hodgkin disease. Primary cutaneous Hodgkin disease without nodal involvement is thus difficult to prove and is very, very rare, if it exists.

Most cases of Hodgkin disease of the skin usually originate in the lymph nodes, from which extension to the skin is either retrograde through the lymphatics or direct. Lesions present as papules or nodules, with or without ulceration. Lesions resembling scrofuloderma may occur. Miliary dissemination to the skin can occur in advanced disease.

Nonspecific cutaneous findings are common in patients with Hodgkin disease. Generalized, severe pruritus may precede other findings of Hodgkin disease by many months or may occur in patients with a known diagnosis. Secondary prurigo nodules and pigmentation may occur as a result of scratching. An evaluation for underlying lymphoma should be considered in any patient with severe itching, no primary skin lesions, and no other cause identified for the pruritus. Acquired ichthyosis, exfoliative dermatitis, and generalized and severe herpes zoster are other cutaneous findings in patients with Hodgkin disease.

Malignant histiocytosis (histiocytic medullary reticulosis)

Most cases considered to be malignant histiocytosis in the past are now considered to be other forms of lymphoma or lymphomas with large components of reactive histiocytes. Very rare cases of true malignancies of histiocytes may still occur and can have cutaneous lesions, most characteristically erythematous nodules. Often, the bone marrow examination in these patients is initially normal, but cases are rapidly progressive and fatal, and the bone marrow becomes involved.

Introcaso CE, et al: Cutaneous Hodgkin disease. J Am Acad Dermatol 2008 Feb; 58(2):295–298.

Leukemia cutis

Clinical features

Cutaneous eruptions seen in patients with leukemia may be divided into specific (leukemia cutis) and nonspecific lesions (reactive and infectious processes). Overall, about 30% of biopsies from patients with leukemia will show leukemia cutis. All forms of leukemia can be associated with cutaneous findings, but skin disease is more common in certain forms of leukemia. Myeloid leukemia with monocytic differentiation involves the skin more commonly than other types of myeloid leukemia. CD68 and lysozyme immunostains can be helpful in distinguishing this form of leukemia. Dermatologic manifestations are commonly seen in patients with acute myelogenous leukemia (AML) and myelodysplastic syndrome (MDS). AML includes types M1–M5. In AML and MDS patients, only about 25% of skin biopsies will show leukemia cutis, the remainder showing complications of the leukemia. These include infections, graft versus host disease, drug reactions, or the reactive conditions associated with leukemia that are sometimes referred to as leukemids. By contrast, in patients with acute lymphocytic leukemia (ALL), chronic myelogenous leukemia (CML), and chronic lymphocytic leukemia (CLL), about 50% of biopsies will show leukemia cutis. Lesion presentation may be subtle, and may include macular erythema, hyperpigmentation, or morbilliform rash.

Specific eruptions

The most common morphology of leukemic infiltrations of the skin in all forms of leukemia is multiple papules or nodules

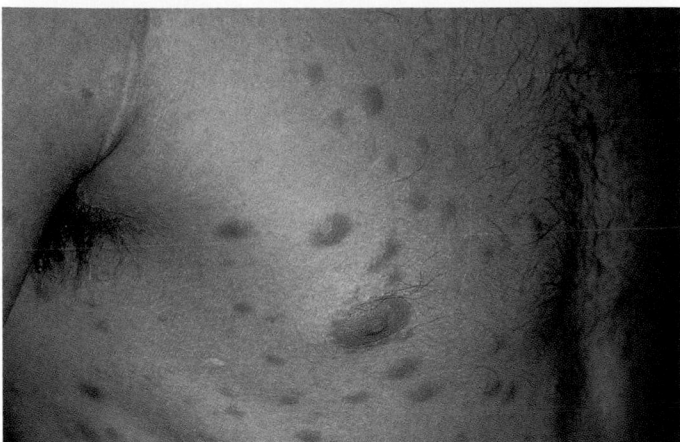

Fig. 32-18 Leukemia cutis.

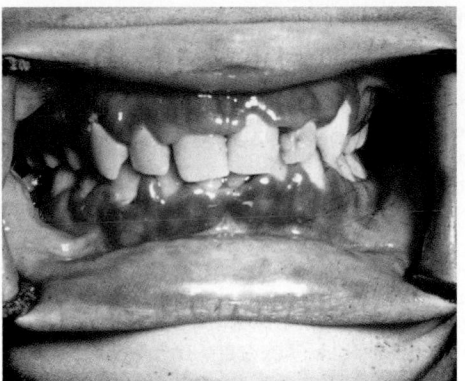

Fig. 32-20 Gingival involvement in leukemia.

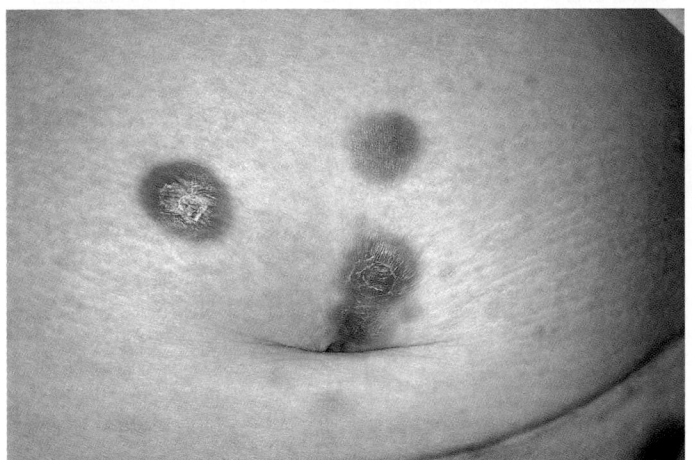

Fig. 32-19 Leukemia cutis.

(60% of cases) or infiltrated plaques (26%). These lesions are usually flesh-colored, erythematous, or violaceous (plum-colored) (Figs 32-18 and 32-19). They are rubbery on palpation and ulceration is uncommon. Extensive involvement of the face may lead to a leonine facies.

Less common manifestations of leukemia cutis are subcutaneous nodules resembling erythema nodosum or panniculitis, arciform lesions (in juvenile CML), ecchymoses, palpable purpura, erythroderma, ulcerations (which may resemble pyoderma gangrenosum or venous stasis ulceration), and urticaria-like, urticaria pigmentosa-like (in ALL), and guttate psoriasis-like lesions. Rare manifestations are a lesion resembling Sister Mary Joseph nodule and cutaneous sarcoidal lesions. Myelogenous leukemia may be complicated by lesions resembling stasis dermatitis or chilblains. Gingival infiltration causing hypertrophy is common in and relatively unique to patients with acute myelomonocytic leukemia (Fig. 32-20).

Leukemia cutis most commonly occurs concomitant with or following the diagnosis of leukemia. The skin may also be a site of relapse of leukemia after chemotherapy, especially in patients who present with leukemia cutis. Uncommonly, leukemia cutis may be identified while the bone marrow and peripheral blood are normal. These patients are classified as "aleukemic leukemia cutis," as they have normal bone marrow evaluations and no circulating blasts. These cases are often misdiagnosed as cutaneous lymphomas and undertreated. They eventually relapse, with full-blown leukemia. The key to the diagnosis is a Leder stain, which will identify the atypical cells as myeloid. Systemic involvement occurs within 3 weeks to 20 months (average 6 months). Leukemia cutis is a poor prognostic finding in patients with leukemia, with 90% of such patients having extramedullary involvement and 40% having meningeal infiltration.

The term congenital leukemia applies to cases appearing within the first 4–6 weeks of life. Leukemia cutis occurs in 25–30% of such cases, the vast majority being congenital myelogenous leukemia. The typical morphology is multiple, red or plum-colored nodules. In about 10% of cases of congenital leukemia cutis (or 3% of all cases of congenital leukemia), the skin involvement occurs while the bone marrow and peripheral blood are normal. Systemic involvement is virtually always identified in 5–16 weeks. Unlike in other forms of leukemia, in congenital leukemia, cutaneous infiltration does not worsen prognosis. Congenital leukaemia cutis has been complicated by disseminated linear calcinosis cutis. Early-onset aleukemic leukemia cutis can occasionally undergo spontaneous regression. One report involved a child with mastocytosis, who also developed a leukemia clone with a t(5; 17)(q35; q12), nucleophosmin (NPM)-retinoic acid receptor-α (RARA) fusion gene.

Granulocytic sarcoma (chloroma)

Granulocytic sarcomas are rare tumors of immature granulocytes. They occur in about 3% of patients with myelogenous leukemia. Granulocytic sarcoma is seen in four settings: in patients with known AML; in patients with CML or MDS as a sign of an impending blast crisis; in undiagnosed patients as the first sign of AML; or after BMT as the initial sign of relapse. Most lesions occur in the soft tissues, periosteum, or bone. Skin lesions represent 20–50% of reported cases. They may be solitary or multiple. They appear as red, mahogany, or violaceous firm nodules with a predilection for the face, scalp, or trunk.

The name chloroma comes from the green color of fresh lesions, which can be enhanced by rubbing with alcohol; this is caused by the presence of myeloperoxidase. This appearance is variable, so the preferred term is now granulocytic sarcoma.

The diagnosis is not difficult if the diagnosis of leukemia has been established. Such patients are treated with appropriate chemotherapy. However, if the skin lesion is the initial manifestation of leukemia, and the blood and bone marrow are normal, the lesion may be misdiagnosed as a large-cell lymphoma. The treatment of such patients is controversial, but most go on to develop AML within months, so chemotherapy is often given.

Hairy cell leukemia

Skin involvement is rare in hairy cell leukemia, and violaceous papules and nodules, which are the characteristic morphology of other forms of leukemia cutis, are extremely rare in hairy cell leukemia. Rather, a diffuse erythematous, nonpruritic eruption occurs, often in the setting of a systemic mycobacterial infection or a drug reaction. This may progress to erythroderma or a severe blistering eruption. Stopping the offending medication usually leads to resolution of the eruption. This is especially common in patients treated with 2-chlorodeoxyadenosine and allopurinol. The former treatment alone does not lead to these severe skin reactions, suggesting that the allopurinol is the cause. Patients with hairy cell leukemia also develop lesions of pustular vasculitis of the dorsal hands, a neutrophilic dermatitis closely related to bullous Sweet syndrome. This is sometimes termed a "vasculitis" in the oncology literature.

Nonspecific conditions associated with leukemia (leukemids)

Leukemia and its treatment are associated with a series of conditions that may also be seen in patients without leukemia, but which are seen frequently enough in leukemic patients to be recognized as a complication of that condition or its treatment.

When a dermatologist or dermatopathologist is consulted to evaluate a patient with leukemia and skin lesions, the differential diagnosis usually includes four groups of conditions: drug reactions, leukemia cutis, an infectious complication, and a reactive condition. Drug reactions include all forms of reactions, but are most commonly erythema multiforme, morbilliform reactions, or acral erythema. Infections may present in many ways but are usually purpuric papules, pustules, or plaques, if they are caused by bacteria or fungi. Ulceration is typical. Herpes simplex and herpes zoster should be considered in all erosive, ulcerative, or vesicular lesions. The reactive conditions include a group of neutrophilic dermatoses with considerable clinical overlap. These include Sweet syndrome, pyoderma gangrenosum, neutrophilic hidradenitis, and leukocytoclastic vasculitis. Transient acantholytic dermatosis and eosinophilic reactions resembling insect bites may occur, most commonly in patients with CLL. In CLL a pruritic and unremitting exfoliative erythroderma is a unique feature. A granulomatous rosacea-like leukemid and cutaneous reactive angiomatosis have also been described in patients with leukemia.

Evaluation of these patients must be complete, and extensive diagnostic tests and empiric treatment are often pursued until the diagnosis is established. In the acute setting, a clinical diagnosis is made based on morphology. Possible infectious complications are covered by appropriate antibiotics, especially if the patient is febrile or the diagnosis of a herpesvirus infection is made. A skin biopsy is often diagnostic. For herpes infections, a direct fluorescent antibody test should be done, as the results are virus-specific and rapid, so appropriate treatment can be given quickly. Once the diagnostic tests return, the therapy is tailored to the appropriate condition. Except for herpes infections, a skin biopsy is often required. If infection is considered, a portion of the biopsy should be sent for culture.

Angulo J, et al: Leukemia cutis presenting as localized cutaneous hyperpigmentation. J Cutan Pathol 2008 Jul; 35(7):662–665.
Cho-Vega JH, et al: Leukemia cutis. Am J Clin Pathol 2008 Jan; 129(1):130–142.
Cibull TL, et al: Myeloid leukemia cutis: a histologic and immunohistochemical review. J Cutan Pathol 2008 Feb; 35(2):180–185.
D'Orazio JA, et al: Spontaneous resolution of a single lesion of myeloid leukemia cutis in an infant: case report and discussion. Pediatr Hematol Oncol 2008 Jun; 25(5):457–468.
Hattori T, et al: Leukemia cutis in a patient with acute monocytic leukemia presenting as unique facial erythema. J Dermatol 2008 Oct; 35(10):671–674.
Hejmadi RK, et al: Cutaneous presentation of aleukemic monoblastic leukemia cutis—a case report and review of literature with focus on immunohistochemistry. J Cutan Pathol 2008 Oct; 35(Suppl 1):46–49.
Kanegane H, et al: Spontaneous regression of aleukemic leukemia cutis harboring a NPM/RARA fusion gene in an infant with cutaneous mastocytosis. Int J Hematol 2009 Jan; 89(1):86–90.
Mariñas EA, et al: Cutaneous reactive angiomatosis associated with chronic lymphoid leukemia. Am J Dermatopathol 2008 Dec; 30(6):604–607.
Remková A, et al: Acute vasculitis as a first manifestation of hairy cell leukemia. Eur J Intern Med 2007 May; 18(3):238–240.
Skiljević D, et al: Granulomatous rosacea-like leukemid in a patient with acute myeloid leukemia. Vojnosanit Pregl 2008 Jul; 65(7):565–568.
Stern M, et al: Leukemia cutis preceding systemic relapse of acute myeloid leukemia. Int J Hematol 2008 Mar; 87(2):108–109.
Weinel S, et al: Therapy-related leukaemia cutis: a review. Australas J Dermatol 2008 Nov; 49(4):187–190.

Cutaneous myelofibrosis

Myelofibrosis is a chronic myeloproliferative disorder characterized by a clonal proliferation of defective multipotential stem cells in the bone marrow. Overproduction and premature death of atypical megakaryocytes in the bone marrow produce excess amounts of platelet-derived growth factor, a potent stimulus for fibroblast proliferation and collagen production. Extramedullary hematopoiesis (EMH) is a hallmark of myelofibrosis. Myelofibrosis may coexist with signs of mastocytosis. Blast cells and committed stem cells escape the marrow in large numbers, enter the circulation, and form tumors of the same atypical clone in other organs, especially the spleen, liver, and lymph node. EMH in the skin of neonates is usually caused by intrauterine viral infections. In adults, cutaneous EMH has rarely been reported, characteristically associated with myelofibrosis. Skin lesions are dermal and subcutaneous nodules. Histologically, the cutaneous lesions are composed of dermal and subcutaneous infiltrates of mature and immature myeloid cells, erythroid precursors (in only half of cases), and megakaryocytic cells (which may predominate). There is marked production of collagen fibers in the cutaneous lesions by the mechanism described above. Myelofibrosis must be distinguished from CML, since both have elevated white blood cell counts with immature myeloid forms, defective platelet production, and marrow fibrosis. Both may terminate in blast crisis, and myelofibrosis may rarely convert to CML. CML is associated with the Philadelphia chromosome, whereas chromosomal abnormalities occur in 40% of myelofibrosis cases on various chromosomes.

Haniffa MA, et al: Cutaneous extramedullary hemopoiesis in chronic myeloproliferative and myelodysplastic disorders. J Am Acad Dermatol 2006 Aug; 55(2 Suppl):S28–31.
Miyata T, et al: Cutaneous extramedullary hematopoiesis in a patient with idiopathic myelofibrosis. J Dermatol 2008 Jul; 35(7):456–461.
Turchin I, et al: Unusual cutaneous findings of urticaria pigmentosa and telangiectasia macularis eruptiva perstans associated with marked myelofibrosis. Int J Dermatol 2006 Oct; 45(10):1215–1217.

Hypereosinophilic syndrome

Idiopathic hypereosinophilic syndrome (HES) is defined as eosinophilia with more than 1500 eosinophils/mm^3 for more than 6 months, with some evidence of parenchymal organ involvement; there must also be no apparent underlying disease to explain the hypereosinophilia and usually no evidence of vasculitis. Ninety percent of patients reported have been men, mostly between the ages of 20 and 50. Childhood cases are rare. Presenting symptoms include fever (12%), cough (24%), fatigue, malaise, muscle pains, and skin eruptions. Two pathogenic variants of HES have been defined: m-HES (myeloproliferative HES) and l-HES (lymphocytic HES). M-HES patients are overwhelmingly males, and anemia, thrombocytopenia, elevated serum B_{12} levels, mucosal ulcerations, splenomegaly, and endomyocardial fibrosis are the clinical features. Isolated Loeffler's endocarditis has been reported as a presenting sign. Eosinophil clonality and interstitial deletion on 4q12 result in fusions of *FIP1qL1* and *PDGFRa* genes, forming an F/P fusion protein displaying constitutive activity, are pathogenically related to m-HES cases. Increased mast cells and elevated tryptase levels with myeloid precursors in peripheral blood and myelofibrosis may be found, suggesting that mast cells may be pathogenically related to this form of HES. Leukemia may develop in patients with m-HES. L-HES has been associated with circulating T-cell clones of CD4+ phenotype, which secrete Th2 cytokines, especially IL-5. Females and males are equally affected by l-HES and cutaneous manifestations are observed in virtually all patients. Skin manifestations include urticaria, angioedema, pruritus, eczema, and erythroderma. Splinter hemorrhages and necrotic skin lesions are seen in some HES patients as well. Endomyocardial fibrosis is uncommon, but pulmonary and digestive symptoms are common. Some cases of l-HES are clinically identical to Gleich syndrome or episodic angioedema and hypereosinophilia. Over time some patients with l-HES will develop lymphoma.

Treatment is determined by classifying cases appropriately as m-HES or l-HES. M-HES patients may be treated with corticosteroids, hydroxyurea, IFN-α, and chemotherapeutic agents. Imatinib mesylate (Gleevac, 100 mg/day or less) can be highly effective for m-HES patients with the F/P mutation, as imatinib inhibits the phosphorylation of the F/P protein and leads to apoptosis of cells producing this protein. This has rapidly become first-choice treatment for this subset of patients. Response may be dramatic, with eosinophil levels improving, and skin and gastrointestinal manifestations clearing in days. For l-HES patients, systemic glucocorticoids, and perhaps IFN-α with glucocorticoids, can be used and are usually effective. Monoclonal anti-IL-5 antibody, cyclosporine A, anti-IL-2R-α, infliximab, and CTLA-4-Ig may be treatment options. If lymphoma supervenes, intense chemotherapy and allogenic stem cell transplantation can be considered.

Dahabreh IJ, et al: Management of hypereosinophilic syndrome: a prospective study in the era of molecular genetics. Medicine (Baltimore) 2007 Nov; 86(6):344–354.

Hayashi M, et al: Case of hypereosinophilic syndrome with cutaneous necrotizing vasculitis. J Dermatol 2008 Apr; 35(4):229–233.

Leiferman KM, et al: Dermatologic manifestations of the hypereosinophilic syndromes. Immunol Allergy Clin North Am 2007 Aug; 27(3):415–441.

Sen T, et al: Hypereosinophilic syndrome with isolated Loeffler's endocarditis: complete resolution with corticosteroids. J Postgrad Med 2008 Apr–Jun; 54(2):135–137.

Taverna JA, et al: Infliximab as a therapy for idiopathic hypereosinophilic syndrome. Arch Dermatol 2007 Sep; 143(9):1110–1112.

Angioimmunoblastic lymphadenopathy with dysproteinemia (angioimmunoblastic T-cell lymphoma)

Angioimmunoblastic lymphadenopathy with dysproteinemia (AILD) is an uncommon lymphoproliferative disorder. Patients are middle-aged or elderly and present with fever (72%), weight loss (58%), hepatomegaly (60%), polyclonal hyperglob-ulinemia (65%), and generalized adenopathy (87%). Pruritus occurs in 44% and a rash in 46%. The skin eruption is usually morbilliform in character, resembling an exanthem or a drug reaction. Petechial, purpuric, nodular, ulcerative, and erythro-dermic eruptions have also been reported, and may mimic infection. In about 30% of cases the eruption is associated with the ingestion of a medication. The eruptions usually resolve with oral steroids, misleading the clinician into believing that the eruption was benign. Reversible myelofibrosis has been described. Recent evidence suggests that the neoplastic cells are derived from germinal center T-helper cells, as they express genes unique to this population, including programmed death-1 (*PD-1*) and *CXCL13*.

Histopathologically, there is a patchy and perivascular dermal infiltrate of various types of lymphoid cells, plasma cells, histiocytes (enough to rarely give a "granulomatous" appearance), and eosinophils. The lymphoid cells are usually helper T cells (CD4+). Some portion of the lymphoid cells is atypical in most cases, suggesting the diagnosis. Blood vessels are increased and the endothelial cells are prominent, often cuboidal. Unfortunately, these changes may not be adequate to confirm the diagnosis. However, clonal T-cell gene rearrangement is found in three-quarters of these skin lesions and is the same as the clone in the lymph node. Immunophenotyping of the skin lesions does not give a consistent pattern. At times, the skin lesions will show leukocytoclastic vasculitis on biopsy. Lymph node biopsy is usually required to confirm the diagnosis and exclude progression to lymphoma.

AILD appears to develop in a stepwise fashion. Initially, there is an immune response to an unknown antigen. This immune reaction persists, leading to oligoclonal T-cell proliferation. Monoclonal evolution may occur, eventuating in lymphoma (angioimmunoblastic lymphoma [AILD-L]). These are usually T-cell lymphomas, but B-cell lymphomas can also occur. In the case of AILD-L, skin lesions may contain the neoplastic cells (secondary lymphoma cutis). In up to 50% of cases, multiple unrelated neoplastic cell clones have been identified. Clones identified in the skin may be different from clones found in lymph node. Trisomy 3 or 5, or an extra X chromosome may be found. AILD is an aggressive disease, with mortality ranging from 48% to 72% in various series (average survival time is 11–60 months). The cause of death is usually infection. Epstein–Barr virus and HHV 6 and 8 have been implicated in AILD.

Treatment of AILD has included systemic steroids, methotrexate plus prednisone, combination chemotherapy, fludarabine, 2-chlorodeoxyadenosine, IFN-α, and cyclosporine. Early treatment with systemic steroids during an oligoclonal or pre-lymphomatous stage may induce a long-lasting remission. Asymptomatic patients may not be treated initially but must be watched very closely. More aggressive chemotherapy achieves better remission. None the less, recurrence rates are high, and average survival is between 1 and 3 years.

Matsui K, et al: Angioimmunoblastic T cell lymphoma associated with reversible myelofibrosis. Intern Med 2008; 47(21):1921–1924.

Shah ZH, et al: Monoclonality and oligoclonality of T cell receptor beta gene in angioimmunoblastic T cell lymphoma. J Clin Pathol 2009 Feb; 62(2):177–181.

Yu H, et al: Germinal-center T-helper-cell markers PD-1 and CXCL13 are both expressed by neoplastic cells in angioimmunoblastic T-cell lymphoma. Am J Clin Pathol 2009 Jan; 131(1):33–41.

Sinus histiocytosis with massive lymphadenopathy (Rosai–Dorfman disease)

Sinus histiocytosis with massive lymphadenopathy (SHML), or Rosai–Dorfman disease, usually appears in patients in the first or second decade of life as a febrile illness accompanied

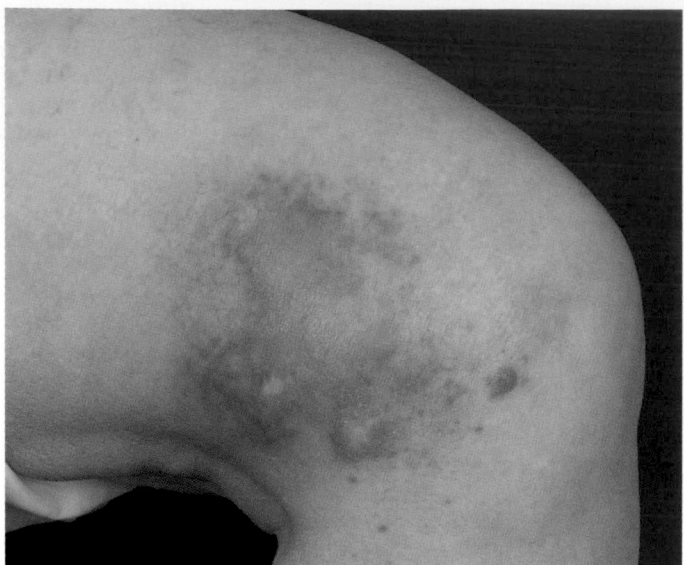

Fig. 32-21 Rosai–Dorfman disease. (Courtesy of Ellen Kim, MD)

by massive cervical (and commonly other) lymphadenopathy, polyclonal hyperglobulinemia, leukocytosis, anemia, and an elevated sedimentation rate. Males and black persons are especially susceptible. Extranodal involvement occurs in 40% of cases, with skin being the most common site. Ten percent of patients with SHML have skin lesions and 3% of patients have disease detectable only in the skin. The terms cutaneous sinus histiocytosis or cutaneous Rosai–Dorfman disease have been applied to these cases. Skin lesions consist of isolated or disseminated yellow–brown papules, pustules, or nodules (Fig. 32-21), or macular erythema. Large annular lesions, resembling granuloma annulare, may occur. Most patients with cutaneous Rosai–Dorfman are older (40–60 years).

Histologically, there is a superficial and deep perivascular infiltrate of lymphocytes and plasma cells. Nodular and diffuse infiltration of the dermis by large, foamy histiocytes is present. A very important diagnostic feature is the finding of intact lymphocytes (and less commonly, plasma cells) in the cytoplasm of the histiocytic cells. This is called emperipolesis. Foamy histiocytes may be seen in dermal lymphatics. The cutaneous histology in some cases may be very nonspecific (except for the finding of emperipolesis), and only on evaluation of lymph node or other organ involvement does the diagnosis become clear. Immunohistochemistry and electron microscopy may be very useful, as the infiltrating cells are positive for CD4, factor XIIIa, and S-100, but do not contain Birbeck granules.

The cause of this condition is unknown, but numerous reports have identified HHV 6 in involved lymph nodes. The condition usually clears spontaneously, so no treatment is required. Numerous agents have been used therapeutically with variable success, but are only indicated if the condition puts the patient at risk for death or a significant complication (usually by compressing a vital organ). Treatments have included radiation, systemic corticosteroids, and thalidomide. Single and multiagent chemotherapy is met with mixed to poor response. To treat skin lesions, cryotherapy, topical steroids, acitretin, and intralesional steroids may be tried.

Kong YY, et al: Cutaneous Rosai–Dorfman disease: a clinical and histopathologic study of 25 cases in China. Am J Surg Pathol 2007 Mar; 31(3):341–350.

Mebazaa A, et al: Extensive purely cutaneous Rosai–Dorfman disease responsive to acitretin. Int J Dermatol 2007 Nov; 46(11):1208–1210.

Merola JF, et al: Cutaneous Rosai–Dorfman disease. Dermatol Online J 2008 May 15; 14(5):8.

Ohnishi A, et al: Cutaneous Rosai–Dorfman disease. J Dermatol 2008 Sep; 35(9):604–605.

Polycythemia vera (erythremia)

Polycythemia vera (PCV) is characterized by an absolute increase of circulating red blood cells, with a hematocrit level of 55–80%. Leukocyte and platelet counts are also increased. The skin changes are characteristic. There is a tendency for the skin to be red, especially on the face, neck, and acral areas. The mucous membranes are engorged and bluish. The phrase "red as a rose in summer and indigo blue in winter" has been ascribed to Osler in describing PCV. Telangiectases, bleeding gums, and epistaxis are frequently encountered. Cyanosis, purpura, petechiae, hemosiderosis, rosacea, and koilonychia may also be present.

In 50% of patients with PCV, aquagenic pruritus occurs. In about two-thirds of patients, this is of limited severity and does not require treatment. The pruritus is typically triggered after a bath or shower, and the feeling induced may be itching, burning, or stinging. It usually lasts 30–60 min and is independent of the water temperature. Pruritus unassociated with water exposure may also occur. There is a concurrent elevation of blood and skin histamine. Pruritus is present in about 20% of patients at presentation and develops in the remaining 30% over the course of their disease. Patients with pruritus have lower mean corpuscular volumes and higher leukocyte counts. Some have suggested that iron deficiency plays a role in PCV-associated pruritus, so a ferritin level and a trial of iron therapy may be indicated. Platelet counts are no different between PCV patients who itch and those who do not.

The treatment of PCV-associated pruritus may be difficult. Initial therapy would include first- or second-generation H_1 antihistamines. Hydroxyzine was reported as the most effective antihistamine by a group of PCV patients. H_2 blockers can be added. Narrow-band UVB has been reported to be effective in 80% of patients. Topical therapy is of limited benefit, but paroxetine (Paxil), 20–60 mg/day, may be dramatically effective. Phlebotomy may be useful in patients with elevated hematocrits, and imatinib mesylate appears effective in many patients.

Abdel-Naser MB, et al: Cutaneous mononuclear cells and eosinophils are significantly increased after warm water challenge in pruritic areas of polycythemia vera. J Cutan Pathol 2007 Dec; 34(12):924–929.

Jones CM, et al: Phase II open label trial of imatinib in polycythemia rubra vera. Int J Hematol 2008 Dec; 88(5):489–494.

Bonus images for this chapter can be found online at

http://www.expertconsult.com

Diseases of the Skin Appendages

33

Diseases of the hair

Normal human hairs can be classified according to cyclical phases of growth. Anagen hairs are growing hairs, catagen hairs are those undergoing transition from the growing to the resting stage, and telogen hairs are resting hairs, which remain in the follicles for variable lengths of time before they fall out (teloptosis). The lag period between loss of the telogen hair and growth of a new anagen hair has been referred to as kenogen.

Anagen hairs grow for about 3 years (1000 days), with a range between 2 and 6 years. The follicular matrix cells grow, divide, and become keratinized to form growing hairs. As the matrix produces the hair shaft, it incorporates substances that may be useful in medical or forensic analysis. Catagen hairs are in a transitional phase, lasting 1 or 2 weeks, in which all growth activity ceases, with the eventual formation of the telogen "club" hair. Many apoptotic cells are present in the outer root sheath of the catagen hair as it involutes. Telogen club hairs are resting hairs, which continue in this state for 3–5 months (about 100 days) before they are released.

Among human hairs plucked from a normal scalp, 85–90% are anagen hairs and 10–15% are telogen hairs. Catagen hairs normally comprise less than 1% of scalp hairs. It has been estimated that the scalp normally contains about 100 000 hairs, and the average number of hairs shed daily is 100–150. The hair growth rate of terminal hairs is about 0.37 mm/day. Contrary to popular belief, neither shaving nor menstruation has any effect on hair growth rate. The average uncut scalp hair length is estimated to be 25–100 cm, although exceptional hairs may be as long as 170 cm (70 inches).

Human hair is also designated as lanugo, vellus, or terminal hair. Lanugo hair is the fine hair present on the body of the fetus. This is replaced by the vellus and terminal hairs. Vellus hairs are fine and usually light-colored, and have a narrow hair shaft thinner than the width of the inner root sheath. Terminal hairs are coarse, thick, and dark, except in blonds. Hair occurs on all skin surfaces except the palms, soles, labia minora, lips, nails, glans, and prepuce. Terminal hairs are commonly present on a man's face, chest, and abdomen, but vellus hairs usually predominate on these sites in women.

Causes of alopecia are generally divided into the broad categories of cicatricial and noncicatricial alopecia. The evaluation should take into account the patient's age and ethnicity. Examination of hair shafts can establish a diagnosis of trichodystrophy. Hair counts, hair pull, and hair pluck (trichogram) can establish the degree of hair shedding, the type of hair that is shed, and the anagen to telogen ratio. Biopsies can also determine anagen to telogen ratio, and provide information regarding the potential for regrowth, as well as providing a diagnosis. Biopsies are particularly valuable in the evaluation of cicatricial alopecia. Often, a correct diagnosis hinges on a synthesis of clinical, histologic, serologic, and immunofluorescent data.

Collado MS, et al: Recent advances in hair cell regeneration research. Curr Opin Otolaryngol Head Neck Surg 2008 Oct; 16(5):465–471.
Harries MJ, et al: Management of primary cicatricial alopecias: options for treatment. Br J Dermatol 2008 Jul; 159(1):1–22.
Piraccini BM, et al: Drug-induced hair disorders. Curr Drug Saf 2006 Aug; 1(3):301–305.
Randall VA: Androgens and hair growth. Dermatol Ther 2008 Sep–Oct; 21(5):314–328.
Shapiro J: Clinical practice. Hair loss in women. N Engl J Med 2007 Oct 18; 357(16):1620–1630.
Somani N, et al: Cicatricial alopecia: classification and histopathology. Dermatol Ther 2008 Jul–Aug; 21(4):221–237.
Unger W, et al: The surgical treatment of cicatricial alopecia. Dermatol Ther 2008 Jul–Aug; 21(4):295–311.

Noncicatricial alopecia

Alopecia areata

Clinical features

Alopecia areata (in French, pelade) is characterized by rapid and complete loss of hair in one or more round or oval patches, usually on the scalp, bearded area, eyebrows, eyelashes, and less commonly, on other hairy areas of the body. Often the patches are from 1 to 5 cm in diameter. A few resting hairs may be found within the patches. Early in the course there may be sparing of gray hair, and white hairs are rarely affected. Sudden whitening of hair may represent widespread alopecia areata in a patient with salt and pepper hair. In about 10% of cases of alopecia areata, especially in long-standing cases with extensive involvement, the nails develop uniform pits that may form transverse or longitudinal lines. Trachyonychia, onychomadesis, and red or spotted lunulae occur, but less commonly. Dermoscopic examination typically demonstrates diffuse, round, or polycyclic perifollicular yellow dots.

Complete loss of scalp hair is referred to as alopecia totalis, and complete loss of all hair as alopecia universalis. In most cases, hair loss is confined to the scalp and is patchy in distribution. Loss may occur confluently along the temporal and occipital scalp (ophiasis) (Fig. 33-1) or on the entire scalp except for this area (sisaipho). Rarely, alopecia areata may present in a diffuse pattern that may mimic pattern alopecia. Clues to the correct diagnosis include a history of periodic regrowth, nail pitting, and the presence of tapered fractures or exclamation point hairs (Fig. 33-2). Alopecia areata generally presents as an anagen effluvium, with an inflammatory insult to the hair matrix resulting in tapering of the hair shaft and in fracture of anagen hairs. As the hair miniaturizes or converts from anagen to telogen, the remaining lower portion of the hair rises above the level of the scalp, producing the exclamation point hair.

Alopecia areata is associated with a higher incidence than usual of atopic dermatitis, Down syndrome, lichen planus, and autoimmune diseases, such as systemic lupus erythematosus

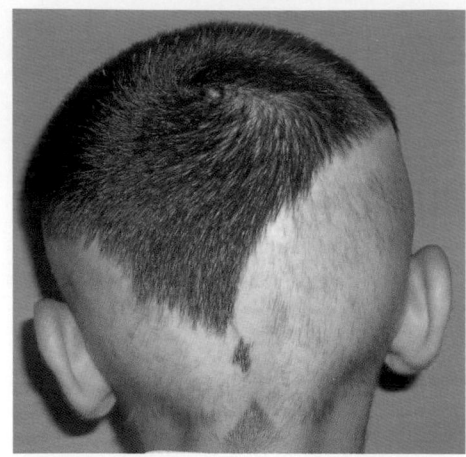

Fig. 33-1 Ophiasis. (Courtesy of Shyam Verma, MD)

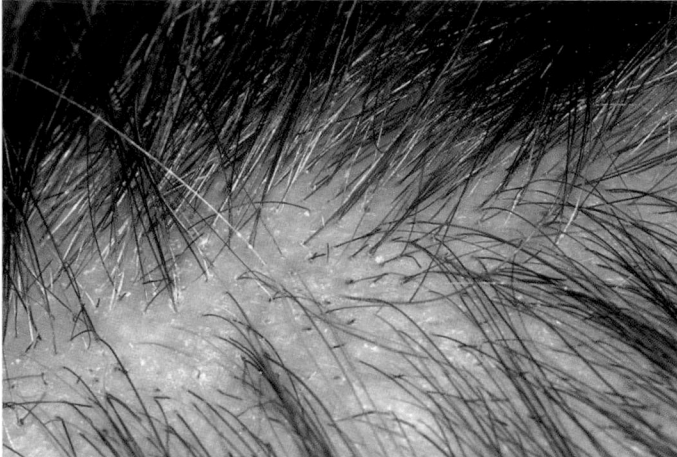

Fig. 33-2 Exclamation point hairs of alopecia areata.

(SLE), thyroiditis, diabetes mellitus, myasthenia gravis, and vitiligo. However, most cases of alopecia areata occur without associated disease, and routine screening for these disorders is of little value unless prompted by signs or symptoms.

Migratory poliosis of the scalp may represent a forme fruste of alopecia areata. Patients with this disorder present with migrating circular patches of white hair, but never lose hair. The histology resembles alopecia areata.

Etiologic factors

The preponderance of evidence supports an autoimmune etiology. Oligoclonal and autoreactive T lymphocytes are present in the peribulbar inflammatory infiltrate, and many patients respond to immune-modulating drugs. Affected alopecia areata scalp skin grafted on to nude mice with severe combined immunodeficiency demonstrates loss of infiltrating lymphocytes and hair growth. In this model, injecting T lymphocytes with scalp homogenate can reproduce the alopecia. Follicular melanocytes substitute for scalp homogenates to produce alopecia areata in this model, providing evidence that follicular melanocytes are the targets for activated T cells in this disease. This hypothesis is also supported by the observations that white hair is rarely affected and regrowing hair is often depigmented.

In early alopecia areata, the perifollicular and intrafollicular inflammatory infiltrate is composed of activated CD4+ and CD8+ T cells, together with macrophages and Langerhans cells. The early phase of hair loss appears to be mediated by

type 1 cytokines, including interleukin (IL)-2, interferon (IFN)-γ, and tumor necrosis factor (TNF)-α. The hair bulb normally represents an area of relative immune privilege during anagen, as evidenced by a very low level of expression of major histocompatibility complex (MHC) class Ia antigens. This immune privilege may prevent antigen recognition by autoreactive CD8+ T cells. Alopecia areata may be related to collapse of this immune privilege. IFN-γ-deficient mice are resistant to alopecia areata.

Onset of disease after Epstein–Barr virus infectious mononucleosis has been reported. Neuropeptides modify immune reactivity and may have a role in the disease. Heredity also plays a part. Overall, nearly 25% of patients have a positive family history; there are reports of twins with alopecia areata. Patients with "early onset, severe, familial clustering alopecia areata" have a unique and highly significant association with the HLA antigens DR4, DR11, and DQ7. The "later onset, milder severity, better prognostic" subsets of patients have a lower frequency of familial disease and do not share these HLA antigens. Familial alopecia areata associated with hereditary thrombocytopenia related to mutations in genes on chromosome 17 has been described. R620W (c.1858C>T, a variant of the protein tyrosine phosphatase nonreceptor 22 gene [PTPN22]) is associated with a variety of autoimmune disorders, including alopecia areata. It is associated with early onset of disease, widespread hair loss, and a positive family history.

Histology

In early disease there is a lymphoid infiltrate in the peribulbar area of anagen or early catagen follicles. Eosinophils may be present in the infiltrate, and lymphocyte-mediated damage to the bulb produces melanin pigment incontinence in the surrounding stroma. The hair structures enter an abnormal catagen phase, followed by telogen. During this phase, the presence of many catagen hairs and pigment casts within the follicular canal can cause histologic confusion with trichotillomania. In alopecia areata, the follicles eventually miniaturize, appearing as small dystrophic anagen hairs high in the dermis, often with a persistent lymphocytic peribulbar infiltrate. The presence of a peribulbar infiltrate helps to distinguish the miniaturized follicles of alopecia areata from those of androgenetic alopecia. Fibrous tract remnants beneath the miniaturized bulbs of alopecia areata may contain lymphoid cells, eosinophils, and melanin pigment. These findings are never present in trichotillomania or androgenetic alopecia. With time, the lymphocytes disappear, but focal eosinophils and pigment remain. Finally, only focal melanin pigment remains in the fibrous tract remnants. Hair fiber granulomas and scarring never occur. Every histologic feature of alopecia areata may be seen in syphilis. The presence of plasma cells is suggestive of syphilis, but plasma cells are also lacking in about one-third of syphilis biopsies. Plasma cells may be present in biopsies from any form of inflammatory alopecia if the biopsy is taken from the occipital scalp, as this site readily recruits plasma cells.

Differential diagnosis

The sharply circumscribed patch of alopecia with exclamation point hairs at the periphery and the absence of scarring are indicative of alopecia areata. Tinea capitis, androgenetic alopecia, early lupus erythematosus, syphilis, congenital triangular alopecia, alopecia neoplastica, and trichotillomania should be kept in mind when alopecia areata is considered. A biopsy will generally help to distinguish alopecia areata from these other entities, except syphilis, which may be indistinguishable. In endemic areas of southwest Asia, *Pheidole* ants shear hair shafts during the night, resulting in overnight loss of clumps of hair. The resulting round patches of hair loss closely mimic alopecia areata.

Treatment

The natural course of the hair loss is highly variable. Some patches will regrow in a few weeks without any treatment. Various treatments can induce growth, but the inherent risks and cost must be weighed against the benefit of earlier regrowth. In his series of 63 consecutive responders to a follow-up questionnaire, Arnold found that, after reassurance only, hair had regrown in all but four patients after 1 year and in all but one after 2 years. The great majority had recovered in 3 months after their only office visit. Therefore, anecdotal reports of success must be interpreted carefully in the light of the high rate of spontaneous recovery.

Intralesional injections of corticosteroid suspensions are the treatment of choice for localized, cosmetically conspicuous patches, such as those occurring in the frontal hairline or involving an eyebrow. Injections of triamcinolone, 2–10 mg/mL, are typically given intradermally or in the superficial subcutaneous tissue. Large volumes and higher concentrations of triamcinolone present a greater risk of atrophy. Injection under significant pressure or with a small-bore syringe increases the likelihood of retinal artery embolization. High-strength topical steroids may be used as a safer first-line therapy, but are less reliable than injections. Several investigators have reported the use of pulsed oral corticosteroids in rapidly progressing or widespread disease. However, long-term treatment is frequently needed to maintain growth, and the attendant risks should be carefully weighed against the benefits. In a study of 66 patients aged 9–60 years, monthly methylprednisolone was administered at a dose of 500 mg/day during 3 days or 5 mg/kg twice a day over 3 days in children. More than 60% of patients with widespread patchy alopecia responded. Half of the patients with alopecia totalis had a good response, while a quarter of those with universal alopecia responded. Patients with ophiasic alopecia areata did not respond.

Induction of contact sensitivity to squaric acid dibutyl ester, dinitrochlorobenzene, and diphencyprone can be useful in refractory cases. In mice, contact immunotherapy is associated with a decrease in cutaneous activated T cells, a reduction in intrafollicular CD8+ lymphocytes, and reduced expression of CD44v3+ and CD44v10+ cells. These results suggest that blockade of leukocyte trafficking and extravasation is an important mechanism of action. Topical or oral methoxsalen and ultraviolet A (PUVA) therapy is an option for refractory or widespread lesions. Short-contact topical anthralin 1% cream (applied for 15–20 min and then shampooed off) can be of benefit. Topical minoxidil may be combined with other treatments or utilized as a single agent. Preliminary results suggest methotrexate and sulfasalazine may be beneficial. Biologics have produced mixed, and largely disappointing, results, and alopecia areata has developed during biologic therapy for other conditions. The 308 nm xenon chloride excimer laser (300–2300 mJ/cm^2/session) has been reported to produce regrowth after 11 and 12 sessions over a 9–11-week period. Periocular pigmentation is associated with use of travoprost for eyelash disease. Therapeutic results are mixed.

Alopecia areata can cause tremendous psychological stress. Education about the disease process, cosmetically acceptable alternatives (especially information about wigs), and research into innovative therapies should all be made available to the patient. In addition to the information conveyed by the dermatologist, an excellent resource is the National Alopecia Areata Foundation (NAAF): E-mail: info@naaf.org, website: www.naaf.org.

Prognosis

The tendency is for spontaneous recovery in patients who are postpubertal at onset. At first, the regrowing hairs are downy and light in color; later, they are replaced by stronger and darker hair with full growth. Predictors of a poor prognosis are the presence of atopic dermatitis, childhood onset, widespread involvement, ophiasis, duration of longer than 5 years, and onychodystrophy. Acute diffuse and total alopecia is a newly defined subtype of alopecia areata that occurs in young adults and has a good prognosis.

Ahmed AM, et al: Familial alopecia areata and chronic thrombocytopenia. J Am Acad Dermatol 2008 May; 58(5 Suppl 1):S75–77.

Avgerinou G, et al: Alopecia areata: topical immunotherapy treatment with diphencyprone. J Eur Acad Dermatol Venereol 2008 Mar; 22(3):320–323.

Bakar O, et al: Is there a role for sulfasalazine in the treatment of alopecia areata? J Am Acad Dermatol 2007 Oct; 57(4):703–706.

Betz RC, et al: The R620W polymorphism in PTPN22 confers general susceptibility for the development of alopecia areata. Br J Dermatol 2008 Feb; 158(2):389–391.

Feletti F, et al: Periocular pigmentation associated with use of travoprost for the treatment of alopecia areata of the eyelashes. J Eur Acad Dermatol Venereol 2007 Mar; 21(3):421–423.

Freyschmidt-Paul P, et al: Interferon-gamma-deficient mice are resistant to the development of alopecia areata. Br J Dermatol 2006 Sep; 155(3):515–521.

Garcia Bartels N, et al: Development of alopecia areata universalis in a patient receiving adalimumab. Arch Dermatol 2006 Dec; 142(12):1654–1655.

Hubiche T, et al: Poor long term outcome of severe alopecia areata in children treated with high dose pulse corticosteroid therapy. Br J Dermatol 2008 May; 158(5):1136–1137.

Joly P: The use of methotrexate alone or in combination with low doses of oral corticosteroids in the treatment of alopecia totalis or universalis. J Am Acad Dermatol 2006 Oct; 55(4):632–636.

Kolde G, et al: Successful treatment of alopecia areata with efalizumab. J Eur Acad Dermatol Venereol 2008 Dec; 22(12):1519–1520.

Lew BL, et al: Acute diffuse and total alopecia: a new subtype of alopecia areata with a favorable prognosis. J Am Acad Dermatol 2009 Jan; 60(1):85–93.

Manolache L, et al: Alopecia areata and relationship with stressful events in children. J Eur Acad Dermatol Venereol 2009 Jan; 23(1):107–109.

McMichael AJ, et al: Alopecia in the United States: outpatient utilization and common prescribing patterns. J Am Acad Dermatol 2007 Aug; 57(2 Suppl):S49–51.

Misery L, et al: Treatment of alopecia areata with sulfasalazine. J Eur Acad Dermatol Venereol 2007 Apr; 21(4):547–548.

Price VH, et al: Subcutaneous efalizumab is not effective in the treatment of alopecia areata. J Am Acad Dermatol 2008 Mar; 58(3):395–402.

Rodriguez TA, et al: Onset of alopecia areata after Epstein-Barr virus infectious mononucleosis. J Am Acad Dermatol 2008 Jul; 59(1):137–139.

Tosti A, et al: Alopecia areata during treatment with biologic agents. Arch Dermatol 2006 Dec; 142(12):1653–1654.

Tosti A, et al: The role of scalp dermoscopy in the diagnosis of alopecia areata incognita. J Am Acad Dermatol 2008 Jul; 59(1):64–67.

Telogen effluvium

Telogen effluvium presents with excessive shedding of normal telogen club hairs. This excessive shedding of telogen hairs has several possible mechanisms. It most commonly occurs 3–5 months after the premature conversion of many anagen hairs to telogen hairs induced by surgery, parturition, fever, drugs, dieting, or traction. Local patches of early telogen conversion may be induced by papulosquamous diseases affecting the scalp. Alternatively, follicles may remain in prolonged anagen rather than normally cycling into telogen. This occurs during pregnancy. On delivery, many follicles are then released simultaneously into telogen, and shedding occurs 3–5 months later. Prolongation of telogen also occurs during pregnancy, and results in an initial wave of hair loss soon after delivery or heralding early termination of a pregnancy. Shortening of the anagen phase occurs in pattern (androgenetic) alopecia, and results in telogen effluvium. Normally, anagen lasts about 1000 days and telogen about 100 days. This results in a 10:1 ratio of anagen to telogen hairs in the scalp. With progression of pattern alopecia, anagen shortens, and the ratio of anagen to telogen hairs falls. A greater proportion of hairs is in telogen at any one time, resulting in a chronic increase in telogen shed. Administration of topical minoxidil may produce a telogen effluvium by premature termination of telogen necessary to initiate anagen in responding follicles. This causes early telogen release and a brief telogen effluvium.

Whatever the cause of the telogen loss, the hair is lost "at the root." Each hair will have a visible depigmented club-shaped bulb and will lack a sheath (Fig. 33-3). In most cases, loss is diffuse. Patients commonly have more than one mechanism for telogen hair loss. Patchy or diffuse telogen may be associated with papulosquamous diseases of the scalp. Perceptible thinning of the hair is more common in patients with pre-existing pattern alopecia. In patients with pattern alopecia, shortening of the hair cycle results in increased telogen shed. Superimposed papulosquamous disease, iron deficiency, or thyroid disease can result in even more telogen shed and accentuates the pattern loss.

Trichodynia is a common symptom in patients with telogen effluvium, as it is in pattern hair loss. Trichodynia often coexists with signs of depression, obsessive personality disorder, and anxiety.

Telogen shed may be estimated by the pull test: grasping 40 hairs firmly between thumb and forefinger, followed by a slow pull that causes minimal discomfort to the patient. A count of more than 4–6 club hairs is abnormal, but the result is influenced by recent shampooing (a count of 2–3 hairs being abnormal in a freshly shampooed scalp), combing, and the phase of telogen effluvium (whether it is resolving or entering a chronic phase). The clip test may also be useful; 25–30 hairs are cut just above the scalp surface and mounted. Indeterminate and telogen hairs are short and of small diameter. Many hairs of this type may be present in telogen effluvium or pattern alopecia. Trichogram evaluation (50 hairs plucked with a Kelly clamp with rubber drains over the teeth) can also provide information on the anagen to telogen ratio.

Age, sex, race, and genetic factors influence the normal average daily hair loss in an individual. A full head of hair numbers about 100 000; of these, approximately 100–150 are lost daily. In telogen effluvium, estimates of loss vary from 150 to more than 400. Patients may be instructed to collect and count the hair daily; however, they should make sure they collect all small hairs and those that come out in washing and in the bed, as well as those present on the comb or brush. When the pull test is positive, hair shed counts are not needed. An alternative is to collect all hairs lost during a 1 min combing session. For this technique, developed by Dr Jeffrey Miller, the patient combs for 1 min prior to shampooing on 3 consecutive days. The patient is instructed to comb from the vertex to the anterior hairline. The normal range of lost hairs with this technique is 10–15. Loss of more than 50 is common in telogen effluvium. Serial 1 min hair counts can be performed to monitor progress.

Telogen effluvium is commonly related to protein or other nutrient deprivation (Fig. 33-4). Assessment of dietary habits and determination of iron saturation and ferritin are the simplest ways to determine nutritional status. Iron replacement is advisable if saturation or ferritin is low, but in one study iron replacement alone did not result in resolution of telogen effluvium. Iron may merely serve as a marker for overall nutritional status. Patients with evidence of deficiency should be given supplements to correct the identified deficiency and encouraged to eat a varied diet. Sources of blood loss, such as menstrual bleeding and gastrointestinal blood loss, should be investigated. Hypothyroidism, allergic contact dermatitis to hair dyes, and renal dialysis with secondary hypervitaminosis A may also be associated with telogen effluvium. Drug-induced telogen effluvium has been noted with the use of aminosalicylic acid, amphetamines, bromocriptine, captopril, carbamazepine, cimetidine, coumarin, danazol, enalapril, etretinate, levodopa, lithium carbonate, metoprolol, metyrapone, pramipexole, propranolol, pyridostigmine, and trimethadione. Postnatal telogen effluvium of infants may occur between birth and the first 4 months of age. Usually, regrowth occurs by 6 months of age. Telogen counts by Kligman in six

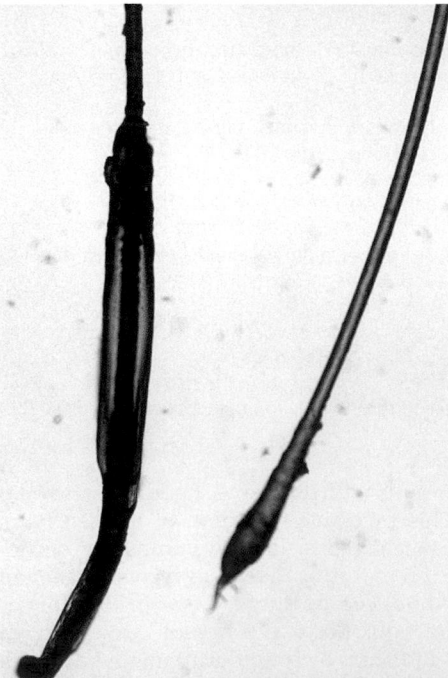

Fig. 33-3 Anagen and telogen hair (anagen hair has a pigmented bulb and is surrounded by a gelatinous root sheath; telogen hair has a nonpigmented bulb and lacks a root sheath).

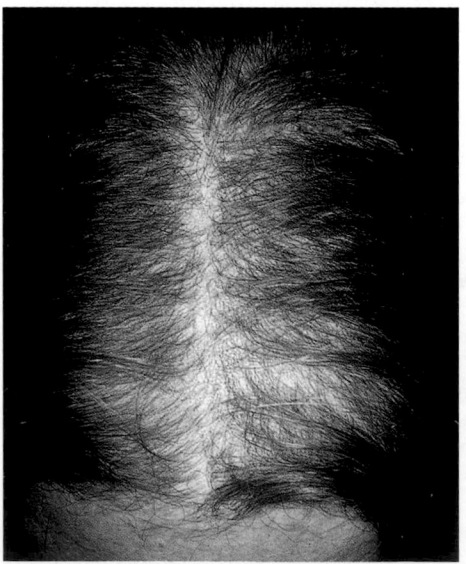

Fig. 33-4 Telogen effluvium secondary to crash dieting.

infants varied from 64% to 87%. He also found a tendency for the alopecia to occur in the male-pattern distribution. Idiopathic chronic telogen effluvium has been described by Whiting in a group of 355 patients (346 women and 9 men) with diffuse generalized thinning of scalp hair. Most were 30–60 years old, and their hair loss started abruptly, with increased shedding and thinning. There was a fluctuating course and diffuse thinning of the hair all over the scalp, accompanied by bitemporal recession. He found high telogen counts on horizontal sections of scalp biopsies and considers these patients to have a chronic form of telogen effluvium. This chronic form may respond to 5% minoxidil solution.

If a 4 mm punch biopsy is performed, 25–50 hairs are normally present for inspection in transverse (horizontal) sections. If more than 12–15% of terminal follicles are in telogen, this indicates a significant shift from anagen to telogen. Pattern (androgenetic alopecia) demonstrates miniaturization, variable hair shaft diameter, and an increased proportion of telogen hairs. Traction alopecia and trichotillosis (trichotillomania) result in an increased number of catagen and telogen hairs. Pigment casts, empty anagen follicles, trichomalacia, and catagen hairs help distinguish these entities from simple telogen effluvium.

No specific therapy is required for most patients with telogen effluvium. In the majority of cases the hair loss will stop spontaneously within a few months and the hair will regrow. Drug-induced telogen effluvium responds to discontinuation of the offending agent. The prognosis is good if a specific event can be pinpointed as a probable cause. Papulosquamous scalp disorders may precipitate telogen hair loss and should be addressed. Iron and thyroid status should be determined if the course is prolonged or if history or physical examination suggests an abnormality. Patients should be encouraged to eat a balanced diet. In a mouse model, sonic stress can produce catagen. This model may be useful in the study of agents for the treatment of telogen effluvium.

Bedocs LA, et al: Adolescent hair loss. Curr Opin Pediatr 2008 Aug; 20(4):431–435.

Katz KA, et al: Telogen effluvium associated with the dopamine agonist pramipexole in a 55-year-old woman with Parkinson's disease. J Am Acad Dermatol 2006 Nov; 55(5 Suppl):S103–104.

Millikan L: Hirsutism, postpartum telogen effluvium, and male pattern alopecia. J Cosmet Dermatol 2006 Mar; 5(1):81–86.

Piraccini BM, et al: Drug-induced hair disorders. Curr Drug Saf 2006 Aug; 1(3):301–305.

Ramos-e-Silva M, et al: Hair, nail, and pigment changes in major systemic disease. Clin Dermatol 2008 May–Jun; 26(3):296–305.

Anagen effluvium

Anagen effluvium usually results from hair shaft fracture. It is frequently seen following the administration of cancer chemotherapeutic agents, such as the antimetabolites, alkylating agents, and mitotic inhibitors. These agents result in temporary shutdown of the hair matrix with resultant tapering of the shaft (Pohl–Pinkus constrictions). Trichograms reveal tapered fractures. Only anagen hairs are affected. The 10% of scalp hairs in telogen have no matrix and are unaffected. The loss tends to be diffuse but not complete. It may resemble pattern alopecia. Severe loss is frequently seen with doxorubicin, the nitrosureas, and cyclophosphamide. When high doses are given, loss of anagen hairs becomes most apparent clinically in 1–2 months. The hair shafts are abruptly narrowed at the time of maximum drug effect, and when the very thin portion reaches the surface, the hair shafts all break at about the same time. With cessation of drug therapy, the follicle resumes its normal activity within a few weeks; the process is entirely reversible. It is apparent that mitotic inhibition merely stops the reproduction of matrix cells but does not perma-

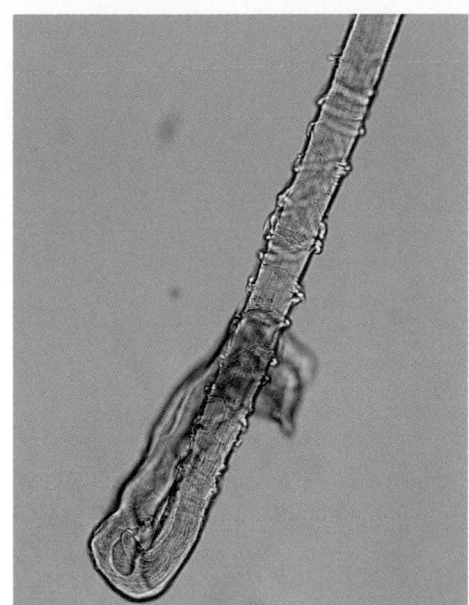

Fig. 33-5 Loose anagen hair with "rumpled sock" cuticle.

nently destroy the hair. A pressure cuff applied around the scalp during chemotherapy and scalp hypothermia have been reported to prevent such anagen arrest, but as the scalp may be a site of metastasis, it may be better not to spare the scalp from the effects of chemotherapy. Topical minoxidil has been shown to shorten the period of baldness by an average of 50 days.

In addition to the cytotoxic chemotherapeutic agents, various agents, such as isoniazid INH, thallium, and boron may induce anagen effluvium. Anagen effluvium with tapered fractures also occurs in alopecia areata and syphilis. In these diseases, an inflammatory insult to the hair bulb results in Pohl–Pinkus constrictions and tapered fracture.

Anagen loss may also occur at the root. Loose anagen syndrome, described by Price in 1989, is a disorder in which anagen hairs may be pulled from the scalp with little effort. It occurs mostly in blond girls and usually improves with age. The syndrome appears to be related to a defect in the hair cuticle. Instead of anchoring the hair firmly, the cuticle simply folds back like a rumpled sock (Fig. 33-5), allowing the hair shaft to be extracted. Woolly hair can be associated with loose anagen hair syndrome. A keratin mutation, E337K in K6HF, was identified in three of nine families studied. Colobomas have also been associated with loose anagen hair.

Anagen hairs may be easily extracted from active areas of lupus erythematosus and lichen planopilaris. They commonly lack the root sheath that normally surrounds a plucked anagen hair (Fig. 33-6). Anagen effluvium has also been described in lesions of pemphigus.

Trüeb RM: Chemotherapy-induced anagen effluvium: diffuse or patterned? Dermatology 2007; 215(1):1–2.

Yun SJ, et al: Hair loss pattern due to chemotherapy-induced anagen effluvium: a cross-sectional observation. Dermatology 2007; 215(1):36–40.

Pattern alopecia (androgenetic alopecia)

Male-pattern baldness

Male-pattern alopecia or male-pattern androgenetic alopecia (common baldness) shows itself during the teens, twenties, or early thirties with gradual loss of hair, chiefly from the vertex and frontotemporal regions. The process may begin at any time after puberty, and the presence of "whisker" or kinky hair may be the first sign of impending male-pattern alopecia. The anterior hairline recedes on each side, in the

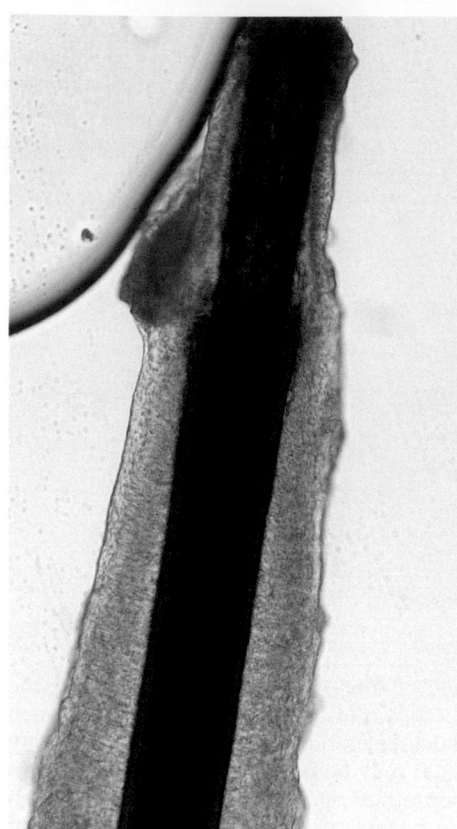

Fig. 33-6 Stain for citrulline demonstrates the inner root sheath (red) surrounded by an outer root in a plucked anagen hair from a normal scalp.

Geheimratswinkeln ("professor angles"), so that the forehead becomes high. Eventually, the entire top of the scalp may become devoid of hair. Several patterns of this type of hair loss occur, but the most frequent is the biparietal recession with loss of hair on the vertex. The rate of hair loss varies among individuals. Sudden hair loss may occur in the twenties and then proceed relentlessly, though very slowly, for a number of years. The follicles produce finer and lighter hairs with each hair cycle until terminal hairs are eventually replaced by vellus hairs. During evolution of the process, hair shafts vary significantly in diameter. The parietal and occipital areas are usually spared permanently from this process of progressive miniaturization.

Early-onset male-pattern alopecia is related to the androgen receptor gene. There is no doubt that inherited factors and the effect of androgens such as dihydrotestosterone on the hair follicle are important. Arguments for regarding the inheritance as polygenic include the high prevalence, gaussian curve of distribution in the population, increased risk with number of affected relatives, increased risk in relatives of severely affected women compared with mildly affected, and greater import of an affected mother than an affected father. The possibility that the early onset (before the age of 30) and later onset (after the age of 50) forms may be inherited separately by single genes is also hypothesized.

Male-pattern alopecia is dependent on adequate androgen stimulation and appears to be related to the androgen receptor gene. Eunuchs do not develop baldness if they are castrated before or during adolescence. If they are given androgen therapy, baldness may develop. The 5-α reduction of testosterone is increased in the scalp of balding individuals, yielding increased dihydrotestosterone. Androgen-inducible transforming growth factor (TGF)-β1 derived from dermal papilla

cells appears to mediate hair growth suppression. In congenital 5-α-reductase deficiency, the type 2 isoenzyme is lacking and baldness does not occur. Pattern alopecia does occur in males with X-linked ichthyosis, indicating that steroid sulfatase is not critical for the production of alopecia.

Progressive shortening of the anagen phase of hair growth is noted as the hair shaft diameter decreases, so hairs are not only narrowing, but are becoming shorter. A higher proportion of telogen hairs in the affected area results in greater telogen shed. There may also be an increase in the duration of the lag phase between telogen and anagen (the kenogen lag phase).

Histologically, a decrease in anagen and increase in telogen follicles is present. Follicular miniaturization and variability in shaft diameter are noted. These features are particularly evident in transverse sections. Below the level of the miniaturized or telogen follicle, a vascular or fibromucinous fibrous tract remnant is present. These tracts appear numerous in cross-section. Many mast cells may be noted in the fibrous tract remnant, but inflammatory cells are absent. Sebaceous glands may be enlarged, and hair thinning may be associated with solar elastosis. Sparse lymphoid inflammation with spongiosis may be noted at the level of the follicular infundibulum. This may represent associated seborrheic folliculitis. A sparse lymphoid infiltrate may also be noted at the level of the hair bulge.

Miniaturized human hair follicles grafted on to immunodeficient mice can quickly regenerate and grow as well as or better than terminal follicles from the same individual. This suggests that even advanced pattern alopecia may be reversible. Unfortunately, available pharmacologic interventions produce little effect in advanced pattern alopecia.

Minoxidil, an oral hypotensive drug that causes hypertrichosis when given systemically, is available as topical solutions (Rogaine). Minoxidil promotes the survival of dermal papilla cells, prolongs anagen phase, and results in enlargement of shaft diameter. Clinically, apparent success is best in early cases (less than 10 years) of limited extent (bald area of less than 10 cm diameter on the vertex) in whom pretreatment hair density is above 20 hairs/cm². Minoxidil is available without a prescription as a 2% or a 5% solution. With the 2% solution, 26% of men studied showed moderate to dense regrowth, while 33% showed minimal regrowth after 4 months. Studies show a 45% increase in hair weight with the 5% solution compared to the 2% solution. In those who respond, regrowth can occur as early as 2 months after the first application. Those who respond must continue to use minoxidil indefinitely to maintain a response.

Finasteride, a type 2 5-α-reductase inhibitor, given as a 1 mg tablet daily, is effective in preventing further hair loss and in increasing the hair counts to the point of cosmetically appreciable results in men aged 18–41 with mild to moderate hair loss at the vertex, in the anterior midscalp, and in the frontal region. It has been shown to stop hair loss in up to 90% of men for at least 5 years. Approximately 65% of men demonstrate hair regrowth. As with monoxidil, continued use of the product is required to sustain benefits. Hair patterning on the temples is not improved. It has been shown to lower dihydrotestosterone in the scalp and the serum of treated patients. Hair growth will be evident only after 6 months or more on the drug. If no effect is seen after 12 months, further treatment is unlikely to be of benefit. In one study, regimens that included finasteride were more effective than minoxidil alone, and therapeutic efficacy was enhanced by combining the two drugs. Short-term side effects related to finasteride are infrequent; however, the need to take this medication indefinitely suggests that study of long-term side-effect profiles is critical. A prostate cancer prevention trial with a different dosage form of the same drug showed a decrease in the incidence of cancer. However, those cancers that did occur in the treatment group had a higher average Gleason score. This could be because only lower-grade cancers were prevented. Dutasteride blocks both type 1 and type 2 5-α-reductase, and is effective in the treatment of male-pattern hair loss. Other treatments that show some promise in preliminary studies include fluridil (a topical antiandrogen that suppresses the human androgen receptor) and hormone-enriched topical cell culture medium. Hair transplantation using micrografts of hair follicles from the occipital area to the anterior scalp may satisfactorily recreate hairlines and give excellent cosmetic results.

Female-pattern alopecia (androgenetic alopecia in women)

Women generally have diffuse hair loss throughout the apical scalp with the part wider anteriorly. There is typically sparing of the frontal hairline, although a subset of women exhibits a "male" pattern of temporal recession. Although maintenance of the frontal hairline is the rule in women, a progressive decrease in hair density from the vertex to the front of the scalp does occur. The midline part is an important clinical clue, revealing a "Christmas tree pattern" of hair loss with the part tapering from the anterior to posterior scalp. The BASP classification has been suggested as a single hair loss classification scheme for use in men and women. It is based on basic (BA) types representing the shape of the anterior hairline, and specific (SP) types representing the density of hair on distinct areas (frontal and vertex). This is important because patients of either sex may demonstrate male or female patterns of alopecia. Phototrichograms and measurement of shaft diameter can be used to assess female-pattern alopecia. The same basic changes—reduced hair density and diameter, and diminished anagen and increased telogen hair—occur in women as in men. Sebaceous gland hyperplasia may be present, but is less common than in men. Transverse histologic sections demonstrate variability in the size of hair follicles (anisotrichosis).

The cause is now believed to be a genetic predisposition with an excessive response to androgens. Both women and men with pattern alopecia have higher levels of 5-α-reductase and androgen receptor in frontal hair follicles compared to the levels in occipital follicles. There is also evidence suggesting a hierarchy of androgen sensitivity within follicular units. Follicular miniaturization relates to unrepaired DNA damage and a reduced proliferation rate of matrix keratinocytes. Smoking may be an independent risk factor. Most women with pattern alopecia have normal menses and fertility. If other evidence of androgen excess is present, such as hirsutism, menstrual irregularities, or acne, or if the onset is sudden, evaluation as outlined for hirsutism (see below) should be performed. Men with spinal and bulbar muscular atrophy (Kennedy disease), an X-linked neurodegenerative disease caused by an expansion of a polymorphic tandem CAG repeat within the androgen receptor gene, have a decreased incidence of pattern alopecia.

Topical minoxidil is of benefit. Although some data suggest that 5% minoxidil may be of greater benefit than 2% minoxidil, the evidence is mixed. Given the higher cost of 5% minoxidil, the 2% formulation may be the best choice for many women. Oral antiandrogens, including spironolactone and cyproterone acetate, have been used to treat androgenetic alopecia in women. In one study, cyproterone acetate was more effective than minoxidil when there were other signs of hyperandrogenism, hyperseborrhea, and menstrual abnormalities, and when the body mass index was high. When these other factors were absent, minoxidil was the more effective treatment.

Treatment with finasteride is of no benefit for most women, although the subset with temporal recession may show some benefit. Finasteride treatment is contraindicated in women who may become pregnant. Hair transplantation, wigs, or interwoven hair may give satisfactory cosmetic results. In a pilot study, topical melatonin appeared to prolong anagen phase and may prove to be of some benefit. In some women, telogen effluvium may produce worsening of pre-existing pattern alopecia. Reversible causes of telogen effluvium, such as seborrheic dermatitis, nutrient deficiency, and thyroid disease, should be addressed.

Camacho FM, et al: Value of hormonal levels in patients with male androgenetic alopecia treated with finasteride: better response in patients under 26 years old. Br J Dermatol 2008 May; 158(5): 1121–1124.

Carlson JA, et al: Female-patterned alopecia in teenage brothers with unusual histologic features. J Cutan Pathol 2006 Nov; 33(11):741–748.

El-Domyati M, et al: Proliferation, DNA repair and apoptosis in androgenetic alopecia. J Eur Acad Dermatol Venereol 2009 Jan; 23(1):7–12.

Hong JB, et al: A woman with iatrogenic androgenetic alopecia responding to finasteride. Br J Dermatol 2007 Apr; 156(4):754–755.

Lee WS, et al: A new classification of pattern hair loss that is universal for men and women: basic and specific (BASP) classification. J Am Acad Dermatol 2007 Jul; 57(1):37–46.

Olsen EA, et al: The importance of dual 5alpha-reductase inhibition in the treatment of male pattern hair loss: results of a randomized placebo-controlled study of dutasteride versus finasteride. J Am Acad Dermatol 2006 Dec; 55(6):1014–1023.

Rogers NE, et al: Medical treatments for male and female pattern hair loss. J Am Acad Dermatol 2008 Oct; 59(4):547–566.

Sewell LD, et al: "Anisotrichosis": a novel term to describe pattern alopecia. J Am Acad Dermatol 2007 May; 56(5):856.

Sinclair R, et al: Men with Kennedy disease have a reduced risk of androgenetic alopecia. Br J Dermatol 2007 Aug; 157(2):290–294.

Su LH, et al: Association of androgenetic alopecia with smoking and its prevalence among Asian men: a community-based survey. Arch Dermatol 2007 Nov; 143(11):1401–1406.

Yazdabadi A, et al: The Ludwig pattern of androgenetic alopecia is due to a hierarchy of androgen sensitivity within follicular units that leads to selective miniaturization and a reduction in the number of terminal hairs per follicular unit. Br J Dermatol 2008 Dec; 159(6):1300–1302.

Trichotillomania (trichotillosis)

Trichotillomania is the compulsive practice of plucking hair from the scalp, brows or eyelashes. Typical areas are irregular patches of alopecia that contain hairs of varying length. The scalp has a rough texture, resulting from the short remnants of broken-off hairs. Trichotillomania is seen mostly in girls under the age of 10, but boys, or adults of either sex, may engage in the practice also. Some patients relate exquisite pain localized to a follicle that can only be relieved by plucking the hair.

When speaking with a patient with characteristic areas of alopecia, it has been suggested that it be asked not if but rather how removal of the hair is done. If this fails to uncover a history of hair pulling, shaving a 3 cm² area in the involved part of the scalp will result in hairs too short for plucking, and normal regrowth in the "skin window" within 3 weeks. Finally, a biopsy, especially if cut horizontally, may demonstrate empty anagen follicles, catagen hairs, pigment casts within the infundibulum, trichomalacia, and hemorrhage. Alopecia areata shares many of these histologic features, and care must be taken to search for the presence of peribulbar lymphocytes or inflammatory cells within the fibrous tract remnants.

Trichotillomania is usually a manifestation of an obsessive–compulsive disorder, but may also be associated with depression or anxiety. It may be associated with compulsive swallowing of the plucked hairs (trichophagia), and may result in formation of a gastric bezoar. Behavior modification, psychotherapy, and appropriate psychopharmacologic medication (such as serotonin-reuptake inhibitors) may be helpful. Valproic acid, quetiapine and naltrexone have been reported as effective in some patients.

Adewuya EC, et al: Trichotillomania: a case of response to valproic acid. J Child Adolesc Psychopharmacol 2008 Oct; 18(5):533–536.

Crescente JA Jr, et al: Quetiapine for the treatment of trichotillomania. Rev Bras Psiquiatr 2008 Dec; 30(4):402.

De Sousa A: An open-label pilot study of naltrexone in childhood-onset trichotillomania. J Child Adolesc Psychopharmacol 2008 Feb; 18(1):30–33.

Other forms of noncicatricial alopecia

Alopecia syphilitica may have a typical moth-eaten appearance on the occipital scalp (Fig. 33-7), may show a generalized thinning of the hair, or may resemble alopecia areata. Other areas such as the eyebrows, eyelashes, and body hair may be involved. The alopecia may be the first sign of syphilis.

Follicular mucinosis (alopecia mucinosa) most commonly occurs on the scalp or beard area and manifests as a boggy red plaque or hypopigmented patch with hair loss. Comedone-like lesions may exude mucin when expressed. Biopsy demonstrates deposition of mucin in the outer root sheath and sebaceous glands. The mucin stains as hyaluronic acid, rather than epithelial sialomucin. Primary cases (unassociated with underlying disease) usually occur as localized lesions of the head or neck. Young people are primarily affected. The secondary type is associated with mycosis fungoides-type cutaneous T-cell lymphoma or a chronic inflammatory skin disease. Lesions associated with mycosis fungoides are generally widespread and chronic, and occur in older patients.

Vascular or neurologic alopecia, most often of the lower extremities, may be seen in diabetes mellitus or atherosclerosis. In meralgia paresthetica there may be alopecia of the anesthetic area of the outer thigh.

Endocrinologic alopecia may occur in various endocrinologic disorders. In hypothyroidism the hair becomes coarse, dry, brittle, and sparse. The proportion of telogen hairs has been shown to be 3–7 times higher than the normal 10%. In hyperthyroidism the hair becomes extremely fine and sparse. Oral contraceptives have been implicated in some instances of androgenetic alopecia. It develops in predisposed women who are usually taking androgenic progestogens. It is advisable to discontinue the androgen-dominant pill and substitute an estrogen-dominant oral contraceptive. Some women develop telogen effluvium 2–4 months after discontinuing anovulatory agents, which is analogous to postpartum alopecia.

Congenital alopecia occurs either as total or partial loss of hair, or a lack of initial growth, accompanied usually by other ectodermal defects of the nails, teeth, and bone. The hair is light and sparse, and grows slowly. Congenital triangular alopecia (Fig. 33-8) and aplasia cutis congenita are examples of congenital localized absence of hair, while hidrotic ectodermal dysplasia is an example of a diffuse abnormality of hair associated with dental and nail changes.

Lipedematous alopecia consists of thickening of the scalp that gives the impression of thick cotton batting. The hair may be normal or shortened and sparse. Biopsy shows an increase in thickness of the subcutaneous fat and variable lymphoid inflammation. This disease appears to affect black persons primarily.

González-Guerra E, et al: Lipedematous alopecia: an uncommon clinicopathologic variant of nonscarring but permanent alopecia. Int J Dermatol 2008 Jun; 47(6):605–609.

Cicatricial alopecia

Cicatricial alopecia appears as areas of hair loss with absence of follicular ostia (Fig. 33-9). Acute lesions may appear as erythematous plaques, perifollicular papules, keratotic follicular

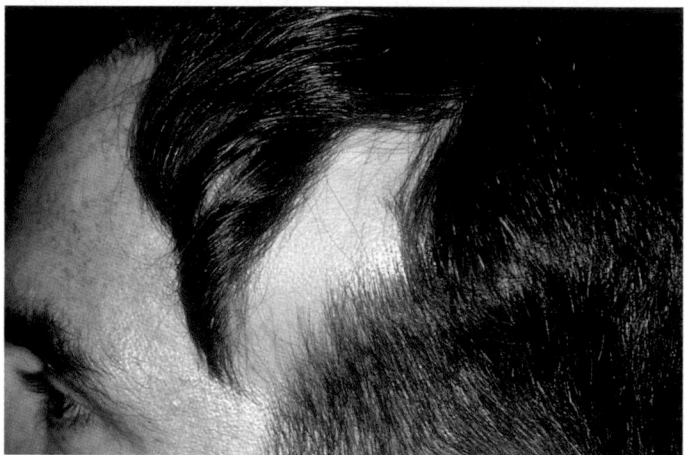

Fig. 33-8 Triangular alopecia. (Courtesy of Brooke Army Medical Center Teaching File)

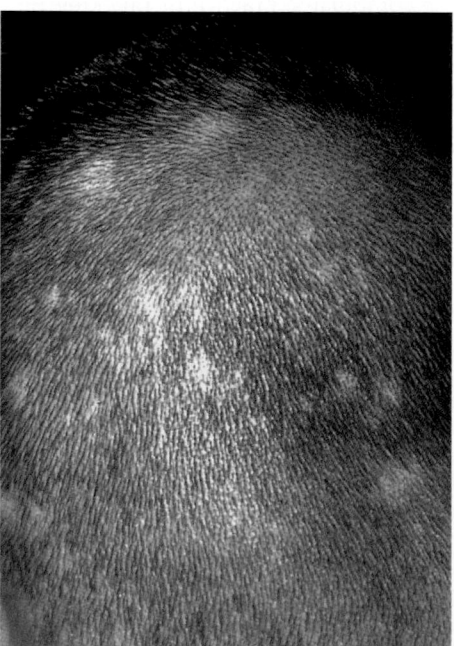

Fig. 33-7 Syphilitic alopecia. (Courtesy of Brooke Army Medical Center Teaching File)

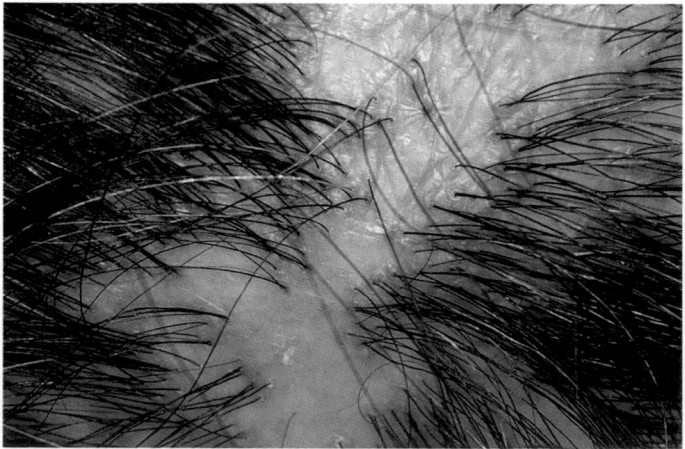

Fig. 33-9 Loss of follicular ostia in scarring alopecia.

spines, or pustules. Deep inflammatory lesions may be boggy or may resemble noncicatricial areata clinically. The inflammatory nature of the lesion may only be evident on biopsy.

Discoid lupus erythematosus, lichen planopilaris, sarcoidosis, and folliculitis decalvans are the most common inflammatory causes of cicatricial alopecia. Chronic bacterial and fungal infections may produce inflammatory alopecia that mimics primary scarring alopecia. For example, fungal folliculitis may mimic lupus erythematosus.

Biopsy can confirm the diagnosis and provide prognostic information regarding the potential for new growth. A 4 mm punch biopsy will provide the pathologist with an adequate specimen. Smaller specimens are of limited value. The punch should be placed parallel to the direction of hair growth to avoid transecting follicles, and the punch should be advanced to the deep subcutaneous fat. The biopsy site will typically bleed profusely, but a 4 mm-wide strip of gel foam advanced into the defect will generally provide rapid hemostasis. Sutures are rarely necessary, and as the scar from a sutured biopsy site generally stretches back to the original dimensions of the biopsy, suturing provides little benefit to the patient.

Where to biopsy, how many biopsies to obtain, and how to process the tissue depend on the suspected diagnosis and the preference of the pathologist. In all cases, a pathologist experienced in the interpretation of scalp biopsies is an advantage. The pathologist may prefer vertical or transverse (horizontal) sectioning of the specimen. Each has advantages. Every follicular unit in the specimen will be demonstrated in transverse sections. Vertical sections are superior for demonstrating changes in the surface epidermis, dermoepidermal junction, superficial dermis, and subcutaneous fat. In general, the features of androgenetic (pattern) alopecia, telogen effluvium, and trichotillomania are better demonstrated in transverse (horizontal) sections through the specimen. Alopecia areata and syphilitic alopecia are well demonstrated in transverse sections if serial step sections are obtained to demonstrate deeper planes of section or if the block is cut horizontally in a bread-loaf fashion prior to embedding. They are equally well demonstrated with serial vertical sections through the block. Lupus erythematosus and lichen planopilaris are more easily demonstrated in serial vertical sections.

The diagnostic yield can be enhanced by pairing vertical and transverse sections. If two biopsies are done, one specimen can be bisected vertically for direct immunofluorescence (DIF) and hematoxylin and eosin (H&E) processing. It is most easily split by laying it on its side and bisecting it with a 15 blade pushed cleanly through the specimen in a single downward motion. Sawing at the specimen will not produce a satisfactory result. One-half of the bisected specimen is placed in formalin, and the other half in immunofluorescent media. The second specimen can be bisected for transverse sections in the clinic or left for the laboratory to bisect after processing. If it is to be bisected in the clinic, it should be placed on its side. The 15 blade should be pushed downward through the specimen in a single motion at the level of the mid-dermis. All pieces for vertical and transverse sections may be placed in a single bottle to be embedded in a single cassette.

In many forms of cicatricial alopecia, a biopsy of an active inflammatory lesion will be most diagnostic. In lupus erythematosus, the biopsy must be from a lesion of several months' duration in order to demonstrate hyperkeratosis, follicular plugging, basement membrane thickening (Fig. 33-10), and dermal mucin. Only biopsies from established lesions of lupus will demonstrate reliable immunofluorescence.

When biopsies of the most active area of alopecia have failed to yield a definite diagnosis, a biopsy from a scarred area may provide additional information. Scars show loss of elastic tissue with the Verhoeff–van Gieson stain. The pattern of

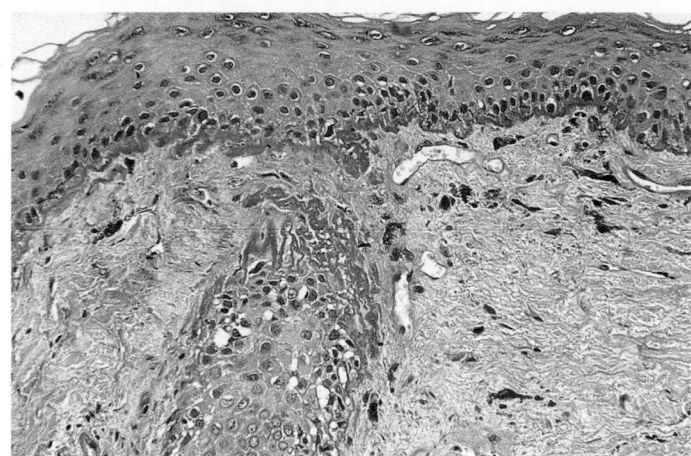

Fig. 33-10 Basement membrane thickening in lupus erythematosus (periodic acid–Schiff [PAS] stain).

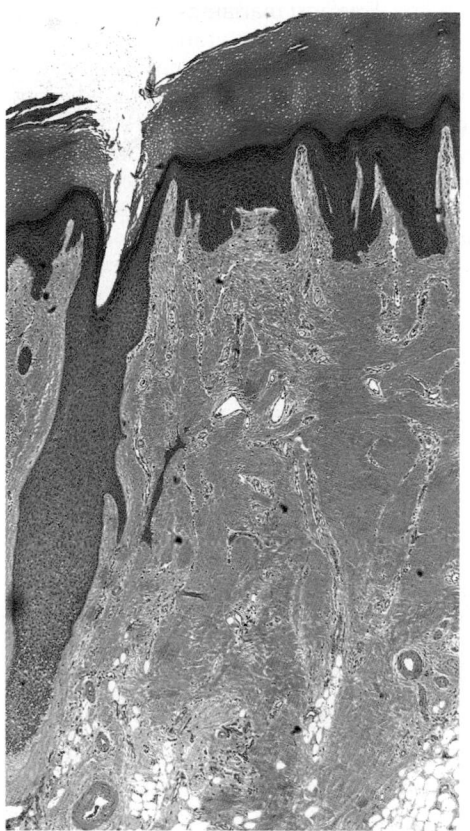

Fig. 33-11 Scarring alopecia (H&E stain).

elastic tissue loss is the "footprint" of the preceding inflammatory process (Figs 33-11 and 33-12). Lichen planopilaris and folliculitis decalvans both affect the infundibulum. Both result in wedge-shaped superficial dermal scars. Discoid lupus erythematosus results in scarring of both the follicular units and the intervening dermis. Morphea does not produce a scar, but rather hyalinization of collagen bundles with preservation of the elastic fibers. In idiopathic pseudopelade, the fibrous tract remnants are widened, but the elastic tissue sheath at the periphery of the fibrous tract is preserved.

Most patients with cicatricial alopecia experience gradual progression of the alopecia, and the prolonged course of the disease may lead to inappropriate therapeutic complacency. The progressive destruction of hairs will result in ever-expanding areas of permanent alopecia. Therefore, cicatricial alopecia must be treated aggressively and early to avoid

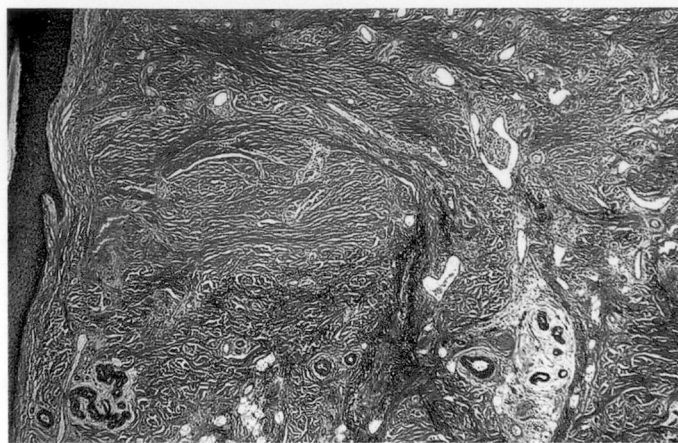

Fig. 33-12 Scarring alopecia (elastic stain). Normal elastic fibers (black) indicate the nonscarred portions of the dermis.

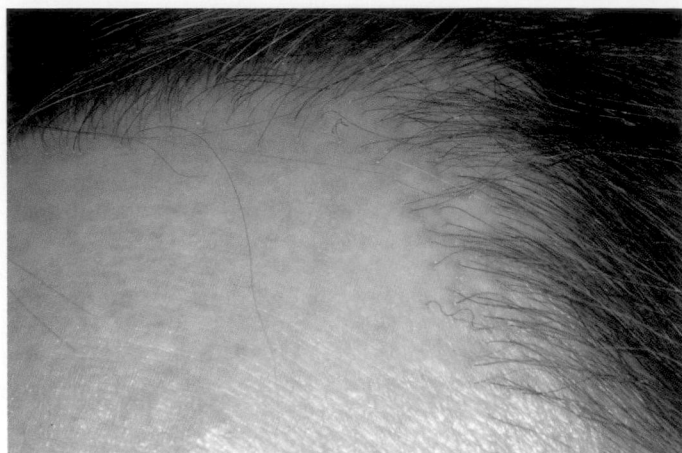

Fig. 33-13 Frontal fibrosing alopecia. (Courtesy of Don Adler DO)

permanent disfigurement. Surgical revision of the hairless plaque is an option for stable end-stage alopecia, but unless the underlying disease is controlled, surgery may only lead to a flare of the underlying disease with progression of hair loss. Therapy may be forestalled by the inability to establish a definite diagnosis. To help guide therapy for patients who defy diagnosis, work groups of the North American Hair Research Society have proposed a classification scheme based on the type and pattern of inflammation. Some forms of destructive alopecia are lymphocyte-mediated, while some are suppurative processes. The type of infiltrate and the portion of the pilosebaceous unit affected can be used to guide therapy. This classification system may also allow patients to enroll in clinical trials, even in the absence of a definite diagnosis.

Lymphoid-mediated disorders

Lupus erythematosus

Chronic cutaneous lupus of the scalp (discoid lupus erythematosus [DLE]) is a common cause of cicatricial alopecia. In active disease, anagen hairs may be easily extracted from the involved area. Usually, erythema, atrophy, follicular plugging, and mottled hyperpigmentation and hypopigmentation are present. Patients with chronic cutaneous lupus of the scalp may or may not have accompanying SLE or skin lesions of DLE on other parts of the body. The external ear canal and concha should always be examined, as they are common sites for discoid lesions. Occasionally, alopecia occurs in a plaque of tumid lupus. Lupus panniculitis may occasionally result in alopecia in the absence of surface skin changes. SLE is often associated with discoid lesions of the scalp. Patients with SLE may also have short miniaturized "lupus hairs" on the anterior scalp.

Biopsy of early lesions of DLE is often nondiagnostic. Patchy lymphoid inflammation and perifollicular mucinous fibrosis may be the only histologic findings. Focal vacuolar interface dermatitis may or may not be noted. Active established lesions, present for several months, have a higher diagnostic yield. Active established lesions usually demonstrate hyperkeratosis, follicular plugging, vacuolar interface dermatitis, basement membrane zone thickening, pigment incontinence, and dermal mucin. Perivascular and periadnexal lymphoid infiltrates are patchy and involve the eccrine coil and fibrous tract remnants. Fibrous tract involvement creates dense vertical columns of lymphocytes. The underlying subcutaneous tissue may demonstrate nodular lymphoplasmacytic infiltrates and fibrin or hyaline rings around necrotic fat. Hypertrophic lesions of chronic cutaneous lupus erythematosus often demonstrate lichenoid dermatitis. DIF may be nonspecific, but active established lesions typically demonstrate a "full house"

(continuous granular deposition of IgG, IgA, IgM, and C3) at the dermoepidermal junction. When present, this pattern is particularly helpful in distinguishing lichenoid hypertrophic lupus erythematosus from lichen planopilaris. Burnt-out lesions of DLE demonstrate loss of elastic fibers throughout the dermis, which differs from the focal peri-infundibular wedge-shaped scars of lichen planopilaris. In systemic lupus, there may be follicular atrophy associated with pronounced dermal mucinosis.

Chronic cutaneous lupus may respond to intralesional or potent topical corticosteroids, but systemic therapy is frequently required. Antimalarials, retinoids, dapsone, thalidomide, sulfasalazine, mycophenolate mofetil, and methotrexate have been used successfully. Topical tazarotene and topical calcineurin inhibitors are generally disappointing.

Lichen planopilaris

Lichen planopilaris presents with perifollicular erythema and progressive scarring. Small follicular papules may be noted, or the lesion may resemble the ivory white irregular patches of pseudopelade. In some patients, typical polygonal flat-topped papules are present on the wrists and ankles, and lacy white lesions are noted on the oral and genital mucosa. Widespread follicular papules may be present on the trunk or extremities. In most patients, however, only the scalp is involved. Frontal fibrosing alopecia appears to be a variant of lichen planopilaris. Most patients are older women with bandlike frontotemporal alopecia (Fig. 33-13). Graham Little–Piccardi–Lassueur syndrome includes cicatricial alopecia on the scalp, keratosis pilaris in the skin of the trunk and extremities, and noncicatricial hair loss in the pubis and axillae. It has been described in association with complete androgen insensitivity syndrome, a condition that also presents with noncicatricial alopecia in the axillary and pubic hair.

Diagnostic biopsies demonstrate lichenoid interface dermatitis of the follicular unit and sometimes the intervening epidermis. The entire fibrous tract may be filled with cytoid bodies (Fig. 33-14). The changes commonly occur focally and may be best visualized with serial vertical sections. Perifollicular mucinous fibrosis is common and focal perifollicular lymphoid infiltrates tend to involve the infundibulum (the infiltrates of lupus erythematosus tend to involve the isthmus). DIF may be negative or may reveal cytoid bodies and shaggy linear fibrin at the dermoepidermal junction.

Lichen planopilaris responds to oral and intralesional corticosteroids. Topical corticosteroids may be adequate in a few patients, but the activity of the disease waxes and wanes, and slow progression should not lead to therapeutic complacency. Oral retinoids can be effective. Alternative therapies

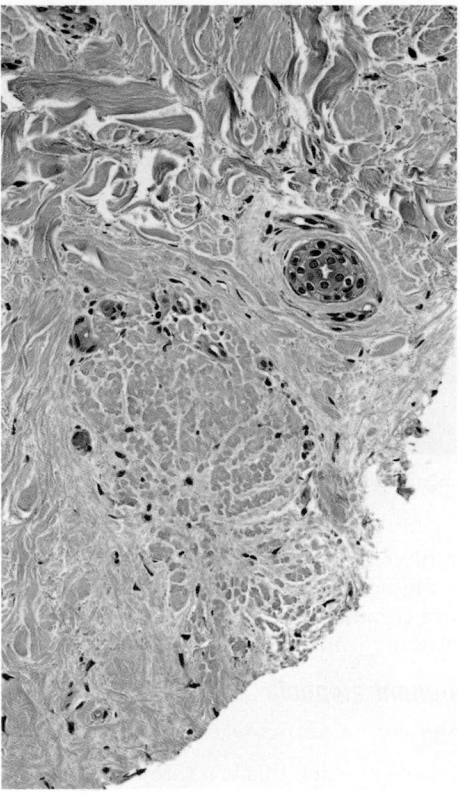

Fig. 33-14 Lichen planopilaris, note cytoid bodies completely fill the fibrous tract remnant.

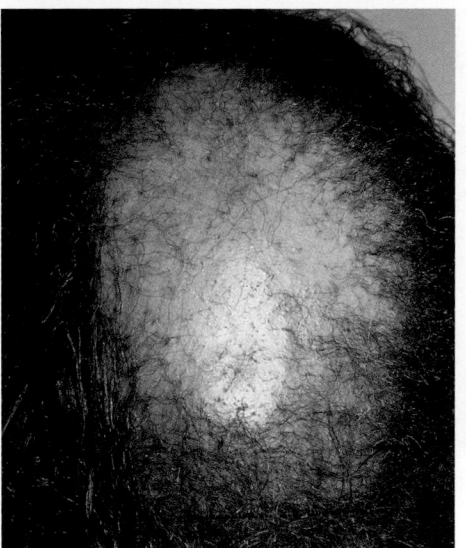

Fig. 33-15 Central centrifugal cicatricial alopecia.

include the other oral agents used to treat lupus; however, there are fewer data regarding their use in lichen planopilaris. As in lupus, topical tazarotene and topical macrolactams are generally disappointing. Biologics have been suggested as therapy, but onset of lichen planopilaris has been noted during etanercept therapy.

Hot comb alopecia and central centrifugal cicatricial alopecia

Hot comb alopecia was reported in the late 1960s as a scarring alopecia seen in black women who straightened their hair with hot combs for cosmetic purposes. It develops characteristically on the crown and spreads peripherally to form a large oval area of partial hair loss. The hot petrolatum used with the iron was thought to cause thermal damage to the hair follicle. However, Sperling et al reported a similar-appearing scarring alopecia in both men and women who did not report the use of hot combs. Some authors now regard hot comb alopecia, central centrifugal cicatricial alopecia (CCCA), and idiopathic pseudopelade to be one entity or overlapping entities that can be indistinguishable.

CCCA is seen most commonly in African American women, is slowly progressive, usually begins in the crown, and advances to the surrounding areas (Fig. 33-15). The term is often used as a broad category that includes cases once classified as hot comb alopecia and central elliptical pseudopelade in white women. Some patients will demonstrate crops of crusts at the periphery of the patches, a feature of folliculitis decalvans. Treatment of CCCA is difficult and often unsatisfactory. Discontinuation of chemical and heat processing, and reduction of traction are routinely recommended, but the effectiveness of these recommendations has yet to be substantiated. Cases with overlapping features of folliculitis decalvans may respond to long-term antibiotic therapy and topical corticosteroids. In such overlapping cases, the histology shows a lymphocytic infiltrate during the chronic stage, but periodic crops of pustules demonstrate a neutrophilic folliculitis.

Neutrophil-mediated disorders

Folliculitis decalvans

Folliculitis decalvans presents with crops of pustules that result in cicatricial alopecia. Successive crops of pustules, crusts, or erosions lead to expansion of the alopecic patches. Staphylococci are sometimes cultured from the lesions, and some authors have suggested that folliculitis decalvans merely represents a chronic staphylococcal infection. It is more likely that follicular destruction is the result of an abnormal suppurative immune response. Staphylococci and other organisms probably play a role in inciting the response. The lesions often respond to long-term treatment with tetracycline. The improvement may reflect the antineutrophil effects of the drug or its antimicrobial effects. Many patients also respond to other forms of antistaphylococcal therapy, but the lesions generally recur after the antibiotic is discontinued. Chronic antibiotic treatment generally results in a continued response. Some sustained responses have been noted after combination therapy with rifampin and clindamycin. Rifampin alone has been used, but may promote the emergence of resistance. Selenium sulfide shampoo and topical corticosteroids may be useful as adjunctive therapy. Oral retinoids, oral and topical fusidic acid, and oral zinc sulphate have sometimes produced sustained responses.

A variant of folliculitis decalvans occurs in African American patients who present with pseudofolliculitis of the beard, acne keloidalis nuchae, and scarring alopecia in the vertex and parietal scalp. The scalp demonstrates ingrown hairs, crops of pustules or crusts, and permanent scarring alopecia. While pseudofolliculitis barbae is generally accepted to be the result of ingrown hairs, the pathogenesis of acne keloidalis nuchae remains in question. Histologically, ingrown hairs are common in advanced lesions. Early lesions may not demonstrate the hair. Some patients merely develop small papules on the nape of the neck, while others develop pustules, crusts, and progressive alopecia. This latter group overlaps with folliculitis decalvans.

Acne necrotica

Acne necrotica presents with discrete excoriated follicular papules in the scalp. Biopsy demonstrates an inflammatory crust and suppurative folliculitis. Usually there is no associated scarring alopecia, but occasional cases overlap with folliculitis decalvans.

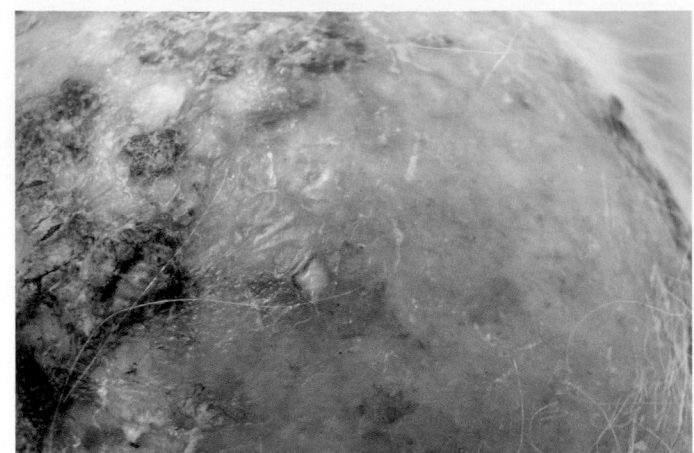

Fig. 33-16 Erosive pustular dermatitis.

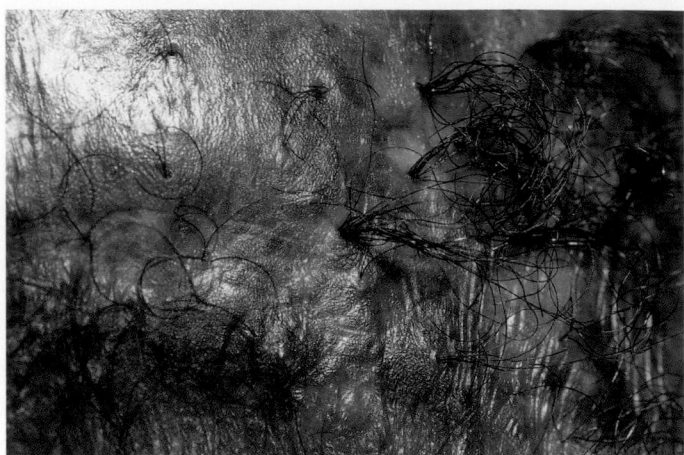

Fig. 33-18 Tufted doll's hairs, cicatricial alopecia.

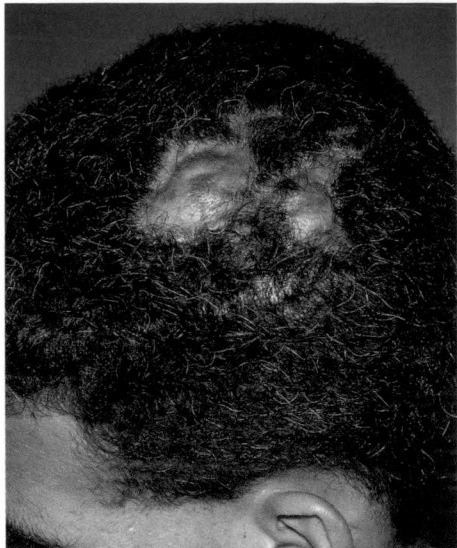

Fig. 33-17 Dissecting cellulitis.

Erosive pustular dermatitis of the scalp

This often presents as expanding eroded patches with moist granulation tissue (Fig. 33-16). The lesions often follow trauma or a surgical procedure and tend to be chronic and progressive. They respond best to class I topical corticosteroids.

Dissecting cellulitis (perifolliculitis capitis abscessens et suffodiens of Hoffman)

This often coexists with acne conglobata and hidradenitis suppurativa. It may also occur with folliculitis decalvans. The lesions are deep, boggy, and suppurative (Fig. 33-17). They may respond to tetracyclines, retinoids, and intralesional corticosteroids.

Tufted folliculitis

Tufted folliculitis presents with doll's hair-like bundling of follicular units. It is seen in a wide range of scarring conditions, including chronic staphylococcal infection, chronic lupus erythematosus, lichen planopilaris, Graham Little syndrome, folliculitis decalvans (Fig. 33-18), acne keloidalis nuchae, immunobullous disorders, and dissecting cellulitis. Compound hairs (two or more hairs sharing a common

infundibulum) occur physiologically on the scalp and legs. They are common in the occipital scalp. Recurrent staphylococcal infection is more common in patients with many compound hairs and commonly leads to tufted folliculitis.

Other forms of permanent alopecia

Pseudopelade of Brocq

Also known as alopecia cicatrisata, this is a rare form of cicatricial alopecia in which destruction of the hair follicles produces multiple round, oval, or irregularly shaped, hairless, cicatricial patches of varying sizes. They are usually coin-sized and are white or slightly pink in color, with a smooth, shiny, marble-like or ivory, atrophic, "onion skin" surface. Interspersed in the patches may be a few spared follicles with hairs growing from them. A clinical inflammatory stage is completely absent. No pustules, crusts, or broken-off hairs are present. The onset is, as a rule, insidious, with one or two lesions appearing on the vertex. The condition affects females three times more commonly than males, and has a prolonged course. In advanced cases large irregular patches are formed by coalescence of some of the many small macules, a pattern referred to as "footprints in the snow." The alopecia is permanent and the disease is slowly progressive. Histologically, the majority of patients with clinical lesions of pseudopelade demonstrate true scarring (indicated by loss of elastic tissue) in a wedge-shaped pattern in the superficial dermis. The pattern is similar to that seen in lichen planopilaris and suggests that many cases classified as pseudopelade represent an end stage of lichen planopilaris. A subset of patients, however, demonstrates no perifollicular or interfollicular scarring at all. This subset has been called idiopathic pseudopelade. It shows significant clinical overlap with CCCA. In these patients, the dermis is contracted into a thin band of dense collagenous tissue. Elastic fibers are intact and quite thick as a result of elastic recoil related to dermal contraction. Fibrous tract remnants are wide and hyalinized with an intact elastic sheath. Lymphoid and neutrophilic inflammation is absent, but loss of the inner and outer root sheaths with subsequent hair fiber granuloma formation is noted. Sebaceous glands are decreased or absent, as they are in most forms of permanent alopecia. DIF is negative.

The end stage of many forms of cicatricial alopecia can resemble pseudopelade clinically, but, like lichen planopilaris, they demonstrate distinct patterns of elastic tissue loss in the dermis. Folliculitis decalvans is distinguished by periodic crops of pustules or crusts at the periphery of the alopecic patches. It produces superficial wedge-shaped scars similar to those of lichen planopilaris.

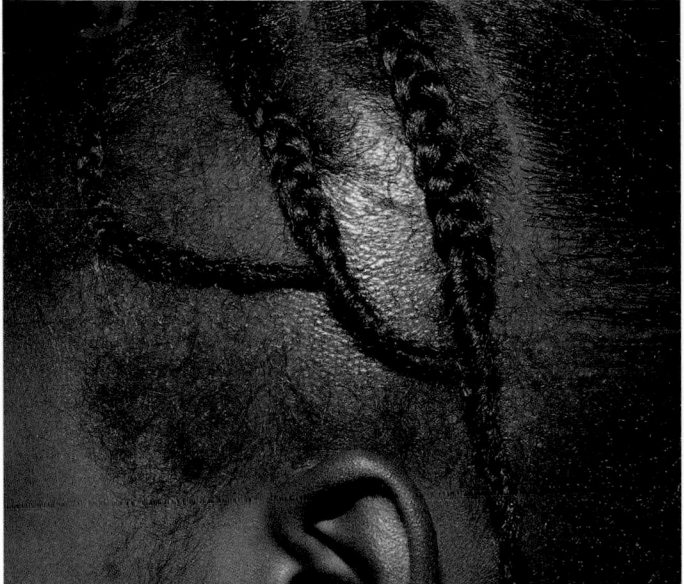

Fig. 33-19 Traction alopecia.

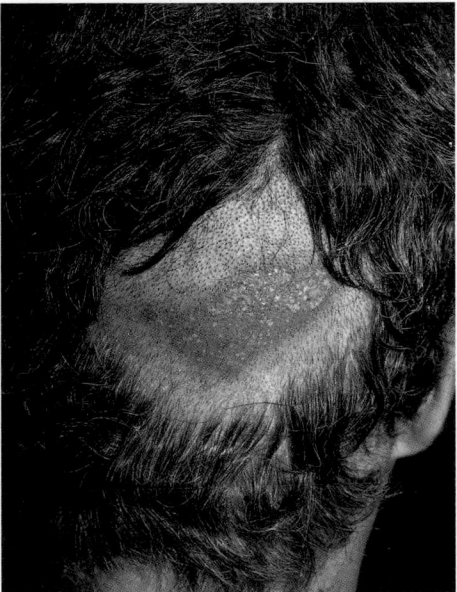

Fig. 33-20 Pressure alopecia with scalp demonstrating pressure-induced geometric pressure necrosis.

Topical and intralesional corticosteroids and long-term tetracycline in anti-inflammatory doses may be tried but are not often successful. The disease usually reaches an inactive end stage after many years.

Traction alopecia

Traction alopecia occurs from prolonged tension on the hair, either from wearing the hair tightly braided or in a ponytail, pulling the hair to straighten it, rolling curlers too tightly, or from the habit of twisting the hairs with the fingers. Traction alopecia most commonly involves the periphery of the scalp, especially the temples and above the ears (Fig. 33-19).

Sarcoidosis

Sarcoidosis of the scalp presents with diffuse or patchy hair loss. The involved scalp is often indurated and a raised peripheral border may be present. The lesions are often red–brown in color and may have an apple jelly appearance with diascopy. Biopsy reveals noncaseating granulomas. Treatment is as for other forms of sarcoidosis.

Pressure alopecia

Pressure alopecia occurs in adults after prolonged pressure on the scalp during general anesthesia, with the head fixed in one position. It may also occur in chronically ill persons after prolonged bed rest in one position (Fig. 33-20), which causes persistent pressure on one part of the scalp. It probably arises because of pressure-induced ischemia.

Tumor alopecia

Tumor alopecia refers to hair loss in the immediate vicinity of either benign or malignant tumors of the scalp. Syringomas, nerve sheath myxomas, and steatocystoma multiplex are benign tumors that may be limited to the scalp and cause alopecia. Alopecia neoplastica is the designation given to hair loss from metastatic tumors, most often from breast or renal carcinoma (Fig. 33-21).

Keratosis pilaris atrophicans

Keratosis pilaris atropicans includes many forms of keratosis pilaris with cicatricial alopecia. Variants include keratosis pilaris atrophicans faciei, atrophoderma vermiculatum, keratosis follicularis spinulosa decalvans, and ichthyosis follicularis.

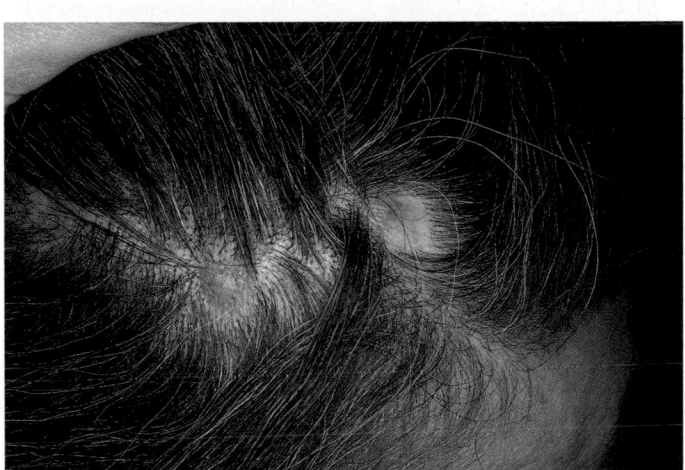

Fig. 33-21 Alopecia neoplastica.

Keratosis pilaris atrophicans faciei (ulerythema ophryogenes, keratosis pilaris rubra atrophicans faciei, folliculitis rubra, lichen pilare, or xerodermie pilaire symmétrique de la face) begins in infancy as follicular papules with perifollicular erythema. Initially, the lesions are restricted to the lateral eyebrows. With time, they spread to involve the cheeks and forehead. There may be associated keratosis pilaris on the extremities and buttocks. The condition may also be associated with an atopic diathesis, ectodermal dysplasia, or Noonan syndrome.

Atrophoderma vermiculatum (acne vermoulanti, honeycomb atrophy, folliculitis ulerythema reticulata, ulerythema acneiforme, folliculitis ulerythematous reticulata, atrophodermia reticulata symmetrica faciei, atrophoderma reticulatum) presents with erythematous follicular papules on the cheeks in childhood. With time, the lesions develop into pit-like depressions (reticulate atrophy). Autosomal-dominant inheritance has been described. This condition generally spares the scalp and eyebrows.

Keratosis follicularis spinulosa decalvans is a rare X-linked disorder described by Siemens in 1926. The gene has been mapped to Xp21.2–p22.2. It begins in infancy with keratosis pilaris localized on the face, and then evolves to more diffuse involvement. Progressive cicatricial alopecia occurs on the scalp, eyebrows, and sometimes eyelashes. The alopecia starts during childhood, and active disease may remit during the early teenage years. Corneal and conjunctival inflammation, corneal dystrophy, and blepharitis occur, and photophobia is usually a prominent finding.

Ichthyosis follicularis also demonstrates extensive spiny follicular hyperkeratosis, permanent alopecia, and photophobia. Palmar plantar keratosis, nail deformities, atopy, and recurrent cheilitis have been described.

Atrichia with papular lesions

Atrichia with papular lesions is a rare autosomal-recessive disorder with early onset of atrichia, followed by a papular eruption appearing within the first years of life. The condition has been linked to chromosome 8p21 and mutations have been detected in what is now referred to as the hairless gene. It is discussed in more detail in Chapter 27.

Alzolibani AA, et al: Pseudopelade of Brocq. Dermatol Ther 2008 Jul–Aug; 21(4):257–263.

Elston DM, et al: Vertical and transverse sections of alopecia biopsy specimens: combining the two to maximize diagnostic yield. J Am Acad Dermatol 1995; 32:454.

Elston DM, et al: Elastic tissue in scars and alopecia. J Cutan Pathol 2000; 27:147.

Elston DM, et al: A comparison of vertical versus transverse sections in the evaluation of alopecia biopsy specimens. J Am Acad Dermatol 2005; 53:267.

Harries MJ, et al: Management of primary cicatricial alopecias: options for treatment. Br J Dermatol 2008 Jul; 159(1):1–22.

Hordinsky M: Cicatricial alopecia: discoid lupus erythematosus. Dermatol Ther 2008 Jul–Aug; 21(4):245–248.

Kang H, et al: Lichen planopilaris. Dermatol Ther 2008 Jul–Aug; 21(4):249–256.

Otberg N, et al: Folliculitis decalvans. Dermatol Ther 2008 Jul–Aug; 21(4):238–244.

Shapiro J: Cicatricial alopecias. Dermatol Ther 2008 Jul–Aug; 21(4):211.

Somani N, et al: Cicatricial alopecia: classification and histopathology. Dermatol Ther 2008 Jul–Aug; 21(4):221–237. Review.

Unger W, et al: The surgical treatment of cicatricial alopecia. Dermatol Ther 2008 Jul–Aug; 21(4):295–311.

Whiting DA, et al: Central centrifugal cicatricial alopecia. Dermatol Ther 2008 Jul–Aug; 21(4):268–278.

Hair color

Melanin in the hair follicles is produced in the cytoplasm of the melanocytes. Organelles involved include the endoplasmic reticulum, ribosomes, and Golgi apparatus. Melanocytes producing hair pigment are associated with the hair matrix, and melanogenesis occurs only during anagen. This cyclic melanin synthesis distinguishes follicular melanogenesis from the continuous melanogenesis of the epidermis. With age, cyclic melanocytic activity in the follicular unit declines. By 40 years of age most individuals show evidence of graying. Graying results primarily from a reduction in tyrosinase activity within hair bulb melanocytes. Defective migration of melanocytes from a diminishing reservoir in the outer root sheath may play a role. Physiologic graying may also be related to reactive oxygen species-mediated damage to nuclear and mitochondrial DNA in bulbar melanocytes. The melanocortin 1 receptor gene (MCR1) is closely related to red hair, freckling, and sun sensitivity.

The pigment in black and dark brown hair is composed of eumelanin, whereas in blond and red hair it is pheomelanin. In black hair the melanocytes contain the densest melanosomes. Brown hair differs only by its smaller melanosomes. Light brown hair consists of a mixture of the melanosomes of

dark hair and the incomplete melanosomes of blond hair. Many of the melanosomes in blond hair develop only on the matrix fibers and not in the spaces between the fibers.

Red hair shows incomplete melanin deposits on the matrix fibers to produce a blotchy-appearing melanosome. Pheomelanin is distinguished by its relatively high content of sulfur, which results from the addition of cysteine to dopaquinone along the biosynthetic pathway of melanin synthesis.

In gray hair (canities), melanogenic activity is decreased as a result of fewer melanocytes and melanosomes, as well as a gradual loss of tyrosinase activity. Graying of the scalp hair is genetically determined and may start at any age. Usually, it begins at the temples and progresses with time. The beard usually follows, with the body hair graying last. Premature whitening of scalp hair is usually caused by vitiligo, sometimes without recognized, or actually without, lesions of glabrous skin.

Early graying (before age 20 in white or before age 30 in black persons) is usually familial; however, it may occur in progeria, Rothmund–Thomson syndrome, Böök syndrome, and Werner syndrome.

In poliosis, gray or white hair occurs in circumscribed patches. This may occur in Waardenburg syndrome and piebaldism, Tietz syndrome, Alezzandrini syndrome, neurofibromatosis, and tuberous sclerosis. Poliosis is also found in association with regressing melanoma, vitiligo, and Vogt–Koyanagi syndrome, and may be seen in alopecia areata when the new hairs grow. Migratory poliosis without hair loss may represent a forme fruste of alopecia areata.

Green hair has been traced to copper in the water of a swimming pool. This occurs only in blond or light hair, and may be treated with topical EDTA, penicillamine-containing shampoos, or 1.5% aqueous 1-hydroxyethyl diphosphonic acid. Tars and chrysarobin stain light-colored hair brown.

Changes in hair color occur in various disorders. The hair is blond in phenylketonuria and homocystinuria. Light hair is also seen in oasthouse disease (familial methionine malabsorption), Menkes kinky hair syndrome, and albinism. In Griscelli and Chédiak–Higashi syndromes the hair has a silvery sheen. In kwashiorkor the hair assumes a red–blond color and may demonstrate periodic banding (flag sign, segmental heterochromia). Alternating light and dark bands may also occur in iron deficiency anemia and with courses of sunitinib. In vitamin B_{12} deficiency and with IFN therapy, whitening may occur. The disorder has been called canities segmentata sideropenica. It responds completely to iron supplementation. Triparanol is associated with hypopigmented hair. Minoxidil (by changing vellus to terminal hairs) causes darkening of hair; another hypotensive agent, diazoxide, gives the hair a reddish tint. Chloroquine therapy may cause hair whitening, usually in redheads and blonds, but not in brunettes. Pigmentation of the eyelashes and irides has been described with latanoprost. Xanthotrichia (yellow hair) has been noted with selenium sulfide and dihydroxyacetone.

Many black patients with acquired immunodeficiency syndrome (AIDS) have experienced softening, straightening, lightening, and thinning of their hair. Patients with human immunodeficiency virus (HIV)-1 infection may also experience elongated eyelashes and telogen effluvium.

Hartmann JT, et al: Sunitinib and periodic hair depigmentation due to temporary c-KIT inhibition. Arch Dermatol 2008 Nov; 144(11): 1525–1526.

Prevost N, et al: Xanthotrichia (yellow hair) due to selenium sulfide and dihydroxyacetone. J Drugs Dermatol 2008 Jul; 7(7):689–691.

Vaughn MR, et al: A comparison of hair colour measurement by digital image analysis with reflective spectrophotometry. Forensic Sci Int 2009 Jan 10; 183(1–3):97–101.

Hair structure defects

Examination of hairs for structural defects is greatly facilitated by a method devised by Shelley: putting a piece of double-stick tape on a microscope slide and aligning 5 cm segments of hair in parallel on it. Dermoscopy can be useful in assessing hair morphology. Microscopic mounts of hairs are best examined under a dissecting microscope or polarized light. Gold-coating and scanning electron microscopy can also be done on hairs so mounted. Hairs from multiple body sites may need to be sampled. This has been documented in Netherton syndrome where scalp hair can be normal while eyebrow hair demonstrates the characteristic hair shaft defect.

Boussofara L, et al: Netherton's syndrome: the importance of eyebrow hair. Dermatol Online J 2007 Jul 13; 13(3):21.
Cheng AS, et al: The genetics of hair shaft disorders. J Am Acad Dermatol 2008 Jul; 59(1):1–22.
Whiting DA, et al: Office diagnosis of hair shaft defects. Semin Cutan Med Surg 2006 Mar; 25(1):24–34.

Hair casts (pseudonits)

Hair casts represent remnants of the inner root sheath. They often occur in great numbers and may mimic nits in the scalp. While nits are firmly cemented to the hair shaft, hair casts slide freely along the shaft. Taeb et al reviewed 36 published cases and distinguished two groups: girls between 2 and 8 years of age with diffuse involvement and no scalp disease, and children and adults with psoriasis, lichen planus, seborrheic dermatitis, or trichotillomania. Keipert made a similar distinction, separating a large group of cases with some keratinizing disorder of the scalp and dark, oddly shaped masses of keratin adherent to or surrounding the hairs, which he called parakeratotic hair casts; and lighter-colored tubular casts, 2–4 mm long, which he called peripilar hair casts. Taeb et al found 0.025% tretinoin lotion effective. False hair casts may occur as a result of hair spray or deodorant concretions. Immunoglobulin casts and cutaneous spicules have been noted in multiple myeloma.

Miller JJ, et al: Hair casts and cutaneous spicules in multiple myeloma. Arch Dermatol 2006 Dec; 142(12):1665–1666.

Pili torti

Also known as twisted hairs, pili torti is a malformation of hair characterized by twisting of the hair shaft on its own axis (Fig. 33-22). The hair shaft is segmentally thickened, and light and dark segments are seen. Scalp hair, eyebrows, and eyelashes may be affected. The hairs are brittle and easily broken.

In the classic type, unassociated with other disorders, onset is usually in early childhood; by puberty, it has usually improved. Clinically, it may be associated with patchy alopecia and short, broken hairs. It usually follows a dominant inheritance pattern, though recessive and sporadic cases have been reported. Acquired cases have been described in young women with anorexia nervosa. Pili torti may be seen with associated abnormalities. The Björnstad syndrome consists of congenital deafness of the cochlear type, with pili torti. Both autosomal-dominant and autosomal-recessive inheritance patterns have been described. *BCS1L* mutations cause the Björnstad syndrome. The gene encodes an ATPase necessary for the assembly of complex III in mitochondria. *BCS1L* mutations also cause lethal conditions, including the complex III deficiency and the GRACILE syndrome, with severe multisystem and neurologic manifestations.

Pili torti also may occur in citrullinemia (argininosuccinate synthetase deficiency), Menkes kinky hair syndrome, Bazex

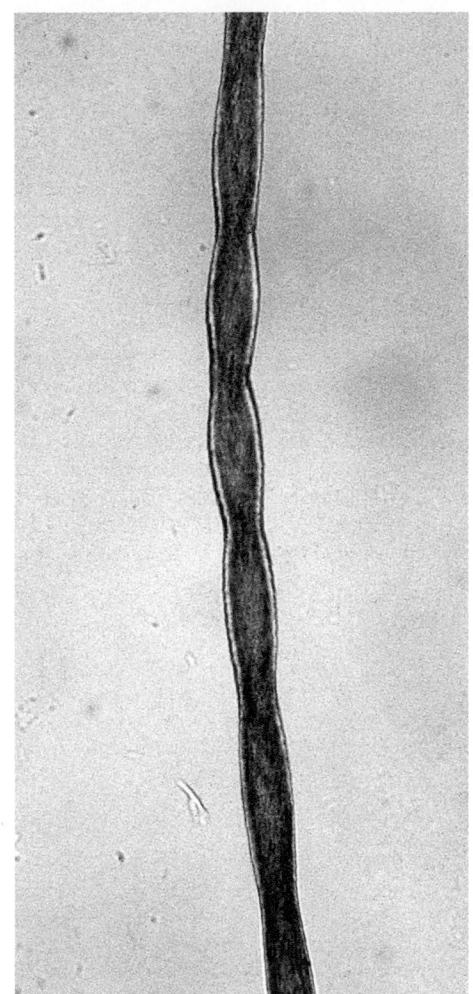

Fig. 33-22 Pili torti.

follicular atrophoderma syndrome, ectodermal dysplasias, Crandall syndrome (pili torti, nerve deafness, hypogonadism), Netherton syndrome (along with bamboo hair), with isotretinoin and etretinate therapy, in anorexia nervosa, and in trichothiodystrophy.

Laron syndrome is an autosomal-recessive disease with primary insulin-like growth factor 1 deficiency and primary growth hormone insensitivity. Affected children have sparse hair and frontal recession. Pili torti et canaliculi, tapered hair, and trichorrhexis nodosa have been noted.

Hinson JT, et al: Missense mutations in the BCS1L gene as a cause of the Björnstad syndrome. N Engl J Med 2007 Feb 22; 356(8):809–819.

Menkes kinky hair syndrome

Pili torti, and often monilethrix and trichorrhexis nodosa, are all common in the hairs in this sex-linked recessively inherited disorder. It has also been called steely hair disease, because the hair resembles steel wool. The characteristic ivory color of the hair appears between 1 and 5 months of age. Drowsiness, lethargy, convulsive seizures, severe neurologic deterioration, and periodic hypothermia ensue with death at an early age. Hairs become wiry, sparse, fragile, and twisted about their long axes. Osteoporosis, and dental and ocular abnormalities are common. The skin is pale and the face pudgy, and the upper lip has an exaggerated "Cupid's bow" configuration. The occipital horn syndrome, primarily a connective tissue disorder, is a milder variant of Menkes syndrome. Patients have a deficiency of serum copper and copper-dependent enzymes, resulting from mutations in the *ATP7A* gene. The gene encodes a trans-Golgi membrane-bound copper transporting P-type ATPase. Loss of this protein activity blocks the export of dietary copper from the gastrointestinal tract and causes the copper deficiency. Low serum copper and ceruloplasmin are characteristic, but are not seen in all patients. They are particularly variable in the first weeks of life. Other tests helpful for screening include the ratio of catechols, such as dihydroxyphenylalanine to dihydroxyphenylglycol. High levels of the catechols DOPA, dihydrophenylacetic acid, and dopamine, and low levels of dihydroxyphenylglycol are characteristic. Studies of copper egress in cultured fibroblasts have also been used. Early detection allows for genetic counseling and the institution of copper histidine treatment, which is being studied and has shown promising results in some infants. Pamidronate treatment is associated with an increase in bone mineral density in children with Menkes disease. In zebra fish, antisense morpholino oligonucleotides directed against the splice-site junctions of two mutant calamity alleles were able to correct the molecular defect. This is a promising area for research.

Bertini I, et al: Menkes disease. Cell Mol Life Sci 2008 Jan; 65(1):89–91.
Madsen EC, et al: In vivo correction of a Menkes disease model using antisense oligonucleotides. Proc Natl Acad Sci U S A 2008 Mar 11; 105(10):3909–3914.
Rudolph V, et al: Copper trafficking and extracellular superoxide dismutase activity: kinky hair, kinky vessels. Hypertension 2008 Nov; 52(5):811–812.

Uncombable hair syndrome

First reported in 1973 by Dupré et al as cheveux incoiffables (undressable hairs) and by Stroud and Mehergan as spunglass hair, the microscopic abnormality of a triangular cross-sectional appearance with a longitudinal groove gives the disease its other name, pili triangulati et canaliculi.

Clinically, the defect is noted in the first few years of life as dry, blond, shiny hair that stands straight out from the scalp and cannot be combed (Fig. 33-23). On light microscopy it may appear quite normal when viewed lengthwise, but on horizontal sectioning and on scanning electron microscopy it shows the longitudinal grooves that make it abnormally rigid. These depressions are sometimes seen in unaffected persons, so that 50% of hairs need to be affected for the condition to be clinically detectable.

Autosomal-dominant, autosomal-recessive, and sporadic forms have been described. Uncombable hair has been associated with angel-shaped phalango-epiphyseal dysplasia. It has also been seen in combination with retinal dystrophy, juvenile cataract, and brachydactyly. It has also been reported in a patient who acquired the abnormality at age 39 after an episode of diffuse alopecia treated with spironolactone. Although there are usually no associated ectodermal defects, isolated cases have been reported in which uncombable hair is one component of several clustered findings. Until more experience is available in the literature, grouping of these cases into new syndromes is premature.

Some patients have responded clinically to biotin, 0.3 mg orally three times a day. Some cases improve spontaneously in late childhood.

Anderson HF, et al: Uncombable hair syndrome. Cutis 2008 Jul; 82(1):20, 31–32.
Jarell AD, et al: Uncombable hair syndrome. Pediatr Dermatol 2007 Jul–Aug; 24(4):436–438.
Schena D, et al: Uncombable hair syndrome, mental retardation, single palmar crease and arched palate in a patient with neurofibromatosis type I. Pediatr Dermatol 2007 Sep–Oct; 24(5):E73–E75.

Monilethrix

Monilethrix, also known as beaded hairs, is a rare hereditary disease. It is characterized by dryness, fragility, and sparseness of the scalp hair (Fig. 33-24), with fusiform or spindle-shaped swellings of the hair shaft separated by narrow atrophic segments. The hair tends to break at the delicate internodes. There is an occasional rupture at the node and longitudinal fissuring of the shaft, which also involves the nodes.

The disease is often associated with keratosis pilaris of the extensor surfaces, temples, and back of the neck. Hair on regions other than the scalp may be affected. Leukonychia may occur. Inheritance of monilethrix is an autosomal-dominant trait. It has been described in association with Menkes syndrome. Mutations in *desmoglein 4* are seen in monilethrix and in localized autosomal-recessive hypotrichosis, a disorder that shares clinical features with monilethrix but lacks the characteristic hair shaft changes. Several cases of monilethrix have been linked to the type II keratin gene cluster on chromosome 12q13. Causative heterozygous mutations of

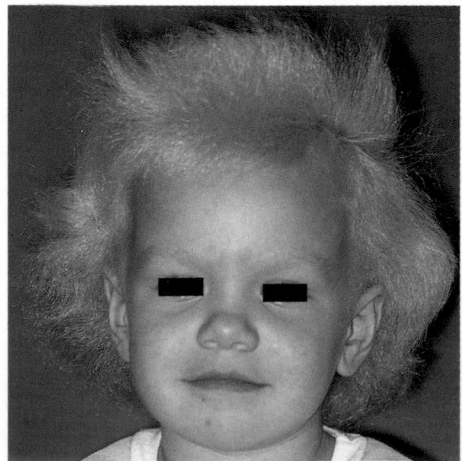

Fig. 33-23 Uncombable hair syndrome.

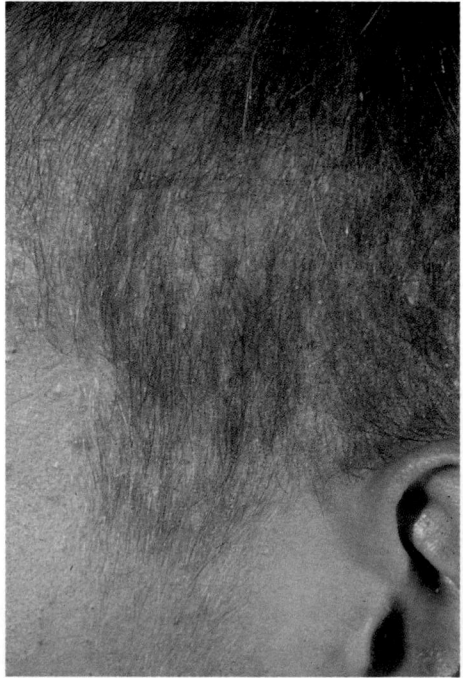

Fig. 33-24 Monilethrix.

a highly conserved glutamic acid residue of the type II hair keratins hHb6 and hHb1 occur. Both hHb1 and hHb6 are largely coexpressed in cortical trichocytes of the hair shaft, confirming that monilethrix is a disease of the hair cortex. Improvement of the hair may occur during pregnancy, but after delivery the hair returns to its original state. Improvement may also occur with age and there may be seasonal improvement during the summer. Improvement with acitretin has been reported.

Trichorrhexis nodosa

The affected hair shafts fracture easily and may have small white nodes arranged at irregular intervals. These nodes are the sites of fraying of the hair cortex. The splitting into strands produces a microscopic appearance suggestive of a pair of brooms stuck together end to end by their bristles. The hairs soon break at these nodes (Fig. 33-25). The number of these nodes along one hair shaft varies from one to several, depending on its length. These fractured hairs are found mostly on the scalp, often in just a small area or areas, but other sites such as the pubic area, axillae, and chest may be involved.

Several categories or types of trichorrhexis nodosa have been described. Proximal trichorrhexis nodosa involves the proximal shafts of the hairs of black patients who traumatize their hair with styling or chemicals. The involved hairs break a few centimeters from the skin surface, resulting in patches of short hair. It appears to occur in genetically predisposed patients. Distal trichorrhexis nodosa affects primarily Asians and white patients; it occurs several inches from the scalp, and is associated with trichoptilosis, or longitudinal splitting, known as split ends. Acquired localized trichorrhexis nodosa is a common type in which the defect occurs in a localized area, a few centimeters across. A number of diseases accompany this type of trichorrhexis nodosa in which pruritus is a prominent symptom; scratching and rubbing may be the cause. Among such diseases are circumscribed neurodermatitis, contact dermatitis, and atopic dermatitis.

The occurrence of trichorrhexis nodosa in some patients with argininosuccinicaciduria has suggested an etiologic connection. Trichorrhexis nodosa has been described in Menkes kinky hair syndrome, Netherton syndrome, hypothyroidism, ectodermal dysplasia, the syndrome of intractable infant diarrhea, and trichothiodystrophy. Trichoschisis, a clean transverse fracture across the hair shaft, is more commonly present in trichothiodystrophy. The curly hair that may result from isotretinoin therapy has been attributed to extensive trichorrhexis nodosa. Because trauma may induce this hair shaft

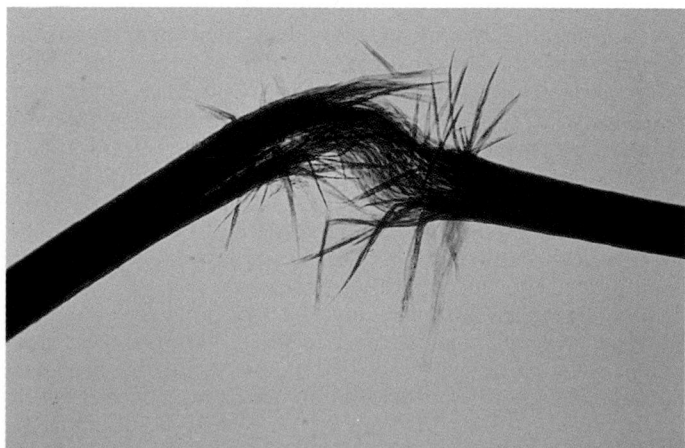

Fig. 33-25 Trichorrhexis nodosa.

abnormality, the specificity of this finding in the above conditions may simply be fortuitous.

Treatment is directed toward the avoidance of trauma to the hair.

Trichorrhexis invaginata

Also known as bamboo hair, trichorrhexis invaginata is caused by intussusception of the hair shaft at the zone where keratinization begins. The invagination is caused by softness of the cortex in the keratogenous zone. The softness may be caused by inadequate conversion of –SH to S–S proteins in the cortex. The patient with bamboo hair will have nodose ball-and-socket deformities, with the socket forming the proximal and the ball part forming the distal portion of the node along the hair shaft. This type of hair is associated with Netherton syndrome. Occasionally, only the proximal half of the abnormality is seen; this has been called golf tee hairs.

Trichorrhexis invaginata associated with congenital ichthyosiform erythroderma or ichthyosis linearis circumflexa constitutes Netherton syndrome. Atopic manifestations and high IgE levels are commonly present. The bamboo hairs may be present not only on the scalp but also on the eyebrows, eyelashes, and rarely in other hairy areas. Hair sparsity is noted all over the body. The bamboo hairs may become normal within a few years. Other reported findings include pili torti, trichorrhexis nodosa, moniliform hairs, urticaria, angioedema, growth retardation, recurrent infections, multiple epithelial neoplasms, and mental retardation. An autosomal-recessive mode of inheritance has been suggested, although reported cases involving women far outnumber men. Pathogenic mutations have been identified in serine protease inhibitor Kazal-type 5 (*SPINK5*) on chromosome 5q32, a gene encoding lymphoepithelial Kazal-type-related inhibitor (*LEKTI*), a serine protease inhibitor involved in skin barrier formation and immunity. PUVA has been reported to help the circumflex linear ichthyosis, while etretinate has been reported both to exacerbate and to improve skin findings.

Menne et al reported the bamboo hair defect in very thin, probably vellus, hairs in a 7-year-old boy with short, thin, brittle scalp hairs and no eyebrows. They termed this a cane-stick deformity.

Pili annulati (ringed hair, spangled hair)

Pili annulati is an unusual disease in which the hair seems banded by alternating segments of light and dark color when seen in reflected light. The light bands are caused by clusters of abnormal air-filled cavities, which scatter light, and reduplicated lamina densa in the region of the root bulb.

Hair growth is normal in patients with pili annulati, although it is rarely associated with trichorrhexis nodosa-like breaks of the hair shaft. There are no other associated abnormalities of skin or other organ systems. It is inherited by autosomal-dominant mode, begins in infancy, and requires no treatment, since the spangled appearance of the hair is not unattractive (Fig. 33-26). The condition has been reported to disappear following recovery from alopecia totalis.

Pili pseudoannulati

This anomaly of human hair mimics pili annulati. The two differ in that the light bands in pili annulati are caused by internal effects, whereas the bright segments in pili pseudoannulati are caused by reflection and refraction of light by flattened, twisted surfaces of hair. This latter type is a variant of normal hair.

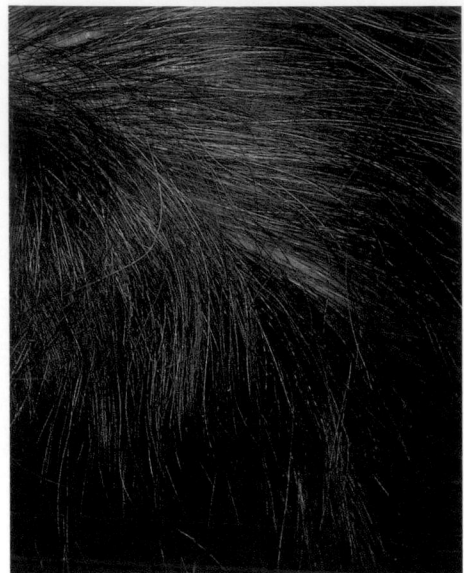

Fig. 33-26 Spangled hair of pili annulati.

Kinking hair

Acquired progressive kinking of the hair, first described and named by Wise and Sulzberger in 1932, involves a structural abnormality of kinking and twisting of the hair shaft at irregular intervals. The main recognized variant of this disorder begins in men in their late teens or early twenties on the frontotemporal or vertex regions, and then progresses to both the parietal and frontal areas. Usually straight, light brown hair becomes curly, frizzy, and lusterless.

When this occurs in the androgen-dependent areas of young men it is a precursor of male-pattern hair loss; usually these men have a strong family history of androgenetic alopecia. Treatment with topical minoxidil has not prevented development of hair thinning. "Whisker" hairs, the short dark hairs that grow anterior to the ears in young people who eventually develop androgenic alopecia, is felt to be a variant of acquired kinking of the hair.

Acquired hair kinking has been described in other clinical situations. Some reports detail prepubertal patients or women, as well as men, in whom kinking develops in non-androgen-dependent areas. In these reports alopecia has not developed, and the curly, frizzy hair may remain present or revert to its previous condition.

Widespread kinking of the hair may be induced by drugs, notably retinoids, and it may also occur in patients with AIDS.

Woolly hair

Woolly hair is present at birth and is usually most severe during childhood, when it is often impossible to brush the hair. In adult life there is a variable amelioration in the condition. There is a clear distinction between the appearance of the affected and nonaffected members of a family. Both autosomal-dominant and autosomal-recessive inheritance have been described. Woolly hair nevus has partial scalp involvement by woolly hair, which has a markedly reduced diameter. Naxos' disease is an autosomal-recessive syndrome with arrhythmogenic right ventricular cardiomyopathy, diffuse nonepidermolytic palmoplantar keratoderma, and woolly hair. Hair abnormalities are a reliable marker for subsequent heart disease. The disease is caused by a mutation in the gene encoding plakoglobin. Carvajal syndrome is a familial cardiocutaneous syndrome consisting of woolly hair, palmoplantar

keratoderma, and heart disease. It is caused by a recessive deletion mutation in desmoplakin.

Woolly hairs tend to unite into tight locks, whereas the hairs of black persons remain individual. The hair may not grow beyond a length of 12 cm, but may attain a normal appearance in adult life. In the familial group the eyebrows and hairs on the arms, legs, and pubic and axillary regions may be short and pale. There are no associated cutaneous or systemic diseases. A Dutch kindred has been described with premature loss of curly, brittle hair, premature loss of carious teeth, nail dystrophy, and acral keratoderma. It has been designated the curly hair-acral keratoderma-caries syndrome.

The microscopic findings of woolly hair include a decreased diameter, an ovoid shape on cross-section, a pili torti-like twisting about a longitudinal axis, trichorrhexis nodosa, and pili annulati.

Plica neuropathica (felted hair)

This is a curling, looping, intertwisting, and felting or matting of the hair in localized areas of the scalp. Predisposing factors include kinky hairs, changes in hair care, and a neurotic mental state. Plica polonica is an older name for this condition.

Burkhart CG, et al: Trichorrhexis nodosa revisited. Skinmed 2007 Mar–Apr; 6(2):57–58.

Clarke JT, et al: Acquired kinking of the hair caused by acitretin. J Drugs Dermatol 2007 Sep; 6(9):937–938.

Fichtel JC, et al: Trichorrhexis nodosa secondary to argininosuccinicaciduria. Pediatr Dermatol 2007 Jan–Feb; 24(1):25–27.

Liu CI, et al: Rapid diagnosis of monilethrix using dermoscopy. Br J Dermatol 2008 Sep; 159(3):741–743.

Rudnicka L, et al: Trichoscopy: a new method for diagnosing hair loss. J Drugs Dermatol 2008 Jul; 7(7):651–654.

Schaffer JV, et al: Mutations in the desmoglein 4 gene underlie localized autosomal recessive hypotrichosis with monilethrix hairs and congenital scalp erosions. J Invest Dermatol 2006 Jun; 126(6):1286–1291.

Schweizer J: More than one gene involved in monilethrix: intracellular but also extracellular players. J Invest Dermatol 2006 Jun; 126(6):1216–1219.

Schweizer J, et al: Hair follicle-specific keratins and their diseases. Exp Cell Res 2007 Jun 10; 313(10):2010–2020.

Shimomura Y, et al: Mutations in the desmoglein 4 gene are associated with monilethrix-like congenital hypotrichosis. J Invest Dermatol 2006 Jun; 126(6):1281–1285.

Zlotogorski A, et al: An autosomal recessive form of monilethrix is caused by mutations in DSG4: clinical overlap with localized autosomal recessive hypotrichosis. J Invest Dermatol 2006 Jun; 126(6):1292–1296.

Pseudofolliculitis barbae

Pseudofolliculitis barbae are hairs that, after appearing at the surface, curve back and pierce the skin as ingrowing hairs. This results in inflammatory papules and pustules, which may scar (Fig. 33-27). In severe cases, large deforming keloids may result in the beard area. Pseudofolliculitis of the beard is seen in more than 50% of black men, who must sometimes give up shaving to alleviate the disorder. A single-nucleotide polymorphism, giving rise to a disruptive Ala12Thr substitution in the 1A α-helical segment of the companion layer-specific keratin K6hf appears to be partially responsible for the phenotype. White persons are uncommonly affected; however, it is more common in renal transplant recipients. Tenderness responds to mid-strength topical steroids. The use of clippers or chemical depilatories, glycolic acid lotion, and adjunctive antibiotic therapy may be helpful. Benzoyl peroxide 5%/clindamycin 1% gel has been shown to be effective in double-blind evaluation. Laser hair removal with the long-pulse Nd:YAG laser is

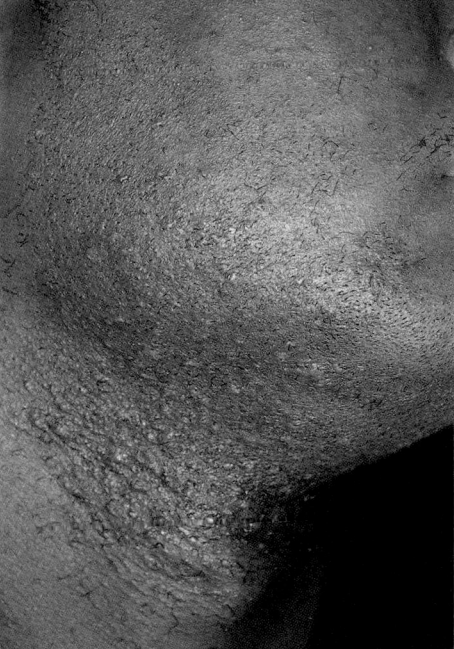

Fig. 33-27 Pseudofolliculitis barbae.

suitable for a wide range of skin types. The diode laser has also been used.

Lally A, et al: Hypertrophic pseudofolliculitis in white renal transplant recipients. Clin Exp Dermatol 2007 May; 32(3):268–271.
Quarles FN, et al: Pseudofolliculitis barbae. Dermatol Ther 2007 May–Jun; 20(3):133–136.
Schulze R, et al: Low-fluence 1,064-nm laser hair reduction for pseudofolliculitis barbae in skin types IV, V, and VI. Dermatol Surg 2009 Jan; 35(1):98–107.

Pili multigemini

This rare malformation is characterized by the presence of bifurcated or multiple divided hair matrices and papillae, giving rise to the formation of multiple hair shafts within the individual follicles (Fig. 33-28). It sometimes follows lines of Blaschko. Mehregan et al reported a patient with cleidocranial dysostosis and extensive pili multigemini over the heavily bearded chin and cheek areas. There is no treatment.

Pili bifurcati

In this disorder, bifurcation is found in short segments along the shafts of several hairs. Each branch of the bifurcation is covered with its own cuticle. It has been seen in association with the trisomy 8 mosaic syndrome. Pili bifurcati differs from pili multigemini in which a single follicular matrix produces two different-sized hair shafts with separate cuticles that do not fuse again. Trichoptilosis is characterized by split distal ends that are never surrounded by a complete cuticle.

Lester L, et al: The prevalence of pili multigemini. Br J Dermatol 2007 Jun; 156(6):1362–1363.

Trichostasis spinulosa

Trichostasis spinulosa is a common disorder of the hair follicles that clinically gives the impression of blackheads (Fig. 33-29), but the follicles are filled with funnel-shaped, horny plugs within which are bundles of vellus hairs (Fig. 33-30). The hairs are round at their proximal ends and shredded distally. The disease occurs primarily on the nose and forehead, but

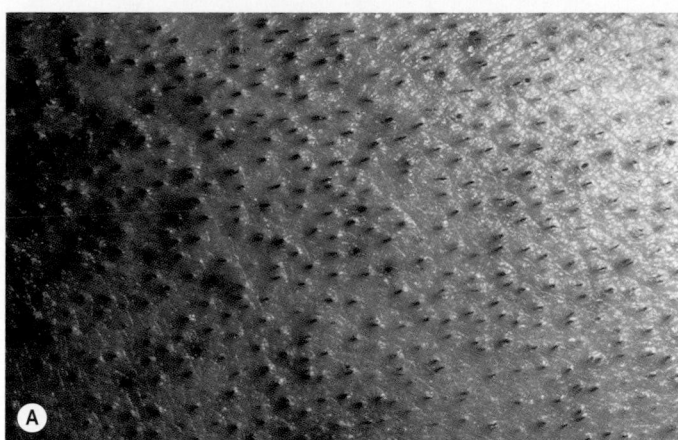

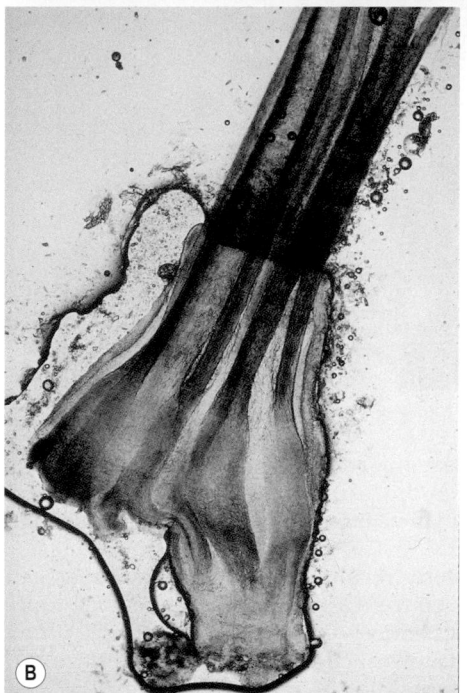

Fig. 33-28 A, Pili multigemini of beard. B, Multiple hair shafts in single follicle.

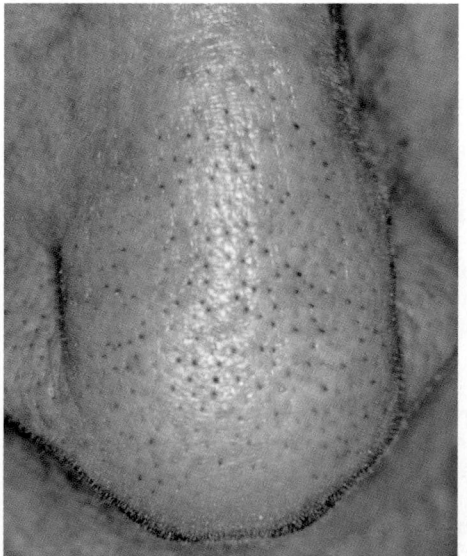

Fig. 33-29 Trichostasis spinulosa.

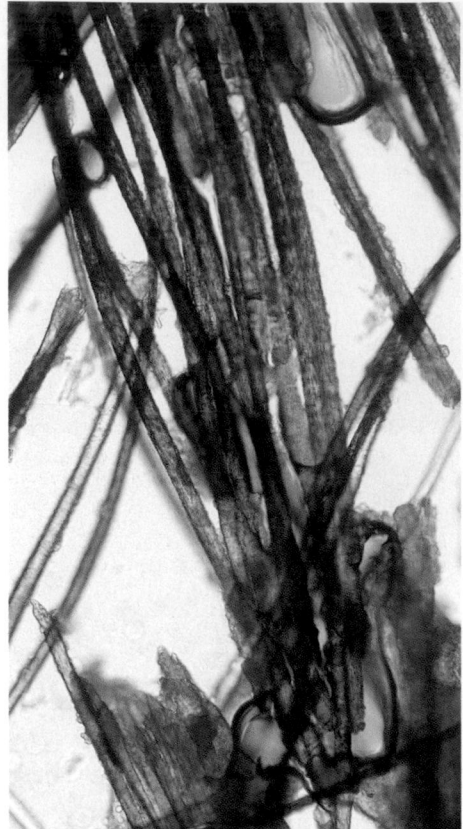

Fig. 33-30 Trichostasis spinulosa.

may also occur on the trunk and be accompanied by pruritus. Dermoscopy or microscopy can be used to establish the diagnosis. The condition may be more common in patients in renal failure.

Trichostasis spinulosa results from retention of telogen hairs, which are derived from a single hair matrix. It is primarily caused by a hyperkeratosis of the follicular infundibulum, which leads to a partial obstruction of the follicular orifice and thus does not permit shedding of small telogen hairs.

The plugs may be removed with hydroactive adhesive (Biore) pads. Keratolytics are also effective after using a wax depilatory. The pulsed diode laser has been used successfully, and application of 0.05% tretinoin solution, applied daily for 2 or 3 months, may also produce satisfactory results.

Elston DM, et al: Treatment of trichostasis spinulosa with a hydroactive adhesive pad. Cutis 2000; 66:77.

Janjua SA, et al: Trichostasis spinulosa: possible association with prolonged topical application of clobetasol propionate 0.05% cream. Int J Dermatol 2007 Sep; 46(9):982–985.

Pozo L, et al: Dermoscopy of trichostasis spinulosa. Arch Dermatol 2008 Aug; 144(8):1088.

Intermittent hair-follicle dystrophy

Birnbaum et al reported a disorder of the hair follicle leading to increased fragility of the shaft, with no identifiable biochemical disturbance. The prevalence of this disorder is unknown.

Bubble hair deformity

Bubble hairs appear as areas of hair with altered texture. Fragility has been reported. The hairs may be curved or straight and stiff. Small, bubble-like defects are found within the hair shafts on light and electron microscopy. The condition is produced by overheating of wet hair with a malfunctioning hair dryer, analogous to the popping of popcorn. All damp hair will develop bubbles of gas when exposed to high heat.

Hypertrichosis

Hypertrichosis is an overgrowth of hair not localized to the androgen-dependent areas of the skin. Several forms exist. Many cases are induced by medications, including minoxidil, cyclosporine, and efalizumab. The excessive hair growth can be managed with bleaching, trimming, shaving, plucking, waxing, chemical depilatories, and electrosurgical epilation. Laser treatment with long-pulse Nd:YAG, diode, ruby, long- and short-pulse alexandrite lasers, and intense pulsed light sources can be effective. Skin type must be considered when choosing a laser system. The greatest experience in dark skin types has been with the long-pulse Nd:YAG laser.

Localized acquired hypertrichosis

Eyelash trichomegaly can occur with erlotinib, latanoprost, and intentionally with bimatoprost. Dermal tumors, such as melanocytic nevi, smooth muscle hamartomas, meningiomas, or Becker nevi, may have excessive terminal hair growth. Repeated irritation, trauma, occlusion under a cast, eczematous states, topical steroid use, linear melorheostotic scleroderma, lymphedema associated with filariasis, the Crow–Fukase (POEMS) syndrome, and pretibial myxedema may be other situations in which there is a localized increase in hair growth. Porphyrias generally show a localized hypertrichosis over the malar area, such as in porphyria cutanea tarda or variegate porphyria; however, in the Gunther variety of erythropoietic porphyria it may be generalized or more diffuse in nature.

Localized congenital hypertrichosis

Hypertrichosis cubiti (hairy elbows) consists of long vellus hair on the extensor surfaces of the distal third of the upper arm and the proximal third of the forearm bilaterally. It is a progressive, excessive growth of lanugo hairs that often begins in infancy; the hairs may reach a length of 10 cm. Later they become coarser, but regression has been observed during adolescence. There appear to be familial cases and a sporadic form. Short stature and some developmental abnormalities are present in some cases; however, there is no need for endocrine studies or other evaluation. The condition appears to be of cosmetic significance only.

Other causes of localized congenital hypertrichosis include congenital nevocytic nevi, anterior cervical hypertrichosis, and simple nevoid hypertrichosis. Localized hypertrichosis may be a sign of underlying spinal dysraphism when it occurs over the sacral midline.

Generalized congenital hypertrichosis (congenital hypertrichosis lanuginosa)

This rare type of excessive and generalized hairiness is a fully penetrant X-linked dominant trait. The entire body is covered with fine vellus hairs 2–10 cm long (Fig. 33-31). The scalp hair appears to be normal. Except for the palms and soles, all other areas are covered. Congenital hypertrichosis lanuginosa may be associated with dental anomalies and gingival fibromatosis. This type of hairiness has attracted considerable attention over the centuries. Hair removal by laser may be quite useful.

Other cases of congenital generalized hypertrichosis may be secondary to drug ingestion by the mother. The fetal hydantoin syndrome is characterized by hypertrichosis, depressed nasal bridge, large lips, a wide mouth, and a short, webbed

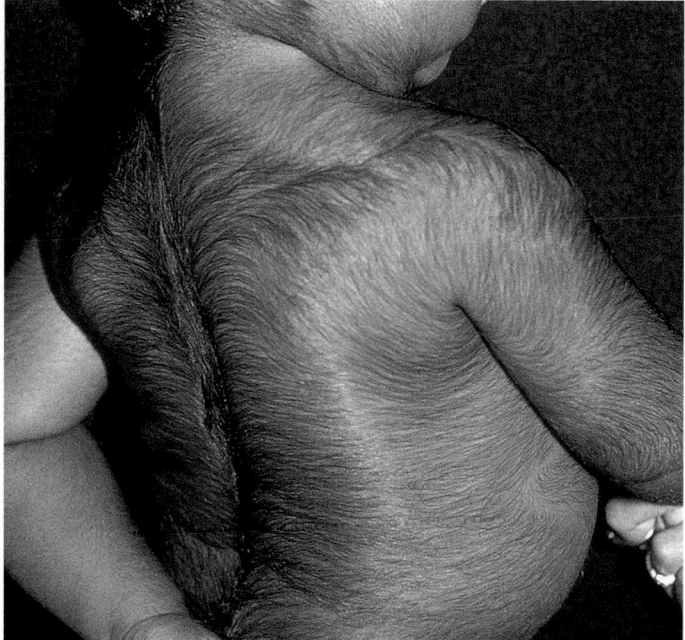

Fig. 33-31 Hypertrichosis lanuginosa. (Courtesy of Brooke Army Medical Center Teaching File)

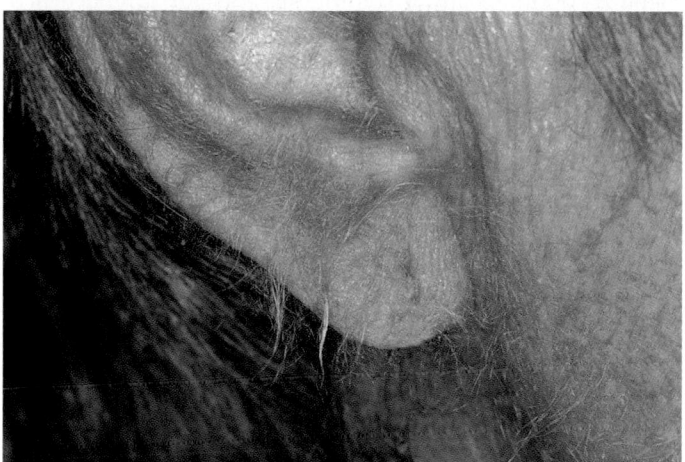

Fig. 33-32 Hypertrichosis lanuginosa associated with an internal malignancy (malignant down).

neck. The fetal alcohol syndrome includes hypertrichosis, a small face, capillary hemangiomas, and physical and mental retardation. A case of generalized hypertrichosis and multiple congenital defects was reported by Kaler et al in a baby born to a mother who used minoxidil throughout pregnancy. Fetal valproate syndrome is characterized by generalized hypertrichosis sparing the palms and soles, coarse facies, gum hypertrophy, hypotonia, club feet and club hands, and abnormal dermatoglyphics.

Generalized or patterned acquired hypertrichosis

These cases include those caused by acquired hypertrichosis lanuginosa, those associated with various syndromes, and those secondary to drug intake. Acquired hypertrichosis lanuginosa (Fig. 33-32) is an ominous sign of internal malignancy. Syndromes associated with increased hair growth include lipoatrophic diabetes, stiff skin syndrome, Down syndrome, Rubenstein–Taybi syndrome, Laband syndrome, Cornelia de Lange syndrome, Hurler syndrome, leprechaunism, Winchester syndrome, the Schynzel–Giedier syndrome, and hypertrichosis

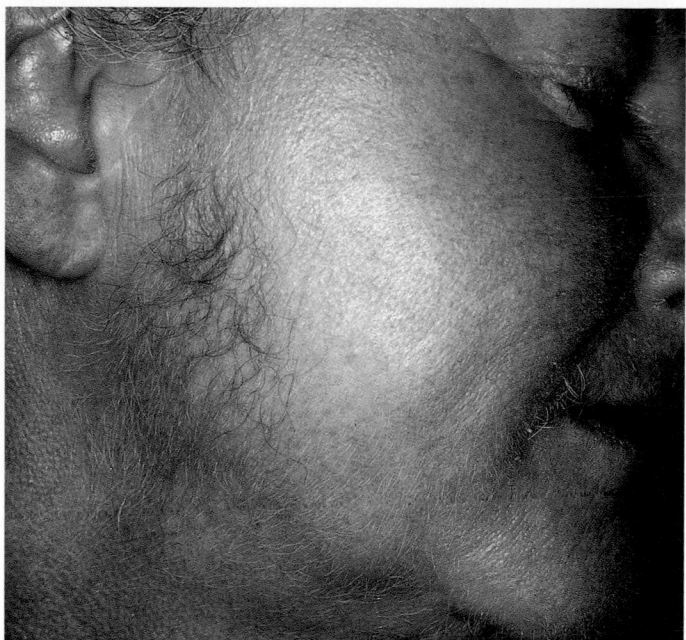

Fig. 33-33 Hirsutism.

with acromegalic features. Drugs associated with hypertrichosis include minoxidil, cyclosporine, diphenylhydantoin, diazoxide, streptomycin, penicillamine, corticosteroids, danazol, psoralens, hexachlorobenzene, PUVA, topical bimatoprost, topical steroids, and topical androgens.

Márquez G, et al: A case of trichomegaly of the eyelashes and facial hypertrichosis induced by erlotinib (Tarceva). Int J Dermatol 2009 Jan; 48(1):97–98.

Mendiratta V, et al: Hypertrichosis lanuginosa congenita. Pediatr Dermatol 2008 Jul–Aug; 25(4):483–484.

Papadopoulos R, et al: Trichomegaly induced by erlotinib. Orbit 2008; 27(4):329–330.

Rallis E, et al: Efalizumab-induced hypertrichosis. Br J Dermatol 2008 May; 158(5):1158–1159.

Hirsutism

Clinical features

Hirsutism is an excess of terminal hair growth in women in a pattern more typical of men. Androgen-dependent growth areas affected include the upper lip, cheeks (Fig. 33-33), chin, central chest, breasts, lower abdomen, and groin. This altered growth pattern of the hair may be associated with other signs of virilization, which include temporal balding, masculine habitus, deepening of the voice, clitoral hypertrophy, and amenorrhea. Acne is an additional sign of hyperandrogenism.

Pathogenesis

When virilization accompanies hirsutism, especially when progression is rapid, a neoplastic cause is likely. In the absence of virilization, a neoplastic cause is extremely unlikely. Most medically significant hirsutism is related to the polycystic ovarian syndrome (PCOS, hyperinsulinemic hyperandrogenism with anovulation). In a study of 873 patients with medically significant hirsutism, PCOS was present in 82%. Idiopathic hirsutism was present in 4.7%, and 6.75% of the patients had elevated androgen levels and hirsutism with normal ovulation.

Ethnic variation should be considered when evaluating hirsutism. Women of Southwest Asian, Eastern European and southern European heritage commonly have facial, abdominal, and thigh hair; whereas Asian and Indian women generally have little terminal hair growth in these areas.

In women, androgen biosynthesis occurs in the adrenal and ovary. Testosterone and the androgen precursor androstenedione are secreted by the ovary. The adrenal contributions are preandrogens: dehydroepiandrosterone (DHEA), DHEA sulfate, and androstenedione. They require peripheral conversion in the skin and liver to testosterone.

Testosterone is converted to dihydrotestosterone, the androgen that promotes androgen-dependent hair growth, in the hair follicle by 5-α-reductase. Receptor molecules in the end organ are necessary for binding and hormone action at that level. Because testosterone is normally bound to carrier molecules in the plasma at a 99% level, and it is the unbound testosterone that is active, the levels of free testosterone correlate with clinical evidence of androgen excess.

Hirsutism may result from excessive secretion of androgens from either the ovary or the adrenal gland. The excessive secretion may be from functional excesses or, rarely, from neoplastic processes. Ovarian causes include PCOS (Stein–Leventhal syndrome), and a variety of ovarian tumors, both benign and malignant. PCOS is defined by anovulation (fewer than nine periods a year or periods longer than 40 days apart) with clinical evidence of hyperandrogenism. Ovarian cysts are not required for the diagnosis, and laboratory and imaging studies are not required to establish the diagnosis. The pathogenesis of PCOS may relate to insulin resistance with resultant elevated insulin levels leading to ovarian overproduction of androgens. Prevalence rates of PCOS for black and white women in the US are 8.0% and 4.8%, respectively.

Ovarian tumors include unilateral benign microadenomas, arrhenoblastomas. Leydig cell tumors, hilar cell tumors, granular/theca cell tumors, and luteomas are rare causes of hirsutism. In tumor-associated hirsutism, the onset is usually rapid, occurs with other signs of virilization, and begins between the ages of 20 and 40.

Adrenal causes include congenital adrenal hyperplasia (CAH) and adrenal tumors, such as adrenal adenomas and carcinomas. The adrenogenital syndrome or CAH is an autosomal-dominant disorder that may result from deficiencies of the following enzymes: 21-hydroxylase (most common form), 11β-hydroxylase, or 3β-hydroxy steroid dehydrogenase. Onset is generally in childhood, with ambiguous genitalia, precocious growth, and virilism. Nonclassic (adult-onset) CAH may present with hirsutism.

Pituitary causes include Cushing's disease, acromegaly, and prolactin-secreting adenomas. Prolactin-secreting microadenomas have a 20% incidence of hirsutism and acne. Prolactin elevations may be seen in patients with PCOS. Other conditions in which prolactin levels may be elevated and that may lead to hirsutism include hypothyroidism, phenothiazine intake, and hepatorenal failure.

Other causes of hirsutism include the exogenous intake of androgens. End-organ hypersensitivity may be a mechanism in patients with a normal evaluation. Drugs such as minoxidil, diazoxide, corticosteroids, and phenytoin, which have been reported to cause hirsutism, generally cause hypertrichosis—a generalized increase in hair that is not limited to the androgen-sensitive areas.

Evaluation

Most hirsutism is related to ethnic heritage or PCOS. 21-Hydroxylase-deficient nonclassic adrenal hyperplasia, the hyperandrogenic insulin-resistant acanthosis nigricans syndromes, and androgen-secreting tumors are relatively uncommon causes. A careful history and physical examination are

essential. The history should focus on onset and progression, virilization, menstrual and pregnancy history, and family/racial background. Physical examination may reveal signs of Cushing's disease, hypothyroidism, or acromegaly. Other signs to be evaluated are the distribution of muscle mass and body fat, clitoral dimensions, voice depth, and galactorrhea.

Laboratory evaluation is controversial. In the authors' opinion, testing is of value only when it affects management. If this is accepted, there is no mandatory hormonal testing for stable hirsutism in patients who have no signs of virilization. A diagnosis of PCOS does not require laboratory confirmation. Determination of serum lipids and testing for glucose intolerance may be the most important laboratory evaluations in patients with PCOS, as they have the greatest impact on management and long-term prognosis. When the history and physical examination suggest the possibility of a neoplasm, laboratory evaluation should include a total testosterone level. A dehydroepiandrosterone sulfate level is commonly performed if an adrenal cause is suspected. A 24 h urine cortisol test is the gold standard for the diagnosis of Cushing's disease. Measurement of thyroid-stimulating hormone (TSH), growth hormone, and somatomedin C levels are indicated if the history and physical examination suggest hypothyroidism or acromegaly.

Dexamethasone suppression tests are recommended by some authorities, but the results often do not affect management. A baseline 17-hydroxyprogesterone and adrenocorticotropic hormone (ACTH) stimulation test can screen for late-onset CAH, but steroid replacement has not been proved to result in better outcomes than empiric treatment with antiandrogens. Baseline 17-hydroxyprogesterone may be normal in some women with nonclassic 21-hydroxylase deficiency, and ACTH stimulation may result in overdiagnosis of the syndrome. An exaggerated 17-hydroxyprogesterone response to ACTH stimulation is common in PCOS at a pharmacologic dose (250 μg) but not at a physiologic dose (1 μg) of ACTH. An ovarian origin of hirsutism can be identified by a buserelin test in 30% of patients with hirsutism and by dexamethasone in 22% of patients, but data proving that buserelin challenge results in better outcomes are lacking. A prolactin level will screen for prolactin-secreting tumors, but will also lead to further expensive testing in many patients ultimately diagnosed with PCOS. A prolactin level should be obtained in any patient with galactorrhea, but is of limited value as a routine screening test for patients with hirsutism alone.

If signs of acromegaly, Cushing's disease, or virilization are present clinically, referral to an endocrinologist is recommended. The presence of major menstrual irregularities is also an indication for referral to an endocrinologist or gynecologist. Although 90% of women with hirsutism have an elevated testosterone level, elevations above 200 ng/dL and rapid onset or progressive virilization suggest serious underlying disease. A major elevation in the DHEA sulfate level (greater than 7000 ng/mL) suggests an adrenal neoplasm, and imaging of the adrenal gland is recommended. Many patients with late-onset CAH will have normal screening DHEA sulfate. Patients with prolactin levels above 20 ng/mL should likewise be referred for further evaluation with an MRI or CT scan. Polymorphisms in the gene coding for sex hormone-binding globulin have been identified in some families with hirsutism, but such testing does not affect management.

Treatment

Various forms of mechanical, chemical, and laser epilation can be performed, as for hypertrichosis. Spironolactone with various oral contraceptives, cyproterone acetate plus ethinyl estradiol, gonadotropin-releasing hormone agonists such as leuprolide and nafarelin, flutamide, finasteride, and topical eflornithine have been used successfully alone and in various combinations to treat hirsutism. The optimal combination and dosage remain to be determined. Finasteride at doses of 2.5–5 mg/day has been shown to decrease hair number and diameter in women with hirsutism. The combination of spironolactone, 100 mg/day, plus finasteride, 5 mg/day, has been shown to be superior to spironolactone, 100 mg/day, alone. An analysis of the current literature suggested that spironolactone alone, 100 mg/day, is superior to finasteride alone, 5 mg/day, and low-dose cyproterone acetate alone, 12.5 mg/day for the first 10 days of a cycle, in the treatment of hirsutism. As spironolactone is commonly used at a dose of 100 mg twice a day, further studies are needed comparing this higher dose with other modes of therapy. In a prospective, randomized study of Diane 35 (cyproterone acetate [CPA], 2 mg, and ethinyl estradiol, 35 µg), Diane 35 plus spironolactone, and spironolactone alone, all treatments were well tolerated. Combination therapy resulted in superior measured endocrine responses, but the authors concluded that spironolactone alone was the most cost-effective treatment. The choice of an oral contraceptive (OC) is also controversial. Third-generation OCs result in a significant increase in sex hormone-binding globulin and decrease in free testosterone, but both second- and third-generation OCs are clinically effective in treating hirsutism. When flutamide is used, initial treatment with 250 mg/day is followed by a long maintenance treatment period using 125 mg/day.

Insulin sensitizers are being studied in the treatment of hirsutism, particularly PCOS. The best data to date are for metformin. Metformin therapy has been shown to control menstrual cycles and improve fertility in women with PCOS. It causes a decline in testosterone and insulin levels. Oligomenorrheic women with an increased luteinizing hormone (LH) to follicle-stimulating hormone (FSH) ratio and lower testosterone levels respond best. Spironolactone, 50 mg/day, was superior to metformin, 1000 mg/day, in the treatment of hirsutism and menstrual cycle frequency in a study of 82 adolescent and young women with PCOS. Doses of 200 mg/day are commonly used to treat hirsutism. At this dose, menstrual irregularities induced by the drug are common, and it may be best used in combination with an OC pill. Yasmin, which contains the progestogen drospirenone, has been shown to provide good cycle control for women with PCOS, with an improvement in acne but not in other symptoms of the syndrome. Good correlation has been noted between an increase in ovulation frequency with clomiphene citrate and the chance of pregnancy in women with PCOS. Other options include acarbose, gonadotrophins, and laparoscopic ovarian drilling. Infertility is best managed by a specialist in this field. Empiric treatment with an antiandrogen may be as good as steroid replacement for the management of hirsutism in patients with nonclassic CAH.

Abbas M, et al: The use of metformin as first line treatment in polycystic ovary syndrome. Ir Med J 2008 Feb; 101(2):51–53.

Blume-Peytavi U, et al: Medical treatment of hirsutism. Dermatol Ther 2008 Sep–Oct; 21(5):329–339.

Demirci C, et al: Congenital adrenal hyperplasia. Dermatol Ther 2008 Sep–Oct; 21(5):340–353.

Dikensoy E, et al: The risk of hepatotoxicity during long-term and low-dose flutamide treatment in hirsutism. Arch Gynecol Obstet 2009 Mar; 279(3):321–327.

Kircher C, et al: Acarbose for polycystic ovary syndrome. Ann Pharmacother 2008 Jun; 42(6):847–851.

Lin-Su K, et al: Congenital adrenal hyperplasia in adolescents: diagnosis and management. Ann N Y Acad Sci 2008; 1135:95–98.

Lujan ME, et al: Diagnostic criteria for polycystic ovary syndrome: pitfalls and controversies. J Obstet Gynaecol Can 2008 Aug; 30(8):671–679.

Minozzi M, et al: Treatment of hirsutism with myo-inositol: a prospective clinical study. Reprod Biomed Online 2008 Oct; 17(4):579–582.

Norman RJ, et al: Polycystic ovary syndrome. Lancet 2007 Aug 25; 370(9588):685–697.

Rosenfield RL: What every physician should know about polycystic ovary syndrome. Dermatol Ther 2008 Sep–Oct; 21(5):354–361.

Somani N, et al: The clinical evaluation of hirsutism. Dermatol Ther 2008 Sep–Oct; 21(5):376–391.

Wanitphakdeedecha R, et al: Physical means of treating unwanted hair. Dermatol Ther 2008 Sep–Oct; 21(5):392–401.

Trichomycosis axillaris

Discrete nodules, 1–2 mm in size and attached firmly to the hair shafts of the axillary or pubic areas, characterize trichomycosis. The color of the nodules may be yellow (Fig. 33-34), red, or black. Hyperhidrosis of the affected regions is usually present. A yellowish discoloration of the axillae is sometimes noted. Large numbers of *Corynebacterium* are present in the concretions. The disorder may coexist with erythrasma and pitted keratolysis. Treatment with topical antibiotic preparations, such as topical clindamycin or erythromycin, or naftifine, which has antibacterial properties, combined with any modality that will decrease the hyperhidrosis, is effective, but shaving is faster.

Rho NK, et al: A corynebacterial triad: prevalence of erythrasma and trichomycosis axillaris in soldiers with pitted keratolysis. J Am Acad Dermatol 2008 Feb; 58(2 Suppl):S57–S58.

Associated hair follicle diseases

Pityriasis amiantacea (tinea amiantacea)

Thick, asbestos-like (amiantaceous), shiny scales on the scalp characterize pityriasis amiantacea. The silvery-white or dull

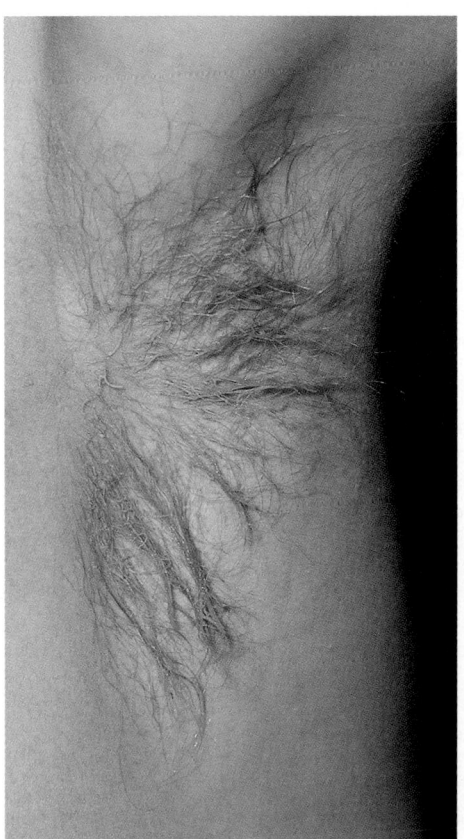

Fig. 33-34 Trichomycosis axillaris. (Courtesy of Anthony Slagel, MD)

gray crusting may be localized or, less often, generalized over the entire scalp. The proximal parts of the hairs are matted together by the laminated crusts. There are no structural changes in the hair, but in some patches where the crusting is thick, there may be some purulent exudate under the crust and temporary alopecia such as occurs after some cases of furunculosis of the scalp.

The cause is most often severe or untreated seborrheic dermatitis or psoriasis. In a prospective study of 85 patients, psoriasis was documented in 35% and processes suggesting seborrheic dermatitis or atopic dermatitis occurred in another 35%. Tinea capitis was the eventual diagnosis in 13%. Staphylococcus was found in 96.5%, compared with 15% of controls. The patient should shampoo daily or every other day with selenium sulfide suspension, or a tar- or steroid-containing shampoo, for a couple of weeks. Prior application of peanut oil or a keratolytic a few hours before shampooing facilitates removal of the scales and crusts. With such debridement, followed by topical steroid solution in Caucasians or steroid ointment in African Americans, the secondary bacterial infection usually resolves without the need for oral antistaphylococcal therapy.

Abdel-Hamid IA, et al: Pityriasis amiantacea: a clinical and etiopathologic study of 85 patients. Int J Dermatol 2003; 42:260.
Gordon D, et al: Dermacase: tinea or pityriasis amiantacea. Can Fam Physician 2009; 55:165.

Folliculitis nares perforans

Perforating folliculitis of the nose is characterized by small pustules near the tip of the inside of the nose. The lesion becomes crusted, and when the crust is removed it is found that the bulbous end of the affected vibrissa is embedded in the inspissated material. The affected hairs are typical of those occurring inside the nostril. *Staphylococcus aureus* may at times be cultured from the pustules. The hair should be removed and antibiotic ointment such as mupirocin applied.

White SW, et al: Pseudofolliculitis vibrissae. Arch Dermatol 1981; 117:368.

Acquired perforating dermatosis

Perforating folliculitis, Kyrle's disease, and acquired perforating collagenosis are designations that have been supplanted by the more inclusive term acquired perforating dermatosis. The condition is not uncommon and is most often associated with renal failure or diabetes or both. Between 4% and 10% of dialysis patients develop umbilicated dome-shaped papules on the legs, or less often on the trunk, neck, arms, or scalp, with variable itchiness (Fig. 33-35). Early lesions may be pustular; late lesions resemble prurigo nodularis both clinically and histologically. There is a central hyperkeratotic cone that projects into the dermis, so that when it is removed, a pitlike depression remains. Usually the papules are discrete, but they may coalesce to form circinate plaques. Coalescing verrucous plaques are frequently seen, especially on the lower extremities. Koebner phenomenon may also be observed, in which case plaques or elevated verrucous streaks are formed. The latter are seen primarily in the antecubital and popliteal spaces. Atrophic scars are seen on involution of these lesions.

Histologically, the epidermis becomes edematous, the granular layer disappears, and parakeratosis develops. Eventually, the epidermis becomes atrophic, with disruption of the sites over the papillae. Through these sites necrobiotic connective tissue, degenerating inflammatory cells, and collagen bundles are extruded into a cup-shaped epidermal depression.

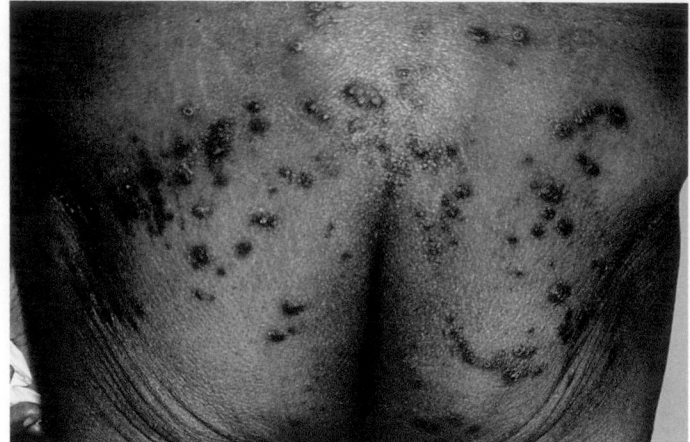

Fig. 33-35 Acquired perforating disease in uremia. (Courtesy of Curt Samlaska, MD)

The condition is felt to be a response to trauma, usually scratching or rubbing in response to the pruritus of the associated renal failure or dry skin. Other predisposing conditions reported include HIV infection, sclerosing cholangitis or other liver diseases, hypothyroidism, hyperparathyroidism, Hodgkin disease, in areas of healed herpes zoster, and as a reaction to laser hair removal or TNF-α inhibitors.

Ultraviolet treatment of either PUVA or UVB type helps the pruritus of renal disease and improves the perforating disorder. Hydration of the skin with a soaking tub bath in plain water, followed immediately (without drying) by triamcinolone ointment, is also useful. Topical retinoic acid (0.1% cream), allopurinol, doxycycline, isotretinoin, and etretinate have been effective in flattening lesions. HIV-infected patients may respond well to thalidomide. The disease may remit promptly after renal transplantation.

Doshi SN, et al: Koebnerization of reactive perforating collagenosis induced by laser hair removal. Laser Surg Med 2003; 32:177.
Gilaberte Y, et al: Perforating folliculitis associated with tumor necrosis factor-alpha inhibitors administered for rheumatoid arthritis. Br J Dermatol 2007; 156:368.
Hoque SR, et al: Acquired reactive perforating collagenosis. Br J Dermatol 2006; 154:759.
Iyoda M, et al: Acquired reactive perforating collagenosis in a nondiabetic hemodialysis patient. Am J Kidney Dis 2003; 42:E11.
Mahajan S, et al: Perforating folliculitis with jaundice in an Indian male: a rare case with sclerosing cholangitis. Br J Dermatol 2004; 150:614.
Ohe S, et al: Treatment of acquired perforating dermatosis with narrow band UVB. J Am Acad Dermatol 2004; 50:892.
Rivard J, et al: Ultraviolet phototherapy for pruritus. Dermatol Ther 2005; 18:344.
Saray Y, et al: Acquired perforating dermatosis. J Eur Acad Dermatol Venereol 2006; 20:679.

Reactive perforating collagenosis

Reactive perforating collagenosis is an inherited condition characterized by pinhead-sized, skin-colored papules that grow to a diameter of 4–6 mm and develop a central area of umbilication in which keratinous material is lodged (Fig. 33-36). The discrete papules may be numerous and involve sites of frequent trauma such as the backs of the hands, forearms, elbows, and knees. The lesion reaches a maximum size of about 6 mm in 4 weeks and then regresses spontaneously in 6–8 weeks.

It is believed that this is caused by a peculiar reaction of the skin to superficial trauma. Koebnerization is often observed. Young children are most frequently affected. Most reports

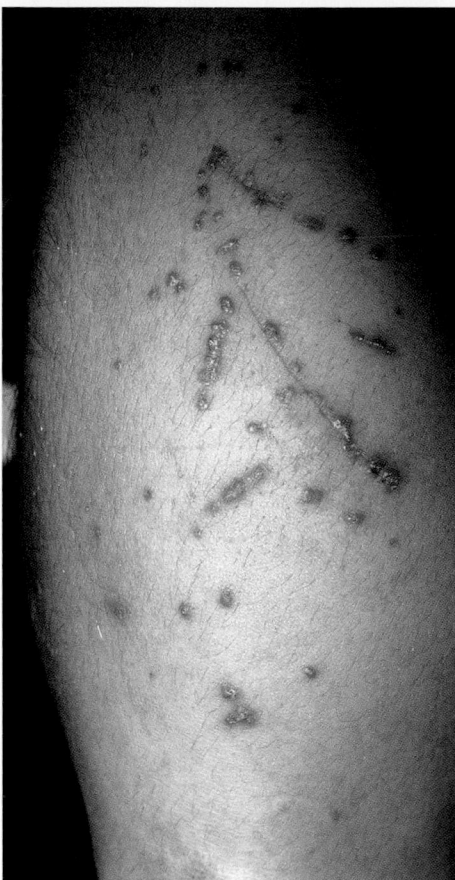

Fig. 33-36 Reactive perforating collagenosis.

Histologically, a slight hyperkeratosis occurs, with epidermal hyperpigmentation and dilation of the upper dermal vessels. The hair follicles may be enlarged in the infundibular area and the sebaceous glands may be hypertrophic. A lymphocytic infiltration surrounds the adnexa.

Ermertcan AT, et al: Erythromelanosis follicularis faciei et colli associated with keratosis pilaris in two brothers. Pediatr Dermatol 2006; 23:31.

Sardana K, et al: An observational analysis of erythromelanosis follicularis faciei et colli. Clin Exp Dermatol 2008; 33:333.

Disseminate and recurrent infundibulofolliculitis

Hitch and Lund described a disseminate follicular eruption on the torso of a black man that involved all the pilosebaceous structures. The lesions were irregularly shaped papules pierced by a hair. They likened the eruption to cutis anserina viewed through a magnifying glass. The eruption is mildly pruritic at times, and is chronic, with recurrent exacerbations. The papules are uniform, and 1 or 2 mm in diameter; they involve all the follicles in the affected areas, which are usually the upper trunk and neck, though the entire trunk and proximal extremities may be involved. Rarely, pustules may occur.

Histologically, the infundibular portion of the follicles is chiefly affected, and the lesions are inflammatory rather than hyperkeratotic. Edema, lymphocytic and neutrophilic infiltration, and slight fibroblastic infiltration surround the affected follicles.

Treatment with topical steroids, isotretinoin, or PUVA may be effective.

Aroni K, et al: Disseminate and recurrent infundibulofolliculitis: response to isotretinoin. J Drugs Dermatol 2004; 3:434.

Hinds GA, et al: A case of disseminate and recurrent infundibulofolliculitis responsive to treatment with topical steroids. Dermatol Online J 2008; 14:11.

Lichen spinulosus

Lichen spinulosus (keratosis spinulosa) is chiefly a disease of children and is characterized by minute filiform horny spines, which protrude from follicular openings independent of any papules. The spines are discrete and grouped. The lesions appear in crops and are symmetrically distributed over the trunk, limbs, and buttocks (acne corne). There is a predilection for the neck, buttocks, abdominal wall, popliteal spaces, and the extensor surfaces of the arms. Little or no itching is present. Occasional cases of a generalized form in adults with HIV infection or alcoholism have been reported.

Histologic evaluation shows simple inflammatory changes and follicular hyperkeratosis. The lesions may respond to keratolytics and emollients, such as salicylic acid, lactic acid, or urea gels or ointments. Tretinoin or tacalcitol creams are other alternatives. The lesions tend to involute at puberty.

Foreman SB, et al: Lichen spinulosus. Arch Dermatol 2007; 143:122.

Kim SH, et al: Successful treatment of lichen spinulosus with topical tacalcitol cream. Pediatr Dermatol 2010; (epub).

Disorders of the sweat glands

Hyperhidrosis

Hyperhidrosis, or excessive sweating, may be localized to one or several areas or it may be more generalized. True generalized hyperhidrosis is rare, and even hyperhidrosis caused by systemic diseases is usually accentuated in certain regions.

support an autosomal-recessive mode of inheritance; however, a family in which it appeared to be inherited by autosomal dominance has been reported.

No specific treatment is indicated, since the lesions involute spontaneously. Tretinoin 0.1% cream may be effective.

Ramesh V, et al: Familial reactive perforating collagenosis. J Eur Acad Dermatol Venereol 2007; 21:766.

Traumatic anserine folliculosis

Traumatic anserine folliculosis is a curious gooseflesh-like follicular hyperkeratosis that may result from persistent pressure and lateral friction of one skin surface on another. Such friction is often caused by habitual pressure on the elbows, chin, jaw, or neck, often while watching television. Two-thirds of patients who develop this are atopic.

Padilha-Gonalves A: Traumatic anserine folliculosis. J Dermatol 1979; 6:365.

Erythromelanosis follicularis faciei et colli

Erythromelanosis follicularis faciei et colli is an erythematous pigmentary disease involving the follicles. A reddish-brown, sharply demarcated, symmetrical discoloration involves the preauricular and maxillary regions. At times the pigmentation may be blotchy. In addition, follicular papules and erythema are present. Under diascopic pressure the reddish-brown area, containing telangiectases, becomes pale and the light brown pigmentation becomes more apparent. Pityriasiform scaling and slight itching may occur. Keratosis pilaris on the arms and shoulders is frequently found. It preferentially affects Asian and Indian patients.

Palmoplantar hyperhidrosis (emotional hyperhidrosis)

This type of hyperhidrosis is usually localized to the palms, soles, and/or axillae, and may be worse during warm temperatures. Patients with palm and sole hyperhidrosis may also have axillary hyperhidrosis, but only 25% of patients with axillary hyperhidrosis have palmoplantar hyperhidrosis. The hands may be cold and show a dusky hue. The soggy keratin of the hyperhidrotic soles is frequently affected by pitted keratolysis and has a foul odor. Sweating may be intermittent; in these cases anxiety, stress, or fear may trigger it. When sweating is constant, usually emotion is not as important.

This type of sweating can be autosomal-dominantly inherited. Its onset is in childhood for the palmar type and adolescence for axillary disease. It tends to improve with age. Sweating typically ceases during sleep.

Gustatory hyperhidrosis

Certain individuals regularly experience excessive sweating of the forehead, scalp, upper lip, perioral region, or sternum a few moments after eating spicy foods, tomato sauce, chocolate, coffee, tea, or hot soups. Gustatory sweating may be idiopathic or caused by hyperactivity of the sympathetic nerves (Pancoast tumor or postoperatively), sensory neuropathy (diabetes mellitus or subsequent to zoster), parotitis or parotid abscess, and surgery or injury of the parotid gland (auriculotemporal syndrome of von Frey). Frey syndrome occurs in one-third or more of patients following parotid surgery. Fortunately, only 10% of affected patients require treatment.

Other localized forms of hyperhidrosis

Localized sweating can occur over lesions of blue rubber bleb nevus, glomus tumors, and hemangiomas (sudoriferous hemangioma), and in POEMS syndrome, Gopalan syndrome, complex regional pain syndrome, as a result of spinal cord tumors (especially when unilateral palmar hyperhidrosis is the complaint), and pachydermoperiostosis.

Generalized hyperhidrosis

Febrile diseases, vigorous exercise, or a hot, humid environment, such as a tropical milieu, may induce generalized hyperhidrosis. Hyperthyroidism, acromegaly, diabetes mellitus, pheochromocytoma, hypoglycemia, salicylism, substance abuse, lymphoma, carcinoid syndrome, pregnancy, and menopause may also produce generalized hyperhidrosis. Additional causes of hyperhidrosis include concussion, Parkinson's disease, other disturbances of the sympathetic nervous system, and metastatic tumors producing a complete transection of the spinal cord. Drugs such as anticholinesterases, antidepressants of the selective serotonin-reuptake inhibitor or tricyclic types, antiglaucoma agents, bladder stimulants, opioids, and sialogogs may cause hyperhidrosis.

Treatment

The therapy of generalized hyperhidrosis is aimed at treating the underlying systemic disease. Virtually all cases of hyperhidrosis seen by dermatologists are of the palmoplantar or axillary types, and the treatments discussed below relate primarily to these conditions.

Topical medication Topical aluminum chloride or aluminum chlorhydroxide are the most commonly used agents for hyperhidrosis. For the axillae, application of a 10–35% solution nightly to a very dry axilla (blown dry with a hair dryer) is usually very effective. To limit irritation, lower concentrations should be tried first. Also, it should be washed off in 6–8 h. Occlusion is usually not required. In palmar hyperhidrosis the application of aluminum chloride nightly in up to a 50% concentration, alone or occluded with plastic gloves, has pro-

duced good results for some patients. If topical treatment is effective when performed nightly, the frequency may be reduced to as little as once or twice a week with continued benefit.

Iontophoresis Iontophoresis with plain tap water is an alternative for patients for whom topical treatments fail. It is frequently effective, using either a Drionic device or a Fischer unit. Treatments generally require 20–30 min sessions each day or twice a day. Once response has occurred, treatments may be used intermittently (as little as once every 2 weeks) for maintenance. Use of glycopyrrolate 0.01% and aluminum chloride 2% in the iontophoresis medium may hasten the response. A new dry-type iontophoresis has been described but is not readily available.

Botulinum toxin Injection of botulinum A toxin into 4 cm^2 areas on the palms, soles, or axillae dramatically reduces sweating at the treated areas to at least 25% and often to less than 10% of baseline rates. Dosages vary according to the type of botulinum toxin A and the site of treatment. Grunfeld et al offer a complete review of injection techniques and tips. Complications are rare but include some grip weakness when higher doses are used in the palms. This problem, the expense, and the painful injections limit its use in the palms and soles especially. The hypohidrosis continues for an average of 7 months, with some patients continuing to have substantial benefit at 16 months after one injection. Repeated injections generally do not lose efficacy and result in similar response and complication rates. This form of treatment should be offered to all patients who fail topical treatments before surgical modalities are considered. Frey syndrome remits for 1–1.5 years in nearly every patient treated. This treatment may be considered for other rare forms of localized hyperhidrosis. Myobloc (botulinum toxin B) is also effective, but with more limited duration of response.

Internal medication The use of anticholinergic agents such as propantheline bromide, oxybutynin (available in an extended-release formulation which may result in lower efficacy), and glycopyrrolate may be helpful. The dosage of each is regulated by the patient's tolerance and response. Often, sweating is suppressed just as anticholinergic side effects reach intolerable levels, and this approach has to be abandoned. Side effects of acetylcholine-blocking agents may also cause or aggravate such conditions as glaucoma and convulsions. The effects on sweating generally last 4–6 h, and many patients prefer to use the medication to ensure dryness for special occasions only, rather than as continuous treatment. Other agents reported to reduce localized hyperhidrosis include diltiazem and clonidine.

Surgical treatment Axillary hyperhidrosis may be effectively controlled by excision of the most actively sweating portion of the axillary skin, followed by undercutting and subcutaneous resection of the sweat glands for 1–2 cm on each side of the elliptical excision. This procedure is virtually always effective. Alternatively, liposuction or surgical ultrasonic aspiration removal may be used. The most important preoperative consideration is the accurate mapping of the most active sweating areas of the axillae. The responsible eccrine glands are not necessarily located in the same areas as the axillary hair and are often in a reasonably limited area. Mapping may be performed with cobalt chloride or starch iodide.

Upper thoracic sympathectomy has been found to be effective in excessive palmar sweating when all other measures have failed. Sympathetic denervation of the upper extremities is performed via endoscopy by reversibly clipping or performing resection of the fourth thoracic sympathetic ganglion. Acute surgical complications occur in less than 2% but include chronic pain, infection, pneumothorax, hemothorax, bleeding, pneumonia, and even death. Sweating of the hands is stopped completely. Only 60% of patients are satisfied, however, since compensatory and gustatory hyperhidrosis occurs in more than two-thirds of patients. This may be severe and as debilitating as the original problem. Topical glycopyrrolate may sometimes help alleviate compensatory hyperhidrosis, but it does not decrease with time. Horner syndrome may rarely result. Endoscopic thoracic sympathetic block at T4 is being evaluated as another alternative.

Anliker MD, et al: Tap water iontophoresis. Curr Probl Dermatol 2002; 30:48.

Bajaj V, et al: Use of oral glycopyrronium bromide in hyperhidrosis. Br J Dermatol 2007; 157:118.

Cheshire WP, et al: Disorders of sweating. Semin Neurol 2003; 23:399.

Cheshire WP, et al: Drug-induced hyperhidrosis and hypohidrosis. Drug Saf 2008; 31:109.

Cladellas E, et al: A medical alternative to the treatment of compensatory hyperhidrosis. Dermatol Ther 2008; 21:406.

Cohen JL, et al: Diagnosis, impact, and management of focal hyperhidrosis. Facial Plast Surg Clin North Am 2007; 15:17.

De Bree R, et al: Repeated botulinum toxin type A injections to treat patients with Frey syndrome. Arch Otolaryngol Head Neck Surg 2009; 135:287.

Grunfeld A, et al: Botulinum toxin for hyperhidrosis. Am J Clin Dermatol 2009; 10:87.

Hornberger J, et al: Recognition, diagnosis, and treatment of primary focal hyperhidrosis. J Am Acad Dermatol 2004; 51:274.

Klein A: Complications with the use of botulinum toxin. Dermatol Clin 2004; 22:197.

Krogstad AL, et al: Daily pattern of sweating and response to stress and exercise in patients with palmar hyperhidrosis. Br J Dermatol 2006; 154:1118.

Liu Y, et al: Surgical treatment of primary palmar hyperhidrosis. Eur J Cardiothorac Surg 2009; 35:398.

Mijnhout GS, et al: Oxybutynin. Neth J Med 2007; 65:356.

Na GY, et al: Control of palmar hyperhidrosis with a new "dry-type" iontophoretic device. Dermatol Surg 2007; 33:57.

Ojimba TA, et al: Drawbacks of endoscopic thoracic sympathectomy. Br J Surg 2004; 91:264.

Reisfeld R, et al: Evidence-based review of the nonsurgical management of hyperhidrosis. Thorac Surg Clin 2008; 18:157.

Seo SH, et al: Tumescent superficial liposuction with curettage for treatment of axillary hyperhidrosis. J Eur Acad Dermatol Venereol 2008; 22:30.

Sugimura H, et al: Thoracoscopic sympathetic clipping for hyperhidrosis. J Thorac Cardiovasc Surg 2009; 137:1370.

Talarico-Filho S, et al: A double-blind, randomized, comparative study of two type A botulinum toxins in the treatment of primary axillary hyperhidrosis. Dermatol Surg 2007; 33:S44.

Vor Kamp T, et al: Hyperhidrosis. Surgeon 2010; 8:287.

Walles T, et al: Long term efficiency of endoscopic thoracic sympathicotomy. Interact Cardiovasc Thorac Surg 2009; 8:54.

Wolina U, et al: Tumescent suction curettage versus minimal skin resection with subcutaneous curettage of sweat glands in axillary hyperhidrosis. Dermatol Surg 2008; 34:709.

Anhidrosis (hypohidrosis)

Anhidrosis is the absence of sweating. Hypohidrosis, or reduced sweating, is part of the spectrum of these disorders. Dysfunction in any step in the normal physiologic process of sweating can lead to decreased or absent sweating. It may be localized or generalized. Generalized anhidrosis occurs in anhidrotic ectodermal dysplasia, miliaria profunda (tropical asthenia), Sjögren syndrome, Fabry syndrome, hereditary sensory neuropathy (type IV) with anhidrosis, and in some patients with diabetic neuropathy, thyroid dysfunction, and multiple myeloma. A large number of drugs may cause hypohidrosis. These include anticholinergics, antidepressants of the tricyclic type, antiepileptics, antihistamines, antihypertensives, antipsychotics, antiemetics, antivertigo drugs, bladder antispasmodics, gastric antisecretory drugs, muscle

relaxants, neuromuscular paralytics, and opioids. Anhidrosis may follow infections, be part of a neurodegenerative disorder, occur as a symptom related to toxin exposure, be a paraneoplastic phenomenon, or be secondary to autoimmune inflammation. Atopic dermatitis is frequently associated with reduced sweating and pruritus when sweating is triggered. Patients with psoriasis may have similar symptoms, but less frequently.

Anhidrosis with pruritus is a rare syndrome of young adults. Severe itching occurs whenever they are stimulated to sweat. No sweat is delivered to the skin surface, but when the body temperature is raised by about 0.5°C, fine papules appear at each eccrine orifice. The associated pruritus is so severe that patients feel completely incapacitated and distracted. Cooling immediately resolves the symptoms. This may represent one form of tropical asthenia or a mild form of the autonomic neuropathies described below. The natural history is unknown, but spontaneous resolution may occur after several years. These patients are frequently misdiagnosed as having cholinergic urticaria.

Segmental anhidrosis may be associated with tonic pupils (Holmes–Adie syndrome); this is called Ross syndrome. Patients have heat intolerance and segmental areas of anhidrosis on the trunk, arms, or legs. Loss of deep tendon reflexes in the arms, trunk, and legs is consistently seen. Compensatory segmental hyperhidrosis of functionally intact areas may occur. A selective degeneration of the cholinergic sudomotor neurons is the hypothesized abnormality.

Autonomic neuropathies associated with antibodies to nicotinic acetylcholine receptors may cause a variety of symptoms related to dysfunction of systems controlled by autonomic nerves. There is a spectrum of abnormalities ranging from severe autonomic failure characterized by orthostatic hypotension, gastrointestinal dysmotility, anhidrosis, bladder dysfunction, and sicca syndrome to isolated anhidrosis and heat intolerance. In this condition a biopsy may reveal an inflammatory infiltrate surrounding the eccrine glands, and some patients respond to pulse steroids or immunosuppressants. It may also spontaneously resolve.

Anhidrosis localized to skin lesions occurs regularly over plaques of tuberculoid leprosy. This is also true of segmental vitiligo (but not generalized type), in the hypopigmented streaks of incontinentia pigmenti, in lesions of syringolymphoid hyperplasia with alopecia and anhidrosis, and on the face and neck of patients with the rare Bazex syndrome consisting of follicular atrophoderma, basal cell carcinomas, and hypotrichosis, an X-linked dominant disorder.

Cheshire WP, et al: Drug-induced hyperhidrosis and hypohidrosis. Drug Saf 2008; 31:109.

Hagemann G, et al: Adie's pupil in the Ross syndrome. N Engl J Med 2000; 355:e5.

Nolano M, et al: Ross syndrome. Brain 2006; 129:2119.

Ogino J, et al: Idiopathic acquired generalized anhidrosis due to occlusion of proximal coiled ducts. Br J Dermatol 2004; 150:589.

Palm F, et al: Successful treatment of acquired idiopathic generalized anhidrosis. Neurology 2007; 68:532.

Sandroni P, et al: Other autonomic neuropathies associated with ganglionic antibodies. Auton Neurosci 2009; 146:13.

Sommer C, et al: Selective loss of cholinergic sudomotor fibers causes anhidrosis in Ross syndrome. Ann Neurol 2002; 52:247.

Thami GP, et al: Acquired idiopathic generalized anhidrosis. Clin Exp Dermatol 2003; 28:262.

Vernino S, et al: Autonomic ganglia, acetylcholine receptor antibodies, and autoimmune ganglionopathy. Auton Neurosci 2009; 146:3.

Bromhidrosis

Also known as fetid sweat, osmidrosis and malodorous sweating, bromhidrosis is chiefly encountered in the axillae. Bacterial decomposition of apocrine sweat, producing fatty acids with distinctive offensive odors, is considered to be the cause. Often, patients who complain of offensive axillary sweat actually have no offensive odor; the complaint represents a delusion, paranoia, phobia, or a lesion of the central nervous system. Intranasal foreign body and chronic mycotic infection in the sinuses are additional causes. True bromhidrosis is usually not recognized by the patient.

Fish odor syndrome should be considered in patients presenting with complaints of offensive odor. It is caused by excretion of trimethylamine (which smells like rotten fish) in the eccrine sweat, urine, saliva, and other secretions. This chemical is produced from carnitine and choline in the diet and is normally metabolized in the liver. An autosomal-dominant defect in the ability to metabolize trimethylamine because of a defect in flavin-containing mono-oxygenase 3 is the cause of this syndrome. Dietary reduction of foods high in carnitine and choline is beneficial.

Antibacterial soaps and many commercial deodorants are quite effective in controlling axillary malodor. Frequent bathing, changing of underclothes, shaving of the axillae, and topical application of aluminum chloride (Drysol) are all helpful measures. Surgical removal of the glands either by excision or tumescent liposuction is possible, as in axillary hyperhidrosis, but this is rarely indicated. Botulinum toxin A injections in the axilla have controlled body odor in this site as well in the pubic area.

Plantar bromhidrosis is produced by bacterial action on eccrine sweat-macerated stratum corneum. Hyperhidrosis is the chief associated factor, and pitted keratolysis is often present. Careful washing with an antibacterial soap and the use of dusting powders on the feet are helpful in eliminating bromhidrosis. Use of topical antibiotics, such as clindamycin, may be beneficial. Previously described measures to control plantar hyperhidrosis should be instituted. Botulinum toxin A is likely to be effective.

Arseculeratne G, et al: Trimethylaminuria (fish odor syndrome). Arch Dermatol 2007; 143:81.

Heckman M, et al: Amelioration of body odor after intracutaneous axillary injection of botulinum toxin A. Arch Dermatol 2003; 139:57.

Lee JB, et al: A case of foul genital odor treated with botulinum toxin A. Dermatol Surg 2004; 30:1233.

Seo SH, et al: Tumescent superficial liposuction with curettage for treatment of axillary bromhidrosis. J Eur Acad Dermatol Venereol 2008; 22:30.

Chromhidrosis

Chromhidrosis, or colored sweat, is an exceedingly rare functional disorder of the apocrine sweat glands, frequently localized to the face or axilla. It has been less often noted on the abdomen, chest, breasts, thighs, groin, genitalia, and lower eyelids. The colored sweat may be yellow (most common), blue, green, or black. The colored secretion appears in response to adrenergic stimuli, which cause myoepithelial contractions. Colored apocrine sweat fluoresces and is caused by lipofuscin. Treatment with botulinum toxin A or topical capsaicin has been reported to be effective.

Eccrine chromhidrosis is caused by the coloring of the clear eccrine sweat by dyes, pigments, or metals on the skin surface. Examples are the blue–green sweat seen in copper workers and the "red sweat" seen in flight attendants from the red dye in the labels in life-vests. Brownish staining of the axillae and undershirt may occur in ochronosis. Bile secretion in eccrine sweat occurs in patients with liver failure and marked hyperbilirubinemia. Small, round, brown or deep-green macules occur on the palms and soles.

Gandhi V, et al: Apocrine chromhidrosis localized to the areola in an Indian female treated with topical capsaicin. Indian J Dermatol Venereol Leprol 2006; 72:382.

Matarasso SL: Treatment of facial chromhidrosis with botulinum toxin type A. J Am Acad Dermatol 2005; 52:89.

Polat M, et al: Apocrine chromhidrosis. Clin Exp Dermatol 2009; 39:e373.

Fox–Fordyce disease

Fox–Fordyce disease is rare, occurring mostly in women during adolescence or soon afterward. It may occasionally be familial in nature. It is characterized by conical, flesh-colored or grayish, intensely pruritic, discrete follicular papules in areas where apocrine glands occur. The axillae and areolae are the primary sites of involvement, but the umbilicus, pubes, labia majora, and perineum may be affected. Apocrine sweating does not occur in affected areas, and hair density may be decreased. In some cases there is no itching. Ninety percent of cases occur in women between the ages of 13 and 35, but the disease may present postmenopausally or in males. Pregnancy invariably leads to improvement.

Histologically, Fox–Fordyce disease is characterized by obstruction of the follicular ostia by orthokeratotic cells. An inflammatory infiltrate of lymphocytes surrounds the upper third of the hair follicles and upper dermal vessels. There is an associated spongiosis of the infundibulum at the site of entrance of the apocrine duct into the hair follicle. In one case, detached apoeccrine cells obstructed the duct. Foam cells have been noted to be a histologic marker, as many of the above findings are either nonspecific or difficult to demonstrate. Localized axillary xanthomatosis has been postulated to be either a variant of Fox–Fordyce disease or a type of verruciform xanthoma.

No form of therapy is universally effective for Fox–Fordyce disease. Oral contraceptive pills, topical tretinoin or adapalene, topical pimecrolimus or weak corticosteroid creams, intralesional steroids, topical clindamycin solution, benzoyl peroxide, isotretinoin, and UV phototherapy have all been effective in small numbers of patients. Excision or liposuction-assisted curettage may be successful in axillary sites.

Chae KM, et al: Axillary Fox–Fordyce disease treated with liposuction-assisted curettage. Arch Dermatol 2002; 138:452.

Bormate AB Jr, et al: Perifollicular xanthomatosis as a hallmark of axillary Fox–Fordyce disease. Arch Dermatol 2008; 144:1020.

Ghislain P-D, et al: Itchy papules of the axillae. Arch Dermatol 2002; 138:259.

Kamada A, et al: Apoeccrine sweat duct obstruction as a cause for Fox–Fordyce disease. J Am Acad Dermatol 2003; 48:453.

Pock L, et al: Pimecrolimus is effective in Fox–Fordyce disease. Int J Dermatol 2006; 45:1134.

Scroggins L, et al: Fox–Fordyce disease in daughter and father. Dermatology 2009; 218:176.

Granulosis rubra nasi

Granulosis rubra nasi is a rare familial disease of children, occurring on the nose, cheeks, and chin. It is characterized by diffuse redness, persistent hyperhidrosis, and small dark red papules that disappear on diascopic pressure. The tip of the nose is red or violet. There may be a few small pustules. Hyperhidrosis precedes the erythema (Fig. 33-37). The tip of the nose is cold and is not infiltrated. The disease disappears spontaneously at puberty without leaving any traces. The cause is unknown. Histologically, blood vessels are dilated and there is an inflammatory infiltrate about the sweat ducts.

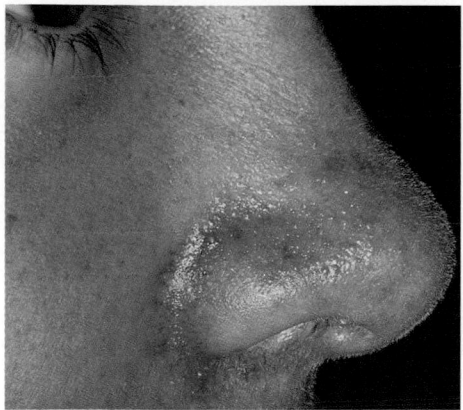

Fig. 33-37 Early granulosis rubra nasi.

Treatment is with local preparations for relief of the inflammation, and reassurance that with puberty there is usually involution of the process.

Akhdari N: Granulosis rubra nasi. Int J Dermatol 2007; 46:396.

Hidradenitis

Hidradenitis is a term used to describe diseases in which the histologic abnormality is primarily an inflammatory infiltrate around the eccrine glands. This group includes neutrophilic eccrine hidradenitis and idiopathic plantar hidradenitis (recurrent palmoplantar hidradenitis).

Neutrophilic eccrine hidradenitis

Ninety percent of patients with neutrophilic eccrine hidradenitis (NEH) have a malignancy. It has been described primarily in patients with acute myelogenous leukemia (AML); however, other leukemias, lymphomas, and uncommonly solid tumors may be present. It usually begins about 10 days after the start of chemotherapy. While the majority of patients have been treated with cytarabine, it has not been uniformly linked to any chemotherapeutic agent and may occur in patients who have not been treated. Patients with AML in remission have been reported to develop NEH with associated sclerodermoid changes that herald a relapse of the leukemia. Granulocyte colony-stimulating factor (G-CSF), imatinib mesylate, zidovudine, acetaminophen, and various antibiotics have also been implicated as triggers for this neutrophilic dermatosis.

The lesions are typically erythematous and edematous papules and plaques of the extremities, trunk, face (periorbital), and palms (in decreasing frequency). Pigmentation, purpura, or pustules may be present within the papules and plaques. Fever and neutropenia are often present. Histologically, there is a dense neutrophilic infiltrate around and infiltrating eccrine glands. Necrosis of sweat glands may be present, with or without the inflammatory infiltrate. Syringosquamous metaplasia may occur. This finding can also occur in fibrosing alopecia, in burn scars, adjacent to various nonmelanoma skin cancers and ischemic and surgical ulcers, in alopecia mucinosa, and in ports of radiation therapy.

The lesions may recur with repeated courses of chemotherapy, but many do not. Resolution over 1–4 weeks (average, 10 days) usually occurs. Nonsteroidal anti-inflammatory drugs or oral corticosteroids may hasten the healing. Prophylactic administration of dapsone prevented recurrence in one patient.

Infectious neutrophilic hidradenitis may present as a recurrent, pruritic, papular eruption. *Serratia*, *Enterobacter cloacae*, *Nocardia*, and *Staphylococcus aureus* have been implicated, and appropriate antibiotics for bacterial agents are curative. The diagnosis is confirmed by histologic evaluation and culture of affected tissue (surface cultures may not be adequate). Additionally, many HIV-infected patients have developed neutrophilic eccrine hidradenitis.

Recurrent palmoplantar hidradenitis

Recurrent palmoplantar hidradenitis is primarily a disorder of healthy children and young adults. Lesions are primarily painful, subcutaneous nodules on the plantar surface, resembling erythema nodosum. Rarely, palmar lesions also occur. In some children *Pseudomonas* infection may be the cause (pseudomonal hot foot, see Chapter 14). Children may present refusing to walk because of plantar pain. The condition is typically recurrent, and may be triggered by exposure to wet shoes or cold, damp weather. The use of oral and topical steroidal preparations may be beneficial.

Antonovich DD, et al: Infectious eccrine hidradenitis caused by *Nocardia*. J Am Acad Dermatol 2004; 50:315.
Crawford GH, et al: Erythematous facial plaques in a patient with leukaemia. Arch Dermatol 2003; 139:531.
Rubinson R, et al: Palmoplantar eccrine hidradenitis: seven new cases. Pediatr Dermatol 2004; 21:466.
Shih IH, et al: Childhood neutrophilic eccrine hidradenitis. J Am Acad Dermatol 2005; 52:963.
Srivastava M, et al: Neutrophilic eccrine hidradenitis masquerading as facial cellulitis. J Am Acad Dermatol 2007; 56:693.
Yasukawa K, et al: Neutrophilic eccrine hidradenitis with sclerodermoid change heralding the relapse of AML. Dermatology 2007; 215:261.

Diseases of the nails

Several general references are available that review a wide spectrum of nail changes.

Andre J, et al: Pigmented nail disorders. Dermatol Clin 2006; 24:329.
Baran R, et al: Baran and Dawber's Diseases of the Nails and Their Management. Oxford: Blackwell Science, 2008.
Bodman MA: Nail dystrophies. Clin Podiatr Med Surg 2004; 21:663.
DeBerker D: Childhood nail diseases. Dermatol Clin 2006; 24:355.
Holzberg M: Common nail disorders. Dermatol Clin 2006; 24:349.
Iorizzo M, et al: Nail cosmetics in nail disorders. J Cosmet Dermatol 2007; 6:53.
Kovich OI, et al: Clinical pathologic correlations for diagnosis and treatment of nail disorders. Dermatol Ther 2007; 20:11.
Nandedkar-Thomas MA, et al: An update on disorders of the nails. J Am Acad Dermatol 2005; 52:877.
Piraccini BM, et al: Drug-induced nail diseases. Dermatol Clin 2006; 24:387.
Rich P, Scher R: Atlas of Nail Diseases. New York: Pantheon, 2003.
Scher R, Daniel CR (eds): Nails. Philadelphia: Elsevier, 2005.
Tosti A, et al: The nail in systemic diseases. Dermatol Clin 2006; 24:341.

Nail-associated dermatoses

Numerous dermatoses are associated with characteristic, sometimes specific, nail changes. Many are considered elsewhere.

Lichen planus of nails

The reported incidence of nail involvement in lichen planus varies from less than 1% to 10%. Lichen planus of the nails may occur without skin changes, but 25% with nail disease will have lichen planus at other locations. Although it may occur at any age, most commonly it begins during the fifth or sixth decade of life. The nail plate may be markedly thinned, and at times distinct papules of lichen planus may involve the nailbed. Twenty-nail dystrophy (trachyonychia) may be the

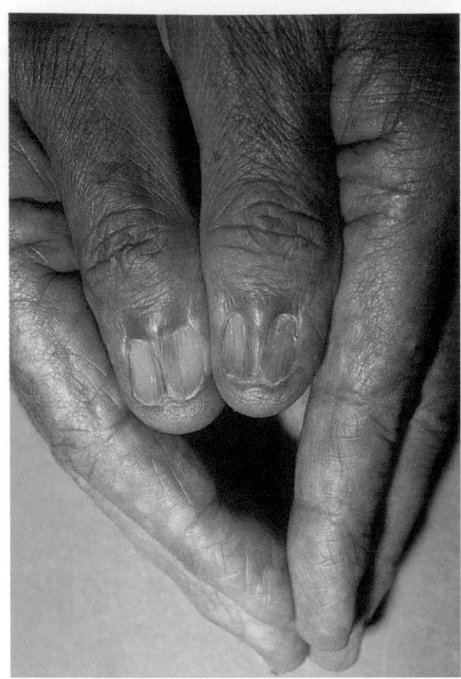

Fig. 33-38 Pterygium caused by lichen planus. (Courtesy of Lawrence Lieblich, MD)

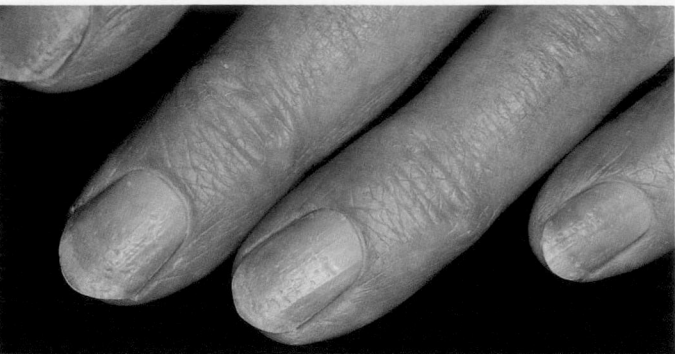

Fig. 33-39 Pitting caused by psoriasis.

Scheinfeld NS: Trachyonychia: a case report and review of manifestations, associations, and treatments. Cutis 2003; 71:299.
Tosti A, et al: Nail lichen planus in children: clinical features, response to treatment and long term follow-up. Arch Dermatol 2001; 137:1027.

Psoriatic nails

Nail involvement in psoriasis is common, with reported incidences varying from 10% to 78%. Older patients, those with active exacerbations of disease, and those with psoriatic arthritis are more likely to express nail abnormalities. In the nail plate there may be pits (Fig. 33-39), or much less often, furrows or transverse depressions (Beau's lines), crumbling nail plate, or leukonychia, with a rough or smooth surface. Splinter hemorrhages are found in the nailbed, with reddish discoloration of a part or all of the nailbed, and horny masses. In the hyponychium, subungual hyperkeratosis, oil spots, and a yellowish–green discoloration may occur in the area of onycholysis. Onychomycosis may be closely simulated. The severity of nail disease may correlate with the severity of skin and joint disease. Pustular psoriasis may produce onycholysis, with lakes of pus in the nailbed or in the perionychial areas. Rarely, anonychia may result. Other papulosquamous diseases may affect the nails like psoriasis, with the exception of nail pitting. Reiter's disease, pityriasis rubra pilaris, Sézary syndrome, and acrokeratosis paraneoplastica produce as a rule hypertrophic nails with subungual hyperkeratosis.

Psoriatic nail disease may be a solitary finding or be part of a widespread skin and nail involvement. The treatment options selected depend on the degree of cutaneous and nail involvement. (See Chapter 10 for additional information and therapeutic options.) Successful systemic treatment of psoriasis will usually also improve or clear the nail changes. Methotrexate, PUVA, cyclosporine, the biologics, or acitretin may be effective. All local therapies have limitations. Intralesional injection of triamcinolone acetonide suspension, 3–5 mg/mL, with a 30-gauge needle is frequently helpful. Digital nerve block facilitates adequate injection. Topical 5-fluorouracil (5-FU) applied to the proximal nailfold has been reported to be effective. It is best to avoid the free edge of the nail when applying 5-FU, as it may cause distal onycholysis. Topical cyclosporine and topical tazarotene 0.1% gel may also be helpful. Topical calcipotriol improves about 50% of patients with localized pustular psoriasis of the nails and may be used as a maintenance treatment after successful intervention with systemic retinoids.

sole manifestation of lichen planus. Other nail changes are irregular longitudinal grooving and ridging of the nail plate, thinning of the nail plate, pterygium formation (Fig. 33-38), shedding of the nail plate with atrophy of the nailbed, subungual keratosis, or even onychopapilloma, erythronychia (red streaks), subungual hyperpigmentation, and nail degloving. This latter sign is a newly described entity where there is partial or total shedding of the nail or the entire nail apparatus. The surrounding skin may also slough. This may be caused by trauma, ischemia and gangrene, or severe dermatologic disease such as toxic epidermal necrolysis or lichen planus.

The histologic changes of lichen planus may be evident in any individual nail constituent or a combination of them. The one most frequently involved is the matrix.

Treatment is mostly unsatisfactory. Intralesional injection of corticosteroids may be of help in some patients. Digital nerve blocks should be considered before infiltration of the matrix or nailbed. Topical corticosteroids under polyethylene occlusive dressings are usually inadequate. Clobetasol combined with tazarotene may be successful. Oral prednisone (0.5–1 mg/kg for 3 weeks) or oral retinoids in combination with topical steroids applied to the involved sites has been successful in some patients. Tosti et al reported that typical lichen planus of the nails in children responded to 0.5–1 mg/kg/month of intramuscular triamcinolone acetonide given for 3–6 months, until the proximal half of the nail was normalized. Disease recurred in only two patients during the follow-up period. While twenty-nail dystrophy was not treated, patients spontaneously improved; those with idiopathic atrophy of the nails were unchanged. (See Chapter 12 for additional therapeutic considerations.)

Baran R, et al: Nail degloving, a polyetiologic condition with 3 main patterns. J Am Acad Dermatol 2008; 58:232.
De Berker DA, et al: Localized longitudinal erythronychia. Arch Dermatol 2004; 140:1253.
Okiyama N, et al: Squamous cell carcinoma arising from lichen planus of nail matrix and nail bed. J Am Acad Dermatol 2005; 53:908.
Piraccini BM, et al: Nail lichen planus. Eur J Dermatol 2010; 20:489.
Richert B, et al: Nail bed lichen planus associated with onychopapilloma. Br J Dermatol 2007; 156:107.

Cassell S, et al: Therapies for psoriatic nail disease. J Rheumatol 2006; 33:1452.
De Berker D: Management of psoriatic nail disease. Semin Cutan Med Surg 2009; 28:39.
Diluvio L, et al: Childhood nail psoriasis. Pediatr Dermatol 2007; 24:332.
Jiaravuthisan MM, et al: Psoriasis of the nail. J Am Acad Dermatol 2007; 57:1.

Noiles K, et al: Nail psoriasis and biologics. J Cutan Med Surg 2009; 13:1.

Piraccini BM, et al: Pustular psoriasis of the nails. Br J Dermatol 2001; 144:1000.

Salomon J, et al: Psoriatic nails: a prospective clinical study. J Cutan Med Surg 2003; 7:317.

Tosti A, et al: Evaluation of the efficacy of acitretin therapy for nail psoriasis. Arch Dermatol 2009; 145:269.

Darier's disease

Longitudinal, subungual, red or white streaks, associated with distal wedge-shaped subungual keratoses, are the nail signs diagnostic for Darier–White disease. Keratotic papules on the dorsal portion of the nailfold may clinically resemble acrokeratosis verruciformis, but histologically have features of Darier's disease. Other nail findings include splinter hemorrhages and leukonychia. All of these findings are less pronounced on the toenails.

Baran R, et al: An effective surgical treatment for nail thickening in Darier's disease. J Eur Acad Dermatol Venereol 2005; 19:689.

Dc Berker DA, et al: Localized longitudinal erythronychia. Arch Dermatol 2004; 140:1253.

Clubbing

Clubbing is divided into two types: idiopathic and acquired, or secondary. The changes occur not only in the nails but also in the terminal phalanges. The nails bulge and are curved in a convex arc in both transverse and longitudinal directions. The eponychium is thickened. The angle formed by the dorsal surface of the distal phalanx and the nail plate (Lovibond's angle) is approximately 160°; however, with clubbing this angle is obliterated and becomes 180° or greater (Fig. 33-40). There is no diamond-shaped window when the dorsal surfaces of the corresponding finger of each hand are opposed (Schamroth's sign). The soft tissues of the terminal phalanx are bulbous and of are mobile when pressure is applied over the matrix. Thickening of the nailbed is present and can be assessed reliably by a plain radiograph of the index finger.

Idiopathic clubbing is either of the isolated dominantly inherited type or of the pachydermoperiostosis type with its associated findings. In the hereditary isolated type, a homozygous missense mutation in exon 6 of the human *HPGD* gene encoding NAD(+)-dependent 15-hydroxyprostaglandin dehydrogenase (15-PGDH) has been identified. Secondary (acquired) clubbing is usually a consequence of pulmonary, cardiac, thyroid, hepatic, or gastrointestinal disease. Around 36% of HIV patients has been documented to express clubbed nails. Typically, there is periostitis, with periosteal new bone formation in the phalanges, metacarpals, and distal ulna and radius. This is called hypertrophic osteoarthropathy and is responsible for the painful clubbing. It typically occurs in men with bronchogenic carcinoma. Unilateral or asymmetrical clubbing may also occur in Takayasu arteritis and sarcoidosis.

Dever LL, et al: Digital clubbing in HIV-infected patients. AIDS Patient Care STDS 2009; 23:19.

Moriera AL, et al: Clubbed fingers. Clin Anat 2008; 21:314.

Myers KA, et al: The rational clinical examination. Does this patient have clubbing? JAMA 2001; 286:1972.

Pallarés-Sanmartin A, et al: Validity and reliability of the Schamroth sign for the diagnosis of digital clubbing. JAMA 2010; 304:159.

Spicknall KE, et al: Clubbing. J Am Acad Dermatol 2005; 52:1020.

Tariq M, et al: Mutation in the HPGD gene encoding NAD+dependent 15-hydroxyprostaglandin dehydrogenase underlies isolated congenital nail clubbing. J Med Genet 2009; 46:14.

Shell nail syndrome

Cornelius et al described a shell nail in association with bronchiectasis. The nail resembles a clubbed nail, but the nailbed is atrophic instead of being a bulbous proliferation of the soft tissue.

Cornelius CE: Shell nail syndrome. Arch Dermatol 1969; 100:118.

Koilonychia (spoon nails)

Spoon nails are thin and concave, with the edges everted so that if a drop of water were placed on the nail, it would not run off (Fig. 33-41). Koilonychia may result from faulty iron metabolism and is one of the signs of Plummer–Vinson syndrome, as well as of hemochromatosis. Spoon nails have been observed in coronary disease, syphilis, polycythemia, and acanthosis nigricans. Familial forms are also known to occur. Other associations include psoriasis, lichen planus, Raynaud disease, scleroderma, acromegaly, hypothyroidism and hyperthyroidism, monilethrix, palmar hyperkeratoses, and steatocystoma multiplex. A significant number of cases are idiopathic. Manual trauma in combination with cold exposure may result in seasonal disease. Sherpas are Tibetan people living in the Nepalese Himalayas, who often serve as porters on mountain-climbing expeditions. Chronic cold exposure, in combination with hypoxemia, may contribute to the high frequency with which koilonychia is observed among them.

Gao XH, et al: Familial koilonychia. Int J Dermatol 2001; 40:290.

Kumar G, et al: Koilonychia, or spoon-shaped nails, is generally associated with iron-deficiency anemia. Ann Emerg Med 2007; 49:243.

Congenital onychodysplasia of the index fingers

Congenital onychodysplasia of the index fingers is defined by the presence of the condition at birth, index finger involvement (unilateral or bilateral), variable distortion of the nail or lunula, and polyonychia, micronychia, anonychia, hemionychogryphosis, or malalignment. It may also involve adjacent fingers, such as the middle fingers and thumbs. An underlying bone dysplasia may be present beneath the involved nail. Cases have occurred in an autosomal-dominant pattern; other proposed causes include in utero ischemia or exposure to teratogens.

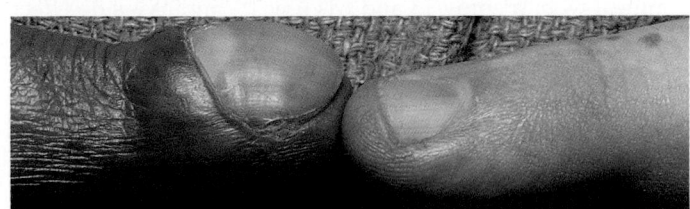

Fig. 33-40 Clubbing. (Courtesy of Lawrence Lieblich, MD)

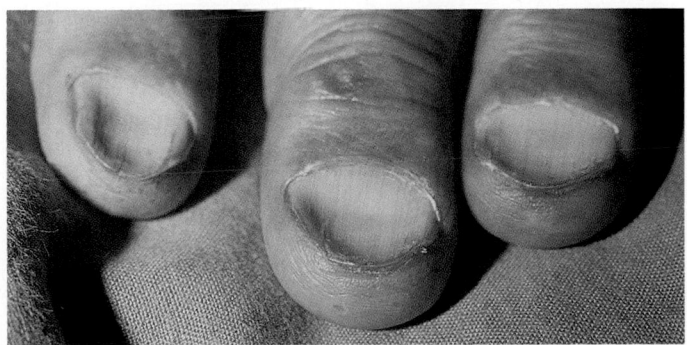

Fig. 33-41 Koilonychia.

De Smet L: Congenital onychodysplasia of the index finger. Genet Couns 2000; 11:37.

Prais D, et al: Prevalence and new phenotypic and radiologic findings in congenital onychodysplasia of the index finger. Pediatr Dermatol 1999; 16:201.

Trachyonychia

The nails may become opalescent, thin, dull, fragile, and finely ridged longitudinally (and as a result, distally notched). When this involves all 20 nails, it is referred to as twenty-nail dystrophy. This latter presentation may be seen at any age from 1½ years to adulthood, although it is most commonly diagnosed in children. It can be idiopathic or caused by alopecia areata, psoriasis, lichen planus, atopy, ichthyosis vulgaris, or other inflammatory dermatoses. Familial forms exist. In some cases spongiosis may be found on nail biopsy. Trachyonychia has also been reported associated with autoimmune processes such as selective IgA deficiency, vitiligo, sarcoidosis, and graft versus host disease. Unilateral involvement may occur in complex regional pain syndrome. Thus it is caused by a heterogenous group of inflammatory conditions. Tazarotene alone or in association with topical steroids may improve the condition. Childhood cases may resolve spontaneously; in one study 50% cleared within 6 years.

Blanco FP, et al: Trachyonychia. J Drugs Dermatol 2006; 5:469.

Grover C, et al: Longitudinal nail biopsy: utility in 20-nail dystrophy. Dermatol Surg 2003; 29:1125.

Pucevich B, et al: Unilateral trachyonychia in a patient with reflex sympathetic dystrophy. J Am Acad Dermatol 2008; 58:320.

Sakata S, et al: Follow up of 12 patients with trachyonychia. Australas J Dermatol 2006; 47:166.

Scheinfeld NS: Trachyonychia: a case report and review of manifestations, associations, and treatments. Cutis 2003; 71:299.

Soda R, et al: Treatment of trachyonychia with tazarotene. Clin Exp Dermatol 2005; 30:301.

Onychauxis

In onychauxis the nails are thickened but without deformity (simple hypertrophy). Simple thickening of the nails may be the result of trauma, acromegaly, Darier's disease, psoriasis, or pityriasis rubra pilaris. Some cases are hereditary.

Treatment involves periodic partial or total debridement of the thickened nail plate by mechanical or chemical (40% urea paste) means. Matricectomy and nail ablation are options, as they are in onychogryphosis, congenital nail dystrophies, and chronic painful nails such as recalcitrant ingrown toenails or splits within the medial or lateral third of the nail.

Baran R, et al: Matricectomy and nail ablation. Hand Clin 2002; 18:696.

Singh G, et al: Nail changes and disorders among the elderly. Indian J Dermatol Venereol Leprol 2005; 71:386.

Onychogryphosis

Hypertrophy may produce nails resembling claws or a ram's horn. Onychogryphosis may be caused by trauma or peripheral vascular disorders but is most often caused by neglect (failure to cut the nails for very long periods). It is most commonly seen in the elderly.

Some recommend avulsion of the nail plate with surgical destruction of the matrix with phenol or the CO_2 laser, if the blood supply is good.

Baran R, et al: Matricectomy and nail ablation. Hand Clin 2002; 18:696.

Mohrenschlager M, et al: Onychogryphosis in elderly persons. Cutis 2001; 68:233.

Onychophosis

A common finding in the elderly, onychophosis is a localized or diffuse hyperkeratotic tissue that develops on the lateral or proximal nailfolds, within the space between the nailfolds and the nail plate. It may involve the subungual area, as a direct result of repeated minor trauma, and most frequently affects the first and fifth toes. The use of comfortable shoes should be encouraged. The areas involved should be debrided and treated with keratolytics. Emollients are also helpful.

Singh G, et al: Nail changes and disorders among the elderly. Indian J Dermatol Venereol Leprol 2005; 71:386.

Anonychia

Absence of nails, a rare anomaly, may be the result of a congenital ectodermal defect, ichthyosis, severe infection, severe allergic contact dermatitis, self-inflicted trauma, Raynaud phenomenon, lichen planus, epidermolysis bullosa, or severe exfoliative diseases. Permanent anonychia has been reported as a sequel of Stevens–Johnson syndrome. It may also be found in association with congenital developmental abnormalities, such as microcephaly, and wide-spaced teeth (autosomal-recessive inheritance), the autosomal-dominant Cooks syndrome (bilateral nail hypoplasia of digits 1–3, the absence of nails of digits 4 and 5 of the hands, total absence of all toenails, and absence or hypoplasia of the distal phalanges of the hands and feet), DOOR syndrome (deafness, onycho-osteodystrophy, mental retardation), and the glossopalatine syndrome (abnormal mouth, tongue being attached to the temporomandibular joint).

It may also present as an autosomal-recessive disorder with anonychia as the solitary finding. It has been found to be caused by a mutation in the *R-spondin 4* gene. R-spondins are secreted proteins that activate the Wnt/β-catenin signaling pathway. *R-spondin 4* is exclusively expressed in the mesenchyme underlying the digit tip epithelium in embryonic mice.

Al Hawsawi K, et al: Anonychia congenita totalis. Int J Dermatol 2002; 41:397.

Bruchle NO, et al: RSPO4 is the major gene in autosomal-recessive anonychia and mutations cluster in the furin-like cysteine-rich domains of the Wnt signaling ligand R-spondin4. J Invest Dermatol 2008; 128:791.

Ishii Y, et al: Mutations in R-spondin 4 underlie inherited anonychia. J Invest Dermatol 2008; 128:867.

Ozdemir O, et al: Total anonychia congenita. Genet Couns 2004; 15:43.

Pall A, et al: Twenty-nail anonychia due to lichen planus. J Dermatol 2004; 31:146.

Onychoatrophy

Faulty underdevelopment of the nail may be congenital or acquired. The nail is thinned and small. Vascular disturbances, epidermolysis bullosa, lichen planus, Darier's disease, multicentric reticulohistiocytosis, and Hansen's disease may cause onychoatrophy. It is also seen in congenital syndromes such as Apert, Goltz, Turner, Ellis–van Creveld, nail–patella, dyskeratosis congenita, cartilage–hair hypoplasia, progeria, hypohidrotic ectodermal dysplasia, incontinentia pigmenti, popliteal web, trisomy 13 and trisomy 18, and as a side effect of etretinate therapy.

Al Hawsawi K, et al: Anonychia congenita totalis. Int J Dermatol 2002; 41:397.

Onychomadesis

Onychomadesis is a periodic idiopathic shedding of the nail beginning at its proximal end. The temporary arrest of the

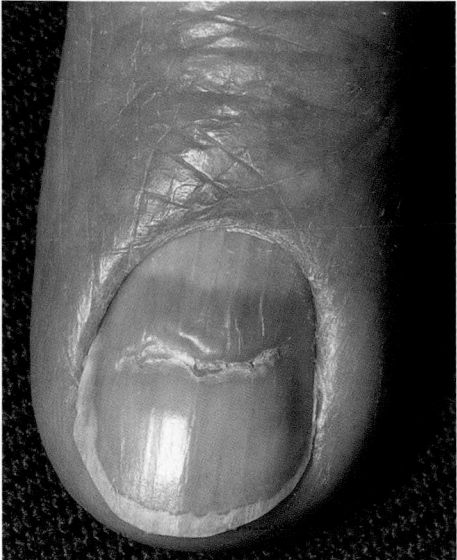

Fig. 33-42 Beau's lines.

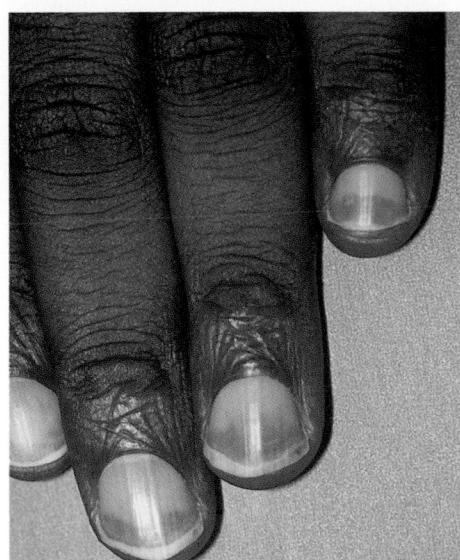

Fig. 33-43 Half and half nails.

function of the nail matrix may cause onychomadesis. Neurologic disorders, peritoneal dialysis, cutaneous T-cell lymphoma, Kawasaki's disease, pemphigus vulgaris, drug allergy, and keratosis punctata palmaris et plantaris have been reported causes. It may appear as a periodic finding in runners. Immobilization from casting for fractures may cause onychomadesis and pyogenic granuloma formation. Medications such as antineoplastic agents, azithromycin, and retinoids may cause onychomadesis also.

Bodman MA: Nail dystrophies. Clin Podiatr Med Surg 2004; 21:663.

Mehra A, et al: Idiopathic familial onychomadesis. J Am Acad Dermatol 2000; 43:349.

Patel NC, et al: Neonatal onychomadesis with candidiasis limited to affected nails. Pediatr Dermatol 2008; 25:641.

Piraccini BM, et al: Drug-induced nail diseases. Dermatol Clin 2006; 24:387.

Tosti A, et al: Onychomadesis and pyogenic granuloma following cast immobilization. Arch Dermatol 2001; 137:231.

Beau's lines

Beau's lines are transverse furrows that begin in the matrix and progress distally as the nail grows (Fig. 33-42). They are ascribed to the temporary arrest of function of the nail matrix. Although usually found to be bilateral, unilateral Beau's lines may occur. Various systemic and local traumatic factors may cause this. They may result from almost any systemic illness or major injury, such as a broken hip. Some specific associations are childbirth, measles, paronychia, acute febrile illnesses, high altitude exposure, and drug reaction. When the process is intermittent, the nail plate may resemble corduroy. Shelley "shoreline" nails appear to be a very severe expression of essentially the same transient growth arrest. They have been reported in all 20 nails of a newborn.

Guhl G, et al: Beau's lines and multiple periungual pyogenic granulomas after long stay in an intensive care unit. Pediatr Dermatol 2008; 25:278.

Mortimer NJ, et al: Beau's lines. N Engl J Med 2004; 351:1778.

Piraccini BM, et al: Drug-induced nail diseases. Dermatol Clin 2006; 24:387.

Half and half nails

Half and half nails show the proximal portion of the nail white and the distal half red, pink, or brown, with a sharp line of demarcation between the two halves (Fig. 33-43). Seventy-six percent of hemodialysis patients and 56% of renal transplant patients have at least one type of nail abnormality. Half and half nails are the most frequent, affecting 20% of hemodialysis patients. Absence of lunula, splinter hemorrhage, and half and half nails were significantly more common in hemodialysis patients, while leukonychia was significantly more common in transplant patients.

Salem A, et al: Nail changes in chronic renal failure patients under haemodialysis. J Eur Acad Dermatol Venereol 2008; 22:1326.

Saray Y, et al: Nail disorders in hemodialysis patients and renal transplant recipients: a case control study. J Am Acad Dermatol 2004; 50:197.

Muehrcke's lines

Muehrcke described narrow white transverse bands occurring in pairs as a sign of chronic hypoalbuminemia. The lines may resolve when serum albumin is raised to or near normal (Fig. 33-44). Unlike Mees' lines, the disturbance appears to be in the nailbed, not in the nail plate. Similar lines have been reported in patients with normal albumin levels who are receiving chemotherapy. In a case of unilateral Muehrcke's lines associated with trauma, it was suggested that edema effects this change by inducing microscopic separation of the normally tightly adherent nail from its bed.

Alam M, et al: Muehrcke's lines in a heart transplant recipient. J Am Acad Dermatol 2001; 44:316.

Chen W, et al: Nail changes associated with chemotherapy in children. J Eur Acad Dermatol Venereol 2007; 21:186.

Morrison-Bryant M, et al: Muehrcke's lines. N Engl J Med 2007; 30:917.

Mees' lines

Mees described single or multiple white transverse bands in 1919 as a sign of inorganic arsenic poisoning. They have also been reported in thallium poisoning, septicemia, dissecting aortic aneurysm, parasitic infections, chemotherapy, and both acute and chronic renal failure.

Chauhan S, et al: Mees' lines. Lancet 2008; 372:1410.

Hall AH: Chronic arsenic poisoning. Toxicol Lett 2002; 128:69.

Lu CI, et al: Short-term thallium intoxication. Arch Dermatol 2007; 143:93.

Uede K, et al: Skin manifestations in acute arsenic poisoning from the Wakayama curry-poisoning incident. Br J Dermatol 2003; 149:757.

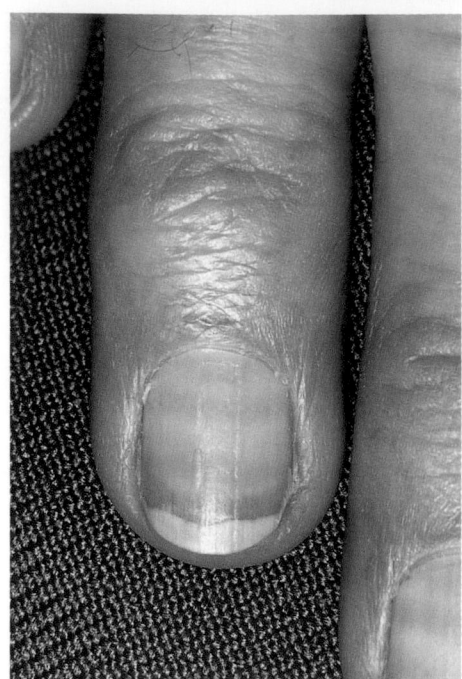

Fig. 33-44 Muehrke's lines.

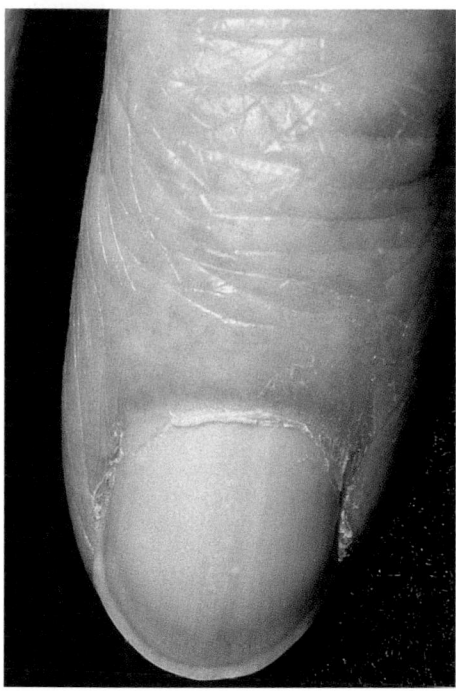

Fig. 33-45 Terry nails.

Zhao G, et al: Clinical manifestations of acute thallium poisoning. Eur Neurol 2008; 60:292.

Terry nails

In Terry nails the distal 1–2 mm of the nail shows a normal pink color (Fig. 33-45), while the entire nail plate or proximal end has a white appearance as a result of telangiectases in the nailbed. These changes have been noted in 25% of hospitalized patients, most commonly those with cirrhosis, chronic congestive heart failure, and adult-onset diabetes, and in very elderly patients.

Blyumin M, et al: Terry nails. Cutis 2005; 76:172.

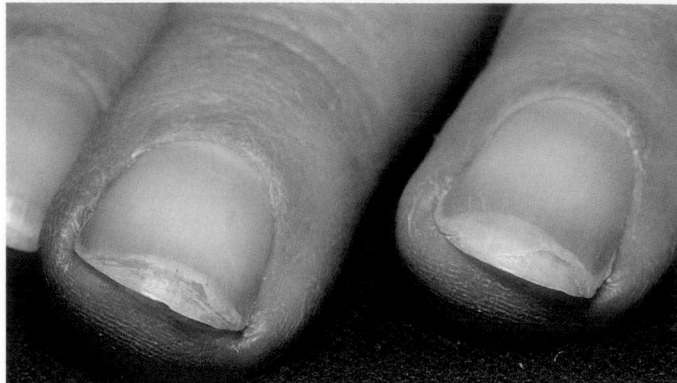

Fig. 33-46 Onychoschizia.

Onychorrhexis (brittle nails)

Brittleness with breakage of the nails may result from frequent soap and water exposure, nail polish remover, hypothyroidism, anorexia or bulimia, or after oral retinoid therapy. It affects up to 20% of the population, women twice as often as men. Fragilitas unguium (nail fragility) is part of this process. In a series of 35 patients treated with biotin, 63% showed clinical improvement. The nail plate thickness in patients treated with biotin increases by 25%. Daily application of white petrolatum after soaking in water is also helpful.

Uyttendaele H, et al: Brittle nails: pathogenesis and treatment. J Drugs Dermatol 2003; 2:48.
Van de Kerkhof PC: Brittle nail syndrome. J Am Acad Dermatol 2005; 53:644.

Onychoschizia

Splitting of the distal nail plate into layers at the free edge (Fig. 33-46) is a very common problem among women and represents a dyshesion of the layers of keratin, possibly as a result of dehydration. Longitudinal splits may also occur. Patients with biotinidase deficiency may manifest onychoschizia, along with total or partial alopecia and an eczematous or desquamating periorificial eruption. Hypotonia, seizures, and developmental delay in children and depression in adults are the most common systemic abnormalities. Lack of treatment may result in loss of hearing and vision.

Nail polish should be discontinued; nail buffing can be substituted. Frequent application of emollients may be helpful. Biotin has also been shown to be effective in doses up to 2.5 mg/day, or 2–4 times that much in deficient patients.

Redondo-Mateo J, et al: Facial erythema and onychoschizia. Arch Dermatol 2005; 141:1457.

Stippled nails

Small, pinpoint depressions in an otherwise normal nail characterize this type of nail change. This may be an early change seen in psoriasis. Stippled nails are also seen with some cases of alopecia areata, in early lichen planus, psoriatic or rheumatoid arthritis, chronic eczematous dermatitis, perforating granuloma annulare, and in some individuals with no apparent disease. The deeper, broader pits are more specific for psoriasis. The pitting in alopecia areata tends to be shallower and more regular, suggesting a "Scotch plaid" (tartan) pattern.

Tosti A, et al: Prevalence of nail abnormalities in children with alopecia areata. Pediatr Dermatol 1994; 11:12.

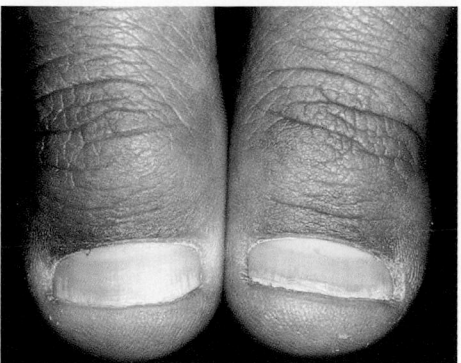

Fig. 33-47 Racquet nails.

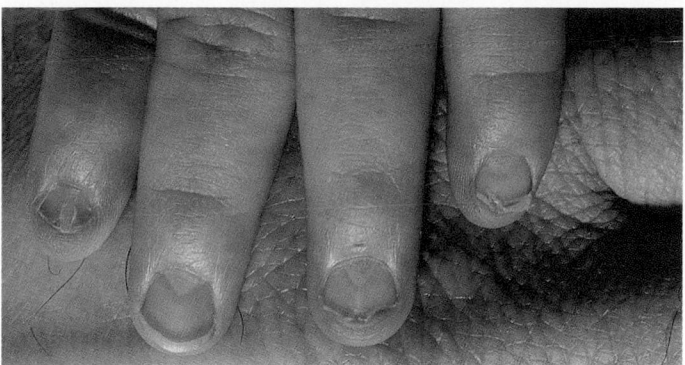

Fig. 33-48 Nail–patella syndrome. (Courtesy of Marshall Guill, MD)

Racquet nails (nail en raquette)

In racquet nails, the end of the thumb is widened and flattened, the nail plate is flattened as well, and the distal phalanx is abnormally short (Fig. 33-47). Racquet nails occur on one or both thumbs and are apparently inherited as an autosomal-dominant trait.

Baran R, et al: Baran and Dawber's Diseases of the Nails and Their Management. Oxford: Blackwell Scientific, 2008.

Chevron nail (herringbone nail)

This entity appears to be a rare transient fingernail ridge pattern of children. The ridges arise from the proximal nailfold and converge in a V-shaped pattern toward a midpoint distally.

Parry EJ: Chevron nail/herringbone nail. J Am Acad Dermatol 1999; 40:497.
Zaiac MN, et al: Chevron nail. J Am Acad Dermatol 1998; 38:773.

Hapalonychia

Softened nails result from a defect in the matrix that makes the nails thin and soft so that they can be easily bent. This type of nail change is attributed to malnutrition and debility. It may be associated with myxedema, rheumatoid arthritis, anorexia, bulimia, Hansen's disease, Raynaud phenomenon, oral retinoid therapy, or radiodermatitis.

Baran R, et al: Baran and Dawber's Diseases of the Nails and Their Management. Oxford: Blackwell Scientific, 2008.

Platonychia

The nail is abnormally flat and broad. It may be seen as part of an autosomal-dominant condition in which multiple nail abnormalities are present in many members of a large family.

Hamm H, et al: Isolated congenital nail dysplasia: a new autosomal dominant condition. Arch Dermatol 2000; 136:1239.

Nail–patella syndrome (hereditary osteo-onychodysplasia, Fong syndrome)

Nail–patella syndrome comprises numerous anomalies and is characterized by the absence or hypoplasia of the patella and congenital nail dystrophy. Triangular lunulae are characteristic (Fig. 33-48). Other bone features are thickened scapulae, hyperextensible joints, radial head abnormalities, and posterior iliac horns. The skin changes may also include webbing of the elbows. Eye changes such as cataracts, glaucoma, and heterochromia of the iris may also be present.

Hyperpigmentation of the pupillary margin of the iris ("Lester iris") is a characteristic finding in about half the cases. Patients with nail–patella syndrome may exhibit glomerulonephritis with urinary findings of albuminuria, hematuria, and casts of all kinds, especially hyaline casts. They may be predisposed to developing hemolytic–uremic syndrome, edema, and hypertension. Sixty percent of patients have renal abnormalities, and 20% suffer from renal failure. It is an autosomal-dominant trait localized to the distal long arm of chromosome 9. Limb and kidney defects seen in L1M-homeodomain protein Lmx1b mutant mice are similar to those present in patients with nail–patella syndrome. Mutations of the human *LMX1B* gene result in this syndrome.

Bongers EM, et al: Nail–patella syndrome. Overview on clinical and molecular findings. Pediatr Nephrol 2002; 17:703.
Dyer JA, et al: Multiple triangular lunula unguis. Mo Med 2007; 104:506.
Granata A, et al: Nail–patella syndrome and renal involvement. Clin Nephrol 2008; 69:377.
Lee BH, et al: Clinico-genetic study of nail–patella syndrome. J Korean Med Sci 2009; 24(Suppl):S82.
Schulz-Butulis BA, et al: Nail–patella syndrome. J Am Acad Dermatol 2003; 49:1086.

Onychophagia

Nail biting is a common compulsive behavior that may markedly shorten the nail bed, sometimes damages the matrix, and at times leads to pterygium formation. It is a difficult habit to cure. If there is strong motivation, habit reversal training with awareness training, competing response training, and social support may help. Psychopharmacologic intervention with medications, such as serotonin-reuptake inhibitors, and hypnosis are other options.

Ravindran AV, et al: Obsessive–compulsive spectrum disorders. Can J Psychiatry 2009; 54:331.
Tanaka OM, et al: Nailbiting, or onychophagia. Am J Orthod Dentofacial Orthop 2008; 134:305.
Twohig MP, et al: Evaluating the efficacy of habit reversal: comparison with a placebo control. J Clin Psychiatry 2003; 64:40.

Onychotillomania

Onychotillomania is a compulsive neurosis in which the patient picks constantly at the nails or tries to tear them off. Like onychophagia, this obsessive–compulsive disorder may be treated by biofeedback, cognitive–behavioral methods, hypnosis, or psychopharmacologic agents.

Inglese M, et al: Onychotillomania. Cutis 2004; 73:171.
Lin YC, et al: Onychotillomania, major depressive disorder and suicide. Clin Exp Dermatol 2006; 31:597.
Shenefelt PH: Biofeedback, cognitive–behavioral methods and hypnosis in dermatology. Dermatol Ther 2003; 16:114.

Onycholysis

Onycholysis is a spontaneous separation of the nail plate, usually beginning at the free margin and progressing proximally. Rarely, the lateral borders may be involved, with spread confined to these. Less often, separation may begin proximal to the free edge, in an oval area 2–6 mm broad, with a yellowish-brown hue ("oil spot"). This is a lesion of psoriasis; ordinary distal onycholysis is also commonly due to psoriasis. The nail itself is smooth and firm with no inflammatory reaction. Underneath the nail a discoloration may occur from the accumulation of bacteria, most commonly *Pseudomonas*, or yeast, most commonly *Candida*. Color changes, such as green (a result of pyocyanin from *Pseudomonas*), black, or blue may be seen. One or more nails may be affected.

Onycholysis is noted most commonly in women, probably secondary to traumatically induced separation. It is common in patients with hand dermatitis. Keratinization of the distal nailbed, chronic exposure to irritants, untreated dermatitis, and secondary infection with *Candida albicans* are potential reasons for the failure of the nail to reattach itself.

Systemic causes are many: hyper- and hypothyroidism, pregnancy, porphyria, pellagra, and syphilis. Onycholysis has also been associated with atopic dermatitis, eczema, lichen planus, congenital abnormalities of the nails, trauma induced by clawing, pinching, stabbing (manicuring), and foreign-body implantation. It may be caused by mycotic, pyogenic, or viral (herpes) infections. Women should be checked for vaginal candidiasis, because that anatomic location may be the source of the infection opportunistically invading and aggravating onycholysis. Chemical causes may include the use of solvents, nail polish base coat, nail hardeners containing formalin derivatives, artificial fingernails, and allergic or irritant contact dermatitis from their use. Rarely, photo-onycholysis may occur during or soon after therapy with tetracycline derivatives, psoralens, fluoroquinolones, or chloramphenicol, and subsequent exposure to sunlight. Chemotherapeutic agents and systemic retinoids may induce onycholysis. On rare occasions it may be a sign of subungual exostoses, squamous cell carcinoma, or metastasis. Autosomal-dominant hereditary forms are also known.

Trauma and chemical irritants should be completely avoided and the nailbed should be kept completely dry. The affected portion of the nail should be kept clipped away. Drying by exposing the nailbed in this way will rid the area of *Pseudomonas* and assist greatly in eliminating *Candida*. The combination of drying and topical steroids to minimize inflammation will often allow for reattachment of the nail and improvement or cure. Usually, this process takes 3–6 months or more to occur.

Anoop TM, et al: Plummer's nails. Onycholysis. N Z Med J 2008; 121:66.
Baran R, et al: Photoonycholysis. Photodermatol Photoimmunol Photomed 2002; 18:202.
Helsing P, et al: Onycholysis induced by nail hardener. Contact Dermatitis 2007; 57:280.
Hogeling M, et al: Onycholysis associated with capecitabine in patients with breast cancer. J Cutan Med Surg 2008; 12:93.
Piraccini BM, et al: Drug-induced nail diseases. Dermatol Clin 2006; 24:387.

Median nail dystrophy (dystrophia unguis mediana canaliformis, solenonychia)

Median nail dystrophy consists of longitudinal splitting or canal formation in the midline of the nail. The split, which often resembles a fir tree, occurs at the cuticle and proceeds outward as the nail grows (Fig. 33-49). Trauma has been sus-

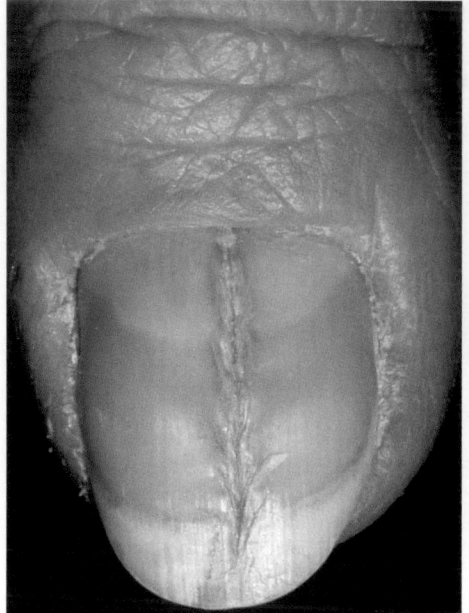

Fig. 33-49 Median nail dystrophy.

pected of being the chief cause. Repeated typing with the nail tip on personal digital assistants or Blackberry™-type devices has been reported to cause a median nail dystrophy. Some cases will resolve with avoidance of trauma; however, many will persist for years despite scrupulous care. The deformity may result from a papilloma or glomus tumor in the nail matrix, producing a structure like a tube (solenos) distal to it. Familial cases and an onset with isotretinoin therapy are other associations.

Olszewska M, et al: The PDA nail. Am J Clin Dermatol 2009; 10:193.
Sweeney SA, et al: Familial median canaliform nail dystrophy. Cutis 2005; 75:161.

Pterygium unguis

Pterygium unguis forms as a result of scarring between the proximal nailfold and matrix. The classic causative example is lichen planus. It has been reported to occur as a result of sarcoidosis, porokeratosis of Mibelli, peripheral circulatory disturbances, and Hansen's disease. Onychomatricoma may uncommonly simulate pterygium, but histologic examination will confirm the nature of this benign tumor.

Kim DS, et al: Pterygium unguis formation in porokeratosis of Mibelli. Br J Dermatol 2007; 156:1384.
Perrin C, et al: Onychomatricoma with dorsal pterygium. J Am Acad Dermatol 2008; 59:990.
Richert BJ, et al: Pterygium of the nail. Cutis 2000; 66:343.

Pterygium inversum unguis

Pterygium inversum unguis is characterized by adherence of the distal portion of the nailbed to the ventral surface of the nail plate (Fig. 33-50). The condition may be present at birth or acquired, and may cause pain with manipulation of small objects, typing, and close manicuring of the nail. It is a condition resulting from the extension of the zone of the nailbed that normally contributes to the formation of the nail plate. This eventually leads to a more ventral and distal extension of the hyponychium. The most common forms of pterygium inversum unguis are the acquired secondary forms caused by systemic connective tissue diseases, particularly progressive systemic sclerosis and SLE.

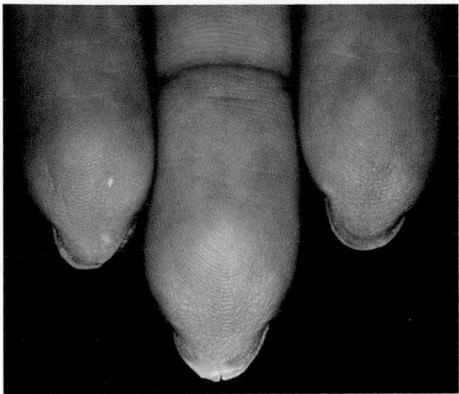

Fig. 33-50 Pterygium inversum unguis.

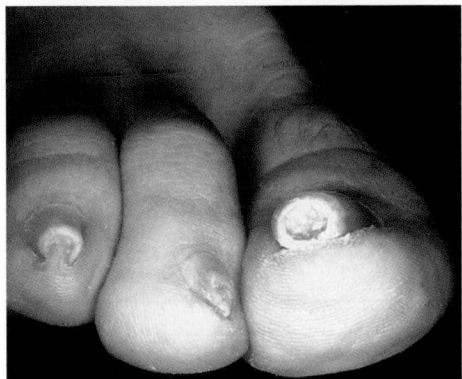

Fig. 33-51 Pincer nails.

Paley K, et al: Pterygium inversum unguis secondary to acrylate allergy. J Am Acad Dermatol 2008; 52(2 Suppl):S53.

Vadmal M, et al: Pterygium inversum unguis associated with stroke. J Am Acad Dermatol 2005; 53:501.

Hangnail

Hangnail is an overextension of the eponychium (cuticle), which becomes split and peels away from the proximal or lateral nailfold. These lesions are painful and annoying, so that persistent cuticle biting frequently develops. Trimming these away with scissors is the best solution. The use of emollient creams to keep the cuticle soft is also recommended.

Lee HJ, et al: Minor cutaneous features of atopic dermatitis in South Korea. Int J Dermatol 2000; 39:337.

Pincer nails

Pincer nails, trumpet nails, or omega (from the shape of the Greek letter) nails are alternative terms for a common toenail disorder in which the lateral edges of the nail slowly approach one another, compressing the nailbed and underlying dermis (Fig. 33-51). It may less often occur in the fingernails and, surprisingly, is usually asymptomatic. Uncommonly, pain, recurrent or chronic infections, or even underlying osteomyelitis may complicate this condition. It may be an autosomal-dominantly inherited condition, acquired after trauma, or associated with Kawasaki's disease, renal disease, lupus erythematosus or use of β-blockers.

Some treatment success has been obtained with the use of commercial plastic braces after flattening of the nail. Urea ointment under occlusion, various surgical approaches, or chemical matricectomy with phenol and surgical nailbed repair have also been reported to be effective.

Bostanci S, et al: Pincer nail deformity. Int J Dermatol 2004; 43:316.

Kim KD, et al: Nail plate separation and splint fixation: a new non-invasive treatment of pincer nails. J Am Acad Dermatol 2003; 48:791.

Mutaf M, et al: A new surgical technique for the correction of pincer nail deformity. Ann Plast Surg 2007; 58:496.

Pang HN, et al: Pincer nails complicated by distal phalangeal osteomyelitis. J Plast Reconstr Aesthet Surg 2009; 62:254.

Onychocryptosis (unguis incarnatus, ingrown nail)

Ingrown toenail is one of the most frequent nail complaints. It occurs chiefly on the great toes, where there is an excessive lateral nail growth into the nailfold, leading to this painful, inflammatory condition. The lateral margin of the nail acts as a foreign body and may cause exuberant granulation tissue. Unguis incarnatus may be caused by wearing improperly fitting shoes and by improper trimming of the nail at the lateral edges so that the anterior portion cuts into the flesh as it grows distally. Drugs such as isotretinoin, lamivudine, and indinavir may induce periungual granulation tissue mimicking onychocryptosis.

In mild cases, soaking the foot in warm soapy water and insertion of a cotton pad, dental floss, or a flexible plastic tube beneath the distal corner of the offending nail may make surgery unnecessary. When surgical intervention is necessary, simple removal of the lateral portion of the nail plate can produce significant relief. Another simple operation involves removal of the overhanging lateral nailfold so that the nail does not cut into it. When healed, the nail edge resembles that of the thumb, and an excellent functional result occurs. The nail is not altered, since it is not touched.

Partial or complete nail avulsion with ablation of the nail matrix will prevent recurrence. Ablation can be accomplished surgically, with phenol, 10% sodium hydroxide, or with a CO_2 laser. When phenol is used, the proximal nailfold should be incised and reflected to avoid burning the nailfold. As an alternative, it can be left in place and injected with a corticosteroid to reduce the subsequent inflammation. Liquid nitrogen spray to the area of tissue and nail involved for a freeze time of 20–30 s has been successful in some patients, but may be painful and is reserved for patients in whom other surgical approaches are not appropriate.

Retronychia

Retronychia is an unusual event associated with ingrowing of the nail plate into the proximal nail fold. It then induces a chronic paronychia. The cause in the few cases reported has been trauma, usually of the great toe. An incomplete shedding of the nail plate results in the new growing nail pushing the old partially detached nail plate up and backwards into the proximal nail fold. Avulsion is curative.

Akasakal AB, et al: Decompression for the management of onychocryptosis. J Dermatolog Treat 2004; 15:108.

Andreassi A, et al: Segmental phenolization for the treatment of ingrowing toenails. J Dermatolog Treat 2004; 15:179.

Baumgartner M, et al: Retronychia. Dermatol Surg 2010; (epub).

Dahdah MJ, et al: Retronychia. J Am Acad Dermatol 2008: 58:1051.

Heidelbaugh JJ, et al: Management of the ingrown toenail. Am Fam Physician 2009; 79:303.

Kim YJ, et al: Nail-splinting technique for ingrown nails. Dermatol Surg 2003; 29:745.

Ozdemir E, et al: Chemical matricectomy with 10% sodium hydroxide for the treatment of ingrowing toenails. Dermatol Surg 2004; 30:26.

Persichetti P, et al: Wedge excision of the nail fold in the treatment of ingrown toenail. Ann Plast Surg 2004; 52:617.

Rounding C, et al: Surgical treatments for ingrowing nails. Cochrane Database Syst Rev 2005; (2):CD001541.

Woo S-H, et al: Surgical pearl: nail edge separation with dental floss for ingrown toenails. J Am Acad Dermatol 2004; 50:939.

Nail discolorations

Andre J, et al: Pigmented nail disorders. Dermatol Clin 2006; 24:329.

Leukonychia or white nails

Four forms of white nail are recognized: leukonychia punctata, leukonychia striata, leukonychia partialis, and leukonychia totalis. The punctate (Fig. 33-52) variety is common in completely normal persons with otherwise normal nails. Leukonychia striata, transverse white parallel line, may be hereditary, of traumatic origin, or associated with systemic diseases such as HIV or Kawasaki's, or with drugs such as those used in chemotherapy. Partial leukonychia may occur with tuberculosis, nephritis, complex regional pain syndrome, Hodgkin disease, chilblains, metastatic carcinoma, or Hansen's disease, or be idiopathic.

Leukonychia totalis may be hereditary and is of a simple autosomal-dominant type. It may also be associated with typhoid fever, Hansen's disease, cirrhosis, ulcerative colitis, nail biting, use of emetine, complex regional pain syndrome, cytostatic agents, and trichinosis. Leukonychia may result from abnormal keratinization, with persistence of keratohyalin granules in the nail plate.

A syndrome comprising leukonychia totalis, multiple sebaceous cysts, and renal calculi in several generations has been reported. Other reports have linked total leukonychia with deafness or with koilonychia; however, it is most often inherited as an isolated finding.

Antonarakis ES: Acquired leukonychia totalis. N Engl J Med 2006; 355:e2.

Beard R, et al: Leukonychia striata in Kawasaki disease. J Pediatr 2008; 152:889.

De D, et al: Hereditary leukonychia totalis. Indian J Dermatol Venereol Leprol 2007; 73:355.

De Carvalho VO, et al: Transverse leukonychia and AIDS. Arch Dis Child 2006; 91:326.

Dunman I, et al: Unusual cases of acquired leukonychia totalis and partialis secondary to reflex sympathetic dystrophy. J Eur Acad Dermatol Venereol 2007; 21:1445.

Longitudinal erythronychia

Longitudinal red bands in the nail plate that commence in the matrix and extend to the point of separation of the nail plate and nailbed may occur on multiple nails with inflammatory conditions such as lichen planus or Darier's disease, or as an isolated finding. When only a localized single or bifid streak is present, this may signal a benign or malignant tumor of the matrix. The fingernails of middle-aged persons are most commonly affected, with the thumbnail being most frequently involved. There may be a distal keratosis seen, as with Darier, human papilloma virus (HPV) infection, or a squamous cell carcinoma. Excision of this distal keratosis, however, usually does not result in cure or diagnostic findings; biopsy of the affected matrix is necessary. Since this may lead to a scar with a permanent split of the nail plate, observation may be indicated. As in longitudinal melanonychia, if the band broadens over time, then an excisional biopsy is indicated, as this may be secondary to an amelanotic melanoma.

Baran R, et al: Idiopathic polydactylous longitudinal erythronychia. Br J Dermatol 2006; 155:219.

de Berker DAR, et al: Localized longitudinal erythronychia. Arch Dermatol 2004; 140:1253.

Jellinek NJ: Longitudinal erythronychia. J Am Acad Dermatol 2010; (epub).

Melanonychia

Black or brown pigmentation of the normal nail plate is termed melanonychia. It may be present as a normal finding on many digits in black patients, as a result of trauma, systemic disease, or medication, or as a postinflammatory event from such localized events as lichen planus or fixed drug reaction. Pigmentation of the nails may occur with acanthosis nigricans, Addison's disease, Peutz–Jeghers syndrome, and vitamin B_{12} deficiency, after adrenalectomy for Cushing syndrome, as a part of Laugier–Hunziker syndrome (pigmentation of the nails associated with buccal and lip hyperpigmentation), with PUVA or ionizing radiation treatment, and as a drug-induced melanocyte activation with such medications as chemotherapy, antimalarials, minocycline, antivirals (zidovudine [Fig. 33-53] or lamivudine), or metals (gold, arsenic, thallium, or mercury). Drugs may induce both transverse and longitudinal bands, with multidrug chemotherapy causing the majority of the former. Friction may cause longitudinal pigmented bands in the toenails, and subungual hemorrhage or black nail caused

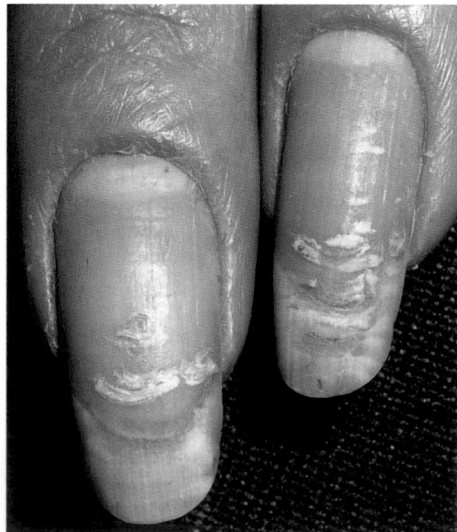

Fig. 33-52 Leukonychia punctata.

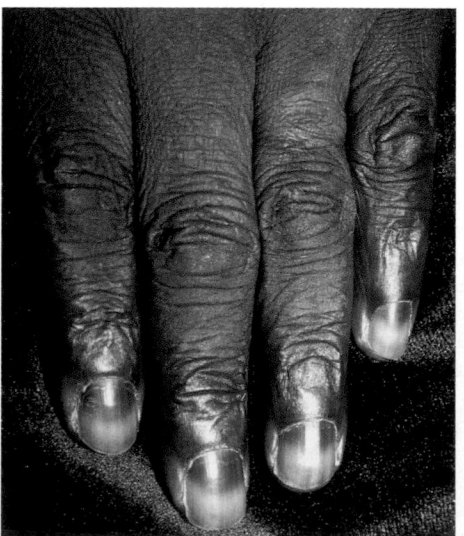

Fig. 33-53 Zidovudine-induced hyperpigmentation of the nail.

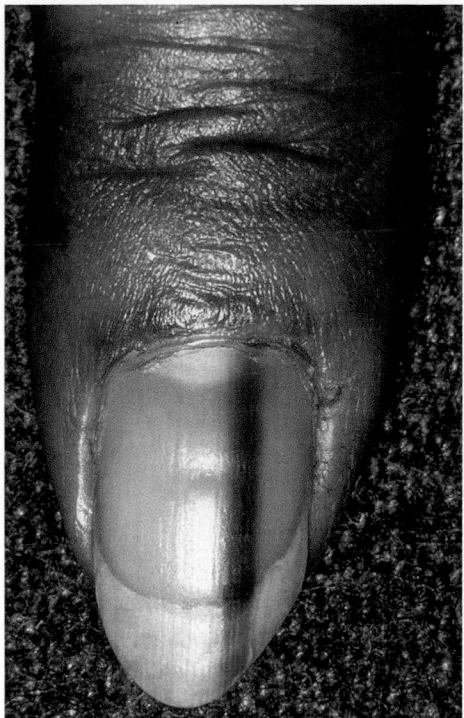

Fig. 33-54 Longitudinal melanonychia.

by *Proteus mirabilis* or *Trichophyton rubrum* may enter into the differential diagnosis of a dark nail.

Longitudinal black or brown banding of the nails has been reported to occur in 77–96% of black persons and 11% of Asians. It is a rare finding in white children; however, it is not uncommon in white adults. In a series by Duhard, the prevalence of melanonychia was 12.6 in 100 in a white hospitalized population, and 1.4 in 100 in 4400 white clinic-based patients. The risk increased with age, the peak occurring between the ages of 56 and 65.

When only one nail is affected by melanonychia striata (a single longitudinal band of brown or black color [Fig. 33-54]), a tumor of the nail matrix is the most important consideration. The location in the matrix can be inferred from the location of the pigment in the nail plate when viewed end-on. Dorsal nail-plate pigmentation results from a proximal matrix lesion. Ventral nail-plate pigmentation is the result of a lesion in the distal matrix.

Tosti et al studied 100 white adult patients with a single band of longitudinal melanonychia of unknown cause. Biopsies revealed melanocytic hyperplasia in 65, nevi in 22, melanocytic activation in 8, and melanoma in 5. Whereas they were unable to ascertain any clear clinical criteria that would exclude melanoma, they recommended a biopsy of any adult with the appearance of a longitudinal band of pigment in only one nail without a clear relation to a definite cause. Other reasons to biopsy include a band that has a triangular shape (one that is wider at the proximal part compared with the distal part), a blurred lateral border of the band, a lack of homogeneity of the pigmentations (bands or lines of different color), or pigmentation of the periungual skin (Hutchinson's sign). The latter is not pathognomonic, however, as Bowen's disease may produce this appearance, and pigmentation of the nail matrix and proximal nailbed may reflect through the nailfold (pseudo-Hutchinson's sign). Finally, dermoscopic features that suggest melanoma are a brown coloration of the background and the presence of irregular coloration, spacing, or thickness of longitudinal lines or disruption of their parallelism. Retracting the proximal nailfold to expose the origin of the streak at the matrix allows selection of the best biopsy site. The recommended biopsy is one that includes the whole lesion; this may be accomplished by the tangential matrix excision, which may leave minimal scarring in some cases, or more certainly this is accomplished by longitudinal excision.

Recommendations for prepubertal children, however, are different. Longitudinal melanonychia that appears in children is usually benign in nature, and it is recommended that since an ungual melanocytic band can appear at an age when other nevi appear, the majority can be followed. If the lesion is alarming in its appearance, especially if it is widening or darkening, sampling the whole lesion via tangential matrix or longitudinal excision is, however, necessary.

Abimelec P: Tips and tricks in nail surgery. Semin Cutan Med Surg 2009; 28:55.

Andre J, et al: Pigmented nail disorders. Dermatol Clin 2006; 24:329.

Goettmann-Bonvallot S, et al: Longitudinal melanonychia in children. J Am Acad Dermatol 1999; 41:17.

Izumi M, et al: Subungual melanoma. J Dermatol 2008; 35:695.

Lambiase MC, et al: Bowen disease of the nail bed presenting as longitudinal melanonychia: detection of human papillomavirus type 56 DNA. Cutis 2003; 72:305.

Ledbetter LS, et al: Melanonychia associated with PUVA therapy. J Am Acad Dermatol 2003; 48:S31.

Piraccini BM, et al: Drug-induced nail diseases. Dermatol Clin 2006; 24:387.

Richert B, et al: New tools in nail disorders. Semin Cutan Med Surg 2009; 28:44.

Smith DF, et al: Longitudinal melanonychia. Arch Dermatol 2003; 139:1209.

Tosti A, et al: Dealing with melanonychia. Semin Cutan Med Surg 2009; 28:49.

Green nails

When onycholysis is present, a green discoloration may occur in the onycholytic area as a result of an infection with *Pseudomonas aeruginosa* (see Chapter 14). The color change may also occur as transverse green stripes. The stripes are ascribed to intermittent episodes of infection. Green nails may also result from copper in tap water.

Hengge UR, et al: Green nails. N Engl J Med 2009; 360:1125.

Staining of the nail plate

Nicotine, dyes (including hair dyes and nail polish), potassium permanganate, mercury compounds, hydroquinone, elemental iron, mepacrine, photographic developer, anthralin, chrysarobin, glutaraldehyde, or resorcin may cause nail-plate staining. This is only a partial list; a complete listing is given in the article by Jeanmougin et al. A helpful diagnostic maneuver to distinguish nail-plate staining from exogenous sources and nail-plate pigmentation from melanin or endogenous chemicals is to scrape the surface of the nail plate several times firmly with a glass slide or scalpel blade. Exogenous stains frequently scrape off completely if the agent has not penetrated the entire nail plate. If the stain follows the curvature of the lunulae, it is probably endogenous; if it follows the curvature of the proximal and lateral nailfolds, it is exogenous.

Coulson IH: "Fade out" photochromonychia. Clin Exp Dermatol 1993; 18:87.

Jeanmougin M, et al: Nail dyschromia. Int J Dermatol 1983; 22:279.

Red lunulae

Dusky erythema confined to the lunulae has been reported in association with alopecia areata. Twenty percent of patients with SLE have been reported to have this abnormality. It may also be seen in patients on oral prednisone for severe rheumatoid arthritis or dermatomyositis, in cardiac failure, cirrhosis, lymphogranuloma venereum, psoriasis, vitiligo, chronic urticaria, lichen sclerosus et atrophicus, CO₂ poisoning, chronic obstructive pulmonary disease, twenty-nail dystrophy, and reticulosarcoma. The cause may be vascular congestion.

Cohen PR: Red lunulae: case report and literature review. J Am Acad Dermatol 1992; 26:292.

Tunc SE, et al: Nail changes in connective tissue diseases. J Eur Acad Dermatol Venereol 2007; 21:497.

Spotted lunulae

This distinctive change occurs with alopecia areata.

Cohen PR: The lunula. J Am Acad Dermatol 1996; 34:943.

Purpura of the nail beds

Purpura beneath the nails usually results from trauma. Causes of toe involvement include physical pressure on the toes, such as that seen in surfboarding caused by a windsurfer trying to maintain his/her balance, or exogenous pressure exerted from poorly fitting shoes. It may simulate a melanoma if the patient does not communicate the acuteness at onset.

Adams BB: Dermatologic disorders of athletes. Sports Med 2002; 32:309.

Blue nails

A blue discoloration of the lunulae is seen in argyria and cases of hepatolenticular degeneration (Wilson's disease). The blue color in the latter is probably related to the changes in copper metabolism by the patient. It has also been reported in hemoglobin M disease and hereditary acrolabial telangiectases. Lunular blue color, as well as blue discoloration of the whole nailbed, occurs with some therapeutic agents, especially 5-FU, minocycline, imipramine, mepacrine and other antimalarials, hydroxyurea, phenolphthalein, and azidothymidine. Blue discoloration may also result from subungual hematoma, blue nevi, and melanotic whitlow. Blue nails are a normal variant finding in Black people.

Dalle S, et al: A blue–gray subungual discoloration. Arch Dermatol 2007; 143:937.

Glaser DA, et al: Blue nails and acquired immunodeficiency syndrome: not always associated with azidothymidine use. Cutis 1996; 57:243.

Kalouche H, et al: Blue lunulae. Australas J Dermatol 2007; 48:182.

Kim Y, et al: A case of generalized argyria after ingestion of colloidal silver solution. Am J Ind Med 2009; 52:246.

Piraccini BM, et al: Drug-induced nail abnormalities. Am J Clin Dermatol 2003; 4:31.

Yellow nail syndrome

The yellow nail syndrome is characterized by marked thickening and yellow to yellowish-green discoloration of the nails often associated with systemic disease, most commonly lymphedema and compromised respiration. The nails are typically overcurved both transversely and longitudinally, grow very slowly (less than 0.2 mm/week), are often subject to onycholysis, and lose both lunulae and cuticles (Fig. 33-55). Lymphedema, pleural effusions, chronic pulmonary infections, and chronic sinusitis most commonly precede the nail changes. Other less frequently associated conditions include autoimmune disorders, immunodeficiency states, the use of gold or d-penicillamine, and malignancies. In the latter cases, treatment of the underlying lymphoma or solid tissue tumor has resulted in improvement of the nail findings. Individual

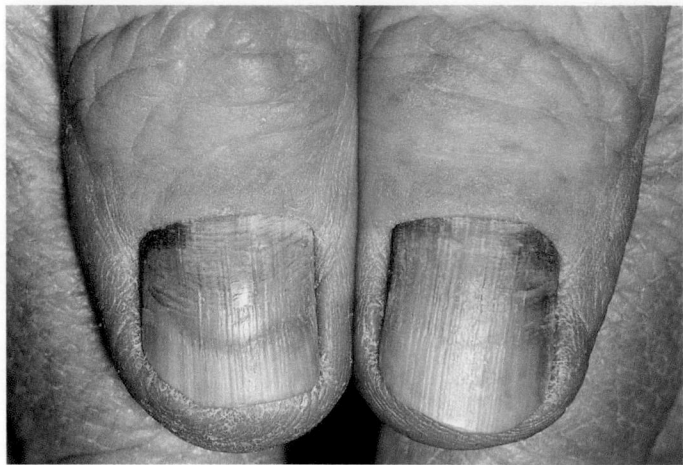

Fig. 33-55 Yellow nail syndrome.

clinical responses have been seen with oral zinc or 800 IU/day of d-α-tocopherol alone or in combination with itraconazole. While approximately 30–50% of patients experience spontaneous improvement in the condition of their nails, fluconazole taken in combination with vitamin E cured or improved all 13 patients treated by Baran et al.

Baran R, et al: Combination of fluconazole and alpha-tocopherol in the treatment of yellow nail syndrome. J Drugs Dermatol 2009; 8:276.

Elmariah SB, et al: Yellow nail syndrome. Dermatol Online J 2008; 14:17.

Hoque SR, et al: Yellow nail syndrome. Br J Dermatol 2007; 156:1230.

Maldonado F, et al: Yellow nail syndrome. Chest 2008; 134:375.

Tosti A, et al: Systemic itraconazole in the yellow nail syndrome. Br J Dermatol 2002; 146:1067.

Neoplasms of the nailbed

Various benign and malignant neoplasms may occur in or overlying the nail matrix and in the nailbed. Signs heralding such neoplasms are paronychia, ingrown nail, onycholysis, pyogenic granuloma, nail-plate dystrophy, longitudinal erythronychia, bleeding, and discolorations. Symptoms of pain, itching, and throbbing may also occur with various neoplasms.

Benign tumors of the nails include verruca, pyogenic granuloma, fibromas, nevus cell nevi, myxoid cysts, angiofibromas (Koenen tumors), onychopapillomas, and epidermoid cysts. Pyogenic granuloma-like lesions may occur during treatment with isotretinoin, lamivudine, indinavir, or the epidermal growth factor receptor inhibitor family of drugs. Glomangioma is readily recognized by exquisite tenderness in the nailbed. Enchondroma of the distal phalanx often presents as a paronychia. Subungual exostoses may also present as an inflammatory process, but more commonly resemble a verruca at the start. Most of these are on the great toe, and radiographic evaluation will aid in the diagnosis of these last two entities. Onychopapillomas are benign tumors of the nail bed which usually present as longitudinal erythronychia. Tender swelling of the distal finger with nail distortion and radiographic evidence of solitary lytic changes can be caused by intraosseous epidermoid cysts.

Onychomatricoma is a benign tumor of the nail matrix. It presents as a yellow thickened plate growing out from under the proximal nailfold and then extending distally in a longitudinal band (Fig. 33-56). There is an increased transverse curvature of the nail and splinter hemorrhages often are seen in the proximal nail. Uncommonly, it can appear as a cutaneous horn emanating from the proximal nailfold, with dorsal

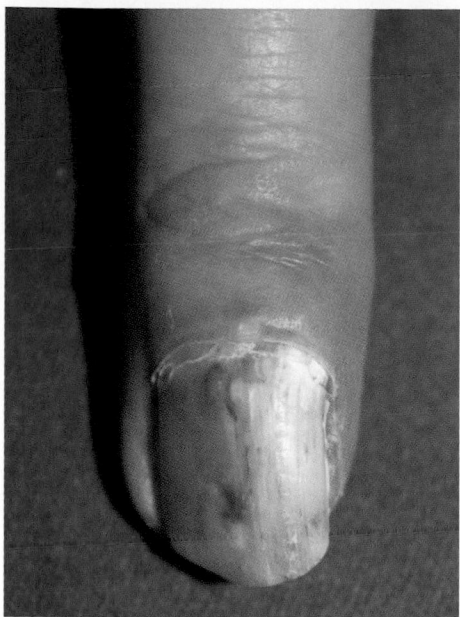

Fig. 33-56 Onychomatricoma.

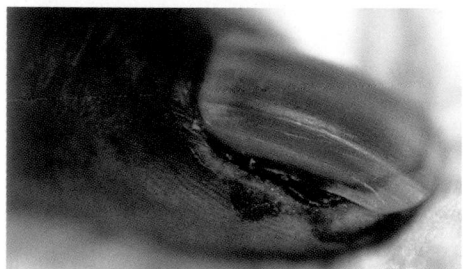

Fig. 33-57 Bowen's disease.

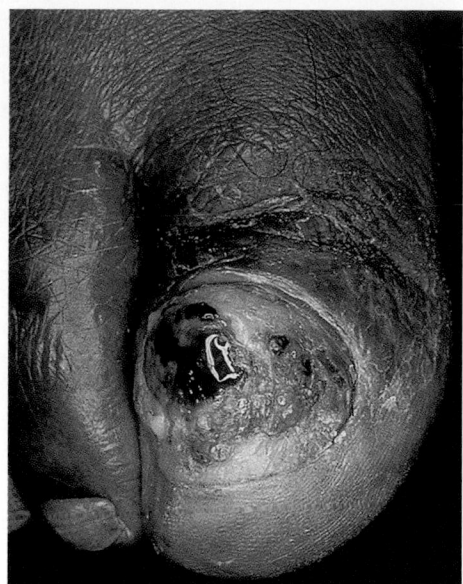

Fig. 33-58 Subungual melanoma.

pterygium formation. Biopsy at the matrix origin will permit diagnosis.

Bowen's disease and squamous cell carcinoma of the nailbed are uncommon. Radiographs may reveal lytic changes in the distal phalanx. Metastases are rare. Mohs surgery is the treatment of choice. When they occur on more than one digit, they are proven to be secondary to HPV infection. Bowen's disease may be pigmental (Fig. 33-57). When keratoacanthoma occurs, there is often lysis of underlying bone, which fills in after excision of the tumor. Basal cell carcinoma may occur, but is uncommon in this location.

Subungual melanoma (Fig. 33-58) is frequently diagnosed late in the course of growth, since it simulates onychomycosis or subungual hematoma, with which it is confused. Amelanotic melanoma may occur and may be mistaken for granuloma pyogenicum. Although melanoma is rare among Japanese, periungual and subungual melanoma is more frequently found in Japanese than in other ethnic populations. Discussion of melanoma in this location may be found in Chapter 30 and in the melanonychia section of this chapter.

Onycholemmal carcinoma is a slowly growing malignant tumor of the nail bed epithelium. It is composed of small cysts filled with eosinophilic amorphous keratin. The cyst wall is lined with atypical keratinocytes. No granular layer is seen. Also solid nests and strands of atypical keratinocytes fill the dermis and may invade the bone. Mohs excision or even disarticulation of the digit may be necessary.

Evaluation of these masses may be carried out by plain x-ray, looking for bone lysis or other changes. MRI by both T1-weighted spin-echo images and turbo spin-echo T2-weighted images may offer excellent diagnostic information about these tumors as well.

Afshar A, et al: A rare metastasis in the hand. J Hand Surg Am 2007; 32:393.
Alessi E, et al: Onycholemmal carcinoma. Am J Dermatopathol 2004; 26:397.
Choi JH, et al: Subungual keratoacanthoma. Skeletal Radiol 2007; 36:769.
Criscione V, et al: Onychopapilloma presenting as longitudinal leukonychia. J Am Acad Dermatol 2010; 63:541.
de Berker DAR, et al: Localized longitudinal erythronychia. Arch Dermatol 2004; 140:1253.
Figus A, et al: Squamous cell carcinoma of the lateral nail fold. J Hand Surg Br 2006; 31:216.
Guarneri C, et al: Solitary asymptomatic nodule of the great toe. Int J Dermatol 2005; 44:245.
Hu JC, et al: Cutaneous side effects of epidermal growth factor receptor inhibitors. J Am Acad Dermatol 2007; 56:317.
Inaoki M, et al: Onycholemmal carcinoma. J Cutan Pathol 2006; 33:577.
Izumi M, et al: Subungual melanoma. J Dermatol 2008; 35:695.
Koc O, et al: Subungual glomus tumour. Australas Radiol 2007; 51 Spec No:B107.
Koch A, et al: Polydactylous Bowen's disease. J Eur Acad Dermatol Venereol 2003; 17:213.
Orsini RC, et al: Basal cell carcinoma of the nail unit. Foot Ankle Int 2001; 222:675.
Perrin C, et al: Onychomatricoma with dorsal pterygium. J Am Acad Dermatol 2008; 59:990.
Samlaska CP, et al: Intraosseous epidermoid cysts. J Am Acad Dermatol 1992; 27:454.
Song M, et al: Surgical treatment of subungual glomus tumor. Dermatol Surg 2009; 35:786.
Suga H, et al: Subungual exostosis. Ann Plast Surg 2005; 55:272.
Tosti A, et al: Dealing with melanonychia. Semin Cutan Med Surg 2009; 28:49.
Turowski CB, et al: Human papillomavirus-associated squamous cell carcinoma of the nail bed in African-American patients. Int J Dermatol 2009; 48:117.

Bonus images for this chapter can be found online at http://www.expertconsult.com

Disorders of the Mucous Membranes

34

Lesions on the mucous membranes may be more difficult to diagnose than lesions on the skin, and not merely because they are less easily and less often seen. There is less contrast of color and greater likelihood of alterations in the original appearance because of secondary factors, such as maceration from moisture, abrasion from food and teeth, and infection. Vesicles and bullae rapidly rupture to form grayish erosions, and the epithelium covering papules becomes a soggy lactescent membrane, easily rubbed off to form an erosion. Grouping and distribution are less distinctive in the mouth than on the skin, and not infrequently it is necessary to establish the diagnosis by observing the character of any associated cutaneous lesions or by noting subsequent developments.

Abdollahi M, et al: Current opinion on drug-induced oral reactions. J Contemp Dent Prac 2008; 9:1.
Greenberg M, et al (eds): Burket's Oral Medicine. Hamilton: BC Decker, 2008.
Huber MA: White oral lesions, actinic cheilitis and leukoplakia. Clin Dermatol 2010; 28:262.
Prabhu SR, et al (eds): Textbook of Oral Diagnosis. Oxford: Oxford University Press, 2009.
Rogers RS III (ed.): Diseases of the mucous membranes. Dermatologic Clinics 2003; 21:1.

Cheilitis

Cheilitis exfoliativa

The term cheilitis exfoliativa has been used to designate a primarily desquamative, mildly inflammatory condition of the lips, of unknown cause, and also a clinically similar reaction secondary to other disease states. The former is a persistently recurring lesion that produces scaling and sometimes crusting; it most often affects the upper lip. The recurrent exfoliation leaves a temporarily erythematous and tender surface.

In the latter form, the lips are chronically inflamed and covered with crusts that from time to time tend to desquamate, leaving a glazed surface on which new crusts form. Fissures may be present, and there may be burning, tenderness, and some pain. The lower lip is more often involved, with the inflammation limited to the vermilion part. The cheilitis may be secondary to seborrheic dermatitis, atopic dermatitis, psoriasis, retinoid therapy, pyorrhea, long-term actinic exposure, or the habit of lip-licking (Fig. 34-1). Uncommonly, the initial or only manifestation of atopic dermatitis may be a chronic cheilitis. Irritating or allergenic substances in lipsticks, dentifrices, and mouthwashes may be causative factors. Dyes in lipsticks may photosensitize. Candidiasis may be present. Cheilitis may be part of the Plummer–Vinson syndrome or Sjögren syndrome. Cheilitis is not uncommon in patients with acquired immune deficiency syndrome (AIDS), and it is a known common complication of protease inhibitor therapy. These and other uncommon causes of cheilitis are discussed in more detail within the specific entities.

The only uniformly effective treatment is the elimination of causes when they can be found. Topical tacrolimus ointment, pimecrolimus cream, or low-strength corticosteroid ointments and creams are usually helpful. If the underlying etiology is determined, specific therapy may be instituted. When there are fissures, petrolatum or zinc oxide ointment may be useful.

Connolley M, et al: Exfoliative cheilitis successfully treated with topical tacrolimus. Br J Dermatol 2004; 151:241.
Garcia-Silva J, et al: Protease inhibitor-related paronychia, ingrown toenails, desquamative cheilitis and cutaneous xerosis. AIDS 2000; 14:1289.
Leland L, et al: Exfoliative cheilitis managed with antidepressant medication. Dent Update 2004; 31:524.
Mani SA, et al: Exfoliative cheilitis. J Can Dent Assoc 2007; 73:629.

Allergic contact cheilitis

The vermilion border of the lips is much more likely to develop allergic contact sensitivity reactions than is the oral mucosa. Allergic cheilitis is characterized by dryness, fissuring, edema, crusting, and angular cheilitis. Over 90% of patients are women and over half of the reactions are due to lipsticks. While patch testing with standard allergens will reveal a relevant positive in approximately 25–30% of patients, about 1 in 5 will only react to their own product. It may result from use of topical medications, dentifrices and other dental preparations, antichap agents, lipsticks, and sunscreen-containing lip balms; from contact with cosmetics, nail polish, rubber, and metals; or from eating foods such as mangoes. Fragrance and nickel are the most commonly identified individual sensitizers.

Treatment includes discontinuation of exposure to the offending agent and administration of topical tacrolimus, pimecrolimus, or corticosteroid preparations.

Chan EF, et al: Contact dermatitis to foods and spices. Am J Contact Dermat 1998; 9:71.
Francalanci S, et al: Multicentre study of allergic contact cheilitis from toothpastes. Contact Dermatitis 2000; 43:216.
Freeman S, et al: Cheilitis. Am J Contact Dermat 1999; 10:198.
Jacob SE, et al: Allergic contact dermatitis to propolis and carnauba wax from lip balm and chewable vitamins in a child. Contact Dermatitis 2008; 58:242.
Schena D, et al: Contact allergy in chronic eczematous lip dermatitis. Eur J Dermatol 2008; 18:688.
Strauss RM, et al: Allergic contact cheilitis in the UK. Am J Contact Dermat 2003; 14:75.
Zug KA, et al: Patch-testing North American lip dermatitis patients. Dermatitis 2008; 19:202.

Actinic cheilitis

Actinic cheilitis is an inflammatory reaction of the lips to chronic excessive sunlight exposure over many years. The lower lip, which is usually the only one involved, becomes

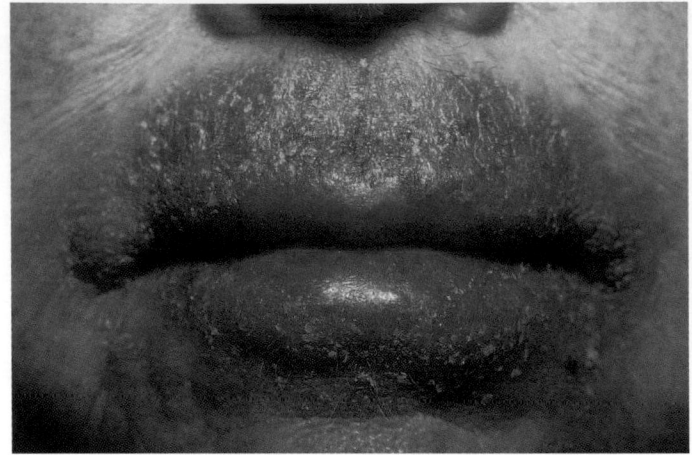

Fig. 34-1 Cheilitis secondary to lip-licking.

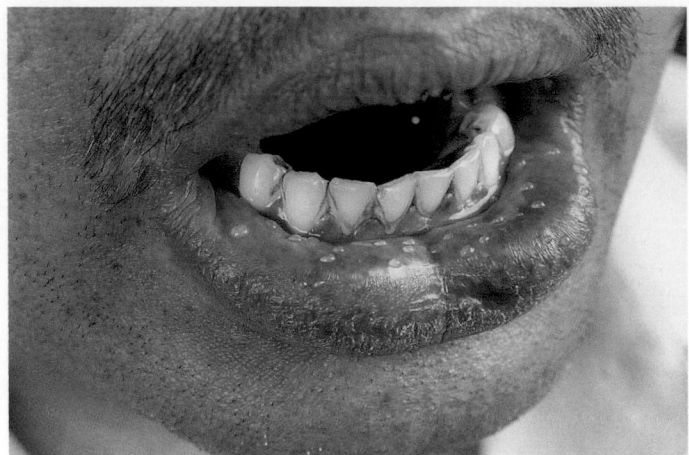

Fig. 34-3 Cheilitis glandularis. (Courtesy of Shyam Verma, MD)

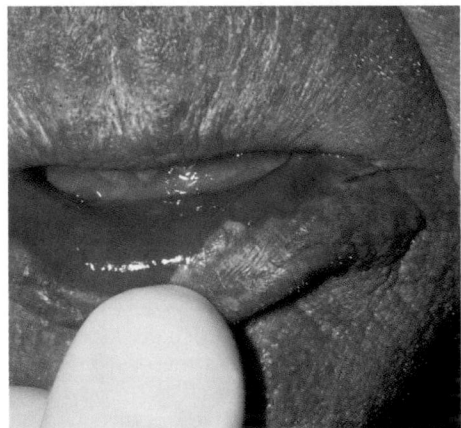

Fig. 34-2 Actinic cheilitis.

scaly, fissured, atrophic, and at times eroded and swollen; leukoplakia and even squamous cell carcinoma may develop (Fig. 34-2). Painful erosions may occur; actual ulceration is very rare unless carcinoma has developed. Hereditary polymorphous light eruption can resemble chronic actinic cheilitis, but it has no malignant potential.

Avoiding sun exposure and the use of sunscreen containing lip pomades suffice to minimize further damage. A biopsy should be performed on any suspicious, thickened areas that persist; preferably, a shave technique should be used to avoid scarring.

Cryosurgical treatment may be effective, particularly for localized lesions. In cases with diffuse involvement, application of topical 5-fluorouracil (5-FU), imiquimod, or photodynamic therapy may be curative. Treatment with a CO_2 or Er:YAG laser, dermabrasion, or electrodesiccation may be required for severe disease and provides excellent results. Long-term follow-up is necessary; one study of 43 patients showed that 15% of CO_2-treated lesions developed squamous cell carcinoma over an average follow-up time of 29 months. Should treatment fail, vermilionectomy of the lower lip may be necessary. Excision of the exposed vermilion mucous membrane with advancement of the labial mucosa to the skin edge of the outer lip is effective, but this is performed less frequently since the advent of laser therapy. Refer to Chapter 29 for more information on actinic cheilitis.

Castineiras I, et al: Actinic cheilitis. J Dermatolog Treat 2010; 21:49.
Castineiras I, et al: Dermabrasion for actinic cheilitis. Dermatol Surg 2008; 34:848.

Cavalcante AS, et al: Actinic cheilitis. J Oral Maxillofac Surg 2008; 66:498.
Dufresne RG Jr, et al: Dermabrasion for actinic cheilitis. Dermatol Surg 2008; 34:848.
Kodama M, et al: Photodynamic therapy for the treatment of actinic cheilitis. Photodermatol Photoimmunol Photomed 2007, 23:209.
Markopoulos A, et al: Actinic cheilitis. Oral Dis 2004; 10:212.
Orenstein A, et al: A new modality in the treatment of actinic cheilitis using the Er:YAG laser. J Cosmet Laser Ther 2007; 9:23.
Rossi R, et al: Photodynamic therapy. Dermatol Ther 2008; 21:412.
Smith KJ, et al: Topical 5% imiquimod for the therapy of actinic cheilitis. J Am Acad Dermatol 2002; 47:497.

Cheilitis glandularis

Cheilitis glandularis is characterized by swelling and eversion of the lower lip, patulous openings of the ducts of the mucous glands, cysts, and general enlargement of the lips (Fig. 34-3). Mucus exudes freely to form a gluey film that dries over the lips and causes them to stick together during the night. When the lip is palpated between the thumb and index finger, the enlarged mucous glands feel like pebbles beneath the surface. The lower lip is the site of predilection.

In general, two types are recognized: cheilitis glandularis simplex and cheilitis glandularis apostematosa. (Apostematosa means "with abscess formation.") The latter type probably stems from the simplex form by the development of infection. Cheilitis glandularis is a chronic inflammatory reaction that is due to an exuberant response to chronic irritation, or to atopic, factitious, or actinic damage.

On biopsy, there is a moderate histiocytic, lymphocytic, and plasmacytic infiltration in and around the glands. Some believe it to be a disorder of ductal ectasia. Cheilitis glandularis has been reported to eventuate in squamous cell carcinoma, but these cases may be attributed to chronic sun exposure, which frequently precedes cheilitis glandularis.

Treatment depends on the nature of the antecedent irritation; in most cases, treatment as described for actinic cheilitis is appropriate. Surgical debulking may be necessary. Intralesional triamcinolone may be beneficial in some cases, as may the combination of minocycline and tacrolimus ointment.

Bovenschen JH: Novel treatment for cheilitis glandularis. Acta Derm Venereol 2009; 89:99.
Nico MM, et al: Cheilitis glandularis. J Am Acad Dermatol 2010; 62:233.
Stoopler ET, et al: Cheilitis glandularis. Oral Surg Oral Med Oral Pathol Oral Radiol Endod 2003; 95:312.
Verma S: Cheilitis glandularis. Br J Dermatol 2003; 148:362.

Angular cheilitis

Angular cheilitis is synonymous with perlèche. Fissures radiate downward and outward from the labial commissures. It is an intertriginous dermatitis caused by excessive wetness or dryness. It is often complicated by secondary infection with *Candida albicans* or *Staphylococcus aureus*.

The disease usually occurs in elderly people who wear dentures, but it may develop simply from an overhanging of the upper lip and cheek, and recession and atrophy of the alveolar ridges in old age. Measuring the facial dimensions with a ruler and tongue blade will help with objective assessment of the importance of decreased vertical facial dimension in the development of perlèche. If the distance from the base of the nose to the lower edge of the mandible is greater than or equal to 6 mm less than the distance from the center of the pupil to the parting line of the lips, the vertical dimension is decreased. In these circumstances, drooling is usually a factor. In children, angular cheilitis occurs commonly in thumb suckers, gum chewers, and lollipop eaters. Other inciting factors include riboflavin deficiency, anorexia nervosa, Down syndrome, intraoral candidiasis, especially in patients with diabetes, AIDS, chronic mucocutaneous candidiasis, Sjögren syndrome, orthodontic treatment, drug-induced xerostomia, and atopic dermatitis.

Opening the "bite" by improving denture fit, capping teeth, replacing lost teeth, or increasing denture height, combined with topical use of nystatin and iodochlorhydroxyquin in hydrocortisone ointment, is usually effective when the condition is associated with anatomically predisposing factors. Stubborn cases typically respond to a slightly stronger corticosteroid, such as desonide, in combination with a topical anticandidal agent. Injection of collagen or insertion of Softform implants to obliterate the angular creases may be beneficial. Therapy for underlying diseases should be maximized. If *S. aureus* is present, mupirocin ointment may be needed. Excision of the region, followed by a rotating flap graft, is another therapeutic option, but surgery should be reserved for resistant cases.

Adedigba MA, et al: Patterns of oral manifestations of HIV/AIDS among 225 Nigerian patients. Oral Dis 2008; 14:341.

Cross DL, et al: Angular cheilitis occurring during orthodontic treatment. J Orthod 2008; 35:229.

Lu DP: Prosthodontic management of angular cheilitis and persistent drooling. Compend Contin Educ Dent 2007; 28:572.

Sharon V, et al: Oral candidiasis and angular cheilitis. Dermatol Ther 2010; 23:230.

Soy M, et al: Cutaneous findings in patients with primary Sjögren's syndrome. Clin Rheumatol 2007; 26:1350.

Strumia R: Dermatologic signs in patients with eating disorders. Am J Clin Dermatol 2005; 6:165.

Plasma cell cheilitis

This is also referred to as plasma cell orificial mucositis or, when the gingival is the site of involvement, plasma cell gingivitis. It is characterized by a sharply outlined, infiltrated, dark red plaque with a lacquer-like glazing of the surface of the involved area.

This lesion has the same microscopic features as Zoon balanitis plasmacellularis. There is plasma cell infiltration in a bandlike pattern. Plasma cell cheilitis is not a response that is specific for any stimulus but rather represents a reaction pattern to any one of a variety of stimuli. Successful therapies include application of topical tacrolimus ointment or clobetasol propionate ointment twice a day.

Plasmoacanthoma

Plasma cell cheilitis and plasmoacanthoma have been reported in the same patient and are believed to represent a spectrum

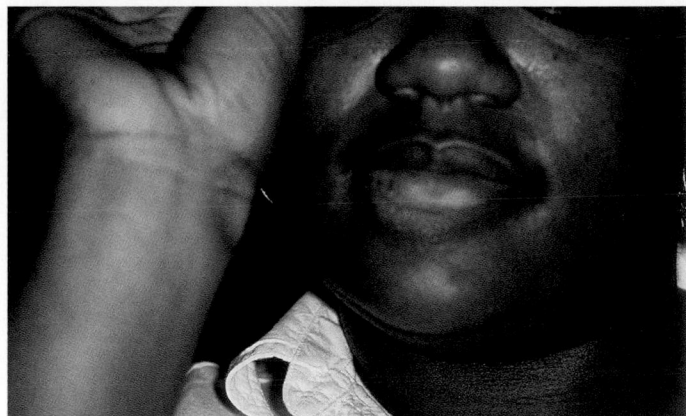

Fig. 34-4 Fixed drug eruption.

of the same disease. Plasmoacanthoma is a verrucous tumor with a plasma cell infiltrate involving the oral mucosa, particularly along the angles. Other locations may occur, such as the perianal, periumbilical, or inguinal areas and toe webs. *C. albicans* has been found within the tissue, suggesting that it may be implicated as a cause of this disease. Excision, destruction, anticandidal preparations, and intralesional steroids are all options for treatment.

Farrier JN, et al: Plasma cell cheilitis. Br J Oral Maxillofac Surg 2008; 46:679.

Rocha N, et al: Plasma cell cheilitis. J Eur Acad Dermatol Venereol 2004; 18:96.

Senol M, et al: Intertriginous plasmacytosis with plasmoacanthoma. Int J Dermatol 2008; 47:265.

Tseng JT, et al: Plasma cell cheilitis. Clin Exp Dermatol 2009; 34:174.

Drug-induced ulcer of the lip

Painful or tender, well-defined ulcerations without induration on the lower lip may heal after withdrawal of oral medications. The causative drugs may be phenylbutazone, chlorpromazine, phenobarbital, methyldopa, or thiazide diuretics.

Solar exposure appears to be a predisposing causative influence; in some cases this reaction may represent a fixed drug photoeruption. On rare occasions, fixed drug eruptions may also involve the lip; usually the culprit is naproxen, one of the oxicams, or trimethoprim–sulfamethoxazole (Fig. 34-4).

Ozkaya-Bayazit E: Specific site involvement with fixed drug eruptions. J Am Acad Dermatol 2003; 49:1003.

Pemberton MN, et al: Fixed drug eruption to oxybutynin. Oral Surg Oral Med Oral Pathol Oral Radiol Endod 2008; 106:e19.

Other forms of cheilitis

Several diseases discussed elsewhere may affect the lips, including lichen planus, lupus erythematosus, atopic dermatitis, and psoriasis. A high percentage of patients with Down syndrome have cheilitis of one or both lips. Lip-biting may be a factor.

Oral and cutaneous Crohn's disease

Crohn's disease is a chronic granulomatous disease of any part or parts of the bowel, to which the names terminal ileitis, regional enteritis, and granulomatous colitis have also been given. Patients with Crohn's disease may develop inflammatory hyperplasia of the oral mucosa, with metallic dysgeusia and gingival bleeding. Reported typical changes include diffuse oral swelling, focal mucosal hypertrophy and fissuring (cobble-stoning), persistent ulceration, polypoid lesions, indurated fissuring of the lower lip, angular cheilitis, granulomatous cheilitis, or pyostomatitis vegetans. Oral involvement occurs in 10–20% of cases of Crohn's disease, and 90% have granulomas on biopsy. Males with early-onset disease are most often affected. Concomitant involvement of the anal and esophageal mucosa is common.

Many cases of Crohn's disease with other cutaneous manifestations have been reported, notably pyoderma gangrenosum (more closely associated with ulcerative colitis) and erythema nodosum, polyarteritis nodosa, pellagra, pernicious anemia, an acrodermatitis-like eruption, urticaria, and necrotizing vasculitis. Direct extension to perianal skin may occur.

Metastatic Crohn's disease denotes noncaseating granulomatous skin lesions in patients with Crohn's disease. In the absence of bowel involvement, the diagnosis cannot be made. Genital swelling or condyloma-like lesions, leg ulceration, pyogenic granuloma-like lesions of the retroauricular skin, or erythematous nodules, plaques, or ulcers in other locations are the morphologic appearances seen.

Treatment of the gastrointestinal manifestations with sulfasalazine, metronidazole, systemic corticosteroids, infliximab, or immunosuppressive medications such as cyclosporine, azathioprine, mycophenolate mofetil, and methotrexate can improve the cutaneous findings. Several delivery systems use only the active ingredient of sulfasalazine, mesalamine. These include Asacol, Pentasa, Rowasa, and olsalazine, and they may be useful in treating the skin involvement of Crohn's disease. A mouthwash containing triamcinolone acetonide, tetracycline, and lidocaine may provide symptomatic and objective improvement. Cutaneous ulcerated granulomas and erythematous plaques caused by Crohn's disease may respond to high-potency topical corticosteroids or tacrolimus ointment. Curettage and zinc by mouth have resulted in healing in several reported patients. Dietary manipulation is another measure that can be helpful in select individuals. The course is often prolonged over several years.

Emanuel PO, et al: Metastatic Crohn's disease. J Cutan Pathol 2008; 35:457.

Ephgrave K: Extra-intestinal manifestations of Crohn's disease. Surg Clin North Am 2007; 87:673.

Farhi D, et al: Significance of erythema nodosum and pyoderma gangrenosum in inflammatory bowel diseases. Medicine (Baltimore) 2008; 87:281.

Harty S, et al: A prospective study of the oral manifestations of Crohn's disease. Clin Gastroenterol Hepatol 2005; 3:866.

Komatsuda A, et al: Cutaneous polyarteritis nodosa in a patient with Crohn's disease. Mod Rheumatol 2008; 18:639.

Mignogna MD, et al: Oral Crohn's disease. Am J Gastroenterol 2008; 103:2954.

Ojha J, et al: Gingival involvement in Crohn's disease. J Am Dent Assoc 2007; 138:1574.

Paradisi A, et al: Cutaneous Crohn disease mimicking anal condylomata in a child. J Am Acad Dermatol 2010; 63:165.

Yuksel I, et al: Mucocutaneous manifestations of inflammatory bowel disease. Inflamm Bowel Dis 2009; 15:546.

Pyostomatitis vegetans

Pyostomatitis vegetans, an inflammatory stomatitis, is most often seen in association with ulcerative colitis but may also occur in other inflammatory bowel diseases, such as Crohn's disease. Edema and erythema with deep folding of the buccal mucosa characterize it, together with pustules, small vegetating projections, erosions, ulcers, and fibrinopurulent exudates (Fig. 34-5). Eroded pustules fuse into shallow ulcers, resulting in characteristic "snail-track" ulcers. It has also been associated with sclerosing cholangitis. Several cases have been reported without any underlying systemic disorder.

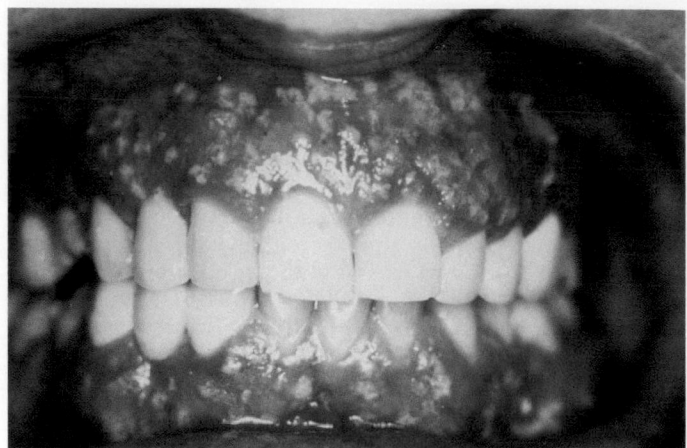

Fig. 34-5 Pyostomatitis vegetans. (Courtesy of Charles Casima, MD)

Histologically, there are dense aggregates of neutrophils and eosinophils. At times, crusted erythematous papulopustules that coalesce into asymmetrical annular plaques may occur with or after the oral lesions. These associated skin lesions favor the axilla, groin, and scalp, and are termed pyodermatitis vegetans. Topical corticosteroids or tacrolimus ointment may be effective; systemic steroids or infliximab, however, are usually necessary.

Gonzalez-Moles MA, et al: Pyostomatitis vegetans. J Eur Acad Dermatol Venereol 2008; 22:252.

Ko HC, et al: Two cases of pyodermatitis-pyostomatitis vegetans. J Dermatol 2009; 36:293.

Lourenco SV, et al: Oral manifestations of inflammatory bowel disease. J Eur Acad Dermatol Venereol 2010; 24:204.

Wechaniak AE, et al: Treatment of pyostomatitis vegetans with topical tacrolimus. J Am Acad Dermatol 2005; 52:722.

Yasuda M, et al: Pyodermatitis-pyostomatitis vegetans associated with ulcerative colitis. Dermatology 2008; 217:146.

Cheilitis granulomatosa

Cheilitis granulomatosa is characterized by a sudden onset and progressive course, terminating in chronic enlargement of the lips. Usually, the upper lip becomes swollen first; several months may elapse before the lower lip becomes swollen. Usually only enlargement is present, without ulceration, fissuring, or scaling. The swelling remains permanently. It may be a part of the Melkersson–Rosenthal syndrome when associated with facial paralysis and plicated tongue.

The cause is unknown. Histologically, it is characterized by an inflammatory reaction of lymphocytes, histiocytes, and plasma cells, and by tuberculoid granulomas consisting of epithelioid and Langerhans giant cells. In the differential diagnosis, solid edema, angioedema, cheilitis glandularis, sarcoidosis, oral Crohn's disease, infectious granulomas, contact allergy and Ascher syndrome must be considered. This may be the presenting sign in a patient who will develop Crohn's disease or sarcoidosis at a later time.

Treatment with intralesional injections of corticosteroids is sometimes successful. In the firmly established case, surgical repair of the involved lip through a mucosal approach and, in some cases, concomitant intralesional steroid treatment give best results. Other anecdotally effective medications include tetracyclines, roxithromycin, hydroxychloroquine, clofazimine, and sulfasalazine.

Cernik C, et al: Asymptomatic, edematous upper lip in a 39-year-old woman. Arch Dermatol 2009; 145:77.

Chiu CS, et al: Cheilitis granulomatosa associated with allergic contact dermatitis to betel quid. Contact Dermatitis 2008; 58:246.

Lopez-Urbano MJ, et al: Granulomatous cheilitis. J Investig Allergol Clin Immunol 2009; 19:68.

Praessler J, et al: Persistent non-tender swelling of the upper lip. Am J Clin Dermatol 2007; 8:251.

Ratzinger G, et al: Cheilitis granulomatosa and Melkersson–Rosenthal syndrome. J Eur Acad Dermatol Venereol 2007; 21:1065.

Melkersson–Rosenthal syndrome

Melkersson in 1928 and Rosenthal in 1930 described a triad consisting of recurring facial paralysis or paresis, soft nonpitting edema of the lips, and scrotal tongue. Attacks usually start during adolescence, with permanent or transitory paralysis of one or both facial nerves, repeated migraines, and recurring edema of the upper lip, cheeks, and occasionally the lower lip and circumoral tissues. Swelling of the skin and mucous membranes of the face and mouth is the dominant finding and most important diagnostic feature (Fig. 34-6). In order of frequency, the swelling occurs first on the upper lip, then the lower lip, and then other regions. Chronic eyelid swelling may occur.

Extrafacial swellings appear on the dorsal aspect of the hands and feet, and in the lumbar region. The pharynx and respiratory tract may be involved, with thickening of the mucous membrane. The relapsing condition produces an overgrowth of connective tissue, edema, and atrophy of the muscle fibers, with permanent deformities of the lips, cheeks, and tongue.

The cause is unknown. The association at times with megacolon, otosclerosis, and craniopharyngioma supports the theory of a neurotrophic origin. It may be familial.

Histopathologic evaluation shows a tuberculoid type of granuloma with lymphedema and a banal perivascular infiltrate. In the differential diagnosis, a number of diseases characterized by edema of the lips must be considered. Ascher syndrome consists of swelling of the lips with edema of the eyelids (blepharochalasis) and is inherited. Melkersson-Rosenthal syndrome must also be differentiated from the acute swellings produced by angioedema, trauma, and infections of all sorts. Lymphangioma, hemangioma, neurofibroma, and sarcoidosis are some of the diseases to be considered on a clinical basis.

Melkersson–Rosenthal syndrome is frequently seen in an incomplete form, and other granulomatous diseases may present as swellings of the lips or oral–facial tissues. It is worthwhile considering these as a group called orofacial granulomatosis so that various underlying disease states or etiologic factors will not be missed when evaluating such patients. Oral Crohn's disease, patients who will develop typical Crohn's or sarcoidosis in the future, cheilitis granulomatosa, sarcoidosis, granulomatous infiltrates associated with tooth infections, and patients with food or contact allergic reactions should all be considered.

There is no satisfactory treatment, although intralesional injections of corticosteroids may be beneficial. Decompression of the facial nerve may be indicated in those patients with recurrent attacks of facial palsy. Surgery alone or combined with intralesional steroid injections may be more successful than either alone. Odontogenic infection has been reported to initiate this condition and antibiotic therapy for this may lead to remission. Clofazimine, thalidomide, and prednisone combined with minocycline or tetracycline have been reported to improve individual patients.

Kakimoto C, et al: Melkersson–Rosenthal syndrome. Otolaryngol Head Neck Surg 2008; 138:246.

Kondratiev S, et al: Melkersson-Rosenthal syndrome presenting as chronic eyelid swelling. Ophthalmic Surg Lasers Imaging 2010; 9.1.

Kruse-Losler B, et al: Surgical treatment of persistent macrocheilia in patients with Melkersson–Rosenthal syndrome and cheilitis granulomatosa. Arch Dermatol 2005; 141:1085.

Mignogna MD, et al: The multiform and variable patterns of onset of orofacial granulomatosis. J Oral Pathol Med 2003; 32:200.

Fordyce's disease (Fordyce spots)

Fordyce spots are ectopically located sebaceous glands, clinically characterized by minute orange or yellowish pinhead-sized macules or papules in the mucosa of the lips, cheeks, and, less often, the gums. Similar lesions may occur on the areola, glans penis, and labia minora. Prominent lip involvement may result in a lipstick-like mark left on the rim of a glass mug after consuming a hot beverage (Meffert's sign). Involvement of the labial mucosa with pseudoxanthoma elasticum may simulate Fordyce spots.

Because the anomaly is asymptomatic and inconsequential, treatment should be undertaken only if there is a significant cosmetic problem. The CO_2 laser, electrodesiccation and curettage, bichloracetic acid, photodynamic therapy, and isotretinoin are therapeutic options.

Chen PL, et al: Fordyce spots of the lip responding to electrodesiccation and curettage. Dermatol Surg 2008; 34:960.

Elston DM, et al: Fordyce spots. Cutis 2001; 68:24, 49.

Ocampo-Candiani J, et al: Treatment of Fordyce spots with CO_2 laser. Dermatol Surg 2003; 29:869.

Stomatitis nicotina

Also known as smoker's keratosis and smoker's patches, stomatitis nicotina is characterized by distinct umbilicated papules on the palate. The ostia of the mucous ducts appear as red pinpoints surrounded by milky white, slightly umbilicated asymptomatic papules. The intervening mucosa becomes white and thick and has a tendency to desquamate in places, leaving raw, beefy-red areas. Ulceration and the formation of aphthous ulcers may occur.

This condition is attributed to heavy smoking in middle-aged men, although it has also been reported in nonsmokers who habitually drink hot beverages. Heat may be the causative event. Indeed, the most severe cases are associated with the type of tobacco use that produces intense heat—pipe and reverse smoking.

Treatment consists of abstaining from the use of tobacco or ingestion of hot liquids.

Mirbod SM, et al: Tobacco-associated lesions of the oral cavity. J Can Dent Assoc 2000; 66:252.

Taybos G: Oral changes associated with tobacco use. Am J Med Sci 2003; 326:179.

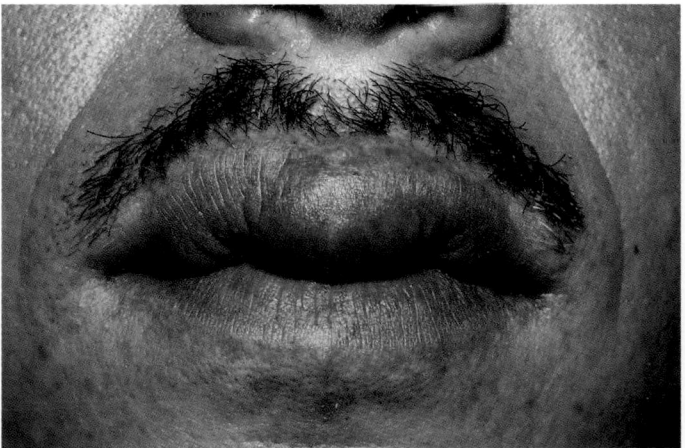

Fig. 34-6 Melkersson–Rosenthal syndrome. (Courtesy of Curt Samlaska, MD)

Torus palatinus

Torus palatinus is a bony protuberance in the midline of the hard palate, marking the point of junction of the two halves of the palate. It is asymptomatic. Exostoses also commonly occur in the floor of the mouth, involving the inner surface of the mandible.

Piera-Navarro N, et al: Clinical evaluation of hard tissue proliferations of the mouth. Med Oral 2002; 7:97.
Tran KT, et al: Torus palatinus. N Engl J Med 2007; 356:1759.

Fissured tongue

Also known as furrowed tongue, scrotal tongue, or lingua plicata, fissured tongue is a congenital and sometimes familial condition in which the tongue is generally larger than normal and there are plicate superficial or deep grooves, usually arranged so that there is a longitudinal furrow along the median raphe, reminiscent of scrotal rugae (Fig. 34-7).

Fissured tongue is seen in Melkersson–Rosenthal syndrome and in many patients with Down syndrome. Individual case reports have been seen in association with pachyonychia congenita, pemphigus vegetans, and Cowden syndrome. Geographic tongue occurs together with fissured tongue in 50% of patients, and both are more commonly present in psoriasis patients than nonpsoriatics.

The condition gives rise to no difficulty, and treatment is not necessary, except that the deep furrows should be kept clean by use of mouthwashes. Herpetic geometric glossitis may mimic fissured tongue, but is painful, affects predominately immunocompromised individuals, and is centered on the back of the dorsal tongue.

Byrd JA, et al: Glossitis and other tongue disorders. Dermatol Clin 2003; 21:123.
Mirowski GW, et al: Herpetic geometric glossitis in an immunocompetent patient with pneumonia. J Am Acad Dermatol 2009; 61:139.
Zargari O: The prevalence and significance of fissured tongue and geographic tongue in psoriatic patients. Clin Exp Dermatol 2006; 31:192.

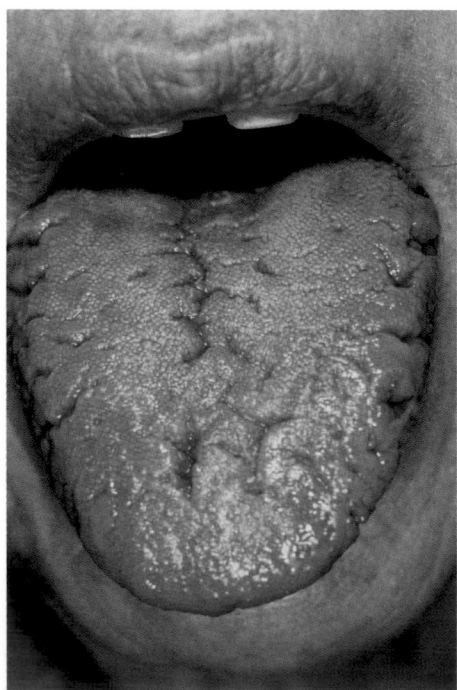

Fig. 34-7 Fissured tongue.

Geographic tongue

Geographic tongue is also known as lingua geographica, transitory benign plaques of the tongue, glossitis areata exfoliativa, and benign migratory glossitis. In some patients it is a manifestation of atopy, and in others, of psoriasis. However, in most it is an isolated finding.

The dorsal surface of the tongue is the site usually affected. Geographic tongue begins with a small depression on the lateral border or the tip of the tongue, smoother and redder than the rest of the surface. This spreads peripherally, with the formation of sharply circumscribed ringed or gyrate red patches, each with a narrow yellowish-white border, making the tongue resemble a map. The appearance changes from day to day; patches may disappear in one place and manifest themselves in others. The disease is characterized by periods of exacerbation and quiescence. The lesion may remain unchanged in the same site for long periods. The condition is frequently unrecognized because it produces no symptoms except for the occasional complaint of glossodynia.

There are two clinical variants of geographic tongue. In one type, discrete, annular "bald" patches of glistening, erythematous mucosa with absent or atrophic filiform papillae are noted. Another type shows prominent circinate or annular white raised lines that vary in width up to 2 mm. The clinical appearance and histopathologic findings of the tongue lesions in pustular psoriasis, reactive arthritis (Reiter syndrome), and geographic tongue are identical; when the tongue lesions occur with psoriasis or reactive arthritis, the name annulus migrans has been suggested for this entity (Fig. 34-8). It has been reported as being acquired in patients with AIDS or as a result of lithium therapy.

Histologically, the main features are marked transepidermal neutrophil migration with the formation of spongiform pustules in the epidermis and an upper dermal mononuclear infiltrate.

Although treatment is not usually necessary, a 0.1% solution of tretinoin solution (Retin-A) applied topically has produced clearing within 4–6 days.

Byrd JA, et al: Glossitis and other tongue disorders. Dermatol Clin 2003; 21:123.
Miloglu O, et al: The prevalence and risk factors associated with benign migratory glossitis lesions in 7619 Turkish dental outpatients. Oral Surg Oral Med Oral Pathol Oral Radiol Endod 2009; 107:e29.
Shulman JD, et al: Prevalence and risk factors associated with geographic tongue among US adults. Oral Dis 2006; 12:381.
Zargari O: The prevalence and significance of fissured tongue and geographic tongue in psoriatic patients. Clin Exp Dermatol 2006; 31:192.

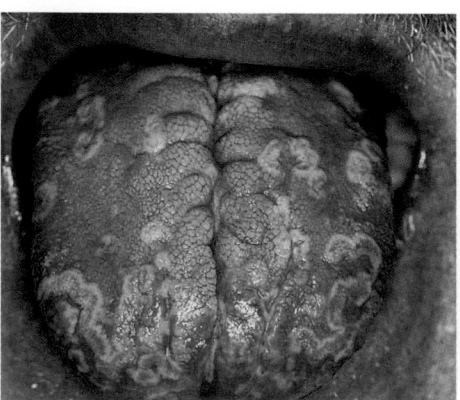

Fig. 34-8 Annulus migrans.

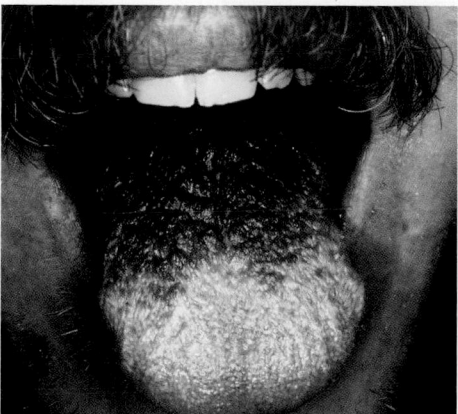

Fig. 34-9 Black hairy tongue.

Black hairy tongue

Black or brown hairy tongue occurs on the dorsum of the tongue anterior to the circumvallate papillae, where black, yellowish, or brown patches form, consisting of hairlike intertwining filaments several millimeters long (Fig. 34-9). The "hairs" result from a benign hyperplasia of the filiform papillae of the anterior two-thirds of the tongue, resulting in retention of long conical filaments of orthokeratotic and parakeratotic cells. It occurs far more frequently in men than in women.

Black hairy tongue may be associated with several conditions that may be predisposing factors in its causation: smoking, use of oral antibiotics, psychotropic drugs, and presence of *Candida* on the surface of the tongue.

This lesion may be differentiated both clinically and histologically from oral hairy leukoplakia, which is seen in human immunodeficiency syndrome (HIV)-infected patients. Hairy leukoplakia is usually seen on the lateral surface of the tongue at first in corrugated patches, then with time as solid white plaques that are adherent. Microscopic examination reveals acanthosis, parakeratosis, irregular projections of keratin, and vacuolated keratinocytes with Epstein–Barr virus present within them.

A toothbrush may be used to scrub off the projections, either alone, with 1–2% hydrogen peroxide, or after application of Retin-A gel, 40% aqueous solution of urea, or papain (meat tenderizer). Such predisposing local factors as smoking, antibiotics, and oxidizing agents should be eliminated, if possible, and scrupulous oral hygiene should be maintained.

Korber A, et al: Black hairy tongue. N Engl J Med 2006; 354:67.
Pigatto PD, et al: Black hairy tongue associated with long-term oral erythromycin use. J Eur Acad Dermatol Venereol 2008; 22:1269.
Taybos G: Oral changes associated with tobacco use. Am J Med Sci 2003; 326:179.

Smooth tongue

Also known as bald tongue or atrophic glossitis, the smooth glossy tongue is often painful and results from atrophy of the filiform and eventually the fungiform papillae (Fig. 34-10). When present with vitamin B_{12} deficiency, it has been termed Moeller or Hunter glossitis. It begins with the tip and lateral surfaces of the tongue becoming intensely red, well-defined irregular patches in which the filiform papillae are absent or thinned and the fungiform papillae are swollen. The disease is chronic and the patches are painful and sensitive so that eating may be difficult and taste impaired. With time, the entire tongue becomes smooth and a leukoplakia may result. Treatment of pernicious anemia with vitamin B_{12} therapy will

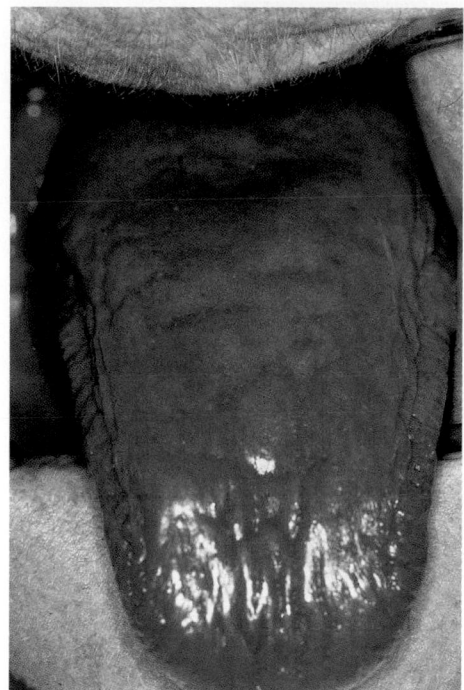

Fig. 34-10 Smooth tongue in Plummer–Vinson syndrome.

result in improvements in the appearance and sensitivity of the tongue.

Atrophic glossitis is also a distinctive sign of pellagra; it results from a deficiency of niacin or its precursor, tryptophan. The sides and tip of the tongue are erythematous and edematous, with imprints of the teeth. Eventually, the entire tongue assumes a beefy-red appearance. Small ulcers appear, and all the mucous membranes of the mouth may be involved. Later, the papillae become atrophied to produce a smooth, glazed tongue, as seen in pernicious anemia. Burning or pain in the ulcers may be present. Increased salivary flow early in the disease may lead to drooling and angular cheilitis. In malabsorption syndrome, riboflavin deficiency, anorexia nervosa, alcoholism, and sprue, similar changes may be noted. Vitamin B complex is curative.

Patients with iron-deficiency anemia, alone or when combined with esophageal webs (Plummer–Vinson syndrome), folic acid deficiency, syphilis, amyloidosis, celiac disease, Sjögren syndrome, and Riley–Day syndrome, may all manifest smooth tongue. Candidiasis may result in tongue pain and a partial or total atrophic appearance, along with a red or magenta color, on the dorsum of the tongue. In such cases, anticandidal therapy results in rapid improvement.

Atmatzidis K, et al: Plummer–Vinson syndrome. Dis Esophagus 2003; 16:154.
Byrd JA, et al: Glossitis and other tongue disorders. Dermatol Clin 2003; 21:123.
Lee HJ, et al: A smooth, shiny tongue. N Engl J Med 2009; 360:e8.
Lehman JS, et al: Atrophic glossitis from vitamin B_{12} deficiency. J Periodontol 2006; 77:2090.
Terai H, et al: Atrophic tongue associated with *Candida*. J Oral Pathol Med 2005; 34:397.

Eruptive lingual papillitis

Lacour and Perrin first described this acute, self-limiting inflammatory stomatitis in 1997. It affects children of both sexes equally, with a mean age of onset of 3½ years. It has a seasonal distribution, with the majority of cases occurring in the spring. Fever (40%), difficulties in feeding (100%), and intense salivation (60%) are common symptoms. The tongue

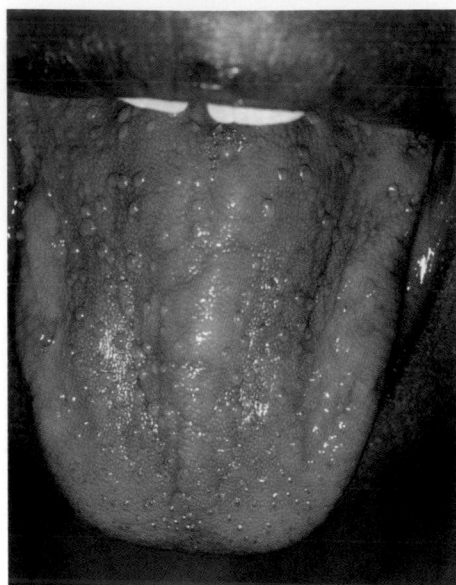

Fig. 34-11 Eruptive lingual papillitis.

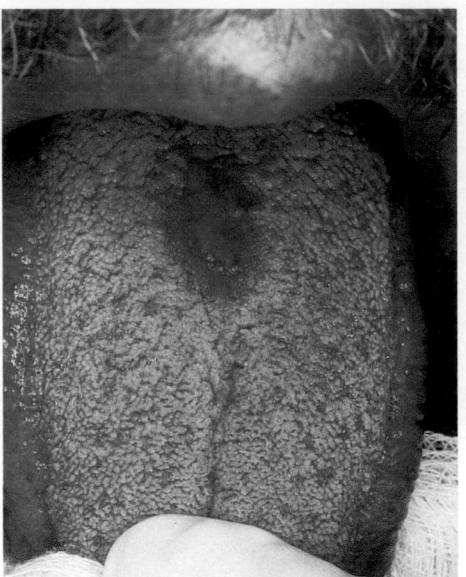

Fig. 34-12 Median rhomboid glossitis.

examination reveals inflammatory hypertrophy of the fungiform papillae on the tip and dorsolateral sites (Fig. 34-11). Additional signs include submandibular or cervical adenopathy (40%) and angular cheilitis (10%). Associated skin eruptions have not been described. Spontaneous involution occurs in a mean of 7 days with a range of 2–15 days. Recurrence is noted in 13%. It is felt to be the result of a viral infection, and the 50% transmission among family members further supports this theory.

Brfannon RB, et al: Transient lingual papillitis. Oral Surg Oral Med Oral Pathol Oral Radiol Endod 2003; 96:187.

Lacour JP, et al: Eruptive familial lingual papillitis. Pediatr Dermatol 1997; 14:13.

Roux O, et al: Eruptive lingual papillitis with household transmission. Br J Dermatol 2004; 150:299.

Median rhomboid glossitis

Median rhomboid glossitis is characterized by a shiny oval or diamond-shaped elevation, invariably situated on the dorsum in the midline immediately in front of the circumvallate papillae (Fig. 34-12). The surface is abnormally red and smooth. In some instances, a few pale yellow papules surmount the elevation. On palpation the lesion feels slightly firm, but it usually causes no symptoms. It persists indefinitely, with little or no increase in size. There is no relationship to cancer. One report noted its presence a patient with pachyonychia congenita.

It may result from abnormal fusion of the posterior portion of the tongue, but it is nearly always chronically infected with *Candida*. If there is palatal inflammation above the inflamed part of the tongue, AIDS should be suspected and an HIV test obtained. Histologically, the changes are those of a simple, chronic inflammation with fibrosis, and usually with fungal hyphae in the parakeratin layer. Treatment with oral antifungals, such as itraconazole, may lead to improvement.

Bae GY, et al: A case of median rhomboid glossitis. J Dermatol 2003; 30:423.

Karen JK, et al: Pachyonychia congenita associated with median rhomboid glossitis. Dermatol Online J 2007; 13:21.

McCullough MJ, et al: Oral candidosis and the therapeutic use of antifungal agents in dentistry. Aust Dent J 2005; 50(4 Suppl 2):S36.

Nelson BL, et al: Median rhomboid glossitis. Ear Nose Throat J 2007; 86:600.

Eosinophilic ulcer of the oral mucosa

Eosinophilic ulcer occurs most commonly on the tongue, but may occur anywhere in the oral mucosa. It is characterized by an ulcer with indurated and elevated borders that is usually covered by a pseudomembrane. It develops rapidly, most commonly on the posterior aspect of the tongue, and spontaneously resolves in a few weeks. A traumatic cause has been postulated for this benign, self-limited disorder. The histopathologic findings show a predominantly eosinophilic infiltrate in company with some histiocytes and neutrophils.

In some multifocal, recurrent cases, CD30+ cells have been reported. These patients may have the oral counterpart of primary cutaneous CD30+ lymphoproliferative disease, or may simply be a simulator of this disorder. HIV-infected patients may develop ulcerations of the oral mucosa, resulting from a variety of infectious agents, such as herpes simplex virus (HSV), candidiasis, and histoplasmosis. However, 5 of the 16 patients they reported had no evidence of infection and simply showed eosinophilic infiltrates below the ulcer.

Ada S, et al: Eosinophilic ulcer of the tongue. Australas J Dermatol 2007; 48:248.

Segura S, et al: Eosinophilic ulcer of the oral mucosa. Br J Dermatol 2006; 155:460.

Segura S, et al: Eosinophilic ulcer of the oral mucosa. Oral Dis 2008; 14:287.

Caviar tongue

William Bean gave the picturesque name caviar tongue to the purplish venous ectasias so commonly found on the undersurface of the tongue after the age of 50. They are attributed to elastic tissue deterioration with aging and may be associated with Fordyce angiokeratomas of the scrotum. Phleboliths or thrombophlebitis may occasionally complicate this condition.

Kocsard E, et al: The histopathology of caviar tongue. Dermatologica 1970; 140:318.

Cutaneous sinus of dental origin (dental sinus)

In dental (or odontogenous) sinus, chronic periapical infection about a tooth produces a burrowing, practically asymptomatic,

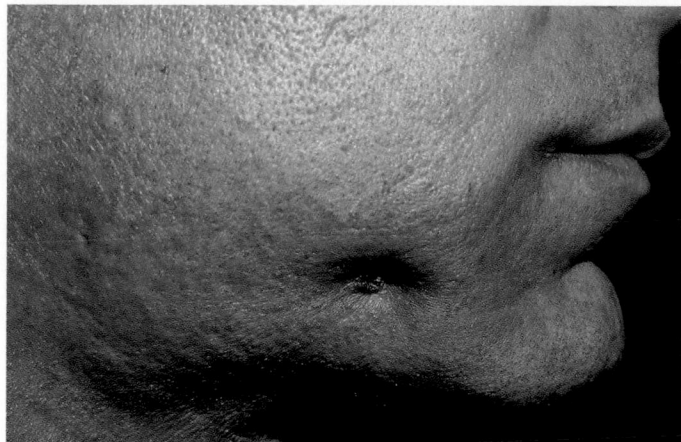

Fig. 34-13 Odontogenic sinus.

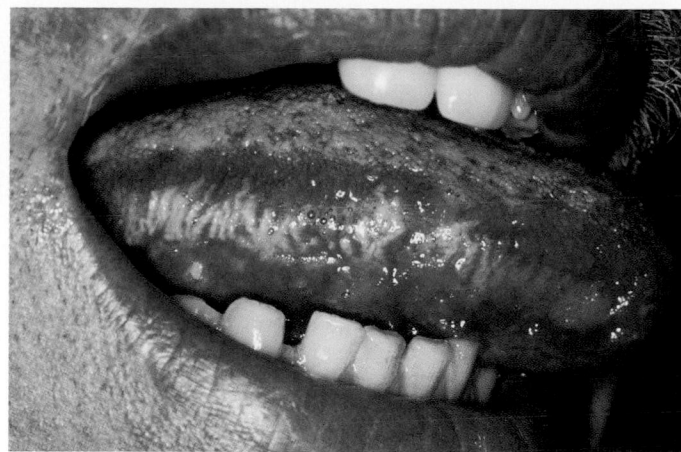

Fig. 34-14 Oral hairy leukoplakia of HIV.

occasionally palpable, cordlike sinus tract that eventually appears beneath the surface of the gum, palate, or periorificial skin. It forms a fistulous opening with an inflamed red nodule at the orifice. It may appear anywhere from the inner ocular canthus to the neck but is most often seen on the chin or along the jawline (Fig. 34-13). Bilateral involvement has been reported. Dental radiography is diagnostic. Pyogenic granuloma, actinomycosis, squamous cell carcinoma, osteomyelitis of the mandible, congenital fistulas, the deep mycoses, bisphosphonate-related osteonecrosis of the jaw, and foreign body reactions must be considered in the differential diagnosis.

Treatment requires the removal of the offending tooth or root canal therapy of the periapical abscess.

Barrowman RA, et al: Cutaneous sinus tracts of dental origin. Med J Aust 2007; 186:264.

Mittal N, et al: Management of extra oral sinus cases. J Endod 2004; 30:541.

Pasternak-Junior B, et al: Diagnosis and treatment of odontogenic cutaneous sinus tracts of endodontic origin. Int Endod J 2009; 42:271.

Soares JA, et al: Conservative treatment of patients with periapical lesions associated with extraoral sinus tracts. Aust Endod J 2007; 33:131.

Truong SV, et al: Bisphosphonate-related osteonecrosis of the jaw presenting as a cutaneous dental sinus track. J Am Acad Dermatol 2010; 62:672.

Neoplasms

Many tumors may involve the oral cavity. Most are discussed elsewhere in this book, and several are uncommon entities that affect specialized oral structures, such as the many subtypes of benign and malignant proliferations that occur in the major and minor salivary glands. These will not be covered further here, and only a few selected neoplasms will be presented.

Leukoplakia

Clinical features

Leukoplakia presents as a whitish thickening of the epithelium of the mucous membranes, occurring as lactescent superficial patches of various shapes and sizes that may coalesce to form diffuse sheets. The surface is generally glistening and opalescent, often reticulated, and may even be somewhat pigmented. The white pellicle is adherent to the underlying mucosa and attempts to remove it forcibly cause bleeding. At times it is a thick, rough, elevated plaque. The lips, gums, cheeks, and edges of the tongue are the most common sites, but the lesion

may arise on the anus and genitalia. Leukoplakia is found chiefly in men over the age of 40.

Biopsy of these white lesions may reveal orthokeratosis or parakeratosis with minimal inflammation, or there may be evidence of varying degrees of dysplasia. There is a benign form that is usually a response to chronic irritation and that has very little chance of conversion into the precancerous dysplastic form. Premalignant leukoplakia, with atypical cells histologically, is present in only about 10–20% of leukoplakia. Unfortunately, it is not possible to predict clinically which lesions will be worrisome histologically, except that if ulceration, red areas, or erosions are scattered throughout, the lesion is most likely precancerous. Therefore, biopsy is indicated.

When the lesion occurs on the lip, leukoplakia is closely related to chronic actinic cheilitis, which consists of a circumscribed or diffuse keratosis, almost invariably on the lower lip. It is preceded by an abnormal dryness of the lip and may be caused by smoking (especially pipe smoking) or chronic sun exposure. This type of leukoplakia is distinguished from squamous cell carcinoma of the lip by the absence of infiltration, from lichen planus and psoriasis of the lips and mouth by the absence of lesions elsewhere, and from lupus erythematosus by the absence of telangiectases. Biopsy is necessary, however, to differentiate these conditions fully.

Intraoral leukoplakia appears to progress to squamous cell carcinoma in not more than 1% per year. In time, an extensive, thick, white pellicle may cover the tongue or oral mucosa. In old lesions the epithelium may be desquamated and there may be fissures or ulcerations. Such changes are associated with more or less hyperemia and tenderness, and with a tendency to bleed after slight trauma. If transformation to carcinoma occurs, it generally follows a 1 to 20-year lag time, with the exception that immunosuppressed transplant patients may have a rapid course of transformation.

Oral hairy leukoplakia is a term used to describe white, corrugated plaques that occur primarily on the sides of the tongue of patients with AIDS (Fig. 34-14). This is a virally induced lesion, discussed in Chapter 19, which has a characteristic histology.

Leukoplakia of the vulva usually occurs in obese women after menopause as grayish white, thickened, pruritic patches that may become fissured and edematous from constant rubbing and scratching. Secondary infection with edema, tenderness, and pain may occur. It is differentiated from lichen planus by the absence of discrete, rectangular, or annular flat papules of violaceous hue in the mucosa outside the thickened patches, about the anus, on the buccal mucosa, or on the skin. Leukoplakia of the vulva is most frequently confused with lichen sclerosus et atrophicus and other vulval atrophies. On the penis, though leukoplakia may occur, a similar precancerous process called erythroplasia (of Queyrat) is usually seen instead.

Etiology

Numerous factors are involved in the cause of leukoplakia. It may develop as a result of tobacco smoking, use of smokeless tobacco, areca, qat, or betel nut chewing, reverse smoking, alcohol, poorly fitting dentures, sharp and chipped teeth, or improper oral hygiene. Extensive involvement of the lips and oral cavity with leukoplakia may exist for years without any indication of carcinoma. On the other hand, small, inflamed patches may be the site of a rapidly growing tumor, which, with relatively insignificant local infiltration, may involve the cervical lymphatics. Carcinoma in leukoplakia usually begins as a localized induration, often about a fissure, or as a warty excrescence or a small ulcer. There is a 6–10% transformation rate of intraoral leukoplakia into squamous cell carcinoma. Predictors of a higher risk of squamous cell carcinoma development include older age, female sex, nonsmokers, large size, presence on the lateral or ventral tongue, floor of the mouth, or retromolar/soft palate complex, erythroleukoplakia, and a nonhomogeneous morphology.

The degree of epithelial atypia may be considered in staging the risk of developing malignancy. Aneuploid leukoplakia has a high rate of transformation into aggressive squamous cell carcinoma, and the cancers derived from it are more likely to be lethal.

Treatment

It must be remembered that cancer develops frequently on histologically dysplastic leukoplakia, so that its complete removal should be the goal in each case—first by conservative measures, then by surgery or destruction, if necessary. The use of tobacco should be stopped, and proper dental care obtained. Fulguration, simple excision, cryotherapy, and CO_2 laser ablation are effective methods of treatment. Medical therapies that have been the subject of randomized clinical trials may lead to temporary resolution of the lesions, but relapses and adverse effects are common and there is no evidence that they prevent the transformation to malignancy.

Leukoplakia with tylosis and esophageal carcinoma

Leukoplakia associated with tylosis and esophageal carcinoma is extremely rare but may occur.

Epidermization of the lip

Relatively smooth leukokeratosis of the lower vermilion, blending evenly into the skin surface distally and having a steep, sharp, irregular proximal margin, may easily be mistaken clinically for precancerous leukoplakia. Histologically, it shows only hyperkeratosis, without parakeratosis or cellular atypia. A shallow shave excision suffices to cure it and to rule out precancerous leukoplakia; no fulguration is required.

Erythroplakia

The term erythroplakia is applied to leukoplakia that has lost (or has not developed) the thick keratin layer that makes leukoplakia white; it is the usual pattern in mucocutaneous junctions. A focal red patch with no apparent cause should be suspected of being precancerous when found on the floor of the mouth, soft palate, or buccal mucosa, or under the tongue (Fig. 34-15). Histologically, there is cellular atypia, pleomorphism, hyperchromatism, and increased mitotic figures.

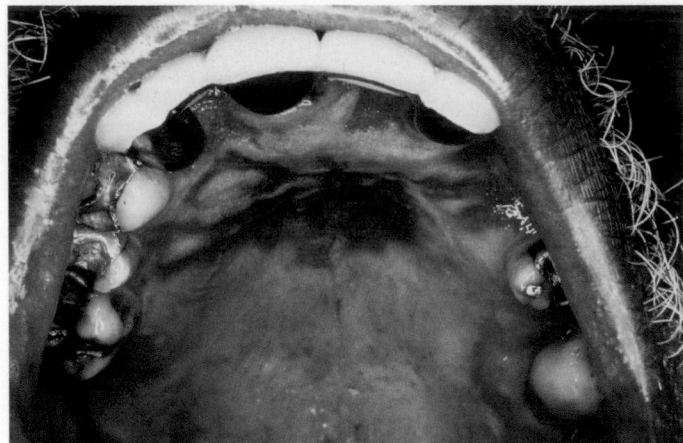

Fig. 34-15 Erythroplakia.

Carcinoma in situ or invasive carcinoma is found in 90% of lesions.

Oral florid papillomatosis

Oral florid papillomatosis is a confluent papillomatosis covering the mucous membranes of the oral cavity. The distinctive picture is that of a white mass resembling a cauliflower, covering the tongue and extending on to the other portions of the mucous membranes, including the oropharynx, larynx, and trachea. Usually there is no lymphadenopathy.

The course of the disease is progressive. Many lesions eventuate in squamous cell carcinoma, whereas others continue for many years, the patient dying of some intercurrent disease. Oral florid papillomatosis should be regarded as a verrucous carcinoma, which has been defined as a distinctive, slowly growing, fungating tumor representing a well-differentiated squamous cell carcinoma in which metastases occur very late or not at all. The histologic features are those of papillomatosis, acanthosis, and varying degrees of dysplasia of the epithelium, without disruption of the basement membrane. It is reasonable to expect the eventual development of epidermoid carcinoma in most patients. Esophageal involvement and keratotic papules of the extremities may occur. In the differential diagnosis, leukoplakia, proliferative verrucous leukoplakia, candidiasis, acanthosis nigricans, and condyloma acuminatum should be considered. The recommended treatment is surgical excision; however, it is often followed by recurrence and spread. Recombinant interferon-α 2a in combination with a CO_2 laser has also been used.

Proliferative verrucous leukoplakia

Proliferative verrucous leukoplakia is a slowly progressive condition that begins as multifocal sites of hyperplasia of the oral mucous membranes and proceeds to thicken and enlarge until squamous cell carcinoma results (Fig. 34-16). Women outnumber men 4:1. Initially flat, usually white patches are present, but the lesions relentlessly become warty, exophytic masses. The patches may involve the lips and chin. Seventy percent develop squamous cell carcinoma (most frequently of the palate and gingiva), with 40% of the total dying of proliferative verrucous leukoplakia-associated carcinoma. It has been irregularly associated with human papillomavirus (HPV)-16 infection, and risk factors for squamous cell carcinoma of the oral cavity are usually not present. Treatment is difficult because of the multifocal nature of the lesions. Aggressive early surgical therapy is best. Many patients develop recurrence after only a short interval. Laser treatment

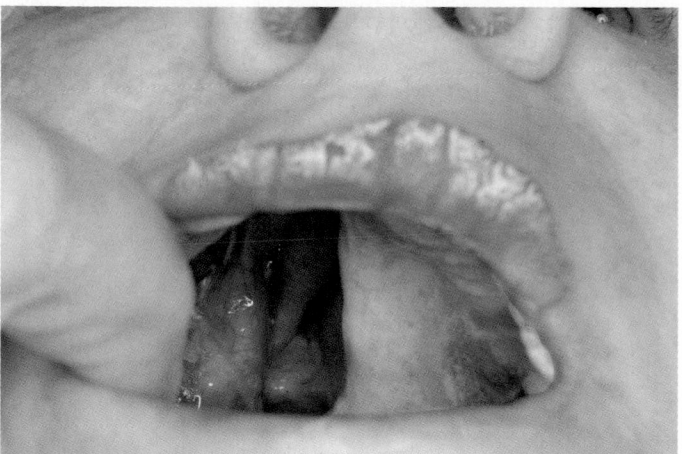

Fig. 34-16 Proliferative verrucous leukoplakia, three sites of SCC: lip and twice in the palate.

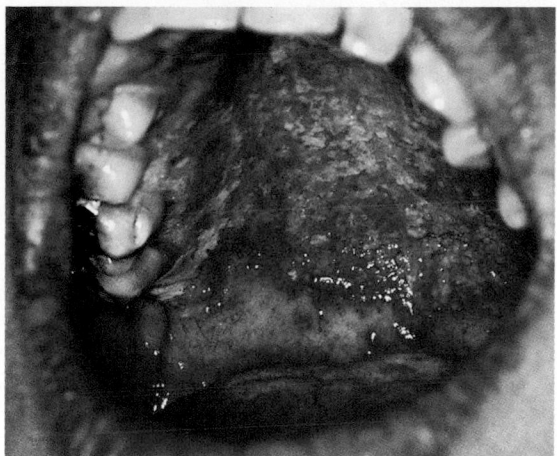

Fig. 34-18 Acquired dyskeratotic leukoplakia.

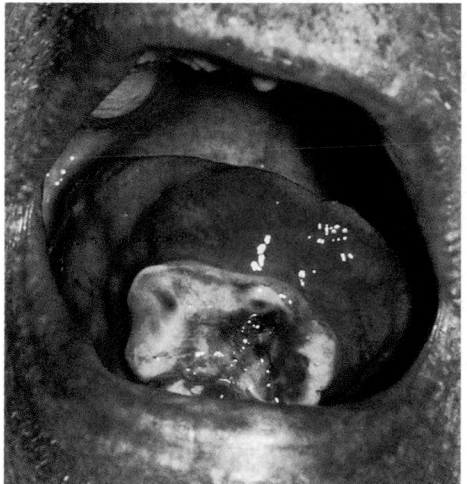

Fig. 34-17 Oral squamous cell carcinoma.

or photodynamic therapy should be considered primary options.

Squamous cell carcinoma

Squamous cell carcinoma is the most common oral malignancy, comprising 2–3% of all new cancers. With nearly 30 000 yearly cases in the US, it is the tenth most common malignancy. It occurs primarily in older men. The most frequent sites are the lower lip, tongue, soft palate, and floor of the mouth (Fig. 34-17). Squamous cell carcinoma of the lip develops from actinic damage, with 95% of the cases involving the lower lip. Intraoral lesions frequently develop from leukoplakia or erythroplakia, at sites of frequent irritation, or from long-standing mucosal inflammatory disease such as ulcerative lichen planus. About 20% of oral squamous cell cancers have an associated focus of leukoplakia; these tend to be diagnosed at a less advanced stage than those where no associated leukoplakia exists. Verrucous carcinomas occur in the oral mucosa as they do on the skin. Tobacco-smoking, the use of smokeless tobacco, areca, qat, or betel nut-chewing, and reverse smoking are risk factors for the development of intraoral squamous cell carcinoma. Alcohol has not been shown to be an independent risk factor. They may also complicate xeroderma pigmentosa (the tip of the tongue), dyskeratosis congenita, dystrophic epidermolysis bullosa, erosive lichen planus, and oral submucous fibrosis. Unfortunately, the survival rate has remained at 50% for many years because disease is often discovered late, after it has metastasized to the cervical lymph nodes. Exfoliative cytology is a practical and accurate aid to oral cancer screening.

Bagan J, et al: Proliferative verrucous leukoplakia. Oral Dis 2010; 16:328.

Brennan M, et al: Management of oral epithelial dysplasia. Oral Surg Oral Med Oral Pathol Oral Radiol Endod 2007; 103(Suppl):S19 e1.

Cabay RJ, et al: Proliferative verrucous leukoplakia and its progression to oral carcinoma. J Oral Pathol Med 2007; 36:255.

Casiglia J, Woo SB: A comprehensive review of oral cancer. Gen Dent 2001; 49:72.

El-Wajeh YA, et al: Qat and its health effects. Br Dent J 2009; 206:17.

Greer RO: Pathology of malignant and premalignant epithelial lesions. Otolaryngol Clin North Am 2006; 39:249.

Haya-Fernandez MC, et al: The prevalence of oral leukoplakia in 138 patients with oral squamous cell carcinoma. Oral Dis 2004; 10:346.

Hernandez G, et al: Rapid progression from oral leukoplakia to carcinoma in an immunosuppressed liver transplant recipient. Oral Oncol 2003; 39:87.

Ishii J, et al: Management of oral leukoplakia by laser surgery. J Clin Laser Med Surg 2004; 22:27.

Jacob BJ, et al: Betel quid without tobacco as a risk factor for oral precancers. Oral Oncol 2004; 40:697.

Kademani D: Oral cancer. Mayo Clin Proc 2007; 82:878.

Lodi G, et al: Interventions for treating oral leukoplakias. Cochrane Database Syst Rev 2006; 4:CD001829.

Lodi G, et al: Management of potentially malignant disorders. J Oral Pathol Med 2008; 37:63.

Napier SS, et al: Natural history of potentially malignant oral lesions and conditions. J Oral Pathol Med 2008; 37:1.

Reichart PA, et al: Oral erythroplakia. Oral Oncol 2005; 41:551.

Rhodus NL: Oral cancer. Dent Clin North Am 2005; 49:143.

Scheifele C, et al: The sensitivity and specificity of the OralCDx technique: evaluation of 103 cases. Oral Oncol 2004; 40:824.

Schwartz RA: Verrucous carcinoma of the skin and mucosa. J Am Acad Dermatol 1995; 32:1.

Sciubba JJ: Oral Cancer. Am J Clin Dermatol 2001; 2:239.

Sudbo J, et al: The influence of resection and aneuploidy on mortality in oral leukoplakia. N Engl J Med 2004; 350:1405.

Thoma G, et al: Risk factors for multiple oral premalignant lesions. Int J Cancer 2003; 107:285.

Trivedy CR, et al: The oral health consequences of chewing areca nut. Addict Biol 2002; 7:115.

van der Hem PS, et al: The results of CO_2 laser surgery in patients with oral leukoplakia: a 25 year follow up. Oral Oncol 2005; 41:31.

Acquired dyskeratotic leukoplakia

James and Lupton reported a patient with acquired dyskeratotic leukoplakia, which manifested as distinctive white plaques on the palate, gingivae, and lips (Fig. 34-18). There were similar lesions of the genitalia of the patient. Histologically, there was a unique finding of clusters of dyskeratotic cells in the prickle-cell layer in all affected sites.

Aggressive laser treatment was followed by recurrence. Use of etretinate afforded some improvement, but the condition continues unabated after 20 years.

James WD, et al: Acquired dyskeratotic leukoplakia. Arch Dermatol 1988; 124:117.

White sponge nevus

The mouth, vagina, or rectum may be the site of this spongy, white overgrowth of the mucous membrane, with acanthosis, vacuolated prickle cells, and acidophilic condensations in the cytoplasm of keratinocytes, which have been shown by electron microscopy to be aggregated tonofilaments. The buccal mucosa is the most common site of involvement. There are no extramucosal lesions. Progression of the disorder generally stops at puberty. The disease is inherited as an autosomal-dominant disorder. A mutation in the mucosal keratin pair *K4* and *K13* has been identified as the inherited defect. HPV-16 DNA has been identified in some patients, the significance of which remains to be determined. Antibiotics, particularly tetracycline, may give significant improvement. A 0.25% aqueous preparation of tetracycline as a mouth rinse, 5 mL swished in the mouth for 1 min twice daily, has been successful.

López Jornet P: White sponge nevus. Pediatr Dermatol 2008; 25:116.
Nishizawa A, et al: A de novo missense mutation in the keratin 13 gene in oral white sponge naevus. Br J Dermatol 2008; 159:974.
Otobe IF, et al: White sponge naevus. Clin Exp Dermatol 2007; 32:749.
Zhang JM, et al: Two new mutations in the keratin 4 gene causing oral white sponge nevus in Chinese family. Oral Dis 2009; 15:100.

Melanocytic oral lesions

A wide variety of melanocytic lesions appear on the mucous membranes. Nevi of the oral mucosa in general are very uncommon. Among the melanocytic nevi of the cellular type, the intramucosal type is the most frequent, with the compound nevus next and the junction nevus occurring only rarely. Ephelis, lentigo, blue nevus, and labial melanotic macules are other types of focal hyperpigmentation. Ephelides darken on sun exposure and are usually limited to the lower lip. The blue nevus has dendritic cells in the submucosa. Lentigines show acanthosis of rete ridges on biopsy. Oral melanotic macules are solitary, sharply demarcated, flat, pigmented lesions that occur chiefly in young women, do not change on sun exposure, and show only acanthosis and basal-layer melanin on biopsy.

Oral melanoacanthoma is a simultaneous proliferation of keratinocytes and melanocytes. It is most commonly observed in young black patients (average age, 23) on the buccal mucosa. It seems to be a reactive process, usually following trauma and resolving spontaneously in 40% of patients.

Melanoma occurs uncommonly, mostly in older patients. It is recognized by being larger than the usual benign pigmented lesion and more irregular in shape, with a tendency to ulcerate and bleed. A peripheral areola of erythema and satellite pigmented spots may be present. There is a striking predilection for palatal (or, less often, gingival) involvement. The overall prognosis is poor (less than 5% survival at 5 years) because the lesions are usually deeply invasive by the time they are discovered. Whereas oral nevi are uncommon, biopsy of solitary pigmented oral lesions is indicated when the clinical diagnosis is uncertain. Biopsy of a pigmented tumor will occasionally reveal a squamous cell carcinoma.

Buchner A, et al: Relative frequency of solitary melanocytic lesions of the oral mucosa. J Oral Pathol Med 2004; 33:550.

Carlos-Bregni R, et al: Oral melanoacanthoma and oral melanotic macule. Med Oral Pathol Oral Cir Bucal 2007; 12:E374.
Femiano F, et al: Oral malignant melanoma. J Oral Pathol Med 2008; 37:383.
Gaeta GM, et al: Oral pigmented lesions. Clin Dermatol 2002; 20:286.
Gondivkar SM, et al: Primary oral melanoma. Quintessence Int 2009; 40:41.
Lisboa Castro J, et al: Pigmented oral squamous cell carcinoma. Int J Surg Pathol 2009; 17:153.
Medina JE, et al: Current management of mucosal melanoma of the head and neck. J Surg Oncol 2003; 83:116.
Meleti M, et al: Oral pigmented lesions of the oral mucosa and perioral tissues. Oral Surg Oral Med Oral Pathol Oral Radiol Endod 2008; 105:606.
Ojha J, et al: Intraoral cellular blue nevus. Cutis 2007; 80:189.

Melanosis

Pigmentation of the oral cavity tends to occur most frequently in black persons. In other races, the darker the skin, the more mucosal pigmentation may be expected. Oral melanosis may occur with Albright syndrome, Peutz–Jeghers syndrome, Carney complex, Laugier–Hunziker disease, and Addison's disease, or rarely, as an idiopathic process with no associated disease.

James et al reported a patient with inflammatory acquired oral hyperpigmentation that first occurred at age 30 with numerous distinct pigmented macules, similar to those seen in Peutz–Jeghers syndrome. However, the condition progressed rapidly to a diffuse oral hyperpigmentation (Fig. 34-19). This appeared to be caused by an undefined inflammation, and slow partial resolution occurred after several years of observation.

In the differential diagnosis of oral hyperpigmentation, these other entities should be included. The amalgam tattoo is a focal, brownish-blue macule incurred from fragments of dental silver or amalgam being implanted into the gums (Fig. 34-20).

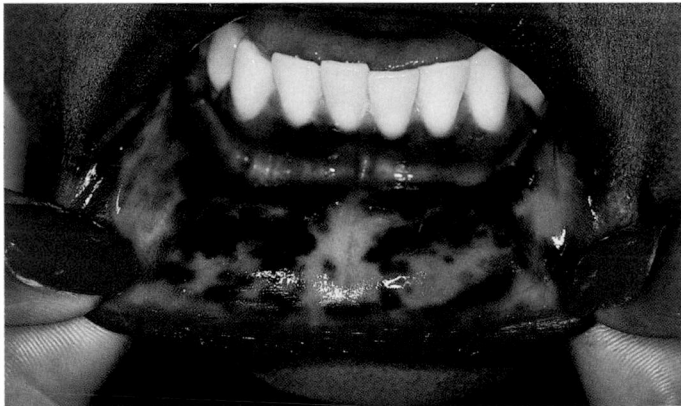

Fig. 34-19 Oral melanosis.

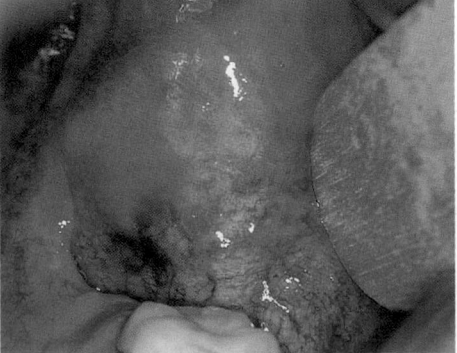

Fig. 34-20 Amalgam tattoo.

Heavy-metal poisoning may also induce such lesions. Bismuth, lead, and cis-platinum may produce a pigmented line along the gums near their margin. A multitude of medications will cause pigmentation. Amodiaquine, chloroquine, oral contraceptives, phenothiazines, phenolphthalein, quinacrine, quinidine, thallium, tobacco, and zidovudine are among the most common of these.

Abdollahi M, et al: A review of drug-induced oral reactions. J Contemp Dent Pract 2003; 15:10.

James WD, et al: Inflammatory acquired oral hyperpigmentation. J Am Acad Dermatol 1987; 16:220.

Laporta VN, et al: Minocycline-associated intra-oral soft-tissue pigmentation. J Clin Periodontol 2005; 32:119.

Meleti M, et al: Oral pigmented lesions of the oral mucosa and perioral tissues. Oral Surg Oral Med Oral Pathol Oral Radiol Endod 2008; 105:606.

Osseous choristoma of the tongue

Osseous choristoma of the tongue presents as a nodule on the dorsum of the tongue containing mature lamellar bone without osteoblastic or osteoclastic activity. This does not recur after simple excision.

Naik VR, et al: Choristoma of the base of the tongue. Indian J Pathol Microbiol 2009; 52:86.

Peripheral ameloblastoma

This is a neoplasm of the gingivae, which appears most often on the lower jaw. The mean age at onset is the early fifties and men outnumber women. It presents as a growing pink to red sessile or pedunculated mass. Excision is followed by recurrence in 19% of the cases, but the lesion is benign. Basal cell carcinoma can be simulated histologically.

Curran AE, et al: Peripheral desmoplastic ameloblastoma. J Oral Maxillofac Surg 2008; 66:820.

Vanoven BJ, et al: Peripheral ameloblastoma of the maxilla. Am J Otolaryngol 2008; 29:357.

Trumpeter's wart

Trumpeter's wart is a firm, fibrous, hyperkeratotic, pseudoepitheliomatous nodule on the upper lip of a trumpet player. A similar callus may grow on the lower lip of trombone players.

Gambichler T, et al: Skin conditions in instrumental musicians. Contact Dermatitis 2008; 58:217.

Epulis

The term epulis means any benign lesion situated on the gingiva. The majority of these are reactive processes that display varying degrees of fibrosis, inflammation, and vascular proliferation on biopsy. Giant cell epulis (peripheral giant cell granuloma) is a solitary, bluish-red, 10–20 mm tumor occurring on the gingiva between or about deciduous bicuspids and incisors. Lesions may be induced by dental implants. Similar lesions may occur in the autosomal-dominantly inherited syndrome, cherubism. Histologically, they resemble giant cell tumor of the tendon sheath.

Salum FG: Pyogenic granuloma, peripheral giant cell granuloma and peripheral ossifying fibroma. Minerva Stomatol 2008; 57:227.

Scarano A, et al: Peripheral giant cell granuloma associated with a dental implant. Minerva Stomatol 2008; 57:529.

Pyogenic granuloma

Pyogenic granuloma is an exuberant overgrowth of granulation tissue, frequently occurring in the oral cavity, most often involving the gingiva. It may also occur on the buccal mucosa, lips, tongue, or palate. It is a red to reddish-purple, soft, nodular mass that bleeds easily and grows rapidly, but is usually not painful. When it develops during pregnancy, it is called pregnancy tumor or granuloma gravidarum. Surgical excision, pulsed dye or Nd:YAG lasers, and cryosurgery offer effective methods of treatment.

Gordon-Nunez MA, et al: Oral pyogenic granuloma. J Oral Maxillofac Surg 2010; 68:2185.

Jafarzadeh H: Oral pyogenic granuloma. J Oral Sci 2006; 48:167.

Granuloma fissuratum

Granuloma fissuratum is a circumscribed, firm, whitish, fissured, fibrous granuloma occurring in the labioalveolar fold. The lesion is discoid, smooth, and slightly raised, about 1 cm in diameter. The growth is folded like a bent coin, so that the fissure in the bend is continuous on both sides with the labioalveolar sulcus. Symptoms are slight. It is an inflammatory fibrous hyperplasia that usually results from chronic irritation caused by poorly fitting dentures. In the dental literature it is called epulis fissuratum, particularly when there is a deep cleft traversing the lesion. Treatment is by surgical extirpation, CO_2 laser ablation, or electrodesiccation after biopsy.

Bhattacharyya I: Epulis fissuratum. Todays FDA 2008; 20:15.

Angina bullosa haemorrhagica

The sudden appearance of one or more blood blisters of the oral mucosa characterizes this entity. There is no associated skin or systemic disease. The blisters may be recurrent, occur most often in the soft palate, and usually present in middle-aged or elderly patients. No treatment is necessary.

Sera D, et al: Angina bullosa haemorrhagica. Eur J Dermatol 2010; 20:509.

Yip HK: Angina bullosa haemorrhagica. Gen Dent 2004; 52:162.

Mucocele

The term mucocele refers to a lesion that occurs as a result of trauma or obstruction of the minor salivary ducts. The most common type is the mucous extravasation phenomenon, which is usually seen inside the lower lip because it is caused by trauma from biting (Fig. 34-21). The inside of the upper lip and buccal mucosa are uncommonly involved. It presents as a soft, rounded, translucent projection; it commonly has a bluish tint. The lesion varies from 2 to 10 mm in diameter. It is painless, fluctuant, and tense. Incision of it, or sometimes merely compression, releases sticky, straw-colored fluid (or bluish fluid if hemorrhage has occurred into it). Usually, the

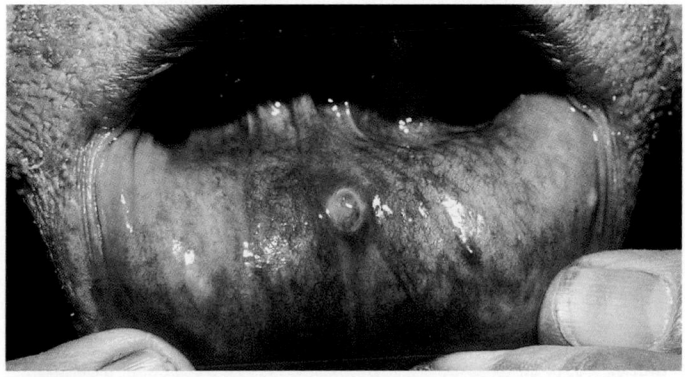

Fig. 34-21 Mucocele.

lesions are solitary; however, multiple superficial mucoceles have been reported to occur with graft versus host disease and lichenoid inflammation. In these cases topical steroids may help prevent recurrences.

The cause is rupture of the mucous duct, with extravasation of sialomucin into the submucosa to produce cystic spaces with inflammation. Granulation tissue formation is followed by fibrosis. Excisional biopsy will document the diagnosis and eliminate the problem. Cryotherapy and laser ablation have also been reported to be successful.

There are true mucous retention cysts where there is true obstruction of the duct leading to an epithelial-lined cavity. They are seen more in the posterior portions of the oral mucosa. A ranula (from Rana, the frog genus) is a mucocele of the floor of the mouth.

Two other cysts that may be present in the mouth are the parotid duct cyst, which occurs in musicians who use wind instruments (the cyst develops opposite the upper second molar on the buccal mucosa), and the dermoid cyst, which may occur on the floor of the mouth, especially in the sublingual area.

Balasubramaniam R, et al: Superficial mucoceles in chronic graft-versus-host disease. Gen Dent 2009; 57:82.
Nico MM, et al: Mucocele in pediatric patients. Pediatr Dermatol 2008; 25:308.
Silva A Jr, et al: Superficial mucocele of the labial mucosa. Gen Dent 2004; 52:424.

Acute necrotizing ulcerative gingivostomatitis (trench mouth, Vincent's disease)

Acute necrotizing ulcerative gingivitis (ANUG) is characterized by a rapid onset of characteristic punched-out ulcerations appearing on the interdental papillae and marginal gingivae. A dirty white pseudomembrane may cover the ulcerations. The lesions may spread rapidly and involve the buccal mucosa, lips, and tongue, as well as the tonsils, pharynx, and entire respiratory tract. The slightest pressure causes pain and bleeding. There is a characteristic foul, fetid odor that is always present. ANUG may lead to loss of attachment of the gingiva and alveolar bone (necrotizing ulcerative periodontitis).

Trench mouth begins in a nidus of necrotic tissue, which provides an anaerobic environment for the infection by fusospirochetal organisms (*Bacteroides fusiformis*) in association with *Borrelia vincentii* and other organisms. Poor dental hygiene, smoking, poor nutrition, ingestion of methylenedioxymethamphetamine (ecstasy), and immunosuppression are predisposing factors. It may be seen as a component of the oral infections and inflammatory lesions that occur in immunocompromised HIV-infected patients.

Acute herpetic gingivostomatitis, primary HSV infection, may be confused with ANUG. Young children are susceptible to this severe febrile stomatitis with lymphadenitis. It is not primarily gingival in location and does not cause necrosis of the interdental papillae. Noma is a form of fusospirillary gangrenous stomatitis occurring in children with low resistance and poor nutrition. The onset is often triggered by measles. At the onset there is ulceration of the buccal mucosa; this rapidly assumes a gangrenous character and extends to involve the skin and bones, with resultant necrosis. It may end in the patient's death.

Treatment consists of thorough dental hygienic measures under the supervision of a dentist. Penicillin with debridement is the treatment of choice. Use of a 3% hydrogen peroxide mouthwash is also helpful.

Brazier WJ, et al: Ecstasy related periodontitis and mucosal ulceration. Br Dent J 2003; 194:197.

Buchanan JA, et al: Necrotizing stomatitis in the developed world. Clin Exp Dermatol 2006; 31:372.
Euwonwu CO, et al: Noma (cancrum oris). Lancet 2006; 368:147.
Feller L, et al: Necrotizing periodontal diseases in HIV-seropositive subjects. J Int Acad Periodontol 2008; 10:10.
Golayan MO: The epidemiology, etiology, and pathophysiology of acute necrotizing ulcerative gingivitis associated with malnutrition. J Contemp Dent Pract 2004; 5:28.
Salama C: Fusospirochetosis causing necrotic oral ulcers in patients with HIV infection. Oral Surg Oral Med Oral Pathol Oral Radiol Endod 2004; 98:321.

Acatalasemia

Acatalasemia (Takahara's disease) is a rare disease in which the enzyme catalase is deficient in the liver, muscles, bone marrow, erythrocytes, and skin. There are several forms. The absence of catalase leads to progressive gangrene of the mouth, with recurrent ulcerations resulting from increased susceptibility to infection by anaerobic organisms.

Nearly 60% of affected individuals develop alveolar ulcerations, beginning in childhood. The mild type of the disease is characterized by rapidly recurring ulcers. In the moderate type, alveolar gangrene develops, with atrophy and recession of the alveolar bone, so that the teeth fall out spontaneously. In the severe type, widespread destruction of the jaw occurs. After puberty, all lesions heal, even in individuals who have the severe type.

There is no gross difference in appearance between the blood of an acatalasic patient and that of a normal individual, but when hydrogen peroxide is added to a sample of blood, acatalasic blood immediately turns blackish-brown and the peroxide does not foam. Normal blood remains bright and causes the peroxide to foam exuberantly because of the presence of erythrocyte catalase.

Acatalasia is a rare peroxisomal disorder and is inherited as an autosomal-recessive trait. Treatment consists of extraction of the diseased teeth and the use of antibiotics to control the harmful effects of the offending bacteria.

Ogata M: Acatalasemia. Hum Genet 1991; 86:331.
Perner H, et al: Acatalasemia—Takahara's disease. Hautarzt 1999; 50:590.

Cyclic neutropenia

Cyclic, or periodic, neutropenia is characterized by a decrease of circulating neutrophils and dermatologic manifestations. At regular intervals (21 days), neutropenia and mouth ulcerations develop, usually accompanied by fever, malaise, and arthralgia. Ulcerations of the lips, tongue, palate, gums, and buccal mucosa may be extensive. The ulcers are irregularly outlined and are covered by a grayish-white necrotic slough. The anterior teeth may show a grayish-brown discoloration. Premature alveolar bone loss and periodontitis occur. In addition, opportunistic cutaneous infections, such as abscesses, furuncles, noma, pyomyositis, and cellulitis, may develop during the neutropenic stage. Urticaria and erythema multiforme have been reported.

There is a cyclic depression of neutrophils occurring at intervals of 12–30 days (average, 21 days) and lasting 5–8 days. The neutrophils in the peripheral blood regularly fall to low levels or completely disappear. Some cases have been associated with agammaglobulinemia. The cause of cyclic neutropenia is a germline mutation of the gene encoding neutrophil elastase (*ELANE*). This is thought to produce apoptosis of bone marrow progenitor cells. Both the autosomal-dominant disease and sporadic cases have this abnormality. Severe congenital neutropenia is caused by a mutation in the same gene but at a different site. The latter condition predisposes to the development of myelodysplasia and acute myelogenous leukemia, while cyclic neutropenia does not.

In the differential diagnosis are other periodic fever syndromes, including periodic fever, aphthous stomatitis, pharyngitis and adenopathy (PFAPA) syndrome, Mediterranean fever, Hibernian fever and hyperimmunoglobulin D syndrome, tumor necrosis factor receptor-associated periodic syndrome (TRAPS), and pyogenic sterile arthritis, pyoderma gangrenosum and acne (PAPA) syndrome. All share a predisposition to the development of aphthous-like oral ulcerations. PFAPA syndrome is defined clinically and is characterized by 4 days of high fevers (over 40°C) that recur at regular intervals every 2–8 weeks, separated by wellbeing between episodes. Associated with fevers are aphthous stomatitis (70%), pharyngitis (72%), and cervical adenitis (88%). The disease is not familial, begins before 5 years of age, and responds to small doses of prednisone for 1–2 days. Tonsillectomy has been reported to cure it.

Use of recombinant human granulocyte colony-stimulating factor (G-CSF) has been successful in the treatment of cyclic neutropenia patients. If the potential side effects limit use of this therapy, cyclosporine has been reported to be effective also. Administering antibiotics during infections seems to expedite recovery. Careful attention to oral hygiene, including plaque control, helps improve mouth lesions and reduces the risk of infections. Death may occur from pneumonia, sepsis, gangrenous pyoderma, or granulocytopenia.

Femiano F: Oral aphthous-like lesions, PFAPA syndrome. J Oral Pathol Med 2008; 37:319.

Jacobs Z, et al: Periodic fever syndromes. Curr Allergy Asthma Rep 2010; (epub).

Kanazawa N, et al: Autoinflammatory syndromes with a dermatological perspective. J Dermatol 2007; 34:601.

Scully C, et al: Recurrent oral ulceration. Oral Surg Oral Med Oral Pathol Oral Radiol Endod 2008; 106:845.

Shiohara M, et al: Ela2 mutations and clinical manifestations in familial congenital neutropenia. J Pediatr Hematol Oncol 2009; 31:319.

Recurrent intraoral herpes simplex infection

Recurrent intraoral infection with HSV is characterized by numerous small, discrete vesicles occurring in one or a few clusters. The site of involvement is a key feature in suspecting the diagnosis. The keratinized or masticatory mucosa (the palate, gingiva, and tongue) is affected. The grouped vesicles rupture rapidly to form punctate erosions with a red base. Smears from the base prepared with Wright stain will show giant multinucleated epithelial cells. Immunofluorescent tests and viral cultures are also confirmatory.

The differential diagnosis of this uncommon manifestation of HSV includes oral herpes zoster, herpangina, and oral aphthosis. The latter two involve nonattached mucosa, whereas recurrent HSV involves mucosa fixed to bone. Differentiation from zoster is made on clinical grounds or by culture and immunofluorescent testing.

Chronic progressive ulcerative and nodular intraoral herpes are seen occasionally in HIV-infected patients, or those with leukemia or neutropenia (Fig. 34-22). Mucosal toxicity to chemotherapy may be mimicked. Solitary painful erosions of the tongue or attached mucosa should be tested for HSV in such patients. Additionally, herpetic geometric glossitis, linear longitudinal, cross-hatched, or branching fissures of the dorsal tongue, usually along the central area, may occur. This may be quite painful and limit oral intake. While it usually affects only immunocompromised patients, at least one immunocompetent patient has been affected.

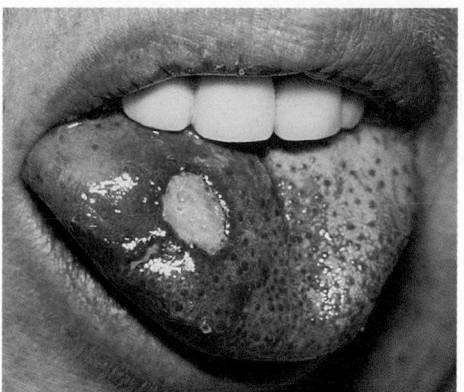

Fig. 34-22 Chronic herpes in a patient on cancer chemotherapy.

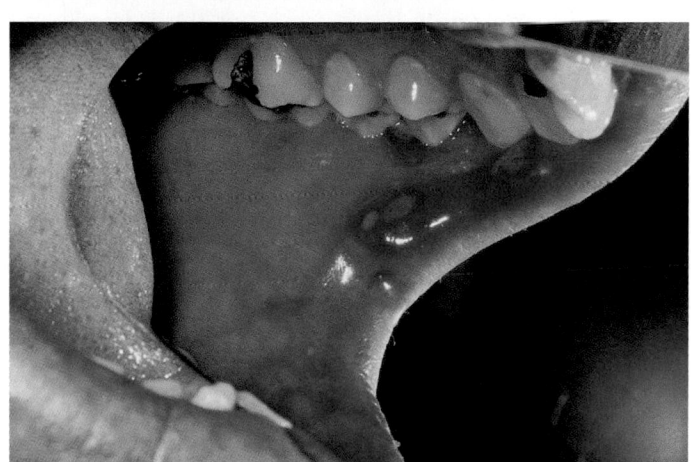

Fig. 34-23 Aphthous stomatitis.

Arduino PG, et al: Herpes simplex virus type 1 infection. J Oral Pathol Med 2008; 37:107.

Druce AJ, et al: Acute oral ulcers. Dermatol Clin 2003; 21:1.

Mirowski GW, et al: Herpetic geometric glossitis in an immunocompetent patient with pneumonia. J Am Acad Dermatol 2009: 61:139.

Woo SB, et al: Management of recurrent oral herpes simplex infections. Oral Surg Oral Med Oral Pathol Oral Radiol Endod 2007; 103(Suppl): S12.e1.

Recurrent aphthous stomatitis (canker sores, aphthosis)

Clinical features

Aphthous stomatitis is a painful, recurrent disease of the oral mucous membrane. It begins as small, red, discrete, or grouped papules, which in a few hours become necrotizing ulcerations. They are small, round, shallow, white ulcers (aphthae), generally surrounded by a ring of hyperemia (Fig. 34-23). As a rule, they are tender; they may become so painful that they interfere with speech and mastication. They are mostly about 5 mm in diameter but may vary in size from 3 to 10 mm. When larger, they are called major aphthae. A third subcategory, herpetiform aphthae, consists of small 1–3 mm lesions grouped into a coalescing larger plaque, which may take 1–4 weeks to resolve. Usually, 1–5 lesions occur per attack; however, they may occur in any number. They are located in decreasing frequency on the buccal and labial mucosa, edges of the tongue, buccal and lingual sulci, and soft palate. There is a marked predilection for the nonkeratinized mucosa (any not bound to underlying periosteum). This and the fact that they are rarely confluent, even when they occur as small crops of 1 or 2 mm lesions (herpetiform aphthae), help to distinguish them from the uncommon recurrent intraoral HSV infection. Aphthae may also occur on the vagina, vulva, penis, anus, and even the conjunctiva. When they involve the oral and genital mucosa and are nearly always present in numbers greater than or equal to three, the term complex aphthosis is applied.

The lesions tend to involute in 1–2 weeks, but recurrences are common. These recurrences may be induced by trauma, such as self-biting, toothbrush injury, and dental procedures, spicy foods, citrus, fresh pineapple, walnuts, allergy, emotional stress, or hormonal changes in women, such as in menstruation, pregnancy, menarche, and menopause. A familial predisposition has also been described as familial epidemic aphthosis.

Recurrent aphthous stomatitis is the most common lesion of the oral mucosa, affecting from 10% to 20% of the population. It starts commonly in the second or third decade and patients may experience recurrent bouts of lesions several times yearly for many decades. When present in neonates or young children, autoinflammatory syndromes should be considered. In PFAPA syndrome, the high fevers and associated findings occur with striking periodicity every 4 weeks, last 4–6 days, and resolve only to recur the following month. The children are otherwise well. One or two doses of prednisone (2 mg/kg) abort the attack and tonsillectomy may cure it. Aphthous oral ulcerations may also be seen in familial Mediterranean fever, TRAPS, hyperimmunoglobulinemia D and periodic fever, PAPA syndrome, and the newly defined deficiency of the interleukin-1-receptor antagonist (DIRA) syndrome.

Ulcerations such as these may also be the presenting sign in Behçet syndrome, HIV infection, malabsorption syndromes, gluten-sensitive enteropathy, pernicious anemia, cyclic neutropenia, neutropenia, ulcerative colitis, and Crohn's disease. History, physical examination, complete blood count, and long-term follow-up documenting the recurrent course in the absence of other symptoms will secure the diagnosis. Some patients have aphthosis associated with low folate, B$_{12}$ or iron levels, so testing should include evaluation of these.

Etiologic factors

Although individual patients often suspect that one of the factors mentioned above is responsible for precipitating their recurrence, infectious or immunologic causation is favored by investigators. The true cause is unknown.

Histologically, the lesion consists of a lymphocytic inflammatory infiltration with occasional plasma cells and eosinophils, which suggests delayed hypersensitivity.

Diagnosis

Aphthous stomatitis must be differentiated from mucous patches of early syphilis, candidiasis, Vincent angina, the avitaminoses (particularly pellagra and scurvy), erythema multiforme, pemphigus, cicatricial pemphigoid, lichen planus, primary HSV infection of the mouth, recurrent labial herpes, and recurrent intraoral HSV infection.

Treatment

No permanent cure is available. Several topical agents will lessen the pain. A mixture of equal parts of elixir of Benadryl and Maalox, held in the mouth for 5 min before meals, is soothing. Kaolin may also be added to the mixture. Lidocaine (Xylocaine Viscous) 2% solution, keeping 1 teaspoonful in the mouth for several minutes, is helpful in allaying pain. Another useful topical anesthetic is dyclonine hydrochloride (Dyclone) 0.5% applied to the lesions. A large number of reasonably effective over-the-counter remedies are also available. Triggers, such as spicy foods, citrus, walnuts, pineapple, and other irritating substances should be avoided.

One may use other measures to shorten the course and induce healing of lesions. A mixture of equal parts of fluocinonide ointment and Orabase, applied to the ulcers three or four times a day, is effective in aiding the healing of existing ulcers; however, it does not prevent new ulcers. Some patients object to the thick, sticky texture of Orabase and prefer fluocinonide gel. Clobetasol ointment can also be very effective. Intralesional steroids and short 3- or 4-day courses of oral steroids may help, particularly for indolent or large lesions. Nonsteroidal alternatives include 5 mL of an oral suspension containing 250 mg of tetracycline; this is held in the mouth for 2 min and then swallowed. This is done four times daily for 1 week. Amlexanox 5% oral paste (Aphthasol) is a useful topical therapy both to induce healing and to relieve pain. Sucralfate suspension, alone or compounded with a topical steroid, may be useful, as has been described in peptic ulcer disease and the ulcerations of Behçet's disease.

To try to prevent new lesions, known triggers for the individual patient should be avoided as much as possible. Colchicine at 0.6 mg per day for 1 week, then increasing to 1.2 or even 1.8 mg per day, is recommended. If this is ineffective or gastrointestinal or other side effects limit dosage, dapsone may be added to colchicine or substituted for it. It is given in steadily increasing doses of 25 mg for 3 days, then 50 mg for 3 days, then 75 mg for 3 days, then 100 mg for 7 days. If the blood count is normal, no side effects are present, and the disease is not controlled, further increases to 125 or even 150 mg may be given. Thalidomide is another effective alternative, but caution regarding teratogenicity and neurotoxicity is necessary if this is to be considered. One method is thalidomide, 300 mg/day to start, 200 mg/day after 10 days, and 100 mg/day after 2 months. Relapses are treated with 100 mg/day for 12 days.

Several investigators have reported finding low folate, iron, or B$_{12}$ levels in about 20% of aphthosis patients investigated, but others do not see this with such high frequency. Still, it is worth investigating, as correction of the abnormality clears or improves the condition in most cases where an abnormality exists. Two studies document improvement with cyanocobalamin, even of those without abnormalities.

Aksentijevich I, et al: An autoinflammatory disease with deficiency of the interleukin-1-receptor antagonist. N Engl J Med 2009; 360:2467.

Berlucchi M, et al: Update on treatment of Marshall's syndrome (PFAPA syndrome). Ann Otol Rhinol Laryngol 2003; 112:365.

Bruce AJ, et al: Acute oral ulcers. Dermatol Clin 2003; 21:1.

Femiano F, et al: Guidelines for diagnosis and management of aphthous stomatitis. Pediatr Infect Dis J 2007; 26:728.

Glucan E, et al: Cyanocobalamin may be beneficial in the treatment of recurrent aphthous stomatitis even when vitamin B$_{12}$ levels are normal. Am J Med Sci 2008; 336:379.

Hello M, et al: Use of thalidomide for severe recurrant aphthous stomatitis. Medicine (Baltimore) 2010; 89:176.

Lynde CB, et al: Successful treatment of complex aphthosis with colchicine and dapsone. Arch Dermatol 2009; 145:273.

Sampaio IC, et al: Two siblings with PFAPA syndrome. Pediatr Infect Dis 2009; 28:254.

Scully C, et al: Oral mucosal disease: recurrent aphthous stomatitis. Br J Oral Maxillofac Surg 2008; 46:198.

Scully C, et al: Auto-inflammatory syndromes and oral health. Oral Dis 2008; 14:690.

Shetty C, et al: Current role of thalidomide in HIV-positive patients with recurrent aphthous ulcerations. Gen Dent 2007; 55:537.

Zunt SL: Recurrent aphthous stomatitis. Dermatol Clin 2003; 21:33.

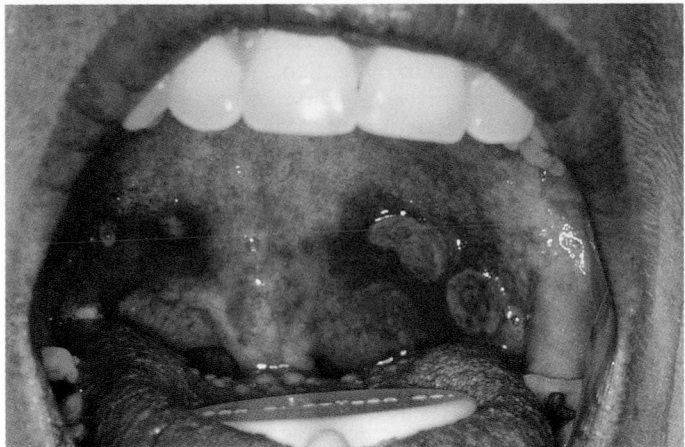

Fig. 34-24 Major aphthae.

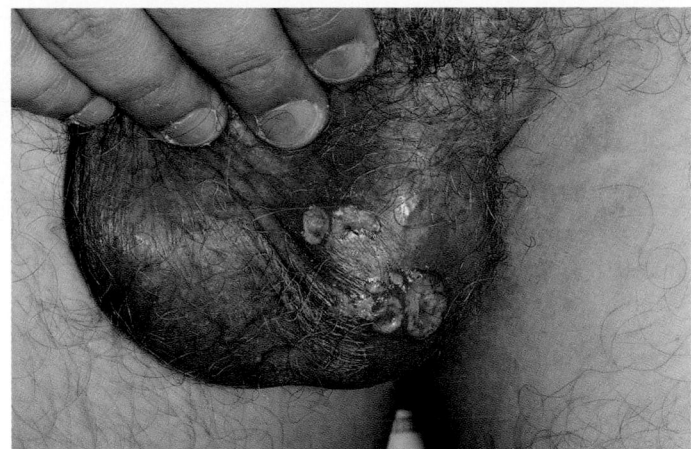

Fig. 34-25 Behçet disease.

Major aphthous ulcer (periadenitis mucosa necrotica recurrens)

In Sutton's disease, a major aphthous ulcer begins as a small shotlike nodule on the inner lip, buccal mucosa, or tongue, which breaks down into a painful, sharply circumscribed ulcer with a deeply punched-out and depressed crater. It may at times begin in the faucial pillars or oropharynx (Fig. 34-24). It may persist for 2–12 weeks before healing with a soft, pliable scar. There are seldom more than 1–3 lesions present at one time. However, remissions tend to be short, and new lesions may appear before old ones have quite healed. The term major aphthous ulcers has supplanted the unwieldy Latin name for this disease.

The cause is unknown, but evidence favors an immunologic or infectious etiology. These painful lesions are frequently present in HIV-infected patients who may experience similar lesions in the esophagus, rectum, anus, and genitals.

Treatment is difficult, and the general measures discussed under recurrent aphthae should be employed. Intralesional or systemic steroids in short courses, which may be effective, are often given. If recurrences are such that systemic steroids are prescribed for more than two or three short courses per year, alternative oral medications such as colchicine, dapsone, or thalidomide may be tried.

Boldo A: Major recurrent aphthous ulceration. Conn Med 2008; 72:271.

Chung JY, et al: Recurrent scarring ulcers of the oral mucosa. Arch Dermatol 1997; 133:1162.

Shetty C, et al: Current role of thalidomide in HIV-positive patients with recurrent aphthous ulcerations. Gen Dent 2007; 55:537.

Behçet syndrome (oculo-oral-genital syndrome)

Clinical features

Behçet syndrome consists of recurrent oral aphthous ulcerations that recur at least three times in one 12-month period in the presence of any two of the following: recurrent genital ulceration, retinal vasculitis or anterior or posterior uveitis, cutaneous lesions (erythema nodosum; pseudofolliculitis or papulopustular lesions; or acneiform nodules in postadolescent patients who are not receiving corticosteroid treatment), or a positive pathergy test.

Oral lesions occur on the lips, tongue, buccal mucosa, soft and hard palate, tonsils, and even in the pharynx and nasal cavity. The lesions are single or multiple, 2–10 mm or larger in diameter, and sharply circumscribed, with a dirty grayish base and a surrounding bright red halo. Other patients show deep ulcerations that leave scars resembling those caused by Sutton major aphthous ulcers. The lesions are so painful that eating may be difficult. A foul mouth odor is in most cases markedly noticeable.

Genital lesions occur in men on the scrotum (Fig. 34-25) and penis or in the urethra, and in women, on the vulva, cervix, or vagina; they may be found in both sexes on the genitocrural fold, anus, or perineum, or in the rectum. These ulcerations are similar to those seen in the mouth. In addition, macules, papules, and folliculitis may develop on the scrotum. Lesions in women may lead to deep destruction of the vulva. Swellings of the regional nodes and fever may accompany oral and genital attacks.

The ocular lesions start with intense periorbital pain and photophobia. Retinal vasculitis is the most classic eye sign and the chief cause of blindness. Conjunctivitis may be an early accompaniment of uveitis, and hypopyon a late one. Iridocyclitis is frequently seen. Both eyes are eventually involved. Untreated disease leads to blindness from optic atrophy, glaucoma, or cataracts.

Neurologic manifestations are mostly in the central nervous system and resemble most closely those of multiple sclerosis. Remissions and exacerbations are the rule. Thrombophlebitis occurs with some frequency. Thrombosis of the superior vena cava may also occur. Arthralgia is most often present in the form of polyarthritis.

Unfortunately, the international criteria include nonspecific common cutaneous lesions (pseudofolliculitis, papulopustular or acneiform lesions). Demonstration of either leukocytoclastic vasculitis or a neutrophilic vascular reaction on histologic examination of a lesion would make the cutaneous criteria more specific.

There is a relatively high prevalence of Behçet's disease in the Far East and Mediterranean countries, whereas in the US and Western Europe it is much less common. In large series of patients from areas of high prevalence, men with an age of onset in the thirties predominate. They tend to have a worse prognosis than women. Mangelsdorf et al reported on 25 patients seen in a university dermatology referral practice in the US; 22 of their patients were young women with a high frequency of mucocutaneous lesions and a low prevalence of ocular involvement. This may reflect referral bias or could indicate that the disease is less severe in the US.

On histologic examination, the early lesions show a leukocytoclastic vasculitis. There is perivascular infiltration, which is chiefly lymphocytic in older lesions, with endothelial proliferation that obliterates the lumen. The cause of Behçet's disease has been postulated to have an infectious, immunologic, and/or genetic basis but the evidence is still inconclusive for any of these.

Diagnosis

Usually the disease starts with one oral ulceration, followed by others. It may take years before additional lesions develop. Therefore, the diagnosis requires two classic signs in addition to oral ulcerations. In women anal and genital lesions predominate, often with subsequent involvement of the eyes.

Behçet's disease must be differentiated from herpetic or aphthous stomatitis, pemphigus, oral cancer, and Stevens–Johnson syndrome (erythema multiforme). A skin puncture or pathergy test may be used to investigate patients further; however, it is not reliable in that it may be negative in otherwise well-documented cases. It is done by injecting 0.1 mL of normal saline solution into the skin or by simply pricking the skin with a sterile needle. A pustule appears at the site within 24 h. If results are negative, the test should be repeated at 2–5 points before results are accepted. Pathergy has been observed in patients with Behçet's disease, pyoderma gangrenosum, Sweet syndrome, and bowel-associated dermatosis–arthritis syndrome.

Treatment

Usually, the ulcerations heal spontaneously. Mild mouthwashes and toothpastes and restricted use of the toothbrush should be prescribed when there are oral lesions. With regard to treating the symptoms and healing of the aphthae, local treatments as described for aphthae may be used. Sucralfate suspension has been studied in Behçet oral and genital ulcers, and was found to decrease pain and healing time. On the whole, the therapeutic problem of aphthosis is not the healing of the individual lesions but the prevention of new attacks. For that purpose, several options exist, none of which is optimal. Colchicine, 0.6 mg twice a day, may be started for 2 weeks. In the absence of response and gastrointestinal side effects, the dose may be increased to three times a day. Although this may not totally alleviate the mucocutaneous lesions, it may decrease their recurrence rate by 50% or more. Dapsone may be substituted or added to this for improvement of response. The usual therapeutic final dose is 100 mg/day. Thalidomide has been found to be effective in many patients. One dosing method is thalidomide, 200 mg twice a day for 5 days, and 100 mg twice a day for 15–60 days. It has no effect on iridocyclitis. Of course, long-term treatment will commonly be complicated by neurotoxicity and the teratogenicity of this medication is well known.

Methotrexate, in a weekly oral dose of 7.5 to 20 mg, should be reserved for severe refractory cases, as should more aggressive systemic treatments such as systemic corticosteroids, azathioprine, chlorambucil, cyclosporine, interferon-α, tumor necrosis factor antagonists, and cyclophosphamide.

The long-term outlook is for intermittent recurrent flares that may be life-long. Blindness, neurologic impairment, and vascular thromboses are potential serious complications.

Almonznino G, et al: Infliximab for the treatment of resistant oral ulcers in Behçet's disease. Clin Exp Rheumatol 2007; 25:S99.

Alpsoy E, et al: Mucocutaneous lesions of Behçet's disease. Yonsei Med J 2007; 48:573.

Calamia KT, et al: Behçet's disease. Curr Rheumatol Rep 2008; 10:349.

Calamia KT, et al: Epidemiology and clinical characteristics of Behçet's disease in the US. Arthritis Rheum 2009; 61:600.

Evereklioglu C: Managing the symptoms of Behçet's disease. Expert Opin Pharmacother 2004; 5:317.

Lin P, et al: Behçet's disease. J Clin Rheumatol 2006; 12:282.

Mangelsdorf HC, et al: Behçet's disease. J Am Acad Dermatol 1996; 34:745.

Mendes D, et al: Behçet's disease—a contemporary review. J Autoimmun 2009; 32:178.

Oh SH, et al: Comparison of the clinical features of recurrent aphthous stomatitis and Behçet's disease. Clin Expt Dermatol 2009; 34:e208.

Rogers RS 3rd: Pseudo-Behçet's disease. Dermatol Clin 2003; 21:49.

Uzun S, et al: The clinical course of Behçet's disease in pregnancy. J Dermatol 2003; 30:499.

Yurdakul S, et al: Behçet syndrome. Curr Opin Rheumatol 2004; 16:38.

Bonus images for this chapter can be found online at
http://www.expertconsult.com

Fig. 34-1 Benign oral leukoplakia.

Fig. 34-2 Torus palatinus.

Cutaneous Vascular Diseases

35

Raynaud phenomenon and Raynaud's disease

Raynaud phenomenon occurs in the presence of an associated disease, usually collagen vascular disease, and often systemic sclerosis/scleroderma. This is also called secondary Raynaud's phenomenon. Raynaud's disease (or primary Raynaud's disease) occurs in the absence of such disease. In a series of 165 patients with Raynaud, 51 had primary disease (Raynaud's disease). A defined connective tissue disease was present in about one-third of the remaining patients, but 54 had undefined connective tissue disease (35 with positive antinuclear antibody [ANA] titer). In another study of 142 patients with idiopathic Raynaud phenomenon followed for more than 10 years, 14% progressed to a definite connective tissue disease. The initial presence of ANAs, thickening of fingers, older age at onset, and female sex were predictors of connective tissue disease. In a larger study of 586 patients with Raynaud, followed by sequential nailfold capillary microscopy and autoantibody determinations, these two investigations were able, in 80% of cases, to identify the 12.6% of patients who went on to develop systemic sclerosis. The absence of nailfold capillaroscopic findings is also predictive of primary Raynaud's disease (no associated systemic disease). Laser Doppler perfusion imaging may enhance the evaluation of vascular damage from Raynaud's. Technetium digital blood flow scintigraphy may aid in the early diagnosis of Raynaud's of either the primary or the secondary type.

Many of the studies on pathogenesis and therapy in Raynaud are conducted on patients with systemic sclerosis/scleroderma, so it may not be possible to translate these findings to patients with Raynaud's disease. However, it appears that cold exposure is a major trigger of vasospasm in all Raynaud's patients. There appears to be an exaggerated sympathetic response to cold. This may be due to both excessive vasoconstrictor tone and a weak systemic vasodilatation process, centrally mediated at least in part. The abnormal sympathetic response may also explain why some patients say that "stress" triggers Raynaud attacks. High homocysteine levels have been detected in patients with both primary and secondary Raynaud's disease. Patients with systemic sclerosis and Raynaud's phenomenon have elevated levels of endothelin (ET-1), and this correlated with both nailfold capillaroscopic findings and more advanced disease.

Raynaud phenomenon

Raynaud phenomenon is produced by an intermittent constriction of the small digital arteries and arterioles. The digits have sequential pallor, cyanosis, and rubor. The involved parts are affected in paroxysms by the attacks of ischemia, which cause them to become pale, cold to the touch, and numb. The phenomenon is more frequently observed in cold weather. When exposed to cold, the digits become white (ischemic), then blue (cyanotic), and finally red (hyperemic). In time, the parts may fail to regain their normal circulation between attacks and become persistently cyanotic and painful. If this phenomenon persists over a long period, punctate superficial necrosis of the fingertips develops (Fig. 35-1); later, even gangrene may occur.

Raynaud phenomenon occurs most frequently in young to middle-aged women. It occurs with scleroderma, dermatomyositis, lupus erythematosus, mixed connective tissue disease (MCTD), Sjögren syndrome, rheumatoid arthritis, and paroxysmal hemoglobinuria. Scleroderma was the underlying diagnosis in more than half of patients in one series. Occlusive arterial diseases, such as embolism, thromboangiitis obliterans, arteriosclerosis obliterans, and large-vessel vasculitis (Takayasu's disease), may be present. In addition, various diseases of the nervous system, including cervical rib, scalenus anticus syndrome, and complex regional pain syndrome (reflex sympathetic dystrophy), may produce the disorder. Physical trauma, such as hand-transmitted vibration as occurs with pneumatic hammer operation, can induce a syndrome identical to Raynaud's and has been termed "vibration white finger" or "hand–arm vibration syndrome". Pianists and typists may also develop this phenomenon. Raynaud's is a well-recognized complication following cold injury, especially frostbite. Pharmacological agents, such as bleomycin, ergot, β-blockers (including eyedrops), cyclosporine, interferon (IFN)-α and β, vinyl polychloride exposure, and cocaine, may also be the cause. The clumping of red blood cells is believed to be responsible for the induction of Raynaud phenomenon, with high titers of circulating cold agglutinins. It may occur in cryoglobulinemia and polycythemia vera. Patients with cancer may develop Raynaud's as a paraneoplastic phenomenon. Endocrine disorders, such as acromegaly, pheochromocytoma, carcinoid, and hypothyroidism, may present with or be associated with Raynaud's. Raynaud's of the nipple is a variant of Raynaud's that is difficult to diagnose. It presents with severe pain during lactation, and must be distinguished from nipple candidiasis and eczema. Patients report the onset of symptoms during pregnancy, and when asked, will say that the symptoms are triggered by cold and accompanied by biphasic or triphasic color changes of the nipple. Nifedipine can be highly effective in this condition and is safe for use during lactation, since little is found in the breast milk.

Simple tests and physical examination will generally distinguish between Raynaud's disease and Raynaud phenomenon. Sclerodactyly, digital pitted scars, puffy fingers with telangiectases, positive ANA, subcutaneous calcifications, basilar lung fibrosis, and changes on nailfold capillary microscopy (avascular "skip" areas with irregularly dilated capillary loops) are signs of connective tissue disease. An anticentromere antibody is an indicator of CREST (Calcinosis, Raynaud's syndrome, Esophageal dysmotility, Sclerodactyly, Telangiectasia) syndrome. Measuring rewarming after cold exposure can distinguish hand–arm vibration syndrome

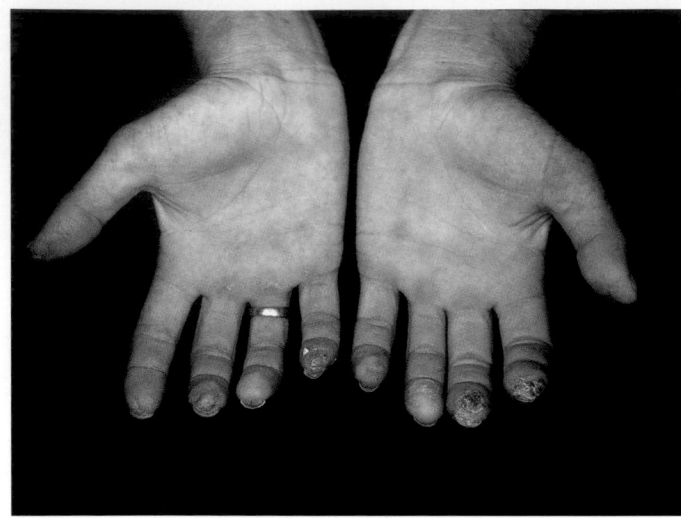

Fig. 35-1 Raynaud phenomenon with fingertip necrosis.

(HAVS) from Raynaud's. HAVS patients will all rewarm their hand temperature by >2.2°C in the first 30 seconds, and will rewarm their hand temperature by 5°C in the same time period as normal persons (less than 5 min 30 sec); in Raynaud's patients, rewarming averages 7 min and is always longer than 5 min 30 sec.

Raynaud's disease (primary Raynaud's disease)

Raynaud's disease is a primary disorder of cold sensitivity primarily seen in young women. The intermittent attacks of pallor, cyanosis, hyperemia, and numbness of the fingers are identical to those in Raynaud phenomenon. The disease is usually bilateral, and gangrene occurs in less than 1% of cases.

The diagnosis requires the absence of the diseases enumerated under Raynaud phenomenon. Although some suggest that Raynaud's disease should be present for 2 years before being classified as a primary process, it may take as long as 11 years for some systemic disorders to manifest. Overall, fewer than half of patients presenting with Raynaud symptoms will prove to have a connective tissue disease. The prognosis is good for primary Raynaud's disease.

Treatment

Treatments have often been studied only in patients with Raynaud's phenomenon and digital ulceration, so not all treatments can be assumed to be effective in primary Raynaud's disease or Raynaud's secondary to other causes. If an underlying cause if found, treatment of that associated condition will often lead to improvement of the Raynaud's. In both primary and secondary Raynaud's, exposure to cold should be avoided. This includes avoidance of exposure to cold not only of the extremities but also of other parts of the body, since vasospasm may be induced by reduction of core body temperature. Warm gloves should be worn whenever possible. Residence in a warm climate is helpful. Trauma to the fingertips should be avoided. Smoking is absolutely contraindicated. An attack of Raynaud's may be broken at times by swinging the affected arm in a wide circle from the shoulder—the "windmill" maneuver. The use of standard nitroglycerin paste has had minimal efficacy and can produce systemic side effects. A new form of topical nitroglycerin, known as MQX-503, has been reported to improve Raynaud's while having the same side effects as placebo. Alternative treatments, including ginkgo and other herbal medications, have limited efficacy when compared to the standard treatments below, and cannot be recommended for patients with significantly symptomatic disease.

Calcium channel-blockers are the first-line therapy used in Raynaud's due to their efficacy and low side-effect profile. Prolonged-release amlodopine or nifedipine is usually recommended. Two-thirds of treated patients will respond favorably. The phosphodiesterase inhibitor sildenafil has been effective in both reducing the frequency of Raynaud's episodes and in healing digital ulcers. It has become the second-line agent of choice. Tadalafil has not been compared to sildenafil, but has not been effective in secondary Raynaud's in scleroderma, and substitution of tadalafil for sildenafil for cost savings may not be appropriate in the treatment of Raynaud's. An angiotensin II-receptor type I antagonist (losartan) or selective serotonin-reuptake inhibitors (fluoxetine or venlafaxine) may be useful in refractory cases. Quinapril is not effective, suggesting that not all angiotensin-converting enzyme (ACE) inhibitors are effective in Raynaud's. Intravenous biweekly N-acetylcysteine has been effective in reducing the number of attacks and was relatively side effect-free. The use of statins (specifically atorvastatin) in patients with Raynaud's due to systemic sclerosis/scleroderma was associated with a reduction in Raynaud's-associated symptoms. This may be through the vasoprotective actions of statins, since statin administration was associated with reduction of circulating markers of vascular injury, which are commonly elevated in scleroderma patients. Bosentan, an endothelin receptor (ETA and ETB) antagonist, significantly reduces the frequency of Raynaud's attacks and reduces new digital ulcers. Iloprost, a prostaglandin analog, has substantial efficacy in scleroderma-associated Raynaud's and digital ulceration, when given intravenously but not orally. Oral cisaprost has minimal or no efficacy. Treprostinil and epoprostenol have preliminary data supporting their benefit.

In cases that are refractory to the medical treatments outlined above, surgical modalities can be considered. If single digits are involved, botulinum toxin injections in the palm around each involved neurovascular bundle may lead to dramatic and, at times, immediate pain reduction. Ulcerations of the affected digits heal following the injections. The duration of response is often months to years, and can be repeated with similar efficacy. Local digital sympathectomy can be effective, and avoids amputation of chronically ulcerated digits. Cervical sympathectomy and endoscopic thoracic sympathectomy may give initial relief, but Raynaud's symptoms often recur after 1 year to 18 months. However, despite the return of the Raynaud's symptoms, digital ulceration is markedly reduced. Compensatory hyperhidrosis is a common complication of thoracic sympathectomy.

Allen D, et al: Paraneoplastic Raynaud's phenomenon in a breast cancer survivor. Rheumatol Int 2009 Jun 11 (Epub ahead of print).

Anderson JE, et al: Raynaud's phenomenon of the nipple: a treatable cause of painful breastfeeding. Pediatrics 2004; 113:c360.

Batthish M: Raynaud's phenomenon as a presenting feature of hypothyroidism in an 11-year-old girl. J Rheumatol 2009; 36:203.

Blagojevic J, Matucci-Cerinic M: Are statins useful for treating vascular involvement in systemic sclerosis? Nat Clin Pract Rheumatol 2009; 5:70.

Bovenzi M: A longitudinal study of vibration white finger, cold response of digital arteries, and measure of daily vibration exposure. Int Arch Occup Environ Health 2009 Sep 4 (Epub ahead of print).

Brueckner CS, et al: Effect of sildenafil on digital ulcers in systemic sclerosis—analysis from a single centre pilot study. Ann Rheum Dis 2009 Nov 8 (Epub ahead of print).

Choi WS, et al: To compare the efficacy and safety of nifedipine sustained release with Ginkgo biloba extract to treat patients with primary Raynaud's phenomenon in South Korea: Korean Raynaud study (KOARA study). Clin Rheumatol 2009; 28:553.

Chung L, et al: MQX-503, a novel formulation of nitroglycerin, improves the severity of Raynaud's phenomenon. Arthritis Rheum 2009; 60:870.

De Angelis R, et al: Raynaud's phenomenon: clinical spectrum of 118 patients. Clin Rheumatol 2003; 22:279.

Delgado S, et al: Bacterial analysis of breast milk: a tool to differentiate Raynaud's phenomenon from infectious mastitis during lactation. Curr Microbiol 2009; 59:59.

Dorafshar AH, et al: Reoperative digital sympathectomy in refractory Raynaud's phenomenon. Plast Reconstr Surg 2009; 123:36e.

Fregene A, et al: Botulinum toxin type A: a treatment option for digital ischemia in patients with Raynaud's phenomenon. J Hand Surg Am 2009; 34:446.

Friedman EA, et al: The effects of tadalafil on cold-induced vasoconstriction in patients with Raynaud's phenomenon. Clin Pharmacol Ther 2007; 81:503.

Funauchi M, et al: Effects of bosentan on the skin lesions: an observational study from a single center in Japan. Rheumatol Int 2009; 29:769.

Gargh K, et al: A retrospective clinical analysis of pharmacological modalities used for symptomatic relief of Raynaud's phenomenon in children treated in a UK paediatric rheumatology centre. Rheumatology (Oxford) 2009 Oct 1 (Epub ahead of print).

Gayraud M: Raynaud's phenomenon. Joint Bone Spine 2007; 74:e1.

Gliddon AE, et al: Prevention of vascular damage in scleroderma and autoimmune Raynaud's phenomenon: a multi-center, randomized, double-blind, placebo-controlled trial of the angiotensin-converting enzyme inhibitor quinapril. Arthritis Rheum 2007; 56:3837.

Herrick AL: A local approach to Raynaud phenomenon. Nat Rev Rheumatol 2009; 5:246.

Heymann WR: Sildenafil for the treatment of Raynaud's phenomenon. J Am Acad Dermatol 2006 Sep; 55:501.

Khan MI, et al: Efficacy of cervicothoracic sympathectomy versus conservative management in patients suffering from incapacitating Raynaud's syndrome after frost bite. J Ayub Med Coll Abbottabad 2008; 20:21.

Koenig M, et al: Autoantibodies and microvascular damage are independent predictive factors for the progression of Raynaud's phenomenon to systemic sclerosis. Arthritis Rheum 2008; 58:3902.

Kuwana M, et al: Long-term beneficial effects of statins on vascular manifestations in patients with systemic sclerosis. Mod Rheumatol 2009; 19:530.

Kwon SR, et al: Diagnosis of Raynaud's phenomenon by (99m) Tc-hydroxymethylene diphosphonate digital blood flow scintigraphy after one-hand chilling. J Rheumatol 2009; 36:1663.

Lambova SN, Muller-Ladner U: The role of capillaroscopy in differentiation of primary and secondary Raynaud's phenomenon in rheumatic diseases: a review of the literature and two case reports. Rheumatol Int 2009; 29:1263.

Lazzerini PE, et al: Homocysteine and Raynaud's phenomenon: a review. Autoimmun Rev 2009 Aug 15 (Epub ahead of print).

Malenfant D, et al: The efficacy of complementary and alternative medicine in the treatment of Raynaud's phenomenon: a literature review and meta-analysis. Rheumatology (Oxford) 2009; 48:791.

Mariotti A, et al: Finger thermoregulatory model assessing functional impairment in Raynaud's phenomenon. Ann Biomed Eng 2009 Sep 4 (Epub ahead of print).

Mondelli M, et al: Sympathetic skin response in primary Raynaud's phenomenon. Clin Auton Res 2009; 19:355.

Morino C, et al: Raynaud's phenomenon of the nipples: an elusive diagnosis. J Hum Lact 2007; 23:191.

Nagy Z, et al: Nailfold digital capillaroscopy in 447 patients with connective tissue disease and Raynaud's disease. J Eur Acad Dermatol Venereol 2004; 18:62.

Neumeister MW, et al: Botox therapy for ischemic digits. Plast Reconstr Surg 2009; 124:191.

Pope J, et al: Iloprost and cisaprost for Raynaud's phenomenon in progressive systemic sclerosis. Cochrane Database Syst Rev 2000; (2):CD000953.

Rosato E, et al: Laser Doppler perfusion imaging is useful in the study of Raynaud's phenomenon and improves the capillaroscopic diagnosis. J Rheumatol 2009; 36:2257.

Rosato E, et al: The treatment with N-acetylcysteine of Raynaud's phenomenon and ischemic ulcers therapy in sclerodermic patients: a prospective observational study of 50 patients. Clin Rheumatol 2009; 28:1379.

Salem KM, et al: Analysis of rewarming curves in Raynaud's phenomenon of various aetiologies. J Hand Surg Eur Vol 2009; 34:621.

Schiopu E, et al: Randomized placebo-controlled crossover trial of tadalafil in Raynaud's phenomenon secondary to systemic sclerosis. J Rheumatol 2009; 36:2264.

Sulli A, et al: Raynaud's phenomenon and plasma endothelin: correlations with capillaroscopic patterns in systemic sclerosis. J Rheumatol 2009; 36:1235.

Sunderkotter C, et al: Comparison of patients with and without digital ulcers in systemic sclerosis: detection of possible risk factors. Br J Dermatol 2009; 160:835.

Wasserman A, Brahn E: Systemic sclerosis: bilateral improvement of Raynaud's phenomenon with unilateral digital sympathectomy. Semin Arthritis Rheum 2009 Oct 29 (Epub ahead of print).

Wu YJ, et al: Vascular response of Raynaud's phenomenon to nifedipine or herbal medication (duhuo-tisheng tang with danggui-sini tang): a preliminary study. Chang Gung Med J 2008; 31:492.

Ziegler S, et al: Long-term outcome of primary Raynaud's phenomenon and its conversion to connective tissue disease: a 12-year retrospective patient analysis. Scand J Rheumatol 2003; 32:343.

Erythromelalgia

Also called erythermalgia and acromelalgia, erythromelalgia is a not uncommon condition. The population-based incidence is 1.3 per 100 000 per year: 2.0 per 100 000 in women and 0.6 per 100 000 in men per year. Erythromelalgia is an easily recognized clinical syndrome characterized by paroxysmal vasodilation affecting the feet, with burning, localized pain, redness, and high skin temperature. Infrequently, the hands (Fig. 35-2), face, and ears may be involved. The burning paroxysms may last from a few minutes to several days, and are usually triggered by an increase in environmental temperature or exercise. The average patient has 1–2 attacks per week, but in some patients, the attacks are much more frequent. Often, relief can only be obtained by immersing the burning feet in ice water. Over 20% of patients will have evidence of cold injury, and more than 1% will suffer gangrene or undergo amputation. Quality of life is severely impacted by this condition.

Erythromelalgia can be considered primary, secondary, and familial. For treatment purposes, secondary cases of erythromelalgia should be carefully divided into those associated with myeloproliferative diseases, often with elevated platelets, and others. Mycloproliferative diseases complicated by erythromelalgia include polycythemia vera, thrombotic thrombocytopenic purpura, and various forms of thrombocythemia. Administration of romiplostim, a thrombopoiesis-stimulating protein, has resulted in erythromelalgia. Low-dose aspirin is effective therapy for erythromelalgia associated with platelet abnormalities. If this fails, other methods to reduce the platelet count should be considered.

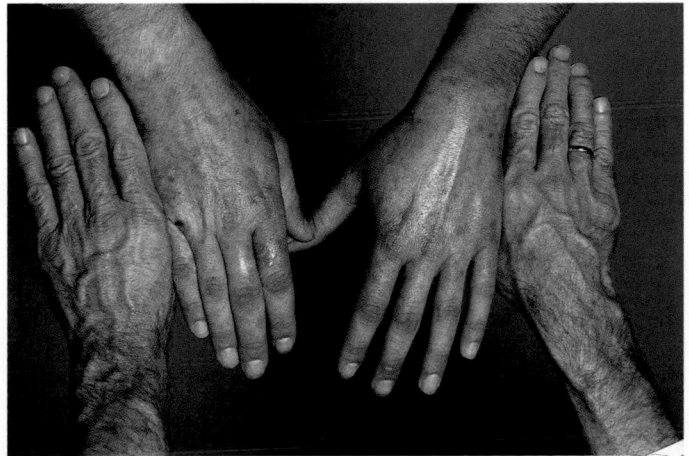

Fig. 35-2 Erythromelalgia of the hands (normal hands lateral to the patient's).

Acquired erythromelalgia has been reported secondary to topical exposure to isopropyl alcohol and after mushroom poisoning with *Clitocybe acromelalga* and *Clitocybe amoenolens*. Medications that have induced erythromelalgia include calcium channel-blockers (both nifedipine and verapamil), ergot derivatives such as bromocriptine and pergolide, and cyclosporine. There may be a long period of treatment (years) with these agents before the appearance of the erythromelalgia. Stopping the offending medication usually leads to improvement of symptoms within weeks.

In the vast majority of cases seen by dermatologists, erythromelalgia is probably a neurological disorder. It can be seen in various neurological conditions or diseases associated with neurological sequelae, such as peripheral neuropathy, myelitis, multiple sclerosis, autoimmune small-fiber axonopathy, or diabetes mellitus. Two patients with autoimmune disease and idiopathic thrombocytopenic purpura developed erythromelalgia and responded to intravenous immunoglobulin (IVIG) therapy. Erythromelalgia is sometimes associated with Raynaud phenomenon, both disorders of abnormal neurovascular function. In many cases, no associated neurological disease may be detected by routine neurological examination, but careful neurological testing will reveal evidence of a small-fiber neuropathy in the majority of such cases.

Inherited, familial, or hereditary erythromelalgia usually has its onset in childhood or adolescence (early or late onset). Familial cases have an autosomal-dominant inheritance pattern. Familial erythromelalgia is now known to be an "inherited neuronal ion channelopathy." The mutation is in the gene *SCN9A*, which encodes a peripheral sodium channel Na$_V$1.7. This is a mainly peripheral sodium channel with robust expression in dorsal root ganglion neurons and sympathetic ganglion neurons, especially those with nociceptive function. This sodium channel acts as a "threshold" channel and sets the gain in nociceptors. Many mutations in the affected gene have been mapped. Gene mutations causing erythromelalgia occur in areas that affect the structure of the actual channel by substituting amino acids in this critical location. The mutations causing erythromelalgia are gain-of-function mutations. The amount of gain of function correlates with the age of onset of the disease, more significant mutations having earlier onset. The nature of the mutation also affects the binding of medications to the channel, so various mutations may have different responses to same medication, depending on whether that mutation allows the drug to bind to the channel. Other gain-of-function mutations in the *SCN9A* gene cause "paroxysmal extreme pain disorder" (formerly called familial rectal pain syndrome). This disorder has prominent autonomic manifestations that include skin flushing (sometimes with only half of the face turning red [harlequin color change]), syncope with bradycardia, and severe burning pain—most commonly rectal, ocular, or mandibular. One mutation in Na$_V$1.7 produced a clinical syndrome with features of both erythromelalgia and paroxysmal extreme pain disorder. Autosomal-recessive nonsense mutations that cause loss of function of the Na$_V$1.7 channel result in the inability to sense pain. These patients are otherwise neurologically normal.

When severe, erythromelalgia is a life-altering disease, and aggressive management is warranted. Patients may benefit from referral to special clinics for pain management or pain rehabilitation. At times, simple measures such as immersion in cool water may stop pain crises. Biofeedback can be of benefit. In general, no more than 50% of patients with erythromelalgia of the neuropathic type will respond to any one medication, so the treatment must be tailored to each patient, and often combinations of agents are used. Topical amitriptyline 1% and ketamine 0.5% in a gel are safe topical options, and are especially reasonable for affected thin-skinned areas, such

as the face or ears, where penetration would be optimal. Oral amitriptyline, sertraline, nortriptyline, and venlafaxine have shown benefit in some multiple patients. Oral magnesium in extremely high doses (>1 g per day in liquid form) was beneficial in one patient. Mexiletine, carbamazepine, and the combination of carbamazepine and gabapentin are also reported to be effective in individual patients. Neurosurgical intervention has been used in the most severely affected, carefully selected cases that have failed medical management.

Red ear syndrome

Red ear syndrome describes a rarely reported disorder characterized by relapsing attacks of redness and burning affecting both ears, but usually only one ear at a time. The attacks are more common in the winter and are precipitated by touching, movements, and exposure to warmth. Associated conditions include neural disorders of the trigeminal and glossopharyngeal nerves, migraines, and lupus erythematosus. It is unclear if red ear syndrome is a disease sui generis or is actually erythromelalgia of the ears. Treatment with oral and topical tricyclics has been beneficial. Red ear syndrome must be distinguished from the springtime variant of polymorphous light eruption seen in young males with cold exposure, relapsing polychondritis (the lobe is also involved in red ear syndrome), cellulitis, and borrelial lymphocytoma.

Badeloe S, et al: Secondary erythromelalgia involving the ears probably preceding lupus erythematosus. Int J Dermatol 2007; 46:6.

Berk DR, Eisen AZ: Erythromelalgia of the ears: an unusual variant and response to therapy. J Drugs Dermatol 2008; 7:285.

Berlin AL, et al: Coexistence of erythromelalgia and Raynaud's phenomenon. J Am Acad Dermatol 2004; 50:456.

Brill TJ, et al: Red ear syndrome and auricular erythromelalgia: the same condition? Clin Exp Dermatol 2009 Jun 1 (Epub ahead of print).

Buttaci CJ: Erythromelalgia: a case report and literature review. Pain Med 2006; 7:534.

Catterall WA, et al: Inherited neuronal ion channelopathies: new windows on complex neurological diseases. J Neurosci 2008; 28:11768.

Chan MK, et al: Erythromelalgia: an endothelial disorder responsive to sodium nitroprusside. Arch Dis Child 2002; 87:229.

Cheng X, et al: Mutation I136V alters electrophysiological properties of the Na(v)1.7 channel in a family with onset of erythromelalgia in the second decade. Mol Pain 2008; 4:1.

Choi JS, et al: Mexiletine-responsive erythromelalgia due to a new Nav1.7 mutation showing use-dependent current fall-off. Exp Neurol 2009; 21:383.

Cohen JS: High-dose oral magnesium treatment of chronic, intractable erythromelalgia. Ann Pharmacother 2002; 36:255.

Cohen JS: Transdermal therapy for erythromelalgia. Arch Dermatol 2006; 142:1508.

Coppa LM, et al: Erythromelalgia precipitated by acral erythema in the setting of thrombocytopenia. J Am Acad Dermatol 2003; 48:973.

David MD, et al: Thermoregulatory sweat testing in patients with erythromelalgia. Arch Dermatol 2006; 142:1583.

Davis MD, et al: Erythromelalgia: vasculopathy, neuropathy, or both? A prospective study of vascular and neurophysiologic studies in erythromelalgia. Arch Dermatol 2003; 139:1337.

DiCaudo DJ, et al: Alleviation of erythromelalgia with venlafaxine. Arch Dermatol 2004; 140:621.

Drenth JP, et al: Primary erythermalgia as a sodium channelopathy: screening for *SCN9A* mutations: exclusion of a causal role of *SCN10A* and *SCN11A*. Arch Dermatol 2008; 144:320.

Durosaro O, et al: Intervention for erythromelalgia, a chronic pain syndrome: comprehensive pain rehabilitation center, Mayo Clinic. Arch Dermatol 2008; 144:1578.

Estacion M, et al: Nav1.7 gain-of-function mutations as a continuum: A1632E displays physiological changes associated with erythromelalgia and paroxysmal extreme pain disorder mutations and produces symptoms of both disorders. J Neurosci 2008; 28:11079.

Firmin D, et al: Treatment of familial erythromelalgia with venlafaxine. J Eur Acad Dermatol Venereol 2007; 21:836.

Fisher TZ, et al: A novel Nav1.7 mutation producing carbamazepine-responsive erythromelalgia. Ann Neurol 2009; 65:733.

Han C, et al: Early- and late-onset inherited erythromelalgia: genotype-phenotype correlation. Brain 2009; 132:1711.

Iqbal J, et al: Experience with oral mexiletine in primary erythromelalgia in children. Ann Saudi Med 2009; 29:316.

Jackson AL, Oates JA: A patient with adult erythermalgia: evidence suggesting an autoimmune etiology. Am J Med Sci 2008; 335:320.

Kalgaard OM, et al: Prostacyclin reduces symptoms and sympathetic dysfunction in erythromelalgia in a double-blind randomized pilot study. Acta Derm Venereol 2003; 83:442.

Kluger N, et al: Romiplostim-induced erythromelalgia in a patient with idiopathic thrombocytopenic purpura. Br J Dermatol 2009; 161:482.

Lampert A, et al: A pore-blocking hydrophobic motif at the cytoplasmic aperture of the closed-state Nav1.7 channel is disrupted by the erythromelalgia-associated F1449V mutation. J Biol Chem 2008; 283:24118.

Lampert A, et al: Erythromelalgia mutation L823R shifts activation and inactivation of threshold sodium channel Nav1.7 to hyperpolarized potentials. Biochem Biophy Res Commun 2009; 390:319.

Michiels JJ, et al: Platelet-mediated erythromelalgic, cerebral, ocular and coronary microvascular ischemic and thrombotic manifestations in patients with essential thrombocythemia and polycythemia vera: a distinct aspirin-responsive and coumadin-resistant arterial thrombophilia. Platelets 2006; 17:528.

Misery L, et al: Severe neurological complications of hereditary erythermalgia. J Eur Acad Dermatol Venereol 2007; 21:1446.

Mork C, et al: The prostaglandin E1 analog misoprostol reduces symptoms and microvascular arteriovenous shunting in erythromelalgia—a double-blind, crossover, placebo-compared study. J Invest Dermatol 2004; 122:587.

Nanayakkara PWB, et al: Verapamil-induced erythermalgia. Neth J Med 2007; 65:349.

Natkunarajah J, et al: Treatment with carbamazepine and gabapentin of a patient with primary erythermalgia (erythromelalgia) identified to have a mutation in the SCN9A gene, encoding a voltage-gated sodium channel. Clin Exp Dermatol 2009 Jun 17 (Epub ahead of print).

Paticoff J, et al: Defining a treatable cause of erythromelalgia: acute adolescent autoimmune small-fiber axonopathy. Anesth Analg 2007; 104:438.

Pipili C, Cholongitas E: Erythromelalgia in a diabetic patient managed with gabapentin. Diabetes Res Clin Pract 2008; 79:e15.

Reed KB, Davis MDP: Incidence of erythromelalgia: a population-based study in Olmsted County, Minnesota. J Eur Acad Dermatol Venereol 2009; 23:13.

Saviuc PF, et al: Erythromelalgia and mushroom poisoning. J Toxicol Clin Toxicol 2001; 39:403.

Sheets PL, et al: A Nav1.7 channel mutation associated with hereditary erythromelalgia contributes to neuronal hyperexcitability and displays reduced lidocaine sensitivity. J Physiol 2007; 581:1019.

Thami GP, et al: Erythromelalgia induced by possible calcium channel blockade by cyclosporin. BMJ 2003; 326:910.

Young FB: When adaptive processes go awry: gain-of-function in SCN9A. Clin Genet 2008; 73:34.

Livedo reticularis, livedo racemosa

Livedo reticularis is the term used to describe a netlike, mottled or reticulated, pink or reddish-blue discoloration of the skin, mostly on the extremities, especially the legs. It is more prominent with exposure to cold, and may vanish with warming. It is commonly seen on the lower extremities in young children and women. The pathogenic basis is reduced blood flow through and lowered oxygen tension in the venous plexus of the skin. Cutis marmorata is another name for livedoid physiologic mottling of skin exposed to cold. For clinical purposes, it is best to separate livedo reticularis (a benign condition in most cases) from fixed livedo reticularis, better known as livedo racemosa. Livedo racemosa forms irregular networks, and broken circular segments that are fixed and do not vary appreciably with temperature changes (Fig. 35-3). The lesions are usually asymptomatic. If necrosis or purpura occurs over the livedoid areas, the terms necrotizing livedo and "retiform

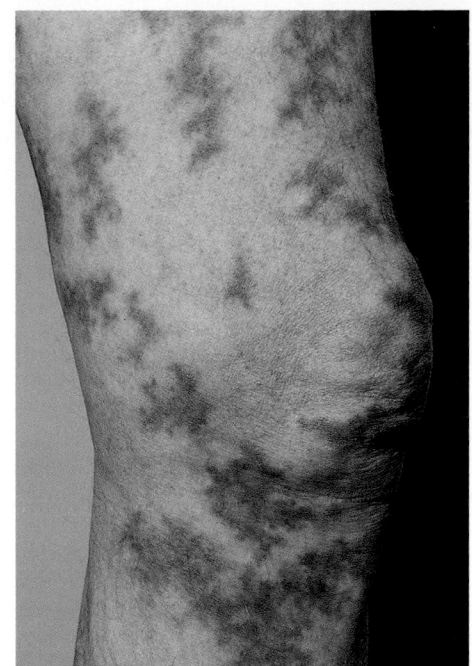

Fig. 35-3 Livedo racemosa.

purpura" respectively may be used. Livedo racemosa and livedo with purpura or necrosis are almost always associated with significant systemic disease that requires treatment. Unfortunately, the literature does not always accurately separate these entities, and patients may present with variable livedo (resembling livedo reticularis) and later develop more fixed lesions. In addition, some patients who have more variable livedo may have serious underlying disease that may require evaluation and treatment. These patients may not be easily identifiable initially on physical examination features alone. In this section, the term livedo will be used to describe this cutaneous finding and its association with other conditions. When livedo reticularis is seen, the clinician should consider the following categories of diseases as possibly causal: physiologic, hypercoagulable states (including myelodysplasias, cancer, and antiphospholipid and Sneddon syndromes), vasculitis (especially medium- and large-vessel), emboli, medications, and neurologic disorders.

Drugs may cause livedo. Amantadine (Symmetrel) may be not uncommonly associated with livedo reticularis. Quinidine and quinine may be associated with a photosensitivity that is livedoid in appearance, but on biopsy an interface dermatitis will be present. Minocycline can cause livedo, and this is a marker for the development of an antineutrophil cytoplasmic antibody (ANCA)-positive vasculitis in these patients. The medication must be stopped immediately. Other medications associated with livedo include gemcitabine, heparin (perhaps associated with heparin-induced antiplatelet antibodies), IFN-β, and bismuth.

Neurological disorders can create livedo reticularis by altering innervation and consequently blood flow in the skin. Brain injury, multiple sclerosis, diabetes mellitus, poliomyelitis, and Parkinson's disease are some examples.

Many of the syndromes with fixed livedo (livedo racemosa) have important systemic implications. These conditions can be either primary thrombotic processes or vascular inflammatory processes. If the vessels of the skin are affected, are the vessels in other organs, specifically the central nervous system (CNS) and kidneys, at risk? Sneddon syndrome usually occurs in young to middle-aged women. They present with livedo, and then develop cerebrovascular infarcts. The prognosis is poor.

Frequently, patients have antiphospholipid antibodies (up to 85%) and may have enough features to be diagnosed with systemic lupus erythematosus (SLE). They would be accurately diagnosed as having antiphospholipid antibody syndrome. Other connective tissue diseases, such as dermatomyositis, rheumatoid arthritis, and systemic sclerosis, may have antiphospholipid/anticardiolipin antibodies and hence feature livedo. For this reason, patients with SLE and livedo are apt to have more severe disease manifestations, such as renal disease, vasculitis, and anticardiolipin antibodies, even in the absence of fullblown Sneddon syndrome. Headache may be the presenting symptom in these patients, and the misdiagnosis of migraine may initially be entertained. Not all patients with Sneddon syndrome can be diagnosed as having antiphospholid antibody syndrome, however, and their optimal evaluation and management is unclear. Other significant disorders with livedo as a skin manifestation include thrombotic processes (hypercoagulable states, type I cryoglobulinemia), microangiopathic hemolytic anemias (thrombotic thrombocytopenic purpura, hemolytic uremic syndrome, and disseminated intravascular coagulopathy), medium- and large-vessel vasculitides, and septicemia. Moyamoya disease is a rare, chronic cerebrovascular occlusive condition characterized by progressive stenosis of the arteries in the circle of Willis. Patients present with ischemic strokes or cerebral hemorrhages. Both idiopathic moyamoya disease and disease connected with factor V Leiden mutation have been associated with livedo reticularis. Divry–van Bogaert syndrome, with livedo racemosa, seizures, and significant CNS disease, may be related to moyamoya or Sneddon syndrome.

Oxalosis may lead to livedo reticularis from deposition of oxalate crystals in and around blood vessel walls. The characteristic crystals are seen on biopsy. Calciphylaxis, with calcium deposits in vessels and tissue, may cause livedo by a still unclear mechanism. Other possible causes of livedo include cryofibrinogenemia, Graves' disease (associated with anticardiolipin antibodies), atrial myxoma, tuberculosis (perhaps as a complication of vascular inflammation—vascular-based tuberculid), and syphilis.

Asherson RA, et al: Unusual manifestations of the antiphospholipid syndrome. Clin Rev Allergy Immunol 2003; 25:61.

Gibbs MB, et al: Livedo reticularis: an update. J Am Acad Dermatol 2005; 52:1009.

Kraemer M, et al: The spectrum of differential diagnosis in neurological patients with livedo reticularis and livedo racemosa. A literature review. J Neurol 2005; 252:1155.

Miesbach W, et al: Recurrent life-threatening thromboembolism and catastrophic antiphospholipid syndrome in a patient despite sufficient oral anticoagulation. Clin Rheumatol 2004; 23:256.

Richards KA, et al: Livedo reticularis in a child with moyamoya disease. Pediatr Dermatol 2003; 20:124.

Shoenfeld Y, et al: Features associated with epilepsy in the antiphospholipid syndrome. J Rheumatol 2004; 31:1344.

Sladden MJ, et al: Livedo reticularis induced by amantadine. Br J Dermatol 2003; 149:656.

Tebbe B: Clinical course and prognosis of cutaneous lupus erythematosus. Clin Dermatol 2004; 22:121.

Tektonidou MG, et al: Antiphospholipid syndrome nephropathy in patients with systemic lupus erythematosus and antiphospholipid antibodies: prevalence, clinical associations, and long-term outcome. Arthritis Rheum 2004; 50:2569.

Tietjen GE, et al: Migraine is associated with livedo reticularis: a prospective study. Headache 2002; 42:263.

Tietjen GE, et al: Livedo reticularis and migraine: a marker for stroke risk? Headache 2002; 42:352.

Cholesterol emboli

Cholesterol emboli resulting from severe atherosclerotic disease, usually of the abdominal aorta, may cause unilateral

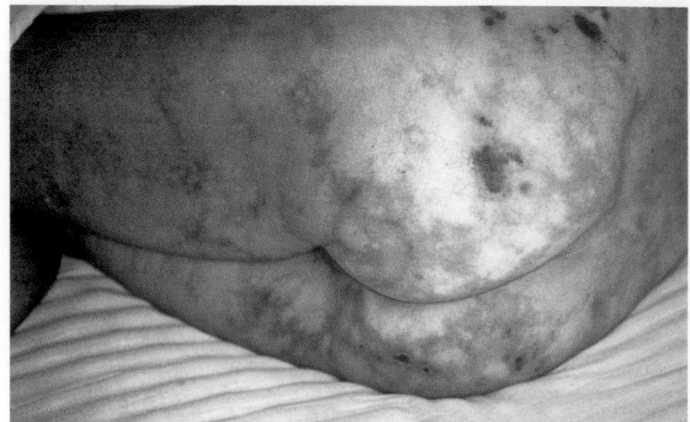

Fig. 35-4 Livedo reticularis secondary to cholesterol emboli.

or bilateral livedo of the lower extremities. The livedo may not be present with the patient supine, and may only be present when the legs are dependent. Patients frequently have concomitant cyanosis (blue toes), purpura, nodules, ulceration, or gangrene (Fig. 35-4). Pain often accompanies the skin lesions. Acute renal failure occurs in up to 75% and about one-third of patients will have characteristic skin lesions. An eosinophilia on complete blood count is present in 80% of cases. Older men with severe atherosclerotic disease are at greatest risk. They are often on anticoagulant therapy, and many have recently undergone vascular surgery or instrumentation. Slightly more than 1% of left heart catheterizations are complicated by cholesterol emboli. The differential diagnosis includes vasculitis, septic staphylococcal emboli resulting from endocarditis or an infected aneurysm, and periarteritis nodosa. Mortality is around 75% at 1 year. Deep biopsy with serial sections may demonstrate the characteristic cholesterol clefts within thrombi. Frozen section evaluation with polarized microscopy is particularly sensitive. Livedo reticularis of recent onset in an elderly person warrants consideration of this diagnosis.

Fukumoto Y, et al: The incidence and risk factors of cholesterol embolization syndrome, a complication of cardiac catheterization: a prospective study. J Am Coll Cardiol 2003; 42:211.

Hagiwara N, et al: Renal cholesterol embolism in patients with carotid stenosis: a severe and underdiagnosed complication following cerebrovascular procedures. J Neurol Sci 2004; 222:109.

Evaluation of the patient with possible cutaneous vascular disorders

In the evaluation of patients who present with livedo, purpura, or ulceration, a broad differential diagnosis must be considered. Among the diseases considered should be primary pathology of the cutaneous vasculature. In general, these vascular disorders of the skin are divided into two main groups: vasculitis and vasculopathy. Vasculitis includes disorders in which the primary damage in the blood vessels occurs due to inflammatory cells infiltrating and damaging the vessel walls. As a consequence of inflammation within vessels, the clotting cascade is triggered and thrombosis may be seen adjacent to and in the late stages of healing vasculitic lesions. In vasculopathy, the primary process is thrombosis. This is usually due to a hypercoagulable state. Once thrombosis occurs, inflammatory cells enter the vessel and vessel wall in an attempt to re-establish local circulation. Thus late in the process of a primary thrombotic process, vascular inflammation is seen and can be misinterpreted as a "vasculitis." Emboli can be considered thrombotic events and late lesions from embolic lesions may also be inflammatory and misleading histologically. All these processes—vasculitis, vasculopathy, and emboli—alter cutaneous blood flow and can be accompanied by livedo. If vessels lose competence they may leak, creating purpura, and if vasculitis, vasculopathy, or emboli are severe enough or affect a large enough vessel, the viability of the overlying skin is compromised, and necrosis and ulceration may occur. Complicating this situation is the fact that patients may have both a vasculitis and a hypercoagulable state, resulting in biopsies that, at times, are pathogenically discordant. A patient with an inherited or acquired disorder of coagulation and a drug-induced cutaneous vasculitis would be a not uncommon example. The above discussion makes it clear that this area of differential diagnosis is a difficult one for even the most skilled dermatologist. Careful sampling of early lesions, with large and deep biopsies if necessary, may be required to find the "primary" vascular pathology. Since vasculitis may be a focal process, step sections may be required to find the diagnostic features. In addition, the diagnosis proposed must be interpreted in the context of other elements of the patient's medical condition, such as medications, infections, underlying diseases, and involvement of other organ systems besides the skin.

Livedoid vasculopathy

Synonyms for livedoid vasculopathy include livedoid vasculitis, atrophie blanche, segmental hyalinizing vasculitis, livedo reticularis with summer/winter ulceration, and PURPLE (painful purpuric ulcers with reticular pattern of the lower extremities). The vasculopathy is characterized clinically by early focal, painful purpuric lesions of the lower extremities that frequently ulcerate and heal slowly (Fig. 35-5). The ulcers heal, with small, stellate and reticulated, white scars, referred to as atrophie blanche (Fig. 35-6). The ulcers may be ringed by telangiectasis and hemosiderin-induced hyperpigmentation. Livedo racemosa may be present on the affected extremity or be more widespread. About two-thirds to three-quarters of the patients are female; the mean age of onset is 45 years. The condition is bilateral in 80% of patients and ulceration occurs in 70%.

Histologically, livedoid vasculopathy is characterized by hyaline thrombi within small and at times medium vessels in the dermis. Perivascular hemorrhage may be present. Leukocytoclastic vasculitis is *not* found, and the biopsies can be described as showing "intravascular thrombosis without inflammation." Focal lymphocytic intravascular and perivascular inflammation may be seen, but this is considered second-ary to the thrombotic process, rather than a primary and pathogenic component of the disease. By direct immunofluorescence, fibrin, C3, and IgM are often found in the vessel walls, but these are again considered secondary to the thrombosis. In biopsies of older lesions, recanalizing vessels may demonstrate endothelial proliferation. Biopsy of the atrophie blanche-like lesions may show lobular vascular proliferation, as observed in chronic stasis dermatitis. In about 15% of patients, an initial biopsy does not reveal diagnostic histology and a second biopsy is required. After two biopsies, diagnostic pathology is found in 98% of patients.

The pathogenic etiology is considered to be a hypercoagulable state that results in spontaneous thrombosis of superficial skin vessels. The thrombosis results in low tissue oxygen tension, with local hypoxia and skin damage. However, the hypercoagulable state can be identified with current testing technology in only about 40% of patients. In livedoid vasculopathy, testing should include anticardiolopin antibody, lupus anticoagulant, factor V Leiden gene mutation (usually heterozygous), protein C, S, or antithrombin III heterozygous deficiency, prothrombin G20210A gene mutation, cryoproteins, and homocysteine level. The finding of methylene-tetrahydrofolate reductase (MTHFR) deficiency with or without hyperhomocysteinemia has been reported in livedoid vasculopathy, but the pathogenic significance of this is unclear. Plasminogen activator inhibitor-1 (*PAI-1*) mutation with increased PAI-1 plasma levels has been found in some patients with livedoid vasculopathy. PAI-1 is an important inhibitor of fibrinolysis, and elevated levels are associated with an increased risk of thrombosis.

Not surprisingly, underlying connective tissue disease, carcinomas, myeloma, lymphoma, venous insufficiency, deep venous thrombosis, and cerebrovascular accident have been seen in association with livedoid vasculopathy. These are all conditions associated with a prothrombotic state in some patients. Mononeuropathy multiplex has been reported in association with livedoid vasculopathy.

There is a broad differential diagnosis for livedoid vasculopathy, since many conditions can cause livedo reticularis with ulceration of the lower extremity. The conditions that must be excluded include small-vessel vasculitis (especially

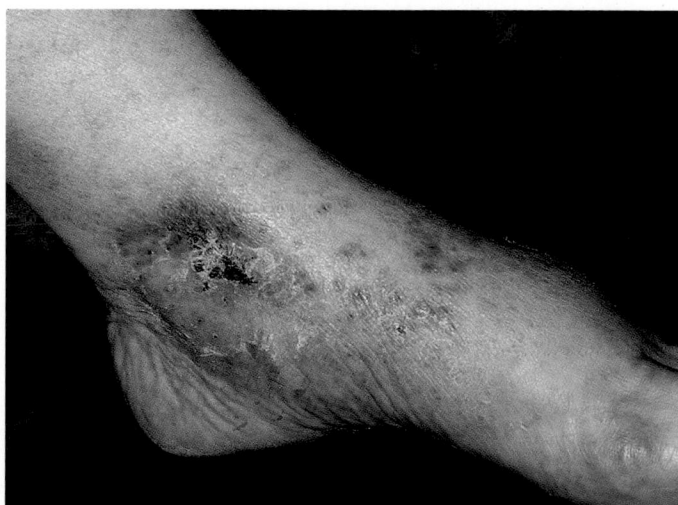

Fig. 35-5 Livedoid vasculopathy.

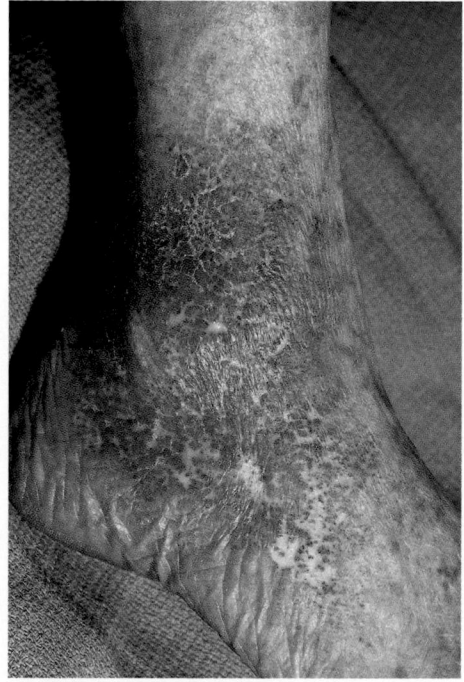

Fig. 35-6 Atrophie blanche.

that associated with hepatitis C virus and essential mixed cryoglobulinemia or a connective tissue disease), microscopic polyarteritis, polyarteritis nodosa (PAN) (both cutaneous and systemic), peripheral vascular disease, erythema induratum mimicking PAN, and hydroxyurea-associated leg ulceration.

The treatment of livedoid vasculopathy is directed at treating the hypercoagulable state. About one-third of patients are smokers, and this should be stopped. Patients with venous insufficiency should be managed with elevation, compression, and bandaging as appropriate. These patients may improve with this local therapy alone. If venous insufficiency ulcerations with an atrophie blanche appearance are slow to heal, consideration for treatment with the livedoid vasculopathy therapeutic ladder should be considered. Agents demonstrated to be effective in livedoid vasculopathy (in order of their recommended use) include: low-dose aspirin, oral pentoxifylline, oral dipyridamole, folic acid and a B complex multivitamin (in patients with MTHFR mutation and elevated homocysteine), danazol or stanazol (to increase endogenous antithrombotic proteins), heparin (low molecular weight or regular), and warfarin. Warfarin may be slightly superior to heparin. No treatment is universally beneficial in all patients, and treatment may need to be tailored to individual response and disease activity. In patients with connective tissue diseases (and antiphospholipid antibodies) hydroxychloroquine may be beneficial. In refractory cases, tissue plasminogen activator infusion, IVIG, and rituximab can be considered. Hyperbaric oxygen may accelerate ulcer healing. Other treatments that have been reported as effective include PUVA, niacin, iloprost, and ketanserin. Systemic immunosuppressives usually are of no benefit in cases with true livedoid vasculopathy. If there is a dramatic response to steroids, another diagnosis should be sought.

Anavekar ND, Kelly R: Heterozygous prothrombin gene mutation associated with livedoid vasculopathy. Australas J Dermatol 2007; 48:120.

Boyvat A, et al: Livedoid vasculopathy associated with heterozygous protein C deficiency. Br J Dermatol 2000; 143:840.

Browning CE, Callen JP: Warfarin therapy for livedoid vasculopathy associated with cryofibrinogenemia and hyperhomocysteinemia. Arch Dermatol 2006; 142:75.

Calamia KT, et al: Livedo (livedoid) vasculitis and the factor V Leiden mutation: additional evidence for abnormal coagulation. J Am Acad Dermatol 2002; 46:133.

Callen JP: Livedoid vasculopathy: what it is and how the patient should be evaluated and treated. Arch Dermatol 2006; 142:1481.

Cardoso R, et al: Livedoid vasculopathy and hypercoagulability in a patient with primary Sjögren's syndrome. Int J Dermatol 2007; 46:431.

Davis MD, Wysokinski WE: Ulcerations caused by livedoid vasculopathy associated with a prothrombotic state: response to warfarin. J Am Acad Dermatol 2008; 58:512.

Deng A, et al: Livedoid vasculopathy associated with plasminogen activator inhibitor-1 promoter homozygosity (4G/4G) treated successfully with tissue plasminogen activator. Arch Dermatol 2006; 142:1466.

Frances C, Barete S: Difficult management of livedoid vasculopathy. Arch Dermatol 2004; 140:1011.

Gotlib J, et al: Heterozygous prothrombin G20210A gene mutation in a patient with livedoid vasculitis. Arch Dermatol 2003; 139:1081.

Hairston BR, et al: Treatment of livedoid vasculopathy with low-molecular-weight heparin: report of 2 cases. Arch Dermatol 2003; 139:987.

Hairston BR, et al: Livedoid vasculopathy. Arch Dermatol 2006; 142:1413.

Irani-Hakime NA, et al: Livedoid vasculopathy associated with combined prothrombin G20210A and factor V (Leiden) heterozygosity and MTHFR C677T homozygosity. J Thromb Thrombolysis 2008; 26:31.

Juan WH, et al: Livedoid vasculopathy: long-term follow-up results following hyperbaric oxygen therapy. Br J Dermatol 2006; 154:251.

Kavala M, et al: A case of livedoid vasculopathy associated with factor V Leiden mutation: successful treatment with oral warfarin. J Dermatolog Treat 2008; 19:121.

Magy N, et al: Livedoid vasculopathy with combined thrombophilia: efficacy of iloprost. Rev Med Interne 2002; 23:554.

Meiss F, et al: Livedoid vasculopathy: the role of hyperhomocysteinemia and its simple therapeutic consequences. Eur J Dermatol 2006; 16:159.

Mimouni D, et al: Cutaneous polyarteritis nodosa in patients presenting with atrophie blanche. Br J Dermatol 2003; 148:789.

Ravat FE, et al: Response of livedoid vasculitis to intravenous immunoglobulin. Br J Dermatol 2002; 147:166.

Toth C, et al: Mononeuropathy multiplex in association with livedoid vasculitis. Muscle Nerve 2003; 28:634.

Tsai TF, et al: Polymorphisms of MTHFR gene associated with livedoid vasculopathy in Taiwanese population. J Dermatol Sci 2009; 54:214.

Zeni P, et al: Successful use of rituximab in a patient with recalcitrant livedoid vasculopathy. Ann Rheum Dis 2008; 67:1055.

Calciphylaxis

Calciphylaxis is an increasingly reported syndrome that is potentially fatal. It occurs most commonly in the setting of chronic renal failure, often with type 2 diabetes, and obesity. Women outnumber men 3:1 to 4:1. About 1–4% of patients on hemodialysis and 4% of patients on peritoneal dialysis develop calciphylaxis. About half of calciphylaxis patients are diabetic and more than half have a body mass index (BMI) of >30. Every gain in the BMI of 1 point over 30 increases the risk for calciphylaxis by 10%. Calciphylaxis occurs on the background of extensive calcification of the media of medium-sized and small arterioles. Parathyroid hormone (PTH) levels are often abnormal (either high or low), and calciphylaxis may also be seen in the setting of primary hyperparathyroidism, as well as secondary hyperparathyroidism of renal failure. Tumors may also produce PTH-related proteins and be associated with calciphylaxis. In about 20% of calciphylaxis patients, the Ca X PO4 product will be greater than 70, a sensitive but not specific marker for calciphylaxis. The arteriolar calcification is a chronic process due to many metabolic factors and signaling molecules that cause vascular smooth-muscle cells to transform to an osteogenic phenotype. Thus the vascular calcification in calciphylaxis and most cases of calcific uremic arteriolopathy is due to local deposition of calcium in the blood vessels by the vascular smooth muscles cells. It is *not* metastatic or dystrophic calcification. Liver disease and systemic corticosteroid therapy increase the risk for development of calciphylaxis by 2–3-fold.

Calciphylaxis begins as fixed livedo reticularis (livedo racemosa). Areas within the livedo become increasingly violaceous and eventually purpuric, bullous, and necrotic. Subcutaneous nodules may herald the onset of the livedo and be associated with it. Affected tissue in calciphylaxis has reduced tissue oxygenation. Lesions affect the legs below the knees in 90% of cases. More proximal lesions, and lesions of the fatty areas of the thighs, buttocks, and abdomen occur in about two-thirds of cases. Severe pain is a cardinal feature of calciphylaxis, often requiring narcotic analgesia for control. Ischemic myopathy may occur in severe cases, and muscle pain may precede the appearance of the skin lesions. Necrotic skin lesions are very resistant to healing and infection of open wounds with septicemia is a common cause of death. The 1-year survival of all calciphylaxis patients is about 40%, and only 10% in patients with both proximal and distal disease.

An optimum biopsy to confirm the diagnosis of calciphylaxis should be adjacent to the necrotic area where there is erythema or early purpura. Ideally, it should be deep and large enough to identify diagnostic features. This may require an incisional rather than a simple punch biopsy. Since vascular calcification is common in all patients with chronic renal failure, this alone cannot confirm the diagnosis. In addition, there should be evidence of tissue damage (necrosis), extravascular calcification, and thrombosis in the arterioles of the dermis and subcutaneous tissue.

The pathogenesis of calciphylaxis is still being elucidated. In most cases, it occurs on the background of extensive calcification of arterioles of the skin. The calcification triggers intimal proliferation and narrows the arterioles. Gradually or rather suddenly, the patient will develop areas of livedo and necrosis. This heralds the onset of vascular thrombosis. The mechanism that triggers this thrombotic phase of calciphylaxis and the appearance of the skin lesions is unclear. Some of these may be prothrombotic states, such as female gender, warfarin administration, trauma, the presence of cancer, edema, and anatomic location. The skin overlying fatty areas, such as the medial thighs, abdomen, and breasts of women, is particularly susceptible to thrombotic diseases such as diffuse dermal angiomatosis and warfarin and heparin necrosis. This may be caused by low blood flow or the reduced circulation due to tethering and kinking of vessels due to gravity. In some patients, low protein C levels are identified. Human immunodeficiency virus (HIV) infection and cryofibrinogenemia have also been associated. A useful model to consider pathogenically is that calciphylaxis is analogous to atherosclerotic myocardial disease. There is a gradual and progressive abnormality of the vasculature, with narrowing of the vessel lumen (by plaque in the case of atherosclerosis and by intimal calcification in the case of calciphylaxis). The acute symptomatology is triggered by thrombosis of the narrowed vessel, leading to occlusion of the vessel and downstream anoxia and necrosis. As in atherosclerotic disease, treatment for calciphylaxis should be directed at early prevention of intimal calcification. Unlike atherosclerosis, however, it is unclear how to prevent intimal calcification in the setting of renal disease.

Penile calciphylaxis is a particularly painful variant. The glans penis develops a deep necrotic ischemic ulceration. The risk factors are diabetes and renal failure. Penectomy is often required for pain management. One case resembled temporal arteritis.

Much of the treatment for calciphylaxis is directed at altering abnormal calcium metabolism. Low calcium dialysis, oral phosphate binders, cinacalcet, bisphosphonates, and intravenous sodium thiosulfate have all been used with some success. Once the ulcerations are present, gentle debridement is associated with healing and increased survival. Painful ulcers may also respond to hyperbaric oxygen therapy. Parathyroidectomy is best reserved for cases refractory to the above regimens and a marked elevation of PTH.

Al-Absi AI, et al: Case report: medial arterial calcification mimicking temporal arteritis. Am J Kidney Dis 2004; 44:e73.

Asobie N, et al: Calciphylaxis in a diabetic patient provoked by warfarin therapy. Clin Exp Dermatol 2008; 33:342.

Funabiki M, et al: Sudden onset of calciphylaxis: painful violaceous livedo in a patient with peritoneal dialysis. Clin Exp Dermatol 2009; 34:622.

Guldbakke KK, Khachemoune A: Calciphylaxis. Int J Dermatol 2007; 46:231.

Hackett BC, et al: Calciphylaxis in a patient with normal renal function: response to treatment with sodium thiosulfate. Clin Exp Dermatol 2009; 34:39.

Hanafusa T, et al: Intractable wounds caused by calcific uremic arteriolopathy treated with bisphosphonates. J Am Acad Dermatol 2007; 57:1021.

Hayden MR, et al: Vascular ossification—calcification in metabolic syndrome, type 2 diabetes mellitus, chronic kidney disease, and calciphylaxis—calcific uremic arteriolopathy: the emerging role of sodium thiosulfate. Cardiovasc Diabetol 2005; 4:4.

Hussein MR, et al: Calciphylaxis cutis: a case report and review of literature. Exp Mol Pathol 2009; 86:134.

Kalajian AH, et al: Calciphylaxis with normal renal and parathyroid function: not as rare as previously believed. Arch Dermatol 2009; 145:451.

Kyritsis I, et al: Combination of sodium thiosulphate cinacalcet, and paricalcitol in the treatment of calciphylaxis with hyperparathyroidism. Int J Artif Organs 2008; 31:742.

Li JZ, Huen W: Images in clinical medicine. Calciphylaxis with arterial calcification. N Engl J Med 2007; 357:1326.

Mwipatayi BP, et al: Calciphylaxis: emerging concept in vascular patients. Eur J Dermatol 2007; 17:73.

Nigwekar SU, et al: Calciphylaxis from nonuremic causes: a systematic review. Clin J Am Soc Nephrol 2008; 3:1139.

Ohta A, et al: Penile necrosis by calciphylaxis in a diabetic patient with chronic renal failure. Intern Med 2007; 46:985.

Pallure V, et al: Cinacalcet as first-line treatment for calciphylaxis. Acta Derm Venereol 2008; 88:62.

Schliep S, et al: Successful treatment of calciphylaxis with pamidronate. Eur J Dermatol 2008; 18:554.

Weenig RH, et al: Calciphylaxis: natural history, risk factor analysis, and outcome. J Am Acad Dermatol 2007; 56:569.

Woods M, et al: Penile calciphylaxis. J Am Acad Dermatol 2006; 54:736.

Marshall–White syndrome and Bier spots

The marbled mottling produced in the forearm and hand by occluding the brachial artery with a tight sphygmomanometer cuff is characterized initially, and chiefly, by pale macules 1–2 cm in diameter. These were described by Bier in 1898 and are known as Bier spots. Wilkin re-examined this phenomenon with laser Doppler velocimetry and concluded that the red spots on the hand are caused by relative vasodilation, with vasoconstriction in the pale areas.

Wilkin JK, et al: Bier's spots reconsidered: a tale of two spots, with speculation on a humerus vein. J Am Acad Dermatol 1986; 14:411.

Purpura

Purpura is the term used to describe extravasation of blood into the skin or a mucous membrane. It presents as distinctive brownish-red or purplish macules a few millimeters to many centimeters in diameter. Several terms are used to describe various clinical manifestations of purpura.

Petechiae are superficial, pinhead-sized (<3 mm), round, hemorrhagic macules, bright red at first, then brownish or rust-colored. They are most commonly seen in the dependent areas, are evanescent, occur in crops, regress over a period of days, and most often imply a disorder of platelets rather than a coagulation factor disorder. These disorders typically give rise to ecchymoses or hematomas rather than petechiae. Petechiae may also be a sign of vasculitis.

Ecchymoses are better known as bruises or "black and blue marks." These extravasations signify a deeper and more extensive interstitial hemorrhage, which forms a flat, irregularly shaped, bluish-purplish patch. Such patches gradually turn yellowish and finally fade away. They are characteristic of scurvy.

Vibices (singular, vibex) are linear purpuric lesions.

Hematoma designates a pool-like collection of extravasated blood in a dead space in tissue that, if of sufficient size, produces a swelling that fluctuates on palpation. Hematomas are usually walled off by tissue planes.

Pathogenesis

Purpura may result from hyper- and hypocoagulable states, vascular dysfunction, and extravascular causes, including idiopathic thrombocytopenic purpura, thrombotic thrombocytopenic purpura, disseminated intravascular coagulation (DIC), drug-induced thrombocytopenia, bone marrow failure, congenital or inherited platelet function defects, acquired platelet function defects (aspirin, renal or hepatic disease, or gammopathy), and thrombocytosis secondary to myeloproliferable diseases. Most of these disorders produce findings of nonpalpable purpura. Ecchymosis predominates in procoagulant defects, such as hemophilia, anticoagulants, vitamin K deficiency, and hepatic disease resulting in poor procoagulant synthesis. There is often a component of trauma. Increased frequency of ecchymotic skin can be the result of poor dermal support of blood vessels, most often localized to the area of trauma, and may result from actinic (senile) purpura, topical or systemic corticosteroid therapy, scurvy, systemic amyloidosis, Ehlers–Danlos syndrome, or pseudoxanthoma elasticum.

Primarily prothrombotic disorders form characteristic "retiform" purpura or purpura associated with livedo reticularis. These include disorders in which fibrin, cryoglobulin, or other material occludes vessels. Representative causes include monoclonal cryoglobulinemia, cryofibrinogenemia, DIC, purpura fulminans, protein C/S deficiency, warfarin-induced necrosis, heparin necrosis, cholesterol emboli, oxalate crystal occlusion, and antiphospholipid syndrome.

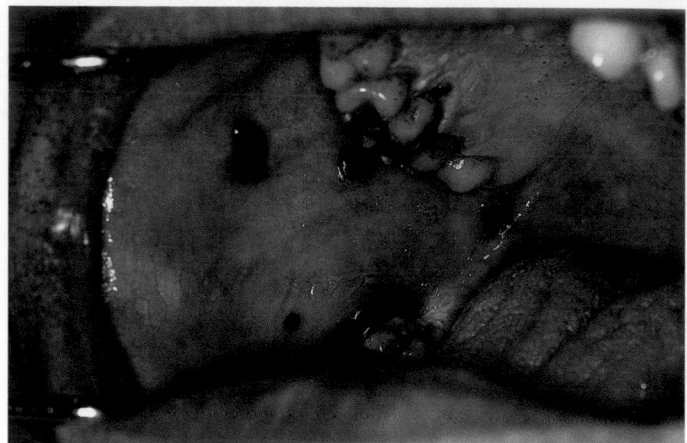

Fig. 35-7 Oral hemorrhagic bullae as the presenting complaint in immune thrombocytopenic purpura.

Evaluation

A history and physical examination are often all that is necessary. A family history of bleeding or thrombotic disorders, duration of symptoms, use of drugs and medications that might affect platelet function and coagulation, as well as a review of medical conditions that may result in altered coagulation, should be documented. Physical examination should stress the size, type, and distribution of purpura; a search for telangiectases; a joint examination; and an evaluation of skin elasticity, unusual scars, and unusual body habitus. Correlation of purpura morphology with pathogenesis allows for a more focused approach.

A complete blood cell count and differential can be used to assess for microangiopathic anemia, screen for myeloproliferative disorders, and assess the number and morphology of platelets. A bleeding time is the preferred method of assessing platelet function. The partial thromboplastin time (PTT) and the prothrombin time (PT) are tests to evaluate abnormal coagulation states.

Thrombocytopenic purpura

Thrombocytopenic purpura may be classified into two large categories: states resulting from accelerated platelet destruction and states resulting from deficient platelet production. Accelerated platelet destruction may be immunologic or nonimmunologic. The former may be due to antibodies (autoimmune or drug-induced thrombocytopenia), isoantibodies (congenital or post-transfusion), immune complex disease, or other immunologic processes, such as erythroblastosis fetalis, neonatal lupus, scleroderma, other connective tissue diseases, or acquired immunodeficiency syndrome (AIDS). The group of thrombocytopenias with accelerated platelet destruction includes thrombotic thrombocytopenic purpura and DIC. Deficient platelet production may be related to diseases such as aplastic anemia and leukemia.

Immune thrombocytopenic purpura (immune thrombocytopenia)

Immune thrombocytopenic purpura (ITP) was also known as idiopathic thrombocytopenic purpura or Werlhof's disease. It is an autoimmune disease characterized by an isolated thrombocytopenia (platelet count <100 000). The causative antibodies are directed at molecules on the platelet surface, leading to their premature sequestration and destruction, primarily in the spleen. ITP is called primary in the absence of another cause, or secondary if there is a causal association, e.g.

"secondary ITP (SLE-associated)." Bleeding symptoms are minimal or absent in a large proportion of cases. Cutaneous manifestations can include an acute or gradual onset of petechiae or ecchymoses in the skin and mucous membranes, especially in the mouth. Epistaxis, conjunctival hemorrhages, hemorrhagic bullae in the mouth (Fig. 35-7), and gingival bleeding may occur. Melena, hematemesis, and menorrhagia are also present, and the latter may be the first sign of this disease in young women. Chronic leg ulcers occasionally develop.

Bleeding can occur when the platelet count drops below 50 000/mm³. Post-traumatic hemorrhage, spontaneous hemorrhage, and petechiae may appear. The risk of serious hemorrhage is greatly increased at levels below 10 000/mm³. The gravest complication is intracranial hemorrhage. ITP may be fatal, but most mortality in adults occurs secondary to treatment complications. Bleeding time is usually prolonged and coagulation time is normal, whereas the clot retraction is abnormal and capillary fragility is increased. Increased numbers of megakaryocytes are found in the bone marrow.

The age of onset determines the clinical manifestations and course. In children the onset is often acute and follows a viral illness in 50–60% of patients. Parvovirus B19 is frequently complicated by thrombocytopenia, which may be ITP or simply a consequence of reduced bone marrow production of platelets. The average lag between purpura and the preceding infection is usually 2 weeks (range 1–4). Most of these cases resolve spontaneously. Since children are at much less risk of developing serious hemorrhagic complications, a more conservative management approach may be taken. A few patients will develop chronic thrombocytopenia, and deaths, usually from cerebral hemorrhage, have been reported. In a series of 332 children with ITP, 58 (17%) had episodes of major hemorrhage. One death resulted from sepsis. In another series of 427 cases, 323 (72%) had mild to benign disease. Roughly 85% of children who undergo splenectomy experience remission. More than half of the remaining patients spontaneously remit within 15 years.

The chronic form occurs most often in adults, is persistent, and has a female to male ratio of between 2:1 and 4:1. Secondary ITP is more common in adults. HIV, hepatitis C, and autoimmune disease are the most common associated diseases. Treatment of the associated disease may lead to improvement of the thrombocytopenia. Breast cancer has been associated with ITP, with a parallel course in one-third of cases. Other malignancies have also been associated with ITP. *Helicobacter pylori* infection as a cause of ITP is controversial, but testing for *H. pylori* antibodies and treatment for infection have limited toxicity so could be considered.

ITP in the elderly is more difficult to manage. Patients more frequently have major bleeding complications, more complications from immunosuppressive agents, especially corticosteroids, and more complications from splenectomy. Corticosteroids have a particularly low response rate in elderly ITP patients. Danazol has demonstrated reasonable safety and efficacy in the elderly.

The differential diagnosis of ITP includes drug-induced thrombocytopenia, myelodysplasia, thrombotic thrombocytopenic purpura, and congenital/hereditary thrombocytopenia. The goal of treatment for ITP is to raise the platelet count above 20 000 to 30 000 and to stop all bleeding symptoms. Platelet transfusions are indicated if there is significant bleeding or if the platelet count is dangerously low. If the platelet count is above 20 000–30 000, the patient may be closely monitored. The treatment of ITP has changed with the availability of new treatment approaches. Initial treatment is a short course of corticosteroids, either for 1–2 weeks or as monthly pulses. IVIG or anti-D may be given with this treatment. If the patient relapses or has persistent symptoms, systemic corticosteroids are given with any of the following: rituximab, anti-D, IVIG, or a thrombopoietin agonist. Splenectomy can be considered a second-line treatment, although age >60 years makes this treatment less desirable. Danazol can be added as a second-line agent, especially in the elderly. When second-line treatments have failed in patients with chronic and persistent or worsening disease, immunosuppression with mycophenolate mofetil, azathioprine, cyclosporine, vincristine, lymphoma-type chemotherapeutic regimens, and even autologous transplantation could be considered.

Aktepe OC, et al: Human parvovirus B19 associated with idiopathic thrombocytopenic purpura. Pediatr Hematol Oncol 2004; 21:421.

Aledort LM, et al: Prospective screening of 205 patients with ITP, including diagnosis, serological markers, and the relationship between platelet counts, endogenous thrombopoietin, and circulating antithrombopoietin antibodies. Am J Hematol 2004; 76:205.

Daou S, et al: Idiopathic thrombocytopenic purpura in elderly patients: a study of 47 cases from a single reference center. Eur J Intern Med 2008; 19:447.

de Latour RP, et al: Breast cancer associated with idiopathic thrombocytopenic purpura: a single center series of 10 cases. Am J Clin Oncol 2004; 27:333.

George JN: Definition, diagnosis and treatment of immune thrombocytopenic purpura. Haematologica 2009; 94:759.

Kuter DJ, et al: Efficacy of romiplostim in patients with chronic immune thrombocytopenic purpura: a double-blind randomised controlled trial. Lancet 2008; 371:395.

Maloisel F, et al: Danazol therapy in patients with chronic idiopathic thrombocytopenic purpura: long-term results. Am J Med 2004; 116:590.

Rodeghiero F, et al: Standardization of terminology, definitions and outcome criteria in immune thrombocytopenic purpura of adults and children: report from an international working group. Blood 2009; 113:2386.

Vesely SK, et al: Management of adult patients with persistent idiopathic thrombocytopenic purpura following splenectomy: a systematic review. Ann Intern Med 2004; 140:112.

Drug-induced thrombocytopenia

Thrombocytopenic purpura resulting from drug-induced antiplatelet antibodies may be caused by drugs such as heparin, sulfonamides (antibiotics and hydrochlorthiazide), digoxin, quinine, quinidine, chlorothiazides, penicillin, cephalosporins, minocycline, acetaminophen, nonsteroidal anti-inflammatory drugs (NSAIDs), statins, fluconazole, protease inhibitors, H_2 blockers, antiplatelet agents, rifampin, and lidocaine.

Heparin-induced thrombocytopenia (HIT) is associated with life-threatening arterial and venous thrombosis and, to a lesser extent, hemorrhagic complications. The platelet count usually begins to fall 4–14 days after starting heparin, more commonly in a patient with prior exposure to the medication. Platelet counts drop to about 50% of their pre-HIT level, usually with a nadir of about 50 000, and rarely 10 000. HIT is mediated by an antibody to the platelet factor 4 (PF4)–heparin complex. The antibody cross-links FcγRII receptors on the platelet surface, resulting in platelet activation, aggregation, and simultaneous activation of blood-coagulation pathways. Tests for HIT antibodies include immunoassays (such as enzyme-linked immunoassay [ELISA]) and functional tests.

Treatment for drug-induced thrombocytopenia consists of removal of the offending agent. Corticosteroids are helpful in moderately high dosage (60 mg/day prednisone) and are usually only necessary as a brief course. When a clinical diagnosis of HIT is made, heparin should be stopped immediately and treatment with an alternative anticoagulant should be started, if required. In patients with thrombosis, warfarin therapy can begin when the platelet count has normalized.

Blackmer AB, et al: Fondaparinux and the management of heparin-induced thrombocytopenia: the journey continues. Ann Pharmacother 2009; 43:1636.

Chong BH, Isaacs A: Heparin-induced thrombocytopenia: what clinicians need to know. Thromb Haemost 2009; 101:279.

Grossjohann B, et al: Ceftriaxone causes drug-induced immune thrombocytopenia and hemolytic anemia: characterization of targets on platelets and red blood cells. Transfusion 2004; 44:1033.

Picker SM, et al: Pathophysiology, epidemiology, diagnosis and treatment of heparin-induced thrombocytopenia (HIT). Eur J Med Res 2004; 9:180.

Russell KN, et al: Acute profound thrombocytopenia associated with readministration of eptifibatide: case report and review of the literature. Pharmacotherapy 2009; 29:867.

Selleng K, et al: Heparin-induced thrombocytopenia in intensive care patients. Semin Thromb Hemost 2008; 34:425.

Shantsila E, et al: Heparin-induced thrombocytopenia: a contemporary clinical approach to diagnosis and management. Chest 2009; 135:1652.

Syed S, Reilly RF: Heparin-induced thrombocytopenia: a renal perspective. Nat Rev Nephrol 2009; 5:501.

Wirth SM, et al: Evaluation of a clinical scoring scale to direct early appropriate therapy in heparin-induced thrombocytopenia. J Oncol Pharm Pract 2009 Aug 19 (Epub ahead of print).

Zondor SD, et al: Treatment of drug-induced thrombocytopenia. Expert Opin Drug Saf 2002; 1:173.

Thrombotic microangiopathy

The diagnosis of a thrombotic microangiopathy is made in the presence of a microangiopathic hemolytic anemia and thrombocytopenia in the absence of another plausible explanation. Thrombotic thrombocytopenic purpura and hemolytic uremic syndrome are the two major diseases in this group. Certain drugs, such as cyclosporine, quinine, ticlopidine, clopidogrel, mitomycin C, docetaxel, trastuzumab, and bleomycin, have been associated with a thrombotic microangiopathy.

Thrombotic thrombocytopenic purpura

Also known as Moschcowitz syndrome, thrombotic thrombocytopenic purpura (TTP) was in the past diagnosed with the pentad of thrombocytopenia, hemolytic anemia, renal abnormalities, fever, and disturbances of the CNS. Many cases, however, do not have renal disease, and CNS findings are not required for the diagnosis. The diagnosis of TTP requires only a Coombs-negative hemolytic anemia and thrombocytopenia with platelet aggregation in the microvasculature. Most patients will develop neurological findings. Fever is present in 75%. Multiple ecchymoses and retiform purpura may be found on the skin. The presence of schistocytes on a blood smear is the morphologic hallmark of the disease, and a schistocyte count of greater than 1% in the absence of other known causes of thrombotic microangiopathy strongly suggests a diagnosis of TTP. Tests may show a decreased hematocrit and decreased platelets, an elevated lactate dehydrogenase, and elevated indirect bilirubin. A delay in diagnosis may lead to a mortality rate as high as 90%.

Biopsies demonstrate hemorrhage and fibrin occlusion of vessels. Inflammation is absent. Studies of plasma samples from patients with active TTP have often shown the presence of unusually large von Willebrand factor (VWF) multimers. The underlying cause of TTP is a congenital or acquired deficiency of the VWF cleaving protease, ADAMTS13. VWF is secreted by the endothelial cell in long multimers, which should be cleaved into monomers by ADAMTS13 and released into the circulation. Instead, multimers circulate and extend from the surface of the endothelial cells in the microvasculature. Platelets adhere to these multimers and the surface of the endothelial cell, leading to microvascular thrombosis.

TTP is divided into two forms, idiopathic and congenital (Upshaw–Schulman syndrome). Congenital TTP is less common (<10% of cases), and usually presents in infancy or childhood with jaundice and thrombocytopenia. Some patients with a congenital deficiency of ADAMTS13 do not present until adulthood or may even remain asymptomatic. The course is frequently relapsing TTP at regular intervals. Idiopathic TTP is a rare disease (about 10 per million per year). Females represent 70% of cases and black people have a nine-fold risk of developing idiopathic TTP. Idiopathic TTP is due to an autoantibody directed against ADAMTS13 that can be detected in up to 85% of cases. Neurological symptoms are the most frequent presentation, and range from confusion to seizures or coma.

Until exchange plasmapheresis was instituted as the treatment of choice, 80% of these patients died; now, 80% survive. Plasma exchange therapy is the primary treatment. It clears the VWF multimers, reduces the autoantibody, and replenishes the inhibited ADAMTS13. Plasma exchange is usually continued daily until clinical symptoms improve and the platelet count is above 150 000. In conjunction with plasma exchange, glucocorticoids may be given, although their success is variable. Cyclosporine and rituximab have been used in refractory cases, with promising results. Splenectomy may be used in refractory cases. Congenital TTP is usually much easier to treat, with only small amounts of normal plasma infusion required to provide the missing ADAMTS13 and stop the clotting.

Hemolytic uremic syndrome

Hemolytic uremic syndrome (HUS) has many similarities to TTP but is now considered a distinct entity, both clinically and pathogenically. HUS is most commonly a disease of childhood. Patients have a microangiopathic hemolytic anemia, often following a diarrheal illness caused by Shiga toxin (Stx)-producing *Escherichia coli*. The annual incidence is 6.1 cases per 100 000. It is the most common cause of acute renal injury requiring transplantation in children aged 1–5. *Streptococcus pneumoniae* infection can also be followed by HUS. Cases of HUS not following such infections are called "atypical HUS."

Fever is usually absent in HUS cases. Renal insufficiency occurs in all patients and is the hallmark of HUS. Neurological disease can occur but affects less than half of cases.

The pathogenic mechanism of typical HUS is endothelial damage due to the bacterial toxin and subsequent complement activation on the endothelial surface. The affected vessels are thickened, endothelial cells are detached, and the vascular lumen is narrowed and occluded by platelet thrombi. The renal vessels are at particular risk, since the subendothelial membrane is exposed and this membrane is particularly at risk for complement-mediated damage. In atypical and familial HUS, similar complement activation via the alternative pathway (through C3b) occurs on endothelial surfaces, leading to endothelial damage and intravascular thrombosis.

In atypical and familial HUS, mutations in the alternative complement cascade have been identified. Complement factor H (CFH) mutations are most common and many patients are heterozygotes. The abnormal CFH complexes with the normal CFH, inactivating it. CFH is the major downregulator of the alternative complement cascade as it degrades C3b. Loss of CFH activity allows for unopposed C3b activity and complement activation. Other mutations are in complement factor I (CFI), which cleaves c3B and C4b. Mutations in membrane cofactor protein (MCP), a cofactor for CFI, in C3 itself, in complement factor B (a component of C3b), and in thrombomodulin can also cause atypical HUS. The type of mutation determines the clinical course of atypical HUS, with CFH, CFI, CFB, and thrombomodulin mutations having rates of death or end-stage renal disease of more than 50%. Recurrence of HUS occurs in more than three-quarters of patients with CFH and CFI mutations. Some patients are compound heterozygotes with mutations in two different genes noted above. About 6% of patients have an autoantibody to CFH and have "autoimmune HUS."

Although HUS is a disorder caused by a genetic deficiency in most cases, onset may not occur until middle age. About 67% of atypical HUS occurs during childhood, with almost all patients with anti-CFH antibodies diagnosed before age 16. Oral contraceptives may trigger HUS in 8% of patients with CFH and 20% of patients with CFI mutations.

HUS is treated with plasma exchange as soon as the diagnosis is made. Corticosteroids, azathioprine, mycophenolate mofetil, and rituximab may be used in atypical HUS. The role of cadaver kidney transplantation in atypical HUS is unclear due to the high rate of recurrence and loss of the graft. The likelihood for a successful outcome following transplantation is dependent on mutation type.

Bouw MC, et al: Thrombotic thrombocytopenic purpura in childhood. Pediatr Blood Cancer 2009; 53:537.

Burns ER, et al: Morphologic diagnosis of thrombotic thrombocytopenic purpura. Am J Hematol 2004; 75:18.

Cataland SR, et al: Demographic and ADAMTS13 biomarker data as predictors of early recurrences of idiopathic thrombotic thrombocytopenic purpura. Eur J Haematol 2009 Aug 10 (Epub ahead of print).

Davies M, et al: Successful vaginal delivery in a patient with extreme thrombotic thrombocytopenic purpura at term. J Obstet Gynaecol 2009; 29:765.

De S, et al: Severe atypical HUS caused by CFH S1191L—case presentation and review of treatment options. Pediatr Nephrol 2009 Oct 24 (Epub ahead of print).

Elliott MA, et al: Rituximab for refractory and or relapsing thrombotic thrombocytopenic purpura related to immune-mediated severe ADAMTS13-deficiency: a report of four cases and a systematic review of the literature. Eur J Haematol 2009; 83:365.

Ferrari S, et al: IgG subclass distribution of anti-ADAMTS13 antibodies in patients with acquired thrombotic thrombocytopenic purpura. J Thromb Haemost 2009; 7:1703.

Feys HB, et al: ADAMTS13 in health and disease. Acta Haematol 2009; 121:183.

Feys HB, et al: Mutation of the H-bond acceptor S119 in the ADAMTS13 metalloprotease domain reduces secretion and substrate turnover in a patient with congenital thrombotic thrombocytopenic purpura. Blood 2009; 114:4749.

Itala M, et al: Excellent response of refractory life-threatening thrombotic thrombocytopenic purpura to cyclosporine treatment. Clin Lab Haematol 2004; 26:65.

Jhaveri KD, et al: Treatment of refractory thrombotic thrombocytopenic purpura using multimodality therapy including splenectomy and cyclosporine. Transfus Apher Sci 2009; 41:19.

Kamiya K, et al: Rituximab was effective on refractory thrombotic thrombocytopenic purpura but induced a flare of hemophagocytic syndrome in a patient with systemic lupus erythematosus. Mod Rheumatol 2009 Sep 26 (Epub ahead of print).

Kremer Hovinga JA, et al: Splenectomy in relapsing and plasma-refractory acquired thrombotic thrombocytopenic purpura. Haematologica 2004; 89:320.

Lotta LA, et al: ADAMTS13 mutations and polymorphisms in congenital thrombotic thrombocytopenic purpura. Hum Mutat 2009 Oct 21 (Epub ahead of print).

Marques MB: Thrombotic thrombocytopenic purpura and heparin-induced thrombocytopenia: two unique causes of life-threatening thrombocytopenia. Clin Lab Med 2009; 29:321.

Noris M, Remuzzi G: Atypical hemolytic-uremic syndrome. N Engl J Med 2009; 361:1676.

Patel A, et al: Thrombotic thrombocytopenic purpura: the masquerader. South Med J 2009; 102:504.

Prestidge C, Wong W: Ten years of pneumococcal-associated haemolytic uraemic syndrome in New Zealand children. J Paediatr Child Health 2009 Oct 26 (Epub ahead of print).

Siau K, Varughese M: Thrombotic microangiopathy following docetaxel and trastuzumab chemotherapy: a case report. Med Oncol 2009 Oct 22 (Epub ahead of print).

van Goor H, et al: Adamalysins in biology and disease. J Pathol 2009; 219:277.

Yomtovian R, et al: Rituximab for chronic recurring thrombotic thrombocytopenic purpura: a case report and review of the literature. Br J Haematol 2004; 124:787.

Nonthrombocytopenic purpura (dysproteinemic purpura)

Cryoglobulinemia and cryofibrinogenemia

The term cryoglobulinemia refers to the presence in the serum of proteins that precipitate at temperatures below 37°C and redissolve on rewarming. These tend to be chronic conditions, unless the underlying disease process is treated. Abnormal serum proteins behaving as cryoglobulins and cryofibrinogens may be IgG, IgM, or both. Type I cryoglobulinemia occurs most frequently in multiple myeloma and macroglobulinemia, and is of a monoclonal IgM, IgG, or Bence Jones cryoglobulin form. Type II cryoglobulins are monoclonal and have rheumatoid factor-like activity. They are autoantibodies to the constant region of IgG. They occur in many connective tissue diseases and may also be due to the B-cell proliferation seen in hepatitis C virus (HCV) infection. Mixed cryoglobulinemia (type III), in which the cryoglobulins are of various classes, are associated with HCV infection in more than 90% of cases.

Purpura is most apt to occur on exposed surfaces after cold exposure. It may be of sudden onset and may clear rapidly once the patient is kept warm. Marked brown hyperpigmentation of the dorsal feet, at times in a livedoid pattern, may suggest this diagnosis. Cryoglobulinemia can be the cause of chronic leg ulcers (Fig. 35-8). An unusual clinical presentation of type I cryoglobulinemia in association with multiple myeloma is follicular hyperkeratosis of the central face, especially the nose.

In monoclonal disease, the biopsy reveals amorphous, jelly-like, eosinophilic material in the vessel lumen. In types II and III cryoglobulinaemia, a skin biopsy reveals classic leukocytoclastic vasculitis, and less commonly features of polyarteritis nodosa.

Treatment of type I cryoglobulinemia is to address the associated myeloproliferative disorder. Thalidomide was beneficial in one patient with a type I cryoglobulin, retiform purpura and clonal plasma cell expansion. For cryoglobulinemia associated with HCV or connective tissue disease, options include plasmapheresis, IVIG, systemic steroids, immunosuppressors, and colchicine. Simple plasma exchange can be helpful, but cryofiltration apheresis is the best method to remove cryoproteins in the treatment of cryoprecipitate-induced diseases.

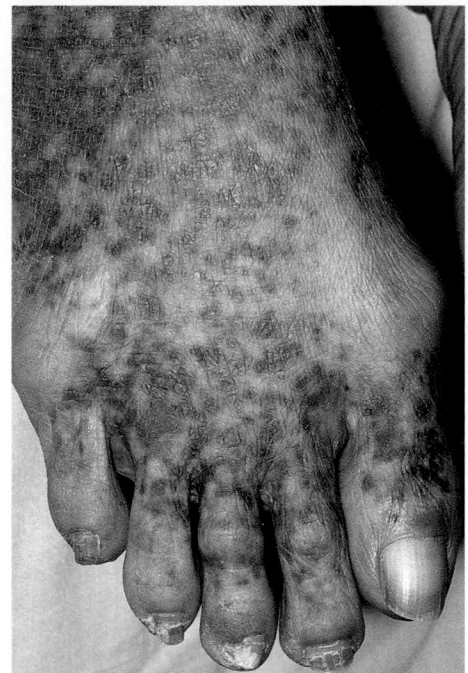

Fig. 35-8 Cryoglobulinemia.

Reduction of the HCV viral load is the long-term solution in HCV-associated cases and can result in disappearance of the cryoglobulins. IFN treatment produced an exacerbation of vasculitis in one reported patient. Mixed cryoglobulinemia with renal, neurologic, and cardiac disease refractory to other treatments can respond to rituximab.

In contrast to cryoglobulinemia, cryofibrinogenemia is rarely symptomatic. The precipitating cryofibrinogen is a cold insoluble complex of fibrin, fibrinogen, and fibrin split products with albumin, cold insoluble globulin, factor VIII, and plasma proteins. Associated collagen–vascular disorders, infections, and malignancies are significantly more frequent in patients with combined cryofibrinogen and cryoglobulin than in those with isolated cryofibrinogenemia. Cryofibrinogen has been associated with calciphylaxis in the setting of renal disease, and livedoid vasculopathy when accompanied by other prothrombotic risks. Familial primary cryofibrinogenemia manifests as painful purpura with slow-healing ulcerations and edema of both feet during the winter months.

Amdo TD, et al: An approach to the diagnosis and treatment of cryofibrinogenemia. Am J Med 2004; 116:332.

Auzerie V, et al: Leg ulcers associated with cryoglobulinemia: clinical study of 15 patients and response to treatment. Arch Dermatol 2003; 139:391.

Batisse D, et al: Sustained exacerbation of cryoglobulinemia-related vasculitis following treatment of hepatitis C with peginterferon alfa. Eur J Gastroenterol Hepatol 2004; 16:701.

Blain H, et al: Cryofibrinogenaemia: a study of 49 patients. Clin Exp Immunol 2000; 120:253.

Cavallo R, et al: Rituximab in cryoglobulinemic peripheral neuropathy. J Neurol 2009; 256:1076.

Charles ED, Dustin LB: Hepatitis C virus-induced cryoglobulinemia. Kidney Int 2009; 76:818.

da Silva Fucuta Pereira P, et al: Long-term efficacy of rituximab in hepatitis C virus-associated cryoglobulinemia. Rheumatol Int 2009 Aug 25 (Epub ahead of print).

De Rosa FG, Agnello V: Observations on cryoglobulin testing: I. The association of cryoglobulins containing rheumatoid factors with manifestation of cryoglobulinemic vasculitis. J Rheumatol 2009; 36(9):1953.

De Rosa FG, et al: Observations on cryoglobulin testing: II. The association of oligoclonal mixed cryoglobulinemia with cirrhosis in patients infected with hepatitis C virus. J Rheumatol 2009; 36:1956.

Della Rossa A, et al: Hyperviscosity syndrome in cryoglobulinemia: clinical aspects and therapeutic considerations. Semin Thromb Hemost 2003; 29:473.

Ferri C, et al: Mixed cryoglobulinemia: demographic, clinical, and serologic features and survival in 231 patients. Semin Arthritis Rheum 2004; 33:355.

Harati A, et al: Skin disorders in association with monoclonal gammopathies. Eur J Med Res 2005; 10:93.

Lo KY, et al: Hepatitis C virus-associated type II mixed cryoglobulinemia vasculitis complicated with membranous proliferative glomerulonephritis. Ren Fail 2009; 31:149.

Rayhill SC, et al: Positive serum cryoglobulin is associated with worse outcome after liver transplantation for chronic hepatitis C. Transplantation 2005; 80:448.

Requena L, et al: Follicular spicules of the nose: a peculiar cutaneous manifestation of multiple myeloma with cryoglobulinemia. J Am Acad Dermatol 1995; 32:834.

Resnik KS: Intravascular eosinophilic deposits—when common knowledge is insufficient to render a diagnosis. Am J Dermatopathol 2009; 31:211.

Rongioletti F, et al: The histological and pathogenetic spectrum of cutaneous disease in monoclonal gammopathies. J Cutan Pathol 2008; 35:705.

Sampson A, Callen JP: Thalidomide for type 1 cryoglobulinemic vasculopathy. Arch Dermatol 2006; 142:972.

Siami FS, et al: Cryofiltration apheresis in the treatment of cryoprecipitate induced diseases. Ther Apher 1997; 1:58.

Tallarita T, et al: Successful combination of rituximab and plasma exchange in the treatment of cryoglobulinemic vasculitis with skin ulcers: a case report. Cases J 2009; 2:7859.

Waldenström hyperglobulinemic purpura (purpura hyperglobulinemica)

Waldenström hyperglobulinemic purpura presents with episodic showers of petechiae occurring mainly on the lower extremities. The dorsum of the feet is intensely involved, and the petechiae diminish on the ascending parts of the feet (Fig. 35-9). A diffuse "peppery" distribution is commonly noted, resembling Schamberg's disease. The petechiae may be induced or aggravated by prolonged standing or walking, or by wearing constrictive garters or stockings.

Serum protein electrophoresis demonstrates a broad-based peak (polyclonal hypergammaglobulinemia). The bulk of the protein increase is IgG, though occasionally increased amounts of IgA are also found. IgM is usually normal or decreased. Rheumatoid factor in varying amounts is present in almost all patients. Antithyroglobulins, increased erythrocyte sedimentation rate (ESR), leukopenia, antinuclear factors, and proteinuria may be found. Almost 80% of patients with hypergammaglobulinemic purpura of Waldenström have antibodies to Ro/SSA.

Hyperglobulinemic purpura occurs most commonly in women and is frequently seen with Sjögren syndrome and rheumatoid arthritis. Adverse fetal outcomes in these women may be associated with the associated autoantibodies (SSA/SSB). Hyperglobulinemic purpura may also be a primary chronic benign illness. When it is associated with hepatitis C, it has a predilection for men, and has manifestations that usually last longer than those associated with Sjögren syndrome.

In about one-third of patients, leukocytoclastic vasculitis is present. Patients with leukocytoclastic vasculitis have a higher prevalence of articular involvement, peripheral neuropathy, Raynaud phenomenon, renal involvement, ANA, rheumatoid factor, and anti-Ro/SSA antibodies. The course of the disease is essentially benign, but chronic. Rare deaths are related to associated cryoglobulin disease. Hyperglobulinemic purpura may be a manifestation or harbinger of connective tissue or hematopoietic diseases, and rarely, progression to myeloma has been reported.

Patients often improve with support stockings. Steroids should be reserved for severe disease. Indomethacin and hydroxychloroquine may be of value in the treatment of milder disease, especially in patients who have connective tissue disease or are SSA/B (Ro/La)-positive. Aspirin and colchicine have been used with some success.

Al-Mayouf SM, et al: Hypergammaglobulinaemic purpura associated with IgG subclass imbalance and recurrent infection. Clin Rheumatol 2000; 19:499.

Jolly EC, et al: "Benign" hypergammaglobulinemic purpura is not benign in pregnancy. Clin Rheumatol 2009; 28:S11.

Maeda-Tanaka M, et al: Juvenile-onset hypergammaglobulinemic purpura and fetal congenital heart block. J Dermatol 2006; 33:714.

Malaviya AN, et al: Hypergammaglobulinemic purpura of Waldenström: report of 3 cases with a short review. Clin Exp Rheumatol 2000; 18:518.

Ramos-Casals M, et al: Cutaneous vasculitis in primary Sjögren syndrome: classification and clinical significance of 52 patients. Medicine (Baltimore) 2004; 83:96.

Waldenström macroglobulinemia

Waldenström macroglobulinemia (WM) is a lymphoplasmacytic lymphoma of B lymphocytes, with proliferation of monoclonal lymphocytes in bone marrow, lymph nodes, and spleen. Lymphadenopathy, hepatosplenomegaly, and anemia are characteristic. Elevated levels of IgM in the circulation define this unique and rare lymphoproliferative disease, and the IgM is responsible for some of the skin manifestations of this disorder. Elderly men are predominately affected, and there is a strong familial predisposition. The cutaneous manifestations of WM can be divided into two categories: nonspecific and specific. Nonspecific manifestations are related to the hyperviscosity syndrome created by the circulating IgM, and include purpura of the skin and mucous membranes. The purpura may be surmounted by giant tense bullae. Bleeding of the gums and epistaxis can occur. The IgM may behave as a cryoglobulin, resulting in purpura, livedo, cutaneous ulcerations, and vasculitis. Urticaria (some patients satisfying the diagnostic criteria for Schnitzler's syndrome), disseminated xanthoma, and amyloid deposition can be seen. Specific skin lesions are of two types: specific skin deposits of aggregates of the IgM (IgM storage lesions), and cutaneous infiltrates with neoplastic lymphoid cells. The specific skin lesions usually occur once the diagnosis of WM is already known, but uncommonly the skin

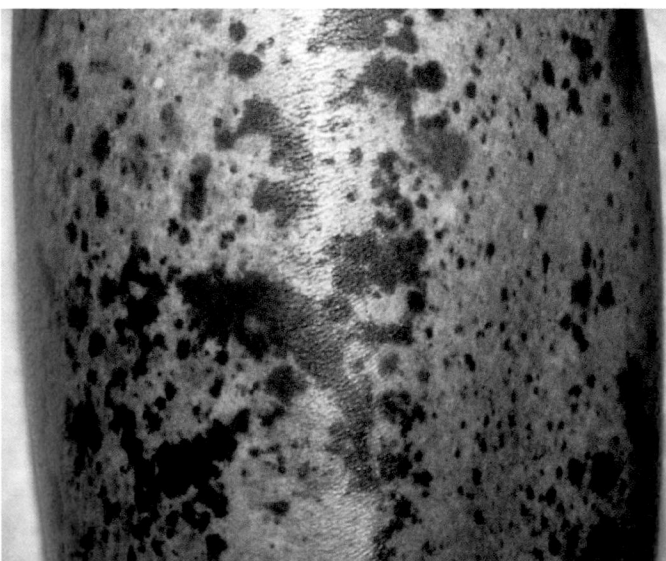

Fig. 35-9 Waldenström hyperglobulinemic purpura.

lesions are the first clue to the diagnosis. The specific IgM deposits present clinically as subepidermal blisters (clinically and histologically resembling bullous amyloidosis) or translucent 1–3 mm papules. They are found most commonly on the lower extremity, even on the sole. Slight hyperkeratosis may be seen over the papules. Histologically, the papules are composed of dermal nodular homogenous and fissured pink deposits with a tendency to involve newly formed vessels. They are periodic acid-Schiff (PAS)-positive, but negative for Congo red. Direct immunofluorescence will identify the dermal globules as being composed of IgM and is a useful diagnostic approach. When WM results in specific cutaneous lymphoid aggregates, the presentation is very nonspecific. Small red–brown to violaceous macules, papules, nodules, or plaques may be present, usually on the face. Rosacea is often initially entertained as a diagnosis. Widespread skin involvement with a "deck-chair" sign (sparing the abdominal skin folds) has been reported.

The natural history of WM is that of an indolent myelodysplasia. Treatment is directed at reducing the volume of neoplastic cells and should be managed by an oncologist. Most indolent and asymptomatic patients are followed or treated only when clinical disease occurs. Given the risk of secondary neoplasms, fludarabine is avoided, unless other options are not possible. Combinations of cyclophosphamide, systemic steroids, and rituximab or bortezomib, systemic steroids and rituximab are initial therapeutic options. Plasmapheresis can be effective in controlling acute symptoms of hyperviscosity syndrome. Rituximab is not used as a monotherapy in WM patients with hyperviscosity, as they may experience a flare of their disease. Soluble CD27 can be used as a marker to determine response to therapy.

Abdallah-Lotf M, et al: Cutaneous manifestations as initial presentation of Waldenström's macroglobulinemia. Eur J Dermatol 2003; 13:90.

Autier J, et al: Cutaneous Waldenström's macroglobulinemia with "deck-chair" sign treated with cyclophosphamide. J Am Acad Dermatol 2005; 52:45.

Chan I, et al: Cutaneous Waldenström's macroglobulinaemia. Clin Exp Dermatol 2003; 28:491.

Ciccarelli BT, et al: Soluble CD27 is a faithful marker of disease burden and is unaffected by the rituximab-induced IgM flare, as well as by plasmapheresis, in patients with Waldenström's macroglobulinemia. Clin Lymphoma Myeloma 2009; 9:56.

Colvin JH, et al: Cutaneous lymphoplasmacytoid lymphoma (immunocytoma) with Waldenström's macroglobulinemia mimicking rosacea. J Am Acad Dermatol 2003; 49:1159.

Harnalikar M, et al: Keratotic vascular papules over the feet: a case of Waldenström's macroglobulinaemia-associated cutaneous macroglobulinosis. Clin Exp Dermatol 2009 Oct 23 (Epub ahead of print).

Libow LF, et al: Cutaneous Waldenström's macroglobulinemia: report of a case and overview of the spectrum of cutaneous disease. J Am Acad Dermatol 2001; 45(6 Suppl):S202.

Murota H, et al: Improvement of recurrent urticaria in a patient with Schnitzler syndrome associated with B-cell lymphoma with combination rituximab and radiotherapy. J Am Acad Dermatol 2009; 61:1070.

Pascal L, et al: Bortezomib and Waldenström's macroglobulinemia. Expert Opin Pharmacother 2009; 10:909.

Rajkumar SV, et al: Monoclonal gammopathy of undetermined significance, Waldenström macroglobulinemia, AL amyloidosis, and related plasma cell disorders: diagnosis and treatment. Mayo Clin Proc 2006; 81:693.

Rongioletti F, et al: The histological and pathogenetic spectrum of cutaneous disease in monoclonal gammopathies. J Cutan Pathol 2008; 35:705.

Stone MJ: Waldenström's macroglobulinemia: hyperviscosity syndrome and cryoglobulinemia. Clin Lymphoma Myeloma 2009; 9:97.

Tedeschi A, et al: Fludarabine-based combination therapies for Waldenström's macroglobulinemia. Clin Lymphoma Myeloma 2009; 9:67.

Treon SP: How I treat Waldenström macroglobulinemia. Blood 2009; 114:2375.

Wolgamot GM, et al: Firm papules on lower extremities of 52-year-old male. Am J Dermatopathol 2005; 27:313.

Yokote T, et al: Cutaneous infiltration with Waldenström macroglobulinemia. Leuk Res 2006; 30:1207.

Purpura secondary to clotting disorders

Hereditary disorders of blood coagulation usually result from a deficiency or qualitative abnormality of a single coagulation factor, as in hemophilia or von Willebrand's disease. Acquired disorders commonly result from multiple coagulation factor deficiencies, as in liver disease, biliary tract obstruction, malabsorption, or drug ingestion. Acquired clotting disorders may also involve platelet abnormalities, as in DIC. Hemorrhagic manifestations are common and may be severe, especially in hereditary forms. Ecchymoses and subcutaneous hematomas are common, especially on the legs. Severe hemorrhage may follow trauma, and hemarthrosis is frequent. Other hemorrhagic manifestations include respiratory obstruction resulting from hemorrhage into the tongue, throat, or neck; epistaxis; gastrointestinal and genitourinary tract bleeding; and, rarely, CNS hemorrhage.

Harley JR: Disorders of coagulation misdiagnosed as nonaccidental bruising. Pediatr Emerg Care 1997; 13:347.

Sham RL, et al: Evaluation of mild bleeding disorders and easy bruising. Blood Rev 1994; 8:98.

Drug- and food-induced purpura

Drug-induced purpura may be related to platelet destruction, vessel fragility, interference with platelet function, or vasculitis. Drug-induced thrombocytopenic purpura was discussed earlier in this chapter. Examples of purpurogenic drugs are: aspirin and other NSAIDs, allopurinol, thiazides, gold, sulfonamides, cephalosporins, hydralazine, phenytoin, quinidine, ticlopidine, and penicillin. Combinations of diphenhydramine and pyrithyldione can induce purpuric mottling and areas of necrosis. Cocaine-induced thrombosis with infarctive skin lesions is associated with skin popping.

Topical EMLA cream can induce purpura within 30 min of application, a result of a toxic effect on the capillary endothelium. Agave ingestion can induce purpura and vasculitic-like lesions due to a direct toxic effect on the endothelium. Purpura has been associated with the use of acetaminophen in patients afflicted with infectious mononucleosis. Small-vessel vasculitis, including urticarial vasculitis, has been caused by the ingestion of tartrazine dye. Pseudoephedrine can induce a pigmented purpura-like reaction. Patch testing reproduced the eruption. Purpuric contact dermatitis is rare and usually caused by rubber chemical or textile dyes.

Aster RH: Can drugs cause autoimmune thrombocytopenic purpura? Semin Hematol 2000; 37:229.

D'Addario SF, et al: Minocycline-induced immune thrombocytopenia presenting as Schamberg's disease. J Drugs Dermatol 2003; 2:320.

Diaz-Jara M, et al: Pigmented purpuric dermatosis due to pseudoephedrine. Contact Dermatitis 2002; 46:300.

Dlott JS, et al: Drug-induced thrombotic thrombocytopenic purpura/hemolytic uremic syndrome: a concise review. Ther Apher Dial 2004; 8:102.

Neri I, et al: Purpura after application of EMLA cream in two children. Pediatr Dermatol 2005; 22:566.

O'Flynn G, et al: Evaluation of a cocktail of three bacteriophages for biocontrol of Escherichia coli O157:H7. Appl Environ Microbiol 2004; 70:3417.

Verma GK, et al: Purpuric contact dermatitis from footwear. Contact Dermatitis 2007; 56:362.

Purpura fulminans

Also known as purpura gangrenosa, this is a severe, rapidly fatal reaction. There are three forms of the disease:

1. that associated with infection and DIC
2. hereditary deficiency of protein C or S
3. that which follows a febrile illness that leads to an acquired protein S deficiency.

The most common form is that which is associated with an infectious illness, usually bacterial septicemia, but sometimes a viral infection (varicella). Asplenic patients, who are at risk for pneumococcal or meningococcal sepsis, are also predisposed to purpura fulminans. Neonates with homozygous protein C or protein S deficiencies may suffer purpura fulminans (Fig. 35-10). Some patients develop transient deficiencies of proteins C and S in response to infection. A number of cases of purpura fulminans associated with infections and factor V Leiden mutation, with normal protein C and protein S levels, have been reported. Meningococcemia, streptococcal sepsis, *Capnocytophaga* sepsis (from dog bite), staphylococcal septicemia, and urosepsis are the most common causes. Rickettsial disease and malaria may present as purpura fulminans. Active HHV-6 replication with acquired protein S deficiency and purpura fulminans has been described. Purpura fulminans presents as the sudden appearance of large ecchymotic areas, especially prominent over the extremities, progressing to acral hemorrhagic skin necrosis. (Fig. 35-11). The term "symmetrical peripheral gangrene" is used to describe cases when acral gangrene is present. Fever, shock, and DIC usually accompany the skin lesions, which on biopsy show noninflammatory necrosis, with platelet–fibrin thrombi occluding the blood vessels.

Other disease, such as the fibrinolysis syndrome, may have purpura fulminans as part of the symptom complex. An acquired form has been reported secondary to alcohol and acetaminophen ingestion, as well as from diclofenac or propylthiouracil. When purpura fulminans occurs in the setting of SLE, the catastrophic antiphospholipid antibody syndrome (CAPS) must be considered (Fig. 35-12). Purpura fulminans has been reported as a presenting feature of the Churg–Strauss syndrome and other ANCA-positive vasculitides.

Management is usually supportive, with treatment of the underlying disease process (antibiotics for the septicemia) and replacement therapy using fresh frozen plasma. Protein C and antithrombin replacement is useful in treating patients shown to have deficiencies. Plasmapheresis has been used in nonbacterial cases. Heparin anticoagulation can be used. Despite these measures, amputations (often multiple extremities) and deaths continue to occur in patients with severe disease. The use of pressors to maintain blood pressure during the septic episode may contribute to reduced peripheral circulation and peripheral tissue damage. Fasciotomy during the initial management of these patients may reduce the depth of soft-tissue involvement and the extent of amputations.

Akman A, et al: Unusual location of purpura fulminans associated with acquired protein C deficiency and administration of propylthiouracil. Clin Exp Dermatol 2009; 34:e463.

Betrosian AP, et al: Meningococcal purpura fulminans in a patient with systemic lupus erythematosus: a mimic for catastrophic antiphospholipid antibody syndrome? Am J Med Sci 2004; 327:373.

Boccara O, et al: Nonbacterial purpura fulminans and severe autoimmune acquired protein S deficiency associated with human herpesvirus-6 active replication. Br J Dermatol 2009; 161:181.

Culpeper KS, et al: Purpura fulminans. Lancet 2003; 361:384.

Davis MD, et al: Presentation and outcome of purpura fulminans associated with peripheral gangrene in 12 patients at Mayo Clinic. J Am Acad Dermatol 2007; 57:944.

de Souza AL, et al: Purpura fulminans without meningitis: a rare condition? Am J Med 2007; 120:e17.

Dhainaut JF, et al: Protein C/activated protein C pathway: overview of clinical trial results in severe sepsis. Crit Care Med 2004; 32(5 Suppl):S194.

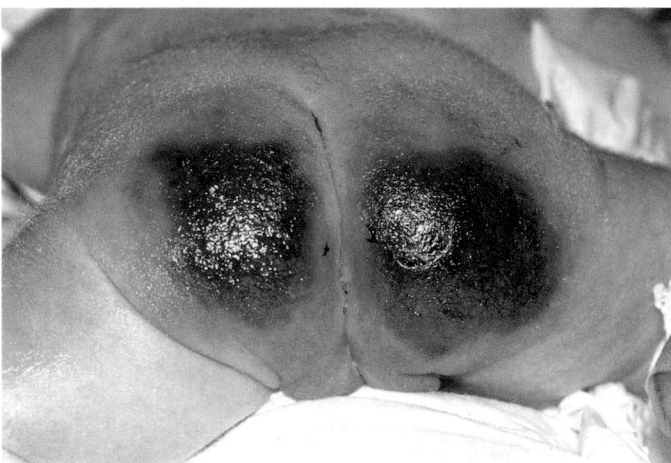

Fig. 35-10 Neonatal purpura fulminans secondary to homozygous protein C deficiency.

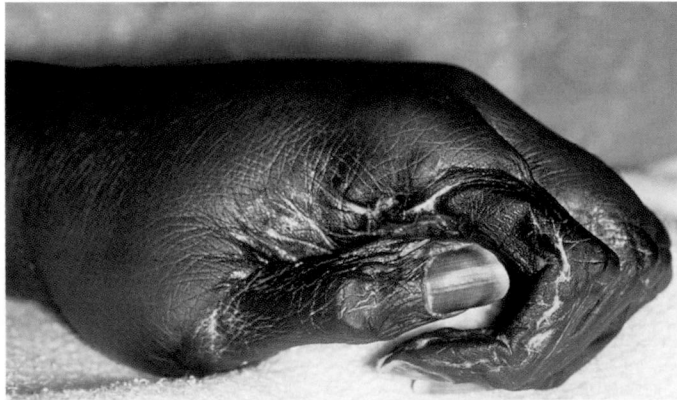

Fig. 35-11 Purpura fulminans.

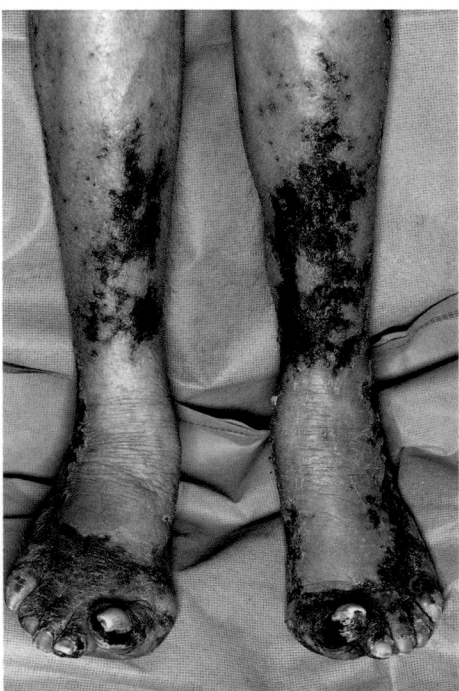

Fig. 35-12 Catastrophic antiphospholipid antibody syndrome.

Edlich RF, et al: Modern concepts of the diagnosis and treatment of purpura fulminans. J Environ Pathol Toxicol Oncol 2008; 27:191.

Fourrier F, et al: Combined antithrombin and protein C supplementation in meningococcal purpura fulminans: a pharmacokinetic study. Intensive Care Med 2003; 29:1081.

Ghosh SK, et al: Symmetrical peripheral gangrene: a prospective study of 14 consecutive cases in a tertiary-care hospital in eastern India. J Eur Acad Dermatol Venereol 2009 Jun 9 (Epub ahead of print).

Ghosh SK, et al: Purpura fulminans: a cutaneous marker of disseminated intravascular coagulation. West J Emerg Med 2009; 10:41.

Hassan Z, et al: Purpura fulminans: a case series managed at a regional burn center. J Burn Care Res 2008; 29:411.

Jaconelli T, Psirides A: Medical image. A fulminant rash: purpura fulminans. N Z Med J 2009; 122:3558.

Kato Y, et al: Purpura fulminans: an unusual manifestation of severe falciparum malaria. Intensive Care Med 2007; 33:1168.

Krzelj V: Response to hyperbaric oxygen therapy for purpura fulminans. Pediatr Emerg Care 2005; 21:485.

Lalitha AV, et al: Spectrum of purpura fulminans. Indian J Pediatr 2009; 76:87.

Regnault V, et al: Anti-protein S antibodies following a varicella infection: detection, characterization and influence on thrombin generation. J Thromb Haemost 2005; 3:1243.

Staquet P, et al: Detection of *Neisseria meningitidis* DNA from skin lesion biopsy using real-time PCR: usefulness in the aetiological diagnosis of purpura fulminans. Intensive Care Med 2007; 33:1168.

Stein RH, et al: Purpura fulminans. Int J Dermatol 2003; 42:130.

Warner PM, et al: Current management of purpura fulminans: a multicenter study. J Burn Care Rehabil 2003; 24:119.

Watt SG, et al: Purpura fulminans in paroxysmal nocturnal haemoglobinuria. Br J Haematol 2007; 137:271.

Zenz W, et al: Use of recombinant tissue plasminogen activator in children with meningococcal purpura fulminans: a retrospective study. Crit Care Med 2004; 32:1777.

Disseminated intravascular coagulation

Up to two-thirds of patients with disseminated intravascular coagulation (DIC) have skin lesions, which may be the initial manifestation of the syndrome. Minute, widespread petechiae, ecchymoses, ischemic necrosis of the skin, and hemorrhagic bullae are the usual findings. Purpura fulminans may supervene and progress to symmetrical peripheral gangrene. DIC may be initiated by a variety of disorders, including septicemic hypotension, hypoxemia, acidosis, malignancies, chemotherapy, obstetric crises, antiphospholipid antibody syndrome, SLE, arthropod envenomation, and leukemia. Long-term treatment with granulocyte colony-stimulating factor (G-CSF) has also been reported to precipitate DIC. Children with kaposiform hemangioendotheliomas are at risk for consumptive coagulopathy (Kasabach–Merritt syndrome).

DIC is the result of widespread intravascular coagulation in which certain coagulation factors are consumed faster than they can be replaced. Laboratory findings include decreased platelets, decreased fibrinogen (only in severe cases; normal in 57% of cases), elevated PT/PTT (50–60% of cases), and increased fibrin degradation products and D-dimers. Control of the underlying disease is the paramount consideration, and often antibiotics or surgical drainage of loculated infection may lead to spontaneous resolution of DIC. Bleeding is treated with platelet transfusion in the presence of thrombocytopenia and fresh frozen plasma to correct coagulation factor abnormalities. Heparin is considered when thrombosis in the form of venous, arterial, or widespread microvascular thrombosis (purpura fulminans) is present. Protein C concentrate may benefit patients with severe sepsis and DIC.

Levi M, et al: Guidelines for the diagnosis and management of disseminated intravascular coagulation. British Committee for Standards in Haematology. Br J Haematol 2009; 145:24.

Okabayashi K, et al: Hemostatic markers and the sepsis-related organ failure assessment score in patients with disseminated intravascular coagulation in an intensive care unit. Am J Hematol 2004; 76:225.

Congenital fibrinogen disorders

Deficiencies of fibrinogen are classified as reductions in quantity (afibrinogenemia or hypofibrinogenemia) or in quality (dysfibrinogenemia). Afibrinogenemia occurs at a rate of about 1 per million in the population. It may present at birth with umbilical cord bleeding. Epistaxis, menorrhagia, hemarthrosis (but much less than in hemophilia and with far fewer musculoskeletal sequelae), trauma, and surgery-related bleeding can occur. The severity of the bleeding tendency is highly variable from patient to patient, some suffering no bleeding problems at all. Pregnancy complications include recurrent miscarriage and peripartum hemorrhage. Ironically, due to the loss of the antithrombotic effect of fibrinogen, thrombotic events are increased in afibrinogenemia. Arterial and venous thrombosis can occur. Patients with hypofibrinogenemia are more numerous, and in general are less symptomatic and only occasionally require treatment. Hypofibrinogenemia can be associated with pregnancy losses and rarely liver disease due to accumulation of abnormal fibrinogen in the endoplasmic reticulum of hepatocytes. Dysfibrinogenemia is asymptomatic in 55% of cases, 25% exhibit bleeding tendencies, and 20% have a tendency to thrombosis. This represents only 0.8% of patients with deep venous thrombosis, so screening for this condition is not cost-effective, unless there is a family history. Mutations in the fibrinogen gene cluster cause all three of these fibrinogen disorders.

Asselta R, et al: Molecular genetics of quantitative fibrinogen disorders. Cardiovasc Hematol Agents Med Chem 2007; 5:163.

de Moerloose P, Neerman-Arbez M: Congenital fibrinogen disorders. Semin Thromb Hemost 2009; 35:356.

Vu D, Neerman-Arbez M: Molecular mechanisms accounting for fibrinogen deficiency: from large deletions to intracellular retention of misfolded proteins. J Thromb Haemost 2007; 5:125.

Blueberry muffin baby

Originally coined to describe the characteristic appearance of the purpuric lesions observed in newborns with congenital rubella, the term blueberry muffin baby is associated with many disorders that produce extramedullary erythropoiesis. The eruption consists of generalized dark blue to magenta, nonblanchable, indurated, round to oval, hemispheric papules ranging from 1 to 7 mm. Lesions favor the head, neck, and trunk.

Etiologic factors include congenital infections (toxoplasmosis, rubella, cytomegalovirus, and parvovirus B19), hemolytic disease of the newborn (Rh incompatibility, blood group incompatibility), hereditary spherocytosis, twin transfusion syndrome, neuroblastoma, rhabdomyosarcoma, Langerhans cell histiocytosis, and congenital leukemia. Patients with multiple vascular disorders, such as hemangiopericytoma, hemangioma, blue rubber bleb nevus, and glomangioma, may be mistaken for "blueberry muffin" baby. Evaluation should include a peripheral blood cell count, hemoglobin level, TORCH serologies, viral cultures, and a Coombs test. A skin biopsy may also be helpful in determining the cause.

Brisman S, et al: Blueberry muffin rash as the presenting sign of Aicardi–Goutieres syndrome. Pediatr Dermatol 2009; 26:432.

Gaffin JM, Gallagher PG: Picture of the month. Blueberry muffin baby (extramedullary hematopoiesis) due to congenital cytomegalovirus infection. Arch Pediatr Adolesc Med 2007; 161:1102.

Holland KE, et al: Neonatal violaceous skin lesions: expanding the differential of the "blueberry muffin baby." Adv Dermatol 2005; 21:153.

Mehta V, et al: Blueberry muffin baby: a pictorial differential diagnosis. Dermatol Online J 2008; 14:8.

Sankilampi U, et al: Congenital Langerhans cell histiocytosis mimicking a "blueberry muffin baby." J Pediatr Hematol Oncol 2008; 30:145.

Miscellaneous purpuric manifestations

Deep venous thrombosis

Deep venous thrombosis (DVT) is a common medical condition that can result in immediate (pulmonary embolism) or long-term consequences (venous insufficiency, postphlebitic syndrome). Risk factors include female gender, obesity, immobilization, low atmospheric pressure, winter season, and the presence of cancer. In 35% of cancer-associated cases, the thrombosis is the first sign of the cancer. The use of erythropoiesis-stimulating agents doubles the risk of venous thromboembolism (VTE) for cancer patients. Hereditary mutations that result in a hypercoagulable state also increase the risk for VTE. The left leg is more often affected than the right. The mean age is 52 years. Significant superficial vein thrombosis is considered a risk factor for DVT. The risk of pulmonary embolism from DVT is the major concern. Treatment includes preventive strategies (exercise, weight control, and prophylaxis for high-risk settings—postoperative, post-stroke, and immobilized cancer patient).

Bates SM, et al: Clinical practice. Treatment of deep-vein thrombosis. N Engl J Med 2004; 351:268.

Brown HK, et al: The influence of meteorological variables on the development of deep venous thrombosis. Thromb Haemost 2009; 102:676.

Canonico M, Scarabin PY: Hormone therapy and risk of venous thromboembolism among postmenopausal women. Climacteric 2009;12:76.

Coss E, et al: 57-year-old woman with acute lower extremity pain and swelling. Mayo Clin Proc 2009; 84:e1.

Doggen CJ: High coagulant factors & venous thrombosis. Blood 2009; 114:2854.

Fanikos J, et al: Long-term complications of medical patients with hospital-acquired venous thromboembolism. Thromb Haemost 2009; 102:688.

Hershman DL, et al: Patterns of use and risks associated with erythropoiesis-stimulating agents among Medicare patients with cancer. J Natl Cancer Inst 2009; 101:1633.

Kucher N, et al: Lack of prophylaxis before the onset of acute venous thromboembolism among hospitalized cancer patients: the SWIss Venous ThromboEmbolism Registry (SWIVTER). Ann Oncol 2009 Oct 14 (Epub ahead of print).

Lyman GH, Khorana AA: Cancer, clots and consensus: new understanding of an old problem. J Clin Oncol 2009; 27:4821.

Millar JA: Selection of medical patients for prophylaxis of venous thromboembolism based on analysis of the benefit–hazard ratio. Intern Med J 2009; 39:606.

Pai N, et al: Differences in etiological and clinical manifestations in upper extremity and lower limb deep venous thrombosis patients from India. Clin Appl Thromb Hemost 2009 Nov 10 (Epub ahead of print).

Piazza G, Goldhaber SZ: Physician alerts to prevent venous thromboembolism. J Thromb Thrombolysis 2009 Nov 4 (Epub ahead of print).

Shrier I, et al: Effect of early physical activity on long-term outcome after venous thrombosis. Clin J Sport Med 2009; 19:487.

Spyropoulos AC, et al: Rates of venous thromboembolism occurrence in medical patients among the insured population. Thromb Haemost 2009; 102:951.

Vedantham S: Deep venous thrombosis: the opportunity at hand. Am J Roetgenol 2009; 193:922.

Superficial thrombophlebitis

Painful induration with erythema, often in a linear or branching configuration forming cords, is the classic presentation of

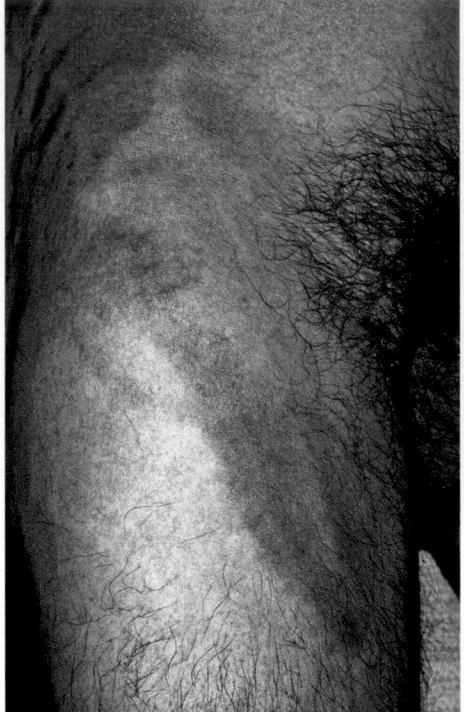

Fig. 35-13 Superficial migratory thrombophlebitis.

superficial venous thrombosis (Fig. 35-13). Patients may also exhibit indurated subcutaneous nodules and overlying purpura or brown discoloration indicative of postinflammatory hyperpigmentation.

Primary hypercoagulable states that may be associated with superficial thrombophlebitis include deficiencies of antithrombin III, heparin cofactor II, protein C, protein S, and factor XII; disorders of tissue plasminogen activator; abnormal plasminogen; dysfibrinogenemia; and lupus anticoagulant. Secondary hypercoagulable states include varicosities, malignancy (Trousseau syndrome), pregnancy, oral contraceptive use, infusion of prothrombin complex concentrates, Behçet's disease, thromboangiitis obliterans, acute thrombophlebitis of superficial veins of the breast (Mondor's disease), septic thrombophlebitis, psittacosis, secondary syphilis, intravenous catheters, intravenous drugs (sugar solutions, protein hydrolysates, calcium, potassium, hypertonic concentrates, diazepam, nitrogen mustard, acridinylaniside, dacarbazine, and carmustine), and street drugs (cocaine, bulking agents such as paregoric, quinine, dextrose, sucrose, and lactose).

In the evaluation of superficial thrombophlebitis, one should consider the possibility of underlying deep venous disease. Superficial femoral vein involvement should alert the physician to underlying deep venous disease requiring anticoagulation. Lesser saphenous vein thrombophlebitis is also frequently associated with underlying DVT. Elliptic biopsies across the palpable cord may be required to exclude other considerations such as sarcoidal granulomas, cutaneous polyarteritis nodosa, Kaposi sarcoma, and vasculotropic metastasis.

Treatment is directed at the underlying cause. Leg elevation and local heat will help to promote the dissolution of clots, which may take up to 8–12 weeks to resolve. Heparin therapy may reduce the incidence of thromboembolic complications in high-risk individuals.

Mondor's disease

Mondor's disease occurs three times more frequently in women than in men, and most patients are between 30 and 60

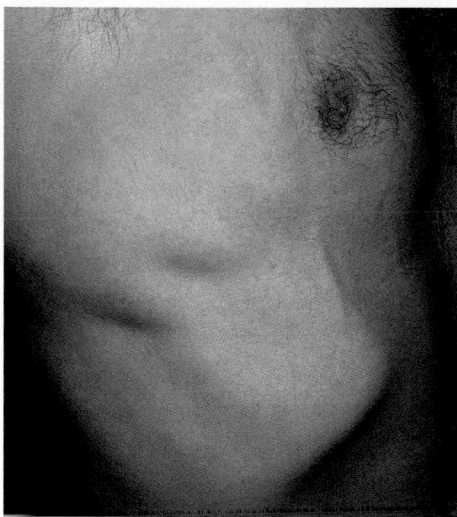

Fig. 35-14 Mondor's disease.

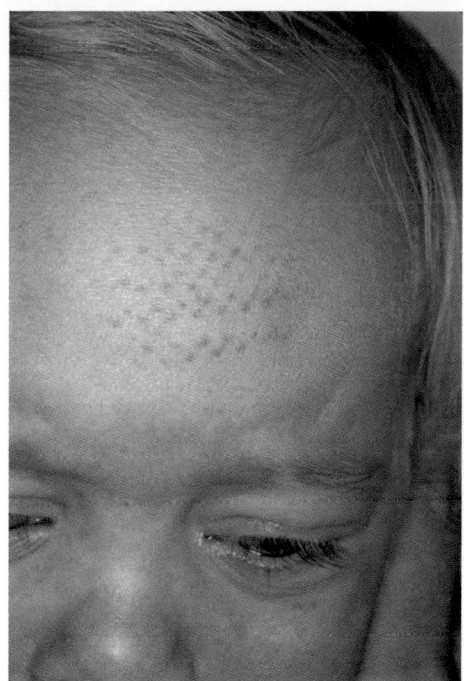

Fig. 35-15 Child abuse, purpura of the face from the sole of a shoe.

years of age. The sudden appearance of a cordlike thrombosed vein along the anterior–lateral chest wall is characteristic (Fig. 35-14). It is at first red and tender and subsequently changes into a painless, tough, fibrous band. There are no systemic symptoms. Both sides of the chest have the same rate of involvement. Mondor's disease may be associated with strenuous exercise, pregnancy, intravenous drug abuse, jellyfish stings, breast cancer, and breast surgery. The condition represents a localized thrombophlebitis of the veins of the thoracoepigastric area. The veins involved are the lateral thoracic, thoracoepigastric, and superior epigastric. In the end stage, a thick-walled vein remains that has a hard, ropelike appearance and, on occasion, may result in a furrowing of the breast. Exceptionally, a vein coursing up the inside of the upper arm and across or into the axilla may be thrombosed, leading to the "axillary web syndrome." Similar string-like phlebitis findings have been described in the penis, antecubital fossa, groin, and abdomen.

Treatment is symptomatic, with hot, moist dressings and analgesics or NSAIDs. The disease process runs its course in 3 weeks to 6 months.

Craythorne E, et al: Axillary web syndrome or cording, a variant of Mondor disease, following axillary surgery. Arch Dermatol 2009; 145:1199.
de Godoy JM, et al: The association of Mondor's disease with protein S deficiency: case report and review of literature. J Thromb Thrombolysis 2002; 13:187.
Kraus S, et al: Mondor's disease of the penis. Urol Int 2000; 64:99.
Samlaska CS, James WD: Superficial thrombophlebitis. I. Primary hypercoagulable states. J Am Acad Dermatol 1990; 22:975.
Samlaska CS, James WD: Superficial thrombophlebitis. II. Secondary hypercoagulable states. J Am Acad Dermatol 1990; 23:1.

Postcardiotomy syndrome

Between 2 and 3 weeks after pericardiotomy, fever, pleuritis, pericarditis, or arthritis may appear, together with petechiae on the skin and palate. This syndrome may be confused with infectious mononucleosis and bacterial endocarditis.

Orthostatic purpura (stasis purpura)

Prolonged standing or even sitting with the legs lowered (as in a bus, airplane, or train) may produce edema and a purpuric eruption on the lower extremities. Elevation of the legs and the use of elastic stockings are helpful preventive strategies.

Obstructive or traumatic purpura

Purpura may be evoked by mechanical obstruction to the circulation, with resulting stress on the small vessels. This may be encountered in cardiac decompensation, or after convulsions, vomiting episodes, the Valsalva maneuver, pertussis, or sexual climax. Nonpalpable purpura has been reported in association with the use of a mucus-clearing device, which requires the patient to exhale forcefully through a flutter valve (flutter valve purpura). Local obstruction of the blood flow with purpura may result from compression of the veins by tumors or a gravid uterus or by occlusions from thrombosis.

Purpuric lesions in children bring into question the possibility of the battered child (Fig. 35-15). Bruises and ecchymoses on the genital area, buttocks, or hands are suggestive of an abused child. Linear lesions on accessible areas raise the question of factitial disease. Ecchymoses of bizarre shapes may also correspond to trauma inflicted during religious rituals or cultural practices. Coin-rubbing and cupping performed as remedies for common diseases are examples. "Passion purpura" on the palate may result from fellatio, or on the neck or upper arms (a "hickey") from biting and sucking. Facial, cheek, and periorbital purpura can be postictal and may be mistaken for spousal abuse. Bathtub suction-induced purpura occurs on the lower back location in a U-shaped distribution. It may be mistaken for abuse.

Baselga E, et al: Purpura in infants and children. J Am Acad Dermatol 1997; 37:673.
Ely SF, et al: Asphyxial deaths and petechiae: a review. J Forensic Sci 2000; 45:1274.
Jaffe FA: Petechial hemorrhages. A review of pathogenesis. Am J Forensic Med Pathol 1994; 15:203.
Knoell KA, et al: Flutter valve purpura. J Am Acad Dermatol 1998; 9:292.
Landers MC, et al: Bathtub suction-induced purpura. Pediatr Dermatol 2004; 21:146.
Reis JJ, et al: Postictal hemifacial purpura. Seizure 1998; 7:337.

Paroxysmal nocturnal hemoglobinuria (PNH)

This acquired intravascular hemolytic anemia usually occurs in young adults, median age 40 years. It is an acquired clonal disorder resulting from a somatic mutation in a multipotent hematopoietic stem cell that produces all the bone marrow-derived cell lines (neutrophils, lymphocytes, platelets, and erythrocytes). The clinical manifestations are intravascular hemolysis, smooth muscle dystonia due to depletion of tissue nitric oxide (abdominal pain, esophageal spasm, fatigue, erectile dysfunction), and life-threatening venous thrombosis. Some cases occur after recovery from aplastic anemia. Widespread cutaneous thrombosis, with initial erythematous cutaneous plaques progressing to hemorrhagic bullae, can occur. Vascular thrombi are found on biopsy. The cause of PNH is a mutation in an X-linked gene, phosphatidylinositol glycan class A (*PIGA*). The product of this gene is the first step in the biosynthesis of all GPI anchors on the surface of hematopoietic cells. Erythrocytes in PNH lack two GPI-anchored proteins, CD55 and CD59, which prevent complement activation on the erythrocyte surface. CD55 accelerates the rate of breakdown of membrane-bound C3 convertase, and CD59 reduces the number of membrane attack complexes that are formed. The diagnosis of PNH can be made by detecting the loss of CD55 and CD59 through monoclonal antibody tests. The FLAER (fluorescent aerolysin) flow cytometry test is now commonly used to diagnose PNH. Hematopoietic stem-cell transplantation may be curative, after either ablative or non-ablative conditioning regimens. Eculizumab, a humanized monoclonal antibody against C5, inhibits terminal complement activation. It stabilizes hemoglobin levels and reduces transfusion requirements in PNH patients.

Brodsky RA: Narrative review. Paroxysmal nocturnal hemoglobinuria: the physiology of complement-related hemolytic anemia. Ann Intern Med 2008; 148:587.

Haspel RL, Hillmen P: Which patients with paroxysmal nocturnal hemoglobinuria (PNH) should be treated with eculizumab? ASH evidence-based review 2008. Hematology Am Soc Hematol Educ Program 2008:35.

Hillmen P: The role of complement inhibition in PNH. Hematology Am Soc Hematol Educ Program 2008:166.

Parker CJ: Bone marrow failure syndromes: paroxysmal nocturnal hemoglobinuria. Hematol Oncol Clin North Am 2009; 23:333.

White JM, et al: Haemorrhagic bullae in a case of paroxysmal nocturnal haemoglobinuria. Clin Exp Dermatol 2003; 28:504.

Paroxysmal hand hematoma (Achenbach syndrome)

Spontaneous focal hemorrhage into the palm or the volar surface of a finger may result in transitory localized pain, followed by rapid swelling and localized bluish discoloration. The lesion resolves spontaneously within a few days. Spontaneous hemorrhage from an arteriole appears to be responsible. The acute nature, purpuric findings, and rapid resolution are distinguishing features of Achenbach syndrome.

Robertson A, et al: Paroxysmal finger haematomas (Achenbach's syndrome) with angiographic abnormalities. J Hand Surg [Br] 2002; 27:391.

Easy bruising syndromes

Young women who bruise easily despite normal coagulation profiles and normal platelet counts may have antiplatelet antibodies. Otherwise, specific platelet function defects should be suspected. Bernard–Soulier syndrome is a rare inherited disorder characterized by giant platelets, thrombocytopenia, and a prolonged bleeding time. It is caused by genetic defects of the glycoprotein Ib–IX complex that constitutes the VWF

receptor. Sebastian syndrome consists of giant platelets, leukocyte inclusions, and thrombocytopenia. Fechtner syndrome is a rare type of familial thrombocytopenia associated with large platelets, leukocyte inclusions, and features of Alport syndrome. The May–Hegglin anomaly consists of easy bruising with giant platelets and Dohle-like cytoplasmic inclusions in granulocytes. The inclusions appear as electron-dense long rods and needles oriented along the long axis of the spindle. All four of these syndromes are due to abnormalities in the *MYH-9* gene. Glanzmann thrombasthenia, with dysfunctioning alphaIIbeta3 receptor, is a platelet storage pool defect causing similar clinical findings.

Balderramo DC, et al: Sebastian syndrome: report of the first case in a South American family. Haematologica 2003; 88:ECR17.

Hadjkacem B, et al: Bernard–Soulier syndrome: novel nonsense mutation in GPIbbeta gene affecting GPIb–IX complex expression. Ann Hematol 2009; 88:465.

Matzdorff AC, et al: Perioperative management of a patient with Fechtner syndrome. Ann Hematol 2001; 80:436.

Nurden AT, et al: Genetic testing in the diagnostic evaluation of inherited platelet disorders. Semin Thromb Hemost 2009; 35:204.

Nurden P, Nurden AT: Congenital disorders associated with platelet dysfunctions. Thromb Haemost 2008; 99:253.

Sachs UJ, et al: Bernard–Soulier syndrome due to the homozygous Asn-45Ser mutation in *GPIX*: an unexpected, frequent finding in Germany. Br J Haematol 2003; 123:127.

Salles II, et al: Inherited traits affecting platelet function. Blood Rev 2008; 22:155.

Simon D, et al: Platelet function defects. Haemophilia 2008; 14:1240.

Painful bruising syndrome (autoerythrocyte sensitization, Gardner–Diamond syndrome, psychogenic purpura)

Painful bruising syndrome is a distinctive localized purpuric reaction occurring primarily in young to middle-aged women who usually manifest personality disorders. There may be depression, anxiety, hysterical or masochistic character traits, or inability to deal with hostile feelings. A recurrent type of eruption, it is characterized by extremely painful and tender, ill-defined ecchymoses about the extremities (Fig. 35-16) and sometimes on the face or trunk. The lesions evolve in a few hours and resolve within 5–8 days. New lesions may appear in crops. Emotional upsets are generally associated with the appearance of these painful purpuric lesions. Some patients will report a premonition as to when they will develop new

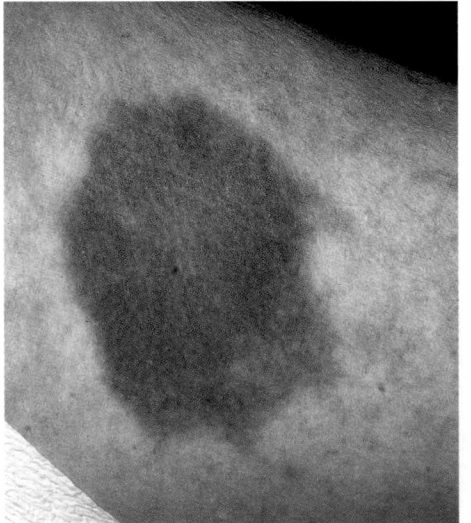

Fig. 35-16 Gardner–Diamond syndrome.

lesions a few hours ahead of time by the tingling and burning sensation at the site of a future lesion. Extracutaneous somatic symptoms are common, such as headache, paresthesias, transient paresis, syncope, diplopia, abdominal distress, diarrhea, nausea and vomiting, and arthralgia.

Gardner and Diamond reported that intracutaneous injections of erythrocyte stroma evoked typical lesions. Since then, many have reported similar reactions to autologous whole blood, packed or washed red cells, or fractions of erythrocyte stroma. These are hard to assess, because similar reactions have been reported to substances as diverse as hemoglobin, phosphatidyl serine, histamine, histidine, trypsin, purified protein derivative (PPD), autologous serum, and platelets. Blinded, controlled testing, trying to avoid factitial trauma, has given mixed responses. Abnormalities in tissue plasminogen activator-dependent fibrinolysis, thrombocytosis, and anticardiolipin antibodies have also been implicated. Most now believe this syndrome is psychosomatic and artifactual. The most effective treatment is to address the underlying psychological dysfunction. Improvement of the underlying psychopathology usually leads to disappearance of the cutaneous manifestations.

Archer-Dubon C, et al: Two cases of psychogenic purpura. Rev Invest Clin 1998; 50:145.

Datta S, et al: A case of psychogenic purpura in a female child. J Indian Med Assoc 2009; 107:104.

Moll S: Psychogenic purpura. Am J Hematol 1997; 55:146.

Panconesi E, et al: Stress, stigmatization and psychosomatic purpuras. Int Angiol 1995; 14:130.

Uthman IW, et al: Autoerythrocyte sensitization (Gardner–Diamond) syndrome. Eur J Haematol 2000; 65:144.

Yucel B, et al: Dissociative identity disorder presenting with psychogenic purpura. Psychosomatics 2000; 41:279.

Pigmentary purpuric eruptions (progressive pigmentary dermatosis, progressive pigmenting purpura, purpura pigmentosa chronica)

The pigmented purpuric eruptions (PPE) are a group of common dermatoses of unknown pathogenesis.

The most common variant of progressive pigmentary dermatosis is Schamberg's disease. The typical lesions are thumbprint-sized and composed of aggregates of pinhead-sized petechiae resembling grains of cayenne pepper on a background of golden-brown hemosiderin staining. The lesions commonly begin on the lower legs, with slow proximal extension (Fig. 35-17). These lesions seldom itch. The favored sites are around the lower shins and ankles, but lesions may be more widespread and occasionally affect the upper extremities or trunk.

Majocchi's disease is also known as purpura annularis telangiectodes. The early lesions are 1–3 cm annular patches composed of dark red telangiectases with petechiae and hemosiderin staining. Central involution and peripheral extension produce ringed, semicircular, target-like, or concentric rings, such as are seen on the cross-cut section of a tree trunk. The eruption begins symmetrically on the lower extremities, spreads up the legs, and may extend on to the trunk and arms. Involution of individual patches is slow and, because new lesions continue to form, may continue indefinitely. The lesions are asymptomatic.

Gougerot–Blum syndrome (pigmented purpuric lichenoid dermatitis) is characterized by minute, rust-colored to violaceous, lichenoid papules that tend to fuse into plaques of various hues between red, violaceous, and brown (purpura with lichenoid dermatitis). Favorite locations are the legs, thighs, and lower trunk. The chief difference between this and Schamberg's disease is the deeper color and the presence of

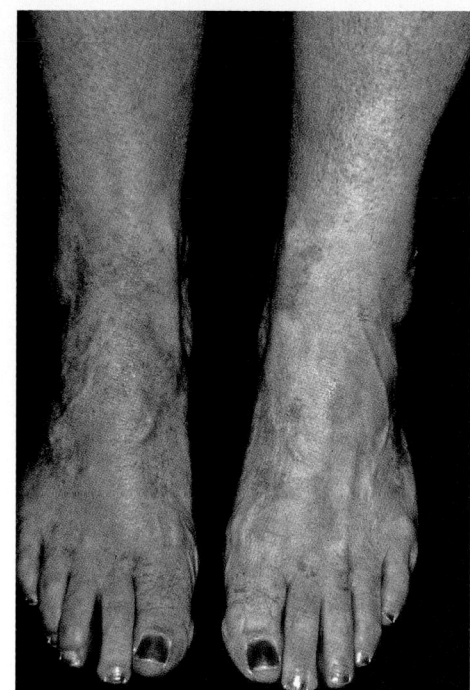

Fig. 35-17 Schamberg's disease.

induration, both of which relate to the presence of a lichenoid band of lymphoid inflammation. Similar lesions have also occurred during IFN therapy for hepatitis C.

Ducas and Kapetanakis pigmented purpura is scaly and eczematous. The eczematous patches also demonstrate petechiae and hemosiderin staining. Pruritus is common, and the lesions are often more extensive than the other pigmented purpuras. It is distinguished histologically by the presence of spongiosis. Purpuric pityriasis rosea may resemble Ducas and Kapetanakis purpura.

Lichen aureus is characterized by the sudden appearance of one or several golden or rust-colored, closely packed macules or lichenoid papules. The macules may be grouped into a patch and may occur on any part of the body, but the vast majority of lesions occur on the feet or lower leg. The patches are usually solitary and asymptomatic, but may occasionally be painful. Adults predominate, but children may also be affected.

Rare variants of the pigmented purpuric dermatoses are the linear or zosteriform type and the transitory type. These tend to be more transient than the other variants. A single case of evolution to linear morphea has been reported.

Histologically, all forms of pigmenting purpura demonstrate superficial perivascular lymphocytic (and at times granulomatous) infiltrate associated with extravasation of red cells and, in later lesions, hemosiderin deposition. The degree of hemosiderin deposition may be variable and insufficient to confirm the diagnosis histologically. The infiltrating cells are primarily CD4+ lymphocytes. There may be a lichenoid band of lymphoid inflammatory cells (Gougerot–Blum type) or spongiosis (Ducas and Kapetanakis type). An iron stain (Perl, Prussian blue, ferricyanide) is sometimes used to demonstrate the hemosiderin deposition.

Cutaneous T-cell lymphoma may begin with clinical lesions that resemble pigmented purpura. In addition, lesions of pigmented purpuric dermatosis may demonstrate clonality. Patients with more widespread lesions above the knee are much more likely to have clonal infiltrates and eventually meet histological criteria for the diagnosis of cutaneous T-cell lymphoma.

In most cases of pigmented purpuric dermatosis, the etiology is unknown. Patients with stasis dermatitis and venous insufficiency may develop lesions that bear a superficial clinical resemblance to Schamberg's disease. Their lesions are more diffuse and do not form well-circumscribed macules. Oral medications can induce eruptions that closely resemble Ducas–Kapetanakis purpura. These include acetaminophen, aspirin, glipizide, IFN-α, and medroxyprogesterone injections. Stopping the offending medication will lead to resolution of the eruption. Pigmented purpuric contact dermatitis may simulate a PPE. Inciting allergens include nickel sulfate, fragrance mix, and Disperse Blue dyes. Patch testing on the back may be negative, but a positive response may be seen when the offending allergen is applied to a lesion. As with pigmenting drug eruptions, pigmented purpuric contact dermatitis should be suspected when the lesions are more widespread (sites other than the legs) and especially if they have an eczematous character.

Anecdotal reports of benefit from topical steroids make a therapeutic trial for 4–6 weeks reasonable. Oral rutoside, 50 mg twice a day, and ascorbic acid, 500 mg twice a day, have cleared a few patients. PUVA and narrow-band ultraviolet (UV) B have demonstrated efficacy and should be considered when the above modalities fail. Immunosuppressive therapy with cyclosporine and methotrexate has also been effective, but is usually not warranted in such a pauci-symptomatic disorder. If immunosuppression is considered, CTCL (cutaneous T-cell lymphoma) must be excluded, and patch testing and drug withdrawal should have been undertaken.

Abe M, et al: Transitory pigmented purpuric dermatoses in a young Japanese female. J Dermatol 2008; 35:525.

Bell HK, et al: Localized morphoea preceded by a pigmented purpuric dermatosis. Clin Exp Dermatol 2003; 28:369.

Engin B, et al: Patch test results in patients with progressive pigmented purpuric dermatosis. J Eur Acad Dermatol Venereol 2009; 23:209.

Georgala S, et al: Persistent pigmented purpuric eruption associated with mycosis fungoides: a case report and review of the literature. J Eur Acad Dermatol Venereol 2001; 15:62.

Gupta G, et al: Capillaritis associated with interferon-alfa treatment of chronic hepatitis C infection. J Am Acad Dermatol 2000; 43(5 Pt 2):937.

Hamada T, et al: A case of zosteriform pigmented purpuric dermatosis. Arch Dermatol 2007; 143:1599.

Hoesly FJ, et al: Purpura annularis telangiectodes of Majocchi: case report and review of the literature. Int J Dermatol 2009; 48:1129.

Komericki P, et al: Pigmented purpuric contact dermatitis from Disperse Blue 106 and 124 dyes. J Am Acad Dermatol 2001; 45:456

Lin W-L, et al: Granulomatous variant of chronic pigmented purpuric dermatoses: report of four new cases and an association with hyperlipidaemia. Clin Exp Dermatol 2007; 32:513.

Magro CM, et al: Pigmented purpuric dermatosis. Am J Clin Pathol 2007; 128:218.

Rose RF, et al: Pigmented purpuric dermatosis as a delayed reaction to medroxyprogesterone acetate. J Eur Acad Dermatol Venereol 2008; 22:1150.

Sardana K, et al: Pigmented purpuric dermatoses: an overview. Int J Dermatol 2004; 43:482.

Ugajin T, et al: Mycosis fungoides presenting as pigmented purpuric eruption. Eur J Dermatol 2005; 15:489.

Purpuric agave dermatitis

Agave americana is a large, thick, long-leaved, subtropical plant with a striking blue–gray color. It is commonly used in ornamental beddings in the southwestern US. The plant grows up to 2 metres in diameter and may overgrow the surrounding landscape. As these plants are very deep-rooted and difficult to remove, some individuals have attempted removal with the help of a chain saw. A striking purpuric dermatosis occurs in a pattern corresponding to the splatter of the plant's sap.

Histologically, there is vascular damage at the level of the capillary and postcapillary venule, with a sparse infiltrate of neutrophils and karyorrhectic debris, suggesting low-grade leukocytoclastic vasculitis. Papulovesicular lesions have also been described. The plant's sap contains calcium oxalate crystals, as well as various acrid oils and saponins. The causative component is unknown.

Cherpelis BS, et al: Purpuric irritant contact dermatitis induced by *Agave americana*. Cutis 2000; 66:287.

Ricks MR, et al: Purpuric agave dermatitis. J Am Acad Dermatol 1999; 40(2 Pt 2):356.

VASCULITIS

Vasculitis is a clinicopathologic process characterized by inflammation and necrosis of blood vessels. Since the clinical morphology correlates with the size of the affected blood vessel(s), these disorders are classified by the blood vessel(s) affected. Diseases may involve vessels of overlapping size. In general, small-vessel disease (affecting postcapillary venules) causes urticarial lesions and palpable purpura; small-artery disease manifests as subcutaneous nodules; medium-sized arteries with necrosis of major organs, livedo, purpura, and mononeuritis multiplex; and large-vessel disease with symptoms of claudication and necrosis.

Classification

Numerous classification schemes have been proposed, all of which have limitations. It is important to remember that infectious and thrombotic conditions, which "classically" show thrombosis of vessels histologically, may also at times show true leukocytoclastic vasculitis. Hence, infectious, embolic, and thrombotic causes of vessel damage must always be considered before unequivocally diagnosing a case as an "inflammatory" vasculitis. Leukocytoclastic vasculitis is also commonly seen adjacent to suppurative folliculitis and at the base of chronic ulcers. The discovery of the association of some forms of small- and medium-vessel vasculitides with positive ANCAs has made their diagnosis and classification much easier (Box 35-1).

Carlson JA, Chen KR: Cutaneous vasculitis update: small vessel neutrophilic vasculitis syndromes. Am J Dermatopathol 2006; 28:486.

Fiorentino DF: Cutaneous vasculitis. J Am Acad Dermatol 2003; 48:311.

Grzeszkiewicz TM, Fiorentino DF: Update on cutaneous vasculitis. Semin Cutan Med Surg 2006; 25:221.

Sunderkotter C, Sindrilaru A: Clinical classification of vasculitis. Eur J Dermatol 2006; 16:114.

Small-vessel vasculitis

Cutaneous small-vessel vasculitis (cutaneous leukocytoclastic vasculitis)

The vast majority of cases of cutaneous leukocytoclastic vasculitis (LCV) follow an acute infection or exposure to a new medication. Palpable purpura is the hallmark of this disease, with lesions ranging from pinpoint to several centimeters in diameter (Fig. 35-18). Annular, vesicular, bullous, or pustular lesions may develop. Small ulcerations may develop, but when ulceration is prominent, one must suspect either a vasculitis of larger vessels (small to medium arterioles) or the presence of both a vasculitis and a hypercoagulable state. Lesions of LCV predominate on the ankles and lower legs, affecting mainly dependent areas or areas under local pressure. Edema, especially of the ankles, is usually noted. In the hospitalized or bedridden patient, the buttocks and posterior

Box 35-1 Classification of vasculitis

I. Cutaneous small-vessel (postcapillary venule)
- **A.** Idiopathic cutaneous small-vessel vasculitis
- **B.** Henoch–Schönlein purpura
- **C.** Acute hemorrhagic edema of infancy
- **D.** Urticarial vasculitis
- **E.** Cryoglobulinemic vasculitis
- **F.** Erythema elevatum diutinum
- **G.** Granuloma faciale
- **H.** Other diseases with leukocystoclastic vasculitis: drug-induced vasculitis, malignancy (lymphoreticular more common than solid tumor), connective tissue diseases, hyperglobulinemic purpura, inflammatory bowel disease, bowel-associated dermatitis–arthritis syndrome (bowel bypass), HIV infection, and neutrophilic dermatoses (Bchçct; Sweet; erythema nodosum leprosum; septic vasculitis; autoinflammatory conditions–familial Mediterranean fever, and serum sickness)

II. Medium-vessel
- **A.** Polyarteritis nodosa
  - **1.** Benign cutaneous forms
  - **2.** Systemic form

III. Mixed size (medium and small) vessel disease
- **A.** Connective tissue disease associated (usually rheumatoid vasculitis)
- **B.** Septic vasculitis
- **C.** ANCA-associated
  - **1.** Microscopic polyangiitis
  - **2.** Wegener granulomatosis
  - **3.** Allergic granulomatosis (Churg–Strauss)
  - **4.** Occasional drug-induced (most are postcapillary venule only)

IV. Large-vessel vasculitis
- **A.** Giant-cell arteritis
- **B.** Takayasu arteritis

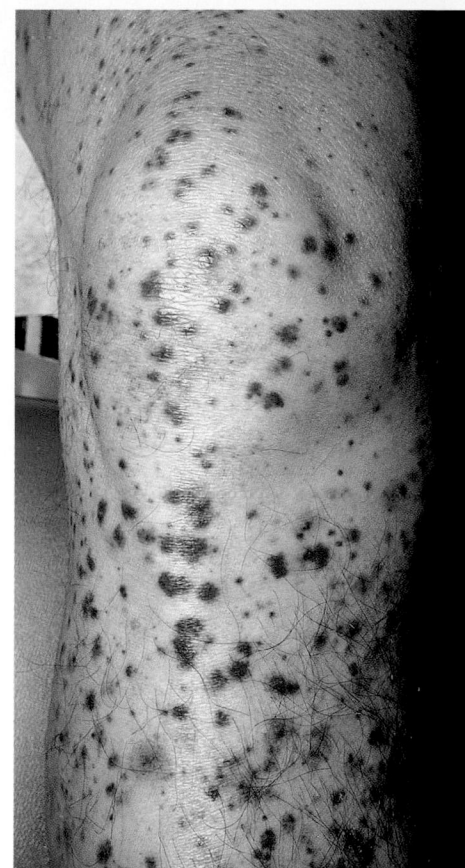

Fig. 35-18 Leukocytoclastic vasculitis, palpable purpura.

thighs are dependent areas and may be the initial or primary site of involvement. Mild pruritus, fever, and malaise may occur. Arthralgias or, less commonly, frank arthritis may be seen. Other systemic involvement is rare and should raise the consideration of another diagnosis. Although, in general, systemic involvement is not found or is minimal, serious systemic disease can accompany cutaneous LCV and should be looked for in every patient.

The lesions usually resolve within 3–4 weeks, with residual postinflammatory hyperpigmentation. Ten percent of cases of cutaneous LCV may have recurrences. A persistent underlying cause must be sought in cases that are chronic.

Histology

There is angiocentric segmental inflammation of the postcapillary venule, with expansion of the vessel wall, fibrin deposition, and infiltration by neutrophils that show fragmentation of their nuclei (karyorrhexis or leukocytoclasia). Endothelial cell swelling is common, but endothelial necrosis suggests more serious illness (including septic vasculitis, ANCA-associated vasculitis). Vascular thrombosis may be present. The presence of tissue eosinophilia favors a medication as the cause. Immunofluorescence and ultrastructural studies have shown the presence of immunoglobulins, complement components, and fibrin deposits within postcapillary venule walls if the biopsy is taken within the first 24 h. Later, fibrin is prominent, but immunoglobulin deposits may have been destroyed. An important exception is Henoch–Schönlein purpura, which

usually demonstrates prominent IgA deposits, even in more advanced lesions.

Pathogenesis

Cutaneous small-vessel vasculitis is felt to be caused by circulating immune complexes. These complexes lodge in vessel walls and activate complement. Various inflammatory mediators are produced, contributing to endothelial injury. Cocaine use may cause or exacerbate small-vessel vasculitis.

Etiology

Most cases of cutaneous LCV are post-infectious or drug-induced. Drugs in virtually every class have been reported as causing LCV, and the time from when the medication was started to the onset of the eruption may be hours to years, making any ingested agent a possible cause. A host of infectious agents, such as β-hemolytic *Streptococcus* group A, *Mycoplasma*, and rarely *Mycobacterium tuberculosis* may cause palpable purpura. Patients with lymphoproliferative neoplasms, as well as solid tumors (lung, colon, genitourinary, and breast cancer) may experience cutaneous small-vessel vasculitis at some time during the course of their disease. A recurrence of the LCV may mark the return of a treated malignancy. Cutaneous LCV may be the initial manifestation of a medium or mixed-vessel vasculitis.

Clinical evaluation

The clinical evaluation is critical in separating those cases of benign cutaneous vasculitis (usually following an infection or induced by a medication) from those cases associated with more serious underlying disease or which have significant systemic involvement. It may not be possible on initial physical examination to separate the more benign-behaving cases from those associated with more serious disease. The history should focus on possible infectious disorders, prior associated diseases, drugs ingested, and a thorough review of systems. Screening laboratory tests may help to elucidate the underlying cause or extent of organ involvement. When the history suggests a recent drug and the patient is clinically well, nothing more than a urinalysis may be required. A complete blood count, urinalysis, strep throat culture or ASO titer, hepatitis B and C serologies, and ANA and rheumatoid factor are a reasonable initial screen for patients with no obvious cause for their vasculitis. Serum protein electrophoresis, serum complements, ANCAs, and cryoglobulins may be required in some cases. A skin biopsy should be performed to confirm the diagnosis of LCV. Direct immunofluorescence should be performed to identify Henoch–Schönlein purpura.

Treatment

The initial treatment of most cases of leukocytoclastic vasculitis in patients who are clinically well and have a normal urinalysis should be nonaggressive, since the majority of cases are acute and self-limited, affect only the skin, and do not threaten progressive deterioration of internal organs. Rest and elevation of the legs is likely to be helpful. Analgesics and avoidance of trauma and cold are prudent general measures. An identified antigen or drug should, of course, be eliminated and any identified infectious, connective tissue, or neoplastic disease treated.

A variety of systemic treatments may be required for severe, intractable, or recurrent disease, especially if significant organ involvement is present. For disease limited to the skin, NSAIDs can be considered for the arthralgias. Colchicine, 0.6 mg 2–3 times a day, or dapsone, 50–200 mg/day, as trials of 2–3 weeks each, may be useful for chronic vasculitis. Low doses of colchicine and dapsone may be combined, if either medication alone is unsuccessful or effective doses of either drug cannot be reached. Although one controlled trial suggested that colchicine was ineffective in LCV, even in that trial a portion of the patients did respond and flared when the drug was stopped. Oral antihistamines, by blocking the vasodilation induced by histamine, may reduce immune complex trapping and improve LCV. Systemic corticosteroids, in doses ranging from 60 to 80 mg/day, are recommended for patients with serious systemic manifestations or necrotic lesions. Usually, a brief course leads to resolution, and chronic treatment is rarely required. In refractory patients immunosuppressive agents, such as mycophenolate mofetil, 2–3 g/day; methotrexate, 5–25 mg/week; or azathioprine, 50–200 mg/day (2–3.5 mg/kg/day), may be considered. Azathioprine dosing is based on thiopurine methyltransferase levels. In more difficult cases, cyclophosphamide, monthly intravenous pulses of steroids or cyclophosphamide, or cyclosporine, 3–5 mg/kg/day, may be effective. The tumor necrosis factor (TNF)-blockers, especially infliximab and to a lesser degree etanercept, may be effective in cutaneous small-vessel vasculitis. These agents may also cause vasculitis. Rituximab has been effective in refractory cases.

Bahrami S, et al: Tissue eosinophilia as an indicator of drug-induced cutaneous small-vessel vasculitis. Arch Dermatol 2006; 142:155.

Drago F, et al: Cutaneous vasculitis induced by cyclo-oxygenase-2 selective inhibitors. J Am Acad Dermatol 2004; 51:1029.

Fain O, et al: Vasculitides associated with malignancies: analysis of sixty patients. Arthritis Rheum 2007; 57:1473.

Fiorentino DF: Cutaneous vasculitis. J Am Acad Dermatol 2003; 48:311.

Greco F, et al: Cutaneous vasculitis associated with *Mycoplasma pneumoniae* infection: case report and literature review. Clin Pediatr (Phila) 2007; 46:451.

Kim HM, et al: Cutaneous leukocytoclastic vasculitis with cervical tuberculous lymphadenitis: a case report and literature review. Rheumatol Int 2006; 26:1154.

Mang R, et al: Therapy for severe necrotizing vasculitis with infliximab. J Am Acad Dermatol 2004; 51:321.

McCain ME, et al: Etanercept and infliximab associated with cutaneous vasculitis. Rheumatology 2002; 41:116.

McIlwain L, et al: Hypersensitivity vasculitis with leukocytoclastic vasculitis secondary to infliximab. J Clin Gastroenterol 2003; 36:411.

Nousari HC, et al: Annular leukocytoclastic vasculitis associated with monoclonal gammopathy of unknown significance. J Am Acad Dermatol 2000; 43:955.

Sais G, et al: Colchicine in the treatment of cutaneous leukocytoclastic vasculitis. Results of a prospective, randomized controlled trial. Arch Dermatol 1995; 131:1399.

Solans-Laque R, et al: Paraneoplastic vasculitis in patients with solid tumors: report of 15 cases. J Rheumatol 2008; 35:294.

Cutaneous vasculitis and connective tissue disease

Patients with various connective tissue diseases (SLE, Sjögren's syndrome, rheumatoid arthritis [RA], and dermatomyositis) may develop cutaneous vasculitic lesions. Vasculitis in the setting of connective tissue disease may be associated with significant internal organ involvement, especially of the peripheral and central nervous system and the kidneys (glomerulonephritis). Ischemic digital infarcts are seen in addition to palpable purpura. Ulceration of vasculitic lesions is not uncommon and may be particularly difficult to manage in the patient with RA. The prevalence of vasculitis in patients with RA has decreased with improved treatment of RA. Treatment is the same as for cutaneous LCV, along with management of the underlying connective tissue disease.

Genta MS, et al: Systemic rheumatoid vasculitis: a review. Semin Arthritis Rheum 2006; 36:88.

Piqué E, et al: Leukocytoclastic vasculitis presenting as an erythema gyratum repens-like eruption on a patient with systemic lupus erythematosus. J Am Acad Dermatol 2002; 47:S254.

Subtypes of small-vessel vasculitis

Henoch–Schönlein purpura

Henoch–Schönlein purpura (HSP) is characterized by purpura, arthralgias, and abdominal and renal disease. Typically, mottled purpura appears on the extensor aspects of the extremities, which become hemorrhagic within a day and start to fade in about 5 days (Fig. 35-19). New crops may appear over a period of a few weeks. Urticarial lesions, vesicles, necrotic purpura, and hemangioma-like lesions may also be present at some stages. It occurs primarily in male children, with a peak age between 4 and 8 years; however, adults may also be affected. A viral infection or streptococcal pharyngitis is the usual triggering event. *H. pylori* infection has been implicated in some childhood and adult cases.

In about 40% of cases, the cutaneous manifestations are preceded by mild fever, headache, joint symptoms, and

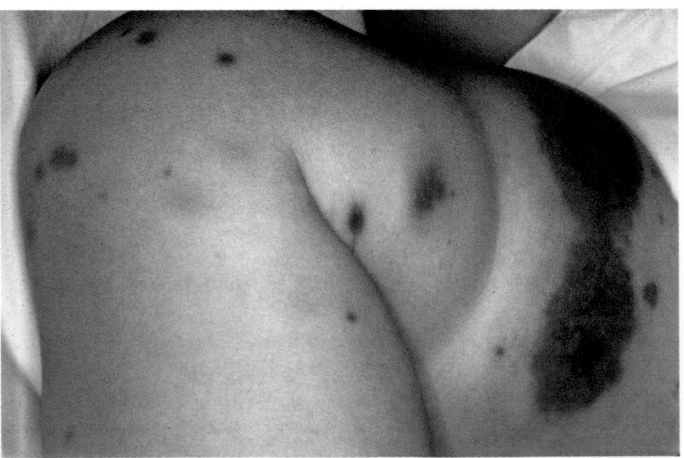

Fig. 35-19 Henoch–Schönlein purpura.

abdominal pain for up to 2 weeks. Arthralgia progressing to arthritis produces periarticular swelling around the knees and ankles. There may be pulmonary hemorrhage, which can be fatal. Abdominal pain and gastrointestinal bleeding may occur at any time during the disease; severe abdominal pain may even suggest—or portend—an acute surgical abdomen. Paralytic ileus may occur. Vomiting, rebound tenderness, and distension are other manifestations. Gastrointestinal radiographs may show "spiking" or a marbled "cobble-stone" appearance. Renal involvement manifests as microscopic or even gross hematuria, and may occur in 25% or more of patients. The long-term prognosis in children with gross hematuria is very good; however, progressive glomerular disease and renal failure may develop in a small percentage, so that careful follow-up is necessary for those with hematuria.

IgA, C3, and fibrin depositions have been demonstrated in biopsies of both involved and uninvolved skin by immunofluorescence techniques. Since IgA immune complexes persist longer in vasculitis, they are easier to identify than the IgG/M-containing immune complexes in other forms of LCV. In patients with abdominal pain suggestive of HSP but with no skin lesions, one can inject histamine (as used as a control by the allergists) into the skin and biopsy the area 4 h later. This "histamine trap test" may identify IgA in vessels and confirm the diagnosis of HSP.

In adults, HSP is not rare. Adult patients have IgA glomerulonephritis or other renal abnormalities in more than 50% of cases. Purpura above the waist in adults was more common in patients with glomerulonephritis. In adult patients with HSP and upper gastrointestinal symptoms (gastritis), a search for *H. pylori* infection should be undertaken. If an association with *H. pylori* can be confirmed, treatment of the gastrointestinal infection may lead to resolution of the HSP. HSP in adults can be associated with an underlying malignancy. Males represent 90% or more of malignancy-associated HSP cases. Solid tumors are seen in more than half of cases (especially non-small-cell lung cancer, prostate cancer, and renal cancer). Forty percent of cases have a hematological malignancy. About half of the cases present within 1 month of the diagnosis of the malignancy.

Treatment is supportive. The usual duration of illness is 6–16 weeks. Between 5% and 10% of patients will have persistent or recurrent disease. Dapsone, 50 to 200 mg/day, or colchicine, 0.6 mg/day to 1.2 mg twice a day, can be used initially if treatment is required and skin lesions are the primary concern. For abdominal pain, an H_2 blocker and/or corticosteroids (prednisone at 1 mg/kg/day) can be effective. Corticosteroids are more effective for abdominal pain than is analgesia. The value of systemic corticosteroids in the treatment of renal disease is controversial, but they may be used preventively or to treat active nephritis. IVIG can be used in refractory skin disease and persistent abdominal pain, and to arrest rapidly progressive glomerulonephritis. NSAIDs are best avoided, as they may cause renal or gastrointestinal complications.

Blanco R, et al: Henoch–Schönlein purpura as clinical presentation of a myelodysplastic syndrome. Clin Rheumatol 1997; 16:626.

Egan CA, et al: Relapsing Henoch–Schönlein purpura associated with *Pseudomonas aeruginosa* pyelonephritis. J Am Acad Dermatol 1999; 41:381.

Hoshino C: Adult onset Schönlein–Henoch purpura associated with *Helicobacter pylori* infection. Intern Med 2009; 48:847.

Mytinger JR, et al: Henoch–Schönlein purpura associated with *Helicobacter pylori* in a child. Pediatr Dermatol 2008; 25:630.

Paller AS, et al: Pulmonary hemorrhage: an often fatal complication of Henoch–Schoenlein purpura. Pediatr Dermatol 1997; 14:299.

Piette WW: What is Schönlein–Henoch purpura, and why should we care (editorial)? Arch Dermatol 1997; 133:438.

Reinauer S, et al: Schönlein–Henoch purpura associated with gastric *Helicobacter pylori* infection. J Am Acad Dermatol 1995; 33:876.

Tancrede-Bohin E, et al: Schönlein–Henoch purpura in adult patients. Arch Dermatol 1997; 133:438.

Trapani S, et al: Severe hemorrhagic bullous lesions in Henoch–Schönlein purpura: three pediatric cases and review of the literature. Rheumatol Int 2009 Jul 16 (Epub ahead of print).

Zurada JM, et al: Henoch–Schönlein purpura associated with malignancy in adults. J Am Acad Dermatol 2006; 55:S65.

Acute hemorrhagic edema of infancy

Also known as Finkelstein's disease, Seidlmayer syndrome, medallion-like purpura, infantile postinfectious iris-like purpura and edema, and purpura en cocarde avec oedème, acute hemorrhagic edema (AHE) of infancy affects children under the age of 2 with a recent history of an upper respiratory illness (75%), a course of antibiotics, or both. The children are often nontoxic in appearance. There is abrupt onset of large cockade, annular, or targetoid purpuric lesions involving the face, ears, and extremities (Fig. 35-20). Scrotal purpura may also occur. Early in the course there may first be acral edema, with subsequent proximal spread. The edema is nontender and may be asymmetrical. A low-grade fever is common, and involvement of internal organ systems (joint pains, gastrointestinal symptoms, and renal involvement) is rare. Routine laboratory tests are unremarkable. Spontaneous recovery without sequelae occurs within 12–20 days. The differential diagnosis includes HSP, meningococcemia, erythema multiforme, urticaria, and Kawasaki's disease. There are some similarities between HSP and AHE (postinfectious, seasonal, favors males), but it is different in that it favors younger children (<2 years), resolves more quickly, lacks IgA on direct immunofluorescence in most cases, and is rarely associated with systemic symptoms. In one family, a child under 4 developed AHE while the sibling aged 16 developed HSP following the same pharyngitis. From a clinical point of view, the most urgent need is to exclude the possibility of septicemia, especially meningococcemia.

Goraya JS, Kaur S: Acute infantile hemorrhagic edema and Henoch–Schönlein purpura: is IgA the missing link? J Am Acad Dermatol 1999; 47:801.

Ince E, et al: Infantile acute hemorrhagic edema: a variant of leukocytoclastic vasculitis. Pediatr Dermatol 1995; 12:224.

Karremann M, et al: Acute hemorrhagic edema of infancy: report of 4 cases and review of the current literature. Clin Pediatr (Phila) 2009; 48:323.

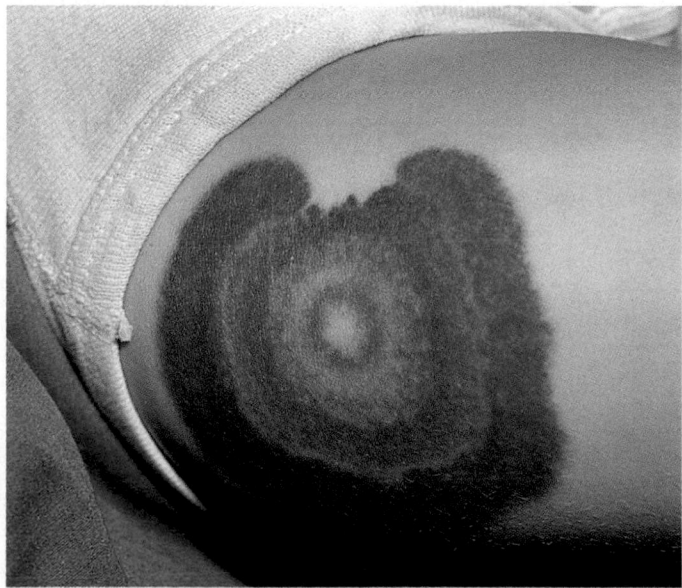

Fig. 35-20 Acute hemorrhagic edema, typical large annular hemorrhagic plaques.

Kuroda K, et al: Acute haemorrhagic oedema of infancy associated with cytomegalovirus infection. Br J Dermatol 2002; 147:1254.

Millard T, et al: Acute infantile hemorrhagic oedema. J Am Acad Dermatol 1999; 41:837.

Urticarial vasculitis

A significant percentage of patients (reported as high as 5–10%, but probably less) with fixed urticarial lesions will have vasculitis histologically. This is termed "urticarial" vasculitis (Fig. 35-21). This urticarial morphology is maintained throughout the course of the illness. Microscopic hemorrhage into the urticarial plaques may occur, resulting in a bruise-like appearance as the lesions fade. Determination of the serum complement levels (CH50, C3, C4, and anti-C1q precipitins) is critical in the evaluation of urticarial vasculitis. Patients with normal complement levels usually have a leukocytoclastic vasculitis, which is idiopathic, limited to the skin, self-resolving, and best considered a subset of cutaneous small-vessel vasculitis. Hypocomplementemic urticarial vasculitis is a distinctive syndrome seen virtually always in women. Clinical features include arthritis (50%), arthralgias, angioedema, eye symptoms, asthma and obstructive pulmonary disease (20%), and gastrointestinal symptoms (20%). Glomerulonephritis may be present. A rare subset of patients with hypocomplementemic urticarial vasculitis has Jaccoud's arthropathy and serious valvular heart disease.

Underlying diseases associated with all forms of urticarial vasculitis include gammopathies (IgG and IgM gammopathy), SLE, Sjögren syndrome, serum sickness, and viral infections, especially hepatitis C. Patients with hypocomplementemic urticarial vasculitis can have anti-C1q antibodies directed against the collagen-like region of that molecule, a feature used to define this disease. Patients with SLE may also have these autoantibodies. Many patients with hypocomplementemic urticarial vasculitis will have positive ANAs, and up to one-quarter will have positive anti-dsDNA antibodies. The vast majority (96%) will have a positive "lupus band test." Over time, more than 50% will meet the criteria for the diagnosis of SLE. For this reason, some consider hypocomplementemic urticarial vasculitis a form of SLE. Patients with HCV infection may develop hypocomplementemic or normocomplementic urticarial vasculitis without a detectable cryoglobulin.

Three clinical features distinguish the skin lesions of urticarial vasculitis from true urticaria:

1. The lesions are often painful, rather than pruritic.
2. The lesions last longer than 24 h and are fixed, rather than migrating.
3. On resolving, there is postinflammatory purpura or hyperpigmentation.

More difficult is the distinction of urticarial vasculitis from neutrophilic urticaria, as patients with the latter condition can have painful, more persistent lesions. Histologic evaluation is critical.

Histologically, patients with hypocomplementemic urticarial vasculitis will show both leukocytoclastic vasculitis and diffuse interstitial neutrophils. Eosinophils are more likely to be seen in patients with neutrophilic urticaria or normocomplementemic urticarial vasculitis. Sweet syndrome shows a more intense dermal infiltrate with marked upper dermal edema. Sweet syndrome and vasculitis share the presence of karyorrhexis. While virtually all biopsies of idiopathic urticaria demonstrate neutrophils, karyorrhexis is usually distinctly absent. In neutrophilic urticaria, neutrophils will be found in the dermis and in the vessel walls (moving from the vascular compartment into the skin). Finding neutrophils in the vessel walls alone without fibrinoid necrosis of vessel walls and leukocytoclasia is insufficient to make the diagnosis of urticarial vasculitis. Most patients with urticarial lesions with neutrophilic infiltrates and normal complements have neutrophilic urticaria rather than urticarial vasculitis.

Other neutrophilic disorders that are in the differential diagnosis of urticarial vasculitis include mixed cryoglobulinemia, Schnitzler syndrome, the autoinflammatory syndromes (CIAS-1/NALP-3 mutations), and neutrophilic dermatosis associated with connective tissue disease. Mixed cryoglobulinemia will be seen most frequently in the context of HCV infection and may present with urticarial, purpuric, or even necrotic/ulcerative lesions. Vasculitis should be seen on biopsy. The other three conditions all can have cutaneous lesions that are urticarial and clinically very similar. They tend to have less dermal edema than is typical of either urticaria or Sweet syndrome. Histologically, they lack vasculitis but show tissue neutrophilia with leukocytoclasia. Schnitzler is diagnosed by the finding of an IgM monoclonal gammopathy. The autoinflammatory syndromes are diagnosed by their characteristic features and genetic testing. In some patients with adult-onset Still disease or SLE, transient macules and papules coalescing into plaques may be seen. This condition has been termed "neutrophilic urticarial dermatitis", but its pathogenesis remains unknown. In the setting of such neutrophilic urticarial lesions, ferritin measurement and a workup for SLE are appropriate.

The treatment of hypocomplementemic urticarial vasculitis is directed at the symptomatology and severity of the disease. Indomethacin has been particularly effective. Antihistamines, dapsone, and colchicine may be tried. The addition of pentoxifylline to dapsone may be effective. Antimalarials can be beneficial, as would be expected in this autoimmune connective tissue disease. Immunosuppressive therapy with prednisone and the steroid-sparing agent mycophenolate mofetil (2 g/day) can be considered in refractory and severe cases.

Amano H, et al: Hypocomplementemic urticarial vasculitis with Jaccoud's arthropathy and valvular heart disease: case report and review of the literature. Lupus 2008; 17:837.

Chang S, Carr W: Urticarial vasculitis. Allergy Asthma Proc 2007; 28:97.

Davis MDP, et al: Clinicopathologic correlation of hypocomplementemic and normocomplementemic urticarial vasculitis. J Am Acad Dermatol 1998; 38:899.

Fiorentino DF: Cutaneous vasculitis. J Am Acad Dermatol 2003; 48:311.

Hamid S, et al: Urticarial vasculitis caused by hepatitis C virus infection. J Am Acad Dermatol 1998; 39:278.

Hunt DP, et al: Pulmonary capillaritis and its relationship to development of emphysema in hypocomplementaemic urticarial vasculitis syndrome. Sarcoidosis Vasc Diffuse Lung Dis 2006; 23:70.

Kieffer C, et al: Neutrophilic urticarial dermatosis. Medicine 2009; 88:23.

Nurnberg W, et al: Urticarial vasculitis syndrome effectively treated with dapsone and pentoxifylline. Acta Derm Venereol 1995; 75:54.

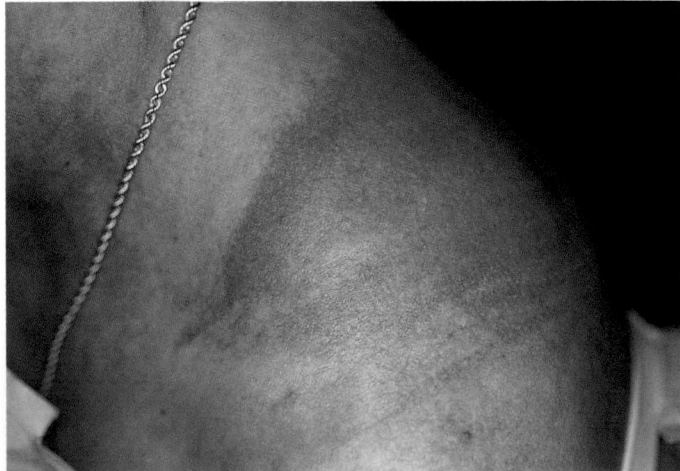

Fig. 35-21 Urticarial vasculitis.

Saadoun D, et al: Anti-C1q antibodies in hepatitis C virus infection. Clin Exp Immunol 2006; 145:308.

Shaw D, et al: Hypocomplementaemic urticarial vasculitis associated with non-Hodgkin lymphoma and treatment with intravenous immunoglobulin. Br J Dermatol 2007; 157:392.

Toprak O, et al: Hypocomplementaemic urticarial vasculitis syndrome and acute renal failure with cryoglobulin(–) hepatitis C infection. Nephrol Dial Transplant 2004; 19:2680.

Worm M, et al: Mycophenolate mofetil is effective for maintenance therapy of hypocomplementaemic urticarial vasculitis. Br J Dermatol 2000; 143:1324.

Cryoglobulinemic vasculitis

About 15% of patients with a circulating cryoprecipitable protein are symptomatic and have cryoglobulinemic vasculitis. They typically have mixed cryoglobulinemia. Mixed cryoglobulinemia follows a benign course in half of cases, but in about one-third liver or renal failure occurs. Fifteen percent of cases develop malignancy, usually B-cell lymphoma, and less frequently hepatocellular or thyroid cancer. By far the most common cause of cryoglobulinemic vasculitis is HCV infection, but autoimmune diseases and lymphoproliferative disorders can also be associated with cryoglobulinemic vasculitis. Cryoglobulinemic vasculitis usually presents with macular or palpable purpura, typically confined to the lower extremities. Lesions may be limited or severe. Two-thirds of patients show confluent areas of hemosiderosis of the feet and lower legs, characteristic of prior episodes of purpura. While only 30% of patients report an exacerbation with cold exposure, up to 50% will have Raynaud phenomenon and cold-induced acrocyanosis of the ears. Other morphologies include ecchymoses, livedo reticularis, urticaria, and ulcerations. Widespread systemic vasculitis occurs in about 10% of patients. Neuropathy and other neurologic complications occur in 40% of patients. Arthralgias, xerostomia, and xerophthalmia are frequent complaints. Laboratory evaluation will reveal a cryoglobulin, hypocomplementemia (90%), and a positive rheumatoid factor (70%). ANCAs are rarely positive. A skin biopsy will show LCV.

The treatment of cryoglobulinemic vasculitis is the treatment of the underlying disease if possible. In the case of HCV infection, this usually is IFN-α plus ribavirin. Cryoglobulinemic vasculitis associated with HCV may also be flared by IFN treatment. Colchicine, dapsone, IVIG, infliximab, and rituximab (an anti-CD20 monoclonal antibody) can be attempted. In severe cases plasmapheresis may be beneficial.

Batisse D, et al: Sustained exacerbation of cryoglobulinaemia-related vasculitis following treatment of hepatitis C with peginterferon alfa. Eur J Gastroenterol Hepatol 2004; 16:701.

Cacoub P, et al: Anti-CD20 monoclonal antibody (rituximab) treatment for cryoglobulinemic vasculitis: where do we stand? Ann Rheum Dis 2008; 67:283.

Chandesris MO, et al: Infliximab in the treatment of refractory vasculitis secondary to hepatitis C-associated mixed cryoglobulinaemia. Rheumatology 2004; 43:532.

De Blasi T, et al: Cryoglobulinemia-related vasculitis during effective anti-HCV treatment with PFG-interferon alfa 2b. Infection 2008; 36:285.

Enomoto M, et al: Entecavir to treat hepatitis B-associated cryoglobulinemic vasculitis. Ann Intern Med 2008; 149:912.

Farri C, et al: Mixed cryoglobulinemia: demographic, clinical, and serologic features and survival in 231 patients. Semin Arthritis Rheum 2004; 33:355.

Kawakami T, et al: Remission of hepatitis B virus-related cryoglobulinemic vasculitis with entecavir. Ann Intern Med 2008; 149:911.

Nemni R, et al: Peripheral neuropathy in hepatitis C virus infections with and without cryoglobulinaemia. J Neurol Neurosurg Psychiatry 2003; 74:1267.

Roccatello D, et al: Long-term effects of anti-CD20 monoclonal antibody treatment of cryoglobulinaemic glomerulonephritis. Nephrol Dial Transplant 2004; 19:3054.

Scarpato S, et al: Plasmapheresis in cryoglobulinemic neuropathy: a clinical study. Dig Liver Dis 2007; 39:S136.

Tallarita T, et al: Successful combination of rituximab and plasma exchange in the treatment of cryoglobulinemic vasculitis with skin ulcers: a case report. Cases J 2009; 2:7859.

Macular lymphocytic arteritis (lymphocytic thrombophilic arteritis)

This is a rarely reported condition that affects predominantly non-Caucasian females. It presents with multiple ill-defined brown macules on the lower legs resembling postinflammatory hyperpigmentation. Histologically, a vessel in the subcutaneous fat is infiltrated with lymphocytes but there is no destruction of the vessels. Neutrophils are absent.

Golfer's and exercise-related "vasculitis"

This syndrome, which occurs mostly in hot weather, affects primarily older men (age >50). Golfing or exercise with prolonged walking is the trigger. The syndrome is characterized by asymptomatic or pruritic, burning, or stinging, purpuric, macular or slightly raised papules and plaques, predominately just above the sock line near the ankles. Mild ankle swelling may be present. The lesions resolve in under 3 days in most patients. Histologically, true LCV is not seen, but erythrocytes and neutrophils are present in the affected tissue. About half of the patients are on antithrombotic agents. This syndrome probably represents a form of purpura due to anticoagulation and prolonged erect posture rather than a true vasculitis.

Kelly RI, et al: Golfer's vasculitis. Australas J Dermatol 2005; 46:11.

Saleh Z, Mutasim DF: Macular lymphocytic arteritis: a unique benign cutaneous arteritis, mediated by lymphocytes and appearing as macules. J Cutan Pathol 2009; 36:1269.

Erythema elevatum diutinum

A rare condition, erythema elevatum diutinum (EED) is considered to be a chronic fibrosing leukocytoclastic vasculitis. Classically, multiple orange to yellow papules and plaques develop over the joints (Fig. 35-22), particularly the elbows, knees, hands, and feet. Lesions may also involve the buttocks and areas over the Achilles tendon. Petechiae and purpura can be associated with early lesions. More rarely, large plaques

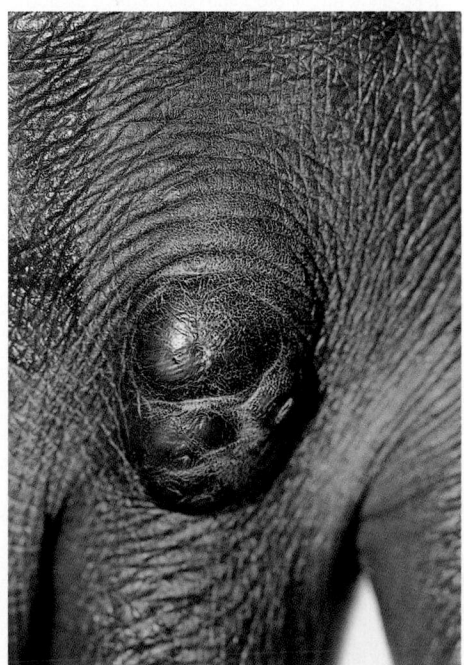

Fig. 35-22 Erythema elevatum diutinum.

with nodules at the periphery may affect the trunk and extremities. Scattered nodules on the trunk with no acral lesions constitute another rare variant. With time, the papules take on a doughy to firm consistency and develop a red or purple color. In HIV infection, skin-colored or red nodules affect the soles, producing lesions resembling keloids, Kaposi sarcoma, or bacillary angiomatosis. Pruritus, arthralgias, and pain have been reported; however, most patients are asymptomatic. Some patients with EED will develop pyoderma gangrenosum-like ulcerations, which in one case presented as a phagedenic penile ulceration. Systemic complications are rare, but an unusual and potentially rapidly destructive keratitis can lead to blindness. EED has been associated with HIV infection, SLE, Sjögren syndrome, lymphoma, breast cancer, lymphoepithelioma-like carcinoma, dermatitis herpetiformis, and celiac disease. IgA monoclonal gammopathy may be detected. Chronic and recurrent streptococcal infections cause exacerbations of the disease in some patients. These may all represent conditions with persistent circulating immune complexes that might trigger a chronic vasculitis. Pathogenically, ANCAs (60% IgA and 33% IgG) are found in EED. ANCA-positive vasculitides, such as Wegener granulomatosis, have rarely been reported to have EED-like lesions.

Histologically, early lesions are a leukocytoclastic vasculitis, but with prominent interstitial neutrophils. Well-formed lesions are composed of nodular and diffuse mixed infiltrates of neutrophils and nuclear dust, eosinophils, histiocytes, and plasma cells that often extend into the subcutaneous fat. The prominence of eosinophils; the chronicity of the process, which results in an onion skin-like perivascular fibrosis; and the admixture of plasma cells and many lymphocytes are the hallmarks of EED. Erythrocyte extravasation may lead to extracellular cholesterol crystals in long-standing cases.

Dapsone is the treatment of choice. Patients with celiac disease may respond to a gluten-free diet. Tetracycline and nicotinamide, sulfapyridine, colchicine, antimalarials, and intralesional or systemic steroids have all been reported as effective in a limited number of cases. Intermittent plasma exchange has been used successfully in patients with IgA paraproteinemia. The interstitial keratitis also responds to dapsone. Unfortunately, the late nodular lesions may not resolve with dapsone treatment.

Aldave AJ, et al: Peripheral keratitis associated with erythema elevatum diutinum. Am J Ophthalmol 2003; 135:389.

Ayaoub N, et al: Antineutrophil cytoplasmic antibodies of IgA class in neutrophilic dermatoses with emphasis on erythema elevatum diutinum. Arch Dermatol 2004; 140:931.

Barzegar M, et al: An atypical presentation of erythema elevatum diutinum involving palms and soles. Int J Dermatol 2009; 48:73.

Chow RK, et al: Erythema elevatum diutinum associated with IgA paraproteinemia successfully controlled with intermittent plasma exchange. Arch Dermatol 1996; 132:1360.

Di Giacomo TB, et al: Erythema elevatum diutinum presenting with a giant annular pattern. Int J Dermatol 2009; 48:290.

Farley-Loftus R, et al: Erythema elevatum diutinum. Dermatol Online J 2008; 14:13.

Futei Y, Konohana I: A case of erythema elevatum diutinum associated with B-cell lymphoma: a rare distribution involving palms, soles and nails. Br J Dermatol 2000; 142:116.

Golmia A, et al: The development of erythema elevatum diutinum in a patient with juvenile idiopathic arthritis under treatment with abatacept. Clin Rheumatol 2008; 27:105.

Grabbe J, et al: Erythema elevatum diutinum—evidence for disease-dependent leucocyte alterations and response to dapsone. Br J Dermatol 2000; 143:415.

Hatzitolios A, et al: Erythema elevatum diutinum with rare distribution as a first clinical sign of non-Hodgkin's lymphoma: a novel association? J Dermatol 2008; 35:297.

High W, et al: Late-stage nodular erythema elevatum diutinum. J Am Acad Dermatol 2003; 49:764.

Kavanagh GM, et al: Erythema elevatum diutinum associated with Wegener's granulomatosis and IgA paraproteinemia. J Am Acad Dermatol 1993; 28:846.

Liu TC, et al: Erythema elevatum diutinum as a paraneoplastic syndrome in a patient with pulmonary lymphoepithelioma-like carcinoma. Lung Cancer 2009; 63:151.

Mitamura Y, et al: Nodular scleritis and panuveitis with erythema elevatum diutinum. Am J Ophthalmol 2004; 137:368.

Muratori S, et al: Erythema elevatum diutinum and HIV infection: a report of five cases. Br J Dermatol 1999; 141:335.

Pai HS, et al: Erythema elevatum diutinum in association with celiac disease. Int J Dermatol 2009; 48:787.

Shimizu S, et al: Erythema elevatum diutinum with primary Sjögren syndrome associated with IgA antineutrophil cytoplasmic antibody. Br J Dermatol 2008; 159:733.

Soubeiran E, et al: Erythema elevatum diutinum with unusual clinical appearance. J Dtsch Dermatol Ges 2008; 6:303.

Tasanen K, et al: Erythema elevatum diutinum in association with coeliac disease. Br J Dermatol 1997; 136:624.

Tomasini C, et al: Infantile erythema elevatum diutinum: report of a vesiculo-bullous case. Eur J Dermatol 2006; 16:683.

Wahl CE, et al: Erythema elevatum diutinum. Am J Dermatopathol 2005; 27:397.

Wayte JA, et al: Pyoderma gangrenosum, erythema elevatum diutinum and IgA monoclonal gammopathy. Australas J Dermatol 1995; 36:21.

Yoshii N, et al: Erythema elevatum diutinum manifesting as a penile ulcer. Clin Exp Dermatol 2007; 32:211.

Granuloma faciale

Characterized by brownish-red, infiltrated papules, plaques (Fig. 35-23), and nodules, granuloma faciale involves the facial areas, particularly the nose. Healthy, middle-aged (mean 53 years) white men (male to female ratio, 5:1) are most typically affected. Childhood cases have been reported. Extrafacial disease occurs in up to 20% of cases, usually affecting the upper trunk and extremities.

The pathology of granuloma faciale is similar to that of EED, with focal leukocytoclastic vasculitis, diffuse dermal neutrophilia with leukocytoclasia, tissue eosinophilia, and perivascular fibrosis.

A variety of treatment options are available. Intralesional corticosteroids are the recommended first approach. Cryotherapy in combination with intralesional corticosteroids has been shown to be very effective. Topical corticosteroids may also be useful. Although controlled clinical trials are lacking, dapsone, colchicine, or antimalarials could be considered if the patient remains unresponsive. Laser treatment with pulsed dye and argon lasers has been effective in multiple cases, making it a reasonable consideration as first-line treatment.

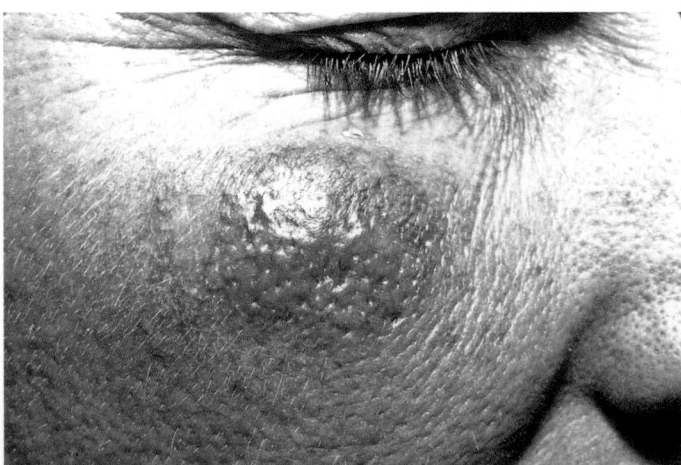

Fig. 35-23 Granuloma faciale.

Ammirati CT, et al: Treatment of granuloma faciale with the 585-nm pulsed dye laser. Arch Dermatol 1999; 135:903.

Dowlati B, et al: Granuloma faciale: successful treatment of nine cases with a combination of cryotherapy and intralesional corticosteroid injection. Int J Dermatol 1997; 36:548.

Marcoval J, et al: Granuloma faciale: a clinicopathological study of 11 cases. J Am Acad Dermatol 2004; 51:269.

van de Kerkhof PC: On the efficacy of dapsone in granuloma faciale. Acta Derm Venereol 1994; 74:61.

Welsh JH, et al: Granuloma faciale in a child successfully treated with the pulsed dye laser. J Am Acad Dermatol 1999; 41:351.

Zargari O: Disseminated granuloma faciale. Int J Dermatol 2004; 43:210.

Polyarteritis nodosa

Polyarteritis nodosa (PAN) is characterized by necrotizing vasculitis affecting primarily the small to medium-sized arteries. There are two major forms, the benign cutaneous and the systemic, although even long-standing benign cutaneous PAN can evolve into systemic disease. There are ten diagnostic criteria for systemic PAN:

1. livedo racemosa
2. polymorphonuclear arteritis
3. leg pain/myopathy/weakness
4. mono-/polyneuropathy
5. positive hepatitis B virus (HBV) serology
6. weight loss >4 kg
7. testicular pain/tenderness
8. diastolic blood pressure >90 mmHg
9. elevated BUN/creatinine
10. arteriographic abnormality.

Separating systemic PAN from microscopic polyangiitis (MPA) can be difficult, and the skin manifestations clinically and histologically are of no benefit in this regard.

PAN is 2–4 times more common in men than in women and the mean age of presentation is 45–50 years. A cutaneous vasculitis identical to PAN has been seen in intravenous drug abusers (see below) and in association with SLE, inflammatory bowel disease, hairy cell leukemia, familial Mediterranean fever, and Cogan syndrome (nonsyphilitic interstitial keratitis and vestibulo-auditory symptoms). Infectious associations include hepatitis B, hepatitis C, and antecedent streptococcal infections. Vascular-based tuberculids (erythema induratum, nodular tuberculid) may have histology identical to PAN. The proportion of PAN cases associated with HBV is currently about 5–7% of cases overall, but this percentage is falling with HBV immunization. The identification of associated hepatitis virus infection has therapeutic and prognostic implications.

The skin is involved in up to 50% of patients with the systemic form of PAN, with wide-ranging findings. The most striking and diagnostic lesions (15% of patients) are 5–10 mm subcutaneous nodules occurring singly or in groups, distributed along the course of the blood vessels, above which the skin is normal or slightly erythematous (macular arteritis). These nodules are often painful and may pulsate and, in time, ulcerate (Fig. 35-24). Common sites are the lower extremities, especially below the knee. Ecchymoses and peripheral gangrene of the fingers and toes may also be present. Livedo reticularis in combination with subcutaneous nodules strongly suggests the diagnosis of PAN. Palpable purpura with histologic features of cutaneous LCV may be seen in PAN in 20% of patients. Urticaria is present in 6% of cases of PAN. HBV-associated PAN is associated with cutaneous findings in only 30% of cases.

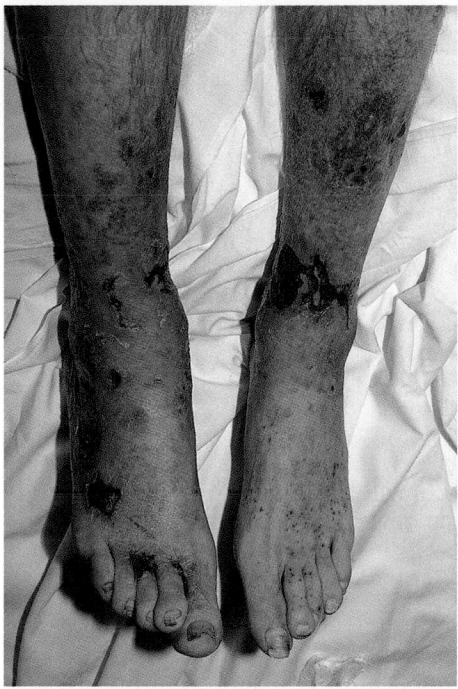

Fig. 35-24 Polyarteritis nodosa with multiple leg ulcerations.

Classic systemic PAN may involve the vessels throughout the entire body. It has a particular predilection for the skin, peripheral nerves, gastrointestinal tract, and kidneys. Hypertension (due to renal involvement in 80%), tachycardia, fever, edema, and weight loss (>70%) are cardinal signs of the disease. Arthralgia/arthritis (up to 75%), myocardial and intestinal infarctions, and peripheral neuritis (75%) are also seen. Mononeuritis multiplex, most often manifested as foot drop, is a hallmark of PAN. Involvement of the meningeal, vertebral, and carotid arteries may lead to hemiplegia and convulsions. The lungs and spleen are rarely involved. Aneurysms develop, which may result in multiorgan infarcts. A Five Factor Score (FFS) has been validated, with 1 point each for proteinuria, renal insufficiency, gastrointestinal tract involvement, CNS involvement, and cardiomyopathy. The 5-year survival for patients with FFS scores of 0, 1, and >2 are 88%, 75%, and 54% respectively. Prior to the use of systemic immunosuppressives, the mortality for systemic PAN exceeded 90%.

A leukocytosis of as high as 40 000/mm^3 may occur, with neutrophilia to 80%; thrombocytosis, progressive normocytic anemia, and an elevated sedimentation rate and C-reactive protein (CRP) may also be found. Hepatitis B and C studies should be performed. Urinary abnormalities, such as proteinuria, hematuria, and casts, are present in 70% of patients. The prevalence of ANCA positivity is related to how one diagnoses PAN as opposed to MPA. ANCAs are more commonly found in MPA than in PAN, and in both diseases p-ANCA is the predominant type. HBV-associated PAN is rarely, if ever, ANCA-positive.

The histology is that of an inflammatory necrotizing and obliterative panarteritis that attacks the small and medium-sized arteries. Focal vasculitis forms nodose swellings that become necrotic, producing aneurysms and rupture of the vessels. Hemorrhage, hematoma, and ecchymosis may result. Obliteration of the lumen may occur, with ischemic necrosis of surrounding tissue. Characteristically, the arteries are affected at their branching points.

The mainstay of diagnosis is the presence of these histologic features and the constellation of clinical findings. The preferable site for biopsy is an accessible area such as skin, muscle, or testis. If these are not involved, angiography may detect aneurysmal dilations as small as 1 cm wide in the renal, hepatic, or other visceral vessels.

Treatment

Untreated classic PAN can be fatal, death usually being due to renal failure or cardiovascular or gastrointestinal complications. Death generally occurs early in the course of the disease. Patients with HBV- or HCV-associated PAN should be given IFN and other antiviral treatments as their initial therapy. For PAN not associated with HBV or HCV, treatment with corticosteroids and cytotoxic agents has increased the 5-year survival rate to more than 75%. Corticosteroids in the range of 1 mg/kg/day are given initially. Once the disease remits, the dose should be reduced. After an average of 3–6 months, with the patient in remission, the steroids are slowly tapered to discontinuation.

Cyclophosphamide is given with steroids or sometimes as a single agent. Initially, 2 mg/kg/day as a single dose is recommended. Twice this amount may be required for severely ill patients. The oral dose is then adjusted to maintain the white blood cell count between 3000 and 3500/mm^3 and the neutrophil count above 1500 cells/mm^3. When the disease has been quiescent for at least 1 year, the cyclophosphamide may be tapered and stopped. On average, 18–24 months of therapy are required. Pulsed intravenous cyclophosphamide is associated with a lower incidence of toxicity, especially the long-term risk of malignancy. Plasma exchange may be used for acute crises or treatment failures with corticosteroids and cyclophosphamide. Ulcerations in PAN can be very painful due to the associated neuropathy. They should be managed like nonhealing leg ulcers.

Cutaneous polyarteritis nodosa

About 10% of patients present with PAN localized to the skin and with limited systemic involvement. Neuropathy occurs in 20%. Subcutaneous nodules (80%), livedo (70%), and ulceration (44%) are the characteristic cutaneous features that should lead to suspicion of cutaneous PAN. Atrophie blanche-like lesions around the ankles may be the sole cutaneous manifestation of cutaneous PAN. Plaques on the trunk and proximal extremities expanding slowly and centrifugally are another manifestation. At the periphery of the plaques is a ring of 1–2 cm subcutaneous nodules. Cutaneous PAN has a better prognosis and will require less aggressive therapy, patients rarely suffering the systemic renal, gastrointestinal, and cardiovascular complications of systemic PAN. This form of PAN is the most common childhood pattern of PAN. Whether there are two clear subsets of patients, cutaneous and systemic PAN, or rather a spectrum of disease is controversial. Patients with "cutaneous" PAN must be followed carefully and regularly evaluated to exclude the development of systemic involvement, which may appear as long as two decades after the initial diagnosis.

The diagnosis of cutaneous PAN is made by biopsy of a subcutaneous nodule. An excisional biopsy is recommended, as the vasculitis is focal. The affected arteriole is at the junction of the dermis and subcutaneous tissue or in the subcutaneous fat. Adjacent to the affected vessel there is an inflammatory panniculitis, and inadequate evaluation of the biopsy or too small a sample may lead to the erroneous diagnosis of a panniculitis. Also distal to the affected arteriole, thrombosis usually occurs. If the biopsy is inadequate in depth or size, this bland thrombosis without inflammation is seen and the erroneous diagnosis of a "vasculopathy" will be made. Cutaneous PAN has been associated with HBV surface antigenemia, HCV infection, Crohn's disease, Takayasu arteritis, relapsing polychondritis, streptococcal infections, tuberculosis, and medica-

tions (minocycline). Typically, the only laboratory abnormality is an elevated erythrocyte sedimentation rate (ESR) or CRP. In some cases, a p-ANCA may be present. Most patients respond well to aspirin, NSAIDs, prednisone, pentoxifylline, sulfapyridine, or methotrexate, alone or in some combination. In childhood cutaneous PAN, since streptococcal infection is common, penicillin treatment may be used. In refractory cases, IVIG may be used.

Asano Y, et al: High-dose intravenous immunoglobulin infusion in polyarteritis nodosa: report on one case and review of the literature. Clin Rheumatol 2006; 25:396.

Bauzá A, et al: Cutaneous polyarteritis nodosa. Br J Dermatol 2002; 146:694.

Chan PT, et al: Inflammatory plaque with peripheral nodules: a new specific finding of cutaneous polyarteritis nodosa. J Am Acad Dermatol 2009; 60:320.

Diaz-Perez JL, et al: Cutaneous polyarteritis nodosa. Semin Cutan Med Surg 2007; 26:77.

Fathalla BM, et al: Cutaneous polyarteritis nodosa in children. J Am Acad Dermatol 2005; 53:724.

Fein H, et al: Cutaneous arteritis presenting with hyperpigmented macules: macular arteritis. J Am Acad Dermatol 2003; 49:519.

Fortin PR, et al: Prognostic factors in systemic necrotizing vasculitis of the polyarteritis nodosa group: a review of 45 cases. J Rheumatol 1995; 22:78.

Guillevin L, et al: Prognostic factors in polyarteritis nodosa and Churg–Strauss syndrome: a prospective study in 342 patients. Medicine (Baltimore) 1996; 75:17.

Guillevin L, et al: Short-term corticosteroids then lamivudine and plasma exchanges to treat hepatitis B virus-related polyarteritis nodosa. Arthritis Rheum 2004; 51:482.

Komatsuda A, et al: Cutaneous polyarteritis nodosa in a patient with Crohn's disease. Mod Rheumatol 2008; 18:639.

Kumar L, et al: Benign cutaneous polyarteritis nodosa in children below 10 years of age: a clinical experience. Ann Rheum Dis 1995; 54:134.

Matsumura Y, et al: A case of cutaneous polyarteritis nodosa associated with ulcerative colitis. Br J Dermatol 2000; 142:561.

Mimouni D, et al: Cutaneous polyarteritis nodosa in patients presenting with atrophie blanche. Br J Dermatol 2003; 148:789.

Pak H, et al: Purpuric nodules and macules on the extremities of a young woman: cutaneous polyarteritis nodosa. Arch Dermatol 1998; 134:232.

Pennoyer JW, et al: Ulcer associated with polyarteritis nodosa treated with bioengineered human skin equivalent (Apligraf). J Am Acad Dermatol 2002; 46:145.

Rogalski C, Sticherling M: Panarteritis cutanea benigna—an entity limited to the skin or cutaneous presentation of a systemic necrotizing vasculitis? Report of seven cases and review of the literature. Int J Dermatol 2007; 46:817.

Schaffer JV, et al: Perinuclear antineutrophilic cytoplasmic antibody-positive cutaneous polyarteritis nodosa associated with minocycline therapy for acne vulgaris. J Am Acad Dermatol 2001; 44:198.

Segelmark M, Selga D: The challenge of managing patients with polyarteritis nodosa. Curr Opin Rheumatol 2007; 19:33.

Sheth AP, et al: Cutaneous polyarteritis nodosa of childhood. J Am Acad Dermatol 1994; 31:561.

Siberry GK, et al: Cutaneous polyarteritis nodosa. Arch Dermatol 1994; 130:884.

Soufir N, et al: Hepatitis C virus infection in cutaneous polyarteritis nodosa. Arch Dermatol 1999; 135:1001.

ANCA-positive small-vessel vasculitides

Antineutrophil cytoplasmic antibodies (ANCAs) have become an important laboratory finding used in the diagnosis and, in some cases, the prognosis of systemic vasculitis. ANCAs occur in three patterns: cytoplasmic (c-ANCA); perinuclear (p-ANCA); and atypical ANCA. c-ANCA is associated with antibodies directed against proteinase 3 (PR3). Antibodies against myeloperoxidase result in the p-ANCA pattern, but antibodies against other antigens may also give this pattern. Atypical ANCAs are not directed against myeloperoxidase or

PR3. Most laboratories now perform specific tests to determine whether positive ANCAs are reactive against myeloperoxidase or PR3. Anti-PR3 antibodies are relatively specific for Wegener granulomatosis and microscopic polyangiitis. Antibodies against myeloperoxidase are less specific and can be found in microscopic polyangiitis, Churg–Strauss syndrome, and drug-induced vasculitis. Usually, either anti-myeloperoxidase or anti-PR3 antibodies are found, but not both. If both patterns are found, drug-induced vasculitis should be suspected. ANCAs have been used to delineate a group of small-vessel vasculitides called "ANCA small-vessel vasculitides" or ANCA-SVV. These include microscopic polyangiitis, Wegener granulomatosis, and Churg–Strauss syndrome. These diseases have overlapping features, but characteristically demonstrate pulmonary hemorrhage and/or necrotizing glomerulonephritis (pulmonary–renal syndrome). Conversely, 60% of patients with the pulmonary–renal syndrome will have ANCA-SVV. With ANCA testing, ANCA-SVV can be diagnosed with 85% sensitivity and 98% specificity. While ANCAs are usually negative in Takayasu arteritis, giant-cell arteritis, Kawasaki's disease, and Behçet disease, positive ANCAs can be found in cryoglobulinemia and other forms of skin-limited vasculitis, in 20% of patients with SLE, and in a higher percentage of patients with RA. ANCAs are used in the setting of vasculitis with systemic features or in situations where the clinical findings suggest ANCA-SVV. ANCA testing does not replace other tests or, more importantly, histologic confirmation of the presence of vasculitis. While the ANCA-SVVs are of unknown etiology, in multiple cases a solid tumor has been identified at the time of the diagnosis of the vasculitis, and Wegener granulomatosis and microscopic polyangiitis are the two most frequent forms of ANCA-positive vasculitis. Thrombophlebitis occurs in about 8% of persons with an ANCA-positive vasculitis.

Microscopic polyangiitis

With the advent of ANCA serologies and clarification of the features of microscopic polyangiitis (MPA), this diagnosis is becoming increasingly more common. There is a north–south gradient in incidence, with southern European countries having 3–4 times as many cases. Most patients with MPA have systemic symptoms, such as fever, weight loss, myalgias, and arthralgias, which can present with an acute flu-like illness or can evolve for months to years before a more explosive phase of their disease. These cases have been termed "slowly progressive MPA." Most patients with MPA will have or develop segmental necrotizing and crescentic glomerulonephritis (80–90%), with pulmonary involvement in 25–65% of cases. Pulmonary capillaritis, which can be complicated by hemorrhage, occurs in 12–29% of MPA patients. The skin is involved in 44% of cases of MPA. Purpura as papules, macules, or ecchymoses (retiform purpura) is present in 26% of cases and cutaneous ulceration may result. Urticarial lesions occur in 1% of cases. Patients with MPA may present with skin lesions as their initial clinical findings. Livedo is seen in two-thirds of such patients. Skin biopsies of macules, papules, petechiae, or sites adjacent to ecchymoses may reveal a necrotizing LCV in the reticular dermis. Palisading and neutrophilic granulomatous dermatitis was found on a skin biopsy of the elbow of an MPA patient.

Vasculitic neuropathy is common (58%) and eye disease may occur. Eosinophilia and asthma are not seen. ANCAs are positive in 70% of cases, p-ANCA more frequently than c-ANCA. MPA is separated from PAN by the presence of glomerulonephritis, pulmonary symptoms, and the absence of hypertension and microaneurysms. ANCAs are less frequently positive in PAN.

MPA is managed like other forms of ANCA-SVV, with systemic corticosteroids and often cytotoxic agents from the disease onset. If the disease is localized, sulfamethoxazole/trimethoprim with corticosteroids may be considered. In generalized but non-organ-threatening disease, methotrexate may be added to the corticosteroids. Cyclophosphamide is usually used in the early induction phase of treatment (6–12 months) as monthly pulses (as opposed to daily treatment). Lower-toxicity immunosuppressives (methotrexate, azathioprine, mycophenolate mofetil) may be used as maintenance or in milder cases. IVIG and anti-TNF agents (infliximab) may be considered in refractory cases. Relapses are frequent; the 5-year survival is about 75% and 7-year survival is 62%.

Bosch X, et al: Treatment of antineutrophil cytoplasmic antibody-associated vasculitis: a systematic review. JAMA 2007; 298:655.

Greenfield JR, et al: ANCA-positive vasculitis induced by thioridazine: confirmed by rechallenge. Br J Dermatol 2002; 147:1265.

Guilleven L, et al: Microscopic polyangiitis: clinical and laboratory findings in eighty-five patients. Arthritis Rheum 1999; 42:421.

Irvine AD, et al: Microscopic polyangiitis. Arch Dermatol 1997; 133:474.

Jacobs-Kosmin D, et al: Pantoprazole and perinuclear antineutrophil cytoplasmic antibody-associated vasculitis. J Rheumatol 2006; 33:629.

Kawakami T, et al: Cutaneous manifestations in patients with microscopic polyangiitis: two case reports and a minireview. Acta Derm Venereol 2006; 86:144.

Kawakami T, et al: Clinical and histopathologic features of 8 patients with microscopic polyangiitis including two with a slowly progressive clinical course. J Am Acad Dermatol 2007; 57:840.

Kluger N, et al: Comparison of cutaneous manifestations in systemic polyarteritis nodosa and microscopic polyangiitis. Br J Dermatol 2008; 159:615.

Maejima H, et al: Microscopic polyangiitis presenting urticarial erythema and Henoch–Schönlein purpura: two case reports. J Dermatol 2004; 31:655.

Niiyama S, et al: Dermatological manifestations associated with microscopic polyangiitis. Rheumatol Int 2008; 28:593.

Penas PF, et al: Microscopic polyangiitis: a systemic vasculitis with a positive p-ANCA. Br J Dermatol 1996; 134:542.

Watz H, et al: Bronchioloalveolar carcinoma of the lung associated with a highly positive pANCA-titer and clinical signs of microscopic polyangiitis. Pneumologie 2004; 58:493.

Wegener granulomatosis

Wegener granulomatosis is a syndrome consisting of necrotizing granulomas of the upper and lower respiratory tract, generalized necrotizing angiitis affecting the medium-sized blood vessels, and focal necrotizing glomerulitis. By far the most common initial manifestation, present in 90% of patients, is the occurrence of rhinorrhea, severe sinusitis, and nasal mucosal ulcerations, with one or several nodules in the nose, larynx, trachea, or bronchi. Fever, weight loss, and malaise occur in these patients, who are usually 40–50 years of age and more often male than female (1.3:1). Obstruction in the nose may also block the sinuses. The nodules in the nose frequently ulcerate and bleed. The parenchymal involvement of the lungs produces cough, dyspnea, and chest pain. Granulomas may occur in the ear and mouth, where the alveolar ridge becomes necrotic, and ulceration of the tongue and perforated ulcers of the palate develop. The combination of nasal and palatal involvement may lead to saddle-nose deformity. The "strawberry gums" appearance of hypertrophic gingivitis is characteristic, and biopsy from these lesions may be diagnostic (Fig. 35-25).

Cutaneous findings occur in 45% of patients. Nodules may appear in crops, especially along the extensor surfaces of the extremities. The firm, slightly tender, flesh-colored or violaceous nodules may later ulcerate. These may be mistaken for ulcerating rheumatoid nodules. The necrotizing angiitis of the skin may present as a palpable purpura, petechial or

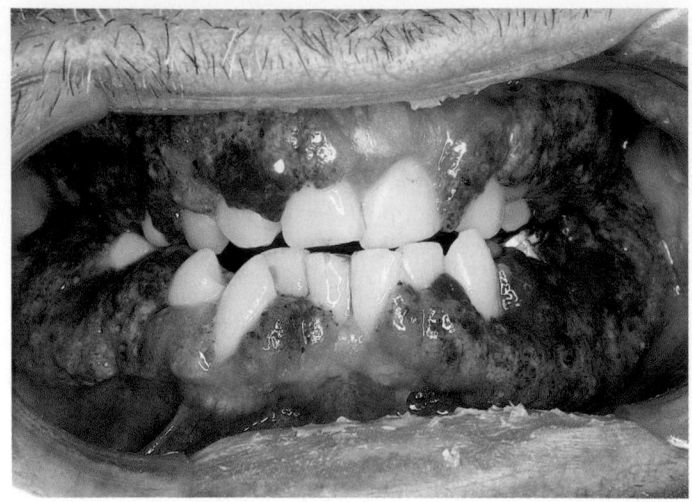

Fig. 35-25 Wegener granulomatosis, strawberry gingiva.

hemorrhagic pustular eruption, subcutaneous nodules, or ulcers. Livedo reticularis is rare in Wegener granulomatosis. Patients may present with pyoderma gangrenosum-like lesions and several patients have been reported presenting with features of temporal arteritis. The condition previously described as "malignant pyoderma" is now felt to represent Wegener granulomatosis.

Limited forms involving the upper respiratory tract without renal involvement may also occur and have a better prognosis. Cutaneous findings can be associated with limited disease. Focal necrotizing glomerulitis occurs in 85% of patients. It may be fulminant from the outset or may become more severe as the disease progresses. Renal failure was the most frequent cause of death before cyclophosphamide treatment. Other organs frequently involved include the joints (arthralgia in two-thirds); eyes (conjunctivitis, episcleritis, and proptosis) in 58%; and CNS and cardiac involvement in 22% and 12% of patients, respectively.

Histologically, the cutaneous lesions may demonstrate an LCV, with or without granulomatous inflammation. Granulomatous vasculitis may be seen. Palisaded granulomas with multinucleated giant cells and a central core of neutrophils and debris are a characteristic finding. Often, if the lesions are ulcerated, they are nonspecific histologically. Biopsy of another affected organ may be required to confirm the diagnosis. The early detection of Wegener granulomatosis has improved with the availability of ANCA testing, as 75–80% of patients are c-ANCA (anti-PR3)-positive.

Untreated Wegener granulomatosis has a mean survival time of 5 months and a 90% mortality over 2 years. Cyclophosphamide therapy has dramatically changed the prognosis. Treatment recommendations are cyclophosphamide, 2 mg/kg/day, and prednisone, 1 mg/kg/day, followed by tapering of the prednisone to an alternate-day regimen. Complete remission is achieved in up to 93% of patients and lasts an average of 4 years for still living patients. In more limited disease, patients may respond to methotrexate alone or methotrexate in combination with prednisone. After initial induction therapy and a remission, methotrexate, azathioprine, leflunomide, or mycophenolate mofetil may be used instead of cyclophosphamide. Treatment should be continued for at least 1 year. Trimethoprim–sulfamethoxazole may decrease the relapse rate and can be considered for long-term treatment of patients with limited upper respiratory tract involvement in remission in combination with conventional immunosuppressive protocols. The benefit of long-term sulfamethoxazole/trimethoprim is due to its reduction of

nasal carriage of *Staphylococcus aureus*, an accepted trigger of Wegener granulomatosis. In refractory cases, IVIG and anti-TNF therapy (infliximab) may be used. Tacrolimus, 0.1 mg/kg/day, was successful in treating a pyoderma gangrenosum-like ulceration in a patient with Wegener granulomatosis.

Bartolucci P, et al: Efficacy of the anti-TNF-alpha antibody infliximab against refractory systemic vasculitides: an open pilot study on 10 patients. Rheumatology 2002; 41:1126.
De Groot K, et al: Wegener's granulomatosis: disease course, assessment of activity and extent and treatment. Lupus 1998; 7:285.
Frances C, et al: Wegener's granulomatosis. Arch Dermatol 1994; 130:861.
Gürses L, et al: Wegener's granulomatosis presenting as neutrophilic dermatosis: a case report. Br J Dermatol 2000; 143:207.
Manchanda Y, et al: Strawberry gingiva: a distinctive sign in Wegener's granulomatosis. J Am Acad Dermatol 2003; 49:335.
Micali G, et al: Cephalic pyoderma gangrenosum (PG)-like lesions as a presenting sign of Wegener's granulomatosis. Int J Dermatol 1994; 33:477.
Nishino H, et al: Wegener's granulomatosis associated with vasculitis of the temporal artery. Mayo Clin Proc 1993; 68:194.
Rozin A: Infliximab efficiency in refractory Wegener's granulomatosis. Rheumatology 2003; 42:1124.
Wenzel J, et al: Successful treatment of recalcitrant Wegener's granulomatosis of the skin with tacrolimus (Prograf). Br J Dermatol 2004; 151:927.

Churg–Strauss syndrome

Churg–Strauss syndrome (CSS) occurs in three phases. The initial phase, often lasting many years, consists of allergic rhinitis, nasal polyps, and asthma. The average age of onset of the asthma is 35 years in CSS (as opposed to allergic asthma, which often presents in childhood). After 2 to 12 years, a debilitated asthmatic begins to experience attacks of fever and eosinophilia (20–90%), with pneumonia and gastroenteritis (second phase). After a few more months or years, but on average 3 years after the initial symptoms, a diffuse angiitis involves the lungs, heart, liver, spleen, kidneys, intestines, and pancreas. Mononeuritis multiplex is common. Triggers of this third phase have included vaccination, desensitization, leukotriene inhibitors, azithromycin, inhaled fluticasone, or rapid discontinuation of corticosteroids. Renal involvement is less common than in Wegener granulomatosis or microscopic polyangiitis. A fatal outcome is likely in most untreated patients, with congestive heart failure resulting from granulomatous inflammation of the myocardium being the most frequent cause of death. Increased rates of arterial and venous thrombosis are seen in CSS, perhaps related to the dense infiltrates of eosinophils.

Cutaneous lesions are present in two-thirds of patients. Palpable purpura is seen in nearly 50% of patients. Subcutaneous nodules on the extensor surfaces of the extremities and on the scalp are seen in 30%. Firm, nontender papules may be present on the fingertips. These may resemble lesions seen with septic emboli or atrial myxoma, but show vasculitis on biopsy. Urticaria, solar urticaria, and livedo reticularis can occur in CSS. Plaques with the histologic features of eosinophilic cellulitis (Well syndrome) can be seen.

Laboratory studies are significant for a peripheral eosinophilia, which correlates with disease severity. ANCAs are frequently positive (55–70%), most commonly for anti-myeloperoxidase (p-ANCA) and less frequently for anti-PR3 (c-ANCA), and tend to correlate with disease severity.

Histologically, a small-vessel vasculitis is present that involves not only superficial venules, but also larger and deeper vessels. The tissue is often diffusely infiltrated with eosinophils, and granulomas may be present. Palisaded granulomas differ from those in Wegener granulomatosis in that they generally lack multinucleated giant cells and the core contains eosinophils. In some patients, flame figures, similar to those in Well syndrome, are noted in the dermis.

Corticosteroids alone may be used in patients with CSS and an FFS (see PAN above) of 0. Cyclophosphamide alone or in combination with corticosteroids should be used in cases of neuropathy, refractory glomerulonephritis, myocardial disease, severe gastrointestinal disease, and CNS involvement. Methotrexate and other immunosuppressives can be used as a steroid-sparing agent, especially to maintain a remission. IFN-α, mycophenolate mofetil, and the anti-TNF agents (infliximab and etanercept) have also been used successfully in CSS.

Abe R, et al: Disseminated subcutaneous nodules alone as manifestations of Churg–Strauss syndrome. Int J Dermatol 2008; 47:532.

Abe-Matsuura Y, et al: Allergic granulomatosis (Churg–Strauss) associated with cutaneous manifestations. J Dermatol 1995; 22.46.

Ames PR, et al: Eosinophilia and thrombophilia in Churg–Strauss syndrome: a clinical and pathogenetic overview. Clin Appl Thromb Hemost 2009 Oct 14 (Epub ahead of print).

Assaf C, et al: Churg–Strauss syndrome: successful treatment with mycophenolate mofetil. Br J Dermatol 2004; 150:596.

Black JG, et al: Montelukast-associated Churg–Strauss vasculitis: another associated report. Ann Allergy Asthma Immunol 2009; 102:351.

Chen KR, et al: Granulomatous arteritis in cutaneous lesions of Churg–Strauss syndrome. J Cutan Pathol 2007; 34:330.

Davis MDP, et al: Cutaneous manifestations of Churg–Strauss syndrome. J Am Acad Dermatol 1997; 37:199.

Drage LA, et al: Evidence for pathogenic involvement of eosinophils and neutrophils in Churg–Strauss syndrome. J Am Acad Dermatol 2002; 47:209.

Fisher K, et al: Cutaneous Churg–Strauss granuloma in a child. J Cutan Pathol 2009; 36:910.

Govoni M, et al: Churg–Strauss syndrome and Wells syndrome: coincidence or pathogenetic association? A new case report. Clin Exp Rheumatol 2007; 25:S41.

Jaworsky C: Leukotriene receptor antagonists and Churg–Strauss syndrome: an association with relevance to dermatopathology? J Cutan Pathol 2008; 35:611.

Kranke B, et al: Macrolide-induced Churg–Strauss syndrome in a patient with atopy. Lancet 1997; 350:1551.

Lee SC, et al: Wells syndrome associated with Churg–Strauss syndrome. J Am Acad Dermatol 2000; 43:556.

Louthrenoo W, et al: Childhood Churg–Strauss syndrome. J Rheumatol 1999; 26:1387.

Nepal M, Padma H: Fluticasone-associated cutaneous allergic granulomatous vasculitis: an underrecognized but important cause of drug-induced cutaneous Churg–Strauss syndrome. South Med J 2008; 101:761.

Oh MJ, et al: Churg–Strauss syndrome: the clinical features and long-term follow-up of 17 patients. J Korean Med Sci 2006; 21:265.

Shimauchi T, et al: Solar urticaria as a manifestation of Churg–Strauss syndrome. Clin Exp Dermatol 2007; 32:209.

Tatsis E, et al: Interferon-alpha treatment of four patients with the Churg–Strauss syndrome. Ann Intern Med 1998; 129:370.

Vanoli M, et al: A case of Churg–Strauss vasculitis after hepatitis B vaccination. Ann Rheum Dis 1998; 57:256.

Cocaine-associated vasculitis

There are numerous reports of various forms of cutaneous vasculitis associated with the intravenous or intranasal use of cocaine. Skin lesions have included typical LCV, as well as larger-vessel vasculitis resembling PAN. Localized nasal lesions with vasculitis resembling Wegener granulomatosis have been observed in patients using inhaled cocaine. This has been termed "cocaine-induced pseudovasculitis" or "cocaine-induced midline destructive lesions" to try to distinguish it from true Wegener granulomatosis. In addition, patients using cocaine may develop more widespread cutaneous and sys-temic vasculitis affecting kidneys, lungs, and testes. The cutaneous lesions resemble LCV, but ecchymotic lesions and skin necrosis were more prominent in these patients than in the typical LCV patient. Purpura and necrosis of the earlobe were especially common and characteristic. Agranulocytosis, not a typical feature of ANCA-positive vasculitis, was also found. These patients have an elevated c-ANCA (PR3-ANCA), similar to patients with true Wegener granulomatosis. However, the c-ANCA in patients with cocaine-induced vasculitis reacts with human neutrophil elastase (HNE-ANCA). Patients with Wegener granulomatosis and microscopic polyangiitis are negative for HNE-ANCA.

Street cocaine is commonly contaminated with pharmaceutical agents. Surprisingly, levamisole has been found in the cocaine seized by law enforcement in up to 30% of cases in the US and 100% in Italy. Levamisole therapy is associated with ecchymotic purpura and necrosis, with a predilection for the ears. It also causes agranulocytosis and c-ANCA positivity. It is therefore unclear whether the vasculitic lesions seen in recreational cocaine users are due to the cocaine or to the levamisole excipient or both. In every patient presenting with a cutaneous or systemic vasculitis, a detailed history of recreational drug use must be obtained, and toxicology screening should be considered in any patient with vasculitis having the features outlined above, especially agranulocytosis or cutaneous necrosis, or failure to respond to appropriate therapy. In these patients, stopping of the drug may lead to a gradual improvement of the vasculitis, although initial immunosuppressive therapy may be required. Treatment to eradicate nasal *S. aureus* should be considered if there are prominent nasal findings.

Barbano G, et al: Disseminated autoimmune disease during levamisole treatment of nephrotic syndrome. Pediatr Nephrol 1999; 13:602.

Fucci N: Unusual adulterants in cocaine seized on Italian clandestine market. Forensic Sci Int 2007; 172:e1.

Kinzie E, et al: Levamisole found in patients using cocaine. Ann Emerg Med 2009; 53:546.

Menni S, et al: Ear lobe bilateral necrosis by levamisole-induced occlusive vasculitis in a pediatric patient. Pediatr Dermatol 1997; 14:477.

Neynaber S, et al: PR3-ANCA-positive necrotizing multi-organ vasculitis following cocaine abuse. Acta Derm Venereol 2008; 88:594.

Rachapalli SM, Kiely PD: Cocaine-induced midline destructive lesions mimicking ENT-limited Wegener's granulomatosis. Scand J Rheumatol 2008; 37:477.

Rongioletti F, et al: Purpura of the ears: a distinctive vasculopathy with circulating autoantibodies complicating long-term treatment with levamisole in children. Br J Dermatol 1999; 140:948.

Wiesner O, et al: Antineutrophil cytoplasmic antibodies reacting with human neutrophil elastase as a diagnostic marker for cocaine-induced midline destructive lesions but not autoimmune vasculitis. Arthritis Rheum 2004; 50:2954.

Zhu NY, et al: Agranulocytosis after consumption of cocaine adulterated with levamisole. Ann Intern Med 2009; 150:287.

Giant-cell arteritis/temporal arteritis

Giant-cell arteritis is a systemic disease of people over the age of 50 years (mean age >70), favoring women (2:1). It is uncommon in African Americans and favors whites. Its best-known location is the temporal artery, where it is known as temporal arteritis, cranial arteritis, and Horton's disease. It is characterized by a necrotizing arteritis with granulomas and giant cells, which produce unilateral headache and exquisite tenderness in the scalp over the temporal or occipital arteries in 50–75% of patients. Temporal headaches are characteristically constant, severe, and boring. Ear and parotid pain and mastication-induced jaw claudication may occur. Fever, anemia, and a high sedimentation rate (>50) are usually present. Proximal,

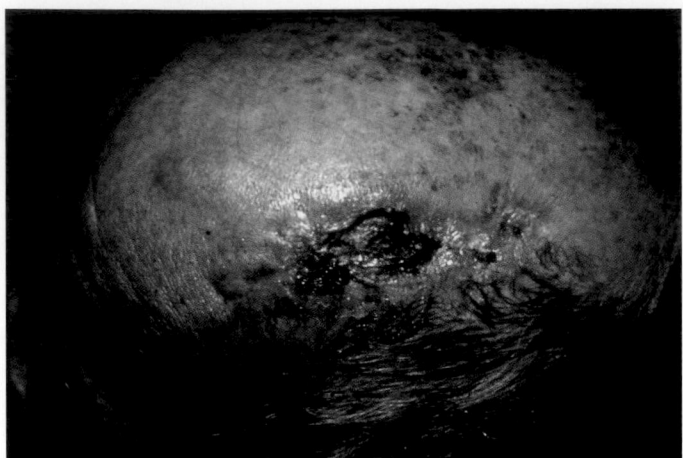

Fig. 35-26 Giant cell arteritis with scalp necrosis.

symmetrical, and severe morning and even day-long stiffness, soreness, and pain occur in 50% of patients (associated polymyalgia rheumatica). It is rarely fatal. Blindness may develop and is the most feared complication of the disease. Many patients who develop visual loss have premonitory symptoms allowing for the diagnosis and intervention, which may prevent permanent visual loss.

The cutaneous manifestations may be only inflammatory. The affected artery becomes evident as a hard, pulsating, tender, tortuous bulge under red or cyanotic skin. Another manifestation is necrosis of the scalp (Fig. 35-26). The lesions may first appear as ecchymoses. Later, they may become vesicular or bullous and are followed by gangrene. Urticaria, purpura, alopecia, tender nodules, prurigo-like nodules, and livedo reticularis may be seen. Lingual artery involvement may cause an accompanying red, sore, or gangrenous tongue. Nasal septal perforation may develop. Actinic granuloma may be associated. Actinic damage of the arterial elastic tissue of the temporal artery may be possible due to its superficial location. The elderly Caucasian is at greatest risk, and when lesions are biopsied, at times only the external half of the artery that received solar radiation is involved. Temporal arteritis may be an actinically induced disease.

Polymyalgia rheumatica (PMR) has a significant clinical association with giant-cell arteritis. Prompt treatment may forestall serious disease. About 10% of central retinal artery occlusions are due to giant-cell arteritis. ESRs are elevated in more than 90% of patients with giant-cell arteritis. Temporal artery biopsy is generally diagnostic, provided that at least a 2 cm segment is provided. Even arteries that are normal to palpation may show diagnostic findings. Magnetic resonance angiography is a noninvasive diagnostic method that may aid in confirming the clinical suspicion and identify the best site to biopsy. Not all patients with arteritis of the temporal artery have giant cell arteritis, as temporal arteritis may be a manifestation or part of the systemic vasculitides such as PAN, Wegener granulomatosis, or microscopic polyarteritis. Pathogenically, the presence of TNF polymorphisms in patients with PMR and temporal arteritis suggests a genetic predisposition.

Treatment is usually begun with prednisone, 60 mg/day, and continued for 1 month or until all reversible clinical and laboratory parameters (such as the ESR) have returned to normal. The disease is quite steroid-responsive and tapering to a dose of 7.5–10 mg/day is usually possible. Daily therapy seems to be important and is usually necessary for a minimum of 1–2 years. Most patients achieve complete remission that is often maintained after therapy is withdrawn. Anti-TNF agents may be used in refractory cases, but relapses occur when treatment is stopped, and corticosteroid therapy is usually required.

Andonopoulos AP, et al: Experience with infliximab (anti-TNFα monoclonal antibody) as monotherapy for giant cell arteritis. Ann Rheum Dis 2003; 62:1116.
Botella-Estrada R, et al: Magnetic resonance angiography in the diagnosis of a case of giant cell arteritis manifesting as scalp necrosis. Arch Dermatol 1999; 135:769.
Carlson JA, Chen KR: Cutaneous vasculitis update: neutrophilic muscular vessel and eosinophilic, granulomatous, and lymphocytic vasculitis syndromes. Am J Dermatopathol 2007; 29:32.
Hamidou MA, et al: Temporal arteritis associated with systemic necrotizing vasculitis. J Rheumatol 2003; 30:2165.
Marcos O, et al: Tongue necrosis in a patient with temporal arteritis. J Oral Maxillofac Surg 1998; 56:1203.
Tsianakas A, et al: Scalp necrosis in giant cell arteritis: case report and review of the relevance of this cutaneous sign of large-vessel vasculitis. J Am Acad Dermatol 2009; 61:701.

Takayasu arteritis

Known also as aortic arch syndrome and pulseless disease, Takayasu arteritis is a thrombo-obliterative process of the great vessels stemming from the aortic arch, occurring generally in young women (female to male ratio, 9:1) in the second or third decade of life. It is more common in Japan, Southeast Asia, India, and South America. Radial and carotid pulses are typically obliterated. Most skin changes are due to the disturbed circulation. There may be loss of hair and atrophy of the skin and its appendages, with underlying muscle atrophy. Occasional patients with cutaneous necrotizing or granulomatous vasculitis of small vessels have been reported. Erythematous nodules with or without livedo, simulating erythema nodosum or erythema induratum, may rarely occur. Pyoderma gangrenosum-like ulcerations are well described in Japan. Pyoderma gangrenosum lesions precede the diagnosis of the arteritis by an average of 3 years. These lesions are more commonly generalized and in three-quarters of cases occur on the upper extremities.

Treatment of Takayasu arteritis with prednisone, 1 mg/kg/day tapered in 8–12 weeks to 20 mg/day or less, is recommended. Methotrexate may be used for its steroid-sparing effects. With active medical and surgical intervention, the aggressive course of this disease can be modified. The pyoderma gangrenosum-like lesions are also treated with systemic steroids, but azathioprine, cyclophosphamide, mycophenolate mofetil, cyclosporine, and tacrolimus have also been effective.

Ohta Y, et al: Inflammatory diseases associated with Takayasu's arteritis. Angiology 2003; 54:339.
Pascual-Lopez M, et al: Takayasu's disease with cutaneous involvement. Dermatology 2004; 208:10.
Skaria AM, et al: Takayasu arteritis and cutaneous necrotizing vasculitis. Dermatology 2000; 200:139.
Ujiie H, et al: Pyoderma gangrenosum associated with Takayasu's arteritis. Clin Exp Dermatol 2004; 29:357.

Malignant atrophic papulosis

Papulosis atrophicans maligna, also known as Degos' disease, is a potentially fatal obliterative arteritis syndrome. Some affected patients have a long benign course with skin lesions only, while in others, death occurs within a few years. Degos' disease occurs 2–3 times more frequently in men than in women, often presenting between the ages of 20 and 40. Familial kindreds are well reported. In patients with the more aggressive variant, survival averages 2–3 years after the disease has developed.

Skin lesions are usually the first sign of the disease. Clinically, Degos' disease is characterized by the presence of pale rose, rounded, edematous papules occurring mostly on the trunk. Similar lesions may occur on the bulbar conjunctiva and oral mucosa. Palms, soles, and face are spared, but the penis may be involved. Over days to weeks, the lesions become umbilicated, with a central depression, which enlarges. The center becomes distinctively porcelain-white, while the periphery becomes livid red and telangiectatic. Central atrophy occurs eventually. The eruption proceeds by crops in which only a few new lesions appear at any one time. One patient was reported to develop panniculitis. Lesions characteristic of Degos' disease may be seen in patients with lupus erythematosus, dermatomyositis, scleroderma, and Wegener granulomatosis.

Systemically, ischemic infarcts involve the intestines, producing acute abdominal symptoms, which include epigastric pain, fever, and hematemesis. Death is usually due to fulminating peritonitis caused by multiple perforations of the intestine. Less commonly, death occurs from cerebral infarctions.

Wedge-shaped necroses brought on by the occlusion of arterioles and small arteries account for the clinical lesions. Proliferation of the intima and thrombosis constitute the typical histologic picture. The thrombosing process is usually pauci-inflammatory, although neutrophils or lymphocytes may be found associated with the thrombosis. The overlying dermis, which is infarcted, contains abundant mucin, especially early in the lesion's evolution. Adnexae are typically necrotic and the depressed central portion may be noted histologically.

The etiology of this disease is unknown, but based on the infarctive nature of the lesions and the universal presence of arteriolar thrombosis, a hyperthrombotic state or endothelial abnormality is suggested. While most patients have not had abnormalities identified, abnormal platelet aggregation and abnormal coagulation have been identified in some cases. Antiphospholipid antibodies and anticardiolipin antibodies have been present in some patients, and a Leiden factor V mutation in one patient. Parvovirus B19 infection was associated with a fatal case in an adult.

Administration of immunosuppressives has not been beneficial. IVIG has been of therapeutic benefit in one case, but failed in another. Ingestion of low-dose acetylsalicylic acid alone or in combination with dipyridamole (Persantine) has been effective in some patients. Heparin, as described by Degos, has been helpful, and should be considered if antiplatelet therapy is ineffective. Nicotine patches, 5 mg/day, were effective in one case. In severe crises, fibrinolytic therapy should be considered. The prognosis is guarded in patients with systemic involvement.

Cebeci Z, et al: Degos' disease. Ophthalmology 2009; 116:1415.
Chung HY, et al: Degos' disease: a rare condition simulating rheumatic diseases. Clin Rheumatol 2009; 28:861.
Cuchillero RMO, et al: Benign cutaneous Degos' disease. Clin Exp Dermatol 2003; 28:145.
De Breucker S, et al: Inefficacy of intravenous immunoglobulins and infliximab in Degos' disease. Acta Clin Belg 2008; 63:99.
Dyrsen ME, et al: Parvovirus B19-associated catastrophic endothelialitis with a Degos-like presentation. J Cutan Pathol 2008; 35:20.
Guhl G, et al: Wegener's granulomatosis: a new entity in the growing differential diagnosis of Degos' disease. Clin Exp Dermatol 2009; 34:e1.
High WA, et al: Is Degos' disease a clinical and histological end point rather than a specific disease? J Am Acad Dermatol 2004; 50:895.
Hohwy T, et al: A fatal case of malignant atrophic papulosis (Degos' disease) in a man with factor V Leiden mutation and lupus anticoagulant. Acta Derm Venereol 2006; 86:245.
Kanekura T, et al: A case of malignant atrophic papulosis successfully treated with nicotine patches. Br J Dermatol 2003; 149:660.
Katz SK, et al: Malignant atrophic papulosis (Degos' disease) involving three generations of a family. J Am Acad Dermatol 1997; 37:480.
Kim DW, et al: Degos disease (malignant atrophic papulosis) as a fatal cause of acute abdomen: report of a case. Surg Today 2008; 38:866.
Liu CM, et al: Lesions resembling malignant atrophic papulosis in a patient with progressive systemic sclerosis. Cutis 2005; 75:101.
Moss C, et al: Degos disease: a new simulator of non-accidental injury. Dev Med Child Neurol 2009; 51:647.
Powell J, et al: Benign familial Degos' disease worsening during immunosuppression. Br J Dermatol 1999; 141:524.
Requena L, et al: Degos' disease in a patient with acquired immunodeficiency syndrome. J Am Acad Dermatol 1998; 38:852.
Saglik E, et al: Malignant atrophic papulosis: endocardial involvement and positive anticardiolipin antibodies. J Eur Acad Dermatol Venereol 2006; 20:602.
Scheinfeld N: Degos' disease is probably a distinct entity: a review of clinical and laboratory evidence. J Am Acad Dermatol 2005; 52:375.
Scheinfeld N: Malignant atrophic papulosis. Clin Exp Dermatol 2007; 32:483.
Shahshahani MM, et al: A case of Degos disease with pleuropericardial fibrosis, jejunal perforation, hemiparesis, and widespread cutaneous lesions. Int J Dermatol 2008; 47:493.
Tan WP, et al: Generalized red papules with gastrointestinal complications. Clin Exp Dermatol 2007; 32:615.
Thomson KF, Highet AS: Penile ulceration in fatal malignant atrophic papulosis (Degos' disease). Br J Dermatol 2000; 143:1320.
Torrelo A, et al: Malignant atrophic papulosis in an infant. Br J Dermatol 2002; 146:916.
Zhao WH, et al: A fatal case of malignant atrophic papulosis. Eur J Dermatol 2009; 19:193.
Zhu KJ, et al: The use of intravenous immunoglobulin in cutaneous and recurrent perforating intestinal Degos disease (malignant atrophic papulosis). Br J Dermatol 2007; 157:206.

Thromboangiitis obliterans (Buerger's disease)

Thromboangiitis obliterans (TAO) is a nonatherosclerotic segmental occlusive disease affecting the arteries of multiple extremities. It is most often seen in men between the ages of 20 and 40 who smoke heavily. Smoking and, rarely, the use of smokeless tobacco are intimately tied to Buerger's disease. Various diagnostic criteria have been proposed. They usually include: age younger than 45 (or 50); history of tobacco use; distal extremity involvement (infrapopliteal segmental arterial occlusion with sparing of the proximal vasculature); frequent distal upper extremity involvement (Raynaud or digital ulcers); consistent angiographic findings; superficial thrombophlebitis; exclusion of autoimmune disease, diabetes mellitus, and hypercoagulable or embolic states.

The vasomotor changes in early cases may be transitory or persistent; they produce blanching, cyanosis, burning, and tingling. Superficial thrombophlebitis in the leg and foot occurs in 38% of cases and 44% of patients may have Raynaud phenomenon. The color of the part may change when it is elevated or lowered below heart level, being red when dependent and white when elevated. Pain is a constant symptom, coming at first only after exercise and subsiding on resting. Instep and foot claudication is the classic complaint. Ultimately, the dorsalis pedis and posterior tibial pulses disappear, followed by others. In TAO, skin supplied by affected arterioles tends to break down, with central necrosis and ulceration, and eventual gangrene (Fig. 35-27). Gastrointestinal involvement has been reported. Exposure to cold may cause exacerbations, and more cases are identified in the winter than any other season.

Arteriography should be carried out to investigate for central atherosclerotic disease, which may be operable, rather than the inoperable distal damage of Buerger's disease. A characteristic tapering and occlusion of the major arteries with "corkscrew" collateral arteries is found in Buerger's disease on angiography. A vasculo-occlusive syndrome similar to Buerger's disease has been reported in cannabis smokers, but venous thrombophlebitis does not occur. The pathogenic mechanism of the vascular occlusion in Buerger's disease is unknown. In one report G20210A prothrombin mutations, the majority homozygotic, were found, but these findings have not been reproduced.

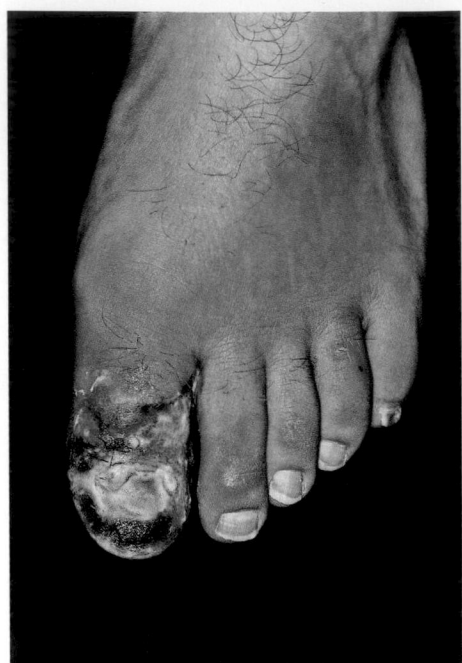

Fig. 35-27 Buerger's disease.

The most important therapeutic aspect is the cessation of smoking. Even one or two cigarettes/day, smokeless tobacco, or nicotine replacement may keep the disease active. Intravenous iloprost (a prostaglandin analog) may help the patient with critical limb ischemia get through an acute episode. Oral iloprost is ineffective. Sympathectomy can provide temporary relief. Autologous transplantation of bone marrow mononuclear cells into the calf muscle has benefited patients with TAO and other forms of limb ischemia. G-CSF-mobilized peripheral blood mononuclear cells have had similar efficacy. In patients who stop smoking and do not have gangrene, major amputations are rare. In continued smokers, at least 43% will require amputations. Implantation of a spinal cord stimulator may be tried.

Boda Z, et al: Stem cell therapy: a promising and prospective approach in the treatment of patients with severe Buerger's disease. Clin Appl Thromb Hemos 2009; 15:552.

Cazalets C, et al: Cannabis arteritis: four new cases. Rev Med Interne 2003; 24:127.

De Vriese AS, et al: Autologous transplantation of bone marrow mononuclear cells for limb ischemia in a Caucasian population with atherosclerosis obliterans. J Intern Med 2008; 263:395.

Espinoza LR: Buerger's disease: thromboangiitis obliterans 100 years after the initial description. Am J Med Sci 2009; 337:285.

Faizer R, Forbes TL: Buerger's disease. J Vasc Surg 2007; 46:812.

Kakihana A, et al: Improvement of cardiac function after granulocyte-colony stimulating factor-mobilized peripheral blood mononuclear cell implantation in a patient with non-ischemic dilated cardiomyopathy associated with thromboangiitis obliterans. Intern Med 2009; 48:1003.

Kobayashi M, et al: Ischemic intestinal involvement in a patient with Buerger's disease: case report and literature review. J Vasc Surg 2003; 38:170.

Laohapensang K, et al: Seasonal variation of Buerger's disease in northern part of Thailand. Eur J Vasc Endovasc Surg 2004; 28:418.

Malecki R, et al: Thromboangiitis obliterans in the 21st century—a new face of disease. Atherosclerosis 2009; 206:328.

Manfredini R, et al: Thromboangiitis obliterans (Buerger's disease) in a female mild smoker treated with spinal cord stimulation. Am J Med Sci 2004; 327:365.

Matsushita M, et al: Buerger's disease in a 19-year-old woman. J Vasc Surg 2003; 38:175.

Olin JW: Thromboangiitis obliterans (Buerger's disease). N Engl J Med 2000; 343:864.

Arteriosclerosis obliterans

Arteriosclerosis obliterans is an occlusive arterial disease most prominently affecting the abdominal aorta, and the small and medium-sized arteries of the lower extremities. The symptoms are due to ischemia of the tissues. There is intermittent claudication manifested by pain, cramping, numbness, and fatigue in the muscles on exercise; these are relieved by rest. There may be "rest pain" at night when in bed. Also, sensitivity to cold, muscular weakness, stiffness of the joints, and paresthesia may be present. Sexual impotence is common and there is an increased frequency of coronary artery disease.

Impaired to absent pulses (dorsalis pedis, posterior tibial, or popliteal arteries) may be found on physical examination, confirming the diagnosis. The feet, especially the toes, may be red and cold. Striking pallor of the feet on elevation and redness when dependent are compatible findings. Decreased to absent hair growth may be observed on the legs. Ulceration and gangrene may supervene. If present, they usually begin in the toes and are quite painful. Arteriography may be indicated as a preliminary to corrective surgery (arterial grafts). Occasionally, subclavian atherosclerosis may give rise to these signs in the distal upper extremity, producing painful nails and loss of digital skin. Diabetes mellitus, smoking, and hyperlipidemia are risk factors for the development of atherosclerosis.

Claudication and diminished blood pressure in the affected extremity are findings that may lead to earlier diagnosis and thus to curative surgical intervention. Usually, bypass of the affected artery or sympathectomy, or both, are the preferred treatment. Balloon angioplasty or stent placement may also be effective. When critical limb ischemia is present, injection of stem cells into the calf muscle may be beneficial.

Kerdel FA, et al: Subclavian occlusive disease presenting as a painful nail. J Am Acad Dermatol 1984; 10:523.

Matsumoto K, et al: Insulin resistance and arteriosclerosis obliterans in patients with NIDDM. Diabetes Care 1997; 20:1738.

Diffuse dermal angiomatosis

Diffuse dermal angiomatosis (DDA) is a not uncommon disorder that preferentially affects women. The most common location is the breast, especially the dependent portion. Affected women tend to have large, pendulous breasts, and are usually older than 45 years of age. Patients may have had a reduction mammoplasty (often decades before), and the disease tends to localize adjacent to the scar from that procedure. The clinical lesions may be reticulated groups of telangiectasias, ischemic (retiform) purpura, or ulceration, or some combination. The erythematous/telangiectatic plaques are slightly palpable but not usually indurated. The nipple and areola are spared. The affected patients often have multiple risk factors for a hypercoagulable state or premature atherosclerosis. These include a personal history of atherosclerotic cardiovascular disease, obesity, smoking, hypertension, mutations in the thrombolytic pathway (analogous to those seen in livedoid vasculopathy), and a strong family history for premature atherosclerotic disease-related cardiovascular events. The areas involved are very similar to those affected by other prothrombotic disorders such as warfarin necrosis and heparin necrosis—skin with overly abundant adipose tissue. The breast is most commonly affected, but the abdomen and medial thighs are also sites of predilection. Usually, only one site is affected, but if the breast is involved, the process can be bilateral. Surgical procedures on the affected area may lead to ulceration that is very painful and slow to heal. Because a surgical procedure triggered the ulceration, a mistaken diagnosis of pyoderma gangrenosum may be entertained.

Histologically, a diffuse dermal proliferation of endothelial cells and bland blood vessels occupies much of the dermis. Atypical cells and atypical vascular shapes (as seen in angiosarcoma and Kaposi sarcoma) are not seen. The dermal cells stain for markers of endothelial cells The pathogenesis is felt to be local chronic ischemia, which may either lead to vascular proliferation (angiomatosis), or if acute and severe, may lead to retiform purpura or ulceration. The fatty areas are poorly oxygenated (worse in the obese patient), and the pendulous nature of the breasts may stretch or tether the vessels, further compromising the circulation. Inherited and acquired hypercoagulable risk factors (smoking, atherosclerosis, and so on) contribute to the pathogenesis.

The treatment involves reversing the contributing factors. This includes stopping smoking, weight reduction, and antithrombotic medications such as low-dose aspirin, 81 mg per day, and pentoxifylline, 400 mg BID. Reduction mammoplasty may lead to resolution. Atherosclerosis of the arteries serving the affected area may be found, and vascular surgery to enhance circulation may lead to improvement. One patient has been successfully treated with isotretinoin. Isotretinoin has a fibrinolytic effect, which may be the mechanism by which it improved DDA in this one patient.

McLaughlin ER, et al: Diffuse dermal angiomatosis of the breast: response to isotretinoin. J Am Acad Dermatol 2001; 45:462.

Pichardo RO, et al: What is your diagnosis? Diffuse dermal angiomatosis secondary to anticardiolipin antibodies. Am J Dermatopathol 2002; 24:502.

Quatresooz P, et al: Diffuse dermal angiomatosis: a previously undescribed pattern of immunoglobulin and complement deposits in two cases. Am J Dermatopathol 2006; 28:150.

Villa MT, et al: The treatment of diffuse dermal angiomatosis of the breast with reduction mammaplasty. Arch Dermatol 2008; 144:693.

Yang H, et al: Diffuse dermal angiomatosis of the breast. Arch Dermatol 2006; 142:343.

Mucocutaneous lymph node syndrome (Kawasaki's disease)

The typical presentation is an irritable, ill-appearing, febrile infant or child younger than 5 years old. Clinical findings (four of which, plus fever for 5 days, are diagnostic of Kawasaki syndrome) include a skin eruption; stomatitis (injected pharynx, strawberry tongue) and fissuring cheilitis; edema of the hands and feet; conjunctival injection; and cervical lymphadenitis. The skin eruption is polymorphous and may be macular, morbilliform, urticarial, scarlatiniform, erythema multiforme-like, pustular, or erythema marginatum-like. An early finding (within the first week) is the appearance of an erythematous, desquamating perianal eruption in about two-thirds of patients. Periorbital edema has been reported. Fifteen to 20% of children with Kawasaki's disease (KD) and fever will not have one or more of the other cardinal features. These cases are termed "incomplete KD." These patients are still at risk for cardiac disease.

Numerous cutaneous and systemic complications have been reported as accompanying or following KD. Pincer nail deformities may appear and resolve spontaneously. Intestinal pseudo-obstruction may occur. Facial nerve paralysis has been described, and a severe peripheral vasculitis with vasospasm, digital ischemia, and gangrene can occur. Numerous children have developed guttate or plaque psoriasis 10–20 days after the KD had begun. The presumed mechanism is the triggering of psoriasis by the superantigens associated with the acute illness.

The acute illness evolves over 10–20 days. A week or two following the acute illness, the fingers and toes desquamate, starting around the nails (Fig. 35-28). Coronary artery aneu-

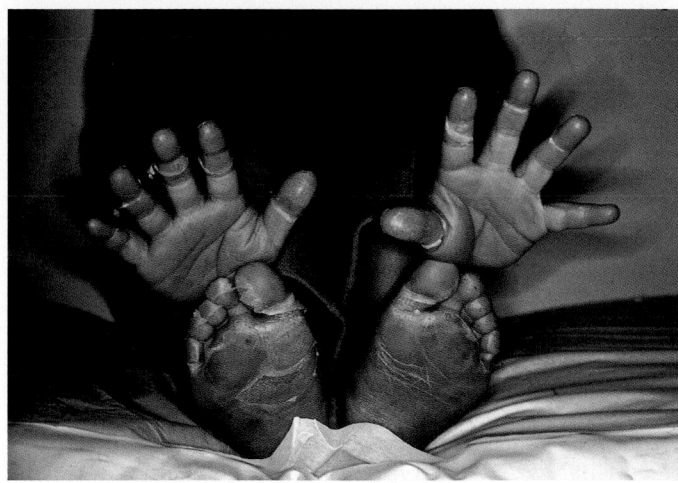

Fig. 35-28 Desquamation in Kawasaki's disease.

rysms occur in 20–25% of untreated children and 3–5% of treated children. This is the most common cause of acquired cardiac disease in young children. The cardiac involvement, which, in addition to aneurysms, can include decreased left ventricular function, arrhythmias, mitral regurgitation, and pericardial effusion, may lead to immediate cardiac complications, the major cause of morbidity and mortality. In addition, over time, those with aneurysms can develop coronary artery stenosis, and as a result acute cardiac events can occur in young adulthood.

Pathogenesis

A viral or infectious pathogenesis is attractive for the following reasons:

1. Cases were rare before 1950.
2. KD affects children older than 3 months but younger than 8 years.
3. Seasonal peaks occur in the winter and spring.
4. Focal epidemics have been reported.
5. Oligoclonal IgA immune responses are found, suggesting a respiratory portal of entry of an infectious agent.

There are increased superantigens in the stool of children with KD. A KD-like illness has been described with group A meningococcal septicemia. An infectious pathogenesis, therefore, remains the most plausible etiologic hypothesis.

It has long been suspected that there is a genetic basis for KD. The disease is 10–20 times more common in persons from Northeast Asia (Japan and Korea), where rates of up to 1 per 150 children are reported. When these Asians move to the US, they still have this high rate of increased susceptibility. The risk of a sibling developing KD is increased tenfold. Children of parents who had KD in childhood have a twofold increased risk of developing KD. A recent genome-wide search of almost 1000 KD cases and family members found strong linkage to five genes, three of which form a single functional network. The central gene of this network is *CAMK2D*, which encodes a serine/threonine kinase expressed in cardiomyocytes and vascular endothelial cells. These genes are already known to be involved in cardiac and inflammatory pathways. The transcripts of these genes were also markedly suppressed during KD. The previously reported genetic associations for KD were not found in this study, including the *ITPKC* gene mutation.

Coronary arterial disease occurs after day 10 of the illness (subacute phase), in combination with thrombocythemia (up to 1 million). This combination of an altered endovascular surface and too many platelets, plus abnormal blood flow in the coronary aneurysms, leads to thrombosis and occlusion of the vessels and the subsequent cardiac events.

Treatment

IVIG is the cornerstone of therapy, given in a single dose of 2 g/kg infused over 10–12 h. Response to treatment is best if given during the first 5–6 days of the illness; however, children with persistent fever beyond this period may benefit from later treatment. Aspirin is used to reduce inflammation and platelet aggregation. The dose is 80–100 mg/kg/day in four divided doses. Once the child has been afebrile for 3–7 days, the aspirin dose is decreased to a single daily dose of 3–5 mg/kg. If the child remains febrile, a second 2 g/kg dose of IVIG should be given. A single dose of infliximab, 5 mg/kg, has been reported to be effective in refractory cases, but response, as with other treatments, is not universal. If there is no response to the second IVIG dose, systemic steroid therapy is commonly given. Angioplasty, thrombolytic therapy, or coronary artery bypass surgery may be required for patients with coronary disease.

Ahn SY, et al: Treatment of intravenous immunoglobulin-resistant Kawasaki disease with methotrexate. Scand J Rheumatol 2005; 34:136.

Ayusawa M, et al: Revision of diagnostic guidelines from Kawasaki disease (the 5th revised edition). Pediatr Int 2005; 47:232.

Burgner D, et al: A genome-wide association study identifies novel and functionally related susceptibility loci for Kawasaki disease. PLoS Genet 2009; 5:e1000319.

Burns JC, Glodé MP: Kawasaki syndrome. Lancet 2004; 364:533.

Burns JC, et al: Infliximab treatment for refractory Kawasaki syndrome. J Pediatr 2005; 146:662.

Fretzayas A, et al: Meningococcal group A sepsis associated with rare manifestations and complicated by Kawasaki-like disease. Pediatr Emerg Care 2009; 25:190.

Garty B, et al: Guttate psoriasis following Kawasaki disease. Pediatr Dermatol 2001; 18:507.

Harnden A, et al: Kawasaki disease. BMJ 2009; 338:1133.

Larralde M, et al: Kawasaki disease with facial nerve paralysis. Pediatr Dermatol 2003; 20:511.

Miura M, et al: Coronary risk factors in Kawasaki disease treated with additional gammaglobulin. Arch Dis Child 2004; 89:776.

Muta H, et al: Early intravenous gamma-globulin treatment for Kawasaki disease: the nationwide surveys in Japan. J Pediatr 2004; 144:496.

Pannaraj PS, et al: Failure to diagnose Kawasaki disease at the extremes of the pediatric age range. Pediatr Infect Dis J 2004; 23:789.

Thapa R, et al: Neonatal Kawasaki disease with multiple coronary aneurysms and thrombocytopenia. Pediatr Dermatol 2007; 24:662.

Yamauchi H, et al: Optimal time of surgical treatment for Kawasaki coronary artery disease. J Nippon Med Sch 2004; 71:279.

Yoon SY, et al: Plaque type psoriasiform eruption following Kawasaki disease. Pediatr Dermatol 2007; 24:336.

Telangiectasia

Telangiectasia are fine linear vessels coursing on the surface of the skin; the name given to them collectively is telangiectasia. Telangiectasia may occur in normal skin at any age, in both sexes, and anywhere on the skin and mucous membranes. Fine telangiectases may be seen on the alae nasi of most adults. They are prominent in areas of chronic actinic damage. In addition, persons long exposed to wind, cold, or heat are subject to telangiectasia. Calcium channel-blockers may lead to telangiectatic lesions in a generalized or photodistribution and contribute to the appearance of photoaging. Telangiectasias may also be found on the legs as a result of heredity, varicosities, pregnancy, and birth control pill use.

Telangiectases can be found in conditions such as radiodermatitis, xeroderma pigmentosum, lupus erythematosus, scleroderma and the CREST syndrome, rosacea, pregnancy, cirrhosis of the liver, AIDS, poikiloderma, basal cell carcinoma, necrobiosis lipoidica diabeticorum, lichen sclerosus et atrophicus, sarcoid, lupus vulgaris, keloid, adenoma sebaceum, Kaposiform hemangioendothelioma, angioma serpiginosum, angiokeratoma corporis diffusum, hereditary benign telangiectasia, Cockayne syndrome, ataxia-telangiectasia, and Bloom syndrome.

Altered capillary patterns on the finger nailfolds (cuticular telangiectases) are indicative of collagen vascular disease, such as lupus erythematosus, scleroderma, or dermatomyositis. They may infrequently be present in rheumatoid arthritis. These disorders are reviewed in Chapter 8.

Beaubien ER, et al: Kaposiform hemangioendothelioma. J Am Acad Dermatol 1998; 38:799.

Cooper SM, Wojnaraowska F: Photo-damage in Northern European renal transplant recipients is associated with the use of calcium channel blockers. Clin Exp Dermatol 2003; 28:588.

Grabczynska SA, Cowley N: Amlodipine-induced photosensitivity presenting as telangiectasia. Br J Dermatol 2000; 142:1255.

Huh J, et al: Localized facial telangiectasias following frostbite injury. Cutis 1996; 57:97.

Ioulios P, et al: The spectrum of cutaneous reactions associated with calcium antagonists: a review of the literature and the possible etiopathogenic mechanisms. Dermatol Online J 2003; 9:6.

Kanekura T, et al: Lichen sclerosus et atrophicus with prominent telangiectasia. J Dermatol 1994; 21:447.

Silvestre JF, et al: Photodistributed felodipine-induced facial telangiectasia. J Am Acad Dermatol 2001; 45:323.

Generalized essential telangiectasia

Generalized essential telangiectasia (GET) is characterized by the appearance of telangiectasia over a large segment of the body without preceding or coexisting skin lesions. Lesions tend to appear first on the legs and progress caudad. Women are more commonly affected, with the condition starting between age 20 and 50. Characteristic features include:

1. widespread cutaneous distribution
2. progression or permanence of the lesions
3. accentuation in dependent areas and by dependent positioning
4. absence of coexisting epidermal or dermal changes, such as atrophy, purpura, depigmentation, or follicular involvement

The telangiectases may be distributed over the entire body or localized to some large area, such as the legs, arms, and trunk. They may be discrete or confluent. Distribution along the course of the cutaneous nerves may occur. Systemic symptoms are absent, although conjunctival telangiectasias can also be seen. GET is usually not believed to be associated with an increased risk of epistaxis, but gastrointestinal bleeding has been reported. Families with this disorder, inherited as an autosomal-dominant trait, have been reported. The cause of essential telangiectasia is unknown. Treatment is with vascular lasers, if required.

Collagenous vasculopathy, a condition favoring middle-aged males, is clinically similar to GET but histologically distinct. Histologically, markedly dilated subepidermal vessels are present. These blood vessels have thickened vascular walls and perivascular hyaline. Type IV collagen staining accentuates the superficial vessels.

Ali MM, et al: Generalized essential telangiectasia with conjunctival involvement. Clin Exp Dermatol 2006; 31:781.

Davis TL, et al: Collagenous vasculopathy: a report of three cases. J Cutan Pathol 2008; 35:967.

Gambichler T, et al: Generalized essential telangiectasia successfully treated with high-energy, long-pulse, frequency-doubled Nd:YAG laser. Dermatol Surg 2001; 27:355.

Long D, Marshman G: Generalized essential telangiectasia. Australas J Dermatol 2004; 45:67.

Unilateral nevoid telangiectasia

In unilateral nevoid telangiectasia (UNT), fine, thread-like telangiectases develop in a unilateral, sometimes dermatomal (or following the lines of Blaschko) distribution. Spider angiomas may also be present. The most common distribution is unilateral or bilateral involvement of the third and fourth cervical dermatomes. The condition is rare in men; in affected women, it starts in adulthood. The familial form (very rare) favors males, is autosomal-dominant, and appears postnatally. UNT is associated with conditions that have increased levels of estrogen: puberty, pregnancy, oral contraceptive use, HCV infection, and cirrhosis. Treatment with pulse dye laser can be effective.

Dadlani C, et al: Unilateral nevoid telangiectasia. Dermatol Online J 2008; 14:3.

Derrow AE, et al: Acquired unilateral nevoid telangiectasia in a 51-year-old female. Int J Dermatol 2008; 47:1331.

Hynes LR, et al: Unilateral nevoid telangiectasia: occurrence in two patients with hepatitis C. J Am Acad Dermatol 1997; 36:819.

Karakas M, et al: Unilateral nevoid telangiectasia. J Dermatol 2004; 31:109.

Kreft B, et al: Unilateral nevoid telangiectasia syndrome. Dermatology 2004; 209:215.

Sardana K, et al: Unilateral nevoid telangiectasia syndrome. J Dermatol 2001; 28:453.

Sharma VK, Khandpur S: Unilateral nevoid telangiectasia—response to pulsed dye laser. Int J Dermatol 2006; 45:960.

Taskapan O: Acquired unilateral nevoid telangiectasia syndrome (letter). J Am Acad Dermatol 1998; 39:138.

Woollons A, et al: Unilateral naevoid telangiectasia syndrome in pregnancy. Clin Exp Dermatol 1996; 21:459.

Hereditary hemorrhagic telangiectasia (Osler's disease)

Also known as Osler–Weber–Rendu disease, hereditary hemorrhagic telangiectasia (HHT) is characterized by small tufts of dilated capillaries scattered over the mucous membranes and the skin. These slightly elevated lesions develop mostly on the lips, tongue, palate, nasal mucosa, ears, palms, fingertips, nailbeds, and soles. They may closely simulate the telangiectases of the CREST variant of scleroderma, which may be distinguished by the lack of other features of CREST syndrome and by anticentromere antibodies, which are not found in HHT. Diagnostic criteria have been proposed and include:

1. epistaxis—spontaneous, recurrent nosebleeds
2. telangiectases—multiple at characteristic sites (lips, oral cavity, fingers, nose) (Fig. 35-29)
3. visceral lesions—gastrointestinal bleeding, pulmonary, hepatic, cerebral, or spinal arteriovenous malformation (AVM)
4. family history—one affected first-degree relative.

The presence of three of the four criteria indicates a definite diagnosis, while two of four indicate a possible diagnosis. There are at least three variants, HHT1 and HHT2, and a third associated with juvenile polyposis.

Frequent nosebleeds and melena are experienced because of the telangiectasia in the nose and gastrointestinal tract. Epistaxis is the most frequent and persistent sign. Worsening epistaxis may herald high-output cardiac failure from AVMs. Pregnancy can also exacerbate HHT. Gastrointestinal bleeding is the presenting sign in up to 25% of cases; however, 40–50% develop gastrointestinal bleeding some time during the course of their disease. Chronic persistent anemia requiring iron and

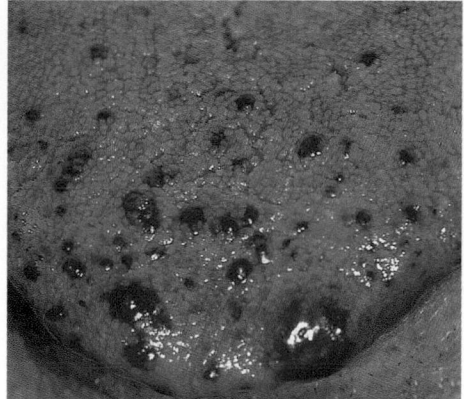

Fig. 35-29 Hereditary hemorrhagic telangiectasia.

blood transfusions is characteristic of severe cases. The spleen may be enlarged. Pulmonary and CNS AVMs may appear later in life. Liver failure can result from diffuse intrahepatic shunting—hepatic artery to vein, bypassing the liver parenchyma. Retinal arteriovenous aneurysms occur only rarely. Other sites of bleeding may be the kidney, spleen, bladder, liver, meninges, and brain. The risk of cerebral hemorrhage from cerebral AVMs, cerebral abscesses, and pulmonary hemorrhage from pulmonary AVMs is probably high enough that asymptomatic patients should be screened for the presence of cerebral and pulmonary AVMs. Because of the risk of cerebral abscess, some have advocated antibiotic prophylaxis for dental and contaminated skin procedures.

The telangiectases tend to increase in number in middle age; however, the first appearance on the undersurface of the tongue and floor of the mouth is at puberty. Pulmonary or intracranial arteriovenous fistulas and bleeding in these areas may be a cause of death.

HHT is inherited as an autosomal-dominant trait. The vascular abnormalities found in HHT consist of direct arteriovenous connections without an intervening capillary bed. Affected patients have mutations in one of three genes, most commonly in two, endoglin (*ENG*) or ALK-1 (*ACVRL1*). They encode a homodimeric integral membrane glycoprotein, which is a transforming growth factor (TGF)-β receptor. HHT1 is associated with *ENG* mutations, and HHT2 with *ACVRL1* mutations. HHT1 patients have a higher prevalence of pulmonary AVMs, while HHT2 patients tend to have a milder phenotype and later age of onset, but increased liver manifestations. Patients with HHT and juvenile polyposis have mutations in the *MADH4* gene, a downstream effector of TGF-β signaling. TGF-β is a potent stimulator of vascular endothelial growth factor (VEGF) production. VEGF leads to disorganized and tortuous vessels, as seen in HHT. VEGF levels are increased in patients with HHT.

Treatment is directed at controlling the specific complication, and identifying and treating AVMs before they become symptomatic. The tendency to epistaxis has been reduced by estrogen therapy and some recommend oral contraceptives for affected postpubertal females. Dermoplasty of the bleeding nasal septum may be performed by replacing the mucous membrane with skin from the thigh or buttock. Repeated laser treatments of the nasal and gastrointestinal mucosa are often required. Topical tranexamic acid has been used to control epistaxis. Bleeding episodes are treated supportively with iron and red blood cell transfusions. Interventional radiology with selective embolization can treat pulmonary and CNS AVMs and episodes of bleeding, avoiding invasive surgeries. In patients with liver failure or high-output heart failure due to liver AVMs, liver transplantation may be required. Blocking

VEGF with thalidomide (or more effectively with lenalidomide) can reduce gastrointestinal bleeding and transfusion dependence. Bevacizumab, a monoclonal inhibitor of VEGF, has dramatically improved some severely ill HHT patients, reducing the size and flow of their hepatic AVMs, reversing heart and liver failure, and reducing transfusion requirement.

Abdalla SA, et al: Visceral manifestations in hereditary haemorrhagic telangiectasia type 2. J Med Genet 2003; 40:494.

Al-Saleh S, et al: Screening for pulmonary and cerebral arteriovenous malformations in children with hereditary haemorrhagic telangiectasia. Eur Respir J 2009; 34:875.

Bose P, et al: Bevacizumab in hereditary hemorrhagic telangiectasia. N Engl J Med 2009; 360:2143.

Bowcock SJ, Patrick HE: Lenalidomide to control gastrointestinal bleeding in hereditary haemorrhagic telangiectasia: potential implications for angiodysplasias? Br J Haematol 2009; 146:220.

Faughnan ME, et al: International Guidelines for the Diagnosis and Management of Hereditary Hemorrhagic Telangiectasia. J Med Genet 2009 Jun 29 (Epub ahead of print).

Fernandez-Fernandez FJ: Hereditary haemorrhagic telangiectasia: from symptomatic management to pathogenesis based treatment. Eur J Hum Genet 2009 Nov 4 (Epub ahead of print).

Flieger D, et al: Dramatic improvement in hereditary hemorrhagic telangiectasia after treatment with the vascular endothelial growth factor (VEGF) antagonist bevacizumab. Ann Hematol 2006; 85:631.

Fuchizaki U, et al: Hereditary haemorrhagic telangiectasia (Rendu–Osler–Weber disease). Lancet 2003; 362:1490.

Gallione CJ, et al: A combined syndrome of juvenile polyposis and hereditary haemorrhagic telangiectasia associated with mutations in MADH4 (SMAD4). Lancet 2004; 363:852.

Garcia-Tsao G, et al: Liver disease in patients with hereditary hemorrhagic telangiectasia. N Engl J Med 2000; 343:931.

Goussous T, et al: Hereditary hemorrhagic telangiectasia presenting as high output cardiac failure during pregnancy. Cardiol Res Pract 2009; 2009:437237.

Haneen S, et al: Mutation analysis of "Endoglin" and "Activin receptor-like kinase" genes in German patients with hereditary hemorrhagic telangiectasia and the value of rapid genotyping using an allele-specific PCR-technique. BMC Med Genet 2009; 10:53.

Kanna B, Das B: Hemorrhagic pericardial effusion causing pericardial tamponade in hereditary hemorrhagic telangiectasia. Am J Med Sci 2004; 327:149.

Khalid SK, et al: Worsening of nose bleeding heralds high cardiac output state in hereditary hemorrhagic telangiectasia. Am J Med 2009; 122:779.e1.

Klepfish A, et al: Intranasal tranexamic acid treatment for severe epistaxis in hereditary hemorrhagic telangiectasia. Arch Intern Med 2001; 161:767.

Lee JB, et al: The diagnostic quandary of hereditary haemorrhagic telangiectasia vs. CREST syndrome. Br J Dermatol 2001; 145:646.

Mager JJ, Westermann CJJ: Value of capillary microscopy in the diagnosis of hereditary hemorrhagic telangiectasia. Arch Dermatol 2000; 136:732.

Mei-Zahav M, et al: Symptomatic children with hereditary hemorrhagic telangiectasia: a pediatric center experience. Arch Pediatr Adolesc Med 2006; 160:596.

Mitchell A, et al: Bevacizumab reverses need for liver transplantation in hereditary hemorrhagic telangiectasia. Liver Transpl 2008; 14:210.

Leg ulcers

Leg ulcers are a common medical condition, affecting 3–5% of the population over the age of 65. The cause of chronic leg ulceration is venous insufficiency alone in 45–60% of cases, arterial insufficiency in 10–20%, diabetes mellitus in 15–25%, or combinations in 10–15%. Smoking and obesity increase the risk for ulcer development and persistence, independent of the underlying cause. Defining the cause of the leg ulceration is important in treating the leg ulcer.

The wound healing response is complex, involving intricate interactions between different cell types, structural proteins, growth factors, and proteinases. Normal wound repair consists of three phases—inflammation, proliferation, and remodeling—that occur in a predictable sequence.

Venous diseases of the extremities

Stasis dermatitis

Stasis dermatitis presents as erythema and a yellowish or light-brown pigmentation of the lower third of the lower legs, especially in the area just superior to the medial malleolus. An associated eczematous dermatitis may occur. The dermatitis may be weepy or dry, scaling or lichenified; it is almost invariably hyperpigmented by melanin and hemosiderin. Varicose veins are usually present, though they need not be numerous or conspicuous. Stasis dermatitis is a cutaneous marker for venous insufficiency. The approach to management should be two-fold: relief of symptoms and treatment of the underlying venous insufficiency. Patients with pruritus and an eczematous component should be treated with emollients and topical corticosteroids. The daily use of elevation and support stockings is strongly recommended.

Venous insufficiency and obesity-associated mucinosis

Localized areas of mucin deposition can be observed directly over the perforators on the lower extremity. These present as blushed, red–blue, partially compressible, agminated papules. On biopsy, deposits of dermal mucin against a background of the changes of venous insufficiency are seen. In the setting of morbid obesity and lower extremity edema, pretibial translucent papules can appear and merge into plaques. The plaques are composed of dermal mucin (hyaluronic acid). The diagnosis of "pretibial myxedema" is usually made, but thyroid functions are normal. With weight loss the lesions improve, suggesting that they were due to the lower extremity edema/venous insufficiency of obesity.

Venous insufficiency ulceration

Stasis dermatitis and venous ulceration result from increased pressure in the venous system of the lower leg. The most common cause is insufficiency of the valves in the deep venous system and lower perforating veins of the lower leg. With each contraction of the calf, blood should be pumped to the heart via this "muscle pump." Intact valves in the lower leg are required to prevent this "pumped" blood from refluxing out through the perforators into the superficial system. Increased flow through the superficial system results in enlargement of the superficial venous plexus and the appearance of "varicose veins." Increased pressure on the iliac veins from pregnancy or obesity, or simple inactivity may also result in the appearance of "venous insufficiency," as well. The valvular insufficiency results in disorder in the venous and capillary circulation in the leg. Valve insufficiency may occur from prior thrombophlebitis or congenital "weakness." Prolonged standing without walking or contracting the calf muscles, sitting for long periods, anemia, zinc deficiency, and a defective fibrinolytic system may accelerate the process. If a history of thrombophlebitis is present, an evaluation for a hypercoagulable state, such as a deficiency of Leiden factor V, should be considered.

Edema and fibrosis develop in the skin over the medial aspect of the ankle and lower third of the shin (Fig. 35-30). Following minor trauma, a macular hemorrhage appears. This is the premonitory sign of an impending ulceration. Venous

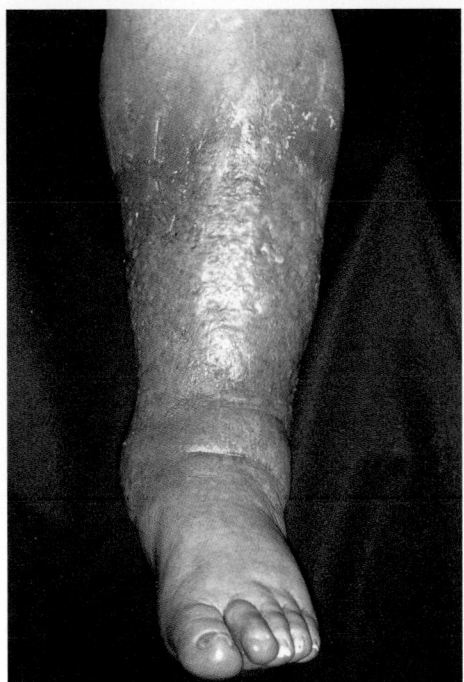

Fig. 35-30 Stasis dermatitis, venous insufficiency.

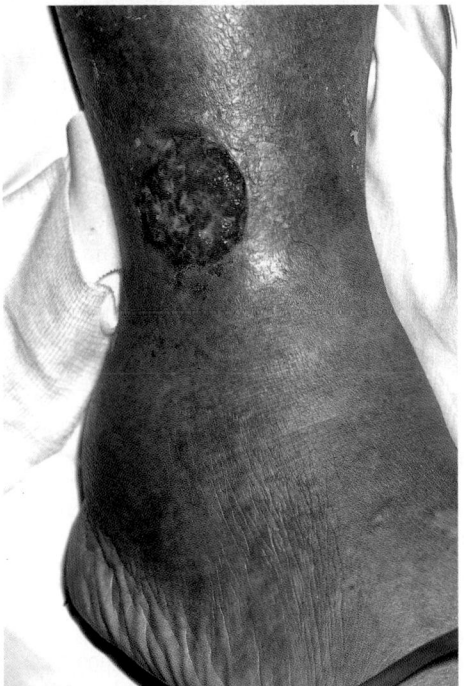

Fig. 35-31 Venous leg ulcer.

ulcers usually occur on the lower medial aspect of the leg. They may appear on the background of stasis dermatitis with lipodermatosclerosis (Fig. 35-31). Venous ulcerations can be painful, but not as painful as pyoderma gangrenosum or arterial or embolic ulcerations. The ulcer tends to be round or oblong and has a characteristic yellow, fibrinous base. Multiple lesions may occur.

In most cases, the diagnosis of a venous ulceration can be made on clinical grounds. If there is no clear history or physical findings of venous insufficiency, venous rheography can be performed. An ABI (ankle:brachial index, or ratio of blood pressure in the leg to the arm) should be performed, especially in cases where peripheral pulses are diminished and hair on the lower legs is lost. This will identify coexistent arterial disease. More extensive vascular studies may be necessary to identify the presence and extent of arterial disease or focal venous valvular incompetence or congenital absence. In leg ulcers of the lower medial leg, even if cutaneous findings of venous insufficiency are absent, venous insufficiency will still be the most common cause of the ulcer. Lesions in atypical locations, those that do not respond appropriately to therapy, and those in which venous rheography is normal may require a biopsy to exclude other causes, including a cutaneous neoplasm. Additional workup may also be required to identify other, less common causes of leg ulcers, such as cholesterol emboli, atherosclerotic disease, diabetes mellitus, sickle cell disease, vasculitis, infection, and pyoderma gangrenosum.

Despite extensive research and the marketing of many new products and devices for the treatment of leg ulcers, very little has changed in their management over the last decades. Treatment is primarily to improve venous return and reduce edema. Compression therapy is the mainstay of treatment. This involves the use of pressure wraps, such as Unna boots covered with Coban or elastic wraps. Elevation of the leg above the heart, for as much of the time as is possible (a minimum of 2 h twice a day), is also beneficial. Elastic support of the legs must be continued after the ulcer heals. Other causes of edema, such as cardiac failure, must be addressed. The avoidance of long, cramped sitting (in airplanes or vehicles) or prolonged standing is advisable. Diuretics are overused and not proven to be of benefit. If there is a central cause of fluid retention (cirrhosis, heart failure, renal failure), diuretics may be beneficial, but otherwise they are best avoided. Avoidance of trauma is important. Pentoxifylline, 400–800 mg three times a day, in addition to compression, is beneficial in healing refractory venous ulcerations. A cooperative patient and a patient physician are necessary in the long-term management of venous disease. Topical anti-infectives are usually not necessary (except metronidazole gel to prevent anaerobic overgrowth). There is a high risk of allergic contact dermatitis from other topical antibiotics. Oral antibiotics should only be used to treat associated invasive infection. A rim of erythema commonly surrounds an ulcer. Expanding erythema, an enlarging ulcer, or increasing pain or tenderness may be signs of infection. Surface cultures and Gram stains may demonstrate colonizing, but not pathogenic, bacteria. Biopsy for histology and tissue homogenate culture is the most effective way to demonstrate a true invasive pathogen.

Many treatment options have been developed for chronic ulcers. Unfortunately, conclusive comparative studies between the various treatment alternatives are lacking. All are to be used in combination with compression treatment. Occlusive and semipermeable biosynthetic wound dressings can be very effective when combined with compression. They can speed healing, reduce pain, make dressing changes infrequent, and help debridement. If a hard eschar is present over the ulcer when first seen, a dressing will assist in its removal. Early in the treatment of an ulcer, a highly inflammatory and exudative phase occurs. This will often wash off the semipermeable dressing and may require the use of fenestrated dressings and even the application of absorbent padding over the dressing for the first few weeks. The patient will interpret this increased wound exudate, which is normal and indicates the conversion of a non-healing to a healing wound, as an infection. He/she should be appropriately educated before such dressings are applied. Dressings containing dilute acetic acid or silver may help reduce bacterial overgrowth in the wound, but fail to decrease the time to healing. However, metronidazole gel 0.75% instilled into the wound will help to reduce the amount of wound exudate (by eliminating anerobic bacteria) and remove the smell of the wound exudate. The smell of achronic leg ulcer may reduce the patient's quality of life. Becaplermin (Regranex) is expensive, but promotes wound healing. Granulation tissue formation is enhanced. It may be useful in wounds that are unable to develop a granulation tissue base despite local care and conservative debridement. Weekly debridement of the anesthetic dead fibrinous tissue can be useful in stimulating granulation tissue at the base of slow-to-heal venous ulcerations. Injection of granulocyte–macrophage colony-stimulating factor (GM-CSF) into the ulcer base may also stimulate refractory ulcers to heal. It is very expensive. Grafts and skin substitutes should be reserved for refractory ulcers that have failed conservative therapy. In more than 90% of cases, only simple but persistently applied measures are required. Enhanced compliance, longer elevation, and removal of leg edema are the first steps in attempting to heal refractory leg ulcers. If these are not optimized, expensive dressing and medications will not lead to healing. The role of vascular surgery or venous ablation in the healing of leg ulcers is controversial.

Risk factors that predict failure to heal within 24 weeks of limb compression therapy include a large wound area, history of venous ligation or stripping, history of hip or knee replacement, ABI <0.80, fibrin on 50% or more of the wound surface, and the presence of the ulcer for an extended time. For every 6 months of duration, the ulcer healing time doubles.

Arterial insufficiency (ischemic) ulcer

Ischemic ulcers are mostly located on the lateral surface of the ankle or the distal digits. The initial red, painful plaque breaks down into a painful superficial ulcer with a surrounding zone of purpuric erythema. Granulation tissue is minimal, little or no infection is present, and a membranous inactive eschar forms over the ulcer. Patients at risk are those with long-standing hypertension, smokers, diabetics, and those with hyperlipidemia. The presence of an arterial ulceration identifies patients at increased risk for limb loss.

Signs and symptoms indicating that arterial disease is the cause of the ulceration include thinning of the skin, absence of hair, decreased or absent pulses, pallor on elevation, coolness of the extremity, dependent rubor, claudication on exercise, and pain on elevation (especially at night) relieved on dependency. In progressive disease, the diagnosis of thromboangiitis obliterans, or Buerger's disease, should be considered. Patients with arterial insufficiency are also at risk for cholesterol emboli, another arterial cause of lower leg ulceration. Eosinophilia, palpable peripheral pulses, sudden onset, and associated renal insufficiency are clues to the diagnosis of cholesterol emboli.

The diagnosis of arterial insufficiency can usually be confirmed by physical examination and careful palpation of the pulses in the legs. For more accurate evaluation, take the blood pressure in the arm and leg. They should be nearly identical. The ratio of the popliteal to brachial pressure is called the ABI. If it is less than 0.75, arterial insufficiency exists; if less than 0.5, the insufficiency is substantial.

Surgical intervention may be required to heal the ulceration. If the blood supply cannot be improved, little can be done, except to prevent infection by the measures described under venous ulcers. The area should be protected from injury and cold, and smoking and tight socks should be avoided. Hyperbaric oxygen may be of some use, but it is limited by availability and cost.

Neuropathic ulcers

Foot ulcers in diabetics are usually related to sensory neuropathy. Offloading the ulcer is the primary principle of management. Necrotic tissue should be debrided back to bleeding viable tissue. As the foot is typically insensate, this can be done in the office without the need for anesthetic. Associated osteomyelitis is best treated by removal of the infected bone. Consultation with or referral to a podiatrist or orthopedic surgeon may be indicated. Various shoes and padded boots can be used to offload different areas of the foot. An orthotics consultation is usually indicated. Clinical infection should be treated, but simple colonization typically does not require treatment. After the ulcer heals, a shoe of appropriate depth and width will help to prevent recurrence. Frequent foot inspections for the presence of "hot spots," as well as debridement of dystrophic nails, are important facets of prevention of leg ulcers in diabetics.

Baldursson B, et al: Venous leg ulcers and squamous cell carcinoma. Br J Dermatol 1995; 133:571.

Choucair M, et al: Compression therapy. Dermatol Surg 1998; 24:141.

Davies C: Use of Doppler ultrasound in leg ulcer assessments. Nurs Stand 2001; 15:72.

Falanga V, et al: Rapid healing of venous ulcers and lack of clinical rejection with an allogeneic cultured human skin equivalent. Arch Dermatol 1998; 134:293.

Fletcher A, et al: A systematic review of compression treatment for venous leg ulcers. BMJ 1997; 315:576.

Grossman D, et al: Activated protein C resistance and anticardiolipin antibodies in patients with venous leg ulcers. J Am Acad Dermatol 1997; 37:409.

Groves RW, Schmidt-Lucke JA: Recombinant human GM-CSF in the treatment of poorly healing wounds. Adv Skin Wound Care 2000; 13:107.

Hafner J, et al: Leg ulcers in peripheral arterial disease (arterial leg ulcers): impaired wound healing above the threshold of chronic critical limb ischemia. J Am Acad Dermatol 2000; 43:1001.

Jull A, et al: Pentoxifylline for treatment of venous leg ulcers: a systematic review. Lancet 2002; 359:1550.

Maessen-Visch MB, et al: The prevalence of factor V Leiden mutation in patients with leg ulcers and venous insufficiency. Arch Dermatol 1999; 135:41.

Margolis DJ, et al: Risk factors associated with failure of a venous leg ulcer to heal. Arch Dermatol 1999; 135:920.

Mekkes JR, et al: Causes, investigation and treatment of leg ulceration. Br J Dermatol 2003; 148:388.

Michaels JA, et al: Randomized controlled trial and cost-effectiveness analysis of silver-donating antimicrobial dressings for venous leg ulcers (VULCAN) trial. Br J Surg 2009; 96:1147.

Padberg F, et al: Does severe venous insufficiency have a different etiology in the morbidly obese? Is it venous? J Vasc Surg 2003; 37:79.

Pennington M, et al: Cholesterol embolization syndrome: cutaneous histopathological features and the variable onset of symptoms in patients with different risk factors. Br J Dermatol 2002; 146:511.

Pugashetti R, et al: Dermal mucinosis as a sign of venous insufficiency. J Cutan Pathol 2009 Jul 10 (Epub ahead of print).

Rico T, et al: Vascular endothelial growth factor delivery via gene therapy for diabetic wounds: first steps. J Invest Dermatol 2009; 129:2084.

Rongioletti F, et al: Obesity-associated lymphoedematous mucinosis. J Cutan Pathol 2009; 36:1089.

Samson RH, et al: Stockings and the prevention of recurrent venous ulcers. Dermatol Surg 1996; 22:373.

Siddiqui FH, et al: Recombinant granulocyte macrophage colony stimulating factor (rhu-GM-CSF) in the treatment of extensive leg ulcers: a case report. Surgery 2000; 127:589.

Sultan MJ, McCollum C: Don't waste money when dressing leg ulcers. Br J Surg 2009; 96:1099.

Teepe RG, et al: Randomized trial comparing cryopreserved cultured epidermal allografts with hydrocolloid dressings in healing chronic venous ulcers. J Am Acad Dermatol 1993; 29:982.

Tokuda Y, et al: Chronic obesity lymphoedematous mucinosis: three cases of pretibial mucinosis in obese patients with pitting oedema. Br J Dermatol 2006; 154:157.

Valencia IC, et al: Chronic venous insufficiency and venous leg ulceration. J Am Acad Dermatol 2001; 44:401.

LYMPHEDEMA

Lymphedema is the swelling of soft tissues in which an excess amount of lymph has accumulated. Chronic lymphedema is characterized by long-standing, nonpitting edema. A working classification of lymphedema is shown in Box 35-2.

The most prevalent worldwide cause of lymphedema is filariasis. In the US the most common cause is postsurgical. If lymphedema is long-standing, a verrucous appearance to the affected extremity develops (elephantiasis verrucosa nostra).

Lymphedema of the lower extremity must be distinguished from "lipedema." This syndrome is characterized by bilateral, symmetrical lower extremity enlargement due to subcutaneous fat deposition. The buttocks to the ankles are affected in women, starting at puberty with gradual progression. The feet are spared in lipedema but usually involved in lower extremity lymphedema. Lipedema does not respond to compression therapy. The skin fold at the base of the second toe is too thick to pinch in lymphedema but normal in lipedema (Stemmer's sign). Verrucous changes do not occur in lipedema but do occur in lymphedema. Women with lipedema will have tenderness to pressure on the affected area. There is frequently a family history of lipedema. Magnetic resonance imaging (MRI)

will separate the two entities if the diagnosis cannot be confirmed on a clinical basis.

Types

Lymphedema is classified by clinical type (Box 35-2). Primary types include congenital, and early- and late-onset types. Other primary types of lymphedema are associated with characteristic features or syndromes. Some cutaneous disorders are associated with or are a complication of primary lymphedema. Secondary lymphedema can occur from numerous causes, including neoplasia and its treatment, infections, and physical factors.

Lymphedema praecox

Lymphedema praecox develops in females between the ages of 9 and 25. Swelling appears around the ankle and then extends upward to involve the entire leg. With the passage of time, the leg becomes painful, with a dull, heavy sensation. Once this stage has been reached, the swollen limb remains swollen, as fibrosis has occurred. Primary lymphedema is caused by a defect in the lymphatic system. Lymphangiography demonstrates hypoplastic lymphatics in 87%, aplasia in approximately 5%, and hyperplasia with varicose dilation of the lymphatic vessels in 8%.

Nonne–Milroy–Meige syndrome (hereditary lymphedema)

Milroy hereditary edema of the lower legs is characterized by a unilateral or bilateral lymphedema present at birth and inherited as an autosomal-dominant trait. The edema is painless, pits on pressure, is not associated with any other disorder, and persists throughout life (Fig. 35-32). It may involve the genitalia and produce lymphangiectasias superficially. Chylous discharge can occur. The face and arm may also be involved. Most frequently, the lymphedema is unilateral, and females are predominantly affected.

Treatment of this particular type of edema is extremely difficult, since the disease is an anomaly of the lymph-draining vessels. Decongestive physiotherapy can be considered. In some cases, surgical procedures to remove affected tissue can

---

Box 35-2 Classification of lymphedema

Primary lymphedema
- Congenital lymphedema (Milroy's disease)
- Lymphedema praecox
- Lymphedema tarda

Syndromes associated with primary lymphedema
- Yellow nail syndrome
- Turner syndrome
- Noonan syndrome
- Pes cavus
- Phakomatosis pigmentovascularis
- Distichiasis–lymphedema
- Emberger syndrome
- WILD syndrome
- Hypotrichosis-telangiectasia-lymphedema syndrome

Cutaneous disorders sometimes associated with primary lymphedema
- Yellow nails
- Hemangiomas
- Xanthomatosis and chylous lymphedema
- Congenital absence of nails

Secondary lymphedema
- Postmastectomy lymphedema
- Melphalan isolated limb perfusion
- Malignant occlusion with obstruction
- Extrinsic pressure
- Factitial lymphedema
- Postradiation therapy
- Following recurrent lymphangitis/cellulitis
- Lymphedema of upper limb in recurrent eczema
- Granulomatous disease
- Rosaceous lymphedema
- Primary amyloidosis

Complications of lymphedema
- Cellulitis of lymphedema
- Elephantiasis nostra verrucosa
- Ulceration
- Lymphangiosarcoma

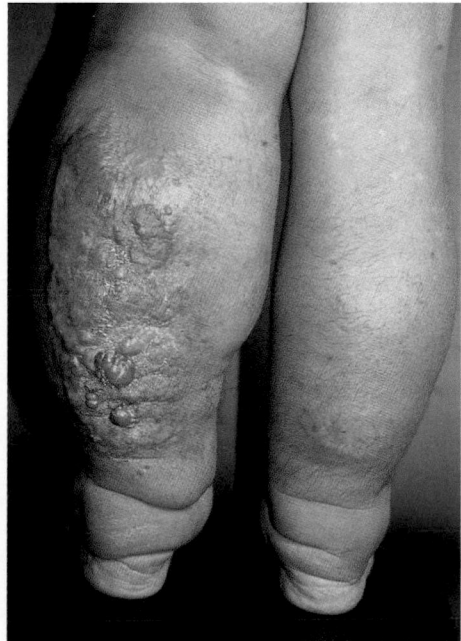

Fig. 35-32 Milroy's disease. (Courtesy of Lawrence Lieblich, MD)

be performed. This condition may be linked to a mutation in *flt4*, the gene for VEGFR3.

Lymphedema–distichiasis syndrome

The association of distichiasis (double row of eyelashes) and late-onset lymphedema is a form of hereditary lymphedema called lymphedema-distichiasis syndrome, or Meige syndrome. It is an autosomal-dominant syndrome with the appearance of bilateral lymphedema, beginning between the ages of 8 and 10 in affected boys, and 13 and 30 in affected girls. Lymphatic vessels are increased (not hypoplastic or absent, as in other forms of congenital lymphedema) in the affected legs. Associated findings are varicose veins in 50% by age 64; congenital ptosis (31%); and congenital heart disease (6.8%), cleft palate (4%), scoliosis, and renal abnormalities. There may be phenotypic heterogeneity in this syndrome, as different types of mutation may lead to slightly different phenotypes, especially with regard to the ancillary features associated with the syndrome. This syndrome is due to a mutation in the FOXC2 transcription factor. This factor is expressed in developing eyelids, lymphatics, lymphatic valves, and other tissues with abnormalities in this syndrome.

Emberger syndrome

Emberger syndrome is primary lymphedema associated with myelodysplasia. This genetic syndrome presents with lymphedema of one or both lower limbs and often the genitalia between infancy and puberty. Myelodysplastic syndrome and/or acute myeloid leukemia developing in adolescence or childhood are preceded by pancytopenia with a high incidence of monosomy 7 in the bone marrow. Associated features include mild skeletal abnormalities, deafness, and multiple warts.

WILD syndrome (Warts, Immunodeficiency, Lymphedema, anogenital Dysplasia)

Lymphedema appears in early childhood and may progress to involve all 4 extremities and the genitalia. Widespread flat warts appear during childhood resembling the numerous flat warts seen in epidermodysplasia verruciformis. The anogenital region develops numerous warts and anogenital dysplasia. Helper T cells are reduced.

Hypotrichosis-telangiectasia-lymphedema syndrome

Lymphedema appears in childhood. Vascular dilations and telangiectasias appear on the palms and soles. Both autosomal recessive and autosomal dominant patterns of inheritance occur, but both forms are due to mutations in the SOX18 gene.

Primary lymphedema associated with yellow nails and pleural effusion (yellow nail syndrome)

Lymphedema is confined mostly to the ankles and occurs in about 60% of patients with this syndrome. The nails show a distinct yellowish discoloration and thickening. Recurrent pleural effusion or bronchiectasis may be a feature.

Secondary lymphedema

In some malignant diseases, involvement of the axillary or pelvic lymph nodes will produce blockage and lymphedema. Malignant disease of the breast, uterus, prostate, skin, bones, or other tissues may cause such changes. Hodgkin disease and, especially, Kaposi sarcoma (KS) may be accompanied by significant lymphedema well beyond the amount expected from the degree of skin involvement by the KS. Such patients require chemotherapy, as this is the hallmark of lymphatic involvement by the KS. Chronic lymphedema is frequently seen after mastectomy and the removal of the axillary nodes; it may occur after varying lengths of time.

Postmastectomy lymphangiosarcoma (Stewart–Treves syndrome)

This type of vascular malignancy usually arises in chronic postmastectomy lymphedema. The lesions are bluish or reddish nodules arising on the arm. Similarly, primary or secondary lymphedema of the lower extremity may be complicated by angiosarcoma. Angiosarcoma arising in a lymphedematous extremity often presents with multiple lesions. Metastasis and death commonly result. Early aggressive surgical treatment with amputation may be life-saving. The treatment of breast cancer with lumpectomy and local radiation therapy may be complicated by angiosarcoma of the breast with minimal or no associated lymphedema. This is called cutaneous postradiation angiosarcoma of the breast. This form of angiosarcoma also frequently results in metastasis and death.

Postinflammatory lymphedema

The lymphedematous extremity may be caused by and worsened by repeated bacterial cellulitis/lymphangitis. It is these recurrent infectious episodes, when they complicate filariasis, that cause the elephantiasis. Streptococcal cellulitis following venectomy in patients who had undergone coronary bypass surgery is a well-documented cause. However, almost any chronic or recurrent infection can cause this. Chronic antibiotic therapy can halt the progression by preventing the attacks of bacterial cellulitis.

Bullous lymphedema

Commonly misdiagnosed as an immunobullous disease, bullous lymphedema usually occurs with poorly controlled edema related to heart failure and fluid overload. Compression results in healing.

Factitial lymphedema

Also known as hysterical edema, lymphedema can be produced by wrapping an elastic bandage, cord, or shirt around an extremity, and/or holding the extremity in a dependent and immobile state. Self-inflicted causes of lymphedema are usually difficult to prove and may occur in settings of known causes of lymphedema, such as postphlebitic syndrome or surgical injury to the brachial plexus. Factitial lymphedema caused by blunt trauma localized to the dorsum of the hand or forearm is referred to as Secretan syndrome or l'oedème bleu, respectively. It often is unilateral and there may be significant purpura. Effective care of such patients requires psychiatric intervention. Occupational causes must be excluded.

Podoconiosis

Podoconiosis, or mossy foot, is a non-infectious form of lymphedema. It is restricted to tropical regions in Central Africa, Central America, and North India. It occurs in persons walking barefoot in soil of volcanic origin. This soil has high concentrations of aluminum, silicon, beryllium, zirconium, magnesium, and iron. Apparently, colloid-sized particles of the dust penetrate the sole, and migrate to lymph nodes ingested in macrophages. Lymphatic drainage is impaired by fibrosis of lymphatic channels, induced by the microscopic deposits of the substances. Males and females are equally affected, and in endemic areas up to 5% of the population can develop the disease. Moving into an endemic area from a non-endemic area can lead to the condition appearing over the next 5 years. Podoconiosis begins in childhood or adolescence with mild swelling of the feet. Burning of the feet occurs at night. The dorsal surface of the foot itches, and is rubbed and lichenified. Increased skin markings and finally marked hyperkeratosis due to repeated infections result. This closely resembles elephantiasis verrucosa cutis. The condition is usually asymmetrical. Podoconiosis is prevented by wearing shoes. Elevation, compression, and local wound care all aid in this condition. Extensive surgery, as done for filariasis, has had disappointing results.

Other causes

Occupational persistent hand edema in divers, related to the constrictive action of the divers' suits and pricks from sea urchin spines, can occur.

Evaluation

The diagnosis is usually based on a classic presentation; however, in the early stages the disease may require further investigation. Considerations include isotopic lymphoscintigraphy, indirect and direct lymphography, MRI, computed tomography, and ultrasonography.

Treatment

Most cases are treated conservatively by means of various forms of compression therapy, complex physical therapy, pneumatic pumps, and compressive garments. Chronic antibiotic treatment may be beneficial in patients suffering repeated episodes of erysipelas or cellulitis. In diabetics with insensate feet, the frequency of infection can be reduced by wearing properly fitting shoes. Volume-reducing surgery and lymphatic microsurgery are rarely performed, although a few centers consistently report favorable results. It is best to refer these patients to a center versed in the treatment of these complicated conditions, to optimize patient compliance and customize therapy to the patient's lifestyle.

Allen PJ, et al: Lower extremity lymphedema caused by acquired immune deficient syndrome-related Kaposi's sarcoma. J Vasc Surg 1995; 22:178.

Ameen M, et al: Clinicopathological case 2: lymphoedema–distichiasis syndrome. Clin Exp Dermatol 2003; 28:463.

Angelini G, et al: Occupational traumatic lymphedema of the hands. Dermatol Clin 1990; 8:205.

Badger C, et al: Physical therapies for reducing and controlling lymphoedema of the limbs. Cochrane Database Syst Rev 2004; 4:CD003141.

Bastien MR, et al: Treatment of lymphedema with a multicompartmental pneumatic compression device. J Am Acad Dermatol 1989; 20:853.

Billings SD, et al: Cutaneous angiosarcoma following breast-conserving surgery and radiation. Am J Surg Pathol 2004; 28:781.

Campisi C, Boccardo F: Microsurgical techniques for lymphedema treatment: derivative lymphatic-venous microsurgery. World J Surg 2004; 28:609.

Cerri A, et al: Lymphangiosarcoma of the pubic region: a rare complication arising in congenital non-hereditary lymphedema. Eur J Dermatol 1998; 8:511.

Downes M, et al: Vascular defects in a mouse model of hypotrichosis-lymphedoma-telangiectasia syndrome indicate a role for SOX18 in blood vessel maturation. Hum Mol Genet 2009; 18:2839.

Durr HR, et al: Stewart–Treves syndrome as a rare complication of hereditary lymphedema. Vasa 2004; 33:42.

Fonder MA, et al: Lipedema, a frequently unrecognized problem. J Am Acad Dermatol 2007; 57:S1

Harel L, et al: Lymphedema praecox seen as isolated unilateral arm involvement. J Pediatr 1997; 130:492.

Irrthum A, et al: Mutations in the transcription factor gene SOX18 underlie recessive and dominant forms of hypotrichosis-lymphedema-telangiectasia. Am J Hum Genet 2003; 72:1470.

Johnson SM, et al: Lymphedema–distichiasis syndrome: report of a case and review. Arch Dermatol 1999; 135:347.

Joseph A, et al: The efficacies of affected-limb care with penicillin diethylcarbamazine, the combination of both drugs or antibiotic ointment, in the prevention of acute adenolymphangitis during bancroftian filariasis. Ann Trop Med Parasitol 2004; 98:685.

Makrilakis K, et al: Successful octreotide treatment of chylous pleural effusion and lymphedema in the yellow nail syndrome. Ann Intern Med 2004; 141:246.

Maldonado F, Ryu JH: Yellow nail syndrome. Curr Opin Pulm Med 2009; 15.371.

Miller TA, et al: Staged skin and subcutaneous excision for lymphedema: a favorable report of long-term results. Plast Reconstr Surg 1998; 102:1486.

Moorjani N, et al: Pleural effusion in yellow nail syndrome: treatment with bilateral pleuro-peritoneal shunts. Respiration 2004; 71:298.

Mortimer PS: Managing lymphedema. Clin Dermatol 1995; 13:499.

Nenoff P, et al: Podoconiosis-non-filarial geochemical elephantiasis—a neglected tropical disease. JDDG 2010; 8:7.

Radhakrishnan K, Rockson SG: The clinical spectrum of lymphatic disease. Ann N Y Acad Sci 2008; 1131:155.

Ruocco V, et al: Lymphedema: an immunologically vulnerable site for development of neoplasms. J Am Acad Dermatol 2002; 47:124.

Schissel DJ, et al: Elephantiasis nostras verrucosa. Cutis 1998; 62:77.

Tosti A, et al: Systemic itraconazole in the yellow nail syndrome. Br J Dermatol 2002; 146:1064.

Yalcin E, et al: Yellow nail syndrome in an infant presenting with lymphedema of the eyelids and pleural effusion. Clin Pediatr 2004; 43:569.

Bonus images for this chapter can be found online at
http://www.expertconsult.com

Fig. 35-1 Raynaud disease.

Fig. 35-2 Photo-induced livedo reticularis secondary to quinidine.

Fig. 35-3 Hematoma.

Fig. 35-4 Purpura secondary to vomiting.

Fig. 35-5 Pigmented purpuric dermatosis.

Fig. 35-6 Leukocytoclastic vasculitis, concentration of lesions along the dividing line between the dorsal foot and sole (Wallace line).

Fig. 35-7 Henoch–Schönlein purpura.

Fig. 35-8 Hereditary hemorrhagic telangiectasia.

Fig. 35-9 Hereditary hemorrhagic telangiectasia.

Fig. 35-10 Stasis dermatitis, venous insufficiency.

Fig. 35-11 Elephantiasis verrucosa nostra.

Fig. 35-12 Distichiasis. (Courtesy of Curt Samlaska, MD)

36 Disturbances of Pigmentation

The visible pigmentation of the skin or hair is a combination of the amount of melanin, type of melanin (eumelanin versus pheomelanin), degree of vascularity, presence of carotene, and thickness of the stratum corneum. Other materials can be deposited abnormally in the skin, leading to pigmentation. Eumelanin is the primary pigment producing brown coloration of the skin. Pheomelanin is yellow or red, and is also produced solely in melanocytes. Melanin is formed from tyrosine, via the action of tyrosinase, in the melanosomes of melanocytes. There are hundreds of genes expressed only in melanosomes and apparently important in melanin production and delivery. Melanosomes are lysosome-related organelles. Melanosome formation and the end result, pigmentation, require both the adequate manufacture of melanin and the appropriate transport of melanosomes within the melanocyte. The melanosomes are transferred from a melanocyte to a group of 36 keratinocytes called the epidermal melanin unit, to which they provide melanin. The variations in skin color between persons and races are related to the degree of melanization of melanosomes, their number, and their distribution in the epidermal melanin unit. Disorders of loss or reduction of pigmentation may be related to loss of melanocytes or the inability of melanocytes to produce melanin or transport melanosomes correctly. Wood's light examination is often performed to evaluate lesions of hyper- or hypopigmentation. Hyperpigmented lesions that enhance with Wood's light usually have increased epidermal melanocyte number or activity. If the lesions do not enhance, the melanin is located in the dermis. Wood's light will markedly enhance depigmented lesions (complete loss of pigment), but does not enhance lesions with partial pigment loss (hypopigmentation).

Barral DC, Seabra MC: The melanosome as a model to study organelle motility in mammals. Pigment Cell Res 2004; 17:111.
Dell'Angelica EC: Melanosome biogenesis: shedding light on the origin of an obscure organelle. Trends Cell Biol 2003; 13:503.
Rees JL: Genetics of hair and skin color. Annu Rev Genet 2003; 37:67.
Setaluri V: The melanosome: dark pigment granule shines bright light on vesicle biogenesis and more. J Invest Dermatol 2003; 121:650.

Pigmentary demarcation lines

Pigmentary demarcation boundaries of the skin can be classified into six groups, as follows:
1. Group A: Lines along the outer upper arms with variable extension across the chest.
2. Group B: Lines along the posteromedial aspect of the lower limb (Fig. 36-1).
3. Group C: Paired median or paramedian lines on the chest, with midline abdominal extension.
4. Group D: Medial, over the spine.
5. Group E: Bilaterally symmetrical, obliquely oriented, hypopigmented macules on the chest.
6. Group F: Facial pigmentary demarcation lines.

More than 70% of black patients have one or more lines; they are much less common in white patients. Type B lines often appear for the first time during pregnancy.

Pigmentary demarcation lines must be distinguished from the much rarer condition, acquired dermal melanocytosis. This primarily affects Asian and Hispanic women (male to female ratio, 1:17). It often first appears during pregnancy or the therapeutic use of estrogen/progesterone. Lesions present as blue–gray patches, with superimposed brown macules affecting the face, trunk, or extremities. Lesions do not enhance with Wood's light. They may be localized (following trauma) or more diffuse. Biopsy shows melanocytes in the dermis, similar to the findings in Mongolian spot, nevus of Ota, and nevus of Ito.

Bonci A, Patrizi A: Pigmentary demarcation lines in pregnancy. Arch Dermatol 2002; 138:127.
Rubin AI, et al: Acquired dermal melanocytosis: appearance during pregnancy. J Am Acad Dermatol 2001; 45:609.
Ruiz-Villaverde R, et al: Pigmentary demarcation lines in a pregnant Caucasian woman. Int J Dermatol 2004; 43:911.

Abnormal pigmentation

Hemosiderin hyperpigmentation

Pigmentation due to deposits of hemosiderin occurs in purpura, hemochromatosis, hemorrhagic diseases, and stasis dermatitis. Clinically, hemosiderin hyperpigmentation is distinguished from postinflammatory dermal melanosis by a golden brown hue, as opposed to the brown or gray–blue pigmentation of epidermal and dermal melanin, respectively. At times, a biopsy is required to distinguish melanin- from hemosiderin-induced hyperpigmentation. Some medications (including minocycline) deposit in the skin and complex with both iron and melanin, making uniquely colored (usually blue–gray) deposits.

Postinflammatory hyperpigmentation (postinflammatory pigmentary alteration—PIPA)

Any natural or iatrogenic inflammatory condition can result in hyper- or hypopigmentation. Postinflammatory dyspigmentation is more frequent in persons with Fitzpatrick skin types IV, V, and VI, especially those of skin types IV and V. It is equally common in males and females. Hyperpigmentation may result from two mechanisms:
1. increased epidermal pigmentation via increased melanocyte activity
2. dermal melanosis from melanocyte damage and melanin dropout from the epidermis into the dermis.

Wood's light examination will distinguish these two patterns of postinflammatory hyperpigmentation. Lesions of hyperpigmentation tend to be tan to brown (Fig. 36-2), and may have

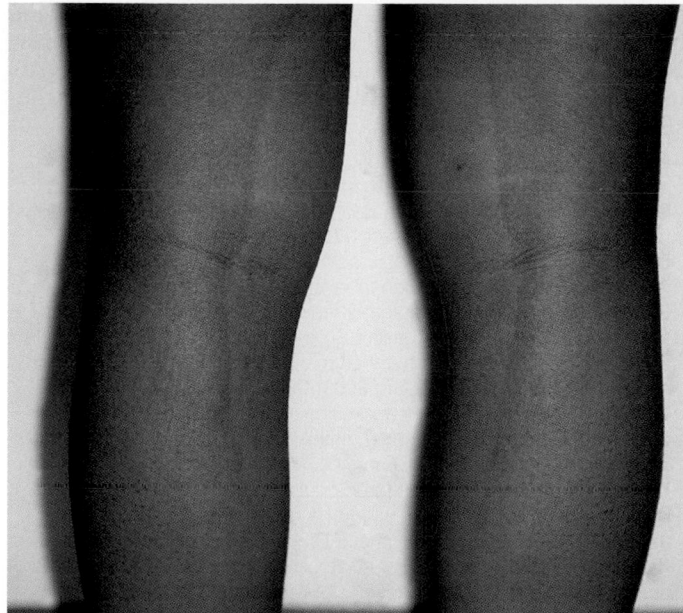

Fig. 36-1 Pigmentary demarcation lines.

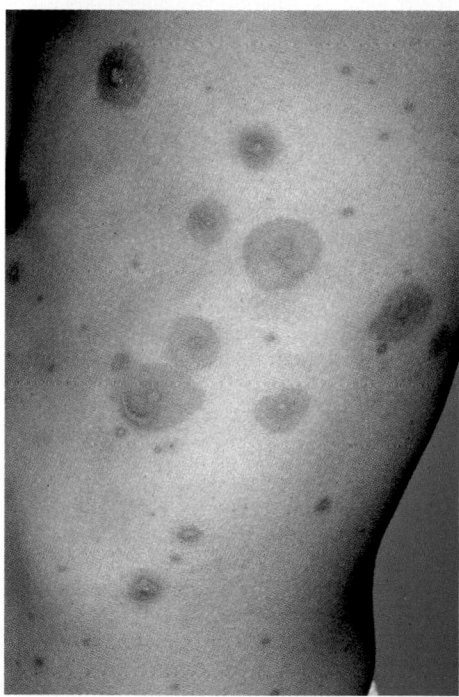

Fig. 36-2 Postinflammatory hyperpigmentation from varicella.

a gray hue (due to dermal melanin). Hypopigmented lesions are prominently lighter than the surrounding area. Histologically, there is melanin in the upper dermis and around upper dermal vessels, located primarily in macrophages (melanophages). The pattern of the dermal melanosis does not predict whether the lesion will be lighter or darker as a result of the prior inflammatory process—hence the tendency of pathologists to provide a diagnosis of "postinflammatory pigmentary alteration" in such cases. Postinflammatory dyspigmentation is addressed initially by treating the underlying skin disease, if possible. The resolution of pityriasis alba with mild topical steroids and moisturizers is an example of resolution of postinflammatory hypopigmentation by treating the cause. This should be the sole approach in hypopigmented lesions after inflammation. For hyperpigmented lesions, hydroquinone may be used in hyperpigmented cases that

enhance with Wood's light. Tretinoin application may enhance the effect of hydroquinone. Laser treatments and chemical peels must be done with extreme caution, as increased pigmentation may result. For additional management approaches, see the section on melasma below.

Grimes PE: Management of hyperpigmentation in darker racial ethnic groups. Semin Cutan Med Surg 2009; 28:77.

Lacz NL, et al: Postinflammatory hyperpigmentation: a common but troubling condition. Int J Dermatol 2004; 43:362.

Ortonne JP, et al: Latest insights into skin hyperpigmentation. J Invest Dermatol Symposium Proceedings 2008; 13:10.

Melasma (chloasma)

Melasma is a very common disorder. It tends to affect darker-complexioned individuals, especially East, West, and Southeast Asians, Hispanics, and black persons who live in areas of intense sun exposure and have Fitzpatrick skin types IV and V. Subtle melasma, as identified by ultraviolet (UV) light examination, may be seen in up to 30% of middle-aged Asian females. Men are also affected, especially those from Central America, who may have prevalence rates as high as 35%. Guatemalan men seem to be at greater risk than Mexican men, and speaking a native tongue is also a risk factor, suggesting a genetic component associated with indigenous heritage.

The pathogenesis of melasma is not known. However, many observations strongly suggest that sun exposure is the primary trigger. Melasma affects the face, a sun-exposed area, and worsens in the summer. Melasma patients have lower MED (minimal erythema dose) to UV light, and pigment more easily with UV exposure. There is an association between the number of melanocytic nevi and the development of vitiligo. The number of nevi, in addition to being familial, is also related to sun exposure. The prevalence of melasma increases with age in both men and women. Solar elastosis is more marked in areas of melasma, compared to unaffected facial skin. At the cellular level, areas of melasma have higher levels of inducible nitric oxide synthase and phosphorylated Akt, an element of the nuclear factor kappa B (NF-κB) pathway. The role of sunlight in inducing melasma may be to cause elevated levels of nitric oxide via the NF-κB pathway. Inducible nitric oxide stimulates tyrosinase activity of melanocytes, increasing local melanin production. This results in the clinically evident hyperpigmentation in sun-exposed sites.

After sun exposure, the second most important triggers for melasma are female hormones. Melasma is more common and severe in women than men. It occurs frequently during pregnancy, with oral contraceptives use, or with hormone replacement therapy (HRT) at menopause. Discontinuing the use of contraceptives or HRT rarely clears the pigmentation and it may last for many years after the drugs are discontinued. In contrast, melasma of pregnancy usually clears within a few months of delivery. Melasma may be seen in other endocrinologic disorders, and with dilantin therapy.

Melasma is characterized by brown patches, typically on the malar prominences and forehead. The forearms may also be affected. There are three clinical patterns of facial vitiligo: centrofacial, malar, and mandibular. The centrofacial and malar patterns comprise the majority of patients (Fig. 36-3), but most patients have multiple types, making this classification not very useful therapeutically. The pigmented patches are usually quite sharply demarcated. While melasma has classically been classified as epidermal- or dermal-based on the presence or absence of Wood's light enhancement, respectively, most cases show both epidermal and dermal melanin. Dermal melanophages are a normal finding in sun-exposed Asian skin. Independent of Wood's light findings, a therapeutic trial of

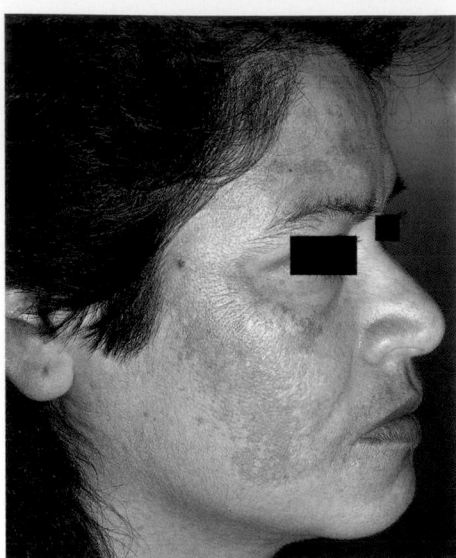

Fig. 36-3 Melasma of the cheek.

some form of hypopigmenting agent should be recommended if the patient requests it.

A number of topical therapies are available. Exposure to sunlight should be avoided and a complete sunblock with broad-spectrum UVA coverage should be used daily. Bleaching creams with hydroquinone are the gold standard and are moderately efficacious; they contain from 2% (available over the counter) to 4% hydroquinone. Tretinoin cream may be added to increase efficacy. While tretinoin alone may reduce melasma, it may also increase pigmentation via its irritant effect. The combination of hydroquinone and tretinoin, administered in conjunction with a topical steroid, has been called "Kligman's formula" and is excellent. This is available as a commercial product, Triluma, used once a day. The efficacy of this product has been reported to be superior to any combination of two of its ingredients, with a more rapid and complete response with the triple combination. Glycolic acid is at times added to hydroquinone to enhance its efficacy. In some patients with melasma, 4% hydroquinone is insufficient and higher doses of hydroquinone must be compounded. Satellite pigmentation and local ochronosis are potential complications from use of these higher-concentration preparations. Mequinol, azelaic acid, kojic acid, licorice extract, ellagic acid, glucosamine, niacinamide, vitamin C, vitamin E, phytosterol, glycyrrhetinic acid, pidobenzone 4%, and arbutin are other therapies with efficacy. Many of these agents are added to cosmetic products for skin lightening, and may be combined, as they act on different steps of melanogenesis.

Various surgical procedures, such as peels and light-based treatments, have been proposed as effective for melasma. Most patients who undergo surgical procedures have been previously treated with hydroquinone, and this therapy is frequently continued or is used in preparation for the surgical treatment. Peels are usually given in a series. It is suggested that repeated peels with glycolic acid, low-concentration TCA, and salicylic acid, when combined with pretreatment with hydroquinone, enhance the improvement obtained with hydroquinone alone, but comparative trials are lacking. The use of surgical modalities for the treatment of melasma should be approached with caution. These products are all irritants and these therapies may be complicated by hyperpigmentation, irritation, hypopigmentation, and even scarring, if not used appropriately. Since these treatments are not standardized from one report to another, the literature is not compara-

ble, and the variable results may be in part technique-dependent. Intense pulse light, fractional resurfacing, erbium:YAG resurfacing, 578 nm copper bromide, and Q-switched Nd:YAG have all been reported as effective. However, results are inconsistent, and complications may result.

Adalatkhah H, et al: Melasma and its association with different types of nevi in women: a case-controlled study. BMC Dermatology 2008; 8:3.

Balkrishnan R, et al: Improved quality of life with effective treatment of facial melasma: the pigment trial. J Drugs Dermatol 2004; 3:377.

Ertam I, et al: Efficiency of ellagic acid and arbutin in melasma: a randomized, prospective, open-label study. J Dermatol 2008; 35:570.

Goldberg DJ, et al: Histologic and ultrastructural analysis of melasma after fractional resurfacing. Lasers Surg Med 2008; 40:134.

Grimes PE: Management of hyperpigmentation in darker racial ethnic groups. Semin Cutan Med Surg 2009; 28:77.

Guevara IL, Pandya AG: Safety and efficacy of 4% hydroquinone combined with 10% glycolic acid, antioxidants, and sunscreen in the treatment of melasma. Int J Dermatol 2003; 42:966.

Hantash BM, Jimenez F: A split-face, double-blind, randomized and placebo-controlled pilot evaluation of a novel oligopeptide for the treatment of recalcitrant melasma. J Drugs Dermatol 2009; 8:732.

Hernandez-Barrera R, et al: Solar elastosis and presence of mast cells as key features in the pathogenesis of melasma. Clin Exp Dermatol 2008; 33:305.

Hurley ME, et al: Efficacy of glycolic acid peels in the treatment of melasma. Arch Dermatol 2002; 138:1578.

Jo HY, et al: Co-localization of inducible nitric oxide synthase and phosphorylated Akt in the lesional skins of patients with melasma. J Dermatol 2009; 36:10.

Kim MJ, et al: Punctate leucoderma after melasma treatment using 1064-nm Q-switched Nd:YAG laser with low pulse energy. J Eur Acad Dermatol Venereol 2009; 23:960.

Li YH, et al: Efficacy and safety of intense pulsed light in treatment of melasma in Chinese patients. Dermatol Surg 2008; 34:693.

Nanda S, et al: Efficacy of hydroquinone (2%) versus tretinoin (0.025%) as adjunct topical agents for chemical peeling in patients of melasma. Dermatol Surg 2004; 30:385.

Ortonne JP, Bissett DL: Latest insights into skin hyperpigmentation. J Investig Dermatol Symp Proc 2008; 13:10.

Pichardo R, et al: Prevalence of melasma and its association with quality of life among adult male migrant Latino workers. Int J Dermatol 2009; 48:22.

Rendon M, et al: Successful treatment of moderate to severe melasma with triple-combination cream and glycolic acid peels: a pilot study. Cutis 2008; 82:372.

Rendon MI: Utilizing combination therapy to optimize melasma outcomes. J Drugs Dermatol 2004; 3:S27.

Sarvjot V, et al: Melasma: a clinicopathological study of 43 cases. Indian J Pathol Microbiol 2009; 52:357.

Scherdin U, et al: Skin-lightening effects of a new face care product in patients with melasma. J Cosmet Dermatol 2008; 7:68.

Sharquie KE, et al: Topical 10% zinc sulfate solution for treatment of melasma. Dermatol Surg 2008; 34:1346.

Varma S, Roberts DL: Melasma of the arms associated with hormone replacement therapy. Br J Dermatol 1999; 141:592.

Wanitphakdeedecha R, et al: Treatment of melasma using variable square pulse Er:YAG laser resurfacing. Dermatol Surg 2009; 35:475.

Zanieri F, et al: Melasma: successful treatment with pidobenzone 4% (K5lipogel). Dermatol Ther 2008; 21:S18.

Pigmented anomalies of the extremities

This group of disorders is linked by the similar clinical features (reticulate pigmented macule) and characteristic histology—adenoid pigmented proliferations of the rete ridges of the interfollicular and infundibular follicular epidermis. Patients may have features of several different syndromes, making classification difficult. They probably represent at least three distinct disorders, but since the genetic cause has not been found for all these conditions, their uniqueness cannot be proven. Interestingly, dermatopathia pigmentosa is due to a mutation in the keratin 14 gene, and Dowling–Degos disease is due to a similar mutation in keratin 5. Keratin 5 and 14 are a keratin pair highly expressed and required for structural integrity of the basal cell layer. Also the rare EB subtype, EB simplex with mottled pigmentation, is also due to a mutation in keratin 14. These genetic clues can explain how slightly different syndromes can have similar phenotypes, since the genetic defects are in proteins that interact in vivo.

Dyschromatosis symmetrica hereditaria (DSH) (reticulate acropigmentation of Dohi)

Originally described and still reported primarily in the Japanese, acropigmentation of Dohi has been found to affect individuals from Europe, India, and the Caribbean. It is also referred to as dyschromatosis symmetrica hereditaria (DSH) or symmetrical dyschromatosis of the extremities. It is inherited most commonly as an autosomal-dominant trait, although autosomal-recessive kindreds have been reported. Patients develop progressive hyperpigmented and hypopigmented macules, often mixed in a reticulate pattern, concentrated on the dorsal extremities, especially the dorsal hands and feet. The lesions vary in size from pinpoint to pea-sized. Freckle-like macules can present on the face. Lesions appear in infancy or early childhood and commonly stop spreading before adolescence. The pigmentary lesions last for life. The autosomal-dominant form of DSH is due to a mutation in the *DSRAD* gene, which encodes a double-stranded RNA-specific adenosine deaminase, an RNA editing enzyme. There is no association between the site of the mutation in this gene and the clinical phenotype.

Alfadley A, et al: Reticulate acropigmentation of Dohi: a case report of autosomal recessive inheritance. J Am Acad Dermatol 2000; 43:113.
Li M, et al: A novel mutation of the *DSRAD* gene in a Chinese family with dyschromatosis symmetrica hereditaria. Clin Exp Dermatol 2004; 29:533.
Obieta MP: Familial reticulate acropigmentation of Dohi: a case report. Dermatol Online J 2006; 12:16.
Oyama M, et al: Dyschromatosis symmetrica hereditaria (reticulate acropigmentation of Dohi): report of a Japanese family with the condition and a literature review of 185 cases. Br J Dermatol 1999; 140:491.
Suzuki N, et al: Mutation analysis of the *ADAR1* gene in dyschromatosis symmetrica hereditaria and genetic differentiation from both dyschromatosis universalis hereditaria and acropigmentatio reticularis. J Invest Dermatol 2005; 124:1186.

Dyschromatosis universalis hereditaria (DUH)

Dyschromatosis universalis hereditaria is a rare autosomal or autosomal-recessive genodermatosis characterized by reticulate hyper- and hypopigmented macules in a generalized distribution (Fig. 36-4). Lesions appear in childhood, often in the first few months of life. The palms, soles, and mucous membranes of the mouth and tongue may be diffusely pigmented, with hypopigmented macules interspersed. Most DUH patients do not show other symptoms and are otherwise well. Uncommonly reported associations include ocular and auditory abnormalities, photosensitivity, developmental delay, and short stature. In different kindreds the causal gene has been reported on chromosome 6 or 12, making this syndrome genetically distinct from DSH and Dowling–Degos disease.

Al Hawasai K, et al: Dyschromatosis universalis hereditaria: report of a case and review of the literature. Pediatr Dermatol 2002; 19:523.
Bukhari IA, et al: Dyschromatosis universalis hereditaria as an autosomal recessive disease in five members of one family. J Eur Acad Dermatol Venereol 2006; 20:628.
Kenani N, et al: Dyschromatosis universalis hereditaria: two cases. Dermatol Online J 2008; 14:16.

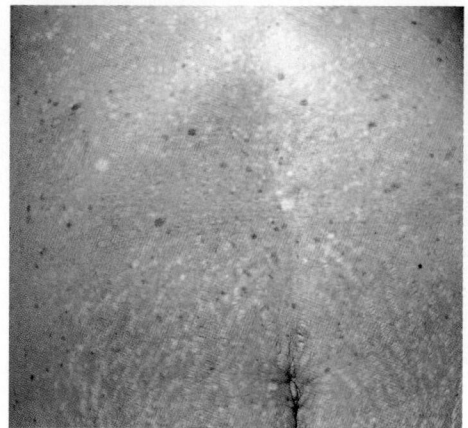

Fig. 36-4 Dyschromatosis universalis hereditaria.

Nuber UA, et al: Dyschromatosis universalis hereditaria: familial case and ultrastructural skin investigation. Am J Med Genet A 2004; 125:261.
Sethuraman G, et al: Dyschromatosis universalis hereditaria. Clin Exp Dermatol 2002; 27:477.
Stuhrmann M, et al: Dyschromatosis universalis hereditaria: evidence for autosomal recessive inheritance and identification of a new locus on chromosome 12q21–q23. Clin Genet 2008; 73:566.

Reticular pigmented anomaly of the flexures (Dowling–Degos disease)

Reticular pigmented anomaly of the flexures is a rare autosomal-dominant pigmentary disorder; it is sometimes called Dowling–Degos disease or dark dot disease. Pigmentation usually appears at puberty or in early adolescence, but may present later in adulthood. The skin lesions primarily affect the axillae, neck, and inframammary/sternal areas. In some cases, the dorsal hands are involved. The pigmentation is reticular; at the periphery, discrete, brownish-black macules surround the partly confluent central pigmented area. In more mildly affected patients the pigmentation is dappled. The pigmentation progresses very gradually. There are frequently acneiform, pitted scars, sometimes pigmented, about the mouth. Comedonal and cystic lesions have been described on the flexures and in the axilla. Hidradenitis suppurativa-like lesions in the groin and axilla may occur. Patients may complain that the condition is worse during hot weather. Squamous cell carcinoma of the buttocks or perianal area has been described.

Histologically, in addition to the typical lentiginous adenoid proliferations of the rete ridges, small horn cysts may be present, so that the pattern resembles that of a reticulated seborrheic keratosis. Comedones may be present. Erbium:YAG laser has treated the pigmented lesions of the chest.

Dowling–Degos disease is caused by mutations in the keratin 5 gene. The reported mutations have been proposed as altering function of the initiation codon, or premature termination of the keratin 5 polypeptide. Similar mutations occur in Galli–Galli disease, suggesting that the two conditions represent variants of the same disorder, rather than separate diseases.

Galli–Galli disease

Galli–Galli disease is now recognized as a variant of Dowling–Degos disease, also caused by mutations in the keratin 5 gene. The skin lesions are 1–2 mm, slightly keratotic, red to dark brown papules, which are focally confluent in a reticulate pattern (Fig. 36-5). The skin lesions favor skinfolds but other skin sites may also be involved. The neck, axillae, upper

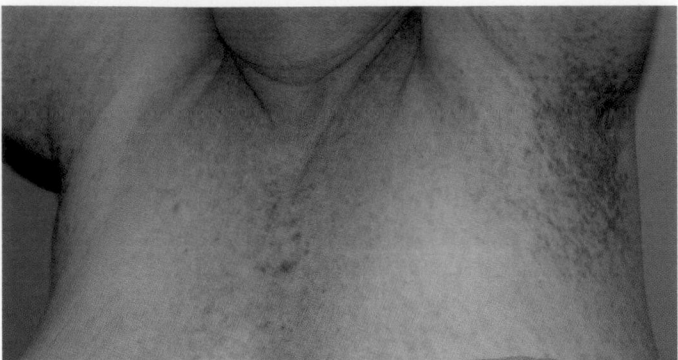

Fig. 36-5 Galli–Galli disease.

extremities, dorsal hands, trunk, groin, and even the scrotum and lower extremities may be affected. Histologically, there is prominent digitate downgrowth of the rete ridges, identical to that seen in Dowling–Degos disease. The characteristic histologic feature is a suprabasilar cleft and suprapapillary thinning of the epidermis. There is no dyskeratosis, as is seen in Grover's disease.

Braun-Falco M, et al: Galli–Galli disease: an unrecognized entity or an acantholytic variant of Dowling–Degos' disease? J Am Acad Dermatol 2001; 45:760.

El Shabrawi-Caelen L, et al: The expanding spectrum of Galli–Galli disease. J Am Acad Dermatol 2007; 56:S86.

Gilchrist H, et al: Galli–Galli disease: a case report with review of the literature. J Am Acad Dermatol 2008; 58:299.

Hanneken S, et al: Systematic mutation screening of KRTS supports the hypothesis that Galli-Galli disease is a variant of Dowling-Degos disease. Br J Dermatol 2010; 163:197.

Kossard S, Krivanek J: Dowling–Degos' disease—a heat aggravated variant. Australas J Dermatol 2001; 42:214.

Loo WJ, et al: Hidradenitis suppurativa, Dowling–Degos and multiple epidermal cysts: a new follicular occlusion triad. Clin Exp Dermatol 2004; 29:622.

Muller CS, et al: Changing a concept—controversy on the confusing spectrum of the reticulate pigmented disorders of the skin. J Cutan Pathol 2009; 36:44.

Sprecher E, et al: Galli–Galli disease is an acantholytic variant of Dowling–Degos disease. Br J Dermatol 2007; 156:572.

Wu YH, Lin YC: Generalized Dowling–Degos disease. J Am Acad Dermatol 2007; 57:327.

Reticulate acropigmentation of Kitamura

Reticulate acropigmentation of Kitamura is a rare autosomal-dominant disease, which initially was recognized in Japan, but now has been seen in many countries, usually in persons of color. The characteristic presentation is pigmented, angulated, irregular, freckle-like lesions with atrophy, arranged in a reticulate pattern on the dorsal feet and hands. Lesions start in the first to second decade, gradually progress, and slowly darken over time. The axillae and groin may be affected, as can the skin of the trunk and more proximal extremities. Linear irregular breaks in the dermatoglyphics of the palms are characteristic and help to distinguish this disorder from the other "reticulate flexural anomalies."

Kocaturk E, et al: Reticulate acropigmentation of Kitamura: report of a familial case. Dermatol Online J 2008; 14:7.

Dermatopathia pigmentosa reticularis

Dermatopathia pigmentosa reticularis (DPR) is an autosomal-dominant disorder characterized by the triad of generalized reticulate hyperpigmentation (Fig. 36-6), noncicatricial alopecia, and onychodystrophy. Additional associations include loss of dermatoglyphics, hypo- or hyperhidrosis, pigmented

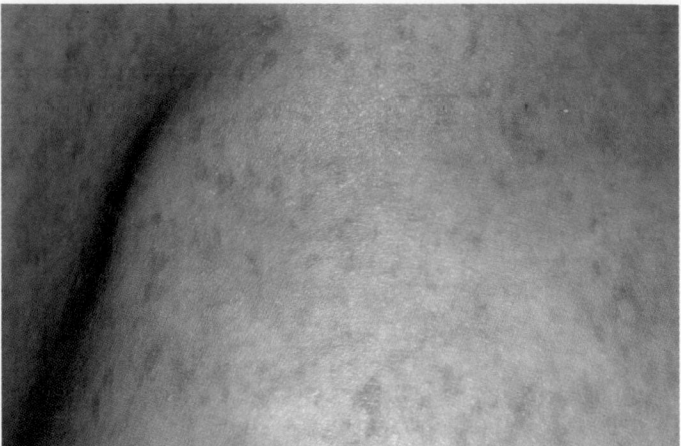

Fig. 36-6 Dermatopathia pigmentosa reticularis.

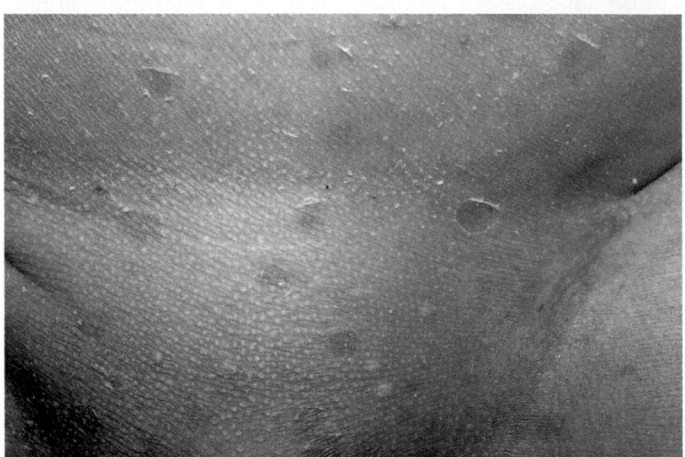

Fig. 36-7 Transient neonatal pustulosis.

lesions of the oral mucosa, palmoplantar hyperkeratosis, and nonscarring blisters on the dorsa of the hands and feet. Wiry scalp hair and digital fibromatosis have also been reported. Dental anomalies are not a feature of DPR. Some members of families affected by Naegeli–Franceschetti–Jadassohn syndrome (NFJS) have clinical features identical to DPR. Both NFJS and DPR are due to mutations in the E1/V1 encoding region of the keratin 14 gene, which would lead to premature termination at the translation initiation site of keratin 14. NFJS and DPR are now best considered variants of the same genetic disorder. EB simplex with mottled pigmentation also has a mutation in keratin 14, explaining the presence of blistering in DPR and mottled pigmentation in this unique form of EB.

Brar BK, et al: Dermatopathia pigmentosa reticularis. Pediatr Dermatol 2007; 24:566.

Goh BK, et al: A case of dermatopathia pigmentosa reticularis with wiry scalp hair and digital fibromatosis resulting from a recurrent KRT14 mutation. Clin Exp Dermatol 2009; 34:340.

Lugassy J, et al: Naegeli–Franceschetti–Jadassohn syndrome and dermatopathia pigmentosa reticularis: two allelic ectodermal dysplasias caused by dominant mutations in KRT14. Am J Hum Genet 2006; 79:724.

Tunca M, et al: Early-onset gastric carcinoma in a man with dermatopathia pigmentosa reticularis. Int J Dermatol 2008; 47:641.

Transient neonatal pustular melanosis

Also called transient neonatal pustulosis, this disorder is present at birth. Newborns present with 1–3 mm flaccid, superficial fragile pustules (Fig. 36-7). Some of the pustules may have already resolved in utero, leaving pigmented macules.

Lesions affect the chin, neck, forehead, back, and buttocks, but can occur anywhere. In dark-skinned infants, pigmented macules may persist for weeks or months after the pustules have healed, whereas in affected lighter-skinned neonates, dyspigmentation less commonly occurs. The condition is observed in 4.4% of black and 0.6% of white newborns.

Histologically, there are intracorneal or subcorneal aggregates predominantly of neutrophils, but eosinophils may also be found. Dermal inflammation is composed of a mixture of neutrophils and eosinophils. The differential diagnosis includes erythema toxicum neonatorum, neonatal acne, and acropustulosis of infancy.

Van Praag MC, et al: Diagnosis and treatment of pustular disorders in the neonate. Pediatr Dermatol 1997; 14:131.

Peutz–Jeghers syndrome

Peutz–Jeghers syndrome (PJS) is characterized by hyperpigmented macules on the lips and oral mucosa, and polyposis of the small intestine. The dark brown or black macules appear typically on the lips, especially the lower lip, in infancy or early childhood (Fig. 36-8). Similar lesions may appear on the buccal mucosa, tongue, gingiva, and genital mucosa; macules may also occur around the mouth, on the central face, and on the backs of the hands, especially the fingers, toes, and tops of the feet. More than two-thirds of patients have lesions on the hands and feet, and 95% have perioral lesions. Skin lesions grow in size and number until puberty, after which they begin to regress. Similar pigmentation may be seen in the bowel.

The associated polyposis involves the small intestine by preference (64%), but hamartomatous polyps may also occur in the stomach (49%), colon (49%), and rectum (32%). The polyposis of the small intestine may cause repeated bouts of abdominal pain and vomiting. Bleeding is common; intussusception is frequent (47%).

Patients with PJS have a 15-fold greater lifetime cancer risk (85–93%) than the general population. The greatest risk is for gastrointestinal malignancy of the colon (39% of patients), stomach (29% of patients), and small intestine (13% of patients). Cancers begin to appear around age 30 years. Cancers occur in both the gastrointestinal tract and extraintestinal sites. Pancreas (36%), breast (can be bilateral, 54%), ovary (21%), lung, cervix, uterus, and thyroid carcinomas may develop. Sertoli–Leydig cell stromal tumors occur in 9% of PJS males,

and sex cord tumors with annular tubules can occur in female PJS patients. Patients with PJS lacking an *STK11/LKB1* mutation have a 40% risk of cholangiocarcinoma.

The syndrome is transmitted as a simple mendelian dominant trait. Between 50 and 70% of families with PJS have a germline mutation of the *STK11/LKB1* tumor suppressor gene on chromosome 19p13. The gene product is a serine–threonine kinase involved in signal transduction in the mTOR pathway. Patients have one inactive copy of this gene. Patients with truncation of the gene rather than a missense mutation are more severely affected, suggesting a phenotype/genotype correlation.

Laugier–Hunziker syndrome and Cronkhite–Canada syndrome should be considered in the differential diagnosis. Laugier–Hunziker syndrome presents with mucosal pigmentation and pigmented nail streaks. Cronkhite–Canada syndrome consists of melanotic macules on the fingers and gastrointestinal polyposis. Also there is generalized, uniform darkening of the skin, extensive alopecia, and onychodystrophy. The polyps that occur are usually benign adenomas and may involve the entire gastrointestinal tract. A protein-losing enteropathy may develop and is associated with the degree of intestinal polyposis. Onset is typically after age 30 in this sporadically occurring, generally benign condition. Hypogeusia is the dominant initial symptom, followed by diarrhea and ectodermal changes. Seventy-five percent of all cases have been reported from Japan. Zinc therapy may improve the hypogeusia and other symptoms.

Barnard J: Screening and surveillance recommendations for pediatric gastrointestinal polyposis syndromes. J Pediatr Gastroenterol Nutr 2009; 48:S75.

Baudendistel TE, et al: Clinical problem-solving. The leading diagnosis—a 23-year-old black woman presented to the emergency department with diffuse, colicky abdominal pain of 1 hour's duration. N Engl J Med 2007; 357:2389.

Campos-Munoz L, et al: Dermoscopy of Peutz–Jeghers syndrome. J Eur Acad Dermatol Venereol 2009; 23:730.

Cureton E, Kim S: Images in clinical medicine. Peutz–Jeghers syndrome. N Engl J Med 2007; 357:e9.

Flutter L, Mulik R: Peutz–Jegher syndrome. Arch Dis Child 2008; 93:163.

Heymann WR: Peutz–Jeghers syndrome. J Am Acad Dermatol 2007; 57:513.

Hezel AF, Bardeesy N: LKB1; linking cell structure and tumor suppression. Oncogene 2008; 27:6908.

Katajisto P, et al: LKB1 signaling in mesenchymal cells required for suppression of gastrointestinal polyposis. Nat Genet 2008; 40:455.

Kilic-Okman T, et al: Breast cancer, ovarian gonadoblastoma and cervical cancer in a patient with Peutz–Jeghers syndrome. Arch Gynecol Obstet 2008; 278:75.

Lynch HT, et al: Hereditary colorectal cancer syndromes: molecular genetics, genetic counseling, diagnosis and management. Fam Cancer 2008; 7:27.

Santos P, et al: Perioral pigmentation: what is your diagnosis? Dermatol Online J 2008; 14:16.

Saranrittichai S: Peutz–Jeghers syndrome and colon cancer in a 10-year-old girl: implications for when and how to start screening? Asian Pac J Cancer Prev 2008; 9:159.

Velez A, et al: Two novel LKB1 mutations in Colombian Peutz–Jeghers syndrome patients. Clin Genet 2009; 75:304.

Wong SS, et al: Peutz–Jeghers syndrome associated with primary malignant melanoma of the rectum. Br J Dermatol 1996; 135:439.

Yoo JH, et al: A novel de novo mutation in the serine-threonine kinase STK11 gene in a Korean patient with Peutz–Jeghers syndrome. BMC Med Genet 2008; 9:44.

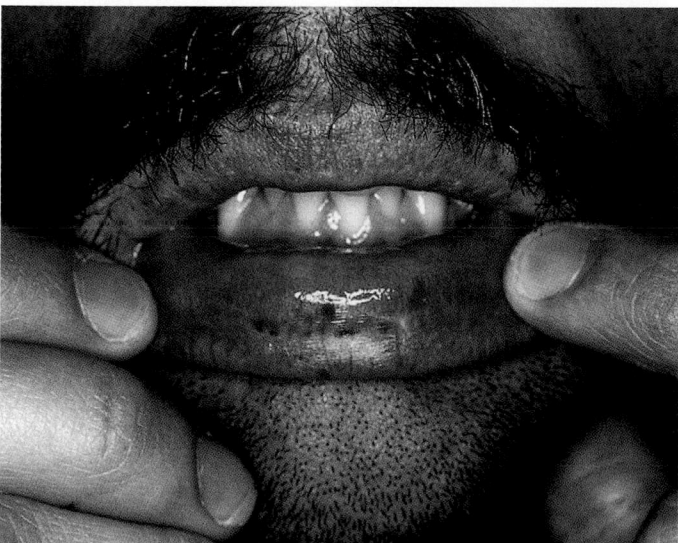

Fig. 36-8 Peutz–Jeghers syndrome, macular pigmentation of the lower lip.

Riehl melanosis

Riehl melanosis describes the pigmentation that occurs following photoallergic contact dermatitis, usually from fragrances and essential oils in cosmetics. This term is no longer used.

Miyoshi K, et al: Riehl's melanosis-like eruption associated with Sjögren's syndrome. J Dermatol 1997; 24:784.

Seike M, et al: Coexistence of Riehl's melanosis and lichen planus. J Dermatol 2003; 30:132.

Serrano G, et al: Riehl's melanosis. J Am Acad Dermatol 1989; 21:1057.

Tar melanosis (melanodermatitis toxica lichenoides)

Tar melanosis is an occupational dermatosis that occurs among tar handlers after several years' exposure. Severe widespread itching develops and is soon followed by the appearance of reticular pigmentation, telangiectases, and a shiny appearance of the skin. In addition, there is a hyperhidrotic tendency. Small, dark, lichenoid, follicular papules become profuse on the extremities, particularly the forearms. Bullae are sometimes observed. This represents a photosensitivity or phototoxicity induced by tar. This condition is rarely observed with current occupational protections.

Lebwohl M, et al: Tar melanosis. Mt Sinai J Med 1995; 62:412.

Familial progressive hyperpigmentation

Familial progressive hyperpigmentation (FPH) is characterized by patches of hyperpigmentation, present at birth, which increase in size and number with age. Later, hyperpigmentation appears in the conjunctivae and the buccal mucosa. Eventually, a large portion of the skin and mucous membranes becomes involved. Inheritance is in an autosomal-dominant pattern with variable penetrance. A focus in a small village in Germany has recently been reported. FPH is differentiated from other hyperpigmentations mainly by the presence of bizarre, sharply marginated patterns of hyperpigmented skin. A gain-of-function mutation in *c-KIT* has been described in an affected kindred.

Betts CM, et al: Progressive hyperpigmentation: case report with a clinical, histological, and ultrastructural investigation. Dermatology 1994; 189:384.

Wang ZQ, et al: Gain-of-function mutation of *KIT* ligand on melanin synthesis causes familial progressive hyperpigmentation. Am J Hum Genet 2009; 84:672.

Zanardo L, et al: Progressive hyperpigmentation and generalized lentiginosis without associated systemic symptoms: a rare hereditary pigmentation disorder in south-east Germany. Acta Derm Venereol 2004; 84:57.

Periorbital hyperpigmentation

Dark circles around the eyes are not uncommon, often familial, and frequently found in individuals with dark pigmentation or Mediterranean ancestry. Atopic patients may also exhibit periorbital pigmentation (allergic shiners). There are probably multiple pathogenic factors involved, including epidermal hypermelanosis, dermal melanosis, increased vasculature, and normal anatomic variants. Since there are multiple etiologies, treatment is often ineffective.

Metallic discolorations

Pigmentation may develop from the deposit of fine metallic particles in the skin. The metal may be carried to the skin by the bloodstream or may permeate into it from surface applications. Discolorations from medications containing silver and gold are discussed in Chapter 6.

Arsenic

Acute arsenic poisoning is associated with flushing on day 1 of exposure, and facial edema on days 2–5. A morbilliform eruption appears on days 4–6. Hepatic dysfunction occurs simultaneously with the appearance of an eruption of discrete red–brown, erythematous papules in the intertriginous areas (areas of friction) of the lower abdomen, buttocks, and lateral upper chest. It regresses after 2–3 weeks, at times accompanied by acral desquamation. Three months after exposure, Mee's lines, total leukonychia, Beau's lines, and onychodystrophy may be seen. Periungual pigmentation occurs in up to half of acutely poisoned patients at 3 months.

Arsenic is an elemental metal that is ubiquitous, existing in nature as metalloids, alloys, and a variety of chemical compounds. These various forms of arsenic may be deposited into water, soil, and vegetation, producing serious health risks. In West Bengal, India, an estimated 200 000 people have arsenic-induced skin disorders and more than 1 million Indians are drinking arsenic-laced water from contaminated wells. Arsenic-contaminated water sources are a worldwide health concern also affecting countries such as Japan, Chile, Taiwan, and Mongolia. It is not known what are safe levels of arsenic in drinking water.

Industries using arsenical compounds place their workers at risk of exposure. Use of arsenic pesticides and exposure to sodium arsenite, used as a veterinary pesticide exposing sheep-dip workers, has resulted in chronic arsenism. In the US arsenic is used for pesticides, rodenticides, herbicides, insecticides, desiccants, feed additives, and wood preservatives. Pressure-treated lumber, particularly the marine-treated plywood, exposes carpenters and shipbuilders. The largest risk from wood products, however, occurs when pretreated wood is burned and the arsenic fumes are inhaled. Electroplating silver may also require arsenic. Another potential source of exposure during the 1960s was American tobacco, resulting mostly from the use of arsenic-containing insecticides.

The most common form of arsenic exposure worldwide is chronic, from contaminated wells and ground water. In areas of exposure, even young children can demonstrate cutaneous stigmata. Skin lesions occur only when arsenic concentrations are 200 µg/L or more. Two characteristic forms of skin disease occur. Cutaneous hyperpigmentation is the most common and earliest side effect. The hyperpigmentation is usually diffuse, most prominent on the trunk. Patchy hyperpigmentation may be accentuated in the inguinal folds, on the areolae, and on palmar creases. This can simulate Addison's disease. Areas of hypopigmentation may be scattered in the hyperpigmented areas, giving a "raindrop" appearance. Focal melanotic macules may also be present. The pigmentation may resolve or persist indefinitely. Punctate keratoses on the palms and soles are characteristic. Diffuse palmoplantar keratoderma may rarely occur. Blackfoot disease—arsenic-induced peripheral vascular disease that can lead to vasospasm and peripheral gangrene—and a severe peripheral neuropathy can also occur with chronic arsenic ingestion. Risk factors for development of clinically evident arsenic-induced disease include: concentration of arsenic contamination in exposure source (usually water), and malnutrition/low body mass index (BMI). There is significant variation in prevalence of skin disease from arsenic exposure in different racial groups and different individuals. There is evidence that polymorphisms in arsenic-metabolizing (methylation) pathways, specifically converting monomethylarsonic acid to dimethylarsinic acid, may explain these risk differences. Arsenic exposure is also associated with a significant reduction in circulating helper T cells, perhaps contributing to increased cancer risk. One study identified polymorphisms in the *XPD* gene as a risk factor for arsenic-induced skin lesions. Histologically, the arsenical keratosis on the palms and soles shows hyperkeratosis, parakeratosis, acanthosis, and papillomatosis. Approximately 6–7% of hyperkeratotic skin lesions will demonstrate basilar atypia, and about 1% will show cancer. Arsenic exposure leads to the development of nonmelanoma skin cancers. Bowen's disease represents the majority of arsenic-induced skin cancers and may appear on sun-exposed or sun-protected skin. Basal cell carcinomas are frequent, are usually multiple, are most common on the trunk, and can be in sun-protected sites. Squamous cell carcinoma may also occur. Acitretin may improve "arsenical" keratoses. Arsenic exposure results in increased risk for lung, liver, and renal carcinoma.

Ahsan T, et al: Chronic arsenic poisoning. J Pak Med Assoc 2009; 59:105.

Chakraborti D, et al: Status of groundwater arsenic contamination in the state of West Bengal, India: a 20-year study report. Mol Nutr Food Res 2009; 53:542.

Elmariah SB, et al: Invasive squamous-cell carcinoma and arsenical keratoses. Dermatol Online J 2008; 14:24.

Li X, et al: Arsenic methylation capacity and its correlation with skin lesions induced by contaminated drinking water consumption in residents of chronic arsenicosis area. Environ Toxicol 2009 Sep 18 (Epub ahead of print).

Liao WT, et al: Differential effects of arsenic on cutaneous and systemic immunity: focusing on CD4+ cell apoptosis in patients with arsenic-induced Bowen's disease. Carcinogenesis 2009; 30:1064.

Lin GF, et al: Association of XPD/ERCC2 G23591A and A35931C polymorphisms with skin lesion prevalence in a multiethnic, arseniasis-hyperendemic village exposed to indoor combustion of high arsenic coal. Arch Toxicol 2009 Oct 16 (Epub ahead of print).

Pilsner JR, et al: Folate deficiency, hyperhomocysteinemia, low urinary creatinine, and hypomethylation of leukocyte DNA are risk factors for arsenic-induced skin lesions. Environ Health Perspect 2009; 117:254.

Rahman MM, et al: Chronic exposure of arsenic via drinking water and its adverse health impacts on humans. Environ Geochem Health 2009; 31:189.

Ratnaike RN: Acute and chronic arsenic toxicity. Postgrad Med J 2003; 79:391.

Rossman TG, et al: Evidence that arsenite acts as a cocarcinogen in skin cancer. Toxicol Appl Pharmacol 2004; 198:394.

Schuhmacher-Wolz U, et al: Oral exposure to inorganic arsenic: evaluation of its carcinogenic and non-carcinogenic effects. Crit Rev Toxicol 2009; 39:271.

Sengupta SR, et al: Pathogenesis, clinical features and pathology of chronic arsenicosis. Indian J Dermatol Venereol Leprol 2008; 74:559.

Smith AH, Steinmaus CM: Health effects of arsenic and chromium in drinking water: recent human findings. Annu Rev Public Health 2009; 30:107.

Tomi NS, et al: A silver man. Lancet 2004; 363:532.

Valenzuela OL, et al: Association of AS3MT polymorphisms and the risk of premalignant arsenic skin lesions. Toxicol Appl Pharmacol 2009; 239:200.

Waalkes MP, et al: Arsenic exposure in utero exacerbates skin cancer response in adulthood with contemporaneous distortion of tumor stem cell dynamics. Cancer Res 2008; 68:8278.

Watson K, Creamer D: Arsenic-induced keratoses and Bowen's disease. Clin Exp Dermatol 2004; 29:46.

Xia Y, et al: Well water arsenic exposure, arsenic induced skin-lesions and self-reported morbidity in Inner Mongolia. Int J Environ Res Public Health 2009; 6:1010.

Lead

Chronic lead poisoning can produce a "lead hue," with lividity and pallor, and a deposit of lead in the gums may occur: the "lead line" (Fig. 36-9).

Iron

In the past, soluble iron compounds were used in the treatment of allergic contact and other dermatitides. In eroded

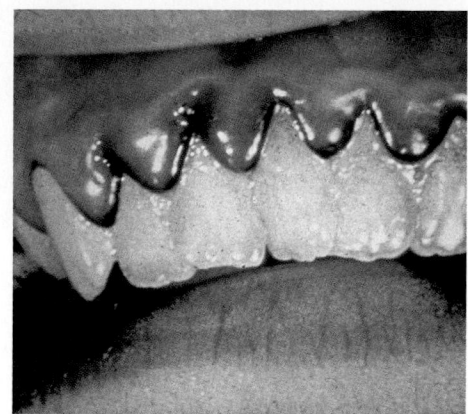

Fig. 36-9 Lead line.

areas, iron was sometimes deposited in the skin, like a tattoo. The use of Monsel solution can produce similar tattooing, so aluminum chloride is now preferred. If Monsel is used to minimize tattooing, it is best applied with a cotton-tipped applicator barely moistened with the solution, then rolled across a wound that has just been blotted dry.

Hemochromatosis

Hemochromatosis is a disorder caused by mutations in at least five different genes involved in iron absorption. It is very common in the white European population, where the majority of the mutations are at two genetic loci, C282Y and H63D, allowing for widespread genetic screening. At least four different phenotypes are described. Many of the patients with the most common genetic defects do not develop any disease (perhaps 25% of men and 6% of women). Men are affected more frequently and at an earlier age (usually between 30 and 50 years). With widespread genetic testing, the age of diagnosis has been decreased, and the number of asymptomatic affected females has dramatically increased. The characteristic cutaneous manifestation is gray to brown mucocutaneous hyperpigmentation. This is enhanced in sun-exposed areas of the forearms, dorsal hands, and face, as well as in the inguinal area. The mucous membranes are pigmented in up to 20% of patients. The percentage of affected males with pigmentation is around 30% and in women fewer than 10% of diagnosed patients have skin changes. Other skin changes that can be seen include koilonychia and localized ichthyosis. Alopecia is common and pruritus can occur. Porphyria cutanea tarda may be present due to inhibition of uroporphyrinogen decarboxylase in the liver by iron overload. In patients with chronic venous insufficiency, the risk of lower leg ulceration is increased six-fold in those also carrying the C282Y mutation, leading some to suggest that this test should be ordered in at-risk patients at the initial stages of venous insufficiency. Biopsy of affected hyperpigmented skin shows dermal iron deposition, but the visible pigmentation is actually increased epidermal melanin in the basal cell layer.

The most seriously affected organ is the liver. Hepatomegaly and elevated liver function tests are signs of hepatic iron overload. Cirrhosis and hepatocellular carcinoma may develop, but are now uncommon with early diagnosis and treatment. The endocrine system is also affected, with diabetes mellitus, impotence, and amenorrhea being most common. Arthropathy is seen in about 50% of women and 40% of men. Cardiac abnormalities include heart failure and arrhythmias. Consuming alcohol and smoking, as well as coexistent hepatitis C infection, all make it more likely that persons with genetic predisposition will develop clinical disease.

Laboratory evaluation should be pursued in persons with appropriate clinical findings suggesting the diagnosis of hemochromatosis. Levels of plasma iron and the serum iron-binding protein are elevated. The transferrin saturation (TS = serum iron/total iron-binding capacity) is a useful screening measure. A score of 45 or less is normal, except in premenopausal women when greater than 35 may be considered abnormal. High serum ferritin levels are also present. Genotyping is now performed in persons with a TS greater than 45 and an elevated ferritin, and confirms the diagnosis. Liver biopsy is reserved for persons with elevated liver function tests, a ferritin greater than 1000, or age over 40.

Four different genes cause autosomal-recessive hemochromatosis and one causes autosomal-dominant disease. The most common autosomal-recessive form is due to a mutation in the *HFE* gene, most frequently C282Y, and less commonly H63D. The incidence of homozygosity for C282Y is 5 in 1000 persons of northern European descent, making it ten times more common than cystic fibrosis. Compound heterozygotes (C282Y/H63D) also develop disease. Two autosomal-recessive forms of juvenile hereditary hemochromatosis are described, due to mutations in the *Hemojuvelin* and *Hepcidin* genes, respectively. Mutations in the transferrin receptor 2 gene lead to a form of autosomal-recessive adult-onset hemochromatosis. Ferroportin mutation leads to an adult-onset form of autosomal-dominant hemochromatosis.

All forms of hemochromatosis are treated with phlebotomy until satisfactory iron levels are attained. Vitamin C supplementation must be avoided, as it can worsen the disease. Raw seafood should be avoided because *Vibrio vulnificus* infection may occur. Phlebotomy can prevent cirrhosis. Once cirrhosis is present, phlebotomy does not prevent the development of hepatocellular carcinoma, which occurs in 30% of patients.

Limdi JK, Crampton JR: Hereditary haemochromatosis. Q J Med 2004; 97:315.
Pietrangelo A: Hereditary hemochromatosis—a new look at an old disease. N Engl J Med 2004; 350:2383.
Scotet V, et al: Impact of HFE genetic testing on clinical presentation of hereditary hemochromatosis: new epidemiological data. BMC Med Genet 2005; 6:24.
Zamboni P, et al: Hemochromatosis C282Y gene mutation increases the risk of venous leg ulceration. J Vasc Surg 2005; 42:309.

Titanium

A titanium-containing ointment caused yellowish papules on the penis in a patient. Titanium screws used for orthopedic procedures, if they come in close proximity to the skin, can cause cutaneous blue–black hyperpigmentation.

Akimoto M, et al: Metallosis of the skin mimicking malignant skin tumor. Br J Dermatol 2003; 149:653.
Dupre A, et al: Titanium pigmentation. Arch Dermatol 1985; 121:656.

Canthaxanthin

The orange–red pigment, canthaxanthin, is present in many plants (notably algae and mushrooms) and in bacteria, crustaceans, sea trout, and feathers. When ingested for the purpose of simulating a tan, its deposition in the panniculus imparts a golden orange hue to the skin. Stools become brick red and the plasma orange, and golden deposits appear in the retina. Its use is not recommended, since it may be associated with liver and retinal damage.

Lober CW: Canthaxanthin: the "tanning" pill. J Am Acad Dermatol 1985; 13:660.

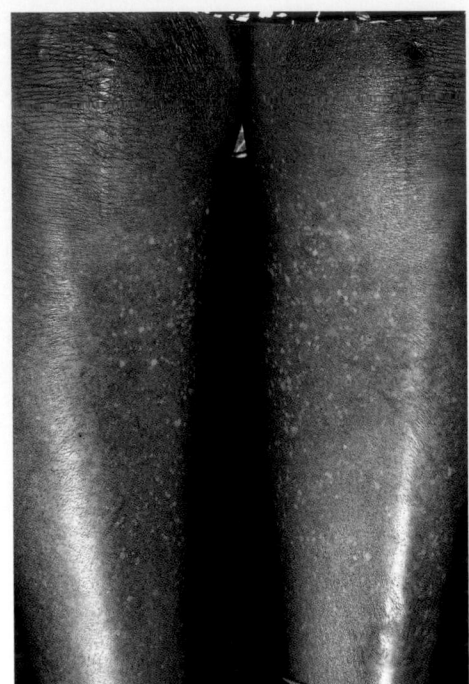

Fig. 36-10 Idiopathic guttate hypomelanosis.

Idiopathic guttate hypomelanosis (leukopathia symmetrica progressiva)

Idiopathic guttate hypomelanosis is a very common acquired disorder that affects women more frequently than men. It usually occurs after age 40 and its prevalence increases with age. The lesions occur chiefly on the shins (Fig. 36-10) and forearms, suggesting that sun exposure plays a role. Widespread lesions have occurred in patients receiving UVB therapy. Individual lesions are small (2–5 mm on average), hypopigmented macules. They usually number between 10 and 30, but numerous lesions may occur. Lesions spare the trunk and face. The lesions are irregularly shaped and very sharply defined, like depigmented ephelides. Histologically, there is epidermal atrophy and reduced numbers of hypoactive melanocytes. Cryotherapy can improve the appearance of the lesions.

Arrunategui A, et al: HLA-DQ3 is associated with idiopathic guttate hypomelanosis, whereas HLA-DR8 is not, in a group of renal transplant patients. Int J Dermatol 2002; 41:744.
Kaya TI, et al: Idiopathic guttate hypomelanosis: idiopathic or ultraviolet induced? Photodermatol Photoimmunol Photomed 2005; 21:270.

Vitiligo

Vitiligo usually begins in childhood or young adulthood, with a peak onset between 10 and 30 years. About half of cases begin before the age of 20. The prevalence ranges from 0.5% to 1%. Although females are disproportionately represented among patients seeking care, it is not known whether they are actually more commonly affected or simply are more likely to seek medical care. Vitiligo has developed in recipients of bone marrow transplant or lymphocyte infusions from patients with vitiligo.

Clinical features

Vitiligo is an acquired pigmentary anomaly of the skin manifested by depigmented white patches surrounded by a normal

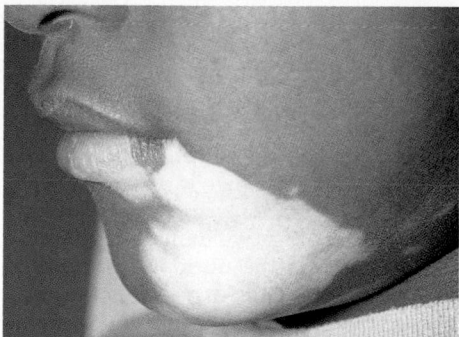

Fig. 36-11 Localized vitiligo.

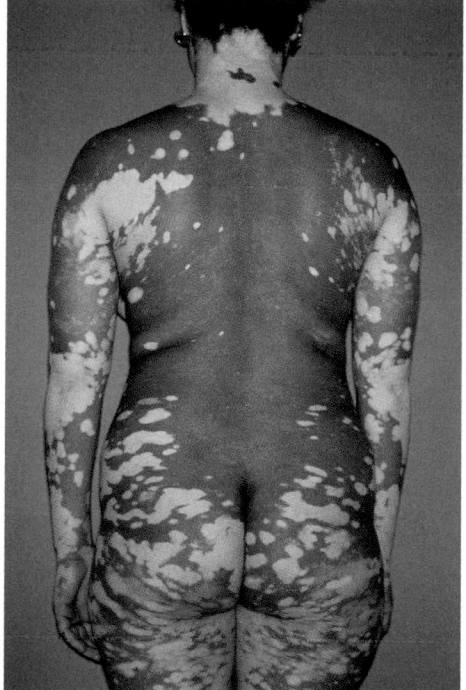

Fig. 36-12 Vitiligo, generalized.

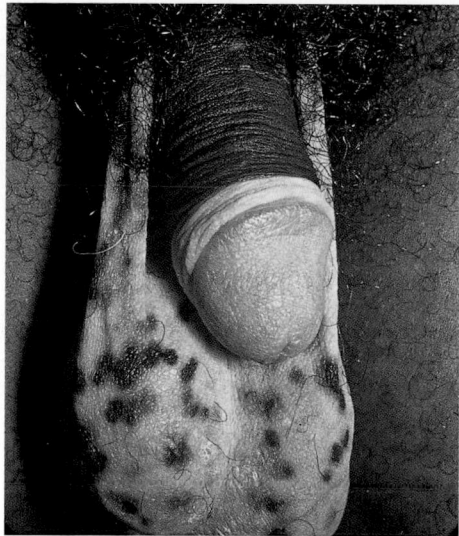

Fig. 36-13 Penile vitiligo.

or a hyperpigmented border. There may be intermediate tan zones or lesions halfway between the normal skin color and depigmentation—so-called trichrome vitiligo. Blue–gray hyperpigmented macules representing melanin incontinence may be present focally. The hairs in the vitiliginous areas usually become white also. Very rarely, the patches may have a red, inflammatory border. The patches are of various sizes and configurations, but the margins are usually smooth, except in the case of segmental vitiligo.

Six types have been described, according to the extent and distribution of the involved areas: localized (Fig. 36-11); or focal (single or a few macules in one anatomic area, often the trigeminal area, especially in children); segmental; generalized (common symmetric); universal (Fig. 36-12); acrofacial; and mucosal. The generalized pattern is most common. Involvement is symmetrical. The most commonly affected sites are the face, upper part of the chest, dorsal aspects of the hands, axillae, and groin. There is a tendency for the skin around orifices to be affected: namely, the eyes, nose, mouth, ears, nipples, umbilicus, penis, vulva, and anus. Lesions appear at areas of trauma, so vitiligo favors the elbows and knees. Universal vitiligo applies to cases where the entire body surface is depigmented. The acrofacial type affects the distal fingers and facial orifices (lips and tips). Focal vitiligo may affect one nondermatomal site (such as the glans penis) (Fig. 36-13), or

asymmetrically affects a single region. It is to be distinguished from the segmental form of vitiligo, which is treatment-resistant, has an earlier onset, and is less frequently associated with other autoimmune phenomena. It represents 5% of adult vitiligo and 20% of childhood vitiligo. Segmental vitiligo often has a dermatomal or quasi-dermatomal distribution.

In patients with vitiligo, local loss of pigment may occur around nevi and melanomas, the so-called halo phenomenon. Vitiligo-like leukoderma occurs in about 1% of melanoma patients. In those with previously diagnosed melanoma, this suggests metastatic disease. Paradoxically, however, as the reaction indicates an autoimmune response against melanocytes, patients who develop it have a better prognosis than patients without leukoderma. Lesions of vitiligo are hypersensitive to UV light and burn readily when exposed to the sun. With repeated sun exposure, lesions of vitiligo can tolerate additional UV exposure (photoadaptation), allowing for increasing doses of therapeutic UV phototherapy.

Ocular abnormalities are increased in patients with vitiligo, including iritis and retinal pigmentary abnormalities. Patients have no visual complaints. Eight percent of patients with idiopathic uveitis have vitiligo or poliosis. The conditions most frequently associated with vitiligo are other "autoimmune" diseases. These include type 1 diabetes mellitus, pernicious anemia, Hashimoto thyroiditis, Graves' disease, Addison's disease, and alopecia areata, which in total affect 32% of family members of patients with vitiligo. If a family history of autoimmune disease is obtained, the vitiligo patient (except those with segmental vitiligo) should be tested for serum antithyroglobulin and antithyroid peroxidase antibodies, since autoimmune thyroid disease is the most common autoimmune disease to be present in vitiligo patients. Additional screening should be directed by signs and symptoms. Vitiligo occurs in 13% of patients with the autoimmune polyendocrinopathy–candidiasis–ectodermal dystrophy (APECED) syndrome, caused by mutations in the autoimmune regulator gene (AIRE). Polymorphisms in the AIRE gene are found more commonly in vitiligo patients than controls.

Although familial aggregation of vitiligo is seen—up to 30% of vitiligo patients have an affected relative—it is not inherited as an autosomal-dominant or recessive trait, but rather seems to have a multifactorial genetic basis. In addition to the autoimmune pathogenic hypothesis, which is most likely, oxidant/antioxidant and neural theories have been proposed. Several of these mechanisms may simultaneously be pathogenic in vitiligo.

The psychologic effect of vitiligo should not be underestimated. Patients are frequently anxious or depressed because of the appearance of their skin and the way it affects their social interactions. This is true for both children and adults. Young adults with childhood vitiligo have persistent health-related quality of life impairment. Referring the patient to a mental health professional or the National Vitiligo Foundation (www.nvfi.org) may be helpful in this situation.

Histopathology

There is a complete absence of melanocytes. Usually, there is no inflammatory infiltrate, but lichenoid or spongiotic inflammation may be detected at the edge of a substantial number of vitiligo lesions. This explains the scaling or hyperpigmentation sometimes observed around lesions of vitiligo.

Differential diagnosis

Vitiligo must be differentiated from morphea and lichen sclerosus, both of which are hypopigmented but associated with a change in the skin texture. Pityriasis alba has a fine scale, is slightly papular, and is poorly defined. Tinea versicolor favors the center back and chest, and has a fine scale; yeast and hyphal forms are demonstrable with potassium hydroxide (KOH) examination. The tertiary stage of pinta might easily lead to diagnostic confusion, but a travel history and serologic testing will help elucidate the diagnosis. Chemical leukoderma (see below) may closely resemble vitiligo.

Treatment

Vitiligo can be a frustrating condition to treat. Spontaneous repigmentation occurs in no more than 15–25% of cases. Response is typically slow, and response rates are low in some anatomic areas. Since vitiligo is common, many studies have been published regarding therapeutic options. However, they are often of poor quality, or have markedly different results when performed at different centers. Persons of different Fitzpatrick phototypes may have different rates of response when facial vitiligo is treated. In addition, some forms of treatment, such as phototherapy, may actually worsen the appearance of the vitiligo initially by pigmenting surrounding skin, accentuating the depigmented areas. This is particularly true in persons of lower Fitzpatrick phototypes (I and II). The anatomic location of the lesion predicts the likelihood of response, independent of the modality used for therapy. Facial vitiligo has an excellent prognosis, with many patients achieving cosmetically significant improvement. The dorsal hands and feet, by contrast, respond to most forms of treatment only about 10–20% of the time. Truncal vitiligo demonstrates an intermediate response.

The major problem for the vitiligo patient is appearance. With regard to vitiligo in persons of low Fitzpatrick phototypes (I and II), non-treatment is an option. These patients are treated with sun protection, supplemented with cosmetic camouflage as required. The newer self-tanning creams are useful for light-skinned and olive-complexioned patients with acral lesions. Phototherapy may more dramatically increase the risk of skin cancer in those with lower Fitzpatrick phototypes, suggesting that alternative approaches should be considered. In addition, mucosal vitiligo (of the lips), and periungual and dorsal hand vitiligo currently have essentially no reproducibly effective form of medical therapy. Camouflage is, therefore, an important therapeutic modality for the vitiligo patient. Dihydroxyacetone is a brown dye that stains the skin. In lower concentrations it can be used in lower phototypes, as it is a golden or tan color (self-tanning products). In high concentrations it is dark brown and can be used in patients with type V and VI phototypes to camouflage their lesions. As it is a stain, it does not rub off, but needs to be reapplied because it is sloughed off from the epidermis (every 5–10 days). Covermark, Dermablend, Dermacolor, Keromask, Veil Cover, and PerfectCover are trademarks that specialize in cosmetic products for patients with dyspigmentations, including vitiligo. These products can be amazingly effective in making the vitiliginous skin blend completely into the normal surrounding skin. However, it is technically difficult for patients to match their skin color without instruction. In the beginning, vitiligo patients using these products will benefit by consulting an aesthetician trained in medical camouflage. Once applied, the products tend to rub off. Application of Cavilon "No Sting Barrier Film" as a spray over the camouflage cosmetic may prevent the product from rubbing off during daily activities.

Topical treatment is appropriate for limited skin areas (<10–20% body surface area [BSA]). Occlusion of all forms of topical therapy may enhance efficacy. Topical potent to superpotent steroids are used for a 2-month trial. Up to 80% of patients with facial vitiligo will achieve >90% repigmentation. This usually occurs diffusely, not perifollicularly, as occurs on the trunk. On the trunk only 40% of patients achieve >90% repigmentation. Treatment should be limited to 4–6 months and the patient must be monitored for acne, atrophy, and telangiectasias.

Topical pimecrolimus cream and tacrolimus ointment 0.1% have been particularly efficacious in treating facial vitiligo. In some series they have been as effective as superpotent topical steroids and avoid the complications of atrophy and acne induced by topical steroids. Patients who initiate treatment in the summer have a higher rate of response. Continual application may be required, as patients who discontinue treatment may suffer the appearance of new lesions. With topical therapies, new areas of vitiligo appear in untreated areas, suggesting there is no systemic effect. Topical pimecrolimus may enhance the efficacy of narrow-band UVB (NBUVB) in repigmenting facial, but not non-facial vitiligo. Topical calcipotriene and other vitamin D analogs have had variable results. Alone these agents lack efficacy. When they are used in combination with other treatments, some studies have demonstrated additive benefit and others no benefit. Therefore, these agents cannot be recommended.

NBUVB twice weekly has become the preferred form of phototherapy to treat vitiligo. It avoids the need for prolonged eye protection and the occasional psoralen-induced nausea. About half of patients will achieve more than 75% repigmentation of the face, trunk, proximal arms, and legs. Hand and foot lesions repigment in less than 25% of patients. Children may have slightly higher response rates than adults. In patients with >20% BSA involvement, only about 5% will show complete repigmentation with phototherapy. Long courses of treatment may be required. PUVA therapy can also be used to treat vitiligo, but is less effective than NBUVB. Repigmentation from phototherapy may begin after 15–25 treatments; however, significant improvement may take as many as 100–200 treatments (6–24 months). On average, maximum improvement is seen after about 9 months of therapy. If follicular repigmentation has not appeared after 3 months, phototherapy treatments should be discontinued. Known photosensitivity, porphyria, and systemic lupus erythematosus are contraindications to phototherapy.

Topical application of 8-methoxypsoralen at a concentration of 0.01–0.1%, followed by UVA exposure, may lead to repigmentation. Topical PUVA is used for focal or limited lesions. Inadvertent burns with blistering are frequent complications during treatment in the US, even when the patient is treated by professionals. For this reason, topical PUVA has been very difficult for the patient to carry out at home. Topical PUVA, however, is widely used in India with success, suggesting that, in the right hands, this treatment can be effective.

Excimer laser phototherapy can be as effective as NBUVB, and the response is more rapid. It can be used on limited areas, avoiding whole-body UV exposure. While 25% of treated patches repigment completely, treatment-resistant areas (elbows, knees, wrists, dorsal hands and feet) have only a 2% rate of at least 75% repigmentation. The addition of topical steroid treatment to excimer laser may enhance efficacy.

In certain situations, the use of systemic immunosuppressives may be appropriate in the treatment of vitiligo. This is usually in the setting of very rapidly progressive disease, with the goal of reducing the total amount of pigment loss. Systemic corticosteroids are usually used and are tapered over several months. Twice weekly dexamethasone, at a dose of 10 mg, is one such regimen. Once the disease is arrested, the patient can be converted to phototherapy. The long-term use of systemic immunosuppressives is not recommended. They initially may control the disease, but with chronic use, unacceptable toxicity often develops.

Surgical treatments can be applied to limited lesions if the above methods do not prove beneficial, but these are time-consuming. They are recommended primarily in patients with treatment-resistant vitiligo. Patients must have stable disease (no new lesions, or expansion of lesions for 1 year). Surgical procedures are not effective in patients who exhibit Koebner phenomenon or have active vitiligo. Given its expense, surgical treatment should be reserved for exposed skin sites covering less than 2–3% of BSA. Minigrafting, transplantation of autologous epidermal cell suspension, and ultra thin epidermal grafts have all been used. UV phototherapy is often given following the surgical procedure.

Systemic immunosuppressives, specifically high-dose corticosteroids, can arrest rapidly progressive vitiligo. However, they cannot be used long-term due to toxicity, so another form of therapy must be sought once the vitiligo has been arrested.

Total depigmentation

If more than 50–80% of the body surface area is affected by vitiligo, the patient can consider depigmentation. This form of treatment should be considered permanent and the goal is total depigmentation. Limited areas (such as those exposed daily) may be treated, but satellite and distant depigmentation may occur, so the action of the medication cannot be limited to the applied area. Monobenzone (monobenzyl ether of hydroquinone) 20% is applied twice a day for 3–6 months to residual pigmented areas. Up to 10 months may be required to complete the treatment. About 1 in 6 patients treated experiences acute dermatitis, usually confined to the still-pigmented areas, but this rarely limits treatment. Once the patient achieves a uniform depigmented appearance, he/she is very satisfied. Topical 20% 4-methoxyphenol cream (mequinol, monomethylether of hydroquinone) can also be used for depigmentation. The Q-switched laser selectively destroys melanocytes and can also achieve depigmentation. It can be combined with a topical depigmenting agent for added efficacy.

Chemical leukoderma (occupational vitiligo)

Chemical leukoderma is an acquired, depigmented dermatosis caused by repeated exposure to chemicals. It is frequently misdiagnosed as vitiligo. Patients with vitiligo or a family history of vitiligo are at much greater risk of developing chemical leukoderma. The diagnostic criteria are:

1. acquired vitiligo-like depigmented lesions
2. history of repeated exposure to a specific chemical compound
3. patterned vitiligo-like macules conforming to site of exposure
4. confetti macules.

The majority of cases are caused by exposure to aromatic or aliphatic derivatives of phenols and catechols, including paratertiary butylphenol (adhesive in shoes), amylphenol, butylcatechol, and alkyl phenols. However, sulfhydryls, mercurials, arsenics, cinnamic aldehyde, p-phenylenediamine, chloroquine, and azelaic acid have also been incriminated. Some of these compounds have a structure similar to tyrosine and may be converted by tyrosine-related protein-1 to compounds toxic to the melanocyte. This process is considered to be different from depigmentation following allergic contact dermatitis. The clinical pattern may be very similar to idiopathic vitiligo, but lesions tend to be concentrated in areas of repeated contact with the incriminated substance. The first recognized cases of occupational vitiligo occurred in individuals who worked in rubber garments or wore gloves that contained monobenzyl ether of hydroquinone. This compound may still contaminate some rubber products. Phenolic antiseptic detergents used in hospitals and in industrial cleaners have caused chemical leukoderma in janitorial and housekeeping employees. Adhesives and glues containing incriminated chemicals may be found in shoes, wristbands, adhesive tape, and rubber products used in brassieres, girdles, panties, or condoms. Self-sticking bindis (the cosmetic used by many Indian women on the forehead) have been reported to induce leukoderma from the adhesive material. Also, electrocardiograph electrodes may cause similar round hypopigmented spots at the site of contact.

The most common location for chemical leukoderma is the face (40% of cases), followed by the hands and feet. The scalp is rarely affected. Hair dye (at the rim of the scalp but not on the scalp), deodorant (axilla), detergent, adhesives (face, bindis), rubber sandals (feet), black socks and shoes (feet), and rubber condoms (penis) are the exposures associated with lesions in various anatomic regions. Pruritus occurs in more than 20% of patients (a rare complaint in vitiligo patients). The clinical lesions are sharply marginated macules and patches, often with confetti or pea-sized macules seen at the periphery. This clinical pattern is atypical for idiopathic vitiligo and should suggest the diagnosis of chemical leukoderma. More than 25% of patients have lesions outside the area of contact with the incriminated chemical. In about 10% of patients, new vitiliginous lesions will continue to develop, even after exposure to the chemical is stopped. Treatment is avoidance and measures used for idiopathic vitiligo (see above). Chemical leukoderma in a person without vitiligo has a good prognosis, with repigmentation in up to 75% of cases. If a person with vitiligo develops a chemical leukoderma, repigmentation only occurs in 20% of cases. Histologically, the vitiliginous areas of a chemical leukoderma show an absence of melanocytes identical to lesions of true vitiligo.

Akimoto S, et al: Multiple actinic keratoses and squamous cell carcinomas on the sun-exposed areas of widespread vitiligo. Br J Dermatol 2000; 142:824.

Alajlan A, et al: Transfer of vitiligo after allogeneic bone marrow transplantation. J Am Acad Dermatol 2002; 46:606.

Attili VR, Attili SK: Lichenoid inflammation in vitiligo—a clinical and histopathologic review of 210 cases. Int J Dermatol 2008; 47:663.

Au WY, et al: Generalized vitiligo after lymphocyte infusion for relapsed leukaemia. Br J Dermatol 2001; 145:1015.

Austin M: Fighting and living with vitiligo. J Am Acad Dermatol 2004; 51:S7.

Basak PY, et al: The role of helper and regulatory T cells in the pathogenesis of vitiligo. J Am Acad Dermatol 2009; 60:256.

Chen YF, et al: Treatment of vitiligo by transplantation of cultured pure melanocyte suspension: analysis of 120 cases. J Am Acad Dermatol 2004; 51:68.

Cockayne SE, et al: Vitiligo treated with topical corticosteroids: children with head and neck involvement respond well. J Am Acad Dermatol 2002; 46:964.

Esfandiarpour I, et al: The efficacy of pimecrolimus 1% cream plus narrow-band ultraviolet B in the treatment of vitiligo: a double-blind placebo-controlled clinical trial. J Dermatolog Treat 2009; 20:14.

Falabella R, Barona MI: Update on skin repigmentation therapies in vitiligo. Pigment Cell Melanoma Res 2009; 22:42.

Fenton JS, et al: Vitiligo: nonsurgical treatment options and the evidence behind their use. J Drugs Dermatol 2008; 7:705.

Gawkrodger DJ, et al: Guideline for the diagnosis and management of vitiligo. Br J Dermatol 2008; 159:1051.

Ghosh S, Mukhopadhyay S: Chemical leucoderma: a clinico-aetiological study of 864 cases in the perspective of a developing country. Br J Dermatol 2009; 160:40.

Godse KV: Comparison of two diluents of 1% methoxsalen in the treatment of vitiligo. Indian J Dermatol Venerol Leprol 2008; 74:298.

Grimes PE: White patches and bruised souls: advances in the pathogenesis and treatment of vitiligo. J Am Acad Dermatol 2004; 51:S5.

Grimes PE, et al: Topical tacrolimus therapy for vitiligo: therapeutic responses and skin messenger RNA expression of proinflammatory cytokines. J Am Acad Dermatol 2004; 51:52.

Halder RM, Chappell JL: Vitiligo update. Semin Cutan Med Surg 2009; 28:86.

Hartmann A, et al: Occlusive treatment enhances efficacy of tacrolimus 0.1% ointment in adult patients with vitiligo: results of a placebo-controlled 12-month prospective study. Acta Derm Venereol 2008; 88:474.

Hexsel CL, et al: A clinical trial and molecular study of photoadaptation in vitiligo. Br J Dermatol 2009; 160:534.

Hsu S: Camouflaging vitiligo with dihydroxyacetone. Dermatol Online J 2008; 14:23.

Lepe V, et al: A double-blind randomized trial of 0.1% tacrolimus vs 0.05% clobetasol for the treatment of childhood vitiligo. Arch Dermatol 2003; 139:581.

Linthorst Homan MW, et al: Impact of childhood vitiligo on adult life. Br J Dermatol 2008; 159:915.

Martin-Garcia RF, et al: Chloroquine-induced, vitiligo-like depigmentation. J Am Acad Dermatol 2003; 48:981.

Mulekar SV, et al: Treatment of vitiligo on difficult-to-treat sites using autologous noncultured cellular grafting. Dermatol Surg 2009; 35:66.

Natta R, et al: Narrowband ultraviolet B radiation therapy for recalcitrant vitiligo in Asians. J Am Acad Dermatol 2003; 49:473.

Nicolaidou E, et al: Narrowband ultraviolet B phototherapy and 308-nm excimer laser in the treatment of vitiligo: a review. J Am Acad Dermatol 2009; 60:470.

Njoo MD, et al: Treatment of generalized vitiligo in children with narrow-band (TL-01) UVB radiation therapy. J Am Acad Dermatol 2000; 42:245.

Njoo MD, et al: Depigmentation therapy in vitiligo universalis with topical 4-methoxyphenol and the Q-switched ruby laser. J Am Acad Dermatol 2000; 42:760.

Nordlund JJ, et al: Dermatitis produced by applications of monobenzone in patients with active vitiligo. Arch Dermatol 1985; 121:1141.

Olssom MJ: What are the needs for transplantation treatment in vitiligo, and how good is it? Arch Dermatol 2004; 140:1273.

Passeron T, et al: Topical tacrolimus and the 308-nm excimer laser: a synergistic combination for the treatment of vitiligo. Arch Dermatol 2004; 140:1065.

Radakovic-Fijan S, et al: Oral dexamethasone pulse treatment for vitiligo. J Am Acad Dermatol 2001; 44:814.

Sassi F, et al: Randomized controlled trial comparing the effectiveness of 308-nm excimer laser alone or in combination with topical hydrocortisone 17-butyrate cream in the treatment of vitiligo of the face and neck. Br J Dermatol 2008; 159:1186.

Silverberg NB, et al: Tacrolimus ointment promotes repigmentation of vitiligo in children: a review of 57 cases. J Am Acad Dermatol 2004; 51:760.

Suga Y, et al: Medical pearl: DHA application for camouflaging segmental vitiligo and piebald lesions. J Am Acad Dermatol 2002; 47:436.

Taieb A, Picardo M: Clinical practice. Vitiligo. N Engl J Med 2009; 260:160.

Tanioka M, Miyachi Y: Camouflaging vitiligo of the fingers. Arch Dermatol 2008; 144:809.

Tanioka M, Miyachi Y: Camouflage for vitiligo. Dermatol Ther 2009; 22:90.

Tazi-Ahnini R, et al: The autoimmune regulator gene (AIRE) is strongly associated with vitiligo. Br J Dermatol 2008; 159:591.

van Geel N, et al: Double-blind placebo-controlled study of autologous transplanted epidermal cell suspensions for repigmenting vitiligo. Arch Dermatol 2004; 140:1203.

Vogt–Koyanagi–Harada syndrome

Vogt–Koyanagi–Harada syndrome (VKHS) is a disease complex affecting the eyes, skin, auditory system, and central nervous system (CNS). It affects primarily pigmented races and is rare in white persons. It is more common in females, and affects all ages. The disease occurs in four phases. First is the prodromal phase or meningoencephalitic phase, with fever, malaise, headache, nausea, and vomiting. The CNS involvement can include meningismus, headaches, mental status changes, cerebrospinal fluid pleocytosis, tinnitus, and dysacusis. Recovery is usually complete. The second stage, the uveitic phase, is characterized by anterior and/or posterior uveitis and inflammation of many other parts of the eye. The third or convalescent phase begins 3 weeks to 3 months after the uveitis appears, usually as it begins to improve. This stage is characterized by frontal non-cicatricial alopecia, vitiligo, and poliosis of scalp, eyebrows, eyelashes, and hairs of the axillae. The skin lesions must begin after the ocular symptoms to be considered diagnostic. The fourth phase is one of recurrent attacks of uveitis. Most ocular complications occur as a result of this stage of the disease, and include permanent decreased visual acuity, cataracts, and glaucoma.

VKHS is a cell-mediated autoimmune disease with the autoantigen(s) felt to be solely expressed in melanin-containing cells. The target antigens may be the tyrosinase family proteins, as immunization of mice with several of these proteins can induce a syndrome similar to VKHS. Supporting this hypothesis are the rare observations that vitiligo, erythroderma, interferon therapy for hepatitis C, and melanoma can all be associated with the appearance of VKHS. Aggressive immunosuppressive therapy with systemic steroids and immunomodulatory medications (cyclosporine, azathioprine, mycophenolate, tacrolimus, infliximab) may preserve ocular function and prevent ocular complications. Th17 CD4+ cells stimulated by high levels of interleukin (IL)-23 and secreting IL-17 are present in VKHS patients with active uveitis. IL-23 is important in the production and maintenance of autoimmune diseases, and IL-17 is one of the most important effector cytokines in autoimmune diseases. At least four patients with psoriasis and VKHS have been reported.

Aisenbrey S, et al: Vogt–Koyanagi–Harada syndrome associated with cutaneous malignant melanoma: an 11-year follow-up. Graefe's Arch Clin Exp Ophthalmol 2003; 241:996.

Andreoli CM, Foster CS: Vogt–Koyanagi–Harada disease. Int Ophthalmol Clin 2006; 46:111.

Chi W, et al: IL-23 promotes CD4+ T cells to produce IL-17 in Vogt–Koyanagi–Harada disease. J Allergy Clin Immunol 2007; 119:1218.

Kluger N, et al: Vogt–Koyanagi–Harada syndrome associated with psoriasis and autoimmune thyroid disease. Acta Derm Venerol 2008; 88:397.

Liu X, et al: Inhibitory effect of cyclosporin A and corticosteroids on the production of IFN-gamma and IL-17 by T cells in Vogt–Koyanagi–Harada syndrome. Clin Immunol 2009; 131:333.

Niccoli L, et al: Efficacy of infliximab therapy in two patients with refractory Vogt–Koyanagi–Harada disease. Br J Ophthalmol 2009; 93:1553.

Paredes I, et al: Immunomodulatory therapy for Vogt–Koyanagi–Harada patients as first-line therapy. Ocul Immunol Inflamm 2006; 14:87.

Rao NA, et al: Vogt–Koyanagi–Harada disease diagnostic criteria. Int Ophthalmol 2007; 27:195.

Rathinam SR, et al: Vogt–Koyanagi–Harada syndrome after cutaneous injury. Ophthalmology 1999; 106:635.

Sylvestre DL, et al: Vogt–Koyanagi–Harada disease associated with interferon alpha-2b/ribavirin combination therapy. J Viral Hep 2003; 10:467.

Tsuruta D, et al: Inflammatory vitiligo in Vogt–Koyanagi–Harada disease. J Am Acad Dermatol 2001; 44:129.

Wong SS, et al: Vogt–Koyanagi–Harada disease: extensive vitiligo with prodromal generalized erythroderma. Dermatology 1999; 198:65.

Alezzandrini syndrome

Alezzandrini syndrome is a very rare condition characterized by a unilateral degenerative retinitis, followed after several months by ipsilateral vitiligo on the face and ipsilateral poliosis. Deafness may also be present.

Hoffman MD, Dudley C: Suspected Alezzandrini's syndrome in a diabetic patient with unilateral retinal detachment and ipsilateral vitiligo and poliosis. J Am Acad Dermatol 1992; 26:496.

Leukoderma

Postinflammatory leukoderma may result from many inflammatory dermatoses, such as pityriasis rosea, psoriasis, herpes zoster, secondary syphilis, and morphea. Sarcoidosis, tinea versicolor, mycosis fungoides, scleroderma, and pityriasis lichenoides chronica may all present with hypopigmented lesions (only rarely are these actually depigmented), as may Hansen's disease. Burns, scars, postdermabrasion, and intralesional steroid injections with depigmentation are other examples of leukoderma.

Friedman SJ, et al: Perilesional linear atrophy and hypopigmentation after intralesional corticosteroid therapy. J Am Acad Dermatol 1988; 19:537.

Oculocutaneous albinism

Oculocutaneous albinism (OCA) is an autosomal-recessively inherited trait with reduction or absence of melanin in skin, hair, and eyes. Eye problems are frequently present, including moderate to severe impairment of visual acuity, nystagmus, strabismus, and photophobia. The cutaneous phenotype of the various forms of albinism is broad, but the ocular phenotype is reasonably constant in most forms. Genetic disorders of pigment cells can now be defined as caused by:

1. disruption of melanoblast migration to target tissues during development (Waardenburg syndrome and piebaldism)
2. disruption of melanin synthesis (oculocutaneous albinism)
3. disruption of melanosome formation (Chédiak–Higashi and Hermansky–Pudlak syndromes)
4. disruption of melanosome transport and melanin transfer to keratinocytes (Griscelli syndrome).

The most serious sequelae of albinism are gross visual disturbances and the increased risk for the development of skin cancer. A number of syndromes associated with albinism can also cause premature mortality due to impairment of the functioning of other involved organs and systems.

Disorders of melanin synthesis

The four genetic forms of non-syndromal OCA are all caused by disruption of melanin synthesis and all autosomal-recessive disorders. Their prevalence varies widely around the world, but is estimated to be about 1 in 17 000. That means that about 1 in 70 persons carries a gene for OCA. Given the phenotypic overlap of the various forms of OCA, genetic testing is recommended to establish the diagnosis. Since both parents are obligate carriers and two-thirds of healthy siblings are at risk for being carriers, genetic counseling is recommended. Carriers are asymptomatic. All persons with OCA and their parents should be educated regarding aggressive sun protection with sunscreens, appropriate clothing, and sun avoidance. Vitamin D supplementation may be required. As adults, patients should be examined for skin lesions suspicious for melanoma and nonmelanoma skin cancer.

Oculocutaneous albinism 1

OCA1 results from mutations in the tyrosinase gene and accounts for approximately 40% of OCA worldwide. It is the most severe form of albinism, and is the most common type of albinism in Japanese, non-Hispanic Caucasians, and a mixed race European population, with a prevalence of about 1 in 40 000. Affected patients are homozygous for the mutant gene or are compound heterozygotes for different mutations in the tyrosinase gene (TYR). OCA1 is divided into two forms: OCA1A and OCA1B. At birth these are indistinguishable. OCA1A is the most severe form, with complete absence of tyrosinase activity and complete absence of melanin in the skin and eyes. Visual acuity is decreased to 20/400. The hair, eyelashes, and eyebrows are white, and the skin is white and does not tan. Irises are light blue to pink and fully translucent. Amelanotic nevi may be present. In OCA1B, tyrosinase activity is greatly reduced but not absent. Affected patients may show an increase in skin, hair, and eye color beginning at age 1–3 years, and can tan. Iris color may also darken over time. OCA1B was originally called "yellow mutant" albinism. Temperature-sensitive OCA (OCA1-TS) is considered a variant of OCA1B; it results from mutations in the tyrosinase gene that produce an enzyme with limited activity below 35°C (95°F) and no activity above this temperature. Affected patients have white hair, skin, and eyes at birth. At puberty, dark hair develops in cooler acral areas. Visual acuity is not as severely affected in OCA1B.

Oculocutaneous albinism 2

OCA2 has a prevalence of 1 in 36 000 in white Europeans, but as much as 1 in 4000 in some parts of Africa. It is the most common form of OCA, accounting for approximately 50% of OCA worldwide. OCA2 was formerly called "tyrosinase-positive" albinism, or "brown OCA." Inheritance is autosomal-recessive and results from mutations in the OCA2 gene, formerly known as the P gene. The OCA2 gene encodes an integral melanosomal protein that is important for normal biogenesis of melanosomes and for normal processing and transport of melanosomal proteins such as tyrosinase and tyrosinase-related protein 1 (TYRP1). The cutaneous phenotype of OCA2 patients is broad, ranging from nearly normal pigmentation to virtually no pigment. Newborns have pigmented hair. Nevi and ephelides are common. Pink irises are usually not seen. Visual defects are not as severe as in OCA1. Pigmentation increases with age and visual acuity improves from infancy to adolescence. Prader–Willi and Angelman syndromes are caused by deletions in the chromosomal region contiguous to and sometimes including the OCA2 gene. One percent of patients with these syndromes also have OCA2.

Oculocutaneous albinism 3

OCA3 is caused by mutations in the *TYRP1* gene. TRYP1 protein is an enzyme in the melanin biosynthesis pathway that oxidizes dihydroxyindole carboxylic acid (DHICA) monomers into melanin. Mutations in this enzyme result in delayed maturation and early degradation of tyrosine. This form of OCA has been most commonly found in African patients and was called "rufous" or red OCA. It has also been seen in a large Pakistani family and a Caucasian patient. Patients have red hair and reddish-brown skin. Visual abnormalities may not be detectable.

Oculocutaneous albinism 4

OCA4 is due to mutations in the *MATP* gene encoding a membrane-associated transporter protein, predicted to span the membrane 12 times and to function as a transporter. Patients are hypopigmented to a variable degree, and are phenotypically identical to patients with OCA2. Visual acuity is decreased and nystagmus is found in many but not all patients. This has also been reported in a Turkish patient, as well as German, Japanese, and Korean OCA patients.

Disorders of melanosome formation

These are multisystem syndromes that are associated with albinism. These syndromes are caused by genes that function in intracellular organelle formation and movement in a variety of specialized cell types, such as melanocytes, neurons, immune cells, monocytes, platelets, and type II epithelial cells in lungs. The silver hair of some of these syndromes may demonstrate pigment clumping, allowing the diagnosis to be suspected.

Chédiak–Higashi syndrome

Chédiak–Higashi syndrome (CHS) is a progressively degenerative, fatal disease characterized by partial oculocutaneous albinism (decreased skin, eye, and hair pigment), giant intracellular granules, pigment clumping in hair shafts, and a bleeding diathesis due to absent or reduced platelet-dense bodies. It presents in childhood, usually with life-threatening infections of the skin and lungs. Common pathogens are *Staphylococcus aureus*, streptococcus, Gram-negative organisms, *Candida*, and *Aspergillus*. Immunoglobulins, antibody production, and phagocytosis are normal, but neutropenia is common and leukocytes display impaired migration. Natural killer cells are decreased in function. The hair of these patients is blond and sparse. The ocular albinism is accompanied by nystagmus and photophobia. In darker-skinned races, affected patients are lighter-skinned than their parents and siblings, and may have speckled hyper- and hypopigmentation.

CHS results from mutations in the *SHS1* gene, the exact biological function of which is unknown. The gene must be important in lysosome and lysosome-related organelle trafficking or size regulation. Melanosomes are giant, and platelets, eosinophils, basophils, and monocytes have giant intracellular granules that are azurophilic.

In 85% of cases a lymphohistiocytosis syndrome occurs, referred to as the "accelerated phase." It is fatal and caused by the unfettered proliferation of lymphocytes creating a lymphoma-like situation with fever, anemia, neutropenia, hepatosplenomegaly, and lymphadenopathy. Liver function tests and serum ferritin may be elevated. Bone marrow transplantation (BMT) prior to the onset of this phase may be lifesaving, and also prevents the infections. Unfortunately, even with BMT, if CHS patients survive into adulthood they develop progressive neurological involvement.

Hermansky–Pudlak syndrome

Hermansky–Pudlak syndrome (HPS) is an autosomal-recessive disorder consisting of oculocutaneous albinism, a hemorrhagic diathesis secondary to the absence of dense bodies in platelets, and accumulation of a ceroid-like material in the reticuloendothelial system, visceral organs, oral mucosa, and urine. Patients with this disorder have a history of easy bruisability, epistaxis, gingival bleeding, hemoptysis, and bleeding after various surgical procedures and childbirth. Major bleeding occurs in 40% of HPS patients. The hypopigmentation is due to impaired melanosome formation, trafficking, or transfer to keratinocytes.

Currently, eight human genes (*HPS1–8*) have been identified, which, when independently mutated, lead to a clinical picture consistent with HPS. It is anticipated that more HPS genes will be identified in humans, since in mice there are at least 14 non-allelic genes that, when singly defective, give rise to HPS. While the HPS subtypes 1–8 all share the clinical signs and symptoms noted above, a few subtypes either lack some of or have additional unique features that serve to distinguish them from the other HPS subtypes. Seven of the eight genes causing HPS (not *HPS2*) are parts of distinct complexes that are called biogenesis of lysosome-related organelle complexes, or BLOCs. Mutations in any member of a BLOC tend to create a similar clinical phenotype. There are three known BLOCs, and mutations in most of the BLOC subunits cause a variant of HPS.

The most common subtype is HPS1, which, together with HPS4, comprises 50% of the known worldwide cases of HPS. One in 21 Puerto Ricans has a mutation (usually a 16-base pair [bp] duplication) in the *HPS1* gene. HPS accounts for 80% of albinos in Puerto Rico, and 1 in 1800 Puerto Ricans in the northwest region of the country has HPS. HPS1 and HPS4 are clinically very similar, since they together form the BLOC3 complex (Fig. 36-14). These are the two most severe forms of HPS. Skin pigmentation can vary from total lack to lighter hair and skin coloring than in other members of the family. Ocular changes similar to those of OCA can occur, including iris transillumination, hypopigmented retina, visual impairment, horizontal nystagmus, and strabismus. Atypical nevi, acanthosis nigricans-like lesions in the axillae and neck, and trichomegaly also occur. Solar damage, as evidenced by solar lentigines, actinic keratoses, and nonmelanoma skin cancers, occurs in 80% of patients with the 16-bp duplication in HPS1. Interstitial pulmonary fibrosis, inflammatory bowel disease, renal failure, and cardiomyopathy are late complications, and can cause premature mortality between the ages of 20 and 50 years. Sixty percent of patients with HPS have pulmonary symptoms, starting at a mean age of 35 years. Pirfenidone, an antifibrotic

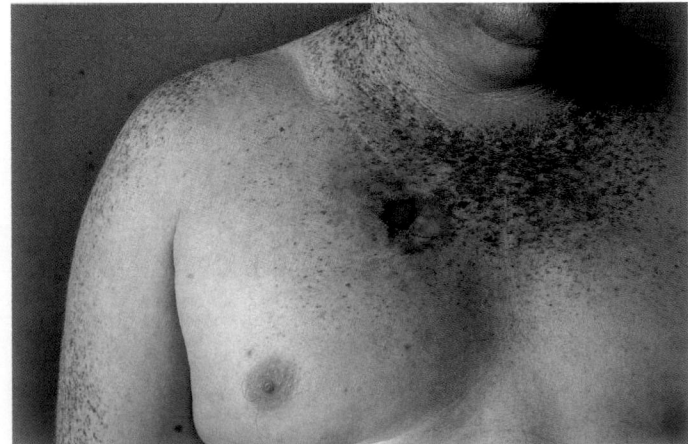

Fig. 36-14 Hermansky–Pudlak syndrome, freckling of the "V" of the neck and a basal cell carcinoma in a Puerto Rican man.

agent, can slow the progression of pulmonary fibrosis in HPS1 patients with significant residual lung function (initial forced ventilatory capacity >50%). Lung transplantation can be considered.

HPS2 is caused by a mutation in the gene (*AP3B1*) coding for the 3βA subunit of AP3, a molecule necessary for normal protein trafficking to the lysosome. HPS2 is notable for immunodeficiency and persistent neutropenia, with patients suffering recurrent bacterial infections of the upper respiratory system and middle ear, possibly due to the lack of antigen presentation by the CD1b molecule, since CD1b fails to gain access to the lysosome. Initially, patients may be misdiagnosed as having CHS due to pigment dilution and recurrent infections. However, the large intracellular granules of CHS are absent. Mild pulmonary fibrosis and a mild hearing defect can be associated with HPS2.

HPS3, HPS5, and HPS6 have mild clinical findings, without reported pulmonary or gastrointestinal involvement. They are due to mutations in three proteins that make up BLOC2.

HPS 7 and 8 are very rare and present with a phenotype of oculocutaneous albinism and a bleeding tendency due to platelet dysfunction. The HPS7 gene (*DTNBP1*) encodes dysbindin; the HPS8 gene is *BLOC1S3*.

Disorders of melanocyte transport

Griscelli syndrome

Griscelli syndrome (GS) is a rare autosomal-recessive disorder with mild skin and hair hypopigmentation, immunological impairment, lymphohistiocytosis, or defects in the central nervous system. Patients do not have a bleeding tendency. There are three forms of GS. GS1 is caused by mutations in the *MYO5A* gene encoding the actin-associated myosin Va motor protein. Patients have primary neurological dysfunction but no immunological disease. They have silver hair. GS1 and Elejalde syndrome are felt to be the same disease. GS2 is due to mutations in the *RAB27A* gene. Patients have silver hair, infections, and lymphohistiocytosis. Leukocytes infiltrating the brain can cause secondary neurological disease, but patients have no primary neural defects. GS3 is cause by mutations in *Melanophilin* and results only in cutaneous hypopigmentation. The three genes responsible for GS all form a protein complex essential for the capture and local movement of melanosomes in the actin-rich periphery of melanocytes.

Al-Khenaizan S: Hyperpigmentation in Chédiak–Higashi syndrome. J Am Acad Dermatol 2003; 49(5 Suppl):S244.

Emanuel PO, et al: Griscelli syndrome. Skinmed 2007; 6:147.

Gronskov K, et al: Oculocutaneous albinism. Orphanet J Rare Dis 2007; 2:43.

Huizing M, et al: Disorders of lysosome-related organelle biogenesis: clinical and molecular genetics. Annu Rev Genomics Hum Genet 2008; 9:359.

Lazarchick J, et al: Chédiak–Higashi syndrome. Blood 2005; 10:4162.

Tager AM, et al: Case records of the Massachusetts General Hospital. Case 32-2009: a 27-year-old man with progressive dyspnea. N Engl J Med 2009; 361:1585.

Toro J, et al: Dermatologic manifestations of Hermansky–Pudlak syndrome in patients with and without a 16-base pair duplication in the HPS1 gene. Arch Dermatol 1999; 135:774.

Wei A, et al: A comprehensive analysis reveals mutational spectra and common alleles in Chinese patients with oculocutaneous albinism. J Invest Dermatol 2009 Oct 29 (Epub ahead of print).

Wei ML: Hermansky-Pudlak syndrome: a disease of protein trafficking and organelle function. Pigment Cell Res 2006; 19:19.

Disorders of melanoblast migration and survival

These disorders cause "spotting," i.e. patches of white hair and/or unpigmented skin.

Waardenburg syndrome

Four genotypic variants of Waardenburg syndrome exist, with overlapping phenotypic features; all are autosomal-dominant. Types 1 and 3 are caused by mutations in the *PAX3* gene, encoding a transcription factor. Type 2 is caused by mutations in the *MITF* gene, also encoding a transcription factor, and type 4 is due to either a heterozygous mutation in the *SOX10* gene (encoding a transcription factor), or homozygous mutations in the endothelin-3 (*EDN3*) or the endothelin B receptor (*EDNR3*) gene. These mutations impair the ability of melanoblasts to reach their final target sites (inner ear, eye, skin) during embryogenesis.

Patients with this syndrome have features of piebaldism, with a white forelock, hypopigmentation, premature graying, and other characteristic findings including synophrys, congenital deafness, dystopia canthorum (broad nasal root), and ocular changes, including heterochromia iridis (Fig. 36-15). Types 1 and 3 are both characterized by dystopia canthorum; in type 1, white forelock and depigmented skin patches are more frequent; while in type 3, limb anomalies occur. In type 2, no dystopia canthorum is observed, but hearing loss and heterochromia iridis are more frequently found. Type 4 Waardenburg's syndrome is identical to type 3, except that it is associated with Hirschprung disease.

Piebaldism

Piebaldism is a rare, autosomal-dominant syndrome with variable phenotype, presenting at birth. The characteristic clinical features are a white forelock and patchy absence of skin pigment (Fig. 36-16). The depigmented lesions are static and characteristically occur on the anterior and posterior trunk, mid-upper arm to wrist, mid-thigh to mid-calf, and shins. A characteristic feature of piebaldism is the presence of hyperpigmented macules within the areas lacking pigmentation and also on normally pigmented skin. The depigmented lesions may repigment spontaneously, or especially after injury. The white forelock is a triangular or diamond-shaped midline white macule on the frontal scalp or forehead, and is the only

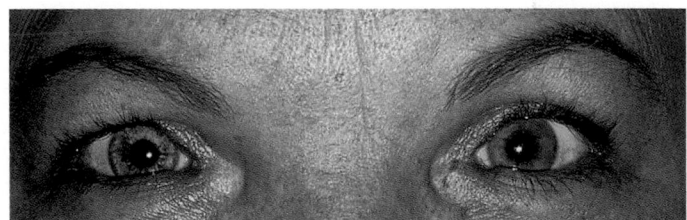

Fig. 36-15 Waardenburg syndrome with heterochromia iridis.

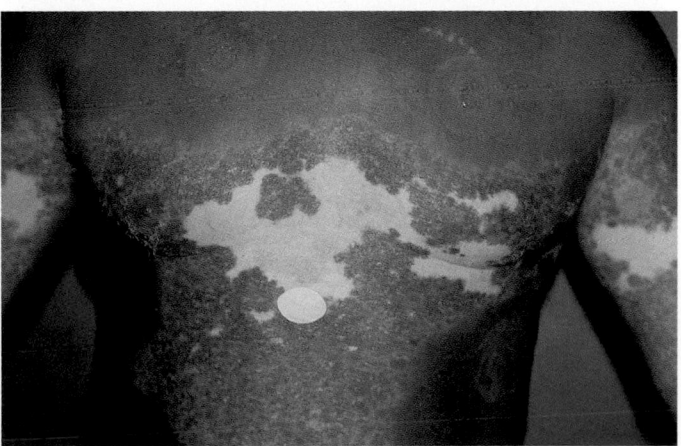

Fig. 36-16 Piebaldism, vitiligo-like depigmentation.

manifestation in 80–90% of patients. The medial portions of the eyebrows and eyelashes may be white. Histologically, melanocytes are completely absent in the white macules.

Piebaldism is caused by mutations in the *KIT* gene (gene product kit proto-oncogene), encoding a cell surface receptor for the steel factor, an embryonic growth factor. The phenotypic differences between families are caused by different locations of mutations in the gene. A mild phenotype occurs in cases associated with mutations in the ligand-binding region, whereas more severe phenotypes occur from mutations in the tyrosine kinase region of the receptor. The white lesions may respond to camouflage cosmetics or surgical corrections (see discussion under vitiligo). Hirschprung disease and neurofibromatosis type I have rarely been associated with piebaldism.

Cross–McKusick–Breen syndrome

Also known as Cross syndrome, oculocerebral hypopigmentation syndrome, or hypopigmentation and microphthalmia, this extremely rare disorder is characterized by white skin, blond hair with a yellow–gray metallic sheen, small eyes with cloudy corneas, jerky nystagmus, gingival fibromatosis, and severe mental and physical retardation.

Spritz RA: Molecular basis of human piebaldism. J Invest Dermatol 1994; 103(Suppl):137.

Thomas I, et al: Piebaldism: an update. Int J Dermatol 2004; 43:716.

Bonus images for this chapter can be found online at

http://www.expertconsult.com

Fig. 36-1 Dermatopathia pigmentosa reticularis.

Fig. 36-2 Vitiligo, characteristic periorificial location.

Fig. 36-3 Hemochromatosis.

Fig. 36-4 Idiopathic guttate hypomelanosis.

Fig. 36-5 Piebaldism, white forelock.

Dermatology has always been a surgically oriented specialty. While procedures such as curettage, biopsy, destruction, and excision have been key components of the field, the practice has evolved to include a greater number and extent of surgical procedures. This progression can be attributed to a variety of factors. Dermatologists have a greater understanding of cutaneous pathology, which places them in a unique role to manage complex surgical procedures. In addition, outpatient dermatologic surgery has been shown to be cost-effective, safe, and efficacious, and to deliver a greater degree of patient convenience, particularly when compared to other fields. With this in mind, the American Board of Dermatology mandates certain surgical exposure and experience for all residents in dermatology residency programs. Furthermore, with the recent Accreditation Council for Graduate Medical Education (ACGME) accreditation of Procedural Dermatology fellowships, dermatologic surgery has become recognized as a mainstream medical option for patients. While the practice of dermatologic surgery can be the subject of entire textbooks, the following chapters provide a survey of procedures, indications, and appropriate management within the spectrum of the field.

Preparation for surgery

A thorough and complete preoperative evaluation is required prior to performing any surgical procedure. A detailed medical history must be obtained, including information on drug allergies, current medications (including herbal or natural supplements), presence of a pacemaker or implantable cardioverter/defibrillator, recently implanted prosthetics, history of prior wound infection or perioperative bleeding, and history of endocarditis, or cardiac valvular or congenital malformation.

Anticoagulants

Much has been written regarding the role of antiplatelets and/or anticoagulants and surgical bleeding. Dermatologists are frequently presented with the dilemma of whether to discontinue blood thinners in the setting of surgery. Data and multiple reviews have shown that continuous treatment with blood thinners perioperatively in patients undergoing Mohs and cutaneous surgery is not associated with an increase in surgical complications leading to significant morbidity. In contrast, discontinuation of these medications may increase the risk of catastrophic cerebral and cardiovascular complications. Kovich and Otley reported a series of thrombotic complications in a group of patients who had discontinued aspirin or warfarin prior to surgery; these included stroke, transient ischemic attack, myocardial infarction, pulmonary embolus, and death. Multiple authors feel that the potential adverse effects of discontinuing essential medical blood thinners far outweigh the potential side effects of surgical bleeding (i.e.

managing a postoperative hematoma). In fact, despite some surgeons' claims to the contrary, several studies have demonstrated that blinded surgeons are unable to identify intraoperatively which patients are taking anticoagulation medication based on the subjective amount of surgical oozing. As such, it is recommended that patients be maintained on all medically necessary blood thinners during cutaneous surgery. Patients taking aspirin for primary prevention may discontinue use 2 weeks prior to any surgical procedure.

Herbal supplements are becoming increasingly popular with patients who are looking for a "natural" option to traditional medication. Patients may not readily volunteer the fact that they are taking these supplements, either because they do not characterize them as medication or out of fear that physicians will not be accepting of alternative treatments. Therefore, it is important to ask patients specifically if they are taking any supplements. Ginkgo, garlic, ginseng, ginger, and vitamin E may increase the risk of perioperative bleeding. As these herbal supplements are not medically necessary, patients should discontinue them for several weeks prior to undergoing dermatologic surgery.

Ah-Weng A: Preoperative monitoring of warfarin in cutaneous surgery. Br J Dermatol 2003; 149:386–389.

Dinehart SM, Henry L: Dietary supplements: altered coagulation and effects on bruising. Dermatol Surg 2005; 31:819–826.

Dixon AJ, et al: Bleeding complications in skin cancer surgery are associated with warfarin but not aspirin therapy. Br J Surg 2007 Nov; 94(11):1356–1360.

Hurst EA, et al: Bleeding complications in dermatologic surgery. Semin Cutan Med Surg 2007; 26:40–46.

Kovich O, Otley CC: Thrombotic complications related to discontinuation of warfarin and aspirin therapy preoperatively for cutaneous operation. J Am Acad Dermatol 2003; 48:233–237.

Lewis KG, Dufresne RG Jr: A meta-analysis of complications attributed to anticoagulation among patients following cutaneous surgery. Dermatol Surg 2008; 34:160–164.

Otley CC: Perioperative evaluation and management in dermatologic surgery. J Am Acad Dermatol 2006 Jan; 54(1):119–127. Review.

Syed S, et al: A prospective assessment of bleeding and international normalized ratio in warfarin-anticoagulated patients having cutaneous surgery. J Am Acad Dermatol 2004; 51:955–957.

West SW, et al: Cutaneous surgeons cannot predict blood-thinner status by intraoperative visual inspection. Plast Reconstr Surg 2002; 110:98–103.

Antibiotic prophylaxis

Dermatologists performing cutaneous surgery are often faced with the decision of whether to prescribe prophylactic antibiotics. The main issues surrounding antibiotic prophylaxis are prevention of surgical site infections and reduction of the risk of endocarditis or contamination of prosthetic devices in high-risk patients. While there is a trend in medicine towards evidence-based approaches, this is often overlooked by many dermatologists when it comes to antibiotic prophylaxis. While reducing infection is one objective in the use of antibiotics, dermatologists must take into consideration the risks of such treatment, including adverse drug reaction, serious drug reactions, drug interactions, development of resistant strains of bacteria, and increased cost.

Surgical site infection

Determining the indications for antibiotic prophylaxis for surgical site infections requires an understanding of the various types of wound that the dermatologist may encounter. Wounds are categorized into four groups:

1. Clean wounds (class I) are created on normal skin using clean or sterile technique. Examples include excision of neoplasms, noninflamed cysts, biopsies, and most cases of Mohs surgery. The majority of dermatologic surgery falls into this category. The infection rate of these wounds is less than 5%. Of note, this incidence is based on general surgery cases, which are often of longer duration and a greater extent than most dermatologic procedures. This explains the lower actual infection rate in dermatologic surgery, which is in the 1–3% range.

2. Clean-contaminated wounds (class II) are created on contaminated skin or any mucosal or moist intertriginous surface, such as the oral cavity, upper respiratory tract, axilla, or perineum. The infection rate of these wounds is 10%.

3. Contaminated wounds (class III) involve visibly inflamed skin with/without nonpurulent discharge and have an infection rate of 20–30%. Examples included inflamed cysts or traumatic wounds.

4. Infected wounds (class IV) have contaminated foreign bodies, purulent discharge, or devitalized tissue. Examples included necrotic tumors, ruptured cysts, or active hidradenitis suppurativa. These wounds have an infection rate of 40%.

Clean (class I) wounds, which constitute the vast majority of dermatologic surgery procedures, do not require antibiotic prophylaxis.

Although antibiotic prophylaxis in clean-contaminated (class II) wounds is not a clear issue, most cases do not require routine antibiotics. It is preferable to treat infections should they arise (as they are not a common occurrence, even in class II wounds), rather than expose all patients to antibiotics and the increased rate of drug-related adverse events. The exception to this would be those surgery cases that violate mucosal membranes (i.e. oral, nasal, or anogenital mucosa), and patients with heavily colonized skin (i.e. atopic dermatitis or infected skin), as well as those patients in whom a wound infection would result in significant morbidity.

In contaminated (class III) and infected (class IV) wounds, antibiotics serve a therapeutic, rather than a prophylactic, role and should be used routinely in these cases.

Antibiotic selection and timing

In order to be achieve optimal prophylaxis, antibiotics ought to be in the bloodstream, and thus at the surgical site, at the time of incision. Antibiotics given at the conclusion of the procedure are not as effective in preventing infection, as they are not incorporated into the coagulum of the wound. Once the surgical wound is closed, the risk of infection decreases significantly. As the majority of dermatologic procedures are of short duration, a single preoperative dose of antibiotics 1 h before the start of the case is sufficient. In rare cases with an extended dermatologic procedure, a second dose of antibiotics can be administered 6 h postoperatively.

The choice of antibiotic is based on the surgical site's most likely causative organism (Table 37-1). *Staphylococcus aureus* is the most common wound infection in cutaneous surgery.

Table 37-1 Antibiotic prophylaxis for heavily colonized or high-risk patients

Situation	Antibiotic	Regimen (1 h preoperative dose)
Skin	Cephalexin	1 g orally
	Dicloxacillin	1 g orally
	Clindamycin	300 mg orally
	Vancomycin	500 mg IV
Oral/respiratory mucosa	Cephalexin	1 g orally
	Amoxicillin	1 g orally
	Clindamycin	300 mg orally
Gastrointestinal/ genitourinary mucosa	Cephalexin	1 g orally
	Trimethoprim/ sulfamethoxazole	1 double-strength tablet orally
	Ciprofloxacin	500 mg orally

Other pathogens that need to be considered in some situations include *Streptococcus viridans* (oral mucosa) and *Escherichia coli* (perineal and genital location).

First-generation cephalosporins are an ideal initial choice for the treatment of wound infection because of their coverage of staphylococcal organisms, common Gram-negative organisms such as *E. coli*, and certain *Proteus* species. They are rapidly absorbed when taken orally and have good tissue penetration. The estimated cross-reactivity in penicillin-allergic patients is 5–10%.

Isoxazolyl penicillins, such as dicloxacillin and nafcillin, can also be used as they provide coverage for most strains of streptococci and β-lactamase-producing bacterial strains such as *S. aureus*. Aminopenicillins, such as ampicillin and amoxicillin, have better Gram-negative, enterococcal, and group A streptococcal coverage. However, they are not effective against β-lactamase-producing bacteria, and thus are more commonly used in procedures involving oral mucosa.

Clindamycin, macrolides (i.e. erythromycin or azithromycin), trimethoprim-sulfamethoxazole, and ciprofloxacin can all be considered in patients with a penicillin or cephalosporin allergy, with the specific choice based on the site of surgery and thus the presumed causative organism. Vancomycin is generally limited to those cases where methicillin-resistant *S. aureus* (MRSA) is suspected, as it requires intravenous administration and adjustment in patients with impaired renal function.

Treatment of wound infection

Postoperative surgical site infection is quite uncommon in dermatologic surgery procedures, with an incidence of 1–3%. Infections typically present 4–7 days after surgery with increased erythema, tenderness, warmth, and purulent drainage. Sutures can be removed to allow for drainage of exudate. In cases where infection leads to dehiscence, the wound can be packed or allowed to heal by second intention. Scar revision can be performed at a later date. A culture should be performed prior to initiating empiric antibiotics to determine sensitivities.

S. aureus is the most common pathogen, and cephalexin or dicloxacillin is an appropriate first-line treatment. Those patients with a penicillin allergy can be treated with clindamycin. Although this antibiotic has been associated with colitis, the short courses that are typically used with surgical site infection generally do not present a problem. In those communities or institutions with a high incidence of MRSA, antibiotic choice can be modified based on community sensitivities (e.g. doxycycline or trimethoprim-sulfamethoxazole). Ciprofloxacin can be used for those infections with a higher likelihood of Gram-negative or *Pseudomonas* organisms (e.g.

ear). Antibiotic choice should be modified based on culture results.

Endocarditis prophylaxis

The American Heart Association (AHA) updated its recommendations on infective endocarditis (IE) prophylaxis in 2007. The overall conclusions were that bacteremia from daily activities is much more likely to cause IE than bacteremia associated with dental procedures, and that far fewer patients are now recommended to have antibiotic prophylaxis. Antibiotic prophylaxis has been limited to patients with the conditions listed in Box 37-2. All other cardiac conditions, including mitral valve prolapse and other forms of congenital heart disease, no longer require prophylaxis for any procedure.

Antibiotic prophylaxis is reasonable when procedures involve manipulation of gingival tissue, perforation of oral mucosa, or incision or biopsy of the respiratory mucosa, or are performed on infected skin, but only in patients with underlying cardiac conditions associated with the highest risk of adverse outcome, as outlined in the box below. Antibiotic prophylaxis solely to prevent infective endocarditis is not recommended for gastrointestinal or genitourinary procedures. The AHA reaffirmed its 1997 statement regarding medical procedures, including incision or biopsy of surgically scrubbed skin, that do not require antibiotic prophylaxis. Antibiotic prophylactic regimens for those selected high-risk patients should be a single dose of antibiotic administered 1 h before the procedure (Table 37-3).

There are no formal guidelines regarding the use of antibiotics in patients with orthopedic prosthetic devices undergoing dermatologic surgery. However, guidelines for dental procedures in patients with joint replacement can be extrapolated to certain procedures. Patients with joint replacement probably do not need prophylactic antibiotics for clean wounds. If mucosa is invaded, prophylaxis may be appropriate and reasonable in the small number of patients who might be at high risk of joint infection. Consultation with orthopedic surgery is appropriate in determining whether antibiotic prophylaxis is necessary.

American Dental Association, American Academy of Orthopedic Surgeons: Antibiotic prophylaxis for dental patients with total joint replacements. J Am Dent Assoc 2003 Jul; 134(7):895–899.

Amici JM, et al: A prospective study of the incidence of complications associated with dermatologic surgery. Br J Dermatol 2005; 153:967–971.

Hurst EA, et al: Infectious complications and antibiotic use in dermatologic surgery. Semin Cutan Med Surg 2007; 26:47–53.

Maragh SL, et al: Antibiotic prophylaxis in dermatologic surgery: updated guidelines. Dermatol Surg 2005; 31:83–91.

Messingham MJ, Arpey CJ: Update on the use of antibiotics in cutaneous surgery. Dermatol Surg 2005; 31:1068–1078.

Otley CC: Perioperative evaluation and management in dermatologic surgery. J Am Acad Dermatol 2006 Jan; 54(1):119–127. Review.

Wilson W, et al: Prevention of infective endocarditis: guidelines from the American Heart Association: a guideline from the American Heart Association Rheumatic Fever, Endocarditis, and Kawasaki Disease Committee, Council on Cardiovascular Disease in the Young, and the Council on Clinical Cardiology, Council on Cardiovascular Surgery and Anesthesia, and the Quality of Care and Outcomes Research Interdisciplinary Working Group. Circulation 2007; 116:1736–1754.

Wright TI, et al: Antibiotic prophylaxis in dermatologic surgery: advisory statement 2008. J Am Acad Dermatol. 2008 Sep; 59(3):464–473.

Preoperative antisepsis

Many surgical preparations are available. Alcohol is commonly used for minor clean procedures, such as biopsies. However, since it has only weak antimicrobial activity, it is not recommended for more extensive procedures.

Chlorhexidine has a broad spectrum against Gram-positive and Gram-negative organisms, a rapid onset of activity, sustained residual activity even after being wiped off, and is nonstaining. Chlorhexidine has been reported to cause both

---

Box 37-2 Cardiac conditions associated with the highest endocarditis risk

- Prosthetic cardiac valve or prosthetic material used for cardiac valve repair
- Previous infectious endocarditis
- Congenital heart disease (CHD)*
  - Unrepaired cyanotic CHD, including palliative shunts and conduits
  - Completely repaired congenital heart defect with prosthetic material or device, during the first 6 months after the procedure
  - Repaired CHD with residual defects at the site or adjacent to the site of a prosthetic patch or prosthetic device (which inhibit endothelialization)
- Cardiac transplantation recipients who develop cardiac valvulopathy

*Except for conditions listed above, antibiotic prophylaxis is not recommended for any other form of CHD.
Adapted from Wilson et al. (2007)

Table 37-3 Endocarditis prophylaxis regimen (single dose 1 h prior to procedure)

Situation	Agent	Adults	Children
Able to take oral medication	Amoxicillin	2 g	50 mg/kg
Unable to take oral medication	Ampicillin *or*	2 g IM/IV	50 mg/kg IM/IV
	Cefazolin or ceftriaxone	1 g IM/IV	50 mg/kg IM/IV
Allergic to penicillins or ampicillin and able to take oral medication	Cephalexin* *or*	2 g	50 mg/kg
	Clindamycin *or*	600 mg	20 mg/kg
	Azithromycin or clarithromycin	500 mg	15 mg/kg
Allergic to penicillins or ampicillin and unable to take oral medication	Cefazolin or ceftriaxone* *or*	1 g IM/IV	50 mg/mg IM/IV
	Clindamycin	600 mg IM/IV	20 mg IM/IV

*Cephalosporins should not be used in patients with a history of anaphylaxis, angioedema, or urticaria with penicillins or ampicillin.
Adapted from Wilson et al. (2007)

ototoxicity and keratitis from direct tympanic or ocular contact. However, this is mainly in patients under general anesthesia who cannot respond to immediate irritation associated with ocular contact, a problem that is avoided in most dermatologic procedures performed under local anesthesia.

Betadine and all iodine-containing preparations have an excellent bactericidal activity within several minutes of application. However, they are often irritating to the skin, leave a residual color, can be absorbed in premature infants, and must dry before the procedure if they are to act as an effective antimicrobial agent.

Hexachlorophene is not bactericidal against many Gram-negative organisms. It has the potential for neurotoxicity in children and teratogenicity in pregnancy. Hydrogen peroxide has no significant antiseptic properties, and thus it is not suitable for sterile skin preparation.

If hair must be removed prior to surgery, this should be done in a manner that does not leave open skin (i.e. cuts or scratches), which can serve as a conduit for infection. Preoperative shaving has been associated with a higher rate of bacterial infection secondary to cutting of the skin surface.

Thornton Spann C, et al: Topical antimicrobial agents in dermatology. Clin Dermatol 2003; 21:70–77.

Anesthesia

Anesthetics work by blocking sodium influx into neurons and preventing depolarization and blockage of action potential. Small unmyelinated C-fibers, which carry pain and temperature sensation, are more easily blocked than larger myelinated A-fibers, which carry pressure sensation and motor function. This difference translates clinically, with patients under local anesthesia not experiencing pain from the sharp incision, but still maintaining the sensation of pressure during the procedure.

All local anesthetics have a similar structure, consisting of three parts: an aromatic hydrophobic ring, an intermediate chain, and an amine end. The aromatic hydrophobic portion is lipophilic and facilitates diffusion through nerve cell membranes, correlating to the potency of the anesthesia. The hydrophilic amine end contributes to the aqueous solubility of the anesthetic and is involved in binding of the molecule to the sodium channel. The intermediate chain consists of either an amide or an ester. Amides are metabolized by hepatic microsomal enzymes, while esters are metabolized in plasma by pseudocholinesterase and excreted by the kidney.

The choice of anesthetic is based on a variety of factors, including patient allergy, renal or hepatic impairment, and type of procedure being performed. The workhorse anesthetic of dermatologic surgery is lidocaine, due to its rapid onset of action and intermediate duration of action. Longer-acting anesthetics, such as bupivacaine, have a delayed onset of action, but can be used in special procedures or in combination with lidocaine to maximize duration of anesthesia.

All local anesthetics, with the exception of cocaine and prilocaine, cause vasodilatation due to relaxation of smooth muscle. As a result, patients experience increased surgical bleeding and shorter duration of action as the anesthesia is cleared from the surgical site due to vasodilatation. Epinephrine, which causes vasoconstriction, is often added to local anesthetics to decrease bleeding, increase duration of anesthesia, and reduce systemic side effects due to systemic absorption. Concentrations of 1:100 000 to 1:400 000 are typically used, with lower concentrations having fewer side effects while still maintaining clinical efficacy. As the vasoconstrictive effect of epinephrine takes 15 min for onset, the surgeon must allow adequate time prior to starting the procedure. Epinephrine is a strong α- and β-adrenergic receptor agonist, and has an absolute contraindi-

cation in hyperthyroidism and pheochromocytoma. Large amounts of epinephrine must be used cautiously in patients with severe hypertension or narrow-angle glaucoma, and in pregnancy. Patients taking β-blockers, monoamine oxidase inhibitors, tricyclic antidepressants, and phenothiazines are more sensitive to epinephrine. While the subject of much controversy, epinephrine is safe to use in well-vascularized areas, such as the ear, nose, and genitals. Reports of necrosis are likely due to excessive volume being placed, which can cause a physical tamponade of vessels, rather than being a direct result of epinephrine.

Sodium bicarbonate (8.4%) can be added (1:10 ratio) in order to reduce the pain and burning associated with the lower pH of lidocaine with epinephrine. However, sodium bicarbonate can reduce epinephrine activity with time, thus requiring freshly mixed preparations on a regular basis.

Side effects

The most common side effect of local anesthetic is injection site pain. Buffering with sodium bicarbonate, using a small-gauge needle (i.e. 30 gauge), using ice or vibratory distraction at the injection site, injecting slowly into the subcutaneous tissue (rather than the dermis), warming the anesthesia, minimizing the number of injections, and placing subsequent injections in an already anesthetized location can minimize the pain associated with local anesthesia. Vasovagal reactions are common during anesthesia administration. Patients should lie flat during the injection to reduce this occurrence. Cold compresses and placing the patient in a Trendelenburg position can help if symptoms occur.

Maximum dosage of anesthesia has traditionally been accepted as 5 mg/kg of 1% plain lidocaine and 7 mg/kg of 1% lidocaine with epinephrine. These numbers have been based on old industry-based studies, not found in the medical literature. Experience with tumescent liposuction has taught that dosages up to 55 mg/kg are well tolerated and safe in certain clinical situations. Bupivacaine has a greater risk of cardiac toxicity than lidocaine, because of its longer duration of action.

Most true allergic reactions to local anesthetics have been reported with esters. The metabolite *p*-aminobenzoic acid (PABA) is responsible for ester allergies. There is no cross-reactivity between ester and amide classes of anesthetics, so allergy to one type does not preclude the use of the other. True systemic amide allergy is extremely rare. Thorough questioning of patients who report allergy often reveals a vasovagal reaction or epinephrine sensitivity. If local anesthetic use is precluded, intradermal injection with diphenhydramine can be used. Drowsiness can be a side effect when large doses of this agent are used. Bacteriostatic saline, with the benzyl alcohol preservative acting as the anesthetic agent, is often sufficient to provide the brief anesthesia needed to perform small procedures.

Topical anesthetics can be effectively used for many laser procedures, as well as decreasing pain associated with pin-pricks of local anesthesia. These products require an extended time of application and/or occlusion in order to penetrate the stratum corneum and work effectively. The level of anesthesia obtained with these topical agents is often inconsistent. They are more effective on mucosa, due to the absence of the corneal barrier. There are numerous lidocaine-containing products in a variety of preparations. Eutectic mixture of 2.5% lidocaine and 2.5% prilocaine (EMLA, AstraZeneca, Wilmington, DE) has also been used extensively. Prilocaine-induced methemoglobinemia has been reported in children due to the increased systemic absorption of prilocaine from certain topical products.

Direct application of ice can reduce injection site pain. Ethyl chloride spray rapidly chills the skin and can be used for small curettage procedures or needle insertion. Refrigerated forced air or water-chilled sapphire crystals can help reduce pain associated with laser procedures. Ophthalmic solutions of proparacaine 0.5% or tetracaine 0.5% can provide rapid anesthesia and are useful when placing corneal shields.

Amin SP, Goldberg DJ: Topical anesthetics for cosmetic and laser dermatology. J Drugs Dermatol 2005; 4:455–461.

Koay J, Orengo I: Application of local anesthetics in dermatologic surgery. Dermatol Surg 2002; 28:143–148.

Anatomy

A thorough understanding of anatomy is critical when performing dermatologic surgery. The vascular supply, sensory and motor innervation, and muscles of facial expression all play a role in the successful surgical outcome (Figs 37-1 to 37-3; Box 37-4).

Several key danger zones are worthy of mention. The temporal branch of the facial nerve is at greatest risk for injury when it runs superficial to the deep temporalis fascia as it crosses the zygomatic arch. Care must be taken to undermine bluntly in a plane above the SMAS (superficial muscular aponeurotic system). Injury to the temporal nerve results in brow ptosis and inability to raise the eyebrow. The danger zone for the marginal mandibular nerve lies where it crosses over the body of mandible, just anterior to the masseter muscle. Injury to the marginal mandibular nerve causes asymmetrical ipsilateral lip elevation and inability to show the lower teeth. The spinal accessory nerve is at risk in a region of the neck

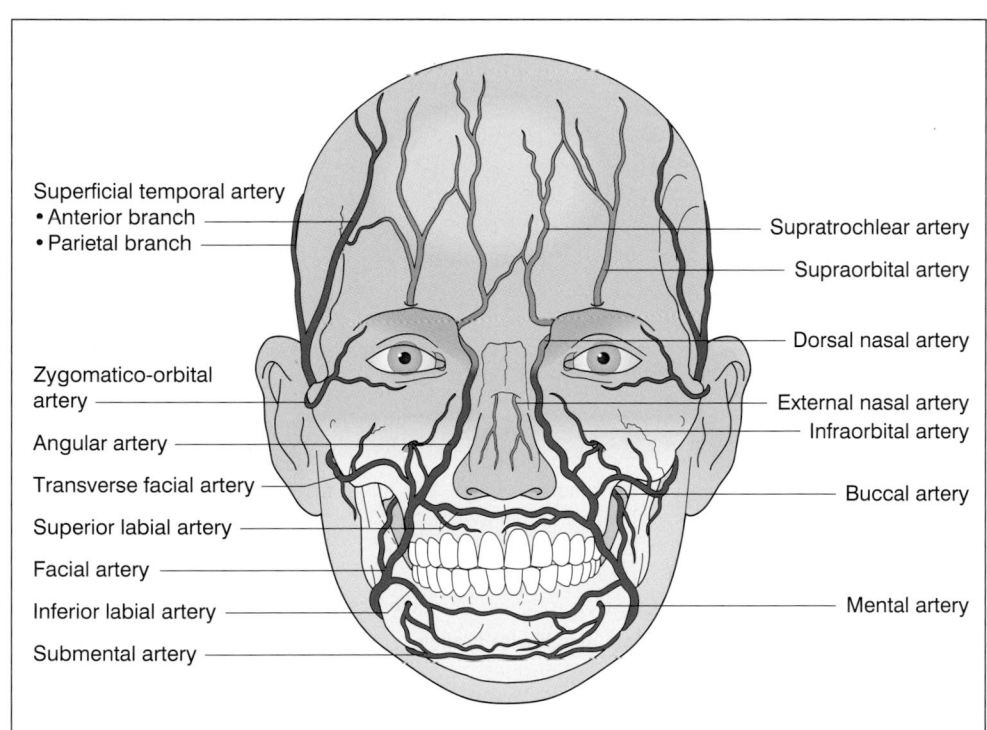

Fig. 37-1 Arterial supply of the face. Light pink designates arteries derived from the internal carotid artery; dark pink, from the external carotid artery. With permission from Bolognia JL, Jorizzo JL, Rapini RP (eds): Dermatology. 2nd edn. London: Mosby, 2008.

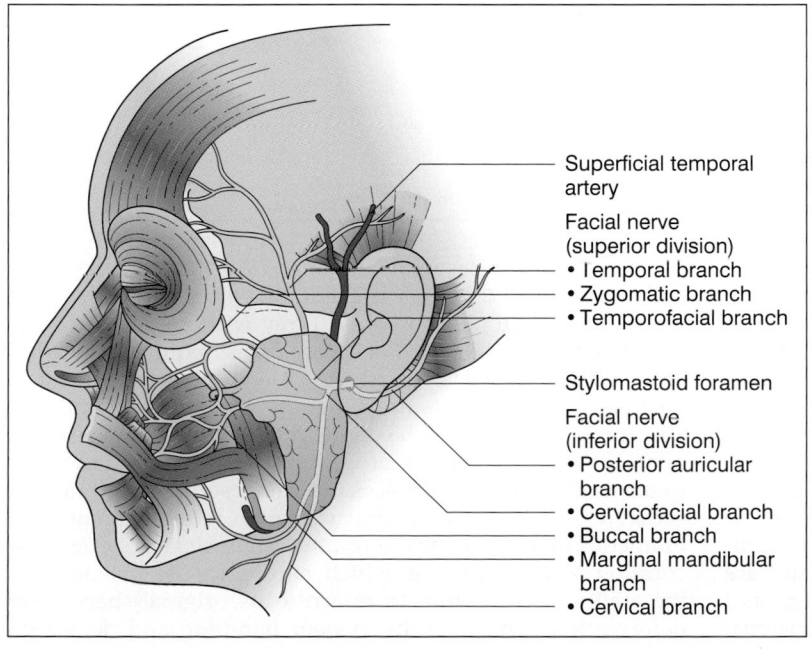

Fig. 37-2 The facial (motor) nerve. With permission from Bolognia JL, Jorizzo JL, Rapini RP (eds): Dermatology. 2nd edn. London: Mosby, 2008.

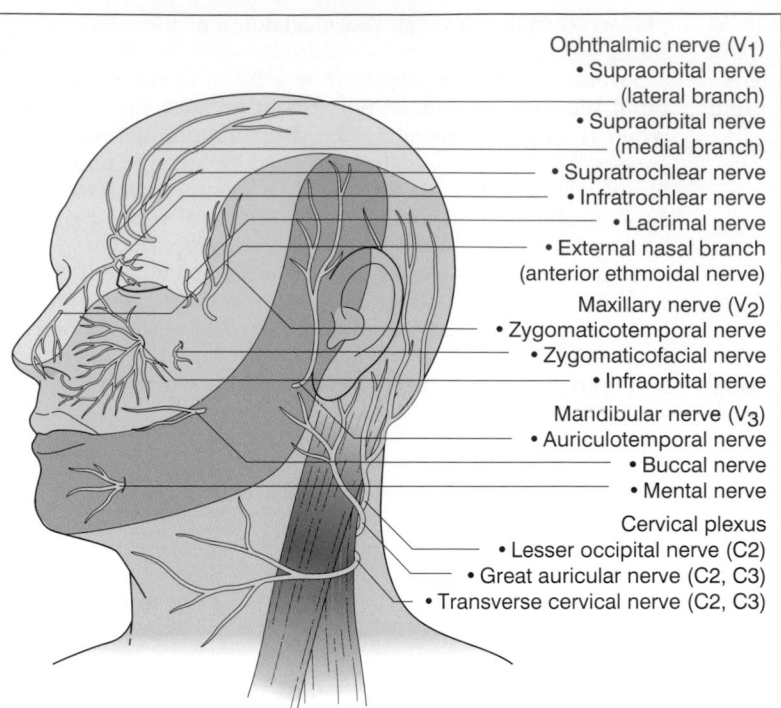

Fig. 37-3 The trigeminal (cranial nerve V) and cervical plexus cutaneous sensory nerves. The concha and external auditory canal are variably innervated by branches of the vagus, glossopharyngeal, and facial nerves. With permission from Bolognia JL, Jorizzo JL, Rapini RP (eds): Dermatology. 2nd edn. London: Mosby, 2008.

Ophthalmic nerve (V₁)
- Supraorbital nerve (lateral branch)
- Supraorbital nerve (medial branch)
- Supratrochlear nerve
- Infratrochlear nerve
- Lacrimal nerve
- External nasal branch (anterior ethmoidal nerve)

Maxillary nerve (V₂)
- Zygomaticotemporal nerve
- Zygomaticofacial nerve
- Infraorbital nerve

Mandibular nerve (V₃)
- Auriculotemporal nerve
- Buccal nerve
- Mental nerve

Cervical plexus
- Lesser occipital nerve (C2)
- Great auricular nerve (C2, C3)
- Transverse cervical nerve (C2, C3)

Box 37-4 Innervation of the muscles of facial expression via cranial nerve VII (the facial nerve)

Temporal branch
- Frontalis muscle (m.)
- Corrugator supercilii m.
- Orbicularis oculi m. (upper portion)
- Auricular m. (anterior and superior; also known as the temporoparietalis m.)

Posterior auricular branch
- Occipitalis m.
- Auricular m. (posterior)

Zygomatic branch
- Orbicularis oculi m. (lower portion)
- Nasalis m. (alar portion)
- Procerus m.
- Upper lip muscles
  - Levator anguli oris m.
  - Zygomaticus major m.

Buccal branch
- Buccinator m. (muscle of mastication)
- Depressor septi nasi m.

- Nasalis m. (transverse portion)
- Upper lip muscles
  - Zygomaticus major and minor m.
  - Levator labii superioris m.
  - Orbicularis oris m.
  - Levator anguli oris m.
- Lower lip muscles (orbicularis oris m.)

Marginal mandibular branch
- Lower lip muscles
  - Orbicularis oris m.
  - Depressor anguli oris m.
  - Depressor labii inferioris m.
  - Mentalis m.
- Risorius m.
- Platysma m. (upper portion)

Cervical branch
- Platysma m.

With permission from Bolognia JL, Jorizzo JL, Rapini RP (eds): Dermatology. 2nd edn. London: Mosby, 2008.

---

delineated by the clavicle inferiorly, the sternocleidomastoid muscle anteriorly, and the trapezius muscle laterally and posteriorly. Damage to the nerve causes a winged scapula, inability to shrug the shoulder, difficulty abducting the shoulder, shoulder drop, and chronic shoulder pain.

Equipment

The choice of instruments and suture depends on the procedure being performed. Most simple, in-office biopsies are performed in a "clean" rather than sterile manner, and require minimal instrumentation. More complex excisional

and reconstructive surgery is generally performed with sterile technique and employs a surgical tray with a wider range of instruments (Box 37-5). For procedures requiring sutures, absorbable material is used for deeper, layered closures, whereas surface sutures are generally nonabsorbable or fast-absorbing (Box 37-6). The large number of suture choices relates to both the type of procedure performed and the anatomic location treated. Choices include absorbable and nonabsorbable, synthetic and nonsynthetic, monofilament and braided. There are a variety of other characteristics one must consider when choosing which suture to use. Memory is the ability of the suture to return to its original shape after deformation, which results in poor handling and decreased

Box 37-5 Cutaneous surgical instruments and supplies

- Scalpel handle (flat No. 3)
- Blade (No. 15)
- Needle holder (appropriate size)
- Sharp curved iris scissors, tissue-cutting scissors
- Blunt undermining scissors
- Skin hook (dull-tipped, 2–4-prong)
- Hemostats
- Forceps (1 × 2 teeth, with suture platform)
- Skin preparatory scrub in sterile basin
- Sterile towels
- Sterile gauze and cotton-tipped swabs
- Hyfrecator cover
- Suture
- Suture scissors
- Blade remover

Box 37-6 Examples of common skin suture material

Absorbable

Gut (chromic, plain)	twisted
Polyglycolic acid (Dexon®)	braided
Polygalactin 910 (Vicryl®)	braided
Polydioxanone (PDS®)	monofilament
Polytrimethylene carbonate (Maxon®)	monofilament
Poliglecaprone 25 (Monocryl®)	monofilament
Glycomer 631 (Biosyn®)	monofilament

Nonabsorbable

Silk	braided
Nylon (Ethilon®, Dermalon®)	monofilament
Nylon (Surgilon®, Nurolon®)	braided
Polypropylene (Prolene®, Surgipro®)	monofilament
Polyester (Ethibond®, Mersilene®, Dacron®)	braided
Polybutester (Novafil®)	monofilament

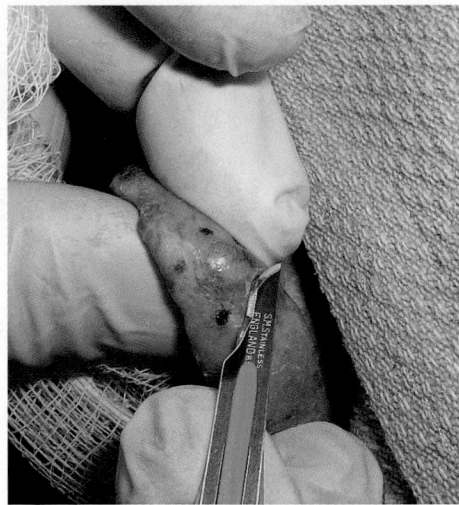

Fig. 37-4 Shave biopsy. Lesion is pinched up with thumb and finger and biopsy performed with sweeping strokes.

knot security. Plasticity is the ability of the suture to retain its new shape after it has been stretched. Elasticity is the ability of a suture to return to its original length and shape after stretching, an important factor to consider in relation to the resulting edema associated with surgery. The coefficient of friction is the ease with which the suture slides through tissue and is directly related to knot security. Capillarity is the ability of the suture to wick away fluid, with braided sutures having an increased tendency to trap fluid and bacteria. All have appropriate applications and a detailed discussion is beyond the scope of this chapter.

In general, for procedures requiring buried suture, a synthetic braided suture is a common choice. The 50% tensile strength for this class of suture is about 3 months. Additionally, it is less palpable under the skin. For procedures on the trunk and extremities (i.e. areas under tension), a monofilament absorbable suture may be a better choice, as the tensile strength may last for a greater length of time. The thicker skin in these areas may hide the palpability of this class of suture, making it more acceptable to patients. Epidermal approximation in more delicate areas is more appropriately closed with smaller 5-0 or 6-0 sutures. Absorbable sutures (e.g. gut) may be considered in sensitive areas where suture removal may be painful or difficult (e.g. eyelids) or in children. Facial sutures are often taken out in 4–7 days to decrease the chance of forming track marks from epithelialization of the suture puncture site, whereas sutures on the scalp, neck, and body are often left in for approximately 2 weeks. Running subcuticular sutures can

be left in for 3 weeks to add tensile strength to wounds without the risk of suture marks.

Biopsies

When performing a skin biopsy, the clinician should consider the lesion characteristics, reason for biopsy (i.e. diagnostic versus cosmetic), and site. Shave biopsies can range from a superficial scissor snip of an epidermal growth to deep shave excisions of papillary dermal processes. Punch biopsies are most often used for dermal lesions, sampling deeper than shave biopsies, but requiring sutures. Excisional biopsies remove an entire clinical lesion and are the biopsy of choice for pigmented lesions suspicious for melanoma. Incisional biopsies remove a portion of a clinical lesion and are often performed on larger plaques or patches when an excisional biopsy is not cosmetically acceptable or feasible. A wedge biopsy is a deep incisional biopsy that can sample pathologic tissue and adjacent normal tissue, and is especially useful for pathologic diagnosis of certain inflammatory conditions (e.g. panniculitis, fasciitis).

Shave biopsies are best suited to pedunculated, papular, or otherwise exophytic lesions. Using a deep or rolled shave, samples can also be obtained of macular or indurated lesions, provided the necessary histologic changes reside in the epidermis or papillary dermis. Infiltration of local anesthesia distends and elevates the lesion, increases skin turgor, affords greater resistance to the blade, and facilitates undercutting the lesion. Using either a 15-blade scalpel or a razor blade, which can be flexed to achieve the desired depth, a horizontal incision is made and the lesion removed with sweeping strokes (Fig. 37-4). Hemostasis is attained with 35% aluminum chloride solution.

Sharp scissor biopsy is best suited to pedunculated lesions. Iris or Gradle scissors are used to snip the base of the lesion. In many cases, this can be done without anesthesia. Chemical hemostasis, electrocautery, or simple pressure can be used to control bleeding.

The dermatologic punch is commonly used for both excisional and incisional biopsies (Fig. 37-5). When performing a punch biopsy, the skin should be stretched perpendicular to the relaxed skin tension lines. The elliptical wound resulting from the release of the tension can be suture-closed in a linear fashion without redundancy or puckering associated with circular wounds. The punch is placed on the skin perpendicular to the surface. While the surgeon applies gentle pressure, it is

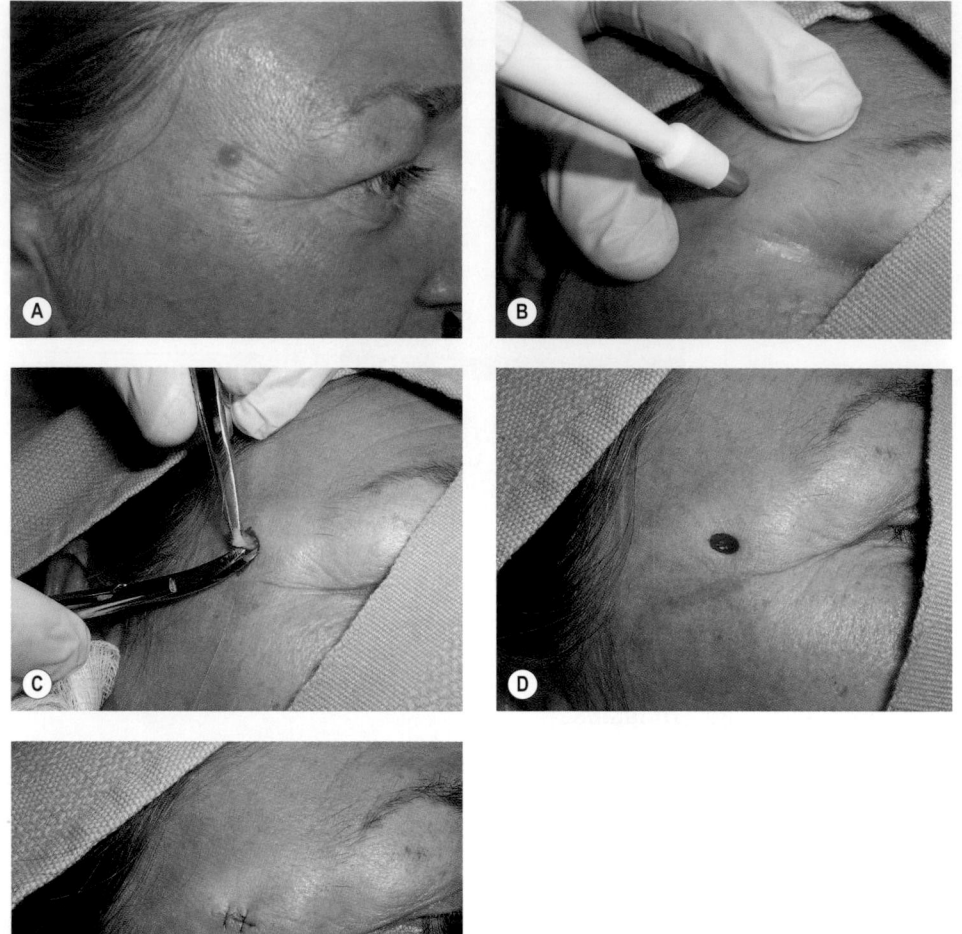

Fig. 37-5 Punch biopsy. A, Lesion to be removed. B, Skin stretched perpendicular to relaxed skin tension lines and punch inserted with twisting motion. C, Specimen is carefully grasped and removed. D, Resultant elliptical defect. E, Sutures in place.

rotated back and forth and advanced to the hub. The specimen is carefully grasped to avoid crush artifact and the base is cut. Sutures are typically placed to achieve hemostasis, but punch sites that are allowed to heal by second intention have been shown to heal with a similar cosmetic outcome.

A variation of the punch biopsy can be used to remove larger subcutaneous nodules. Narrow-hole extrusion is a surgical technique that uses a punch biopsy to make a small cutaneous portal through which larger benign growths (e.g. lipoma) can be extruded (Fig. 37-6). This technique allows the evacuation of large subcutaneous growths with a relatively small surface incision.

Suture technique

Proper suture placement is essential to obtain the desired final result. Sutures are used to close any dead space, reduce bleeding, provide tensile strength and minimize tension to facilitate wound healing, and achieve epidermal wound approximation to maximize cosmetic outcome. Instrument-tied knots are the most common sutures used in dermatologic surgery. Various suturing techniques can be employed, based on factors such as size, anatomic location, and thickness of the surgical wound.

Buried subcutaneous sutures are used for larger or deeper wounds to reduce the chance of wound dehiscence. Proper placement is key to achieving eversion of the wound edges

and decreasing tension (Fig. 37-7). The stitch is in the dermis and fat, with the knot cut short and buried to reduce tissue reaction and "spitting" sutures.

Simple epidermal interrupted sutures are one of the most versatile stitches used in dermatology. They are best used for closure of small punch biopsies, or for larger layered excision or flap repairs. They are especially useful in high-tension wounds, as a single suture can be removed and the surgeon can assess the wound for any dehiscence. For wound edges with a step off the opposing epidermal edges, the surgeon places the suture more superficially at the higher side and deeper on the lower side to even the edges (Fig. 37-8).

The vertical mattress suture is useful for reducing tension, closing dead space, and achieving wound eversion (Fig. 37-9). It can function as both the buried and the superficial suture. As this suture has a high tendency to leave track marks and strangulate the skin, it must be used strategically and removed sooner than traditional sutures. The horizontal mattress suture reduces tension and can be used as a retention suture when attempting to close larger wounds (Fig. 37-10). It can cause strangulation and necrosis of poorly vascularized tissue and should be used with caution when closing flaps.

Running sutures can be used for epidermal closure in wounds under little tension and with closely approximated wound edges. Placement is much faster than simple interrupted sutures, as knots are only used at each end of the wound. The running locked suture is a variant of the simple

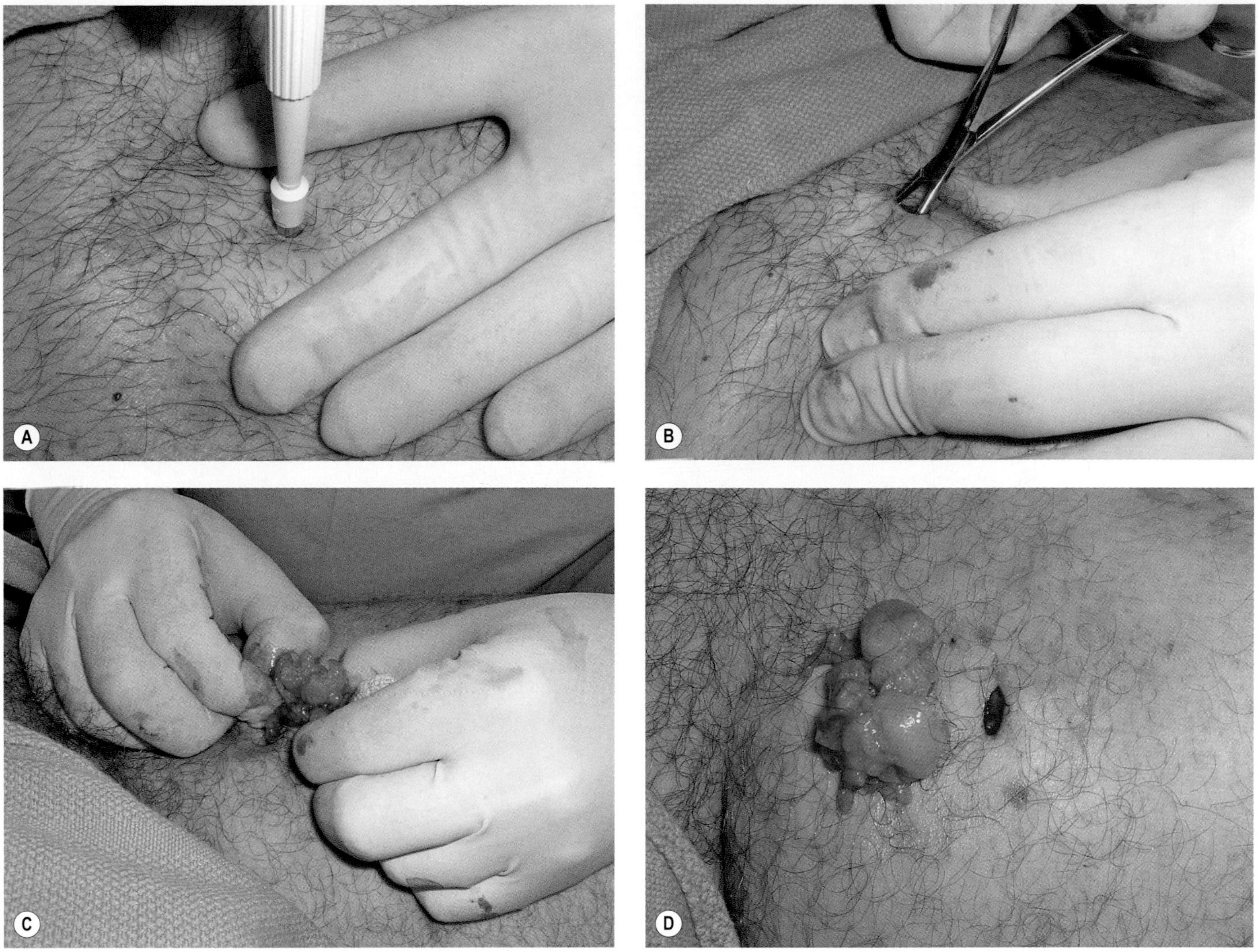

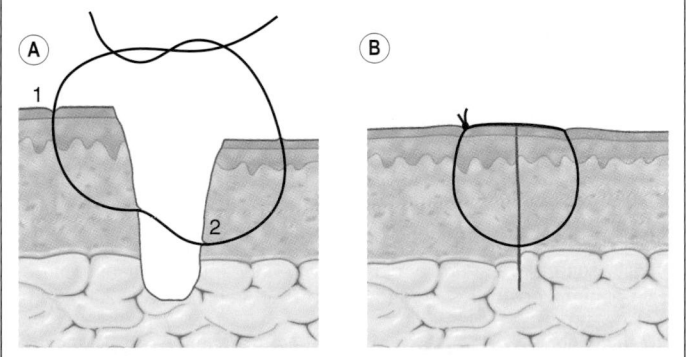

Fig. 37-6 Narrow-hole extrusion of lipoma. A, 4 mm punch in center of lipoma. B, Hemostat used to loosen lipoma. C, Extrusion of lipoma through narrow hole. D, Entire lipoma removed.

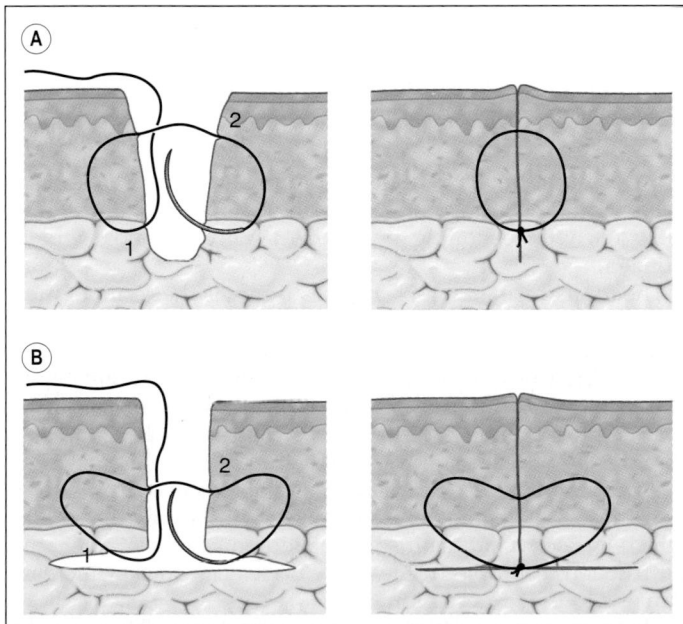

Fig. 37-7 Buried dermal sutures. Numbers indicate entry points of the needle. A, Conventional buried suture placement results in mild wound eversion. B, Buried vertical mattress suture placement results in moderate to significant wound eversion. With permission from Robinson JK, Hanke CW, Sengelmann RD, Siegel DM (eds): Surgery of the Skin. Philadelphia: Mosby, 2005.

Fig. 37-8 Step-off correction. A, To correct a step-off deformity, place a simple interrupted suture superficially on the higher wound edge (1) and deeply on the lower wound edge (2). Numbers indicate entry points of the needle. B, Tying this suture results in even wound edges. With permission from Robinson JK, Hanke CW, Sengelmann RD, Siegel DM (eds): Surgery of the Skin. Philadelphia: Mosby, 2005.

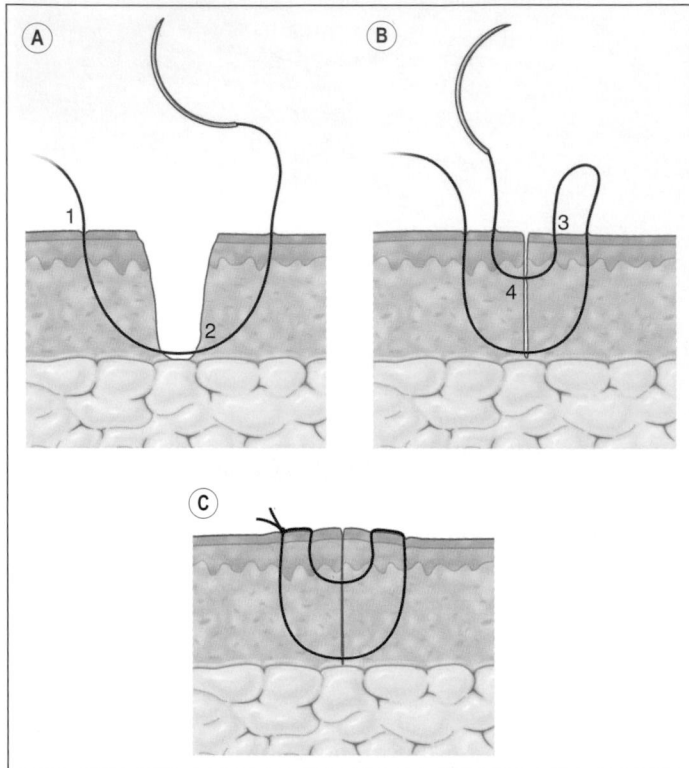

Fig. 37-9 Placement of the vertical mattress stitch. A, The needle is placed 5–10 mm from the wound edge, and a deeply seated simple interrupted suture is placed (1)(2). Numbers indicate entry points of the needle. B, The needle is redirected back across the wound more superficially, penetrating the skin edge 2–4 mm from the wound on both sides (3). C, Final appearance of this suture after tying. With permission from Robinson JK, Hanke CW, Sengelmann RD, Siegel DM (eds): Surgery of the Skin. Philadelphia: Mosby, 2005.

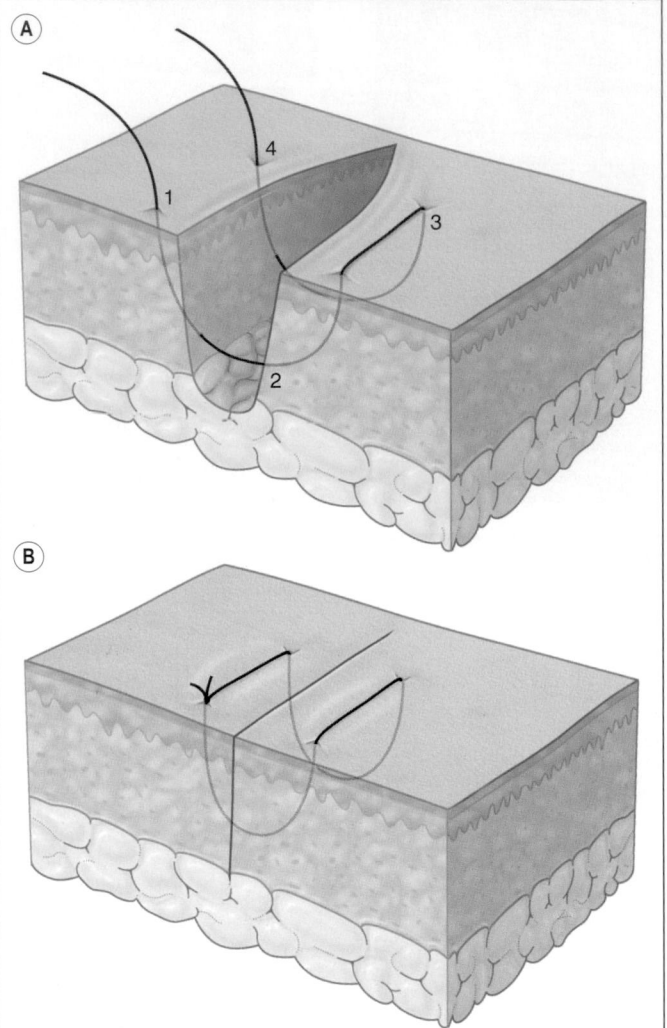

Fig. 37-10 Horizontal mattress suture. A, To place this suture, begin with a widely spaced simple interrupted suture (1) (2). Numbers indicate entry points of the needle. Move laterally down the wound 3–5 mm, and place another interrupted suture in the opposite direction as the first (3) (4). B, The appearance of this suture when tied. With permission from Robinson JK, Hanke CW, Sengelmann RD, Siegel DM (eds): Surgery of the Skin. Philadelphia: Mosby, 2005.

running suture and involves passing the needle through the previous loop (Fig. 37-11). This technique creates pressure along the wound edge and can be used in highly vascularized regions for additional hemostasis.

Running subcuticular sutures typically use a non-absorbable suture and are used for trunk and extremity closures where sutures are left for 2–3 weeks. Since the suture is buried, it can be left in place for a longer period of time without developing cross-hatch marks (Fig. 37-12) A single loop coming out in the middle of larger wounds can help facilitate removal of the suture. Alternatively, absorbable suture can be used and eliminate the need for removal.

Christenson LJ, et al: Primary closure vs second-intention treatment of skin punch biopsy sites: a randomized trial. Arch Dermatol 2005 Sep; 141(9):1093–1099.

Krunic AL, et al: Running combined simple and vertical mattress suture: a rapid skin-everting stitch. Dermatol Surg 2005 Oct; 31(10): 1325–1329.

Lee KK, et al: Surgical revision. Dermatol Clin 2005 Jan; 23(1):141–150, vii.

Moy RL, et al: A review of sutures and suturing techniques. J Dermatol Surg Oncol 1992 Sep; 18(9):785–795.

Cryosurgery

Cryosurgery is used for the treatment of numerous benign, premalignant, and malignant skin lesions. This modality is extensively employed by almost every dermatologist, owing to its ease of use, cost-effectiveness, and versatility. Postoperative wound care is relatively simple and complica-

tions are infrequent. Although a number of cryogens have been used (including ethyl chloride, CO_2, and NO), liquid nitrogen, with a boiling point of –195.6°C, is most widely utilized.

The mechanism of injury in cryosurgery is the result of multiple factors, including mechanical damage to cells resulting from intracellular and extracellular ice crystal formation, exposure to high electrolyte concentrations in surrounding nonfrozen or thawing fluid, recrystallization patterns during thaw, and ischemia caused by vascular stasis and damage. Rapid freezing causes intracellular ice crystals that are more destructive than the extracellular crystals formed during slow freezing. Tissue damage is maximized with a slow thaw time, which causes increased solute gradients and greater cell destruction. Multiple freeze–thaw cycles can further increase damage to the target lesion.

There are several techniques for cryosurgery. The simplest is the use of a cotton-tipped applicator. Varying the amount of pressure applied and the length of contact of the applicator to the skin can control the depth of freeze. Additionally, the volume of liquid nitrogen can be increased or decreased by

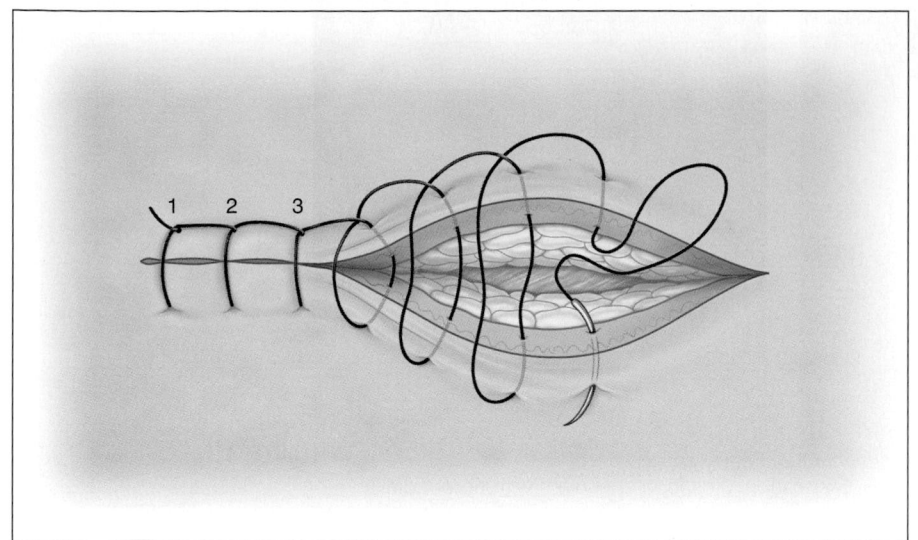

Fig. 37-11 Running block suture. A running simple suture is placed, passing the needle through the loop created by the last suture. This locking suture facilitates hemostasis. Numbers indicate entry points of the needle. With permission from Robinson JK, Hanke CW, Sengelmann RD, Siegel DM (eds): Surgery of the Skin. Philadelphia: Mosby, 2005.

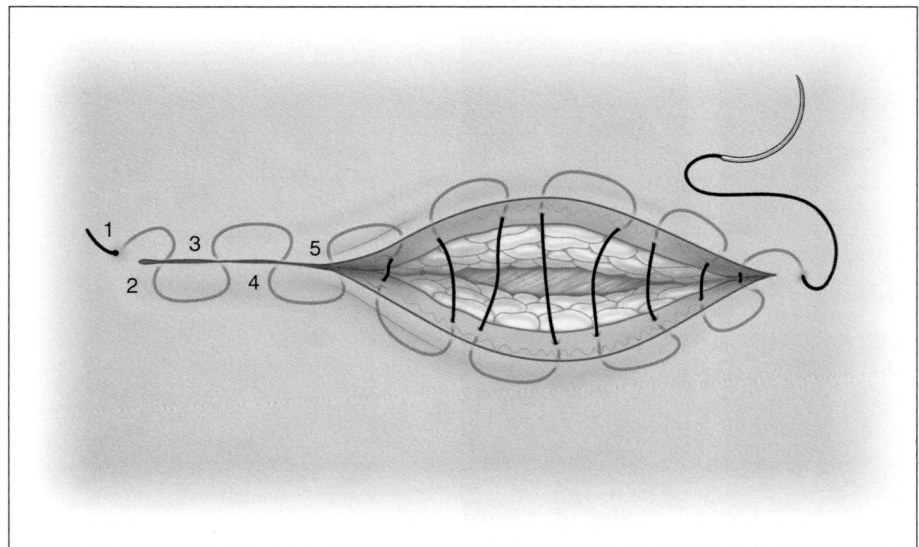

Fig. 37-12 Running subcuticular suture. Multiple horizontally placed dermal sutures are placed in succession on alternating wound edges. This results in epidermal and dermal closure without visible suture marks. Numbers indicate entry points of the needle. With permission from Robinson JK, Hanke CW, Sengelmann RD, Siegel DM (eds): Surgery of the Skin. Philadelphia: Mosby, 2005.

adding or removing cotton from the applicator tip. As viruses have been shown to survive in liquid nitrogen, cotton-tipped applicators should never be reintroduced to the storage container. Rather, a small amount of liquid nitrogen should be transferred to an individual container and discarded after use.

Spray application is one of the most commonly used methods of cryosurgery. This technique uses a hand-held liquid nitrogen spray unit with an adjustable nozzle to vary the size of the stream delivered. An insulating cone or a disposable otoscope speculum can be used to focus the delivery of liquid nitrogen, resulting in a deeper freeze and finer control with less damage to uninvolved skin (Fig. 37-13).

Basal cell carcinomas (BCCs) can be treated effectively with cryosurgery. Freezing to reach a target temperature of approximately −50°C, as measured by a thermocouple, is appropriate for management of these tumors. This translates to a thaw time of approximately 60 sec, with a freeze margin of approximately 5 mm (Fig. 37-14). It is important to recognize that the pain associated with such treatment requires local anesthesia. In a review of published data, Kokoszka et al found a recurrence rate of less than 10% for primary small, noninfiltrating (i.e. superficial and nodular) BCC treated with cryosurgery. Some have suggested that initially treating the tumor with curettage, followed by cryosurgery, can lead to cure rates consistent with curettage and electrodesiccation. However, Kuijpers et al have suggested that standard excision provides higher cure rates than curettage and cryosurgery, and recommend that excision be used as the preferred treatment for BCC, due to the higher cure rate, better cosmetic outcome, and faster healing rates.

Side effects of cryosurgery are similar to those of other ablative procedures (e.g. curettage and electrodesiccation), and include blistering, crusting, pain, a 3–4-week healing period, and scarring. As melanocytes are more susceptible to thermal damage than keratinocytes, hypopigmentation can often be seen, especially in individuals with darker skin tones. While

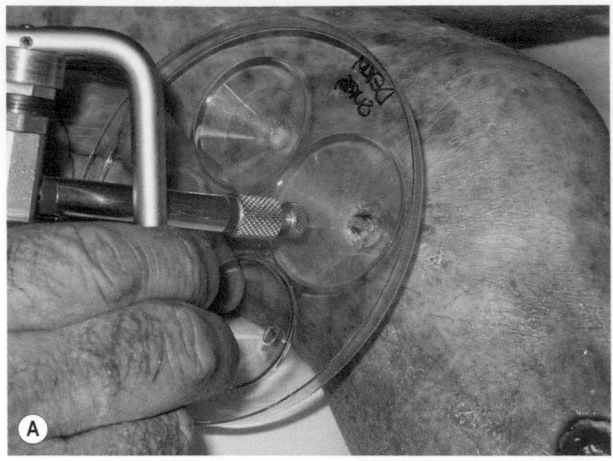
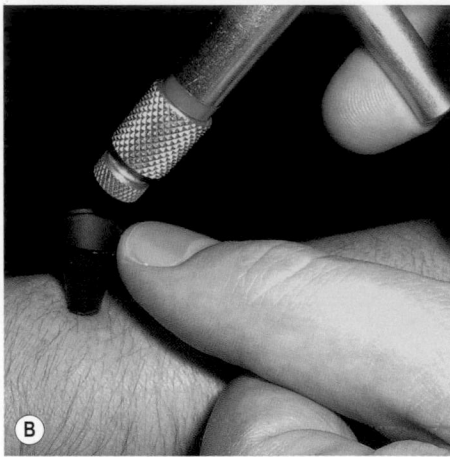

Fig. 37-13 A, Cryoplate with multiple sized openings. B, Disposable otoscope speculum with tip cut off.

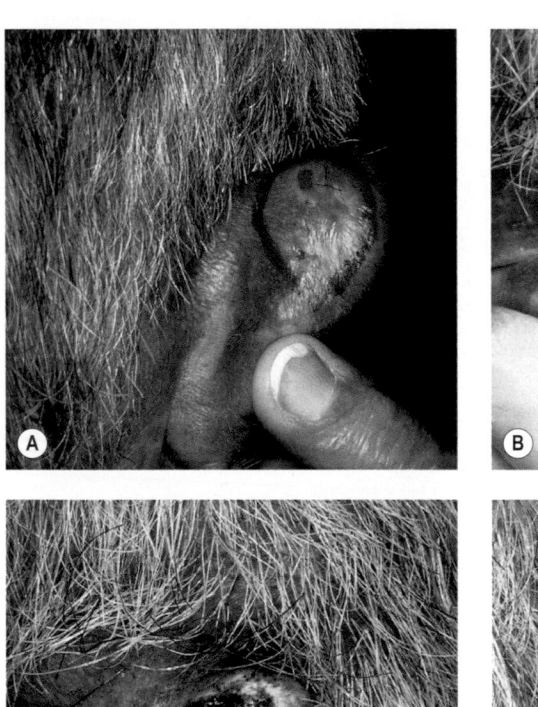
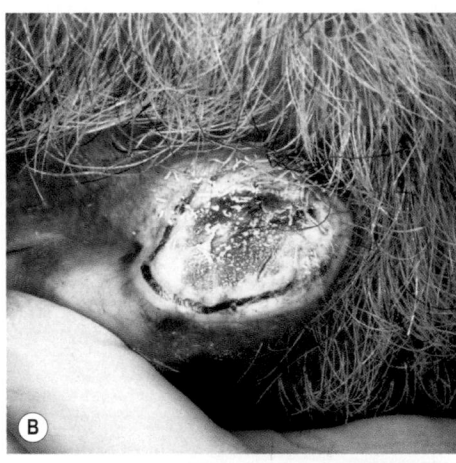
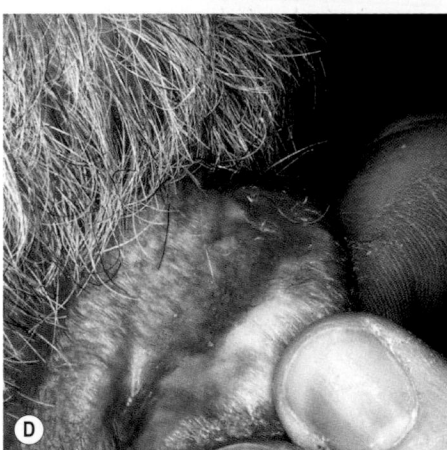

Fig. 37-14 Cryosurgery. A, Basal cell carcinoma on the posterior helix. B, Cryosurgery to neoplasm. C, 1 week later, with necrosis and sloughing of treatment area. D, Final result several months later.

pigment alterations are more frequently seen with longer freeze–thaw times, these changes can be observed even with very brief treatment cycles. A self-limited hyperplastic or pseudoepitheliomatous healing response may occur approximately 2–4 weeks after freezing. Nerve injury can occur during cryosurgery. Anatomic locations with superficial nerves (e.g. lateral aspects of the fingers, ulnar groove of the elbow, pre- and post-auricular skin) are especially susceptible to this complication. Techniques to limit this risk include tenting the skin up and away from the nerve, ballooning the skin with lidocaine, or sliding the skin back and forth over the underlying fascia during treatment to limit exposure to the underlying nerve. Alopecia can occur when treating hair-bearing areas.

Both atrophic and hypertrophic scars can be seen following cryosurgery.

Kokoszka A, Scheinfeld N: Evidence-based review of the use of cryosurgery in treatment of basal cell carcinoma. Dermatol Surg 2003; 29:566.

Kuijpers DI, et al: Surgical excision versus curettage plus cryosurgery in the treatment of basal cell carcinoma. Dermatol Surg 2007; 33:579–587.

Lindemalm-Lundstam B, Dalenbäck J: Prospective follow-up after curettage-cryosurgery for scalp and face skin cancers. Br J Dermatol 2009; 161:568–576.

Nordin P: Curettage-cryosurgery for non-melanoma skin cancer of the external ear: excellent 5-year results. Br J Dermatol 1999; 140:291.

Curettage

The curette has long been a standard tool in the dermatologist's surgical management of neoplasm. This round, semi-sharp knife is available in sizes from 0.5 to 10 mm, allowing for the removal of a variety of lesions. Since it is not as sharp as a scalpel, the curette does not easily cut through normal skin. Therefore, it is best suited for use on soft or friable lesions, such as warts, seborrheic and actinic keratoses, the papules of molluscum contagiosum, or selected basal and squamous cell carcinomas. The proper selection of lesion, location, and the size of the curette, combined with the surgeon's technique, all play a role in both the therapeutic and cosmetic outcome.

The skin should be stabilized with the nondominant hand while the curette is held like a pencil. Curettage should be performed in a centripetal manner (from the outside in) to avoid stripping sun-damaged skin and creating a larger wound. To ensure complete destruction, curettage should be performed in multiple directions to produce symmetrical wound margins. A large curette is used for initial debulking, followed by a smaller curette to remove any residual foci or extensions. Curettage is complete when the "gritty," firm sensation of normal dermis is felt and slight punctate dermal bleeding occurs.

Curettage, combined with electrodesiccation (C&E), is widely used for the treatment of BCC and squamous cell carcinomas (SCC) (Fig. 37-15). Silverman et al reviewed the cure rates of primary BCC treated with C&E over a 27-year period at New York University. The result of the study stratified low-, middle-, and high-risk anatomic locations and the risk of recurrence following C&E of primary BCC. Low-risk anatomic sites (neck, trunk, and four extremities) had a 5-year recurrence rate of 3.3%. Middle-risk sites (scalp, forehead, pre- and post-auricular, and malar areas) had an overall recurrence rate of 12.9%, but this was reduced to 5% when limited to noninfiltrative carcinomas of less than 1 cm. High-risk sites (nose, paranasal, nasolabial groove, ear, chin, mandibular, perioral, periocular areas) had an overall recurrence rate of 17.5%, but a more acceptable 5% recurrence rate was achieved when treatment was limited to lesions of less than 6 mm.

In addition to size and anatomic location, the histologic subtype is an important factor in the effectiveness of C&E. Infiltrative and micronodular BCC are not appropriate for C&E, while it can be considered a therapeutic option in superficial and nodular subtypes. SCC in situ may be appropriately treated with C&E, while in most circumstances invasive SCC would not typically be amenable to this modality.

There is little agreement regarding the requisite number of cycles of C&E. Indeed, treating all lesions identically with a particular number of cycles may lead to overtreatment of some lesions and undertreatment of others. In general, accepted therapy employs three cycles to treat most malignant lesions. However, smaller superficial malignancies may be treated with fewer cycles; the rationale is to improve cosmetic outcome, while still achieving acceptable cure rates. None the less, the success of C&E relies on the surgeon's ability to identify by feel and appearance the tissue to be ablated. Finally, C&E should be replaced by excision if curettage extends into subcutaneous tissue. As such, lesions that have been previously biopsied using a punch that has extended into the subcutaneous fat may be less amenable to C&E.

Barlow JO, et al: Treatment of basal cell carcinoma with curettage alone. J Am Acad Dermatol 2006 Jun; 54(6):1039–1045.
Goldman G: The current status of curettage and electrodesiccation. Dermatol Clin 2002; 20:569.
Rodriguez-Vigil T, et al: Recurrence rates of primary basal cell carcinoma in facial risk areas treated with curettage and electrodesiccation. J Am Acad Dermatol 2007; 56:91–95.
Sheridan AT, Dawber RP: Curettage, electrosurgery and skin cancer. Australas J Dermatol 2000; 41:19.
Silverman MK, et al: Recurrence rates of treated basal cell carcinomas. Part 2: Curettage-electrodesiccation. J Dermatol Surg Oncol 1991; 17:720.

Electrosurgery

Electrosurgery comprises a variety of surgical techniques, applications, and apparatus. In general, the tissue effect is created by heat delivered to or generated in the tissue as a result of an electrical current. Various forms of electrosurgery are routinely used by dermatologists for applications such as destruction, hemostasis, excisions, and cosmetic procedures. An understanding of the different modalities and their applications can improve surgical outcome (Fig. 37-16).

Electrocautery

Electrocautery is most often performed today with battery-powered, hand-held, disposable units. Direct current is passed through a metal treatment tip. Resistance to the flow of current causes heat to be generated, which can be adjusted by the intensity of the current. Hemostasis is achieved by direct heating of the tissue; no electrical current passes through the patient. As such, this device may be considered in patients with implantable cardiac devices sensitive to electric current.

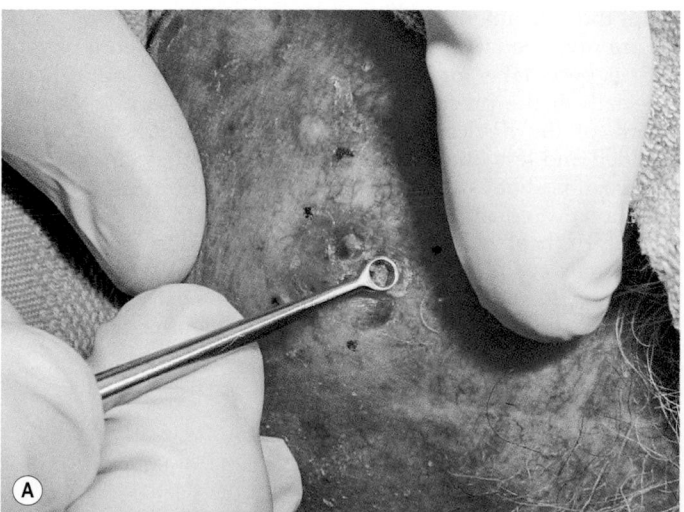 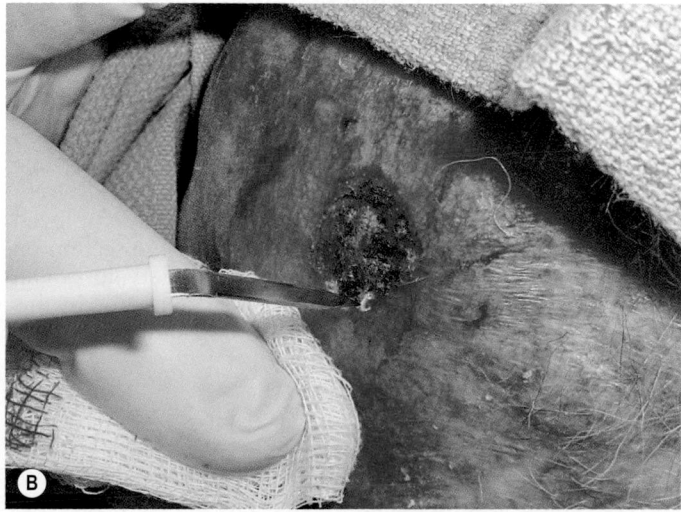

Fig. 37-15 Curettage and electrodesiccation. A, Curettage of squamous cell carcinoma in situ. B, Electrodesiccation immediately following.

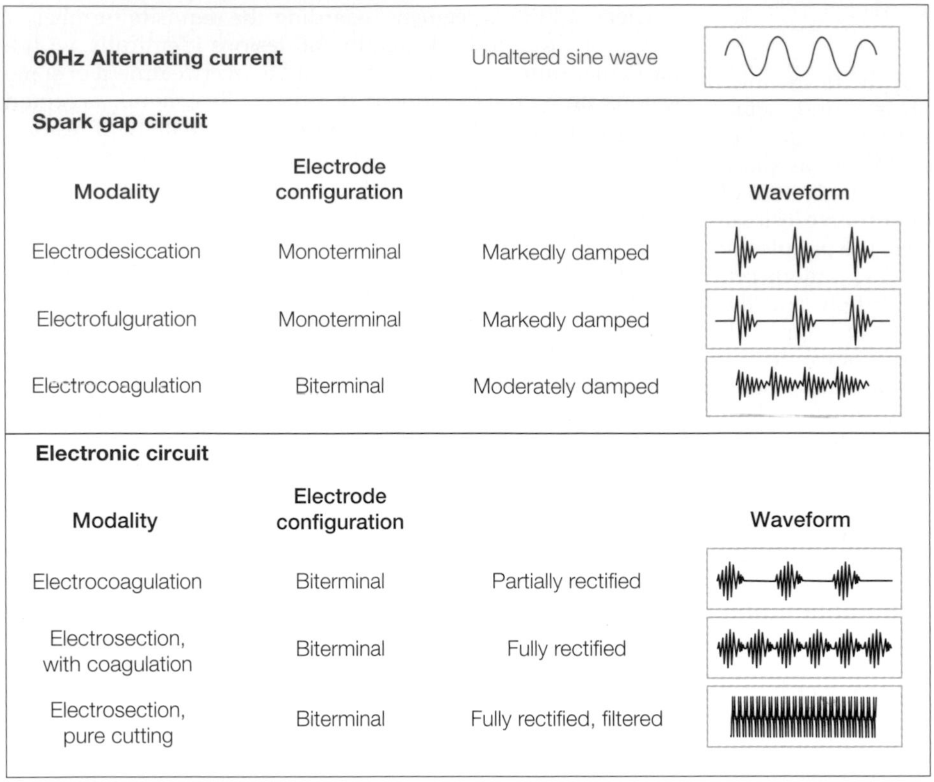

60Hz Alternating current		Unaltered sine wave	

Spark gap circuit

Modality	Electrode configuration	Waveform	
Electrodesiccation	Monoterminal	Markedly damped	
Electrofulguration	Monoterminal	Markedly damped	
Electrocoagulation	Biterminal	Moderately damped	

Electronic circuit

Modality	Electrode configuration	Waveform	
Electrocoagulation	Biterminal	Partially rectified	
Electrosection, with coagulation	Biterminal	Fully rectified	
Electrosection, pure cutting	Biterminal	Fully rectified, filtered	

Fig. 37-16 Electrosurgery waveforms.

Electrodesiccation and electrofulguration

Electrodesiccation (from the Greek desiccate, meaning "dry") and electrofulguration (from the Greek fulgur, meaning "lightning") represent the most commonly employed uses of electrosurgery in dermatology. In electrodesiccation, the electrode tip is in contact with the tissue; with electrofulguration, a 1–2 mm separation between the tip and the tissue produces a spark. Electrodesiccation causes a deeper wound, while electrofulguration is more superficial.

A highly damped (decreasing amplitude) waveform of high voltage and low amperage is produced by a spark-gap generator. As this is a monoterminal current, a grounding electrode on the patient is not required. Electrodesiccation/fulguration produces superficial destruction, as the carbonization on the treated surface limits damage to deeper tissue.

This type of electrosurgery has numerous applications in the daily practice of dermatology. Superficial, small dermal tumors, such as syringomas or seborrheic keratoses, may be treated with electrodesiccation. Insertion of the fine epilating needle into the tumor is followed by the application of low current until a surface bubbling occurs. The small amount of char is then removed with a curette, resulting in a smooth surface appearance. In addition, skin tags, warts, and fine telangiectases may all be effectively removed by this technique. Electrodesiccation or fulguration is commonly employed in treatment of many BCCs and SCCs (see above section on curettage). It is also useful in excisional surgery to obtain hemostasis. The field must be dry, since the destruction by this current is superficial and will not be transmitted through blood.

Electrocoagulation

Electrocoagulation employs moderately damped current with a lower voltage and higher amperage. The patient is incorporated into a biterminal circuit. Electrocoagulation causes greater tissue damage and deeper penetration than electrodessication or electrofulguration.

Electrosection

Electrosection employs an undamped, low-voltage, high-amperage current in a biterminal fashion. This technique has the advantage of cutting with simultaneous hemostasis. As such, it is used for bloodless excisional surgery of protuberant masses and growths, such as rhinophyma. There is vaporization of tissue with little heat spread. Care must be taken with this technique, as maintaining an appropriate depth can be difficult, given the ease with which the device can cut through skin. When the device is properly used, fine surgical excisions can be produced, with minimal trauma to surrounding tissue and excellent hemostasis. Various handpiece attachments, including scalpels, needles, wire loops, and balls, can further adapt the instrument to the specific procedure.

Care must be taken when using electrosurgery in a patient with a pacemaker or implantable cardioverter-defibrillator, especially if the procedure is performed within a few centimeters of the device. Although modern devices are better shielded and less likely to respond to external electrical interference, it is always prudent to deliver current in short bursts. Additionally, consideration should be given to the use of electrocautery (heat only, no electrical transmission) or a bipolar device (current transmitted between two tips) when treating these patients. Yu et al recently reviewed the use of electrosurgery in patients with cardiac devices and offer a complete discussion of the subject.

Aferzon M, Millman B: Excision of rhinophyma with high-frequency electrosurgery. Dermatol Surg 2002; 28:735.

Matzke TJ, et al: Pacemakers and implantable cardiac defibrillators in dermatologic surgery. Dermatol Surg 2006; 32:1155–1162.

Rex J, et al: Surgical management of rhinophyma: report of eight patients treated with electrosection. Dermatol Surg 2002; 28:347.

Wagner RF Jr: Medical and technical issues in office electrolysis and thermolysis. J Dermatol Surg Oncol 1993; 19:575.

Yu SS, et al: Cardiac devices and electromagnetic interference revisited: new radiofrequency technologies and implications for dermatologic surgery. Dermatol Surg 2005; 31:932.

Excisional technique

The fusiform or elliptical excision is the workhorse procedure used to treat invasive skin cancers, as well as benign skin lesions needing extirpation (Fig. 37-17). The basic principle of

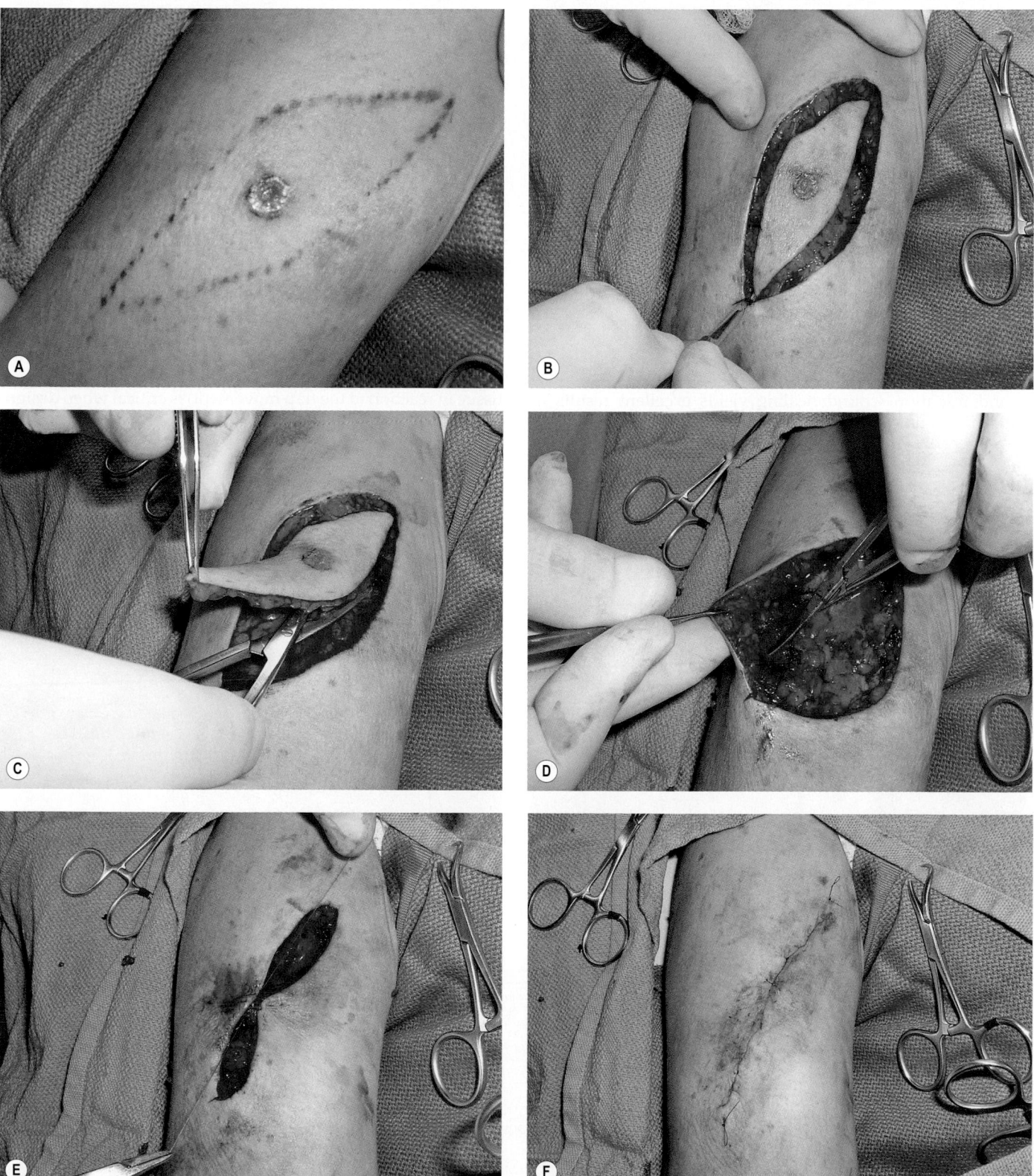

Fig. 37-17 Elliptical excision. A, Ellipse is designed along relaxed skin tension lines with a 3:1 length to width ratio. B, Incision made into subcutaneous tissue. C, Removal using tissue scissors in even plane. D, Blunt undermining of skin edges using skin hook. E, Buried interrupted tension-bearing absorbable sutures placed. F, Epidermal approximation using nonabsorbable running subcuticular sutures, with interruption in center of wound for easier removal.

the fusiform ellipse is excision of a specimen oriented with its longest axis along skin tension lines and its width not exceeding one-third of its length. The ellipse can be curved in a crescentic or "lazy S" pattern to align the final scar better with skin tension lines. If the procedure is performed with the correct dimensions (usually a length to width ratio of 3:1) and a 30° angle at each pole, standing cutaneous cones at the two extremes of the excision are generally avoided. Standing cutaneous cones represent excess tissue bunching at the poles of a skin closure and should be "sewn out" or excised by triangulation or M-plasty if needed. Undermining, using sharp or blunt dissection of the skin from underlying subcutaneous tissue, reduces wound tension and helps with wound edge eversion.

Skin flaps and grafts

Choosing whether to close a wound by linear closure, local skin flap, or skin graft, or allowing it to heal by second intention can be complex. Important considerations include patient concerns, local tissue movement, adjacent anatomic structural preservation and function, and cosmesis.

Second intention

Second intention wound healing yields excellent results in appropriate clinical settings. As there is contraction in wound healing, wounds that are adjacent to a free margin may result in a pull and distortion. This may affect surrounding anatomic structures (e.g. pull on a nasal rim or eyelid). The wounds may heal with hypertrophic or pigmentary changes. However, there are areas and situations where allowing a wound to heal by second intention is appropriate. These include superficial wounds in concave areas (e.g. medial canthus, conchal bowl, and junction between the nose and cheek), partial thickness wounds involving the mucosa of the lip, or certain clinical situations, such as elderly or frail patients with decreased cosmetic concerns (Fig. 37-18). Wound care is simple and postoperative restrictions are minimal.

Flaps

Local skin flaps are geometric segments of tissue contiguous with a skin defect that are advanced, rotated, or transposed to close a wound. Advantages of flaps include better approximation of skin texture and color, hiding incision lines, redirecting tension vectors, and covering exposed cartilage and bone. Flap survival is based on the preservation of the random blood supply along the pedicle. Consideration of both the primary movement of the flap (the actual movement of the flap into the defect) and secondary movement (movement of surrounding tissue in reaction to the flap movement) is critical when designing the repair (Fig. 37-19).

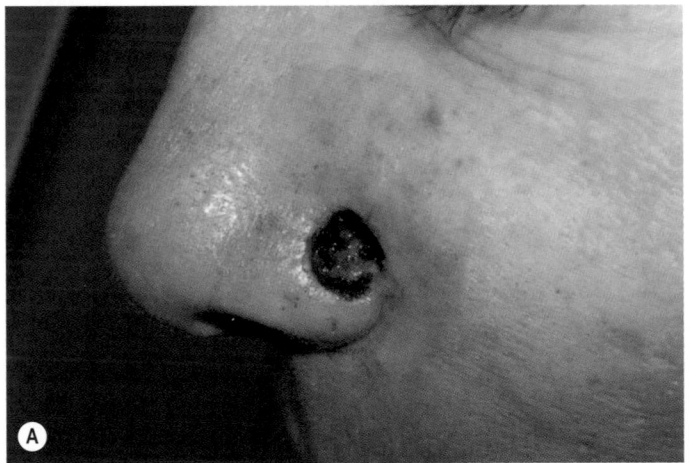
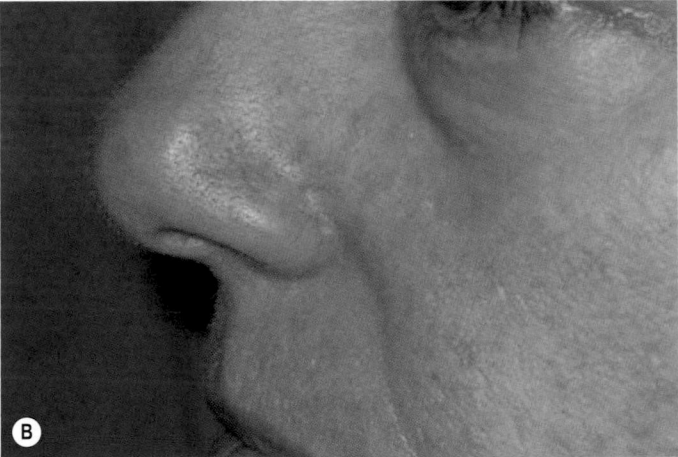

Fig. 37-18 Second intention. A, Mohs defect. B, Final result 9 months later.

Fig. 37-19 Advancement flap movement.

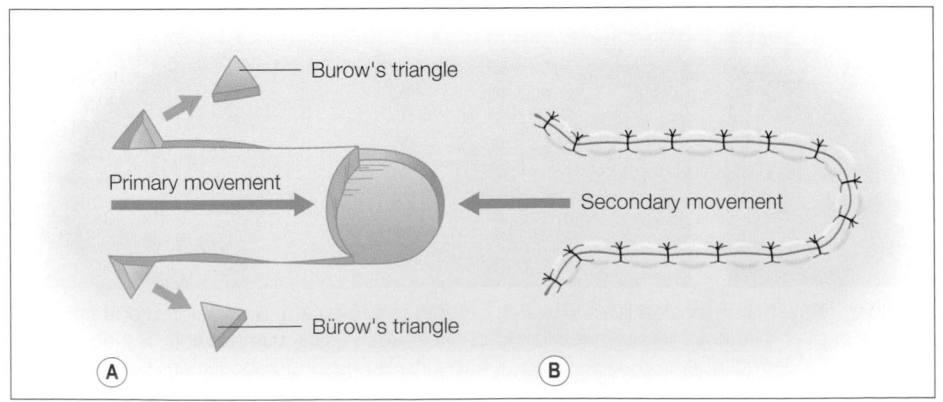

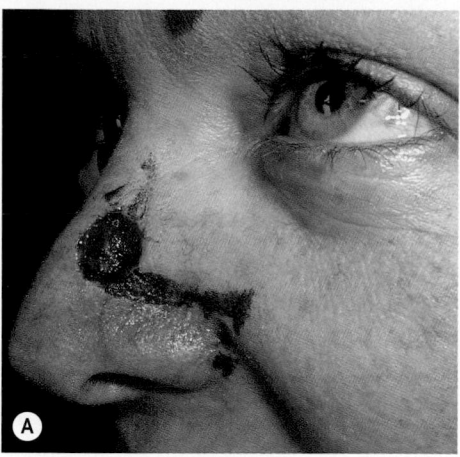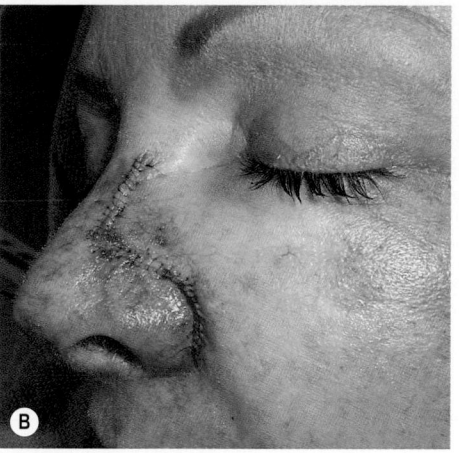

Fig. 37-20 Single arm advancement flap. A, Advancement flap designed on nasal sidewall. B, Final wound closure.

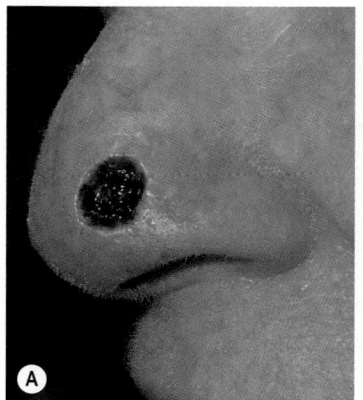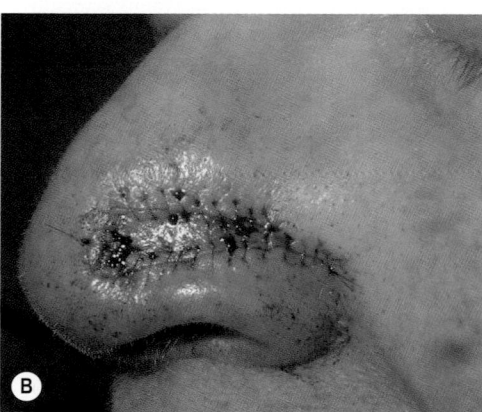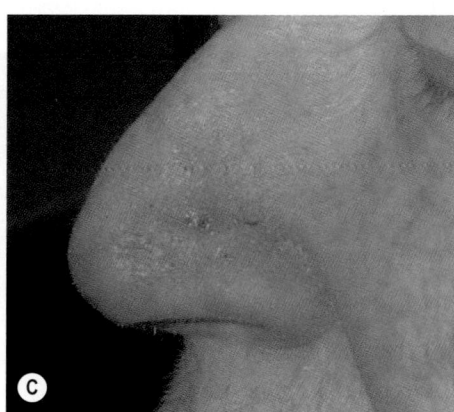

Fig. 37-21 Island pedicle flap. A, Mohs defect. B, Final wound closure. C, 6 weeks postoperatively.

Advancement flap

An advancement flap moves almost entirely in one linear direction (Fig. 37-20). The classic advancement flap involves the creation of a rectangular pedicle, which slides into position over the primary surgical defect. The key suture advances the flap and closes the primary defect. Tissue redundancies at the base of the flap can be removed by triangulation. As survival of the distal tip of the flap depends on blood supply from the base, a maximum length : width ratio of 3:1 should be designed.

If insufficient movement is obtained with a single advancement flap, a bilateral advancement (O-H) can be employed, such that each flap advances to cover half the defect. This repair can be used in eyebrow or helical rim repairs. Single arm advancement flaps (O-L) and bilateral single arm advancement flaps (O-T) are similar to classic advancement flaps, except that only a single incision is made and the standing cone is removed by triangulation. These flaps have the advantage of a larger pedicle providing blood supply and allow a linear portion of the flap to be hidden in an existing rhytid for better cosmetic outcome. Common sites for single arm advancement flaps include the nasal sidewall, helical rim, upper lip, forehead, and eyebrow.

The island pedicle flap is a specific variant of an advancement flap (Fig. 37-21). This flap depends on a subcutaneous vascular pedicle for its blood supply and has all of the epidermal connections severed by incisions. Care must be taken in designing island pedicle flaps as the incision lines surrounding the flap can result in a patch-like appearance in the final

outcome. The best cosmetic results are achieved when at least one of the incision lines can be hidden in a existing rhytid or anatomic boundary.

Rotation flap

The rotation flap can conceptually be considered a variation of the advancement flap, in that it slides into position in much the same way, albeit in an arcuate manner. Tension vectors from this pulling action are directed along the arc of rotation in reverse fashion (Fig. 37-22). Rotation flaps are often used to close large defects when there is insufficient tissue laxity (Fig. 37-23). The flap has the advantage of good survival secondary to the large pedicle and the ability to recruit skin from a great distance. A back cut can be used to reduce pivotal restraint and provide greater tissue movement, but may compromise the vascular pedicle. Variations include bilateral rotation flap (O-Z) (Fig. 37-24) or dorsal nasal rotation flap (Fig. 37-25).

Transposition flaps

In the case of the transposition flap, the flap is elevated, transposed over intervening tissue, and sutured into the primary defect (Fig. 37-26). The tension vector is redirected across the closure of the secondary defect (i.e. the area originally occupied by the flap). This is especially helpful for defects that are adjacent to anatomic free margins. The key suture closes the secondary defect, and the flap is then lifted

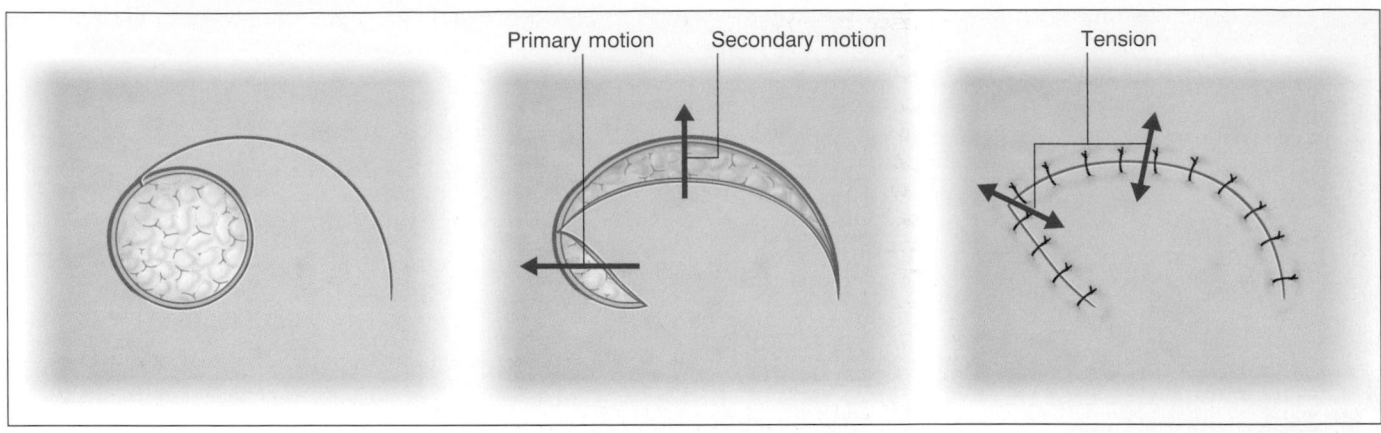

Fig. 37-22 Rotation flap movement. With permission from Robinson JK, Hanke CW, Sengelmann RD, Siegel DM (eds): Surgery of the Skin. Philadelphia: Mosby, 2005.

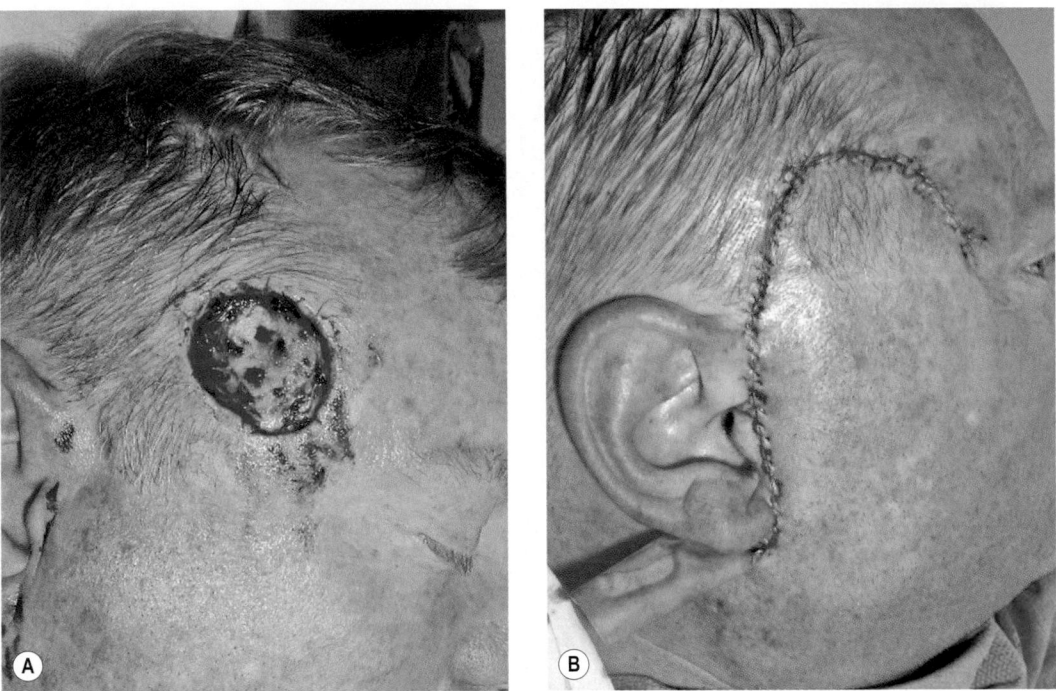

Fig. 37-23 Rotation flap. A, Rotation flap designed with M-plasty. Redundant skin from cheek is borrowed to repair defect. B, Final closure.

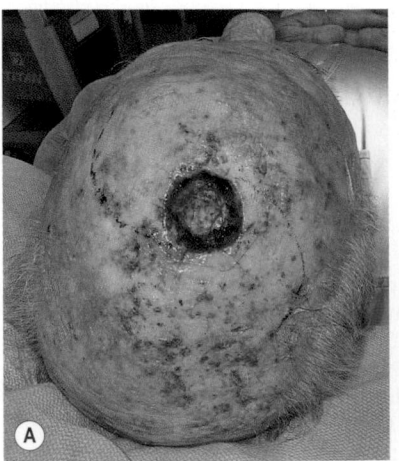
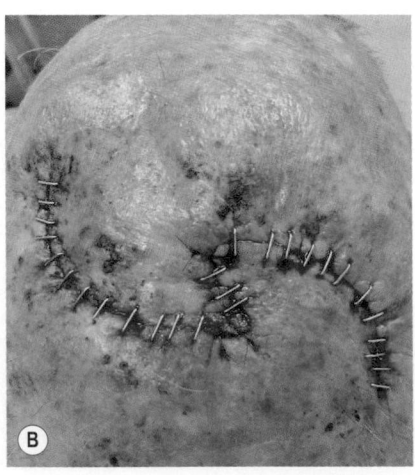

Fig. 37-24 O-Z rotation flap. A, Flap designed. B, Final wound closure.

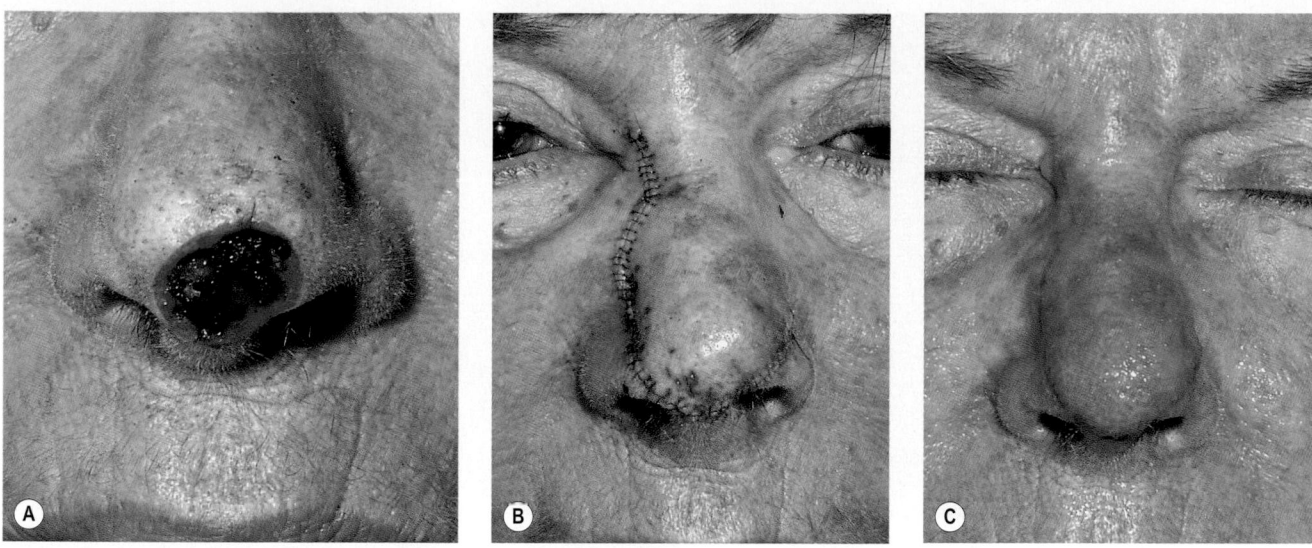

Fig. 37-25 Dorsal nasal rotation flap. A, Mohs defect. B, Final wound closure. C, 8 weeks postoperatively.

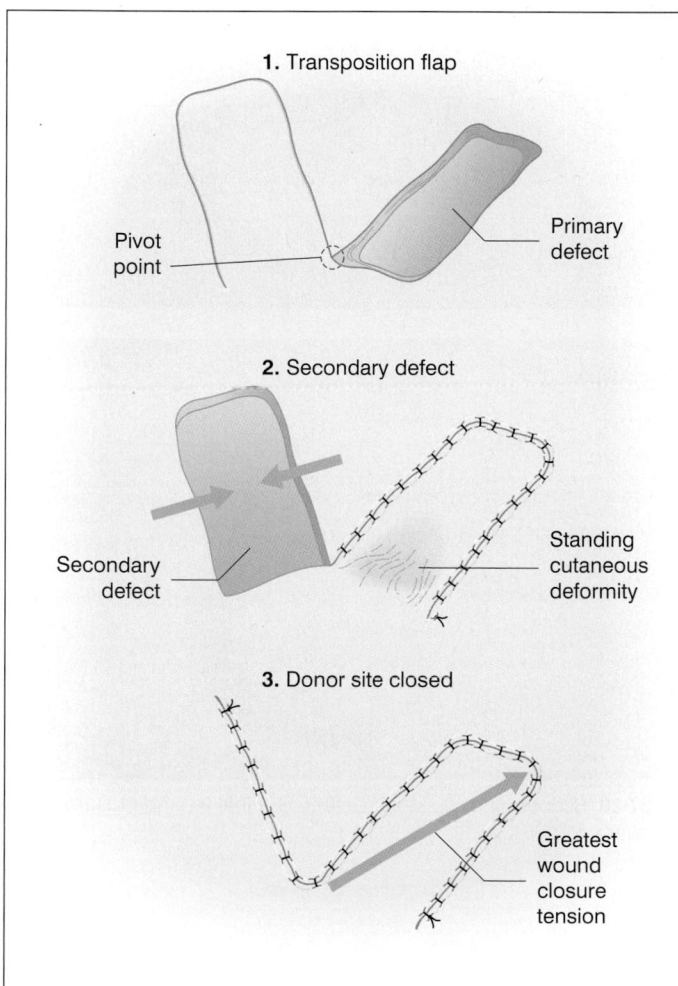

1. Transposition flap

Pivot point

Primary defect

2. Secondary defect

Secondary defect

Standing cutaneous deformity

3. Donor site closed

Greatest wound closure tension

Fig. 37-26 Transposition flap movement.

and transposed into position over the primary defect. The prototype of this flap is the rhombic flap (Fig. 37-27). Other examples include bilobed flaps (Fig. 37-28), nasolabial/melolabial flaps, banner flap, Z-plasty, and Webster's 30° flap (Fig. 37-29).

Choice of a particular type of flap must take multiple factors into consideration, including location of defect, availability of tissue movement, surrounding structures, effects of tissue movement, and blood supply. Full discussion of flaps is beyond the scope of this chapter and is available in multiple referenced texts. The successful design and execution of flap repairs can be complex, and requires appropriate and extensive training.

Skin grafts

Skin grafts are employed when primary closure or flap closure is not an available option. By definition, a graft is completely excised from the donor site and is devitalized (i.e. no intrinsic blood supply). Success is predicated on the reattachment of vascular supply to the graft from the defect. Grafts offer the advantage of fewer incision lines, as compared to local flaps. However, the lack of color and texture match due to the remote donor location of grafts is a potential disadvantage.

Grafts can be categorized as full, split, or composite. Choice of when to use each of these depends on the depth of the defect, vascular supply, and concern about skin cancer recurrence. Full-thickness skin grafts have a full dermis and are the most common grafts used in dermatologic surgery. The graft is defatted, trimmed to fit the defect, anchored in place with peripheral and basting sutures, and secured with a tie-over dressing. Common donor sites include pre-auricular cheek, post-auricular crease, conchal bowl, upper eyelid, upper inner arm, or clavicle. Full-thickness grafts can produce an excellent cosmetic result if executed properly (Fig. 37-30). However, the increased skin thickness results in an increased metabolic demand and a higher rate of necrosis and failure.

Imbibition occurs during the first 24–48 h after graft placement. The graft is sustained by passive diffusion of nutrients from the wound bed during this stage. It becomes edematous, and the fibrin network attaches the graft to the bed. Inosculation is the next stage, with revascularization from linkage of dermal vessels in graft to wound bed. Neovascularization occurs from capillary ingrowth to the graft from recipient base and sidewalls. Full circulation can be restored in 7 days and depends on the graft thickness and vascularity of the wound bed.

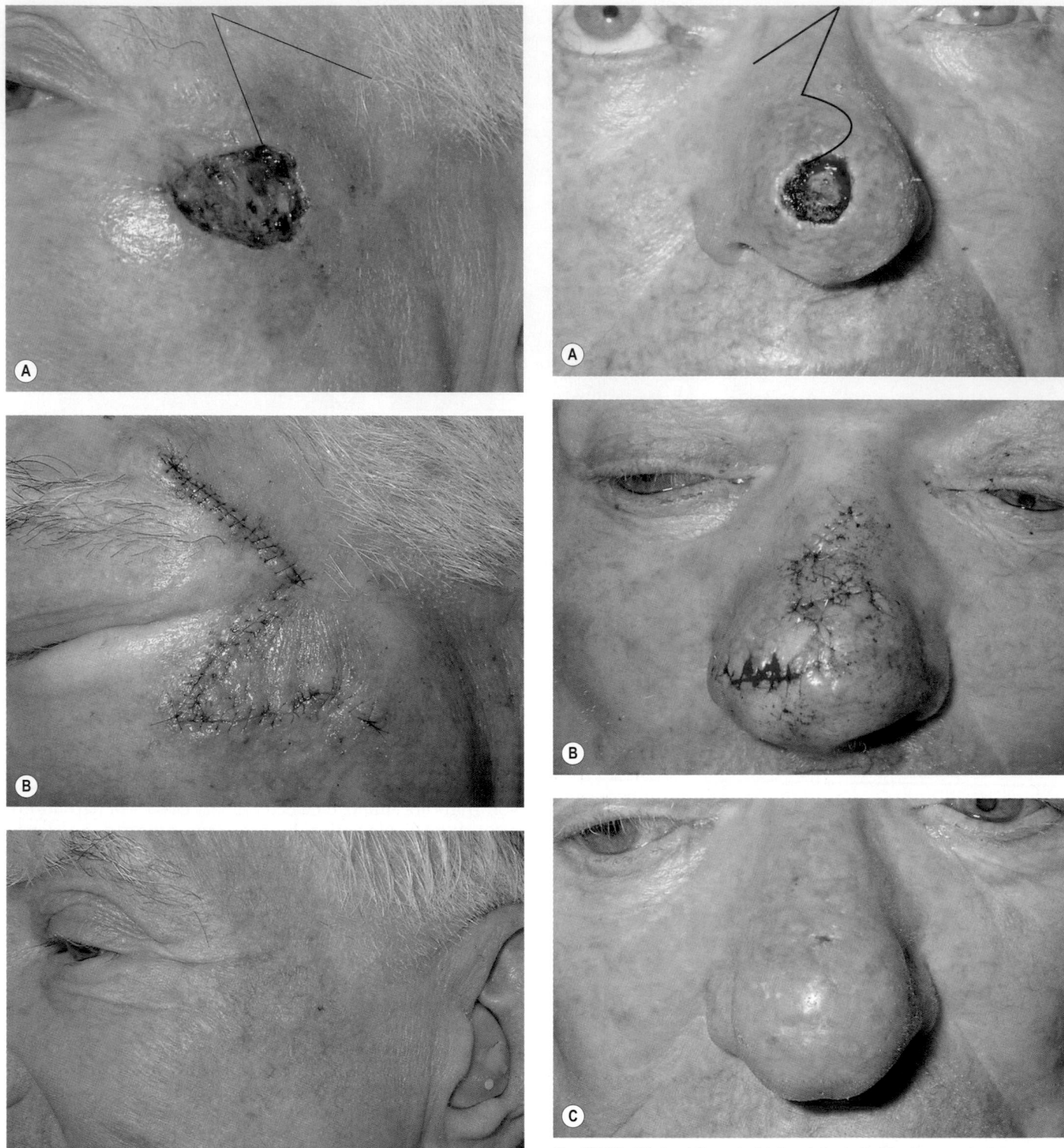

Fig. 37-27 Transposition flap. A, Mohs defect. B, Final wound closure. C, 3-month follow-up.

Fig. 37-28 Bilobed flap. A, Mohs defect. B, Final wound closure. C, 6-week follow- up.

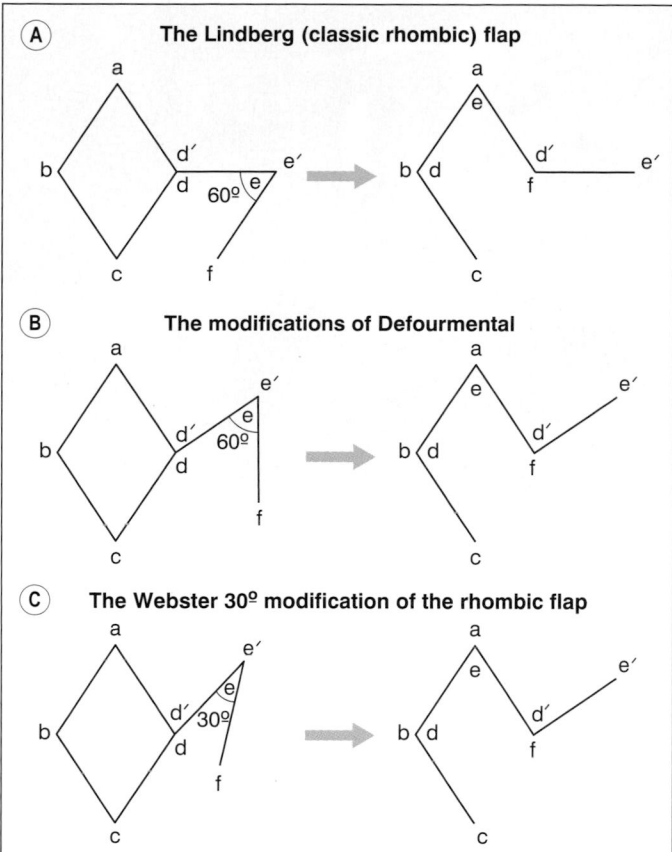

Fig. 37-29 Variations of transposition flap.

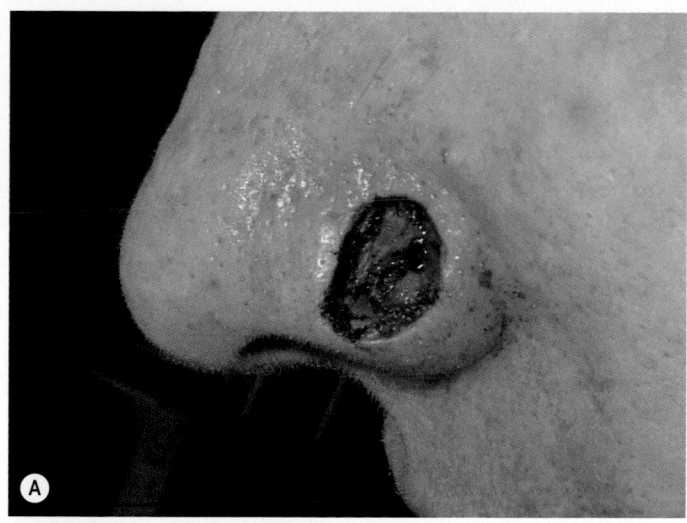

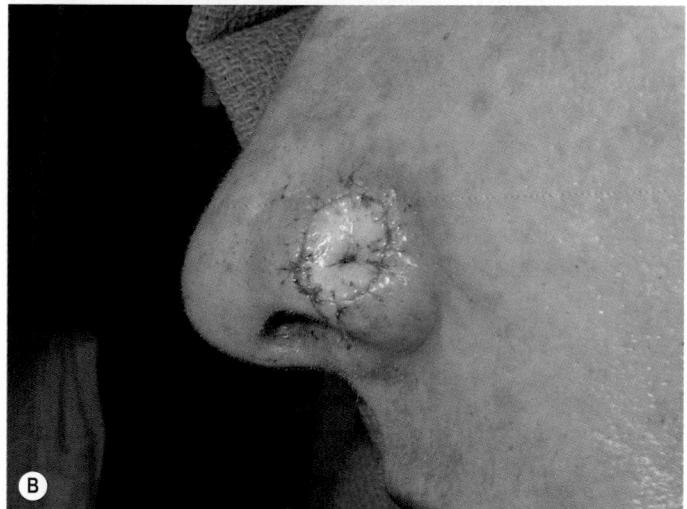

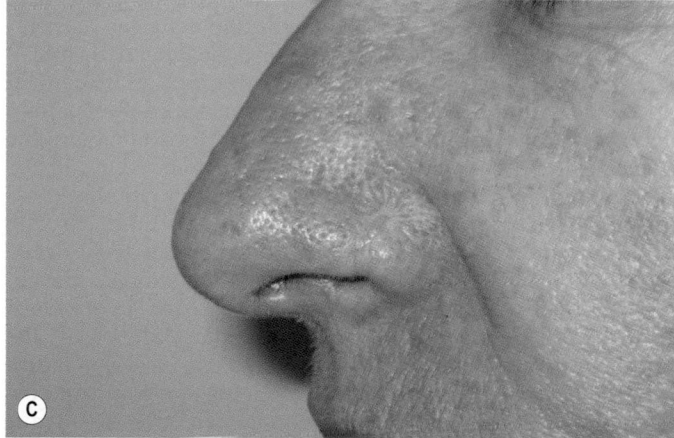

Fig. 37-30 Full-thickness skin graft. A, Mohs surgery defect. B, Final wound closure. C, 3-year follow-up.

Split-thickness skin grafts have only a partial dermis and are useful for covering large areas or for improved surveillance in tumors with a high risk of recurrence. Small grafts can be harvested freehand with No. 15 blade or with a hand-held Weck blade using various guards to determine graft thickness (Fig. 37-31), while larger grafts can be obtained using a power dermatome (Fig. 37-32). Grafts can be meshed in order to provide coverage for larger defects. In comparison to full-thickness skin grafts, split-thickness grafts have a higher rate of survival and shorter healing time, do not require repair of the donor site, and are a good choice for poorly vascularized areas due to lower metabolic demand. However, they have a higher degree of contraction, lack skin appendages, and provide a poorer cosmetic match.

Composite grafts most commonly consist of skin and underlying structure (e.g. cartilage), and are predominately used to repair such wounds as full-thickness alar rim defects. These grafts have an increased nutrient requirement and thus are more likely to fail. Free cartilage grafts can be used for reconstruction of the ear and nasal ala or tip.

Adams DC, Ramsey ML: Grafts in dermatologic surgery: review and update on full- and split-thickness skin grafts, free cartilage grafts, and composite grafts. Dermatol Surg 2005; 31:1055–1067.

Goldman GD: Rotation flaps. Dermatol Surg 2005; 31:1006–1013.

Krishnan R, et al: Advancement flaps: a basic theme with many variations. Dermatol Surg 2005; 31:986–994.

Leonard AL, Hanke CW: Second intention healing for intermediate and large postsurgical defects of the lip. J Am Acad Dermatol 2007; 57:832–835.

Mott KJ, et al: Regional variation in wound contraction of Mohs surgery defects allowed to heal by second intention. Dermatol Surg 2003 Jul; 29(7):712–722.

Pipitone MA, Gloster HM Jr: Repair of the alar groove with combination partial primary closure and second-intention healing. Dermatol Surg 2005 May; 31(5):608–609.

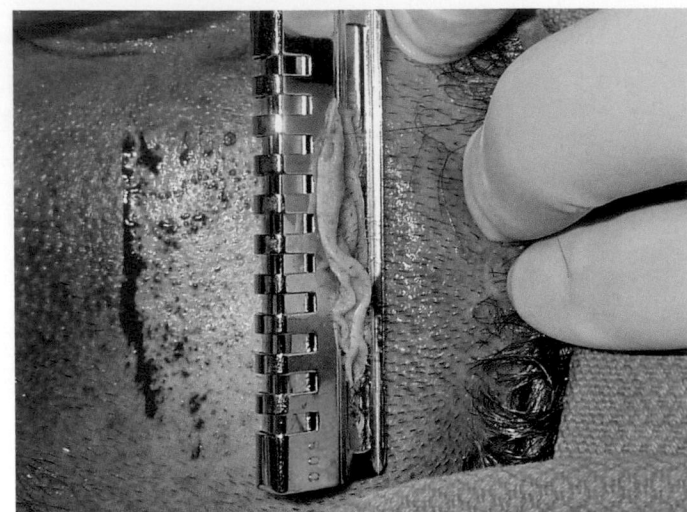

Fig. 37-31 Harvesting of split-thickness skin graft. Mastoid process is an excellent source. Hair will regrow at donor site and hide the wound. Hairs remaining in the graft are above the level of the bulb and will not persist once the graft takes.

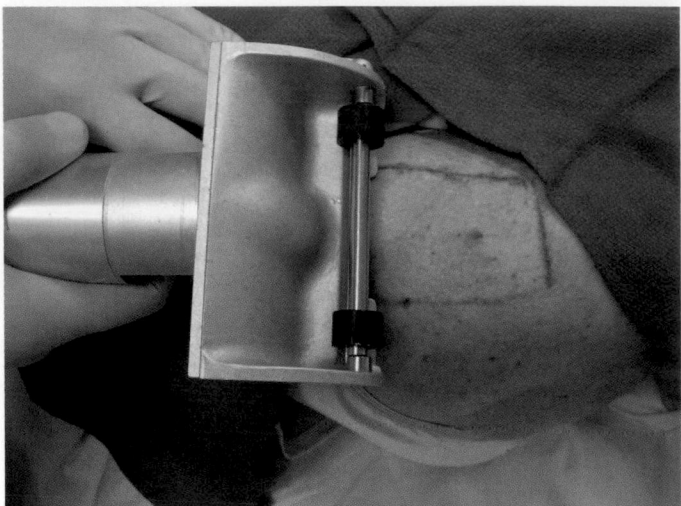

Fig. 37-32 Harvesting of split-thickness skin graft with powered dermatome.

Rohrer TE, Bhatia A: Transposition flaps in cutaneous surgery. Dermatol Surg 2005; 31:1014–1023.

Mohs micrographic surgery

Frederic Mohs initially developed this technique at the University of Wisconsin in the 1930s as a means for margin control during surgical excision of skin cancer. The original technique used zinc chloride paste to fix tissue in vivo, followed by surgical excision. Drs Theodore Tromovitch and Samuel Stegman modified this technique in the 1970s to a fresh-frozen tissue variant that continues to be used today. While the basic surgical principles in Mohs micrographic surgery are similar to those used in standard excision, there are unique challenges encountered with Mohs surgery. A complete understanding of pathology, anatomy, cutaneous oncology, advanced surgical reconstruction, and management of surgical complications is critical to a successful patient outcome. Any dermatologist performing Mohs micrographic surgery should be well trained in this technique and all the accompanying challenges of surgical and postoperative care.

Mohs micrographic surgical excision is a tissue-sparing technique that employs frozen-section control of 100% of the surgical margin. This evaluation of the entire surgical margin using horizontal sections (not vertical, as used in standard sectioning), combined with precise mapping, allows for the highest cure rate of cutaneous neoplasms (Fig. 37-33). In addition, the sparing of normal adjacent tissue can improve cosmesis and decrease the risk of functional defects in a sensitive anatomic location. Any tumor that has a contiguous growth pattern would be a candidate for Mohs micrographic surgical excision. Immunohistochemical stains can be used in specific cases to help identify residual tumor.

There are multiple indications for Mohs micrographic surgical excision (Box 37-7, Fig. 37-34). Mohs surgery provides cure rates of 99% for primary BCCs, and 95% for recurrent BCCs. SCCs on the skin and lip treated with Mohs surgery have a 5-year recurrence rate of 3.1% (versus 10.9% for other modalities). SCC on the ear treated with Mohs surgery has a 5-year recurrence rate of 5.3% (versus 18.7% for other modalities). Locally recurrent SCC also had a reduced recurrence rate when treated with Mohs surgery, as compared to other modalities (10% versus 23.3%). Other tumors that can be successfully

Box 37-7 Indications for Mohs surgery

- Recurrent or incompletely excised nonmelanoma skin cancer
- Tumors with aggressive histologic subtypes (i.e. infiltrative, morpheaform, micronodular, perivascular, or perineural involvement)
- Tumors with poorly defined clinical margins
- High-risk location >0.4 cm (H-zone of the face, eyes, ears, nose)
- Large tumors (>1.0 cm on face; >2.0 cm on trunk or extremities)
- Cosmetically and functionally important areas, including genital, anal, perianal, hand, foot, and nail units
- Tumors arising in immunosuppressed patients
- Tumors arising in previously irradiated skin or scar
- Genetic conditions with increased risk of neoplasms (i.e. basal cell nevus syndrome or xeroderma pigmentosa)

treated by Mohs surgery include dermatofibrosarcoma protuberans, atypical fibroxanthoma, and microcystic adnexal carcinoma. Mohs micrographic surgical excision of melanoma continues to be debated. Bricca et al demonstrated comparable 5-year local recurrence rates, metastasis rates, and disease-specific survival rates in head and neck melanomas treated with Mohs micrographic surgery, as compared to standard excision. In contrast, Walling et al showed that staged excision for melanoma resulted in lower recurrence rates and similar-sized defects compared to Mohs surgery.

Bricca GM, et al: Cutaneous head and neck melanoma treated with Mohs micrographic surgery. J Am Acad Dermatol 2005; 52:92.

Leibovitch I, et al: Cutaneous squamous cell carcinoma treated with Mohs micrographic surgery in Australia I. Experience over 10 years. J Am Acad Dermatol 2005 Aug; 53(2):253–260.

Leibovitch I, et al: Basal cell carcinoma treated with Mohs surgery in Australia II. Outcome at 5-year follow-up. J Am Acad Dermatol 2005 Sep; 53(3):452–457.

Rowe DE, et al: Long-term recurrence rates in previously untreated (primary) basal cell carcinoma: implications for patient follow-up. J Dermatol Surg Oncol 1989; 15:315.

Rowe DE, et al: Mohs surgery is the treatment of choice for recurrent (previously treated) basal cell carcinoma. J Dermatol Surg Oncol 1989; 15:424.

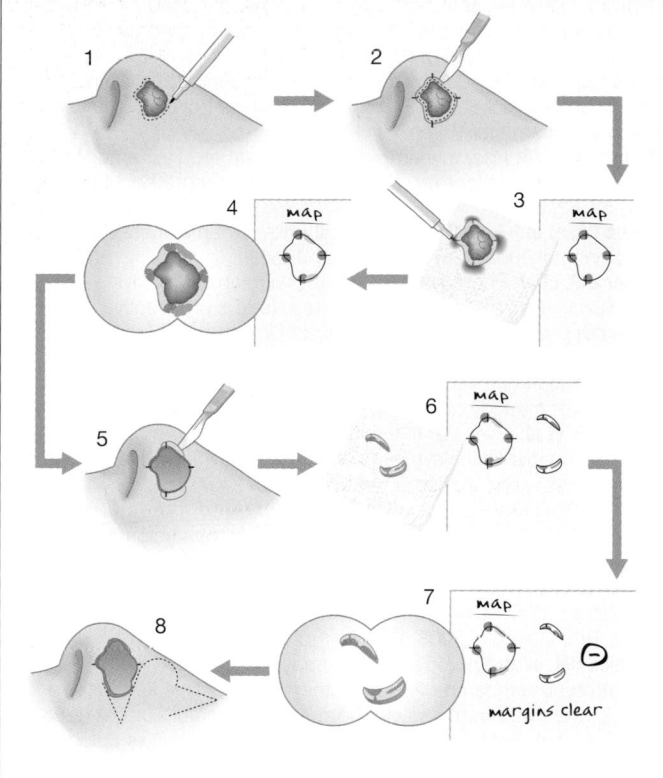

Fig. 37-33 The Mohs surgery process.

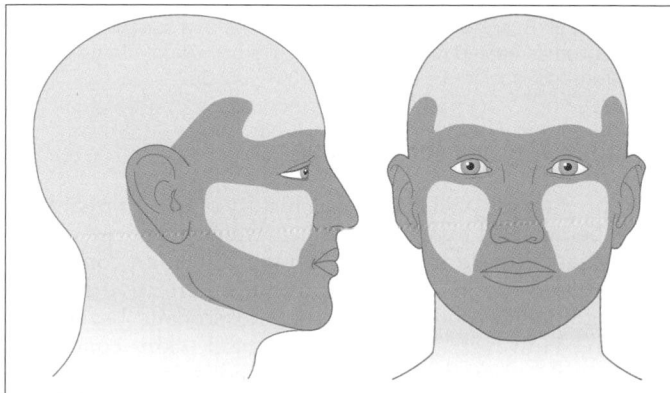

Fig. 37-34 H-zone of the face.

Rowe DE, et al: Prognostic factors for local recurrence, metastasis, and survival rates in squamous cell carcinoma of the skin, ear, and lip. Implications for treatment modality selection. J Am Acad Dermatol 1992; 26:976.

Thomas CJ, et al: Mohs micrographic surgery in the treatment of rare aggressive cutaneous tumors: the Geisinger experience. Dermatol Surg 2007 Mar; 33(3):333–339.

Thosani MK, et al: Current progress of immunostains in Mohs micrographic surgery: a review. Dermatol Surg 2008 Dec; 34(12):1621–1636.

Walling HW, et al: Staged excision versus Mohs micrographic surgery for lentigo maligna and lentigo maligna melanoma. J Am Acad Dermatol 2007 Oct; 57(4):659–664.

Photodynamic therapy

Photodynamic therapy (PDT) involves the activation of a photosensitizer by visible light in the presence of oxygen, resulting in the creation of reactive oxygen species, which selectively destroy the target tissue.

The first requirement for PDT is delivery of either a systemic or a topical photosensitizing drug. Systemic photosensitizing molecules are large, lipophilic molecules that require intravenous administration to reach the target site. One of the major disadvantages of these systemic drugs is the prolonged period of phototoxicity. Examples include porfimer sodium and hematoporphyrin derivative. The benzoporphyrin derivative monoacid ring A (verteporfin) has a shorter period of photosensitivity (<72 h) compared to other systemic agents.

Topical agents offer the advantage of limiting photosensitivity to the application site and have become widely used in dermatology. Delta-aminolevulinic acid (ALA) is the most commonly used photosensitizing agent used in dermatology. It is applied and left on the skin for a sufficient period of time to allow for accumulation within the target cells. ALA is subsequently converted to the photosensitizer, protoporphyrin IX (PpIX), which can then be stimulated through the controlled use of a light source. Tumor cells are thought to be selectively targeted by increased penetration of ALA through the abnormal epidermis overlying the tumor cells. In addition, the iron-deficient, rapidly proliferating tumor cells have an increased production of PpIX as compared to normal epidermal cells, resulting in selective photosensitivity and damage to the target site. Methyl aminolevulinate (mALA) is also used as a topical photosensitizing agent. Gentle scraping or curettage prior to application is performed to increase penetration. Once absorbed, mALA is converted to ALA within the target tissue.

The second requirement of PDT is an appropriate light source to activate the photosensitizer. The light source must match the absorption peak of the photosensitizer. Lasers, intense pulsed light devices, or an incoherent light source can be used. Red light uses the 630 nm peak of PpIX as its target, and has a deeper penetration, which is appropriate for dermal processes. Blue light targets the 417 nm peak and has a more superficial penetration, making it an appropriate choice for the treatment of epidermal lesions like actinic keratoses.

Following absorption of light, the photosensitizer is converted from a stable ground state to an excited triplet state. The excited triplet state electrons interact with tissue oxygen, creating singlet oxygen. Singlet oxygen causes oxidative damage to cellular membranes (i.e. mitochondria and other cellular organelles) and direct cell death, the key mechanism of action in topical PDT. This entire process occurs over the course of microseconds. In comparison, PDT using systemic photosensitizers predominantly causes destruction of target sites via vascular injury that leads to tissue ischemia.

Actinic keratosis

Numerous studies have demonstrated the efficacy of PDT in the treatment of actinic keratoses, with overall clearance rates ranging from 50 to 70% for a single treatment, and up to 90% with additional treatment sessions. Facial lesions tend to respond better than acral or extremity lesions. Initial studies have demonstrated that topical ALA applied for 14–18 h, followed by activation with a variety of light sources (i.e. blue light, red light, pulsed dye laser, intense pulsed light, and so on), is an effective treatment for actinic keratoses on the scalp and face. More recent studies have shown that short incubation periods of 1–3 h with ALA are an effective protocol for the treatment of actinic keratoses, vastly improving the convenience of this therapy. Kurwa et al demonstrated similar reduction in actinic keratoses with a single ALA PDT and red light treatment, as compared to a 3-week course of twice a day topical 5-fluorouracil (5-FU) (70% versus 73% reduction).

mALA may offer several advantages over ALA, including improved skin penetration due to its increased lipophilic quality, greater selectivity for neoplastic cells, and possibly less pain and discomfort associated with treatment. However, there are no comparative studies for ALA and mALA PDT in the treatment of actinic keratosis. Pariser et al showed that mALA, applied for 3 h followed by noncoherent red light, resulted in an almost 90% response rate in the treatment of actinic keratosis. Szeimies et al demonstrated a similar response rate for mALA PDT compared to cryotherapy, but PDT gave better cosmetic results and had a higher degree of patient satisfaction.

Given the absence of stratum corneum on the lips and the increased penetration of topical ALA, PDT has been used effectively for the treatment of actinic cheilitis. This may be an option in patients with recalcitrant disease. Alexiades-Armenakas et al demonstrated about a 70% clearance with an excellent cosmetic result using ALA PDT activated by the long-pulsed dye laser in patients with refractory actinic cheilitis.

Basal cell carcinoma

Studies suggest that topical PDT for the treatment of BCC can have initial clearing and excellent cosmetic results, with cure rates ranging from 64 to 97%. However, despite the initial success, BCCs treated with PDT often have a higher recurrence rate with long-term follow-up. In addition, comparative studies of PDT and traditional surgical treatments (e.g. excision or Mohs surgery) are limited or lacking.

Superficial BCC tends to have better response rates than nodular BCC, likely due to the limited penetration of both ALA and the activating light into the deeper portion of the dermis for nodular tumors. Pre-treatment with curettage for thicker lesions may help to facilitate penetration of ALA and may result in improved cure rates. Infiltrative tumors have an even higher recurrence rate, suggesting that PDT should not be considered a first-line treatment for this histologic subset of BCC.

Subsets of patients with numerous and extensive BCC (e.g. basal cell nevus syndrome) may be unique cases where PDT can be considered for nodular or more extensive tumors, due to the tissue-sparing and chemopreventative advantages over traditional surgical treatments.

Squamous cell carcinoma in situ

SCC in situ is quite responsive to PDT. Multiple studies demonstrate an initial cure rate in a range of 54–100%, with quite a variable long-term efficacy. Red light should be used over blue light, as it penetrates more deeply and thus more effectively treats adnexal extensions. In a randomized study, Salim et al compared topical ALA PDT with 5-FU. At 1-year follow up, PDT achieved an 82% clinical response rate compared to 48% with 5-FU. Varma et al showed initial clearing in 88% of Bowen's disease lesions using ALA PDT with red light; however, at 12-month follow-up, complete response decreased to 69% (compared to initial response of 95% and 12-month response of 82% for superficial BCC).

There are few reports of the use of PDT for invasive cutaneous SCC. Given the limited success in treating these tumors and potential for metastatic spread, PDT is not recommended as standard therapy for invasive SCC.

Alexiades-Armenakas MR, Geronemus RG: Laser-mediated photodynamic therapy of actinic cheilitis. J Drugs Dermatol 2004; 3:548.

Braathen LR, et al: Guidelines on the use of photodynamic therapy for nonmelanoma skin cancer: an international consensus. J Am Acad Dermatol 2007 Jan; 56(1):125–143.

Calzavara-Pinton PG, et al: Methylaminolaevulinate-based photodynamic therapy of Bowen's disease and squamous cell carcinoma. Br J Dermatol 2008 Jul; 159(1):137–144.

Kurwa HA, et al: A randomized paired comparison of photodynamic therapy and topical 5-fluorouracil in the treatment of actinic keratoses. J Am Acad Dermatol 1999; 41:414.

MacCormack MA: Photodynamic therapy in dermatology: an update on applications and outcomes. Semin Cutan Med Surg 2008 Mar; 27(1):52–62.

Morton CA, et al: Guidelines for topical photodynamic therapy: update. Br J Dermatol 2008 Dec; 159(6):1245–1266.

Pariser DM, et al: Photodynamic therapy with topical methyl aminolevulinate for actinic keratosis: results of a prospective randomized multicenter trial. J Am Acad Dermatol 2003; 48:227.

Piacquadio DJ, et al: Photodynamic therapy with aminolevulinic acid topical solution and visible blue light in the treatment of multiple actinic keratoses of the face and scalp. Arch Dermatol 2004; 140:41.

Rhodes LE, et al: Five-year follow-up of a randomized, prospective trial of topical methyl aminolevulinate photodynamic therapy vs surgery for nodular basal cell carcinoma. Arch Dermatol 2007 Sep; 143(9):1131–1136.

Salim A, et al: Randomized comparison of photodynamic therapy with topical 5-fluorouracil in Bowen's disease. Br J Dermatol 2003; 148:539.

Sotiriou E, et al: Actinic cheilitis treated with one cycle of 5-aminolaevulinic acid-based photodynamic therapy: report of 10 cases. Br J Dermatol 2008 Jul; 159(1):261–262.

Szeimies RM, et al: Photodynamic therapy using topical methyl 5-aminolevulinate compared to cryotherapy for actinic keratosis: a prospective, randomized study. J Am Acad Dermatol 2002; 47:258.

Tierney E, et al: Photodynamic therapy for the treatment of cutaneous neoplasia, inflammatory disorders, and photoaging. Dermatol Surg 2009 May; 35(5):725–746.

Touma D, et al: A trial of short incubation, broad-area photodynamic therapy for facial actinic keratoses and diffuse photodamage. Arch Dermatol 2004; 140:33.

Varma S, et al: Bowen's disease, solar keratoses and superficial basal cell carcinomas treated by photodynamic therapy using a large-field incoherent light source. Br J Dermatol 2001; 144:567.

Radiation therapy for skin cancer

Radiation therapy (XRT) has a long history of use for treatment of both benign and malignant skin conditions. The use of ionizing radiation in dermatologic therapy of benign conditions has decreased markedly, owing to highly effective medical therapies and the potential genetic and somatic hazards of radiation. However, XRT for malignant skin conditions remains an important primary and adjuvant therapeutic modality. When used in the proper clinical situation, XRT can provide effective treatment while sparing normal tissue and eliminating the need for surgical reconstruction.

XRT is an appropriate primary treatment for skin cancer in patients who refuse surgery or are poor surgical candidates. In contrast, patients who are relatively young should not be candidates for XRT due to the increased risk of developing additional primary tumors within the radiation field and the long-term cosmetic complications associated with this therapy. Tumors located on the eyelids, nose, ears, and lips do well with XRT, while lesions on the extremities are better treated by surgical excision. Treatment of primary BCC with XRT can produce cure rates of more than 90%, while primary SCC may have slightly lower cure rates. It is important to stress that Mohs micrographic surgical excision of primary tumors can achieve cure rates of 97–99%, often with excellent long-term cosmetic outcomes.

XRT may also be considered if margins show microscopic evidence of residual tumor following surgical excision. Recurrent BCC and SCC that had been treated previously by nonradiologic methods can be treated by radiation, although not with the same success as primary tumors. Caccialanza et al demonstrated an 84% 5-year cure rate for recurrent BCC and

SCC in a group of nearly 250 recurrent tumors, with almost all having an acceptable cosmetic result. Locke et al showed that primary tumors treated with radiation had a response rate of 93%, as compared to 80% for recurrent neoplasms. Mohs micrographic surgical excision of recurrent nonmelanoma skin cancer produces higher cure rates (95%).

Several studies indicate that recurrence of nonmelanoma skin cancer after primary XRT may be more aggressive and invasive than recurrence after primary surgical treatment. Smith et al demonstrated that BCCs that recurred following primary radiation therapy had deeper subcutaneous tissue invasion and larger percentage increase between clinical pre-operative tumor area and final postoperative defect area, as compared to recurrent tumors that had initially been treated with other modalities.

XRT offers a valuable adjunctive treatment option for particularly aggressive perineural SCC and BCC. Detection of single-cell tumor spread may be particularly difficult following excisional surgery. In addition, perineural carcinoma may spread more rapidly along nerve sheaths than by contiguous growth. Given the increased risk of metastasis and recurrence in this group of tumors, adjuvant XRT should be considered as prophylactic treatment following surgical excision.

Caccialanza M, et al: Radiotherapy of recurrent basal and squamous cell skin carcinomas: a study of 249 re-treated carcinomas in 229 patients. Eur J Dermatol 2001; 11:25.

Han A, Ratner D: What is the role of adjuvant radiotherapy in the treatment of cutaneous squamous cell carcinoma with perineural invasion? Cancer 2007 Mar 15; 109(6):1053–1059.

Jambusaria-Pahlajani A, et al: Surgical monotherapy versus surgery plus adjuvant radiotherapy in high-risk cutaneous squamous cell carcinoma: a systematic review of outcomes. Dermatol Surg 2009 Apr; 35(4):574–585.

Locke J, et al: Radiotherapy for epithelial skin cancer. Int J Radiat Oncol Biol Phys 2001; 51:748.

Silverman MK, et al: Recurrence rates of treated basal cell carcinomas. Part 4: X-ray therapy. J Dermatol Surg Oncol 1992; 18:549.

Smith SP, et al: Use of Mohs micrographic surgery to establish quantitative proof of heightened tumor spread in basal cell carcinoma recurrent following radiotherapy. J Dermatol Surg Oncol 1990; 16:1012.

Veness MJ: The important role of radiotherapy in patients with non-melanoma skin cancer and other cutaneous entities. J Med Imaging Radiat Oncol 2008 Jun; 52(3):278–286.

Wang Y, et al: Indications and outcomes of radiation therapy for skin cancer of the head and neck. Clin Plast Surg 2009 Jul; 36(3):335–344.

38 | Cutaneous Laser Surgery

Almost no area of dermatology is changing as rapidly as that of cutaneous laser surgery. Development of new lasers, as well as improvements in existing lasers, continues to advance the field. As a result of this progress, laser surgery has become an effective therapeutic modality for a variety of dermatologic conditions.

Laser principles

"Laser" is an acronym for light amplification by stimulated emission of radiation. The first laser, a ruby laser, was operated in 1960 by Theodore Maiman. Medical applications were quickly recognized, and Leon Goldman pioneered their dermatologic use.

While technology has advanced through the years, several distinctive characteristics have remained in all lasers. As compared to other light sources, laser light is defined as monochromatic (only one wavelength), collimated (i.e. nondivergent), and coherent (i.e. in phase, with peaks and troughs of the light all aligned) (Fig. 38-1). Laser energy is measured in joules (J). Fluence is defined as the amount of energy delivered per unit

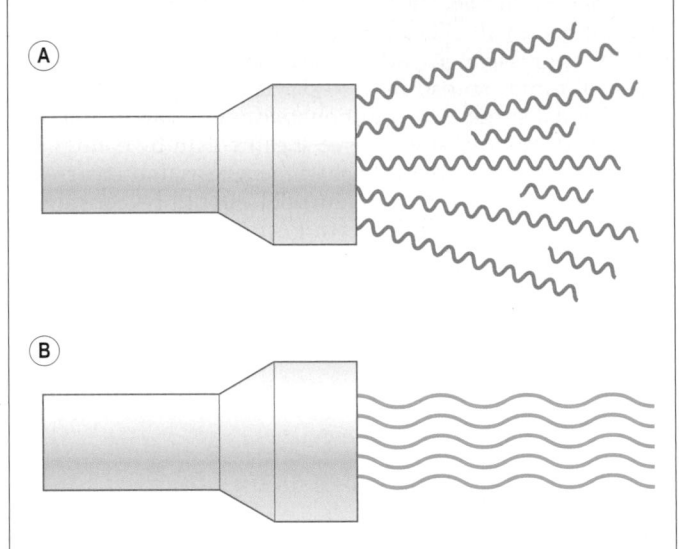

Fig. 38-1 Laser characteristics. In contrast to A, B demonstrates laser light that is both collimated and coherent.

Table 38-1 Dermatologic lasers

Laser	Wavelength (nm)	Color	Applications
Argon	488–514	Blue–green	Vascular lesions
Intense pulsed light (IPL)	515–1200	Green–red and infrared	Vascular lesions, pigmented lesions, epilation, photodamage
Potassium titanyl phosphate (KTP)	532	Green	Vascular lesions, pigmented lesions
Q-switched Nd:YAG (frequency-doubled)	532	Green	Vascular lesions, pigmented lesions, tattoo—red
Copper vapor	578/511	Yellow–green	Vascular lesions, pigmented lesions
Flashlamp pumped pulsed dye (PDL)	585–600	Yellow	Vascular lesions
Q-switched ruby	694	Red	Deep and superficial pigmented lesions; tattoo—black, blue, green
Long pulsed ruby	694	Red	Epilation
Q-switched alexandrite	755	Infrared	Tattoo—blue, black, green
Long pulsed alexandrite	755	Infrared	Epilation
Diode	810	Infrared	Epilation
Q-switched Nd:YAG	1064	Infrared	Deep and superficial dermal pigment; tattoo—black, blue
Long pulsed Nd:YAG	1064	Infrared	Epilation, vascular lesion
Er:YAG	2940	Infrared	Superficial skin resurfacing and destruction of superficial growths
Carbon dioxide	10 600	Infrared	Skin resurfacing and destruction of warts, keloids, superficial cancers, and benign growth

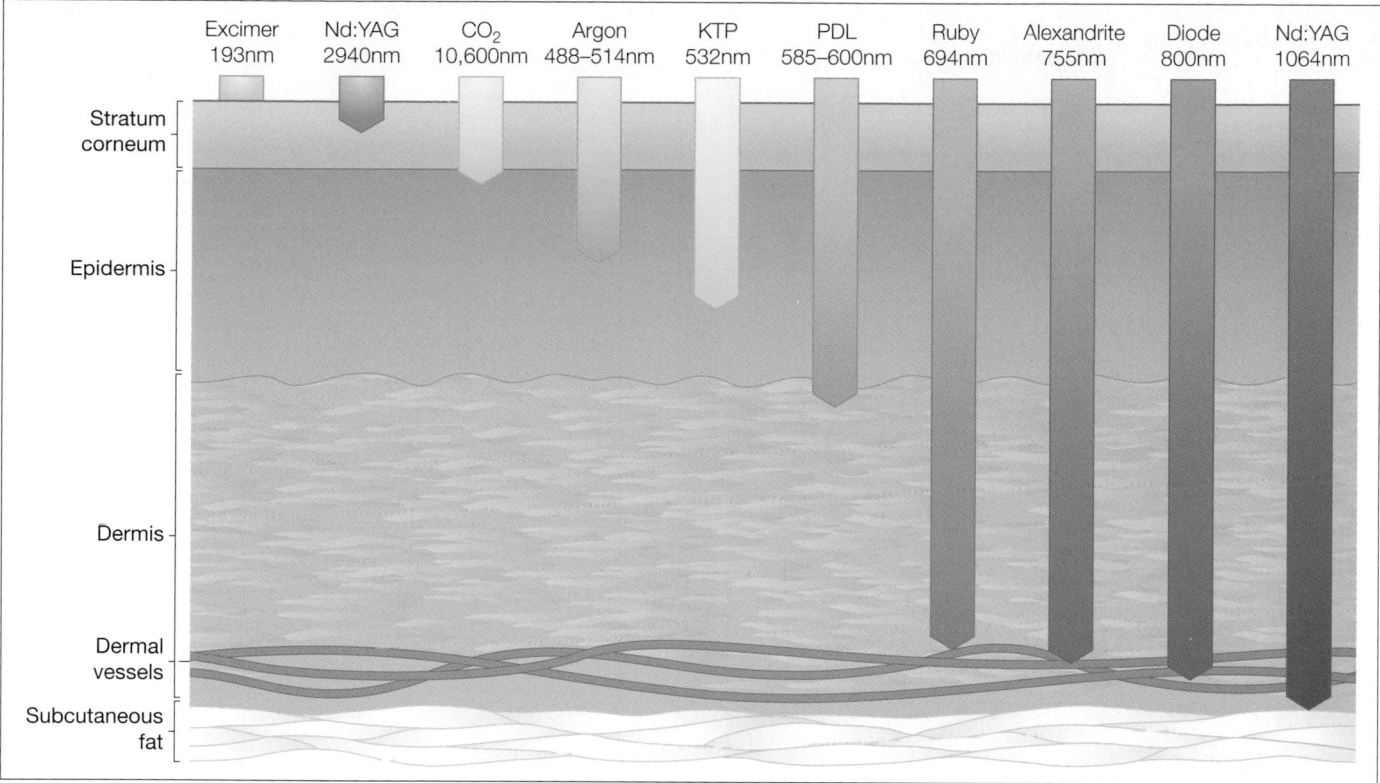

Fig. 38-2 Laser penetration.

area (J/cm^2). Power is the rate at which energy is delivered and is measured in watts (1 watt is defined as 1 J/sec).

The wavelength is determined by the active medium of each particular laser. Active medium can consist of a gas (e.g. argon or CO_2), liquid (e.g. dye), or a solid (e.g. ruby or yttrium-aluminum-garnet crystal) (Table 38-1). The choice of wavelength is determined by the target tissue and depth of penetration required (Fig. 38-2).

Continuous wave lasers emit a constant beam of light with long, constant exposure. Quasi-continuous wave lasers shutter the continuous beam into short segments, producing interrupted emissions of constant laser emission. Pulsed lasers produce short, high-energy pulses of light. Q-switched (quality-switched) lasers are able to generate extremely high-energy pulses over very short (i.e. nanoseconds) pulse durations and are used primarily for treating pigmented lesions.

Light can interact with incident targets in one of several ways: reflected, scattered, transmitted, or absorbed (Fig. 38-3). Approximately 5% of the laser light is reflected from the epidermis and not absorbed. Transmitted light passes unaltered through the tissue. Light is scattered by the various skin structures, molecules, and cells, thus limiting its depth of penetration and effect on tissue. In these first three cases, the light has no effect on the target tissue. However, when absorbed, the light energy is transformed into heat. In most cases of laser therapy, it is the heat generated by absorption that produces the desired effect. One notable exception is photodynamic therapy (see Chapter 37).

The concept of selective photothermolysis was originally promoted by Parish and Anderson, and is the basis for all laser tissue interactions. Lasers in cutaneous surgery are selected by matching their particular wavelength with the absorption spectrum of a desired target. The target structures that absorb laser light are defined as chromophores, with the most common in the skin being water, hemoglobin, and melanin (Fig. 38-4). The goal is to deliver a wavelength that is specifically absorbed

Table 38-2 Pulse durations and targets of selective photothermolysis

Chromophore	Diameter	TRT	Typical laser pulse duration
Tattoo ink particle	0.1 µm	10 ns	10 ns
Melanosome	0.5 µm	250 ns	10–100 ns
PWS vessels	30–100 µm	1–10 ms	0.4–20 ms
Terminal hair follicle	300 µm	100 ms	3–100 ms
Leg vein	1 mm	1 s	0.1 s

PWS, port-wine stain; TRT, thermal relaxation time.

by the chromophore, inducing heat build-up and destruction of that target.

In an ideal situation, that wavelength would have little or no absorption by surrounding structures. By controlling exposure times and energy delivered (fluence), the amount of heat build-up can be confined to the desired target with minimal or no damage to surrounding structures from heat dissipation (a property defined as thermal relaxation). A target's thermal relaxation time is defined as the time required for the heated tissue to dissipate half the absorbed heat, and is related to the size and shape of the target structure. Selective photothermolysis is achieved by ensuring that the laser pulse duration is equal to or less than the thermal relaxation time of the target tissue. Thus, larger structures (e.g. hair follicles) have a longer thermal relaxation time and are best treated with longer pulse widths, as compared to smaller structures (e.g. melanosomes), which have a shorter thermal relaxation time and can be treated with much shorter pulse durations (Table 38-2).

The beam diameter of the laser, or spot size, is a factor in depth of penetration of the laser. Small spot sizes produce

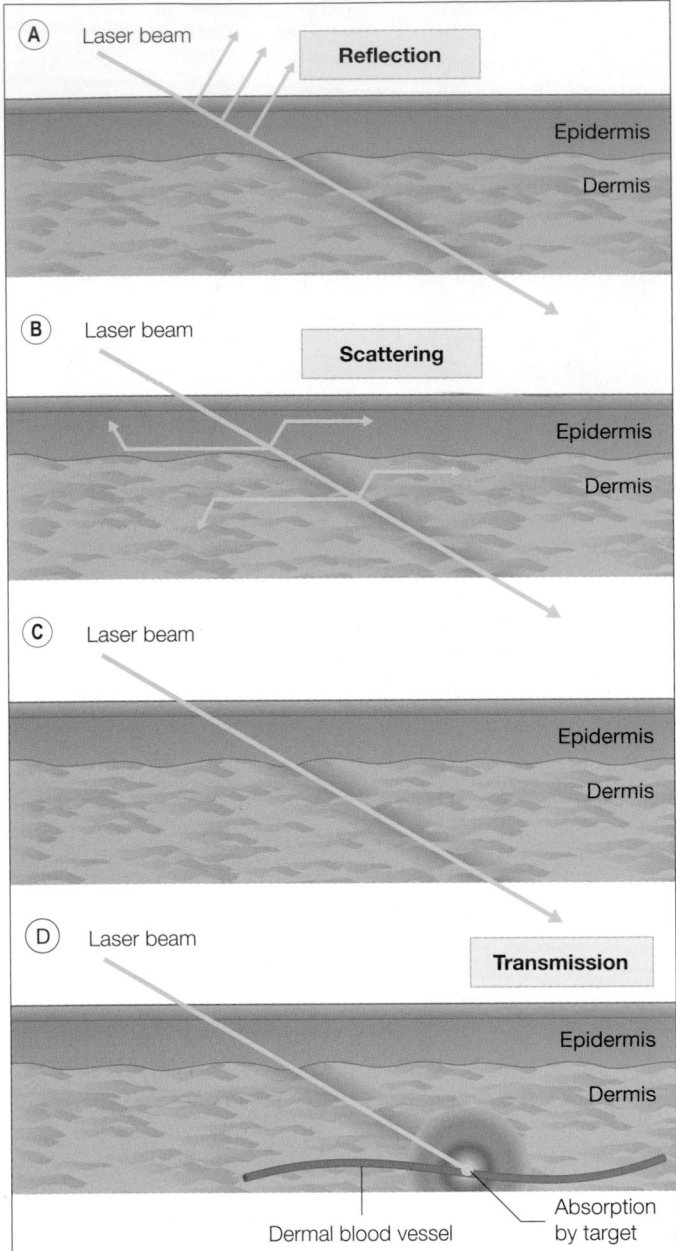

Fig. 38-3 Laser interaction with skin.

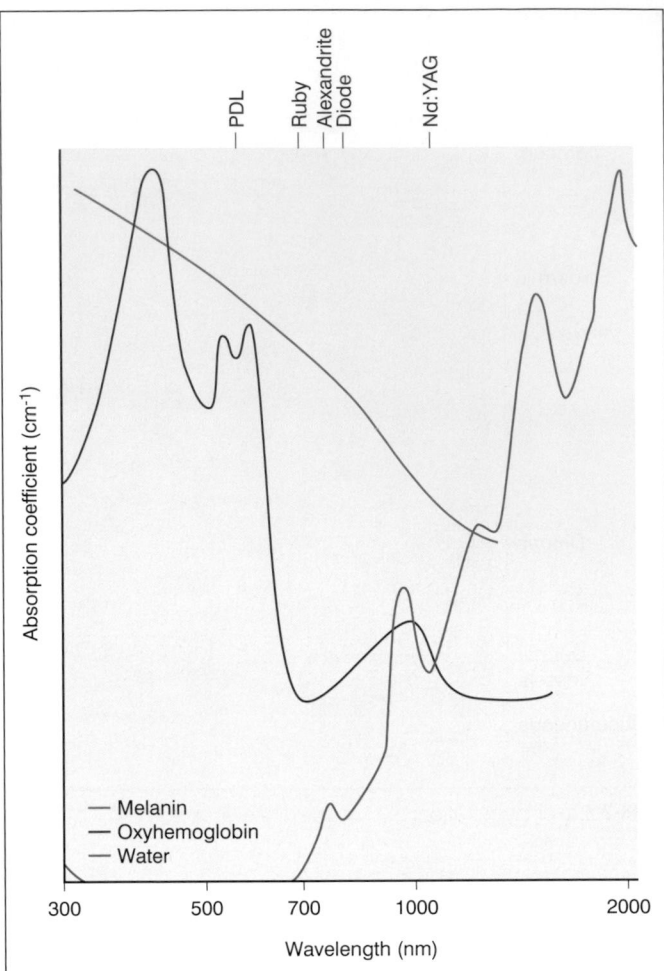

Fig. 38-4 Absorption spectra. The heterogenous absorption spectra of chromophores allow selective photothermolysis to work. Modified with permission from Bolognia JL, Jorizzo JL, Rapini RP, et al (eds): Dermatology, 2nd edn. London: Elsevier, 2008.

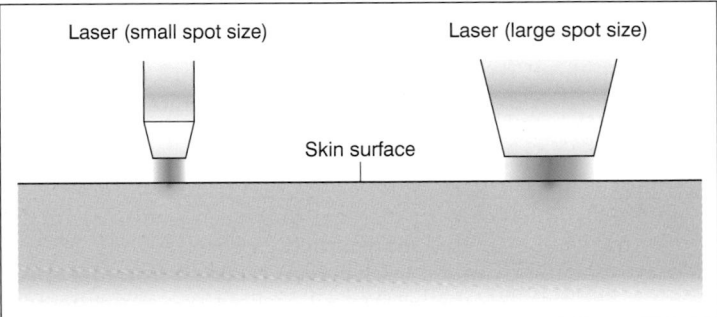

Fig. 38-5 The effects of spot size on scattering. The larger spot size allows more photons to remain within a beam's diameter, whereas with a smaller spot size a greater fraction of photons scatters outside the beam and is ineffective. Thus, a beam of a given wavelength penetrates to a deeper level with a larger spot size. Reproduced with permission from Bolognia JL, Jorizzo JL, Rapini RP, et al (eds): Dermatology, 2nd edn. London: Elsevier, 2008.

significantly more scatter of the laser outside of the effective beam, thus resulting in smaller effective treatment areas. In contrast, larger spot sizes produce more photons that remain within the beam diameter, resulting in higher fluences at a given depth. Therefore with any given wavelength, a larger beam diameter results in a deeper level of penetration (Fig. 38-5).

Epidermal melanin and heat transfer from dermal structures can result in inadvertent epidermal heating and injury. By selectively cooling the overlying skin, while still maintaining sufficient dermal heat to damage the target, the laser surgeon can reduce the chances of epidermal injury. Precooling, parallel cooling, and postcooling have all been used to protect the skin. Dynamic cooling devices use a cryogen spray to cool the skin before and after laser exposure. Contact cooling with a chilled sapphire tip can be used throughout the treatment, and is especially useful for parallel cooling. Forced cooled air provides less effective cooling as compared to other methods, but can be useful in reducing pain associated with laser treatment. Direct application of ice can also be used for postcooling.

The laser is a technologically advanced instrument. However, as with any surgery, side effects can occur. Hypertrophic scar-

ring and pigmentary changes are the most common, but infection, pain, and lack of efficacy are possible. Appropriate instruction and supervision in the use of lasers must be obtained by dermatologic surgeons in order to ensure optimum safety and surgical outcome.

Anderson RR, Parrish JA: Selective photothermolysis: precise microsurgery by selective absorption of pulsed radiation. Science 1983; 220:524.

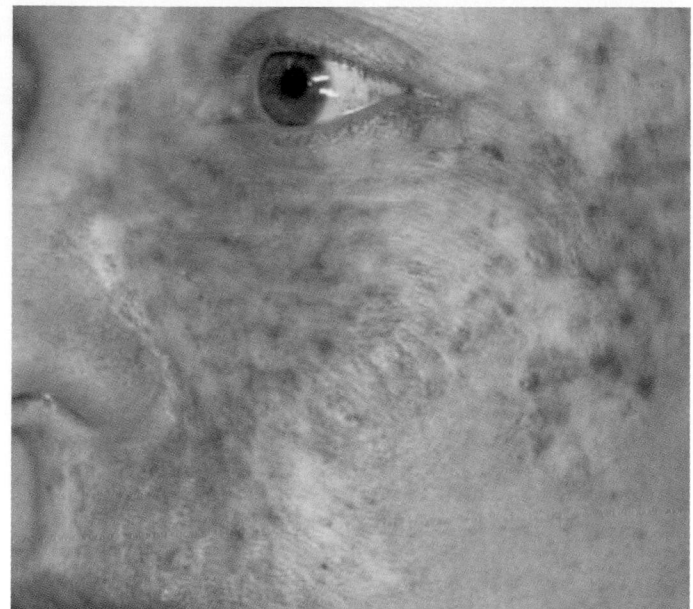

Fig. 38-6 Argon laser. Port wine stain treated with an argon laser. Note the significant scarring and pigmentation changes.

Carroll L, Humphreys TR: LASER–tissue interactions. Clin Dermatol 2006 Jan–Feb; 24(1):2–7.

Tanzi EL, Lupton JR, Alster TS: Lasers in dermatology: four decades of progress. J Am Acad Dermatol 2003 Jul; 49(1):1–31.

Laser treatment of vascular lesions

A number of congenital and acquired vascular lesions can be effectively treated with laser. Given the variety of choices available, the laser surgeon must have a complete understanding of the inherent differences in wavelengths, pulse durations, and the vessel size of the particular lesion being targeted. Over the years, lasers have become more selective and treatment of vascular lesions is more effective.

Argon laser

The argon laser was one of the first lasers used for the treatment of vascular and pigmented lesions. Because its wavelengths (488 and 514 nm) do not precisely correspond to absorption peaks of either hemoglobin or melanin, and also because of its continuous wave nature, thermal damage to surrounding tissue may be significant (Fig. 38-6). Other lasers have been developed that have largely replaced the argon laser, due to their greater efficacy and improved side effect profile (i.e. less scarring and dyspigmentation). In addition, the newer technology has resulted in smaller and more reliable laser devices.

Copper vapor/copper bromide laser

These devices, with wavelengths of 578 and 511 nm, were effective in treating vascular and pigmented lesions. Due to technical concerns regarding size of the device, reliability, and cost of maintenance, they have been replaced by several of the lasers discussed below.

Pulsed dye laser

The pulsed dye laser (PDL) was the first laser developed specifically to take advantage of the theory of selective photothermolysis. The laser medium is a rhodamine dye, which initially was developed to deliver a wavelength of 577 nm, coinciding with a specific hemoglobin absorption peak. Older lasers used a wavelength of 585 nm, but for various technical and clinical reasons, the wavelength has evolved in the current generation of PDL to be 595 nm. Initial pulse durations were of the order of 500 μs/pulse. This was based on calculations that the target, hemoglobin, had a thermal relaxation time of 1 ms or less. These parameters resulted in immediate postoperative purpura lasting up to 2 weeks.

Newer configurations of the laser allow for pulse durations from 0.45 to 40 ms, based on newer understandings of thermal relaxation times in the context of the size of the target (e.g. capillaries vs. larger vessels) and clinical effects (purpuric vs. nonpurpuric treatments). By using longer pulse durations, more gentle and uniform heating results in reduced or absent post-treatment purpura (more acceptable to patients) than the earlier PDL configurations, while still maintaining clinical efficacy.

The PDL is an extremely useful instrument for the treatment of vascular lesions. These lasers have traditionally been used for port wine stains, telangiectasias, erythematotelangiectatic rosacea, and hemangiomas. The risk of scarring and pigment change is very slight, and infants as young as a few weeks old can be treated. The newer long pulsed and longer wavelength lasers allow for treatment of larger and deeper vessels. By associating these treatments with surface cooling devices, the epidermis can be protected, which allows for the delivery of greater energy in a safer and less painful manner.

PDL is the treatment of choice for port wine stains. A series of treatments every 4–6 weeks is required for maximum benefit, with gradual improvement after each session. While most patients will show improvement, total clearance of lesions is extremely rare (Fig. 38-7). Rate of improvement is related to anatomic location, with lesions on the extremity having less of a response than facial lesions. Size also plays a role in the response rate of port wine stains. Smaller lesions have greater rate of improvement as compared to larger lesions. Treatments are typically performed with short pulse durations, with resulting purpura lasting for 10–14 days. When the treatment is performed with proper cooling and appropriate technique, the risk of atrophic scarring and pigmentary alterations is extremely low. Redarkening of treated port wine stains following treatment with PDL has been shown over time, and may necessitate repeat treatments years later.

Ulcerated hemangiomas have been successfully treated by PDL. In addition, following spontaneous resolution of infantile hemangiomas, PDL can be used for any persistent telangiectasias. However, PDL has a limited depth of penetration and thus is not effective in the treatment of deeper components of hemangiomas that are likely to continue to proliferate despite laser therapy. The use of PDL for treatment of superficial hemangiomas in the proliferative phase remains controversial. Some studies have demonstrated that early treatment with PDL results in improved clearing. However, others have advocated that the natural course of hemangiomas is of regression, and that potential risk of ulceration and atrophy from PDL treatment is not warranted for uncomplicated lesions.

Erythematotelangiectatic rosacea is a common condition characterized by persistent facial erythema, telangiectasias, and flushing. PDL has been shown to be an effective and safe treatment option (Fig. 38-8). The long pulsed PDL has the advantage of purpura-free treatment, which is better tolerated by patients desiring cosmetic improvement.

PDL has been effectively used for the treatment of warts, producing similar cure rates as traditional therapy. Several reports address the use of PDL for hypertrophic scars. Manuskiatti and Fitzpatrick demonstrated that PDL, intralesional corticosteroid, and 5-fluorouracil (5-FU) produced similar beneficial effects in the treatment of hypertrophic sternotomy scars. The mechanism of action in both incidences

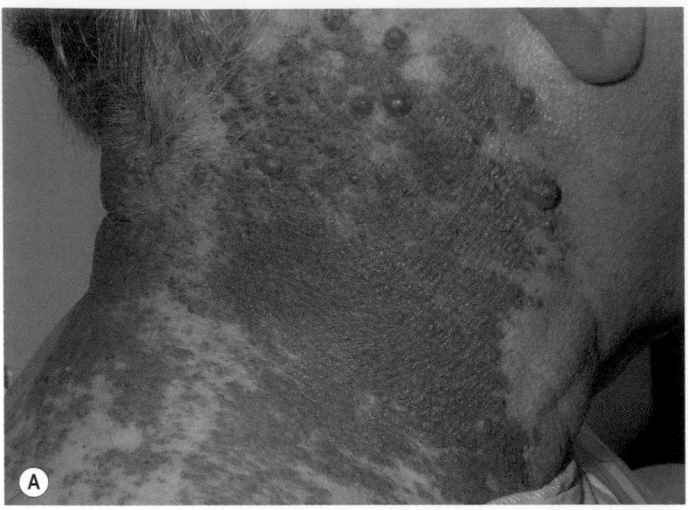
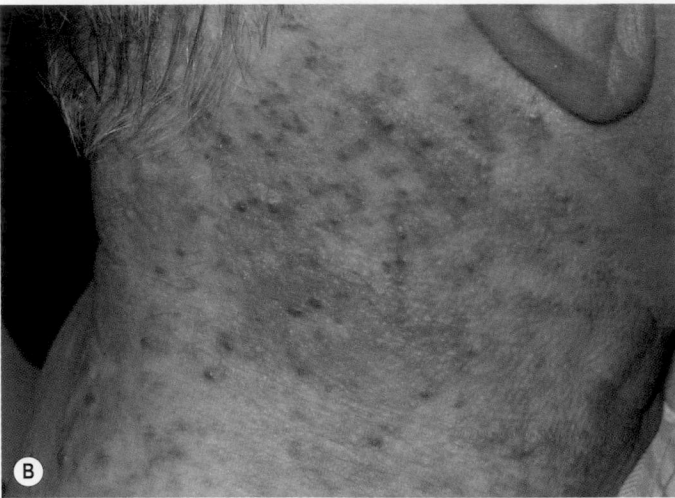

Fig. 38-7 Port wine stain. A, Prior to treatment. B, After eight treatments with the pulsed dye laser.

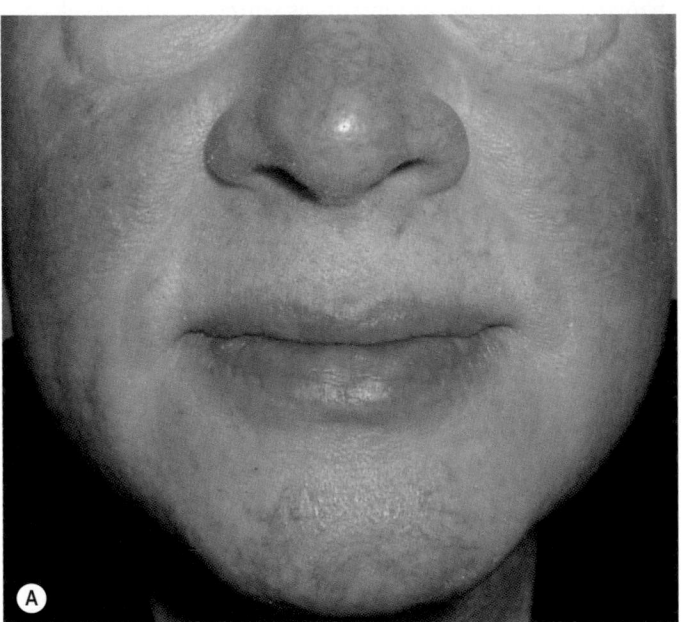
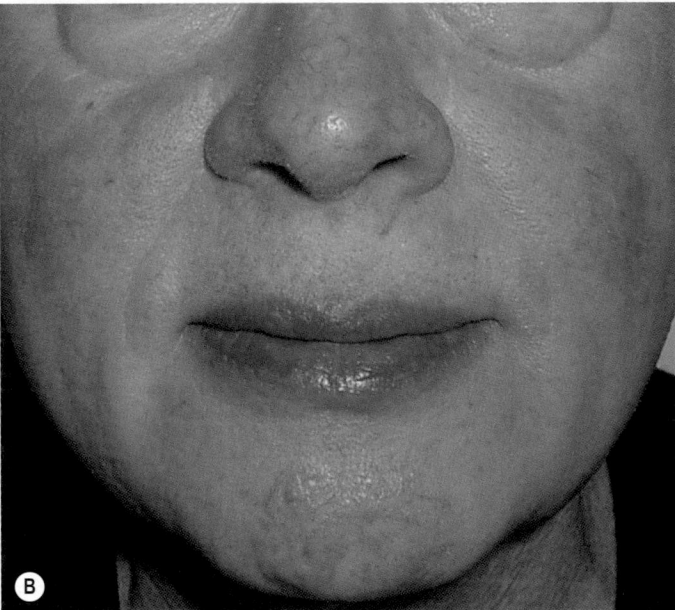

Fig. 38-8 Rosacea. A, Prior to treatment. B, After two treatments with subpurpuric pulsed dye laser.

is not clear. It may be related to injury to vessels supporting the lesions or simply to heat-related injury. As with other treatment modalities for these two conditions, results are variable.

KTP (potassium titanyl phosphate) laser

The KTP laser produces a visible green beam of 532 nm. Since there is significant hemoglobin and melanin absorption of this wavelength, KTP can be used to treat both vascular and superficial pigmented lesions (see below). The KTP laser is actually an Nd:YAG laser that emits a wavelength of 1064 nm. The beam is passed through a crystal of KTP that reduces the wavelength by 50%, producing the 532 nm wavelength.

Pulsed KTP lasers have pulse durations ranging from 1 to 100 ms. The advantage of these lasers is the strong absorption of their wavelength by hemoglobin. In addition, purpura is not present with the longer pulse widths. The 532 nm wavelength has a limited depth of penetration, making it an excellent choice for the treatment of fine facial vessels. However, it can be absorbed by epidermal pigment to a greater degree

than other longer wavelength vascular lasers, which increases the possibility of pigmentary complications. KTP lasers can be quite compact, allowing for easy transport between various locations. With few moving parts they are relatively maintenance-free.

These lasers are best suited to treatment of individual telangiectasias of the face, cherry angiomas, and small spider angiomas. Since individual vessels must be traced out using a narrow beam diameter, there are limitations to the number of vessels treated in any given session.

Long pulsed infrared lasers

Lasers are now being used to take advantage of the broad oxyhemoglobin absorption band in the near-infrared range. Long pulsed lasers include the alexandrite (755 nm), diode (800 nm, 940 nm), and neodymium:yttrium-aluminum-garnet (Nd:YAG; 1064 nm). These lasers are best used for larger and deeper vessels, such as large-vessel venous malformations, vascular blebs in port wine stains, blue reticular veins, and lower extremity spider veins (Fig. 38-9).

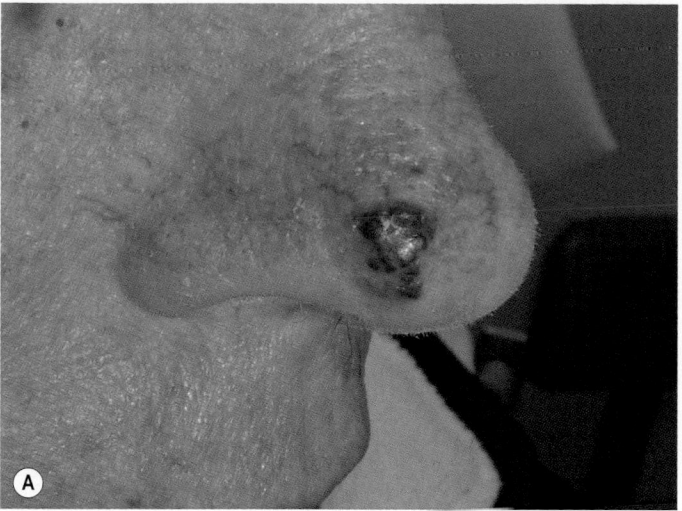
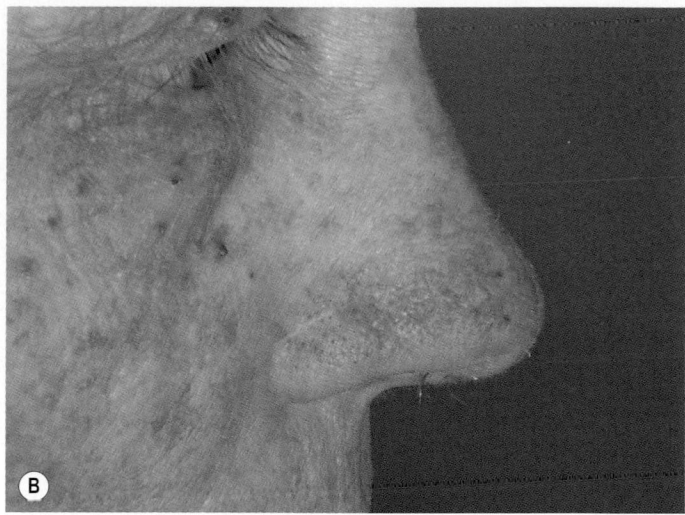

Fig. 38-9 Venous lake. A, Prior to treatment. B, After two treatments with the long pulsed Nd:YAG laser.

Intense pulsed light

The intense pulsed light (IPL), while technically not a laser, is a device that uses a flashlamp that emits a noncoherent broad spectrum of light (from 400 to 1200 nm) at various pulse durations and intervals. By employing filters to eliminate the lower wavelengths, light from 560 nm and above can be used to treat various cutaneous conditions. This technology has the advantage of treating more than one specific chromophore at a time and is especially useful in improving both vascular and pigmentary changes commonly seen in photodamaged skin (see below). In addition, it has a relatively large beam size and rapid pulse rate, allowing for the treatment of a large area in a relatively short amount of time.

IPL has been used for the treatment of facial telangiectasia and rosacea. There is generally no purpura when appropriate settings are used, but care must be taken to avoid dyspigmentation and blistering in darker skin types. As with other light sources, a series of treatment sessions spaced out every 4–6 weeks are typically required for maximum improvement.

Bekhor PS: Long-pulsed Nd:YAG laser treatment of venous lakes: report of a series of 34 cases. Dermatol Surg 2006 Sep; 32(9):1151–1154.

Clark C, et al: Treatment of superficial cutaneous vascular lesions: experience with the KTP 532 nm laser. Lasers Med Sci 2004; 19(1):1–5.

Faurschou A, et al: Pulsed dye laser vs. intense pulsed light for port-wine stains: a randomized side-by-side trial with blinded response evaluation. Br J Dermatol 2009 Feb; 160(2):359 364.

Galeckas KJ: Update on lasers and light devices for the treatment of vascular lesions. Semin Cutan Med Surg 2008 Dec; 27(4):276–284.

Groot D, et al: Algorithm for using a long-pulsed Nd:YAG laser in the treatment of deep cutaneous vascular lesions. Dermatol Surg 2003; 29:35.

Huikeshoven M, et al: Redarkening of port-wine stains 10 years after pulsed-dye-laser treatment. N Engl J Med 2007 Mar 22; 356(12):1235–1240.

Kono T, et al: Treatment of resistant port-wine stains with a variable-pulse pulsed dye laser. Dermatol Surg 2007 Aug; 33(8):951–956.

Manuskiatti W, Fitzpatrick RE: Treatment response of keloidal and hypertrophic sternotomy scars: comparison among intralesional corticosteroid, 5-fluorouracil, and 585-nm flashlamp-pumped pulsed-dye laser treatments. Arch Dermatol 2002; 138:1149.

Neuhaus IM, et al: Comparative efficacy of nonpurpuragenic pulsed dye laser and intense pulsed light for erythematotelangiectatic rosacea. Dermatol Surg 2009 Jun; 35(6):920–928.

Robson KJ, et al: Pulsed-dye laser versus conventional therapy in the treatment of warts: a prospective randomized trial. J Am Acad Dermatol 2000; 43:275.

Schellhaas U, et al: Pulsed dye laser treatment is effective in the treatment of recalcitrant viral warts. Dermatol Surg 2008 Jan; 34(1):67–72.

Schroeter CA, et al: Effective treatment of rosacea using intense pulsed light systems. Dermatol Surg 2005 Oct; 31(10):1285–1289.

Stier MF, et al: Laser treatment of pediatric vascular lesions: port wine stains and hemangiomas. J Am Acad Dermatol 2008 Feb; 58(2):261–285.

Tan SR, Tope WD: Pulsed dye laser treatment of rosacea improves erythema, symptomatology, and quality of life. J Am Acad Dermatol 2004 Oct; 51(4):592–599.

Uebelhoer NS, et al: A split-face comparison study of pulsed 532-nm KTP laser and 595-nm pulsed dye laser in the treatment of facial telangiectasias and diffuse telangiectatic facial erythema. Dermatol Surg 2007 Apr; 33(4):441–448.

Witman PM, et al: Complications following pulsed dye laser treatment of superficial hemangiomas. Lasers Surg Med 2006 Feb; 38(2):116–123.

Laser treatment for pigmented lesions

Highly pigment-selective Q-switched lasers are used extensively in the treatment of both epidermal and dermal pigmented lesions. In most cases, the target chromophore is the melanosome. These tiny structures have a very short thermal relaxation time (250–1000 nsec), and the development of Q-switching allows for production of extremely high energies and short nanosecond pulse durations. As a result, these lasers can produce damage to the selected target while minimizing injury to surrounding tissue.

Q-switched lasers are used to treat epidermal pigmented lesions and tattoos. The delivery of tremendous amounts of energy over a very short period of time produces pressure waves. This photoacoustic effect results in shock waves that shatter the larger ink particles into smaller fragments. Repeated treatments are necessary for complete response. Q-switched lasers include the ruby (694 nm), alexandrite (755 nm), and Nd:YAG, in both a frequency doubled (532 nm) and standard (1064 nm) mode (Table 38-3). Because of the longer wavelength, the Nd:YAG laser penetrates much more deeply and therefore is more useful in treating more deeply seated or thicker lesions compared to shorter wavelength Q-switched lasers.

Less pigment-selective lasers can be used in some clinical settings. The variable pulsed KTP laser can be used to treat epidermal pigmentation, such as lentigines, ephelides, thin seborrheic keratoses, and dermatosis papulosis nigra. As the KTP laser has a limited depth of penetration, it is not effective in the treatment of deeper dermal lesions. Long pulsed ruby, alexandrite, and Nd:YAG lasers can also be used to treat pigmented lesions; however, they are not as effective as their Q-switched counterparts.

Non-pigment-specific ablative lasers have been used in the treatment of pigmented lesions and tattoos. Carbon dioxide (10 600 nm) and erbium:YAG lasers (2940 nm) target water. They non-selectively remove the entire epidermis and a variable level of dermis tissue, and any associated pigment present.

Epidermal pigmented lesions

Lentigines are hyperpigmented macules composed of an increased number of basal melanocytes. These lesions can be

Table 38-3 Q-switched lasers

Laser type	Wavelength	Pulse duration
QS Nd:YAG (frequency doubled)	532 nm	5–7 nsec
QS ruby	694 nm	25–40 nsec
QS alexandrite	755 nm	50–100 nsec
QS Nd:YAG	1064 nm	5–7 nsec

effectively treated with a variety of laser and light sources owing to their superficial position in the skin. Q-switched lasers can be used to treat solar lentigines and those associated with syndromes (e.g. Peutz–Jeghers) (Figs 38-10 and 38-11). Variable pulsed KTP provides effective treatment. IPL is an excellent choice for patients with widespread photodamage consisting of both vascular and pigmentary changes.

Café-au-lait macules and Becker's nevus can be treated with Q-switched lasers. Unfortunately, treatment often results in variable clinical efficacy. Short-term lightening or clearing with multiple treatments is frequently seen, but recurrence is common.

Dermal pigmented lesions

Nevus of Ota and nevus of Ito are dermal melanocytoses that can be effectively treated with Q-switched lasers. A series of treatments can significantly improve or even clear the lesion (Fig. 38-12). These treatments are generally well tolerated and the results are long-lasting.

Melasma is an acquired hypermelanosis that is often associated with sun exposure, pregnancy, and oral contraceptives. First-line treatment includes strict sun protection, discontinuing any offending systemic medication, and the use of topical agents such as hydroquinone and retinoids. Laser treatment is

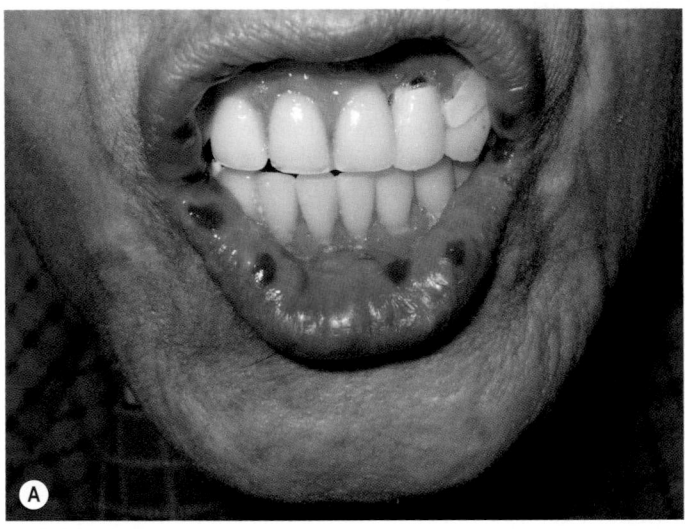
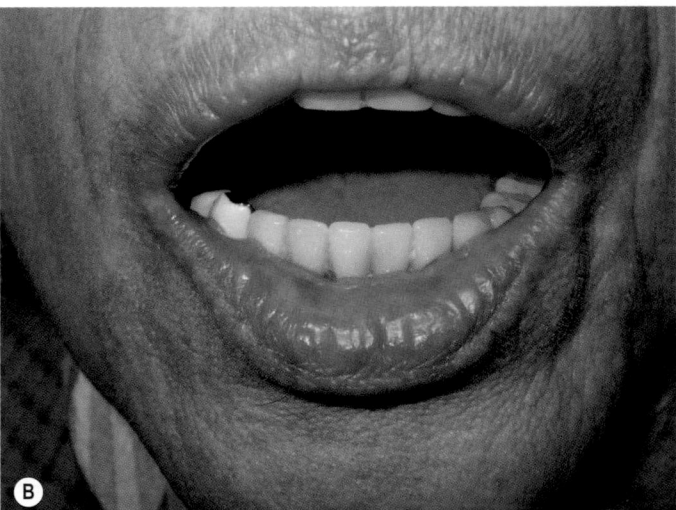

Fig. 38-10 Labial melanotic macules. A, Prior to treatment. B, After single treatment with a Q-switched 532 nm laser.

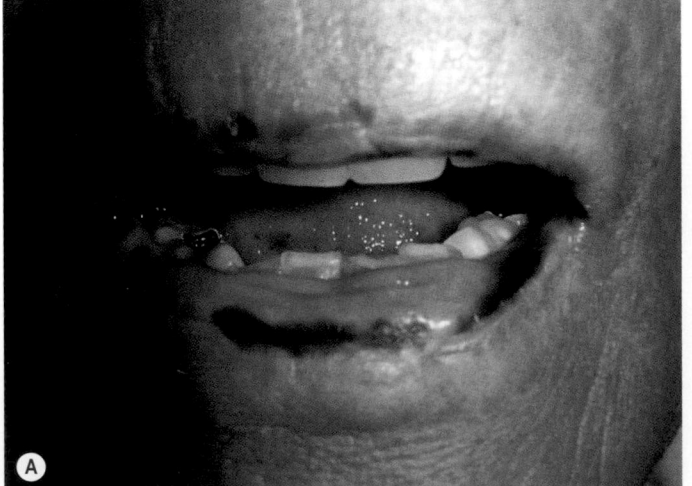
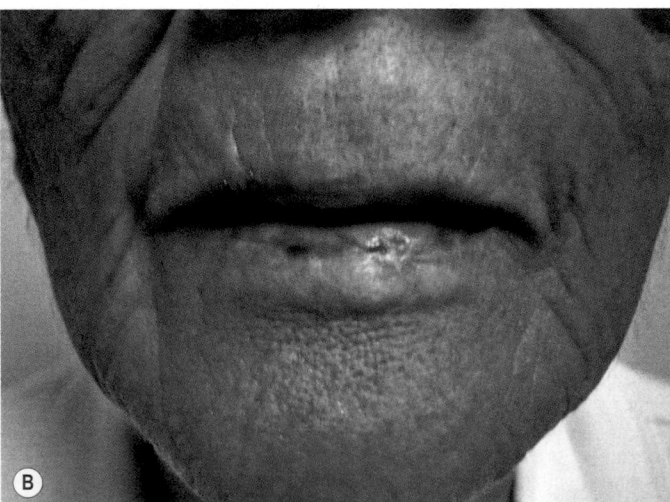

Fig. 38-11 Peutz–Jeghers syndrome. A, Prior to treatment. B, After treatment with a Q-switched ruby laser.

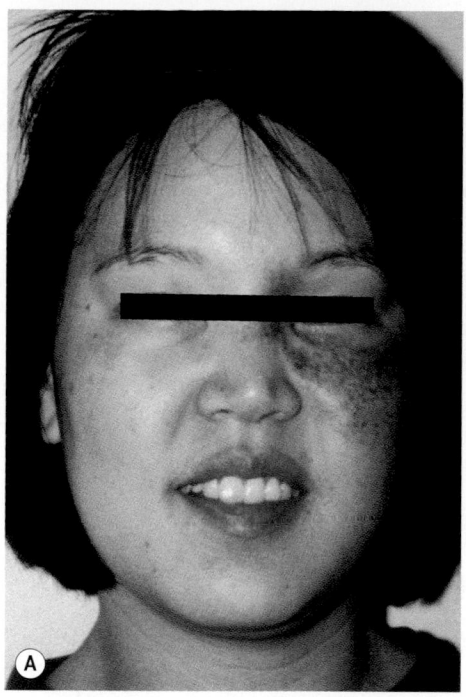
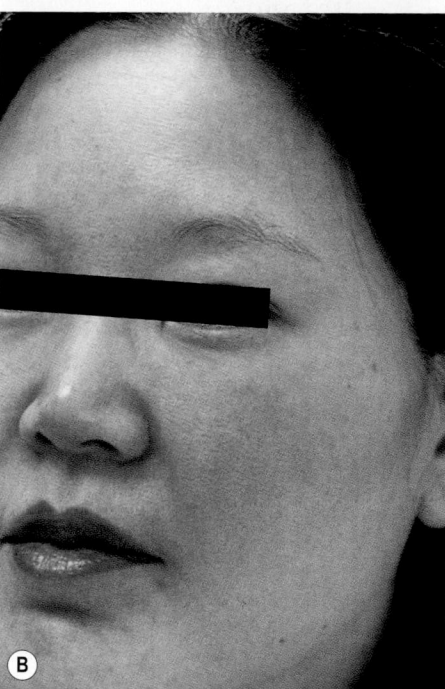

Fig. 38-12 Nevus of Ota. A, Prior to treatment. B, After treatment with a Q-switched ruby laser.

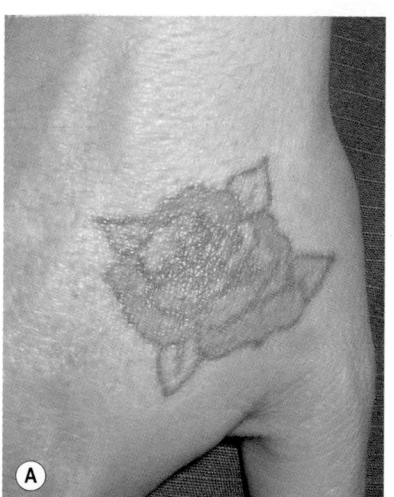
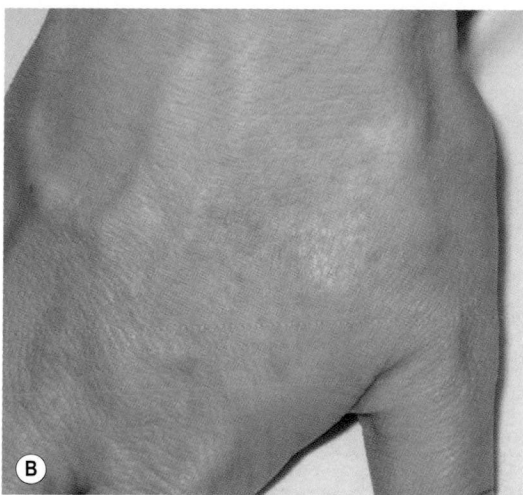

Fig. 38-13 Tattoo. A, Prior to treatment. B, After six treatments with Q-switched ruby and Q-switched Nd:YAG laser.

often ineffective, and recurrence is commonly seen in those cases with initial improvement.

Post-inflammatory hyperpigmentation does not generally respond to Q-switched laser. Recurrence or worsening is typically seen due to additional epidermal injury associated with laser treatment.

Tattoos

Pigmentation to mark the skin for decorative purposes has been used by humans for thousands of years and remains a popular practice today. As a result of the increasing number of people with tattoos, it should come as no surprise that many patients desire removal. Regardless of the type of tattoo (i.e. cosmetic, medical, and traumatic), effective treatment can be frequently offered.

In the past, tattoos were removed by a variety of non-selective destructive techniques, including excision, derm-abrasion, cryosurgery, and ablative laser. While effective in eliminating the ink, these techniques produced significant scarring. With the advent of newer technology that is more specific and less traumatic, these destructive modalities are not generally employed today.

Currently, Q-switched lasers are the first-line treatment for tattoo removal. The delivery of high energy in very short pulse durations causes fragmentation of the tattoo ink particle, which is then eliminated from the body via phagocytosis of macrophages and lymphatic drainage. Repeat treatments are required to achieve maximum benefit (Fig. 38-13).

Patients frequently inquire as to the number of treatment sessions needed for maximum improvement. Unfortunately, a precise answer is difficult to provide and depends on the amount of ink, size of tattoo, location, and color being treated. Amateur tattoos typically have less ink and generally have a better response to laser treatment. In contrast, multicolored professional tattoos have a more unpredictable response and require more treatments (sometimes 10–15 or more) to achieve maximum benefit. The choice of which laser to use is dependent on the specific tattoo color being targeted (Table 38-4).

Tattoo complications

Textural changes can occur as a result of the repetitive injury associated with laser treatment (Fig. 38-14). Epidermal injury can be seen with excessive fluences and with short treatment intervals. By spacing out treatment sessions, lowering fluences, and using longer wavelengths to protect the epidermis, this can often be avoided.

Hypopigmentation is sometimes seen in patients with darker skin types (Fig. 38-15). Much like textural changes, pigmentary changes are more common with shorter wavelengths (i.e. ruby and alexandrite), which can cause more epidermal damage. Similar precautions can be used to minimize these changes.

Paradoxical darkening of flesh, brown, or white tattoos (with red and yellow ink less frequently) can occur immediately following treatment with Q-switched lasers. The reduction of rust-colored ferric oxide to black-colored ferrous oxide or the white-colored titanium^{4+} dioxide to blue titanium^{3+} dioxide is felt to be responsible for the color change. This reaction is typically seen is cosmetic tattoos used for lip liners, eyebrows, etc. However, as many brightly colored tattoos have some white in them, caution must be taken in these circumstances (Fig. 38-16). Test treatment should be done if there is a potential for paradoxical darkening. The darkened tattoo can be treated with the appropriate QS wavelength, but response is unpredictable and requires numerous treatments.

Despite appropriate treatment, tattoos may not respond completely. This may be due to the color, ink density, anatomic location, age of tattoo, etc. Appropriate preoperative counseling is required before embarking on any treatment course.

Table 38-4 Tattoo colors and pigments and lasers used for treatment

Color/Etiology	Pigment	Laser
Traumatic	Lead, asphalt, carbon, gunpowder	QS ruby; QS alexandrite; QS Nd:YAG (1064 nm)
Amateur black	India ink, carbon	QS ruby; QS alexandrite; QS Nd:YAG (1064 nm)
Professional black	Carbon, iron oxide, logwood extract	QS ruby; QS alexandrite; QS Nd:YAG (1064 nm)
Blue	Cobalt aluminate (azure blue)	QS ruby; QS alexandrite; QS Nd:YAG (1064 nm)
Green	Chromium oxide (casalis green), hydrated chromium sesquioxide (guignet green), malachite green, lead chromate, ferro-ferric cyanide, curcumin green, phthalocyanine dyes (copper salts with yellow coal tar dyes)	QS ruby; QS alexandrite
Red	Mercury sulfide (cinnabar), cadmium selenide (cadmium red), sienna (red ochre; ferric hydrate and ferric sulfate), azo dyes	QS Nd:YAG (532 nm)
Yellow	Cadmium sulfide (cadmium yellow), ochre, curcumin yellow	QS Nd:YAG (532 nm)
Brown	Ochre	Tan/light brown: QS Nd:YAG (532 nm) Dark brown: QS ruby; QS alexandrite; QS Nd:YAG (1064 nm)
Violet	Manganese violet	QS Nd:YAG (532 nm)
White	Titanium dioxide, zinc oxide	QS Nd:YAG (532 nm)
Flesh	Iron oxides	QS Nd:YAG (532 nm)

Adapted from Bolognia JL, Jorizzo JL, Rapini RP (eds): Dermatology. 2nd edn. London: Elsevier, 2008.

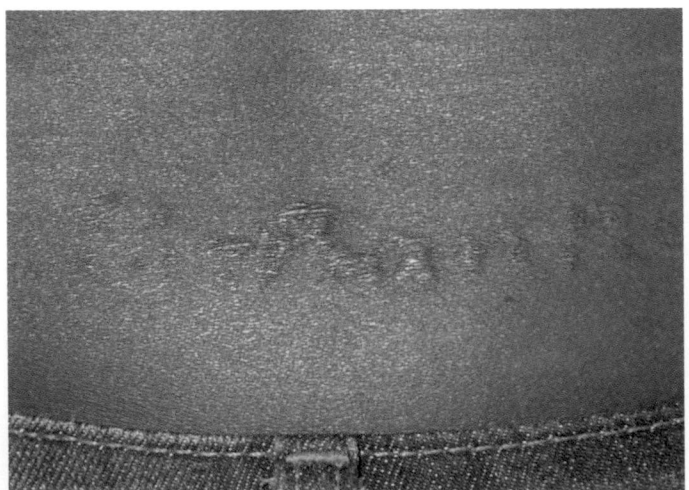

Fig. 38-14 Textural changes secondary to Q-switched laser treatment.

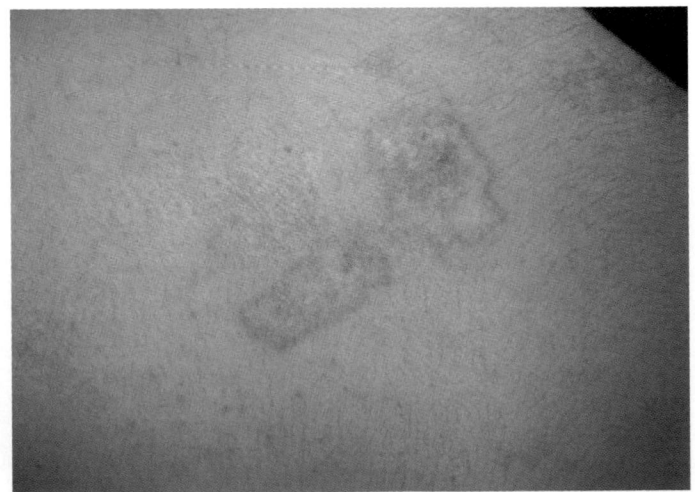

Fig. 38-15 Hypopigmentation secondary to Q-switched laser treatment.

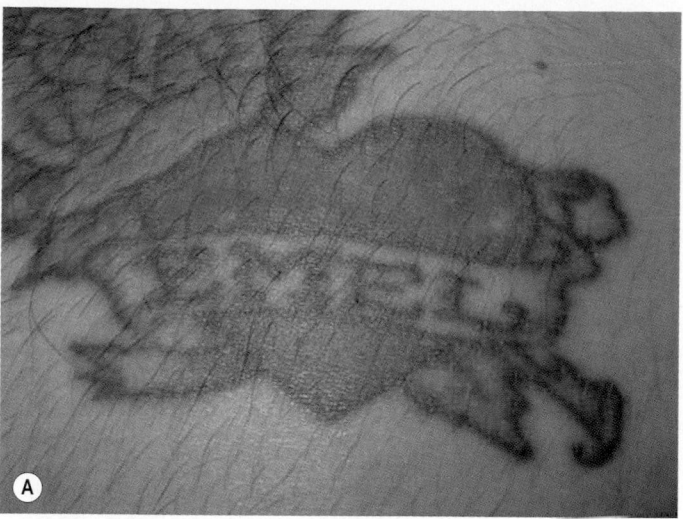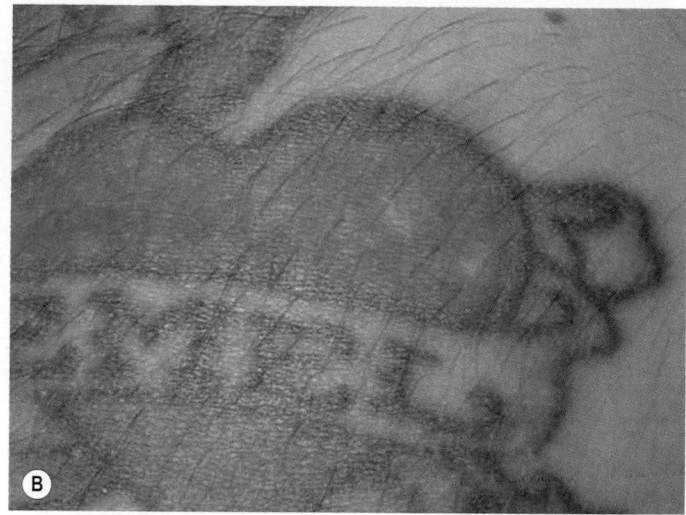

Fig. 38-16 Paradoxical darkening of red tattoo following single test pulse with Q-switched 532 nm laser. A, Prior to treatment. B, Following treatment of darkening with Q-switched Nd:YAG laser.

Treatment of gunpowder traumatic tattoos can result in microexplosions and scars. Care must be taken when treating these patients.

Bernstein EF: Laser treatment of tattoos. Clin Dermatol 2006 Jan–Feb; 24(1):43–55.

Dawson E, et al: Adverse events associated with nonablative cutaneous laser, radiofrequency, and light-based devices. Semin Cutan Med Surg 2007 Mar; 26(1):15–21.

Fusade T, et al: Treatment of gunpowder traumatic tattoo by Q-switched Nd:YAG laser: an unusual adverse effect. Dermatol Surg 2000 Nov; 26(11):1057–1059.

Holzer AM, et al: Adverse effects of Q-switched laser treatment of tattoos. Dermatol Surg 2008 Jan; 34(1):118–122.

Kono T, et al: Use of Q-switched ruby laser in the treatment of nevus of Ota in different age groups. Lasers Surg Med 2003; 32(5):391–395.

Park JM, et al: Combined use of intense pulsed light and Q-switched ruby laser for complex dyspigmentation among Asian patients. Lasers Surg Med 2008 Feb; 40(2):128–133.

Sadighha A, et al: Efficacy and adverse effects of Q-switched ruby laser on solar lentigines: a prospective study of 91 patients with Fitzpatrick skin type II, III, and IV. Dermatol Surg 2008 Nov; 34(11):1465–1468.

Suchin KR, Greenbaum SS: Successful treatment of a cosmetic tattoo using a combination of lasers. Dermatol Surg 2004 Jan; 30(1):105–107.

Trafeli JP, et al: Use of a long-pulse alexandrite laser in the treatment of superficial pigmented lesions. Dermatol Surg 2007 Dec; 33(12):1477–1482.

Varma S, et al: Tattoo ink darkening of a yellow tattoo after Q-switched laser treatment. Clin Exp Dermatol 2002 Sep; 27(6):461–463.

Wang CC, et al: A comparison of Q-switched alexandrite laser and intense pulsed light for the treatment of freckles and lentigines in Asian persons: a randomized, physician-blinded, split-face comparative trial. J Am Acad Dermatol 2006 May; 54(5):804–810.

Wang HW, et al: Analysis of 602 Chinese cases of nevus of Ota and the treatment results treated by Q-switched alexandrite laser. Dermatol Surg 2007 Apr; 33(4):455–460.

Xi Z, et al: Q-switched alexandrite laser treatment of oral labial lentigines in Chinese subjects with Peutz–Jeghers syndrome. Dermatol Surg 2009 Jul; 35(7):1084–1088.

Laser hair removal

Laser hair removal is widely used for the permanent reduction of hair and is one of the most popular laser procedures performed. Hair removal lasers target the melanin within the follicle and, given the size of the target chromophore, longer pulse durations are required to generate enough heat to damage the bulbar stem cells. Patients with dark hair and

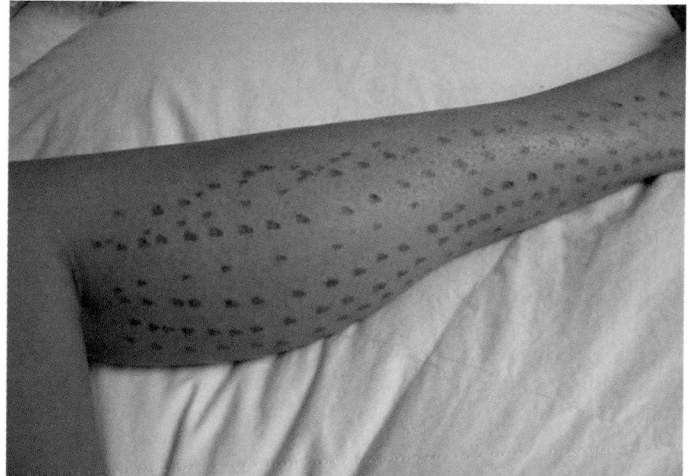

Fig. 38-17 Epidermal burns secondary to laser hair removal performed by an unlicenced provider at a medi-spa.

lightly pigmented skin are the best candidates for treatment, while white, blond, and gray hairs generally respond poorly.

In order to maintain a target, patients must avoid waxing, electrolysis, or plucking of hairs prior to laser treatment. Shaving prior to laser treatment is acceptable (and is mandatory immediately prior to treatment to avoid epidermal injury); it will not interfere with efficacy. Only hairs in the anagen growth phase are permanently injured. Therefore, sufficient time must elapse between treatments for hair to regrow and provide an appropriate chromophore for subsequent laser treatment, generally 6–8 weeks.

Currently used devices for hair removal include the long pulsed ruby, alexandrite, diode, and Nd:YAG lasers, and the IPL. Multiple treatments are required for maximum benefit. In addition, these longer pulsed lasers can produce a significant reduction in both hair and papules/pustules in patients with pseudofolliculitis barbae and folliculitis decalvans.

Complications are rare with proper patient selection and treatment parameters. Excessive fluences or insufficient cooling can result in epidermal injury (Fig. 38-17). Caution must be employed in treating patients with increased skin pigmentation due to sun tanning, as pigmentary changes and cutaneous burns can occur. As melanin is the target for these lasers, care must be taken in treating more darkly pigmented patients to avoid epidermal damage. In this patient population, the longer pulsed Nd:YAG laser has allowed safe treatment with fewer complications, owing to the deeper penetration and reduced melanin absorption of this wavelength. Paradoxical hypertrichosis as a result of laser hair treatment has been reported. The etiology is unclear, but the condition seems to occur more frequently in darker skin types.

Alajlan A, et al: Paradoxical hypertrichosis after laser epilation. J Am Acad Dermatol 2005 Jul;53(1):85–88.

Bouzari N, et al: Laser hair removal: comparison of long-pulsed Nd:YAG, long-pulsed alexandrite, and long-pulsed diode lasers. Dermatol Surg 2004 Apr; 30(4 Pt 1):498–502.

Davoudi SM, et al: Comparison of long-pulsed alexandrite and Nd:YAG lasers, individually and in combination, for leg hair reduction: an assessor-blinded, randomized trial with 18 months of follow-up. Arch Dermatol 2008 Oct; 144(10).1323–1327.

El Bedewi AF: Hair removal with intense pulsed light. Lasers Med Sci 2004; 19(1):48–51.

McGill DJ, et al: A randomised, split-face comparison of facial hair removal with the alexandrite laser and intense pulsed light system. Lasers Surg Med 2007 Dec; 39(10):767–772.

Rao J, Goldman MP: Prospective, comparative evaluation of three laser systems used individually and in combination for axillary hair removal. Dermatol Surg 2005 Dec; 31(12):1671–1676.

Sadick NS, Laughlin SA: Effective epilation of white and blond hair using combined radiofrequency and optical energy. J Cosmet Laser Ther 2004; 6:27.

Schroeter CA, et al: Hair reduction using intense pulsed light source. Dermatol Surg 2004; 30:168.

Tanzi EL, Alster TS: Long-pulsed 1064-nm Nd:YAG laser-assisted hair removal in all skin types. Dermatol Surg 2004 Jan; 30(1):13–17.

Weaver SM 3rd, Sagaral EC: Treatment of pseudofolliculitis barbae using the long-pulse Nd:YAG laser on skin types V and VI. Dermatol Surg 2003 Dec; 29(12):1187–1191.

Ablative laser resurfacing

Both CO_2 and erbium:YAG (Er:YAG) lasers are absorbed by water. Since water makes up 72% of the skin, they effectively ablate the skin to varying depths depending on the energy delivered. They can be used therapeutically to treat conditions such as warts, adnexal tumors, and skin cancers. In addition to these medical indications, ablative lasers can also be employed to remove very superficial external layers and resurface the skin for cosmetic enhancement (i.e. photorejuvenation, acne scarring, etc.). Despite all the efforts to produce nonablative resurfacing technology, ablative lasers remain unparalleled in producing meaningful and dramatic rejuvenation.

Early systems employed a continuous wave mode of emission, which led to a greater degree of thermal damage and risk of scarring. Newer, high-energy, ultra-pulsed and computerized scanning systems have allowed a greater degree of control with laser ablation, resulting in more predictable outcomes.

Carbon dioxide lasers

The CO_2 laser emits an invisible infrared beam of 10 600 nm and can be used in continuous-wave or super-pulsed mode. Water nonselectively absorbs laser energy, turning it instantly into steam, and producing ablative and thermal damage. Used in the super-pulsed mode, the laser beam can be delivered in short bursts, allowing thermal destruction of the epidermis and papillary dermis while limiting deeper thermal damage. Delivery in this mode is more uniform and markedly faster when the optomechanical scanner is employed. Super-pulsed CO_2 lasers are extremely effective for the treatment of actinic damage and photoaging. The thermal injury causes conformational changes within the collagen, leading to clinical tightening. As such, ablative laser resurfacing produces significant improvement in wrinkling, scarring, and skin tone.

Side effects include postinflammatory pigmentary changes, especially in patients with Fitzpatrick skin types III–VI.

Treatment with hydroquinone at the first sign of hyperpigmentation can effectively reduce the hyperpigmentation. Hypopigmentation is frequently seen following resurfacing and is often due to the contrast between treated and untreated skin. In order to minimize the aesthetic impact, the entire face should be treated or, if this is not possible, regional subunits to avoid a clear line of demarcation. Scarring and textural changes can rarely be seen. Prolonged erythema can last from 3 to 10 months. Infections (bacterial, viral, and fungal) have all been reported with resurfacing. Prophylactic antiviral agents are typically started on the day of the procedure, even in patients with no history of orolabial herpes simplex virus (HSV) infection. Antibiotic and antifungal treatment can be started if patients develop infection. Given the morbidity of the postoperative course and prolonged recovery associated with ablative resurfacing, patients must be properly counseled during the preoperative visit.

Used in the quasi continuous-wave mode, the CO_2 laser is an excellent therapeutic choice for very large plantar and periungual warts that have failed to respond to routine office modalities. Both a cutting mode and a defocused ablative mode can be used with these systems to excise the visible verrucae effectively and to treat any residual human papillomavirus in surrounding skin.

The CO_2 laser is also a treatment option for earlobe keloids. Other benign lesions amenable to CO_2 laser ablation include xanthelasma, rhinophyma, and syringomas. Various malignant and premalignant lesions are also effectively treated by laser ablation, including actinic cheilitis and superficial basal and squamous cell carcinomas.

Erbium:yttrium-aluminum-garnet laser

The Er:YAG laser emits an invisible near-infrared beam of 2940 nm, resulting in significantly more efficient absorption by water (16 times) and a more explosive ablative effect, as compared to the CO_2 laser. As such, the Er:YAG laser results in tissue ablation with less surrounding thermal damage. In addition, this wavelength is close to a collagen absorption peak, thus allowing for greater collagen ablation than the CO_2 laser. The decreased thermal injury and collagen ablation is an advantage for treatment of scars, photodamaged skin, rhytids, and rhinophyma (Figs 38-18 and 38-19). Some maintain that healing may be slightly faster, with less risk of prolonged erythema and scarring. None the less, the depth of injury produced (regardless of technology used) is the primary determinant for the healing process and incidence of side effects, not the laser used.

As compared to the photocoagulation effects of the CO_2 laser, the decreased thermal damage produced by the Er:YAG can result in poor hemostasis. To address this limitation, certain Er:YAG systems have a coagulation feature to limit the amount of intraoperative bleeding. In addition, the collagen-tightening effect may not be as pronounced as with the CO_2 laser. However, when similar clinical injuries and depth are achieved, studies have shown that the Er:YAG and CO_2 lasers have comparable photorejuvenating effects, and similar postoperative healing times and complication profiles.

Fractional resurfacing

Fractional photothermolysis is a technique whereby an ablative laser is administered in a pixilated pattern over a grid. These lasers created small columns of thermal injury, or micro-thermal zones (MTZ), which are separated by areas of untreated skin. As only 15–25% of the skin surface is typically ablated during a treatment session, this technology allows for more rapid re-epithelialization, as compared to the confluent

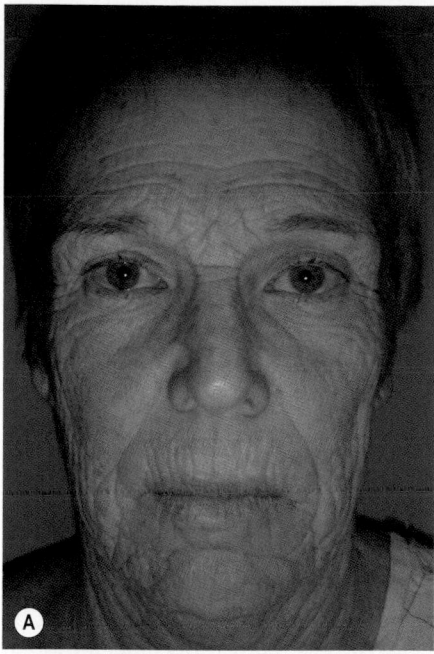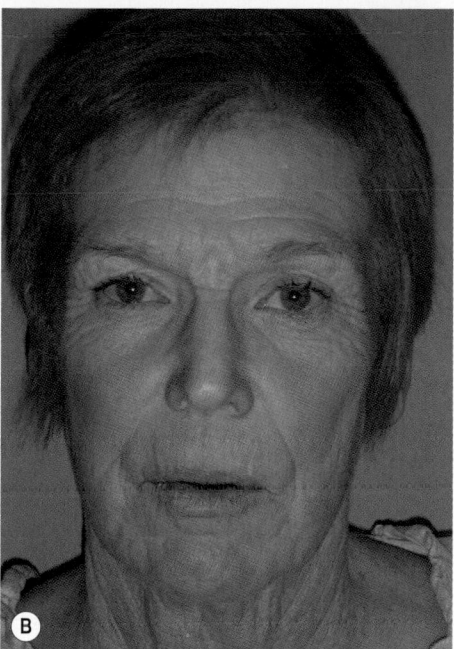

Fig. 38-18 Er:YAG ablative resurfacing. A, Prior to treatment. B, Six months following full-face resurfacing. (Courtesy of Roy Grekin, MD)

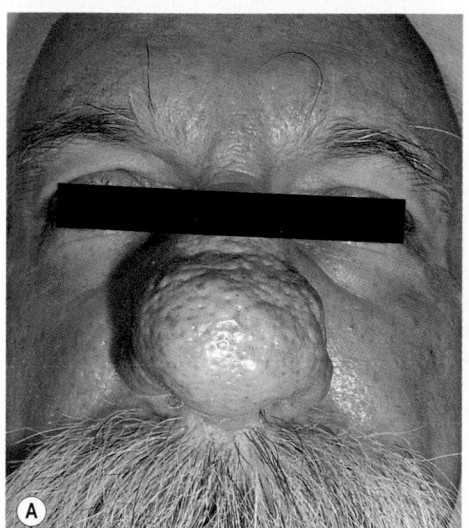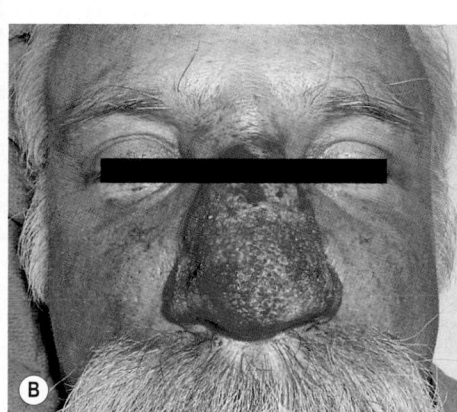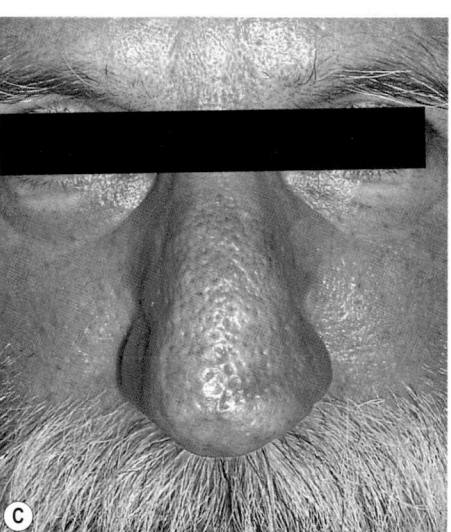

Fig. 38-19 Rhinophyma. A, Prior to treatment. B, Immediately following treatment with an Er:YAG laser. C, Final result 3 months later, with marked improvement in shape and appearance.

patch of laser-induced injury typically created with traditional ablative resurfacing. The injury created by MTZ results in the stimulation of collagen synthesis and cutaneous remodeling, much in the same manner as traditional resurfacing but to a proportionately lesser degree.

Fractional resurfacing has been used for the treatment of photoaging, with the advantage of more rapid healing, reduced erythema and swelling, and fewer side effects. An additional advantage is the ability to treat any anatomic location, including hands, chest, neck, and arms. However, patients often need multiple treatment sessions in order to achieve maximum benefit and the final result is not nearly as impressive as with traditional ablative resurfacing. In addition, the cumulative down time required with multiple treatments may exceed that of a single ablative resurfacing treatment, thus negating the perceived benefit of fractional resurfacing.

Brightman LA, et al: Ablative and fractional ablative lasers. Dermatol Clin 2009 Oct; 27(4):479–489, vi–vii.

Chapas AM, et al: Successful treatment of acneiform scarring with CO_2 ablative fractional resurfacing. Lasers Surg Med 2008 Aug; 40(6):381–386.

Graber EM, et al: Side effects and complications of fractional laser photothermolysis: experience with 961 treatments. Dermatol Surg 2008 Mar; 34(3):301–305.

Hedelund L, et al: Ablative versus non-ablative treatment of perioral rhytides. A randomized controlled trial with long-term blinded clinical evaluations and non-invasive measurements. Lasers Surg Med 2006 Feb; 38(2):129–136.

Madan V, et al: Carbon dioxide laser treatment of rhinophyma: a review of 124 patients. Br J Dermatol 2009 Oct; 161(4):814–818.

Manstein D, et al: Fractional photothermolysis: a new concept for cutaneous remodeling using microscopic patterns of thermal injury. Lasers Surg Med 2004; 34:426–438.

Riggs K, et al: Ablative laser resurfacing: high-energy pulsed carbon dioxide and erbium:yttrium-aluminum-garnet. Clin Dermatol 2007 Sep–Oct; 25(5):462–473.

Rostan EF, et al: Laser resurfacing with a long pulse erbium:YAG laser compared to the 950 ms CO2 laser. Lasers Surg Med 2001; 29:136–141.

Tanzi EL, Alster TS: Single-pass carbon dioxide versus multiple-pass Er:YAG laser skin resurfacing: a comparison of postoperative wound healing and side-effect rates. Dermatol Surg 2003 Jan; 29(1):80–84.

Tierney EP, et al: Review of fractional photothermolysis: treatment indications and efficacy. Dermatol Surg 2009 Oct; 35(10):1445–1461.

39 Cosmetic Dermatology

Dermatologists have been leaders in the field of cosmetic surgery. Many procedures, products, and technologies in cosmetic dermatologic surgery have been developed and researched by dermatologists. Patients are increasingly turning to dermatologists for the management of cosmetic issues. As a result, the specialty must continue to be at the forefront of cosmetic procedures and remain committed to advancing the field through innovation and scientific progress.

Soft-tissue augmentation

Soft-tissue augmentation has been gaining in popularity in recent years as patients seek cosmetic improvement without undergoing invasive procedures. There are numerous fillers available to correct soft-tissue contour abnormalities and provide cosmetic enhancement. While they provide numerous advantages over surgical techniques, the temporary nature of most fillers requires repeated treatment to maintain a desired outcome. While some patients find the temporary nature of these agents to be less than ideal, one must also consider that undesired outcomes of treatment are also temporary. In the last few years, there has been an increase in the number of available agents. In Europe there are as many as 30 different filler choices. In contrast, in the US the Food and Drug Administration (FDA) has approved fewer, although recently several new products have become available.

Bovine collagen

Bovine-derived collagen has been used for over 20 years and is the gold standard against which all filler substances are compared. There are currently three FDA-approved products for use in soft-tissue augmentation: Zyderm I®, Zyderm II®, and Zyplast® (Allergan, Irvine, CA). The source for all three types is a closed herd in the US, and there have been no cases of bovine spongiform encephalopathy associated with these products. All are composed of 95% type I collagen and the remainder type III collagen, suspended in buffered saline and 0.3% lidocaine.

Zyderm I® consists of 35 mg/mL of collagen, while Zyderm II® has a higher concentration of 65 mg/mL of collagen. Zyplast® is cross-linked with glutaraldehyde, making it more resistant to proteolytic degradation, which provides longer duration. All three products come preloaded into syringes and are stored at 4°C.

Bovine collagen hypersensitivity occurs in about 3% of the population, making skin testing a requirement prior to using these products. Additionally, 1–2% of patients with a negative skin test will subsequently develop an allergic reaction following treatment. Therefore, many dermatologists recommend a second skin test after an initial negative test. Patients may also develop allergy after multiple treatments. Therefore, in patients with a span between treatments of more than 2 years, repeated skin testing is indicated.

Zyderm I® and Zyderm II® are injected into the superficial dermis, while Zyplast® is placed deeper. A combination of threading, fanning, and serial puncture injection techniques with a 30-gauge needle can be used. Anesthesia may not be required, as the product already contains lidocaine, although regional nerve blocks may be helpful in sensitive patients or when injecting the lips. Slight overcorrection is recommended with bovine collagen, as it tends to reduce in volume due to the amount of water in the product.

Patients can expect 2–5 months of improvement, depending on the location of placement. Dynamic rhytids (e.g. due to muscular activity) have a shorter duration of correction, as opposed to more static conditions (e.g. acne scars). Zyplast® may have a longer duration due to its relative protection from enzymatic degradation. However, it must be placed deeper in the dermis to avoid a beaded surface appearance and is therefore less useful for correction of superficial rhytids.

Complications with bovine collagen include delayed hypersensitivity reactions. Although this is extremely rare, allergic reactions can occur in 1% of patients who have had two negative skin tests. This presents as swollen granulomas or sterile abscesses at the treatment site. While self-limiting, these reactions can take up to a year to resolve. Intralesional steroid injections, antibiotics, and systemic anti-inflammatory drugs can be considered for treatment. Zyplast® placed in the glabellar complex has resulted in vascular occlusion and necrosis. This may be due to the deeper placement required with this product and the associated adverse pressure-related effects on cutaneous vasculature.

Human collagen

One of the main shortcomings of bovine collagen is the risk of hypersensitivity reaction. Synthetic human collagen has been developed as an alternative that does not require multiple skin testing and can be administered immediately. There has been no documented cross-reaction between bovine and bioengineered human collagen, allowing patients with a documented allergy to bovine collagen to be treated safely with human collagen.

Cosmoderm 1® and 2®, and Cosmoplast® (Allergan, Irvine, CA) are FDA-approved bioengineered human collagen derived from neonatal foreskin. Synthetic human collagen has a very similar formulation to its bovine counterpart and is packaged in similar concentrations. Cosmoderm 1® has a concentration of 35 mg/mL and is in phosphate-buffered saline with 0.3% lidocaine. Cosmoderm 2® has a concentration of 65 mg/mL and Cosmoplast® has 35 mg/mL of human-derived collagen and is cross-linked with glutaraldehyde.

All products have the same indications, are injected in a similar manner to their bovine counterparts, and have similar cosmetic results and longevity

Porcine collagen

Porcine collagen (Evolence®, Ortho–McNeil–Janssen Pharmaceuticals, Titusville, NJ) is now FDA-approved in the US. It consists of porcine collagen composed of 35 mg/mL type I collagen that was derived from porcine tendons with ribose used as a cross-linker. Since porcine-derived collagen is similar to human collagen, there is no significant risk of allergy, and skin testing is not required prior to treatment. The product is stored at room temperature and injected into the mid-dermis with a 30-gauge needle. Initial studies suggest that it has a longer duration than either bovine or human collagen. At the time of publication, the manufacturer announced that it was discontinuing the production and marketing of the product.

Hyaluronic acid

Hyaluronic acid, a polysaccharide, is a natural component of human connective tissue. A member of the family of glycosaminoglycans, hyaluronic acid is composed of repeating disaccharide units. This molecule has the advantage of being identical across all species. As such, hypersensitivity reactions should not occur and skin testing is not required prior to treatment. However, Friedman et al demonstrated a local hypersensitivity reaction in 1 in every 1400 patients treated, although the incidence has declined with the introduction of a more purified product.

Hyaluronic acid avidly binds water and patients may experience redness, swelling, and bruising in the first few days after treatment. Most of the volume is maintained following placement, making overcorrection unnecessary when injecting. Hyaluronic acid products consist of a clear gel and most contain no lidocaine, often necessitating the use of local anesthesia and regional blocks for patient comfort. Recent preparations of hyaluronic acid now include lidocaine, thus eliminating the need for adjuvant anesthesia and making them significantly more comfortable for patients. Hyaluronic acid fillers can produce a more durable aesthetic improvement as compared to collagen, often lasting from 5 to 8 months (Fig. 39-1).

There are two types of hyaluronic acid filler substance. Streptococcal-derived is the most common, and includes Restylane® and Perlane® (Medicis, Scottsdale, AZ), Juvederm®

(Allergan, Irvine, CA), and Prevelle® (Mentor, Santa Barbara, CA). An alternative source is the rooster comb, which includes Hylaform® gel (Inamed, Santa Barbara, CA), although its use is fading in comparison to other products with greater longevity. These fillers come in prepackaged syringes and do not require refrigeration.

The characteristics and viscosity of the different products are largely determined by the size and concentration of the molecule within each preparation. Restylane® contains 20 mg/mL of hyaluronic acid with a particle size of 100 000/mL and is injected with a 30-gauge needle. Perlane® also has a concentration of 20 mg/mL, but a much larger particle size of 8000/mL, and requires a larger 27-gauge needle. Juvederm® is available in two formulations, Ultra and Ultra Plus. Both have a concentration of 24 mg/mL, with Ultra Plus have more crosslinkage, making it more appropriate for deeper folds. The denser products are effective for the treatment of deeper contour abnormalities.

Hyaluronic acids tend to produce more swelling and bruising than collagen. Proper preoperative consultation is necessary to ensure that the patient understands this and does not have upcoming social engagements. Improper placement of hyaluronic acid too superficially can result in a blue discoloration or nodule on the skin surface. An incision with a large-gauge needle or number 11 blade and expression of the product can be performed. Hyaluronidase injections can dissolve the product if either a reaction or unevenness results, a considerable advantage over other filler substances.

Poly-L-lactic acid

Microparticles of poly-L-lactic acid (Sculptra®, Sanofi Aventis/Dermik, Bridgewater, NJ) are used as an injectable implant to replace diffuse volume loss, rather than the small-volume injections of other fillers. This product is currently FDA-approved for correcting facial lipoatrophy in patients with human immunodeficiency virus (HIV) and more recently for aesthetic treatment of lines and contour deficiencies.

Poly-L-lactic acid is a biodegradable, biocompatible, and immunologically inert product that does not require skin testing. Polylactic acid has been used as absorbable suture material (e.g. Vicryl®). Polylactic acid is absorbed gradually in the skin, inducing a fibroblastic response and de novo collagen synthesis. Multiple treatment sessions at 4–6-week intervals are often required to achieve the final result (Fig. 39-2). Since correction is dependent upon the formation of new collagen, patients must be counseled that an immediate effect does not occur with this product. Results can last for up to 2 years.

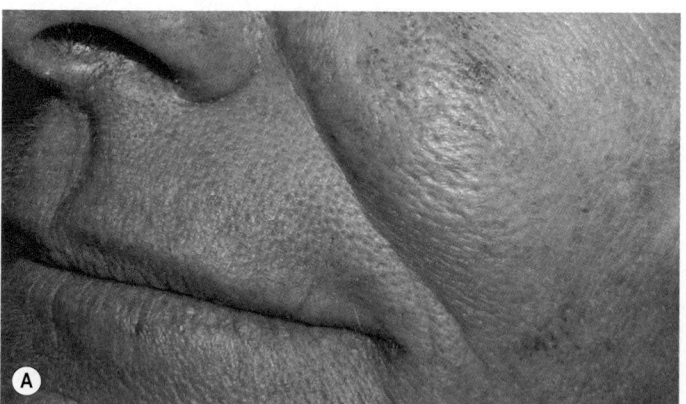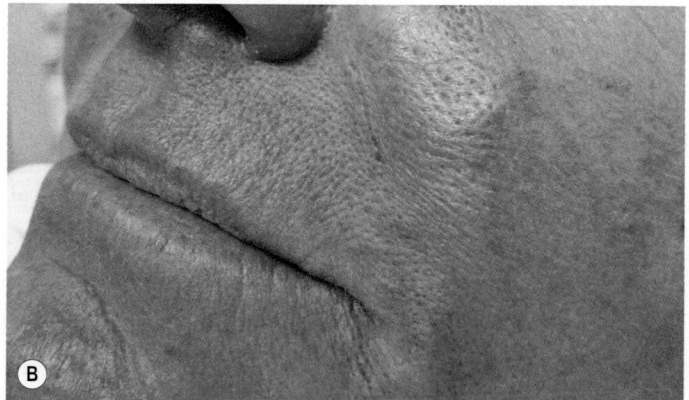

Fig. 39-1 Hyaluronic acid filler, nasolabial fold. A, Prior to treatment. B, Immediately following placement of hyaluronic acid with marked improvement and reduction of rhytids.

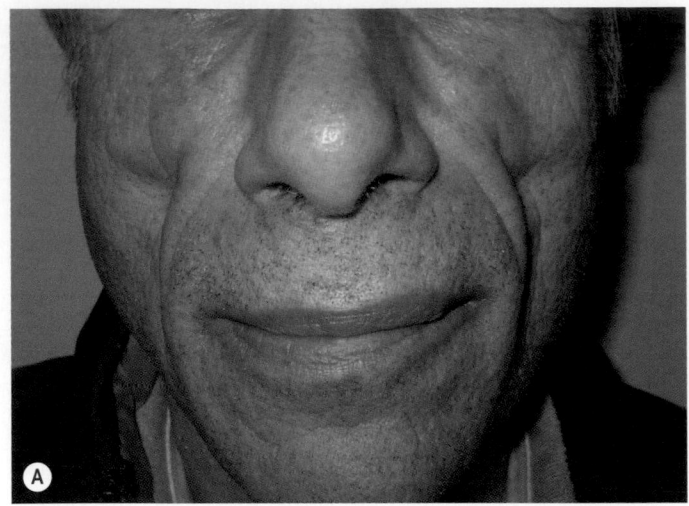
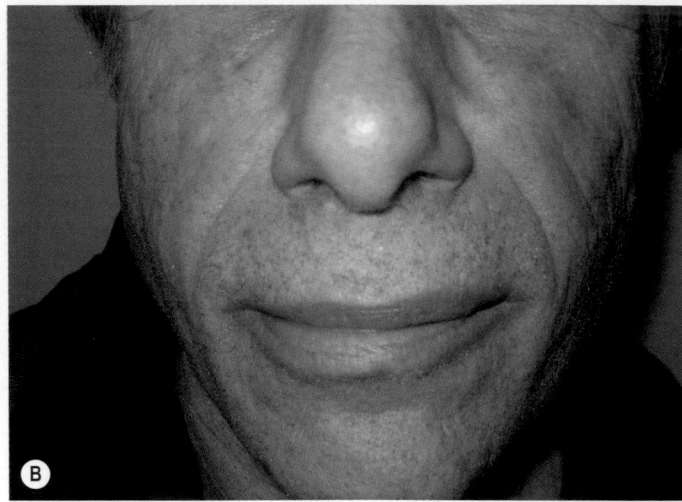

Fig. 39-2 Poly-L-lactic acid for HIV lipoatrophy. A, Prior to treatment. B, Following five treatments.

Poly-L-lactic acid comes packaged as a freeze-dried powder and must be reconstituted for a minimum of 4 hours prior to injection to ensure adequate hydration of the particles. Lidocaine can be added to the vial to reduce injection pain. The product is injected using a 25-gauge needle at the level of the deep dermis and subcutaneous junction in a fanning or cross-hatch fashion. Post-injection massage for several days can help reduce nodules.

Side effects include delayed foreign body granulomas at injection sites. Intralesional 5-fluorouracil (5-FU) or triamcinolone, 10 mg/mL, may be used for the treatment of these papules.

Calcium hydroxylapatite

Calcium hydroxylapatite (Radiesse®, BioForm, San Mateo, CA) consists of fine particles (25–45 µm) of material traditionally used to reconstruct bone. Once injected into the dermal–subcutaneous junction, the particles act as a scaffolding for autologous collagen synthesis. The ensuing fibrotic reaction results in soft-tissue correction that can last for 9–12 months. It is FDA-approved for correction of moderate to severe folds and wrinkles such as nasolabial folds, and for HIV facial lipoatrophy.

Injections can be quite painful and local anesthesia is generally used. Calcium hydroxylapatite is injected into the deep dermis and subcutaneous junction with a threading technique using a 27-gauge needle. It comes prepackaged in syringes and can be stored at room temperature.

Nodules are more commonly seen when calcium hydroxylapatite is injected into the lips, thereby discouraging its use in the treatment of hypolabium. Experience with this product is limited and long-term risks are not well known. Caution must be exercised, as any product that requires a fibrotic reaction in order to be effective can result in a granulomatous reaction and an untoward result. As calcium is radiopaque, the product may be detected and interfere with radiological imaging.

Autologous fat transplantation

Autologous lipotransfer allows for soft-tissue augmentation without the risk of allergy, rejection, or infectious transmission. Unlike other filler techniques, fat transfer is truly a grafting procedure. As such, its success is predicated on the survival of the transferred adipocytes. Fat is harvested from a choice of

donor sites, typically the abdomen, buttock, thigh, or knee. There is no consensus as to the advantages of harvesting with a liposuction cannula, syringe extraction with a large-bore needle, or open surgical method. The fat is then separated from anesthetic fluid and blood, and injected through a large-bore needle (16- to 18-gauge) into the desired location. Any remaining fat can be frozen at −70°C for use at a later time, with varying claims regarding loss of efficacy.

The variable rate of graft survival, the recipient site reaction (i.e. bruising, swelling), and the added morbidity of a donor site are limiting factors in patient satisfaction with this technique. In some instances, partial survival results in uneven correction that may require additional treatments. Some argue that multiple smaller-volume injections spaced out over 2–3 treatments are more effective than single large-volume lipotransfer. If the fat survives, it can provide a very natural correction. However, local factors such as motor activity and gravitational effects will mitigate against permanent correction. This technique is not useful for the correction of superficial rhytids, and mainly corrects deeper defects such as nasolabial folds, hypolabium, buccal depression, and deep scars.

Silicone

Silicone has been used in the past for soft-tissue augmentation by dermatologists. This product was never FDA-approved and issues of purity and safety limited its widespread use. In 1994 it was removed from the market by the FDA. Recently, 1000 centistoke liquid silicone (Silikon 1000®, Alcon Labs, Fort Worth, TX) has been approved by the FDA for the treatment of retinal detachment. It is currently being used off-label as a permanent filler for HIV-associated facial lipoatrophy, scars, and rhytids.

The potential for delayed and severe complications with this permanent filler, as well as legal concerns and restrictions, has limited its use. Adverse reactions associated with silicone injections include granuloma formation and migration of implant, which are compounded by the permanent nature of the product. Many of the past reported complications of silicone injection were the result of using either an impure and nonmedical-grade substance or an improper technique with large-volume injections. A multisession, microdroplet technique, placing multiple depot injection of 0.01 mL of product into the deep dermis in 1–3 mm intervals, significantly reduces the complication rate. An additional consideration is that the current FDA-approved product is more concentrated than the previous silicone products. Further study is needed to evaluate the long-term safety and efficacy of silicone oil injections for correction of soft-tissue contour deficiencies.

Polymethylmethacrylate

Artefill® (Suneva Medical, San Diego, CA) is an FDA-approved suspension containing 20% polymethylmethacrylate (PMMA) microspheres of 30–40 microns in diameter suspended in 80% bovine collagen for soft-tissue augmentation. The carrier collagen provides initial correction and is degraded over several months, leaving the PMMA microspheres. PMMA serves as a permanent framework for connective tissue deposition and can produce long-term correction.

Technique is critical to successful outcomes. If injected too deeply, the implant is ineffective, while superficial placement can cause prolonged erythema. Granuloma formation and hypertrophic scarring can occur and have been reported as a delayed reaction. Intralesional triamcinolone can be used for treatment of these reactions. One patient who developed a delayed foreign body granuloma 6 years after injection with PMMA was successfully treated with a 24-week course of 600 mg/day of allopurinol. Since the product contains bovine collagen, skin testing is required prior to use.

Expanded polytetrafluoroethylene

Expanded polytetrafluoroethylene (ePTFE) is a synthetic solid material that is soft and pliable, is not degraded, and has the advantage of being permanent. The material is placed through a small skin incision and positioned in the desired location. Areas commonly treated with this include lip margins or the muscular portion of the vermillion for enhancement, nasolabial folds, and soft-tissue depressions. Some complications associated with ePTFE include extrusion, migration, shrinkage, and hardening.

Alcalay J, et al: Late-onset granulomatous reaction to Artecoll. Dermatol Surg 2003; 29:859.

Bachmann F, et al: The spectrum of adverse reactions after treatment with injectable fillers in the glabellar region: results from the injectable filler safety study. Dermatol Surg 2009; 35:1629–1635.

Baumann LS, et al: JUVEDERM vs. ZYPLAST Nasolabial Fold Study Group. Comparison of smooth-gel hyaluronic acid dermal fillers with cross-linked bovine collagen: a multicenter, double-masked, randomized, within-subject study. Dermatol Surg 2007 Dec; 33(Suppl 2):S128–135.

Benedetto AV, Lewis AT: Injecting 1000 centistoke liquid silicone with ease and precision. Dermatol Surg 2003; 29:211.

Butterwick KJ, et al: Fat transplantation using fresh versus frozen fat: a side-by-side two-hand comparison pilot study. Dermatol Surg 2006 May; 32(5):640–644.

Cohen SR, et al: Five-year safety and efficacy of a novel polymethylmethacrylate aesthetic soft tissue filler for the correction of nasolabial folds. Dermatol Surg 2007 Dec; 33(Suppl 2):S222–230.

Friedman PM, et al: Safety data of injectable nonanimal stabilized hyaluronic acid gel for soft tissue augmentation. Dermatol Surg 2002; 28:491.

Glaich AS, et al: Injection necrosis of the glabella: protocol for prevention and treatment after use of dermal fillers. Dermatol Surg 2006 Feb; 32(2):276–281.

Jones DH, et al: Highly purified 1000-cSt silicone oil for treatment of human immunodeficiency virus-associated facial lipoatrophy: an open pilot trial. Dermatol Surg 2004 Oct; 30(10):1279–1286.

Lemperle G, et al: Soft tissue augmentation with Artecoll: 10-year history, indications, techniques, and complications. Dermatol Surg 2003 Jun; 29(6):573–587.

Levy RM, et al: Treatment of HIV lipoatrophy and lipoatrophy of aging with poly-L-lactic acid: a prospective 3-year follow-up study. J Am Acad Dermatol 2008 Dec; 59(6):923–933.

Lowe NJ, et al: Injectable poly-L-lactic acid: 3 years of aesthetic experience. Dermatol Surg 2009 Feb; 35(Suppl 1):344–349.

Markey AC, Glogau RG: Autologous fat grafting: comparison of techniques. Dermatol Surg 2000; 26:1135.

Matarasso SL: Injectable collagens: lost but not forgotten—a review of products, indications, and injection techniques. Plast Reconstr Surg 2007 Nov; 120(6 Suppl):17S–26S.

Narins RS, et al: A randomized, double-blind, multicenter comparison of the efficacy and tolerability of Restylane versus Zyplast for the correction of nasolabial folds. Dermatol Surg 2003; 29:588.

Narins RS, et al: Twelve-month persistency of a novel ribose-cross-linked collagen dermal filler. Dermatol Surg 2008 Jun; 34(Suppl 1):S31–39.

Reisberger EM, et al: Foreign body granulomas caused by polymethylmethacrylate microspheres: successful treatment with allopurinol. Arch Dermatol 2003; 139:17.

Reszko AE, et al: Late-onset subcutaneous nodules after poly-L-lactic acid injection. Dermatol Surg 2009 Feb; 35(Suppl 1):380–384.

Sadick NS, et al: A multicenter, 47-month study of safety and efficacy of calcium hydroxylapatite for soft tissue augmentation of nasolabial folds and other areas of the face. Dermatol Surg 2007 Dec; 33(Suppl 2):S122–126.

Sclafani AP, Fagien S: Treatment of injectable soft tissue filler complications. Dermatol Surg 2009; 35:1672–1680.

Shoshani O, et al: The role of frozen storage in preserving adipose tissue obtained by suction-assisted lipectomy for repeated fat injection procedures. Dermatol Surg 2001; 27:645.

Tzikas TL: A 52-month summary of results using calcium hydroxylapatite for facial soft tissue augmentation. Dermatol Surg 2008 Jun; 34(Suppl 1):S9–15.

Botulinum toxin

The use of botulinum toxin (BTX) in dermatology has increased rapidly over the years, and at present is the most common cosmetic procedure performed in the US. In 2002, the FDA approved BTX for the treatment of dynamic glabellar frown lines. Although BTX is most commonly approved for relaxation of dynamic rhytids in the upper third of the face, advanced treatment techniques for additional anatomic sites have been developed and are currently used off label.

Produced by *Clostridium botulinum*, there are seven different serotypes of BTX: A, B, C1, D, E, F, and G. These serotypes inhibit the release of acetylcholine from the presynaptic motor neuron, resulting in chemodenervation and paralysis of the treated muscle. Over time, new nerve terminals form and create new neuromuscular junctions with the muscle fibers, which gradually restore motor function.

BTX type A (Botox Cosmetic® (onabotulinumtoxinA), Allergan, Irvine, CA; Dysport® (abobotulinumtoxinA), Medicis, Scottsdale, AZ) is the most commonly used serotype. Its mechanism of action is via the cleavage of SNAP-25, a presynaptic membrane protein required for fusion of neurotransmitter-containing vesicles. Effect is generally noted 2–5 days after treatment with BTX-A, but the delay can be as long as 2 weeks in some cases. Results can last from 3 to 6 months. For dosing purposes, 1 U of Botox® is equivalent to about 3–5 U of Dysport®. There has been a paucity of studies that directly compare Botox® and Dysport®.

The only other serotype that is currently available commercially is BTX type B (Myobloc® (rimabotulinumtoxinB), Solstice Neurosciences, Malvern, PA). Its mechanism of action is via the cleavage of a vesicle-associated membrane protein (VAMP), also known as synaptobrevin. This serotype has more rapid onset of effect than BTX-A. In addition, differences in potency suggest that approximately 100 U of Myobloc® are equivalent to 1 U of Botox®.

Given the efficacy, experience and safety profile of Botox®, it has emerged as the leading choice of botulinum toxin amongst practitioners and all further discussion of BTX-A will refer to Botox®. BTX-A is distributed in vials as a vacuum-dried powder, which is reconstituted with 1.0–5.0 mL of saline. Many physicians feel that the dilution of BTX does not a make a significant difference in patient outcome and studies appear to confirm this notion. Others argue that higher concentrations with smaller injection volumes reduce the amount of unintended diffusion. It is more important to use the same dilution every time to ensure that the physician does not have to do "mental math" and to reduce confusion with each new vial of BTX.

Despite package insert recommendations, experience suggests that there is little loss of potency over several weeks following reconstitution with preserved saline. The use of preserved saline for reconstitution reduces the burning and pain associated with injection due to the anesthetic properties of the benzyl alcohol in preserved saline.

BTX-A is predominantly used in dermatology for treatment of dynamic rhytids on the upper third of the face. The key to successful treatment is understanding the anatomy involved in facial expression, rather than performing the procedure by rote. Having the patient frown, squint, and raise their brows prior to treatment helps identify the active target muscles and serves as a guide for proper placement.

Glabellar frown lines

Currently, treatment of glabellar frown lines is the only FDA-approved cosmetic indication for BTX-A. These lines result from contraction of the corrugator supercilii, which pulls the brows medially, and the procerus, which pulls the brow inferiorly. In addition, by inactivating the brow depressors, unopposed action of the brow elevators (e.g. frontalis) can result in a slight but noticeable brow lift.

Approximately 20–35 U of BTX-A are typically injected into the corrugators and procerus in a five-point injection method (Figs 39-3 and 39-4). Male patients and those with larger muscle mass may require a higher number of units (i.e. 40–60). By having the patient furrow the brow, one can identify the origin and insertion of the corrugator supercilii. By grasping with the thumb and index finger, the physician can isolate the muscle and ensure accurate toxin placement.

If toxin diffuses through the orbital septum into the orbit, weakening of the levator palpebrae can result in upper lid

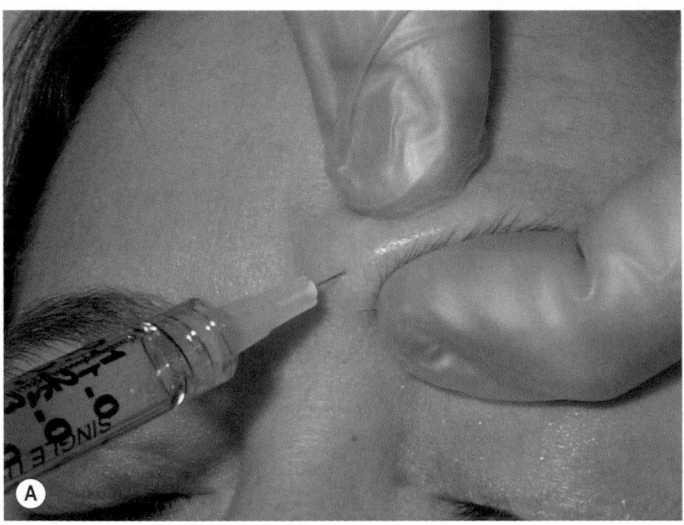
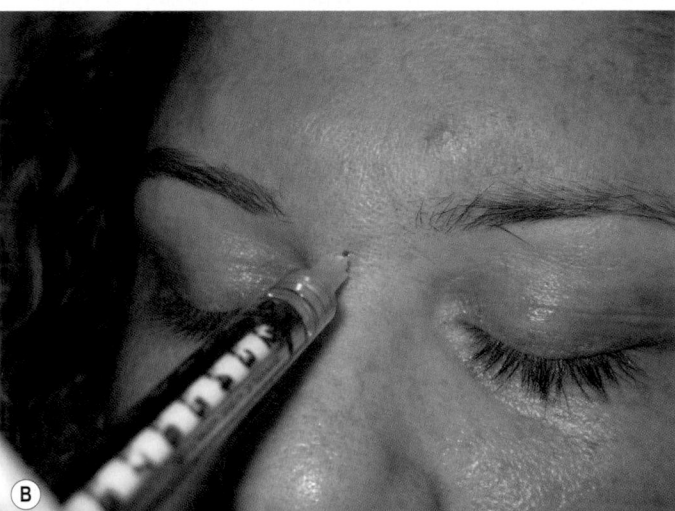

Fig. 39-3 Botulinum toxin injection technique for glabellar complex. A, Patient frowns and muscle is grasped between thumb and index finger; the injection is placed directly into the belly of the corrugator supercilii. B, Injection into the procerus muscle.

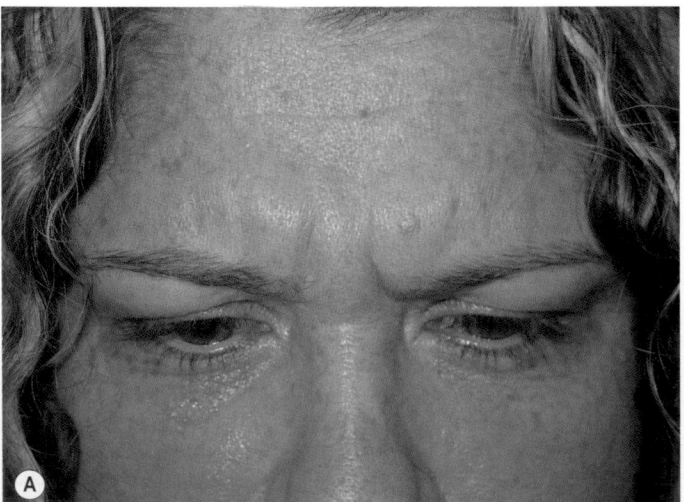
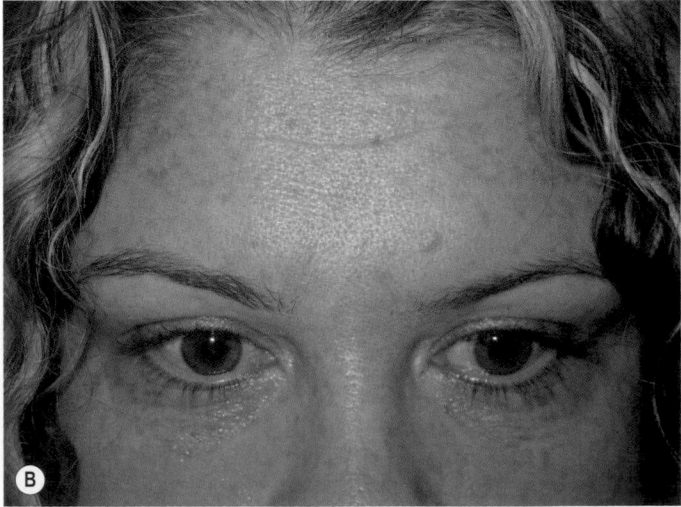

Fig. 39-4 Botulinum toxin for glabellar frown furrow. A, Glabellar lines with frowning. B, Patient attempting to frown after botulinum toxin.

ptosis. Care should be taken to inject 1 cm above the superior bony orbital rim to reduce risk of diffusion of toxin and the resulting complication. The use of α-adrenergic agonist eye drops, such as apraclonidine 0.5% or phenylephrine 2.5%, can stimulate Müller's muscles in the lid, providing some relief until the effects of the BTX dissipate.

Horizontal forehead lines

Horizontal forehead lines are caused by contraction of the frontalis muscle, which produces elevation and movement of the eyebrows. Care must be taken when treating this area with BTX-A to avoid ptosis or "heaviness" of the brow. Extra caution should be used in men with low-set brows or older patients who use their frontalis to raise their eyebrows to assist with vision.

Since the lower portion of the frontalis is primarily responsible for brow elevation, injections are often limited to the upper half or two-thirds of the muscle. Between 10 and 25 U, delivered in multiple superficial injections across the forehead, are typically used for this area.

If upper lateral fibers of the frontalis remain totally untreated, the increased resting muscle tone will raise the lateral edge of the eyebrow, creating a quizzical look (Fig. 39-5). Injecting a small amount of BTX-A in the upper lateral brow can help correct this.

Crow's feet

Crow's feet are rhytids that extend radially from the lateral canthus and are produced by contraction of the lateral orbicularis oculi. Even with successful treatment with BTX-A, rhytids may still persist due to upward motion of the cheek when the patient smiles. Proper preoperative counseling is required to prevent frustrated patients.

Superficial blebs are raised approximately 1 cm lateral to the lateral canthus (Fig. 39-6). Between 8 and 12 U of BTX-A are placed around each orbit. Care should be taken to orient the needle away from the globe as a safety precaution, in case the patient moves unexpectedly.

Bruising is common in this location due to the thin nature of the skin and the presence of numerous periocular superficial veins. Purpura can be minimized by injecting superficially, ensuring proper illumination and stretching of the skin to help identify the veins, and limiting the total number of injections. Diffusion into the zygomaticus major and minor, leading to ipsilateral lip ptosis and asymmetric smile, can occur with overzealous treatment of the inferior portion of the orbicularis oculi.

Other locations

Other sites that can be treated with BTX-A include platysmal bands, diagonal creases along the nasal sidewall (i.e. "sniff lines" or "bunny lines"), mental crease, and depressor anguli oris (for frowning of the lateral corners of the mouth). Care must be taken when treating the lower third of the face to avoid complications with mouth and lip control. Excessive or misplaced BTX-A in the platysmal bands can cause dysphagia, dysphonia, and neck weakness.

Hyperhidrosis

In addition to cosmetic uses, BTX-A is FDA-approved for the treatment of axillary hyperhidrosis. Prior to treatment, a Minor's starch-iodine test is used to document both the severity and location of excessive sweating (Fig. 39-7). Effective treatment can be achieved with doses of 50 U/axilla. Intradermal injections are spaced in a grid 1 cm apart over the entire area. Anhidrosis is achieved within 1 week and typically lasts for 6–12 months. Side effects are generally limited to injection site bruising.

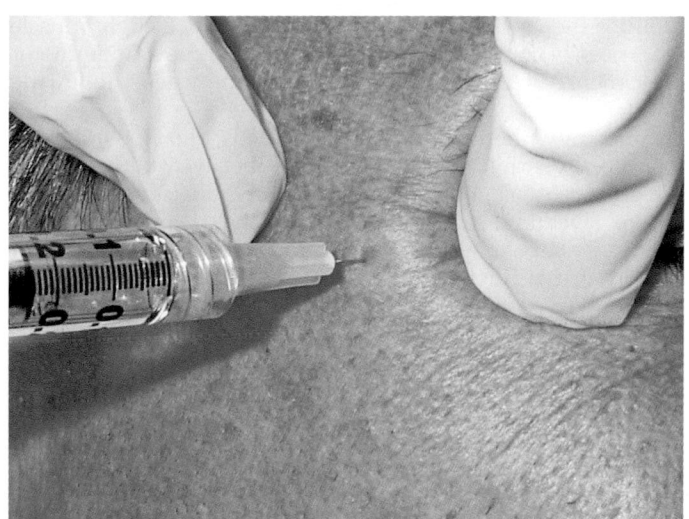

Fig. 39-6 Botulinum toxin injection technique for crow's feet, superficial injection approximately 1 cm from the orbital rim.

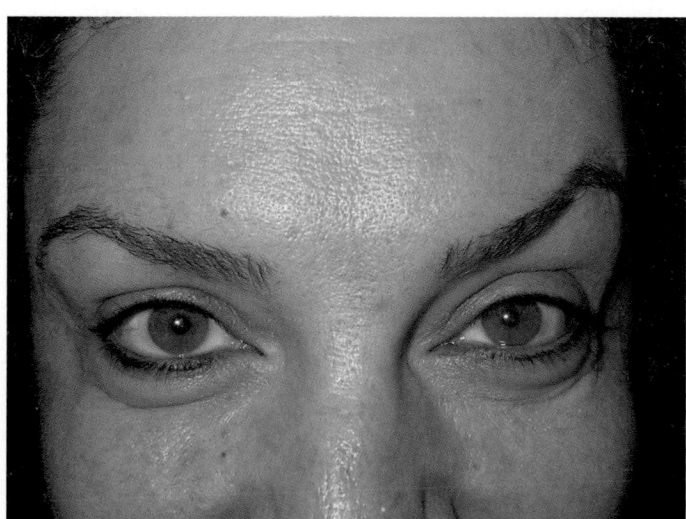

Fig. 39-5 Botulinum toxin complication. "Quizzical" brow look.

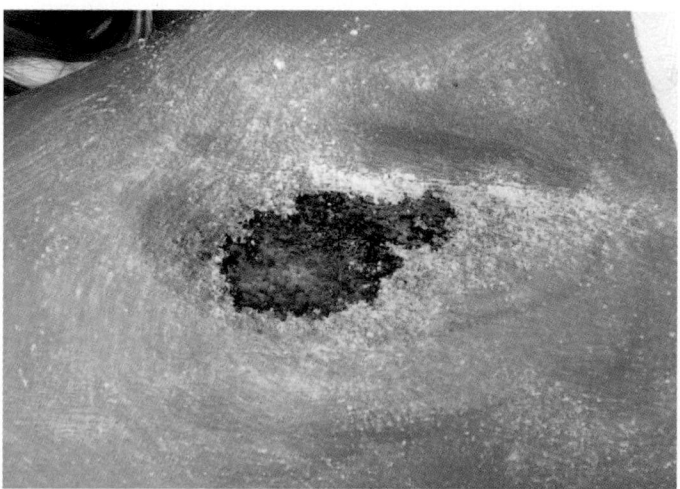

Fig. 39-7 Starch-iodine test, developing positive test with darkening in areas of hyperhidrosis.

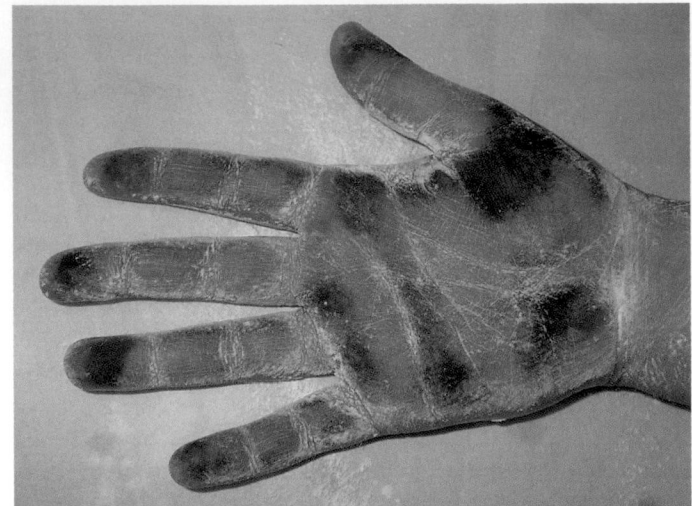

Fig. 39-8 Starch-iodine test, partial response to botulinum toxin.

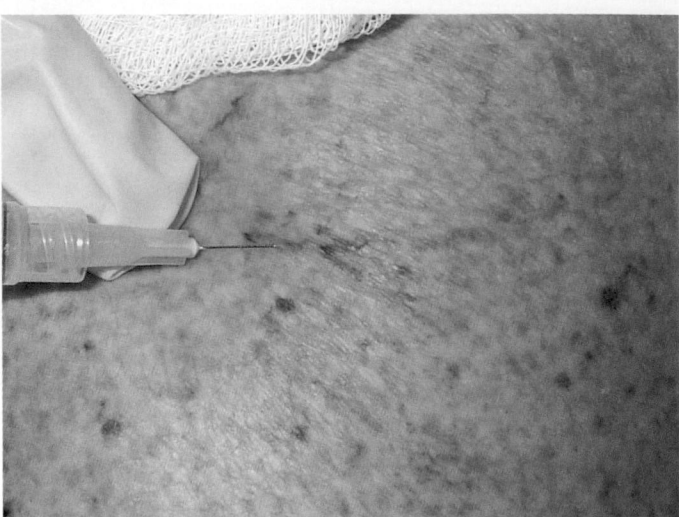

Fig. 39-9 Sclerotherapy, injection technique using fine needle to cannulate vein.

Treatment of palmar hyperhidrosis with BTX-A is more complicated than treating the axilla. Higher doses, typically 100–150 U/palm, are required due to the greater surface area involved and the limited diffusion of the toxin in acral skin. Pain is more significant when treating the palm and typically requires the use of wrist nerve blocks. Lastly, a slight muscle weakness of the hands, manifested by the loss of fine motor movement, is typically seen for several weeks following treatment.

Frequently, there are focal areas of activity following treatment for hyperhydrosis. However, as the sweat diffuses over the entire surface, patients often describe a false sensation of severe sweating and complain that the treatment "didn't work." By repeating the starch-iodine test, the focal areas of activity can be identified and directed touch-up can be performed (Fig. 39-8).

Absar MS, Onwudike M: Efficacy of botulinum toxin type A in the treatment of focal axillary hyperhidrosis. Dermatol Surg 2008 Jun; 34(6):751–755.

Alam M, et al: Pain associated with injection of botulinum A exotoxin reconstituted using isotonic sodium chloride with and without preservative: a double-blind, randomized controlled trial. Arch Dermatol 2002; 138:510.

Baumann L, Black L: Botulinum toxin type B (Myobloc). Dermatol Surg 2003; 29:496.

Carruthers J, Carruthers A: Aesthetic botulinum A toxin in the mid and lower face and neck. Dermatol Surg 2003; 29:468.

Hayton MJ, et al: A review of peripheral nerve blockade as local anaesthesia in the treatment of palmar hyperhidrosis. Br J Dermatol 2003; 149:447.

Hexsel DM, et al: Multicenter, double-blind study of the efficacy of injections with botulinum toxin type A reconstituted up to six consecutive weeks before application. Dermatol Surg 2003; 29:523.

Lowe NJ, et al: North American Botox in Primary Axillary Hyperhidrosis Clinical Study Group. Botulinum toxin type A in the treatment of primary axillary hyperhidrosis: a 52-week multicenter double-blind, randomized, placebo-controlled study of efficacy and safety. J Am Acad Dermatol 2007 Apr; 56(4):604–611.

Monheit GD, Cohen JL: Reloxin Investigational Group. Long-term safety of repeated administrations of a new formulation of botulinum toxin type A in the treatment of glabellar lines: interim analysis from an open-label extension study. J Am Acad Dermatol 2009 Sep; 61(3):421–425.

Naumann M, et al: Botulinum toxin type A is a safe and effective treatment for axillary hyperhidrosis over 16 months: a prospective study. Arch Dermatol 2003; 139:731.

Pena MA, et al: Complications with the use of botulinum toxin type A for cosmetic applications and hyperhidrosis. Semin Cutan Med Surg 2007 Mar; 26(1):29–33.

Solish N, et al: Canadian Hyperhidrosis Advisory Committee. A comprehensive approach to the recognition, diagnosis, and severity-based treatment of focal hyperhidrosis: recommendations of the Canadian Hyperhidrosis Advisory Committee. Dermatol Surg 2007 Aug; 33(8):908–923.

Varicose and telangiectatic veins

Sclerotherapy

Patients frequently seek treatment of telangiectasias and reticular veins in the lower extremities. The treatment of choice for telangiectatic and reticular veins is sclerotherapy (Fig. 39-9). Despite recent technologic advances, laser treatment for lower extremity telangiectasias should be reserved for those vessels which cannot be cannulated with a needle. In addition, laser therapy can be considered in patients who have failed to respond to sclerotherapy or had significant complications from sclerotherapy.

Sclerotherapy solutions

There are three broad classes of sclerosing agent available to dermatologists: hyperosmotic agents, detergents, and chemical irritants (Table 39-1). Hyperosmotic agents cause endothelial cell damage via dehydration, and detergents disrupt the cellular membrane, while chemical irritants act as a corrosive and lead to endothelial injury.

Hypertonic saline is an FDA-approved agent that is commonly used in sclerotherapy. Used at concentrations of 10–30%, this agent has the advantage of a complete lack of allergenicity when used alone. The disadvantage of hypertonic saline is pain associated with injections and ulcerogenic potential. Often, anesthetic agents such as lidocaine are added to the mixture to minimize the discomfort involved, both by decreasing the concentration of the saline and by the direct anesthetic effect.

Hypertonic saline (10%) mixed with dextrose (25%) is another hyperosmolar agent that has been used in vein sclerosing. This agent has the advantages of low allergenicity and decreased pain compared to higher concentrations of plain hypertonic saline. However, this mixture is currently not FDA-approved and is a relatively weak sclerosant as compared to other options available.

Sodium tetradecyl sulfate (STS) is a detergent sclerosant that has been FDA-approved for over 50 years. Typical concentrations used for superficial telangiectasias are 0.1–0.2% and for

Table 39-1 Sclerotherapy agents

Agent	Class	FDA-approved	Comments
Hypertonic saline	Hyperosmotic	Yes	No allergenicity, painful
Hypertonic saline (10%) + dextrose (25%)	Hyperosmotic	No	Lower allergenicity, painful
Sodium tetradecyl sulfate	Detergent	Yes	Can be used as foam, painless except with extravascular injection
Polidocanol	Detergent	Yes	Painless, can be used as foam
Sodium morrhuate	Detergent	Yes	High risk of allergic reaction
Chromated glycerin	Chemical irritant	No	Weak agent
Polyiodinated iodine	Chemical irritant	No	Highly caustic

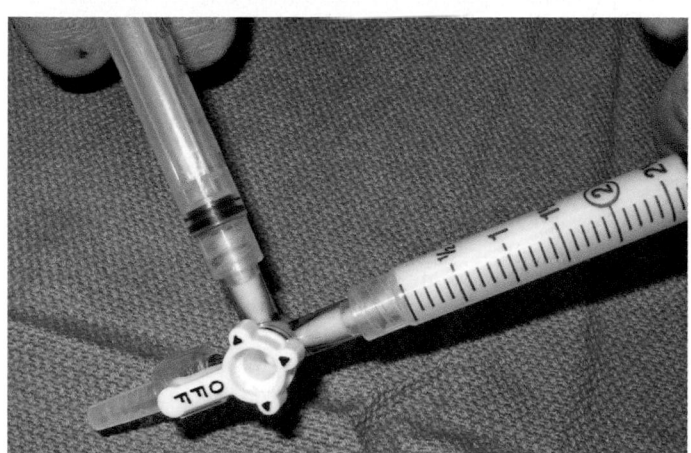

Fig. 39-10 Sclerosing foam, sodium tetradecyl sulfate foam made by mixing air with liquid using a three-way stopcock and two syringes.

reticular veins 0.2–0.5%. One advantage of STS is the lack of pain with injections; however, extravascular injection can be painful. Also, as with all detergents, STS can be made into a foam. This is typically done with a three-way stopcock and a syringe filled with air (Fig. 39-10). Foam can increase contact between the agent and the vessel wall, can result in more effective sclerosis at a lower concentration, and allows treatment of larger-caliber vessels. One disadvantage is the isolated reports of anaphylaxis and death associated with STS.

Polidocanol (Asclera® Merz Aesthetics, San Mateo, CA), a detergent, has recently gained FDA-approved for use in sclerotherapy. It possesses many of the same advantages as STS, including lack of pain with injection and the ability to be used as a foam. Goldman demonstrated comparable efficacy and a similar adverse event profile between polidocanol and STS.

Sodium morrhuate is a detergent approved by the FDA for treatment of varicose veins. However, this sclerosing agent is not generally used for the treatment of cutaneous telangiectasias due to its highly caustic nature and higher anaphylaxis potential.

Glycerin and polyiodide iodine are chemical irritants used as sclerosing agents. Though not FDA-approved for sclerotherapy, these act as corrosive agents and cause a direct injury to the vessel endothelium. Leach and Goldman report a significant decrease in bruising, swelling, and post-procedural hyperpigmentation with glycerin as compared to STS.

Sclerotherapy complications

Side effects and complications can be associated with all types of sclerotherapy agent. Ulceration can occur despite the meticulous technique of the dermatologist and regardless of the sclerosing agent used. Extravasation of sclerosing solution from the vein may occur, or injection into a dermal arteriole or arteriovenous anastomosis may result in cutaneous necrosis. If it is suspected that extravasation has occurred, injection of normal saline to dilute the sclerosing agent may prevent ulceration. Alternatively, application of 2% nitroglycerin ointment may prove beneficial. If ulceration does occur, conservative wound management should be undertaken until healed.

Hyperpigmentation along the course of treated veins has been reported to occur in 10–30% of patients. This pigmentation is due to hemosiderin deposition and has been reported with a variety of sclerosing agents, including hypertonic saline, polidocanol, and STS. Pigmentation often improves with time, with approximately 70% improvement over a 6-month period. Treatment options include trichloracetic acid, hydroquinone, retinoic acid cream, intense pulsed light, and laser treatments. Tafazzoli et al report excellent results with the Q-switched ruby laser.

Telangiectatic matting is the appearance of fine telangiectatic blush at the site of previously treated veins. This has been reported in 10–15% of patients treated with sclerotherapy. Risk factors associated with this include estrogen therapy, obesity, and a family history of telangiectasia. Low injection pressures and limiting the amount of sclerosant per injection site may help reduce the incidence of telangiectatic matting. Spontaneous resolution often occurs within 3–12 months. Treatment options include intense pulsed light, pulsed dye laser, and injection of sclerosant into the matted vessels.

Arterial injection of sclerosant is the most feared complication of vein sclerosing. While extremely rare, it has considerable associated morbidity and necessitates timely action. Classically, the patient reports significant pain immediately following injection, accompanied by pallor and cyanosis. If arterial injection occurs, the physician should immediately apply ice and attempt to dilute the vessel with injections of normal saline. Procaine can be used to inactivate STS. Intravenous heparin and thrombolysis should be considered.

Ambulatory phlebectomy

Ambulatory phlebectomy is an outpatient procedure used to remove varicose veins employing skin hooks via a series of stab incisions made along the course of the varicosity. Tumescent anesthesia is commonly used during this technique and has the added benefit of compression of the vein and reduction of blood loss. Various hooks and clamps are used to remove the vein (Fig. 39-11).

Incision sites heal with minimal scarring. Adverse effects are generally quite limited and consist of minor pain and bruising. Infection and nerve damage are extremely rare.

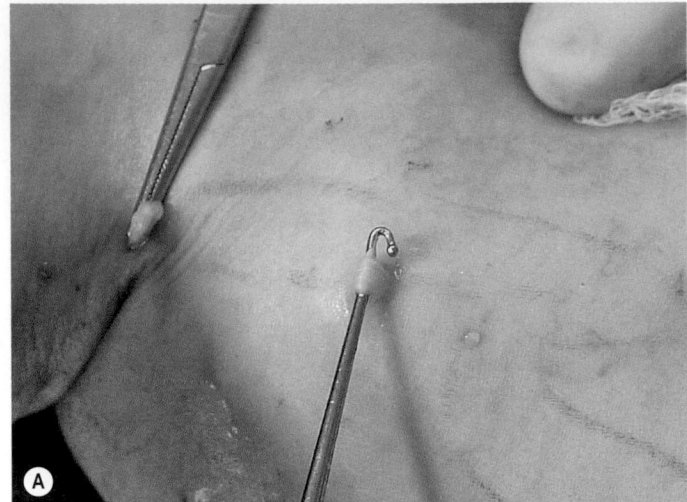

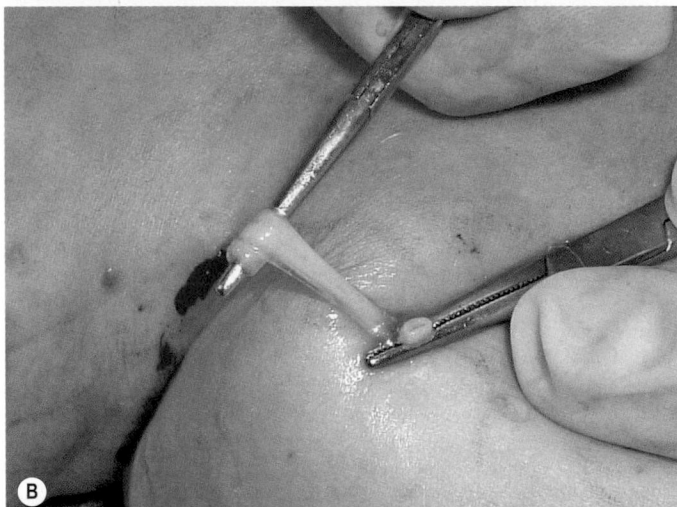

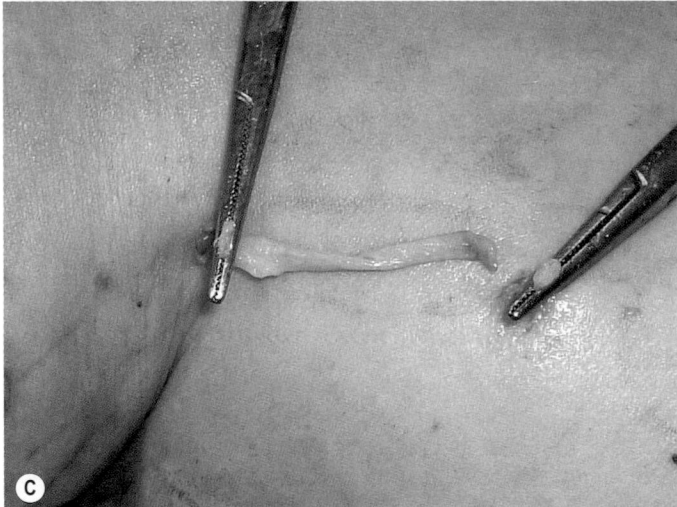

Fig. 39-11 Ambulatory phlebectomy. A, Hook used to secure the vein. B, Vein is clamped on either side and severed. Clamp is then used to remove the vein using a rolling and pulling technique. C, Removed vein segment. The distal end can be tied off using absorbable suture, or additional segments can be removed using the same technique.

Endovenous ablation

Endovenous ablation should be considered in patients with greater saphenous incompetence and is rapidly replacing traditional vein stripping. In patients with lower extremity tel-

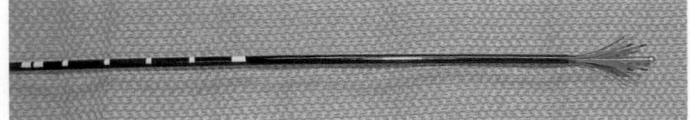

Fig. 39-12 Endovenous ablation, a radiofrequency catheter with deployable electrodes at the tip causes thermal destruction of the vein wall.

angiectasia and reticular veins, prior assessment of underlying saphenous reflux is necessary to prevent recurrence following treatment of the visible varicosities.

Radiofrequency or laser (using 810 nm or 1320 nm) can be used to heat and damage veins (Fig. 39-12). Either method results in vein wall shrinkage and subsequent vessel thrombosis and occlusion. Tumescent anesthesia allows the procedure to be performed painlessly, surrounds and compresses the vein for greater contact between the catheter and vessel wall, and distends the skin away from the heat source, preventing cutaneous damage. A catheter is placed under ultrasound guidance and guided to the sapheno-femoral junction. The catheter is slowly withdrawn along the length of the vein, and the thermal injury leads to vessel occlusion.

The most frequent complications include ecchymosis and pain. Thermal burns of the skin are infrequently seen when tumescent anesthesia is properly used. Nerve injury is uncommon and paresthesias are often temporary. Deep vein thrombosis has been documented, but pulmonary embolism is extremely rare when the technique is performed properly.

Brasic N, et al: Endovenous laser ablation and sclerotherapy for treatment of varicose veins. Semin Cutan Med Surg 2008 Dec; 27(4):264–275.

Davis LT, Duffy DM: Determination of incidence and risk factors for postsclerotherapy telangiectatic matting of the lower extremity: a retrospective analysis. J Dermatol Surg Oncol 1990; 16:327.

Goldman MP: Treatment of varicose and telangiectatic leg veins: double-blind prospective comparative trial between aethoxyskerol and sotradecol. Dermatol Surg 2002; 28:52.

Goldman MP, et al: Intravascular 1320-nm laser closure of the great saphenoid vein: a 6- to 12-month follow-up study. Dermatol Surg 2004; 30:1380.

Merchant RF, et al: Four-year follow-up on endovascular radiofrequency obliteration of great saphenous reflux. Dermatol Surg Feb 2005; 31(2):129–134.

Leach BC, Goldman MP: Comparative trial between sodium tetradecyl sulfate and glycerin in the treatment of telangiectatic leg veins. Dermatol Surg 2003; 29:612.

Lupton JR, et al: Clinical comparison of sclerotherapy versus long-pulsed Nd:YAG laser treatment for lower extremity telangiectases. Dermatol Surg 2002; 28:694.

McCoy S, et al: Sclerotherapy for leg telangiectasia: a blinded comparative trial of polidocanol and hypertonic saline. Dermatol Surg 1999; 25:381.

Munavalli GS, Weiss RA: Complications of sclerotherapy. Semin Cutan Med Surg 2007 Mar; 26(1):22–28.

Nijsten T, et al: Minimally invasive techniques in the treatment of saphenous varicose veins. J Am Acad Dermatol 2009 Jan; 60(1):110–119.

Ramelet AA: Phlebectomy. Technique, indications and complications. Int Angiol 2002; 21:46.

Rao J, et al: Double-blind prospective comparative trial between foamed and liquid polidocanol and sodium tetradecyl sulfate in the treatment of varicose and telangiectatic leg veins. Dermatol Surg 2005 Jun; 31(6):631–635.

Tafazzoli A, et al: Q-switched ruby laser treatment for postsclerotherapy hyperpigmentation. Dermatol Surg 2000; 26:653.

Tessari L, et al: Preliminary experience with a new sclerosing foam in the treatment of varicose veins. Dermatol Surg 2001; 27:58.

Uurto I, et al: Single-center experience with foam sclerotherapy without ultrasound guidance for treatment of varicose veins. Dermatol Surg 2007 Nov; 33(11):1334–1339.

Van Den Bos RR, et al: Endovenous laser ablation-induced complications: review of the literature and new cases. Dermatol Surg 2009 Aug; 35(8):1206–1214.

Weiss RA, Munavalli G: Endovenous ablation of truncal veins. Semin Cutan Med Surg 2005 Dec; 24(4):193–199.

Weiss RA, Weiss MA: Controlled radiofrequency endovenous occlusion using a unique radiofrequency catheter under duplex guidance to eliminate saphenous varicose vein reflux: a 2-year follow-up. Dermatol Surg 2002; 28:38.

Liposuction

Liposuction is used for the removal of local areas of adipose and to improve body contour. It is not a treatment for obesity and should not be used as a weight loss mechanism. The most common areas treated are the abdomen and thighs, neck, jowls, knees, ankles, and breasts (Fig. 39-13). Additional conditions, such as gynecomastia, buffalo hump, lipoma, lipodystrophy, and axillary hyperhidrosis, can be treated by liposuction.

The most common technique employed by dermatologists involves infiltrating the treated area with dilute anesthesia and aspirating the fat via cannulas attached to a vacuum. The choice of cannula can determine the amount of fat aspirated, with more aggressive cannulas having a larger bore, being more pointy, and having multiple, larger holes placed near the tip. Tumescent anesthesia typically consists of 0.05–0.1% lidocaine with 1:1 000 000 epinephrine and sodium bicarbonate. The total safe concentration of lidocaine that can be used is 55 mg/kg. The benefits of tumescent anesthesia are the ability to perform the procedure comfortably under local anesthesia, hemostasis, and hydrodissection of adipocytes, which facilitates aspiration.

Much discussion has been raised regarding the safety of office-based liposuction. It is important to stress that the serious complications seen in liposuction are associated with general anesthesia, and not with procedures performed with local tumescent anesthesia. While there have been reports of deaths occurring during liposuction, no reports have occurred when patients were treated with tumescent anesthesia alone. Office-based tumescent liposuction performed by dermatologic surgeons is safe and has a lower complication rate than hospital-based procedures.

Coleman WP 3rd, et al: Guidelines of care for liposuction. J Am Acad Dermatol 2001; 45:438.

Housman TS, et al: The safety of liposuction: results of a national survey. Dermatol Surg 2002; 28:971.

Lawrence N: Current issues in liposuction. Adv Dermatol 2003; 19:171.

Chemical peels

Superficial peel

Peels are categorized by the level of injury they cause. Superficial peels cause wounding to the epidermis and may reach the papillary dermis. These peels are well tolerated by patients who require limited "down time" after treatment. Superficial peels are used in the treatment of photoaging, actinic keratoses, solar lentigines, and pigmentary dyschromias. Given the limited nature of the injury induced by these peels, patients often need multiple treatments on a weekly or monthly basis to reach a desired result. However, patients need to be properly counseled regarding the limited benefit of superficial peels, as they cannot provide the improvement in wrinkles and deep furrows that may be possible with deeper injury peels.

Alpha-hydroxy acids (AHA), such as glycolic acid and lactic acid, are naturally occurring agents found in foods. The depth of injury is determined by the pH, the concentration of the acid, the amount applied, and the length of treatment time. Glycolic acid, in concentrations up to 70%, is commonly used for melasma, acne, and photoaging. Following rapid application to the entire face, it must be neutralized with sodium bicarbonate or plain water. Glycolic acid has been used in combination with 5-FU for the treatment of actinic keratoses.

Salicylic acid, a beta-hydroxy acid, can be used in concentrations of 20–30% for the treatment of acne and mild photoaging. It is especially useful as an adjunctive treatment for acne due to both the keratolytic and comedolytic properties of salicylic acid. It is also used in combination with other agents as part of the Jessner's solution. Following application, patients experience some mild stinging and discomfort. A whitening of the skin, termed frosting, from the precipitation of salicylic acid crystals is noted within several minutes of application. Salicylic acid does not require neutralization, although cool compresses after application can soothe the skin.

Trichloroacetic acid (TCA) in concentrations of 10–25% is used extensively as a superficial peel. The depth of injury is related to the concentration and the number of applications, with repeated coats of a low-concentration TCA leading to greater penetration. The agent is applied, and erythema and a white frost are noted within 1 minute. Patients experience a burning sensation. Hand-held fans and post-procedure cool compresses can reduce discomfort. TCA does not require neutralization after application.

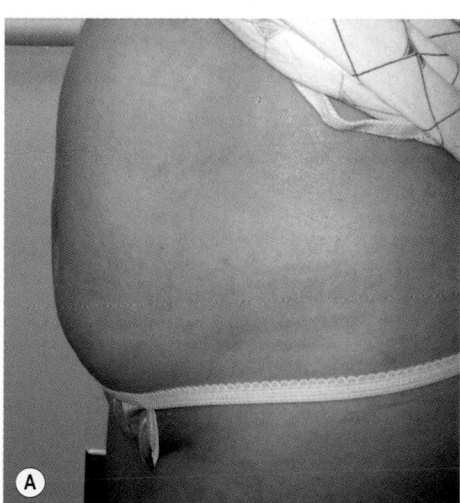
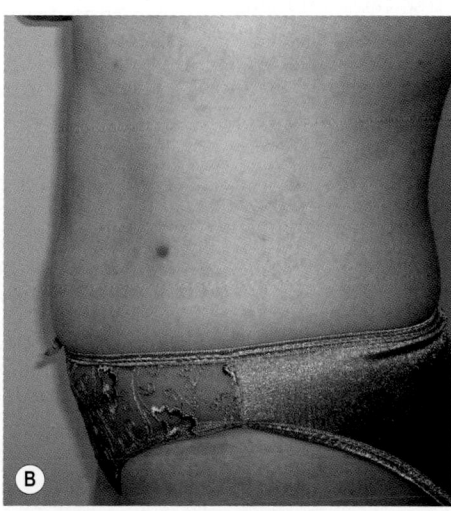

Fig. 39-13 Tumescent liposuction. A, Prior to treatment of abdomen. B, Following treatment.

Table 39-2 Jessner's solution

Resorcinol	14 g
Salicyclic acid	14 g
85% lactic acid	14 g
95% ethanol qs ad	100 mL

Jessner's solution combines resorcinol, salicylic acid, and lactic acid in ethanol (Table 39-2). This superficial peel has keratolytic activity and is commonly used for acne or hyperkeratotic lesions. It is self-neutralizing, and multiple applications can be performed to obtain a deeper injury.

Solid CO_2 (dry ice) has been used alone and in combination with TCA to obtain a deeper peel. It has been proposed as an effective treatment for acne scars and as a way to potentiate the effect of TCA to achieve a deeper peel.

Medium-depth peel

Medium-depth chemical peeling is defined as a controlled wound to the epidermis and deep papillary dermis, often with some extension into the upper reticular dermis. In contrast to the multiple treatments that are often performed with superficial peels, medium-depth peels are generally done as a single procedure due to the more significant injury produced. These peels cause epidermal necrosis and dermal injury, which results in increased collagen production during the wound healing process over the next several months. Medium-depth peels are indicated for the treatment of mild to moderate photodamage, rhytids, pigmentary dyschromias, actinic keratoses, solar lentigines, and other epidermal growths. Lawrence et al demonstrated a similar efficacy with Jessner's/35% TCA medium-depth peel as compared to 5-FU in the treatment of widespread facial actinic keratoses.

The classic medium-depth peel is 50% TCA. However, it is generally not used as a single-agent peel due to the unpredictable results and increased incidence of complications: namely, scarring and dyspigmentation. Rather, combining 35% TCA with an initial application of another agent, such as Jessner's solution or glycolic acid, can produce a medium-depth injury without the complications associated with higher concentrations of TCA alone. As a result of the damage to the epidermis produced with the initial peel, the TCA is able to penetrate deeper and produce a more significant and even result.

Deep peel

Deep chemical peels are defined as those that cause an injury down to the mid-reticular dermis. These peels are indicated for patients with moderate to severe photodamage and advanced rhytids. These peels produce significant injury and patients have an extended period of healing following treatment.

Baker–Gordon formula phenol peel is the traditional deep peel (Fig. 39-14). Undiluted 88% phenol does not produce a deep or consistent injury because it causes complete coagulation of epidermal keratin proteins, thus blocking further penetration. The Baker–Gordon formula (Table 39-3) reduces the concentration of phenol to 55%; the croton oil acts as a keratolytic and potentiates the depth of penetration of the phenol. Cardiac monitoring is required since phenol can produce arrhythmias. Intravenous fluids are given before and during

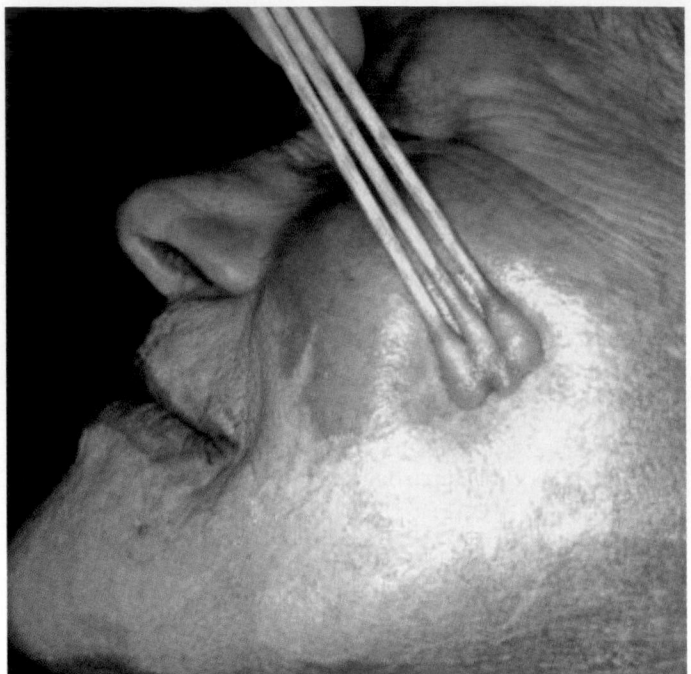

Fig. 39-14 Baker–Gordon phenol peel, white frosting following application. (Courtesy of Richard G. Glogau, MD)

Table 39-3 Baker–Gordon formula

88% liquid phenol, USP	3 mL
Tap water	2 mL
Septisol® liquid soap	8 drops
Croton oil	3 drops

the peel to limit the serum concentrations of phenol. In addition, the face is divided into smaller cosmetic units which are treated individually. An approximately 15 minute wait is required between treating each subunit, spreading the entire procedure over 1–2 hours, and further limiting the systemic concentration of phenol. Following application, occlusive tape can be applied if a deeper wound is desired.

Al-Waiz MM, Al-Sharqi AI: Medium-depth chemical peels in the treatment of acne scars in dark-skinned individuals. Dermatol Surg 2002 May; 28(5):383–387.

Fulton JE, Rahimi AD: Dermabrasion using CO_2 dry ice. Dermatol Surg 1999; 25:544.

Kligman D, Kligman AM: Salicylic acid peels for the treatment of photoaging. Dermatol Surg 1998; 24:325.

Landau M: Cardiac complications in deep chemical peels. Dermatol Surg 2007 Feb; 33(2):190–193.

Lawrence N, et al: A comparison of the efficacy and safety of Jessner's solution and 35% trichloroacetic acid vs 5% fluorouracil in the treatment of widespread facial actinic keratoses. Arch Dermatol 1995; 131:176.

Lee HS, Kim IH: Salicylic acid peels for the treatment of acne vulgaris in Asian patients. Dermatol Surg 2003; 29:1196.

Marrero GM, Katz BE: The new fluor-hydroxy pulse peel. A combination of 5-fluorouracil and glycolic acid. Dermatol Surg 1998; 24:973.

Monheit GD: Medium-depth chemical peels. Dermatol Clin 2001; 19:413.

Sarkar R, et al: The combination of glycolic acid peels with a topical regimen in the treatment of melasma in dark-skinned patients: a comparative study. Dermatol Surg 2002 Sep; 28(9):828–832.

Note: Page numbers followed by b indicate boxes, f indicate figures and t indicate tables.